DISEASES OF SWINE 9TH EDITION

9TH EDITION

DISEASES OF
SWINE

EDITED BY

Barbara E. Straw

Jeffery J. Zimmerman

Sylvie D'Allaire

David J. Taylor

with 128 authoritative contributors
selected for their recognized leadership in this field

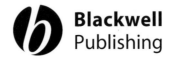

Blackwell
Publishing

©2006 Blackwell Publishing
All rights reserved.

Blackwell Publishing Professional
2121 State Avenue, Ames, Iowa 50014, USA

Orders:	1-800-862-6657
Office:	1-515-292-0140
Fax:	1-515-292-3348
Web site:	www.blackwellprofessional.com

Blackwell Publishing Ltd
9600 Garsington Road, Oxford OX4 2DQ, UK
Tel.: +44 (0)1865 776868

Blackwell Publishing Asia
550 Swanston Street, Carlton, Victoria 3053, Australia
Tel.: +61 (0)3 8359 1011

Authorization to photocopy items for internal or personal use, or the internal or personal use of specific clients, is granted by Blackwell Publishing, provided that the base fee of $.10 per copy is paid directly to the Copyright Clearance Center, 222 Rosewood Drive, Danvers, MA 01923. For those organizations that have been granted a photocopy license by CCC, a separate system of payments has been arranged. The fee code for users of the Transactional Reporting Service is ISBN-13: 978-0-8138-1703-3; ISBN-10: 0-8138-1703-X/2006 $.10.

ISBN-13: 978-0-8138-1703-3
ISBN-10: 0-8138-1703-X

First edition, 1958; second edition, 1964; third edition, 1970; fourth edition, 1975; fifth edition, 1981; sixth edition, 1986; seventh edition, 1992; eighth edition, 1999; ninth edition, 2006.

Library of Congress Cataloging-in-Publication Data

Diseases of swine / edited by Barbara E. Straw ... [et al.].— 9th ed.
    p. cm.
  Includes bibliographical references and index.
  ISBN-13: 978-0-8138-1703-3 (alk. paper)
  ISBN-10: 0-8138-1703-X (alk. paper)
  1. Swine—Diseases. I. Straw, Barbara E.

SF971.D57 2006
636.4′0896—dc22

                                        2005013060

Every effort has been made to ascertain permission requirements for previously published material appearing in this edition of *Diseases of Swine*. The editors and publisher regret any oversight or error in this regard and will be happy to include corrected attributions in the book's next printing.

The last digit is the print number: 9 8 7 6 5 4 3 2 1

Contents

Contributing Authors

Numbers in parentheses beside names refers to chapters.

C. L. Afonso (29)
United States Department of Agriculture
Agricultural Research Service
Plum Island Animal Disease Center
Box 848
Greenport, NY 11944
USA

Gordon M. Allan (14)
Veterinary Sciences Division
Stoney Road
Stormont
Belfast BT4 3SD
Northern Ireland

Glen W. Almond (6)
College of Veterinary Medicine
North Carolina State University
4700 Hillsborough Street
Raleigh, NC 27606
USA

Sandra F. Amass (68)
Dept. of Veterinary Clinical Sciences
Purdue University
VCS/Lynn, 625 Harrison Street
West Lafayette, IN 47907-1248
USA

David E. Anderson (70)
Dept. of Veterinary Clinical Sciences
College of Veterinary Medicine
The Ohio State University
601 Vernon L. Tharp Street
Columbus, OH 43210-1089
USA

C. A. Baldwin (32)
Veterinary Diagnostic and Investigational Laboratory
College of Veterinary Medicine
University of Georgia
Tifton, GA 31793-3000
USA

Ron O. Ball (58)
Dept. of Agricultural, Food and Nutritional Sciences
University of Alberta
Edmonton, Alberta, T6G 2P5
Canada

Laura Batista (6)
Faculty of Veterinary Medicine
University of Montreal
P.O. Box 5000
St. Hyacinthe, Quebec J2S 7C6
Canada

Angela Baysinger (68)
Department of On Farm Food Safety
Farmland Foods
Route 2, Box 45
Bruning, NE 68322
USA

D. A. Benfield (24)
Ohio Agricultural Research and Development Center
The Ohio State University
1680 Research Services Building
Wooster, OH 44691
USA

Patricia C. Blanchard (10)
California Animal Health and Food Safety Laboratory
University of California-Davis
18830 Road 112
Tulare, CA 93274
USA

Janice C. Bridger (19)
Dept. of Pathology & Infectious Disease
The Royal Veterinary College
Royal College Street
London, NW1 OTU
United Kingdom

Ian H. Brown (28)
Veterinary Laboratories Agency – Weybridge
New Haw, Addlestone
Surrey KT15 3NB
United Kingdom

Ranald D. A. Cameron (8)
University of Queensland
7 Teague Street, Indooroopilly
Brisbane, Queensland 4068
Australia

C. Cargill (53)
Livestock Systems Alliance
Roseworthy Campus
University of Adelaide
Roseworthy, SA 5371
Australia

Thomas L. Carson (60)
Veterinary Diagnostic Laboratory
Diagnostic and Production Animal Medicine
College of Veterinary Medicine
Iowa State University
Ames, IA 50011
USA

Kin-Chow Chang (61)
Molecular Medicine Laboratory
Institute of Comparative Medicine
University of Glasgow Veterinary School
Bearsden Road, Glasgow G61 1QH
Scotland

Greg M. Cronin (51,62)
Animal Welfare Science Centre
Department of Primary Industries
Werribee Centre East
600 Sneydes Rd
Werribee VIC 3030
Australia

Ross S. Cutler (62)
Ross Cutler and Associates Ptx Ltd
140 The Parade
Ocean Grove, Victoria 3226
Australia

Sylvie D'Allaire (6,63)
Faculty of Veterinary Medicine
University of Montreal
P.O. Box 5000
St. Hyacinthe, Quebec J2S 7C6
Canada

Peter R. Davies (53,69)
Dept. of Veterinary Population Medicine
College of Veterinary Medicine
University of Minnesota
1988 Fitch Ave
St. Paul, MN 55108
USA

Scott A. Dee (9)
Dept. of Veterinary Population Medicine
University of Minnesota
385 AnSci/Vet Med Bldg, 1988 Fitch Ave
St. Paul, MN 55108
USA

M. F. de Jong (34)
Animal Health Service
P.O. Box 9 NL 7400 AA Deventer
Netherlands

Cornelius F. M. de Lange (66)
Dept. of Animal & Poultry Science
Ontario Agricultural College
University of Guelph
Guelph, Ontario, N1G 2W1
Canada

Aldo Dekker (31)
Institute for Animal Health & Science
Research Brach, Houtribweg 39
Postbus 65
8200 AB Lelystad
Netherlands

Gustavo Delhon (29)
United States Department of Agriculture
Agricultural Research Service
Plum Island Animal Disease Center
Box 848
Greenport, NY 11944
USA

Catherine E. Dewey (1,5,11,66)
Department of Population Medicine
Ontario Veterinary College
University of Guelph
Guelph, Ontario, N1G 2W1
Canada

Mariano Domingo (14)
Centre de Recerca en Sanitat Animal (CReSA)
Departament de Sanitat i Anatomia Animals
Facultat de Veterinaria
Universitat Autonoma de Barcelona
08193 Bellaterra
Barcelona
Spain

Richard Drolet (9,63)
Faculty of Veterinary Medicine
University of Montreal
P.O. Box 5000
St. Hyacinthe, Quebec J2S 7C6
Canada

J. P. Dubey (52)
USDA, ARS, ANRI
Animal Parasitic Diseases Lab
BARC-East Building 1001, Room 1
Beltsville, MD 20705
USA

G. E. Duhamel (46)
Dept. of Veterinary and Biomedical Sciences
University of Nebraska-Lincoln
Lincoln, NE 68583
USA

Bernard C. Easterday (28)
University of Wisconsin-Madison
School of Veterinary Medicine
2015 Linden Dr
Madison, WI 53706
USA

Neil Edington (16)
Royal Veterinary College
Dept. of Pathology & Infectious Disease
Royal College Street
London, NW1 OTU
United Kingdom

Sandra A. Edwards (67)
School of Agricultural Food and Rural Development
University of Newcastle
Newcastle Upon Tyne NE1 7RU
United Kingdom

W. A. Ellis (41)
Veterinary Research Laboratories
Stoney Road
Stormont
Belfast BT4 3SD
Northern Ireland

François Elvinger (32)
Dept. of Large Animal Clinical Sciences
VA-MD Regional College of Veterinary Medicine
Virginia Polytechnic Institute & State University
Phase II, Duckpond Drive
Blacksburg, VA 24061-0442
USA

Peter R. English (67)
Ardachadh, Upper Lenie
Drummadrochit, Inverness IV63 6XF
Scotland

V. Anthony Fahy (62)
Bendigo Agricultural and Veterinary Center
Box 125
Bendigo, Victoria 3550
Australia

John M. Fairbrother (38)
The Escherichia coli Laboratory
Groupe de Recherche sur les Maladies Infectieuses du Porc
Faculté de Médecine Vétérinaire
Université de Montréal
C.P. 5000
Saint-Hyacinthe, Quebec J2S 7C6
Canada

Chantal Farmer (4)
Centre de R&D sur le Bovin Laitier et el Porc
Agriculture et Agroalimentaire Canada
P.O. Box 90
Lennoxville, Quebec J1M 1Z3
Canada

C. Fellström (48)
Faculty of Veterinary Medicine
Swedish University of Agricultural Sciences
Uppsala
Sweden

William L. Flowers (6)
Dept. of Animal Science
North Carolina State University
Raleigh, NC 27695-7621
USA

David Fraser (67)
Faculty of Agricultural Sciences
University of British Columbia
Vancouver, British Columbia V6T 1Z4
Canada

Robert M. Friendship (54,71)
Dept. of Population Medicine
Ontario Veterinary College
University of Guelph
Guelph, Ontario N1G 2W1
Canada

Ian A. Gardner (10)
Dept. of Medicine and Epidemiology
School of Veterinary Medicine
One Shields Ave
University of California-Davis
Davis, CA 95616
USA

Connie J. Gebhart (44)
Dept. of Pathobiology
College of Veterinary Medicine
University of Minnesota
St Paul, MN 55108
USA

Harold W. Gonyou (64)
Prairie Swine Center Inc.
P.O. Box 21057
Saskatoon, Saskatchewan S7H 5N9
Canada

Marcelo Gottschalk (33,47)
Groupe de Recherche sur les Maladies Infectieuses du Porc
Faculté de Médecine Vétérinaire, Université de Montréal,
Saint-Hyacinthe, Quebec J2S 7C6
Canada

R. W. Griffith (45)
Dept. of Veterinary Microbiology and Preventive Medicine
College of Veterinary Medicine
Iowa State University
Ames, IA 50011
USA

Carlton L. Gyles (38)
Dept. of Pathobiology
Ontario Veterinary College
University of Guelph
Guelph, Ontario N1G 2W1
Canada

Patrick G. Halbur (32)
Dept. of Veterinary Diagnostic & Production Animal
    Medicine
College of Veterinary Medicine
Iowa State University
Ames, IA 50011
USA

David J. Hampson (46,48,65)
School of Veterinary and Biomedical Sciences
Murdoch University
Murdoch, Western Australia 6150
Australia

P. H. Hemsworth (51)
Animal Welfare Science Centre
Univ. of Melbourne and Dept. of Primary Industries
600 Sneydes Rd
Werribee VIC 3030
Melbourne
Australia

Louise M. Henderson (37)
USDA, APHIS, VS, CVB
1800 Dayton Road
Ames, IA 50010
USA

Robert Higgins (47)
Département de Pathologie et Microbiologie,
Faculté de Médecine Vétérinaire, Université de Montréal,
Saint-Hyacinthe, Quebec J2S 7C6
Canada

Phillip G. Hoyt (55)
Dept. of Veterinary Clinical Sciences
School of Veterinary Medicine
Louisiana State University
Baton Rouge, LA 70803
USA

Han Soo Joo (21)
Department of Clinical and Population Sciences
College of Veterinary Medicine
University of Minnesota
St. Paul, MN 55108
USA

Sven Erik Jorsal (7)
Danish Institute for Food and Veterinary Research
Bülowsvej 27
DK 1790 Copenhagen V
Denmark

Peter D. Kirkland (27)
Virology Laboratory
Elizabeth Macarthur Agricultural Institute
PMB 8, Camden, NSW 2570
Australia

Steven B. Kleiboeker (12)
Veterinary Medical Diagnostic Laboratory
University of Missouri
1600 East Rollins
Columbia, MO 65211
USA

Christian Klopfenstein (4)
Centre de Développement du Porc du Québec
2795 Boul. Laurier, Bureau 340
Ste-Foy, Quebec G1V 4M7
Canada

Nick J. Knowles (18,19)
Dept. of Vesicular Disease Control
Institute for Animal Health
Pirbright Laboratory, Ash Road
Pirbright, Woking, Surrey GU24 0NF
United Kingdom

Frank Koenen (17)
Dept. of Virology
Veterinary & Agrochemic Research Center (CODA/CERVA)
Grocselenberg 99
B-1180 Ukkel
Belgium

John Korslund (35)
National Swine Programs Liaison
USDA APHIS VS AHP NCAHP EST
4700 River Road, Unit 43
Riverdale, MD 20373
USA

Jean Le Dividich (65)
INRA-UMRVP
St-Gilles 35590
France

Stéphane P. Lemay (64)
Institut de Recherche et de Développement en
    Agroenvironnement
120-A, Chemin Ste-Foy
Deschambault, Quebec G0A 1S0
Canada

Marie-Frédérique Le Potier (15)
Agence Française de Sécurité Sanitaire des Aliments (AFSSA)
Laboratoire d'Etudes et de Recherches Avicoles et Porcines
Zoopole Beaucemaine-Les Croix, BP 53
22440 Ploufragan
France

David S. Lindsay (52)
Center for Molecular Medicine and Infectious Diseases
Dept. of Biomedical Sciences and Pathobiology
Virginia-Maryland Regional College of Veterinary Medicine
Virginia Tech
1410 Prices Fork Road
Blacksburg, VA 24061-0342
USA

Juan Lubroth (31)
Infectious Disease Group
FAO Animal Health Service
Animal Production & Health Division
Viale delle Terme di Caracalla 00100
Rome
Italy

A. P. MacMillan (35)
Central Veterinary Laboratory
New Haw
Addlestone, Surrey KT15 3NB
England

Guy-Pierre Martineau (4)
Ecole Nationale Vétérinaire de Toulouse
23 Chemin de Capelles
B.P. 87614
Toulouse Cedex 3, 31076
France

Steven McOrist (44)
QAF Industries
Corowa
NSW 2646
Australia

X. J. Meng (32)
Center for Molecular Medicine & Infectious Diseases
Dept. of Biomedical Sciences & Pathobiology
VA-MD Regional College of Veterinary Medicine
Virginia Polytechnic Institute & State University
1410 Price's Fork Road
Blacksburg, VA 24061-0342
USA

William L. Mengeling (23)
4220 Phoenix Street
Ames, IA 50014
USA

Alain Mesplède (15)
Agence Française de Sécurité Sanitaire des Aliments (AFSSA)
Laboratoire d'études et de Recherches Avicoles et Porcines
UR Virologie Immunologie Porcines
Zoopole Beaucemaine-Les Croix, BP 53
22440 Ploufragan
France

D. K. Meyerholz (45)
Dept. of Veterinary Pathology
College of Veterinary Medicine
Iowa State University
Ames, IA 50011
USA

P. S. Miller (57)
Dept. of Animal Science
University of Nebraska
Lincoln, NE 68583-0908
USA

Jan Mousing (7)
Danish Institute for Food and Veterinary Research
Bülowsvej 27, DK-1790 Copenhagen V
Denmark

Michael P. Murtaugh (24)
Dept. of Veterinary Pathobiology
University of Minnesota
1971 Commonwealth Avenue
St. Paul, MN 55108
USA

P. J. O'Brien (58)
Pfizer Global Research and Development
Sandwich Laboratories (ipc330)
Sandwich, Kent, CT13 9NJ
England

Simone R. Oliveira (40)
Veterinary Population Medicine Department
College of Veterinary Medicine
University of Minnesota
244 Vet D L
1333 Gortner Avenue
St. Paul, MN 55108
USA

Christopher W. Olsen (28)
Dept. of Pathobiological Sciences
School of Veterinary Medicine
University of Wisconsin-Madison
2015 Linden Drive
Madison, WI 53706
USA

Fernando Osorio (24)
Dept. of Veterinary & Biomedical Sciences
University of Nebraska-Lincoln
Lincoln, NE 68583-0905
USA

G. D. Osweiler (56)
Dept. of Veterinary Diagnostic & Production Animal
    Medicine
College of Veterinary Medicine
Iowa State University
Ames, IA 50011
USA

Z. K. Pejsak (25)
National Veterinary Research Institute
Partyzantow 57
24-100 Pulawy
Poland

Maurice B. Pensaert (20,22)
Laboratory of Veterinary Virology
Faculty of Veterinary Medicine
Ghent University
Salisburylaan 133
9820 Merelbeke
Belgium

Carlos Pijoan (40,43)
Dept. of Clinical and Population Sciences
College of Veterinary Medicine
University of Minnesota
1988 Fitch Avenue
St. Paul, MN 55108
USA

K. B. Platt (21)
2154 College of Veterinary Medicine
Iowa State University
Ames, IA 50011
USA

John R. Pluske (65)
School of Veterinary and Biomedical Sciences
Murdoch University
Murdoch, Western Australia 6150
Australia

John F. Prescott (71)
Dept. of Pathobiology
Ontario Veterinary College
University of Guelph
Guelph, Ontario N1G 2W1
Canada

Vicki J. Rapp-Gabrielson (40)
Pfizer Animal Health
Veterinary Medicine Research and Development
Building 190 MS 39
7000 Portage Road
Kalamazoo, MI 49001
USA

D. E. Reese (57)
Dept. of Animal Science
University of Nebraska
Lincoln, NE 68583-0908
USA

Dan L. Rock (29)
United States Department of Agriculture
Agricultural Research Service
Plum Island Animal Disease Center
Box 848
Greenport, NY 11944
USA

Luis Rodríguez (31)
United States Department of Agriculture
Agricultural Research Service
Plum Island Animal Disease Center
Box 848
Greenport, NY 11944
USA

James A. Roth (2)
College of Veterinary Medicine
Dept. of Veterinary Microbiology & Preventive Medicine
Iowa State University
2156 Vet Med Bldg
Ames, IA 50011
USA

Linda J. Saif (26,30)
Food Animal Health Research Program
Ohio Agricultural Research & Development Center
The Ohio State University
Wooster, OH 44691
USA

Guy St. Jean (70)
School of Veterinary Medicine
Ross University
P.O. Box 334
Basseterre, St. Kitts
West Indies

José Manuel Sánchez-Vizcaíno (13)
Catedrático del Área de Sanidad Animal
Universidad Complutense
Facultad de Veterinaria
Avenida Puerta de Hierro s/n
28040 Madrid
Spain

Heidi Schleicher (35)
USDA, APHIS, VS, NVSL
Brucella and Mycobacterium Reagents Team
1800 Dayton Ave
Ames, IA 50010
USA

K. J. Schwartz (45)
Dept. of Veterinary Diagnostic & Production Animal
    Medicine
College of Veterinary Medicine
Iowa State University
Ames, IA 50011
USA

Joaquim Segalés (14)
Centre de Recerca en Sanitat Animal (CReSA)
Departament de Sanitat i Anatomia Animals
Facultat de Veterinaria
Universitat Autonoma de Barcelona
08193 Bellaterra
Barcelona
Spain

Karol Sestak (30)
Tulane University Primate Center
Tulane University School of Medicine
18703 Three Rivers Road
Covington, LA 70433
USA

E. W. Skov-Jensen (39)
Staby-Ulfborg-Tim Veterinarians
Bygvaenget 25
DK-6990 Ulfborg
Denmark

W. J. Smith (59)
85 Station Road
Banchory
Aberdeenshire AB31 5YP
Scotland

J. Glenn Songer (36)
Dept. of Veterinary Science and Microbiology
The University of Arizona
Tucson, AZ 85721-0090
USA

Vibeke Sørensen (7)
Danish Institute for Food and Veterinary Research
Bülowsvej 27
DK 1790 Copenhagen V
Denmark

E. Murray Spicer (62)
Bendigo Agricultural and Veterinary Center
Box 125
Bendigo Victoria 3550
Australia

Katharina D.C. Stärk (69)
Swiss Federal Veterinary Office
P.O. Box
CH-3003 Bern
Switzerland

Michael J. Stear (61)
Institute of Comparative Medicine
University of Glasgow Veterinary School
Bearsden Road
Glasgow, G6I 1QH
Scotland

Alberto Stephano (27)
Stephano Consultores, S.C.
Villa de Gaudalupe 234
Villa del Campestre
Leon, Guanajuato, C.P. 37129
Mexico

Gregory W. Stevenson (24,26)
Animal Disease Diagnostic Laboratory
College of Veterinary Medicine
Purdue University
West Lafayette, IN 47907
USA

T. Bonner Stewart (55)
Dept. of Pathobiological Sciences
School of Veterinary Medicine
Louisiana State University
Baton Rouge, LA 70803
USA

William C. Stoffregen (35)
Brucellosis Research Project
Bacterial Diseases of Livestock Research Unit
National Animal Disease Center
USDA-ARS
2300 Dayton Ave., Box 70
Ames, IA 50010
USA

Barbara E. Straw (1,11,59)
Dept. of Large Animal Clinical Science
College of Veterinary Medicine
Michigan State University
East Lansing, MI 48824
USA

David J. Taylor (33,36,50)
Glasgow University Veterinary School
Bearsden Road
Bearsden, Glasgow G61 1QH
Scotland

Eileen L. Thacker (2,42)
2118 Veterinary Microbiology & Preventive Medicine
Iowa State University
Ames, IA 50011
USA

Charles O. Thoen (49)
Dept. of Microbiology, Immunology & Preventive Medicine
College of Veterinary Medicine
Iowa State University
Ames, IA 50011
USA

Jill R. Thomson (3,48)
Scottish Agricultural College Veterinary Services
Bush Estate, Penicuik
Midlothian EH26 OQE
Scotland

Montserrat Torremorell (24)
Pig Improvement Company
3033 Nashville Road
Franklin, KY 42135
USA

Marian J. Truszczyński (25)
National Veterinary Research Institute
Partyzantow 57
24-100 Pulawy
Poland

E. R. Tulman (29)
United States Department of Agriculture
Agricultural Research Service
Plum Island Animal Disease Center
Box 848
Greenport, NY 11944
USA

Kristien Van Reeth (28)
Laboratory of Virology
Faculty of Veterinary Medicine
Ghent University
Salisburylaan 133
9820 Merelbeke
Belgium

Philippe Vannier (15)
Agence Française de Sécurité Sanitaire des Aliments (AFSSA)
Laboratoire d'Etudes et de Recherches Avicoles et Porcines
Zoopole Beaucemaine-Les Croix, BP 53
22440 Ploufragan
France

H. C. Wegener (39)
Head of Research
Danish Veterinary Institute
Copenhagen
Denmark

Carolyn A. Wilson (32)
Division of Cellular and Gene Therapies
Office of Cellular, Tissues, and Gene Therapies
Center for Biologics Evaluation and Research
Food and Drug Administration
8800 Rockville Pike, HFM-725
Bethesda, MD 20892
USA

M. R. Wilson (11)
RR 4
Rockwood, Ontario N0B 2K0
Canada

Richard L. Wood (37)
620 River Oak Drive
Ames, IA 50010
USA

Sang-Geon Yeo (22)
College of Veterinary Medicine
Kyungpook National University
Daegu, 702-701
South Korea

Kyoung-Jin Yoon (16)
Dept. of Veterinary Diagnostic & Production Animal
    Medicine
College of Veterinary Medicine
Iowa State University
Ames, IA 50011-1250
USA

Lijuan Yuan (26)
Food Animal Health Research Program
Ohio Agricultural Research & Development Center
The Ohio State University
1680 Madison Avenue
Wooster, OH 44691
USA

Yuanhui Zhang (64)
Dept. of Agricultural Engineering
University of Illinois
1304 W. Pennsylvania
Urbana, IL 61801
USA

Jeffery J. Zimmerman (24)
Dept. of Veterinary Diagnostic & Production Animal
    Medicine
College of Veterinary Medicine
Iowa State University
Ames, IA 50011-1250
USA

Editor's Note

Diseases and production technologiy are often referred to by different common names in different parts of the world. The following terms have been used interchangably at the authors' discretion: pseudorabies/Aujesky's disease, hog cholera/classical swine fever, pleurisy/pleuritis, specific pathogen free/minimal disease, and weaner pig/nursery pig.

Occasionally, outdated terms will be used when appropriate in a historical context, such as (1) mastitis-metritis-agalactia (MMA) instead of postpartum dysgalac-tia syndrome (PPDS) and (2) stillbirth-mummification, embryonic death-infertility (SMEDI) rather than porcine parvovirus infection.

The officially accepted name changes for bacteria have been used in the text. Some that have changed in recent years include *Actinobaculum suis* (earlier *Actinomyces suis, Eubacterium suis,* and *Corynebacterium pyogenes*) and *Brachyspira hyodysenteriae* (earlier *Serpulina hyodysenteriae* and *Treponema hyodysenteriae*).

Physical Examination, Diagnosis, and Body Systems

1 Herd Examination

Catherine E. Dewey and Barbara E. Straw

The rapid trend toward large, intensive, confinement-rearing swine production units and the emergence of herd managers with high levels of education and specialized swine experience has caused a change in the type of service required from veterinary practitioners. The hobby farmer with a few sows as a sideline enterprise may still require a veterinarian to help castrate piglets, farrow a sow, or examine a pen of ill pigs. Specialized pig farmers generally have little need for these traditional services; however, they do require the assistance of professional consultants who can help them solve complex disease, management, environmental, and production problems. Veterinarians also work with producers to ensure pork safety and the welfare of the pigs under their care.

On large swine units the veterinarian functions as part of a consulting team that may be composed of a nutritionist, engineer, marketing expert, geneticist, and accountant. Veterinarians are uniquely suited to coordinate this team, but this leadership role requires that a veterinarian must keep up-to-date with developments in a wide range of fields. The health management veterinarian must be knowledgeable enough to discuss feeding programs with a nutritionist or a ventilation problem with an engineer. The swine health management veterinarian must also be familiar with the complex biological system of a pig farm to differentiate normal and abnormal states. Finally, the swine veterinarian will use herd-based diagnostic skills to provide modern, cost-effective disease-management programs.

Often the ill-defined production problems on large swine farms are precipitated by such factors as poor housing, infectious disease, or poor management of animals or farm personnel. Educating and motivating the herdsmen rather than concentrating on disease conditions of the pig can solve many of these complex production problems. The task of helping farmers to make long-term decisions, motivating them to carry these out, and demonstrating to them the cost benefits of this advice is difficult, partly because of the long time span involved. Good record-keeping and the use of production targets are the cornerstones of such a program. Likewise, regular visits and ongoing discussions with follow-up written reports go a long way to make health management programs successful. This chapter provides an overview of the expectations of a herd health veterinarian working with a specific unit and offers charts of normal values as a reference.

THE HERD HEALTH VISIT

Understand the Producer's Goals for the Unit

The veterinarian must determine the goals of the herd's owner and manager. The recommendations for one producer who wants to eradicate disease will be different from those given to a producer who wants to develop a treatment and prevention program for the diseases in the barn.

Review Production Records

Examine monthly reproductive records for at least 12 months. Determine which parameters are below target and conduct a more thorough investigation of factors that affect these parameters. Alter target values for all parameters as the production unit changes over time. Averages for some specific parameters are listed in Table 1.1. More detail is found in Chapter 6.

Review nursery and grow/finish records for each barn filled over the past 12 months. If the unit is managed in a continuous flow basis, be sure that the values are biologically plausible. Specifically determine growth rate and compare this to the expected values in slow-, moderate-, and fast-growing pigs (Table 1.2). If the farm keeps accurate feed records, analyze the feed conversion rates and margin over feed as well. An evaluation of payment records from the packing plant will be useful to enhance the return per pig marketed.

Then determine the average and range of morbidity and mortality for each age group of pigs. Examine the causes and timing of morbidity and mortality to deter-

Table 1.1.   Country-specific sow productivity averages based on PigCHAMP records collected in 2002.

	Brazil	Canada	Mexico	Thailand	USA
Farms	119	36	78	23	105
Cull rate (%)	38.3	36.5	39.9	32.9	44.7
Death rate (%)	5.2	4.9	5.0	4.0	8.0
Nonproductive sow days	59.8	57.9	52.7	55.7	74.8
Wean-breed interval (da)	5.8	6.9	5.8	6.8	7.3
Farrowing rate (%)	81.0	79.3	82.5	81.0	71.7
Born alive/litter	10.5	10.8	10.6	9.9	10.3
Stillborn/litter	0.55	0.7	0.56	0.80	0.98
Mummies/litter	0.25	0.22	0.26	0.20	0.24
Lactation length (da)	19.9	20.7	20.2	21.9	18.7

Source: Adapted from Deen and Anil (2003).

mine whether disease control programs continue to be appropriate for the unit. Identify seasonal trends in morbidity and mortality. Average nursing pig mortality rates around the world are estimated to range from 12.7 in the U.K. to 19.7% in the U.S.A. (Barnett et al. 2001). Typically, nursery barn mortality ranges from 2–5% and grower-finisher pig mortality ranges from 0.5–3%. The average sow mortality of 6% has increased over time (Abiven et al. 1998; Deen and Anil 2003). In 2002, mortality by country ranged from a low value of 3.6% in Columbia to a high of 8.0% in the United States based on PigCHAMP records (Deen and Anil 2003). There are also large farm-to-farm differences in sow mortality. In the study by Abiven et al. (1998), annual sow mortality ranged from 0–20%. See Chapter 63 for more details on sow culling and mortality.

Farms that have both stalls and pens for sow housing have a lower culling rate due to reproductive failure, lameness, age, death, and euthanasia than farms that have only pens (Paterson et al. 1997, cited by Barnett et al. 2001). Sows housed in pens for a portion of gestation are expected to have reduced farrowing time (Ferket and Hacker 1985), reduced lameness in gilts (Hale et al. 1984), and less joint damage (Fredeen and Sather 1978).

To complete the record analyses, identify problems and prioritize areas according to those with most economic concern. Make lists of short-term and long-term goals. Record questions that arise from the record analyses to be reviewed during the herd visit. Make copies of reports in either table for graph form. Produce a summary of the findings to be included in the final herd report.

Review Production Flow

Draw a detailed map of the whole production facility or system. For a farrow-to-finish facility this will be the details for one site. If the production system is multisite, include all sites in your production map. To the map add information such as number of barns, number of rooms per barn, number of pens per room, and size of each pen. Finally add the age and weight of pigs as they enter and exit the pens. The production records will provide

expected values for production flow, such as number of sows, pigs weaned per litter, growth rate, and mortality rate. Using this information, determine the maximum number of pigs each pen, room, barn, and site will accommodate. Together with the facility design, determine if there is sufficient space for the anticipated production.

The pen area required per pig is determined by the maximum size and number of pigs housed in the pen (Table 1.3). If pigs are not provided adequate space, growth rate will be reduced as overcrowding begins. To enhance the use of space, some producers over stock a pen with lightweight pigs when they first arrive in a facility and then move 1/4 to 1/3 of the pigs to another pen as they grow. Another option for finisher pigs is to market the heaviest pigs at a slightly lower weight, thus alleviating the potential for overcrowding. A space savings of 3% will be gained if the first group of animals is marketed at 5 kg below the typical weight (Gonyou and Stricklin 1998). An allometric measurement of space allowance takes into consideration the floor area required by the pig over a wide range of weights. Research has shown that using the equation area = k × (body weight) 0.667, where *area* is measured in m^2 and *body weight* in kg, if the coefficient *k* is maintained at 0.33, the pigs will not be overcrowded. More detail about the impact of space on productivity is found in Chapter 64.

The area recommended for sows varies widely from 1.4 to 3.6 m^2/pig due to different housing designs and expectations determined by country (English et al. 1982; Jensen 1984; Barnett et al. 2001). When space is insufficient, sows have reduced reproductive performance and show a chronic stress response. There is a reproductive advantage to providing 3 m^2/pig over 2 m^2/pig (Jensen 1984). Outdoor housed sows will each require 1.1 m^2 (12.8 ft2) on a slab area, 0.7 m^2 (7.7 ft2) in a shed for sleeping and an additional space for cooling in a mud hole or a sprinkler area.

When pigs are housed in large groups, there is additional free space compared to housing smaller groups with the same area per pig (Barnett et al. 2001). If sows are kept in relatively small groups, they need 2.4 to 3.6

Table 1.2. Weights and daily gain by age and relative growth rate.

Age	Slow				Moderate				Ideal			
	Weight		Daily Gain in the Previous 20 Days		Weight		Daily Gain in the Previous 20 Days		Weight		Daily Gain in the Previous 20 Days	
(days)	lb	kg	lb	g	lb	kg	lb	g	lb	kg	lb	g
20	8–10	3.6–4.5			10–12	4.5–5.5			12–14	5.5–6.4		
40	18–22	8.2–10.0	0.50–0.60	227–273	22–26	10.0–11.8	0.60–0.70	273–318	26–30	11.8–13.6	0.70–0.80	318–364
60	33–40	15.0–18.2	0.75–0.90	341–409	40–47	18.2–21.4	0.90–1.05	409–477	47–54	21.4–24.5	1.05–1.20	477–545
80	54–64	24.5–29.1	1.05–1.20	477–545	64–74	29.1–33.6	1.20–1.35	545–614	74–84	33.6–38.2	1.35–1.50	614–682
100	82–95	37.3–43.2	1.40–1.55	636–705	95–108	43.2–49.1	1.55–1.70	705–773	108–122	49.1–55.5	1.70–1.90	773–864
120	110–126	50.0–57.3	1.40–1.55	636–705	126–142	57.3–64.5	1.55–1.70	705–773	142–160	64.5–72.7	1.70–1.90	773–864
140	138–157	62.7–71.4	1.40–1.55	636–705	157–176	71.4–80.0	1.55–1.70	705–773	176–198	80.0–90.0	1.70–1.90	773–864
160	165–187	75.0–85.0	1.35–1.50	614–682	187–209	85.0–95.0	1.50–1.65	682–750	209–235	95.0–106.8	1.65–1.85	750–841
180	191–216	86.8–98.2	1.30–1.45	591–659	216–241	98.2–109.5	1.45–1.60	659–727	241–271	109.5–123.2	1.60–1.80	727–818
20–60			0.63–0.75	284–341			0.75–0.88	341–398			0.88–1.00	398–455
60–180			1.32–1.47	598–667			1.47–1.62	667–735			1.62–1.81	735–822
0–180			1.06–1.20	482–545			1.20–1.34	545–609			1.34–151	609–684

Table 1.3. Recommended space per pig by phase of production.

Phase	Indoor Solid	Indoor Slotted	Outdoor
	Area per pig in m^2 (ft^2)		
Gilts	1.86 (20)	1.49 (16)	2.32 (25)
Sows	2.2 (24)	1.86 (20)	2.32 (25)
Farrow pen	8 (88)	NA	NA
Farrow crate	4.4 (48)	4.4 (48)	NA
Boars	NA	1.86 (20)	NA
Nursing	—	2.0 (22)	—
Nursery 20 kg	.37 (4)	.28 (3)	0.74 (8)
Nursery 40 kg	.37 (4)	.40 (4.4)	0.74 (8)
Grower 60 kg	.56 (6)	.53 (5.8)	1.86 (20)
Finish 80 kg	.74 (8)	.67 (7.2)	1.86 (20)
Finish 110kg	.75 (8)	.75 (8)	1.86 (20)

Source: Adapted from English et al. (1982), Baxter (1984), Patience and Thacker (1989), Gonyou and Stricklin (1998).

m^2/pig. This is important with respect to aggression in sows. If sows are provided sufficient space, group size has little impact on aggression. However, if space is restricted, aggression increases as group size increases. Similarly, rectangular pens are essential if space is restricted; otherwise, square pens will suffice. If gilts are provided with only 1.4 m^2/pig the pen must also include full stalls for feeding.

Providing individual feeding stalls within a large pen has the advantage of allowing both individualized feeding and a safe refuge for subordinate sows (Barnett et al. 2001). Partial stalls also provide similar advantages. The benefit is maximized if the sows are fed in these partial stalls. Another alternative is to build a maze or a series of partitions within the large pen to provide escape zones and sleeping areas for small social groups of sows.

Almost all sows in Europe, the U.K., North America, and Australia farrow in crates (Barnett et al. 2001). Farrowing crates are primarily used to reduce preweaning mortality rates by reducing the sow's ability to lie down quickly thereby reducing crushing. Other features include reducing the space used by the piglet, providing a creep area with supplemental heat and draft reduction and slatted floors to improve hygiene. A farrowing crate area will encompass a total width of 1.8 m and a length of 2.4 m. The slotted area of the floor of a farrowing pen should not exceed 10 mm otherwise newborn pigs will get their feet caught in the hole (English et al. 1982). The back gate of the farrowing crate should be at least 750 mm wide to enable personnel to assist the sow during farrowing (English et al. 1982). The creep area will be offset to allow 0.8 m wide on the side with the supplementary heat and 0.3 m wide on the other side for the pigs to nurse. Sow pens used for farrowing tend to be 6–10 m^2, whereas crates are typically 4 m^2.

Outdoor housing is used for one quarter of sows living in the U.K. and New Zealand, 2–4% of sows in Denmark, 7–9% of sows in France and 5–6% of sows in Australia (Barnett et al. 2001). Welfare issues of concern for these sows include health and disease, predation, access to food and water, protection against weather extremes, mutilations, use of electric fences, paddock rotation, and stocking density. To preserve pastures, producers may use nose rings, which discourage foraging. Huts used as shelter in the cold months must provide 1.3 m^2/sow so that timid sows will enter the shelter. Paddocks must provide shelter from wind and well-drained soil. In Australia, outdoor housing is limited to areas with few days over 30°C and limited rainfall. Sows housed outdoors have a higher variation in back fat, a longer outside claw length and a lower farrowing rate (Barnett et al. 2001).

Access to Feed and Water

Onto the map of the facility, insert number and type of feeders and waterers. Determine whether there are sufficient feeders and waterers for the maximum number and size of pig expected to live in the pen.

Pigs consume 10% of their own body weight in water per day, and more in hot weather. One liter of water weighs 1 kg. Therefore, a 100 kg pig will consume at least 10 liters of water per day (Table 1.4). This is important to determine access to water and for water medication. For more information on medication, see Chapter 71. Pigs drink 80% of their water in conjunction to when they feed. Also, pigs prefer to eat and drink at daybreak, and then off and on throughout the day and the evening, but spend the night sleeping. Nursery pigs eat more frequently than grower pigs, which in turn eat more frequently than finisher pigs. If water or feeder access is limited, submissive pigs will be forced to eat and drink during the night. When access to water is insufficient, there is an increase in aggression (see Chapter 64),

Table 1.4. Recommended water requirements, water flow rate, and feeder space per pig by phase of production.

	Water Requirements l/day	Water Requirements l/minute	Feeder Space/Pig mm (inches)
Restricted feed			
Gestating sows	12–25	2	457–610 (18–24)
Lactating sow	10–30	2	
Boar	20	2	
Nursing	1	0.3	
Nursery	2.8	1	254 (10)
Grower	7–20	1.4	260 (10)
Finish	10–20	1.7	330 (13)
Ad libitum			
Nursery	2.8	1	60 (2.3)
Grower	7–20	1.4	65 (2.5)
Finish	10–20	1.7	76 (3)

Source: Adapted from Baxter (1984); Patience and Thacker (1989); *Swine Care Handbook,* 2003; Muirhead and Alexander (1997).

weight gain is decreased because feed intake is decreased, and there is an increase in the variation in pig body weight by age (see Chapter 66). There should be no more than 4 pigs for each feeder space in an ad libitum feed management system. One water nipple can accommodate 10 to 15 pigs. The waterers and feeders must be spaced adequately so that a pig drinking from one water nipple cannot obstruct the ability of another pig to get to a second water nipple. If water is provided in a trough, there must be 300 mm per 20 finisher pigs or 15 sows (Muirhead and Alexander 1997). Water bowls accommodate 17 to 20 pigs. Farrowing crates need to be equipped with water nipples or bowls for both the sow and the piglets.

Feeding dry sows three times per day is associated with lower sow mortality than feeding twice a day, which in turn was associated with lower mortality than feeding once a day (Abiven et al. 1998). Farms feeding dry meal or wet meal had lower mortality than those feeding pelleted ration, likely due to the decreased occurrence of torsions. Dry sows are typically fed 1.5 times their maintenance requirements which is approximately 0.6 of their ad libitum feed intake (Barnett et al. 2001).

Electronic feeders typically accommodate 40 sows per unit (Barnett et al. 2001). Provided the feeder design is appropriate to discourage vulva biting, these feeders work well in stable groups of sows. In dynamic groups, aggression may continue to be a problem because feeding order cannot be established. This may reduce reproductive performance. Group feeding sows in pens continues to provide an unfair advantage to dominant sows who gain significantly more weight during gestation than submissive sows (Bourns and Edwards 1994).

Temperature

Upper and lower critical temperature is dependent on the floor type, amount of feed provided to pigs, live weight, number of animals in the pen, drafts (or wind speed for outdoor pigs), rain, ability to gain shelter, and—for sows—stage of pregnancy (see Table 1.5). Typically, dry sows are fed 1.5 times their maintenance requirements. The lower critical limit is the temperature below which a pig will use extra feed to maintain its body temperature (Barnett et al. 2001). Pigs provided with straw in the winter months will tolerate a lower temperature. For every 5°C below the lower critical temperature, sows will need to be fed an extra 250 g feed/day. For every 1°C below the lower critical temperature for grower/finisher pigs, each pig will have to consume an extra 3.3 kg of feed to reach market weight.

Pigs held above the upper critical temperature will experience decreased feed intake. For sows, this subsequently results in lower reproductive performance and lower milk production. Boars and sows kept at 23–27°C will have reduced fertility (English et al. 1982). Pigs held above the upper critical temperature should be provided with drip coolers for indoor pigs and wallows for outdoor pigs. If straw is provided, the upper critical temperature will be substantially lower than if pigs sleep on a concrete floor.

Ideally, sows will be kept between 21 and 22°C. Newborn pigs will have a creep area maintained at 28–30 °C. Newly weaned pigs should be kept at 26–28°C depending on their age and size at weaning. Temperature is gradually reduced each week so that they are at 22°C when they are moved to the grower barn (Curtis 1983). Grower/finisher pigs prefer to be kept in 15–20°C. It is essential that temperature does not fluctuate rapidly over time.

Begin the Herd Visit with History-Taking

Ask the manager/owner about his/her concerns. This will ensure that these problem areas are addressed during your discussion and as you walk through the barn. Follow this with a complete history-taking, including the topics covered in the following sections.

Herd Security. Were any animals brought onto the farm recently? What are the quarantine and isolation procedures for new stock? Are there one or more sources of breeding stock, nursery, or grower pigs? What steps are taken to control human and animal traffic? How are animals loaded out of the farm? Are livestock trucks clean on arrival? Take note of the biosecurity protocols used for human traffic. (See Chapter 68 for a complete description of biosecurity concerns.)

Table 1.5. Lower and upper critical temperatures (°C) by size of pig based on feeding level and flooring type.

		Maintenance Units of Feed[a]					
		1	2	3	1	2	3
		Dry Concrete			Straw		
		Temperature degrees celcius					
LCT[b]	Sows	19	10	NA	14	5	NA
	Nursing						
	Nursery 20 kg	26	21	16	23	17	11
	Nursery 40 kg	24	18	13	20	13	7
	Growers 60 kg	22	16	12	18	12	5
	Finishers 80 kg	21	15	12	17	10	4
		Dry Concrete			Slatted Floor		
		Temperature degrees celcius					
UCT[c]	Sows	32	27	NA	30	26	NA
	Nursing 1 kg	37	36	36	35	33	31
	Nursery 5 kg	37	35	34	34	32	30
	Nursery 20 kg	36	35	33	35	32	29
	Nursery 40 kg	36	34	32	34	32	29
	Growers 60 kg	35	33	31	34	31	28
	Finishers 80 kg	35	33	31	34	31	29

Source: Adapted from Bruce (1982), Baxter (1984), Patience and Thacker (1989).

[a]Feed provided at 1, 2, or 3 times maintenance.
[b]Lower critical temperature.
[c]Upper critical temperature.
NA = not available.

Genetics

What is the genetic composition of the herd? What procedures are used to guarantee that proper matings will take place? What selection criteria are used for boars, gilts, and sows? Is there a family or breed relationship between animals experiencing the disease?

Breeding Management. In units using natural mating, what is the boar-to-sow ratio? How frequently are individual boars used? Does mating occur in a pen or is hand mating used? With hand mating, what sanitary precautions are taken between boars? In units using artificial insemination, what percent of females are bred this way? Is semen purchased or collected on farm? What are the handling and storage procedures for the semen? How is estrus detection done? How frequently and at what times are sows and gilts mated? When and how is pregnancy diagnosis done? What is the conception rate for sows and gilts? What is the farrowing rate for sows and gilts? How many females return to estrus 21 days after mating and at other intervals? Have abortions been noted?

Farrowing Performance. Are sows washed prior to entering the farrowing area? Are sows induced to farrow and if so, what is the protocol? How frequently do sows require assistance to farrow? What procedure is used for cross-fostering? What are the size of litters and the total born alive, mummies, and stillbirths? What do piglets weigh at birth and weaning? What is the average and range in lactation length? How often are sows weaned?

Mortality. What is the current state of mortality on the farm? If mortality was not fully described in the records, ask questions relating to the historical pattern of mortality. What is the average and range in mortality by phase of production. Within each phase, when does the mortality occur? Is there a seasonal pattern to mortality? What are the clinical observations in pigs just before they die? What is the appearance of the dead pig? Have these types of mortalities occurred previously? What has been done, if anything, to determine the cause of these mortalities?

Medications and Immunizations. What vaccines are used routinely in the herd? What animals are vaccinated and at what time? Is there a routine worming program for sows, boars, and growing pigs? How are external parasites controlled? What medications are used in the feed? Are drugs used at a growth-promoting or therapeutic level? Is drug usage rotated? What injectable treatments are given to sick pigs? Has the producer completed and maintained a quality assurance program? Are there written standard vaccination and treatment protocols displayed as a reference for all employees?

Feed. Is feed grown on the farm or purchased? Where and how is feed mixing done? What nutrient composition is intended for each class of pig? How is feed stored and delivered to the pigs? What quantity of feed is given to limit-fed pigs, and how is the feed measured?

Disease Outbreak. What was the progression of signs within a pig? How old was the pig when signs started? How long did illness persist? Is recovery complete or is pig unthrifty? In the group affected, what is the morbidity and mortality? Has treatment been used, and to what effect? What is the course of disease within the herd? Did the disease start with an explosive outbreak or was it insidious? What animals were originally affected? What animals has disease spread to? Did the initial disease picture differ from the later signs? Is disease becoming more or less severe? Are any other animals besides pigs affected? What is the distribution of affected animals? Is disease sporadic or endemic? Are affected animals grouped by litter, pen, or building? Is one sex affected to a greater extent than the other? Were any changes in management made prior to the outbreak of the disease? Has this problem occurred before on this farm?

Disease Affecting Pigs in Litters. Are whole litters affected, or is incidence sporadic within litters? Are the biggest or smallest pigs affected? Are litters of gilts or of sows more frequently or severely affected?

"Walk Through" the Barns

It is essential to walk through the barns to observe the pigs for clinical signs of disease, abnormal behaviors, availability of space, water, and feed and also to assess the environment/ventilation. Visit all phases of production even if the producer does not have specific concerns in all areas.

Be sure to talk with all farm employees. Each person will have his/her own concerns and observations. As the veterinarian you can address these problems and encourage the employees to reach their potential. Employees will ask you to examine individual pigs showing specific clinical problems. Although swine health management deals with the group of animals, many of these individuals provide an excellent measurement of the whole. These discussions provide an opportunity to review treatment protocols and euthanasia decisions. The welfare of specific pigs and the decisions about pigs in the hospital pen will be discussed during the walkthrough. People working in the barn need to deal with individual pigs to raise the welfare in the barn.

Details of clinical examination are outlined in the systems chapters. Observe the body condition of the sows and compare this to the descriptions in Table 1.6 and Figure 1.1. Normal values for temperature, respiration, and heart rate are outlined in Table 1.7. Using Table 1.8 as a guide, determine the state of management and the health of the pigs in the farrowing room with undesirable physical problems. Discuss the treatment and

Table 1.6. Body condition evaluation.

Numerical Score	Pelvic Bones (Ilium, Ischium) Tail Head	Loin	Vertebrae	Ribs	Inches (mm) of Backfat
1	Pelvic bones very prominent. Deep cavity around the tail head.	Loin very narrow. Sharp edge on transverse spinal process. Flank very hollow.	Prominent and sharp throughout the length of the back-bone.	Individual ribs very prominent.	0.5 (13) or less
2	Pelvic bones obvious but some slight cover. Cavity around tail head.	Loin narrow. Only very slight cover to edge of transverse spinal process. Flank rather hollow.	Prominent.	Rib cage less apparent. Difficult to see individual ribs.	0.6 (15)
3	Pelvic bones covered.	Edge of transverse spinal processes covered and rounded.	Visible over the shoulder. Some cover farther back.	Covered but can be felt.	0.7 (17)
4	Pelvic bones only felt with firm pressure. No cavity around tail.	Edge of transverse spinal processes felt only with firm pressure.	Felt only with firm pressure.	Rib cage not visible. Very difficult to feel any ribs.	0.8 (20)
5	Pelvic bones impossible to feel. Root of tail set deep in surrounding fat.	Impossible to feel bones. Flank full and rounded.	Impossible to feel vertebrae.	Not possible to feel ribs.	0.9 (23)
6	Pelvic bones impossible to feel. Folds of fat obscure the vulva in sows.	Thick fat cover.	Midline appears as a slight hollow between rolls of fat.	Thick fat cover.	1.0 (25)

Table 1.7. Temperature and respiration and heart rate of pigs of different ages.

Age of Pig	Rectal Temperature (Range ± 0.30°C, 0.5°F)		Respiratory Rate (Breaths/Min)	Heart Rate (Beats/Min)
	°C	°F		
Newborn	39.0	102.2	50–60	200–250
1 hr	36.8	98.3		
12 hr	38.0	100.4		
24 hr	38.6	101.5		
Unweaned piglet	39.2	102.6		
Weaned piglet (20–40 lb) (9–18 kg)	39.3	102.7	25–40	90–100
Growing pig (60–100 lb) (27–45 kg)	39.0	102.3	30–40	80–90
Finishing pig (100–200 lb) (45–90 kg)	38.8	101.8	25–35	75–85
Sow in gestation	38.7	101.7	13–18	70–80
Sow				
24 hr prepartum	38.7	101.7	35–45	
12 hr prepartum	38.9	102.0	75–85	
6 hr prepartum	39.0	102.2	95–105	
Birth of first pig	39.4	102.9	35–45	
12 hr postpartum	39.7	103.5	20–30	
24 hr postpartum	40.0	104.0	15–22	
1 week postpartum until weaning	39.3	102.7		
1 day postweaning	38.6	101.5		
Boar	38.4	101.1	13–18	70–80

prevention of these problems with the employees responsible for that area of the production unit. Examine the nursery, grower, and finisher pigs. Specifically determine if they are managed in an all-in, all-out manner and that the room or barn is properly cleaned and disinfected between groups and allowed to dry for a few days before refilling. The pigs should not vary in body weight by age by more than 10%. There should be no indications of clinical disease, such as skin lesions, diarrhea, coughing, or sneezing. Pigs should not be exhibiting vices and should be dunging in the appropriate area. Commonly observed problems include high pig density (refer to Table 1.3); large variation in body weight; runts or poor-doing pigs; coughing, sneezing, or nasal dis-

Table 1.8. Examination of pigs in the farrowing area.

Characteristic	Desirable	Undesirable
Sows		
Physical condition		
Body condition	Normal weight.	Thin, fat, or obese.
Cleanliness	Sows have been thoroughly washed.	Sows are dirty with caked mud and manure.
Mammary glands	At least 12 prominent, evenly spaced nipples.	Inverted, juvenile, or overcrowded teats; glands hot, red, swollen, painful; abnormal milk.
Vulval discharges	Watery, clear-to-whitish fluid.	Purulent, bloody, or foul-smelling discharge.
Skin	Unblemished. Pink in unpigmented areas.	Burns from the heat lamp. Abrasions or calluses. Anemia. Hyperkeratinization.
Feet and legs	Normal stance and movement.	Splaylegged, foot lesions, difficulty getting up or lying down.
Feed		
Amount	4–6 lb (2–2.5 kg), plus 1 lb (0.5 kg) for each pig in the litter.	Less than the desired level.
Feeder condition	Clean, large capacity, and easily accessible.	Dirty, broken, containing old or moldy feed.
Water	Unlimited supply of fresh water.	Fouled water, inadequate flow or inaccessible.
Environment		
Temperature	Between 60°F and 75°F (16–24°C).	Too cold or too hot.
Floor design	Proper spacing between slats, good traction, nonabrasive.	Slippery material. Sharp edges on slats, uneven slats. Slots sized to trap teats and dewclaws.
Floor condition	Clean and dry.	Dirty, wet, cracked or broken.
Crate design	Right size for sow. Permits good exposure of underline.	Too large, allowing sows to flop over and crush pigs. Bottom bar hinders nursing.
Light	12–14 hr daily at 200 lux.	Too dark.
Baby Pigs		
Physical condition		
Birth weight	Average of 3 lb (1.3 kg) or greater.	Average is less than 3 lb (1.3 kg).
Litter sizes	Litters are matched to rearing capacity of sows.	Wide variation in litter size, with 20% or more containing 8 or fewer pigs.
Weights within the litter	Less than 1 lb (0.5 kg) difference between the largest and smallest pigs.	More than 1 lb (0.5 kg) difference between the largest and smallest pigs.
Skin	Unblemished. Pink in unpigmented areas.	Knee abrasions, facial lacerations, teat necrosis, anemia, exudative epidermitis.
Locomotion	Normal gait and anatomy.	Splayleg, swollen joints, foot lesions, lameness.
Infectious disease	None.	Diarrhea, sneezing, unthriftiness.
Teeth	Clipped on day-old pigs. Gums pink and healthy.	Teeth not clipped. Infected gums.
Tails	Clipped neatly or left long.	Clipped tails are swollen, red, or infected.
Feed		
Feed	Fresh creep feed given daily.	None or stale feed offered.
Water	Fresh water easily accessible to piglets.	None, inaccessible, or foul water.
Environment		
Temperature	Creep area provided with temperature of 85–90°F (29–32°C).	Piling or lying next to the sow. Pigs too hot and avoiding the heat lamp.
Drafts	Air evenly distributed throughout the building.	Incoming air moving directly onto litters of pigs.
Floor design	Good traction for pigs in the nursing area. Uniform spacing of slats. Nonabrasive surface.	Slippery flooring material. Slats laid so that slot length is perpendicular to the sow.
Floor condition	Clean, dry; bedded if appropriate.	Dirty, wet, cracked, broken, or exposed aggregate.
Management		
Flow	All-in/all-out animal flow.	Continuous farrowing.
Building use	All farrowings occur within a few days.	Farrowings are spread out over 1 or 2 weeks.
Farrowing schedule	Pigs weaned at the same time.	Pigs are weaned at various times and ages.
Sanitation		
Cleanliness	Excess manure and afterbirth removed daily	Accumulation of manure in the farrowing crates. Wet bedding. Poor fly control.
"Downtime"	Building is empty for a few days between farrowing batches.	New batch added the same day or the day after the previous batch was weaned.
Washing procedures	High-pressure washer is used to remove all organic material. Porous surfaces sealed or disinfected.	Manure left in cracks and corners. Accumulations of dust and cobwebs.

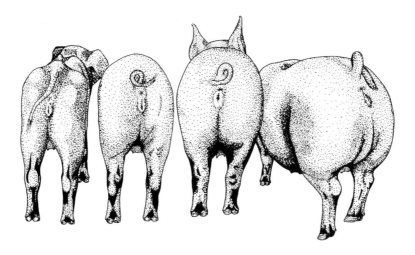

1.1. *Sows just after weaning. Using the criteria in Table 1.6, from left to right their body condition scores are 1, 3, 4, and 6.*

charge; anemia; skin abrasions; diarrhea; rectal prolapse or stricture; hernias; hematomas of the ears; umbilical sucking; and belly nosing. If the environment is not adequate, some problems that may be observed include bitten tails or ears, dunging in the eating or sleeping areas, pigs piling if it is too cold, or pigs panting and lying in the manure if it is too hot. Specific environmental problems include rough or abrasive floor surface or broken slats, inadequate feeder space or plugged feeders, inadequate waterers, plugged nipples, dirty water bowls, inadequate cleaning, manure in the corners of the pen and under the feeders, and cold and drafty barns.

Food Safety

Discuss the medications used in the feed and water, and as injectables to ensure these are essential (see Chapter 71 for more specifics on medications). Arrange to update the Quality Assurance program on the farm to ensure the wholesomeness of the pork being produced. Set up a drug recording and animal tracking system for the unit. Create summaries of standardized treatment plans and vaccination protocols that will be displayed in the farm office. These ensure that all employees follow the same protocols. If feed is mixed on the farm, create similar protocols for all feed that is to be manufactured.

Disease Status

The disease status of the farm can be measured by clinical signs, postmortem examination of dead pigs or those that you cull during your visit, vaccination use, slaughter-check examinations, and serological profiling. Use all or some of these to understand the diseases that are present and those that are causing problems on the farm. Postmortem evaluations must be conducted on at least three pigs during a disease outbreak to ensure that the disease process affecting the group is identified. Untreated pigs in the early phases of the disease provide ideal samples. Live animals must be submitted to diag-

nose enteric illness. More details about disease investigation can be found in other chapters.

Review the disease control measures being used, including vaccinations, antibiotic use, early weaning, multisite production and gilt introductions. Ensure that all vaccinations and antibiotics are essential. Alter the disease control measures if diseases are not being properly controlled.

Serial serological sampling helps determine the epidemiology of the disease within the herd. Blood samples can be taken from 10 pigs in each age category to determine when passive immunity wanes and active immunity is present, or pigs can be individually ear-tagged and then followed over time. Chapter 10 provides more detail about interpretation of tests at the pig and herd levels.

Biosecurity

Determine the biosecurity of the farm with respect to the presence of birds, rodents, and other animal species. Review the movement and access of the facility to people, trucks, incoming feed and pig movement. Identify where biosecurity can be improved, keeping in mind the realistic risks of the current biosecurity system. For detailed information on biosecurity, see Chapter 68.

Welfare

Has the producer enrolled in a welfare assurance program? If there is a formal program in your area, such as the Swine Welfare Assurance Program[SM] available, encourage the producer to participate in the program (Johnson 2004). If such a program does not exist, determine the welfare of the farm and discuss areas for improvement. The specific areas of focus in the SWAP[SM] program include herd health and nutrition, caretaker training, animal observation, body condition scoring, euthanasia, handling and movement, facilities, emergency support, and continuing assessment and education.

Goals

Set short-term goals to address the concerns of the personnel and to work on conditions of immediate economic importance. Discuss long-term goals, including the improvement of production parameters, herd disease status, and personnel issues.

Begin the collection of data for production parameters of importance. Examples include mortality tallies, movement of pigs in and out of barns, and weighing a sample of pigs in and out of the barn.

In large facilities, it is worthwhile to conduct field trials to determine the expected improvements to changes in management or disease control prior to making the change in the whole system.

Follow-up

Schedule a time for a return visit, plan what changes are to be made between now and then, identify the specific outcomes expected, and arrange for further sample collection (i.e., slaughter check or submission of dead pigs to postmortem). Provide a written report summarizing both the successes and problems observed during the review of the records and the herd visit. Outline the expected changes in the form of a checklist so that the producer can refer to these easily. Review this letter prior to the subsequent herd visit.

BLOOD SAMPLING

Blood collection in swine is difficult because of the inaccessibility of good veins and arteries. Many different techniques using various sites have been described. Some of these techniques have some role in experimental work with pigs, but if the practicing veterinarian is to sample blood of a number of pigs with some degree of speed and collect a reasonable volume, the technique of sampling from the jugular vein or the anterior vena cava must be mastered (Brown 1979; Muirhead 1981). Alternatively, some veterinarians prefer to use the orbital sinus for routine blood collection. Appropriate blood collection techniques for various sizes of pig are given in Table 1.9.

Anterior Vena Cava

Depending on the size of the pig, it is restrained either standing by means of a hog snare (Figure 1.2) or manually by holding the front legs (Figure 1.3). The position of the standing pig is important; the head should be raised, the body straight, and the front legs well back. In the standing pig, the jugular groove is traced to its caudal limit just anterior to the thoracic inlet. The needle is inserted at the caudal end of the jugular groove and directed dorsally and somewhat caudomedially along an imaginary line that passes through the top of the opposite shoulder. The location of some of the major veins are shown in Figure 1.4. When drawing blood samples from either the anterior vena cava or the jugular vein, the blood is taken from the right side, since the right vagus nerve provides less innervation to the heart and diaphragm than the left vagus. If the vagus nerve is accidentally punctured, the pig may show dyspnea, cyanosis, and convulsive struggling.

Jugular Vein

The pig is restrained in a standing position as for sampling from the anterior vena cava. The needle is inserted in the jugular groove about 5 cm cranial to the thoracic inlet. The needle is directed dorsally and slightly medially.

Ear Veins

The ear veins are raised by slapping the ear and maintained by a rubber band around the base (Figure 1.5). Venipuncture is done with a quick thrusting stab to prevent the vein from rolling away from the needle. A syringe should be used, since vacutainer collection usually results in collapse of the vein. Alternatively, the ventral ear vein may be incised with a scalpel cut made into and parallel to the vein and the blood collected in a tube as it drips from the incision.

Tail Vessels

Collection from tail vessels is possible only in mature pigs whose tails have not been docked. The tail is held vertically and the needle directed toward the point of junction of the tail with the body (Muirhead 1981).

Table 1.9. Blood collection in swine.

Site	Type of Pig	Needle Size	Quantity	Comments
Anterior vena cava	Up to 100 lb (45 kg)	20 g. 1.5 in. (38 mm)	Unlimited	Danger of damaging the vagus nerve. Vacutainer usable.
	100–250 lb (45–133 kg)	18 g. 2.5 in. (65 mm)		
	Adult	16 g. 3.5 in. (90 mm)		
Jugular vein	Any age	20 g. 1.5 in. (38 mm)	Unlimited	More difficult to do. Vacutainer usable.
Ear veins	Adult pigs	20 g. 1 in. (25 mm); scalpel blade	1–2 mL	Possible hematoma; possible contaminated sample.
Tail	Adult pigs	20 g. 1 in. (25 mm)	5–10 mL	Requires practice. Vacutainer usable.
Orbital sinus	Up to 40 lb (18 kg)	20 g. 1 in. (25 mm)	5–10 mL	Slow. Unaesthetic. Possible postcollection orbital hemorrhage and pressure on the globe.
	40–120 lb (18–54 kg)	16 g. 1.5 in. (38 mm)		
	120 lb–adult (54+ kg)	14 g. 1.5 in. (38 mm)		

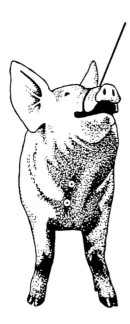

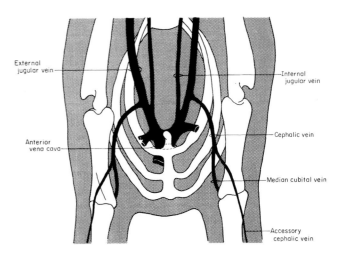

1.4. *Location of some of the major veins in the pig in relation to the skeleton.*

1.2. *Proper restraint for blood sampling from a standing pig. The lower circle indicates the site for sampling from the anterior vena cana; the upper circle indicates the site for sampling from the jugular vein.*

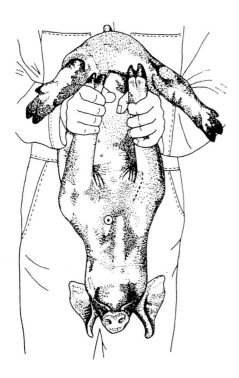

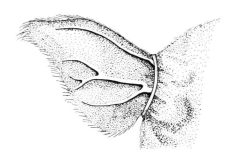

1.5. *Ear veins of a pig raised by rubber band placed at the base of the ear.*

1.3. *Method of restraining pigs weighing less than 20 kg for blood sampling from the anterior vena cava (circle). Location of the cephalic vein is indicated by the dashed line.*

slightly anterioventrally until it punctures the venous sinus. Blood is allowed to drip out of the needle and is collected in an open-top tube (Huhn et al. 1969).

Cephalic Vein

Blood may be withdrawn from the cephalic vein by restraining the pig on its back with the front legs stretched backward and a little outward from the body. The vein is visible under the skin (see Figure 1.4) and is raised with digital pressure (Tumbleson et al. 1968; Sankari 1983).

Miscellaneous Methods

Cardiac puncture (Calvert et al. 1977) and femoral venipuncture techniques (Brown et al. 1978) have been described.

Indwelling Catheters

Indwelling catheters have been used for research that requires repeated blood sampling or minimal excitement of the pig. Investigators have described techniques for placing catheters in the femoral artery and vein (Weirich et al. 1970; Jackson et al. 1972), subcutaneous ab-

Orbital Venous Sinus

Large pigs are restrained by snare and smaller ones held manually, with care to restrain the snout securely. A needle is placed at the medial canthus of the eye just inside the nictitating membrane and advanced medially and

dominal vein and middle sacral artery (Witzel et al. 1973), ear vein (Grün et al. 1973; Brussow et al. 1981), jugular vein (Brown et al. 1973; Wingfield et al. 1974; Ford and Maurer 1978), and uterine vein (Rodriquez and Kunavongkrit 1983).

SAMPLE COLLECTION

Feces are best collected directly from the rectum by hand using a disposable glove. The sample can be kept in the glove after inversion. Urine is collected by catching a midstream sample. Females can be catheterized with the aid of an otoscope or speculum. In barrows it is not possible to exteriorize the penis because of adhesions between the penis and sheath. Procedures for tonsilar swabbing, biopsy, and scraping have been described by Mengeling et al. (1992) and Brown et al. (1995). Briefly, the pig is sedated using a drug with analgesic properties, the jaw is held open with a speculum, and one person provides illumination while another person takes the tonsilar sample. Scraping is best accomplished with a long-handled spoon that has had the bowl sharpened.

REFERENCES

Abiven N, Seegers H, Beaudeau F, Laval A, Fourichon C. 1998. Risk factors for high sow mortality in French swine herds. Prev Vet Med 33:109–119.

Barnett JL, Hemsworth PH, Cronin GM, Jongman EC, Hutson GD. 2001. A review of the welfare issues for sows and piglets in relation to housing. Australian Journal of Agricultural Research 52:1–28.

Baxter S. 1984. The pig's response to the thermal environment. In Intensive Pig Production. Environmental Management and Design, pp. 35–50. London: Granada Publishing.

——. 1984. The pig's influence on its climatic environment. In Intensive Pig Production. Environmental Management and Design, pp. 55–62. London: Granada Publishing.

——. 1984. Space and place. In Intensive Pig Production. Environmental Management and Design, pp. 216–248. London: Granada Publishing.

Bourns F, Edwards AS. 1994. Social rank and feeding behaviour of group housed sows fed competitively or ad libitum. Appl Anim Behv Sci 39:225–235.

Brown CM. 1979. A method for collecting blood from hogs using the thoracic inlet. Vet Med Small Anim Clin 74:361–363.

Brown DE, King GJ, Hacker RR. 1973. Polyurethane indwelling catheters for piglets. J Anim Sci 37:303–304.

Brown JR, Tyeryar EA, Harrington DG, Hilmas DE. 1978. Femoral venipuncture for repeated blood sampling in miniature swine. Lab Anim Sci 28:339–342.

Brown TT, Shin KO, Fuller FJ. 1995. Detection of pseudorabies viral DNA in tonsillar epithelial cells of latently infected pigs. Am J Vet Res 56:587–594.

Bruce JM. 1982. Ventilation and temperature control criteria for pigs. pp. 197–216. In Environmental Aspects of Housing for Animal Production. JA Clark, ed. London: Butterworths.

Brussow VKP, Bergfeld J, Parchow G. 1981. Über mehrjährige Erfahrungen zur Blutgewinnung durch intravenose Dauerkatheter beim Schwein. Monatsh Veterinaermed 36:300–303.

Calvert GD, Scott PJ, Sharpe DN. 1977. Percutaneous cardiac puncture in domestic pigs. Aust Vet J 53:337–339.

Curtis SE. 1983. Thermal-environmental requirements. In Environmental Management in Animal Agriculture, pp.117–122. Ames: Iowa State University Press.

Deen J, Anil SS. 2003. Benchmarking at the global level. Proc AD Leman Swine Conf, Minneapolis, pp. 144–146.

English PR, Smith WJ, MacLean A. 1982. Weaning, mating and pregnancy maintenance. In The Sow—Improving Her Efficiency, p. 240. Ipswich: Farming Press Ltd.

Ferket SL, Hacker RR. 1985. Effect of forced exercise during gestation on reproductive performance of sows. Can J Anim Sci 65:851–859.

Ford JJ, Maurer RR. 1978. Simple technique for chronic venous catheterization of swine. Lab Anim Sci 28:615–618.

Fredeen HT, Sather AP. 1978. Joint damage in pigs reared under confinement. Can J Anim Sci 58:759–773.

Gonyou HW, Stricklin WR. 1998. Effects of floor area allowance and group size on the productivity of growing/finishing pigs. J Anim Sci 76:1326–1330.

Grün E, Hüller G, Möckel HG. 1973. Dauerkatheter am Schweineohr. Monatsh Veterinaermed 28:263–265

Hale OM, Newton GL, Cleveland ER. 1984. Effects of exercise during the growing-finishing period on performance, age at puberty and conception rate of gilts. J Anim Sci 58:541–544.

Huhn RG, Osweiler GD, Switzer WP. 1969. Application of the orbital sinus bleeding technique to swine. Lab Anim Care 19:403–405.

Jackson VMD, Cook DB, Gill G. 1972. Simultaneous intravenous infusion and arterial blood sampling in piglets. Lab Anim Sci 22:552–555.

Jensen P. 1984. Effects of confinement on social interaction patterns in dry sows. Applied Animal Behavior Science 12:93–101.

Johnson AK. 2004. SWAP overview. Proc Am Assoc Swine Vet, Des Moines, pp. 465–470.

Mengeling WL, Lager KM, Volz DM, Brockmeier SL. 1992. Effect of various vaccination procedures on shedding, latency, and reactivation of attenuated and virulent pseudorabies virus. Am J Vet Res 53:2164–2173.

Muirhead MR. 1981. Blood sampling in pigs. Pract 3:16–20.

Muirhead MR, Alexander TJL. 1997. Managing health and disease. In Managing Pig Health and the Treatment of Disease, p. 103. Sheffield: 5 M Enterprises Ltd..

——. 1997. Managing and treating disease in the weaner, grower and finishing periods. In Managing Pig Health and the Treatment of Disease, p. 294. Sheffield: 5 M Enterprises Ltd.

Patience JF, Thacker PA. 1989. Feeding the weaned pig. In Swine Nutrition Guide, pp. 186–187. University of Saskatchewan, Saskatoon: Prairie Swine Centre.

——. 1989. Feeding management of market hogs. In Swine Nutrition Guide, pp. 206–207. University of Saskatchewan, Saskatoon: Prairie Swine Centre.

Rodriquez H, Kunavongkrit A. 1983. Chronical venous catheterization for frequent blood sampling in unrestrained pigs. Acta Vet Scand 24:318–320.

Sankari S. 1983. A practical method of taking blood samples from the pig. Acta Vet Scand 24:133–134.

Swine Care Handbook. 2003. www.porkboard.org/SWAPoem.

Tumbleson ME, Dommert AR, Middleton CC. 1968. Techniques for handling miniature swine for laboratory procedures. Lab Anim Care 18:584–587.

Weirich WE, Will JA, Crumpton CW. 1970. A technique for placing chronic indwelling catheters in swine. J Appl Physiol 28:117–119.

Wingfield WE, Tumbleson ME, Hicklin KW, Mather EC. 1974. An exteriorized cranial vena caval catheter for serial blood sample collection from miniature swine. Lab Anim Sci 24:359–361.

Witzel DA, Littledike ET, Cook HM. 1973. Implanted catheters for blood sampling in swine. Cornell Vet 63:432–435.

2 Immune System

James A. Roth and Eileen L. Thacker

The immune system is comprised of a variety of components that cooperate to defend the host against infectious agents. These components generally can be divided into innate (or nonspecific) immune defense mechanisms and adaptive (or acquired) immune defense mechanisms. The innate defense mechanisms are not antigen specific. They are present in a normal animal and do not require previous exposure to antigen, and they are capable of responding almost immediately to an infectious agent. The major components of the innate immune system are complement, antimicrobial peptides, phagocytic cells (macrophages, neutrophils, and eosinophils), natural killer (NK) cells, and some types of interferon. These components are very important in controlling an infection during the first few days of an initial exposure to an agent. The innate immune system controls infection until the adaptive immune system can be activated and it is important in directing the immune system to produce both antibody and cell-mediated immune responses.

B and T lymphocytes and their products are the components of the adaptive immune response system. This antigen-driven system requires 2–3 weeks to reach optimal functional capacity after the first exposure to antigen. Upon second exposure to antigen, the specific immune response system reaches optimal activity much more rapidly due to the anamnestic, or memory, response. A major mechanism by which B and T lymphocytes enhance resistance to disease is activating the innate defense mechanisms (phagocytic cells, NK cells, and complement) and increasing their efficiency.

Providing immunity at mucosal surfaces and to the newborn piglet are especially difficult challenges for the immune system and for the swine producer. The nature of these special problems are discussed as well as generalities about vaccination to improve immunity at mucosal surfaces and in newborn pigs.

If an animal is immunosuppressed due to stress, a preexisting viral infection, immunotoxicants, or nutritional factors, the innate defense mechanisms may not function optimally. In addition, an adaptive immune response may be slow to develop, and have altered to decreased efficacy and thus be inadequate to control both primary and secondary pathogens. This can result in clinical disease due to an infectious agent that would normally be controlled.

The immune system has potent mechanisms for protecting the pig from infectious and neoplastic diseases. If the immune system is overstimulated or is not appropriately regulated, it may cause hypersensitivity reactions. This can occur in response to infection, vaccination, environmental or dietary antigens, or even against normal host tissues.

PHYSIOLOGY OF THE IMMUNE SYSTEM

Innate Defense Mechanisms

Physical, Chemical, and Microbial Barriers. Physical, chemical, and microbial barriers to infection at body surfaces are a very important part of resistance to disease. These factors include the epithelial cells, bactericidal fatty acids, normal flora, the mucous layer and the flow of mucus, low pH, bile, and numerous enzymes. More detailed information on physical, chemical, and microbial barriers to infection may be found in chapters dealing with specific organ systems.

An important family of molecules that helps form a chemical barrier to limit infection at epithelial surfaces and attack invading bacteria are the antimicrobial peptides. Over 750 antimicrobial peptides have been described in eukaryotes. They are being actively investigated as an alternative to antibiotics for clinical use in antimicrobial therapy. At least 14 antimicrobial peptides have been described in the pig (Brogden et al. 2003). The antimicrobial peptides are relatively small cationic peptides, which vary in structure and antimicrobial activity. They are found predominantly at mucosal surfaces and in phagocytic cells. Some are also found in other tissues. Many have broad spectrum activity against gram-negative bacteria, gram-positive bacteria, and fungal organisms. Some have a more limited spectrum of activity. The concentration of some of the antimicrobial peptides increases in response to inflammation or microbial infection (Brogden et al. 2003).

Complement. The complement system is an enzyme cascade system similar to the coagulation system and is composed of at least 20 serum proteins. In a cascade system the first component is activated, which in turn activates the next component, which in turn activates the next component, etc., until the reaction is completed. Since the sequential steps involve enzymes, the system is greatly amplified as it proceeds. The components of the mammalian complement system can be divided into the classical pathway, the alternative pathway, the mannan-binding (MB) pathway, the membrane attack complex, and regulatory proteins. The complement system is very important in mediating the inflammatory response and controlling bacterial infections. It also plays a prominent role in allergic and hypersensitivity reactions. The classical pathway is triggered primarily by antigen-antibody complexes consisting of IgG and IgM. The alternative pathway may also be activated by antigen-antibody complexes (IgA and IgE) and by certain bacterial products, such as endotoxin or proteases released by tissue damage. The MB pathway recognizes molecules on the surface of bacteria that differ from those present on the host cells. All three pathways end in the splitting of the third component of complement (C3) and start the formation of the membrane attack complex.

The complement system has many important biologic activities. Activation of any of the three pathways causes vasodilation and increased vascular permeability resulting in serum components (including antibody and complement) entering the tissues to help control infection. Complement components produced during activation are chemotactic and attract phagocytic cells to the site of infection. They also coat or opsonize infectious agents to increase their uptake by phagocytic cells. A very important function of the membrane attack pathway of complement is the destruction of cell membranes including some bacterial cell membranes.

The complement system is important for mediating inflammation and controlling bacterial infections. However, since it is so potent it is also capable of causing serious and even life-threatening damage if it is activated in an unregulated fashion. Therefore, there are numerous regulators of complement present in the serum. These regulators help control and stop the complement reaction once it has started.

Toll-like Receptors. Toll-like receptors (TLRs) are a key component of innate immunity (Check 2004; Cullor 1992). TLRs are a family of cell surface molecules that bind to various molecules derived from microbes, such as lipopolysaccharide, peptidoglycans, CpG rich un-

methylated oligonucleotides, and double-stranded RNA. They are the primary method for early detection of and response to microbial invasion. Binding of microbial components to TLRs initiates an inflammatory response that helps activate other aspects of innate immunity and initiate the acquired immune response. Bacterial derived vaccine adjuvants enhance immune response to vaccines through binding to TLRs. At least three TLRs have been described in swine and more are likely to exist (Muneta et al. 2003; Shimosato et al. 2003).

Phagocytic Cells. Phagocytic cells are responsible for engulfing, killing, and digesting invading bacteria. They also play an important role in controlling viral and fungal infections and in killing cancer cells. There are two main types of phagocytic cells: the granulocytes or polymorphonuclear leukocytes, which include neutrophils and eosinophils, and the mononuclear phagocytes, which include the circulating monocytes in the blood and the tissue macrophages. All these cell types are phagocytic and are capable of all the reactions that are described below for neutrophils. In addition, macrophages play an important role in processing antigens and presenting them to lymphocytes to initiate and facilitate the cell-mediated and humoral immune responses.

Granulocytes. Neutrophils are produced in the bone marrow and are released into the blood. The half-life of neutrophils in the blood stream is approximately 8 hours; they then enter the tissues. In the healthy individual the neutrophils are eliminated from the intestinal tract and lungs. Neutrophils migrate into the intestinal tract rapidly in response to *Escherichia coli* infection in the pig (Sellwood et al. 1986). Neutrophils in the circulation tend to marginate in the capillaries by loosely associating with the endothelial cells. In swine, neutrophils seem to have a high affinity for margination in the capillaries of the lung (Ohgami et al. 1989).

The principal function of the neutrophil is the phagocytosis and destruction of invading microorganisms. The neutrophil is well-equipped to perform this function and has several mechanisms for destroying microorganisms. To be effective, the neutrophil must first come into the vicinity of the invading microorganism. This is achieved by the chemotactic attraction of the neutrophil to the site. Chemotactic factors may be produced directly by certain microorganisms, be generated by the cleavage of certain complement components, or be released by sensitized lymphocytes at the site of infection or inflammation. The chemotactic factors will diffuse away from the site to form a gradient. When the chemotactic factors reach a capillary they cause the endothelial cell membrane and the neutrophil membrane to increase the expression of adhesion proteins. The neutrophils then adhere to the endothelial cells and leave the capillary by diapedesis. Once in the tissues, the neutrophils will migrate along the chemotactic factor gradient toward the source of the chemotactic factor and will thus arrive at the site of infection; they may begin to ingest the microorganisms if those agents are susceptible to phagocytic activity. Most pathogenic microorganisms must be opsonized before they can be ingested; bacteria are opsonized by the attachment of specific antibody and/or complement to their surface. The opsonization process facilitates ingestion. When a neutrophil comes into contact with an opsonized particle, it will attempt to surround the particle with pseudopodia and ingest it by the process of phagocytosis. The ingested particle will be within a membrane-bound vesicle called a *phagosome*.

The neutrophil cytoplasm contains two main types of membrane-bound lysosomes or granules: *primary* or *azurophilic granules* and *secondary* or *specific granules*. These lysosomes contain numerous hydrolytic enzymes that have been quantitated in porcine neutrophils (Chibber and Castle 1983) and at least six cationic antibacterial peptides (Brogden et al. 2003; Kokryakov et al. 1993; Shi et al. 1994; Storici et al. 1994; Zanetti et al. 1994) that are important to the bactericidal activity of the neutrophil. After a particle is ingested and is inside a phagosome, the neutrophil will "degranulate"; some of the lysosomes will fuse with the phagosome and release their contents into the phagosome with the ingested particle. The antibacterial peptides act by permeabilizing bacterial membranes. Neutrophils die after a short time at sites of inflammation. The hydrolytic enzymes are released and contribute to the inflammatory response and tissue destruction.

In addition neutrophils have potent bactericidal mechanisms that are due to the oxidative metabolism of the neutrophil. When a neutrophil is stimulated by an opsonized particle a burst of oxidative metabolism results in the production of hydrogen peroxide (H_2O_2), superoxide anion (O_2^-), the hydroxyl radical ($OH\cdot$), and perhaps singlet oxygen ($^1O_2$). All of these components can damage microbial organisms. The H_2O_2 formed after phagocytosis may also react with halide ions in a reaction catalyzed by a myeloperoxidase enzyme that is released from the primary granules. This reaction is one of the most potent bactericidal mechanisms of the neutrophil, and is also potentially fungicidal and virucidal.

Neutrophils also control certain viral infections via a mechanism referred to as antibody-dependent cell-mediated cytotoxicity (ADCC) in which antibodies form a bridge between the neutrophil and the virus-infected target cell. The neutrophil will then attempt to destroy the target cell. The mechanism of this cell destruction is not known but is thought to involve a direct membrane-to-membrane interaction. Porcine neutrophils are very active at ADCC, even in the fetus and newborn (Yang and Schultz 1986; Zarkower et al. 1982).

The eosinophil is capable of the same phagocytic and metabolic functions as the neutrophil, but to a different extent. The eosinophil is not as active as the neutrophil in destroying bacteria but is important in the host's defense against the tissue phase of certain parasitic infections. The eosinophil is geared more toward exocytosis than phagocytosis. That is, rather than ingesting and killing small particles like bacteria, it can efficiently attach to and kill migrating parasites that are too large to be ingested. Eosinophils are also important in helping to control certain types of allergic responses.

Mononuclear Phagocytes. The mononuclear phagocytic system is made up of circulating monocytes, fixed macrophages, wandering macrophages (histiocytes), and dendritic cells. Monocytes are produced in the bone marrow and released into the blood stream where they will circulate before migrating into the tissues to become macrophages and dendritic cells. The fixed macrophages are found lining the endothelium of capillaries (particularly in the lungs) and the sinuses of the spleen, bone marrow, and lymph nodes. Tissue macrophages are important for trapping and removing foreign antigens from the blood stream and lymph. Wandering macrophages are derived from blood monocytes and are found throughout the tissues of the body. In certain locations, they differentiate into specialized types of macrophages, such as the glial cells in the nervous system, Langerhans cells in the skin, and Kupffer cells in the liver. Dendritic cells are specialized cells that originate from myeloid or lymphoid precursors and assist in presenting antigens to lymphocytes, specifically T cells. Immature dendritic cells are located in the various tissues throughout the body. Upon activation, they migrate to the peripheral lymphoid organs where they mature and become important cells in the activation and differentiation of T lymphocytes (Bautista et al. 2002; Carrasco et al. 2001; Johansson et al. 2003; Summerfield et al. 2003).

Macrophages are capable of all the activities described above for neutrophils. Macrophages are said to be the second line of defense. They are slower to arrive at sites of inflammation and are not as aggressive as neutrophils in the first few minutes of contact with microorganisms. However, macrophages are capable of much more sustained activity against pathogens than are neutrophils. They are able to kill certain types of bacteria that are resistant to killing by neutrophils because of this sustained activity. This is especially true if the macrophages have been activated by cytokines secreted by T lymphocytes.

A very important function of macrophages and dendritic cells is the processing of antigen and presentation of antigen to T lymphocytes. This is an essential step in the initiation of a cell-mediated immune response and for facilitating an efficient antibody response by B lymphocytes. The interaction of macrophages and dendritic cells with antigen and T and B lymphocytes is described later.

Alveolar macrophages phagocytize inhaled particles, including low numbers of bacteria that they may encounter (Chitko-McKown et al. 1991). After ingesting the particles they leave the alveolus either through the airways, where they move up the mucociliary escalator, or by migrating out of the alveolus between alveolar epithelial cells and being carried through lymphatic drainage to local lymph nodes. There, they present the antigens they have captured to lymphocytes to initiate an immune response.

Pulmonary intravascular macrophages are found adhered to endothelial cells in the vasculature of the lung (Chitko-McKown and Blecha 1992; Winkler 1988; Winkler and Cheville 1987). They are prominent in pigs and some other species. They are believed to be important in removing infectious agents from the blood of swine. Pulmonary intravascular macrophages are primarily involved in defense against septicemia rather than protection from respiratory disease. Pulmonary intravascular macrophages that are actively clearing bacteria from the bloodstream (especially gram-negative bacteria or free endotoxin), may release cytokines and arachidonic acid metabolites, which contribute significantly to pulmonary inflammation (Bertram 1986; Crocker et al. 1981a,b).

Natural Killer Cells. Natural killer (NK) cells are lymphoid cells of the innate immune system and can kill a variety of nucleated cells without previous antigenic stimulation. NK cells in most species are also called *large granular lymphocytes* because of the presence of granules in their cytoplasm. NK cells in most species are part of the null cell population because they are distinct from B cells, T cells, and macrophages. In most species NK cells have Fc receptors for IgG and can mediate antibody-dependent cell-mediated cytotoxicity (ADCC) against most antibody-coated mammalian cells. When mediating ADCC these cells have been called killer (K) cells.

Natural killer cells in the pig differ markedly from NK cells found in other species. NK activity in swine is mediated by small granular lymphocytes that have the CD2 T cell marker (Duncan et al. 1989; Ferguson et al. 1986) and are, therefore, not null cells (Duncan et al. 1989). Swine NK cells are slower in initiating the lytic process against typical target cells (YAC-1 lymphoma or K-562 myeloid leukemia cells) than cells responsible for NK activity in other species (Ferguson et al. 1986). In swine there is evidence that the NK cell activity and the K cell activity are from two distinct populations of lymphocytes (Kim and Ichimura 1986; Yang and Schultz 1986). Swine NK cells are capable of lysing cells infected with transmissible gastroenteritis virus and pseudorabies virus (Evans and Jaso-Friedmann 1993).

The activity of NK cells in many species is increased in the presence of interferon gamma (IFN-γ) and interleukin (IL)-2. Swine NK cells have been shown to respond to an interferon inducer (poly I:C), IL-2, human interferon alpha, and human IL-1α with enhanced NK activity (Evans and Jaso-Friedmann 1993; Knoblock and Canning 1992; Lesnick and Derbyshire 1988). Therefore, NK cells are an important part of the innate defense mechanisms and also participate in a cell-mediated immune response by enhanced activity through cytokine activation.

Humoral and Cell-Mediated Immunity

Clonal Selection and Expansion. An important concept that is basic to understanding the immune response is the clonal selection process. Each mature T or B lymphocyte in the body has receptors on its surface that it uses to recognize antigens. All of the antigen receptors on one lymphocyte recognize exactly the same antigen (or small group of antigens). All of the lymphocytes that recognize exactly the same antigen make up a "clone" and they have all arisen from the same ancestor cell. There are millions of clones of T and B lymphocytes. Each clone may contain from a few hundred to a few million cells. The lymphocytes are in a resting stage as they circulate through blood, enter the lymph nodes through the postcapillary venules, percolate through the lymph nodes and reenter the bloodstream. In the lymph nodes (or other secondary lymphatic tissues) the lymphocytes come in contact with antigens that have arrived there through the afferent lymphatics and have been trapped by macrophages or dendritic cells. Each lymphocyte responds to only one specific antigen, which it recognizes through its antigen receptor. Therefore, the vast majority of lymphocytes that contact an antigen in the lymph node cannot respond to it. In an animal that never has been exposed to a particular infectious agent before, there are relatively few lymphocytes in each clone that can recognize a particular antigen. The first step, in producing an effective primary immune response is expansion of the clone of lymphocytes that recognize the antigen. The T and B lymphocytes that contact the antigen are stimulated to undergo a series of cell divisions so that within a few days there will be enough lymphocytes in the clone to mount an effective humoral and/or cell-mediated immune response. If the animal has been exposed to the antigen previously, the clone of lymphocytes has already been expanded, so fewer cycles of cell division are required to produce enough lymphocytes to mount an immune response. This can result in protection induced by vaccination or previous exposure even if there is no remaining detectable antibody. The cells present in the expanded clone are called *memory cells*. If the previous exposure has been relatively recent, there still will be circulating antibody and effector T lymphocytes, which can act immediately to control the infection.

Cellular Interactions in the Induction of the Immune Response. The induction of clonal expansion and the immune response requires a complex interaction of macrophages, T lymphocytes, and B lymphocytes. Macrophages attempt to phagocytize and destroy infectious agents. After the infectious agent is partially degraded by the macrophage, antigenic fragments from it appear bound to MHC class II molecules on the macrophage surface where they contact T lymphocytes. Macrophages (and other specialized antigen-presenting cells) have a high density of class II MHC molecules on their surface. T helper (T_H) cells are needed to help initiate the immune response. They can only efficiently recognize foreign antigens that are on a cell surface bound to a class II MHC molecule. Cytotoxic T (T_c) cells are important for killing cells infected with intracellular pathogens and cancer cells. They can recognize only foreign antigens that have been processed intracellularly and transported to a cell surface bound to an MHC class I molecule. Therefore, T_H and T_c cells cannot respond to free soluble antigen or to whole bacteria or viruses. Because the MHC class I and class II molecules play a key role in antigen presentation to T lymphocytes, they are capable of having a significant influence on the nature of the immune response. The MHC molecules in all species are highly polymorphic or differ genetically between individuals. The MHC molecules in swine are called the *swine leukocyte antigen (SLA)* complex molecules. The type of SLA molecules that a pig inherits has some influence on their immune response to pathogens and their ability to resist some infectious diseases (Löfstedt et al. 1983; Lunney 1994).

In addition to antigen and class II MHC molecule contact, the T_H cell also requires the presence of cytokines released by the antigen presenting cell or other T cells and contact with co-stimulatory molecules on the surface of the antigen presenting cell for complete activation. Interleukin-1 (IL-1) is an important molecule released by macrophages that are processing antigen. IL-1 is a protein molecule that is a key mediator of the host response to infection through its ability to induce fever and neutrophilia, among other things. A very important function of macrophage-produced IL-1 is its action on T_H cells to cause them to secrete IL-2, which induces T cells to undergo mitosis and clonal expansion. B cells are also capable of processing antigen and presenting it to T_H cells on MHC II molecules. During secondary immune responses, B cells are thought to be the main type of antigen-presenting cell.

It has been documented that the cytokines secreted by macrophages, dendritic cells, and other T cells play a crucial role in the initiation and maintenance of immune responses against both viral and bacterial pathogens in pigs (Cho and Chae 2003; Thanawongnuwech and Thacker 2003; Thanawongnuwech et al. 2001; Zuckermann et al. 1998). Similar to other species, the $CD4^+$ T cells differentiate into T_H cells (Fischer et al. 2000). The T_H cells differentiate into two cell types known as T_H1 and T_H2 that differ in function and are differentiated only by their cytokine profile. A T_H1 cytokine profile includes the production of IL-2 and interferon gamma (IFN-γ), which activate macrophages and stimulate T_c and B cell proliferation. In contrast, T_H2 cells, which inhibit macrophage activation and promote predominantly B cell activity, produce IL-4 and IL-10. High concentrations of IL-10 are associated with the induction of T regulatory cells or T_H3 cells, which are thought to mediate a form of "tolerance" (Groux 2001). The T_H3 cells actively down-regulate pathological antigen-specific immune responses and are thought to be important in regulation of mucosal immune responses and respiratory tract homeostasis (Groux et al. 1998).

T_H cells are very important in initiating the B cell response resulting in antibody production. B cells contact antigen through immunoglobulins bound to their surface, which act as receptors. Antigens do not have to be presented on MHC class II molecules by macrophages for a B cell to recognize them. An optimal B cell response to antigen requires the help of soluble factors released by T_H cells and contact with co-stimulatory molecules on the T_H cell surface. This T_H cell help is needed for B cell mitosis and clonal expansion and for switching the class of antibody produced from IgM to IgG, IgA, or IgE.

Lymphocyte Subpopulations. Lymphocyte subpopulations are defined by the presence of certain molecules on their surface identified by a CD number that designates similar molecules in all species. CD stands for *cluster of differentiation*. More than 29 CD molecules have been identified on the surface of porcine leukocytes (Haverson et al. 2001). Over 247 CD molecules have been identified on human or mouse leukocytes, and there are probably at least that many on porcine leukocytes also.

Lymphocyte subpopulations in the blood of pigs differ markedly from other species. Young pigs have high blood lymphocyte counts compared to most other mammals (approximately 10^7/ml). Up to 50% of these lymphocytes are null cells, which lack most surface markers characteristic of B or classical T lymphocytes (Duncan et al. 1989; Hirt et al. 1990; Saalmuller and Bryant 1994). These null cells do not recirculate between the blood and lymphatic tissues, and they differ from null cells in other species in that they do not have NK cell activity. The majority of null lymphocytes are gamma delta ($\gamma\delta$) T cells. The T cells which predominate in the blood of man and mice and which recognize peptide antigens presented on MHC molecules are called alpha beta ($\alpha\beta$) T cells. Their antigen receptor is made up of an α and a β chain and they have either a CD4 or CD8 molecule to assist in their interactions with MHC molecules. The antigen receptors on $\gamma\delta$ T cells are made up of a γ and a δ chain. The majority of porcine $\gamma\delta$ T cells do not have CD4 or CD8 molecules associated with them because they recognize intact antigen molecules. Unlike the $\alpha\beta$ T cells, they do not require antigen processing and presentation on MHC molecules (Chien et al. 1996). Pigs and other ungulates have a much higher population of γδ T cells in the blood than other mammals that have been studied. γδ T cells are located predominantly along mucosal surfaces, especially as intraepithelial lymphocytes in the intestine, and are thought to be important in protecting mucosal surfaces from infection and perhaps in oral tolerance (Thielke et al. 2003). γδ T cells proliferate in the intestine and actively recirculate through the intestinal lymphatics to the blood stream and back to the gut (Thielke et al. 2003). The role of the thymus and intestinal epithelium in development of γδ T cells is not understood. A subset of circulating porcine γδ T cells can act as antigen presenting cells and present antigen to T helper cells via MHC II molecules (Takamatsu et al. 2002). Porcine γδ T cells are capable of producing gamma interferon and proliferating in response to recall antigens in vitro and can be cytotoxic (Lee et al. 2004; Takamatsu et al. 2002).

Swine T lymphocytes have at least three unusual properties compared to other species (Lunney and Pescovitz 1987):

- Approximately 25% of swine peripheral blood T cells express both the CD4 and CD8 antigens on their surface. It has been suggested that many of these dual expressing T cells are memory cells; however, the functional significance of having both CD4 and CD8 on the same cells is not known (Pescovitz et al. 1994; Zuckermann and Husmann 1996). Peanut agglutinin has been shown to selectively bind to porcine memory $CD4^+CD8^+$ T cells and could therefore be used to isolate these cells (Hernandez et al. 2002).
- The ratio of $CD4^+$ to $CD8^+$ T cells is normally approximately 0.6 in pigs, which is reversed compared to other species. A normal ratio of $CD4^+/CD8^+$ in humans is 1.5–2.0.
- Resting $CD8^+$ cells in swine preferentially express class II MHC antigens. The significance of these differences between swine T lymphocytes and those of other species is not completely understood.

Lymphocyte Circulation. The lymph node structure and lymphocyte circulation are markedly different in the pig compared to man or other domestic species (Binns 1982). Recirculation of lymphocytes from blood to lymphoid tissues is very important for bringing antigen into contact with lymphocytes for recognition. Circulation of B cells, αβ T cells, macrophages, and dendritic cells through lymph nodes is also important for facilitating cellular interactions needed for the induction of the immune response as described above. Lymphocytes are produced in the bone marrow, but mature in the thymus (αβ T cells) and the secondary lymphoid tissues (B cells) in the pig. T and B lymphocytes circulate in the blood for approximately 30 minutes before entering the tissues. Porcine lymph nodes are structurally in-

verted compared to other domestic species. Lymphatics enter the node through the hilus, and the lymph passes through the node with the lymph leaving through the periphery. The lymph node has a dense medulla, which lacks sinuses and cords. The germinal centers are located in the interior of the node. Other lymphoid organs—such as the Peyer's patches, tonsils, and spleen—are similar to those found in other species (Binns et al. 1986; Pabst and Binns 1986). Lymphocytes in swine and other species enter the lymph nodes through two routes. Lymphocytes that leave the bloodstream and enter the subcutaneous tissues are carried to the lymph node in the afferent lymphatics. Lymphocytes may also directly enter the lymph node by adhering to high endothelial cells in the venules of the lymph node, and then migrating into the node. In other species, the lymphocytes exit the lymph node in the efferent lymphatics and are carried through the thoracic duct back to the circulatory system. In swine, the efferent lymph contains very few lymphocytes. The lymphocytes in the lymph node directly reenter the blood in swine (Binns et al. 1986). In addition to migrating from blood to lymphoid tissues, lymphocytes in swine migrate into most other tissues as well (Binns et al. 1986). Lymphocyte subpopulations in swine show a distinct preference for circulation to either gut-associated lymphoid tissues or surface nodes (Binns et al. 1986). For instance, mesenteric lymph node cells (both T and B lymphocytes) preferentially home to the gut (Salmon 1986). In rodents the majority of the lymphocytes found in the mammary gland also come from gut-associated lymphoid tissue, whereas in swine approximately equal numbers of lymphocytes in the mammary gland come from gut-associated lymphoid tissue and from peripheral lymph nodes. The dual origin of mammary lymphocytes in swine suggests that the local mammary immune response may not depend solely on oral immunization (Salmon 1986, 1987).

Acquired Immune Defense Mechanisms. An important component of lymphocyte activity in host defense is mediated by soluble products released by stimulated lymphocytes. T lymphocytes are the predominant population of cells that secrete a variety of cytokines as well as being cytolytic to abnormal cells. Antibodies produced by B cells are specific for the antigens to which they are induced whereas cytokines are not. The cytokines produced during an immune response play an important role in orchestrating host defense against pathogens partially through their direct activities and partially by enhancing the activity of both the innate immune system (i.e., complement, phagocytic cells, and NK cells) and the adaptive immune response by T_H cells as described earlier.

Cytotoxic T lymphocytes (T_C cells) are an important part of the cell-mediated immune response to virus infection and tumors. T_C cells have the CD8 marker on their surface and recognize only antigen associated with MHC class I molecules on a cell surface. MHC class I molecules present peptide antigens derived from proteins synthesized within the cell, such as viral proteins. The T_C cells directly attack host cells that have foreign antigen (e.g., viral antigen) presented on MHC class I molecules on their surface. These cells do not attack free bacteria or viruses. T_C cell activity specific for hog cholera virus, African swine fever virus, and pseudorabies virus have been demonstrated in pigs that have recovered from infection (Martins et al. 1993; Pauly et al. 1995; Zuckermann et al. 1990). T_C cells kill target cells by making direct contact, releasing granzymes onto the cell surface, and inducing apoptosis (programmed cell death) in the target cells. Production of cytokines, including IL-12 and IFN-γ, by T_H1 cells are required for the activation of T_C lymphocytes and the elimination of cells infected with intracellular pathogens, especially viruses.

Immunoglobulins

Production of Immunoglobulins. B lymphocytes from clones that have never been stimulated by antigen have monomeric IgM antibody molecules on their surface that act as antigen receptors. All of the IgM molecules on one B cell are specific for the same antigen. When a B cell is stimulated by antigen and cytokines produced by T_H cells it begins to undergo mitosis. This results in the formation of many more B cells with IgM receptors that also recognize the same antigen. Some of these newly formed B cells differentiate into plasma cells that secrete IgM. As the antigen-specific IgM antibody concentration begins to increase in the blood, activated T_H cells produce the cytokines that signal the B cells to switch from IgM production to IgG, IgA, or IgE production

(Crawley and Wilkie 2003; Crawley et al. 2003). These B cells then rearrange their genetic material to produce antibody molecules with the same antigenic specificity (i.e., the same light-chain structure and variable portion of the heavy chain) but of a different antibody class (i.e., the constant heavy portion of the antibody molecule is changed). Changing the antibody class gives the antibody molecules different properties. The class of antibody that the T_H cells cause the B cells to switch to depends to a large extent upon the nature of the antigen and the location in the body where the antigen was trapped. T_H cells located in lymph nodes and the spleen tend to induce B cells to switch to IgG production. T_H cells located in Peyer's patches or under other mucosal surfaces tend to induce B cells to switch to IgA and/or IgE production, depending on the nature of the antigen and the genetic predisposition of the individual.

Antibody molecules have a variety of activities in host defense, although they alone cannot kill infectious agents. Antibody molecules can coat infectious agents to prevent them from attaching to or penetrating host cells, they can agglutinate infectious agents to reduce their infectivity, and they can directly bind to and neutralize toxins. A very important function of antibody is that it marks infectious agents for destruction by complement, phagocytic cells, and/or cytotoxic cells.

Classes of Immunoglobulins. Characteristics of the various classes of porcine immunoglobulin were thoroughly reviewed in a previous edition of this book (Porter 1986), and in a recent review article (Crawley and Wilkie 2003).

IgG is the predominant Ig class in the serum of the pig and other species. It accounts for more than 80% of the Ig in serum and colostrum (Table 2.1). The two main

Table 2.1.   Concentration of porcine immunoglobulins (mg/ml) in body fluids.

	IgG	IgG$_2$	IgM	IgA
Adult sow serum	24.3 ± 0.94	14.1 ± 0.49	2.9 ± 0.2	2.1 ± 0.2
Colostrum	61.8 ± 2.5	40.3 ± 1.6	3.2 ± 0.2	9.6 ± 0.6
Milk (24 hours)	11.8 ± 4.8	8.0 ± 3.2	1.8 ± 0.3	3.8 ± 1.0
Milk (48 hours)	8.2 ± 3.2	5.0 ± 1.8	1.8 ± 0.4	2.7 ± 0.6
Milk (3–7 days)	1.9 ± 0.6	1.3 ± 0.3	1.2 ± 0.2	3.4 ± 1.0
Milk (8–35 days)	1.40 ± 0.60	1.00 ± 0.45	0.90 ± 0.25	3.05 ± 0.74
Intestinal fluid				
Piglet	0.002		0.065	0.033
Sow	0.001		0.001	0.091
Urinary tract	4.7			0.77
Follicle				
Diestrus	18.1			0.7
Estrus	25.1			0.7
Uterine secretions				
Diestrus	0.32			0.2
Estrus	0.34			0.12
Cervicovaginal mucus				
Diestrus	6.7		0.6	1.1
Estrus	2.0		0.06	0.6

Used with permission from *Veterinary Clinical Immunology,* R.E.W. Halliwell and N.T. Gorman, editors. W.B. Saunders Company, 1989.

subclasses of IgG are IgG_1 and IgG_2 (Metzger and Fougereau 1968), with IgG_1 predominating in serum and colostrum. IgG_3 and IgG_4 subclasses are found in lesser concentrations.

An 18S Ig has been described that is antigenically similar to IgG_2 and is found in low levels in normal serum and colostrum (Kim et al. 1966). Newborn piglets also possess a 5S IgG, which may not have light chains and may not be functional (Franek and Riha 1964; Stertzl et al. 1960).

IgM accounts for approximately 5–10% of the total Ig in serum and colostrum (refer to Table 2.1). The IgM is a pentamer held together by disulfide bonds and has a sedimentation coefficient of 17.8S (Porter 1969).

The porcine immune system produces far more IgA than any other class of antibody; however, most of the IgA is found on mucosal surfaces, rather than in the serum. IgA is present in swine serum as 6.4S monomers and as 9.3S dimers, which are two monomers bound together with a J chain (Halpern and Koshland 1970; Mestecky et al. 1971; Porter and Allen 1972). IgA at mucosal surfaces is mostly dimeric IgA with a J chain and associated secretory component (see the section on mucosal immunity below).

Porcine IgE has been shown to have the same physicochemical properties as in other species, including the characteristic of losing biologic activity when serum is heated to 56°C (Roe et al. 1993). A polyclonal antisera for porcine IgE inhibited a passive cutaneous anaphylaxis reaction, identified a sparse population of plasma cells in the lamina propria of the gut and mesenteric lymph nodes of parasitized pigs, and reacted with human IgE in Western blotting. Antibodies against human IgE and bovine IgE have been shown to react with a homocytotropic immunoglobulin in swine serum (Barratt 1972; Nielsen 1977).

Polyclonal and Monoclonal Antibodies. Antibody produced by an animal in response to an infection or vaccination is polyclonal and recognizes multiple antigens. Infectious agents are complex antigens with many different antigenic specificities on their surface; therefore, they stimulate many clones of B and T lymphocytes to respond. This results in a heterogenous mixture of antibodies that recognizes a wide variety of surface molecules on the microorganism. This broad spectrum of antibodies that are produced and are present in the serum are most helpful to the animal in overcoming infection. It is sometimes a disadvantage, however, if one wishes to use the serum for developing diagnostic reagents. The polyclonal antibodies produced in response to one infectious agent may cross-react with another infectious agent and thus interfere with the specificity of the assay.

Monoclonal antibodies are commonly produced in research laboratories and often overcome many of the disadvantages of polyclonal antisera for diagnostic and (less commonly) therapeutic purposes. Monoclonal antibodies are the result of expansion of one clone from a single B lymphocyte and therefore are all identical. All of the antibody molecules present in a monoclonal antibody preparation are specific for the same antigenic determinant. This helps reduce the problem of cross-reactivity between microorganisms in diagnostic tests. Monoclonal antibodies produced against a protective antigen on a microorganism could possibly be used in therapy or prevention of disease. Since they can be produced in very high concentrations and purity, a much lower volume of monoclonal antibody compared to a polyclonal antibody solution can be used to immunize animals passively. This reduces the risk of serious reaction to the passively administered antibody and its extraneous protein.

Cytokines. Cytokines are small protein or glycoprotein molecules that are secreted by cells and serve as intercellular signaling molecules. All cells of the immune system are capable of secreting and being influenced by cytokines. Cytokine secretion is usually transient and occurs in response to specific stimuli. The cytokines that are secreted may act locally if they are secreted in low concentrations, or they may have systemic effects if they are secreted in higher concentrations. A cytokine will act only on a cell that has specific receptors for it. Regulation of cytokine receptor expression is an important mechanism for controlling the response to cytokines.

Information regarding cytokine biology has increased rapidly in recent years. Most of the new information on cytokine biology was first developed in mice or humans. However, because of the economic importance of pigs, and their importance in biomedical research, considerable information has been published recently regarding porcine cytokines (Murtaugh 1994; Murtaugh and Foss 1997, 2002) . The porcine cytokines that have been studied are generally similar to their homologue in man or mice. Over 30 porcine cytokines have been described and partially characterized (Murtaugh 1994; Murtaugh and Foss 1997). A currently active field of research studies the various cytokines produced in response to disease (Darwich et al. 2003; Suradhat and Thanawongnuwech 2003; Thanawongnuwech and Thacker 2003). The information obtained from these studies helps us understand both how pathogens cause disease as well as how the immune system functions to control disease.

Cytokines can generally be categorized into four groups based on their functions (Abbas et al. 1994). One group of cytokines is important in mediating innate immunity. This includes the type I interferons (alpha and beta) and the proinflammatory cytokines that include IL-1, IL-6, and tumor necrosis factor α (TNFα). Type I interferon production occurs in response to viral infections by many cell types. Type I interferons can be detected within a few hours of viral infection and make cells resistant to virus infection, increase NK cell activity, and increase the MHC molecule expression on cell surfaces, thus increasing antigen presentation to T cells.

The proinflammatory cytokines (IL-1, IL-6, and TNFα) are produced primarily by macrophages in response to bacterial infection and require no previous exposure. They may also be produced in response to viral, protozoal, or fungal infections, or tissue damage. The proinflammatory cytokines stimulate the liver to produce acute phase proteins and stimulate the release of amino acids from muscle tissue, and may induce cachexia or wasting in chronic infections. In addition, they induce fever, loss of appetite, and fatigue if present in high-enough concentrations. In low levels, these cytokines promote leukocyte adhesion to endothelial cells and diapedesis of leukocytes into the tissues as well as migration of macrophages and dendritic cells to the secondary lymph nodes, resulting in the activation of the adaptive immune response. Their presence in small amounts is required for an effective immune response. However, in large quantities they can induce hypovolemic shock and death.

A second group of cytokines regulate lymphocyte activation, growth, and differentiation. These are produced mainly by the T_H lymphocytes in response to antigen recognition. Four important cytokines in this group are IL-2, IL-4, IL-12 and transforming factor β (TGF-β). IL-2 stimulates T and B cells that have recognized antigen to proliferate. It also activates NK lymphocytes to have increased cytotoxic activity. IL-4 is important for effective IgE-mast cell-eosinophil inflammatory reactions required to control some parasites and may result in allergic symptoms to non-parasite antigens. IL-12 activates NK lymphocytes and induces CD4+ cells to differentiate into T_H1 cells and assists in the maturation of CD8+ cells into T_C cells. TGF-β is primarily a negative regulator of the immune response. It inhibits many activities of lymphocytes and may be a signal for shutting off the immune response.

A third group of cytokines are those that regulate immune-mediated inflammation. They are produced mainly by T_H and T_C cells, and their primary function is to activate or deactivate the cells of the innate immune system. Interferon-gamma (IFN-γ) causes cells to be resistant to virus infection (similar to alpha and beta interferon), and it is also a potent activator of macrophages, neutrophils, and NK cells. TNF-β often acts synergistically with IFN-γ to activate phagocytic cells. TNF-β can also activate endothelial cells resulting in diapedesis of leukocytes into sites of inflammation. IL-5 is secreted by T_H cells and acts to increase eosinophil production and to activate eosinophils resulting in an increased ability to kill parasites. IL-10, secreted by T cells and macrophages is important in suppressing macrophage function and maintaining homeostasis of the respiratory tract.

The fourth group of cytokines stimulate hematopoiesis through the expansion and differentiation of bone marrow progenitor cells. They are called *colony stimulating factors (CSFs)*. IL-3 is a CSF that stimulates the production of all of the types of leukocytes. Granulocyte-macrophage CSF (GM-CSF) stimulates the production of granulocytes and macrophages. Granulocyte CSF (G-CSF) stimulates the production of granulocytes only. The CSFs also may enhance the antimicrobial activities of mature neutrophils and macrophages.

Mucosal Immunity

Providing immunity at mucosal surfaces is a difficult problem due to frequent exposure to infectious agents. The components of the immune system described previously may not function well in the microenvironment on the mucosal surface, and their contribution to protective immunity varies with the mucosal surface. For instance IgG, complement, and phagocytic cells function efficiently in the lower respiratory tract and in the uterus but not in the lumen of the gut.

An important component of immunity at mucosal surfaces is the secretory IgA system, which responds to antigens that enter the body through mucosal surfaces. Specialized epithelial cells called *dome cells* or *M cells* are found overlying aggregations of gut and bronchus associated lymphoid tissues. These dome cells pinocytose antigen and transport it across the epithelial layer. The antigen may then be processed by antigen-presenting cells and presented to T and B lymphocytes.

Lymphocytes in the bloodstream tend to segregate into two populations: those that circulate between the bloodstream and the systemic lymphoid tissues and those that circulate between the bloodstream and lymphoid tissues associated with mucosal surfaces. Because of the nature of the T_H cells, which home to mucosal surfaces, antigens that enter through mucosal surfaces tend to induce an IgA or IgE response. In some cases antigens that enter through the intestinal tract may induce oral tolerance, resulting in suppression of IgG antibody responses.

In the mucosal lymphoid tissues, B cells that have been stimulated by antigen and induced by T_H cells to switch to produce IgA will leave the submucosal lymphoid tissue and reenter the bloodstream. These lymphocytes will exit the bloodstream at submucosal surfaces and locate in the lamina propria where they will differentiate into plasma cells that will secrete dimeric IgA. Many of these cells will return to the same mucosal surface from which they originated, but others will be found at other mucosal surfaces throughout the body. Therefore, oral immunization can result in the migration of IgA precursor cells to the bronchi and subsequent secretion of IgA onto the bronchial mucosa. Oral immunization with live or inactivated *Actinobacillus pleuropneumoniae* has also been shown to result in the trafficking of T cells and IgG positive lymphocytes to the bronchoalveolar space and production of IgA in the bronchoalveolar space (Delventhal et al. 1992; Hensel et al. 1994; Pabst et al. 1995). There is a special affinity for lymphocytes that have been sensitized in the gut of the sow to migrate to the mammary gland to become plasma cells and secrete IgA into the milk.

The dimeric IgA secreted by the plasma cells in the lamina propria will bind to the polyimmunoglobulin receptor on the basal membrane of mucosal epithelial cells. The dimeric IgA and polyimmunoglobulin receptor are then transported to the mucosal surface of the epithelial cell where the polyimmunoglobulin receptor is cleaved. The cleavage product is called the *secretory component* and remains bound to the dimeric IgA. The secretory component is important for protecting the IgA molecule from proteolytic enzymes and also serves to anchor the IgA into the mucous layer so that it forms a protective coating on the mucosal surface.

Secretory IgA plays an important role in immunity at mucosal surfaces by agglutinating infectious agents, preventing attachment of infectious agents to epithelial cells, and neutralizing toxins. Other components of the immune response may also be important in protection against various types of infection at mucosal surfaces. For example, neutrophils in the pig can migrate into the intestinal lumen in large numbers in response to antigen-antibody complexes. The recruitment of neutrophils into the intestinal lumen is dependent upon the presence of antibody that may be circulating IgG antibody (Bellamy and Nielsen 1974), colostral antibody (Sellwood et al. 1986), or locally induced IgA class antibody (Bhogal et al. 1987). The immigration of neutrophils into the lumen of the gut and their subsequent destruction has been shown to result in an increased concentration of lactoferrin, lysozyme, and cationic proteins. These substances may also contribute to immunity to bacterial infections in the gut.

T lymphocytes are important mediators of immunity at mucosal surfaces (Dunkley et al. 1995). This is especially true for respiratory infections caused by facultative intracellular bacterial pathogens. T lymphocytes also play a role in immunity in the intestinal tract. Pigs have high numbers of intraepithelial lymphocytes, which are predominantly $\gamma\delta$ T cells and T_C cells (Salmon 1987; Thielke et al. 2003). The T_C cells in contact with intestinal epithelial cells are likely to be important in destroying virus-infected epithelial cells. The $\gamma\delta$ T cells proliferate in the intestine and recirculate through the lymphatic and blood vessels back to the intestine. They can produce IFN-γ, be cytotoxic, and act as antigen-presenting cells through MHC II molecules (Lee et al. 2004; Takamatsu et al. 2002).

More detailed information on the various aspects of mucosal immunity may be found in chapters in this book dealing with specific organ systems or specific pathogens. The role for lymphocytes in the respiratory immune system of the pig has been reviewed (Pabst and Binns 1994).

Immunity in the Fetus and Neonate

All components of the native and acquired immune systems of the pig develop in utero and are functional at birth. However, they are generally less efficient than in the adult (Hammerberg et al. 1989). Since the normal newborn piglet has not yet been exposed to antigen, humoral and cell-mediated immune responses to infectious agents have not yet been developed. After exposure to infectious agents it will take 7–10 days for a primary antibody or cell-mediated immune response to develop. During this time resistance to infection depends upon the actions of the innate defense mechanisms and antibody, which is passively transferred from the sow to the piglet. In the pig there is virtually no transfer of antibody across the placenta. The epitheliochorial placentation of the sow has several tissue layers between maternal and fetal circulation, which prevents antibody transfer. In the sow, as in other large domestic species, passive transfer of antibody from mother to offspring occurs through the colostrum. The sow concentrates antibody in the colostrum during the last days of gestation. This antibody is largely transferred intact across the gut epithelial cells into the circulation of the newborn piglet. The passive transfer of antibody from sow to piglet in the colostrum and milk is very important for neonatal survival and is discussed in more detail below.

Innate Defense Mechanisms. The newborn piglet has low levels of hemolytic complement activity at birth. The level of hemolytic complement activity is related to the birth weight, with heavier pigs having significantly higher concentrations of complement in the serum (Rice and L'Ecuyer 1963). In colostrum-deprived pigs the hemolytic complement activity gradually increases during the first 36 days of life. Piglets allowed to suckle colostrum have higher titers of hemolytic complement than colostrum-deprived piglets during the first 3 weeks of life. This suggests that some of the complement components that are present in limiting amounts are transferred through the colostrum to the piglet (Rice and L'Ecuyer 1963).

The level of natural interferon alpha production by porcine blood mononuclear cells was shown to be low at birth and to gradually increase until adult age, with a significant increase around puberty (Nowacki et al. 1993).

Phagocytic cells are present in newborn animals but generally have reduced phagocytic activity as compared to adult animals (Osburn et al. 1982). Alveolar macrophages from 1-day-old pigs had reduced oxidative killing mechanisms compared to alveolar macrophages from adult pigs. By 7 days of age, these aspects of alveolar macrophage function had reached adult levels of activity (Zeidler and Kim 1985). Neonatal pigs have low numbers of pulmonary intravascular macrophages, which can increase up to fourteenfold by 30 days of age

(Winkler and Cheville 1987). Since phagocytes depend on complement and/or antibodies to opsonize many infectious agents, the overall efficiency of phagocytosis may be reduced due to inadequate levels of complement and antibodies. Neutrophils from fetal pigs have been shown to have antibody-dependent cell-mediated cytotoxicity activity against chicken red blood cells, which is comparable to that of adult pigs. Neutrophils from neonatal pigs have also been shown to rapidly emigrate into the lumen of the gut in response to the presence of *E. coli* and colostral antibody (Sellwood et al. 1986; Yang and Schultz 1986).

Acquired Immune Mechanisms. The percentage of CD2$^+$, CD4$^+$, and CD8$^+$ T lymphocytes increases with age over the first several weeks of life in specific pathogen-free pigs (Bianchi et al. 1992; Joling et al. 1994). The lymphocyte blastogenic responsiveness to mitogens has been shown to be low after birth and to increase by 4 weeks of age (Becker and Misfeldt 1993). The mucosal lymphoid system is also less developed at birth and matures over the next few weeks of life (Jericho 1970; Ramos et al. 1992).

Natural killer cell activity has been shown to be absent in the peripheral blood of fetal pigs and to be low in pigs of less than 2 weeks of age (Yang and Schultz 1986).

Passive Transfer in the Neonate. Pigs are born with almost no serum antibody and absorb colostrum that is enriched in IgG, IgG$_2$, and IgA as compared to the serum of sows. It has approximately the same concentration of IgM as serum (refer to Table 2.1). When the pig suckles, the colostrum is replaced with milk, which has much lower immunoglobulin content. From 3 days of age until the end of lactation, IgA is the predominant antibody found in sow milk. The percentage of immunoglobulin in the mammary gland derived from serum and locally produced in the mammary gland is different in colostrum and milk and varies with the immunoglobulin class (Table 2.2).

All three major classes of Ig (IgG, IgA, and IgM) are absorbed from the colostrum into the circulation of newborn pigs (Curtis and Bourne 1971; Porter 1969).

Table 2.2. Origin of porcine colostral and milk immunoglobulins (Stokes and Bourne 1989).

	Percent Derived from Plasma (%)	Percent Locally Synthesized (%)
Colostrum		
IgM	85	15
IgG	100	0
IgA	40	60
Milk		
IgM	10	90
IgG	30	70
IgA	10	90

IgA, however, is absorbed less efficiently than the other classes of antibody (Hill and Porter 1974; Porter 1973). This is apparently because much of the IgA in porcine colostrum is dimeric IgA lacking secretory component (Porter 1973). Neonatal colostrum-deprived piglets have been shown to express secretory component in the gut, which tends to localize in the mucus of the crypt areas (Allen and Porter 1973). Because of the affinity of the dimeric IgA and IgM for secretory component, it has been suggested that IgA and IgM are bound in association with secretory component and held in the mucus of the crypt areas and are, therefore, less efficiently absorbed from the colostrum (Butler et al. 1981). The IgA present in sow's milk throughout the suckling period may also bind to the secretory component in the crypt areas and provide relatively continuous protection against intestinal pathogens.

Intestinal absorption of immunoglobulin from the colostrum normally ceases by 24–36 hours after birth. If pigs suckle normally, the efficiency of absorption decreases with a half-life of about 3 hours (Speer et al. 1959). Lecce et al.(1961) found that the period of time that the intestine could absorb antibodies was extended up to 5 days in starved pigs, which were maintained by parental administration of nutrients. Therefore, piglets that have not had an opportunity to eat during the first 24–36 hours may still benefit from colostrum ingestion.

Neonatal pigs have been shown to absorb colostral lymphocytes from their intestinal tract into the blood stream (Tuboly et al. 1988; Williams 1993). By 24 hours cells derived from colostrum were found in the liver, lung, lymph nodes, spleen, and gastrointestinal tissue. Pigs that had absorbed the colostral lymphocytes had higher lymphocyte blastogenic responses to mitogens than control pigs. It is not clear whether the passively transferred lymphocytes also transfer clinically significant cell-mediated or antigen-specific immunity from the sow to the piglet.

HYPERSENSITIVITIES

Hypersensitivities are conditions in which there is an excessive response to an antigen to which the animal has previously been exposed. The clinical signs are due to the immune response to the antigen rather than to a direct action of the antigen or pathogens. Although hypersensitivity conditions can be divided into four types based on their mechanism of action, it is not unusual for clinical hypersensitivity conditions to involve more than one of the four types of hypersensitivity.

Type I or *immediate type* hypersensitivity involves the synthesis of specific IgE antibodies. The IgE molecules preferentially bind to Fc receptors on the surface of tissue mast cells. When the same antigen is encountered subsequently it will bind to the IgE on the mast cell surface (if there is a sufficiently high concentration of IgE specific for the antigen) and cause the mast cell to release numerous pharmacologically active substances, which are responsible for the clinical signs (e.g., histamine, serotonin, kinins, prostaglandins, and others). Type I hypersensitivities may be localized to a particular region or organ or may be systemic (anaphylaxis) (Eyre 1980). Information on naturally occurring localized type I hypersensitivities in pigs is not readily available, although it has been reproduced experimentally (Helm et al. 2003; Roe et al. 1993). Acute systemic anaphylaxis in pigs is due primarily to systemic and pulmonary hypertension, leading to dyspnea and death. In some pigs the intestinal tract may also be involved (Tizard 1987).

A *type II* hypersensitivity response (or *cytotoxic type hypersensitivity*) involves the presence of antibodies directed against cell membrane antigens. These may be normal tissue antigens in the case of autoimmune diseases or foreign antigens (e.g., drugs, viral antigens, or bacterial antigens) that have adhered to the cell surface. Type II hypersensitivities have been reported in pigs in which autoantibodies have formed against erythrocytes, thrombocytes, or neutrophils. This results in a depletion of the respective cell type and the associated clinical signs that one would expect (anemia, bleeding diathesis, or increased susceptibility to infection, respectively). These autoantibodies may arise from blood transfusions, from the use of vaccines that contain blood products, or in multiparous sows that develop antibody against the alloantigens shared by the sire and the fetus. Thrombocytopenia purpura in baby pigs due to passively transferred anti-platelet antibody seems to be rather common. Pigs appear normal at birth, and death usually occurs between 10–20 days of age. The most striking pathologic feature is the presence of hemorrhages in the subcutaneous tissues and internal organs. Castration during the period of thrombocytopenia may greatly increase the death rate.

Antibodies against erythrocytes, thrombocytes, and neutrophils may be present in the same piglet. In one report, 50% of the dams of litters affected with thrombocytopenia purpura had erythrocyte iso-antibodies in their serum (Linklater et al. 1973). Some of the anemia associated with *Mycoplasma haemosuis* (formerly *Eperythrozoon suis*) is due to the development of autoantibodies against the red blood cells induced by the organism (Messick 2004).

A *type III* hypersensitivity (or *immune-complex type hypersensitivity*) involves the presence of antigen-antibody complexes in the circulation or tissue. These immune complexes can fix complement and, therefore, may initiate an inflammatory response, attract neutrophils to the site, and damage cell membranes. The immune complex–mediated glomerulonephritis associated with chronic hog cholera virus, African swine fever virus, and possibly PCV2 infections are examples of this type of hypersensitivity. The immune complexes formed in response to these diseases may also cause polyarteritis nodosa, a systemic vasculitis. Immune complex deposition

in swine kidneys is apparently common. One study evaluated 100 kidneys collected at slaughter with no apparent macroscopic lesions. Ninety-seven of the kidneys had IgG deposits and 98 had C3 deposits as demonstrated by immunocytochemistry. The significance of these immune complex deposits in the kidney is unknown; however, the clinical diagnosis of glomerular disease in swine is rare (Shirota et al. 1986).

A *type IV* hypersensitivity (or *delayed-type hypersensitivity*) is mediated by sensitized T cells releasing cytokines. It does not involve antibody. The tuberculin skin test is a classic type IV hypersensitivity reaction. Delayed-type hypersensitivity is believed to play a role in some cases of food hypersensitivity in pigs. Very little work has been reported on other clinical conditions involving delayed-type hypersensitivity in pigs. Transfer of delayed-type hypersensitivity between genetically matched pigs by transfer of lymphocytes has been demonstrated (Binns et al. 1996).

Food hypersensitivity is thought to be responsible for some cases of post-weaning diarrhea and reduced growth performance in piglets (Stokes et al. 1987; Stokes and Bourne 1989; Li et al. 1990, 1991; Friesen et al. 1993). This apparently involves the formation of both IgG antibodies and a type IV or delayed-type hypersensitivity. Following the introduction of a new protein antigen to the diet, a small proportion (<0.002%) of that protein is absorbed intact inducing an antibody and/or cell-mediated response. Normally, a systemic antibody response (IgG) is suppressed (oral tolerance) and a local mucosal antibody response persists. The local antibody prevents further absorption of the intact protein. Oral tolerance prevents an immune response to most of the proteins that are absorbed. Therefore, following the introduction of new dietary antigen, animals may pass through a brief phase of hypersensitivity before the development of a protected state of tolerance.

In pigs that were weaned abruptly and placed on a soya-containing diet, soya protein was detected in the sera of all animals for up to 20 days postweaning. A delayed-type hypersensitivity skin test reaction to soya proteins was transiently present in the soya-fed group. The changes in gut morphology (crypt hyperplasia and villous atrophy) and the malabsorption associated with early weaning suggested that these changes occur as a result of a transient hypersensitivity to antigen in the postweaning diet. These intestinal changes can facilitate growth and disease production by *E. coli*. Feeding of large amounts of soya prior to the withdrawal of milk prevented the postweaning malabsorption and diarrhea (Stokes et al. 1987).

IMMUNODEFICIENCY AND IMMUNOSUPPRESSION

Primary or secondary immunodeficiencies increase the susceptibility of animals to disease induced by typically low to nonpathogenic microbes. A primary immuno-deficiency is defined as a disorder of the immune system with a genetic basis. A secondary immunodeficiency is a disorder in which the animal is genetically capable of normal immune function, but some secondary factor is impairing resistance to disease.

Clinical findings that are associated with immuno-deficiencies include:

1. Illness from organisms of normally low pathogenicity or from an attenuated live vaccine
2. Recurrent illnesses that are unusually difficult to control
3. Failure to respond adequately to vaccination
4. Unexplained neonatal illness and death affecting more than one animal in a litter
5. A variety of disease syndromes occurring concurrently in a herd

A large number of primary immunodeficiencies have been reported in humans; however, there are no reports of primary immunodeficiencies in pigs. This is probably due to the relatively low value of the individual piglet and the expense and difficulty associated with diagnosing a primary immunodeficiency. In addition, sows and boars that produce nonvigorous litters are not kept in the breeding herd.

A common cause of secondary immunodeficiency is failure of passive transfer of adequate levels of maternal antibody through the colostrum to the piglet. This has been discussed earlier in this chapter. Other potential causes of secondary immunodeficiency (or immuno-suppression) include:

1. Physical or psychological distress
2. Immunosuppressive infectious agents
3. Inadequate nutrition
4. Immunotoxic substances

Physical and Psychological Distress. There is ample evidence that both physical and psychological distress can suppress immune function in animals, leading to an increased incidence of infectious disease. Excess heat or cold, crowding, mixing, weaning, limit-feeding, shipping, noise, and restraint are stressors that are often associated with intensive animal production and have been shown to influence immune function in various species (Kelley 1985). Distress-induced alterations in immune function are mediated by interactions between the neuroendocrine and immune systems. The study of these multisystem interactions initially focused on the secretion and influence of glucocorticoids, which suppress several aspects of immune function. However, pigs are more resistant to the immunosuppessive effects of glucocorticoids compared to some other species (Flaming et al. 1994). It is now recognized that there are many mechanisms by which the neuroendocrine system can

alter immune function; in addition, the immune system is capable of altering the activity of the neuroendocrine system (Breazile 1987; Dunn 1988; Kelley 1988).

Weaning is certainly a stressful event for domestic animals. Piglets are usually separated from the sow, handled, regrouped with unfamiliar pigs, and shifted from a liquid to a solid diet. Weaning at 2, 3, or 4 weeks of age (but not at 5 weeks of age) has been shown to decrease the in vivo and in vitro response of porcine lymphocytes to phytohemagglutinin (Blecha et al. 1983). This is considered to be a measure of the lymphocyte's ability to undergo clonal expansion to initiate an immune response. These same parameters were suppressed in artificially reared neonatal piglets compared to their sow-reared littermates (Blecha et al. 1986; Hennessy et al. 1987). Early weaning of pigs at 3 weeks of age suppressed the ability of mesenteric lymph node cells to produce IL-2 (Bailey et al. 1992). Weaning (at 5 weeks of age) 24 hours after the injection of sheep red blood cells (RBCs) decreased the antibody response to the sheep RBCs. Weaning 2 weeks prior to injecting the sheep RBCs did not decrease the antibody response (Blecha and Kelley 1981). However, successful vaccination strategies at the time of weaning are frequently reported in the field.

Regrouping of pigs at the time of weaning or at 2 weeks after weaning significantly increased their plasma cortisol concentration. However, there were no measurable changes in lymphocyte blastogenesis or antibody responses at the time of elevated plasma cortisol concentration (Blecha et al. 1985).

Crowding or restraint may also stress pigs sufficiently to decrease their immune responsiveness. Housing 8 pigs (11.5–18 kg) per group in pens with 0.13 m^2 of floor space per pig significantly reduced their phytohemagglutinin skin test response as compared to pigs given twice as much space (Yen and Pond 1987). When young pigs were restrained for 2 hours per day over a 3-day period, they had a significantly elevated plasma cortisol concentration, which correlated with a decrease in the size of the thymus gland and with a reduction in the phytohemagglutinin skin test response (Westly and Kelley 1984). Another report indicated that tethering of sows suppressed antibody synthesis to sheep RBCs. It also resulted in a reduction in the amount of antibodies that were transmitted through the colostrum into the blood of the piglets (Kelley 1985).

Immunosuppressive Infectious Agents. Certain infectious agents are capable of suppressing immune function, making the animal more susceptible to secondary infections. For example, infection with *Mycoplasma hyopneumoniae, A. pleuropneumoniae,* virulent or vaccine strains of hog cholera virus, porcine reproductive and respiratory syndrome (PRRS) virus, or pseudorabies virus increases the susceptibility of pigs to *Pasteurella multocida,* increasing the severity of pneumonia (Chung et al. 1993; Done and Paton 1995; Fuentes and Pijoan

1986, 1987; Pijoan and Ochoa 1978; Smith et al. 1973). The mechanism of the immunosuppression induced by these agents has not been completely characterized. A cytotoxin from *A. pleuropneumoniae* is toxic for alveolar macrophages (Chung et al. 1993; Dom et al. 1992; Tarigan et al. 1994). The pseudorabies virus has been shown to replicate in monocytes and alveolar macrophages and to impair their bactericidal and cytotoxic functions (Chinsakchai and Molitor 1992; Iglesias et al. 1989a, b; Iglesias et al. 1992). Porcine parvovirus replicates in alveolar macrophages, as well as lymphocytes, and has been shown to impair macrophage phagocytosis and lymphocyte blastogenesis (Harding and Molitor 1988). Swine influenza virus and PRRS virus also replicate in alveolar macrophages and PRRS virus is lytic to infected macrophages (Bautista et al. 1993; Charley 1983).

PRRS virus and porcine circovirus type 2 (PCV2) both appear to modulate the immune response at many levels. Specific details about the pathogenesis of these two viruses are covered elsewhere in this book. However, it is important to recognize that much of their impact on the swine industry is due to their ability to modulate or alter the ability of the immune system to control other pathogens. The mechanism used by these pathogens to alter the immune response is currently unknown; however, studies have demonstrated that PRRS virus induction of cytokines that induce a $T_H 2$-type of response, as characterized by increased IL-10 levels and decreased IFN-γ production, may play a role in the immunosuppression associated with infection (Thanawongnuwech and Thacker 2003). Thus, although neither of these viruses is classically immunosuppressive, their ability to modulate the immune system allows persistence of the viruses in the host.

In addition to modulation of the immune system by viruses, bacteria including *M. hyopneumoniae, Salmonella typhimurium,* and *S. choleraesuis* have each been shown to alter porcine neutrophil function (Coe et al. 1992; DeBey et al. 1994; Roof et al. 1992a, b) In addition, *M. hyopneumoniae* also appears to induce a preferential $T_H 2$ type of response that may further decrease the ability to control respiratory pathogens (Thanawongnuwech and Thacker 2003; Thanawongnuwech et al. 2000).

Nutritional Influences on Immunity. Both malnutrition and overfeeding may result in impairment of immune function and increased susceptibility to disease due to a deficiency or excess of proteins or calories, or a relative imbalance in vitamin or trace mineral content. Animals under intensive production conditions typically have a completely controlled diet. Therefore, it is very important that the diet, especially the vitamin and trace mineral content, be optimally formulated. Key vitamins and minerals for optimal immune function include vitamins A, C, E, and the B complex vitamins;

copper (Cu); zinc (Zn); magnesium (Mg); manganese (Mn); iron (Fe); and selenium (Se). The balance of these constituents is especially important since an excess or deficiency in one component may influence the availability or requirement for another (Tengerdy 1986).

It is difficult to predict the optimal diet for immune function. There is very little research data in this area for swine. The dietary requirements for optimal immune function may differ from the requirements to avoid deficiencies as judged by traditional methods. Relatively small imbalances of a particular nutrient may suppress immune function, whereas a more severe deficiency must occur before the classical clinical evidence of deficiency of that nutrient is recognized. In addition, stress or the demands of rapid growth may change dietary requirements for optimal immune function.

Dietary and injectable vitamin E and selenium have been evaluated for their influence on antibody levels in young pigs. Dietary vitamin E supplementation increased the antibody response to *E. coli* (Ellis and Vorhies 1976). Supplemental (dietary or injectable) vitamin E and/or selenium treatment in pigs beginning at 4 to 5 weeks of age increased their antibody response to sheep RBCs (Peplowski et al. 1981). Dietary vitamin E and selenium also increased the proliferation response of pig lymphocytes to phytohemagglutinin (Larsen and Tollersrud 1981).

Immunotoxic Substances. In other species, various compounds—including heavy metals, industrial chemicals, pesticides, and mycotoxins—have been shown to be immunosuppressive at very low levels. These compounds may be detrimental to the immune system and predispose animals to infectious diseases at levels that do not cause other symptoms of toxicity (Koller 1979). Very little immunotoxicology research has been conducted in swine. Aflatoxins in the feed of young pigs has been shown to impair immunity to erysipelas, to enhance the severity of clinical signs due to salmonellosis, and to enhance susceptibility to an oral inoculation with *Brachyspira hyodysenteriae* (Cysewski et al. 1978; Joens et al. 1981; Miller et al. 1978).

GENERAL PRINCIPLES OF VACCINATION

For over 100 years scientists have known that animals may develop immunity to diseases if exposed to either the killed infectious agent or a live strain of the agent that has been modified so it does not cause disease. This approach led to the development of many successful vaccines in the early 1900s. However, it soon became apparent that for certain diseases this simple approach was not effective. An animal, for example, might produce antibody in response to vaccination, but still develop the disease, demonstrating that circulating antibody alone is not protective. The challenge of developing vaccines for these diseases is to understand the basis for successful immunity, and then to develop vaccines that induce this type of immunity. It is apparent that different diseases require different types of immunity for protection and the type of vaccine (modified live versus killed), route of administration, and type of adjuvant make a difference in the type of immune response.

General principles regarding vaccine efficacy and vaccine failure will be discussed here. It must be remembered that there are exceptions to these general principles for specific vaccines and specific diseases. Information regarding protective immunity and vaccination for specific diseases may be found in other chapters of this book.

Selective Induction of Different Types of Immunity

It is relatively easy to develop a vaccine that will induce the production of IgG and IgM antibodies in the bloodstream. However, the vaccine may not induce antibodies against the important antigens of the infectious agent, and antibodies alone do not kill infectious agents. Some disease-causing organisms are resistant to control by circulating antibodies. These organisms must be controlled by the cell-mediated immune system or the secretory IgA system. It is more difficult to develop a safe and effective vaccine that induces these types of immunity.

The nature of the vaccine and the route of administration are important for influencing the type of immunity induced. Subcutaneous or intramuscular injection of a killed vaccine will stimulate the immune system to produce both IgM and IgG. However, there is very little production of IgA to protect the mucosal surfaces. In addition, killed vaccines are generally less effective in inducing cell-mediated immunity.

Optimal induction of cell-mediated immunity generally requires a modified live vaccine capable of replicating in the animal or a killed vaccine with a highly effective adjuvant. Modified live vaccine viruses have been attenuated to be of reduced virulence. The attenuation must be shown to be stable; therefore, reversion to virulence is a rare event. New adjuvants and other novel vaccine technologies are being developed that show promise for inducing cell-mediated immunity (Roth and Henderson 2001; Spickler and Roth 2003). There are killed vaccines that have been available for many years and have been effective in controlling certain systemic-type diseases. These are generally diseases that can be controlled by the presence of IgG in the circulation. For those diseases where T cell-mediated immunity is needed for protection, it is important to characterize the response of the various T cell subsets to the vaccine antigens. Several methods exist for evaluating T cell responses to antigens in domestic species (Sandbulte and Roth 2004).

Protecting the animal from infection at mucosal surfaces such as the intestinal tract, respiratory tract, mammary glands, and reproductive tract is especially difficult for the immune system. The antibodies responsible for humoral immunity and the lymphocytes responsible for cell-mediated immunity are predominantly in the blood stream and tissues and they are typically not found on the mucosal surfaces. Therefore, although lymphocytes assist in preventing systemic invasion through the mucosal surface, they are often not very effective at controlling infection on the mucosal surface. Even in the lung and the mammary gland, where IgG and lymphocytes are found in relative abundance, they are not able to function as effectively as in the tissues. Protection on mucosal surfaces is due in large part to secretory IgA, T_C cells, and $\gamma\delta$ T cells, as discussed earlier.

The route of vaccine administration can be important when attempting to induce mucosal immunity. To induce secretory IgA production at mucosal surfaces, it is best for the vaccine to enter the body via a mucosal surface. This can be accomplished by feeding the vaccine to the animal, aerosolizing the vaccine so the animal will inhale it, or by intramammary exposure. If a sow is exposed to an infectious agent in her intestinal tract, she may respond by producing secretory IgA not only in her own intestinal tract, but also in her mammary gland. The sow passes the IgA against the infectious agent to the piglet when it suckles, thus protecting the piglet from infectious agents present in the sow's intestine. This protection will last only as long as the piglet continues to suckle. Enteric infections by many organisms are not controlled by the presence of IgG and IgM in the bloodstream or by a systemic cell-mediated immune response. If a modified live vaccine is given by injection, but goes to a mucosal surface to replicate, it may also induce a secretory IgA response. In addition, killed vaccines for some respiratory pathogens, such as *M. hyopneumoniae* and swine influenza virus, are capable of stimulating an IgA response to challenge.

Vaccination Failure. There are many reasons why animals may develop disease even though they have been vaccinated (Roth 1999). Potential reasons for vaccine failure include:

1. Insufficient time occurred after vaccination to develop immunity.
2. Something happened to the vaccine to make it ineffective.
3. The physiologic status of the animal impaired the response to the vaccine.
4. The animal was immunosuppressed at some point after vaccination.
5. The animal was exposed to an overwhelming challenge dose.
6. The duration of immunity after vaccination was not adequate.
7. Important antigenic differences exist between vaccine and field strains.

8. Interference occurs when multiple vaccines are administered concurrently.

By being aware of these factors, veterinarians and producers can help minimize the occurrence of vaccine failures.

Occurrence of Disease Shortly After Vaccination. The host requires several days after vaccination before an effective immune response will develop. If the animal encounters an infectious agent prior to or near the time of vaccination, the vaccine may not have time to induce immunity. The animal may come down with clinical disease resulting in an apparent vaccination failure. In this situation, disease symptoms will appear shortly after vaccination and may be mistakenly attributed to vaccine agent causing the disease. Modified live vaccine viruses consisting of attenuated virus may be capable of producing disease in immunosuppressed animals.

Alterations in the Vaccine. Improperly handled and administered vaccines may fail to induce the expected immune response in normal, healthy animals. Modified live bacterial and viral vaccines are effective only if the agent in the vaccine is viable and able to replicate in the vaccinated animal. Observing proper storage conditions and proper methods of administration are very important for maintaining vaccine viability. Failure to store the vaccine at refrigerator temperatures or exposure to light may inactivate the vaccine. Even when stored under appropriate conditions, the vaccine loses viability over time. Therefore, vaccines that are past their expiration date should not be used. The use of chemical disinfectants on syringes and needles can inactivate modified live vaccines if there is any residual disinfectant. The use of an improper diluent or the mixing of vaccines in a single syringe may also inactivate modified live vaccines. Diluent for lyophilized vaccines are formulated specifically for each vaccine. A diluent which is appropriate for one vaccine may inactivate a different vaccine. Some vaccines and diluents contain preservatives that may inactivate other modified live vaccines. For these reasons, multiple vaccines should not be mixed in a single syringe unless that particular combination has been adequately tested to insure there is no interference.

Host Factors Contributing to Vaccine Failure. Vaccine failures may occur because a vaccinated animal is not able to respond appropriately to the vaccine. Vaccine failure in young animals may be due to the presence of maternal antibody, which prevents adequate response to vaccination. It can also be due to immunosuppression from a variety of causes, as discussed previously.

Maternal antibodies derived from colostrum are a well-known cause of vaccine failure. These antibodies in the piglets' circulation may neutralize or remove the antigen before it can induce an immune response. Typically, virulent infectious agents are capable of breaking through maternal immunity earlier than modified live or killed vaccines. This means that even if young animals are immunized frequently, there is still often a period when they are vulnerable to infection. Vulnerability occurs between the time that young animals lose their maternal antibody and before they develop their own active immune response. This period can be shortened by the use of less-attenuated modified live vaccines or the use of killed vaccines with high antigenic mass. Overcrowding and poor sanitation exacerbate the problem of inducing immunity in young animals before they come down with clinical disease.

Because only one vaccination is commonly recommended for large domestic animals, the timing of the vaccination is important. If the vaccine is administered too soon, it may be ineffective because of the presence of maternal antibody. If the vaccine is administered after all maternal antibodies are gone from animals in the herd, there may be a prolonged period of vulnerability before they develop their own immune response. Most veterinarians and producers decide that because of time and expense considerations it is impractical to vaccinate young pigs frequently. However, frequent vaccination may be justified in cases of unusually high disease incidence.

Immunosuppression due to a variety of factors including stress, malnutrition, concurrent infection, or immaturity or senescence of the immune system may also lead to vaccination failure. If the immunosuppression occurs at the time of vaccination, the vaccine may fail to induce an adequate immune response. If the immunosuppression occurs sometime after vaccination, disease may occur due to reduced immunity in spite of an adequate response to the original vaccine. Therapy with immunosuppressive drugs (e.g., glucocorticoids) may also cause this to occur.

Another concern is that some modified live vaccines are capable of inducing disease in the immunosuppressed animal. Modified live vaccines are tested for safety in normal, healthy animals. They are not recommended for use in animals with compromised immune systems. Therefore, these vaccines should not be used in animals that are immunosuppressed for any reason. This includes animals in the first few weeks of life unless the vaccine has been specifically tested in animals this young. When it is necessary to vaccinate animals under these conditions, killed vaccines should be used.

Overwhelming Challenge Dose. Most vaccines do not produce complete immunity to disease. They provide an increased ability to resist challenge by infectious agents. If a high challenge dose of organisms is present due to overcrowding or poor sanitation, the immune system may be overwhelmed, resulting in clinical disease.

Vaccine Efficacy. Vaccines that are licensed by the United States Department of Agriculture have been tested to determine that they are safe and effective. However, "effective" is a relative term. It does not mean that the vaccine must be able to induce complete immunity under all conditions that may be found in the field. This would not be realistic since the immune system is not capable of such potent protection under adverse conditions.

To be federally licensed, the vaccine must have been tested under controlled experimental conditions. The vaccinated group must have had significantly less disease than the nonvaccinated control group. This testing is typically done on healthy, nonstressed animals under good environmental conditions and with a controlled exposure to a single infectious agent. Vaccines may be much less effective when used in animals that are under stress, incubating other infectious diseases, or exposed to a high dose of infectious agents due to overcrowding or poor sanitation.

It is important to remember that for most diseases the relationship between the infectious agent and the host is sufficiently complicated that vaccination cannot be expected to provide complete protection. The vaccine can increase the animal's resistance to disease, but this resistance can be overwhelmed if good management practices are not followed.

REFERENCES

Abbas AK, Lichtman AH, Pober JS. 1994. Cellular and Molecular Immunology. Philadelphia: W.B. Saunders Co.

Allen WD, Porter P. 1973. Localisation by immunofluorescence of secretory component and IgA in the intestinal mucosa of the young pig. Immunol 24:365–374.

Bailey M, Clarke CJ, Wilson AD, Williams NA, Stokes CR. 1992. Depressed potential for interleukin-2 production following early weaning of piglets. Vet Immunol Immunopathol 34:197–207.

Barratt ME. 1972. Immediate hypersensitivity to *Metastrongylus* spp. infection in the pig. Immunology 22:601–623.

Bautista EM, Goyal SM, Yoon IJ, Joo SH, Collins JE. 1993. Comparison of porcine alveolar macrophages and CL 2621 for the detection of porcine reproductive and respiratory syndrome (PRRS) virus and anti-PRRS antibody. J Vet Diagn Invest 5:163–165.

Bautista EM, Gregg D, Golde WT. 2002. Characterization and functional analysis of skin-derived dendritic cells from swine without a requirement for in vitro propagation. Vet Immunol Immunopathol 88:131–148.

Becker BA, Misfeldt ML. 1993. Evaluation of the mitogen-induced proliferation and cell surface differentiation anitgens of lymphocytes from pigs 1 to 30 days of age. J Anim Sci 71:2073–2078.

Bellamy JEC, Nielsen NO. 1974. Immune-mediated emigration of neutrophils into the lumen of the small intestine. Infect Immun 9:615–619.

Bertram TA. 1986. Intravascular macrophages in lungs of pigs infected with *Haemophilus pleuropneumoniae*. Vet Pathol 23:681–691.

Bhogal BS, Nagy LK, Walker PD. 1987. Neutrophil mediated and IgA dependent antibacterial immunity against enteropathogenic *Escherichia coli* in the porcine intestinal mucosa. Vet Immunol Immunopathol 14:23–44.

Bianchi ATJ, Zwart RJ, Jeurissen SHM, Moonen-Leusen HWM. 1992. Development of the B- and T-cell compartments in porcine lymphoid organs from birth to adult life: An immunohistological approach. Vet Immunol Immunopathol 33:201–221.

Binns RM. 1982. Organisation of the lymphoreticular system and lymphocyte markers in the pig. Vet Immunol Immunopathol 3:95–146.

Binns RM, Licence ST, Whyte A. 1996. Transfer of T-cell-mediated, antigen-specific delayed type hypersensitivity reactions to naive recipient inbred pigs. Res Vet Sci 60:24–28.

Binns RM, Pabst R, Licence ST. 1986. The behavior of pig lymphocyte populations in vivo. Swine Biomed Res 3:1837–1853.

Blecha F, Kelley KW. 1981. Effects of cold and weaning stressors on the antibody-mediated immune response of pigs. J Anim Sci 53:439–447.

Blecha F, Pollmann DS, Nichols DA. 1983. Weaning pigs at an early age decreases cellular immunity. J Anim Sci 56:396–400.

—— 1985. Immunologic reactions of pigs regrouped at or near weaning. Am J Vet Res 46:1934–1937.

Blecha F, Pollmann DS, Kluber IEF. 1986. Decreased mononuclear cell response to mitogens in artifically reared neonatal pigs. Can J Vet Res 50:522–525.

Breazile JE. 1987. Physiologic basis and consequences of distress in animals. J Am Vet Med Assoc 191:1212–1215.

Brogden KA, Ackermann M, McCray PBJr, Tack BF. 2003. Antimicrobial peptides in animals and their role in host defence. Int J Antimicrob Agents 22:465–478.

Butler JE, Klobasa F, Werhahn E. 1981. The differential localisations of IgA, IgM, and IgG in the gut of suckled neonatal piglets. Vet Immunol Immunopathol 2:53–65.

Carrasco CP, Rigden RC, Schaffner R, Gerber H, Neuhaus V, Inumaru S, Takamatsu H, Bertoni G, McCullough KC, Summerfield A. 2001. Porcine dendritic cells generated in vitro: Morphological, phenotypic and functional properties. Immunology 104:175–184.

Charley B. 1983. Interaction of influenza virus with swine alveolar macrophages: Influence of anti-virus antibodies and cytochalasin B. Ann Virol 134:51–59.

Check W. 2004. Innate immunity depends on toll-like receptors. Am Soc Microbiol News 70:317–322.

Chibber R, Castle AG. 1983. Biochemical characterisation of porcine polymorphonuclear leucocytes: Comparison with human polymorphonuclear leucocytes. Comp Biochem Physiol 75B:335–340.

Chien Y, Jores R, Crowly MP. 1996. Recognition by gamma/delta T cells. In WE Paul, CG Fathman, H Metzger, eds. Annual Review of Immunology. Palo Alto: Annual Reviews Inc., pp. 511–532.

Chinsakchai S, Molitor TW. 1992. Replication and immunosuppressive effects of Pseudorabies virus on swine peripheral blood mononuclear cells. Vet Immunol Immunopathol 30:247–260.

Chitko-McKown CG, Blecha F. 1992. Pulmonary intravascular macrophages: A review of immune properties and functions. Ann Rech Vet 23:201–214.

Chitko-McKown CG, Chapes SK, Brown RE, Phillips RM, McKown RD, Blecha F. 1991. Porcine alveolar and pulmonary intravascular macrophages: Comparison of immune functions. J Leukoc Biol 50:364–372.

Cho WS, Chae C. 2003. Expression of inflammatory cytokines (TNF-alpha, IL-1, IL-6 and IL-8) in colon of pigs naturally infected with *Salmonella typhimurium* and *S. choleraesuis*. J Vet Med A Physiol Pathol Clin Med 50:484–487.

Chung WB, Backstrom L, McDonald J, Collins MT. 1993. *Actinobacillus pleuropneumoniae* culture supernatants interfere with killing of *Pasteurella multocida* by swine pulmonary alveolar macrophages. Can J Vet Res 57:190–197.

Coe NE, Frank DE, Wood RL, Roth JA. 1992. Alteration of neutrophil function in BCG-treated and nontreated swine after exposure to *Salmonella typhimurium*. Vet Immunol Immunopathol 33:37–50.

Crawley A, Wilkie BN. 2003. Porcine Ig isotypes: Function and molecular characteristics. Vaccine 21:2911–2922.

Crawley A, Raymond C, Wilkie BN. 2003. Control of immunoglobulin isotype production by porcine B-cells cultured with cytokines. Vet Immunol Immunopathol 91:141–154.

Crocker SH, Eddy DO, Obenauf RN, Wismar BL, Lowery BD. 1981a. Bacteremia: Host-specific lung clearance and pulmonary failure. J Trauma J 21:215–220.

Crocker SH, Lowery BD, Eddy DO, Wismar BL, Buesching WJ, Obenauf RN. 1981b. Pulmonary clearance of blood-borne bacteria. Surg Gynecol Obstet 153:845–851.

Cullor JS. 1992. Shock attributable to bacteremia and endotoxemia in cattle: Clinical and experimental findings. J Vet Med Assoc 200:1894–1902.

Curtis J, Bourne FJ. 1971. Immunoglobulin quantitation in sow serum, colostrum and milk and the serum of young pigs. Biochem Biophys Acta 236:319–332.

Cysewski SJ, Wood RL, Pier AC, Baetz AL. 1978. Effects of aflatoxin on the development of acquired immunity to swine erysipelas. Am J Vet Res 39:445–448.

Darwich L, Balasch M, Plana-Duran J, Segales J, Domingo M, Mateu E. 2003. Cytokine profiles of peripheral blood mononuclear cells from pigs with postweaning multisystemic wasting syndrome in response to mitogen, superantigen or recall viral antigens. J Gen Virol 84:3453–3457.

DeBey MC, Roth JA, Ross RF. 1994. Enhancement of the increase in intracellular calcium concentration in stimulated neutrophils in Mycoplasma hyopneumoniae. Vet Res Commun 17:249–257.

Delventhal S, Hensel A, Petzoldt K, Pabst R. 1992. Cellular changes in the bronchoalveolar lavage (BAL) of pigs, following immunization by the enteral or respiratory route. Clin Exp Immunol 90:223–227.

Dom P, Haesebrouck F, De Baetselier P. 1992. Stimulation and suppression of the oxygenation activity of porcine pulmonary alveolar macrophages by Actinobacillus pleuropneumoniae and its metabolites. Am J Vet Res 53:1113–1118.

Done SH, Paton DJ. 1995. Porcine reproductive and respiratory syndrome: Clinical disease, pathology and immunosuppression. Vet Rec 136:32–35.

Duncan IA, Binns RM, Duffus WPH. 1989. The null T cell in pig blood is not an NK cell. Immunology 68:392–395.

Dunkley M, Pabst R, Cripps A. 1995. An important role for intestinally derived T cells in respiratory defence. Immunol Today 16:231–236.

Dunn AJ. 1988. Nervous system-immune system interactions: An overview. J Recept Res 8:589–607.

Ellis RP, Vorhies MW. 1976. Effect of supplemental dietary vitamin E on the serologic response of swine to an Escherichia coli bacterin. J Am Vet Med Assoc 168:231–232.

Evans DL, Jaso-Friedmann L. 1993. Natural killer (NK) cells in domestic animals: Phenotype, target cell specificity and cytokine regulation. Vet Res Commun 17:429–447.

Eyre P. 1980. Pharmacological aspects of hypersensitivity in domestic animals: A review. Vet Res Commun 4:83–98.

Ferguson FG, Pinto AJ, Confer FL, Botticelli G. 1986. Characteristics of Yorkshire swine natural killer cells. Swine Biomed Res 3:1915–1924.

Fischer T, Buttner M, Rziha HJ. 2000. T helper 1-type cytokine transcription in peripheral blood mononuclear cells of pseudorabies virus (Suid herpesvirus 1) primed swine indicates efficient immunization. Immunology 101:378–387.

Flaming KP, Goff BL, Frank DE, Roth JA. 1994. Pigs are relatively resistant to dexamethasone induced immunosuppression. Comp Haematol Int 4:218–225.

Franek F, Riha I. 1964. Purification and structural characterisation of 5S gamma globulin in newborn pigs. Immunochemistry 1:49.

Friesen G, Goodband RD, Nelssen JL, Blecha F, Reddy DN, Reddy PG, Kats LJ. 1993. The effect of pre- and postweaning exposure to soybean meal on growth performance and on the immune response in the early-weaned pig. J Anim Sci 71:2089–2098.

Fuentes M, Pijoan C. 1986. Phagocytosis and intracellular killing of Pasteurella multocida by porcine alveolar macrophages after infection with pseudorabies virus. Vet Immunol Immunopathol 13:165–172.

——. 1987. Pneumonia in pigs induced by intranasal challenge exposure with pseudorabies virus and Pasteurella multocida. Am J Vet Res 48:1446–1448.

Groux H. 2001. An overview of regulatory T cells. Microbes Infect 3:883–889.

Groux H, Bigler M, de Vries JE, Roncarolo MG. 1998. Inhibitory and stimulatory effects of IL-10 on human CD8+ T cells. J Immunol 160:3188–3193.

Halliwell REW, Gorman NT. 1989. Veterinary Clinical Immunology. Philadephia: W.B. Saunders Company.

Halpern MS, Koshland ME. 1970. Novel subunit in secretory IgA. Nature 228:1276.

Hammerberg C, Schurig GG, Ochs DL. 1989. Immunodeficiency in young pigs. Am J Vet Res 50:868–874.

Harding MJ, Molitor TW. 1988. Porcine parvovirus: Replication in and inhibition of selected cellular functions of swine alveolar macrophages and peripheral blood lymphocytes. Arch Virol 101:105–117.

Haverson K, Saalmuller A, Alvarez B, Alonso F, Bailey M, Bianchi AT, Boersma WJ, Chen Z, Davis WC, Dominguez J, Engelhardt H, Ezquerra A, Grosmaire LS, Hamilton MJ, Hollemweguer E, Huang CA, Khanna KV, Kuebart G, Lackovic G, Ledbetter JA, Lee R, Llanes D, Lunney JK, McCullough KC, Molitor T, Nielsen J, Niewold TA, Pescovitz MD, de la Lastra JM, Rehakova Z, Salmon H, Schnitzlein WM, Seebach J, Simon A, Sinkora J, Sinkora M, Stokes CR, Summerfield A, Sver L, Thacker E, Valpotic I, Yang H, Zuckermann FA, Zwart R. 2001. Overview of the third international workshop on swine leukocyte differentiation antigens. Vet Immunol Immunopathol 80:5–23.

Helm RM, Ermel RW, Frick OL. 2003. Nonmurine animal models of food allergy. Environ Health Perspect 111(2):239–244.

Hennessy KJ, Blecha F, Pollmann DS, Kluber EF. 1987. Isoprinosine and levamisole immunomodulation in artificially reared neonatal pigs. Am J Vet Res 48:477–480.

Hensel A, Pabst R, Petzoldt K, Petzoldt B. 1994. Oral and aerosol immunization with viable or inactivated Actinobacillus pleuropneumoniae bacteria: Antibody response to capsular polysaccharides in bronchoalveolar lavage fluids (BALF) and sera of pigs. Clin Exp Immunol 96:91–97.

Hernandez J, Garfias Y, Reyes-Leyva J, Chavez R, Lascurain R, Vargas J, Zenteno E. 2002. Peanut and Amaranthus leucocarpus lectins discriminate between memory and naive/quiescent porcine lymphocytes. Vet Immunol Immunopathol 84:71–82.

Hill IR, Porter P. 1974. Studies of bactericidal activity to Escherichia coli of porcine serum and colostral immunoglobulins and the role of lysozyme with secretory IgA. Immunology 26:1239–1250.

Hirt W, Saalmuller A, Reddehase MJ. 1990. Distinct gamma/delta T cell receptors define two subsets of circulating porcine CD2⁻ CD4⁻ CD8⁻ T lymphocytes. Eur J Immunol 20:265–269.

Iglesias G, Pijoan C, Molitor T. 1989a. Interactions of pseudorabies virus with swine alveolar macrophages I: Virus replication. Arch Virol 104:107–115.

——. 1989b. Interactions of pseudorabies virus with swine alveolar macrophages: Effects of virus infection on cell functions. J Leukoc Biol 45:410–415.

——. 1992. Effects of pseudorabies virus infection upon cytotoxicity and antiviral activities of porcine alveolar macrophages. Comp Microbiol Infect Dis 15:249–259.

Jericho KWF. 1970. Intrapulmonary lymphoid tissue of healthy pigs. Res Vet Sci 2:548–552.

Joens LA, Pier AC, Cutlip RC. 1981. Effects of aflatoxin consumption on the clinical course of swine dysentery. Am J Vet Res 42:1170–1172.

Johansson E, Domeika K, Berg M, Alm GV, Fossum C. 2003. Characterisation of porcine monocyte-derived dendritic cells according to their cytokine profile. Vet Immunol Immunopathol 91:183–197.

Joling P, Bianchi ATJ, Kappe AL, Zwart RJ. 1994. Distribution of lymphocyte subpopulations in thymus, spleen, and peripheral blood of specific pathogen free pigs from 1 to 40 weeks of age. Vet Immunol Immunopathol 40:105–117.

Kelley KW. 1985. Immunological consequences of changing environmental stimuli. In Animal Stress. GP Moberg, ed. Bethesda, MD: American Physiological Society, pp. 193–223.

——. 1988. Cross-talk between the immune and endocrine systems. J Anim Sci 66:2095–2108.

Kim YB, Ichimura O. 1986. Porcine natural killer (NK)/killer (K) cell system. Swine Biomed Res 3:1811–1819.

Kim YB, Bradley SG, Watson DW. 1966. Ontogeny of the immune response. I. Development of immunoglobulins in germfree and conventional colostrum-deprived piglets. J Immunol 97:52–63.

Knoblock KF, Canning PC. 1992. Modulation of in vitro porcine natural killer cell activity by recombinant interleukin-1a, interleukin-2 and interleukin-4. Immunology 76:299–304.

Kokryakov VN, Harwig SSL, Panyutich EA, Shevchenko AA, Aleshina GM, Shamova OV, Korneva HA, Lehrer RI. 1993. Protegrins: Leukocyte antimicrobial peptides that combine features of corticostatic defensins and tachyplesins. FEBS Lett 327:231–236.

Koller LD. 1979. Effects of environmental contaminants on the immune system. Adv Vet Sci Comp Med 23:267–295.

Larsen HJ, Tollersrud S. 1981. Effect of dietary vitamin E and selenium on the phytohaemagglutinin response of pig lymphocytes. Res Vet Sci 31:301–305.

Lecce JG, Matrone G, Morgan DO. 1961. Porcine neonatal nutrition: Absorption of unaltered porcine proteins and polyvinyl pyrrolidone from the gut of piglets. J Nutr 73:158.

Lee J, Choi K, Olin MR, Cho SN, Molitor TW. 2004. Gamma delta T cells in immunity induced by *Mycobacterium bovis* bacillus Calmette-Guerin vaccination. Infect Immun 72:1504–1511.

Lesnick CE, Derbyshire JB. 1988. Activation of natural killer cells in newborn piglets by interferon induction. Vet Immunol Immunopathol 18:109–117.

Li DF, Nelssen JL, Reddy PG, Blecha F, Hancock JD, Allee GL, Goodband RD, Klemm RD. 1990. Transient hypersensitivity to soybean meal in the early-weaned pig. J Anim Sci 68:1790–1799.

Li DF, Nelssen JL, Reddy PG, Blecha F, Klemm R, Goodband RD. 1991. Interrelationship between hypersensitivity to soybean proteins and growth performance in early-weaned pigs. J Anim Sci 69:4062–4069.

Linklater KA, McTaggart HS, Imlah P. 1973. Haemolytic disease of the newborn, thrombocytopenic purpura and neutropenia occurring concurrently in a litter of piglets. Br Vet J 129:36–46.

Löfstedt J, Roth JA, Ross RF, Wagner WC. 1983. Depression of polymorphonuclear leukocyte function associated with experimentally induced *Escherichia coli* mastitis in sows. Am J Vet Res 44:1224–1228.

Lunney JK. 1994. Current status of the swine leukocyte antigen complex. Vet Immunol Immunopathol 43:19–28.

Lunney JK, Pescovitz MD. 1987. Phenotypic and functional characterization of pig lymphocyte populations. Vet Immunol Immunopathol 17:135–144.

Martins CLV, Lawman MJP, Scholl T, Mebus CA, Lunney JK. 1993. African swine fever virus specific porcine cytotoxic T cell activity. Arch Virol 129:211–225.

Messick JB. 2004. Hemotrophic mycoplasmas (hemoplasmas): A review and new insights into pathogenic potential. Vet Clin Pathol 33:2–13.

Mestecky J, Zikan J, Butler WT. 1971. Immunoglobulin M and secretory immunoglobulin A: Presence of a common polypeptide chain different from light chains. Science 171:1163.

Metzger JJ, Fougereau M. 1968. Caractérisations biochimiques des immunoglobulines gamma-G et gamma-M porcines. Vet Res Commun 1:37.

Miller DM, Stuart BP, Crowell WA. 1978. Aflatoxicosis in swine: Its effect on immunity and relationship to salmonellosis. Proc Annu Meet Am Assoc Vet Lab Diagn. pp. 135–146.

Muneta Y, Uenishi H, Kikuma R, Yoshihara K, Shimoji Y, Yamamoto R, Hamashima N, Yokomizo Y, Mori Y. 2003. Porcine TLR2 and TLR6: Identification and their involvement in *Mycoplasma hyopneumoniae* infection. J Interferon Cytokine Res 23:583–590.

Murtaugh MP. 1994. Porcine cytokines. Vet Immunol Immunopathol 43:37–44.

Murtaugh MP, Foss DL. 1997. Porcine cytokines and interferons. Handbook of Vertebrate Immunology. London: Academic Press.

——. 2002. Inflammatory cytokines and antigen presenting cell activation. Vet Immunol Immunopathol 87:109–121.

Nielsen KH. 1977. Bovine reaginic antibody III. Cross-reaction of antihuman IgE and antibovine reaginic immunoglobulin antisera with sera from several species of mammals. Can J Comp Med 41:345–348.

Nowacki W, Cederblad B, Renard C, La Bonnardiere C, Charley B. 1993. Age-related increase of porcine natural interferon a producing cell frequency and of interferon yield per cell. Vet Immunol Immunopathol 37:113–122.

Ohgami M, Doerschuk CM, English D, Dodek PM, Hogg JC. 1989. Kinetics of radiolabeled neutrophils in swine. J Appl Physiol 66:1881–1885.

Osburn BI, MacLachlan NJ, Terrell TG. 1982. Ontogeny of the immune system. J Am Vet Med Assoc 181:1049–1052.

Pabst R, Binns RM. 1986. Comparison of lymphocyte production and migration in pig lymph nodes, tonsils, spleen, bone marrow and thymus. Swine Biomed Res 3:1865–1871.

——. 1994. The immune system of the respiratory tract in pigs. Vet Immunol Immunopathol 43:151–156.

Pabst R, Delventhal S, Hensel A, Petzoldt B. 1995. Immunization by the enteral and respiratory route with viable and inactivated bacteria results in a differential increase in lymphocyte subsets in the bronchoalveolar space. Adv Mucosal Immunol 371:1459–1461.

Pauly T, Elbers K, Konig M, Lengsfeld T, Saalmuller A, Thiel H-J. 1995. Classical swine fever virus-specific cytotoxic T lymphocytes and identification of a T cell epitope. J Gen Virol 76:3039–3049.

Peplowski MA, Mahan DC, Murray FA, Moxon AL, Cantor AH, Ekstrom KE. 1981. Effect of dietary and injectable vitamin E and selenium in weanling swine antigenically challenged with sheep red blood cells. J Anim Sci 51:344–351.

Pescovitz MD, Sakopoulos AG, Gaddy JA, Husmann RJ, Zuckermann FA. 1994. Porcine peripheral blood CD4+/CD8+ dual expressing T-cells. Vet Immunol Immunopathol 42:53–62.

Pijoan C, Ochoa G. 1978. Interaction between a hog cholera vaccine strain and *Pasteurella multocida* in the production of porcine pneumonia. J Comp Pathol 88:167–170.

Porter P. 1969. Transfer of immunoglobulins IgG, IgA and IgM to lacteal secretions in the parturient sow and their absorption by the neonatal piglet. Biochem Biophys Acta 181:381–392.

——. 1973. Studies of porcine secretory IgA and its component chains in relation to intestinal absorption of colostral immunoglobulins by the neonatal pig. Immunology 24:163–176.

——. 1986. Immune system. In Diseases of Swine. AD Leman, BE Straw, RD Glock, WL Mengeling, RHC Penny, E Scholl, eds. Ames: Iowa State Univ Press, pp. 44–57.

Porter P, Allen WD. 1972. Classes of immunoglobulins related to immunity in the pig. J Am Vet Med Assoc 160:511.

Ramos JA, Ramis AJ, Marco A, Domingo M, Rabanal R, Ferrer L. 1992. Histochemical and immunohistochemical study of the mucosal lymphoid system in swine. Am J Vet Res 53:1418–1426.

Rice CE, L'Ecuyer C. 1963. Complement titres of naturally and artificially raised piglets. Can J Comp Med Vet Sci 27:157–161.

Roe JM, Patel D, Morgan KL. 1993. Isolation of porcine IgE, and preparation of polyclonal antisera. Vet Immunol Immunopathol 37:83–97.

Roof MB, Kramer TT, Kunesh JP, Roth JA. 1992a. In vivo isolation of *Salmonella choleraesuis* from porcine neutrophils. Am J Vet Res 53:1333–1336.

Roof MB, Roth JA, Kramer TT. 1992b. Porcine salmonellosis: Characterization, immunity and potential vaccines. Compend Contin Ed Vet Pract 14:411–424.

Roth JA. 1999. Mechanistic bases for adverse vaccine reactions and vaccine failures. Adv Vet Med 41:681–700.

Roth JA, Henderson LM. 2001. New technology for improved vaccine safety and efficacy. Vet Clin North Am Food Anim Pract 17:585–597.

Saalmuller A, Bryant J. 1994. Characteristics of porcine T lymphocytes and T-cell lines. Vet Immunol Immunopathol 43:45–52.

Salmon H. 1986. Surface markers of swine lymphocytes: Application to the study of local immune system of mammary gland and transplanted gut. Swine Biomed Res 3:1855–1864.

——. 1987. The intestinal and mammary immune system in pigs. Vet Immunol Immunopathol 17:367–388.

Sandbulte MR, Roth JA. 2004. Methods for analysis of cell-mediated immunity in domestic animal species. J Am Vet Med Assoc 225(4):522–530.

Sellwood R, Hall G, Anger H. 1986. Emigration of polymorphonuclear leucocytes into the intestinal lumen of the neonatal piglet in response to challenge with K88-positive *Escherichia coli*. Res Vet Sci 40:128–135.

Shi J, Ross CR, Chengappa MM, Blecha F. 1994. Identification of a proline-arginine-rich antibacterial peptide from neutrophils that is analogous to PR-39, an antibacterial peptide from the small intestine. J Leukoc Biol 56:807–811.

Shimosato T, Kitazawa H, Katoh S, Tomioka Y, Karima R, Ueha S, Kawai Y, Hishinuma T, Matsushima K, Saito T. 2003. Swine toll-like receptor 9(1) recognizes CpG motifs of human cell stimulant. Biochem Biophys Acta 1627:56–61.

Shirota K, Koyama R, Nomura Y. 1986. Glomerulopathy in swine: Microscopic lesions and IgG or C3 deposition in 100 pigs. Jpn J Vet Sci 48:15–21.

Smith IM, Hodges RT, Betts AO, Hayward AHS. 1973. Experimental infections of gnotobiotic piglets with *Pasteurella septica* (serogroup A) alone or with *Mycoplasma hyopneumoniae*. J Comp Pathol 83:307–321.

Speer VC, Brown H, Quinn L, Catron DV. 1959. The cessation of antibody absorption in the young pig. Immunology 83:632.

Spickler AR, Roth JA. 2003. Adjuvants in veterinary vaccines: Modes of action and adverse effects. J Vet Intern Med 17:273–281.

Stertzl J, Kostka J, Riha I, Mandel I. 1960. Attempts to determine the formation and character of globulin and of natural and immune antibodies in young pigs reared without colostrum. Folia Microbiol 5:29.

Stokes C, Bourne JF. 1989. Mucosal immunity. In Veterinary Clinical Immunology. REW Halliwell, NT Gorman, eds. Philadelphia: W.B. Saunders Company, pp. 164–192.

Stokes CR, Miller BG, Bailey M, Wilson AD, Bourne FJ. 1987. The immune response to dietary antigens and its influence on disease susceptibility in farm animals. Vet Immunol Immunopathol 17:413–423.

Storici P, Scocchi M, Tossi A, Gennaro R, Zanetti M. 1994. Chemical synthesis and biological activity of a novel antibacterial peptide deduced from a pig myeloid cDNA. FEBS Lett 337:303–307.

Summerfield A, Guzylack-Piriou L, Schaub A, Carrasco CP, Tache V, Charley B, McCullough KC. 2003. Porcine peripheral blood dendritic cells and natural interferon-producing cells. Immunology 110:440–449.

Suradhat S, Thanawongnuwech R. 2003. Upregulation of interleukin-10 gene expression in the leukocytes of pigs infected with porcine reproductive and respiratory syndrome virus. J Gen Virol 84:2755–2760.

Tabel H. 1998. Immunology of Mustelidae. In Handbook of Vertebrate Immunology. PP Pastoret, P Griebel, M Bazin, A Govaerts, eds. London: Academic Press, pp. 337–342.

Takamatsu HH, Denyer MS, Wileman TE. 2002. A sub-population of circulating porcine gamma delta T cells can act as professional antigen presenting cells. Vet Immunol Immunopathol 87:223–224.

Tarigan S, Slocombe RF, Browning GF, Kimpton W. 1994. Functional and structural changes of porcine alveolar macrophages induced by sublytic doses of a heat-labile, hemolytic, cytotoxic substance produced by *Actinobacillus pleuropneumoniae*. Am J Vet Res 55:1548–1557.

Tengerdy RP. 1986. Nutrition, immunity and disease resistance. In Proc 6th Int Conf Prod Dis Farm Anim, pp. 175–182.

Thanawongnuwech R, Thacker B, Thacker E. 2000. Cytokine profiles following *M. hyopneumoniae* and PRRSV co-infection using semiquantitative RT-PCR measurement. In Proc 16th Int Pig Vet Soc Cong, p. 173.

Thanawongnuwech R, Young TF, Thacker BJ, Thacker EL. 2001. Differential production of proinflammatory cytokines: In vitro PRRSV and *Mycoplasma hyopneumoniae* co-infection model. Vet Immunol Immunopathol 79:115–127.

Thanawongnuwech R, Thacker EL. 2003. Interleukin-10, interleukin-12, and interferon-gamma levels in the respiratory tract following *Mycoplasma hypopneumoniae* and PRRSV infection in pigs. Viral Immunol 16:357–367.

Thielke KH, Hoffmann-Moujahid A, Weisser C, Waldkirch E, Pabst R, Holtmeier W, Rothkotter HJ. 2003. Proliferating intestinal gamma/delta T cells recirculate rapidly and are a major source of the gamma/delta T cell pool in the peripheral blood. Eur J Immunol 33:1649–1656.

Tizard I. 1987. Veterinary Immunology: An Introduction. 3 ed. Philadelphia: W.B. Saunders Company.

Tuboly S, Bernath S, Glavits R, Medveczky I. 1988. Intestinal absorption of colostral lymphoid cells in newborn piglets. Vet Immunol Immunopathol 20:75–85.

Westly HJ, Kelley KW. 1984. Physiologic concentrations of cortisol suppress cell-mediated immune events in the domestic pig. Proc Soc Exp Biol Med 177:156–164.

Williams PP. 1993. Immunomodulating effects of intestinal absorbed maternal colostral leukocytes by neonatal pigs. Can J Vet Res 57:1–8.

Winkler GC. 1988. Pulmonary intravascular macrophages in domestic animal species: Review of structural and functional properties. Am J Anat 181:217–234.

Winkler GC, Cheville NF. 1987. Postnatal colonization of porcine lung capillaries by intravascular macrophages: An ultrastructural morphometric analysis. Microvasc Res 33:224–232.

Yang WC, Schultz RD. 1986. Ontogeny of natural killer cell activity and antibody dependent cell mediated cytotoxicity in pigs. Dev Comp Immunol 10:405–418.

Yen JT, Pond WG. 1987. Effect of dietary supplementation with vitamin C or carbadox on weanling pigs subjected to crowding stress. J Anim Sci 64:1672–1681.

Zanetti M, Storici P, Tossi A, Scocchi M, Gennaro R. 1994. Molecular cloning and chemical synthesis of a novel antibacterial peptide derived from pig myeloid cells. J Biol Chem 269:7855–7858.

Zarkower A, Eskew ML, Scheuchenzuber WJ, Ferguson FG, Confer F. 1982. Antibody-dependent cell-mediated cytotoxicity in pigs. Am J Vet Res 43:1590–1593.

Zeidler RB, Kim HD. 1985. Phagocytosis, chemiluminescence, and cell volume of alveolar macrophages from neonatal and adult pigs. J Leukoc Biol 37:29–43.

Zuckermann FA, Husmann RJ. 1996. Functional and phenotypic analysis of porcine peripheral blood CD4/CD8 double-positive T cells. Immunology 87:500–512.

Zuckermann FA, Zsak L, Mettenleiter TC, Ben-Porat T. 1990. Pseudorabies virus glycoprotein gIII is a major target antigen for murine and swine virus-specific cytotoxic T lymphocytes. J Virol 64:802–812.

Zuckermann FA, Husmann RJ, Schwartz R, Brandt J, Mateu de Antonio E, Martin S. 1998. Interleukin-12 enhances the virus-specific interferon gamma response of pigs to an inactivated pseudorabies virus vaccine. Vet Immunol Immunopathol 63:57–67.

3 Diseases of the Digestive System

Jill R. Thomson

Diseases of the gastrointestinal tract that affect pigs between neonatal and finishing stages continue to be some of the greatest factors that limit the efficiency and profitability of pig production globally. Advances in effective disease control measures such as development of new vaccines and antimicrobial products have provided new approaches to disease control. However, this is countered by increasing awareness of other issues such as development of antimicrobial resistance, the ban or limitation of the use of antimicrobial growth promoters in some countries, and increasing public awareness and expectation of food safety—particularly in relation to salmonellosis and food residues. Salmonellae surveillance and control have become a major objective in many countries following the schemes initiated in Scandinavia. This has demanded new standards of hygiene and care involving a whole-chain approach to disease control. However, there is also increasing public concern over intensive farming systems and consumer demands for more natural and welfare-friendly methods of farming that allow pigs to express normal rooting behavior through availability of substrate. To these ends, legislation has been introduced in some countries and this is likely to increase, thus presenting new challenges for pig producers and veterinarians in relation to effective control of enteric infections. Organic product is increasing in popularity and requires alternative approaches to enteric disease prevention.

In parallel with these practical issues, there has been substantial ongoing research into the enteric physiology and immunology in the pig. This work provides the foundation for future practical advances in enteric disease control and is briefly reviewed in the following sections. Thereafter there is an overview of enteric diseases (which are covered in depth in other chapters).

ANATOMIC AND HISTOLOGIC FEATURES

The conformation and growth efficiency of the pig has changed dramatically over the years as the result of genetic selection and production of suitable hybrids. However, the gut morphology is apparently unchanged and an area of little focus or attention. The exception is the development of genotypes resistant to F18 and F4 (K88) *Escherichia coli* infections in which pigs do not possess the required receptor for these organisms to cause disease.

Gut maturation occurs rapidly after birth in response to factors such as oxygenation; enteral nutrient presentation; and hormones, particularly cortisol (Sangild 2001). Neonatal hypoxia is associated with intestinal dysfunction and an increased incidence in neonatal enterocolitis (Cohen et al. 1991; Powell et al. 1999). At birth the sudden increase in blood arterial oxygen is a vital factor in gut development. Common occurrences such as delayed parturition or congenital pneumonic infections could be initiating factors for neonatal diarrhea. After birth the small intestine undergoes a rapid growth in response to enteral presentation of nutrients (Burrin et al. 2000). This is stimulated by a wide range of factors such as hormones and growth factors (Sangild 2001). Good intake of milk in the early stages of life is important for rapid gut growth as well as promoting piglet vigor and provision of colostral immunity.

During the first 3–4 weeks of life fetal enterocytes which have high endocytotic activity are gradually replaced by adult type enterocytes devoid of such activity. The process occurs in a proximal-to-distal direction in the intestine and is an important part of intestinal maturation (Baintner 1986). Changes in enterocyte generation influence the expression of brush border enzymes. Lactose activity is high in the newborn pig and steadily decreases to become minimal after weaning, whereas sucrase and maltase activities are low in the newborn but increase after weaning (Pluske et al. 1997). Intestinal maturation can be hastened in the unweaned pig by feeding kidney bean lectin (*Phaseolus vulgaris*) (Pusztai et al. 1999; Biernat et al. 2001; Rådberg et al. 2001). This dietary means of promoting rapid gut maturation could be of value in reducing or preventing postweaning diarrhea problems in pigs in the future.

Weaning is associated with adverse effects, such as abrupt withdrawal of sow's milk, low and variable feed intake, growth stasis, and compromised integrity of the small intestinal epithelium. Changes in gut morphology at weaning include reduced villus height and increased crypt depth (Hampson 1986; Kelly et al. 1991). These adverse effects can be diet-dependent and diet-independent (McCracken et al. 1995). Villus length reduces by 30–40% at days 4 to 7 postweaning but increases back to 94% of original length at 14 days postweaning (Verdonk et al. 2001a). Additionally, a reduction in the length of microvilli occurs at 3–7 days after weaning (Cera et al. 1988). There is a significant relationship between voluntary feed intake and mucosal architecture (Makkink et al. 1994; Pluske et al. 1996b). Low feed intakes or a period of starvation postweaning reduces the villus height throughout the small intestine particularly in the proximal jejunum. To minimize the changes, diets high in milk products, cooked cereals, and low levels of antigenicity are utilized. Raw cereals have a significant adverse effect on gut mucosa as compared with cooked cereals, which are thought to improve postweaning growth (Lawlor et al. 2001). Anorexia at weaning might contribute to local inflammation in the piglet's small intestine (McCracken et al. 1999). With low nutrient intake paracellular transport is higher and this increases over the first 4 days after weaning (Verdonk et al. 2001b). Therefore it would appear that the integrity of the gut mucosa is worse in piglets with low intake levels postweaning due to higher permeability of the tight junctions between cells (paracellular transport route), but permeability of the mucosa cells is not affected. The dietary changes at weaning and the resultant villus atrophy and crypt hyperplasia leads to decreased digestive and absorptive capacities in the intestine (Pluske et al. 1997, Rådberg et al. 2001). Other factors of importance are poor feed consumption, inflammation in response to bacterial metabolites, rotavirus, and hypersensitivity to antigenic components of the diet (Kenworthy 1976; Hampson and Kidder 1986; Kelly 1990). These physiological changes can result in alterations in the number and balance of the enteric bacterial flora often allowing enteropathogenic bacteria to proliferate, resulting in serious postweaning enteropathies such as colibacillosis. The morphological and functional changes in the small intestine of the newly weaned pig have been reviewed by Pluske (2001).

Transport associated stress of pigs has been shown to lower the intestinal pH and result in increased intestinal permeability. Permeability is the highest immediately after transportation and decreases after 2–3 hours of rest (van der Meulen et al. 2001). Translocation of bacteria and/or endotoxins from the gut into the systemic circulation is possible due to increased permeability (Zucker and Krüger 1998; Berg 1999). This might explain the increase in disease problems seen after transportation (Berends et al. 1996).

PHYSIOLOGY AND NUTRITION

The intestinal mucosa receives nutrients from 2 sources—the diet (brush border membrane) and the systemic circulation (baso-lateral membrane). The gut tissues have their own particular nutrient requirements for growth and function. The gastrointestinal tissues in the young growing pig utilize nearly 50% of the dietary amino acid intake and 30–50% of the dietary lysine, leucine, and phenylalanine plus 85% of threonine (Burrin et al. 2001). A substantial proportion of the essential amino acid needs and glucose needs are derived from the arterial circulation rather than from direct dietary sources. The amino acids are utilized in many ways, such as the formation of secretary mucins (Stoll et al. 1998), biosynthesis of other amino acids (Stoll et al. 1999), glutathione (Reeds et al. 1997) and nucleic acids (Perez and Reeds 1998). Nutrient supply for the neonate is derived solely from colostrum and milk. Additionally, colostrum and milk contain a large number of biologically active peptides that have important functions in regulating growth and differentiation of intestinal tissues. Targeted expression of key genes for production of milk peptides holds potential for the future (Kelly and Coutts 1997). On low protein diets, the lysine requirements of the gut remain relatively high and are preferentially met, which limits the systemic availability of lysine for lean tissue growth (Ebner et al. 1994). Exposure to microbial antigens (both pathogenic and nonpathogenic) stimulates a proinflammatory acute-phase response (MacRae 1993; Johnson 1997), which results in the loss of dietary amino acids and reduced deposition of body protein (e.g., reduced growth rate). The use of in-feed antibiotic growth promoters enhances growth rates by limiting this process.

Dietary carbohydrates are comprised of sugars, oligosaccharides, starch, and nonstarch polysaccharides. The enzyme activity responsible for carbohydrate degradation adapts according to the age of the pig and dietary composition. In the young pig there is efficient prececal digestion of lactose during suckling, and sucrose and starch after weaning. Carbohydrates that do not get digested in the small intestine are fermented in the large intestine by a diverse population of anaerobic bacteria. These are mostly nonstarch polysaccharides (NSPs).

Increasing the amount of fermentable carbohydrates and straw in the diet increases the total gastrointestinal tract weight by approximately 8% and 7%, respectively. With fermentable carbohydrates the main weight increase occurs in the colon, whereas with straw it occurs in the stomach and colon (Rijnen et al. 2001).

Most of the starches used in pig diets are highly digestible, with up to 98% of digestion occurring in the small intestine (Glitsø et al. 1998; Bach Knudson and Canibe 2000). Nonstarch polysaccharides (fiber) are present in cereals such as barley, wheat, oats, and rye.

Although there is some digestion of NSPs in the small intestine, the major site of NSP degradation is in the large intestine. Passage of ingesta through the large intestine generally takes from 20–40 hours, allowing time for bacterial degradation. The most common bacterial isolates are *Streptococcus* sp., *Lactobacillus, Fusobacterium, Eubacterium, Bacteroides,* and *Peptostreptococcus* (Moore et al. 1987). Fermentation of carbohydrates and NSPs in the large intestine results in the production of short chain fatty acids, mainly acetate, proprionate and butyrate, and the gases H_2, CO_2, and CH_4. Increasing the level of NSP entering the large intestine results in higher activity of microflora (Bach Knudson et al. 1991; Jensen and Jørgensen 1994), increased production of short chain fatty acids (Giusi-Perier et al. 1989), and increased production of gases (Jensen and Jørgensen 1994). Short chain fatty acids are rapidly absorbed from the large intestine and may provide up to 24% of the maintenance energy requirements for growing pigs (Yen et al. 1991) and potentially even more for adults. The total tract digestibility of NSPs is influenced by a number of complex factors, such as the source of NSPs, the level of inclusion in the diet, the solubility, the degree of lignification, the age and weight of the animal, the transit time, and the microbial composition (Bach Knudson and Jørgensen 2001). Adult animals are more capable of degrading fiber than growing pigs due to the greater intestinal volume and slower transit times. Adaptation to dietary changes in terms of digestibility of NSP residues is considered to take 3–5 weeks (Longland et al. 1993).

In weaner pigs the use of enzyme combinations has been found to increase the apparent ileal digestibility of feeds based on hulless barley, which have high beta-glucan concentrations (Yin et al. 2001). Due to the improved apparent ileal digestibility there was also a reduction in hind gut fermentation. Similarly, the addition of certain enzymes to wheat-based diets of growing pigs has been found to have beneficial effects (Hazzledine and Partridge 1996). There is increasing interest in the role of dietary factors, especially NSP and feed processing methods in so-called nonspecific colitis of pigs (Strachan et al. 2002, Thomson et al. 2004). This condition is thought to be an important precursor to other forms of colitis in pigs although the pathogenesis of this diet-associated form of colitis is poorly understood.

IMMUNOLOGY

For the first 24–48 hours of life the pig intestine is capable of absorbing macromolecules including immunoglobulins by pinocytosis, providing the neonate with passive immunity from colostrum (Weström et al. 1984). Although this process commences prepartum, the major absorptive function occurs postnatally (Sangild et al. 1999). This is a specific maturational process that is timed to maximize immunoglobulin uptake shortly after birth. Piglets born prematurely have a lower capacity for protein absorption than piglets born at full term (Sangild et al. 1997). Therefore fetal maturity is an important factor in successful immunoglobulin uptake from the colostrum.

The intestinal immune system of the young pig is very immature and its slow development may result in increased susceptibility to disease (Stokes et al. 2001). Intestinal lymphoid tissue is present in the form of mesenteric lymph nodes, intestinal Peyer's patches, and lymphocytes distributed through the mucosal lamina propria and intraepithelial sites. In the jejunum there are between 11–26 discrete Peyer's patches containing multiple lymphoid follicles (B lymphocytes) separated by T cells. Plasma cells containing IgM, IgG, and IgA are present in the subepithelial lymphoid dome and between the follicles (Brown and Bourne 1976). The dome region contains dendritic-type cells that express high levels of MHC II antigens. Microfold cells (M cells) that are thought to absorb luminal antigens occur in the overlying lymphoepithelium (Gebert et al. 1994). In the mature pig the intestinal lamina propria is heavily populated with lymphocytes. Plasma cells and B cells predominate in the crypt area, whereas T cells are found mainly in the villi, CD8[+] cells occur in the subepithelial sites, and CD4[+] occur in association with capillary plexuses in the lamina propria (Vega-Lopez et al. 1993). The majority of intraepithelial lymphocytes express CD2, but in mature pigs a high proportion also express CD8 (Stokes et al. 2001).

Functionally the intestinal immune mechanisms play a complex role in preventing and controlling harmful intestinal infections while tolerating many dietary antigens and nonharmful antigens from the intestinal flora. The surface epithelium serves as an effective barrier, providing it remains intact. IgA antibodies play an important defensive role. Significant quantities of dietary protein are absorbed across the intestinal mucosa (Wilson et al. 1989; Telemo et al. 1991). So-called "intestinal tolerance" to dietary proteins has been demonstrated in the pig, where immune responses to the dietary proteins are regulated to prevent inflammatory reaction and tissue damage associated with foreign protein absorption (Bailey et al. 1993). The interaction between the different components of the intestinal immune system is complex, and the basis of inflammation and apoptosis versus down regulation of immune responses is the subject of ongoing research.

Development of the pig's intestinal immune system occurs in response to antigen exposure. Full development of lymphoid tissue can take 7–9 weeks and can be delayed by early weaning at 3–4 weeks of age, as carried out in most modern pig-producing countries (Vega-Lopez et al. 1995). This, among many other factors, predisposes to postweaning diarrhea associated with enterotoxigenic *E. coli* or other pathogens. There is also increasing interest in the role of glutamine in intestinal immune function. Glutamine is an important nitrogen source for enterocytes and plays a key role in maintaining mucosal cell integrity and gut barrier function (den Hond et al. 1999). Key functions of lymphocytes are dependent on glutamine provision (Graham et al. 2000). Glutamine depletion results in immunosuppression, whereas glutamine administration has been found to have significant beneficial effects on the gut mucosal structure and intestinal immune function of piglets after weaning (Pierzynowski et al. 2001). Other studies on enhancing intestinal immune function of piglets at weaning have included feeding nucleotides for 2–4 weeks after weaning. This was found to have an immune enhancing effect on piglets through improving T-cell–mediated responses (Cameron et al. 2001). This is an important area of research because finding cost-effective methods of enhancing immune responses in the young weaner would bring significant benefits to the pig industry.

GUT FLORA

The intestinal flora of the pig is extremely complex and diverse making it difficult to study quantitatively and qualitatively. However this is an area of increasing interest in relation to maintenance of gut health and optimal function. The intestinal microflora of the large intestine has been studied and reviewed by Robinson et al. (1981, 1984).

Marked changes occur in the gut environment (for example, pH and organic acids) and microbial activity along the gastrointestinal tract of pigs (Bach Knudson et al. 1991, 1993). Differences in the diet composition can impose further changes and could affect the diversity of the gut microflora. In an experiment involving diets containing different levels of soluble and insoluble NSP, a medium to high content of NSP resulted in higher microbial diversity in the small intestine (Högberg et al. 2001). The presence of fermentable carbohydrates in the diet stimulates gut microbial activity resulting in the production of organic acids.

The potential value of prebiotics (compounds, other than dietary nutrients, that act as substrates for populations of beneficial microbial organisms in the gut) and probiotics (preparations containing beneficial bacteria) has been the subject of many studies in relation to gut health and prevention of enteric infections. Prebiotics achieve their beneficial effects in two ways. First, compounds such as fructooligosaccharides can be fermented by favorable bacteria (e.g., *Bifidobacteria* and *Lactobacilli*) giving them competitive advantage (Houdjik 1998; Nemcová et al. 1999). Second, mannose-containing compounds added to the diet result in binding with pathogenic bacteria that have mannose-specific lectins in fimbriae—for example, *E. coli* and *Salmonella*. This reduces attachment of pathogenic bacteria to receptor sites on gut mucosal cells (McDonald et al. 2002). Inulin is a natural polymer of fructose extracted from chicory that is considered to have prebiotic properties (Gibson and Roberfroid 1995; Roberfroid et al. 1998). Digestion of inulin in weaned pigs is mainly microbial and takes place in the large intestine. There, it modifies the profile of fermentation metabolites resulting in an increase in N-valerate and propionate and a decrease in acetate and ammonia (Rossi et al. 1997). Using an in vitro adhesion assay for *E. coli*, 5% inulin was found to partially inhibit adhesion of F4 positive *E. coli* to the small intestinal villi. The study also suggested that inulin might have immunomodulatory effects by boosting IgA and IgM antibodies in pigs exposed to foreign proteins (Rossi et al. 2001). In newly weaned pigs, addition of fructooligosaccharide and/or sugar beet pulp to the diet tended to increase the number of intestinal *Bifidobacterium* species and reduce the level of *E. coli*, although there was little difference in the incidence of diarrhea (Kleingebbink et al. 2001). The population of *Bifidobacterium* species is variable in piglets and constitutes less than 1% of the total bacterial population (Mikkelsen and Jensen 2001). Certain plant metabolites may interact with short chain fatty acids to create inhibitory conditions for pathogens such as *E. coli* 0157 (Duncan et al. 1998). The use of prebiotic is likely to be an area of growing scientific interest in the future.

Probiotics work on the principle of competitive exclusion of pathogenic bacteria and have been used successfully, for example, to control *Yersinia* infection in pigs (Asplund et al. 1996). Feeding probiotic bacteria, especially *Lactobacillus* species and *Bifidobacterium* species, may help with controlling enteric infections postweaning when the resident microflora are not yet stable. However, probiotics may also inhibit adherence of enteropathogenic *E. coli* and other gram-negative bacteria to enterocytes through occupying receptor sites (Spencer and Chesson 1994; Mack et al. 1999). This has potential for improved control of a wide range of enteric infections, particularly those of zoonotic importance such as *Salmonella* species and *Campylobacter* species. *Salmonella* infections in pigs are common resulting in clinical salmonellosis or subclinical disease (Lax et al. 1995). Up to 30% of finisher pigs might shed *Salmonella*, thereby presenting risk of carcass contamination at slaughter (Berends et al. 1996). *Campylobacter* is one of the most common causes of human enteric disease and has been isolated from a wide range of raw meats, including pork (Stern et al. 1985; Fricker and Park 1989; Zanetti et al. 1996). The predominant species in pigs is *Campylobacter coli* (Stern et al. 1985; Weitjnes et al. 1993, 1997; Young et al. 2000); however, some pig farms can also have a high prevalence of *Campylobacter jejuni* (Harvey et al. 1999). Contact with the sow during the suckling period results in a high prevalence of *Campylobacter* in piglets, whereas piglets removed from the sow after 24 hours and reared in isolation units have significantly less *Campylobacter* (Harvey et al. 2001).

CONTROL OF ENTERIC INFECTIONS THROUGH DIETARY INTERVENTIONS

Following the European Union ban on the use of the majority of antibiotic growth promoters, alternative measures to control the number and activity of intestinal bacteria have been explored. These include changes in management practices, feeding, hygiene, and the use of products such as probiotics, prebiotics, enzymes, herbs and plant extracts, prefermented feeds, and organic acids (Thomke and Elwinger 1998). Additionally, selective breeding for resistance; improving the pig's immune response through the use of vaccines, cytokines, and other immunomodulatory agents; organic acids; inorganic chemicals—for example, zinc oxide; and use of specific bacteriophages or bacteriocins are also possible (Hampson et al. 2001). The mechanisms by which antimicrobial agents enhance growth and feed efficiency are poorly understood (Commission on Antimicrobial Feed Additives 1997; Anderson et al. 1999). Two of the suggested mechanisms are inhibition of subclinical bacterial infection and less translocation of pathogens, and changing the small intestinal mucosal structure, mainly by increasing villus height promoting uptake of nutrients from the digesta. Finding effective non-antimicrobial alternatives requires a good understanding of the mechanisms that promote the beneficial effects in different age groups of pigs.

Dietary Fiber and Cereals

Different forms of fiber in the diet can influence the composition and metabolic activity of the large intestinal microflora in pigs (Varel et al. 1982; Varel and Pond 1985; Bach Knudson et al. 1991; Jensen and Jørgenson 1994; Reid and Hillman 1999). However, little is known about the ways in which the commensal colonic microflora interacts with pathogenic bacteria; therefore, the basis of dietary control of infectious enteric diseases is not understood. Other ways in which diet could influence pathogenic enteric infections include changing the amount or balance of substrates available for the organism at particular sites, influencing the viscosity, accessibility to receptor sites, and/or intestinal motility. For example, different cereal types and particle sizes have been shown to alter epithelial cell proliferation and lectin binding patterns of the epithelium of the large intestine of pigs (Brunsgaard 1998). The diet can also influence intestinal function. Components in boiled rice inhibit secretion in the small intestine and therefore reduce the magnitude of secretory diarrhea due to pathogens such as enterotoxigenic *E. coli* (Mathews et al. 1999).

One of the most well-recognized examples of dietary effects on enteric pathology is gastric ulceration, in which ulceration of the pars oesophagea occurs particularly in growing and finishing pigs. Such lesions can be associated with reduced growth rates (Ayles et al. 1996) but more importantly can be a cause of gastric hemorrhage and perforation leading to acute illness and death (Friendship 1999). Many studies have demonstrated a strong association between finely ground high wheat diet and gastric ulceration (Accioly et al. 1998). The role of bacteria in the pathogenesis is unclear. The spiral bacterium *Helicobacter heilmannii* has been associated with gastric ulceration in some studies (Barbosa et al. 1995, Queiroz et al. 1996), whereas in other studies, the association was weak or equivocal (Phillips 1999). Experimental inoculation of gnotobiotic pigs with *H. heilmannii* failed to produce lesions of gastric ulceration in pigs fed on a carbohydrate-enriched liquid diet (Krakowa et al. 1998). However inoculation of pigs with *Lactobacillus* sp. and *Bacillus* sp. when fed the same diet did produce ulcers, possibly due to fermentation by these bacteria in the presence of readily available dietary substrate. It is possible that production of short chain fatty acids produced through the fermentation process resulted in ulceration (Krakowa et al. 1998).

Early studies on the influence of diet in postweaning colibacillosis have shown that high concentrations of dietary protein (21%) predispose to the condition (Prohaszka and Baron 1980), whereas highly digestible milk-based weaner diets were associated with reduced postweaning diarrhea (English 1981). Conversely, inclusion of fiber sources was suggested to reduce the severity and incidence of postweaning diarrhea (Bertschinger et al. 1978, Bolduan et al. 1988). Later studies compared the effects of feeding different postweaning diets in experimental *E. coli* challenge model. Diets included a highly digestible cooked rice/animal protein diet with or without the addition of guar gum or 50% pearl barley as sources of additional soluble NSP and a commercial wheat/lupin-based diet (McDonald et al. 1997, 1999, 2001). Significantly more *E. coli* were isolated from the small intestines of piglets fed the soluble NSP supplemented diet and the wheat/lupin-based diet than the highly digestible rice/animal protein diet alone. The reason for the increased *E. coli* numbers in piglets fed the "provocative" diets is uncertain, but factors involving the amount of substrate in the small intestine, the viscosity of the ingesta, the rate of intestinal motility, and different fermentation processes within the small intestine were all potentially significant.

Most work has been done on the influence of diet on swine dysentery. Whereas a cooked rice diet was found to be protective in some studies (Siba et al. 1996) it was not in others (Kirkwood et al. 2000, Lindecrona et al. 2003). Feeding the cooked rice diet to pigs already affected with swine dysentery did not reduce the duration or severity of disease (Durmic et al. 2000). In a study of different cereal types, feeding steam-flaked maize or sorghum reduced the incidence of the disease (Pluske et al. 1996a). Soluble NSP and resistant starch were identified as important factors promoting large intestinal fermentation and bacterial colonization, whereas with the addition of a source of mainly insoluble NSP (oat chaff) the diet remained protective (Pluske et al. 1998). Addition of enzymes to wheat-based diets or the use of heat extrusion to increase digestibility of starch in the small intestine were tested in terms of their potential protective effects in swine dysentery but neither processes prevented colonization (Durmic et al. 2000). Likewise the use of a sorghum-based diet was tested as sorghum is inherently low in soluble NSPs but this diet was not protective against swine dysentery (Durmic 2000). However, the grind size of diets was important, with significantly more pigs developing swine dysentery with coarsely ground wheat or sorghum than with these grains finely ground (Hampson et al. 2001). In porcine colonic spirochetosis, pigs on the cooked rice diet developed infection later and to a lesser extent than pigs on wheat-based diet (Hampson et al. 2000; Lindecrona et al. 2004).

Carriage of *Oesophagostomum dentatum* in pigs is enhanced by diets rich in insoluble fiber (Petkevicius et al. 1997).

Organic Acids and their Salts, Inorganic Compounds, and Fatty Acids

Alternatives to antibiotic inclusion in weaner diets have included the use of organic acids and their salts such as potassium diformate (Roth et al. 1998). Addition of 1.8% potassium diformate to a piglet starter ration decreased the counts of total anaerobic bacteria, lactic acid bacteria, yeasts, and coliforms in the digesta from the stomach, distal small intestine, cecum, and midcolon over a period of 4 weeks after weaning (Canibe et al. 2001). The apparent antimicrobial effects were attributed to the protons and anions formed from formic acid after passing through the bacterial cell wall. These have a disruptive effect on protein synthesis and inhibit bacterial enzymes, thereby reducing bacterial replication (Partenen and Mroz 1999). Other studies agree that coliform counts in the stomach and proximal colon decrease when levels of formic acid increase (Kirchgessner et al. 1992, Gabert et al. 1995), or when potassium diformate is used (Février et al. 2001). Supplementation of weaner diet with organic acids or other salts have been shown to reduce the incidence of postweaning diarrhea and improve growth performance of piglets (Sutton et al. 1991). When the coliform inhibitory effects of various organic acids were compared, the results going from most effective to least effective were benzoic, fumaric, lactic, butyric, formic, and proprionic acid.

Feed supplemented with 2500 ppm zinc oxide has been shown to reduce postweaning diarrhea and has been widely used in commercial pig production, but the mechanism of action is unclear (Holm 1998). In a study of the effects of zinc oxide on the enteric flora, no differences were recorded between the zinc oxide–supplemented group and control group, in terms of the number of coliforms, enterococci, or *Clostridium perfrin-*

gens excreted per gram of feces. However, there was an overall reduction in the diversity of the fecal coliform flora in the zinc oxide–treated pigs. In the second week postweaning zinc oxide treated pigs showed significant increases in growth rate over controls (Melin et al. 2001). However recent European Union (EU) legislation limits the maximum permissible level of zinc inclusion in pig diets to 150 ppm in EU member states (EU regulation No 1334/2003).

Fermented Liquid Feeds

Liquid feeding can improve the feed intake, growth, feed conversion, and health of weaner piglets (Brooks et al. 1996). However, steeping feed in water promotes bacterial proliferation in the feed, which reduces the quality of the feed and presents health risks. Feeding fermented liquid feed has been used as a means of controlling enteric infections through acidification. As part of the diet for newly weaned pigs, fermented liquid feed had beneficial effects on the villus height and ratio of villus height to crypt depth in the proximal jejunum (Scholten et al. 1999), as compared with the diet without fermented liquid wheat. The mechanism is uncertain but it could have been due to a lower pH, increased levels of organic acids, and an altered microbiological status. The use of fermented liquid feed in newly weaned piglets caused a significant reduction in the coliform population in the terminal ileum, cecum, and colon compared with piglets fed dried feed (Jensen and Mikkelsen 1998; Moran et al. 2001). Feed was prepared by inoculating the diet with lactic acid bacteria (*Lactobacillus plantarum)* and steeping it for 5 days at 25°C before feeding. Fermentation prevents bacterial colonization and spoilage of the liquid diet by enteropathogens and other spoilage bacteria. The fermentation temperature is important in relation to bacterial survival. *E. coli* was eliminated more effectively at 37°C than 20°C (Beal et al. 2001). There were also strain differences in terms of *E. coli* survival in fermented liquid feed, with F4 (K88) being the most resistant to killing by fermentation than others (Beal et al. 2001). The effect of temperature has implications for the management of fermented liquid feed systems. Cold-shock proteins help *E. coli* survive at lower temperature (Phadtare et al. 1999). Preferrented diets not only lower the acidity of the diet but also reduce the soluble NSP content of the diet (Hampson et al. 2001).

Piglets showed a significant preference for freshly prepared liquid feed over fermented liquid feed when given the choice (Demeckova et al. 2001). To prevent spoilage, chlorine dioxide added at 300 ppm was found to eliminate coliforms from liquid feeds for young piglets without adversely affecting palatability or growth performance (Demeckova et al. 2001). Chlorine dioxide is a strong oxidizing and phonatizing agent with broad antimicrobial spectrum, being active against bacteria and viruses (Junli et al. 1997). Addition of chlorine dioxide to freshly prepared wet feed did not significantly alter the intake, as compared with nonsanitized freshly prepared wet feed. Chlorine dioxide is reported to kill *E. coli* through loss of permeability control of the outer bacterial cell membrane (Berg et al. 1986).

REHYDRATION OF DIARRHEIC PIGLETS

Oral rehydration fluids are used in piglets with acute diarrhea especially during outbreaks of enterotoxigenic *E. coli* (ETEC) and rotavirus infections. Studies in rats and clinical studies in children have shown that reducing the osmolality of oral rehydration solutions has beneficial effects on the course of diarrhea and the clinical outcome (Thillainayagam et al. 1998). Using an experimental pig model Kiers et al. (2001a) demonstrated that solutions with low osmolality promoted intestinal fluid absorption, although ETEC infection resulted in a decrease in net fluid absorption independent of osmolality, as compared with that of unaffected tissue.

In an experimental model mold-fermented soya bean products were found to be beneficial in maintaining fluid balance during postweaning ETEC infection through preventing fluid loss (Kiers et al. 2001b). The mechanism is uncertain. It might interfere with the attachment of *E. coli* to epithelial cells or modulate the effects of toxin in the intestine.

REGIONAL DISEASES AND PATHOLOGY OF THE DIGESTIVE SYSTEM

The Oral Cavity

There are several recognized congenital defects affecting the oral cavity. Cleft palate and palatoschisis are both multifactorial developmental abnormalities. Cleft palate in piglets has occurred with feeding poisonous plants such as poison hemlock (*Conium maculatum*) or wild tree tobacco (*Nicotiana glauca*) to sows or gilts in early pregnancy (Keeler and Crowe 1983; Panter et al. 1985). Likewise, accidental contamination of sow feed with seeds of *Crotalaria retusa* during pregnancy has resulted in palatoschisis in piglets (Hooper and Scanlan 1977). Brachygnathia superior (shortness of maxillae) is an inherited condition that is progressive and may be confused with progressive atrophic rhinitis. Hypertrophy of the tongue is a rare congenital anomaly in pigs that interfers with normal suckling behavior. Epitheliogenesis imperfecta affects gingiva and tongue and can be seen as irregular, well-demarcated red areas that are devoid of epithelial tissue.

Oral lesions arising from traumatic damage are relatively common. Gingivitis and periodontal inflammation is usually associated with poor teeth clipping technique resulting in damage to the gingival epithelium. Stomatitis and tooth root abscesses may follow. *Fusobacterium necrophorum* is a common isolate from such lesions. Pigs have a diverticulum of the pharynx in the posterior wall immediately above the esophagus. Barley awns and other fibrous materials can lodge there and penetrate the pharynx causing pharyngeal cellulitis. This is usually seen only in young pigs. Stomatitis can also be caused by irritant chemicals, such as caustic or toxic compounds, and by physical burns. Blistering and erosion of the snout epithelium can arise due to sunburn.

A number of important infectious diseases show lesions on the snout and oral tissues. These are primarily the viral vesicular diseases, including foot and mouth disease, swine vesicular disease, and vesicular stomatitis. Lesions include blanching of the epithelium, vesicles, erosions, and epithelial flaps. Sunburn and occasionally parvovirus infection can cause lesions on the snout resembling vesicular diseases. Ulcerative glossitis and stomatitis have been reported in piglets with exudative epidermitis. Piglets may also develop ulcers on the dorsum of the tongue and occasionally on the hard palate associated with *Staphylococcus hyicus* infection (Andrews 1979). Oral erosions and ulcers can also be seen in piglets with congenital swine pox. *Actinobacillus lignieresi* can cause swelling and inflammation of the tongue, with nodule and ulcer formation. Soft tissues of the pharynx and neck can also be affected. Of the parasitic infections, *Trichinella spiralis* can affect the tongue and muscles of mastication. *Gongylonema* species has been found in the mucosa of the tongue in grazing pigs where they cause mild, localized inflammation (Zinter and Migaki 1970).

The tonsils have a strategic role in immune surveillance of the oropharynx. A host of bacterial agents, including *Streptococcus suis* and Pasteurellae, are frequently carried in the tonsils. Crypt inflammation and lymphoid hyperplasia are associated with bacterial infections. Necrotizing tonsillitis occurs in Aujeszky's disease; the tonsils being the site of primary virus replication (Terpstra and Wensvoort 1988). Tonsillitis is also a feature of swine vesicular disease. Hemorrhagic necrotizing tonsillitis can occur in pigs with anthrax.

There are few reported problems concerning the salivary glands in pigs, but sialoadenitis occurs in vitamin A deficiency (Barker et al. 1993). The interlobular ducts of the salivary glands undergo squamous metaplasia leading to salivary stasis, secondary infection, and purulent inflammation. This results in pronounced swelling of salivary glands. Epithelial degeneration of salivary ducts is seen in swine vesicular disease.

The Esophagus

Conditions affecting the esophagus are uncommon but include hyperkeratosis, parakeratosis, mycotic infection, obstructions, and traumatic lesions. Hyperkeratosis and thickening of the epithelium are associated with vitamin A deficiency or chlorinated naphthalene toxicity. Parakeratosis of the esophagus occurs in pigs with cutaneous parakeratosis due to zinc deficiency. Parakeratotic thickening of the epithelium of the distal esophagus, with basal hyperplasia of the epithelium is commonly seen in pigs with ulceration of the pars esophagea of the stomach. Reflux esophagitis is recognized in some pigs with ulceration of the pars oesophagea. The gastric secretion has corrosive effects on the squamous epithelium resulting in mucosal erosion, ulceration, and inflammation.

Mycotic esophagitis caused by *Candida albicans* can occur in suckling piglets and weaners that are immunocompromised and have been given repeated antibiotic treatment or in piglets in which the mucosal flora has been significantly disrupted for some reason.

Obstruction and/or perforation of the esophagus are associated with ingestion of large objects such as stones, potatoes, apples, or corncobs. Perforation can result from ingestion of sharp objects such as fence wire or nails. Inflammation and subsequent stricture are sequelae that affect the esophagus at the site of perforation. Such conditions lead to dysphagia and distension of the esophagus cranial to the site of obstruction or stricture. Encephalitis affecting the medulla oblongata and/or the nuclei or tracts of the cranial nerves involved in swallowing (V, IX, X, XII) also results in dysphagia. Such conditions are very rare in the pig. Nematode parasites (*Gongylonema* species) occasionally occur in the esophageal mucosa leaving serpentine-shaped tracts. However, these parasites do not appear to have any adverse effects in pigs.

The Stomach

Conditions affecting the stomach are mainly physical or functional in nature, the most important being gastroesophageal ulceration affecting the pars oesophagea. The prevalence in growing and finishing pigs varies between farms but it can be high under modern conditions of pig husbandry. The majority of lesions are subclinical, and most studies indicate that mild lesions have little impact on growth or production. Severe ulceration of the pars oesophagea is associated with clinical illness and death. Pigs become anorexic, pale, with intermittent melena, and they die suddenly due to gastric hemorrhage. In such cases, ulcers are substantial lesions. The cause is unclear, but repeated studies have shown that finely ground rations and a high wheat component in the diet are significant factors. Clinically, hemorrhage from gastric ulcers should be differentiated from other causes of melena including proliferative hemorrhagic enteropathy, swine dysentery, and intestinal torsion. This condition is described in more depth in the chapter specifically relating to gastric ulceration (Chapter 54).

Gastric overdistension can occur in adult pigs especially in sows but the cause is uncertain. It is thought to be associated with excessive intake of finely ground grain and water, resulting in excessive fermentation and gaseous distension. Gastric volvulus is thought to be due to rapid intake of large quantities of feed and water followed by physical activity in a competitive group situa-

tion. Clockwise torsion is apparently most common, although torsion can occur in either direction about the long axis of the stomach. The spleen is often involved and becomes extremely enlarged due to blood engorgement (Morin et al. 1984). The stomach becomes massively distended with gas and fluid, and intense mucosal congestion develops. This condition is rapidly fatal. Gastric foreign bodies such as stones are frequently found in stomachs of outdoor sows that are maintained on stony ground. Stone chewing is a regular activity and swallowing of the stones is thought to be accidental. Large quantities of gastric stones have been recorded in some sows, limiting the capacity of feed intake and resulting in loss of body condition.

Gastric venous infarction occurs in pigs, usually in association with severe bacterial infections or toxemia. The lesion can also be seen in classical swine fever. The mucosa in the fundic area becomes reddish black in color and caseous mucosal necrosis may be evident. Thrombosis of capillaries and venules in the mucosa and submucosa with fibrin-plugging is the cause of infarction. Multifocal areas of gastric infarction have also been recorded in cases of porcine dermatitis and nephropathy syndrome (PDNS), due to fibrinoid vasculitis of capillaries. Edema of the stomach wall is a characteristic change in edema disease caused by specific strains of *E. coli*. Edema affects the submucosa, particularly on the greater curvature of the stomach. Other conditions causing gastric edema include hypoproteinemia, arsenic toxicity, and portal hypertension. In these conditions, edematous changes are less pronounced than those of "edema disease."

Gastritis in pigs is most commonly associated with ulceration of the pars oesophagea and the inflammatory sequelae affecting tissue in the cardiac zone of the stomach, as previously mentioned. Candidiasis of the pars oesophagea may occur in association with preulcerative epithelial hyperplasia and parakeratosis. Gastritis could occur due to accidental intake of toxic compounds–such as arsenic, thallium, formalin, bronopol, and phosphatic fertilizers–and by the toxic principles in bitterweed (*Hymenoxon odorata*) or the blister beetle (*Epicanta* sp.). In commercial farming, such conditions are very rare and should be easy to exclude. Mycotic gastritis is occasionally seen in piglets, usually in association with repeated use of antibiotics. Lesions present as multifocal yellowish plaques on the gastric mucosa, with intense congestion of the peripheral gastric mucosa. Fungal hyphae colonize the mucosa and invade tissue and capillaries resulting in thrombosis. Agents are usually zygomycetes such as *Rhizopus*, *Absidia* or *Mucor* species. *Aspergillus* species involvement is rare (Mahanta and Chaudhury 1985).

Parasitic gastritis is now rare in commercial pig farms. Of the parasites that can cause gastritis, *Hyostrongylus rubidus* is of most importance because it is associated with poor growth rates or loss of body condition in adult pigs. Other parasites that can cause mild gastritis in heavy infections include *Ascarops* sp., *Simondsia* sp., and *Physocephalus* sp. The parasite *Gnathostoma* sp. invades the mucosa and undergoes development within inflammatory cysts in the submucosa. In heavy infestations this parasite can cause thickening of the stomach wall.

The Intestinal Tract

Atresia ani is the most common congenital defect of the intestinal tract of pigs and it is believed to be hereditary (Norrish and Rennie 1968). It arises due to failure of perforation of the membrane separating endodermal hindgut from ectodermal anal membrane. Evident at birth, the defect can be corrected by minor surgery unless atresia of the rectum is also present. Persistent Meckel's diverticulum is a rare anomaly in which there is persistence of the omphalomesenteric duct. It presents as a tube of intestinal tissue similar to ileum that branches from the intestine to the umbilicus. Occasionally, it can be involved in abdominal catastrophes such as intestinal strangulation.

Intestinal displacement and obstruction is common in pigs, and a number of different conditions arise.

Rectal prolapse is relatively common in growing pigs and is associated with a number of factors resulting in an increase in intraabdominal pressure. These include persistent coughing, straining associated with enteritis and diarrhea, excessive huddling of pigs kept in cold conditions, pigs gorging on liquid feeding, and feeding of flatulent diets. Feeds high in zearalenone have also been associated with rectal prolapse. Some prolapses resolve spontaneously, but more commonly the tissue becomes traumatized or removed by penmates followed by scar formation as part of the healing process. This results in rectal stricture and progressive obstruction leading to marked distension of the colon (Figure 3.1). Such pigs fail to thrive and die unless corrective action is taken. Rectal stricture can also be a sequel to ulcerative proctitis of ischemic origin caused by *Salmonella enterica* Typhimurium infection. Occasionally, severe intestinal prolapse can accompany vaginal prolapse, via laceration to the vaginal fornix. Intestinal impaction and obstruction can occur in a variety of situations—for example, deaths have occurred in piglets maintained on woodshavings or other fibrous materials such as peat due to impaction of the ileum or colon with such materials (Figure 3.2). On occasions, heavy infestations of *Ascaris suum* have been found to cause small intestinal impaction in piglets. Herniation of the intestine is most commonly associated with a patent umbilicus. Small lesions are of little consequence, but large pendulous lesions become traumatized, with increased risk of intestinal strangulation within the hernia, unless the defect is corrected surgically.

Torsion of the long axis of the mesentery is a common condition in pigs and leads to rapid death. The tor-

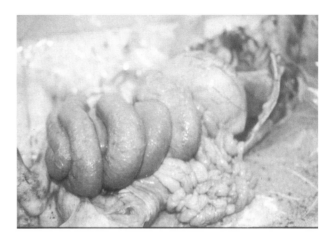

3.1. *Marked distension of the colon in a 2-month-old pig due to recto-anal stricture.*

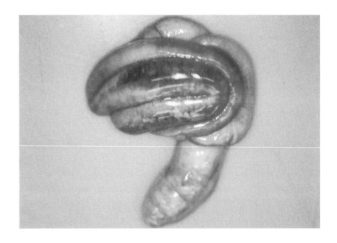

3.2. *Obstruction of the colon in a 10-day-old piglet due to impaction with wood shavings.*

sion may involve small intestine or both small and large intestine (Figure 3.3). Rotation is usually anticlockwise when viewed from the ventrocaudal aspect. Torsion is associated with pigs making sudden unpredictable movements, such as sudden deceleration combined with abrupt changes in direction, particularly when the gut is filled—for example, after feeding or drinking a large volume of water, or when the intestines are gas-filled due to pigs being on a highly fermentable ration. Once torsion occurs, pigs rapidly develop distension of the abdomen. The intestinal loops become very turgid and reddish black in color. The mesenteric vasculature is extremely engorged due to obstruction to the venous return. Other forms of intestinal catastrophe, such as volvulus of a short length of small intestine followed by strangulation of the affected portion, occur more rarely.

Many forms of inflammatory and degenerative changes can affect small and large intestine. In its simplest form, loss of surface enterocytes occurs with enteropathogenic *E. coli* and viral infections, including ro-

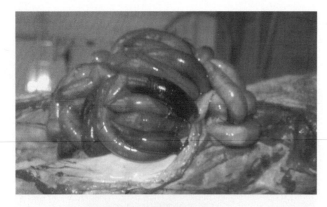

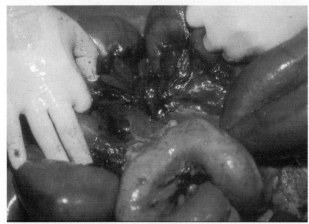

3.3. *Torsion of the small intestine around the root of the mesentery in a 5-month-old pig. Above: Distended, hemorrhagic loops of small intestine containing sanguineous fluid. Below: Root of the mesentery showing the site of the 360° torsion.*

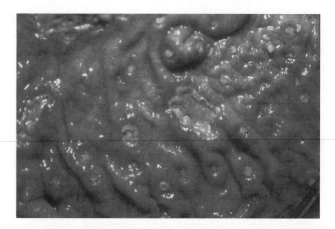

3.4. *Multifocal ulcers in the colonic mucosa of a 4-month-old pig with porcine dermatitis and nephropathy syndrome.*

tavirus and coronaviruses. Fluid exudation is a consequence of this epithelial loss and results in watery diarrhea and dehydration. Villous atrophy is particularly associated with coronavirus and rotavirus infections. Intestinal erosion and necrotizing enteritis in young pigs is often associated with *C. perfringens* type C infection. *Cryptosporidium* (*C. parvum*) infection in neonatal piglets causes villous atrophy, stunting and fusion of villi, with diarrhea due to malabsorption. Intestinal ulceration is associated with salmonellosis and ulcerative typhlocolitis, with swine dysentery. So-called "button ulcers" alert concerns of classical swine fever, but they are also associated with *Salmonella choleraesuis* infection and porcine dermatitis and nephropathy syndrome (Figure 3.4). Similar lesions have also been recorded in pigs infected with bovine viral diarrhea virus (Terpstra and Wensvoort 1988). Degeneration of intestinal crypt epithelium is associated with coccidial infection and bovine viral diarrhea virus infection. In coccidiosis due to *Isospora suis* damage caused by coccidial development in the villous and crypt epithelium will result in villous atrophy, intestinal erosions, and fibrinonecrotic enteritis, mainly affecting the distal jejunum and ileum. Hyperplasia of crypt epithelium is the major feature of

Lawsonia intracellularis infection and leads to thickening of the mucosa in the ileum and/or colon (Figure 3.5). Inflammatory cell infiltration occurs in response to any cause of disruption to the epithelial barrier as well as enteropathogenic infections. Mucosal microabscesses are a feature of yersiniosis; both *Yersinia enterocolitica* and *Y. pseudotuberculosis* affect pigs.

Diseases affecting the intestinal tract are among the most important economic problems affecting pig production. The prevalence of diseases in pigs varies between countries, farming systems and units with different health status. Within farms the disease situation is dynamic and the prevalence can alter quite dramatically between batches for no apparent reason. Multiple enteric infections can occur concurrently, giving rise to complex clinical disease patterns and difficulties in arriving at successful control measures. The major diseases are mentioned only briefly here; detailed descriptions of all are given in other chapters.

In neonatal piglets, enterotoxigenic *E. coli* remains the most important disease, with *C. perfringens* type C causing problems in certain units, most notably in outdoor farming systems (Figure 3.6). Both diseases can be controlled by vaccination of breeding stock provided piglets receive adequate colostrum intake within hours of birth, prior to intestinal "closure." The availability of breeding stock that is genetically resistant to *E. coli* F4 (K88) strains heralds a new and exciting era in the control of enteric disease through genetic selection. Other infections that are commonly reported in the young unweaned pig include rotavirus and coccidiosis (*I. suis*), with cryptosporidia also being implicated in some units. It is rare for *Salmonella* infection to cause significant enteric disease in unweaned pigs though subclinical infection, and shedding can occur as a result of contact with sow feces. The viral diseases transmissible gastroenteritis (TGE) and porcine epidemic diarrhea (PED) cause severe morbidity and mortality in susceptible piglets. Vomiting and wasting disease caused by

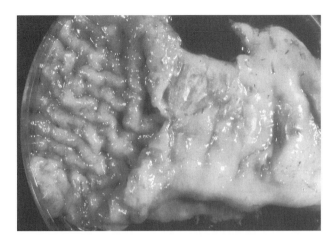

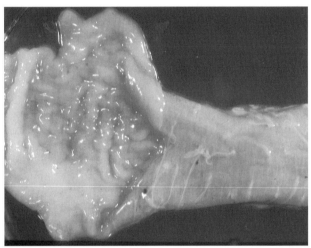

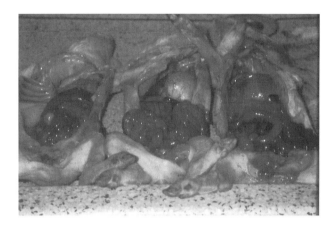

3.6. *Hemorrhagic enteritis in three 10-day-old piglets associated with* Clostridium perfringens *type C.*

3.5. *Ileum from a 2-month-old pig with porcine proliferative enteropathy (PPE) compared with that of a normal age-matched pig. Above: Ileum from a case of PPE showing thickening of the mucosa. Below: Ileum from the unaffected pig showing the normal appearance of the mucosa.*

hemagglutinating encephalomyelitis virus is associated with vomiting and wasting in suckling piglets, but it appears to have reduced in prevalence globally over the last 10–15 years. Porcine adenovirus infection is usually asymptomatic but occasionally is associated with diarrhea and vomiting, with reduced growth rates in piglets from 2–7 weeks of age. Bovine viral diarrhea virus, though a known pathogen of pigs, is rarely reported. *Clostridium difficile* is a recognized cause of necrotizing colitis in suckling piglets and it is also of zoonotic importance. However it appears to be a rare or rarely reported infection of pigs. *Strongyloides* sp. can affect pigs ranging from 10 days of age up to 3 months old. Parasites colonize the anterior half of the small intestine and cause villous atrophy and granulomatous enteritis, resulting in diarrhea and ill thrift.

A number of these preweaning infections are also capable of causing disease in young weaners. Postweaning *E. coli* continues to be a major cause of postweaning diarrhea and mortality, and diseases such as rotavirus, coccidiosis, and cryptosporidiosis can rarely affect

piglets up to 6 weeks of age. The disease patterns in units change dramatically when immunosuppression is a feature. The emergence of postweaning multisystemic wasting syndrome (PMWS), which has occurred in many countries, has dramatically altered patterns of enteric disease. The generalized lymphoid depletion that occurs in weaners with PMWS includes depletion of intestinal Peyer's patches and mesenteric lymph nodes. In units with PMWS, the age range of susceptibility to diseases such as rotavirus, cryptosporidiosis, and coccidiosis increases up to 4–6 weeks, and these enteric diseases play a significant role in the general ill-thrift problems suffered by pigs.

Diarrhea is a feature of PMWS outbreaks and in many instances no enteropathogenic agents are isolated or detected. Histologically the jejunum and ileum may show a viral-type enteropathy, primarily villous atrophy. Whether this is directly related to the disease pathogenesis or whether it is caused by one or more opportunist viruses that are unrecognized as yet remains unknown. Another equally important feature associated with PMWS is mild bacterial-type colitis. Often bacterial cultures fail to show any recognized bacterial pathogen but yield a mixed growth of commensal-type organisms. Histology of the colon shows mixed bacterial infection of crypts and surface epithelium, accompanied by crypt inflammation and goblet cell hyperplasia in chronic cases. This suggests that there is an opportunistic bacterial overgrowth or dysbacteriosis in the colon of affected pigs, possibly associated with altered enteric immune processes.

Through growing and finishing periods the most important economic-limiting diseases continue to be swine dysentery, porcine proliferative enteropathy (PPE), and porcine colonic spirochetosis. In PPE, significant progress has been made with the development of serological tests that can be used for herd profiling and more recently, development of an orally administered vaccine that has proved successful in controlling PPE in commercial units. In contrast, there are no commer-

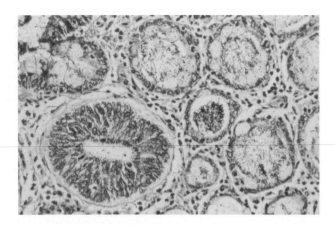

3.7. Colitis in a 10-week-old pig associated with combined Brachyspira pilosicoli *and* Lawsonia intracellularis *infections. Most crypts contain spirochaetes* (S. pilosicoli) *and have normal height of crypt epithelium. One crypt shows hyperplasia of epithelial cells with intracellular curved bacteria* (L. intracellularis) *at the apical pole of the cells.*

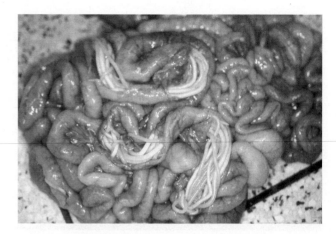

3.8. Small intestine of a 7-week-old piglet heavily infested with Ascaris suum.

cially available serological tests for swine dysentery or porcine colonic spirochetosis, and to date, vaccine studies have proved unsuccessful. The prevalence of *Brachyspira pilosicoli* varies between countries. This infection is becoming increasingly recognized as a cause of diarrhea and reduced growth rates. The infection may also be mild or subclinical. Mixed infections involving *Brachyspira hyodysenteriae, Brachyspira pilosicoli, L. intracellularis, Salmonella* sp., and *Yersinia* sp. are common in grow-finish herds with diarrhea and colitis (Figure 3.7). Achieving the correct diagnosis and finding effective control measures pose significant challenges for the swine veterinarian.

The prevalence of parasitic infections varies considerably between units. Many units have achieved total freedom of enteric parasites, such as *Ascaris suum, Oesophagostomum* sp., *Trichuris* sp., and *Hyostrongylus* sp. However "white spot liver" is commonly reported on abattoir surveys indicating that *A. suum* infection is still a notable health problem in some units (Figure 3.8). *Trichuris suis* and *Oesophagostomum* sp. can be causes of colitis that are often overlooked until nonresponse to antibiotic agents results in further investigation. Rarely, coccidiosis *(I. suis)* can cause acute enteritis and colitis in naive young adult pigs that are introduced into a heavily infected environment. Similarly, the hemorrhagic enteropathy form of PPE can cause acute hemorrhagic diarrhea and deaths in naive young adult pigs introduced into an infected environment. *Eimeria* sp. affect older pigs when exposed to yards and pasture contaminated with oocysts. Some *Eimeria* sp. are considered to be potentially pathogenic, causing villous atrophy and enteritis. *Balantidium coli* is commonly present in the large intestine of pigs. It is a commensal organism but commonly invades the mucosa if other degenerative or necrotizing lesions are present.

In addition to the common endemic diseases already mentioned, the serious epidemic diseases classical swine fever (CSF) and African swine fever (ASF) have an important enteric component. Suspected outbreaks should be reported and investigated appropriately in order to control the outbreak and limit the spread of infection. TGE and PED can cause severe diarrhea in all age groups of pigs in addition to the serious morbidity and mortality that occur in suckling piglets in particular. In Aujeszky's disease, necrotizing enteritis can affect the distal small intestine in addition to the more commonly recognized lesions of necrotizing rhinitis and tonsillitis. Control of TGE, CSF, ASF, and Aujeszky's disease by vaccination is the best method of control in some countries where disease eradication is not possible due to geographic, social, or political reasons or where there is a constant and uncontrollable threat from wildlife vectors.

The Liver

Congenital anomalies affecting the pig liver are rare. One recognized condition is a cystic anomaly affecting bile ducts. The liver is enlarged and shows numerous fluctuating cystic lesions containing bile. The enlarged liver causes abdominal distension and piglets have poor viability.

Traumatic conditions affecting the liver are important. In neonatal piglets, rupture of the liver and fatal hemorrhage is a consequence of trauma, usually inflicted accidentally by the sow. Torsion of one or more liver lobes can affect pigs of any age. It usually affects the left lateral lobe and results in infarction of the lobe. Death occurs due to shock or hepatic rupture and hemorrhage. Hepatosis dietetica is a diet-associated condition in which there is massive hepatic necrosis. Experimentally, concurrent deficiencies of sulphur-containing amino acids, tocopherols, and selenium are required for development of hepatosis dietetica. The pathogenesis is not fully understood but it is thought to be associated with formation of free radicals and their subsequent

Table 3.1. Differential diagnosis of some common enteric diseases of swine.

Cause	Age	Signs	Gross Lesions	Histological Lesions	Laboratory Confirmation—Commonly Used Methods
Escherichia coli (ETEC, EPEC)	Neonatal: 1–4 days old. Postweaning: 1–3 weeks after weaning.	Watery, yellowish diarrhea. Sudden death. Dehydration.	Fluid ingesta, small intestinal congestion, watery content. Stomach usually full of milk.	Mucosal congestion, edema. Bacterial attachment to intestinal epithelium.	Culture, serotype of isolates, PCR. Tissue IHC.
Rotavirus	1 day to 7 weeks old. Most frequent at 2–3 weeks of age.	Watery to pasty diarrhea, may be subclinical. Varying degrees of dehydration.	Fluid ingesta, pale intestines. Sparse stomach contents.	Moderate villous atrophy.	Virus detection: PAGE, PCR, ELISA detection kits. Tissue IHC.
Clostridium perfringens type C	1–14 days (rarely older).	Hemorrhagic/watery diarrhea. Sudden death.	Hemorrhagic intestines, mucosal necrosis.	Mucosal necrosis, hemorrhage. Gram-positive rods associated with lesions.	*C. perfringens* toxin ELISAs on intestinal content. Histopathology.
Cryptosporidium sp.	3 days to weaning.	Mild to moderate yellowish diarrhea. Varying degrees of dehydration.	Fluid ingesta.	None or mild villous atrophy. Cryptosporidial oocysts adjacent to surface epithelium.	Mucosal smear for cryptosporidial oocysts. Histopathology.
Isospora suis	5–21 days (occasionally older).	Watery/yellowish diarrhea. Dehydration.	Fluid ingesta, necrosis of small intestine mucosa.	Villous atrophy, fibrinonecrotic enteritis, intracellular coccidial forms.	Stained mucosal smear for coccidial oocysts. Histopathology: lesions and coccidia, identify coccidia.
Coronaviruses: TGE virus PED virus	All ages.	Watery diarrhea. Rapid dehydration. Vomiting often seen.	Thin-walled pale intestine, sparse content.	Severe villous atrophy.	Virus detection by PCR of gut content, IHC, ISH, or IF of intestinal tissue. Antibody detection by serology.
Lawsonia intracellularis	From approximately 5 weeks old to young adults.	Usually pasty to sloppy diarrhea. In PHE watery hemorrhagic (port wine colored) diarrhea, pale carcass, weakness, ataxia.	Ileitis and/or colitis. Thickened mucosa, sometimes necrotic or ulcerated. In PHE, blood clots in ileum and/or colon, carcass pale.	Crypt epithelial hyperplasia, crypt abscesses. Small curved rods in hyperplastic epithelial cells (silver stain). In PHE, blood exudation into crypts through intact epithelium.	Bacterial detection by PCR on feces or intestinal mucosa. Histopathology, IF, IHC, ISH on tissue. Antibody detection by serology.
Brachyspira hyodysenteriae	From approximately 6 weeks old to adult.	Pasty, sloppy diarrhea, may be mucohemorrhagic. Lethargy.	Typhlo-colitis, fibrinous pseudomembranes, exudation, erosions, ulceration, hemorrhage. Mucoid content in chronic cases.	Epithelial erosions, goblet-cell hyperplasia, inflammation, fibrin exudation, hyperplasia crypts with mucus. Large spirochetes present (silver stain).	Bacterial detection by PCR, culture of feces or tissue. Histopathology, IHC, ISH of tissue.
Brachyspira pilosicoli	From approximately 6 weeks to 4 months old.	Pasty, sloppy diarrhea.	Mild to moderate colitis. Lesions milder than *B. hyodysenteriae*.	Similar to *B. hyodysenteriae* but milder. End-on attachment of spirochetes to surface epithelium seen in some cases.	Bacterial detection by PCR, culture of feces or tissue. Histopathology, IHC, ISH of tissue.

(continued)

49

Table 3.1. Differential diagnosis of some common enteric diseases of swine (*continued*).

Cause	Age	Signs	Gross Lesions	Histological Lesions	Laboratory Confirmation— Commonly Used Methods
Salmonella sp.	All ages after weaning (rarely preweaning).	Variable, watery mucohemorrhagic. Most infections subclinical.	Fibrinous or hemorrhagic, ulcers, lesions in small and/or large intestine.	Diffuse or focal ulcers, neutrophil infiltration, fibrinous thrombi.	Bacterial detection by culture, serotype, phage type. Antibody detection by mix-ELISA.
Oesophagostomum dentatum	From weaning to adult.	Mild, sloppy diarrhea.	Erosions, edema, granulomas in cecum and proximal colon.	Granulomatous typhlocolitis with nematode parasites.	Fecal parasitology, histopathology.
Trichuris suis	From weaning to adult.	Pasty, sloppy occasionally mucohemorrhagic.	Typhlo-colitis, erosions, parasites visible to naked eye.	Erosion/ulceration and inflammation associated with nematode parasites.	Fecal parasitology, gross pathology.
Yersinia sp.	From approximately 6 weeks to 4 months old.	Pasty, sloppy diarrhea.	Mild enteritis and/or colitis.	Mild chronic, active enteritis and/or colitis, microabscesses, granulomas.	Bacterial detection by culture.

EPEC = enteropathogenic *E. coli*; ETEC = enterotoxigenic *E. coli*; IF = immunofluorescence; IHC = immunohistochemistry; ISH = in situ hybridization; PAGE = polyacrylamide gel electrophoresis; PCR = polymerase chain reaction test; PED = porcine epidemic diarrhea; PHE = proliferative hemorrhagic enteropathy; TGE = transmissible gastroenteritis.

adverse effects. It affects rapidly growing pigs and causes sudden death.

Many systemic diseases cause nonspecific changes in the liver, including congestion and inflammatory cell infiltration. Hemorrhages are a feature of septicemia, for example, salmonellosis, especially *S. choleraesuis* infection. Multifocal white nodules, so-called "paratyphoid nodules," are associated with chronic *S. choleraesuis* infection. Parasitism is undoubtedly the most common condition affecting the liver. Migrating *Ascaris suum* larvae cause mechanical damage in the form of hemorrhagic tracts that initiate intense inflammation. Reactive changes, both repair of tissue and hypersensitivity reaction to excretory and secretory products of larvae, cause eosinophil infiltration and fibrosis. "White spot" livers are an economic loss to the farmer (Figure 3.9). In heavy infestations, adult ascarids can migrate up the bile duct or pancreatic duct causing obstruction, jaundice, and cholangitis (Figure 3.10). Other parasitic infections affecting the liver include *Cysticercus tenicollis*, the metacestode of the tapeworm *Taenia hydatigena* (of dogs). Cysts can sometimes be found in the pig peritoneal cavity, often attached to the liver. Immature cysticerci migrate through the liver causing tortuous hemorrhagic tracts before emerging to encyst. *Stephanurus dentatus* infection results in migratory tracts and hepatitis. Portal phlebitis with thrombus formation in the portal vein are additional features following oral infection.

Toxicities affecting the liver can be acute or chronic in nature. Cresol toxicity is caused by exposure to tar compounds that might have been used in construction of piggery buildings, accidental environmental spillage, or "clay pigeons" used as shooting targets. Lesions include severe hepatocellular necrosis leading to sudden death. Chronic cresol toxicity results in jaundice, ascites, and anemia on account of chronic, progressive destruction of hepatic tissue. Iron toxicity occurs occasionally in neonatal piglets, with deaths occurring within 24 hours of iron-dextran administration. Toxicity is associated with marginal or deficient vitamin E and selenium status. Iron-catalyzed lipoperoxidation occurs in liver and muscle resulting in hepatic necrosis and hepatic hemorrhages. Aflatoxicosis is caused by the use of cereals contaminated with *Aspergillus* species or *Penicillium puberulum*. Lesion development is a chronic process in which there is liver hypertrophy and progressive fibrosis. The condition results in reduced growth rates and liver condemnations.

The Pancreas

There has been little focus on pancreatic conditions in pigs. Pancreatic hypoplasia is rare and associated with poor growth in individual weaner pigs. The pancreatic duct can be invaded by *Ascaris suum* in piglets with heavy infestations. This can lead to obstruction of the pancreatic duct resulting in pancreatic necrosis and acute pancreatitis.

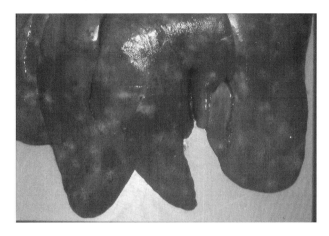

3.9. *"White spot" liver in a 5-month-old pig, associated with* Ascaris suum *larval migration.*

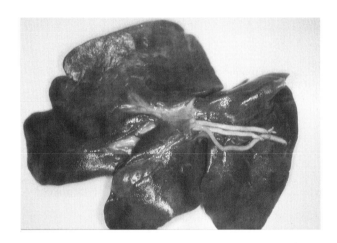

3.10. *Ascaris suum in the common bile duct of a 6-week-old piglet that was heavily infested.*

REFERENCES

Accioly JM, Durmic Z, McDonald DE, Oxberry SL, Pethick DW, Mullan BP, Hampson D.J. 1998. Dietary effects on the presence of ulcers and urease-producing organisms in the stomach of weaner pigs. In Proc 15th Int Pig Vet Soc Congr, vol 3, p. 242.

Anderson DB, McCracken VJ, Aminov RI, Simpson JM, Mackie RI, Verstegen MWA, Gaskins HR. 1999. Gut microbiology and the mechanisms of action of growth-promoting antibiotics in swine. Pig News Info 20:115–122.

Andrews JJ 1979. Ulcerative glossitis and stomatitis associated with exudative epidermitis in suckling swine. Vet Pathol 16:432–437.

Asplund K, Hakkinen M, Bjorkroth J, Nuotio L, Nurmi E. 1996. Inhibition of the growth of *Yersinia enterocolitica* 0:3 by the microflora of the porcine caecum and ileum in an in vitro model. J Appl Bacteriol 81:217–222.

Ayles HL, Friendship RM, Ball RO. 1996. Effects of dietary particle size on gastric ulcers, assessed by endoscopic examination, and relationship between ulcer severity and growth performance of individually fed pigs. J Swine Health Prod 4:211–216.

Bach Knudsen KE, Canibe N. 2000. Breakdown of plant carbohydrates in the digestive tract of pigs fed on wheat or oat based rolls. J Sci Food Agric 80:1253–1261.

Bach Knudsen KE, Jørgensen H. 2001. Intestinal degradation of dietary carbohydrates—From birth to maturity. In Digestive

Physiology of Pigs. JE Lindberg, B Ogle, eds. Wallingford, UK: CAB International, pp. 109–120.

Bach Knudsen KE, Jensen BB, Andersen JO, Hansen I. 1991. Gastrointestinal implications in pigs of wheat and oat fractions. 2. Microbial activity in the gastrointestinal tract. Br J Nutr 65:233–248.

Bach Knudsen KE, Jensen BB, Hansen I. 1993. Oat bran but not a beta-glucan-enriched oat fraction enhances butyrate production in the large intestine of pigs. J Nutr 123:1235–1247.

Bailey M, Miller BG, Telemo E, Stokes CR, Bourne FJ. 1993. Specific immunological unresponsiveness following active primary to proteins in the weaning diets of piglets. Int Archiv Allergy Immunol 101:266–271

Baintner K. 1986. Intestinal Absorption of Macromolecules and Immune Transmission from Mother to Young. Boca Raton, FL: CRC Press, pp. 1–216.

Barbosa AJA, Silva JCP, Nogueira AMMF, Paulino E. Jr, Miranda CR. 1995. Higher incidence of *Gastropirillium* sp. in swine with gastric ulcers of the *pars oesophagea*. Vet Pathol 32:134–139.

Barker IK, Van Dreumel AA, Palmer N. 1993. The alimentary system. In Jubb KVF, Kennedy PC, Palmer N (eds.). Pathology of Domestic Animals (4th ed), Volume 2. London: Academic Press Inc., p. 32.

Beal JD, Moran CA, Campbell A, Brooks PH. 2001. The survival of potentially pathogenic *E. coli* in fermented liquid feed. In Digestive Physiology of Pigs. JE Lindberg, B Ogle, eds. Wallingford, UK: CAB International, pp. 351–353.

Berends BR, Urlings HAP, Snijders JMA, Van Knapen F. 1996. Identification and quantification of risk factors in animal management and transport regarding *Salmonella* spp. in pigs. Int J Food Microbiol 30:37–53.

Berg JD, Roberts PV, Matin A. 1986. Effect of chlorine dioxide on selected membrane funtions of *Escherichia coli*. J Appl Bacteriol 60:213–220.

Berg RD. 1999. Bacterial translocation from the gastrointestinal tract. Adv Exp Med Biol 473:11–30.

Bertschinger HU, Eggenberger E, Jucker H, Pfirter HP. 1978. Evaluation of low nutrient, high fibre diets for the prevention of porcine *Eschericia coli* enterotoxemia. Vet Microbiol 3:281–290.

Biernat M, Gacsalyi U, Rådberg K, Zabielski R, Weström B, Pierzynowski SG. 2001. Effect of kidney bean lectin on gut morphology. A way to accelerate mucosa development. In Digestive Physiology of Pigs. JE Lindberg, B Ogle, eds. Wallingford, UK: CAB International, pp. 46–48.

Bolduan G, Jung H, Schnabel E, Schneider R. 1988. Recent advances in the nutrition of weaner piglets. Pig News Info 9:381–385.

Brooks PH, Geary TM, Morgan DT, Campbell A. 1996. New development in liquid feeding. Pig J 36:43–64.

Brown PJ, Bourne FJ. 1976. Distribution of immunoglobulin staining cells in alimentary tract, spleen and mesenteric lymph node of the pig. Am J Vet Res 37:9–13.

Brunsgaard G. 1998. Effects of cereal type and feed particle size on morphological characteristics, ephithelial cell proliferation, and lectin binding patterns in the large intestine of pigs. J Anim Sci 76:2787–2798.

Burrin DG, Stoll B, Jiang R, Chang X, Hartmann B, Holst JJ, Greeley GH, Reeds PlJ. 2000. Minimal enteral nutrient requirements for neonatal intestinal growth in piglets: How much is enough? Am J Clin Nutr 71:1603–1610.

Burrin DG, Stoll B, van Goudoever JB, Reeds PJ. 2001. Nutrient requirements of intestinal growth and metabolism in the developing pig. In Digestive Physiology of Pigs. JE Lindberg, B Ogle, eds. Wallingford, UK: CAB International, pp. 75–88.

Cameron BF, Wong CW, Hinch GN, Singh D, Nolan JV, Colditz IG. 2001. Effects of nucleotides on the immune function of early-weaned piglets. In Digestive Physiology of Pigs. JE Lindberg, B Ogle, eds. Wallingford, UK: CAB International, pp. 66–68.

Canibe N, Steien SH, Øverland M, Jensen BB. 2001. Effect of formi—LHS on digesta and faecal microbiota, and on stomach alterations of piglets. In Digestive Physiology of Pigs. JE Lindberg, B Ogle, eds. Wallingford, UK: CAB International, pp. 288–290.

Cera KR, Mahan DC, Cross RF, Reinhart GA, Whitmoyer RE 1988. Effect of age, weaning and postweaning diet on small intestinal growth and jejunal morphology in young swine. J Anim Sci 66:574–584.

Cohen IT, Nelson SD, Modley RA, Hirsh MP, Counihan TC, Martin RF 1991. Necrotizing enterocolitis in a neonatal piglet model. J Pediatric Surg 26:598–601.

Commission on Antimicrobial Feed Additives. 1997. Anti microbial feed additives. Government Official reports, SOU 1997:132, Ministry of Agriculture, Stockholm, Sweden.

Demeckova V, Moran CA, Caveney C, Campbell AC, Kuri V, Brooks PH. 2001. The effect of fermentation and/or sanitization of liquid diets on the feeding preferences of newly weaned pigs. In Digestive Physiology of Pigs. JE Lindberg, B Ogle, eds. Wallingford, UK: CAB International, pp. 291–293.

den Hond E, Hiele M, Peeters M, Ghoos Y, Rutgeerts P. 1999. Effect of long-term oral glutamine supplements on small intestinal permeability in patients with Crohn's disease. J Parenteral Enteral Nutr 23:7–11.

Duncan SH, Flint HJ, Stewart CS. 1998. Inhibitory activity of gut bacteria against *Escherichia coli* O157 mediated by dietary plant metabolites. FEMS Microbiology Letters 164:283–288.

Durmic Z. 2000. Evaluation of dietary fibre as a contributory factor in the development of swine dysentery. PhD thesis, Murdoch University, Murdoch, Western Australia.

Durmic Z, Pethick DW, Mullan BP, Schulze H, Accioly J, Hampson DJ. 2000. Extrusion of wheat or sorghum and/or addition of exogenous enzymes to pig diets influences the large intestinal microbiota but does not prevent swine dysentery following experimental infection. J Appl Microbiol 89:678–686.

Ebner S, Schoknecht P, Reeds PJ, Burrin DG. 1994. Growth and metabolism of gastrointestinal and skeletal muscle tissues in protein-malnourished neonatal pigs. Am J Physiol 266:R1736–R1743.

English PR. 1981. Establishing the early weaned pig. In Proc 7th Int Pig Vet Soc Congr, pp. 29–37.

Février C, Gotterbarm G, Jaguelin-Peyraud Y, Lebreton Y, Legouevec F, Aumaître A. 2001. Effects of adding potassium diformate and phytase excess for weaned piglets. In Digestive Physiology of Pigs. JE Lindberg, B Ogle, eds. Wallingford, UK: CAB International, pp. 192–194.

Fricker CR, Park RWA. 1989. A two-year study of the distribution of "thermophilic" campylobacters in human, environmental and food samples from the Reading area with particular reference to toxin production and heat-stable serotype. J Appl Bacteriol 66:477–490.

Friendship RM. 1999. Gastric ulcers. In Diseases of Swine (8th edition). BE Straw, WL Mengeling, S D'Allaire, DJ Taylor, eds. Oxford, UK: Blackwell Scientific Publications, pp. 685–694.

Gabert VM, Sauer WC, Schmitz M, Ahren F, Mosenthin R. 1995. The effect of formic acid and buffering capacity on the ileal digestibilities of amino acids and bacterial populations and metabolites in the small intestine of weanling pigs fed semipurified fish meal diets. Can J Anim Sci 75:615–623.

Gebert A, Rothkotter HJ, Pabst R. 1994. Cytokeratin-18 is an M-cell marker in porcine Peyers-patches. Cell Tissue Res 276:213–221.

Gibson GR, Roberfroid M 1995. Dietary modulation of the human colonic microbiota—Introducing the concept of prebiotics. J Nutr 125:1401–1412.

Giusi-Perier A, Fiszlelewicz M, Rérat A. 1989. Influence of diet composition on intestinal volatile fatty acids and nutrient absorption in unanesthetized pigs. J Anim Sci 67:386–402.

Glitsø LV, Brunsgaard G, Højsgaard S, Sandström B, Bach Knudsen KE. 1998. Intestinal degradation in pigs of rye dietary fibre with different structural characteristics. Br J Nutr 80:457–468.

Graham TE, Sgro V, Friars D, Gibala MJ. 2000. Glutamine ingestion: The plasma and muscle free amino acid pools of resting humans. Am J Physiol Endocrinol Metabolism 278:E83–E89.

Hampson DJ. 1986. Alterations in piglet small intestinal structure at weaning. Res Vet Sci 40:32–40.

Hampson J, Kidder DE. 1986. Influence of creep feeding and weaning on brush border enzyme activities in the piglet small intestine. Res Vet Sci 40:24–31.

Hampson DJ, Robertson ID, La T, Oxberry SL, Pethick DW. 2000. Influences of diet and vaccination on colonisation of pigs with the intestinal spirochaete *Brachyspira (Serpulina) pilosicoli*. Vet Microbiol 73:75–84.

Hampson DJ, Pluske JR, Pethick DW. 2001. Dietary manipulation of enteric disease. In Digestive Physiology of Pigs. JE Lindberg, B Ogle, eds. Wallingford, UK: CAB International, pp. 247–261.

Harvey RB, Anderson RC, Droleskey RE, Genovese KJ, Egan LF, Nisbet DJ. 2001. Reduced *Campylobacter* prevalence in piglets reared in specialized nurseries. In Digestive Physiology of Pigs. JE Lindberg, B Ogle, eds. Wallingford, UK: CAB International, pp. 311–313.

Harvey RB, Young CR, Ziprin RL, Hume ME, Genovese KJ, Anderson RC, Droleskey RE, Stanker LH, Nisbet DJ. 1999. Prevalence of *campylobacter* sp. isolated from the intestinal tract of pigs raised in an integrated swine production system. J Am Vet Med Assoc 215:1601–1604.

Hazzledine M, Partridge GG. 1996. Enzymes in animal feeds—Application, technology and effectiveness. Proc 12th Annu Carolina Swine Nutrition Conf. pp. 12–33.

Högberg A, Melin L, Mattsson S, Lindberg JE, Wallgren P. 2001. Comparison between the ileocaecal and rectal microflora in pigs. In Digestive Physiology of Pigs. JE Lindberg, B Ogle, eds. Wallingford, UK: CAB International, pp. 296–299.

Holm A. 1998. *Escherichia coli*-associated postweaning diarrhea in piglets. Zinc oxide added to feed as an antibacterial agent? Dansk Veterinaertidsskrift 71:1118–1126.

Hooper PT, Scanlan WA. 1977. *Crotalaria retusa* poisoning of pigs and poultry. Aust Vet J 53:109–114.

Houdijk J. 1998. Effects of non-digestible oligosaccharides in young pig diets. PhD thesis, Wageningen Agricultural University, Wageningen, The Netherlands.

Jensen BB, Jørgensen H. 1994. Effect of dietary fibre on microbial activity and microbial gas production in various regions of the gastrointestinal tract of pigs. Appl Environ Microbiol 60:1897–1904.

Jensen BB, Mikkelsen LL. 1998. Feeding liquid diets to pigs. In Garnsworthy PC, Wiseman J (eds.). Recent advances in animal nutrition. Nottingham, UK: Nottingham University Press. pp. 107–126.

Johnson RW. 1997. Inhibition of growth by pro-inflammatory cytokines: An integrated view. J Anim Sci 75:1244–1255.

Junli H, Li W, Nenqi RLX, Fun SR, Guanle Y. 1997. Disinfection effect of chlorine dioxide on viruses, algae and animal planktons in water. Water Res 31:455–460.

Keeler RF, Crowe RW. 1983. Congenital deformities in swine induced by wild tree tobacco (*Nicotiana glauca*). Clin Toxicol 20:49–58.

Kelly D. 1990. Effect of creep feeding on structural and functional changes of the gut of early weaned pigs. Res Vet Sci 48:250–356.

Kelly D, Coutts APG. 1997. Biologically active peptides in colostrum and milk. In Digestive Physiology of Pigs. JP Laplace, C Février, A Barbeau, eds. Proc 7th Int Symp INRA-SRP and EEAP, St-Malo, France, pp. 163–170.

Kelly D, Smyth JA, McCracken KJ. 1991. Digestive development in the early weaned pig. 11. Effect of level of food intake on digestive enzyme activity during the immediate postweaning period. Br J Nutr 6:181–188.

Kenworthy R. 1976. Observations on the effects of weaning in the young pig. Clinical and histopathological studies of intestinal function and morphology. Res Vet Sci 21:69–75.

Kiers JL, Nout MRJ, Rombouts FM, Nabuurs MJA, van der Meulen J. 2001a. Net absorption of fluid in uninfected and ETEC-infected piglet small intestine: Effect of osmolality. In Digestive Physiology of Pigs. JE Lindberg, B Ogle, eds. Wallingford, UK: CAB International, pp. 277–279.

——. 2001b. Protective effect of processed soybean during perfusion of ETEC-infected small intestinal segments of early-weaned piglets. In Digestive Physiology of Pigs. JE Lindberg, B Ogle, eds. Wallingford, UK: CAB International, pp. 261–263.

Kirchgessner M, Gedek B, Wiehler S, Bott A, Eidelsburger U, Roth FX. 1992. Influence of formic acid, calcium formate and sodiumhydrogen-carbonate on the microflora in different segments of the gastrointestinal tract. J Anim Physiol Anim Nutr 68:73–81.

Kirkwood RN, Huang SX, McFall M, Aherne FX. 2000. Dietary factors do not influence the clinical expression of swine dysentery. J Swine Health Prod 8:73–76.

Kleingebbink GAR, Sutton AL, Williams BA, Patterson JA, Richert BT, Kelly DT, Vertegen MWA. 2001. Effects of oligosaccharides in weanling pig diets on performance, microflora and intestinal health. In Digestive Physiology of Pigs. JE Lindberg, B Ogle, eds. Wallingford, UK: CAB International, pp. 269–271.

Krakowa S, Eaton KA, Rings DM, Argenzio RA. 1998. Production of gastrooesophageal erosions and ulcers (GEU) in gnotobiotic swine monoinfected with fermentative commensal bacteria and fed high-carbohydrate diet. Vet Pathol 35:274–282.

Lawlor PG, Flood C, Fitzpatrick E, Lynch PB, Caffrey PJ, Brophy PO. 2001. The effect of weaning diet on the intestinal morphology of young piglets. In Digestive Physiology of Pigs. JE Lindberg, B Ogle, eds. Wallingford, UK: CAB International, pp. 54–56.

Lax AJ, Barrow PA, Jones PW, Wallis TS. 1995. Current perspectives in salmonellosis. Br Vet J 151:351–377.

Lindecrona RH, Jensen TK, Jensen BB, Leser TD, Moller K. 2003. The influence of diet on the development of swine dysentery. Anim Sci 76:81–87.

Lindecrona RH, Jensen TK, Moller K. 2004. Influence of diet on the experimental infection of pigs with *Brachyspira pilosicoli*. Vet Rec 154:264–267.

Longland AC, Low AG, Quelch DB, Bray SP. 1993. Adaptation to the digestion of non-starch polysaccharide in growing pigs fed on cereal or semi-purified basal diets. Br J Nutr 70:557–566.

Mack DR, Michail S, Wie S, McDougall L, Hollingsworth MA. 1999. Probiotics inhibit enteropathogenic E.coli adherence in vitro by inducing intestinal mucin gene expression. Am J Physiol 276:G941–G950.

MacRae JC. 1993. Metabolic consequences of intestinal parasitism. Proceedings of the Nutr Soc 52:121–130.

Mahanta S, Chaudhury B. 1985. Prevalence, pathology and isolation studies on phycomycotic gastric ulcer in neonatal piglets. Sabouraudia: J Vet Med Mycol 23:395–397.

Makkink CA, Negulescu GP, Guixin Q, Verstegen MWA. 1994. Effect of dietary protein source on feed intake, growth, pancreatic enzyme activities and jejunal morphology in newly weaned piglets. Br J Nutr 72:353–368.

Mathews CJ, MacLeod RJ, Zheng SX, Hanrahan JW, Bennett HP, Hamilton JR. 1999. Characterization of the inhibitory effect of boiled rice on intestinal chloride secretion in guinea pig crypt cells. Gastroenterology 116:1342–1347.

McCracken BA, Gaskins HR, Ruwe-Kaiser PJ, Klasing KC, Jewell DE. 1995. Diet-dependent and diet-independent metabolic responses underlie growth stasis of pigs at weaning. J Nutr 125:2838–2845.

McCracken BA, Spurlock ME, Roos MA, Zuckermann FA, Gaskins HR. 1999. Weaning anorexia may contribute to local inflammation in the piglet small intestine. J Nutr 129:613–619.

McDonald DE, Pethick DW, Mullan BP, Pluske JR, Hampson DJ. 2001. Soluble non-starch polysaccharides from pearl barley exacerbate experimental postweaning colibacillosis. In Digestive

Physiology of Pigs. JE Lindberg, B Ogle, eds. Wallingford, UK: CAB International, pp. 280–282.

McDonald DE, Pluske JR, Pethick DW, Hampson DJ. 1997. Interactions of dietary nonstarch polysaccharides with weaner pig growth and post weaning colibacillosis. In Manipulating Pig Production VI. PD Cranwell, ed. Werribee, Australia: Australasian Pig Science Association, p. 179.

McDonald DE, Pethick DW, Pluske JR, Hampson DJ. 1999. Adverse effects of soluble nonstarch polysaccharide (guar gum) on piglet growth and colibacillosis immediately after weaning. Res Vet Sci 67:245–250.

McDonald P, Edwards RA, Greenhalg JED, Morgan CA. 2002. Food additives. In Animal Nutrition (6th ed). Harlow, Essex: Pearson Education Ltd, pp. 616–629.

Melin L, Katouli M, Jensen-Waern M, Wallgren P. 2001. Influence of zinc oxide on faecal coliforms of piglets at weaning. In Digestive Physiology of Pigs. JE Lindberg, B Ogle, eds. Wallingford, UK: CAB International, pp. 294–296.

Mikkelsen LL, Jensen BB. 2001. Bifidobacteria in piglets. In Lindberg JE, Ogle B (eds.). Digestive Physiology of Pigs. CAB International, Wallingford, UK. pp. 285–288.

Moore WEC, Moore LVH, Cato EP, Wilkins TD, Kornegay ET. 1987. Effect of high-fiber and high-oil diets on the fecal flora of swine. Appl Environ Microbiol 53:1638–1644.

Moran CA, Ward G, Beal JD, Campbell A, Brooks PH, Miller BG. 2001. Influence of liquid feed, fermented liquid feed, dry feed and sow's milk fed *ad libitum*, on the "ecophysiology" of the terminal ileum, caecum and colon of the postweaned piglet. In Digestive Physiology of Pigs. JE Lindberg, B Ogle, eds. Wallingford, UK: CAB International, pp. 266–268.

Morin M, Sauvageau R, Phaneuf JB, Teuscher E, Beauregard M, Lagacé A. 1984. Torsion of abdominal organs in sows. A report of 36 cases. Can Vet J 25:440–442.

Nemcová R, Bomba A, Gancarciková S, Herich R, Guba P. 1999. Study of the effect of *Lactobacillus paracasei* and fructooligosaccharides on the faecal microflora in weaning piglets. Berl Münch Tierärztl Wochenschr 112:225–228.

Norrish JG, Rennie JC. 1968. Observations on the inheritance of atresia ani in swine. J Heredity 59:186–187.

Panter KE, Keeler RF, Buck WB. 1985. Induction of cleft palate in newborn pigs by maternal ingestion of poison hemlock (*Conium maculatum*). Am J Vet Res 46:1368–1371.

Partanen KH, Mroz Z. 1999. Organic acids for performance enhancement in pig diets. Nutr Res Reviews 12:1–30.

Perez JF, Reeds PJ. 1998. A novel stable isotopic approach enables the simultaneous determination of protein and RNA synthesis in vivo. J Nutr 128:1562–1569.

Petkevicius S, Bach Knudsen KE, Nanse P, Roepstorff A, Skjoth F, Jensen K. 1997. The impact of diets varying in carbohydrates resistant to endogenous enzymes and lignin on populations of *Ascaris suum* and *Oesophagostomum dentatum* in pigs. J Parasitol 114:555–568.

Phadtare S, Alsina J, Inouye M. 1999. Cold-shock response and cold-shock proteins. Current Opinion Microbiol 2:175–180.

Phillips ND. 1999. Molecular detection and identification of gastric bacteria in pigs. Honors thesis, Murdoch University, Western Australia.

Pierzynowski SG, Valverde Piedra JL, Hommel-Hansen T, Studzinski T. 2001. Glutamine in gut metabolism. In Gut Environment of Pigs. A Piva, KE Bach Knudsen, JE Lindberg, eds. Nottingham, UK: Nottingham University Press, pp. 43–62.

Pluske JR. 2001. Morphological and functional changes in the small intestine of the newly weaned pig. In Gut Environment of Pigs. A Piva, KE Bach Knudsen, JE Lindberg, eds. Nottingham, UK: Nottingham University Press, pp. 1–27.

Pluske JR, Siba PM, Pethick DW, Durmic Z, Mullan BP, Hampson DJ. 1996a. The incidence of swine dysentery in pigs can be re-

duced by feeding diets that limit fermentation in the large intestine. J Nutr 126:2920–2933.

Pluske JR, Williams IH, Aherne FX. 1996b. Villous height and crypt depth in piglets in response to increases in the intake of cows' milk after weaning. Anim Sci 62:145–158.

Pluske JR, Hampson DJ, Williams IH. 1997. Factors influencing the structure and function of the small intestine in the weaned pig: A review. Livest Prod Sci 51:215–236.

Pluske JR, Durmic Z, Pethick DW, Mullan BP, Hampson DJ. 1998. Confirmation of the role of non-starch polysaccharides and resistant starch in the expression of swine dysentery in pigs following experimental infection with *Serpulina hyodysenteriae*. J Nutr 128:1737–1744.

Powell RW, Dyess DL, Collins JN, Roberts WS, Tacchi EJ, Swafford AN Jr, Ferrara JJ, Ardell JL. 1999. Regional blood flow response to hypothermia in premature, newborn, and neonatal piglets. J Pediatric Surg 34:193–198.

Prohaszka L, Baron F. 1980. The predisposing role of high protein supplies in enteropathogenic *Escherichia coli* infections of weaned pigs. Zentralbl Veterinarmed B 27:222–232.

Pusztai A, Ewen SWB, Grant G, Bardocz S. 1999. Effect of lectins on digestion of food and body metabolism. COST-98, Effects of antinutrients on the nutritional value of legume diets 1:22–28.

Queiroz DMM, Rocha GA, Mendes EN, Moura SB, Oliveira AMR, Miranda D. 1996. Association between *Helicobacter* and gastric ulcer disease on the *pars oesophagea* in swine. Gastroenterology 111:19–27.

Rådberg K, Biernat M, Linderoth A, Zabielski R, Pierzynowski SG, Weström BR. 2001. Induced functional maturation of the gut mucosa due to red kidney bean lectin in suckling pigs. In Digestive Physiology of Pigs. JE Lindberg, B Ogle, eds. Wallingford, UK: CAB International, pp. 25–28.

Reeds PJ, Burrin DG, Stoll B, Jahoor F, Wykes LJ, Henry J, Frazer ME. 1997. Enteral glutamate is the preferential source for mucosal glutathione synthesis in fed piglets. Am J Physiol 273:E408–E415.

Reid CA, Hillman K. 1999. The effects of retrogradation and amylose/amylopectin ratio of starches on carbohydrate fermentation and microbial populations in the porcine colon. Anim Sci 68:503–510.

Rijnen MMJA, Dekker RA, Bakker GCM, Verstegen MWA, Schrama JW. 2001. Effects of dietary fermentable carbohydrates on the empty weights of the gastrointestinal tract in growing pigs. In Digestive Physiology of Pigs. JE Lindberg, B Ogle, eds. Wallingford, UK: CAB International, pp. 17–20.

Roberfroid M, Van Loo J, Gibson GR. 1998. The bifidogenic nature of chicory inulin and its hydrolysis products. J Nutr 128:11–19.

Robinson IM, Allison MJ, Bucklin JA. 1981. Characterization of the cecal bacteria of normal pigs. Appl Environ Microbiol 41:950–955.

Robinson IM, Whipp SC, Bucklin JA, Allison MJ. 1984. Characterization of predominant bacteria from the colons of normal and dysenteric pigs. Appl Environ Microbiol 48:964–969.

Rossi F, Ewodo C, Fockedey R, Thielemans MF, Thévis A. 1997. Digestibility and fermentation of inulin in the weaned piglet digestive tract. In Proc Int Symp Non-digestible Oligosaccharides: Healthy Food for the Colon? R Hartemink, ed. Wageningen, The Netherlands, p. 143.

Rossi F, Cox E, Coddeeris B, Portelle D, Wavreille J, Thévis A. 2001. Inulin incorporation in the weaned pig diet: Intestinal coliform interaction and effect on specific systemic immunity. In Digestive Physiology of Pigs. JE Lindberg, B Ogle, eds. Wallingford, UK: CAB International, pp. 299–301.

Roth FX, Windisch W, Kirchgessner M. 1998. Effect of potassium diformate (Formi LHS) on nitrogen metabolism and nutrient digestibility in piglets at graded dietary lysine supply. Agribiological Res 51:167–175.

Sangild PT. 2001. Transitions in the life of the gut at birth. In Digestive Physiology of Pigs. JE Lindberg, B Ogle, eds. Wallingford, UK: CAB International, pp. 3–17.

Sangild PT, Trahair JF, Silver M, Fowden AL. 1997. Luminal fluids affect intestinal enzyme activities in prenatal pigs. Proc Eur Assoc of Anim Prod 88:194–197.

Sangild PT, Trahair JF, Loftager MK, Fowden AL 1999. Intestinal macromolecule absorption in the fetal pig after infusion of colostrum in utero. Paediatric Res 45:595–602.

Scholten RHJ, van der Peet-Schwering CMC, Verstegen MWA, den Hartog LA, Schrama JW, Vesseur PC. 1999. Fermented co-products and fermented compound diets for pigs: A review. Anim Feed Sci Technol 82:1–19.

Siba PM, Pethick DW, Hampson DJ. 1996. Pigs experimentally infected with *Serpulina hyodysenteriae* can be protected from developing swine dysentery by feeding them a highly digestible diet. Epidemiol Infect 116:207–216.

Spencer RJ, Chesson A. 1994. The effects of *Lactobacillus* species on the attachment of enterotoxigenic *Eschericia coli* to isolated porcine enterocytes. J Appl Bacteriol 77:215–220.

Stern NJ, Hernandez MP, Blankenship L, Diebel EE, Doores S, Doyle MP, Ng H, Pierson MD, Sofos NJ, Sveum WH, Westhoff DC. 1985. Prevalence and distribution of *Camplyobacter jejuni* and *Camplyobacter coli* in retail meats. J Food Protection 48:595–599.

Stokes CR, Bailey M, Haverson K. 2001. Development and function of the pig gastrointestinal immune system. In Digestive Physiology of Pigs. JE Lindberg, B Ogle, eds. Wallingford, UK: CAB International, pp. 59–66.

Stoll B, Henry J, Reeds PJ, Yu H, Jahoor F, Burrin DG. 1998. Catabolism dominates the first-pass intestinal metabolism of dietary essential amino acids in milk protein-fed piglets. J Nutr 128:606–614.

Stoll B, Burrin DG, Henry J, Yu H, Jahoor F, Reeds PJ. 1999. Substrate oxidation by the portal drained viscera of fed piglets. Am J Physiol 277:E168–E175.

Strachan WD, Edwards SA, Smith WJ, Chase-Topping M, Gunn G, Hillman K, Stefopoulou SN, Thomson JR. 2002. Association of non-specific colitis with dietary factors in an epidemiological study. In Proc 17th Int Pig Vet Soc Congr, vol 2. p. 214.

Sutton AL, Mathew AG, Scheidt AB, Patterson JA, Kelly DT. 1991. Effects of carbohydrate sources and organic acids on intestinal microflora and performance of the weanling pig. In Proc 5th Int Symp Digestive Physiology in Pigs. MWA Versegren, J Huisman, LA den Hartog, eds. Wageningen, The Netherlands, pp. 442–427.

Telemo E, Bailey M, Miller BG, Stokes CR, Bourne FJ. 1991. Dietary antigen handling by mother and offspring. Scand J Immunol 34:689–696.

Terpstra C, Wensvoort G. 1988. Natural infections of pigs with bovine viral diarrhea virus associated with signs resembling swine fever. Res Vet Sci 45:137–142.

Thillainayagam AV, Hunt JB, Farthing MJ. 1998. Enhancing clinical efficacy of oral rehydration therapy: Is low osmolality the key? Gastroenterology 114:197–210.

Thomke S, Elwinger K. 1998. Growth promotants in feeding pigs and poultry. III. Alternatives to antibiotic growth promotants. Annal Zootechnie 47:245–271

Thomson JR, Edwards SA, Strachan WD, King T, Hazzeldine M. 2004. Effects of dietary raw materials and processing on non-specific colitis in pigs. In Proc 18th Int Pig Vet Soc Congr, vol 2. p. 885.

van der Meulen J, de Graaf GJ, Nabuurs MJA, Niewold TA. 2001. Effect of transportation stress on intramucosal pH and intestinal permeability. In Digestive Physiology of Pigs. JE Lindberg, B Ogle, eds. Wallingford, UK: CAB International, pp. 329–331.

Varel VH, Pond WG 1985. Enumeration and activity of cellulytic bacteria from gestating swine fed various levels of dietary fibre. Appl Environ Microbiol 49:858–862.

Varel VH, Pond WG, Pekas JC, Yen JT. 1982. Influence of high-fibre on bacterial populations in gastrointestinal tracts of obese and lean genotype pigs. Appl Environ Microbiol 44:107–112.

Vega-Lopez MA, Telemo E, Bailey M, Stevens K, Stokes CR. 1993. Immune cell distribution in the small intestine of the pig: Immunohistological evidence for an organised compart-mentalisation in the lamina propria. Vet Immunol Immunopathol 37:49–60.

Vega-Lopez MA, Bailey M, Telemo E, Stokes CR. 1995. Effect of early weaning on the development of immune cells in the pig small intestine. Vet Immunol Immunopathol 44:319–327.

Verdonk JMAJ, Spreeuwenberg MAM, Bakker GCM. 2001a. Nutrient intake level affects histology and permeability of the small intestine in newly weaned piglets. In Digestive Physiology of Pigs. JE Lindberg, B Ogle, eds. Wallingford, UK: CAB International, pp. 332–334.

Verdonk JMAJ, Spreeuwenberg MAM, Bakker GCM, Verstegen MWA. 2001b. Effect of protein source and feed intake level on histology of the small intestine in newly weaned piglets. In Digestive Physiology of Pigs. JE Lindberg, B Ogle, eds. Wallingford, UK: CAB International, pp. 347–349.

Weijtens MJBM, Bijker PGH, van der Plas J, Urlings HAP, Biesheuvel MH. 1993. Prevalence of *Campylobacter* in pigs during fattening: An epidemiological study. Vet Quart 15:138–143.

Weijtens MJBM, van der Plas J, Bijker PGH, Urlings HAP, Koster D, van Logtestijn JG, Huls JHJ Int Veld 1997. The transmission of campylobacter in piggeries: An epidemiological study. J Appl Microbiol 83:693–698.

Weström BR, Svendsen J, Ohlsson BG, Tagesson C, Karlsson BW. 1984. Intestinal transmission of macromolecules (BSA and FITC-labelled dextrans) in the neonatal pig. Biol Neonate 46:20–26.

Wilson AD, Stokes CR, Bourne FJ. 1989. Effect of age of absorption and immune responses to weaning or introduction of novel dietary antigens in pigs. Res Vet Sci 46:180–186.

Yen JT, Nienaber JA, Hill DA, Pond WG. 1991. Potential contribution of absorbed volatile fatty acids to whole-animal energy requirement in conscious swine. J Anim Sci 69:2001–2012.

Yin YL, Baidoo SK, Liu KYG, Schulze H, Simmins PH. 2001. Effect of enzyme supplementation of different quality hulless barley on apparent (ileal and overall) digestibility of nutrients in young pigs. In Digestive Physiology of Pigs. JE Lindberg, B Ogle, eds. Wallingford, UK: CAB International, pp. 145–147.

Young CR, Harvey RB, Anderson RC, Nisbet DJ, Stanker LH. 2000. Enteric colonization following exposure to *Campylobacter* in pigs. Res Vet Sci 65:75–78.

Zanetti F, Varoli O, Stampi S, DeLuca G. 1996. Prevalence of thermophilic *Campylobacter* and *Arcobacter butzleri* in food of animal origin. Int J Food Microbiol 33:315–321.

Zinter DE, Migaki G. 1970. Gongylonema pulchrum in tongues of slaughtered pigs. J Am Vet Med Assoc 157:301–303.

Zucker BA, Krüger M. 1998. Auswirkungen von transportbelastungen auf den endotoxingehalt im blut von schlachtschweinen. Berl München Tierärztl Wochenschr 111:208–210.

4 Diseases of the Mammary Glands

Christian Klopfenstein, Chantal Farmer, and Guy-Pierre Martineau

Inadequate sow milk production leads to reduced piglet growth and, in certain cases, to increased mortality in the litter. The first section of this chapter focus on a good understanding of the normal physiologic processes involved in the initiation and maintenance of sow lactation and on how these processes relate to piglet growth and mortality. Factors affecting the milk production of sows are numerous but they can be synthesized in three major groups:

1. The number of lactocytes (or epithelial cells) producing the milk (see mammary gland)
2. The intensity of milk synthesis by lactocyte (see physiology)
3. The capacity of the other organs and systems to supply the nutrients needed by the mammary gland (see homeorhesis)

The second section of this chapter covers some strategies to increase overall milk production of sows (see manipulating milk production) and the possible etiologies of early lactational problems (see infectious and noninfectious causes of postpartum dysgalactia syndrome) as well as treatment and prevention procedures.

MILK PRODUCTION OF SOWS

Measuring Milk Production
Measuring milk production in the sow is more complicated than in other farm animals. The small teats and the large number of functional mammary glands (12–14) make hand or mechanical milking difficult. Moreover, since milk is not available continually after the colostral phase, milk ejection must be stimulated and sows would have to be milked more than 24 times a day to mimic the piglets (Hernandez et al. 1987). Consequently, sow milk production is usually estimated by taking a number of measurements during the day and extrapolating to the whole day. Seven to eight measurements over a 24-hour period are reported to provide a good estimate of daily milk production (Salmon Legagneur 1965; Mahan et al. 1971). After the colostral phase, milk letdown has to be initiated with exogenous oxytocin (see oxytocin in the treatment section).

Best results are obtained by methods using the piglets to estimate sow milk output. However, in the first part of lactation, when milk production aptitude is greater than the ingestion capacity of the piglets, these methods underestimate the milk production capacity of the mammary gland. In the second part of lactation, when milk supply is a limiting factor for piglet growth, these methods should give a good estimation of the milk production capacity of the sow.

Milking the Sow. Sows can either be hand-milked, which requires a lot of manual labor, or milked with a milking machine. The first sow milking machine was developed following the discovery of the role of oxytocin for milk ejection (Salmon Legagneur 1959). More recently, milking machines have been used to compare milk production between teats (Fraser et al. 1985) and breeds (Grun et al. 1993a). The use of a milking machine has been reported to give much more repeatable estimates of sow milk production than those obtained by hand milking (Fraser et al. 1985); yet, these are not available commercially.

Sow Weight Loss During Suckling Periods. Weighing the sow before and after a suckling period is another recognized but seldom used approach for measuring milk production. Its greatest drawback is a major lack of precision because the weight ratio between milk ejected during each nursing period and sow body weight is approximately 1:1000 (Salmon Legagneur 1956).

Weigh-Suckle-Weigh. The weigh-suckle-weigh (WSW) method has been used extensively during the past years and involves repeated weighing of piglets, preceding and following nursing, for a certain number of sucklings. Apart from the suckling periods, the piglets do not have access to the teats. The general approach is to remove the piglets from the sow 1 hour prior to the first suckling period. The following nursing periods occur at fixed intervals varying between 45 and 60 minutes, and last on average 4–5 minutes. Before each suckling period, the piglets are placed on a cold or wet surface to induce urination and defecation. The piglets can be weighed individually, as half the litter, or as a litter (Barber et al. 1955; Salmon Legagneur 1956; Mahan et al. 1971; Lewis et al. 1978; Noblet and Etienne 1989). The first two estimations should generally be discarded because of their great variability (Speer and Cox 1984). One of the main problems with this technique is to adjust for piglet urinary, fecal, and metabolic losses.

Piglet Growth. Although conceptually simple, measuring piglet growth has not generally been considered sufficiently precise for lactation studies. The first studies reported that piglet growth was a poor predictor of sow milk production ($R^2 < 0.50$) (Salmon Legagneur 1956; Lewis et al. 1978). These low predictions were likely due to the difficulty in adequately estimating sow milk production. Indeed, recent work demonstrated that milk production over different parts of lactation can be adequately predicted by using piglet growth (R^2 between 0.84 and 0.96) (Noblet and Etienne 1989). Based on these equations and other observations, a conversion efficiency of approximately 4.5 g of milk per gram of growth has been estimated (Lewis et al. 1978; Noblet and Etienne 1989).

Body Water Turnover. Milk production can also be estimated by measuring water turnover in the piglet. This method measures the dilution of endogenous water by water absorbed from nursing (MacFarlane et al. 1969). Each piglet receives a known quantity of deuterium-labeled water by parenteral injection, prior to nursing. The difference in isotope concentration preceding and following nursing represents the dilution effect of milk absorption and is directly related to sow milk production. A correlation of 0.96 was found between the estimated and the actual milk intake of artificially reared piglets using this technique (Prawirodigdo et al. 1987).

Pattern of Milk Production

Sow milk production is usually described in four phases: the colostral, ascending, plateau, and descending phases. Sows in modern production units usually do not reach the descending phase because they are weaned during the plateau phase at less than 28 days of lactation.

Typical sow milk production curves are presented in Figure 4.1 (Toner et al. 1996); they are similar to those presented by others (Noblet and Etienne 1986; Shoenherr et al. 1989; Grun et al. 1993b). In the latter publications, the end of the ascending phase was around day 14 postpartum, whereas it was reported to occur later (22–28 days) in some other publications (Elsley 1971;

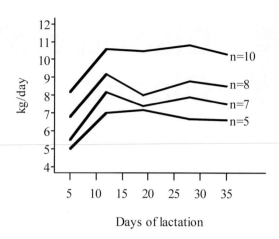

4.1. Pattern of milk production (kg/day) of first-litter sows nursing litters of different sizes (from Toner et al. 1996, reprinted with permission).

Harkins et al. 1989). This discrepancy may be related to differences in breeds, nutrition, and parities of the sows and in the methodology used to estimate milk production.

Colostral Phase. The term *colostrum* describes the mammary secretions obtained during the few days before and/or after parturition. Colostrum usually contains more proteins, mainly immunoglobulins; less fat; and less sugar than the milk produced after initiation of lactation (Dorland 1985). Mammary secretions contain 157, 130, 9, and 6 grams of protein per liter at 0, 6, 12, and more than 12 hours after the first suckling, respectively (Klobasa et al. 1987). Consequently, the colostral phase probably ends between 12 and 24 hours after the first suckling.

Mammary secretions obtained during the first 12 hours postpartum contain large amounts of immunoglobulins (60–80 g/L) (Klobasa et al. 1987). During this short period of time, mammary secretions are continuously available to the piglets, whereas after the colostral phase, milk availability becomes cyclical (de Passillé and Rushen 1989a). Within 48–72 hours postpartum, piglets establish a teat order in which each piglet consistently sucks from one or two specific teats (Fraser 1976; de Passillé et al. 1988; Roychoudhury et al. 1995). Within 48 hours after parturition, any unsuckled mammary gland goes through involution and becomes nonfunctional (Atwood and Hartmann 1993). Consequently, daily milk production and total milk production during lactation are proportional to the number of suckled mammary glands or to the number of piglets in the litter ($R^2 > 0.95$) (Auldist et al. 1998).

Ascending Phase. The ascending phase of lactation (approximately day 0 to 10) is explained by an increase in nursing frequency as well as an increase in the volume of milk obtained at each nursing. Nursing frequency doubled between day 2 and day 10 of lactation (17 vs. 35 nursings/day) (Jensen et al. 1991) and the quantity of milk obtained at each nursing is reported to increase from 29 to 53 g between the first and the third week of lactation (Campbell and Dunkin 1982).

During the ascending phase, sow milk production is adjusted to the needs of the piglets. Indeed, between days 4 and 8, litters of heavier piglets (4.45 kg at day 4) consume more milk (9.1 vs. 7.6 L/day) than litters of lighter piglets (1.92 kg) (King et al. 1997). It is well known that most piglets do not consume much creep feed before they are at least 10 days old (Aumaitre and Salmon Legagneur 1961). During the first 2 weeks of lactation, the heavier piglets at birth (1.39 kg) ingest more milk than their lighter littermates (0.89 kg); however, the milk consumption relative to body weight (g/kg of live weight) is similar for all piglets (Campbell and Dunkin 1982). The larger consumption observed among the heavier piglets was explained by a larger volume ingested at each nursing. It appears that during the ascending phase of lactation, the dynamic equilibrium state between the piglets needs and sow milk nutrient output is so well harmonized that litter size (8 vs. 11) has very little effect on piglet weight before day 7 of lactation (Klopfenstein et al. 1999) (Table 4.1).

Plateau Phase. After day 10 of lactation, milk production is maximal (Figure 4.1) (King et al. 1997); therefore, piglet growth may be inhibited by insufficient milk supply during the later part of lactation, and this inhibition will be greater with longer lactation and in larger litters (Table 4.1). The weight difference between suckling piglets supplemented or not with cow's milk between days 7 and 28 of lactation was 140 g on day 14, 756 g on day 21, and 1761 g on day 28 (Reale 1987). Supplementation with milk replacer from day 3 to weaning also in-

creased average piglet weight by 120 g on day 7, 340 g on day 14, and 910 g on day 21 (Wolter et al. 2002). It was also reported that, in a 21-day lactation, the growth limitation of suckling piglets could be more than 2 kg per pig (Harrell et al. 1993). When piglets are weaned at an early age (14–16 days), which is part of a new management procedure in the swine industry, the limiting effect is likely to be smaller.

Composition of Sow Milk

Sow milk is a complex water solution containing more than 100 different chemical components. The major components are lactose, proteins (casein, alpha-lactalbumin, beta-globulins, serum albumins, immunoglobulins G and A), lipids, lactocytes, leucocytes (neutrophils, eosinophils, lymphocytes, and macrophages), bivalent ions (calcium, phosphorus, and magnesium) and electrolytes (sodium, potassium, and chloride). The relative concentrations of these components vary according to the stage of lactation (Table 4.2). During the colostral phase protein content decreases rapidly mainly because of the fall in the concentrations of immunoglobulins.

Table 4.1. Least-square means of piglet weight (kg) at different ages from randomly chosen litters of different sizes after correction for birth weight (these litters had no mortality for the 28-day lactation period).

		Age of the Piglets (Days)				
Litter Size	n	3	7	14	21	28
8	15	1.87	2.82	4.62	6.42	8.21
9	15	1.85	2.78	4.38	6.18	7.91
10	15	1.87	2.72	4.40	6.18	7.89
11	14	1.88	2.72	4.21	5.60	7.10

Source: Data from a data base of 2000 piglet weights from the Agriculture Canada Research Station, Lennoxville, Quebec.

Table 4.2. Variation of sow milk composition (mean ± std) between the first days (day 1–2) and the plateau phase (day 10–15) of lactation.

Milk Components	Day 1–2	Day 10–15	Difference	Source
Lactose (mmol/L)	160 ± 10	190 ± 10	+30	(Konar et al. 1971)
Sodium (mmol/L)	25 ± 5	18 ± 5	−7	(Konar et al. 1971)
Potassium (mmol/L)	75 ± 5	50 ± 5	−25	(Konar et al. 1971)
Chloride (mmol/L)	25 ± 5	18 ± 5	−7	(Konar et al. 1971)
Calcium (mmol/L)	12 ± 3	50 ± 3	+38	(Perrin 1955)
Phosphate (mmol/L)	12 ± 1	14 ± 1	+2	(Perrin 1955)
Magnesium (mmol/L)	4 ± 1	4 ± 1	0	(Perrin 1955)
Total protein (g/L)	64 ± 6	51 ± 5	−13	(Klobasa et al. 1987)
Lipids (g/L)	65 ± 15	65 ± 15	0	(Klobasa et al. 1987)
Somatic cells (k¢/ml)[2]	1060 ± 790	2012 ± 990	+952	(Schollenberger et al. 1986)
Leucocytes (k¢/ml)[1,2]	748 ± 509	886 ± 519	+138	(Schollenberger et al. 1986)
Lactocytes (k¢/ml)[1,2]	152 ± 103	503 ± 315	+351	(Schollenberger et al. 1986)
Anucleate cells (k¢/ml)[1]	147 ± 160	727 ± 63	+580	(Schollenberger et al. 1986)
% de leucocytes	70	44	−26	(Schollenberger et al. 1986)

Source: adapted from Klopfenstein 2003.

[1]k¢ = 1000 cells.

[2]Somatic cells found in the first colostrum (<12 hours) contains many more cells than milk obtained at day 1–2 (>8000 k¢/ml, 98% leucocytes) (Evans et al. 1982; Magnusson et al. 1991).

[3]Leucocytes are the sum of neutrophils, eosinophils, lymphocytes, and macrophages.

Somatic Cells of Normal Milk. The somatic cell content of mammary secretions from healthy sows is much greater than that in milk of healthy cows: between 1 and 4 million cells per milliliter (M¢/ml) in sows (Evans et al. 1982; Schollenberger et al. 1986; Hurley and Grieve 1988; Magnusson et al. 1991; Drendel and Wendt 1993a; Klopfenstein 2003) compared to less than 1 million cells in cows (Paape et al. 1963). The first mammary secretions obtained at parturition contain many more somatic cells (>8 M¢/ml) than milk obtained later in lactation (Evans et al. 1982; Magnusson et al. 1991). These somatic cells are mainly composed of epithelial cells and leucocytes. The relative concentrations of the various cell types vary with the stage of lactation. In milk collected during the colostral phase, most cells are leucocytes (>98%), whereas during the rest of lactation (days 7, 14, and 28), the cells are predominantly epithelial cells (Evans et al. 1982; Schollenberger et al. 1986; Magnusson et al. 1991).

Somatic Cells of Mastitic Milk. Somatic cells content found in the milk of infected mammary glands is similar (12–35 M¢/ml) to those observed during the colostral phase or during involution (Drendel and Wendt 1993b). Somatic cells found in the milk of infected glands are mainly (>75%) leucocytes. Therefore, during sow lactation, a cellular content over 12 M¢/ml with a increased proportion of leucocytes is an indication of mammary gland alteration. However, during the colostral phase, we cannot, solely based on milk cellular content, discriminate between mammary gland infection and retarded lactogenesis (Drendel and Wendt 1993b).

MAMMARY GLAND

Anatomy

External Structure. The mammary glands of swine are located in two parallel rows along the ventral body wall, from the thoracic region to the inguinal area. In commercial breeds, their number varies generally between 12 and 18 per animal (Labroue et al. 2001) whereas pigs of the Meishan breed can have up to 22 mammary glands (personal communication, L. Maignel, Canadian Center of Swine Improvement, www.ccsi.ca). As suggested by Muirhead (1991), boars and gilts should be retained for breeding only if they have 14 well-placed normal nipples. The rows of teats should be parallel because when the teats diverge from a straight line just before and after the umbilicus, the sows have poor teat presentation therefore limiting accessibility of the teats to the piglets. Sows with poor teat presentation usually have large girth widths, which tends to spread the teat rows apart. Poor teat placement could be a major reason for failure of sows to rear 11 or 12 piglets (Muirhead 1991).

The glands are attached to the ventral body wall by adipose and connective tissue arising from the abdominal fascia. Each mammary gland normally has one teat, or nipple, with two separate teat canals. When the teat sphincter is not visible (inverted teat) it has a 50% chance of remaining blind. Functional supernumerary smaller teats can also be found. Paired vestigial nonfunctional accessory teats, not connected to glandular tissue, may also occur (Molenat and Thibeault 1977; Labroue et al. 2001).

Internal Structure. The microscopic and macroscopic anatomy of the porcine mammary gland has been described by Barone (1978), Schummer et al. (1981), and Calhoun and Stinson (1987). In the nulliparous sow, the mammary gland consists of cell buds distributed among fat and connective tissue, whereas in the lactating gland, the connective tissue is largely displaced by glandular parenchyma. The mammary glands of the lactating sow are composed of a compound tubuloalveolar tissue with the secretory units arranged in lobules. The lobules are lined by epithelial cells, generally described as lactocytes, which synthesize milk. These secreting units are connected by a nonsecreting duct system to an ostium found on the teat. There are usually two complete gland systems within each mammary gland of the pig. The glandular tissue of one system usually interdigitates with the other, although the components of the two systems are independent. Usually, each teat has two openings, one for each glandular system, but sometimes a third ostium can be seen. In these animals, one ostium ends blindly and has no glandular tissue.

The arterial, venous, and lymphatic circulation of the mammary glands in swine is provided on each side of the ventral midline by a network that extends longitudinally from the axillary to the inguinal regions (Barone 1978; Schummer et al. 1981; Lignereux et al. 1996) (Figure 4.2). Moreover, in swine there is a venous anastomosis between the right and left mammary gland of each pair of glands.

Nerve supply to the cranial mammary glands differs from that to the inguinal glands. Cranial mammary glands receive their innervation from the last eight or nine thoracic nerves while inguinal mammary glands receive their innervation mainly from the pudendal nerve (Gandhi and Getty 1969a,b; Ghoshal 1975). A more complete anatomical and histological description of the porcine mammary gland can be found in the seventh edition of *Diseases of Swine* (Smith et al. 1992).

Mammogenesis

The extent of mammary growth is largely related to the number of lactocytes present and has a determinant impact on milk capacity of the sow. Mammary growth starts at the fetal stage but occurs mainly postnatally and, to a greater extent, at the end of gestation; yet it still takes place during lactation.

The mammary glands of newborn piglets have a poorly developed duct system and are largely composed

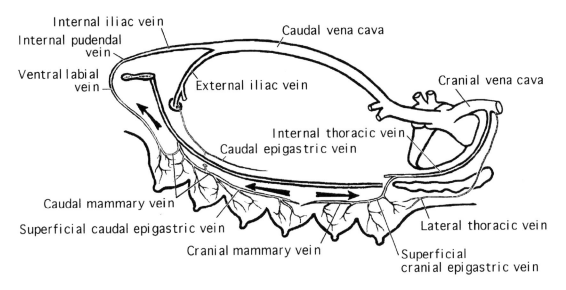

4.2. *Mammary veins of the sow (from Dejean 1971, as modified by Lignereux et al. 1996, reprinted with permission).*

of subcutaneous stromal tissue (Hughes and Varley 1980). Accumulation of mammary tissue and mammary DNA (which is indicative of cell number) is slow until 90 days of age, at which time the rate of accretion of mammary tissue and DNA increases four- to sixfold (Sorensen et al. 2002a). By the time the gilt is mated, the mammary gland is still very small but it consists of an extensive duct system with various budlike outgrowths (Turner 1952).

In pregnant gilts, quantitative development of the mammary glands is slow in the first two-thirds of pregnancy, while almost all accumulation of mammary tissue and DNA takes place in the last third of gestation (Hacker and Hill 1972; Kensinger et al. 1982; Sorensen et al. 2002a). The mammary glands undergo major histological changes as the adipose and stromal tissues are replaced by lobuloalveolar tissue to become the milk secretory apparatus (Hacker and Hill 1972; Kensinger et al. 1982). Both histological changes and differences in DNA concentrations in mammary tissues from gilts indicate increased tissue differentiation between days 75 and 90 of gestation, with maximum cell concentrations present by day 90 (Kensinger et al. 1982).

Allometric mammary gland development occurs mainly during the last 10 days of gestation and continues during lactation (Hurley 2001). Average mammary gland wet weight of gilts was reported to remain fairly stable (approximately 100 g) up to day 110 of gestation and to increase up to 373 g by day 112 (Sorensen et al. 2002a). Average mammary weight of the suckled glands then increased linearly from 381 g on day 5 of lactation up to 593 g on day 21 (57% increase) (Kim et al. 1999). Another study showed that mammary gland wet weight increased by 70, 20, and 30% between day 113 of gestation and day 26 of lactation, for sows of parity 1, 2, and 3, respectively (Beyer et al. 1994). The increase in mammary volume during lactation is mainly the conse-

quence of mammary gland cellular hyperplasia, rather than hypertrophy, as demonstrated by DNA analysis (Kim et al. 1999).

Factors Affecting Mammary Gland Development

Hormones. Estrogens are important for mammogenesis (Kensinger et al. 1986) and the shift in the rate of mammary development occurring at approximately 90 days of age is likely linked to the onset of ovarian activity (Sorensen et al. 2002a). The finding that mammary development is enhanced with the onset of puberty in gilts corroborates this and even suggests that early onset of puberty may be beneficial for mammogenesis in swine (Farmer et al. 2004b). Prolactin was recently shown to have a great impact on the mammary development taking place before puberty. When injected to gilts for a period of 28 days, starting at 75 kg body weight, porcine prolactin stimulates mammary development through an increase in the number of milk secretory cells (Palin and Farmer 2004). The impact of such a treatment on future sow milk yield still needs to be determined.

During pregnancy, the formation of lobuloalveolar cells is related to increases in estrogen and progesterone concentrations in the maternal circulation (Ash and Heap 1975), while concentrations of prolactin remain low (Dusza and Krzymowska 1981). After day 105 of pregnancy, decreasing progesterone and increasing estrogen concentrations are related to a tremendous increase in metabolic activity of the mammary gland (Robertson and King 1974; Knight et al. 1977; Kensinger et al. 1986). The mechanism by which estrogens affect the mammary epithelium is not known; it is possible that they induce prolactin receptors in the mammary gland. There is also a positive association between prolactin levels and mammary wet weight at day 110 of gestation, which may be due to the effect of prolactin on water movement into the gland (Kensinger et al. 1986). Prolactin was recently shown to play an essential role for mammogenesis in pregnant swine. Inhibition of prolactin in the last third of pregnancy drastically decreases mammary development in gilts (Farmer et al. 2000) and the timing of its necessary action for mammogenesis was more specifically identified as being from days 90 to 109 of gestation (Farmer and Petitclerc 2003).

Buttle (1988) reported that ovariectomy, but not removal of the corpora lutea, of gilts at day 60 of gestation delays the onset of lobuloalveolar development in the mammary glands, suggesting that the ovarian stroma or follicles produce a factor stimulating the onset of lobuloalveolar development. Later, Hurley et al. (1991) demonstrated that relaxin replacement therapy after ovariectomy restores mammary parenchymal development. Therefore relaxin plays a major role in promoting mammogenesis in gilts during the last third of pregnancy. Relaxin increases growth of parenchyma and decreases mammary fat pad while having no effect on the cellular composition of mammary parenchyma. The mechanism of action of relaxin on mammary development is unknown, yet it seems likely that it requires estrogen priming as well as interaction with other mammotropic hormones, such as prolactin (Hurley et al. 1991).

Nutrition. Feeding of gilts or sows in the two periods of rapid mammary development (i.e., from 90 days of age until puberty and during the last third of gestation) can have a major impact on the extent of this development. Sorensen et al. (2002b) suggested that a period of ad libitum feeding before puberty is needed to maximize mammary growth in gilts. In accordance, Lyvers-Peffer and Rozeboom (2001) showed that decreasing energy intake of gilts at specific periods between 9 and 25 weeks of age reduces weight of parenchymal tissue and tends to lower mammary DNA at the end of gestation. Farmer et al. (2004b) also demonstrated that a 20% feed restriction, starting at 90 days of age, decreases mammary parenchymal tissue mass by 26% at 210 days of age in gilts. On the other hand, feeding a lower protein diet (14.4% vs. 18.7% crude protein) during that same period of time does not hinder mammary development of gilts, as long as feed intakes of 2.5 and 3.3 kg/day are maintained from 90 to 150 days and from 151 to 200 days of age, respectively.

The last month of pregnancy is critical for the development of milk-secreting tissue. Various studies were conducted to examine the influence of increased energy and protein intakes in this period on mammary development; however, results are controversial. Weldon et al. (1991) reported that increased dietary protein between day 75 and 105 of gestation did not benefit mammary development. Howard et al. (1994) saw no effect of elevated energy intake and fat accretion in gestation on mammary development of pregnant gilts. Kusina et al.

(1995) also reported that even though protein intake in gestation favorably affected milk yield, this increase was not due to an improvement in mammary development. On the other hand, when manipulating the body composition of gilts by changing their protein and energy intakes during pregnancy, it was found that fat gilts produce less milk than lean gilts (7.0 vs. 9.0 L/day) at the same body weight (Head and Williams 1991). When fostering 2-week-old piglets onto gilts that were either fat or lean at the beginning of lactation, lean gilts had a much greater milk output than fat gilts, thereby suggesting that the number of secretory cells at the beginning of lactation can have a very strong effect on the amount of milk produced (Pluske et al. 1995a).

Mammary Gland Involution

Suckled mammary glands of sows undergo dramatic changes during the initial 7 days after weaning, with significant changes occurring even as early as 2 days after weaning (Ford et al. 2003). Mammary gland wet weight decreases from 485.9 g on the day of weaning (at 22 days postpartum) to 151.5 g by 7 days after weaning; mammary DNA also decreases from 838.8 mg to 278.4 mg for this same period of time. These changes in gland wet weight and DNA during the period of mammary gland involution in the sow represent losses of over two-thirds of the parenchymal mass and nearly two-thirds of the cells that were present on the day of weaning (Ford et al. 2003). Mammary gland involution in the sow is a rapid process, which is probably irreversible within 2 or 3 days postweaning, but it is a process that also occurs in early lactation. Indeed, once teat order is established, mammary glands that are not regularly suckled begin to regress through involution. This regression occurs rapidly during the first 7 to 10 days postpartum and seems to be affected by dietary nutrient levels (Kim et al. 2001). Mammary glands that are not suckled during lactation undergo no further reduction in parenchymal tissue during the first 7 days after weaning (Ford et al. 2003). It is of interest to mention that mammary glands that are suckled during lactation are larger than the nonsuckled glands at the end of involution. This may suggest more mammary tissue being available for redevelopment during the subsequent pregnancy and, therefore, greater productivity in the next lactation (Ford et al. 2003). On the other hand, a Norwegian study showed that inactive mammary glands for one or two lactation may have full milk yield in the subsequent lactation (Gut-à Porta et al. 2004).

The abrupt cessation of lactation in sows when milk production is at a maximum (3 to 4 weeks) brings about drastic changes in metabolic activity of the mammary glands and endocrine status. There is a decrease in milk lactose, a transient decrease followed by an increase in milk glucose and increases in plasma lactose and glucose (Atwood and Hartmann 1995), which is due to alterations in the status of the tight junctions between mammary epithelial cells (Figure 4.3). In the week following weaning, the mammary alveoli regress (Hacker 1970) and the secretory glandular mass is replaced by adipose tissue in which a new alveolar system develops in the following pregnancy (Delouis 1986). The absence of stimulation of the mammary glands stops the regular secretion of prolactin (Benjaminsen 1981b) while the concentrations of gonadotropic hormones start to increase, allowing ovarian cycles to resume (Stevenson et al. 1981). It was recently hypothesized that estrogens could affect the mammary involution process; however, the administration of estrogens during the postweaning period did not enhance overall rate of mammary involution in sows when litters were weaned at 21 days of lactation (Ford et al. 2003).

PHYSIOLOGY OF MILK PRODUCTION

Milk Synthesis

Lactocytes are highly specialized cells that have the capacity to synthesize sugars, proteins, and lipids (Akers 2002). One gram of mammary tissue has the potential to produce 1.67 ml of milk per day (Akers 2002). Lactocytes are rich in mitochondria, rough endoplasmic reticulum (RER), and RNA (ribosomal, messenger and transport), and they have a large Golgi apparatus that allows protein and lactose synthesis (Mepham 1987). The cellular concentration of these functional organelles can be used as indicators of intensity of milk component synthesis.

Proteins. Sow milk proteins (50–70 g/L) are mainly constituted of caseins (25–30 g/L), beta-globulins (approximately 5 g/L), IgA (5 g/L), alpha-lactalbumins (approximately 3 g/L) and smaller amounts of other proteins (IgG, IgM, serum albumins, etc.) (Klobasa and Butler 1987; Dodd et al. 1994). Most of these proteins are synthesized from amino acids present in the serum and excreted from the Golgi in the alveoli with lactose, water, and electrolytes (Mepham 1983, 1987; Trottier et al. 1997). The uptake of amino acids by mammary gland tissue was recently studied and reported (Hurley et al. 2000; Jackson et al. 2000; Bryson et al. 2001).

The intensity of protein synthesis by the mammary gland is often estimated by the RNA/DNA ratio. In sows, this ratio is less than 1 at 90 days of gestation, equal to 2 at parturition, and higher than 2.5 on day 4 of lactation (Kensinger et al. 1982). These findings therefore support the idea that the intensity of protein synthesis increases between the end of gestation and parturition but also continues to change at least during the first days of lactation.

Lactose. Lactose is the most predominant molecule in milk and is synthesized in the Golgi apparatus from glucose molecules. The Golgi apparatus is a cellular component that is permeable to glucose and nonpermeable to lactose (Leong et al. 1990). This physical characteristic is one of the fundamental mechanisms allowing the creation of an osmotic gradient essential to milk secretion (Peaker 1978). In sows' milk, the concentration of lactose increases from 89 mmol/L up to 175 mmol/L between parturition and day 7 of lactation, and then remains stable up to day 28 (Klobasa et al. 1987). This supports the idea that the intensity of milk synthesis by lactocytes increases up to day 7 of lactation; however, the extent of protein and of lactose synthesis (milk volume) are not necessarily similar. Indeed, the concentration of milk protein goes down whereas that of lactose increases as lactation proceeds (Klopfenstein 2003) (Table 4.2).

Lipids. The lipids present in sow milk are mainly triglycerides (>95%) and they vary in length because they originate from three different sources: from fatty acids obtained from the digestive tract, from those obtained by tissue lipolysis, or synthesized de novo from glucose and organic acids (Mepham 1987; Migdal 1991).

Minerals. Milk contains many mineral substances (approximately 7 g/L) (Noblet and Etienne 1986). The most common minerals (5–75 mmol/L) are sodium, potassium, chloride, calcium, phosphorus, and magnesium (Park et al. 1994) (Table 4.2). Traces (<1 mmol/L) of sulfur, zinc, boron, copper, aluminum, molybdenum, and manganese can also be found (Park et al. 1994). These minerals are either free in solution or bound to proteins.

Lactogenesis

The initiation of the capacity of the mammary gland to synthesize unique milk components such as lactose, casein, and lipids is termed *lactogenesis* and is often described as a two-phase process. Lactogenesis phase I refers to preparation of the mammary tissue for the synthesis of milk components, and lactogenesis phase II, generally occurring around parturition, describes the start of important milk synthesis and secretion (Hartmann et al. 1995).

Abundant quantities of milk components appear in the alveoli between days 90 and 105 of gestation, thereby indicating the beginning of the lactogenic process (Kensinger et al. 1982). However, hardly any secretion can be obtained from the teats until parturition, and then suddenly, around the time of farrowing, copious mammary secretion can be easily extracted from the glands. This could be related to serum transudation (Figure 4.3) occurring because of the major vascular reorganization taking place at farrowing. Indeed, serum volume increases by more than 20% prior to parturition to supply the uterus (Matte and Girard 1996) and as farrowing proceeds, the excess serum needs to be eliminated and could very well be excreted through the mammary glands. At the end of gestation and during the colostral phase, the junctions between epithelial cells surrounding the alveoli are not tight and allow serum transudate

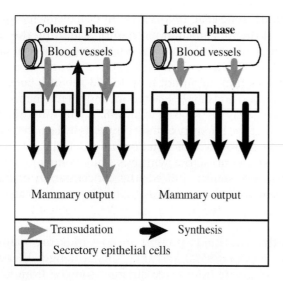

4.3. *Origins of mammary output during the colostral and lacteal phases of lactation in the sow.*

to leak from the bloodstream into the mammary secretions and milk components to leak from the mammary gland alveoli back to the bloodstream (Figure 4.3). Although serum transudation may contribute to the volume of colostrum obtained by the piglets, its contribution is most likely very short in duration.

During the colostral phase, lactose is present in high concentrations in the plasma of sows (>200 mmol/L) (Hartmann et al. 1984), and all the immunoglobulins G found in mammary secretions originate from the plasma (Bourne and Curtis 1973). On the other hand, during lactation, plasma lactose concentrations are low (<100 mmol/L) (Hartmann et al. 1984), and most of the immunoglobulins present in the mammary secretions are synthesized locally (Bourne and Curtis 1973). Similar patterns were found for the plasmatic concentrations of milk whey proteins during the colostral and lactation phases in swine (Dodd et al. 1994).

The onset of milk component synthesis is closely related to the decline in serum progesterone concentrations seen during farrowing (Robertson and King 1974; Hartmann et al. 1984). Moreover, exogenous progesterone administration during late pregnancy delays the beginning of copious milk synthesis in the sow (Whitely et al. 1990). Progesterone withdrawal is therefore considered to be the hormonal signal for the initiation of copious milk synthesis in swine. It is likely that the decrease in progesterone has the function of priming the gland, whereas withdrawal of colostrum from the glands would trigger the initiation of copious milk secretion (Hartmann et al. 1995). Prolactin is also a key hormone for the onset of lactation in sows, as in various other species (Tucker 1985). In the pregnant sow, suppression of the prepartum peak of prolactin inhibits subsequent milk production (Whitacre and Threlfall 1981; Taverne et al. 1982).

Milk Ejection

During the colostral phase, and particularly during parturition and the first hours afterward, colostrum ejection is elicited with ease. At parturition, distension of the cervix for the passage of the piglets and movements of the sow are enough to lead to colostrum ejection (Fraser 1984). Moreover, a sow can cause milk to spurt from the teats by pressing them with her back leg during an attempt to rise (Castren et al. 1989). Colostrum ejections are often as frequent as every 10–20 minutes, and the period of high intramammary pressure, permitting colostrum withdrawal, may be sustained for a minute or more. However, once 50–100 ml of colostrum have been removed, the intramammary pressure is reduced to the point that further withdrawal is more difficult (Fraser 1984).

After the colostral phase, and for the rest of lactation, milk ejection is cyclical, with approximately 24 cycles per day (Whittemore and Fraser 1974; Lewis and Hurnik 1985; Castren et al. 1993). The removal of milk from the alveoli and ductal system of the porcine mammary glands requires a neuroendocrine milk ejection reflex elicited by piglets massaging the udder (Fraser 1980). This reflex consists of an afferent neural pathway and an efferent pathway involving the release of oxytocin and the ejection of milk (Hartmann and Holmes 1989). The activation of neural receptors within the teats of the mammary gland by the nuzzling and suckling of piglets stimulates the release of oxytocin from the posterior pituitary. Oxytocin then stimulates the contraction of myoepithelial cells surrounding the alveolar lumen, thereby forcing milk through the ductal system to the teats (Ellendorf et al. 1982). The amount of oxytocin released during sucklings is not dependent on the massaging time or the number of piglets massaging the udder, but a certain amount of udder stimulation is needed to trigger oxytocin release (Algers et al. 1990). On the other hand, growth rate of piglets is not affected by the peak amplitude in intramammary pressure (Kent et al. 2003), which is linked to oxytocin levels. The increase in circulating oxytocin concentrations can occur up to 30 seconds before milk ejection (Ellendorf et al. 1982), which is very short in duration and lasts only 10–20 seconds (Fraser 1980). Whitely et al. (1985) observed acute episodic releases of relaxin in the blood of sows, both when piglets suckled and after the administration of oxytocin. These authors suggested that relaxin could oppose the action of oxytocin and/or provide a negative feedback on the hypothalamus for the suppression of oxytocin secretion.

During sow lactation not all nursings are successful. Two types of unsuccessful sucklings can be distinguished: those affecting some piglets of a litter and those affecting the whole litter. Among the latter, one must distinguish between sucklings terminated by the piglets and those terminated by the sow (Illmann and Madlafousek 1995). Unsuccessful sucklings affecting the whole litter become more frequent after the colostral phase, both in a natural environment (Castren 1993) and in confinement (Fraser 1977). They are characterized by an absence in rise in intramammary pressure, associated with a lack of increase in plasma oxytocin (Ellendorf et al. 1982). During the first 10 days of lactation the proportion of unsuccessful sucklings is reported to be between 20% and 40% (Fraser 1977; Jensen et al. 1991). Although frequent and requiring a lot of energy from the piglets, ejection failures may be a functional part of nursing in pigs and may play a role in maintaining lactation (Algers 1993). This is supported by the fact that plasma concentrations of lactogenic hormones tend to rise after an unsuccessful nursing (Rushen et al. 1993). On the other hand, an external stress can lead to failed milk ejections; for example, placing sows in a novel environment increases the chance that the subsequent nursing attempt will fail to lead to milk ejection (Rushen et al. 1995). This stress-induced inhibition of milk ejection is not due to increased concentrations of cortisol or adrenocorticotropic hormone (ACTH) but is likely caused by an opioid-mediated inhibition of oxytocin (Rushen et al. 1995). It is of interest to note that even if it increases the chances of unsuccessful sucklings, the stress of a novel environment does not lead to a general increase in the threshold of stimulation of the mammary gland that is required for oxytocin release (Rushen et al. 1995).

Control of Milk Production

Milk Removal. Removal of milk from the mammary glands is of utmost importance in order to maintain milk secretion. Indeed, suckling and milk removal are the major stimulators of mammary growth during lactation in the sow and mammary glands that are underdeveloped at parturition can still grow rapidly in response to suckling (Hurley 2001). As milk is secreted from the mammary epithelial cells into the alveolar lumen, milk components accumulate in the lumen. One of these components is an autocrine factor, termed *feedback inhibitor of lactation* or *FIL* (Peaker and Wilde 1987), which is known to feed back and inhibit further milk secretion from alveolar epithelial cells. Indeed, milk stasis in alveolar spaces is known to be the primary stimulus for the end of lactation and involution of alveoli in swine (Boyd et al. 1995). Removal of milk therefore removes FIL and allows for continued milk secretion. Milk accumulation in the gland also causes an increase in intramammary pressure, which reduces blood flow to the tissue (Hurley 2001). Furthermore, the stimulus of suckling or massaging the mammary glands by the piglets brings about increases in circulating prolactin concentrations in the sow (Spinka et al. 1999), which is a known galactopoietic hormone (Farmer 2001). The importance of milk removal may also be shown by the fact that a drastic increase in nursing stimulus increases milk energy output (Sauber et al. 1994). Moreover, on days 7 and 8 of lacta-

tion, nursing frequency plays a crucial role in adjusting total daily milk output (Spinka et al. 1997). Piglet behavior is therefore important in modulating sow milk production, but the effect of nursing behaviors could be due either to more complete milk removal or to modified hormonal release (Ellendorf et al. 1982).

Nursing Frequency. As described earlier, the increase in nursing frequency is one of the major factors explaining the observed increasing milk production during the ascending phase of milk production. Nursing frequency is approximately 17 per day at parturition, it increases up to 35 per day at the peak of lactation (day 8 to 10), and then it tends to decrease slightly (20 to 30 per day) up to weaning (Jensen et al. 1991; Spinka et al. 1997; Puppe and Tuchscherer 2000; Farmer et al. 2001; Fisette et al. 2004; van den Brand et al. 2004). The slight decrease in nursing frequency in late lactation is indicative of a lower maternal investment.

Nursing frequency seems to be similar between day and night on day 10 of lactation, whereas it decreases during the night on day 17 (van den Brand et al. 2004). Nursing frequency also tends to be greater in sows on a low feeding level. This could easily be explained by the fact that piglets suckled by sows fed a low feeding level have a greater feeding motivation due to the lower milk yield. On the other hand, it is also possible that sows with a low feed intake terminate nursings more often due to their greater restlessness (van den Brand et al. 2004).

Hormonal Control. The activation of neural receptors within the mammary glands by the nuzzling and suckling of piglets stimulates not only the release of oxytocin from the posterior pituitary but also the release of prolactin, growth hormone (GH), ACTH, and thyroid-stimulating hormone from the anterior pituitary. Hormones from the anterior pituitary have the function of maintaining the synthesis of milk from the mammary epithelial cells (Delouis 1986).

The role of GH for milk production can be either direct or indirect (Flint 1995). Its direct role is via its implication as a regulator of nutrient partitioning for milk component synthesis. Its indirect role is via an increase in the concentrations of insulin-like growth factor I (IGF-I), which acts upon the mammary epithelial cells. When circulating levels of GH and IGF-I were reduced in lactation by immunizing sows against GH-releasing factor, milk yield (measured by the WSW method) was significantly decreased yet the growth rate of the piglets was unaltered (Armstrong et al. 1994). It was concluded that GH may have a facilitative, rather than an essential, role in support of lactation in sows.

Until recently, the role of prolactin once lactation is initiated was not clear. It was originally thought that prolactin might be important in the prefarrowing period (Smith and Wagner 1980) but was not essential for milk synthesis in later lactation (Benjaminsen 1981a; Bevers et al. 1983; Mattioli and Seren 1985). Yet, in a recent study where the secretion of prolactin was systematically inhibited at various stages of lactation, the weight gain of piglets was suppressed in the week during which prolactin secretion was suppressed (Farmer et al. 1997). These results therefore clearly demonstrate that prolactin is essential for both the initiation and the maintenance of milk production in sows. This is in agreement with results of Plaut et al. (1989), who showed that the binding of prolactin to its receptor is a major effector of milk production in sows.

Thyroid hormones are required for various metabolic functions, such as oxygen consumption and protein synthesis by the mammary gland, that are closely related to milk production (Tucker 1985). The tripeptide thyrotropin-releasing factor (TRF) also stimulates the release of thyroid hormones and of prolactin in the circulation of sows (Dubreuil et al. 1990), which could lead to a possible involvement in the control of milk production.

HOMEORHESIS

The gestation and lactation periods are two complex physiological processes that imply dynamic changes in behavior and body composition. These dynamic changes are related to modifications in energy, protein, water, and mineral metabolisms, and they are particularly important around the time of farrowing. The dynamic equilibrium between all different characteristics needed to carry through gestation and lactation has been described by the Greek term *homeorhesis* (Bauman and Currie 1980). Although the change from gestation to lactation has an impact on almost all systems of the sow, the present chapter will cover only those that are most crucial for the initiation and maintenance of lactation.

Sow Behavior

Four behavioral changes have been observed between the end of gestation and the beginning of lactation in sows maintained under natural conditions:

1. Approximately 24 hours before parturition, the sow becomes hyperactive and leaves her group in order to build a nest.
2. On the day of parturition and the following day, the sow spends most of her time in or within a few meters of the nest, mainly resting and nursing her piglets. She leaves the nest only to drink or urinate.
3. During the next days (3–10), the sow extends her foraging excursions in time and in distance, while the piglets remain in the nest.
4. After day 10, the sow leaves the nest with her piglets, and the whole family joins the herd (Jensen 1986; Stangel and Jensen 1991; Jensen et al. 1993).

Sows maintained in farrowing crates tend to have similar behaviors (Meunier Salaun et al. 1991; Cronin et al. 1994, 1996; Klopfenstein 2003) (Figure 4.4). The day before farrowing, the number of position changes, the proportion of time spent standing and water intake increase substantially compared to the preceding days (Figure 4.4). After farrowing, sows are very lethargic (95% in lateral recumbency) in their crates and they stand up mainly for feeding. After day 3, sows gradually decrease their time in lateral recumbency to attain less than 50% at day 21.

The nursing behavior of sows changes over the lactation period and is probably related to the milk supply. During the first days after parturition, when milk production is greater than the piglets' needs, most (>85%) of the sucklings are initiated by the sow and are terminated by the piglets. After the fourth week of lactation, when the milk supply becomes limited for the needs of the piglets, most sucklings are initiated by the piglets and terminated by the sow (Jensen 1988; Jensen et al. 1991). Results during the period of midlactation are not as clear. According to the work of Boe (1991), on day 10, 80% of the sucklings are still initiated by the sow, but according to the observations of Jensen et al. (1991), this proportion might be only 55%. The sow terminates the sucklings by leaving the piglets or by rolling over on her belly and hiding her udder to limit access (de Passillé and Rushen 1989a).

Energy Metabolism

The heat excreted by each sow almost doubles between the end of gestation and the beginning of lactation (18 vs. 35 MJ per day) (Noblet and Close 1980; Noblet and Etienne 1987). This increased heat production is the consequence of the intensity of the metabolic activity necessary to sustain milk production. This extra heat production has an impact on rectal temperature and heat stress management during lactation.

Rectal Temperature. The normal rectal temperature of healthy gestating sows is reported to be between 38.3°C and 38.5°C (King et al. 1972; Elmore et al. 1979; Messias de Bragança et al. 1997; Klopfenstein et al. 1997; Klopfenstein 2003), with little variation between studies. After parturition and during lactation, the rectal temperature of sows in crates is reported to increase by 1°C (King et al. 1972; Elmore et al. 1979). Healthy lactating sows have difficulty maintaining stable rectal temperatures, values as low as 38.4°C (Cornette 1950; Ringarp 1960) and as high as 40.5°C (Messias de Bragança et al. 1997) have been reported. These wide variations are most likely the consequence of the heat stress induced by increased internal heat production and high environmental temperatures in farrowing rooms. Consequently, feed intake, room temperature, and type of housing affect the capacity of lactating sows to maintain their body temperature. Restricted-fed sows have lower rectal temperatures than sows fed ad libitum (Moser et al. 1987; Persson et al. 1989; Messias de Bragança et al. 1997). Similarly, GH supplementation, which alters sow metabolism, increased rectal temperature (estimated weekly from days 14 to 35) from 39.1°C to 39.8°C (Toner et al. 1996).

Finally, the expected rectal temperature of lactating primiparous sows is higher than that of multiparous sows (39.6 vs. 39.3°C) (Klopfenstein 2003). This increased rectal temperature observed in lactating sows must be considered as physiological hyperthermia and should not be confused with fever. All these observations suggest that lactating sows housed in confinement are more likely to suffer from heat stress because they are fed ad libitum with high-energy diets, their environment is kept warm for the piglets, and the sows have no access to a cool floor to dissipate the excess heat.

Heat Stress. Lactating sows are extremely vulnerable to heat stress due to their large body size, high metabolic rate (Lynch 1977) and lack of functional sweat glands which prevents dissipation of heat via transpiration (Marzulli and Callahan 1957). They are often exposed to ambient temperatures higher than their upper critical temperature, being in the range of 20–25°C. High temperatures during lactation decrease sow voluntary feed intake (Messias de Bragança et al. 1997; Quiniou and Noblet 1999), increase weight loss, decrease milk production, and hence decrease litter growth rates (Messias de Bragança et al. 1997; Prunier et al. 1997), and also delay the return to estrus of weaned sows (see review by Prunier et al. 1996). Furthermore, sow mortality (and loss of litter) is also associated with high ambient temperatures (D'Allaire et al. 1996) and is largely due to cardiovascular failure.

Fever or Hyperthermia? Fever is defined as an increase in central temperature as a consequence of an increase in the thermoregulatory setpoint (Robinson 1997). Fever is the normal response to systemic infections or to the action of some pyrogenic substances (e.g., endotoxins, interleukins, etc.) (Robinson 1997). Hyperthermia on the other hand, is usually defined as the increase in body temperature observed when the heat production exceeds the heat output capacity (Robinson 1997).

In the lactating sow, there is a lot of confusion on the expected sow normal rectal temperature after farrowing. According to some authors the expected rectal temperature of the healthy lactating sow is 39.5°C (see rectal temperature); others consider that the puerperal sow with a rectal temperature higher or equal to 39.3°C is diseased (see sow rectal temperature and PPDS).

Nutrient Availability

The nutrients required by mammary tissue for milk synthesis come from the diet and from body reserves. Mammary glands are the primary users of absorbed nu-

trients in lactating sows and virtually dictate the dietary nutritional needs (Boyd et al. 1995). Indeed, it was shown that 65–70% of the total energy requirement of a lactating sow is to support milk production (Aherne and Williams 1992). Of the total uptake of plasma metabolites by mammary tissue, glucose accounts for approximately 61%, amino acids 24%, triglyceride fatty acids (TGFA) 12%, and acetate 1% (Spincer et al. 1969). Approximately 53% of the glucose taken up by the mammary gland is partitioned to lactose and 34% is oxidized. The other 13% is used for the synthesis of triglyceride-glycerol, milk fatty acids, and amino acids (Linzell et al. 1969). It is of interest to note that in the presence of both acetate and glucose, sow mammary tissue will preferentially utilize acetate for fatty acid synthesis (Bauman et al. 1970). Therefore it is conceivable that more glucose could be made available for mammary metabolism by raising TGFA levels in the diet (Boyd et al. 1995).

Mammary tissue of lactating sows is very active with respect to transport and metabolism of amino acids. Boyd et al. (1995) ranked each amino acid on the basis of relative uptake by mammary tissue. The order of amino acids was almost identical for mammary uptake and milk composition, but it was also reported that the mammary uptake of branched-chain amino acids (valine, leucine) and arginine may be greater than suggested by the milk amino acid pattern (Boyd et al. 1995; Trottier et al. 1997). Milk production is ultimately energy-dependent, so that the need in amino acid for milk synthesis depends on the amount of dietary energy available (Tokach et al. 1992), thereby reinforcing the importance of glucose sources and of a right balance of nutrients in sow feeding management.

Sow milk contains large amounts of calcium, phosphorus, and magnesium. These bivalent ions found in the milk are transferred from the digestive tract and from bone reserves. Apparent digestive bioavailability of these bivalent ions is known to be low (3–50%) (National Research Council 1998). Intestinal absorption and renal absorption of these minerals is closely regulated by a hormonal system (parathormone, calcitriol, calcitonine), whereas active absorption from the digestive tract requires the synthesis of a transport protein (Greco and Stabenfeldt 1997). After parturition, the availability of bivalent ions may affect initiation of lactation. This problem is well known in cows (Goff 2000) and is often suspected in sows.

Water Availability

Water intake patterns observed between the end of gestation and the beginning of lactation are presented in Figure 4.4. Hourly water intake increases from approximately 1 L/hour at the end of gestation to attain 2.6 L/hour 12 hours before the end of parturition (Klopfenstein 2003). Water intake can be very low in some sows during the first 24 hours following parturition (less than 10 L/day). After this period of transition, water intake increases gradually to attain 20 to 35 L per day during lactation. The increased water intake just prior to farrowing can be due to the occurrence of nesting behavior but is also the consequence of greater water needs. Indeed, during the hours preceding parturition, there is a rapid increase in the water content of the reproductive system to allow the process of parturition (Dobson 1988).

PIGLET GROWTH, MORTALITY, IMMUNITY, AND BEHAVIOR

The newborn piglet is totally dependent on sow's colostrum and milk as a source of protein for growth, energy to maintain body temperature, and immunoglobulins for protection against diseases. Sow milk and colostrum provide the best nutrients for the nutritional needs of the piglets. The biological value of milk protein in swine is very close to 1 (Williams 1995) and the amino acid balance in sow's milk is very similar to that in the lean tissue of pigs (King et al. 1993a).

Piglet Growth

From birth to weaning, piglets from larger litters tend to be lighter than piglets from smaller litters (Dyck and Swierstra 1987; Van der Lende and de Jager 1991; Le Dividich et al. 2004). This difference is the consequence of lower piglet birth weight and, in some cases, of lower milk supply per piglet in large litters. Average piglet birth weight is reported to decrease by approximately 30–40 g for each additional piglet in the litter (Van der Lende and de Jager 1991; Le Dividich et al. 2004). Although average piglet weight decreases with litter size, selection of hyperprolific sows over 10 years had no effect on average piglet weight (Tribout et al. 2003) because it also increased the expected weight of piglets of similar litter sizes. The expected mean birth weight of Large White piglets has not changed (1.45 kg) between 1977 and 1988 although litter size increased from 10.2 to 11.2 piglets. Interestingly, the expected average piglet birth weight for a litter size of 10.7 piglets increased from 1.37 kg to 1.46 kg over the same decade (Tribout et al. 2003).

Growth rate, usually measured as average daily gain (ADG), is related to individual piglet weight at birth (Tyler et al. 1990; Castren et al. 1991; Le Dividich et al. 2004). The expected maximal ADG of a newborn piglet weighing 1.3 kg is lower than that of a piglet with a birth weight of 2.3 kg. It is therefore necessary to take into account initial weight when comparing ADG between piglets. When piglet weights are mathematically corrected for a standard birth weight (1.4 kg), the effect of litter size is absent on day 3, is small on day 7, and becomes greater as lactation proceeds (Table 4.1). These data show that milk production becomes a limiting factor for piglet growth when the sow has attained her maximal milk production capacity (day 10 to 15).

Piglet Mortality

Although swine production is becoming more sophisticated, piglet losses between birth and weaning remain a serious problem for the industry. Preweaning mortalities are often higher than 10% of liveborn piglets and most of these occur during the first week after parturition (English and Morrison 1984; Dyck and Swierstra 1987; de Passillé and Rushen 1989b; Le Cozler et al. 2004). These losses can be explained by litter and piglet characteristics or by inadequate sow milk production.

The effect of litter size on mortality is quadratic. Piglet losses increase only in the largest litters (Guthrie et al. 1987; Fahmy and Bernard 1971; Dyck and Swierstra 1987) and are probably related to an insufficient number of functional mammary glands to supply milk for all the piglets (Chertkov 1986; Bilkei et al. 1994).

The main causes (>75%) of mortality are emaciation and piglet crushing by the sow (English and Morrison 1984; Fraser 1990; Le Cozler et al. 2004). Piglets losses due to emaciation occur mainly on days 4 and 5 after birth as a result of poor nutrition during the first days postpartum (Dyck and Swierstra 1987). Piglets crushed by the sow often had poor gains during the first postnatal days (Dyck and Swierstra 1987). Piglet mortalities are not uniformly distributed between litters. Most of them occur among a few litters (see problem litters) with poorer growth rates during the first days after birth (Pettigrew et al. 1986; Dyck and Swierstra 1987; Thompson and Fraser 1988; de Passillé and Rushen 1989a,b; Fraser and Phillips 1989; Klopfenstein et al. 1995, 1997; Klopfenstein 2003). Most of these problem litters are thought to be the consequence of some inadequate mammary function during the initiation of lactation.

Immune Protection of the Piglet

Newborn piglets rely on colostrum for passive transfer of immunity (Bourne 1976) because there is little or no placental transfer of antibodies in the pig (Rapacz and Hasler Rapacz 1982). The absorption of immunoglobulins from the sow's colostrum causes closure of the intestine for the passage of these large proteins (Klobasa et al. 1991), suggesting that absorption is possible only during the first feedings after birth. Twenty-four hours postnatally, artificially reared piglets receiving 6 hourly feedings of 25 ml of sow colostrum followed by hourly feedings of cow's milk had plasmatic immunoglobulins concentrations similar to those of naturally fed piglets (Klobasa et al. 1991). Increasing the number of hourly feedings of colostrum from 6 to 12, 18, or 24 did not increase the concentrations of plasma immunoglobulins in piglets. On the other hand, allowing the piglets to fast for periods of up to 24 hours after birth before giving them access to their first colostrum intake did not decrease serum immunoglobulins concentrations 12 and 18 hours after feeding (Klobasa et al. 1990). Therefore, closure of the gut system for the passage of immunoglobulins is dependent on the quantity of colostrum ingested rather than on time since birth. Six feedings of colostrum should be sufficient to give adequate immune protection to the piglets.

Passive immunity transfer from the sow to the piglet is essential for protection against diseases. The quantity of IgG ingested by each piglet is affected by birth order due to the rapid changes in colostrum composition taking place between onset of farrowing and birth of the last piglet (Klobasa et al. 2004; Le Dividich et al. 2004). Piglets dying before weaning are reported to have lower plasmatic immunoglobulin concentrations after parturition (Hendrix et al. 1978; Tyler et al. 1990); yet this association disappears when birth weight is used as a covariate (Tyler et al. 1990). Moreover, the probability of dying is not increased among last-born piglets, even though they obtain less immunoglobulins than first-born piglets (Le Dividich et al. 2004). These results, although surprising, can be explained by the fact that most mortalities are the consequence of inadequate nutrition rather than diseases.

Piglet Behavior

The nursing behavior of piglets changes over the lactation period. During the colostral phase, newborn piglets move from teat to teat in a "teat-sampling" process (Hartsock and Graves 1976), enabling them to receive a "free meal" of colostrum (de Passillé and Rushen 1989a; Fraser and Rushen 1992). Udder massaging by the piglets, although frequent during the rest of lactation, is rare during the colostral phase (Castren et al. 1989). The interval between birth and first suckling does not change greatly with birth order (Rohde Parfet and Gonyou 1988).

After the colostral phase, nursing becomes cyclical and the suckling behavior of piglets can then be characterized by four phases (Fraser 1980):

1. Piglets start by vigorously massaging the sow's udder, which is necessary for triggering the oxytocin release. During this phase, piglets often fight and are very noisy. After 1–3 minutes of udder massaging, which is one of the longest periods among mammals, the sow increases her grunting rate, which coincides with the release of oxytocin (Algers et al. 1990).
2. When piglets hear the signal, they become very quiet, keeping the teats in their mouths and waiting for their meal.
3. As soon as milk ejection occurs, the piglets drink the milk with rapid jaw movements.
4. After milk ejection, which lasts only for 10–20 seconds, the piglets continue to massage the udder for a short period of time.

No milk can be obtained by the piglets during either the pre- or postejection massaging phases. Therefore, even if piglets are often seen at the mammary gland, milk is available for only a very short period of time—less than 10 minutes per day (10–20 seconds per milk ejection, 17–30 ejections per day). Failure of milk ejection is indicated by the absence of rapid grunting from the sow and of rapid-mouth movement from the piglets as well as no change in intramammary pressure. Milk ejection failure is due to a lack of pulsatile release of oxytocin during the massaging phase (Ellendorf et al. 1982), which can be brought about by undue stress to the sow.

During the first 8 hours after birth, newborn piglets suckle an average of seven different teats and are often involved in fights (de Passillé and Rushen 1989a). The frequency of teat disputes is not affected by litter size, but piglets suckling many teats are involved in more disputes. Regardless of teat position, the piglet with a teat in its mouth at the beginning of a dispute has a higher probability of winning (de Passillé and Rushen 1989a). Within 48–72 hours postpartum, piglets establish a teat order in which each piglet consistently sucks from one or two specific teats (Roychoudhury et al. 1995). Piglets prefer the anterior teats (Vales et al. 1992), most likely because sows are more responsive to stimulation of these teats than they are to stimulation of the inguinal teats (Fraser 1976). This increased responsiveness could be due to the different nerve supply between front and rear teats (see the section on anatomy). The anatomical and physiological differences between front and rear teats could induce different milk yields. Indeed, piglets suckling the front teats were reported to be heavier at weaning than piglets suckling the caudal teats (Kornblum et al. 1993; Hoy et al. 1995).

MANIPULATING MILK PRODUCTION

Insufficient milk production to meet piglet needs usually occurs when the maximal milk production capacity is attained (7–15 days). This is usually considered a physiological limitation because it affects all sows sooner or later during lactation. Many management strategies have been studied to overcome this physiological limitation and they are discussed in this section.

Feeding Strategies

Milk production requires a great supply of substrates, which come from two sources: the lactation diet and the sow's body reserves. The relative importance of nutrient intake seems to change as lactation progresses. Body reserves might be sufficient in early lactation compared with late lactation to compensate for inadequate nutrient intake (Pettigrew 1995). Accordingly, severe restriction of feed intake during lactation has no impact on litter growth in the first week postpartum, whereas it markedly decreases litter growth during the fourth week of lactation. The size of this reduction depends on the amount of body reserves at farrowing; gilts with lower body reserves being affected most (Mullan and Williams 1989). A survey of 25,000 lactating sows (Koketsu 1994, as reported by Pettigrew 1995) showed that the impact of lactating sows feed intake on litter weight becomes larger as lactation progresses.

The intake of protein/amino acids by lactating sows is critical for their overall lactation performance because of the great nutrient requirements to maintain milk production. Lysine is typically the first limiting amino acid for lactating sows and it was established that 26 g of dietary lysine is needed per kg of litter growth/day (Sohn and Maxwell 1999). When looking at nitrogen balance of lactating sows, Dourmad et al. (1998) demonstrated that, in order to achieve a zero protein balance, 45–55 g/day of crude lysine are required for normal- to high-yielding sows, respectively. Among the branched chain amino acids, both valine and isoleucine, but not leucine, appear to increase milk production as indicated by increased litter weight gain (Kerr 1997, as cited by Sohn et al. 1999). These amino acids can be metabolized to succinyl-CoA and can therefore potentially serve as a source of energy for the mammary gland (Sohn and Maxwell 1999). Indeed, McNamara and Pettigrew (2002) showed that sows can mobilize amino acids from muscle to support mammary growth and milk production, yet they also demonstrated that an increased energy intake can partially relieve the effects of decreased protein intake on milk production.

From various studies designed to determine the relation between milk production and dietary energy, Williams (1995) noted that each suckling piglet grows an extra 1 g/day for each MJ of metabolizable energy consumed by the sow. In recent studies, sows were fed through a stomach cannula in order to override the normal mechanisms that limit feed intake. Matzat et al. (1990) showed a linear relationship between milk output and energy intake of sows, whereas Pluske et al. (1995b) demonstrated a ceiling to milk production from gilts, whereby piglet growth did not respond beyond 75 MJ of metabolizable energy. It therefore seems that gilts and sows might partition energy differently during lactation, and this partitioning is most likely under hormonal regulation. Such a ceiling for lactational performance was also observed in first-parity sows offered increasing amounts of protein (King et al. 1993b).

When attempting to increase sow milk yield, one must keep in mind that as the milk production capacity of a sow is increased, her nutrient requirements for milk synthesis are also elevated. It is therefore important to ensure that lactational feed intake of sows is maximized and that lean-tissue gain during pregnancy is sufficient so that the sows' milk production capacity is not compromised. Various feeding management systems have been used in an attempt to increase sow feed intake. Increasing feed consumption of sows by 8% through wet-feeding had no impact on average daily gains of piglets over an 18-day lactation period (Genest and D'Allaire 1995). Similarly, the use of a bulky diet in gestation increased average lactational feed intake of sows by 8% without improving mean litter weight (Farmer et

al. 1996). Increasing daily feeding frequency from 2 to 3 (Genest and D'Allaire 1995) or 2 to 4 (Farmer et al. 1996) during lactation also had no effect on feed intake. The addition of fat to the sow's diet in order to increase energy density, and energy intake, of sows during lactation was also studied. However, it did not lead to a less-negative energy balance in the sows but resulted in fatter piglets when sows were fed at a high feeding level (van den Brand et al. 2000).

Nursing Interval

Refilling of the mammary glands with milk was reported to be almost complete within 35 minutes after a suckling bout (Spinka et al. 1997), and the frequency of gland emptying was found to play a major role in regulating milk secretion and mammary gland development (Auldist et al. 2000). These last authors increased suckling frequency via cross-suckling, using piglets from another litter, which could not be done commercially. However, it is known that sows within a farrowing room will synchronize their nursings (Wechsler and Brodmann 1996), and this is likely due to the auditory stimulus from the other animals. Experiments were therefore carried out in which the typical sow suckling grunts were recorded and played back to sows and their litters during lactation in an attempt to stimulate nursing frequency. These playbacks can indeed stimulate nursings (Stone et al. 1974). However, the results on piglet growth are variable between studies, with no effect to an 8% increase when a recording of sow suckling grunts was played at 35–42 minute intervals (Cronin et al. 2001; Fisette et al. 2004). On the other hand, playbacks at 35-minute intervals increased mammary parenchymal cell number in sows at the end of lactation (Farmer et al. 2004a). Present results suggest that use of this management practice throughout lactation is not optimal and further work is needed to establish such things as the ideal time in lactation to play these recordings, the optimal interval to be used, and whether there is a habituation effect. It is evident, however, that efforts should be made to encourage greater suckling frequency and to minimize disruption of suckling behavior in farrowing houses in order to maximize sow milk yield.

Exogenous Hormones

The important endocrine control of sow milk yield suggests that exogenous hormones could be used to stimulate milk production. Studies were therefore performed to determine the possible impacts of various peptidic hormones on sow milk yield and piglet performance. Growth hormone (GH) or GH-releasing factor (GHRF) received considerable attention since greater concentrations of GH could allow more nutrients to be utilized for milk synthesis (Farmer 1995). Early studies reported an important increase in milk yield (15–22%), leading to improved piglet growth rates (Harkins et al. 1989). But those results could not be reproduced in further trials

(Smith et al. 1991). Furthermore, Michelchen and Ender (1991) stated that the effect of GH on milk yield is not greater in sows having large litters (13 vs. 8 piglets). The effects of GH on milk composition are also contradictory, whereas reduced voluntary feed intake during lactation and greater body weight and backfat losses of sows receiving GH during lactation are consistent findings in all studies.

The decreased feed intake likely limits the lactation response to GH and leads to an increased use of body reserves to maintain milk production. The addition of 8% fat in the lactation diet could not prevent these losses of backfat in GH-treated sows (Cromvell et al. 1992). Exogenous GH may also have detrimental consequences on sow health (Smith et al. 1991; Cromvell et al. 1992), with some animals dying of bleeding stomach ulcers (Smith et al. 1991) or of apparent heat stress in the peripartal period. It is suggested that sows may be more sensitive to exogenous GH than growing pigs and that the adverse effects of GH in lactating sows may be dose-dependent (Smith et al. 1991). It is apparent that GH does play a role in the regulation of milk yield, but whether this role is an essential or a facilitative one is not known (Armstrong et al. 1994).

The secretion of GH is under the dual control of a GHRF (Guillemin et al. 1982) and a GH-inhibiting factor named somatotropin-release inhibitory factor (SRIF) (Brazeau et al. 1973). Active immunization against SRIF was used as a tool to increase concentrations of GH in sows, but the great variability in animal response to this treatment makes it an unreliable method (Farmer et al. 1990, 1991). The use of GHRF, on the other hand, consistently increases GH concentrations, with sows showing an increased responsiveness to chronic injections (Dubreuil et al. 1987). However, massive doses of GHRF (12 mg thrice daily) did not affect sow milk yield, milk composition, or piglet performance, but decreased weight, backfat thickness, and feed intake of sows on the fourth week of lactation (Farmer et al. 1992). Nevertheless, blood urea was reduced indicating that GHRF-injected sows utilized proteins more efficiently, thereby enabling them to maintain their milk production and litter performance in spite of a decreased feed intake. When combining administration of GHRF with a feeding management designed to optimize feed intake of lactating sows (Farmer et al. 1996), there was only a tendency for piglet weights to be greater. However, the increase in sow feed intake was not as large as expected and was mostly seen in early lactation. It is therefore likely that a management system having a greater effect on sow feed intake is needed for GHRF to exert its maximal effects on milk yield and piglet growth.

Daily intramuscular injections of 50 or 100 mg/sow of thyrotropin-releasing factor (TRF) increased the average daily weight gain of piglets (Wung et al. 1977), but subcutaneous injections of 9 µg/kg given twice daily during lactation had no effect on piglet growth (Dubreuil et al. 1990). Due to its small size, TRF can be absorbed intact by the digestive tract and when 200 mg of TRF were added daily to the feed of sows, piglet weight was increased by 0.7 and 1.1 kg on days 20 and 27 of lactation, respectively, but the weaning to estrus interval went from 4.8 to 36.9 days, making such a treatment totally inadequate for swine producers (Cabell and Esbenshade 1990).

Sows showing spontaneous lactation failure harbor abnormally low concentrations of prolactin (Whitacre and Threlfall 1981). This may explain the 8% increase in litter weight gain observed in gilts (but not sows) receiving a single injection of porcine prolactin on day 1 of lactation (Dusza et al. 1991). Two studies were carried out to determine the effects of chronic injections of prolactin from day 107 of gestation and during lactation, on milk production of sows (Crenshaw et al. 1989; King et al. 1996). Neither of these showed any effect on milk yield and it was postulated that since injections were started before there were any piglets to remove milk from the mammary glands, premature involution of the secretory units of the mammary glands might have taken place (Boyd et al. 1995). In a later study where prolactin was injected to sows from days 2 to 23 of lactation, sow and piglet performances were still unaffected (Farmer et al. 1999). These results also indicated that virtually all prolactin receptors are generally saturated in lactating sows, thereby preventing any beneficial effects of further increasing prolactin concentrations. Studies on the control of prolactin receptor numbers and affinity in lactating sows are therefore needed.

POSTPARTUM DYSGALACTIA SYNDROME

Inadequate and insufficient colostrum and milk production occurs in some sows during the puerperal period usually lasting up to 72 hours after birth of the first piglet. Historically, puerperal lactation problems have been considered to be a cause or a consequence of a pathological condition named as the mastitis-metritis and agalactia syndrome (MMA). As discussed in the first part of this chapter, poor lactation performance can also be explained by three major physiological factors:

1. Inadequate or insufficient mammary gland development
2. Inadequate or insufficient milk synthesis
3. Inadequate adaptation to lactation homeorhesis.

Therefore, postpartum sow lactation problems are more adequately described as postpartum dysgalactia syndrome (PPDS), which is preferred by the authors over the more traditionally used MMA syndrome. Indeed, the latter term has created a lot of confusion because it is assumed that all three symptoms are present in the case of early lactation problems, which is not necessarily the case.

Clinical Signs of PPDS

The primary clinical signs of a sow's inability to produce a sufficient amount of milk and colostrum are piglet growth retardation and increased mortalities. In this chapter, litters with high mortalities and low growth rates during the first days after parturition will be called problem litters. They remain a frequent observation in modern farrowing units, and veterinarians are often consulted to reduce their incidence. Unfortunately, they can be identified with certainty only when the piglets show retarded growth and high mortality, because litter characteristics at birth are poor predictors of future performances. Close observation of the piglets' behavior is one of the best methods for early detection of problem litters (Whittemore and Fraser 1974). These piglets fight more and for longer periods, lose weight, and remain close to the sow between sucklings (Algers and de Passillé 1991).

Early detection of sows with postpartum lactation problems is difficult because most of them do not show any clear clinical signs (Klopfenstein 2003). Temporal variation of sow behavior (Figure 4.4) and body condition were similar among sows nursing litters with poor (≤77 g/kg/day—problem litters) and normal (>77 g/kg/day—normal litters) growth rates between the end of parturition (time 0) and 132 h postpartum (Klopfenstein 2003). In the last study, the major differences between sows nursing problem and normal litters were related to milk composition (Table 4.3). Also, sows nursing problem litters drank less water (−0.36 L/h) and had lower skin temperature (−0.64°C) (Figure 4.4), higher serum phosphate (+0.10 mmol/L), and higher calcium (+0.05 mmol/L) concentrations at hours 36 and 60 of lactation. Rectal temperatures of sows nursing problem litters were similar to those of the others sows at the end of gestation (−96 h) and at the beginning of lactation (12 h, 36 h, 60 h) but were slightly higher at 132 h (39.6 vs. 39.4°C) postpartum. The latter study confirmed that milk production of sows nursing problem litters is dif-ferent compared to the other sows but showed that there is no easy way for the farmer to identify these sows early after parturition. Moreover, in the later study, only 2 sows among the 29 sows nursing problem litters were diseased in the postpartum period. This is a good representation of what is seen in many herds. A few sows presenting PPDS are diseased but many more are apparently normal.

Prevalence of PPDS

Although PPDS is observed in some herds, there is a lot of confusion on the prevalence of postpartum lactation problems due to the subjectivity related to some of the criteria used to identify the affected sows. Indeed the most common criterion used to identify sows affected by lactation problems is based on postpartum rectal temperature. The use of the rectal temperature criteria to classify sows as diseased or normal is adding confusion to our understanding of the pathogenesis of PPDS.

Sow Rectal Temperature and PPDS

For some historical reasons, there seems to be a general consensus that postpartum rectal temperatures higher than 39.3 or 39.5°C categorize sows as being affected by PPDS (Hermansson et al. 1978b; Goransson 1989b; Persson et al. 1989; Madec and Leon 1992; Hoy 2004). However, as discussed previously, this criterion should be seriously questioned because the proposed thresholds are equal or even below the expected rectal temperature of lactating primiparous and multiparous sows (see fever or hyperthermia?).

The use of rectal temperature to classify sows as diseased or normal has led to the publication of paradoxical results. In some instances, litters from sows identified as being "severely affected by early lactation problems (MMA)" because of high rectal temperature (>39.5°C) had better growth rate and lower mortality than litters from nonaffected sows (Furniss 1987; Persson et al. 1989). Moreover, the proposed cut-off to

Table 4.3. Temporal variation of some milk components (least square means) of sows nursing litters with slow (≤ 77 g/kg/day—Problem litters—PL) and normal (>77 g/kg/day—Normal litters—NL) growth rates between the end of parturition (time 0) and 132 hours postpartum (PP).

Milk Components	36 Hours PP		60 Hours PP		132 Hours PP	
	NL	PL	NL	PL	NL	PL
Lactose (mmol/L)	120	120	130	121*	147	141*
Sodium (mmol/L)	23	23	19	23*	16	19*
Potassium (mmol/L)	39	39	36	35	30	30
Chloride (mmol/L)	34	34	33	38*	26	31*
Total protein (g/L)	60	60	56	59*	49	49
Lipids (g/L)	76	76	78	85*	71	71
Leucocytes (k¢/ml)	275	359	319	551*	292	520*
Lactocytes (k¢/ml)	55	75	119	193*	172	298*
% of leucocytes	83	83	73	74	62	64

Source: adapted from Klopfenstein 2003.
*Significant difference between NL and PL (p <0.05)
k¢ = 1000 cells.

classify sows was never adjusted for parity even though the expected rectal temperature of primiparous sows is higher (approximately 0.3°C) than that of multiparous sows (Klopfenstein 2003). Accordingly, it was reported that 43% of gilts and 29% of multiparous sows have postpartum rectal temperatures higher than 39.3°C and it was assumed that all these sows were affected by MMA (Hoy 2003). The belief that higher rectal temperature identifies sows with PPDS is so generally accepted that many researchers use this criterion to identify diseased animals without estimating piglet growth and preweaning mortalities. Many published results on the MMA syndrome where piglet growth and/or litter mortality were not estimated are not included in this chapter since it is very difficult to assess whether the sows classified as "diseased" did in fact have lactation problems.

INFECTIOUS CAUSES OF PPDS

Sows with Clinical Signs of Disease

A number of postpartum lactation problems (<72 hours) are certainly the consequence of some inflammatory process related to localized or systemic infections. Localized tissue infection usually translates into measurable clinical signs such as pain, inflammation (heat), reddening and edema (Cotran et al. 1999). A localized infection can eventually affect the whole animal. Major clinical signs of a diseased sow in the postpartum period are fever (>40°C), lethargy, anorexia and eventually constipation. The main diseases affecting postpartum and lactating sows are urinary tract infections, endometritis, and mastitis. Moreover, severe milk production problems were reported with the porcine respiratory and reproduction syndrome (PRRS) (see Chapter 24). Gross and microscopic pathological evaluation of the reproductive systems of diseased and normal sows in the postpartum period suggest that endometritis is rare (Ringarp 1960; Jones 1976; Middleton-Williams et al. 1977) whereas lactation problems seem to be more frequent in sows with renal infections (Berner 1984, 1988).

Sows that were diseased in the peripartum period have increased circulating serum concentrations of acute phase proteins (haptoglobin-HPT and alpha 1-acid glycoprotein—AGP) and serum cortisol during lactation (Mirko and Bilkei 2004). The concentration of HPT was increased on days 1, 5, and 10 and normal on days 15 and 20 of lactation; AGP was normal on days 1 and 5 and increased on days 10, 15, and 20; serum cortisol concentration was elevated during the whole lactation. Litter performance of the diseased sows of the previous study was very poor (22% mortality) and is certainly related to the incapacity of these sows to produce sufficient amounts of milk.

Mastitis

Mastitis is a clear pathological entity observed in some lactating sows (Ringarp 1960; Middleton-Williams et al.

1977; Hermansson et al. 1978b; Halgaard 1983). The diseased mammary glands are warm to the touch and swollen, with a blotched appearance (Jones 1971). When many glands are involved, the sows often go off feed and have high rectal temperatures (>40°C) (Middleton-Williams et al. 1977; Halgaard 1983). The bacteria isolated from infected glands are mainly coliforms (*Escherichia coli, Klebsiella* sp, *Enterobacter* and *Citrobacter*) and bacteria of the genera *Staphylococcus* sp. and *Streptococcus* sp. (Armstrong et al. 1968; Ross et al. 1981; Persson et al. 1996).

In acute and severe mastitis, necrotic and purulent lesions are present in the mammary glands (Middleton-Williams et al. 1977), milk synthesis is altered and, when many glands are affected, piglet growth is decreased. The suppuration starting at the beginning of the infectious process can become a permanent granuloma that can be observed in culled sows. In one survey in Germany, 23% of 1000 culled sows had granulomatous lesions on some mammary glands (Bollwahn and Meermeier 1989). In another survey in Sweden, the prevalence of granulomatous mastitis in sows from different farms varied from 0 to 50% (mean 16% at weaning). Most affected sows (76%) had only one mammary gland with macroscopic lesions (Hulten et al. 2003). These data show that mastitis can affect many sows but that most of the time severe lesions are found only in a few glands.

In some studies on the importance of mastitis as a pathological entity, it is not always clear whether the sows were selected for the presence of mastitis or because the litter had retarded growth and high mortality. When sows were selected for necropsy on the basis of poor piglet performance, no macroscopic lesions consistent with mastitis were found (Nachreiner et al. 1971). Instead, mammary tissue from sows with problem litters appeared nonfunctional because it did not contain abundant quantities of milk (Martin et al. 1967; Nachreiner et al. 1971). Moreover, the higher cellular content found in the milk of sows nursing problem litters (Table 4.3) was considered to be the consequence of a concentration effect related to lower milk production rather than an indication of mastitis because the proportion of leucocytes (leucocytes/total cells) was similar in the milk of sows nursing problem and normal litters (Klopfenstein 2003). Therefore, we must consider that some problem litters are the consequence of sow mastitis but that many others are likely unrelated to it.

Endotoxemia

The absorption of endotoxins from gram-negative bacteria was proposed as an explanation for early lactation problems. Indeed, some sows (<33%) with problem litters are positive for circulating endotoxins (Morkoç et al. 1983; Pejsak and Tarasiuk 1989). Exogenous administration of gram-negative endotoxins also suppresses serum prolactin concentrations and increases sow rectal temperature and respiratory rate (Nachreiner and Ginther 1974; Elmore et al. 1978; Smith and Wagner 1984, 1985b; Tarasiuk and Pejsak 1986; de Ruijter et al. 1988). However, the effects of injection of endotoxins are of short duration, with sows fully recovering within 8 hours of injection (de Ruijter et al. 1988). Even though a continuous infusion of endotoxins causes severe piglet growth retardation (Ferguson et al. 1984), a single massive dose only retards piglet growth during the 5–8 hours after the injection (Smith and Wagner 1985b). The origin of endotoxins remains unclear, but may be urinary tract inflammation, mastitis, uterine infection, or the intestine.

Sows with Subclinical Forms of Disease

Lactation problems of some sows could be the consequence of a subclinical form of the diseases aforementioned. This hypothesis is very popular because it can explain the disproportion between the number of sows showing clinical signs of disease (rare) and those nursing problem litters (more frequent). This theory is often used as a justification for the common practice of a systematic use of antibiotics and antiinflammatory drugs for the postpartum sow.

NONINFECTIOUS CAUSES FOR PPDS

Mammary Gland Development

Allometric mammary gland development occurs mainly during the last third of gestation and continues during lactation (see mammogenesis). Mammary gland development varies between sows and could certainly explain some lactation problems related to PPDS.

The number of piglets in the litter should always be adjusted to the number of functional mammary glands. Teat malformation, inverted nipples can prevent the piglets from nursing (Labroue et al. 2001). Sows with an insufficient number of functional mammary glands should be culled.

Intensity of Milk Synthesis

Concentrations of milk lactose increase during the first days of lactation (Table 4.3) and this increase is slower among sows affected by PPDS during the first 72 hours after parturition (Klopfenstein 2003). Factors explaining the slower increase in milk synthesis among sows nursing problem litters are not known but could be the consequence of retarded lactogenesis or insufficient mammary gland development at parturition.

Homeorhesis

Sow Behavior. Some sows are aggressive and attempt to bite or crush their piglets soon after parturition, while others refuse mammary access to the piglets. These problems are more characteristic of first-parity sows, and chemical tranquilization is usually sufficient to cause the sow to relax and nursing to proceed normally.

Energy Balance. A recent study showed that serum concentrations of nonesterified fatty acids (NEFA) and glucose are lower in sows nursing litter with high preweaning mortalities (more than 1 piglet dying (Valros et al. 2003). This in conjunction with the well-known detrimental effects of heat stress on sow lactation performance indicates that the capacity of the sow to manage her energy balance is certainly a critical point. Problems of energy balance adjustments after parturition are well documented in cows (Drackley 1999) but have not yet been extensively studied in sows.

Water Balance. Water management around parturition can certainly explain some lactation problems related to PPDS. The shape of the temporal variation in water intake around parturition (Figure 4.4) indeed suggests that water availability prior to parturition is a critical point that needs to be considered in the farrowing room. Postpartum constipation observed in some sows affected by PPDS could be due to insufficient water intake before parturition.

Bivalent Ions Balance. Problems related to metabolic balance adjustment of bivalent ions (calcium, phosphorous and magnesium) are well-described in cows (Goff 2000) and are often suspected in sows. Hermansson et al. (1978a) reported that sows affected by agalactia problems had lower circulating calcium and magnesium concentrations. Klopfenstein (2003) observed higher serum phosphorus and calcium concentrations in sows nursing litters with lower growth rates. Moreover, DeRouchey et al. (2003) were able to increase piglet survivability up to day 10 by feeding sows a diet with a low electrolyte balance from day 109 of gestation and during lactation. This strategy is often used in dairy cows and is known for its beneficial impact on calcium and phosphorus balance in the postpartum cow. The later observations suggest that inadequate adjustment of bivalent ions balance after parturition might explain some lactation problems related to PPDS of sows.

Hormonal Balance. As early as 1967, an endocrine role in the pathogenesis of agalactia was suggested (Martin et al. 1967). Agalactic sows had smaller ovaries and thyroid glands and larger adrenal glands than control sows. In a later study, there was no difference in the size of these three glands but thyroid function was depressed in agalactic sows (Wagner 1972). More recently, it was shown that the hormonal status of first-litter sows with hypogalactia or agalactia differs from that of healthy sows. Concentrations of cortisol both before and after farrowing and prepartum levels of glucose were lower in hypogalactic sows (Samanc et al. 1992). Finally, de Passillé et al. (1993) noted a relationship between poor piglet performance and high concentrations of progesterone in the blood of sows after parturition.

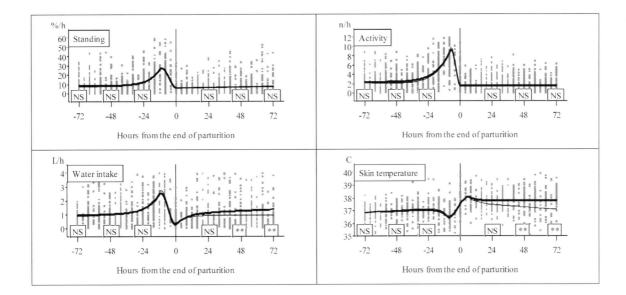

4.4. *Peripartum temporal variation of some behavioral traits and skin temperature of sows nursing litters with slow (≤77 g/kg/day—thin line— Problem litters) and normal growth rates (>77 g/kg/day—thick line—Normal litters). NS = non significant difference, ** = significant difference at p <0.05. Adapted from Klopfenstein 2003.*

Feed Toxicity. Grain contamination with ergot by-products produced by *Claviceps purpurea* has been reported to cause lactation failure in sows (Penny 1970; Anderson and Werdin 1977). Ergot derivates are known to suppress prolactin release (Whitacre and Threlfall 1981; Bevers et al. 1983; Smith and Wagner 1985a), which could in turn inhibit mammary growth and lactation. Diagnosis is based on a history of grain changes and sudden appearance of a great number of affected sows with flaccid mammary glands and carpal erosions but normal rectal temperature. However this condition is rare.

TREATMENT

Every producer wants to maintain the health of the sows and prevent poor litter performance. Veterinarians are placed in a delicate situation when they are called upon to propose treatment for a poorly defined problem for which overtreatment is certainly leading to increased costs of production and unjustified medication overuse. A good strategy to reduce the consequences of PPDS should be based on three levels of intervention:

1. Defining a treatment for the truly diseased postpartum sows
2. Rapidly identifying the problem litters of sows without clinical manifestations and determining a treatment for those sows and piglets
3. Reducing the incidence of problem litters in the herd by addressing the risk factors

The Diseased Sow

The treatment of choice for the diseased sows is antibiotic and/or antiinflammatory treatment to help cure the disease. Moreover, sow treatment must also ensure adequate mammary gland function to sustain piglet growth. In the worst cases, the best strategy is to foster the piglets of the diseased sow to another healthy sow.

Systematic treatment of all sows after farrowing with an antibiotic and sometimes with nonsteroidal antiinflammatory drugs (NSAID) is a common practice in modern farrowing houses. Different strategies for the systematic administration of antibiotics were proposed:

1. Adding antibiotics to the feed from 7 days prepartum to 7 days postpartum, which could decrease piglet mortality by 43% (7.34% vs. 4.18%) and increase weaning weights by 8% (Tabjara et al. 1992)
2. Daily injections of antibiotics for the first 2 days postpartum (Rose et al. 1996)
3. In-feed medication and one injection of antibiotics on the day of parturition (Schoning and Plonait 1990)

Although all these strategies can be used when a whole herd is severely affected by PPDS, systematic treatment of all sows should be only short-term to avoid medication overuse.

Antibiotics. The selection of an antibiotic should be based on its spectrum of activity against bacterial organisms identified in postpartum diseased sows and thought to be related to PPDS. Unfortunately, identifying the most common bacterium related to the diseased sows is often difficult due to the diversity of the clinical signs.

Nonsteroidal Antiinflammatory Drug (NSAID). NSAID treatments seem to have a beneficial effect on health of affected sows. Treatment strategies usually consist of one treatment on the day of parturition and sometimes a second treatment the next day. Drugs that have been proposed are: flunixin (2 mg/kg) (Cerne et al. 1984), tolfenamic acid (2–4 mg/kg) (Rose et al. 1996), meloxicam (0.4 mg/kg) (Hirsch et al. 2003; Hoy and Friton 2004).

Stimulating Milk Production

One of the objectives of the treatment strategy is to stimulate milk flow as rapidly as possible to minimize the consequence of PPDS. Repeated use of oxytocin is certainly the most frequent treatment administered to sows to stimulate milk production.

Oxytocin. Parenteral administration of synthetic oxytocin is a very efficient way to trigger milk ejection. The manufacturers' recommended dose for sows varies from 30 to 50 IU intramuscularly (Canadian Animal Health Institute 2001). In our experience, intramuscular injections of oxytocin do not always trigger the milk ejection process and more predictable results are obtained with intravenous injections of 10 IU. The variable response with intramuscular injections might be related to the product being deposited between muscles or in the fat pad and to the very short half-life of oxytocin. In fact, the short half-life (6–7 minutes) of oxytocin is the reason why it can be administered safely at hourly intervals for at least 6 hours (Knaggs 1967).

Although efficient and considered as safe, repeated use of oxytocin might have some detrimental effects on sows. Indeed, its use was reported to be related to poorer herd performance in some epidemiological studies (Bilkei Papp 1994; Ravel et al. 1996). Moreover, somatic cell counts in sow's milk were found to increase with oxytocin administration, and this was more apparent when oxytocin was injected intramuscularly than intravenously (Garst et al. 1999).

Prolactin Stimulators. Prolactin and prolactin-stimulators were suggested as methods to stimulate milk synthesis of sows affected with PPDS. Purified porcine prolactin is commercially available only in minute quantities. Therefore, most research on PPDS treatment with prolactin has focused on stimulating prolactin release. Administration of various phenothiazine and butyrophenone tranquilizers (e.g., chlorpromazine, acetylpromazine, haloperidol, and azaperone) significantly increases prolactin concentrations in various species; however, they have generally not been effective in stimulating prolactin release in the pig (Smith and Wagner 1985a). Thyroid-stimulating hormone was shown to be effective in increasing prolactin concentrations in swine but for such short duration (<45 minutes) that it is unlikely to be clinically useful (Smith and Wagner 1985a).

Vaccinations

Sow mammary glands initially infected with coliform bacteria do not appear to develop resistance to subsequent infections (Bertschinger and Buhlmann 1990), thereby suggesting that the development of a vaccine for the prevention of coliform mastitis is unlikely. On the other hand, vaccination against urinary tract infections at 4 and 2 weeks before parturition was reported to increase the overall lactation performance of sows (Pejsak et al. 1988).

Supportive Treatment for Piglets

Once problem litters are identified, the main objectives are to avoid piglet dehydration and provide an alternative source of energy. Observations suggest that piglets will drink appreciable amounts of tap water on the first day following birth, particularly if milk supply is limited (Fraser et al. 1988). Water intake is further increased when using a specially designed water dispenser with air bubbles (Phillips and Fraser 1991). It was speculated that under low milk intake conditions, water intake may help prevent dehydration and promote survival of the piglets. Low-birth-weight piglets suckling a sow affected with PPDS need to be transferred rapidly to another sow with good milking capacity. The lower milk production of affected sows will be less detrimental to piglets of heavy birth weight, and most of them may still reach acceptable weaning weights. Moreover, piglets can be efficiently raised with a combination of milk replacers and highly digestible adapted feed.

PREVENTION AND RISK FACTORS

One of the keys in reducing the incidence of problem litters in a herd is the identification and correction of specific risk factors. Factors related to mammary gland development, milk synthesis, and inadequate lactation homeorhesis are certainly crucial. However, because of the complexity of the underlying causes of PPDS, other specific risk factors associated with a high prevalence of problem litters have been described. These factors are not necessarily of an etiologic nature; however, the interplay between some of them will increase the incidence of PPDS. The identified risk factors are mainly related to sow body condition at farrowing, sow constipation, housing and environment.

Sow Body Condition

Maintaining optimal body condition of all sows in the herd is important to reduce the prevalence of PPDS. This is not always easy, because a small error in the amount of feed distributed over the whole gestation period can lead to overweight or underweight sows at the time of parturition (Martineau and Klopfenstein 1996). Sows maintained in pens have more variable body weights, the most aggressive often being overweight while submissive animals are underweight (Martineau 1990; Marchant 1997). Fat sows are also more likely to take longer to farrow (Bilkei 1992; Madec et al. 1992) and to have more stillborn piglets (Zaleski and Hacker 1993; Bilkei Papp 1994).

Sow Constipation

Postpartum constipation was observed in some sows nursing problem litters (Ringarp 1960; Hermansson et al. 1978b). Feeding high-fiber diets in late gestation was therefore proposed and has been widely used in order to decrease the incidence of early lactation problems (Ringarp 1960; Wallace et al. 1974). When fibers are simply added to a diet, the concentrations of the other components are decreased accordingly (Sandstedt et al. 1979; Jensen 1981; Sandstedt and Sjogren 1982; Goransson 1989a,b). As previously discussed, sow water availability is certainly a crucial factor to consider because insufficient water intake just before farrowing can certainly enhance postpartum constipation. Moreover, low postpartum water intake and low activity level of the sows were also proposed as risk factors for early lactation problems (Fraser and Phillips 1989).

Housing and Environment

Housing and general herd management can affect the prevalence of sows affected by PPDS. In one study, there were more litters with starving piglets in herds where the sows farrowed in confinement than when they farrowed on the pasture (Backstrom et al. 1982). Sows are exposed to many changes when they are moved from the gestating room to the farrowing room. Research results, however, do not suggest that these changes are harmful to sows. Indeed, allowing sows to adapt to the new environment for more than a week, rather than only a few days, before parturition was not associated with a lower prevalence of problem litters (Klopfenstein et al. 1995). Stray voltage in the farrowing unit was also suspected as a source of lactation problems (Gillepsie 1984); yet, recent research did not support this hypothesis (Robert et al. 1996). Regular washing of the farrowing unit was reported to be associated with lower preweaning mortality (Ravel et al. 1996).

Sow and piglet management around parturition, although difficult to assess, is known to be extremely important. Supervision and attendance at farrowing time is reported to decrease the number of stillborn piglets and preweaning mortality (Holyoake et al. 1995). Care must be taken to ensure that the sow and piglets are able to drink from the watering system in the farrowing room. Attention must be given to the quality of the environment. Slippery floors are one of the main causes of low activity of lactating sows and may lead to many health problems, including PPDS, and to reduced feed and water intakes. On the other hand, more interventions at farrowing are not always a good practice. Indeed, obstetric aid by either herd managers or veterinarians results in a fourfold increase in the sow's risk of acquiring early lactation problems (Jorsal 1986) and increases the incidence of postfarrowing vulvar discharges and endometritis (Bara and Cameron 1996).

Temperature control in the farrowing room is certainly a crucial factor affecting sow lactation performances (see heat stress). It is essential to provide a localized warm environment for newborn piglets but the temperature requirement of the sow must also be taken into consideration since her zone of thermoneutrality is much lower than that of piglets. In modern swine units, where farrowings are managed as all-in/all-out on a room basis, it is much easier to adjust the temperature according to the physiological state of the sow and her piglets. We generally recommend that room temperature be maintained warm (20–22°C) for the 2–3 days after farrowing to favor piglet survival. However, after this crucial period, room temperature can be gradually decreased to attain 18°C or even 15°C on day 10 of lactation (Farmer et al. 1998). Indeed, when an adequate draft-free heat zone is provided for the piglets, the ambient temperature can be decreased to 15°C on day 8 of lactation with no detrimental effects on sow and litter performances. It is important that the extra heat provided is directed away from the sow and her udder and that it be rapidly removed, when not needed, to favor the sow's well-being and maximize her milk production. One must also keep in mind that position of the heat lamps has an impact on the spatial behavior of neonatal pigs (Titterington and Fraser 1975).

Others

Feeding Strategy. It was hypothesized that a reduced feed consumption in first days of lactation decreases the incidence of lactation failure. However, gradually increasing feed consumption of sows in the first week postpartum instead of feeding ad libitum within 16 hours of farrowing also showed no advantage for litter performance or occurrences of lactation failure (Moser et al. 1987).

Prostaglandins on the Farrowing Day. Prostaglandins are luteolytic agents causing a prepartum decline in progesterone and the release of relaxin from the corpora lutea. They are widely used for the induction of farrowing (Ehnvall et al. 1977), resulting in an immediate and sharp increase in prolactin concentrations lasting approximately 6 hours (Hansen 1979). In some herds with a significant percentage of gilts and sows showing PPDS, induction of parturition with the F series of prostaglandins has proven effective in reducing the incidence of PPDS (Cerne and Jochle 1981; Holtz et al. 1983), whereas it had no effect in other herds (Ehnvall et al. 1977; Hansen 1979). Prostaglandins could be effective in treating PPDS caused by retarded lactogenesis since incomplete luteolysis of corpora lutea can lead to high progesterone concentrations, which inhibit lactogenesis. Moreover, postpartum administration of prostaglandins can have a beneficial effect on uterine involution and prevention of severe clinical endometritis (Waldmann and Heide 1996).

Vitamin E. Some research has suggested a relationship between diets deficient in selenium and vitamin E, and sow lactational problems (Trapp et al. 1970; Whitehair and Miller 1986). The exact mode of action has not been established, but these microelements may give some protection against endotoxins because they both play a role in the maintenance of cellular integrity and in leukocyte function (Elmore and Martin 1986). On the other hand, primary deficiencies are uncommon since vitamin E and selenium are generally supplemented in feed. In fact, increasing dietary levels of vitamin E from 30 to 60 IU did not decrease the prevalence of MMA diagnosed subjectively at parturition based on udder hardness and vulvar discharge (Mahan et al. 2000). In another study, injections of vitamin E (400 IU) and selenium (3 mg) to sows three times during gestation, while they were fed normal levels of these nutrients, increased the survival rate of piglets but did not affect litter weights at weaning (Chavez and Patton 1986).

REFERENCES

Aherne FX, Williams IH. 1992. Nutrition for optimizing breeding herd performance. Vet Clin North Am Food Anim Pract 8:589–608.

Akers RM. 2002. Lactation and the Mammary Gland. Ames: Iowa State University Press.

Algers B. 1993. Nursing in pigs: Communicating needs and distributing resources. J Anim Sci 71:2826–2831.

Algers B, de Passillé AMB. 1991. A new view of piglet mortality (En ny syn pa smagrisdodligheten). Sven Vet Tidn 43:659–663.

Algers B, Rojanasthien S, Uvnas Moberg K. 1990. The relationship between teat stimulation, oxytocin release and grunting rate in the sow. Appl Anim Behav Sci 26:267–276.

Anderson JF, Werdin RE. 1977. Ergotism manifested as agalactia and gangrene in sows. J Am Vet Med Assoc 170:1089–1091.

Armstrong CH, Hooper BE, Martin CE. 1968. Microflora associated with agalactia syndrome of sows. Am J Vet Res 29:1401–1407.

Armstrong JD, Coffey MT, Esbenshade KL, Campbell RM, Heimer EP. 1994. Concentrations of hormones and metabolites, estimates of metabolism, performance, and reproductive performance of sows actively immunized against growth hormone-releasing factor. J Anim Sci 72:1570–1577.

Ash RW, Heap RB. 1975. Oestrogen, progesterone and corticosteroid concentrations in peripheral plasma of sows during pregnancy, parturition, lactation and after weaning. J Endocrinol 64:141–154.

Atwood CS, Hartmann PE. 1993. The concentration of fat, protein and lactose in sow's colostrum from sucked and unsucked glands during lactogenesis II. Aust J Agric Res 44:1457–1465.

——. 1995. Assessment of mammary gland metabolism in the sow. III. Cellular metabolites in the mammary secretion and plasma following weaning. J Dairy Res 62:221–236.

Auldist DE, Morrish L, Eason P, King RH. 1998. The influence of litter size on milk production of sows. Anim Sci 67:333–337.

Auldist DE, Carlson D, Morrish L, Wakeford CM, King RH. 2000. The influence of suckling interval on milk production of sows. J Anim Sci 78:2026–2031.

Aumaitre A, Salmon Legagneur E. 1961. Influence de l'alimentation complémentaire sur la croissance du porcelet avant le sevrage. Ann Zootech 10:127–140.

Backstrom L, Connors J, Price W, Larson R, Morko A. 1982. Mastitis-metritis-agalactia (MMA) in the sow: A field survey of MMA and other farrowing disorders under different gestation and farrowing housing conditions. Proc Int Pig Vet Soc Congr 7:175–175.

Bara MR, Cameron RDA. 1996. The effect of faecal accumulation in farrowing crates and hand farrowing on the incidence of post-farrowing discharges and reproductive performance in sows. Proc Int Pig Vet Soc Congr 14:574–574.

Barber RS, Braude R, Mitchell KG. 1955. Studies on milk production of large white pigs. J Agric Sci 46:97–118.

Barone R. 1978. Splanchnologie, foetus et ses annexes, péritoine et topographie abdominale. Anatomie Comparée des Mammifères Domestiques. École nationale vétérinaire, Lyon.

Bauman DE, Currie WB. 1980. Partitioning of nutrients during pregnancy and lactation: A review of mechanisms involving homeostasis and homeorhesis. J Dairy Sci 63:1514–1529.

Bauman DE, Brown RE, Davies CL. 1970. Pathways of fatty acid synthesis and reducing equivalent generation in mammary gland of rat, sow, and cow. Arch Biochem Biophys 140:237–244.

Benjaminsen E. 1981a. Effect of prolactin suppression on the ovarian activity in the lactating sow. Acta Vet Scand 22:189–197.

——. 1981b. Plasma prolactin in the sow with emphasis on variation in resumption of ovarian activity after weaning. Acta Vet Scand 22:67–77.

Berner H. 1984. Importance of urinary tract infections in development of puerperal endometritis in the sow. Tierarz Umsch 39:450–458.

——. 1988. Cystitis in the diagnosis of metritis-mastitis-agalactia Cystitis in der MMA—Diagnostik. Prakt Tierarzt 69:124–130.

Bertschinger HU, Buhlmann A. 1990. Absence of protective immunity in mammary glands after experimentally induced coliform mastitis. Proc Int Pig Vet Soc Congr 11:175–175.

Bevers M, Willemse AH, Kruip TAM. 1983. The effect of bromocriptine on luteinizing hormones levels in the lactating sow; Evidence for a suppressive action by prolactin and the suckling stimulus. Acta Endocrinol 104:261–265.

Beyer M, Jentsch W, Hoffmann L, Schiemann R, Klein M. 1994. Studies on energy and nitrogen metabolism of pregnant and lactating sows and sucking piglets. 4. Chemical composition and energy content of the conception products, the reproductive organs as well as liveweight gains or losses of pregnant and lactating sows. Arch Anim Nutr 46:7–36.

Bilkei G. 1992. The effect of various treatments on the duration of parturition in sows, with reference to dam body condition. Tierarztl Prax 20:153–158.

Bilkei G, Goos T, Bolcskei A. 1994. Influence of the number of functioning mammary complexes in sows on the litter weight of intensively-reared piglets at four weeks of age. Prakt Tierarzt 75:16–21.

Bilkei Papp G. 1994. Perinatal losses—General condition of sows. III. Experiences obtained with prednisolone pretreatment. Magy Allatorv Lap 49:680–683.

Boe K. 1991. The process of weaning in pigs: When the sow decides. Appl Anim Behav Sci 30:47–59.

Bollwahn W, Meermeier D. 1989. Frequency and diagnosis of chronic udder lesions in breeding sows (abattoir survey). Berl Munch Tierarztl Wochenschr 102:223–227.

Bourne FJ. 1976. Humoral immunity in the pig. Vet Rec 98:499–501.

Bourne FJ, Curtis J. 1973. The transfer of immunoglobulins IgG, IgA and IgM from serum to colostrum and milk in the sow. Immunology 24:157–162.

Boyd RD, Kensinger RS, Harrell RJ, Bauman DE. 1995. Nutrient uptake and endocrine regulation of milk synthesis by mammary tissue of lactating sows. J Anim Sci 73:36–56.

Brazeau P, Vale W, Burgus R, Ling N, Butcher M, Rivier J, Guillemin R. 1973. Hypothalamic polypeptide that inhibits the secretion of immunoreactive pituitary growth hormone. Science 179:77–79.

Bryson JM, Jackson SC, Wang H, Hurley WL. 2001. Cellular uptake of taurine by lactating porcine mammary tissue. Comp Bioch Phys 128:667–673.

Buttle HL. 1988. Role of the ovaries in inducing mammogenesis in pregnant pigs. J Endocrinol 118:41–45.

Cabell SB, Esbenshade KL. 1990. Effect of feeding thyrotropin-releasing hormone to lactating sows. J Anim Sci 68:4292–4302.

Calhoun ML, Stinson AW. 1987. Integuments. In Texbook of Veterinary Histology. Philadelphia: Lea & Febiger, 351 pp.

Campbell RG, Dunkin AC. 1982. The effect of birth weight on the estimated milk intake-growth and body composition of sow-reared piglets. Anim Prod 35:193–197.

Canadian Animal Health Institute. 2001. Compendium of Veterinary Products (7th ed). North American Compendiums Ltd, Hensall, Ont.

Castren H, Algers B, Jensen P, Saloniemi H. 1989. Suckling behaviour and milk consumption in newborn piglets as a response to sow grunting. Appl Anim Behav Sci 24:227–238.

Castren H, Algers B, Saloniemi H. 1991. Weight gain pattern in piglets during the first 24 h after farrowing. Livest Prod Sci 28:321–330.

Castren H, Algers B, de Passillé AMB, Rushen J, Uvnas Moberg K. 1993. Early milk ejection, prolonged parturition and periparturient oxytocin release in the pig. Anim Prod 57:465–471.

Cerne F, Jochle W. 1981. Clinical evaluations of a new prostaglandin analog in pigs: Control of parturition and of the MMA-syndrome. Theriogenology 16:459–467.

Cerne F, Jerkovic I, Debeljak C. 1984. Influence of Finadyne on some clinical signs of MMA. Proc Int Pig Vet Soc Congr 8:290–290.

Chavez ER, Patton KL. 1986. Response to injectable selenium and vitamin E on reproductive performance of sows receiving a standard commercial diet. Can J Anim Sci 66:1065–1074.

Chertkov DD. 1986. Rearing of suckled piglets. Zhivotnovodstvo 8:55–56.

Cornette M. 1950. Septicémie puerpérale de la truie. Rec Méd Vét 126:31–36.

Cotran RS, Kumar V, Collins T. 1999. Acute and chronic inflammation. In Robbins Pathologic Basis of Disease. (6th ed.). RS Cotran, V Kumar, T Collins, SL Robbins, B Schmitt, eds. New York: W.B. Saunders, pp. 50–88.

Crenshaw TD, Grieshop CM, McMurtry JP, Schricker BR. 1989. Exogenous porcine prolactin and somatotropin injections did not alter sow lactation performance [Abstract]. J Dairy Sci 72:258–259.

Cromvell GL, Stahly TS, Edgerton LA, Monegue HJ, Burnell TW, Schenck BB, Schricker BR. 1992. Recombinant porcine somatotropin for sows during late gestation and throughout lactation. J Anim Sci 70:1404–1416.

Cronin GM, Smith JA, Hodge FM, Hemsworth PH. 1994. The behaviour of primiparous sows around farrowing in response to restraint and straw bedding. Appl Anim Behav Sci 39:269–280.

Cronin GM, Simpson GJ, Hemsworth PH. 1996. The effects of the gestation and farrowing environments on sow and piglet behaviour and piglet survival and growth in early lactation. Appl Anim Behav Sci 46:175–192.

Cronin GM, Leeson E, Cronin JG, Barnett JL. 2001. The effect of broadcasting sow suckling grunts in the lactation shed on piglet growth. Asian-Aust J Anim Sci 14:1019–1023.

D'Allaire S, Drolet R, Brodeur D. 1996. Sow mortality associated with high ambient temperatures. Can Vet J 37:237–239.

Delouis C. 1986. Le Porc et son Élevage: Bases Scientifiques et Techniques. Maloine, Paris.

DeRouchey JM, Hancock JD, Hines RH, Cummings KR, Lee DJ, Maloney CA, Dean DW, Park JS, Cao H. 2003. Effects of dietary electrolyte balance on the chemistry of blood and urine in lactating sows and sow litter performance. J Anim Sci 81:3067–3074.

de Passillé AMB, Rushen J. 1989a. Suckling and teat disputes by neonatal piglets. Appl Anim Behav Sci 22:23–38.

——. 1989b. Using early suckling behavior and weight gain to identify piglets at risk. Can J Anim Sci 69:535–544.

de Passillé AMB, Rushen J, Hartsock TG. 1988. Ontogeny of teat fidelity in pigs and its relation to competition at suckling. Can J Anim Sci 68:325–338.

de Passillé AMB, Rushen J, Foxcroft GR, Aherne FX, Schaefer A. 1993. Performance of young pigs: Relationships with periparturient progesterone, prolactin, and insulin of sows. J Anim Sci 71:179–184.

de Ruijter K, Verheijden JHM, Pijpers A, Berends J. 1988. The role of endotoxin in the pathogenesis of coliform mastitis in sows. Vet Q 10:186–190.

Dobson H. 1988. Softening and dilation of the uterine cervix. In Oxford Reviews of Reproductive Biology. JR Clarke, ed. Toronto: Oxford University Press, pp. 491–513.

Dodd SC, Forsyth IA, Buttle HL, Gurr MI, Dils RR. 1994. Milk whey proteins in plasma of sows: variation with physiological state. J Dairy Res 61:21–34.

Dorland WAN. 1985. Dorland's Illustrated Medical Dictionary. (26th ed). Philadelphia: Saunders.

Dourmad JY, Noblet J, Etienne M. 1998. Effect of protein and lysine supply on performance, nitrogen balance, and body composition changes of sows during lactation. J Anim Sci 76:542–550.

Drackley JK. 1999. Biology of dairy cows during the transition period: The final frontier. J Dairy Sci 82:2259–2273.

Drendel C, Wendt K. 1993a. Cell count, lysozyme content, pH and electrical conductivity of sow's milk during lactation. Monatsh Veterinarmed 48:307–313.

——. 1993b. Response of porcine mammary glands to bacterial infection. Monatsh Veterinarmed 48:413–417.

Dubreuil P, Pelletier G, Lapierre H, Couture Y, Morisset J, Gaudreau P, Brazeau P. 1987. Effect of growth hormone-releasing factor (1–29) NH2, and thyrotropin-releasing factor on growth hormone release in lactating sows. Reprod Nutr Dev 27:601–603.

Dubreuil P, Pelletier G, Petitclerc D, Lapierre H, Couture Y, Gaudreau P, Morisset J, Brazeau P. 1990. Influence of growth hormone-releasing factor on sows blood components, milk composition and piglet performance. Can J Anim Sci 70:821–832.

Dusza L, Krzymowska H. 1981. Plasma prolactin levels in sows during pregnancy—Parturition and early lactation. J Reprod Fertil 61:131–134.

Dusza L, Sobczak J, Jana B, Murdza A, Bluj W. 1991. Application of Biolactin-2 (purified porcine prolactin) in stimulation of lactation in sows. Medycyna Weter 47:418–421.

Dyck GE, Swierstra EE. 1987. Causes of piglet death from birth to weaning. Can J Anim Sci 67:543–547.

Ehnvall R, Einarsson S, Larson K, Hard af Segerstad C, Westerberg L. 1977. Prostaglandin-induced parturition in swine—A field study on its accuracy after treatment with different amounts of PGFa. Nord Vet Med 29:376–380.

Ellendorf F, Forsling ML, Poulain DA. 1982. The milk ejection reflex in the pig. J Physiol 333:577–579.

Elmore RG, Martin CE. 1986. Mammary glands. In Diseases of Swine (6th ed). AD Leman, BE Straw, WL Glock, WL Mengeling, HC Penny, E Scholl, eds. Ames: Iowa State University Press.

Elmore RG, Martin CE, Berg JN. 1978. Absorption of Escherichia coli endotoxin from the mammary glands and uteri of early postpartum sows and gilts. Theriogenology 10:439–446.

Elmore RG, Martin CE, Riley JL, Littledike T. 1979. Body temperatures of farrowing swine. J Am Vet Med Assoc 174:620–622.

Elsley FWH. 1971. Nutrition and Lactation in the Sow. Butterworth, London.

English PR, Morrison V. 1984. Causes and prevention of piglet mortality. Pig News Info 5:369–376.

Evans PA, Newby TJ, Stokes CR, Bourne FJ. 1982. A study of cells in the mammary secretions of sows. Vet Immunol Immunopathol 3:515–527.

Fahmy MH, Bernard C. 1971. Causes of mortality in Yorkshire pigs from birth to 20 weeks of age. Can J Anim Sci 51:351–359.

Farmer C. 1995. Increasing growth hormone concentrations in pregnant and lactating sows: Is it beneficial? Pig News Info 16:117N–121N.

———. 2001. The role of prolactin for mammogenesis and galactopoiesis in swine. Livest Prod Sci 70:105–113.

Farmer C, Dubreuil P, Pelletier G, Petitclerc D, Brazeau P. 1990. Active immunization against somatostatin in gestating gilts and the effect of transferred immunity on piglets. Can J Anim Sci 70:211–218.

Farmer C, Dubreuil P, Pelletier G, Petitclerc D, Gaudreau P, Brazeau P. 1991. Effects of active immunization against somatostatin (SRIF) and/or injections of growth hormone-releasing factor (GRF) during gestation on hormonal and metabolic profiles in sows. Dom Anim Endocr 8:415–422.

Farmer C, Petitclerc D, Pelletier G. 1992. The effect of growth hormone-releasing factor (GRF) on the performance of lactating sows. Bulletin Agriculture Canada, Research Branch, No. 15:5–6.

Farmer C, Robert S, Matte JJ. 1996. Lactation performance of sows fed a bulky diet during gestation and receiving growth hormone-releasing factor during lactation. J Anim Sci 74:1298–1306.

Farmer C, Robert S, Rushen J. 1997. Bromocriptine inhibits milk production in sows. Livest Prod Sci 50:165–166.

Farmer C, Robert S, Choiniere Y. 1998. Reducing ambient temperature in farrowing houses with a new controlled-environment system. Can J Anim Sci 78:23–28.

Farmer C, Sorensen MT, Robert S, Petitclerc D. 1999. Administering exogenous porcine prolactin to lactating sows: Milk yield, mammary gland composition, and endocrine and behavioral responses. J Anim Sci 77:1851–1859.

Farmer C, Sorensen MT, Petitclerc D. 2000. Inhibition of prolactin in the last trimester of gestation decreases mammary gland development in gilts. J Anim Sci 78:1303–1309.

Farmer C, Palin MF, Sorensen MT, Robert S. 2001. Lactational performance, nursing and maternal behavior of Upton-Meishan and Large White sows. Can J Anim Sci 81:487–493.

Farmer C, Petitclerc D. 2003. Specific window of prolactin inhibition in late gestation decreases mammary parenchymal tissue development in gilts. J Anim Sci 81:1823–1829.

Farmer C, Fisette K, Robert S, Quesnel H, Laforest JP. 2004a. Use of recorded nursing grunts during lactation in two breeds of sows. II. Effects on sow performance and mammary development. Can J Anim Sci, In press.

Farmer C, Petitclerc D, Sorensen MT, Dourmad JY. 2004b. Impacts of dietary protein level and feed restriction during prepuberty on mammogenesis in gilts. J Anim Sci 82:2343–2351.

Ferguson FG, Confer F, Pinto A, Weber J, Stout T, Kensinger M. 1984. Long-term endotoxin exposure on the sow and neonatal piglet a model for MMA. Proc Int Pig Vet Soc Cong 8:289–289.

Fisette K, Laforest JP, Robert S, Farmer C. 2004. Use of recorded nursing grunts during lactation in two breeds of sows. I. Effects on nursing behaviour and litter performance. Can J Anim Sci, In press.

Flint DJ. 1995. Hormonal regulation of uptake and metabolism of milk precursors in normal lactating mammary gland. J Anim Sci 73:61–71.

Ford JA, Jr., Kim SW, Rodriguez-Zas SL, Hurley WL. 2003. Quantification of mammary gland tissue size and composition changes after weaning in sows. J Anim Sci 81:2583–2589.

Fraser D. 1976. The nursing and suckling behaviour of pigs. I. The importance of stimulation of the anterior teats. Br Vet J 129:324–336.

———. 1977. Some behavioural aspects of milk ejection failure by sows. Br Vet J 133:126–133.

———. 1980. A review of the behavioural mechanism of milk ejection of the domestic pig. Appl Anim Eth 6:247–255.

———. 1984. Some factors influencing the availability of colostrum to piglets. Anim Prod 39:115–123.

———. 1990. Behavioral perspectives on piglet survival. J Reprod Fertil (Suppl) 40:355–370.

Fraser D, Rushen J. 1992. Colostrum intake by newborn piglets. Can J Anim Sci 72:1–13.

Fraser D, Nicholls C, Fagan W. 1985. A sow milking machine designed to compare the yield of different teats. J Agric Eng Res 31:371–376.

Fraser D, Phillips PA, Thompson BK, Peeters Weem WB. 1988. Use of water by piglets in the first days after birth. Can J Anim Sci 68:603–610.

Fraser D, Phillips PA. 1989. Lethargy and low water intake by sows during early lactation: A cause of low piglet weight gains and survival? Appl Anim Behav Sci 24:13–22.

Furniss SJ. 1987. Measurement of rectal temperature to predict "mastitis, metritis and agalactia" (MMA) in sows after farrowing. Prev Vet Med 5:133–139.

Gandhi SS, Getty R. 1969a. Cutaneous nerves of the trunk of the domestic pig with special reference to the spinal nerves. Part II. Cutaneous nerves of the thoracic region. Iowa State J Sci 44:15–30.

———. 1969b. Cutaneous nerves of the trunk of the domestic pig with special reference to the spinal nerves. Part III. Cutaneous nerves of the lumbar-sacral-and coccygeal regions. Iowa State J Sci 44:31–43.

Garst AS, Ball SF, Williams BL, Wood CM, Knight JW, Moll HD, Aardema CH, Gwazdauskas FC. 1999. Influence of pig substitution on milk yield, litter weights, and milk composition of machine milked sows. J Anim Sci 77:1624–1630.

Genest M, D'Allaire S. 1995. Feeding strategies during the lactation period for first-parity sows. Can J Anim Sci 75:461–467.

Ghoshal NG. 1975. Porcine nervous system. Spina nerves. In Sisson and Grossmann's the Anatomy of the Domestic Animal (5th ed). R Getty, ed. Toronto: W.B. Saunders, pp. 1383–1396.

Gillespie TG. 1984. Stray electric voltage. Proc Swine Herd Health Program Conf 260.

Goff JP. 2000. Pathophysiology of calcium and phosphorus disorders. Vet Clin North Am Food Anim Pract 16:319–337.

Goransson L. 1989a. The effect of dietary crude fibre content on the frequency of post partum agalactia in the sow. J Vet Med 36:474–479.

———. 1989b. The effect of feed allowance in late pregnancy on the occurrence of agalactia post-partum in the sow. J Am Vet Med Assoc 36:505–513.

Greco D, Stabenfeldt H. 1997. Endocrine glands and their function. In Textbook of Veterinary Physiology (2nd ed). JG Cunningham, ed. Toronto: W.B.Saunders, pp. 404–439.

Grun D, Reiner G, Dzapo V. 1993a. Investigations on breed differences in milk yield of swine. Part I. Methodology of mechanical milking and milk yield. Reprod Dom Anim 28:14–21.

———. 1993b. Studies on breed differences in milk yield of pigs. II. Milk composition and its effect on piglet development during the suckling period. Reprod Dom Anim 28:22–27.

Guillemin R, Brazeau P, Bohlen P, Esch F, Ling N, Wehrenberg WB. 1982. Growth hormone-releasing factor from a human pancreatic tumor that caused acromegaly. Science 218:585–587.

Gut-à Porta R, Baustad B, Jorgensen A. 2004. Teats and mammary glands in sows in subsequent lactations—A pilot study. Proc Int Pig Vet Soc Congr 18:631.

Guthrie HD, Meckley PE, Young EP, Hartsock TG. 1987. Effect of altrenogest and Lutalyse on parturition control, plasma progesterone, unconjugated estrogen and 13,14-dihydro-15- keto-prostaglandin F2alpha in sows. J Anim Sci 65:203–211.

Hacker RR. 1970. Studies on the development and function of porcine mammary glands. Ph.D. Thesis. Purdue University, West Lafayette, Indiana.

Hacker RR, Hill DL. 1972. Nucleic acid content of mammary glands of virgin and pregnant gilts. J Dairy Sci 55:1295–1299.

Halgaard C. 1983. Epidemiologic factors in puerperal diseases of sows. Nord Vet Med 35:161–174.

Hansen LH. 1979. Reproductive efficiency and incidence of MMA after controlled farrowing using a prostaglandin analogue, cloprostenol. Nord Vet Med 31:122–128.

Harkins M, Boyd RD, Bauman DE. 1989. Effects of recombinant porcine somatotropin on lactational performance and metabolite patterns in sows and growth of nursing pigs. J Anim Sci 67:1997–2008.

Harrell RJ, Thomas MJ, Boyd RD. 1993. Limitations of sow milk yield on baby pig growth. Proc Cornell Nutrition Conf Feed Manufacturers 156–164.

Hartmann PE, Holmes MA. 1989. Sow lactation. In Manipulating Pig Production II. JL Barnett, DP Hennessy, eds. Albury, Australia: Australasian Pig Science Association. pp. 72–97.

Hartmann PE, Thompson MJ, Kennaugh LM, Atwood CS. 1995. Metabolic regulation of sow lactation. In Manipulating Pig Production V. DP Hennessy, PD Cranwell, eds. Werribee, Australia: Australasian Pig Science Association. pp. 26–29.

Hartmann PE, Whitely JL, Willcox DL. 1984. Lactose in plasma during lactogenesis, established lactation and weaning in sows. J Physiol 347:453–463.

Hartsock TG, Graves HB. 1976. Neonatal behavior and nutrition-related mortality in domestic swine. J Anim Sci 42:235–241.

Head RH, Williams IH. 1991. Mammogenesis is influenced by pregnancy nutrition. In Manipulating Pig Production III. Werribee, Australia: Australasian Pig Science Association. p. 33.

Hendrix WF, Kelley KW, Gaskins CT. 1978. Porcine neonatal survival and serum gamma globulins. J Anim Sci 47:1281–1286.

Hermansson I, Einarsson S, Ekman L, Larsson K. 1978a. On the agalactia postpartum in the sow: A hematological and blood chemical study in affected and healthy sows. Nord Vet Med 30:474–481.

Hermansson I, Einarsson S, Larson K, Backstrom L. 1978b. On the agalactia post partum in the sow: A clinical study. Nord Vet Med 30:465–473.

Hernandez A, Diaz J, Avila A, Cama M. 1987. A note on the natural suckling frequency of piglets. Cuban J Agric Sci 21:292–294.

Hirsch AC, Philipp H, Kleemann R. 2003. Investigation on the efficacy of meloxicam in sows with mastitis-metritis-agalactia syndrome. J Vet Pharm Ther 26:355–360.

Holtz W, Hartmann JF, Welp C. 1983. Induction of parturition in swine with prostaglandin analogs and oxytocin. Theriogenology 19:583–592.

Holyoake PK, Dial GD, Trigg T, King VL. 1995. Reducing pig mortality through supervision during the perinatal period. J Anim Sci 73:3543–3551.

Howard KA, Nelson DA, Garcia-Sirera J, Rozeboom DW. 1994. Relationship between body tissue accretion and mammary development in pregnant gilts. J Anim Sci 72 (Suppl. 1):334.

Hoy S. 2003. Investigations on the effects of puerperal diseases in sows on the fertility. Arch Tierzucht 46:341–346.

———. 2004. Puerperal diseases in sows—Impact on performances and influence of different housing factors on frequency. Proc Int Pig Vet Soc Congr 18:849–849.

Hoy S, Friton G. 2004. Preliminary findings of the pharmacoeconomic benefit evaluation of meloxicam (metacam) treatment on litter performance of sows with mma syndrome. Proc Int Pig Vet Soc Congr 18:597–597.

Hoy S, Lutter C, Puppe B, Wahner M. 1995. Correlations between vitality of newborn piglets, teat order, mortality, and liveweight gain up to weaning. Berl Munch Tierarztl Wochenschr 108:224–228.

Hughes PE, Varley MA. 1980. Reproduction in the Pig. London: Butterworths.

Hulten F, Persson A, Eliasson-Selling L, Heldmer E, Lindberg M, Sjogren U, Kugelberg C, Ehlorsson CJ. 2003. Clinical characteristics, prevalence, influence on sow performance, and assessment of sow-related risk factors for granulomatous mastitis in sows. Am J Vet Res 64:463–469.

Hurley WL. 2001. Mammary gland growth in the lactating sow. Livest Prod Sci 70:149–157.

Hurley WL, Grieve RCJ. 1988. Total and differential cell counts and N-acetyl b-D-glucosaminidase activity in sows milk during lactation. Vet Res Comm 12:149–153.

Hurley WL, Doane RM, O'Day Bowman MB, Winn RJ, Mojonnier LE, Sherwood OD. 1991. Effect of relaxin on mammary development in ovariectomized pregnant gilts. Endocrinology 128:1285–1290.

Hurley WL, Wang H, Bryson JM, Shennan DB. 2000. Lysine uptake by mammary gland tissue from lactating sows. J Anim Sci 78:391–395.

Illmann G, Madlafousek J. 1995. Occurrence and characteristics of unsucccesful nursings in mini pigs during the first week of life. Appl Anim Behav Sci 44:9–18.

Jackson SC, Bryson JM, Wang H, Hurley WL. 2000. Cellular uptake of valine by lactating porcine mammary tissue. J Anim Sci 78:2927–2932.

Jensen HM. 1981. Forebyggelse af farefeber (MMA) komplekset vet reduktion af fodret til den draektige sode sidste 3 uger for faring. Dansk Vet Tidsskr 64:659–662.

Jensen P. 1986. Observations on the maternal behaviour of free-ranging domestic pigs. Appl Anim Behav Sci 16:131–142.

———. 1988. Maternal behaviour and mother-young interactions during lactation in free-ranging domestic pigs. Appl Anim Behav Sci 20:297–308.

Jensen P, Stangel G, Algers B. 1991. Nursing and suckling behaviour of semi-naturally kept pigs during the first 10 days postpartum. Appl Anim Behav Sci 31:193–209.

Jensen P, Vestergaard K, Algers B. 1993. Nestbuilding in free-ranging domestic sows. Appl Anim Behav Sci 38:245–255.

Jones JET. 1971. Reflections on post-parturient diseases associated with lactational failure in sows. Vet Res 89:72–77.

———. 1976. Bacterial mastitis and endometritis in sows. Proc Int Pig Vet Soc Congr 4:E6.

Jorsal SE. 1986. Epidemiology of the MMA-syndrome. A field survey in Danish sow herds. Proc Int Vet Pig Soc Congr 9:93–93.

Kensinger RS, Collier RJ, Bazer FW, Ducsay CA, Becker HN. 1982. Nucleic acid, metabolic and histological changes in gilt mammary tissue during pregnancy and lactogenesis. J Anim Sci 54:1297–1308.

Kensinger RS, Collier RJ, Bazer FW. 1986. Effect of number of conceptuses on maternal mammary development during pregnancy in the pig. Dom Anim Endocr 3:237–245.

Kent JC, Kennaugh LM, Hartmann PE. 2003. Intramammary pressure in the lactating sow in response to oxytocin and during natural milk ejections throughout lactation. J Dairy Res 70:131–138.

Kim SW, Osaka I, Hurley WL, Easter RA. 1999. Mammary gland growth as influenced by litter size in lactating sows: Impact on lysine requirement. J Anim Sci 77:3316–3321.

Kim SW, Easter RA, Hurley WL. 2001. The regression of unsuckled mammary glands during lactation in sows: The influence of lactation stage, dietary nutrients, and litter size. J Anim Sci 79:2659–2668.

King GJ, Willoughby RA, Hacker RR. 1972. Fluctuations in rectal temperature of swine at parturition. Can Vet J 13:72–74.

King RH, Rayner CJ, Kerr M. 1993a. A note on the amino acid composition of sow's milk. Anim Prod 57:500–502.

King RH, Toner MS, Dove H, Atwood CS, Brown WG. 1993b. The response of first-litter sows to dietary protein level during lactation. J Anim Sci 71:2457–2463.

King RH, Pettigrew JE, McNamara JP, McMurtry JP, Henderson TL, Hathaway MR, Sower AF. 1996. The effect of exogenous prolactin on lactation performance of first-litter sows given protein-deficient diets during the first pregnancy. Anim Repro Sci 41:37–50.

King RH, Mullan BP, Dunshea FR, Dove H. 1997. The influence of piglet body weight on milk production of sows. Livest Prod Sci 47:169–174.

Klobasa F, Butler JE. 1987. Absolute and relative concentrations of immunoglobulins G, M, and A, and albumin in the lacteal secretion of sows of different lactation numbers. Am J Vet Res 48:176–182.

Klobasa F, Werhahn E, Butler JE. 1987. Composition of sow milk during lactation. J Anim Sci 64:1458–1466.

Klobasa F, Habe F, Werhahn E. 1990. Absorption of colostral immunoglobulins by newborn piglets. I. Influence of the period between birth and the first feed. Berl Munch Tierarztl Wochenschr 103:335–340.

Klobasa F, Werhahn E, Habe F. 1991. Studies on the absorption of colostral immunoglobulins in newborn piglets. III. Influence of the duration of colostrum administration. Berl Munch Tierarztl Wochenschr 104:223–227.

Klobasa F, Schroder C, Stroot C, Henning M. 2004. [Passive immunization in neonatal piglets in natural rearing—Effects of birth order, birth weight, litter size and parity]. Berl Munch Tierarztl Wochenschr 117:19–23.

Klopfenstein C. 2003. Variation temporelle des caractéristiques comportementales et physiologiques des truies qui allaitent les portées à croissance faible et normale en période du péripartum. Thèse de Doctorat. Université de Montréal, Montréal.

Klopfenstein C, D'Allaire S, Martineau GP. 1995. Effect of adaptation to the farrowing crate on water intake of sows. Livest Prod Sci 43:243–252.

Klopfenstein C, Bigras Poulin M, Martineau GP. 1997. La "fièvre chez la truie": Un indicateur des problèmes de lactation en néonatologie porcine? (Reliability of sow 'fever' as an indicator of lactation problems in swine neonatalogy). Journ Rech Porcine France 29:53–58.

Klopfenstein C, Farmer C, Martineau GP. 1999. Mammary glands and lactation problems. In Diseases of Swine (8th ed). BE Straw, WL Mengeling, S D'Allaire, DJ Taylor, eds. Ames: Iowa State University Press, pp. 833–860.

Knaggs GS. 1967. Biological half-life of intravenously injected oxytocin in the circulation of the sow. J Endocrinol 37:229–230.

Knight JW, Bazer FW, Thatcher WW, Franke DE, Wallace HD. 1977. Conceptus development in intact and unilaterally hysterectomized-ovariectomized gilts: Interrelations among hormonal status, placental development, fetal fluids and fetal growth. J Anim Sci 44:620–637.

Konar A, Thomas PC, Rook JAF. 1971. The concentrations of some water-soluble constituents in the milks of cows, sows, ewes and goats. J Dairy Res 38:333–341.

Kornblum E, Molnar S, Guenther KD. 1993. Investigations on the effect of suckling order on piglet growth to 20 days. Zuchtungskunde 65:38–46.

Kusina J, Pettigrew JE, Sower AF, Hathaway MR, White ME, Crooker BA. 1995. The effect of protein (lysine) intake during gestation on mammary development of the gilt. J Anim Sci 73:189.

Labroue F, Caugant A, Ligonesche B, Gaudré D. 2001. Étude de l'évolution des tétines d'apparence douteuse chez la cochette au cours de sa carrière. Journ Rech Porcine France 33:145–150.

Le Cozler Y, Pichodo X, Roy H, Guyomarc'h C, Pellois H, Quiniou N, Louveau I, Lebret B, Lefaucheur L, Gondret F. 2004. Influence du poids individuel et de la taille de la portée à la naissance sur la survie du porcelet, ses performances de croissance et d'abattage et la qualité de la viande. Journ Rech Porcine France 36:443–450.

Le Dividich J, Martineau GP, Thomas F, Demay H, Renoult H, Homo C, Boutin D, Gaillard L, Surel Y, Bouetard R, Massard M. 2004. Acquisition of passive immunity in the piglets and production of colostrum in the sow. Journ Rech Porcine France 36:451–459.

Leong WS, Navaratnam N, Stankiewicz MJ, Wallace AV, Ward S, Kuhn NJ. 1990. Subcellular compartmentation in the synthesis of the milk sugars lactose and alpha-2,3-sialyllactose. Protoplasma 159:144–156.

Lewis AJ, Speer VC, Haught DG. 1978. Relationship between yield and composition of sow's milk and weight gains of nursing pigs. J Anim Sci 47:634–638.

Lewis NJ, Hurnik FJ. 1985. The development of nursing behaviour in swine. Appl Anim Behav Sci 14:225–232.

Lignereux Y, Rossel R, Jouglar JY. 1996. Note sur la vascularisation veineuse des mamelles chez la truie. Rev Med Vet 147:191–194.

Linzell JL, Mepham TB, Annison EF, West CE. 1969. Mammary metabolism in lactating sows: Arteriovenous differences of milk precursors and the mammary metabolism of (14C) glucose and (14C) acetate. Br J Nutr 23:319–332.

Lynch PB. 1977. Effects of environmental temperature on lactating sows and their litters. Ir J Agric Res 16:123–130.

Lyvers-Peffer PA, Rozeboom DW. 2001. The effects of a growth-altering pre-pubertal feeding regimen on mammary development and parity-one lactation potential in swine. Livest Prod Sci 70:167–173.

MacFarlane WV, Howard B, Siebert BD. 1969. Tritiated water in the measurement of milk intake and tissue growth of the ruminant in the field. Nature 221:578–579.

Madec F, Leon E. 1992. Farrowing disorders in the sow: A field study. J Vet Med 39:433–444.

Madec F, Miquet JM, Leon E. 1992. La pathologie de la parturition chez la truie. Étude épidémiologique dans cinq élevages. Rec Méd Vét 168:341–349.

Magnusson U, Rodriguez Martinez H, Einarsson S. 1991. A simple, rapid method for differential cell counts in porcine mammary secretions. Vet Rec 129:485–490.

Mahan DC, Becker DE, Norton HW, Jensen AH. 1971. Milk production in lactating sows and time lengths used in evaluating milk production. J Anim Sci 33:35–37.

Mahan DC, Kim YY, Stuart RL. 2000. Effect of vitamin E sources (RRR- or all-rac-alpha-tocopheryl acetate) and levels on sow reproductive performance, serum, tissue, and milk alpha-tocopherol contents over a five-parity period, and the effects on the progeny. J Anim Sci 78:110–119.

Marchant J. 1997. It's a hard life for sows in these pools of discontent. Pig Farming, April:36–37.

Martin CE, Hooper BE, Armstrong CH, Amstutz HE. 1967. A clinical and pathologic study of the mastitis-metritis-agalactia syndrome of sows. J Am Vet Med Assoc 151:1629–1634.

Martineau GP. 1990. Body building syndrome in sows. Proc Am Assoc Swine Pract Denver, pp. 345–348.

Martineau GP, Klopfenstein C. 1996. Les syndromes corporelles chez la truie. Journ Rech Porcine France 28:331–338.

Marzulli FN, Callahan JF. 1957. The capacity of certain common animals to sweat. J Am Vet Med Assoc 131:80–81.

Matte JJ, Girard CL. 1996. Changes of serum and blood volumes during gestation and lactation in multiparous sows. Can J Anim Sci 76:263–266.

Mattioli M, Seren E. 1985. Effect of bromocriptine treatment during lactational anestrus in pigs. In Endocrine Causes of Seasonal and Lactational Anestrus in Farm Animals. F Ellendorf, F Elsaesser, eds. Boston: Martinus Nijhoff, pp. 165–178.

Matzat PD, Hogberg MG, Fogwell RL, Miller ER. 1990. Lactation performance in high producing sows fed in excess of ad libitum. Report of Swine Research, Michigan State University AS-SW-8904, pp. 36–40.

McNamara JP, Pettigrew JE. 2002. Protein and fat utilization in lactating sows: I. Effects on milk production and body composition. J Anim Sci 80:2442–2451.

Mepham TB. 1983. Biochemistry of Lactation. New York: Elsevier Press.

——. 1987. Physiology of Lactation. Philadelphia: Open University Press.

Messias de Bragança M, Mounier AM, Hulin JC, Prunier A. 1997. La sous-nutrition explique-t-elle les effets d'une température ambiante élevée sur les performances des truies? Journ Rech Porcine France 29:81–88.

Meunier Salaun MC, Gort F, Prunier A, Schouten WGP. 1991. Behavioural patterns and progesterone, cortisol and prolactin levels around parturition in European (Large-White) and Chinese (Meishan) sows. Appl Anim Behav Sci 31:43–59.

Michelchen G, Ender K. 1991. Einfluss von rekombinantem porcinem Somatotropin auf die Aufzuchtleistung von Altsauen (Influence of recombinant porcine somatotropin on litter performance of Landrace sows). Arch Tierzucht 34:313–322.

Middleton-Williams DM, Pohlenz J, Lott-Stolz G, Bertschinger HU. 1977. Untersuchungen uber das matitis-metritis-agalactie-syndrom (milchfieber) der sau. Schweiz Arch Tierheilkd 119:214–223.

Migdal W. 1991. Chemical composition of lipid fraction of the colostrum and milk [of] sows fed rations with rapeseed oil. World Rev Anim Prod 26:21–28.

Mirko CP, Bilkei G. 2004. Acute phase proteins, serum cortisol and preweaning litter performance in sows suffering from periparturient disease. Acta Vet (Beograd) 54:153–161.

Molenat M, Thibeault L. 1977. La chasse aux fausses tétines chez les truies doit être systématique. L'Élevage Porcin 108:33–36.

Morkoç A, Backstrom L, Lund L, Smith AR. 1983. Bacterial endotoxin in blood of dysgalactic sow in relation to microbial status of uterus-milk and intestine. J Am Vet Med Assoc 183:786–789.

Moser RL, Cornelius SG, Pettigrew JE, Hanke HE, Heeg TR, Miller KP. 1987. Influence of postpartum feeding method on performance of the lactating sow. Livest Prod Sci 16:91–99.

Muirhead M. 1991. Underlines often neglected in selecting gilts. Int Pigletter 10:22–23.

Mullan BP, Williams IH. 1989. The effect of body reserves at farrowing on the reproductive performance of first-litter sows. Anim Prod 48:449–457.

Nachreiner RF, Ginther OJ. 1974. Induction of agalactia by administration of endotoxin (Escherichia coli) in swine. Am J Vet Res 35:619–622.

Nachreiner RF, Ginther OJ, Ribelin WE, Carlson IH. 1971. Pathologic and endocrinologic changes associated with porcine agalactia. Am J Vet Res 32:1065–1075.

National Research Council. 1998. Nutrient Requirements of Swine. (10 ed). Washington, D.C.: National Academy Press.

Noblet J, Close WH. 1980. Étude préliminaire sur le métabolisme énergétique de la truie nullipare gravide. Journ Rech Porcine France 12:291–298.

Noblet J, Etienne M. 1986. Effect of energy level in lactating sows on yield and composition of milk and nutrient balance of piglets. J Anim Sci 63:1888–1896.

——. 1987. Metabolic utilization of energy and maintenance requirements in lactating sows. J Anim Sci 64:774–781.

——. 1989. Estimation of sow milk nutrient output. J Anim Sci 67:3352–3359.

Paape MJ, Hafs HD, Snyder WW. 1963. Variation of estimated numbers of milk somatic cells stained with Wright's stain or pyronin y-methyl green stain. J Dairy Sci 46:1211–1216.

Palin MF, Farmer C. 2004. Expression of prolactin receptor, STAT5a, STAT5b and whey acidic protein in mammary tissue of lactating Large White and 50% Meishan sows. J Anim Sci 82 (Suppl. 1):205.

Park YW, Kandeh M, Chin KB, Pond WG, Young LD. 1994. Concentrations of inorganic elements in milk of sows selected for high and low serum cholesterol. J Anim Sci 72:1399–1402.

Peaker M. 1978. Ion and Water Transport in the Mammary Gland. In Lactation. BL Larson, ed. New York: Academic Press, pp. 437–462.

Peaker M, Wilde CJ. 1987. Milk secretion: Autocrine control. News Physiol Sci 2:124–126.

Pejsak Z, Tarasiuk K. 1989. The occurrence of endotoxin in sows with coliform mastitis. Theriogenology 32:335–341.

Pejsak A, Tarasuik K, Jochle W. 1988. Immunoprophylaxis against MMA and/or CM in sows with a vaccine against urinary tract infections (Urovac). Proc Int Vet Pig Soc Congr 10:307.

Penny RHC. 1970. The agalactia complex in the sow: A review. Aust J Biol Sci 46:153–159.

Perrin DR. 1955. The chemical composition of the colostrum and milk of the sow. J Dairy Res 22:103–107.

Persson A, Pedersen E, Gorensen L, Kuhl W. 1989. A long term study on the health status and performance of sows on different feed allowances during late pregnancy. 1-Clinical observations with special reference to agalactia post partum. Acta Vet Scand 30:9–17.

Persson A, Pedersen Morner A, Kuhl W. 1996. A long-term study on the health status and performance of sows on different feed allowances during late pregnancy. III. Escherichia coli and other bacteria, total cell content, polymorphonuclear leucocytes and pH in colostrum and milk during the first 3 weeks of lactation. Acta Vet Scand 37:293–313.

Pettigrew JE. 1995. The influence of substrate supply on milk production in the sow. In Manipulating Pig Production V. DP Hennessy, PD Cranwell, eds. Australasian Pig Science Association, Werribbee, Australia, pp. 129.

Pettigrew JE, Cornelius SG, Moser RL, Heeg TR, Hanke HE, Miller KR, Hagen CD. 1986. Effects of oral doses of corn oil and other factors on preweaning survival and growth of piglets. J Anim Sci 62:601–612.

Phillips PA, Fraser D. 1991. Discovery of selected water dispensers by newborn pigs. Can J Anim Sci 71:223–236.

Plaut KI, Kensinger RS, Griel LC Jr, Kavanaugh JF. 1989. Relationships among prolactin binding, prolactin concentrations in plasma and metabolic activity of the porcine mammary gland. J Anim Sci 67:1509–1519.

Pluske JR, Williams IH, Aherne FX. 1995a. Nutrition of the neonatal pig. In The Neonatal Pig-Development and Survival. MA Varley, ed. Wallingford, U.K.: CAB International, pp. 187–235.

Pluske JR, Williams IH, Cegielski AC, Clowes EC, Zak LJ, Aherne FX. 1995b. Super-alimentation of first litter sows during lactation. In Manipulating Pig Production V. DP Hennessy, PD Cranwell, eds. Australasian Pig Science Association, Werribbee, Australia.

Prawirodigdo S, King RH, Dunkin AC, Dove H. 1987. Estimation of milk intake by pigs using deuterium oxide dilution. In Manipulating Pig Production I. Australasian Pig Science Association, Albury, Australia.

Prunier A, Quesnel H, Messias de Braganca M, Kermabon AY. 1996. Environmental and seasonal influences on the return-to-oestrus after weaning in primiparous sows: A review. Livest Prod Sci 45:103–110.

Prunier A, de Braganca M, Le Dividich J. 1997. Influence of high ambient temperature on performance of reproductive sows. Livest Prod Sci 52:123–133.

Puppe B, Tuchscherer A. 2000. The development of suckling frequency in pigs from birth to weaning of their piglets: A sociobiological approach. Anim Sci 71:273–279.

Quiniou N, Noblet J. 1999. Influence of high ambient temperatures on performance of multiparous lactating sows. J Anim Sci 77:2124–2134.

Rapacz J, Hasler Rapacz J. 1982. Immunogenetic studies of polymorphism, postnatal passive acquisition and development of immunoglobulin gamma (IgG) in swine. Proc World Cong General Appl Livest Prod 2:365–374.

Ravel A, D'Allaire S, Bigras Poulin M. 1996. Influence of management, housing and personality of the stockperson on preweaning performances on independent and integrated swine farms in Québec. Prev Vet Med 29:37–57.

Reale TA. 1987. Supplemental liquid diets and feed flavours for young pigs. M.Sc Thesis. University of Melbourne, Melbourne, Australia.

Ringarp N. 1960. Clinical and experimental investigation into a postparturient syndrome with agalactia in sows. Acta Vet Scand, (Supp 7):1–153.

Robert S, Matte JJ, Farmer C, Girard CL, Martineau GP. 1993. High-fibre diets for sows: Effects on stereotypes and adjunctive drinking. Appl Anim Behav Sci 37:297–309.

Robert S, Matte JJ, Martineau GP. 1996. Sensitivity of reproducing sows and suckling pigs to stray voltage. Am J Vet Res 57:1245–1249.

Robertson HA, King GJ. 1974. Plasma concentrations of progesterone, oestrone, oestradiol-17beta and of oestrone sulphate in the pig at implantation, during pregnancy and at parturition. J Reprod Fertil 40:133–141.

Robinson NE. 1997. Thermoregulation. In Textbook of Veterinary Physiology (2nd ed). JG Cunningham, ed. Toronto: W.B. Saunders, pp. 634–645.

Rohde Parfet KA, Gonyou HW. 1988. Effect of creep partitions on teat-seeking behavior of newborn piglets. J Anim Sci 66:2165–2173.

Rose M, Schnurrbusch U, Heinrotzi H. 1996. The use of cequinome in the treatment of pig respiratory disease and MMA syndrome. Proc Int Pig Vet Soc Congr 14:317–317.

Ross RF, Orning AP, Woods RD, Zimmerman BJ, Cox DF, Harris DL. 1981. Bacteriologic study of sow agalactia. Am J Vet Res 42:949–955.

Roychoudhury R, Sarker AB, Bora NN. 1995. Farrowing and suckling behaviour of Hampshire pigs. Indian J Anim Prod Managmt 11:62–64.

Rushen J, Foxcroft GR, de Passillé AMB. 1993. Nursing-induced changes in pain sensitivity, prolactin, and somatotropin in the pig. Physiol Behav Sci 53:265–270.

Rushen J, Ladewig J, de Passillé AMB. 1995. A novel environment inhibits milk ejection in the pig but not through HPA activity. Appl Anim Behav Sci 45:53–61.

Salmon Legagneur E. 1956. La mesure de la production laitière de la truie. Ann Zootech 2:95–110.

——. 1959. Description et utilisation d'une machine à traire les truies. Ann Zootech 4:345–352.

——. 1965. Quelques aspects des relations nutritionnelles entre la gestation et la lactation chez la truie. Thèse de doctorat. Université de Paris, Paris, France.

Samanc H, Damnjanovic Z, Radojicic B, Stojic V. 1992. Cortisol, triiodothyronine, thyroxine and glucose concentrations in the blood of first litter sows during advanced pregnancy and post partum in relation to hypogalactia and agalactia. Acta Vet (Beograd) 42:109–114.

Sandstedt H, Sjogren U. 1982. Forebuggande atgarder vid hog frekvens av MMA i suggbesattningar. Sven Vet Tidn 34:487–490.

Sandstedt H, Sjogren U, Swahn O. 1979. Foreguggande atgarder mot MMA (agalakti) hos sugga. Sven Vet Tidn 31:193–196.

Sauber TE, Stahly TS, Ewan RC, Williams NH. 1994. Maximum lactational capacity of sows with a high and low genetic capacity for lean tissue growth. J Anim Sci 72:364–364.

Schollenberger A, Degorski A, Frymus T, Shollenberger AD. 1986. Cells of sow mammary secretions. J Vet Med A 33:31–38.

Schoning G, Plonait H. 1990. Herd prophylaxis and treatment of the mastitis-metritis-agalactia syndrome of sows with enrofloxacin (Baytril). Dtsh Tierarztl Wochenschr 97:5–8 10.

Schummer A, Wilkens H, Vollmerhaus B. Habermehl KH. 1981. The Circulatory System, the Skin, and the Cutaneous Organs of the Domestic Mammals. Vol 3. New York: Springer-Verlag, 630 pp.

Shoenherr WD, Stahly TS, Cromvell GL. 1989. The effects of dietary fat or fiber addition on yield and composition of milk of sows housed in a warm or hot environment. J Anim Sci 67:482–488.

Smith BB, Wagner WC. 1980. Lactation physiology in the pig. Proc 9th Int Congr Anim Reprod Artificial Insemination, Madrid, Spain 3:118.

——. 1984. Suppression of prolactin in pigs by Escherichia coli endotoxin. Science 224:605–607.

——. 1985a. Effect of dopamine agonists or antagonists-TRH-stress and piglet removal on plasma concentrations of prolactin in lactating sows. Theriogenology 3:283–296.

——. 1985b. Effect of Escherichia coli endotoxin and TRH on prolactin in lactating sows. Am J Vet Res 46:175–180.

Smith BB, Martineau GP, Bisaillon A. 1992. Mammary glands and lactation problems. In Diseases of Swine (7th ed). AD Leman, BE Straw, WL Mengeling, S D'Allaire, DJ Taylor, eds. Ames: Iowa State University Press, pp. 40–61.

Smith VG, Leman AD, Seaman WJ, Vanravenswaay F. 1991. Pig weaning weight and changes in hematology and blood chemistry of sows injected with recombinant porcine somatotropin during lactation. J Anim Sci 69:3501–3510.

Sohn KS, Maxwell CV. 1999. New technologies for sow nutrition and management—Review. Asian-Aust J Anim Sci 12:956–965.

Sorensen MT, Sejrsen K, Purup S. 2002a. Mammary gland development in gilts. Livest Prod Sci 75:143–148.

Sorensen MT, Vestergaard M, Purup S, Sejrsen K. 2002b. Mammary development, growth and plasma levels of IGF-I and IGF-binding proteins in gilts provided different energy levels from weaning to puberty. J Anim Sci 80 (Suppl. 1):52–52.

Speer VC, Cox DF. 1984. Estimating milk yield of sows. J Anim Sci 59:1281–1285.

Spincer J, Rook JAF, Towers KG. 1969. The uptake of plasma constituents by the mammary gland of the sow. Biochem J 111:727–732.

Spinka M, Illmann G, Algers B, Stetkova Z. 1997. The role of nursing frequency in milk production in domestic pigs. J Anim Sci 75:1223–1228.

Spinka M, Illmann G, Stetkova Z, Krejci P, Tomanek M, Sedlak L, Lidicky J. 1999. Prolactin and insulin levels in lactating sows in relation to nursing frequency. Dom Anim Endocr 17:53–64.

Stangel G, Jensen P. 1991. Behaviour of semi-naturally kept sows and piglets (except suckling) during 10 days postpartum. Appl Anim Behav Sci 31:211–227.

Stevenson JS, Cox NM, Britt JH. 1981. Role of the ovary in controlling luteinizing hormone, follicle stimulating hormone, and prolactin secretion during and after lactation in pigs. Biol Reprod 24:341–353.

Stone CC, Brown MS, Waring GH. 1974. An ethological means to improve swine production. J Anim Sci 39:137.

Tabjara P, Soares M, Richard A. 1992. Genital status and litter performance of sows treated with antibiotics to control MMA. Proc Int Pig Vet Soc Congr 12:473.

Tarasiuk K, Pejsak Z. 1986. Role of Escherichia coli endotoxin in the aetiology of post-partum agalactia in sows Udzial endotoksyny E. coli w etiologii bezmlecznosci poporodowej u loch. Medycyna Weter 42:323–327.

Taverne M, Bevers M, Bradshaw JMC, Dieleman SJ, Willemse AH, Porter DG. 1982. Plasma concentrations of prolactin, progesterone, relaxin and oestradiol-17B in sows treated with progesterone, bromocriptine or indomethacin during late gestation. J Reprod Fertil 65:85–96.

Thompson BK, Fraser D. 1988. Variation in piglet weights: Weight gains in the first days after birth and their relationship with later performance. Can J Anim Sci 68:581–590.

Titterington RW, Fraser D. 1975. The lying behaviour of sows and piglets during early lactation in relation to the position of the creep heater. Appl Anim Eth 2:47–53.

Tokach MD, Pettigrew JE, Crooker BA, Dial GD, Sower AF. 1992. Quantitative influences of lysine and energy intake on yield of milk components in the primiparous sow. J Anim Sci 70:1864–1872.

Toner MS, King RH, Dunshea FR, Dove H, Atwood CS. 1996. The effect of exogenous somatotropin on lactation performance of first-litter sows. J Anim Sci 74:167–172.

Trapp AL, Keahy KK, Whitenack DC, Whitehair CK. 1970. Vitamin E-selenium deficiency in swine: Differential diagnosis and nature of field problems. J Am Vet Med Assoc 157:289–300.

Tribout T, Caritez JC, Gogue J, Gruand J, Billon Y, Bouffaud M, Lafgant H, Le Dividich J, Thomas F, Quesnel H, Gueblez R, Bidanel JP. 2003. Estimation of realised genetic trends in French Large White pigs from 1977 to 1998 for female reproduction traits using frozen semen. Journ Rech Porcine France 35:285–292.

Trottier NL, Shipley CF, Easter RA. 1997. Plasma amino acid uptake by the mammary gland of the lactating sow. J Anim Sci 75:1266–1278.

Tucker HA. 1985. Endocrine and neural control of the mammary gland. In Lactation. BL Larson. ed. Ames: Iowa State University Press, pp. 39–79.

Turner CW. 1952. The Mammary Gland. In The Anatomy of the Udder of Cattle and Domestic Animals. Missouri: Lucas Brothers, pp. 279–314.

Tyler JW, Cullor JS, Thurmond MC, Douglas VL, Parker KM. 1990. Immunologic factors related to survival and performance in neonatal swine. Am J Vet Res 51:1400–1406.

Vales L, Lagreca L, Marotta E, Williams S. 1992. Ethology of suckled piglets: Its suckling behaviour and its relationship with the growing rate. Revta Med Vet B Aires 73:148–154, 156, 158.

Valros A, Rundgren M, Spinka M, Saloniemi H, Rydhmer L, Hulten F, Uvnas-Moberg K, Tomanek M, Krejci P, Algers B. 2003. Metabolic state of the sow, nursing behaviour and milk production. Livest Prod Sci 79:155–167.

van den Brand H, Heetkamp MJW, Soede NM, Schrama JW, Kemp B. 2000. Energy balance of lactating primiparous sows as affected by feeding level and dietary energy source. J Anim Sci 78:1520–1528.

van den Brand H, Schouten WGP, Kemp B. 2004. Maternal feed intake, but not feed composition affects postural behaviour and nursing frequency of lactating primiparous sows. Appl Anim Behav Sci 86:41–49.

Van der Lende T, de Jager D. 1991. Death risk and preweaning growth rate of piglets in relation to the within-litter weight distribution at birth. Livest Prod Sci 28:73–84.

Wagner WC. 1972. Endocrine function in normal and agalactic sows. J Anim Sci 34:270–272.

Waldmann KH, Heide J. 1996. Investigations on uterine contraction post partum and effects of different uterotonicia in puerperal sows. Proc Int Pig Vet Soc Congr 14:614.

Wallace HD, Thieu DD, Combs GE. 1974. Alfalfa meal as a special bulky ingredient in the sow diet at farrowing and during lactation. Res Report-Dept of Animal Science Gainesville Florida.

Wechsler B, Brodmann N. 1996. The synchronization of nursing bouts in group-housed sows. Appl Anim Behav Sci 47:191–199.

Weldon WC, Thulin AJ, MacDougald OA, Johnston LJ, Miller ER, Tucker HA. 1991. Effects of increased dietary energy and protein during late gestation on mammary development in gilts. J Anim Sci 69:194–200.

Whitacre MD, Threlfall WR. 1981. Effects of ergocryptine on plasma prolactin luteinizing hormone and progesterone in the periparturient sow. Am J Vet Res 42:1538–1541.

Whitehair CK, Miller ER. 1986. Nutritional deficiencies. In Diseases of Swine (6th ed.). AD Leman, BE Straw, WL Glock, WL Mengeling, HC Penny, E Scholl, eds. Ames: Iowa State University Press, pp. 746–762.

Whitely JL, Hartmann PE, Willcox DL, Bryant Greenwood GD, Greenwood FC. 1990. Initiation of parturition and lactation in the sow: Effects of delaying parturition with medroxyprogesterone acetate. J Endocrinol 124:465–484.

Whitely JL, Willcox DL, Hartmann PE, Yamamoto SY, Bryant Greenwood GD. 1985. Plasma relaxin levels during suckling and oxytocin stimulation in the lactating sow. Biol Reprod 33:705–714.

Whittemore CT, Fraser D. 1974. The nursing and suckling behavior of pigs II: Vocalization of the sow in relation to suckling behavior and milk ejection. Br Vet J 130:346–356.

Williams IH. 1995. Sow's milk as a major nutrient source before weaning. In Manipulating Pig Production V. DP Hennessy, PD Cranwell, eds. Werribee, Australia: Australasian Pig Science Association. pp. 107–113.

Wolter BF, Ellis M, Corrigan BP, DeDecker JM. 2002. The effect of birth weight and feeding of supplemental milk replacer to piglets during lactation on preweaning and postweaning growth performance and carcass characteristics. J Anim Sci 80:301–308.

Wung SC, Wu HP, Kou YH, Shen KH, Koh FK, Wan WCM. 1977. Effect of thyrotropin-releasing hormone on serum thyroxine of lactating sows and the growth of their suckling young. J Anim Sci 45:299–304.

Zaleski HM, Hacker RR. 1993. Variables related to the progress of parturition and probability of stillbirth in swine. Can Vet J 34:109–113.

5 Diseases of the Nervous and Locomotor Systems

Catherine E. Dewey

Clinical signs of lameness and neurological problems are common in swine herds. Lameness is the second most important cause of culling in breeding-stock animals and hence results in lost opportunity in reproductive performance. Preweaning and postweaning polyserositis and meningitis cause decreases in production. Although cases of nutritional deficiencies and poisonings are rare, they are nonetheless extremely important to diagnose. To diagnose a lameness or neurological problem, begin with a thorough herd evaluation followed by clinical examinations of individual animals. Determine whether the clinical signs are primarily due to the musculoskeletal system or the neurological system to narrow the list of differentials and to focus the clinical examination.

LOCOMOTOR PROBLEMS

Clinical Approach to a Lameness Problem in a Herd

The objectives of the herd examination for a lameness problem include determining the age group(s) affected, the most prominent clinical signs, and the onset and prevalence of the clinical signs. It is essential to examine the affected animals as well as their environment.

To evaluate lameness in the breeding herd, begin by examining the sows in farrowing crates and gestation stalls while they are prone. Record the number of sows that have hoof cracks, hoof wall damage, sole lesions, foot rot, long lateral toes, dewclaw damage, and soft-tissue damage. Most sows will remain prone if you handle their feet gently. Next, encourage all sows to stand. Note the number of sows with clinical lameness, the severity of the lameness, whether the clinical signs involve one or more than one leg, if it is predominantly a forelimb or hindlimb lameness, and the parity and stage of gestation of the sows affected. Palpate joints and soft tissue of the clinically affected legs and lift the leg to examine the foot to determine the primary source of the lameness. Take the sows out of the crates to observe their gait. Describe the severity of the lameness using the following terms: stiffness, weight bearing, resting the leg on the ground or carrying the leg while standing still, weight bearing or carrying the leg during ambulation, and ability to stand and walk without assistance.

Once the stalled animals are observed, examine the sows housed in pens. Note whether the lameness is associated with a specific housing type. Examine the feet of the sows that are lying down, watch the sows move about, and determine the prevalence and severity of the lameness in this group of animals. Specifically look for reluctance to move, degree of difficulty in standing, stiffness, stance with legs under the body, and weight bearing on all limbs.

Depending on the extent of the problem, you may wish to cull a representative group of sows to conduct a complete examination of all joints, feet, and vertebral column. Examine all putative causes of the lameness such as nutrition; relocation of the sows during gestation; and housing conditions, especially floors, including solid versus slatted, slipperiness, roughness, and wetness.

For growing animals, determine the range in severity of clinical signs and whether one or more legs are involved per animal. Examine animals that are acutely and chronically affected, observe their movement, palpate the joints and then each leg looking for heat, swelling, and response to pain. Examine all age groups of animals on the farm, not just those with the most severe signs. The causative factors may be in the environment of younger animals. If the producer has treated pigs, discuss the response to treatment. Finally, select a representative sample of nontreated pigs for a postmortem examination.

Preweaning Pigs

The most common conditions affecting the locomotor system of preweaning pigs will be covered in this section; others can be found in Table 5.1.

Table 5.1.   Lameness in preweaned pigs.

Cause	Clinical Signs	Epidemiology	Pathology
Abrasions of carpi and hooves	Lameness and swollen joints due to abraded skin at carpi and coronary band, and abraded horn at toe	Common, trauma to skin from concrete floors during suckling	Abraded skin
Actinobacillus suis	Listlessness, dyspnea, lameness develops later; pigs may be found dead	Acute septicemia	Petechia on kidneys, pleural effusion, pleuritis, pneumonia, purulent arthritis, omphalophlebitis
Arthritis	Reluctant to stand or move, lameness, one or more joints hot and painful, skin abrasions, poor growth	Widespread, common, sporadic with occasional outbreaks	Synovitis with excessive normal-to-purulent fluid
Hyperostosis	Distal legs thick, firm, red, taut skin; stilted gait; fatal	Rare, widespread, sporadic, inherited	Subcutaneous edema, fibrous tissue, and thickened leg bones

Splayleg. Splayleg is a congenital abnormality causing paresis in newborn pigs. This problem of hindlimb adduction affects approximately 0.4% of live births (Ward 1978). The annual rate in pigs born to German Landrace boars between 1982 and 2000 ranged from 0.26% to 0.69% but did not decrease over time due to selection (Beissner et al. 2003). An examination of 47,323 litters born to German Landrace boars from artificial insemination units showed that the frequency of splayleg was not reduced by selection over a 14-year period (Beissner et al. 2003). The problem is widespread, common, and typically affects only 1–4 pigs per litter and just a few litters at a time. Usually individual herd prevalence is less than 1%; however, sporadic increases occur when the prevalence reaches 8% or higher (Ward and Bradley 1980).

The condition has been associated with low birth weight, slippery floors, *Fusarium* toxicity, choline or methionine deficiency in sow diets, Large White and Landrace pigs, and short gestation lengths (Ward 1978). Farrowing induction may result in a higher prevalence of splayleg especially if producers do not first determine the normal gestation length in their herd. Some studies have suggested that one cause of splayleg was a deficiency in the sow's diet of choline and methionine which are essential for normal myelin production (Cunha 1968; Kornegay and Meacham 1973). The study by Cunha (1968) did not mention the use of controls. However, others have refuted this suggestion (Dobson 1971). In clinical trials on two farms, Dobson (1971) showed that adding 3 g choline and 5 g methionine to the sows' daily ration had no effect on the occurrence of splayleg.

Although some researchers describe muscle hypoplasia as the cause of the clinical signs, myofibrillar hypoplasia is normal in all newborn pigs. At one day of age, myofibrils do not fill the muscle cells completely in splayleg or in normal pigs (Ward and Bradley 1980). Also, the vasculature, nervous supply, neuromuscular bundles, and the myelination of the intramuscular nerves are the same between healthy and affected pigs.

Clinically 3-day-old pigs show improved movement and the myofibrils increase in size, reducing the extra-myofibrillar space. By 6 days of age, the splaylegged pigs do not differ from normal pigs clinically or in the histology of the muscles. In all pigs, myofibrils and nuclei continue to increase in size.

Splayleg is caused by a reduction in the axonal diameter and myelin sheath thickness of the fibers that innervate the hindlimb adductors (Szalay et al. 2001). The pathways from the upper to the lower motor neurons, specifically the lumbar spinal motor neurons are impaired. In affected pigs, nerves at the level of L6 regions near the surface of the spinal cord are somewhat myelinated, whereas deeper areas are unmyelinated. This is particularly obvious in the ventral and lateral funiculi. These areas are responsible for innervation of the hindlimb. Myelination is required for normal impulses to be conducted along nerve fibers. The oligodendroglia form the myelin sheath as the final step in the formation and maturation of the neural pathways. Typically, the lumbar region is myelinated earlier than more rostral sections. It is not known why this problem with myelination occurs in these splaylegged pigs.

Myelin is produced by the fetus' oligodendrocytes. This production appears to occur in two phases. The first peak occurs 2 weeks prior to birth and the second 3 weeks after birth. If pigs live past the first couple of weeks, the myelin sheath is properly developed during this second phase.

Clinically pigs show extreme abduction of the limbs with an inability to stand. Splayleg affects the hindlimb adductors and in severe cases, the forelegs are also involved (Szalay et al. 2001). Clinically signs are similar in the high prevalence periods. Typically half of the affected pigs die due to starvation and overlying, because the pigs have a hard time reaching the udder, retaining hold of the nipple, competing with their littermates and moving out of the sow's lying space. Affected pigs can be kept alive if they are fed artificially, provided with supplemental colostrum and heat, assisted to nurse, crossfostered to reduce competition, and have their limbs taped in a natural standing pose. Pigs that live past the first week of life will recover completely.

Polyarthritis. Polyarthritis is a common problem in preweaned pigs and affects approximately 18% of litters and 3.3% of pigs after 4 days of age (Nielsen et al. 1975). Mortality due to polyarthritis is about 1.4% and is highest in the winter. Most affected pigs will die by 3 weeks of age, but 32% of the pigs do not die until 4–5 weeks of age. There is a lower incidence of polyarthritis in female pigs and in pigs from multiparous sows, small litters, closed herds, and herds that do not have their pigs' teeth clipped or tails docked (Nielsen et al. 1975; Smith and Mitchell 1976). Pigs with polyarthritis are more likely to have necrotizing gingivitis than healthy pigs. Different instruments should be used for the teeth and the tails at processing. Instruments should be disinfected between piglets, and the tail and navel sprayed with a disinfectant (Nielsen et al. 1975).

Haemolytic streptococci cause 65% of the cases but staphylococci and *Escherichia coli* are also frequent causes (Nielsen et al. 1975; Smith and Mitchell 1976). The joint lesions include increased synovial fluid, hyperemia of synovial membranes, fibrinous periarthritis, and joint swelling due to exudate and abscesses. The carpal, elbow, hock, and hip joints are most frequently affected. Often the meninges and brain are congested, and there is turbid cerebrospinal fluid, concurrent pneumonia, endocarditis, and gingivitis (Nielsen et al. 1975). The pathogenesis involves the individual pig's ability to eliminate pyogenic organisms before they multiply in the joints (Nielsen et al. 1975). Early treatment with antibiotics will reduce the duration of illness and mortality. Pigs need to be examined carefully for signs of lameness, particularly at 10 and 18 days of age (Nielsen et al. 1975).

Skin Abrasions. Skin abrasions occurring bilaterally on hindlegs and forelegs are evident within a few hours of birth. Rough floor surfaces increase the chance of skin abrasions and therefore the opportunity for the invasion of microorganisms. Although 98% of 3-day-old pigs have skin abrasions, only 11% of pigs are severely affected and most lesions heal within 2–3 weeks of life (Svendsen et al. 1979; Furniss et al. 1986). The incidence of skin abrasions is highest on old cement floors, intermediate on punch metal and new cement floors, and lowest on plastic-coated woven wire. The incidence increases if the size and shape of the slot is large compared to the piglet's foot size and in litters suckling sows with hypogalactia (Smith and Mitchell 1976). The slot width in farrowing crate floors should not exceed 10 mm.

Postweaning Lameness

Infectious Arthritis. Infectious arthritis causes slaughter condemnations equivalent to 2 whole carcasses and 49.6 partial carcasses per 10,000 pigs slaughtered (Evans and Pratt 1978). Pigs condemned due to arthritis are more likely to have erysipelas or pneumonia than pigs not condemned (Evans and Pratt 1978).

Erysipelothrix rhusiopathiae. *Erysipelothrix rhusiopathiae* affects nursery to adult pigs. It is a widespread but uncommon disease affecting up to 75% of pigs in a pen, with 10% mortality (Buddle 1987). Chronic erysipelas results in a progressively increasing lameness and weight loss over 2–3 weeks, with palpably normal joints. It causes a rheumatoid-like proliferative arthritis in the joints of the long bones, spondylitis, and spondylarthritis. The polyarthritis develops in four stages: hypertrophic villous synovitis, pannus formation and articular surface degeneration, fibrous ankylosis, and bony ankylosis. The disease may stop at one of these stages and the animal will undergo remission; otherwise the disease becomes chronic and the animal becomes unthrifty.

Clinically, the animals shift their weight from leg to leg and may have periods of remission. Early in the disease the joints are swollen, warm, and slightly painful, but in the later stages, joints become firm and nodular, with palpable periarticular enlargements and restricted joint movement (Vaughan 1969). Pigs with erysipelas prefer to lie down and have a stilted gait and poor growth rate (Grabell et al. 1962). Animals support themselves on the tips of their digits and have flexed carpi; hocks are together and feet are under the body, with the back arched. There is no palpable fluid or purulent matter in the joints.

There is moderate improvement after treatment with penicillin. Although it is difficult to isolate *E. rhusiopathiae* from chronic cases, it can be isolated from 65% of lame grower-finisher pigs and it causes large abattoir losses due to polyarthritis.

Mycoplasma hyosynoviae. *Mycoplasma hyosynoviae* is relatively rare and affects up to 10% of the animals, although in some herds 50% of the animals are involved (Buddle 1987). Clinically 3- to 6-month-old pigs experience a sudden onset of lameness over 3–10 days. The organism lives in the respiratory tract and is spread via inhalation (Burch 1986). *Mycoplasma hyosynoviae* causes severe lameness with minimal swelling of stifle, shoulder, elbow, and tarsus joints. Pigs show a shifting lameness, stiff or staggering gait, kneeling, or dog-sitting. Approximately 10–20% will become chronic and progress to recumbency. Pathologic features include fibrinous arthritis, edematous, hyperemic, hypertrophied synovial membrane, and serosanguineous synovial fluid. Treatment with either tiamulin or lincomycin at 10 mg/kg daily for 3 days reduces lameness and improves daily gain (Burch and Goodwin 1984).

Polyserositis. Polyserositis occurs most commonly in 4- to 12-week-old pigs, and more frequently in autumn and winter than in spring and summer (Miniats et al. 1986). *Haemophilus parasuis* is isolated most frequently (36%), followed by *M. hyorhinis* (18%) and then *Streptococcus suis* and *Pasteurella multocida*. These pigs experience peracute death or lameness, inability to rise, swollen joints, and respiratory distress.

Mycoplasma hyorhinis. *Mycoplasma hyorhinis* typically affects pigs at 7 weeks of age and is associated with the decline of passive immunity (Ross and Spear 1973). This is a widespread disease but uncommon and sporadic and results in low morbidity (5–15%) and mortality (<10%) (Buddle 1987). Clinically affected animals carry affected legs because of acute, severe pain. Several joints are moderately hot and swollen, especially carpus, shoulder, tarsus, and stifle (Buddle 1987). There is also polyserositis, causing abdominal breathing and reluctance to move. Occasionally the lesions will spontaneously resolve but more typically pigs experience chronic ill thrift. The gross postmortem lesions include distension of the joint capsule, hyperemia, edema, and fibrin deposits of the synovial membrane (Roberts et al. 1963). The chronic lesions include hyperemia, hypertrophy and yellow discoloration of the synovial membrane, and bone atrophy. The tonsils and mucous membranes of the respiratory tract of sows provide the reservoir for *M. hyorhinis* (Ross and Spear 1973). Typically the organism is introduced with new breeding stock. A synergistic effect of other conditions, such as concurrent *E. coli* infections or poor management, is required to initiate clinical signs (Frus and Feenstra 1994).

***Haemophilus parasuis* (Glasser's Disease).** *Haemophilus parasuis* (Glasser's disease) causes a severe peracute and acute lameness, depression, fever, dyspnea, hot swollen joints, reluctance to stand or move, tremor, paralysis, and sudden death (Nielsen and Danielsen 1975; Smart et al. 1986; Hoefling 1994). Pigs recovering from the acute phase may have chronic arthritis. Experimentally infected pigs will be reluctant to move 36 hours post infection. By 60 hours, they have swollen joints and exhibit lateral recumbence (Vahle et al. 1997).

Haemophilus parasuis is a commensal organism living in the upper respiratory tract of pigs. It can be isolated from the nasal and oral cavities and trachea (Oliveira and Pijoan 2004). *H. parasuis* can cause acute suppurative rhinitis with loss of cilia in the nasal and tracheal mucosa (Vahle et al. 1997). This may be the portal of entry. When *H. parasuis* causes acute septicemia and sudden death, this is due to disseminated intravascular coagulation in response to the bacteria's endotoxin.

The disease is widespread and relatively common. Outbreaks occur due to regrouping pigs, at 1–2 weeks postweaning, and when naive breeding stock are moved to an endemically infected herd.

The prevalence of clinical disease due to *H. parasuis*

in nursery pigs appears to have increased since the 1980s. The change may be due to either the use of off-site early weaning facilities, porcine reproductive and respiratory syndrome virus (PRRSV), or porcine circovirus type 2 (PCV2). Maternal immunity wanes at 6 to 8 weeks of life. Most pigs have not been colonized by the *H. parasuis* bacteria before they are weaned. As maternal immunity wanes, the whole population of nursery pigs is susceptible to infection, which enables outbreaks in these nursery barns (Oliveira et al. 2001). In nurseries affected with PRRSV, pigs often exhibit polyarthritis as well as clinical signs involving other organ systems. In these herds, lameness can affect as many as 80% of the pigs and typically is the result of multiple etiologies, including *H. parasuis*, *S. suis*, *M. hyorhinis*, and *E. rhusiopathiae* (Kern 1994).

If pigs are infected with PRRSV a week before the *H. parasuis* infection, the alveolar macrophages have a marked decrease in their ability to kill the bacteria (Solano et al. 1998). In vitro research conducted by the same laboratory found different results (Segales et al. 1998). One-third of the pigs affected by postweaning multisystemic wasting syndrome in Korea were dually infected by porcine circovirus type 2 and *H. parasuis* (Kim et al. 2002).

Clinical *H. parasuis* is diagnosed by clinical signs; presence of lesions such as fibrinopurulent exudates in the peritoneal, pericardial, and pleural cavities; meningitis; arthritis; and bacterial culture of the organism (Vahle et al. 1997). The bacteria are fastidious and therefore, PCR assays may be used to improve the sensitivity of identifying the bacteria in clinical cases (Oliveira et al. 2003). However, the positive PCR test must be followed by culture for further characterization prior to implementing a control program.

Conventional pig farms typically have multiple strains of *H. parasuis* (Smart et al. 1988). The strains isolated from nasal swabs are often not the same strains isolated from systemically infected pigs from the same farm (Smart et al. 1993). A new indirect hemagglutination test used on 300 isolates from North American submissions to diagnostic laboratories showed that serovars 4, 5, 7, and 13 were the most prevalent (Tadjine et al. 2004). Oliveira et al. (2003) found serovar 4 and nontypable isolates to be the most prevalent in U.S. herds.

If treated early, affected pigs will respond to systemically administered penicillin (Desrosiers et al. 1986). Both commercially available and autogenous vaccines have been used prior to the introduction of breeding stock to reduce incidence of clinical signs (Smart et al. 1986, 1993; Miniats and Smart 1988).

Often *H. parasuis* problems in nursery and grower pigs can be controlled by the use of commercial or autogenous vaccines. However, consistent control of *H. parasuis* has been difficult because of the serovar diversity and the lack of cross protection between strains (Oliveira and Pijoan 2004).

Table 5.2. Lameness in postweaned pigs and adults.

Disease	Clinical Signs	Epidemiology	Pathology
Apophysiolysis	Gradual onset, hind feet slide forward, difficulty in standing, arched back, dog-sitting; progresses to lateral recumbency, crepitation of ischial tuberosity	May be end stage of leg weakness syndrome or may occur independently	Separation of ischial tuba
Asymmetrical hindquarter syndrome	Reduced muscle mass in hip or thigh; normal gait	Rare	Reduced muscle mass in hip or thigh
Back-muscle necrosis	Occurs in 5- to 12-month-old pigs; difficult movement due to swollen, hot, uni- or bilateral lesion of back; chronic muscle atrophy	Rare, sporadic, sudden onset; part of porcine stress syndrome	Pale, soft, exudative necrosis and hemorrhage of back muscles
Epiphysiolysis capitis femoris	Sudden onset of severe lameness in one or both hindlegs; reluctance or inability to stand, dog-sitting, squealing, crepitation and pain over hip, muscle wasting	Part of leg weakness syndrome, often seen in newly weaned gilts	Separation of femoral head at epiphyseal plate
Foot-and-mouth disease	Reluctance to stand or move; depression; fever; small vesicles on snout, coronary band, and teats and between claws; vesicle ruptures leaving hemorrhagic, granular, eroded surfaces; underrunning of hoof horn	Reportable disease; all ages, rapid spread, high morbidity, 5% mortality	Acute deaths in piglets, irregular grayish foci on myocardium
Mastitis, metritis, agalactia	Lameness, heat, front feet painful, digital pulse in fetlock region, stiff gait, reluctance to move	Widespread, common, sporadic, lameness uncommon	Laminitis
Melioidosis	Usually subclinical; occasionally acute septicemia, anorexia, nasal discharge, cough, posterior paresis, death	Zoonotic disease; uncommon, sporadic	Multiple abscesses with caseous, green, purulent matter in subcutis, lymph nodes, lung, spleen, and liver
Osteodystrophia fibrosa	Signs range from mild, shifting lameness to inability to stand; shortened, curved long bones, enlarged joints and facial bones	Absolute or relative calcium deficiency, morbidity up to 100%; secondary hyperthyroidism in grain-fed pigs due to high phosphorus and low calcium	Distorted bones; bone and marrow replaced with fibrous tissue
Trauma	Slight to severe lameness due to sprains and bruising; hoof cracks and cuts	Widespread, common, affects all ages	Referable to clinical signs

Lameness in Growing Pigs and Breeding Animals

The differential diagnosis of lameness in growing and breeding animals includes mainly foot rot, leg injuries, epiphysiolysis, apophysiolysis, osteochondrosis, arthrosis, osteomalacia, fractures, and arthritis (Penny 1979; Wells 1984) (Table 5.2). Leg weakness is a term used to describe lameness due to osteochondrosis, arthrosis, epiphysiolysis, and apophysiolysis. In several studies, osteochondrosis, which is a generalized dyschondroplasia, was found to be the most common cause of lameness in breeding-age animals (Grondalen 1974a; Reiland 1975; Hill et al. 1984; Dewey et al. 1993). The second most important cause of lameness was foot lesions, either foot rot, overgrown claws, or torn dewclaws (Dewey et al. 1993). However, outbreaks of foot problems occur in breeding herds, where up to 100% of the sows are affected (Penny 1979).

Culling Due to Lameness. Lameness is the second most common cause of culling in breeding animals, representing 10–20% of all culled sows (Walker et al. 1966; Reiland 1975; Dagorn and Aumaitre 1978; Karlberg 1979; Friendship et al. 1986; Dewey et al. 1992). In a comparative study of Landrace sows, lameness caused the culling of 20.5% of the low-backfat line, but only 13.8% of the high-backfat line (Grondalen and Vangen 1974). Between 30% and 40% of boars at performance stations and approximately 24% of boars at artificial insemination units are culled for leg weakness; 75% of the latter are less than 18 months of age (Grondalen 1974g; Reiland 1975). Sow herds in France with a lameness prevalence of at least 15% had higher mortality rates than herds with less lameness (Abiven et al. 1998). Lameness is frequently a cause of euthanasia in sows (D'Allaire et al. 1987). In one study, locomotor problems caused 9% of the culling and 28% of sow deaths (D'Allaire et al. 1987). Reiland (1975) examined 230 boars and sows culled for lameness and found few cases of foot rot and concluded that hoof lesions were of secondary importance in leg problems.

The culling rate due to lameness in sows varies from farm to farm, suggesting that leg weakness is a major problem on certain farms. In a survey of Ontario farms, it ranged from 0–38%, with an average of 11%, and was associated with a high culling rate for sows and high proportions of gilts to sows in the breeding herd (Dewey et al. 1992). The culling rate due to lameness in start-up herds (26% ± 13%) was higher than in established herds (8% ± 6%) (Dewey et al. 1992). Herds that are repopulating have a larger proportion of young breeding-age animals and a higher level of culling for lameness.

The housing factors associated with high levels of culling due to lameness were slatted floors for finisher pigs or sows, the use of individual sow stalls, and a high density of pigs in the finishing area. These findings suggest that a change of housing design may result in reducing the culling rate due to lameness and that attention to the way young replacement stock is housed and handled may be very important with respect to subsequent longevity and soundness. Floor type and quality, the size of the space between the slats, the width of the slat, the flooring material, and the type of ground for outdoor housed pigs all impact the prevalence and cause of lameness in pigs. Housing pigs indoors on concrete is associated with lameness in pigs (Barnett et al. 2001). Farms that have both stalls and pens for sow housing had a lower culling rate due to lameness than farms that had only pens (Paterson et al. 1997 cited by Barnett et al. 2001). However, muddy conditions and stones in the paddock cause lameness in pigs housed outdoors (Barnett et al. 2001). Sows housed in pens for a portion of gestation are expected to have reduced farrowing time (Ferket and Hacker 1985), reduced lameness in gilts (Hale et al. 1984), and less joint damage (Fredeen and Sather 1978).

Many sows culled for lameness have more than one problem causing the clinical signs. The primary cause of lameness is likely associated with genetics, predominant feed ingredients, housing type (specifically, intensive versus extensive), floor type, and drainage. Associations between the culling rate due to lameness in sows and various housing factors involving finisher pigs indicate that the environment of the young growing animal may have an effect on the skeletal system that becomes apparent only later in life. This would suggest that managers of herds with higher than acceptable levels of lameness in the sow herd should examine the flooring and housing systems used for the young replacement animals in addition to the sows' environment.

Infectious Arthritis. Infectious arthritis is generally of minor importance as a cause of sow culling and affects 2.5% of culled boars (Grondalen 1974b, e; Grondalen and Vangen 1974; Nakano et al. 1979a). In Reiland's (1975) study of animals culled for lameness, the clinical signs were due to infectious arthritis in 18% of the sows that were less than 18 months of age and in 64% of the sows that were older than 18 months. Most of these animals had spondylitis, osteomyelitis, and/or arthritis of the hock joint which were caused by *E. rhusiopathiae*, streptococci, or *Arcanobacterium pyogenes*. The chronic proliferative arthritis and discospondylitis of the vertebral column were secondary to lesions of osteochondrosis.

If osteotropic bacteria such as streptococci or *Arcanobacterium pyogenes* affect joints with a fracture or epiphysiolysis, the primary lesion cannot be determined (Reiland 1975). In suppurative infectious arthritis, if the bacteria enter the joint by direct penetration, only one joint is involved, but if the bacteria are spread from a septic focus—such as infected hoof lesions, fight wounds, skin abrasions, or uterine infections—polyarthritis ensues. The clinical signs of arthritis are heat, swelling, pain of the affected joint, refusal to bear weight on the leg, pyrexia, and anorexia (Hill et al. 1986).

Osteochondrosis. Osteochondrosis is a noninfectious, degenerative, generalized condition of cartilage. It is manifested as an abnormal differentiation of both physeal and epiphyseal cartilage with secondary bony changes (Reiland 1975; Hill et al. 1985; Palmer 1985). Osteochondrosis is the major cause of leg weakness in growing boars and sows (Grondalen 1974c, i, 1981; Reiland 1975; Nakano et al. 1979a; Palmer 1985). The incidence and severity of lesions due to osteochondrosis increase from 10 to 20 weeks of age or from 60 to 120 kg liveweight (Nakano et al. 1981b; Aherne and Brennan 1985). In animals 4–18 months of age, osteochondrosis affects the weight-bearing joints (Hill et al. 1985).

Predilection Sites. Lesions of osteochondrosis are generally found in several joints in the affected animal. The medial part of the joint is most severely affected (Grondalen 1974a; Reiland 1975; Nakano et al. 1981b). Osteochondrosis can be located in the following areas, listed in descending order of severity of lesions (Reiland 1975; Palmer 1985):

1. Articular-epiphyseal lesions: stifle, elbow, lumbar synovial intervertebral joints, hock, shoulder, and hip
2. Growth plate lesions: distal ulna, distal femur, costochondral junction, femoral head, humeral head, ischiatic tuberosity, and thoracolumbar vertebrae
3. Epiphysiolysis and apophysiolysis lesions: glenoid cavity, ischiatic tuberosity, capital femoral epiphysis, vertebral epiphyses, anconeal process, and distal ulnar epiphysis

Pathogenesis. Osteochondrosis occurs when the mechanism of endochondral bone formation is disturbed in various predilection sites, but its pathogenesis is not clear (Grondalen 1974a; Reiland 1975). It is uncertain which tissue component is abnormal and initiates the onset of the lesions: the chondrocytes, the cartilage matrix, or the blood vessels (Hill 1990). The matrix of cartilage is mainly composed of collagen fibers, water, and proteoglycans, which are protein-glycosamino-glycan (GAG) complexes that exist in free form or in aggregates bound by hyaluronic acid. Failure of endochondral ossification is associated with cell necrosis and reduced amounts of proteoglycans and collagen in the tissue. Osteochondritis dissecans and superficial fractures of the cartilage are associated with clusters of chondrocytes and a less than normal concentration of proteoglycans (Nakano et al. 1979a). More than 98% of the total GAG content of the pig's distal femoral articular cartilage is chondroitin sulfate, and its concentration decreases with increasing age from 3 days to 30 weeks (Nakano et al. 1979b). In normal animals, in the force-bearing areas of the stifle joint, the articular cartilage is thickened and contains more chondroitin sulfate and less collagen than in the non–force-bearing areas, indicating that chondroitin sulfate is used for shock absorption (Nakano et al. 1979a). As the pig grows, the joint cartilage does not mature properly, which leaves the joint surfaces prone to damage from mechanical stress.

Local overloading in the joint is a factor in the pathogenesis of osteochondrosis (Grondalen 1974b, e, i; Nakano et al. 1979a, 1981b; Reiland and Anderson 1979). The lesions may be due to a disturbance of the metaphyseal blood flow caused by a local overloading of one part of the joint (Grondalen 1974d). The mechanical stress in heavy pigs on immature cartilage causes a circulatory disturbance at the osteochondral junction, which contributes to the lesions of dyschondroplasia (Walker et al. 1966; Nakano et al. 1981b). Epiphysiolysis of the femoral head, fractures of bone trabeculae, and worn humeral head cartilage in boars may be due to overloading caused by functionally weak muscles, ligaments, cartilage, or bone or by poor conformation (Grondalen 1974b, f, i; Grondalen and Vangen 1974). This stress causes the joint cartilage to be torn or eroded, leaving exposed bone.

The growth plates that close last are most susceptible to osteochondrosis. Growth plate defects occur when the plate is displaced along the plane of the eosinophilic streaks and then bone unites the epiphysis to the metaphysis, functionally closing the plate (Palmer 1985). Premature closure of the proximal femoral growth plate will lead to a short femoral head and reduced lengthwise growth of the femur, which may cause excessive wear of the acetabular cartilage, subluxation of the femoral head, rupture of the teres ligament, or epiphysiolysis of the femoral head (Grondalen 1974a, b). Osteochondritis dissecans develops when a fissure in the subarticular cartilage extends to the articular surface, creating a flap of cartilage (Palmer 1985).

Growth Rate and Backfat. The modern domestic pig is the product of genetic selection for rapid growth, low feed consumption, long carcass length, low backfat, and high carcass yield of lean meat (Reiland 1975). Bone growth and closure of growth plates occur with age rather than with the weight of the pig or the energy content of the diet (Grondalen 1974e). Pigs reach sexual maturity at 5–6 months of age but do not have a mature skeleton until 18 months of age. Adolescence, the time period between 6 and 18 months, is when the clinical signs of osteochondrosis are seen in the pig. The prevalence of osteochondrosis is related to the pig's rate of gain and backfat thickness, which in turn are functions of both genetics and management practices (Grondalen 1974i; Reiland 1975). Rapid weight gain may increase the mechanical stress on the weight-bearing regions of immature cartilage (Aherne and Brennan 1985). If the growth rate of pigs is slowed by feeding only 50–60% of the feed recommended for their weight range, the clinical signs and the severity of the lesions of osteochondrosis are decreased (Grondalen 1974g; Reiland 1975; Nakano et al. 1979a). There is no evidence that osteochondrosis is related to nutritional excesses or deficiencies. The incidence of osteochondrosis increases with the age and the liveweight of the pig.

Genetics, Breed, and Conformation. Heredity plays a significant role in the leg weakness complex partly due to the inheritance of poor conformational features (Grondalen 1974h, i). Osteochondrotic lesions are correlated with desirable production variables (Grondalen 1974e; Reiland et al. 1978; Webb et al. 1983). The conformation of the pig's body, feet, and legs affects the incidence of osteochondrosis (Aherne and Brennan 1985). Exterior conformation traits that are associated with an increased incidence of osteochondrosis and poor locomotion are long back, narrow lumbar region, broad hams, short hindlegs, cross-legged forelegs, sloping pasterns of the forelegs, and small medial hooves on the hindlegs (Grondalen 1974a, f, g). Choosing replacement stock without these exterior conformation traits may significantly reduce culling due to leg weakness (Grondalen 1974g).

Compression, Overloading, and Physical Stress. Physical stress plays a part in the etiology of osteochondrosis, arthrosis, intervertebral disk degeneration, spondylosis, and epiphysiolysis (Grondalen 1974i; Nakano et al. 1979a). Mechanical stress on the joints leading to lesions of osteochondrosis can be caused by local overloading of cartilage or bone tissue, rapid growth rate or weight gain, poor joint stability, or weak cartilage and bone tissue (Grondalen 1974i). Joint stability is a function of musculature, ligaments, and joint shape.

Clinical Signs. Clinical osteochondrosis is a chronic, progressive, shifting lameness affecting one or more limbs in pigs from 4 to 18 months of age (Reiland 1975; Hill 1990). Affected animals will prefer to spend time lying down, will not bear weight on the affected leg(s), and will favor different legs at different times. By 18 months, the incidence of clinical osteochondrosis decreases, because either the animals have been culled or their lesions have healed (Reiland 1975). The articular cartilage is devoid of nerves, but pain is caused by an increased production of joint fluid and swelling of the joint capsule that occur secondary to the lesions of osteochondrosis (Reiland 1975; Aherne and Brennan 1985).

Animals with severe osteochondrosis or arthrosis of the elbow are often clinically sound unless the lesion is a displaced anconeal process (Grondalen 1974b; Nakano et al. 1982). Osteochondrosis of the stifle causes a severe lameness and is seen in animals less than 1 year of age (Grondalen 1974b). Young sows with a separation of the tuber ischii dog-sit with their hindlegs directed forward, and if forced to rise, they stand for only a short time (Hill et al. 1986). Severe arthrosis of the hock joint, mild arthrosis of the medial condyle of the femur, and repaired lesions of separated tuber ischii all cause little discomfort in sows (Grondalen 1974b). Osteochondrosis of the vertebrae, with or without spondylosis, results in kyphosis (Hill 1990). Proximal femoral epiphysiolysis causes an acute severe lameness, and if the lesion is bilateral, the animal is unable to rise (Hill 1990). Boars that are lame due to osteochondrosis spend a lot of time lying down, show stiffness when moving, and are unable to mount and breed (Grondalen 1974g; Reiland 1975; Nakano et al. 1981a).

Diagnosis. To diagnose osteochondrosis, first rule out all other causes of lameness. Examine suspect animals clinically and then examine a representative sample at postmortem. Sows can be followed to slaughter to examine the feet, stifle, hip and elbow joints, and cut half of the vertebral column. Proximal femoral epiphysiolysis must be differentiated from a femoral fracture, paraplegia due to a lumbosacral fracture, or a spinal canal abscess (Hill 1990). Although the definitive diagnosis of osteochondrosis is made by histologic examination of affected joints, 69% of cases can be diagnosed after clinical and gross postmortem examination (Hill et al. 1984; Dewey et al. 1993).

Gross Postmortem Lesions. Osteochondrosis is manifested as osteochondritis dissecans, epiphysiolysis, deformities of bones, and arthrosis (Palmer 1985). Affected articular cartilage may be invaginated below the level of the surrounding cartilage and may be thick and yellowish or thin and reddish (Grondalen 1974a; Reiland 1975). The border between the cartilage and bone is uneven and its surface may be wrinkled (Reiland 1975).

Joints severely affected with osteochondrosis have an increase in the amount of synovial fluid, ruptures, hemorrhages of the joint capsule and ligaments, thickened joint capsule, and villous proliferation of the synovial membrane (Grondalen 1974b; Nakano et al. 1981b).

A fissure running parallel to the joint surface separates the outer layers of cartilage from the deeper layers or may occur at the osteochondral junction (Grondalen 1974a). The fissure may extend to the articular surface, creating a cartilage flap (Grondalen 1974a; Palmer 1985). Secondary lesions include hemorrhages, connective tissue proliferation and necrosis in the subchondral bone, osteophyte production, and chip bone fractures (Grondalen 1974a; Palmer 1985). Epiphyseal separation can either be complete–as in the head of the femur and the tuber ischii–or partial–as in the distal epiphyseal plate of the ulna (Palmer 1985).

In advanced cases of osteochondrosis, the long bones of the extremities are shorter and the metaphyses are flared. The femoral and humeral heads are flattened and have short necks, and the head is lower than the major trochanter. Premature closure of the distal ulnar growth plate causes a volar deviation of the distal radius, a fractured anconeal process, and a more semicircular, semilunar notch.

Osteochondrosis of the spine occurs in the thoracolumbar region, causing the synovial joint surfaces to vary in shape and size, with the tip of the joint avulsed and connected to the rest of the joint by a fibrous tissue band. In animals older than 18 months, osteophyte production occurs and joints may become ankylosed (Reiland 1975). Intervertebral disks have a nucleus pulposus that is hemorrhagic, granular, yellowish, firm, and almost absent or changed to a homogenous, darkly colored mass. Epiphyseal separation of the tuber ischii is often associated with signs of repair and arthrosis and may cause a fracture through the primary and secondary spongiosa (Grondalen 1974b; Palmer 1985).

Histologic Lesions. Histologic lesions of osteochondrosis involving the growth cartilage of the physis and the epiphysis include foci of metaphyseal dysplasia, eosinophilic streaks, intracartilagenous cavities, and protrusions or invaginations of cartilaginous plates (Grondalen 1974e, g; Reiland 1975; Nakano et al. 1979a; Hill et al. 1984; Palmer 1985). Histologic lesions of osteochondrosis were seen in 94% of culled sows (Dewey et al. 1993).

Treatment. Pigs with a foreleg lameness due to osteochondrosis may respond to 6 weeks of rest in a pen with secure footing, sufficient room for exercise, and freedom from being mounted by other animals. Affected animals need to be rested for 6 weeks prior to being used for breeding. Boars and multiparous sows with clinical signs of the hindlegs or those with a recurring foreleg lameness should be culled. Some boars that are lame due to damaged cartilage become clinically sound when put out on dirt lots (McPhee and Laws 1976; Fredeen and Sather 1978; Nakano et al. 1981a).

A non-steroidal anti-inflammatory drug, meloxicam, was recently approved for use in dogs and cattle and received marketing approval for pigs in Europe (Friton et al. 2003). In double blind, clinical trials, pigs affected with noninfectious causes of lameness had improved lameness scores, improved feed intake, and reduced retreatment rates 4 days after the treatment compared to pigs given a placebo.

Preventing Leg Weakness. Gilts' joints mature with age rather than with weight. Rapidly growing gilts that are fed ad libitum experience joint stress due to their weight. Overfeeding gilts results in increased leg weakness problems and increased culling due to lameness (Jorgensen and Sorensen 1998). Gilts were fed semi–ad libitum (ad libitum for two 30-minute feeding episodes per day), at the recommended Danish standard or 75% of the Danish standard. Sows in the semi–ad libitum group had higher overall leg weakness scores and tended to have weaker pasterns and long accessory digits in the forelimbs. Over the life of the sows twice as many sows were culled for leg weakness in the ad libitum–fed group compared to the other groups. The age sows were culled for lameness was younger in the ad libitum group than the other groups.

A gilt that is moved, exposed to a new floor type, mixed with a new group of animals, or trucked to a new farm will experience stress to her joints. Mating and pregnancy are also potential sources of mechanical stress. Restricted exercise in either a stall or a small pen causes lameness, leg weakness, and poor muscle development. The area per finisher pig and the number of finisher pigs per pen will affect the culling rate due to lameness in sows. Osteochondrosis is associated with rapid weight gain and mechanical stress to joints. Replacement gilts should be selected at the nursery or grower stage. By 150 days of age they should be housed with other gilts in a pen with good secure footing and 10 square feet (1.3 m^2) per animal. Their feed should be restricted and they should be bred on their second or third observed estrus.

Arthrosis. Arthrosis (arthropathy, osteoarthrosis, or osteoarthritis) is a nonspecific, degenerative condition of cartilage that develops in chronic joint disease (Palmer 1985). Lesions of osteoarthrosis include fibrillation of joint cartilage, ulceration of the articular surface, osteophyte production, and thickened synovial membrane and joint capsule (Palmer 1985). Lesions of osteochondrosis that affect the joint surface fill with fibrocartilaginous tissue, which is then replaced by osseous repair tissue (Grondalen 1974b; Nakano et al. 1979a; Palmer 1985). The incidence and severity of arthrosis increases with the increasing age of the animal (Reiland 1975). In Reiland's (1975) study of culled sows, the inci-

dence in sows less than 18 months of age was 7%, and in those older than 18 months, it was 82%. Arthrosis is usually secondary to osteochondrosis (Reiland 1975). Arthrosis of the hock is severe and the incidence is high, but it is of minor significance with respect to clinical lameness (Grondalen 1974b).

Foot Problems. Torn dewclaws, overgrown lateral digits on the hindfeet, or foot rot are either the first or second most important cause of lameness in sows (Smith and Robertson 1971; Penny 1979; Dewey et al. 1993). Dry sows that are housed on partially slatted concrete floors may have their dewclaws torn as their feet slide outward in an attempt to stand. Overgrown lateral digits are seen in animals without exercise, especially those kept on nonabrasive floors such as plastic or steel slats. These sows should have their hooves or dewclaws trimmed on a regular basis. Floors with rough edges or sharp prominences that cause abrasions and floors with poor drainage increase the incidence of foot rot.

Foot Rot. Foot rot begins as a crack in the wall of the hoof which starts at the volar surface and extends two-thirds of the way to the coronary band (Penny 1979). Secondary infection of the crack by *Fusobacterium necrophorum*, *Arcanobacterium pyogenes*, or spirochetes leads to a deep necrotic ulcer of the laminae and coronary band or a necrotic track which may reach the coronary band and form an ulcer (bush foot) or an infection of the deep flexor tendon or phalangeal bones and joints (Vaughan 1969). If the crack does not become infected, it is termed a false sand-crack and does not cause lameness (Hill et al. 1986). Clinically, foot rot causes a unilateral lameness in which the animal is reluctant to bear weight on the affected limb. This contributes to clumsiness and bad mothering in sows and impotentia coeundi in boars (Penny et al. 1963; Hill et al. 1986). Foot rot and associated foot lesions (heel, toe, and sole erosions, white line lesions, and false sand-crack) are seen in 64% of slaughter weight pigs (Penny et al. 1963). In a similar survey done by Backstrom et al. (1980), almost 50% of slaughter pigs had moderate to severe foot lesions, particularly on the pads, sole, and lateral digits.

Lesions of foot rot are commonly seen on the lateral claws of the hindlegs (Simmins and Brooks 1988). Hoof injuries often occur in the lateral claw of animals with uneven claws where the lateral claw is larger than the medial claw (Penny et al. 1963; Vaughan 1969; Grondalen 1974a; Penny 1979). The uneven claw may also cause the animal to stand and walk with an abnormal gait (Penny 1979). Crated animals have fewer hoof lesions than penned animals (Bane et al. 1980). There was a positive, significant, linear relationship between the gross postmortem scores for the foot lesions and the clinical grade and the parity of the sow. The older sows suffered from foot trouble more frequently than the younger sows (Dewey et al. 1993).

Fractures. Fractures occur when animals struggle to free a limb from between slats or under feed troughs or pen rails or when they fall on slippery concrete or during transport (Vaughan 1969; Hill et al. 1986). Clinically there is a sudden onset of severe lameness in one leg, the animal carries the leg, and there is crepitation and pain on palpation (Buddle 1987). The condition is widespread but rare.

Floors

Lameness is associated with many factors and cannot usually be blamed on only one factor. Housing appeared to be an important factor influencing the level of lameness that an individual herd experienced. Floor types affect the incidence of foot and limb disorders (Elliot and Doige 1973; Perrin et al. 1978; Newton et al. 1980; MAFF 1981; Nakano et al. 1981a; Hani and Troxler 1984). A survey of Pig Health Scheme Herds showed that 44% of farms with slatted floors had pigs with injuries, whereas only 28% of farms with solid floors had pigs with injuries caused by flooring (MAFF 1981). Good perforated floors require a durable, low-cost, nonslip, nonabrasive surface and acceptable levels of cleanliness and ease of cleaning (Smith and Mitchell 1976). In sows, lameness is influenced by the floor types used for sows and gilts as well as those used during their rearing period. Concrete floors cause more foot and leg problems than earthen floors or deep straw bedding, and injuries occur more frequently on perforated floors (Nakano et al. 1981b). Perforated floors such as partially slatted or fully slatted concrete or metal slats cause more lameness than solid concrete floors. In the farrowing crates, plastic and steel slats cause more lameness than solid floors. The best floor type for the development of feet and legs is a solid floor with bedding.

It is difficult to obtain the correct balance between nonslipperiness and nonabrasiveness with solid concrete floors. Rough floors are created by using sand of the wrong particle size or by allowing the surface to be broken down by wear or by organic acid in the urine. Poorly laid concrete floors cause abrasions to areas such as the spine of the scapula, the hooves, and the soles. Slippery concrete causes ataxia and tendon swelling, and newly laid concrete causes lameness due to its slippery qualities as well as its surface chemicals. Wet concrete pens cause cracked and bruised soles, which can lead to secondary infections (Penny 1979; MAFF 1981). Substandard concrete may be improved by using bedding, laying a new concrete floor, or coating the concrete with chlorinated rubber, epoxy resin, or polyurethane paints (MAFF 1981).

The floor types associated with culling rates for lameness in sows include steel or plastic slats in the farrowing crates, partially slatted concrete floors and fully slatted concrete floors for sow pens, partially slatted sow stalls with metal slats, and partially slatted concrete floors used for the finisher pigs. The edges of concrete slats are often too rough and the slats may be placed too far apart, causing abrasions of the coronary band and the accessory digits. Plastic slats are too slippery and cause the sow's feet to be overgrown, leading to secondary damage to the accessory digits (MAFF 1981). Foot pad lesions and hoof cracks are positively correlated with hoof and sole length. The hoof length and sole length are the longest on plastic slats, followed by aluminum, steel, and concrete.

Rough concrete floors, sharp-edged concrete slats, and slats of other materials often result in severe foot injuries, which can lead to changes in the way the pig walks. An altered gait may change the joint congruence, causing overloading in the joint and subsequent cartilage damage (Aherne and Brennan 1985). Also, both insecure footing and foot lesions increase the mechanical stress to joints, which in turn increases the incidence of leg weakness (Nakano et al. 1981b). There is an increase in leg weakness on perforated floors (Nakano et al. 1981b; Dewey 1988). Raising pigs on deep straw bedding rather than partially slatted concrete floors decreases the incidence of gait abnormalities and claw injuries and may decrease the incidence of clinical osteochondrosis (Hani and Troxler 1984; Dewey 1988).

There are unique sources of injury related to estrus detection and mating. Specifically, introducing a boar to non-estrus females increases the injury rate. Conducting estrus detection and mating in a specific mating pen reduces the cull rate for injuries. Farms that house sows in stalls for the first 3 weeks postweaning have a lower cull rate than farms that have only pens for sow housing. The prevalence of injuries including those causing lameness is higher in facilities where pigs are fearful of humans (Barnett et al. 2001).

Breeding pens that are too small, have right-angled corners or slippery floors increase the chance for injuries and lameness in boars and sows (Barnett et al. 2001). Dry, nonslip floors in large octagonally shaped pens used only for breeding are preferable (Hemsworth et al. 1989).

Exercise

Pigs given exercise and pigs penned with other animals have significantly better gait scores and less lameness and posterior paresis than pigs denied exercise or individually housed (Elliot and Doige 1973; Grondalen 1974a; Fredeen and Sather 1978). Inactive individually housed animals have a reduction in cortical bone mass and have muscular weakness. Pigs that are exercised have increased muscle strength and are more agile, allowing them surer movement on slippery floors (Elliot and Doige 1973; Grondalen 1974a, g, i). This may be one of the reasons that gilts and sows in loose housing systems are less prone to culling for leg weakness problems. The duration of confinement is correlated positively to the degree of joint damage (Grondalen 1974i; Fredeen and Sather 1978; Hani and Troxler 1984). Boars given exercise have fewer conformational abnormalities such as bowlegs, flexion of the carpus, and sickle hocks than boars that are confined (Perrin and Bowland 1977). Perrin et al. (1978) found that floor type did not influence the degree of joint lesions, but Fredeen and Sather (1978) stated that floor and housing type in the nursing period may increase the piglets' susceptibility to joint damage after weaning.

Diet Causing Locomotor or Neurologic Problems

Diets in modern pig production are typically made of locally grown grains supplemented with a protein source, vitamins, and minerals. Deficient soil or mixing errors in feed manufacture can result in nutritional deficiencies or toxicities (Silvertsen et al. 1992) (Table 5.3).

Table 5.3. Lameness and neurological entities caused by nutritional deficiencies.

Deficiency	Clinical Signs	Epidemiology	Pathology
Copper	Incoordination, paresis, posterior paralysis, excessive flexion of hocks and forelegs, recumbency, occasionally sudden death	Rare: unsupplemented diets, deficient soil	Aortic rupture in sudden deaths
Manganese	Newborns: weak at birth, head tilt, incoordination and poor balance, inability to suckle	Rare: progeny of manganese-deficient sows	
	Growers: shifting lameness, dog-sitting, short bowed legs, thick hocks, weak joints	Rare: progeny of manganese-deficient sows	
	Sows: stillbirths, irregular estrous cycle, return to estrus, dysgalactia	Rare: progeny of manganese-deficient sows	
Niacin	Ataxia, quadriplegia, posterior paralysis, anorexia, reduced growth rate, diarrhea, anemia, dermatitis, alopecia	Unsupplemented corn diets low in tryptophan	Thickened mucosa of colon and cecum
Pantothenic acid	Goose-stepping gait, incoordination, dermatitis with periocular exudate and alopecia, diarrhea	Rare: nonbalanced diets of waste products or corn	Congestion, edema, reddened colon
Selenium (vitamin E and selenium, white muscle)	Affects all ages, especially 30–60 kg: sudden death, ataxia, stiff staggering gait, weakness, paralysis, depression, anorexia, recumbency	Less common, found in selenium-deficient area	Pale areas in muscles, petechiae and white streaks in cardiac muscle, subcutaneous edema
Vitamin A	Newborns: stillbirth, micro- or anophthalmia, cleft palate, edema, high morbidity and mortality	Uncommon	Hydrocephalus, small cranium, herniation of spinal cord in lumbar region, thick epithelial surfaces
	Nursery pigs: progressive neurological dysfunction, incoordination, swaying gait, restlessness, dog-sitting, posterior paralysis, lordosis, blindness, reduced growth	Uncommon	Hydrocephalus, small cranium, herniation of spinal cord in lumbar region, thick epithelial surfaces
Vitamin D	Nursery pigs: enlarged joints and costochondral junctions, decreased average daily gain, stiff gait, lameness	Rare: high morbidity, low mortality	Thick, soft bone cortices, uneven epiphyseal cartilage
Water (salt poisoning)	Peracute: tremors, prostration, running movements, death	Widespread, uncommon, water deprivation, then drinking excessively	Edema of meninges, flattened cerebral cortex, hyperemia, erosions of stomach mucosa
	Acute: repeated seizures at 3–7 minute intervals, twitching face and ears, dog-sitting, head up and back, falling over, violent paddling, salivation then recovery and walking away, apparent blindness, wandering aimlessly	Widespread, uncommon, water deprivation, then drinking excessively	Edema of meninges, flattened cerebral cortex, hyperemia, erosions of stomach mucosa

Biotin. Biotin (vitamin H) is a B vitamin. The bioavailability of biotin in pig feed varies with the major ingredients of the feed (Brooks 1982). Corn is a good natural source of biotin (Bane et al. 1980; Hamilton and Veum 1984), but diets based on cereals such as barley that are low in available biotin may not provide sufficient biotin for horn integrity (Simmins and Brooks 1988). This makes the hoof wall prone to trauma on hard floor surfaces (Bane et al. 1980).

The response of sows with foot lesions to the addition of biotin in the feed is variable because although some may be biotin deficient, there are many causes of foot lesions (Penny et al. 1980; Grandhi and Strain 1980; Brooks 1982; Bryant et al. 1985). Biotin deficiency causes foot lesions due to soft hooves (Penny et al. 1980). Biotin supplementation of feed, 1160 µg/kg during gestation and 2320 µg/kg during lactation compared to 160 µg/kg, decreases the rate of claw lesions in gilts. However, it does not heal lesions in parity 2 and 3 sows with lesions prior to supplementation (Penny et al. 1980). Biotin may also be administered via injection at 250 µg/kg body weight in pregnant animals or 150 µg/kg in lactating animals (Brooks et al. 1977). Supplementary d-biotin at 1 mg/kg feed increases the compressive strength and the hardness of the sidewall regions of the pig's hoof and decreases the hardness of the heel bulb (Webb et al. 1984). The heel bulb acts as a cushion, absorbing energy on contact and spreading the weight of the pig over the area of the foot. Biotin supplementation may reduce the likelihood of injury to the foot and allow an increase of 8% in the floor slot-to-slat ratio from 61% to 69% for 100 kg pigs (Webb et al. 1984). As a preventive measure, pigs weighing 25 kg and more may be given biotin supplementation (Simmins and Brooks 1988).

Osteoporosis. Osteoporosis is caused by an excess resorption of bone and results in endosteal thinning of the trabeculae and cortices (Spencer 1979). In mid-to-late lactation or the early postweaning period, osteoporosis occurs as the sows' bones decalcify to mobilize calcium for milk production. The periosteal surface has a slightly increased mineralization rate. These sows may develop fractures of their vertebrae, femurs, and phalanges. Clinically this occurs as lameness, or "downer" sow syndrome, late in lactation or when the sow is mounted by the boar or another sow. Typically the syndrome occurs late in the first or second lactation or during the postweaning period (Gayle and Schwartz 1980).

The diagnosis is made by identifying thinned cortices. The specific gravity of the bone will be less than 1.018, whereas the specific gravity is 1.022 or more in normal sows (Spencer 1979). A cross section of the sixth rib shows a cortex to total area ratio of less than 0.2 (normal sows have a ratio greater than 0.3). Serum calcium and phosphorus will be within normal levels (Gayle and Schwartz 1980).

Osteoporosis is caused by inadequate levels of dietary calcium, phosphorus, or vitamin D. Recommended daily intake levels for lactating and gestating sows are as follows: calcium, 37.5 g and 10 g; phosphorus, 25 g and 10 g; and vitamin D, 660 IU per kg of feed (Gayle and Schwartz 1980). Reduced exercise from prolonged periods in crates may predispose sows to osteoporosis (Spencer 1979) because of changes in pH and oxygen tension in the bones (Gayle and Schwartz 1980). Demineralization occurs due to the higher levels of parathyroid hormone (PTH) in lactating sows. PTH controls renal synthesis of the active form of vitamin D_3, which is responsible for trabecular bone mobilization. Exertion or slipping of these sows may cause spontaneous fractures of their pelvic bones, femurs, or lumbosacral vertebrae, leading to various degrees of stiffness, lameness, or posterior paralysis (Hill et al. 1986). Fractures in old sows, especially those of the glenoid surface, may be caused by a bone weakened by osteochondrosis (Reiland 1975). Prevention includes adequate dietary vitamins and minerals, lactation limited to 4 weeks, and breeding gilts after 7 months of age (Gayle and Schwartz 1980).

Poisoning

Poisonings occur when pigs consume products in their surroundings, such as rodent bait or excess amounts of compounds normally found in swine feeds (Table 5.4).

Arsanilic Acid. Arsanilic acid is fed to pigs either to promote growth or to treat swine dysentery. Overdoses of arsanilic acid decrease growth rate and cause head tremor, progressive blindness, ataxia, and paresis. Pigs remain bright, alert, and even euphoric. The onset of neurological signs begins 4–6 days after ingesting high levels (1000–2000 g/ton) of arsanilic acid, but at lower levels (600 g/ton) the onset of clinical signs is much slower and growth rate is not depressed. If the drug is removed, the symptoms stop progressing and may regress (Hardin et al. 1968). Other clinical signs are seen in pigs poisoned with 3-nitro-4-hydroxy phenyl arsonic acid (Rice et al. 1980). Symptoms are not visible until the pigs are moved or exercised. After exercise there is trembling of the muscles of the shoulders, hams, and backs followed by violent tremors, incoordination, and extreme agitation and screaming. The seizure lasts for 1 minute, after which the animal lies down and the trembling ceases. Diagnosis is confirmed by identifying arsenicals in the urine. On postmortem examination, the bladder is distended, and there is degeneration of the optic nerves, optic tracts, and peripheral nerves (Hardin et al. 1968).

Insecticide. Organophosphate and organochlorine poisoning occurs in pigs due to inadvertent mixing or spilling of insecticides used for rootworm control in corn crops (Frank et al. 1991). Most pigs (70%) consuming contaminated feed die within hours of ingesting

Table 5.4. Lameness and neurological entities caused by ingested poisons.

Poison	Clinical Signs	Epidemiology	Pathology
Furazolidone	Ataxia, paresis, convulsions, inappetence, vomiting, feed refusal	Rare: overdose of drug concentrate	Hemorrhage, thrombocytopenia
Hygromycin B	Loss of balance, ototoxicity causing ataxia, cataracts causing blindness	Problem if fed continuously; prevent with a schedule of 2 months on, 2 months off	Cataracts
Lead	Salivation, diarrhea, anorexia, hypersensitivity, squealing, tremors, ataxia, enlarged joints, blindness, convulsions, death	Rare: oil used to treat mange	Gastrointestinal reddening
Mercury	Unaware of surroundings, dysphagia, chewing, incoordination, wandering, blindness, loud vocalizations, paresis, tremor, lateral recumbency, paddling, coma, death	Rare: alkylmercurial compounds used as fungicides in grain	Cerebral atrophy, enlarged pale kidney cortex, pale shrunken liver, necrotizing suppurative pharyngitis, focal erosive gastritis
Nitrite	Sudden death without struggling, tremors, weakness, ataxia, recumbency, convulsions, dyspnea, cyanosis, tachycardia, brown mucous membranes	Rare: consumption of preformed nitrite (microbial action on nitrates in whey)	Dark brown blood; endocardial hemorrhage
Phosphorus	Vomiting (smells like garlic), diarrhea with or without blood, abdominal pain, jaundice. Gastrointestinal signs followed by convulsions, coma, death	Rare: consumption of rodent bait	Jaundice, carcass smells like garlic, enlarged mottled liver, catarrhal inflammation of GI tract
Sodium monofluoracetate	Intermittent paddling, tonic-clonic convulsions, persistent vomiting	Rare: consumption of rodent bait	
Vitamin A	Weak hind end, knuckling of pasterns, bowed legs, reluctance to stand, standing with legs under body and back arched, development of short legs, swollen nonpainful joints due to premature closure of epiphyseal plates; thin cortices, slow growth, hyperesthesia, red skin	Rare: oversupplementation (young pigs fed >200,000 μg/kg within 14 days)	Short diaphysis; rotated and enlarged epiphyses of leg bones; pitted articular surfaces; congenital defects of heart, eye, rectovaginal area
Zinc	Enlarged shoulder joints, stiff gait, anorexia, reduced growth rate, rough coat	Rare: dairy products stored in galvanized containers and then fed to pigs	Hemorrhage into joint cavities, arthritis of head of humerus, red mucosa in GI tract

these products. Organophosphates cause pulmonary edema, myocardial hemorrhage, and cholinesterase inhibition, which results in cholinesterase levels of zero in whole blood of affected animals. These chemicals do not persist in the affected animal, so the meat is not hazardous to the consumer. Organochlorines cause convulsions. Although animals recover once the contaminated food is removed, these chemicals persist in meat and milk; therefore, it may not be possible to return the animal to the food chain (Frank et al. 1991). Chemical analysis of the feed is used for the definitive diagnosis. The best preventive measure is to store the chemicals separately from the swine feeds.

Selenium. Selenium is an essential nutrient and is required at 0.3 ppm for growing pigs; however, at more than 4 ppm it becomes toxic (Stowe et al. 1992; Stowe and Herdt 1992). Affected pigs have a decreased feed intake and an incoordinated gait and then become paraplegic or quadriplegic due to segmental spinal cord lesions. They remain bright and alert and occasionally show muscle fasciculation and occasional vomiting. With severe poisonings pigs are in lateral recumbency, show flaccid paralysis, and lose sensation to the skin (Buddle 1987). The diagnosis can be made from a history of feed-mixing error by measuring the selenium levels in the blood, or by identifying spinal cord lesions that include bilaterally symmetrical focal malacia of the gray matter of the ventral horns, a mottled liver, dehydrated carcass, and visceral edema. Once the toxic feed is removed, the majority of pigs will recover but will have a stiff gait and icterus.

Table 5.5. Lameness and neurological entities caused by inhaled toxins.

Poison	Clinical Signs	Epidemiology	Pathology
Carbon dioxide	Anxiety, staggering, coma, death at >400,000 ppm, increased respiratory rate and depth at >50,000 ppm	Rare: inadequate ventilation in winter	Dark colored blood and tissues
Carbon monoxide	Lethargy, incoordination, coma, death due to hypoxia, increased stillbirths and neonatal death, abortion storm	Rare: malfunction of fossil-fuel or gas heaters and poor ventilation	Cherry red blood, bronchodilation
Hydrogen sulfide	Sudden death if >400 ppm; listlessness, incoordination, spasms, coma, respiratory depression, cyanosis	Rare: poor ventilation after agitation of effluent; dangerous for humans, rotten egg smell	Cyanosis, pulmonary edema, congestion, emphysema

***Cassia* sp.** *Cassia* plant species seeds in grain sorghum cause decreased appetite, incoordination, ataxia, staggering, decreased weight gain, and increased mortality in grower pigs (Flory et al. 1992). A similar syndrome is found in chickens, where the plant causes muscle atrophy and pallor.

Inhaled Toxins. Pigs are susceptible to inhaled toxins due to the confinement housing systems. These toxins are described in Table 5.5.

PRIMARY NEUROLOGIC DYSFUNCTION

Clinical Examination

The purpose of the neurological examination is to determine the extent of the neurologic deficits and the location of the lesion. The neurological examination begins with a complete physical examination of the animal(s) involved. Specific history questions include previous illness, behavioral changes, seizures, head tilt, circling, and presence of pain or paresis. After observing the pig in its pen, move the pig into the alleyway, out of its normal surroundings. Allow the pig to become familiar with the area so that you can fully appreciate its behavior. Watch carefully for visual difficulties, proprioceptive loss on slippery floors, purposeful movements, mental status, gait, posture, and evidence of trauma (Kornegay and Seim 1996). Serial examinations are performed to determine the static nature of the clinical signs. Observations may be recorded using the examination form shown in Figure 5.1. Evaluation of cerebral spinal fluid may help differentiate neurologic problems with similar clinical signs (Ebeid et al. 1997).

Specific terminology is used in neurologic examinations to denote loss of function. Plegia and paralysis describe complete loss of sensory and motor function of an extremity. Paresis is partial loss of sensation and complete or partial loss of motor function. Tetraparesis refers to all four limbs, paraparesis to both pelvic limbs, hemiparesis to the front and the hindlimb on one side, and monoparesis to a single limb.

Posture is evaluated in a resting standing position and then after moving the pig into a prone position to determine whether it can regain a normal posture. The clinical signs and their referent lesions are as follows: vestibular abnormalities causing a continuous head tilt; spinal cord lesions, an abnormal truncal posture; proprioceptive deficits, an improper positioning of legs; flaccidity referring to decreased muscle tone, whereas spasticity is an increased muscle tone. Palpate the muscles carefully and systematically, comparing one side to the other. Specifically look for size, tone, strength, normal contour, repetition, and normal motion.

A normal gait requires the neurologic organization of the brain, spinal cord, and peripheral nerves. Proprioceptive abnormalities, which can be caused by a lesion at any level, are seen as knuckling, misplacement of a foot, or scuffing of the hoof. Proprioceptive positioning is tested by flexing the claw so the dorsal position is on the floor and watching how quickly the foot returns to normal positioning. A worn dorsal hoof wall and skin abrasions may signify chronic problems. Paresis, a disruption of the voluntary motor pathways, involves the cerebral cortex, brain stem, and the peripheral nerves. Ataxia is a lack of coordination and usually involves the cerebellum, vestibular system, or spinal cord. Purposeful movement is a conscious attempt to move the animals' legs. Weakly ambulatory or nonambulatory animals drag their legs. In these animals, watch hip movement and pushing with their feet; support the animal with the tail. Lack of purposeful movement suggests severe but possibly reversible spinal cord injury.

Examination of thoracic limbs in lightweight animals can be accomplished by supporting the full weight of the hind end of the animal and allowing the animal to walk forward on one (hopping) or both forelegs (wheelbarrowing). Slow initiation of movement refers to lesions in the cervical spinal cord, brain stem, or cerebral cortex. Exaggerated movements indicate cervical spinal cord, lower brain stem, or cerebellar lesions. The hopping test with poor initiation suggests proprioceptive deficits, but poor movement is due to motor deficits. In the extensor

SIGNALMENT: Age range _____   Numbers affected _____

HISTORY: Duration: ____hours   ____days   ____months
            Onset: ____acute   ____chronic
            Course: ____progressive ____static   ____intermittent

PHYSICAL EXAMINATION: 4 = Exaggerated, clonus   1 = Decreased
                        3 = Exaggerated   0 = Absent
                        2 = Normal   NE = Not evaluated

MENTAL: __ alert   __ depressed   __ disoriented   __ stupor   __ coma
POSTURE: __ normal   __ head tilt   __ tremor   __ falling
GAIT: __ normal   __ ataxic   __ pelvis limbs __ all four   __ circling
PARESIS: __ normal   __ mono   __ para   __ tetra   __ hemi

Postural Reactions	Left Front	Right Front	Left Rear	Right Rear
Hopping				
Extensor postural thrust				
Proprioceptive positioning				
Hemi-standing/walking				
Placing: tactile				
Placing: visual				
Pelvic limb withdrawal				
Forelimb withdrawal				
Crossed extensor				
Anal sphincter				
Wheelbarrowing				

Sensory Exam	Localize	Describe
Cutaneous trunci reflex		
Sensory level		
Hyperpathia		
Superficial pain		
Deep pain		

5.1. *Neurologic clinical examination form (adapted from Kornegay and Seim 1996).*

postural thrust, the thorax is supported and the animal is lowered to the floor so that one can watch for caudal, symmetric walking movements of the hindlegs. Hemi-walking and hemi-standing are performed by supporting the forelimbs and hindlimbs of one side of the body and watching for lateral walking movements. These two tests are evaluated the same way as the wheelbarrow test.

There are two placing tests: tactile placing without vision, where the animal's eyes are covered, and visual placing, where the pig can see the surface it is approaching. Lift the animal and touch the forelegs at or below the carpus to a table; the pig should immediately place the feet on the table or with visual placing should anticipate by reaching for the table. Visual placing requires intact visual pathways to the cerebral cortex and to the motor cortex and motor pathways to the peripheral nerves. Normal tactile placing with abnormal visual placing suggests a sight disorder. The opposite suggests a sensory pathway lesion. Cortical lesions produce a contralateral (opposite) abnormality, but a lesion below the midbrain produces same-side (ipsilateral) deficit.

Spinal Cord Lesions

Vaughan (1969) suggests that the most common cause of posterior paralysis in pigs of all ages is compression of the spinal cord by an abscess that occurs secondary to an infection in the intervertebral disks, vertebral bodies, or paravertebral tissues. Clinical signs begin with incoordination of the hindquarters, which rapidly progresses to flaccid paraplegia, pyrexia, and local swelling of the tissues over the abscess (Vaughan 1969; Buddle 1987). Pigs continue to eat and drink and appear alert. The occurrence is widespread and sporadic, and morbidity is low. Diagnoses are made by identifying the abscess in the spinal canal. In adult animals the most likely causes are an excess load on the disks causing premature disk degeneration or primary osteochondrosis of the vertebrae (Grondalen 1974b). In growing animals spinal cord abscesses are secondary to tail biting. The animals require euthanasia.

To identify a spinal cord lesion, attempt to localize the pain to an extremity or the cervical, thoracolumbar, or lumbosacral areas. Determine whether the pain or paresis is acute or chronic, progressive or static, persistent or intermittent, sharp or dull. The type of pain and paresis can be used to determine whether the spinal injury is extradural, intradural but extramedullary, or intramedullary. Extradural lesions, such as intervertebral disk extrusion, discospondylitis, or vertebral osteomyelitis, present with acute persistent and progressive pain and paresis. Intradural-extramedullary lesions cause chronic dull pain with a slowly progressive paresis. Intramedullary lesions, such as a vascular insult, cause acute sudden but short-lived pain and acute persistent paresis that is not progressive.

Spinal or myotactic reflexes test the sensory and motor components of the reflex arc and the descending motor pathways. It is easier to localize spinal reflexes to the hindlimbs than to the thoracic limbs (Table 5.6). The spinal reflex response can be normal, absent, or depressed, indicating a lower motor neuron (LMN) problem, or exaggerated, indicating an upper motor neuron (UMN) problem. The descending pathways from the brain and spinal cord normally inhibit the reflex, and thus, a UMN problem results in an exaggerated response.

Additional indications of LMN problems include poor strength, flaccid muscle tone, muscle fasciculation, early neurogenic muscle atrophy, and easy bladder expression. UMN problems are associated with variable but strong reflex strength, spastic muscle tone, late disuse muscle atrophy, clonus, difficult bladder expression, and absent root signature. Clonus is sustained quivering

of the muscles after the reflex response, which is palpable but not visual.

The perineal or anal sphincter reflex is tested by stimulating the perineum with forceps (Kornegay and Seim 1996). Contraction of the anal sphincter suggests function of the sacral spinal cord and pudendal nerve. The urinary bladder is innervated by both autonomic (hypogastric and pelvic) and somatic (pudendal) nerves. Spastic bladder outflow and difficult expression (UMN) occur with lesions above S2–S3, whereas lack of sphincter tone and easily expressed bladder occur with lesions of S2–S3 (LMN). Unconscious tail wagging may occur with urination or the anal sphincter reflex and can occur with complete transection of the sacral spinal cord.

The crossed extensor reflex is elicited by pinching the coronary band on the down limb when the pig is in lateral recumbency. Use a gentle stimulus or the animal will attempt to stand. The extension of the upper limb corresponds to a UMN lesion affecting the descending inhibitory pathway of the spinal cord. Panniculus reflex (cutaneous trunci reflex) is the twitching of the cutaneous trunci muscle on both sides of the dorsal midline at the point and cranial to the point of stimulation. Begin testing at the fifth lumbar vertebra and continue cranially. No response will occur one to two segments caudal to the spinal cord lesion.

Deep pain perception tests the functional integrity of the spinal cord. It is the most important prognostic test but should be applied at the end of the physical examination to get reliable responses to the prior tests. Apply painful stimuli to each limb and the tail. The pig will vocalize, look, or attempt to move away. The withdrawal of the limb is not a behavioral response. Spinal cord injuries result in sequential losses of function as follows: first, proprioception, then voluntary motor function, superficial pain sensation, and finally deep pain sensation. The return of function follows the reverse order. The amount of spinal cord compression will be determined by the measurable functional loss. Loss of deep pain sensation indicates a poor prognosis.

Hyperpathia is a behavioral response (vocalization, turning to look, or moving away from examiner) elicited by applying pressure to the spinous processes or paraspinal muscles of the thoracic and lumbar region or the transverse processes of the cervical region. Pain perception occurs at the level of the spinal cord injury. The sensory-level response also helps determine the location of the lesion. Pinpricks are applied to the back from the seventh lumbar vertebra cranially. The part of the back between where the normal behavioral response and the depressed response is observed is two segments caudal to the level of the injury. Lesions can be localized to specific spinal nerves using referent clinical signs and corresponding vertebral bodies (refer to Table 5.6).

Once the location of the lesion has been identified, the signalment, history, and physical examination can be used to determine a list of differential diagnoses (refer to

Table 5.6. Localization of spinal cord lesion by vertebrae site and neurologic response.

Site and Vertebra Number	Spinal Cord Segments	Neurologic Response[a]
Craniocervical: C1–C4	C1–C5	UMN to the forelimbs UMN to the hindlimbs
Caudocervical: C5–T1	C6–T2	LMN to the forelimbs UMN to the hindlimbs
Thoracolumbar: T2–L3	T3–L3	Normal forelimbs UMN hindlimbs
Lumbosacral: L4–L6	L4–S3	Normal forelimbs LMN hindlimbs
Sacral: L5	S1–S3	Normal forelimbs Normal hindlimbs LMN tail and anus

Source: Adapted from Kornegay and Seim (1996).

[a]UMN, upper motor neuron problem; LMN, lower motor neuron problem.

Figure 5.1). General diagnostic categories can be determined using the history of pain or paresis. Infarctions of the spinal cord and fractures of vertebrae cause acute/static pain/paresis. Degenerative, inflammatory, traumatic, or pressure necrosis, such as a spinal cord abscess, causes acute progressive signs. Degenerative or inflammatory processes cause chronic/progressive clinical signs.

Cerebral Cortex and Forebrain

Diseases affecting the cerebral cortex or thalamus (forebrain) cause an altered mental attitude, seizures, blindness with a pupillary light reflex, circling (ipsilateral), compulsive walking, and head pressing (Kornegay and Seim 1996). The four levels of altered mental attitude are

- Depression or a decreased responsiveness
- Stupor, which is unresponsive but arousable
- Coma, which is unresponsive and not arousable
- Mania or delirium with excessive motor activity

Stupor and coma are caused by a problem with the cerebral cortex or the reticular activating system of the brain stem. Mania is due to diseases of the cerebral cortex, particularly the limbic system. Depression may be due to any systemic disease and may not involve the brain. Some causes of abnormal neurological function are listed in Table 5.7; others are described in more detail in this section.

Table 5.7. Diseases causing neurological symptoms in postweaned pigs.

Disease	Clinical Signs	Epidemiology	Pathology
Botulism	Progressive, flaccid paralysis; weakness; incoordination; staggering; recumbency; vomiting; pupillary dilation; deep, labored breathing; salivation; involuntary urination and defecation; death 1–6 days after onset	Rare, sporadic: feeding decomposing food such as garbage or dead fish	No gross lesions
Cerebrospinal angiopathy	Blindness, head tilt, circling	5 weeks postweaning, may be a sequel to edema disease	No gross lesions
Edema disease (enterotoxemic colibacillosis)	Sudden death of best pigs; acute disease; depression, head pressing, difficulty standing, swaying hind end, knuckle over on front end, tremor, paddling, clonic convulsions, flaccid paralysis; characteristic subcutaneous edema of eyelids, conjunctiva, forehead, and throat; residual incoordination	Sporadic, uncommon, outbreaks 2 weeks postweaning, low morbidity, high case fatality rate, caused by specific serotypes of *E. coli*	Subcutaneous edema of eyelids, forehead, throat, ventral abdomen, hocks, elbows, stomach
Hog cholera (swine fever)	Severe systemic illness, depression, fever, anorexia, conjunctivitis, death, weak staggering gait, reddening of skin, watery diarrhea, convulsions and death after 1–3 weeks	Exotic to North America; mortality up to 90%, low-virulence strain mortality 1–60%; spreads easily; only affects pigs	Petechiae of kidneys, larynx, bladder, mucous membranes; infarcts in spleen; hemorrhage of lymph nodes
Listeriosis	Trembling, incoordination, stilted gait on forelegs, posterior paralysis; neonates with septicemia, sudden death	Widespread, rare; organism in soil	Congested lymph nodes, yellow fluid in body cavities, red liver with necrotic foci
Rabies	Sudden onset; progressive disease of incoordination, dullness, prostration, and death within 3 days; alternating periods of pronounced irritation: twitching, snout rubbing, chewing, swallowing, salivating, and recumbency; attacking other pigs or humans; apparent thirst but swallowing difficult; pushing forward and circling in kneeling position	Rare: reportable, zoonotic disease	No gross lesions; submit brain for diagnosis
Stachybotryotoxicosis	Dermatitis of snout, teats of suckling pigs, nasal exudate, depression, vomiting, tremors, anemia, sudden death, abortion	Toxin of *Stachybotrys atra* from hay or straw that depresses erythropoiesis and is epithelionecrotic	

Hydrocephalus. Hydrocephalus is an accumulation of cerebrospinal fluid (CSF) within the brain. It may be congenital or acquired—secondary to encephalitis or meningoencephalitis. Congenital hydrocephalus may be caused by vitamin A deficiency (refer to Table 5.3) or a lethal defect that is inherited as an autosomal recessive trait in Durocs (O'Hara and Shortridge 1966). Clinical signs vary from compulsive walking, head pressing, blindness, and seizures to a more mild form indicated by strabismus and stunted growth. Animals with a primary encephalitis will have signs of multifocal brain involvement.

Hypoglycemia. Hypoglycemia is a common problem in weak newborn pigs who do not nurse regularly. Early clinical signs include tachycardia, tremor, nervousness, vocalization, and irritability. As the hypoglycemia progresses, hypothermia, visual disturbances, mental dullness, confusion, depression, and seizures occur. Other causes of neurologic abnormalities in the newborn pig include congenital tremor and hypoxia (Table 5.8).

Encephalitis. Encephalitis, an inflammation of the brain, causes central vestibular disease.

Teschen Disease. Teschen disease virus causes polioencephalomyelitis, which results in mild fever and depression followed by ataxia and then nervous excitement, including muscle tremor, nystagmus, opisthotonos, and tonic-clonic convulsions (Mills and Nielsen 1968). All ages of pigs are affected and morbidity is up to 50%, with a high mortality in affected pigs.

Talfan Disease. Talfan disease is caused by the enterovirus. It is a widespread virus but clinical signs are uncommon; there is low morbidity and a moderate case fatality rate (Buddle 1987). It affects pigs under 10 weeks of age with fever, hyperesthesia, mild ataxia, and flaccid paralysis (Mills and Nielsen 1968). Affected pigs recover slowly and have a residual reduced growth rate. Both Teschen and Talfan diseases are seen in European countries and affect naive herds.

Eastern Equine Encephalomyelitis. Eastern equine encephalomyelitis virus (EEEV) causes incoordination, depression, seizures, and death in pigs of less than 2 weeks of age (Elvinger et al. 1994). Pathologic lesions include focal necrosis of the cerebral cortex and multifocal my-

Table 5.8. Neurological problems in preweaned pigs.

Cause	Clinical Signs	Epidemiology	Pathology
Congenital tremor	Varies from fine muscle tremor to whole-body shaking to severe muscle spasms causing the pigs to jump or dance; signs are present at birth, increase in severity with stimulation, decrease during sleep, and decrease progressively with age	Widespread, uncommon: depending on cause, may affect most pigs in most litters for 2–3 months or sporadically affect a few pigs in a few litters	
Type A I	Most litters, >40% pigs, high mortality	Hog cholera	Small cerebellum
Type A II	Most litters, >40% pigs, low mortality	Unknown virus	Unknown
Type A III	Few litters, 25% pigs, high mortality, male Landrace	Genetic recessive, Landrace	Small spinal cord
Type A IV	Few litters, 25% pigs, high mortality, defective vision, all Saddlebacks	Genetic recessive, Saddleback	Small spinal cord
Type A V	Most litters, >90% pigs, high mortality, any breed	Trichlorfon toxicity	Small cerebellum
Type B	Variable clinical signs	Unknown cause	Small cerebellum
Hypoglycemia	Hungry squealing pigs, progress to inappetence, huddling, lethargy, shivering, weak squealing when moved, coma, convulsions, death	Common: caused by starvation, sporadic among litters, affects smallest pigs or whole litter if chilled at birth; factors: hypoxia, temperature, teat access, litter size, available milk, housing, and disease	Thin pig with empty stomach
Hypoxia/anoxia	Postpartum central nervous system depression, inability to suck, walking backward or in circles, dog-sitting, reluctance to compete, weak, increased mortality due to starvation, hypothermia, overlying, disease	Common and widespread: associated with dystocia, old, fat, or thin sows, umbilical cord rupture, last pigs in large litter, heat stress, carbon monoxide poisoning	Meconium on pig's body, in mouth and trachea; hemorrhages and edema of thorax, heart, and thymus

ocardial necrosis. Diagnosis is made after a history of mosquito swarming and positive serum virus neutralization tests for EEEV.

Japanese Encephalitis Flavivirus. Japanese encephalitis flavivirus (JEV) is reported to cause encephalitis in pigs occasionally (Yamada et al. 2004). The virus is amplified in the pig and then transmitted via mosquitoes to other species. Researchers observed a nonsuppurative meningoencephalitis in pigs clinically affected by a wasting syndrome thought to be caused by JEV. Subsequently, when researchers injected JEV into SPF, 3-week-old pigs the pigs developed a fever (40–41°C), depression, and hindlimb tremor (Yamada et al. 2004). The JEV caused nonsuppurative encephalitis, neuronal necrosis, neurophagia, glial nodules, and perivascular cuffing. This neurotropism may be age dependent.

Blue Eye Disease. Blue eye disease caused by the pig paramyxovirus causes central nervous system damage and mortality in nursing pigs (Ramirez-Herrera et al. 2001). Morbidity and mortality due to the virus range from 20% to 90% and from 40% to 100%, respectively. Clinically affected pigs show cutaneous hyperexcitability, incoordination, hindlimb paralysis and convulsions. The CNS lesions include focal and diffuse gliosis, perivascular cuffing, glial and neural necrosis, and meningitis. Pigs injected intramusculary with live virus develop protective immunity. However, the infected nerves near the injection site have a decreased inner fiber diameter and myelin sheath disaggregation. The virus appears to reach the CNS in a retrograde fashion.

Porcine Circovirus Type 2 (PCV2). An outbreak of sudden death and acute nervous signs including paddling, tremors, and lateral recumbency occurred in all ages of pigs in one Canadian herd in 2004 (Youssef et al. 2004). PCV2 was identified by immunohistochemistry in the foci of inflammation of the brain and spinal cord in 7 of 10 pigs submitted to the diagnostic laboratory. However, the brain did not test positive for PCV2 by PCR. The tentative diagnosis was viral encephalomyelitis with a secondary bacterial infection due to *S. suis* (2 piglets), *S. equisimilis* (1 piglet) or *Actinobacillus pleuropneumoniae* (1 sow).

Hepatic Encephalopathy. Hepatic encephalopathy may have multifocal lesions in the central nervous system (CNS), but the clinical signs are primarily due to forebrain involvement. Hepatic encephalopathy occurs when neurotoxic substances build up in the bloodstream due to dysfunction of the liver. Clinical signs include blindness, ataxia, head pressing, seizures, and aggression. There will also be signs referable to liver disease, such as anorexia, weight loss, and diarrhea.

Cerebellum

The cerebellum controls unconscious proprioception; hence, dysfunction is seen clinically as truncal ataxia, broad-based stance, dysmetria (either hypermetria or hypometria), and an intention tremor (Kornegay and Seim 1996). Intention tremor is the involuntary trembling caused by intentional movement. Dysmetria is the improper measuring of distance in muscular acts, either overstepping (hypermetria) or underreaching (hypometria).

Cerebellar Hypoplasia. Cerebellar hypoplasia causes pigs to sit with their forelimbs extended or to assume a tripod sitting position. The clinical signs are nonprogressive and other CNS signs are not present.

Vestibular Disease

Vestibular disease is seen clinically as a head tilt involving a deviation of the head from a horizontal plane, or nystagmus, which is an involuntary oscillation of the eyes. Peripheral lesions are not associated with the ascending or descending tracts, so there is no paresis or conscious proprioceptive deficit, animals are not depressed, and nystagmus is always rotatory or horizontal with the fast phase opposite the head tilt and does not vary with head tilt. However, central lesions frequently cause depression, tetraparesis, and nystagmus that varies with head position and may cause other cranial nerve deficits. Most lesions cause ipsilateral clinical signs but the paradoxical vestibular disease causes contralateral signs.

Otitis Media. Otitis media (peripheral vestibular disease) is usually due to progressive external otitis (Kornegay and Seim 1996). The external ear is inflamed and contains debris, and the pig may be sensitive to manipulation of the ear. Vestibular disease causes a head tilt toward the affected side, horizontal nystagmus, and ataxia, which may include circling or falling. The animals remain bright and the appetite is normal (Buddle 1987). The condition is widespread but uncommon and sporadic. Treatment involves parenteral antibiotics and treatment of the primary external otitis.

Otitis media and interna may be common sequelae to *S. suis* infections. Most pigs (20) in a group of 28 diagnosed with meningitis due *S. suis* had either otitis media or interna (Madsen et al. 2001). Exudative otitis interna with a positive immunohistochemistry test for *S. suis* was found in 71% of the pigs. The scala tympani was affected in all of the pigs. Most of these pigs also had a perineuritis along the vestibulocochlear nerve. This nerve is likely a conduit to the CNS infection. Half of the pigs with both ears available for observation were affected bilaterally. This otitis interna can develop by the meningogenic and tympanogenic routes. A chronic, suppurative, otitis media was diagnosed in 34% of the pigs. Pigs recovering from *S. suis* meningitis may have residual hearing and vestibular dysfunction due to chronic otitis interna.

Neuromuscular Diseases

Neuromuscular diseases diffusely involve muscles, neuromuscular junctions, peripheral nerves, or neurons. Clinically, neuromuscular diseases cause diffuse LMN dysfunction, including tetraparesis, hypo- or areflexia, a decrease in muscle tone, and, after a week, neurogenic muscle atrophy. Myopathies can be either inflammatory, infectious, immune-mediated, degenerative, acquired, or inherited.

Congenital Tremor. Congenital tremors (CT) (myoclonia congenita, trembles, jumpy pig disease) is a congenital abnormality caused by hypomyelination or demyelination of the brain and spinal cord. Unlike in splaylegged pigs where the deficit in myelin formation specifically affects the motor system, with CT there is an overall reduction of myelin in the spinal cord (Lamar and Van Sickle 1975).

Affected animals have a generalized tremor involving the entire body, especially the head and limbs (O'Hara and Shortridge 1966; Done 1968; Patterson and Done 1977; Edmonds et al. 1985). The tremor increases in intensity when the pigs are aroused and subsides when the pigs are sleeping (Done 1968). Pigs affected by CT have clonic contractions of the skeletal muscles. Posterior paresis and splayed hindlegs may occur with the tremor. The tremor can be distinguished from the primary head tremor due to cerebellar disease because the tremor becomes less pronounced at rest and more pronounced during excitement. The tremor is due to excessive irritability of the spinal reflexes.

In the Netherlands, CT affects 0.2% of pigs (Smidt 1972). An examination of 47,323 litters born to German Landrace boars from artificial insemination units showed that the frequency of congenital tremor was reduced by selection over a 14-year period (Beissner et al. 2003). The annual rate ranged from 0.23% to 0.01% but was 0.02% in 2000.

There are six categories of CT, which can be inherited or caused by viruses or toxins (refer to Table 5.8). These categories also differ by pathological lesion and prevalence within a herd. Types A and B are distinguished by morphologic changes. Type AI, caused by either the wild type or vaccine hog cholera virus produces hypoplasia, dysgenesis and cortical dysplasia of the cerebellum. The spinal cord is small and has half the normal compliment of myelin (Done 1976a). Both AI and AII produce a smaller white and gray matter areas in cross sections of the spinal cord (Done et al. 1984, 1986). In Type AII, there is significant demyelination, reduced spinal cord lipid content, and depressed and aberrant cerebroside synthesis. Type AIII causes a deficiency of oligodendrocytes with concomitant hypoplasia of the cord and reduced lipid and cellular content. Piglets in-fected by the PR virus and born with CT have demyelination of the cerebellum. Type AV is caused by the ingestion of an antiparasitic drug, Neguvon (metrifonate, trichlorfon) by pregnant sows (Berge et al. 1987). This leads to cerebral, cerebellar, and spinal cord hypoplasia and demyelination and a decrease in the activity of neurotransmitter synthesizing enzymes.

Type AII is transmissible and is the most common form in North America. Typically other CNS functions, such as vision, reflexes, and pain, are normal; however, type AIV causes defective vision (Done 1968).

Hines and Lukert (1994) reproduced CT by inoculating sows with tissue culture fluid from the kidneys of affected pigs. They believed the piglets were infected with porcine circovirus and that this virus caused the deficient myelin. The four sows remained healthy but produced piglets with varying degrees of trembling. In the United States, PCV2 was believed to be associated with CT type AII in four Midwestern farms (Stevenson et al. 2001). The porcine circoviruses isolated from pigs with either clinical congenital tremors type AII or postweaning multisystemic wasting syndrome (PMWS) were examined to determine their genetic similarities (Choi et al. 2002). The samples each came from a different farm. The genomes of the viruses taken from CT and PMWS had 99% sequence identity with one another. Congenital tremors can also be caused by PCV1. This virus shares only 72% nucleotide sequence identity with the PCV2 that causes CT. PCV requires cell division. It is hypothesized that PCV can infect nervous tissues in the fetus only when neural cell division is occurring.

Clinical signs in affected pigs occur within hours of birth. The tremor may be fine or gross, producing twitching of the muscles of the neck and limbs that decreases when the pig is at rest and stops when the pig is sleeping. Pigs with fine tremor continue to walk and nurse. However, gross tremors will affect the ability of the pig to walk, nurse, and compete with littermates. Pigs born with CT may also exhibit splayleg. Mortality in these pigs is caused by starvation, hypothermia or crushing. In animals that survive, the severity of the tremors decrease over time and are usually resolved by 4 weeks of age. Gilt litters are more frequently affected than those of older sows because the females develop immunity to the infectious agents over time. Start-up gilt herds may experience an outbreak of the disease lasting 18 weeks.

Treatment for CT is aimed at reducing mortality. Affected pigs are to be provided with additional heat and assisted to feed. Control of CT depends on identifying and addressing the cause. For types AIII and AIV, eliminating genetic carriers from the herd is important. No affected pigs should be kept for breeding. For AV, trichlorfon is to be avoided in sows. All other types of CT will depend on disease control programs. This may include exposing open sows to the affected piglets so that transfer of infectious agents will occur. The herd is to be considered infectious until there has been a 4-month period with no affected litters (Done 1976b).

A tremor similar to congenital tremor is seen in 3- to 6-month-old pigs (Gedde-Dahl and Standal 1970). Clinically the pigs have a tremor of the head and shoulder that varies in intensity but subsides when the pigs lie down. The problem clusters by litter and occurs more frequently in females. It is associated with high growth rates, lean carcasses, and pale-colored meat.

Seizures

Seizures are involuntary, paroxysmal brain disturbances clinically appearing as uncontrolled muscle activity (Kornegay and Seim 1996). Generalized seizures originate within the cerebral cortex, thalamus, or brain stem and are associated with symmetrical clinical dysfunction. Focal seizures lead to clinical signs that help localize the lesion. Temporolimbic seizures cause behavioral changes such as aggression or biting at the air. Focal motor seizures appear as tonic movements contralateral to the lesion and then within seconds spread to a generalized seizure. Seizures can be caused by encephalitis, neoplasia, or hydrocephalus. Most of the lesions are progressive and usually increase in frequency and severity. Toxins, such as organophosphate and chlorinated hydrocarbons, and internal toxicities, such as hepatic encephalopathy and hypoglycemia, can cause seizures.

Bacterial Meningitis. Bacterial meningitis may cause focal or diffuse CNS problems, which are progressive unless the affected pigs are treated. The problem is widespread, common but sporadic, with a low morbidity and high mortality. It can be associated with overcrowding and inadequate cleaning. Often the first symptom is sudden death. Affected pigs show depression, incoordination, hyperesthesia, tremor, circling, paresis, opisthotonos, recumbency, paddling, nystagmus, convulsions, and death. Postmortem lesions include congestion, edema, and purulent discharge of meninges.

Streptococcus suis. *Streptococcus suis* type 2 is one of the most common causes of meningitis. Additionally, this bacteria causes arthritis, septicemia with sudden death, endocarditis, polyserositis, and pneumonia in pigs (Reams et al. 1994; Madsen et al. 2002b). Of 42 pigs in one study, 27 had meningitis, 19 had polyserositis, 9 had polyarthritis, and 2 had endocarditis (Madsen et al. 2002b). Other lesions included hepatomegaly (17), bronchopneumonia (14), exudative otitis media (12) pleuritis (9), and pericarditis (4).

Clinically the animals exhibit depression, fever, anorexia, incoordination, paralysis, paddling, opisthotonos, tetanic spasms, and death (Buddle 1987). Infection with *S. suis* is widespread and common, often occurs 2 weeks after moving pigs, and is associated with overcrowding and poor ventilation. Affected pigs are

typically in the nursery phase but may range in age from 1 to 22 weeks (Madsen et al. 2002b).

Piglets acquire *S. suis* infection during farrowing from contact with the sow, her feces, and the environment (Gottschalk and Segura 2000). The pharyngeal and palatine tonsils, infected in 52% of the pigs, were the main portals of entry for the bacteria and then the bacteria appeared to spread via the lymph system because they were cultured from the lymph nodes of the upper respiratory tract (Madsen et al. 2002b). In pigs infected experimentally via aerosol, *S. suis* was isolated from the palatine and/or nasalpharyngeal tonsils of all pigs (Madsen et al. 2002a). In systemically infected pigs, the bacterium was also found in the mandibular lymph node. This suggests lymphogenous spread. Additionally, spread of *S. suis* appears to occur hematogenously from the palatine tonsils and intracellularly with the bacteria crossing the blood brain barrier. Bacteria can be found intracellularly in alveolar macrophages and tracheobronchial lymph nodes. The bacteria appear to invade the epithelium of the tonsils. Using porcine brain microvascular endothelial cells researchers have shown that *S. suis* can invade the cells that are component parts of the blood brain barrier (Vanier et al. 2004). This may explain the pathogenesis of meningitis. Interestingly, 7 hours after antibiotic treatment, intracellular viable *S. suis* were still found in porcine brain microvascular endothelial cells (Vanier et al. 2004).

S. suis diagnosis is enhanced by using bacterial culture in combination with immunohistochemistry (Madsen et al. 2002b). Culture rate is highest from the lateral cerebral ventricles or other parts of the brain. Half of the pigs are systemically infected with *S. suis*. The most prominent serotype of *S. suis* diagnosed from clinical cases changes by geographic region and time (Gottschalk and Segura 2000). In Canada, serotype 2 is diagnosed only 15% of the time, whereas in France it is the primary isolate 70% of the time. In Europe, serotypes 9 and 1 are most prominent after serotype 2 (Wisselink et al. 2002). Serotype 14 in the UK and serotypes 1/2 and 5 in Canada appear to be prominent causes of disease.

Effective vaccines against *S. suis* have not been produced because of the variation within and between serotypes and lack of knowledge of the virulence factors (Wisselink et al. 2002). Several types of vaccines have been used, but results have been inconsistent (Smith et al. 1999; Wisselink et al. 2002). (For more information, see Chapter 47.)

There is a high case fatality rate, but if treated early, pigs can recover with no residual clinical signs. Pigs should be removed from the group, put in a warm, dry environment, fed and watered by hand, and treated parenterally for 3–5 days. Of 689 isolates of *S. suis* from diagnostic laboratories and abattoirs in Japan, all were susceptible to amoxicillin and sulfamethoxazole plus trimethoprim (Kataoka et al. 2000). Most were suscepti-

Table 5.9.   Infectious diseases causing neurological problems in preweaned pigs.

Disease	Clinical Signs	Epidemiology	Pathology
Bacterial meningitis	Sudden death, depression, fever, incoordination, hyperesthesia, tremor, circling, paresis, opisthotonos, recumbency, paddling, clonic convulsions	Sporadic but common, low morbidity, high case fatality, secondary to stresses such as overcrowding, continual-flow production, omphalitis	Congestion, edema, purulent exudate in meninges
Hemagglutinating encephalomyelitis (HEV)	4- to 7-day-old pigs, sudden-onset anorexia, depression, hyperesthesia, trembling, incoordination, progressive posterior paralysis, paddling, convulsions, coma and death within 10 days (vomiting, constipation, emaciation)	Virus widespread, rapid spread leads to herd immunity, 2–3 week outbreak, mortality 50–100% in affected litters	Pneumonia, conjunctivitis, corneal opacity
Tetanus	Ataxia progressing to stiff gait, muscle rigidity, erect ears, straight tail, lateral recumbency, opisthotonos, legs extended backward, death; loud noises cause tetanic spasms	Rare, associated with castration	No gross lesions
Toxoplasmosis	Neonates: diarrhea, dyspnea, cough, tremor, weakness, staggering, increased mortality; survivors exhibit ataxia and blindness	Infection might be common in certain areas, but symptoms are rare, associated with cats.	Serofibrinous exudate in cavities; small gray nodules in lungs, liver, spleen, lymph nodes, and fetal membranes; ulcers in small intestine
	Sows: stillbirths, fetal death, prolonged gestation	Infection might be common in certain areas, but symptoms are rare, associated with cats.	Serofibrinous exudate in cavities; small gray nodules in lungs, liver, spleen, lymph nodes, and fetal membranes; ulcers in small intestine

ble to penicillin G, ampicillin, and amoxicillin. Trimethoprim and sulfonamides penetrate the blood-CSF barrier. Penicillin, ampicillin, and cephalosporin will also penetrate the barrier in the presence of meningitis. Other infectious causes of neurologic problems in preweaned pigs are described in Table 5.9.

REFERENCES

Abiven N, Seegers H, Beaudeau F, Laval A, Fourichon C. 1998. Risk factors for high sow mortality in French swine herds. Prev Vet Med 33:109–119.

Aherne FX, Brennan JJ. 1985. Nutrition and leg weakness. Proc Guelph Pork Symposium, pp. 157–163.

Backstrom L, Johnston W, Memon M, Hoefling D. 1980. Diseases in swine recorded by post-slaughter checks at a slaughterhouse in West Central Illinois. Proc Int Pig Vet Soc 6:359.

Bane DP, Meade RJ, Hilley HD, Leman AD. 1980. Influence of d-biotin and housing on hoof lesions. Proc Int Pig Vet Soc 6:334.

Barnett JL, Hemsworth PH, Cronin GM, Jongman EC, Hutson GD. 2001. A review of the welfare issues for sows and piglets in relation to housing. Austr J Agric Res 52:1–28.

Beissner B, Hamann H, Distl O. 2003. Prevalence of congenital anomalies of the pig breeds German Landrace and Pietrain in Bavaria. Zuchtngskunde 75:101–114.

Berge GN, Fonnum F, Brodal P. 1987. Neurotoxic effects of prenatal trichlorfon administration in pigs. Acta Vet Scand 28:321–332.

Brooks PH. 1982. Biotin in pig nutrition. Pig News Inf 3:29–32.

Brooks PH, Smith DA, Irwin VCR. 1977. Biotin supplementation of diets: The incidence of foot lesions, and the reproductive performance of sows. Vet Rec 101:46–50.

Bryant KL, Kornegay ET, Knight JW, Veit HT, Notter DR. 1985. Supplemental biotin for swine. III. Influence of supplementation to corn and wheat based diets on the incidence and severity of toe lesions, hair and skin characteristics, and structural soundness of sows housed in confinement during four parities. J Anim Sci 60:154–162.

Buddle JR. 1987. The T. G. Hungerford VADE MECUM Series for Domestic Animals (Differential Diagnosis). The Diagnosis of the Diseases of Pigs. Series B, Number 8, Nov. Sydney: Univ Sydney Post-graduate Foundation in Veterinary Science.

Burch DGS. 1986. A comparison of the serological findings of two herds infected with Mycoplasma hyosynoviae but with different disease patterns. Proc Int Pig Vet Soc 9:286.

Burch DGS, Goodwin RFW. 1984. Use of tiamulin in a herd of pigs seriously affected with Mycoplasma hyosynoviae arthritis. Vet Rec 8:594–595.

Choi J, Stevenson GW, Kiupel M, Harrach B, Anothayanontha L, Kanitz CL, Mittal SK. 2002. Sequence analysis of old and new strains of porcine circovirus associated with congenital tremors in pigs and their comparison with strains involved with postweaning multisystemic wasting syndrome. Can J Vet Res 66:217–224.

Cunha TJ. 1968. Spraddle hind legs may be a result of choline deficiency. Feedstuffs 40:25–31.

Dagorn J, Aumaitre A. 1978. Sow culling: Reasons for and effect on productivity. Livest Prod Sci 6:167–177.

D'Allaire S, Stein TE, Leman AD. 1987. Culling patterns in selected Minnesota swine breeding herds. Can J Vet Med 51:506–512.

Desrosiers R, Phaneuf JB, Broes A, Robinson Y. 1986. An outbreak of atypical Glasser's disease in Quebec. Proc Int Pig Vet Soc 9:277.

Dewey CE. 1988. An Observational Study of Factors Affecting Lameness in Breeding-Stock Pigs. M.Sc. diss. Univ Guelph, Guelph, Ontario.

Dewey CE, Friendship RM, Wilson MR. 1992. Lameness in breeding age swine—A case study. Can Vet J 33:747–748.

——. 1993. Clinical and postmortem examination of sows culled for lameness. Can Vet J 34:555–556.

Dobson, KJ. 1971. Failure of choline and methionine to prevent splayleg in piglets. Aust Vet J 47(12):587–590.

Done JT. 1968. Congenital nervous diseases of pigs: A review. Lab Anim 2:207–217.

——. 1976a. Developmental disorders of the nervous system in animals. In Advances in Veterinary Science and Comparative Medicine, Vol 20. CH Brandly, EL Jungherr, eds. New York: Academic Press, pp. 69–114.

——. 1976b. The congenital tremor syndrome in pigs. Vet Annu 16:98–102.

Done JT, Woolley J, Upcott DH, Hebert CN. 1984. Porcine congenital tremor type AI: Spinal cord morphometry. Zentralbl Veterinaermed 31:81–90.

——. 1986. Porcine congenital tremor type AII: Spinal cord morphometry. Br Vet J 142:145–150.

Ebeid M, Zimmerman W, Martig J. 1997. Collection and diagnostic value of CSF in the pig. Large Anim Pract 18:32–33.

Edmonds MS, Izquierdo OA, Baker DH. 1985. Feed additives studies with newly weaned pigs: Efficacy of supplemental copper, antibiotics, and organic acids. J Anim Sci 60:462–469.

Elliot JI, Doige CE. 1973. Effects of type of confinement on performance and on the occurrence of locomotory disturbances in market pigs. Can J Anim Sci 53:211–217.

Elvinger F, Liggett AD, Tang K-N, Harrison LR, Cole JR Jr, Baldwin CA, Nessmith WB. 1994. Eastern equine encephalomyelitis virus infection in swine. J Am Vet Med Assoc 205:1014–1016.

Evans DG, Pratt JH. 1978. A critical analysis of condemnation data for cattle, pigs and sheep, 1969 to 1975. Br Vet J 134:476–492.

Ferket SL, Hacker RR. 1985. Effect of forced exercise during gestation on reproductive performance of sows. Can J Anim Sci 65:851–859.

Flory W, Spainhour CB Jr, Colvin B, Herbert CD. 1992. The toxicologic investigation of a feed grain contaminated with seeds of the plant species Cassia. J Vet Diagn Invest 4:65–69.

Frank R, Braun HE, Wilkie I, Ewing R. 1991. A review of insecticide poisonings among domestic livestock in southern Ontario, Canada, 1982–1989. Can Vet J 32:219–226.

Fredeen HT, Sather AP. 1978. Joint damage in pigs reared under confinement. Can J Anim Sci 58:759–773.

Friendship RM, Wilson MR, Almond GW, McMillan I, Hacker RR, Pieper R, Swaminathan SS. 1986. Sow wastage: Reasons for and effect on productivity. Can J Vet Res 50:205–208.

Friton GM, Philipp H, Schneider T, Kleemann R. 2003. Investigation on the clinical efficacy and safety of meloxicam (Metacam) in the treatment of non-infectious locomotor disorders in pigs. Berliner Munchener Tierarztliche Wochenschrift 116:421–426.

Frus NF, Feenstra AA. 1994. Mycoplasma hyorhinis in the etiology of serositis among piglets. Acta Vet Scand 35:93–98.

Furniss SJ, Edwards SA, Lightfoot AL, Spechter HH. 1986. The effect of floor type in farrowing pens on pig injury. I. Leg and teat damage of suckling piglets. Br Vet J 142:434–440.

Gayle LG, Schwartz WL. 1980. Pathologic fractures in young sows during lactation. S West Vet 33:69–71.

Gedde-Dahl TW, Standal N. 1970. A note on a tremor condition in adolescent pigs. Anim Prod 12:665–668.

Gottschalk M, Segura M. 2000. The pathogenesis of the meningitis caused by Streptococcus suis: The unresolved questions. Vet Microbiol 76:259–272.

Grabell I, Hansen HJ, Olsson S, Orstadius EK, Thal E. 1962. Discospondylitis and arthritis in swine erysipelas. Acta Vet Scand 3:33–50.

Grandhi RR, Strain JH. 1980. Effect of biotin supplementation on reproductive performance and foot lesions in swine. Can J Anim Sci 60:961–969.

Grondalen T. 1974a. Osteochondrosis and arthrosis in pigs. I. Incidence in animals up to 120 kg live weight. Acta Vet Scand 15:1–25.

——. 1974b. Osteochondrosis and arthrosis in pigs. II. Incidence in breeding animals. Acta Vet Scand 15:26–42.

——. 1974c. Osteochondrosis and arthrosis in pigs. III. A comparison of the incidence in young animals of the Norwegian Landrace and Yorkshire breeds. Acta Vet Scand 15:43–52.

——. 1974d. Osteochondrosis and arthrosis in pigs. IV. Effect of overloading on the distal epiphyseal plate of the ulna. Acta Vet Scand 15:53–60.

——. 1974e. Osteochondrosis and arthrosis in pigs. VI. Relationship to feed level and calcium, phosphorus, and protein levels in the ration. Acta Vet Scand 15:147–149.

——. 1974f. Osteochondrosis and arthrosis in pigs. VII. Relationship to joint shape and exterior conformation. Acta Vet Scand 15(Suppl):46.

——. 1974g. Leg weakness in pigs. I. Incidence and relationship to skeletal lesions, feed level, protein, and mineral supply, exercise, and exterior conformation. Acta Vet Scand 15:555–573.

——. 1974h. Leg weakness in pigs. II. Litter differences in leg weakness, skeletal lesions, joint shapes, and exterior conformation. Acta Vet Scand 15:574–586.

——. 1974i. Osteochondrosis, arthrosis, and leg weakness in pigs. Nord Vet Med 26:534–537.

——. 1981. Osteochondrosis and arthrosis in Norwegian slaughterpigs in 1980 compared to 1970. Nord Vet Med 33:417–422.

Grondalen T, Vangen O. 1974. Osteochondrosis and arthrosis in pigs. V. A comparison of the incidence in three different lines of the Norwegian Landrace breed. Acta Vet Scand 15:61–79.

Hale OM, Newton GL, Cleveland ER. 1984. Effects of exercise during the growing-finishing period on performance, age at puberty and conception rate of gilts. J Anim Sci 58:541–544.

Hamilton CR, Veum TL. 1984. Response of sow and litters to added dietary biotin in environmentally regulated facilities. J Anim Sci 59:151–157.

Hani H, Troxler J. 1984. Influence of housing systems on incidence and severity of osteochondrosis in fattening pigs: A comparison between open front stable with deep straw bedding and closed stable with partially slatted floor. Proc Int Pig Vet Soc 8:346.

Hardin JDJ, Lewis G, Done JT. 1968. Experimental arsanilic acid poisoning in pigs. Vet Rec 83:560–564.

Hemsworth PH, Barnett JL, Coleman GJ, Hansen C. 1989. A study of the relationships between the attitudinal and behavioural profiles of stockpersons and the level of fear of humans and reproductive performance of commercial pigs. Appl Anim Behav Sci 23:301–314.

Hill MA. 1990. Economic relevance, diagnosis, and countermeasures for degenerative joint disease (osteoarthrosis) and dyschondroplasia (osteochondrosis) in pigs. J Am Vet Med Assoc 197:254–259.

Hill MA, Hilley HD, Feeny DA, Ruth GR, Hansgen DC. 1984. Dyschondroplasias, including osteochondrosis in boars between 25 and 169 days of age: Radiologic changes. Am J Vet Res 35:917–925.

Hill MA, Ruth GR, Hilley HD, Torrison JL, Batent JK, Leman AD. 1985. Dyschondroplasias of growth cartilages (osteochondrosis) in crossbred commercial pigs at 1 and 15 days of age: Radiological, angiomicrographical, and histological findings. Vet Rec 116:40–47.

Hill MA, Hilley HD, Penny RHC. 1986. Skeletal system. In Diseases of Swine, 6th ed. AD Leman, RD Glock, WL Mengeling, RHC Penny, E Scholl, BE Straw, eds. Ames: Iowa State Univ Press, pp. 183–197.

Hines RK, Lukert PH. 1994. Porcine circovirus as a cause of congenital tremors in newborn pigs. Proc Annu Meet Am Assoc Swine Pract, Chicago, p. 344.

Hoefling DC. 1994. The various forms of Haemophilus parasuis. Swine Health Prod 2:19.

Jorgensen B, Sorensen MT. 1998. Different rearing intensities of gilts: II. Effect on subsequent leg weakness and longevity. Livest Prod Sci 54:167–171.

Karlberg K. 1979. Reasons for culling of breeding sows. Nordsk Tidsskr 91:423–426.

Kataoka Y, Yoshida T, Sawada T. 2000. A 10-year survey of antimicrobial susceptibility of *Streptococcus suis* isolates from swine in Japan. J Vet Med Sci 62:1053–1057.

Kern D. 1994. Nursery lameness. Swine Practitioner 2:18–19.

Kim J, Chung H, Jung T, Cho W, Choi C, Chae C. 2002. Postweaning multisystemic wasting syndrome of pigs in Korea: Prevalence, microscopic lesions and coexisting microorganisms. J Vet Med Sci 64:57–62.

Kornegay ET, Meacham TN. 1973. Evaluation of supplemental choline for reproducing sows housed in total confinement on concrete or in dirt lots. J Anim Sci 37:506–509.

Kornegay JN, Seim HB. 1996. Neurology and neurosurgery. In T. G. Hungerford Course for Veterinarians, Proceedings 266, Feb. 12–16, Univ Sydney, Australia.

Lamar CH, Van Sickle DC. 1975. Evaluation of chromatin clumping and myelination of the spinal cord of pigs with congenital tremor. Vet Pathol 12(1):1–5.

Madsen LW, Svensmark B, Elvestad K, Jensen HE. 2001. Otitis interna is a frequent sequela to *Streptococcus suis* meningitis in pigs. Vet Pathol 38:190–195.

Madsen LW, Bak H, Nielsen B, Jensen HE, Aalbaek B, Riising HJ. 2002a. Bacterial colonization and invasion in pigs experimentally exposed to *Streptococcus suis* serotype 2 in aerosol. J Vet Med B 49:211–215.

Madsen LW, Svensmark B, Elvestad K, Aalbaek B, Jensen HE. 2002b. *Streptococcus suis* serotype 2 infection in pigs: New diagnostic and pathogenetic aspects. J Comp Path 126:57–65.

MAFF (Ministry of Agriculture, Fisheries, and Food). 1981. Injuries caused by flooring: A survey in Pig Health Scheme Herds. Pig Vet Soc Proc 8:119–125.

McPhee CP, Laws L. 1976. An analysis of leg abnormalities of boars in the Queensland performance testing station. Aust Vet J 52:123–125.

Mills JHL, Nielsen SW. 1968. Porcine polioencephalomyelitides. Adv Vet Sci 12:33–104.

Miniats OP, Smart NL. 1988. Immunization of primary SPF pigs against Glasser's disease. Proc Int Pig Vet Soc 10:157.

Miniats OP, Smart NL, Metzger K. 1986. Glasser's disease in southwestern Ontario. I. A retrospective study. Proc Int Pig Vet Soc 9:279.

Nakano T, Aherne FX, Thompson JR. 1979a. Effects of feed restriction, sex, and diethylstilbestrol on the occurrence of joint lesions with some histological and biochemical studies of the articular cartilage of growing-finishing swine. Can J Anim Sci 59:491–502.

——. 1979b. Changes in swine knee articular cartilage during growth. Can J Anim Sci 59:167–179.

——. 1981a. Effect of housing system on the recovery of boars from leg weakness. Can J Anim Sci 61:335–342.

——. 1981b. Leg weakness and osteochondrosis in pigs. Pig News Inf 2:29–34.

Nakano T, Thompson JR, Aherne FX, Christian RG. 1982. Observations of abnormalities and age-related changes in the anconeal processes of swine. Am J Vet Res 43:1840–1844.

Newton GL, Boorman CV, Hale OM, Mallinix BG Jr. 1980. Effects of four types of floor slats on certain feet characteristics and performance of swine. J Anim Sci 50:7–20.

Nielsen NC, Bille N, Larsen JL, Svendsen J. 1975. Preweaning mortality in pigs. Nord Vet Med 27:529–543.

Nielsen R, Danielsen V. 1975. An outbreak of Glasser's disease: Studies on etiology, serology, and the effect of vaccination. Nord Vet Med 27:20–25.

O'Hara PJ, Shortridge EH. 1966. Congenital anomalies of the porcine central nervous system. NZ Vet J 14:13–18.

Oliveira S, Pijoan C. 2004. *Haemophilus parasuis*: New trends on diagnosis, epidemiology and control. Vet Microbiol 99:1–12.

Oliveira S, Batista L, Torremorell M, Pijoan C. 2001. Experimental colonization of piglets and gilts with systemic strains of *Haemophilus parasuis* and *Streptococcus suis* to prevent disease. Can J Vet Res 65:161–167.

Oliveira S, Blackall PJ, Pijoan C. 2003. Characterization of the diversity of *Haemophilus parasuis* field isolates by serotyping and genotyping. Am J Vet Res 64:435–442.

Palmer NC. 1985. Bones and joints. In Pathology of Domestic Animals, 3d ed. KVF Jubb, PC Kennedy, NC Palmer, eds. Vol. 1. New York: Academic Press, pp. 1–138.

Patterson DSP, Done JT. 1977. Neurochemistry as a diagnostic aid in the congenital tremor syndrome of piglets. Br Vet J 133:111–119.

Penny RHC. 1979. Genetic, physiological, and anatomical factors contributing to foot and limb disorders in growing and adult pigs including a statistical review of foot and limb disorders in pigs attributable to floors. Pig Vet Soc Proc 4:85–96.

Penny RHC, Osborne AD, Wright AI. 1963. The causes and incidence of lameness in store and adult pigs. Part I: Review. Vet Rec 75:1225–1240.

Penny RHC, Cameron RDA, Johnson S, Kenyon PJ, Smith HA, Bell A. WP, Cole JPL, Taylor J. 1980. Foot rot of pigs: The influence of biotin supplementation on foot lesions in sows. Vet Rec 107:350–351.

Perrin WR, Bowland JP. 1977. Effects of enforced exercise on the incidence of leg weakness in growing boars. Can J Anim Sci 57:245–253.

Perrin WR, Aherne FX, Bowland JP, Hardin RT. 1978. Effects of age, breed, and floor type on the incidence of articular cartilage lesions in pigs. Can J Anim Sci 58:129–138.

Ramirez-Herrera MA, Mendoza-Magana ML, Duenas-Jimenez JM, Mora-Galindo J, Duenas-Jimenez SH. 2001. Electrophysiological and morphological alterations in peripheral nerves by the pig paramyxovirus of Blue Eye Disease in neonatal pigs. J Vet Med B 48:477–487.

Reams RY, Glickman LT, Harrington DD, Thacker HL, Bowersock TL. 1994. *Streptococcus suis* infection in swine: A retrospective study of 56 cases. Part II. Clinical signs, gross and microscopic lesions, and coexisting microorganisms. J Vet Diagn Invest 6:26–334.

Reiland S. 1975. Osteochondrosis in the pig: A morphologic and experimental investigation with special reference to the leg weakness syndrome. Stockholm, Sweden: Akademisk Avhandling.

Reiland S, Anderson K. 1979. Cross breeding experiments with swine: Influences of different combinations of breed on frequency and severity of osteochondrosis. Acta Agric Scand 21:486–489.

Reiland S, Ordell N, Lundeheim N, Olsson SE. 1978. Heredity of osteochondrosis, body condition, and leg weakness in the pig. Acta Pathol 358(Suppl):123–127.

Rice DA, McMurray CH, McCracken RM, Bryson DG. 1980. A field case of poisoning caused by 3-nitro-4-hydroxy phenyl arsonic acid in pigs. Vet Rec 106:312–313.

Roberts ED, Switzer WP, Ramsey FK. 1963. The pathology of *Mycoplasma hyorhinis* arthritis produced experimentally in swine. Am J Vet Res 24:19–31.

Ross RF, Spear ML. 1973. Role of the sow as a reservoir of infection for *Mycoplasma hyosynoviae*. Am J Vet Res 34:373–378.

Segales J, Domingo M, Balasch M, Solano GI, Pijoan C. 1998. Ultrastructural study of porcine alveolar macrophages infected in vitro with porcine reproductive and respiratory syndrome (PRRS) virus, with and without *Haemophilus parasuis*. J Comp Pathol 118:231–243.

Silvertsen T, Overnes G, Karlsen B, Soli N. 1992. Poisoning of domestic animals in Norway in 1990. Norsk Tidsskr 104:173–182.

Simmins PH, Brooks PH. 1988. Supplementary biotin for sows: Effect on claw integrity. Vet Rec 122:431–435.

Smart NL, Miniats OP, Friendship RM, MacInnes J. 1986. Glasser's disease in southwestern Ontario. II: Isolation of *Haemophilus parasuis* from SPF and conventional swine herds. Proc Int Pig Vet Soc 9:280.

Smart NL, Miniats OP, McInnes JI. 1988. Analysis of *Haemophilus parasuis* isolates from southern Ontario swine by restricted endonuclease fingerprinting. Can J Vet Res 52:319–324.

Smart NL, Hurnik D, McInnes JI. 1993. An investigation of enzootic Glasser's disease in a specific pathogen-free grower-finisher facility using restriction endonuclease analysis. Can Vet J 34:487–490.

Smidt WJ. 1972. Congenital defects in pigs. In 7th Int Congr Anim Repro Artificial Insemination, Munich. pp. 1145–1148.

Smith HE, Dmman M, Van der Velde J, Wagenaar F, Wisselink HJ, Stockhofe N, Smits MA. 1999. Identification and characterization of the cps locus of *Streptococcus suis* scrotype 2: The capsule protects against phagocytosis and is an important virulence factor. Infect Immun 67:1750–1756.

Smith WJ, Mitchell CD. 1976. Observations on injuries to suckled pigs confined on perforated floors with special reference to expanded metal. Pig J 1:91–104.

Smith WJ, Robertson AM. 1971. Observations on injuries to sows confined in part slatted stalls. Vet Rec 89:531–533.

Solano GI, Bautista E, Molitor TW, Segales J, Pijoan C. 1998. Effect of porcine reproductive and respiratory syndrome virus infection on the clearance of *Haemophilus parasuis* by porcine alveolar macrophages. Can J Vet Res 62:251–256.

Spencer GR. 1979. Animal model of human disease: Pregnancy and lactational osteoporosis—Animal model: Porcine lactational osteoporosis. Am J Pathol 95:277–280.

Stevenson GW, Kiupel M, Mittal SK, Choi J, Latimer KS, Kanitz CL. 2001. Tissue distribution and genetic typing of porcine circovirus in pigs with naturally occurring congenital tremors. J Vet Diagn Invest 13:57–62.

Stowe HD, Herdt TH. 1992. Clinical assessment of selenium status of livestock. J Anim Sci 70:3928–3933.

Stowe HD, Every AJ, Granger L, Halstead S, Yamini B. 1992. Selenium toxicosis in feeder pigs. J Am Vet Med Assoc 201:292–295.

Svendsen J, Olsson O, Nilsson C. 1979. The occurrence of leg injuries on piglets with the various treatment of the floor surface of the farrowing pen. Nord Vet Med 31:49–61.

Szalay F, Zsarnovszky A, Fekete S, Hullar I, Jancsik V, Hajos F. 2001. Retarded myelination in the lumbar spinal cord of piglets born with spread-leg syndrome. Anat Embryol 2003:53–59.

Tadjine M, Mittal KR, Bourdon S, Gottschalk M. 2004. Development of a new serological test for serotyping *Haemophilus parasuis* isolates and determination of their prevalence in North America. J Clin Microbiol 24:839–840.

Vahle JL, Haynew JS, Andrews JJ. 1997. Experimental reproduction of *Haemophilus parasuis* infection in swine: Clinical, bacteriologic, and morphologic findings. J Vet Diagn Invest 7:476–480.

Vanier G, Segura M, Friedl P, Lacouture S, Gottschalk M. 2004. Invasion of porcine brain microvascular endothelial cells by *Streptococcus suis* serotype 2. Infect Immun 72:1441–1449.

Vaughan LC. 1969. Locomotory disturbance in pigs. Br Vet J 125:354–366.

Walker T, Fell BF, Jones AS, Boyne R, Elliot M. 1966. Observations on "leg weakness" in pigs. Vet Rec 79:472–479.

Ward PS. 1978. The splayleg syndrome in newborn pigs: A review. Part 1. Vet Bull 48:279–399.

Ward PS, Bradley R. 1980. The light microscopical morphology of the skeletal muscles of normal pigs and pigs with splayleg from birth to one week of age. J Comp Pathol 90:421–431.

Webb AJ, Russell WS, Sales DI. 1983. Genetics of leg weakness in performance-tested boars. Anim Prod 36:117–130.

Webb NG, Penny RHC, Johnston AM. 1984. Effect of a dietary supplement of biotin on pig hoof horn strength and hardness. Vet Rec 114:185–189.

Wells GAH. 1984. Locomotor disorders of the pig. In Pract 6:43–53.

Wisselink HJ, Stockhofe-Zurwiede N, Hilgers LAT, Smith HE. 2002. Assessment of protective efficacy of live and killed vaccines based on a non-encapsulated mutant of *Streptococcus suis* serotype 2. Vet Microbiol 84:155–168.

Yamada M, Nakamura K, Yoshii, Kaku Y. 2004. Non-suppurative encephalitis in piglets after experimental inoculation of Japanese encephalitis flavivirus isolated from pigs. Vet Pathol 41:62–67.

Youssef S, DeLay J, Welch K, McEwen B, Josephson G, Carman S. 2004. A confined outbreak of encephalomyelitis in a multi-aged group of pigs. Animal Health Laboratory Newsletter, University of Guelph 8:19.

6 Diseases of the Reproductive System

Glen W. Almond, William L. Flowers, Laura Batista, and Sylvie D'Allaire

REPRODUCTIVE ANATOMY IN THE SOW

Development of the Ovaries and Uterus

Early studies indicated that embryonic gonad in the pig embryo is recognizable at 24–36 days postcoitum (PC) (Christenson et al. 1985). The ovaries of the fetal gilt develop from stromal tissue of the genital ridge and primordial germ cells that migrate to the genital ridge from the embryonic yolk sac. At approximately 31–32 days PC, the fetal gonad in female pigs is differentiated to an ovary with egg nests, which are clusters of primary oocytes within the stromal tissue. Meiosis is common in most ovaries by 50 days PC All germ cells are in egg nests until 60 days PC, at which time primordial follicles are observed (Oxender et al. 1979). Primordial follicles account for the majority of ovarian follicles from 95 days PC to 90 days after birth. Egg nests can still be seen in the gilt's ovaries at birth, and formation of follicles continues during the first few weeks after birth (Morbeck et al. 1992). Primary follicles first appear in the ovaries at 70 days PC and secondary follicles are observed about the time of birth. Tertiary (antral) follicles are rarely observed in pigs younger than 60 days of age; however, one or more tertiary follicles are observed in ovaries from pigs at 60–90 days of age (Oxender et al. 1979). As demonstrated by Greenwald (1978), the number of tertiary follicles peaks at 130 days of age, but most of them (67%) are atretic.

Perhaps the most appropriate summary of prepubertal development includes the following stages: the first stage of development from birth to 70 days, 70 days to 140 days, a variable time of resting stage from 20 weeks until puberty, and the changes associated with puberty (Dyck and Swierstra 1983). The first stage is typified by linear growth proportional to the age of the gilt. The second period commences with the appearance of tertiary follicles and an increase in ovarian and uterine weight relative to body weight. The third period or resting stage is characterized by minimal changes in ovarian follicles, ovarian weight, and uterine weight. Finally, the female pig undergoes significant physiological changes, such as preovulatory growth of follicles and increased oviduct and uterine weight, as the gilt approaches puberty.

Female differentiation of the genital ducts in pigs is comparable to most mammals. The cranial part of the Mullerian duct develops into the oviduct and the middle part develops into the uterus. The caudal part of the Mullerian duct and the urogenital sinus contribute to the vagina and vestibule. During the period from birth to 70 days of age, the uterine wall and endometrium increase in thickness, and the uterine glands commence differentiation. At birth, the uterus comprises three layers (luminal epithelium, stroma, and myometrium) with little organization. The change in the uterine wall thickness is attributed to the profound increase in the development of uterine glands and glandular epithelium and the organization of the myometrium into two layers. Furthermore, folding of endometrium also takes place during this period. It is generally accepted that uterine development during the first 2 months after birth does not require stimulation by ovarian steroids. Nevertheless, development can be altered by treatment of the neonatal gilt with estrogen (Bartol et al. 1993). At approximately 70 to 80 days, uterine growth accelerates. This accelerated growth continues until puberty when there is an abrupt increase in the size of the entire female reproductive tract. It is important to note that morphologic development of the uterine glands, endometrium, and myometrium essentially is complete by approximately 120 days of age even though puberty seldom occurs prior to 150 days.

Rearing Influences on Ovarian and Uterine Function

Numerous studies were conducted to examine the influence of rearing environment on the onset of puberty in female pigs. Most reports focused on advancing the onset of puberty or, conversely, identifying factors that delay puberty. Growth rate and nutrition, genetics, boar exposure, management stimuli, social environment, and climatic environment clearly have the potential to influence the onset of puberty. With some notable exceptions, the studies infer that ovarian and/or uterine function was altered, based on the subsequent reproductive performance, i.e., litter size.

If one considers the three stages of prepubertal development prior to the onset of puberty, it should not be surprising that rearing conditions during the first few weeks after birth can have a permanent effect on the reproductive capacity of the mature gilt and sow. For example, litter size during the suckling period can influence the reproductive traits of pigs. Nelson and Robison (1976) used cross-fostering to rear full-sib gilts in litters of 6 or 14 until weaning at 8 weeks of age. Beyond 8 weeks, gilts were co-mingled and provided access to feed and water ad libitum. Age at puberty did not differ, but ovulation rate, number of embryos in first pregnancy, and number of pigs born alive in the first litter were greater in gilts reared in small than in those reared in large litters (Nelson and Robison 1976; van der Steen 1985). In addition, the administration of low levels of estrogen to gilts from birth to 13 days of age reduced the number of viable conceptuses and lowered embryonic survival, effects attributable to a dysfunctional uterus (Bartol et al. 1993).

Studies that examined the influence of rearing or social environment on puberty have provided controversial results. The number of gilts per pen and stocking density were shown to stimulate, impair, or have no effect on sexual maturation. However, rearing environment cannot be ignored—particularly, its effects on subsequent reproductive performance. This was exemplified when gilts between 2 (30 kg body weight (BW)) and 6 months (100 kg BW) of age were reared as full-sib gilts in low- or high-density pens (Kuhlers et al. 1985). There were no differences in growth rates; however, gilts reared in low-density pens had heavier pituitary glands, adrenal glands, brains, uteri and ovaries at 100 kg and delivered larger litters at first farrowing (Rahe et al. 1987).

Replacement gilts should receive optimal care during the entire prepubertal period, beginning at birth. Replacement gilts should be reared in smaller-sized litters and provided with an environment that encourages above average rate of gain. Replacement gilts should be reared in pens with lower densities.

Follicle Growth

Ovarian follicles undergo a gradual maturation in prenatal pigs during the later stages of gestation and the first few postnatal months. In fact, primordial and primary follicles comprise about 80% of ovarian structures in the pig at birth, but the ovary is unresponsive to gonadotropins as assessed by stimulation of follicle growth (Christenson et al. 1985). Tertiary follicles, capable of endocrine function are observed in the ovaries of gilts between 60–90 days after birth (Dyck and Swierstra 1983). These ovaries are responsive to gonadotropins with increased steroidogenesis and ovulation.

Activation and growth of primordial follicles occur continuously throughout the gilt or sow's life. Continual activation and growth are necessary because follicular development from the primordial stage to the ovulatory stage requires between 80 to 100 days (Morbeck et al. 1992). This 3-month development period is noteworthy and may provide an explanation, at least in part, of how certain factors influence follicle development and ovulation. For example, follicle growth was initiated 3 months prior to a gilt reaching puberty at 180 days of age. Similarly, a follicle that ovulates in a sow after weaning started to grow during the early to mid-trimester of preceding pregnancy.

The prolonged period of follicle growth has significant implications in reproductive management. Perhaps the best example of how management factors alter follicle growth is related to feed intake during lactation. It previously was demonstrated that feed restriction during lactation has detrimental effects on the postweaning performance of sows (Koketsu et al. 1996). Feed restriction during lactation increased weaning-to-estrus interval, impaired early follicle development, and decreased ovulation rate (Miller et al. 1996; Zak et al. 1997). Presumably, changes in metabolism affect follicular development and growth.

In fact, there is considerable evidence that nutritional and metabolic control of follicular growth is mediated by metabolic hormones and growth factors, particularly insulin-like growth factor I (IGF-I) and its binding proteins (IGFBPs) (Cox 1997). During the estrous cycle, the ovulatory population of follicles increases growth between about day 14 and day 16. Between day 16 and estrus, follicular atresia is the fate of approximately 50% of medium-sized follicles. The precise mechanisms that determine whether a follicle grows to an ovulatory diameter or undergoes atresia remain poorly understood; however, follicular atresia is considered a balance between "survival" and atretogenic factors. Factors that favor follicle survival include epidermal growth factor, nerve growth factor, IGF-I, gonadotropins, activin and estrogen, while atretogenic factors include testosterone, gonadotropin releasing hormone (GnRH), and interleukins (Hsueh et al. 1994). It is evident that follicular growth and development is a complex system involving numerous factors and hormones. In addition, the influences of nutritional and metabolic factors on the hypothalamus-hypophyseal-ovarian axis and gonadotropin release must also be considered as important factors in follicular growth (Kemp et al. 1995).

REPRODUCTIVE ENDOCRINOLOGY IN THE SOW

Endocrinology of Puberty

During the prenatal period, luteinizing hormone (LH) and follicle stimulating hormone (FSH) concentrations are low or undetectable before day 80 of gestation, and then acutely increase during the last weeks of gestation (Elsaesser et al. 1976; Colenbrander et al. 1982a). Similarly, estrogen concentrations are low at days 50–60 PC and increase significantly by day 75 (Ford et al. 1979). After birth, blood concentrations of steroids of placental origin decrease rapidly (Elsaesser and Foxcroft 1978). There is negligible secretion of estrogen by the ovary for 2–3 months after birth, and progesterone levels are low from birth to first ovulation (Esbenshade et al. 1982; Karlbom et al. 1982).

After birth, patterns of LH and FSH diverge. Serum concentrations of LH are highest around the time of birth and then decrease gradually, reaching a nadir during the second month of life (Camous et al. 1985; Grieger et al. 1986). In contrast, concentrations of FSH increase from the time of farrowing, plateau at approximately 8 weeks of age, and then gradually decline. A further reduction of FSH occurs near the end of the prepubertal period, coincident with growth of estrogen-secreting follicles.

Although spontaneous steroidogenesis appears to be minimal until just before puberty, the porcine ovary evidently is able to respond to gonadotropins. Using hourly injections of GnRH to stimulate LH release, Pressing et al. (1992) effectively mimicked a high-frequency pattern of LH secretion in gilts at 70, 100, 150, and 190 days of age. Follicular growth and ovulation was stimulated in all gilts 100 days of age or older and some gilts at 70 days of age. Consequently, it is apparent that the integration of the pituitary-ovarian axis is complete in the gilt between 70 and 100 days of age and that spontaneous activation of this axis requires a central signal for onset of puberty.

As puberty approaches, there is an increased pulsatile release of gonadotropins that stimulates the progressive development of ovarian follicles. The gonadotropins act to promote follicular development and consequently steroidogenesis. As the follicles develop, there is increased secretion of estrogen (Esbenshade et al. 1982; Karlbom et al. 1982; Camous et al. 1985). Estrogen peaks immediately prior to the pubertal estrus, which coincides with an increase in LH secretion, characterized by a change in pulse frequency and amplitude and the preovulatory surge of LH (Elsaesser and Foxcroft 1978; Lutz et al. 1984).

Endocrinology of the Estrous Cycle

Ovarian follicles, which are destined to ovulate, grow from approximately 4–5 mm in diameter on day 15 (day 0 = first day of standing estrus) of the estrous cycle to an ovulatory diameter of 8–12 mm (Figures 6.1A and 6.1B). The follicular phase begins when the corpora lutea (CL) regress and is associated with high-frequency, low-amplitude pulses of LH. The higher frequency pulses of LH contribute to maturation of the developing follicles, and there is an associated increase in estradiol and inhibin from these follicles. Estradiol and inhibin suppress FSH. Elevated estradiol acts at the hypothalamus to elicit a prolonged release of GnRH, which triggers the LH surge. In addition, estradiol contributes to estrous behavior and morphological changes in the reproductive tract. The LH surge is necessary to induce ovulation with the subsequent release of ova. Onset of estrus usually coincides with the preovulatory LH surge, and females may be sexually receptive for 1 to 3 days (Figure 6.2). As a general rule, female pigs ovulate at approximately two-thirds of the way through estrus (Soede et al. 1995).

The follicular phase ends at the LH surge, because LH triggers biochemical changes in follicles, leading to a decrease in estradiol and inhibin and an increase in progesterone. After estrus, estradiol, inhibin, and progesterone are low and this leads to a postestrual surge of FSH. This postestrual surge of FSH may be important for promoting growth of follicles to develop for the next follicular phase. Following ovulation, collapsed follicles are 4–5 mm in diameter. Blood rapidly fills the central cavity of the follicles. These blood-filled structures are referred to as corpora hemorrhagica (CH; Figure 6.1C). Luteinization of the follicular remnants results in the formation of multiple CL. Luteinization is a rapid process and the early CL is capable of producing progesterone within a few hours after ovulation. The CL production of progesterone increases by 2–4 days after estrus and continues to increase until a maximum is achieved during mid-diestrus. By day 5–6, the CL have reached their mature diameter of 9–11 mm and the central cavities are completely replaced by luteal tissue (Figure 6.1D). Female pigs are not sexually receptive during these periods of progesterone production.

Failure to initiate pregnancy results in regression of the CL, a decline in serum progesterone concentrations and a return to estrus. Degeneration of the CL typically commences at approximately days 13–15, coinciding with increased concentrations of the luteolysin, prostaglandin-$F_{2\alpha}$ ($PGF_{2\alpha}$). Follicular recruitment begins on days 13–15 and follicles continue to enlarge concomitant with regression of the CL (Figure 6.1A). It is common to observe small follicles of less than 5 mm in the absence of CL in anestrous sows (Figure 6.1E).

Endocrinology of Pregnancy and Parturition

The CL lifespan is extended throughout pregnancy (Figure 6.1F) due to the maternal recognition of pregnancy (days 10–14 after ovulation and successful mating). Both maternal and conceptus factors play important roles in maternal recognition of pregnancy;

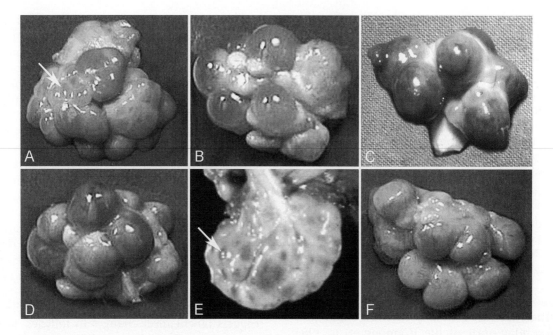

6.1. *Porcine ovaries. A) New follicles (arrow) commencing to develop among corpora lutea. The ovary was collected at approximately day 15–16 of the estrous cycle. B) Large, preovulatory follicles. C) Corpora hemorrhagica (CH). The CH form shortly after ovulation. D) Mature corpora lutea. The ovary was collected during diestrus. E) Ovary collected from an anestrous sow. Note the small follicles (<5 mm; arrow) and the absence of corpora lutea. F) Mature corpora lutea. The ovary was collected from a pregnant sow during midgestation.*

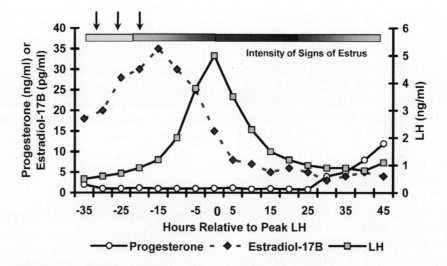

6.2. *Endocrine changes during the periestrous period relative to the peak LH concentrations. Peak LH concentrations typically coincide with the onset of standing estrus. The arrows indicate the period of proestrus, and the bar shows the intensity of signs indicative of estrus.*

however, estrogen, secreted by the conceptuses, may be considered the primary factor that triggers a series of events to maintain the CL of pregnancy. Maternal recognition of pregnancy occurs when developing conceptuses exert an effect that prevents luteolysis (Bazer 1989). In a nonpregnant pig, the uterine endometrium secretes $PGF_{2\alpha}$ in an endocrine fashion, resulting in an increase in the amount of $PGF_{2\alpha}$ reaching the ovary via the utero-ovarian vein and the uterine artery (Figure 6.3). In a pregnant pig, $PGF_{2\alpha}$ is secreted in an exocrine

fashion into the uterine lumen rather than into the utero-ovarian vein. The transition from endocrine to exocrine secretion between day 10 and 12 of pregnancy coincides with the initiation of estrogen secretion by the pig conceptuses (Fisher et al. 1985). In addition, pregnant animals show an increase in secretion of PGE_2, a luteotropic prostaglandin produced by the endometrium or conceptuses. This shifts the ratio of luteotropic to luteolytic prostaglandins in a favorable direction for maintenance of CL function. Furthermore, maternal

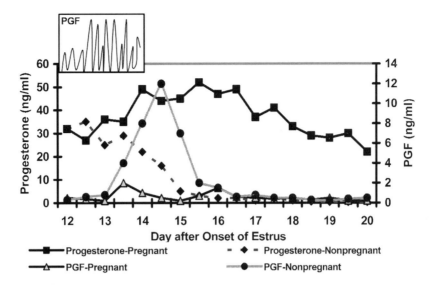

6.3. *Changes in daily concentrations of progesterone and PGF in the utero-ovarian vein of pregnant and nonpregnant gilts (Adapted from Moeljono et al. 1977). The insert illustrates the "pulsatile" nature of the PGF release that is observed if frequent blood samples are collected.*

and conceptus-derived steroid hormones, growth factors, and cytokines, as well as integrins and their ligands, have interrelated roles in mediating adhesion between the conceptus and maternal uterine epithelium (Jaeger et al. 2001). These complex interactions between the conceptus and the uterus are critical to successful implantation in pigs.

Progesterone is required throughout pregnancy in the pig, and the primary source of progesterone is the CL. One corpus luteum is enough to maintain pregnancy, provided that the reduction in CL is done in a stepwise manner (Thomford et al. 1984). Ovariectomy, enucleation of CL or treatment with a luteolytic prostaglandin all cause abortion. The CL are autonomous for the first 2 weeks after estrus and thereafter require only basal LH support to continue to secrete progesterone (First and Bazer 1983). Progesterone concentrations in blood increase to peak values by day 12 after mating and remain elevated, thereby causing myometrial quiescence (Anderson 1987). Hypophyseal luteotropic support is required during most of pregnancy to sustain CL function. Plasma concentrations of estrone sulfate show a transient increase during the fourth week of pregnancy because of production of estrogens by the feto-placental unit. Estrogens then decline until about day 80 when unconjugated estrogens and estradiol-17β increase to peak values just prior to parturition.

As term approaches, a series of endocrine events (Figure 6.4), presumably initiated by the fetal pigs, lead to parturition. Fetuses initiate parturition through fetal pituitary release of adrenocorticotropic hormone (ACTH), which stimulates production of glucocorticoids by the fetal adrenal. Cortisol stimulates increased release of $PGF_{2\alpha}$ from the gravid uterus, which promotes luteolysis and thereby decreases concentrations of progesterone. This facilitates an increased frequency of uter-

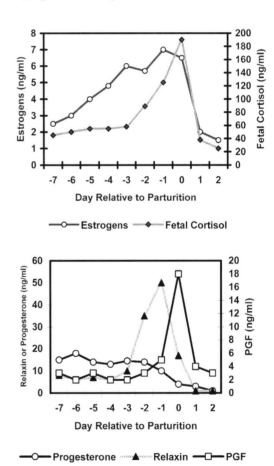

6.4. *Endocrine changes associated with parturition in the female pig (adapted from First and Bosc 1979). Note that the decline in progesterone concentrations is not complete until 1–2 days after parturition.*

ine contractions and the initiation of parturition (First et al. 1982; First and Bazer 1983). The elevated $PGF_{2\alpha}$ concentrations also promote the release of relaxin from the CL and oxytocin from the neurohypophysis.

Relaxin and oxytocin are required for the relaxation of the cervix and promotion of myometrial activity, respectively.

Pseudopregnancy

Pseudopregnancy occurs when CL are maintained beyond the expected time of luteolysis in the absence of viable fetuses. Short pseudopregnancy has been defined as an interestrus interval of at least 3 days beyond normal for a gilt or sow with a minimum duration of at least 23 days (Pusateri et al. 1996). Long pseudopregnancy has been defined as an interestrus interval of more than 50 days. The extended interestrus interval is associated with an extension of luteal function because luteolysis is delayed.

Pseudopregnancy can be induced by treating gilts or sows with estrogen beginning on day 11 or 12 of an estrous cycle. Short-term treatment with estradiol (i.e., treatment on day 11 and 12) will induce short pseudopregnancy in most animals, but longer-term treatment (treatment for 8–9 days beginning on day 11 or 12) is required to induce consistent long pseudopregnancy. Gilts that consume moldy corn contaminated with *Fusarium roseum* that produces zearalenone may show either short or long pseudopregnancy.

Endocrinology of Lactation

Sows experience three reproductive phases after farrowing, namely, the hypergonadotropic phase, the transition phase, and the normalization phase (Britt 1996a). After parturition, the CL regress to form corpora albicantia (CA). The CA gradually regress during lactation and are less than 2 mm in diameter at the time of weaning. During the last few days of pregnancy, follicles develop on the ovary. These follicles initially are present in the first 1 or 2 days of lactation. This hypergonadotropic phase is associated with elevated LH and FSH concentrations, declining estrogens and progesterone (Sesti and Britt 1994) and large, preovulatory sized follicles. Due to suckling-induced inhibition of GnRH secretion and decreased LH and FSH, the large follicles regress within a few days after farrowing. Low levels of gonadotropins, minimal ovarian activity, and low concentrations of estradiol and progesterone characterize the transition phase from day 3 to 14 (Cox et al. 1988; Sesti and Britt 1994). Normalization occurs beyond day 14 when there is an increase in LH and FSH, number of medium and preovulatory sized follicles, and estradiol (Sesti and Britt 1993). Although suckling suppresses estrus by preventing release of GnRH from the hypothalamus, hourly pulses of GnRH will induce estrus and ovulation within 7 days. This attests to the central role the GnRH plays in regulating follicular growth and estrous cycles in both gilts and sows (Cox and Britt 1982).

The uterus is enlarged after farrowing, but involution during this period is rapid with remarkable decreases in weight and length in 2 to 3 days. During the transition phase, the uterus continues to undergo involution, with weight and length reaching a stable plateau by approximately day 14 (Varley 1982).

MANAGEMENT OF REPRODUCTIVE PROCESSES: DETECTION OF ESTRUS

Proestrual Changes

Estrus is the period of sexual receptivity during which sows and gilts display a characteristic pattern of both anatomical changes and behaviors culminating in the immobilization response or standing reflex. The first signs of approaching estrus are increased activity and vocalizations. Sows housed in crates commonly move backward and forward or from side to side within the crate and often attempt to nibble or nose females in adjacent crates. Sometimes these sows will paw at the front door of the crate and chant to animals in adjacent crates. In pens, characteristic activities include sniffing, nuzzling the rear and fore flanks, and attempting to mount or ride other females. Sows attempting to mount or actually riding other females may be either in estrus or approaching estrus.

Reddening and swelling of the vulva usually accompany or occur shortly after the increased activity. The change in size and color of the vulva is the result of an increase in blood flow and retention of fluids. As a result, the external lips of the vulva often are pushed outward exposing a portion of its highly vascular inner lining. Due to these changes, the opening to the vagina often appears to increase in size. In females that are not in heat, the external lips of the vulva are curled inward and block the opening to the vagina giving it a small, puckered appearance. The size and color change of the vulva are greatest just prior to when females will exhibit the immobilization reflex. Reddening and swelling of the vulva often do not appear to occur in older parity sows because the change in color and size are masked by the loose, flabby skin around the vulva caused by repeated deliveries.

The presence of a sticky discharge and enlargement of the clitoris usually occur immediately before and during the standing reflex. When females are in heat, the clitoris is engorged with blood, which causes it to protrude outward and have a bright red color. When females are not in heat, the clitoris is flat and has a pale, light pink color. To observe the clitoris, it is necessary to pull the external lips of the vulva apart and outward. This exposes the internal fold where the lips join and the clitoris is located. Mucus obtained from the inside lining of the vulva from sows that are not in heat has a slimy or slick feel. Just prior to the initiation of the standing reflex, the consistency of the mucus changes and becomes tacky or sticky. Assessment of the consistency of the mucus commonly is referred to as the "thumb check." The thumb check is performed by wiping the inside lining of the vulva with the thumb to obtain a sample of mucus. Then, the thumb and first finger are pressed together and slowly pulled apart. The sample is considered sticky or tacky if small strands of mucus remain connected to both the thumb and pointer as they are drawn apart. In most cases, an engorged clitoris and sticky mucus are good indications that the female is in or within a few hours of exhibiting standing heat.

Standing Reflex

The standing reflex is the most common behavior associated with sexual receptivity and serves as the reference point upon which most breeding regimens are based. Duration of the standing reflex has been reported to be between 46 and 53 hours for sows and 36 and 48 hours for gilts (Signoret et al. 1972; Kemp and Soede 1996). The variation associated with these estimates is considerable, indicating that expression of the standing reflex is influenced by a number of environmental factors (Hemsworth and Barnett 1990). The successful expression and identification of the standing reflex depends upon interactions between internal and external stimuli. High concentrations of estradiol produced by preovulatory follicles are the internal stimuli, while pheromones produced by the boar serve as the external cues. Elevated estradiol levels invoke changes in the central nervous system that gives the female the ability to exhibit the standing reflex. However, it is the presence of the male pheromone, 5-alpha androsterone, that is believed to be the catalyst for the immobilization response (Hughes et al. 1990). Female pheromones may also be involved because the presence of estrual sows has been shown to stimulate and synchronize estrous behaviors in weaned sows and peripubertal gilts (Pearce and Pearce 1992).

The immobilization response requires a tremendous expenditure of energy because it involves the isometric contraction of most of the pig's skeletal muscle. This is why sows exhibiting the standing reflex often appear to quiver or tremble. Most females are only able to maintain this immobilized state for 15–30 minutes before muscles become fatigued (Levis and Hemsworth 1995). When this happens, females enter a period of refractoriness during which they are not able to exhibit a normal standing reflex. This phenomenon is called *habituation* and commonly occurs in situations where sows have continual, fence-line contact with boars. Habituation can be prevented and the standing reflex enhanced by providing short, daily periods of boar exposure or by physical separation of as little as 1 meter (Hemsworth and Barnett 1990).

Pheromones produced by boars are the most potent and effective inducer of the standing reflex in receptive females. Running a boar in front of sows in crates while a breeding technician applies back pressure is a common and effective method of estrous detection. Sows in heat will move forward and assume the standing reflex as the boar moves in front of the crate. When back pressure is applied, females that are truly in heat will actu-

ally push back—a natural response for a sow that is preparing to be mounted by the boar. Sows in crates are probably not in estrus if they try to move away from back pressure, even though they might show some other signs of estrus. In pens, sows will move to the front of the pen as the boar passes. If back pressure is applied and the sow is in heat, then she will exhibit the standing reflex. If back pressure is applied and the sow is not in heat, then she usually will run away from the back pressure. Estrous females housed in pens will sometimes attempt to follow the movement of a boar as he passes in front of their pen. This is due to the fact that sexually receptive females seek out males more so than males finding sows that are in heat.

Ovulatory Dynamics in Relation to Estrus

In general, ovulation in pigs begins 36–44 hours after the onset of estrus and lasts 1–3 hours. Most follicles (68–95%) appear to ovulate over a short period of time, while a minority ovulates over a longer interval. Nevertheless, onset and duration of ovulation are extremely variable within and among herds (Flowers and Esbenshade 1993). For example, in the study of Weitze and co-workers (1992), average duration from the onset of estrus to ovulation was 44.4 hours; but the means for animals in the first and fourth quartiles were 26.2 and 57.9 hours, respectively—a difference of 30 hours. Using real-time ultrasonography, Kemp and Soede (1996) demonstrated that most of the variation associated with the time of ovulation was due to differences in the duration of estrus.

They concluded that ovulation occurs when estrus is about 70% completed; thus, for a gilt that exhibits the standing reflex for 1 day, ovulation would be expected to begin about 17 hours after the onset of estrus, but for one that exhibits a 2-day estrus, ovulation would not begin until 34 hours after onset of estrus.

INSEMINATION

Timing and Frequency

From a physiological perspective, successful breeding regimens consistently create a situation in which an adequate number of viable spermatozoa are present in the oviduct prior to ovulation (Dziuk and Polge 1965). Thus, insemination must be coordinated with ovulation. This is usually accomplished by adjustment of the timing and frequency of matings based on the onset of estrus. However, relationships between ovulation and onset of estrus vary considerably within and among herds (Flowers and Esbenshade 1993). Consequently, reproductive performance could differ considerably among herds using identical mating regimens.

Kemp and Soede (1996) conducted a comprehensive evaluation of the relationship between timing of insemination relative to ovulation and fertility. Time of ovulation was monitored by realtime ultrasonography.

Results indicated that if a mating occurred 0–24 hours prior to ovulation, then fertilization rates were greater than 90%. The insemination dose used in the study was 3 billion spermatozoa that were 24 ± 6 hours old at artificial insemination (AI). Thus it appears that the minimum requirement for the timing and frequency of AI is one mating each day of estrus. Based on this information, one might question the importance of multiple matings within a 24-hour period. Although it is possible that two matings during the 24-hour period before ovulation might result in an improvement in fertilization rates, the 90% in the study of Kemp and Soede (1996) is generally accepted as being close to the maximal rate normally achieved in swine (Polge 1978).

Insemination Dose

Two aspects of insemination dose that affect fertility are the total number of viable spermatozoa and the total volume inseminated. The volume of the insemination dose is an important stimulus for activation of uterine smooth muscle activity, which is responsible for movement of spermatozoa from the site of deposition (cervix) to the site of fertilization (oviduct). Volumes of at least 60–80 ml appear to be required for optimal sperm transport (Baker et al. 1968). A positive relationship exists between number of sperm cells inseminated and number that enter the oviduct when insemination doses are between 1 and 8 billion (Baker et al. 1968). However, the effects of oviductal sperm numbers on litter size and farrowing rate have not been clearly established. Insemination doses between 2 and 5 billion spermatozoa are generally considered sufficient to ensure adequate fertility (Weitze 1991).

Breeding Technician

The technical competence of breeding technicians and reproductive performance within a herd often are assumed to be positively correlated; as the skill level increases, so do farrowing rates and litter size. Documentation that this assumption is true has been provided by two types of studies. In a survey of swine farms experiencing suboptimal reproduction in the southeastern United States, it was estimated that the main problem on 30% of these farms was associated with the skill level of the breeding technicians (Flowers 1996a). Poor detection of estrus was found to be the predominant problem rather than poor insemination or semen handling techniques. It is not appropriate to use these data from a retrospective study as evidence for a cause and effect relationship; however, a prospective study characterized AI breeding technicians within a single commercial swine operation (Flowers 1996a, b). In that study, matings administered by technicians occurred simultaneously within the same production environment. Thus observed differences were due to the influence of the breeding technician and not other confounding factors. Data from this study demonstrated two important concepts: breeding technicians had a large influence on farrowing rates and litter size, and performance of breeding technicians did not remain constant over time. There was a 1036-pig difference in total pigs produced between the best and worst technicians based on 220 sows bred over 13 weeks. If this trend continued for an entire year in this herd, then there would be approximately a 4000-pig difference between the best and worst technician. Farrowing rates of sows supervised by 5 out of 6 technicians exhibited significant fluctuations during the 13-week study. These changes over time could be explained by environmental or animal factors that influenced the entire herd because farrowing rates for some individuals decreased and for others increased. Based on the magnitude of these changes, the ability to monitor reproductive performance of sows on a breeding technician basis would be of great value. However, to accomplish this, record keeping programs must include breeding technician as an independent variable and matings for a given female must be administered by the same individual.

CONTROL OF REPRODUCTIVE PROCESSES

Control of the onset of estrus has been approached along two lines: the induction of ovulation in acyclic, anovulatory females and the regulation of the luteal phase of the estrous cycle in cyclic, ovulatory pigs. The latter approach has utilized suppression of ovarian activity via the administration of oral-active progesterone or synthetic progestins. Presently, the most common exogenous hormone combination for induction of follicle growth and ovulation in acyclic females is a combination of 400 IU of equine chorionic gonadotropin (eCG) and 200 IU of human chorionic gonadotropin (hCG).

Induction and Synchronization of First Estrus in Gilts

To induce puberty successfully in a group of gilts, it is important to know the pubertal status of the group and the usual age of onset of puberty under the conditions on the specific farm. Gilts that are within approximately 1–2 months of natural onset of puberty will respond to treatment with gonadotropins by expressing estrus and continuing to cycle. If gilts are too young, they may express estrus, but then return to an anestrous state. If gilts have already cycled, they usually will not respond to gonadotropin treatment by showing estrus.

Puberty can be induced in gilts by treatment with a single injection of 400 IU of eCG and 200 IU of hCG. Gilts usually show estrus 3–6 days after treatment (Britt et al. 1989). The percentage of gilts that show estrus in a group may vary considerably, but most gilts ovulate even if they do not show estrus (Tilton et al. 1995). The response rate is enhanced if gilts are given daily boar stimulation by direct physical contact beginning at the time of treatment. Gilts respond best if they are held on the finishing floor until the time of injection and are moved and injected on the same day. Failure to respond to this combination may be associated with treating gilts that have already reached puberty.

Synchronization of Second Estrus in Gilts

One can theoretically resynchronize second estrus in treated gilts by giving a luteolytic dose of $PGF_{2\alpha}$ approximately 18 days after the injection of 400 IU of eCG and 200 IU of hCG (Britt 1996b). Pig CL do not undergo luteolysis in response to a single standard luteolytic dose of $PGF_{2\alpha}$ during the first 12 days of the estrous cycle, but beyond the 12th day $PGF_{2\alpha}$ will induce luteolysis. If most gilts in a group are between day 12 and 17 of an estrous cycle, one should be able to synchronize estrus by giving a single injection of $PGF_{2\alpha}$. Most gilts should be beyond day 12 of an estrous cycle 18 days after injection of gonadotropins. If these gilts are given a luteolytic dose of $PGF_{2\alpha}$, their second estrus should be more synchronous than if they remained untreated.

Synchronization of Estrus in Pregnant Gilts

The porcine CL remain unresponsive to the acute administration of $PGF_{2\alpha}$ or its analogs until days 12 to 14 after ovulation. As the porcine CL typically commence natural regression due to endogenous prostaglandins at days 14–17, there is only a transient period when a single treatment with exogenous prostaglandins hastens the onset of estrus. Repeated $PGF_{2\alpha}$ injections between days 5 and 10 will reduce the duration of the estrous cycle; however, the labor and cost preclude this technique from practical application.

In contrast to the relative unresponsiveness of the CL to $PGF_{2\alpha}$ during diestrus, $PGF_{2\alpha}$ is effective for inducing luteolysis, abortion, and prompt return to estrus in pregnant (and pseudopregnant) gilts beyond the second week of pregnancy (Pressing et al. 1987). One method for synchronization is to penmate gilts for 3 weeks and then, treat with $PGF_{2\alpha}$ 2 weeks later (Britt 1996b). This technique is effective, but ages at first farrowing and nonproductive sow days are increased.

Synchronization of Estrus with Progestin

Cyclic gilts can be synchronized by administering a progestin for 14–18 days (Britt 1996b). The progestin inhibits follicular maturation and estrus while permitting the CL to regress naturally. When the progestin is withdrawn, follicles mature and estrus occurs beginning about 3 days later. Several studies demonstrated that feeding altrenogest at the rate of 15–20 mg per day was effective for synchronizing estrus, and subsequent litter size was normal or slightly increased (Davis et al. 1985). Treated gilts exhibit estrus 4–9 days after completion of a 14-day treatment period. The product is administered on an individual gilt basis by top-dressing the animal's daily feed allowance. It is critical that each gilt receives the recommended 15 mg each day, because underfeeding may lead to cystic ovarian degeneration.

Induction of Ovulation in Early Lactation in Sows

Initial studies demonstrated that ovulation was induced in about 75% of sows by giving hCG on the day of farrowing (Britt et al. 1997). These sows form CL that eventually regress spontaneously. If CL were induced by treatment with hCG on the day of farrowing, weaning could occur any time before day 21 but the sow would not be expected to be in heat until day 21 or slightly after. Furthermore, $PGF_{2\alpha}$ could be given after day 14–16 to induce premature luteolysis, and the sow should be in heat 3–5 days later. Despite initial success with this method of synchronization, subsequent reports indicated that the method did not have sufficient reliability for commercial sow farms (Kirkwood et al. 1999).

Induction of Estrus in Weaned Sows

Anestrus after weaning is more likely to occur during the summer and fall and is more common in primiparous than multiparous sows (Britt 1986). Incidence of anestrus can be reduced substantially by treating with gonadotropin at weaning (Bates et al. 1991); therefore, an effective strategy during periods when anestrus is likely to occur at a high rate is to treat sows at weaning with a combination of eCG and hCG. An alternative strategy to treatment of all sows in a group at weaning is selectively to treat those that have not returned to estrus by 7 days after weaning (Britt 1996a); however, there is little experimental evidence supporting the use of gonadotropins for this purpose (Tubbs et al. 1996).

Induction of Parturition

To synchronize farrowing, $PGF_{2\alpha}$ or an analog, is used to induce parturition (Table 6.1). Induction of farrowing creates an opportunity for producers to supervise parturition, reduce stillbirth rates, facilitate cross-fostering of piglets and to decrease variability of piglet weaning ages and lactation lengths. Exogenous $PGF_{2\alpha}$ typically is administered to sows after day 112 of gestation. Prostaglandin-induced farrowing prior to day 110 severely compromises piglet survivability. Some producers prefer to restrict prostaglandin injections to sows that exceed a 114-day or 115-day gestation. Other producers treat all sows with prostaglandin at a specific day (day 112 to 114) of gestation.

The duration of parturition, piglet viability and sow performance during lactation are similar following prostaglandin-induced farrowings and natural delivery (Einarsson et al. 1981; Dial et al. 1987). Prior to implementing an induction program and achieving favorable results, producers need accurate records regarding gestation length and a commitment to supervise farrowings and assist deliveries. The mean interval from $PGF_{2\alpha}$ injection to the onset of parturition was 29.5 hours with a range of 24–32 hours and considerable variation (Pressing 1992), which emphasizes the potential differences in response from farm to farm and from study to

Table 6.1. Interval between oxytocin (OT) injection and onset of farrowing in sows treated with prostaglandin (PGF$_{2\alpha}$ 10 mg) on different days of gestation (adapted from Dial et al. 1987). The OT was given 20 hours after the PGF$_{2\alpha}$ injection. Numbers of interventions required during farrowing also are shown. Data are expressed as means ± SEM.

| | Interval (h) from OT Injection to Farrowing | | | | Interventions per Sow Days 112–114 |
| | Gestation Day of PGF$_{2\alpha}$ Treatment | | | | |
OT Dose (Units)	112	113	114	112–114	
0	11.7 ± 2.8	9.2 ± 1.5	4.3 ± 0.7	8.5 ± 1.2	0.2 ± 0.1
5	14.0 ± 2.3	7.8 ± 2.2	4.3 ± 1.5	8.5 ± 1.5	0.5 ± 0.3
10	11.4 ± 4.1	8.3 ± 2.6	6.7 ± 2.0	8.4 ± 1.5	1.2 ± 0.5
20	11.4 ± 3.2	7.7 ± 2.1	8.0 ± 3.7	9.0 ± 1.5	0.5 ± 0.3
30	4.8 ± 1.4	4.6 ± 1.8	3.5 ± 1.8	4.4 ± 1.1	1.9 ± 0.6

study. The interval from injection to parturition tends to be less with cloprostenol, a PGF$_{2\alpha}$ analog (Pressing 1992); however, in some countries, only the natural prostaglandin is approved for use in swine. The side effects of prostaglandin-induced farrowing include hyperpnea, and increased salivation, urination, and defecation within minutes after injection. Nest-building, rooting, pawing, and bar biting are often evident but subside within 2 hours.

Initial investigations used intramuscular injections of either PGF$_{2\alpha}$ (10 mg) or cloprostenol (175 µg). Subsequent studies demonstrated that the dose could be reduced to 5 mg and 87.5 µg, respectively, with vulvomucosal injections (Friendship et al. 1990). The interval from injection to parturition was similar to the intramuscular injection; however, the undesirable side effects were reduced.

Prostaglandin and Oxytocin Combination. It was proposed that an injection of oxytocin at 20–24 hours after the initial prostaglandin injection would improve synchrony of farrowing during working hours. Treatment with 20–30 IU of oxytocin induced earlier parturition in a larger proportion of sows than 5–10 IU of oxytocin (Table 6.1). The high doses were associated with frequent interruptions of piglet deliveries and dystocia (Dial et al. 1987). With 5–10 IU of oxytocin, few complications occurred during delivery; however, less than 90% of treated animals were induced to farrow during the working day. Thus the low doses of oxytocin cause few problems with parturition; yet they fail to improve the synchrony of parturition, which in turn diminishes the opportunity for supervised farrowings. Clinical reports indicate that vulvomucosal injection of 5 IU of oxytocin is sufficient to induce farrowing without complications.

Other Products. Carazolol, epostane, and clenbuterol were shown to be efficacious in the control of parturition. None of these agents are licensed for use in swine in the U.S. Carazolol, a ß$_{1,2}$-adrenergic blocking agent,

when used in combination with prostaglandins, improved synchronization of farrowing. Carazolol (3 mg/sow), given 20 hours after prostaglandin administration, induced labor within 3 hours, shortened the duration of parturition and did not create adverse side effects (Holtz et al. 1990). This agent also may be used alone (1 mg/100 kg body weight) at the onset of labor to reduce the duration of parturition (Bostedt and Rudloff 1983).

Epostane, a competitive inhibitor of 3ß-hydroxysteroid dehydrogenase, was shown to decrease peripheral levels of progesterone and induce sows to farrow (Martin et al. 1987). The interval from oral administration of 5 and 10 mg/kg body weight to the birth of the first piglet was 31 and 33 hours, respectively. There were no adverse effects reported with epostane-induced farrowings.

Tocolytic agents are used to inhibit rather than hasten the onset of labor. The tocolytic effects of clenbuterol result from its ß$_2$-adrenergic properties. Intravenous or intramuscular administration of clenbuterol (150 µg/sow) during the onset of labor, but before delivery of the first pig, delayed parturition by 15 hours (Zerobin and Kundig 1980). The use of clenbuterol after delivery of one to three piglets interrupted parturition for 3 hours. Detrimental effects were not observed with this dose of clenbuterol; however, repeated, higher doses (300 µg every 6 hours) increased stillbirth rate.

Induction of Abortion

Prostaglandins are effective abortifacients (≥12–14 days after mating) in sows and most sows return to a fertile estrus following the termination of pregnancy (Guthrie and Polge 1978; Pressing et al. 1987). In addition, administration of exogenous PGF$_{2\alpha}$ is luteolytic in pseudopregnant pigs (Smith et al. 1992) and will induce parturition in sows that are carrying mummified fetuses (Hermansson et al. 1981). Both PGF$_{2\alpha}$ (10–15 mg) and cloprostenol (175–500 µg), given once or twice at a 24-hour interval, effectively terminate pregnancy and pseudopregnancy.

PREGNANCY DETECTION

Most pork producers consider pregnancy detection essential to the reproductive efficiency of the sow herd. An ideal pregnancy detection method would have 100% sensitivity and specificity. Testing would take a few seconds per animal and the method would be simple enough that training would be minimal. This "ideal" method would predict pregnancy status prior to the return to estrus at 17–24 days postmating (Almond and Dial 1987). Because an ideal technique is not available, producers rely on one or more techniques for pregnancy diagnosis.

Detection of Estrus

The most common pregnancy detection technique is based on the premise that nonpregnant sows will return to estrus within 17–24 days after breeding. Detection of estrus is improved if the sow's behavior is observed in the presence of a boar, particularly when there is physical contact between the boar and female. The overall accuracy of this technique ranged from 39% (Bosc et al. 1975) to 98% (Almond and Dial 1986). Field reports indicate that most producers identify approximately 50% of nonconceiving sows using this technique. False-positive diagnoses occur when sows are persistently anestrus due to cystic ovarian degeneration (COD), acyclic ovaries, or becoming pseudopregnant. Management factors that interfere with the detection of estrus include housing submissive sows in groups with dominant sows, attempting to detect estrous females in large groups, and assessing estrus without using boar exposure.

Hormone Concentrations

Serum concentrations of progesterone and estrone sulfate were used as indicators of pregnancy. Hormone concentrations are dynamic and collection of samples is restricted to discrete periods during pregnancy.

Progesterone. Regression of the CL typically commences prior to day 15 of the estrous cycle. Following maternal recognition of pregnancy, serum progesterone concentrations are usually greater than 5 ng/ml throughout pregnancy. Thus, serum concentrations of progesterone are high in pregnant sows and gilts during the expected time of return to estrus and low (<5 ng/ml) in sows and gilts that failed to conceive (Ellendorf et al. 1976). The interestrus interval of sows of varying parities ranges from 17 to 24 days, with a mean of 20 to 21 days (Andersson and Einarsson 1980). Therefore, the optimal time to obtain blood samples for progesterone determinations is from 17 to 20 days after mating (Almond and Dial 1987). Using serum progesterone concentrations for pregnancy diagnosis, a sensitivity of more than 97% was achieved, but specificity ranged from 60 to 90% (Larsson et al. 1975; Almond and Dial 1986). False-positive tests occur in animals with delayed or irregular returns to estrus, pseudopregnancies, and COD. False-negative tests may result from laboratory error since it is assumed that ≥5 ng progesterone/ml serum are required for pregnancy maintenance in swine (Ellicott and Dziuk 1973).

Commercial enzyme-linked immunosorbent assays are available for on farm applications, which reduce the need of laboratory-based radioimmunoassays (Glossop et al. 1989). The necessity of collecting blood is a significant limitation of this method; however, enzyme immunoreactive assays (Sanders et al. 1994) and radioimmunoassays were developed for assessing fecal progesterone concentrations. Despite potential applications for these fecal tests, their utility has yet to be determined on commercial farms.

Estrone Sulfate. A high proportion of fetal estrogens is secreted from the uterus into the maternal circulation as estrone sulfate (Robertson et al. 1985). Serum estrone sulfate concentrations cannot be reliably determined until peak levels are reached between 25 and 30 days of gestation (Robertson et al. 1978). At 35 to 45 days, the concentrations decrease to a nadir (Guthrie and Deaver 1979), with a second increase commencing at 70 to 80 days.

Serum estrone sulfate concentrations of >0.5 ng/ml are indicative of pregnancy, whereas <0.5 ng/ml are suggestive of nonpregnant status (Cunningham 1982; Almond and Dial 1986). Using estrone sulfate as a pregnancy test, >97% sensitivity and >88% specificity were obtained when samples were collected between 25 and 30 days of pregnancy (Almond and Dial 1986). False-negative results were obtained in sows or gilts with a delayed rise in estrone sulfate concentrations (Cunningham et al. 1983) or when sows and gilts have less than four pigs in a litter (Almond and Dial 1986). Urinary concentrations of estrone conjugates also were used to predict pregnancy and to diagnose fertility problems (Seren et al. 1983); however, this technique was not developed for commercial application. Quantitative commercial assay kits for the determination of estrone sulfate concentrations in serum or feces from swine are not available. The need to collect blood samples limits the practical application of this technique.

Prostaglandin-F$_{2\alpha}$. The prostaglandin pregnancy test was based on the principles that if serum concentrations of PGF$_{2\alpha}$ are low (<200 pg/ml) or undetectable between days 13 and 15 after mating, the sow can be assumed to be pregnant. The prostaglandin pregnancy test had approximately 90% sensitivity and 70% specificity (Bosc et al. 1975). This method can be conducted during early pregnancy, but it is unreliable for detecting open animals and requires extensive laboratory procedures.

Rectal Palpation

Pregnancy diagnosis by rectal palpation of the sow is practical and highly accurate (Cameron 1977). Sows are examined while standing in gestation crates or pens or while tethered. This technique is based on examination of the cervix and uterus, together with palpation of the middle uterine artery to assess size, degree of tone, and type of pulse. The pelvic canal and rectum are often too small for the procedure to be used on gilts or low parity sows. Despite the potential application of this technique, it has not gained popularity in North America.

Ultrasound Techniques

Doppler Ultrasound. Doppler instruments detect fetal heartbeats or the pulsation of arteries. Approximately 50–100 pulses/minute are detected in the uterine artery, while 150–250 pulses/minute are evident in the umbilical arteries (Swensson 1978). The abdominal probe is positioned on the flank of the animal, lateral to the nipples, and aimed at the sow's pelvis area. The ultrasound waves are emitted and received by transducers and are converted to audible signals. The rectal probe functions similarly, with the exception of the positioning of the transducer. Sensitivity (>85%) and specificity (>95%) did not differ between the rectal and abdominal probes (McCaughey and Rea 1979; Almond and Dial 1986). Optimal results were obtained at 29–34 days (Almond et al. 1985). False-positive results may occur when sows are tested during proestrus or estrus or when animals have active endometritis. False-negative diagnoses occur when examinations are conducted in a noisy environment or if feces become packed around the rectal probe.

Amplitude-Depth (A-mode or Pulse Echo) Ultrasound. Amplitude-depth instruments use ultrasound waves to detect the fluid-filled uterus (Lindahl et al. 1975). From approximately 30 days until 75 days after breeding, the overall accuracy in the determination of pregnancy was commonly >95% (Holtz 1982; Almond et al. 1985). False-negative and uncertain determinations increase from 75 days until farrowing, due to changes in the allantoic fluids and fetal growth. The sensitivity and specificity vary between the different models of amplitude depth instruments (Almond and Dial 1986). Detection of a fluid-filled urinary bladder, pyometra or endometrial edema yields a false-positive test. False-negative results were noted when animals were examined before 28 days of gestation or after day 80 (Holtz 1982).

Real-Time Ultrasonography. Results of initial studies clearly indicated that real-time ultrasonography (RTU) possessed potential for early and accurate pregnancy diagnosis in sows and gilts (Inaba et al. 1983; Jackson 1986). The transducer of RTU probe is placed against the flank of the animal, and the positioning is similar to other pregnancy detection devices. The probe is directed toward the back of the animal, allowing the ultrasound waves to pass through the uterus before returning back to the transducer. Pregnancy is based on the detection

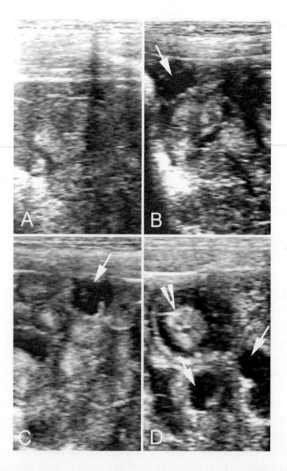

6.5. *These figures illustrate the images observed with real-time ultrasound (linear, 5 mHz probe) at day 21 in a nonpregnant sow (A) and at days 21 (B), 23 (C), and 35 (D) of pregnancy. The circular, black structures, shown with white arrows, are cross-sections of the fluid-filled uterus. A fetus (arrowhead) is evident in the day 35 image.*

of distinct, fluid-filled vesicles in the reproductive tract (Figure 6.5).

For various reasons, such as the purchase price of an instrument, producers and veterinarians were reluctant to use RTU in commercial sow farms. However, the trend to larger sow farms and the decrease in purchase price created opportunities for RTU as a routine pregnancy detection method. On day 21 of gestation, the overall accuracy was 90% and 96% for the 3.5 and 5 mHz probes, respectively (Armstrong et al. 1997). The 5 mHz probe had a greater specificity than the 3.5 mHz probe. It also was evident that technician, day of gestation, instrument, and probe (3.5 vs. 5 mHz and linear vs. sector) influenced the accuracy of RTU. These sources of variation have much less impact when RTU is used at day 28, rather than day 21.

Conclusions. Amplitude depth (a-mode) and doppler instruments typically are used after 30 days postmating and require multiple tests to improve accuracy. Both instruments are inexpensive and neither requires extensive training; however, numerous causes of false-positive and false-negative tests exist with either instrument. Tests for serum progesterone or estrone sulfate require blood samples at specific days of pregnancy. To eliminate blood collection, assay procedures were developed to determine progesterone concentrations in fresh fecal samples. ELISA tests for progesterone concentrations diminished the need for extensive laboratory facilities; however, few producers can justify the time to collect and process samples, and the complexity of these tests preclude their routine use on commercial farms. Rectal palpation is inexpensive, but offers few other advantages over a-mode or doppler instruments, and has not gained popularity in the U.S..

Presently, detection of nonconceiving sows that return to estrus and ultrasound are the most widely used techniques for pregnancy diagnosis. Despite routine use of these traditional methods, many sows either fail to farrow after being considered pregnant or return to estrus at irregular times during a presumed pregnancy. Success of a pregnancy detection program originates from the personnel implementing the program. The most promising technique is RTU; however, cost of the instrument and other factors might interfere with its widespread acceptance by commercial pig producers.

PROBLEMS AT FARROWING

Dystocia

Dystocia along with several other problems that can lead to difficult farrowing (e.g., downer sow) are relatively frequent in sows. Knowledge of the normal process of parturition is essential to determine when there is a need to intervene. Swelling of the vulval lips occurs about 4 days prepartum. The mammary glands become more turbid and tense during the last 2 days before farrowing, with the mammary secretion being serous 48 hours prior to parturition and becoming milky within 24 hours of farrowing. Restlessness and nesting behavior usually start in the 24 hours prefarrowing but recede in the last hour before the first piglet. Intermittent abdominal straining occurs before the birth of the first piglet, but straining is usually mild thereafter except at the moment of expulsion. Farrowing is expected within 20 minutes when a viscid, blood-tinged secretion often containing meconium is observed at the vulva. Duration of parturition is usually less than 3 hours but ranges from 30 minutes to more than 10 hours, with an interval between the birth of piglets averaging 15–20 minutes. Fetal membranes are expulsed in general 4 hours after the birth of the last piglet, from 20 minutes to $12^1/_2$ hours.

Signs of dystocia are anorexia, blood-tinged vulvar discharges, meconium without straining, straining without delivery of piglets, cessation of labor after straining, and the delivery of one or more piglets, exhaustion of the sow, and foul-smelling and discolored vulvar discharge. Primary uterine inertia associated with a decreased contractile activity of the myometrium is uncommon in sows, whereas secondary uterine inertia is much more frequent and results from uterine and maternal exhaustion associated with fetal malpresentation or maternal obstruction. The causes of dystocia are classified into two categories, maternal and fetal dystocia, depending on the origin. Arthur et al. (1989) have reported the following causes of dystocia: uterine inertia without significant cause (37%), breech presentation (14.5%), obstruction of the birth canal (13%), simultaneous presentation of two fetuses (10%), downward deviation of the uterus (9%), and oversized fetuses (4%). In modern sow herds, dystocia may also occur as a result of the use of prostaglandin and oxytocin to induce or control farrowing.

To correct dystocia, farm personnel must act in a timely fashion, since delayed or premature pharmacological or manual intervention may result in piglet death, decreased piglet viability, localized or systemic infections in the sow, or death of the sow. A 20% stillbirth rate is often associated with dystocia. To optimize the success of intervention, sows should be observed at 30-minute intervals once parturition has commenced. At each observation the number of piglets born and the time can be recorded to better assess the interval between the birth of piglets.

Correction of dystocia is achieved by manual examination of the vagina and cervix and removal of the obstruction or malpresented fetuses. Strict hygiene is required and the use of obstetrical gloves and lubricant is recommended. Manual extraction is usually the safest technique to extract fetuses. Caution must be exercised when using forceps, blunt hooks, or cable snares, due to the risk of trauma to the sow's reproductive tract. After removal of the malpresented pigs, the birth canal should be reexamined prior to the administration of oxytocin. High doses (>20 IU) of oxytocin may create a refractory period (3 hours) in which endogenous and exogenous oxytocin fails to stimulate contractions (Einarsson et al. 1975). Injectable antibiotics are warranted if sufficient contamination occurs. Intrauterine infusions of antibiotics or iodine solutions are usually not effective in promoting uterine involution or preventing uterine infections.

Injuries Incidental to Parturition

Hemorrhage may occur postpartum as a result of uterine, vaginal, or vulvar lacerations. Lacerations of the vagina and vulva can be sutured externally, whereas severe uterine lacerations or uterine ruptures are difficult to repair without conducting a laparotomy. The economics of this latter procedure must therefore be considered. Oxytocin treatment promotes uterine contractions and may be beneficial with minor uterine lacerations. Hematomas of the vulva are resolved as the blood and the fluid are resorbed; however, sharp projec-

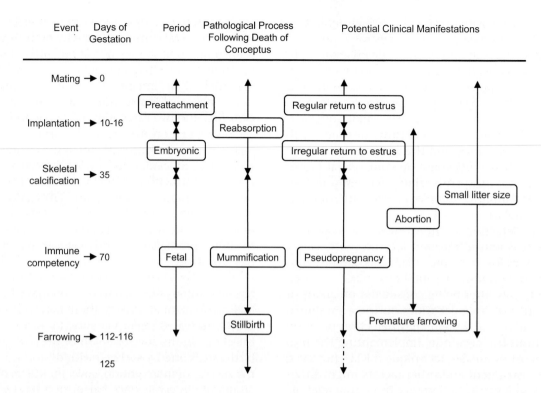

6.6. *Pathological reactions to disease agents according to the stage of reproductive cycle and the associated clinical manifestations.*

tions in farrowing crates increase the danger of lacerating the hematomas.

Vaginal and Uterine Prolapse

Prolapse is often seen shortly before, during or up to several days after farrowing. Factors that have been reported to increase the risk of vaginal or uterine prolapse in sows are genetics, housing, physical trauma to the genital tract following parturition, older parity, and nutrition. The procedures for correction of uterine prolapse are described in Chapter 70.

REPRODUCTIVE FAILURE

Pathological Processes

Diseases can exert their effect on the reproductive system through the general systemic effect on the dam or by infection of the conceptuses or the genital tract. The pathological reactions to disease agents depend on the type of agent and on the stage of reproductive cycle of the animal. The clinical manifestations will vary accordingly, as exemplified in Figure 6.6.

Death of the embryos before implantation, which occurs between 10 to 16 days postcoitus, results in reabsorption of conceptuses and a regular return to estrus for the sow. Four embryos are required at nidation for pregnancy to be initiated otherwise the sow will resume her cyclicity and a regular return to estrus will be observed (Dziuk 1985). Embryos are also reabsorbed when death occurs between 14 to 35 days of gestation. The sow will

have an irregular return to estrus if most of the conceptuses die or will farrow a small litter when only a proportion of embryos dies. The fetal period in swine begins at the onset of skeletal calcification at around 35 days of gestation and continues to parturition. Death of the fetus is followed by mummification or by stillbirth when it occurs in late gestation. Mummies are fetuses that have died in utero and have begun to decompose. Stillbirth results from the expulsion of dead fetus at an age when they could normally survive without undue assistance. Survival before day 109 of gestational age is limited because lung maturation has not been completed by this age. Stillborn pigs die either prepartum or intrapartum and are grossly normal at birth. In a large proportion of the deaths classified as intrapartum, the pigs were actually alive at birth. In true stillborn pigs, lungs will not float when immersed in water.

A combination of mummies and stillborn pigs of variable size is observed when fetuses die at different times of gestation. This is often the consequence of a progressive intrauterine spread of an infectious agent, such as porcine parvovirus. Sows with mummies and stillborn pigs may farrow at the expected time or experience pseudopregnancy when all conceptuses die if they fail to return to normal ovarian cyclicity due to the persistence of the pregnancy CL.

Abortion results from the termination of the pregnancy control mechanisms with subsequent expulsion of all conceptuses. Aborted sows return to estrus within 5–10 days or experience a prolonged anestrus. Abortion may occur from day 14 throughout gestation and is associated with maternal or embryonic/fetal failure. In abortion due to maternal failure fetuses are generally all of the same age. Fetal age beyond 35 days can be estimated using the crown-rump length in the following formula, where X is the crown-rump length in cm (Ullrey et al. 1965):

$$\text{Fetal age in days} = 21.07 + 3.11X$$

Premature farrowing is associated with a high proportion of stillborn and low viability piglets.

Failure to conceive or to initiate and maintain a pregnancy will be expressed as regular or irregular return to estrus, abortion, or pseudopregnancy, all of which may manifest as a lower farrowing rate at the herd level. The specific problems need to be characterized because influencing factors might be different accordingly. Thus it is essential to have an efficient pregnancy detection program to determine as quickly and accurately as possible the reproductive status of the sows.

Several etiologic agents have been associated with abortion, mummification, stillbirth, birth of weak piglets, and decreased farrowing rate.

Infectious Agents

Bacterial reproductive pathogens that can exert an effect on the reproductive tract of pigs include *Brucella suis*, *Leptospira* sp., and *Chlamydia* sp. Mummification is generally not a feature of reproductive bacterial diseases. *Brucella suis* is a primary agent causing abortion at any time of gestation and birth of weak piglets. Early abortions are probably a reflection of exposure via the genital tract at breeding. *Brucella suis* causes severe placentitis and genital infection.

Late-term abortions observed with several serovars of *Leptospira interrogans* result from transplacental infection of fetuses following leptospiremia. Aborted pigs are usually all of the same age although horizontal transmission in utero has been suggested (Fennestad and Borg-Petersen 1966). Some fetuses may be born alive but weak; others are stillborn. Gross lesions in aborted fetuses are usually nonspecific. Histological examination may reveal several spirochetes in the placenta and fetal tissues, namely kidneys. The pathogenesis of infection by *Leptospira* serovar *bratislava* seems to be different. This leptospire causes uterine infection and thus is associated with low conception rate and return to estrus. It is hypothesized that abortion caused by this pathogen is a consequence of transplacental infection by leptospires present in the genital tract rather than following leptospiremia (Ellis et al. 1986). Sow infertility is a common feature in infection by *Leptospira* serovar *bratislava* (Van Til and Dohoo 1991).

Although *Chlamydia* sp. have been associated with late-term abortion and birth of dead or weak pigs, clinically inapparent infection is much more common (Eggemann et al. 2000; Vanrompay et al. 2004).

The role of eperythrozoonosis (*Mycoplasma suis* or *haemosuis*) in reproductive disease is controversial. Some authors have reported anestrus, irregular estrous cycles, abortion, small litters, and stillbirth in seropositive herds (Sisk et al. 1980; Brownback 1981), whereas others did not observe any difference in reproductive parameters between infected and noninfected sows (Zinn et al. 1983).

Several other bacterial diseases—erysipelas, listeriosis, infection with *Actinobacillus pleuropneumoniae*, *Actinobacillus suis*, *Haemophilus parasuis*, and *Lawsonia intracellularis*—induce abortion either through the general effect of fever or by infecting the conceptus. Conceptuses are usually all of the same age and do not show significant lesions. Localized bacterial infection of the genital tract may also interfere with fertilization and viability of gametes, often resulting in regular return to estrus. Several bacterial species have been isolated from infected uteri (see section on vulvar discharge).

Porcine parvovirus is ubiquitous, and infection is enzootic in most swine herds. Outbreaks may occasionally be observed in newly populated herds with several naive animals. Parvovirus has a direct effect on the conceptus by damaging the placenta and a variety of tissues. Tranplacental infection occurs with further intrauterine spread of the virus. Porcine parvovirus infection is characterized by mummified fetuses of different ages, increased returns to estrus, and small litter size, but abortion is unlikely (Mengeling et al. 2000).

The porcine reproductive and respiratory syndrome (PRRS) virus causes abortion at any time of the gestation period, although transplacental infection was initially reported to occur more frequently in the last trimester, resulting in late-term abortions and premature farrowings. Despite lesions observed in the uterus, the precise mechanisms of abortion are still unclear. It may result from the effects of acute illness and fever and from infection of fetuses. It is also suggested that fetuses may die from hypoxia due to arteritis in the umbilical vessels (Lager and Halbur 1996). A combination of mummies, stillborn, and weak piglets is characteristic of PRRS virus infection. They usually occur sequentially within a herd according to the time of infection of the dams.

Exposure to pseudorabies virus during pregnancy may result in reproductive failure. The virus crosses the placenta and infects and kills embryos and fetuses. It also induces infection with lesions in uterus, placenta, and ovaries (Bolin et al. 1985). Lesions in fetuses are characterized by multiple necrotic foci in various tissues, including liver, spleen, lung, and tonsils.

Enteroviruses once were considered to be major causes of reproductive failure. They were attributed to the SMEDI syndrome (stillbirth, mummification, embryonic death, and infertility). Parvovirus had later been identified as the main etiologic agent for this syndrome.

The pathogenesis of reproductive failure following infection by encephalomyocarditis virus is not well understood. Transmission is believed to be transplacental, but pathogenic variability in fetuses has been observed with different isolates and could explain the variability of clinical signs (Kim et al. 1989).

More recently, porcine circovirus type 2, the etiologic agent of postweaning multisystemic wasting syndrome (PMWS), has been associated with late-term abortions and increased stillbirth rate (West et al. 1999).

Swine influenza virus causes abortion, stillbirth, and weak pigs at birth due to fever through a systemic effect on the dam (Vannier 1999). However, it has also been isolated from aborted fetuses, suggesting that the virus could cross the placenta and act as a specific agent causing reproductive problems. However, at present, data are inconsistent to conclude on transplacental infection (Yoon and Janke 2002).

Cytomegalovirus infection, responsible for inclusion body rhinitis, may also manifest itself in some herds as reproductive disorders with embryonic death, mummies of variable age, stillbirth, and weak pigs with high neonatal mortality (Orr et al. 1988). Other viral diseases associated with reproductive failure include blue eye disease, bovine viral diarrhea disease, border disease, transmissible gastroenteritis virus, Japanese B encephalitis, and African and classical swine fever. Abortion, although occurring occasionally, does not seem to be a common feature in blue eye disease, bovine viral diarrhea disease, and border disease (Stephano et al. 1988) and has not been observed with Japanese B encephalitis (Joo and Chu 1999). Reovirus has been isolated from mummies, stillbirths, and aborted fetuses but its role in swine reproductive disease is unclear (Paul and Stevenson 1999).

Menangle virus has been associated with return to estrus, pseudopregnancy, mummification, stillbirth, and congenital deformities but not with abortion (Love et al. 2001). This disease has been observed in only a large farrow-to-finish herd in Australia. The probable source of the infection was a colony of fruit bats that was near the farm. The reproductive problems observed were compatible with transplacental infection, with spreading from fetus to fetus as with porcine parvovirus. Nipah virus causes outbreaks of neurological and respiratory signs. This condition was first seen in late 1998 on several swine farms in Malaysia. Abortion was observed in some sows and was probably due to an acute febrile illness (Singh and Jamaluddin 2002).

Toxoplasma gondii may infect fetuses transplacentally and cause stillbirth and weak piglets at birth. Abortion is uncommon with toxoplasmosis. Abortion and mummies associated with fungal infections, namely *Aspergillus* sp., have been reported but are rare.

Noninfectious Factors

Compared to several other species, the CL in swine are essential for maintenance of pregnancy throughout gestation. Consequently the administration of $PGF_{2\alpha}$ dur-

ing gestation will cause pregnancy cessation with subsequent expulsion and death of the conceptuses. Abortion has been observed following procaine penicillin G injection in pregnant sows. It was hypothesized that the sudden release of toxic amounts of procaine was responsible for the clinical signs, such as fever, vomiting, and shivering (Embrechts 1982). Sows and gilts given feed containing sulfadimethoxine and ormetoprim late in gestation had increased duration of gestation and numbers of stillbirths and weak newborn pigs (Blackwell et al. 1989).

Consumption of grains containing the estrogenic mycotoxin, zearalenone, may result in irregular return to estrus, small litter size, and increased stillbirth rates. Estrogens are luteotropic in swine; therefore, zearalenone will induce anestrus and pseudopregnancy rather than abortion. In prepubertal gilts it will cause swelling of the vulva and prolapse. Fumonisin, a mycotoxin produced by fungi *Fusarium* sp., may produce pulmonary edema. Hence, sows consuming high levels of fumonisin will abort shortly after due to fetal anoxia. Sows fed ergot alkaloids during gestation had piglets with low birth weight and low survival rate, but rarely aborted.

The gestation length influences stillbirth; long gestational period (>117 days) and early induction of parturition (<112 days) are both associated with an increased number of stillborn pigs. Intrapartum deaths of piglets also increase with the duration of farrowing, litter size, and advanced parity of the sow.

High ambient temperature before implantation has been completed, i.e., before day 16, has a detrimental effect on conception rate and early embryonic survival. Also, elevated temperature during the peripartum period may lead to an increase in stillbirth and sow mortality. An increased prevalence of abortion is also observed in early fall and has been attributed to insufficient levels of progesterone and thin sows kept in cold environment. High levels of carbon monoxide in underventilated farrowing facilities may cause an increased stillbirth rate.

Diets deficient in vitamin A, zinc, copper, and iodine during gestation were all reported to increase the incidence of stillbirth.

VULVAR DISCHARGE

Individual cases of vulvar discharge rarely represent a major concern. In contrast, if 5–10% or more of a breeding group show discharges, the problem needs attention. Some vulvar discharges are indicative of normal physiological events, whereas others are pathological and may interfere with fertility and conception. Abnormal discharges originate from either the urinary or the reproductive tract. The diagnostic challenge is to differentiate normal from abnormal discharge and to determine the origin. In that, characterization of the type of discharge and its timing in relation to the estrous cycle will help (Dial and MacLachlan 1988a).

Normal Vulvar Discharges

It is normal to observe discharges following farrowing. They represent the sow's attempts to clear placental remnants and debris from the uterus and usually disappear within 2 days of farrowing. A mucopurulent vulvar discharge is also often seen in pregnant sows during the last 2–3 weeks of gestation. This discharge is associated with mucus production and cellular changes in the vulvovaginal membranes.

Periestrous discharges are considered normal. The high estrogen concentrations result in an increased uterine perfusion and tissue permeability and enhanced leukocyte migration into the uterus. The uterine contractions during proestrus and estrus contribute to physical clearance of uterine contents (De Winter et al. 1996). The discharges contain mucus, vaginal epithelial cells, semen, white blood cells, occasional red blood cells, or any combination of these cells. The quantity of these "normal" discharges is variable.

Abnormal Vulvar Discharges

The presence of fresh blood is common on the vulva of sows or gilts. Vulvar lacerations result from biting by sows (particularly in pen housing), trauma, or the boar. Careful hand-mating or AI procedures reduce the likelihood of breeding-inflicted vulvar lesions.

The presence of a purulent vulvar discharge at 14–20 days (>10 days) after breeding or estrus typically is indicative of metritis or endometritis. The causative agent or agents likely enter the uterus during estrus, either by passive ascension or by active introduction by the boar during mating. Nonspecific endometritis results from infection by bacteria not considered as specific pathogens of the reproductive tract. Several bacterial species have been isolated from these infected uteri, including *Escherichia coli, Streptococcus* sp., *Staphylococcus* sp., *Arcanobacterium pyogenes, Proteus, Klebsiella,* and a variety of others.

Sows inseminated late during estrus, often the third AI, are more susceptible to discharge problems (De Winter et al. 1992). During early metestrus, the protective mechanisms of high estrogen concentrations have dissipated, thereby rendering the animal susceptible to uterine infections. Furthermore, there is a strong correlation between serum progesterone concentrations and the development of endometritis (De Winter et al. 1996). If animals are inseminated as progesterone concentrations begin to increase after ovulation, there is a greater possibility of inducing endometritis. Therefore, some multiple-AI schemes may contribute to problems with endometritis.

Vulvar discharges are often seen in bred or virgin animals on farms with large numbers of replacement gilts, following a startup or repopulation (MacLachlan and Dial 1987). They may be observed after transport and prior to exposure to a boar. Some animals have normal physiological periestrous discharges; however, it is not uncommon to observe isolated cases of virgin animals with endometritis. The causes of discharges in virgin animals remain unclear. In some cases vaginitis is secondary to vulvar biting in the finishing house. Another theory is that many gilts attain puberty prior to transport, and infection of the uterus occurs while the animals are in gilt finishing facilities. Consequently, a discharge is observed 5–8 days prior to their second estrus.

Endometritis also occurs following parturition as a result of dystocia, traumatic injury, abortion, and unhygienic manipulations. The likelihood of subsequent infertility is greater in sows that have a prolonged vulvar discharge following parturition, e.g., more than 6 days (Waller et al. 2002). Pyometra, an acute or chronic suppurative inflammation of the uterus with accumulation of large quantities of pus, is rare in sows.

A purulent vulvar discharge with or without blood may be observed in cases of cystitis/pyelonephritis and should be differentiated from that originating from the genital tract. The discharge usually contains mucus, is associated with urination, especially at the end of the stream, and is not related to the estrous cycle. To confirm urinary tract infections, urinalyses are performed on samples from affected animals, or collection and examination of urinary bladders and kidneys are performed at slaughter. For further details see Chapter 9.

Managing the Discharging Sow

Most discharging sows return to estrus shortly after the initial appearance of the discharge. Attempts to breed these animals at this time are usually futile. One approach is to allow the animals to recycle one more time, if economics and animal flow permit it. Clinical reports have revealed that when sows failed to discharge a second time and were then mated, their conception rates were similar to those of repeat breeders. The other option is to cull any animal with a discharge. Hygiene and management procedures around farrowing, mating, and artificial insemination should be evaluated.

Numerous treatment protocols have been attempted to resolve problems of discharging sows, but their success remains dubious. Medicated feed or injectable antibiotics are common treatments. Precise pathogens involved and their sensitivity to antibiotics are rarely known, so it is often difficult to assess the effectiveness of these treatments (Dial and MacLachlan 1988b).

Some producers infuse the boar's prepuce with extralabel, antibiotic preparations, and systemic antibiotic treatment has been attempted; however, it is unknown whether effective antibiotic concentrations are achieved in the boar's reproductive tract. The prepuce of a boar is rapidly reinfected, and thus, infusion of the prepuce offers only short-term therapy.

OVARIAN CYSTS

Slaughterhouse surveys have demonstrated that 5–10% of sows culled for reproductive problems are affected with cystic ovaries, varying from 1.7–24% (Ryan and Raeside 1991). On several farms on which ultrasonography was used, the incidence of ovarian cysts varied from 0–8% among nonpregnant animals (Gherpelli and Tarocco 1996; Castagna et al. 2004). Multiple large, multiple small, and single cysts occur in the ovaries of sows. They vary in size, from 1–8 cm, and in the extent of luteinization, and may regress spontaneously (Figure 6.7) (Ebbert and Bostedt 1993; Ebbert et al. 1993; Gherpelli and Tarocco 1996; Martinat-Botté et al. 1998). Luteinized cysts are more frequently observed than follicular cysts (Zannoni et al. 2003). In general, sows with ovarian cysts have a greater return to estrus rate than normal sows, 34% vs. 7.7% (Castagna et al. 2004). However, the behavioral and physiological events differ between animals affected with each type of cyst. Most of the multiple large cysts have some luteinized tissue and produce sufficient progesterone to inhibit estrous cyclicity; consequently, such affected sows may be intermittently or permanently anestrous. In contrast, multiple small cysts often produce estrogen, and sows may have irregular estrous cycles or exhibit nymphomania. Anestrus is more frequently observed in sows with a large number of cysts (>10/animal) compared to those with a smaller number, 75% vs. 53% (Ebbert and Bostedt 1993). Single ovarian cysts rarely affect fertility or the estrous cycle of sows.

An impairment or relative deficiency of the preovulatory LH surge is responsible for the failure of ovulation of one or more follicles at estrus, which leads to cystic ovary. Increased incidences of ovarian cysts have been associated with stress, zearalenone toxicity, or corticosteroid and hormonal treatment administered over an extended period, or at an improper phase of the reproductive cycle (Guthrie and Polge 1976; Meredith 1979; Varley 1991; Gherpelli and Tarocco 1996). Sows with cystic ovaries are more frequently observed when lactation length is shorter than 14 days and weaning-to-estrus interval shorter than 3 days (Castagna et al. 2004).

The diagnosis of cystic ovaries generally relies on ultrasonography (Martinat-Botté et al. 1998; Kauffold et al. 2004). Because serum concentrations of progesterone, estradiol, LH, and cortisol are similar in sows affected with ovarian cysts and in diestrous sows, serum hormone concentrations have limited diagnostic value (Almond and Richards 1991).

CONGENITAL DEFECTS AND NEOPLASIA

Defects of the female genital system are common and include cysts of the mesosalpinx; duplication of the vagina; cervix or uterine horns; segmental or complete

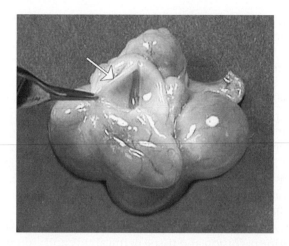

6.7. *Porcine cystic ovary. The cystic structures are fluid filled. The thickened cyst walls (arrow) contain luteinized tissue. The sow failed to exhibit estrus.*

aplasia of the uterus, cervix, vagina, and vulva; and intersexuality. The aplasias, hypoplasias, and duplications appear to have genetic components that can be expressed in varying degrees in different individuals (Wrathall 1975) and may contribute to infertility and perhaps dystocia. Other defects of the female genital system include persistence of the hymen, ovarian aplasia, other ovarian defects, and hypoplasia or malformation of the nipples (Done 1980; Clayton et al. 1981). The incidence of these conditions is low, and in most instances the cause is unknown or suspected to be heritable.

Intersexuality is occasionally observed in pigs. True intersexes, or hermaphrodites, have both testicular and ovarian tissues, whereas pseudohermaphrodites have gonads of one sex and other genital organs of the opposite sex. Pseudohermaphrodites are further subclassified into male or female on the basis of the gonadal tissue. The external genitalia of intersex pigs are usually female in type. In most instances the vulva appears normal, with a variable enlargement of the clitoris, but in some the clitoris is greatly enlarged and the vulva is underdeveloped or prepucelike. Some affected individuals show male behavior, while others show estrus and even become pregnant (Hulland 1964; O'Reilly 1979). Estrus, ovulation, and pregnancy are possible in true hermaphrodites. Reports of female pseudohermaphrodites in pigs are rare. Genetic analyses suggest that pig intersexuality is controlled multigenically.

Neoplasms of the genitalia in sows have not been studied intensively. Investigations of genital tracts at slaughter reveal a low prevalence of neoplasis. The most commonly observed neoplasms were leiomyoma, fibroma, cyst-adenoma, fibroleiomyoma, and carcinoma (Anderson and Sandison 1969; Werdin and Wold 1976; Akkermans and van Beusekom 1984).

INADEQUATE REPRODUCTIVE PERFORMANCE

Reproduction is an extremely complex process and involves many highly specific biological functions. Many factors—such as diet, housing, social surroundings, temperature, disease, and management—influence reproductive performances (Foxcroft and Aherne 2002). There are five major causes of reproductive failure: hormonal imbalances, mating behavior, diseases, structural defects, and management (Leif and Thomson 2002).

Because many of the elements involved in reproduction are interrelated, one problem may give rise to others. Generally by studying records and carrying out clinical observations and pathological tests it is possible to determine precisely where reproductive failure has occurred (Dial 1990). Such failures can be grouped into six categories related to stages in the reproductive cycle: anestrus, estrus and ova production, fertilization, implantation, and maturation. In general, the primary causes of reproductive failure can be identified and corrected; however, the causes of infertility cannot be determined and corrective action taken without collecting reliable information and using it in a meaningful way (Muirhead and Alexander 1997). This information allows us to understand the interrelationships of reproductive failure as related to nonreproductive factors that evade females to express their biological potential.

Definition of Most Commonly Used Parameters of Performance

During the last 15 years, the financial advantage of volume selling and buying has led to an irreversible evolution toward increasingly larger herd sizes. In a climate of increased competition for more discerning markets, the independent producer has been faced with the challenge of either becoming efficient or running the risk of no longer being competitive and no longer having a product desired by the global marketplace. A necessary prelude to being competitive in swine production in general, and in particular in the reproductive area, is a reliable record system that allows producers to monitor both biological and financial performance and to troubleshoot production and financial problems (Dial 1990).

In order to understand and interpret records it is important to have universally accepted definitions for an analyzed parameter so the calculations involved in its computation can be understood. The following is a list of the most common parameters used when troubleshooting reproductive performance:

Adjusted farrowing rate: 100 × total number of females farrowed ÷ (total number of females bred − total number of females removed due to nonreproductive causes) in a specified period of time.

Average parity: average parity of all the females in the breeding herd, including gilts that are part of the inventory.

Conception rate: 100 × (total number of females that conceived between 18–24 days after the first mating ÷ total number of bred females) in a specified period of time.

Farrowing interval: the period of time between two consecutive farrowings of a specified female. On a herd basis this term is the average of the farrowing intervals of a specified group of females in a specific period of time.

Farrowing rate: 100 × (total number of females farrowed ÷ total number of females bred) in a specified period of time.

Gilt pool: group of females that have not been mated but are considered as replacements for the breeding herd.

Irregular return to estrus: the irregular occurrence of estrus from one period to the next. An interestrus interval of more than 24 days.

Litters/crate/year: total number of litters weaned in a year ÷ total number of crates in the farrowing area.

Litters/productive sow/year: average number of litters that a productive female farrows in a year.

Litters/sow/year: average number of litters that a female in inventory farrows in a year when nonproductive days are taken into account.

$$\frac{365 \text{ days} - \text{average nonproductive days/female/year}}{(\text{gestation} + \text{lactation length in days})}$$

Mummies: fetal tissues after bodily fluids have been removed and only the nonabsorbable remains, including calcified skeleton. Mummification normally occurs after 35 days of gestation.

Nonproductive days: number of days when a female is not gestating or lactating. In economical terms nonproductive days include all the days that a female is generating expenses and not income.

Percent repeats: number of females included in a group that have returned to estrus after having been mated.

Pigs/crate/year: number of pigs weaned in a year ÷ total number of crates in the farrowing area.

Pigs weaned/sow/year: total number of pigs that a female in inventory weans in a year.

Regular return to estrus: interestrus interval of 18–24 days.

Stillborn pigs: pigs that die shortly before or during farrowing.

Total number of pigs/litter: Total number of pigs born alive + total number of stillborn pigs + total number of mummies in a litter.

Wean to estrus interval: interval between a weaning and the following estrus.

Targets

Numerous systems are currently available commercially for assessing the biological performance of the breeding herd. Although varying considerably in data entry, report format, and report content, all of the systems provide summaries of breeding, farrowing, and weaning information (Dial 1990). Most provide either time-related or group reports for information relating to fertility, lactation performance, interval from entry or weaning to mating, and piglet survival until weaning. Targets and level at which a corrective intervention should be performed (interference levels) should be included in these production reports (Table 6.2). The value of these parameters should be changed regularly as the herd performances change.

Interrelationships Between Performance Parameters

There are numerous risk factors or differential diagnoses for the different types of reproductive failure. Many can be incriminated or ruled out through examination of records. In fact, although a diagnostic examination of environment, facilities, management, disease status, and nutrition may suggest one or several of them as a cause of reproductive failure, the diagnosis typically must be corroborated through the record analysis. For example, suboptimal total pigs born/litter may involve parity distribution, lactation length, weaning-to-estrus interval, season and ambient temperature, systemic reproductive disease, genetics, nutrition, and breeding management. Both record analysis and flow diagrams are extremely helpful to identify risk factors and explanation of reduced reproductive performance.

Pigs Weaned/Sow/Year. When the productivity of the breeding herd is suboptimal the most widely used measure of the overall biological performance of the breeding herd is pigs weaned/sow/year (Polson et al. 1990a). The two components of pigs weaned/sow/year are litters farrowed/inventoried sow/year and pigs weaned/litter farrowed (Figure 6.8).

Table 6.2. Targets for the reproductive performance of the breeding herd

	Target	Interference Level
Breeding and Gestation		
Age at first service (days of age)	220–240	<220 or >260
Repeat matings (%)	10	>15
Multiple matings (%)	90	<85
Weaning to service interval (days)	4–7	>7
Farrowing rate (%)	≥85	<80%
Regular returns (%)	<6	>8
Irregular returns (%)	<3	>5
Negative pregnancy test (%)	<3	>5
Abortions (%)	<2	>4
Failure to farrow (%)	<1	>3
Adjusted farrowing rate (%)	≥90	≤88
Farrowing		
Total pigs born/litter	≥11.5	<11
Pigs born alive/litter	≥10.5	<10
% stillbirths	<7	>10
% mummies	<3	>5
Litters/productive sow/year	>2.4	<2.3
Litters/sow/year	>2.2	<2.1
Weaning		
Pigs weaned/sow	≥10	≤9.8
Preweaning mortality (%)	<8	>10
Weaning weight at 21 days (kg)	5.5–6.5	<5.0
Pigs weaned/productive sow/year	>24	<23
Pigs weaned/sow/year	>22	<21
Litters/crate/year (3.5-week cycle)	>14.8	<14
Pigs/crate/year	>148	<137
Population (on an annual basis)		
Average parity	3.5	<3 and >4
Replacement rate (%)	≤40	<35 and >45
Culling rate (%)	30–35	<28 and >40
Mortality rate (%)	5–8	>10
Average non productive days (60 day acclimatization period)	≤75	>80

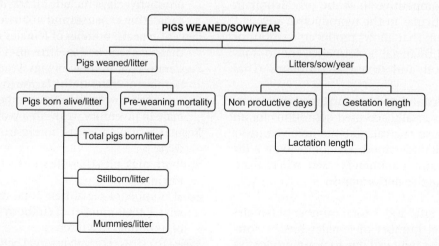

6.8. *Factors related to pigs weaned/sow/year.*

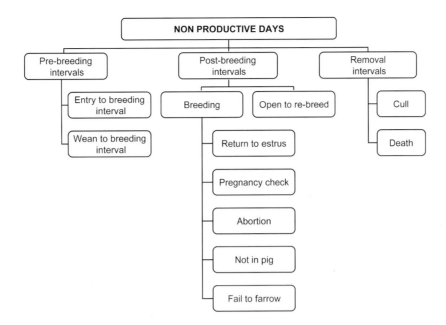

6.9. *Interrelationship between factors influencing nonproductive days.*

The interrelationship between pigs weaned/sow/year shows that litters/female/year greatly influences this interrelationship; however gestation and lactation length cannot be easily reduced or influenced. Therefore improvements in nonproductive days will by far increase pigs weaned/sow/year (Polson et al. 1990b).

Nonproductive Days. Nonproductive days and lactation length are the major factors influencing litters/sow/year. Nonproductive days are influenced largely by time from introduction into the herd or weaning until first mating; time from mating until detection of nonpregnancy status; and time from mating, entry, or weaning until female is culled or dies. Nonproductive days not only must be calculated, but also must be broken down into its different components (Figure 6.9). The risk factors for those elements also must be detailed. Nonproductive days often go unrecognized; however, they are very significant in reducing the productivity of the breeding herd.

Data analysis shows that, in general, the interval from introduction to mating and the interval between the time a female is detected nonpregnant and remating are the most biologically meaningful components of nonproductive days. In order to understand the impact of nonproductive days on the breeding herd performance we can equate 1 nonproductive day to 0.05 pig/sow/year (20 pigs weaned per female per year/365 days). Consequently a decrease of 10 nonproductive days will result in at least 0.5 extra pig/sow/year.

Entry to First Mating Interval. Improved gilt pool management is required to ensure that availability of gilts for service does not limit the ability of herds to achieve their breeding targets. Generally the problem is solved by introducing two or three times as many gilts as required. Gilts must be acclimatized before entering into a herd. This acclimatization allows the gilts to adjust to feed, housing, and management system. Most importantly, it helps to prevent new diseases from entering the recipient herd and to establish procedures that result in a common immune status between the incoming pigs and the receiving herd, without creating infection that perturbs the balance of infectious agents in the receptor herd (Batista 2000). Since the emergence of PRRS, the number of gilts introduced and the period of acclimatization, in general, have increased (Batista et al. 2002). This increase, both in days and inventory, has negatively affected nonproductive days, therefore decreasing the output of the breeding herd. Gilt acclimatization is divided into three periods, as shown in Figure 6.10.

The component that influences this interrelationship the least is isolation. In general a period of 21–30 days is advised (Kuster et al. 2000). Today many different methods of gilt acclimatization are recommended—i.e., introduction of gilts at 5, 30, or 60 kg, followed by a period of time that can range between 4–10 weeks following exposure to different pathogens and or vaccination programs (Batista et al. 2002). Therefore, acclimatization is the most significant component of nonproductive days in the entry to service interval. Finally, the entry to service interval is negatively influenced by delayed puberty. Presently, the relationship between growth performance and age at puberty is well understood. In gilts exposed to boar stimulation from 140 days of age, the minimum age at puberty was around 160 days; this could be achieved at body weights of around 90 kg if gilts were fed appropriately (Beltranena et al.

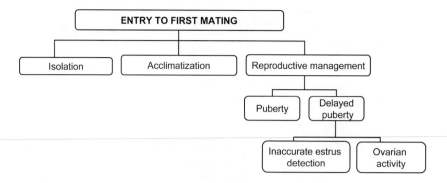

6.10. Components of interval from entry to first mating and its impact on nonproductive days.

1991). Therefore management of the gilt pool plays a very important role in the decrease of nonproductive days in this area.

Farrowing Rate. The factors that cause a sow to fail to conceive are often different than those causing a sow to fail to maintain pregnancy. For example, the number of matings per estrous period affects conception but not pregnancy; in comparison, season primarily influences the capacity of the sow to maintain pregnancy. In order to troubleshoot fertility problems we need to determine whether the returns are regular or irregular. The interrelationship between the different factors affecting farrowing rate are shown in Figure 6.11.

Litter Size. In general, many of the factors influencing fertility have similar effects on total pigs born/litter. Therefore, improvements in fertility appear to be related to an increase in fecundity. When litter size is compromised it is important to review several factors. Classical examples of these interrelationships are litter size by parity, the effect of season and temperature at service

and prior to implantation, the influence of matings per estrous period and timing of matings relative to onset of estrus, the relationship between lactation feed intake and subsequent litter size, etc. (Dial et al. 1992). The main causes for a reduced litter size are presented in Figure 6.12.

Wean to Estrus Interval. Variability in the wean to estrus interval (WEI) is a major problem in the breeding herd management. Delays of the onset of estrus increase nonproductive days. Variation in WEI makes it difficult to meet breeding targets and to concentrate breeding management. Data show that WEI increased rapidly as lactation length was reduced below 17 days, but WEI was relatively unaffected by lactation lengths of 17 to 30 days (Xue et al. 1993). These data also emphasized that the percentage of sows bred by 6 days after weaning was significantly reduced for lactation lengths of 20 days or less. However, ovulation rate and fertilization rate did not appear to be affected by lactation length (Varley 1982). An inadequate nutrient and energy intake will also result in extended wean to estrus interval, lower

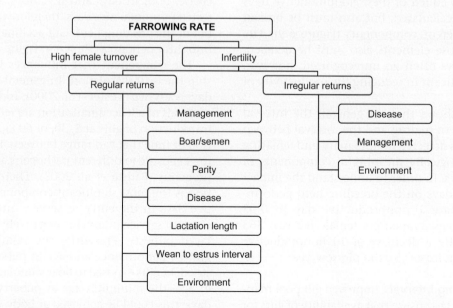

6.11. Interrelationship between the different factors affecting farrowing rate.

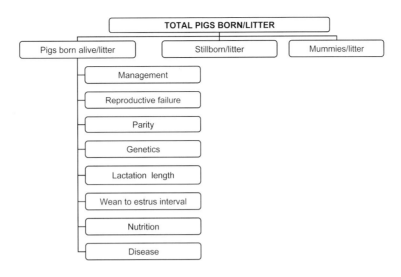

6.12. *Interrelationship between the different factors affecting total pigs born/litter.*

percentage of sows in estrus within 7 days of weaning, reduced pregnancy rate, and reduced embryo survival (Aherne et al. 1999; Quesnel et al. 1998). The factors that affect the extent of WEI are shown in Figure 6.13.

In conclusion, troubleshooting suboptimal reproductive performance requires a structured record analysis in conjunction with the use of flow diagrams that indicate the different factors and their level of importance in contributing to suboptimal reproductive performance. An organized system is less time-consuming, more inclusive, and efficient. This system should also allow validatation of progress and assessment of response to management changes in order to obtain maximal reproductive efficiency of the breeding herd.

REPRODUCTIVE DEVELOPMENT, ANATOMY, AND FUNCTION IN THE BOAR

Development of the male reproductive tract commonly is divided into three distinct periods: early fetal, perinatal, and pubertal. The onset of the early fetal period be-

gins around day 20 postcoitum (PC) with formation of the testicles and ends around day 90 of gestation with the descent of the testicles into the scrotum. The perinatal period encompasses the period of time from just prior to birth through the first month of life. This developmental period is characterized by an increase in the testis-to-body-weight ratio due to Leydig cell differentiation and proliferation. It also has been hypothesized that a large portion of the basis for future spermatogenic capacity of boars is established during this time due to the increased mitotic activity of Sertoli cells characteristic of this developmental phase. The pubertal period begins at around 30 days of age and continues until the boar has reached sexual maturity. During this final stage of maturation, endocrine and cellular aspects characteristic of adult spermatogenesis develop. Mechanisms involved in the development of male reproductive anatomy and function involve complex interactions among the endocrine, neural, and paracrine systems (Colenbrander et al. 1982b). A chronological outline of several key developmental events is presented in Table 6.3.

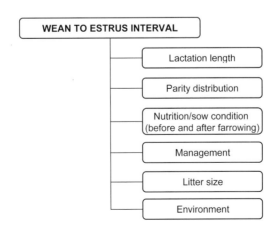

6.13. *Interrelationship between the different factors affecting wean to estrus interval.*

Table 6.3. Summary of key developmental events during sexual maturation of boars.

Period	Time[1]	Event
Early Fetal	21 DPC	Indifferent gonad is present
	26 DPC	Testicular differentiation; primordial germ cell in cords
	27 DPC	Germ cells surrounded by Sertoli cells
	26–35 DPC	Testosterone production begins
	26–50 DPC	Wolffian duct and anlage differentiation; development of secondary sex glands and external genitalia
	30–38 DPC	Leydig cell differentiation andproliferation
	42 DPC	Mitotic activity of Sertoli cells increases
	60–85 DPC	Descent of testes into inguinal canal begins
Perinatal	90 DPC	Sertoli cell tubular length increases
	90 DPC to birth	LH, FSH, and prolactin concentrations increase
	95 DPC to 21 d	Germ cell numbers increase; gonocyte morphology characterized by regular, round shape with centrally located nucleus
	Birth	Testicles completely descended into scrotum
	Birth to 14 d	Testosterone production increases
	Birth to 21 d	Leydig cell differentiation; Leydig cells compose 65% of testicle volume at 3 weeks of age
Pubertal	30 d	Sertoli cell proliferation decreases
	42 d	Sertoli cell junctions appear
	70 d	Germ cell differentiation begins
	91 d	Spermatogonia and pachytene spermatocytes are present and sometimes round spermatids can be seen
	100–120 d	Blood-testis barrier is present
	120 d	Leydig cell development is maximal
	160–180 d	Puberty in most breeds

[1]DPC = days postcoitum; d = days after birth.

Adult Reproductive Function

Hypothalamus and Pituitary Gland. The brain is the component of the male reproductive system that gathers internal signals from within the body and external cues from the environment, integrates them, and regulates physiological and behavioral functions associated with reproduction. The hypothalamus secretes GnRH, which controls the production and secretion of LH and FSH from the pituitary gland. These two hormones are responsible for regulating testicular function (Hafs and McCarthy 1978).

Testes. The primary functions of the testes are to produce spermatozoa and hormones. The majority of the testicular mass is composed of seminiferous tubules, the convoluted network of ducts in which spermatozoa are produced. Sertoli cells, specialized cells involved in the maturation of spermatozoa and hormone production, line the lumen of the seminiferous tubules (Ashdown and Hafez 1993). Leydig cells, blood and lymph vessels, and nerves are located in interstitial spaces between the seminiferous tubules. Important interactions between the Sertoli and Leydig cells regulate virtually every aspect of male reproductive function.

The rete testis comprises a series of tubules that leave the seminiferous tubules and connect to form collecting ducts located in the center of each testis. During spermatogenesis, spermatozoa leave the seminiferous tubules and enter the rete testis during their passage into the epididymis. The rete testis is lined with a nonsecretory epithelium (Hargrove et al. 1977).

Because the testes are located externally, special anatomical systems are needed for effective thermoregulation. The most important component for thermoregulation is the pampiniform plexus, a complex vascular arrangement of testicular arteries and veins in the spermatic cord. The testicular artery forms a convoluted structure in the shape of a cone in which arterial coils are enmeshed with testicular veins. From a functional perspective, this countercurrent heat-exchange mechanism enables arterial blood entering the testis to be cooled by venous blood exiting the testis. In most species, the temperature of arterial blood drops between 2°C and 4°C prior to its entry into the testes (Ashdown and Hafez 1993).

Two groups of muscles, the tunica dartos and cremaster, play an important role in thermoregulation. The tunica dartos lines the inside of the scrotum and controls its proximity to the testis. It contracts during cold weather, pulling the scrotal sac closer to the testis for added insulation, and relaxes during warm weather, allowing the scrotum to recoil into a distal position. The cremaster muscle is located in the spermatic cord and is attached to the thick membranous sac surrounding the testis. It contracts during cold weather, pulling the scrotal sac and testis closer to the body core, and relaxes during warm conditions, allowing the testis to return to its normal position (Robertshaw and Vercoe 1980). Both muscles have an abundant supply of adrenergic neural fibers that respond to temperature sensors located in the central nervous system. In the boar, due to the anatomical relationship between the testis and the body core, the tunica dartos is more important than the cremaster muscle in the regulation of testicular temperature.

Endocrine Activity within the Testes. Leydig cells located in the testicular interstitium and Sertoli cells within the seminiferous tubules are the two primary endocrine-producing cells in the testes. LH released from the anterior pituitary gland stimulates production of androgens from the Leydig cells. The primary androgen produced is testosterone. Testosterone has a variety of important functions in spermatogenesis and male sexual behavior. FSH stimulates the Sertoli cells to produce androgen-binding proteins, convert testosterone to dihydrotestosterone and estrogen, and secrete inhibin (Bartke et al. 1978). Androgen-binding protein forms a complex with androgen and is carried along with the spermatozoa to the epididymis. High local levels of androgen are necessary for the normal function of the epididymal epithelium (Hansson et al. 1976). Inhibin diffuses out of the seminiferous tubules, enters the vascular system, and is transported to the brain, where it has a negative effect on the secretion of FSH. Inhibin production by the testes is an important component of gonadotropin regulation in the male.

In the boar, high quantities of estrogen are found in semen. The source of these estrogens is the Sertoli cells, which convert testosterone to estrogen via the aromatase enzyme. It appears that the primary role of seminal estrogens is to stimulate important reproductive events in the female reproductive tract during breeding (Claus 1990).

Recent investigations have demonstrated that both Sertoli and Leydig cells have receptors for a variety of growth factors, including insulin-like growth factor I (IGF-I), epidermal growth factor (EGF), and transforming growth factor(s) (TGF) (Sharpe 1994). It has been proposed that growth factors may be produced in response to gonadotropin or growth hormone action on testicular tissue and mediate many of the actions of these hormones. In addition, growth factors are believed to be the primary mode in which Sertoli cells and developing spermatozoa regulate each other's secretion of proteins along the length of the seminiferous tubule.

Epididymis. The rete testis enters the efferent ducts, which eventually form a single coiled duct called the epididymis. The epididymis is similar to the seminiferous tubules in that it coils back upon itself many times and forms three distinct sections: the caput (head), corpus (body), and cauda (tail). The convoluted duct of the epididymis is surrounded by a prominent layer of circular muscle fibers and contains pseudostratified columnar, stereociliated epithelium. Masses of spermatozoa are commonly found along the entire lumen of the epididymis (Hemeida et al. 1978).

The primary function of the epididymis is sperm maturation, transport, and storage. Spermatozoa entering the epididymis are neither motile nor fertile. It takes spermatozoa between 9 and 14 days to migrate from the caput to the cauda epididymis, the primary storage site. It has been estimated that the cauda epididymis contains about 75% of the total epididymal spermatozoa (Swierstra 1968). Spermatozoa become motile and acquire fertilizational competence in the corpus epididymis due to the secretion of factors by the cells located in this region. Movement of spermatozoa through the epididymis is thought to be due to the flow of rete fluid, the action of the stereociliated epithelium, and contractions of the circular muscle layer.

Unejaculated spermatozoa are gradually eliminated by excretion into the urine. Spermatozoa that are not excreted in the urine undergo a gradual aging process. Fertilizational competence is lost first and is followed shortly by a decline in motility. The culmination of dying spermatozoa is disintegration (Garner and Hafez 1993). This is the primary reason that ejaculates collected after prolonged sexual rest usually contain a large number of degenerative spermatozoa.

Vas Deferens, Accessory Sex Glands, and Penile Urethra. The remainder of the boar's reproductive tract is relatively nonfunctional until ejaculation is initiated. The vas deferens is a thick, heavily muscled tube through which sperm are transported from the cauda epididymis to the pelvic urethra, at which point the paired genital systems of the boar meet and converge with the urinary tract just anterior to the bladder. Adjacent to the pelvic urethra are three secondary sex glands: the vesicular glands, or seminal vesicles; the prostate gland; and the bulbourethral glands.

The vesicular glands lie lateral to the terminal portion of each vas deferens. In the boar, they are large, lobulated, and relatively diffuse. They often appear to have an orange color. They are responsible for the majority of the fluid volume of boar semen. In addition, they secrete high levels of fructose and citric acid as well as inositol, ergothioneine, several amino acids, and glycerylphosphorylcholine. Most of these compounds are used as energy substrates by ejaculated spermatozoa.

The prostate gland is located cranial to the vesicular glands, with the majority of its body being embedded in the muscle layer surrounding the pelvic urethra. Secretions from the prostate gland during ejaculation are primarily alkaline and contain calcium, acid phosphatase, and fibrinolysin. The primary function of the fluid from the prostate gland is to neutralize the acidic vaginal secretions. Secretions from the prostate gland also are believed to give semen its characteristic odor.

The bulbourethral glands are long, cylindrical glands in the boar located on either side of the pelvic urethra near the ischial arch of the pelvis. The bulbourethral glands secrete the gel fraction of the semen characteristic of porcine ejaculates. Many functions for the gel component of semen have been postulated, but few have been proven.

The terminal portion of the boar's urogenital system is the penile urethra, which is the central tube within the penis. The penile urethra opens into the glans penis. In the boar, the glans penis has a counterclockwise spiral. The glans penis is highly innervated and must be stimulated properly for normal ejaculation to occur. The porcine penis also contains three cavernous bodies, or sinuses, that surround the penile urethra (Ashdown et al. 1981). During erection, blood is pumped into and retained in these areas. In the resting state, the porcine penis is retracted and forms a characteristic "S" fold called the sigmoid flexure.

The free end of the penis in the retracted state resides in the prepuce or sheath. In young prepubertal boars, the glans penis cannot be extended fully because it is fused with the lining of the prepuce. As a boar matures, androgens produced by the testis initiate keratinization of the inner preputial lining, and the penis is eventually freed from its connection with the prepuce. Persistent frenulum is a condition in which strands of tissue do not keratinize fully and are still attached to the penis. When this occurs, the end of the penis curves back toward the prepuce during erection and ejaculation. Removal of these strands of tissue with a pair of sterile scissors corrects this situation.

Near the end of the prepuce is a diverticulum called the preputial sac. Urine, semen, and secreted fluid collect in this sac and are broken down via bacterial action. The contents of the preputial sac are often expelled during detection of estrus or natural matings and are often believed to be the source of the odor associated with mature boars (Ashdown and Hafez 1993).

Erection and Ejaculation

Sexual stimulation results in dilation of the arteries supplying the cavernous penile areas. It has been postulated that parasympathetic fibers originating from the pelvic nerve are responsible for providing the neural signal for dilation and thus the initiation of erection. At the same time vasodilation begins, the ischiocavernosus muscle begins to contract repeatedly, which causes blood to be pumped into the cavernous spaces in the body of the penis. In the boar, no veins drain the distal portion of these spaces, which facilitates the increase in pressure within the penile body and erection. As pressure increases from blood trapped in the cavernous tissue, the retractor penis muscle relaxes, allowing the sigmoid flexure to straighten and the penis to protrude from the sheath (Benson 1994). Several detailed studies demonstrate that erection failures in boars are caused primarily by structural defects rather than psychological problems (Glossop and Ashdown 1986).

Ejaculation is primarily under neural control and involves contractions of smooth muscles. The process is initiated by rhythmic contractions of smooth muscles lining the cauda epididymis and ductus deferens. These contractions are controlled by sympathetic nerves that arise from the pelvic plexis, which is derived from the hypogastric nerve. During ejaculation, the bulbospongiosus muscle compresses the penile bulb and forces blood into the remainder of the cavernous tissue, resulting in a slight enlargement of the glans penis in boars (Setchell et al. 1993).

Spermatogenesis

Spermatogenesis is divided into two basic processes: spermatocytogenesis and spermiogenesis. In a general sense, spermatocytogenesis is the process involved with the mitotic and meiotic divisions of sperm cells, while spermiogenesis refers to the maturational phase of development. Although both hormones are important, it is believed that LH plays a more active role than FSH in spermatocytogenesis, while FSH is the main gonadotropic hormone involved with spermiogenesis (Garner and Hafez 1993).

Spermatocytogenesis. Just prior to puberty in boars, undifferentiated germ cells called gonocytes differentiate to form type A0 spermatogonia. These are the precursor sperm cells from which all other sperm cells originate. There is some evidence that the number of A0 spermatogonia is directly related to the sperm production capacity of males. In adult boars, A0 spermatogonia differentiate into A1 spermatogonia, which divide progressively to form various types of immature sperm cells. The final mitotic division during spermatocytogenesis occurs in primary spermatocytes. Although the average number of mitotic divisions cells undergo between the A1 and primary spermatocyte stages is a subject of some controversy, a figure of 6–8 is commonly used. After the formation of primary spermatocytes, no new DNA synthesis occurs, and the resulting secondary spermatocytes divide to form haploid cells known as spermatids. The entire divisional process of spermatocytogenesis occurs in the testis. It is interesting to note that many of the divisions are actually incomplete in that small cytoplasmic bridges are retained between most cells originating from a common type A1 spermatogonium. Some researchers speculate that these bridges are important in coordinating development of sperm cells as a group (Swierstra 1968).

Spermiogenesis and Spermiation. The round spermatids are transformed into spermatozoa by a series of morphological changes referred to as spermiogenesis. Maturational changes that spermatozoa undergo during spermiogenesis include condensation of nuclear material, formation of the sperm tail, and development of the acrosomal cap and its contents. During most of spermiogenesis, the sperm cells appear to have their heads embedded in Sertoli cells. In reality, the membrane of the Sertoli cell actually is wrapped around the sperm head. Communication and exchange of materials between the Sertoli and developing sperm cells occur via intercellular bridges.

The actual release of spermatozoa into the lumen of the seminiferous tubule is called spermiation. The elongated spermatids are gradually extruded or pushed out of the Sertoli cells into the lumen of the seminiferous tubule until only a small cytoplasmic stalk connects the head of the sperm to the residual body in the Sertoli cell. Breakage of the stalk results in the formation of a cytoplasmic droplet in the neck region of the sperm. These commonly are referred to as proximal cytoplasmic droplets (Garner and Hafez 1993).

Epididymal Maturation. Spermatozoa enter the caput epididymis incapable of fertilization; however, fertility is acquired at some point during transit to the cauda epididymis. It is believed that epididymal secretions contain maturation factors that stimulate biochemical changes within the sperm cells necessary for fertilization. These changes include development of the potential for progressive forward motility; alteration of metabolic mechanisms; loss of the cytoplasmic droplet; and changes in the plasma membrane, acrosomal cap, and nuclear material. It is interesting to note that during storage in the caudal portion of the epididymis, the metabolic activity of mature sperm is actually suppressed by secretion of a "quiescence factor." The entire process of spermatogenesis requires 45–55 days in the boar (Swierstra 1968). The majority of this time is spent in the testicle and involves changes associated with both spermatocytogenesis and spermiogenesis. Maturation in the epididymis is thought to require only 10–14 days.

SEMEN COLLECTION, EVALUATION, AND PROCESSING

Semen Collection
Boar Training. Two things must be accomplished early in the training period if boars are to be taught to mount successfully and be collected from a dummy sow: boars must be forced to focus their attention on the dummy sow upon entry into the collection pen, and boars must associate the collection area and process with a pleasurable experience.

The primary stimulus for initiation of the mounting reflex in boars is an immobile object that resembles another pig (Chenoweth 1981). Therefore, a collection pen that is clean and free of extraneous items forces boars to focus their attention on the dummy sow and supplies the visual stimulus necessary for a successful mount. Similarly, a collection dummy with a strong swine odor supplies the necessary olfactory cues.

A young boar's attention span is limited. Mounting activity usually occurs within the first 5–7 minutes of a training session. Consequently, if mounting or an interest in the collection dummy has not occurred by this time, the probability that such behavior will occur during the current training session is low.

Boars that associate pain or fear with the collection area or collection process are difficult to train. Unpleasant experiences during collection can reduce the sexual activity of trained AI boars. Avoidance of rough handling and loud noises during the training process is critical.

Young, sexually aggressive boars that have not been used in natural mating are the easiest to train. This does not mean that older, sexually experienced boars cannot be taught to mount and be collected from a dummy sow, but the training interval is usually longer and the success rate lower compared to their younger, more inexperienced counterparts. An inverse relationship exists between the age of the boar at the initiation of the training period and the success rate (Reed 1982). When training was initiated at less than 10 months of age, a success rate of 90% resulted. In contrast, only 70% of the boars that were 10 and 18 months old at the beginning of the training period were successfully trained.

Semen Collection. The most common method of semen collection is the gloved hand technique (Almond et al. 1994). Pressure on the glans penis is the primary physiological stimulus for erection and ejaculation. It is often stated that more pressure is required to stimulate an erection than is required for ejaculation. Consequently, it is common for pressure on the end of the penis to be relaxed slightly after an erection has occurred in order to facilitate ejaculation. Routine management practices such as removal of preputial fluid prior to collection and clipping sheath hairs reduce the risk of contamination of semen during collection. Because of anatomical or behavioral abnormalities, some boars release preputial fluid concomitantly with semen during ejaculation, thus contaminating the semen. The preputial sac can be removed surgically to prevent this form of contamination.

Semen Evaluation
Total Number of Spermatozoa. A complete semen evaluation includes determination of total number of spermatozoa and estimations of sperm cell viability and fertility. The two most common pieces of equipment for determination of total numbers of spermatozoa in a sample of the ejaculate are the hemocytometer and the spectrophotometer. The hemocytometer is a special microscope slide. Multiplication of the number of sperm counted by a correction factor and the volume of semen collected yields the total number of spermatozoa. Determination of the total number of spermatozoa with a spectrophotometer is based on the transmittance (or absorbance) of light by a sample of the collected semen. Sperm and other cells block the movement of light through a solution. Samples with high concentrations of spermatozoa will have low transmittances, while the opposite is true for ejaculates with low concentrations. It is important to note that all spectrophotometers must

be calibrated before they can be used to determine spermatozoa concentrations; otherwise, the sperm counts can be overestimated (Flowers 1994). The most common way to do this is to use a hemocytometer. Consequently, the hemocytometer is the standard by which concentrations of spermatozoa are determined. Details concerning the use of hemocytometers and calibration of spectrophotometers are described elsewhere (Almond et al. 1994).

Motility and Morphology of Spermatozoa. The percentage of sperm cells exhibiting progressive forward motility is the most common measurement recorded during semen evaluations. In general, motility is a better estimator of sperm cell viability than of fertility. When motility scores are 60% or greater, there is no clear relationship between in vitro and in vivo estimates of fertility. In contrast, ejaculates with less than 60% motility fertilize fewer eggs in vitro and yield lower farrowing rates in vivo than those above 60%. Consequently, use of ejaculates exhibiting motilities of 60% or higher in AI programs should not compromise reproductive performance (Flowers 1997).

Morphological evaluations are conducted less frequently than motility estimates, yet such evaluations can provide important information about sperm viability and fertility. Abnormalities of the tail and head, the location of the cytoplasmic droplet on the midpiece, and the integrity of the acrosomal membranes can be observed with a light microscope and the proper histological stain (Woelders 1991). Current industry standards for the maximum acceptable levels of primary and secondary abnormalities for porcine spermatozoa used in AI programs are 10% and 20%, respectively (Flowers 1996a, b).

Other Fertility Tests. In addition to the mechanical requirements associated with egg penetration, spermatozoa must also undergo biochemical, metabolic, and molecular changes to acquire fertilizational competence. Table 6.4 summarizes a variety of tests based on one or more of these events. The most promising of these tests attempt to quantify specific aspects of sperm binding to egg membranes or structural changes within sperm membranes. At the present time, many of these tests are still being developed, and their subsequent use within the swine industry remains to be determined.

Semen Processing
Semen Extenders. Semen extenders provide nutritional and metabolic support for stored semen. Generic ingredients used in semen extenders include glucose, electrolytes, buffers, and antibiotics. Glucose is the predominant energy source; electrolytes assist in the regulation of osmotic pressure; buffers are involved in neutralization of metabolic wastes and maintenance of pH; and antibiotics inhibit bacterial growth. An inverse relationship exists between fertility and length of storage for all semen extenders; as the length of storage increases, fertility decreases. The rate at which fertility decreases during storage is primarily a function of the buffering system of the semen extender.

Interactions among several different factors determine the longevity of stored semen. These include individual boar characteristics, semen extender, sperm concentration, and storage temperature. In general, there is an inverse relationship between sperm concentration and length of storage. In other words, an insemination dose of 2 billion sperm cells in a total volume of 80 mL would be expected to have a longer shelf life than one containing 4 billion spermatozoa in the same volume.

Table 6.4. Summary of various measurements used to estimate the fertilizing ability of boar spermatozoa.

Measurement	Rationale	References
Percoll gradients	Velocity of spermatozoa is positively correlated to fertility. Sperm with increased velocities can be separated via Percoll gradients.	Grant et al. 1994
Fluorescent stains	Some fluorescent stains (Hoechst 33258) enter sperm cell if membrane is damaged and stain only dead cells. Others (SYBR-14) enter sperm with a membrane potential and stain only live cells.	Johnson et al. 1996
Sperm chromatic structure	When subjected to acidic conditions and stained with the metachromatic dye acridine orange, double-stranded DNA gives a green fluorescence, while single-stranded DNA (damaged) gives a red fluorescence. Ratio of green to red sperm is related to fertility.	Evenson et al. 1994
Sperm plasma membrane protein profile	Plasma membrane proteins were separated and quantified. Three proteins were positively correlated with sperm binding to egg membranes ($r = 0.38–0.53$). Two proteins were negatively correlated with sperm binding ($r = -0.42$ and -0.37).	Ash et al. 1994
Oocyte membrane-binding assay	Fertile spermatozoa bind to egg membranes. Correlation between egg binding and in vivo fertility from heterospermic inseminations was high ($r = 0.80$).	Berger et al. 1996
Hemizona-binding assay	Oocytes are bisected and the numbers of sperm from different boars binding to each half of the zona pellucida are counted. Within a hemizona pair, increased binding equates to increase fertility.	Fazeli et al. 1995

Source: Reprinted, with permission, from Flowers 1997.

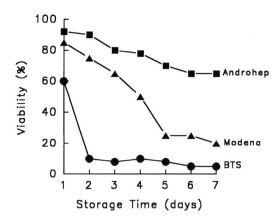

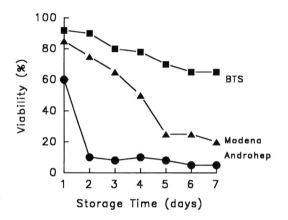

6.14. *Changes in viability of spermatozoa over time for two littermate boars. Spermatozoa from both boars were stored in three different semen extenders. Top panel: Data from boar A. Bottom panel: Data from boar B. Pooled standard errors for A and B were 7.3% and 8.2%, respectively.*

An example of the interaction between individual boar characteristics and semen extender type on sperm cell longevity is illustrated in Figure 6.14. In this example, the viability of semen in storage was optimized by use of one semen extender for one boar and a different extender for a second boar. These data indicate that problems with maintenance of semen viability in vitro may be related to an incompatibility between components of the semen extender and seminal fluids of an individual boar. If such incompatibilities exist, then using different semen extenders may solve the problem.

Semen Extension Procedures. Minimization of any potential differences in temperature, osmolarity, and pH between the extender and semen is necessary to maintain high sperm viability during the dilution process. Temperature differences are minimized by monitoring the temperature of both the extender and the semen and adjusting the temperature of the extender to within 1°C of the semen. Previous studies have demonstrated that a reduction in viability of semen is likely to occur when temperature differences between

the two liquids exceed 2°C. Measurement of osmolarity and pH prior to extension probably is not feasible practically or economically in most situations. However, procedural precautions can be taken to minimize the effects of any differences that may exist. First, it is important to allow sufficient time for the stabilization of the pH and osmolarity of freshly prepared extender before it is mixed with semen. The pH of most semen extenders equillibrate 45–60 minutes after preparation. Second, a two-stage dilution process helps minimize any detrimental effects due to mixing by allowing the semen to equilibrate slowly to any differences in pH or osmolarity that may exist between it and the extender. In a two-stage dilution process, an equal amount of extender is added slowly to semen over a 2- to 5-minute period. The resulting mixture is allowed to equilibrate for at least 5–10 minutes before the remaining volume of extender is added.

REPRODUCTIVE DISEASES OF THE BOAR
Breeding Soundness Examination
Breeding soundness examinations (BSE) are not typically conducted on boars that are used for natural service. Producers and veterinarians often rely on conception or farrowing rates as an indicator of boar fertility; however, the use of heterospermic matings interferes with attempts to identify infertile boars by examining farrowing records. Also, several other factors influence farrowing rates and litter size, and thus, it is difficult to identify problem boars solely by record analysis.

Natural-service boars are selected for BSE when infertility is suspected and following disease or injury, especially if the testes or penis are affected. The clinical history should include the boar's previous libido and mating ability, previous injuries, illnesses, and treatments and information regarding litter size and farrowing rates in females inseminated by the boar.

Abnormal sperm cells may not appear in the ejaculate for several weeks after heat stress or illness because it takes about 7 weeks to complete the entire sperm production process. This makes it difficult to identify causes of infertility in boars without the clinical history.

The body condition and general health of the animal should be assessed, with attention given to the soundness of feet and legs. Physical examination of the external genitalia includes palpation of the testes, epididymis, and prepuce. The testis should be 10–15 cm in length and 6–7 cm in width. Abnormalities, such as abscesses, bites, or scars on the scrotum, should be recorded and the preputial fluid examined for purulent material or blood.

The gloved-hand technique is the most practical method to collect semen from natural-service boars. Instead of using a dummy sow, the boar is exposed to a sow in standing estrus and allowed to mount. The penis is grasped before vulva penetration. At this point, the procedures for semen collection are similar to those used for routine collection from AI boars.

Semen Assessment During the BSE

A complete semen evaluation includes determining the total number of sperm cells and estimating the viability and fertility of sperm cells. There are few differences between semen assessment as part of the BSE and as part of AI programs. However, some components of the evaluation should be emphasized for boars used for natural service:

1. A clean ejaculate has little odor. In contrast, an ejaculate that has been contaminated with preputial fluid or with purulent material has a very distinctive odor.
2. Usually a boar will ejaculate 150–250 mL of semen, but the volume can range from 50 to 500 mL. One must consider the fact that boars without previous experience with gloved-hand collection may not complete ejaculation.
3. Photometers are useful for sperm counts in AI laboratories. However, a hemocytometer and portable microscope should be sufficient for on-farm semen counts.
4. Assessing sperm morphology is time-consuming and requires an above-average microscope with an oil immersion objective. It may be beneficial to stain a sample of sperm cells with eosin-nigrosin and examine the slides at the clinic rather than on the farm. Consider semen with over 30% abnormalities as suspect and reject samples if the percentage of abnormalities exceeds 50%.
5. Assessment of motility is subjective, and motility of sperm cells is highest when temperatures are between 32°C and 38°C. Microscope slides must be within 1–2°C of the semen sample temperature to avoid shocking the sperm cells and reducing motility. The microscope slides can be stored in a portable incubator, or they can be placed on a warming device before dropping the semen onto them. If motility is poor, prepare a second slide, making sure that the slide, the pipette, and the coverslip are at 35°C.

Systemic Infections that Cause Fever

Common causes of poor semen quality include stress and overuse, but overheating of boars is considered the most common cause of abnormal semen. Infectious diseases, wounds, bruising, and cuts on the testes or scrotum can raise the boar's body temperature or the temperature of the injured organ. Because the scrotum plays a role in regulating the temperature of the testes, any defect or abnormal condition of the scrotal area may also have an adverse effect on the production of sperm cells. In general, changes in semen quality after infection are similar to those that occur after boars are exposed to high ambient temperatures.

Abnormal sperm cells may be observed for several weeks after a boar recovers from a disease. The percentage of abnormal sperm cells in an ejaculate depends upon the severity and duration of the illness and the pathogen. Other noninfectious factors affecting semen quality have been reviewed in detail (Almond et al. 1994).

Localized Infections

If the epididymis is infected, there is often swelling of the testes and scrotum. An epididymal infection lowers fertility and should receive immediate attention. Fever, infection, orchitis, or inflammation of the scrotum can cause testicular degeneration of boars with previously demonstrated normal fertility. This condition involves degeneration of the germinal epithelium of the seminiferous tubules and must be diagnosed with a biopsy. Eventually, the testicular tissue will atrophy, resulting in flabby testicles, which may become firm if fibrous growths or calcium deposits accumulate in the testes. Although the boar's libido is unaffected, the ejaculate will have few sperm, sperm motility will be poor, and a high percentage of sperm will be abnormal. If an 8-week rest does not improve the condition, these boars should be culled.

Bacteria that appear to act directly on the function of the testes include *Brucella suis*, *Erysipelothrix rhusiopathiae*, *Mycoplasma hyosynoviae*, *Streptococcus suis*, *Staphylococcus aureus*, and *Escherichia coli*. *Brucella suis* can become localized in the testes and cause inflammation that will impair the boar's ability to manufacture sperm. Brucellosis can also cause testicular degeneration. Erysipelas can cause inflammation and degeneration of the testes. Ubiquitous bacteria, such as *Streptococcus suis*, *Staphylococcus aureus*, and *Escherichia coli*, can localize in the testes. It is not known whether the resulting fertility problems are due to a direct effect on sperm manufacture or to infection of the sow's reproductive tract.

Many viruses, including African swine fever, PPV, and PRRSV, have been shown to infect sows inseminated with contaminated semen. PRRSV can have a marked effect on spermatogenesis, resulting in fewer sperm, impaired motility, and higher percentages of abnormalities for up to 13 weeks after infection (Christopher-Hennings et al. 1995; Preito et al. 1995). Not all affected boars will show clinical signs of PRRS. Under certain circumstances, boars may be included in vaccination protocols intended to control PRRSV. The influence of vaccination, natural infection, or vaccination followed by natural infection on semen quality requires clarification. This confusion is due, at least in part, to apparent differences among the various PRRSV strains in causing disease.

REFERENCES

Aherne FX, Foxcroft GR, Pettigrew JE. 1999. Nutrition of the sow. In Diseases of Swine (8th ed). BE Straw, S D'Allaire, WL

Mengeling, DJ Taylor, eds. Ames: Iowa State University Press, pp. 1029–1043.

Akkermans JP, van Beusekom WJ. 1984. Tumors and tumor-like lesions in the genitalia of sows. Vet Q 6:90–96.

Almond GW, Dial GD. 1986. Pregnancy diagnosis in swine: A comparison of the accuracies of mechanical and endocrine tests with return to estrus. J Am Vet Med Assoc 189:1567–1571.

——. 1987. Pregnancy diagnosis in swine: Principles, applications, and accuracy of available techniques. J Am Vet Med Assoc 191:858–870.

Almond GW, Richards RG. 1991. Endocrine changes associated with cystic ovarian degeneration in sows. J Am Vet Med Assoc 199:883–886.

Almond GW, Bosu WTK, King GJ. 1985. Pregnancy diagnosis in swine: A comparison of two ultrasound instruments. Can Vet J 26:205–208.

Almond GW, Britt JH, Carr J, Flowers WL, Glossop C, Morrow WEM, See MT. 1994. The Swine AI Book. Raleigh, N.C.: Southern Cross Publications.

Anderson LJ, Sandison AT. 1969. Tumours of the female genitalia in cattle, sheep and pigs found in a British abattoir survey. J Comp Pathol 79:53–63.

Anderson LL. 1987. Pigs. In Reproduction in Farm Animals (5th ed). ESE Hafez, ed. Philadelphia: Lea and Febiger, pp. 324–344.

Andersson AM, Einarsson S. 1980. Studies on the oestrus and ovarian activity during five consecutive oestrous cycles in gilts. Acta Vet Scand 21:677–688.

Armstrong JD, Zering KD, White SL, Flowers WL, Woodard TO, McCaw MB, Almond GW. 1997. Use of real-time ultrasound for pregnancy diagnosis in swine. In Proc Am Assoc Swine Pract, pp. 195–202.

Arthur GH, Noakes DE, Pearson H. 1989. Veterinary Reproduction and Obstetrics (6th ed). London: Bailliere Tindall. pp. 193–218.

Ash KL, Berger T, Horner CM, Famula TR. 1994. Boar sperm plasma membrane protein profile: Correlation with the zona-free hamster ova assay. Theriogenology 42:1217–1226.

Ashdown RR, Hafez ESE. 1993. Anatomy of male reproduction. In Reproduction in Farm Animals (6th ed). ESE Hafez, ed. Philadelphia: Lea and Febiger, pp. 3–19.

Ashdown RR, Barnett SW, Ardalani G. 1981. Impotence in the boar. 1. Angioarchitecture and venous drainage of the penis in normal boars. Vet Rec 109:375–382.

Baker RD, Dziuk PJ, Norton HW. 1968. Effect of volume of semen, number of sperm and drugs on sperm transport in artificially inseminated gilts. J Anim Sci 27:88–92.

Bartke A, Hafiez AA, Bex FJ, Dalterio S. 1978. Hormonal interactions in regulation of androgen secretion. Biol Reprod 18:44–54.

Bartol FF, Wiley AA, Spencer TE, Valett JL, Christenson RK. 1993. Early uterine development in pigs. J Reprod Fertil (Suppl) 48:99–116.

Bates RO, Day BN, Britt JH, Clark LK, Brauer MA. 1991. Reproductive performance of sows treated with a combination of pregnant mare's serum gonadotropin and human chorionic gonadotropin at weaning in the summer. J Anim Sci 69:894–898.

Batista L. 2000. Gilt acclimatation: Your insurance for health and production at the farm. In Proc Am Assoc Swine Vet, pp. 289–291.

Batista L, Torremorel M, Pijoan C. 2002. Experimental exposure to porcine reproductive and respiratory syndrome virus (PRRSV) in gilts during acclimatization. J Swine Health Prod 4:147–150.

Bazer FW. 1989. Establishment of pregnancy in sheep and pigs. Reprod Fertil Dev 1:237–242.

Beltranena E, Aherne FX, Foxcroft GR, Kirkwood RN. 1991. Effects of pre- and post-pubertal feeding on production traits at first and second estrus. J Anim Sci 69:886–893.

Benson GS. 1994. Male sexual function: Erection, emission and ejaculation. In The Physiology of Reproduction. E Knobil, JD Neill, eds. New York: Raven Press, pp. 1489–1508.

Berger T, Anderson DL, Penedo MCT. 1996. Porcine sperm fertilizing potential in relationship to sperm functional capacities. Anim Reprod Sci 44:231–233.

Blackwell TE, Werdin RE, Eisenmenger MC, FitzSimmons MA. 1989. Goitrogenic effects in offspring of swine fed sulfadimethoxine and ormetoprim in late gestation. J Am Vet Med Assoc 194:519–523.

Bolin CA, Bolin SR, Kluge JP, Mengeling WL. 1985. Pathologic effect of intrauterine deposition of pseudorabies virus on the reproductive tract of swine in early pregnancy. Am J Vet Res 46:1039–1042.

Bosc MJ, Martinat-Botté F, Nicolle A. 1975. Étude de deux techniques de diagnostic de gestation chez la truie. Ann Zootech 24:651–660.

Bostedt H, Rudloff PR. 1983. Prophylactic administration of the beta-blocker carazolol to influence the duration of parturition in sows. Theriogenology 20:191–196.

Britt JH. 1986. Improving sow productivity through management during gestation, lactation and after weaning. J Anim Sci 63:1288–1296.

Britt JH. 1996a. Biology and management of the early weaned sow. In Proc Am Assoc Swine Pract, pp. 417–426.

——. 1996b. Manipulation of the porcine estrous cycle. In Proc Swine Reprod Symp, Am Soc Therio, pp. 83–91.

Britt JH, Day BN, Webel SK, Brauer MA. 1989. Induction of fertile estrus in prepuberal gilts by treatment with a combination of pregnant mare's serum gonadotropin and human chorionic gonadotropin (P. G. 600™). J Anim Sci 67:1148–1153.

Britt JH, Flowers WL, Armstrong TA. 1997. Induction of ovulation in early weaned sows. In Proc Am Assoc Swine Pract, pp. 33–35.

Brownback A. 1981. Eperythrozoonosis as a cause of infertility in swine. 1981. Vet Med Small Anim Clin 76:375–378.

Cameron RDA. 1977. Pregnancy diagnosis in the sow by rectal examination. Aust Vet J 53:432–435.

Camous S, Prunier A, Pelletier JP. 1985. Plasma prolactin, LH, FSH and estrogen excretion patterns in gilts during sexual development. J Anim Sci 60:1308–1317.

Castagna CD, Peixoto CH, Bortolozzo FP, Wentz I, Neto GB, Ruschel F. 2004. Ovarian cysts and their consequences on the reproductive performance of swine herds. Anim Repro Sci 81:115–123.

Chenoweth P. 1981. Libido and mating behavior in bulls, boars and rams: A review. Theriogenology 16:155–170.

Christenson RK, Ford JJ, Redmer DA. 1985. Maturation of ovarian follicles in the prepubertal gilt. J Reprod Fertil (Suppl) 33:21–36.

Christopher-Hennings J, Nelson EA, Hines RJ, Nelson JK, Swenson SL, Zimmerman JJ, Chase CCL, Yaeger MJ, Benfield DA. 1995. Persistence of porcine reproductive and respiratory syndrome virus in serum and semen of adult boars. J Vet Diagn Invest 7:456–464.

Chung WB, Cheng WF, Wu LS, Yang PC. 2002. The use of plasma progesterone profiles to predict the reproductive status of anestrous gilts and sows. Theriogenology 58:1165–1174.

Claus, R. 1990. Physiological role of seminal components in the reproductive tract of the female pig. J Reprod Fertil (Suppl) 40:117–131.

Clayton GA, Powell JC, Hiley PG. 1981. Inheritance of teat number and teat number and teat inversion in pigs. Anim Prod 33:299–304.

Colenbrander B, van de Wiel DFM, van Rossum-Kok CMJE, Wensing CJG. 1982a. Changes in serum FSH concentrations in the pig during development. Biol Reprod 26:105–109.

Colenbrander B, Frankenhuis MT, Wensing CJG. 1982b. Male sexual development. In Control of Pig Reproduction. DJA Cole, GR Foxcroft, eds. London: Butterworth, pp. 3–24.

Cox NM. 1997. Control of follicular development and ovulation rate in pigs. J Reprod Fert (Suppl) 52:31–46.

Cox NM, Britt JH. 1982. Relationship between endogenous gonadotropin-releasing hormone, gonadotropins and follicular development after weaning in sows. Biol Reprod 27:70–78.

Cox NM, Ramirez JL, Matamoros IA, Bennett WA. 1988. Estrogen induces estrus unaccompanied by a preovulatory surge of luteinizing hormone in suckled sows. Biol Reprod 38:592–596.

Cunningham NF. 1982. Pregnancy diagnosis in sows based on serum oestrone sulphate concentration. Br Vet J 138:543–544.

Cunningham NF, Hattersley JP, Wrathall AE. 1983. Pregnancy diagnosis in sows based on serum oestrone sulphate concentration. Vet Rec 113:229–233.

Davis DL, Stevenson JS, Schmidt WE. 1985. Scheduled breeding of gilts after estrous synchronization with altrenogest. J Anim Sci 60:599–602.

De Winter PJJ, Verdonck M, DeKruif A, Coryn M, Deluyker HA, Devriese LA, Haesebrouck F. 1996. The relationship between the blood progesterone concentration at early metoestrus and uterine infection in the sow. Anim Reprod Sci 41:51–59.

De Winter PJJ, Verdonck M, DeKruif A, Devriese LA, Haesebrouck F. 1992. Endometritis and vaginal discharge in the sow. Anim Reprod Sci 28:51–58.

Dial GD. 1990. Computerized records: Use in troubleshooting reproductive problems of commercial swine herds. In Kansas State University Swine Day. pp. 1–14.

Dial GD, MacLachlan NJ. 1988a. Urogenital infections of swine. Part I. Clinical manifestations and pathogenesis. Comp Cont Ed Pract Vet 10:63–69.

——. 1988b. Urogenital infections of swine. Part II. Pathology and medical management. Comp Cont Ed Pract Vet 10: 529–538.

Dial GD, Almond GW, Hilley HD, Repasky RR, Hagan J. 1987. Oxytocin precipitation of prostaglandin-induced farrowing in swine: Determination of the optimal dose of oxytocin and optimal interval between prostaglandin F2 and oxytocin. Am J Vet Res 48:966–970.

Dial GD, Marsh WE, Polson DD, Vaillancourt JP. 1992. Reproductive failure: Differential diagnosis. In Disease of Swine (7th ed). BE Straw, S D'Allaire, WL Mengeling, DJ Taylor, eds. Ames: Iowa State University Press, pp. 88–137.

Done JT. 1980. Teat deficiences in pigs. Vet Annu 20:246–254.

Dyck GW, Swierstra EE. 1983. Growth of the reproductive tract of the gilt from birth to puberty. Can J Anim Sci 63:81–86.

Dziuk PJ. 1985. Effect of migration, distribution and spacing of pig embryos on pregnancy and fetal survival. J Reprod Fert (Suppl) 33:57–63.

Dziuk PJ, Polge C. 1965. Fertility of gilts following induced ovulation. Vet Rec 77:236–242.

Ebbert W, Bostedt H. 1993. Cystic degeneration in porcine ovaries—First communication: Morphology of cystic ovaries, interpretation of the results. Repro Dom Anim 28:441–450.

Ebbert W, Elsaesser F, Bostedt H. 1993. Cystic degeneration in porcine ovaries—Second communication: Concentrations of progesterone, estradiol-17β and testosterone in cystic fluid and plasma; interpretation of the results. Repro Dom Anim 28:451–463.

Eggemann G, Wendt M, Hoelzle LE, Jager C, Weiss R, Failing K. 2000. Prevalence of chlamydial infections in breeding sows and their correlation with reproductive failure. Dtsch Tierarztl Wochenschr 107:3–10.

Einarsson S, Viring S, Lindell JO. 1975. The effect of prostaglandin-F2 and oxytocin on porcine myometrium in vitro. Zuchthygiene 10:135–179.

Einarsson S, Fischier MN, Karlberg K. 1981. Induction of parturition in sows using prostaglandin F2a or the analogue cloprostenol. Nord Vet Med 33:354–358.

Ellendorff F, Meyer JN, Elsaesser F. 1976. Prospects and problems and fertility diagnosis in the pig by aid of progesterone determination. Br Vet J 132:543–550.

Ellicott AR, Dziuk PJ. 1973. Minimum daily dose of progesterone and plasma concentration for maintenance of pregnancy in ovariectomized gilts. Biol Reprod 9:300–304.

Ellis WA, McParland PJ, Bryson DG, Thiermann AB, Montgomery J. 1986. Isolation of leptospires from genital tract and kidneys of aborted sows. Vet Rec 118:294–295.

Elsaesser F, Foxcroft GE. 1978. Maturational changes in the characteristics of oestrogen-induced surges of luteinizing hormone in immature domestic pig. J Endocrinol 78:455–456.

Elsaesser F, Ellendorff F, Pomerantz DK, Parvizi N, Smidt D. 1976. Plasma levels of luteinizing hormone, progesterone, testosterone and 5a-dihydrotestosterone in male and female pigs during sexual maturation. J Endocrinol 68:347–348.

Embrechts E. 1982. Procaine penicillin toxicity in pigs. Vet Rec 111:314–315.

Esbenshade KE, Paterson AM, Cantley TC, Day BN. 1982. Changes in plasma hormone concentration associated with onset of puberty in the gilt. J Anim Sci 54:320–324.

Evenson DP, Thompson L, Jost L. 1994. Flow cytometric evaluation of boar semen by the sperm chromatin structure assay as related to cryopreservation and fertility. Theriogenology 41:637–651.

Fazeli AR, Holt C, Steenweg W, Bevers MM, Holt WV, Colenbrander B. 1995. Development of a sperm hemizona binding assay for boar semen. Theriogenology 44:17–27.

Fennestad KL, Borg-Petersen C. 1966. Experimental leptospirosis in pregnant sows. J Infect Dis 116:57–66.

First NL, Bazer FW. 1983. Pregnancy and parturition. J Anim Sci (Suppl 2) 57:425–460.

First NL, Bosc MJ. 1979. Proposed mechanisms controlling parturition and induction of parturition in swine. J Anim Sci 48:1407–1421.

First NL, Lohse JK, Nara BS. 1982. The endocrine control of parturition. In Control of Pig Reproduction. DJA Cole, GR Foxcroft, eds. London: Butterworth, pp. 311–342.

Fisher HE, Bazer FW, Fields MJ. 1985. Steroid metabolism by endometrial and conceptus tissues during early pregnancy and pseudopregnancy in swine. J Reprod Fertil 75:69–78.

Flowers WL. 1994. Quality control issues for artificial insemination programs. In Proc Pork Summit '94. A. L. Laboratories, pp. 33–38.

——. 1996a. Successful AI programs. In Proc Swine Reprod Symp. Am Soc Therio, pp. 15–25.

——. 1996b. An update on swine AI. In Proc 16th Tech Conf AI Reprod. National Assoc Anim Breeders, pp. 88–94.

——. 1997. Management of boars for efficient semen production. J Reprod Fertil 52:67–78.

Flowers WL, Esbenshade KL. 1993. Optimizing management of natural and artificial matings in swine. J Reprod Fertil (Suppl) 48:217–228.

Ford JJ, Christenson RK, Maurer RR. 1979. Estrogen concentrations in serum and amniotic and allantoic fluids of fetal pigs. Biol Reprod (Suppl 1) 20:100A.

Foxcroft G. 2003. Working with variance: Hassle or help in developing breeding management programs. In Proc Advances in Pork Production, Banff Pork Seminar, pp. 247–260.

Foxcroft G, Aherne F. 2002. Management of the gilt and first parity sow. In IX Symp Dr. Santiago Martín Rillo: Reproducción e IA de Ganado Porcino, pp. 105–162.

Friendship RM, Templeton CL, Deckert AE. 1990. An evaluation of vulvomucosal injections of prostaglandins for induction of parturition in swine. Can Vet J 31:433–436.

Garner DL, Hafez ESE. 1993. Spermatozoa and seminal plasma. In Reproduction in Farm Animals (6th ed). ESE Hafez, ed. Philadelphia: Lea and Febiger, pp. 165–187.

Gherpelli M, Tarocco C. 1996. A study on the incidence and clinical evolution of the ovarian cysts in the sow. Proc Int Pig Vet Soc Congr 14:587.

Glossop CE, Ashdown RR. 1986. Cavernosography and differential diagnosis of impotence in the boar. Vet Rec 118:357–363.

Glossop CE, Foulkes JA, Whitworth A, Cornwell E. 1989. Use of an on-farm progesterone assay kit to determine pregnancy in sows. Vet Rec 124:115–117.

Grant SA, Long SE, Parkinson TJ. 1994. Fertilizability and structural properties of boar spermatozoa prepared by Percoll gradient centrifugation. J Reprod Fertil 100:477–483.

Greenwald GS. 1978. Follicular activity in the mammalian ovary. In The Vertebrate Ovary. RE Jones, ed. New York: Plenum Press, pp. 639–689.

Grieger DM, Brandt KE, Diekman MA. 1986. Follicular fluid concentrations of estradiol 17b and progesterone and secretory patterns of LH and FSH in prepubertal gilts reared in confinement or outdoors lots. J Anim Sci 62:751–756.

Guthrie HD, Deaver DR. 1979. Estrone concentration in the peripheral plasma of pregnant and nonpregnant gilts. Theriogenology 11:321–329.

Guthrie HD, Polge C. 1976. Control of oestrus and fertility in gilts with accessory corpora lutea by prostaglandin analogues ICI 79,939 and 80,996. J Reprod Fertil 48:427–430.

———. 1978. Treatment of pregnant gilts with a prostaglandin analogue, cloprostenol, to control oestrus and fertility. J Reprod Fertil 52:271–273.

Hafs HD, McCarthy MS. 1978. Endocrine control of testicular function. In Beltsville Symposium in Agricultural Research 3, Animal Reproduction. HW Hawk, ed. New York: Halsted Press. pp. 345–364.

Hansson V, Weddinton SC, French FS, McLean W, Smith A, Hayfeh SN, Ritzen EM, Hagenas L. 1976. Secretion and role of androgen-binding proteins in the testis and epididymis. J Reprod Fertil (Suppl) 24:17–33.

Hargrove JL, MacIndoe JH, Ellis LC. 1977. Testicular contractile cells and sperm transport. Fertil Steril 28:1146–1157.

Hemeida NA, Sack WO, McEntee K. 1978. Ductuli efferentes in the epididymis of boar, goat, ram, bull and stallion. Am J Vet Res 39:1892–1899.

Hemsworth PE, Barnett JL. 1990. Behavioural responses affecting gilt and sow reproduction. J Reprod Fertil (Suppl) 40:343–354.

Hermansson I, Karlberg K, Einarrson S. 1981. Use of a prostaglandin analogue (cloprostenol) for induction of parturition in pigs with prolonged gestation. Nord Vet Med 33:349–353.

Holtz W. 1982. Pregnancy detection in swine by pulse mode ultrasound. Anim Reprod Sci 4:219–226.

Holtz W, Schmidt-Baulain R, Meyer H, Welp C. 1990. Control of prostaglandin-induced parturition in sows by injection of the beta-adrenergic blocking agent carazolol or carazolol and oxytocin. J Anim Sci 68:3967–3971.

Hsueh AJW, Billig H, Tsafriri A. 1994. Ovarian follicle atresia: A hormonally controlled apoptotic process. Endocrine Rev 15:707–724.

Hughes PE, Pearce GP, Paterson AM. 1990. Mechanisms mediating the stimulation effects of the boar on gilt reproduction. J Reprod Fertil (Suppl) 40:323–341.

Hulland TJ. 1964. Pregnancy in hermaphroditism: Clinical management. Can Vet J 5:39–41.

Inaba T, Nakazima Y, Matsui N, Imori T. 1983. Early pregnancy diagnosis in sows by ultrasonic linear electronic scanning. Theriogenology 20:97–101.

Jackson GH. 1986. Pregnancy diagnosis in the sow using real-time ultrasonic scanning. Vet Rec. 119:90–91.

Jaeger LA, Johnson GA, Ka H, Garlow JG, Burghardt RC, Spencer TE, Bazer FW. 2001. Functional analysis of autocrine and paracrine signalling at the uterine-conceptus interface in pigs. Reproduction (Suppl) 58:191–207.

Johnson LA, Maxwell WMC, Dobrinsky JR, Welch GR. 1996. Staining sperm for viability assessment. Reprod Domest Anim 31:37–47.

Jones TC, Hunt RD, King NW. 1997. Genital organ. In Veterinary Pathology (6th ed). Philadelphia: Williams & Wilkins.

Joo HS, Chu RM. 1999. Japanese B encephalitis. In Diseases of Swine (8th ed). BE Straw, S D'Allaire, WL Mengeling, DJ Taylor, eds. Ames: Iowa State University Press, pp. 173–178.

Karlbom I, Einarsson S, Edqvist L. 1982. Attainment of puberty in female pigs: Clinical appearance and patterns of progesterone, oestradiol-17b and LH. Anim Reprod Sci 4:301–312.

Kauffold J, Rautenberg T, Gutjahr S, Richter A, Sobiraj A. 2004. Ultrasonographic characterization of ovaries in non-pregnant first served sows and gilts. Theriogenology 61:1407–1417.

Kemp B, Soede NM. 1996. Relationships of weaning-to-estrus interval to timing of ovulation and fertilization in sows. J Anim Sci 74:944–949.

Kemp B, Soede NM, Helmond FA, Bosch MW. 1995. Effects of energy source in the diet on reproductive hormones and insulin during lactation and subsequent estrus in multiparous sows. J Anim Sci 73:3022–3029.

Kennedy PC, Miller RB. 1992. The female genital system. In Pathology of Domestic Animals (4th ed), vol. 3. KVF Jubb, PC Kennedy, N Palmer, eds. San Diego, CA: Academic Press Inc, pp. 349–470.

Kim HS, Christianson WT, Joo HS. 1989. Pathogenic properties of encephalomyocarditis virus isolates in swine fetuses. Arch Virol 109:51–57.

Kirkwood, RN, Henry SC, Tokach LM, Foxcroft GR. 1999. Human chorionic gonadotropin at parturition fails to consistently induce ovulation in sows. Swine Health Prod 7:69–72.

Koketsu Y, Dial GD, Pettigrew JE, King VL. 1996. Feed intake pattern during lactation and subsequent reproductive performance of sows. J Anim Sci 74:2875–2884.

Kuhlers DL, Jungst SB, Marple DN, Rahe CH. 1985. The effect of pen density during rearing on subsequent reproductive performance in gilts. J Anim Sci 61:1066–1069.

Kuster C, Becton L, Ebert M, Eisenhart M. 2000. Replacement gilt isolation and acclimatization protocols for the control of PRRSV. Proc AD Leman Swine Conf. p 7.

Lager KM, Halbur PG. 1996. Gross and microscopic lesions in porcine fetuses infected with porcine reproductive and respiratory syndrome. J Vet Diagn Invest 8:275–282.

Larsson K, Edqvist LE, Einarsson S, Haggstrom A, Linde C. 1975. Determination of progesterone in peripheral blood-plasma as a diagnostic aid in female swine. Nord Vet Med 27:167–172.

Leif H, Thompson LH. 2002. Managing Swine Reproduction. Circular 1190. University of Illinois at Urbana-Champaign.

Levis DG, Hemsworth PE. 1995. Duration of standing response in estrous gilts. J Anim Sci (Suppl 1) 87:49.

Lindahl IL, Totsch JP, Martin PA, Dzuik PJ. 1975. Early diagnosis of pregnancy in sows by ultrasonic amplitude-depth analysis. J Anim Sci 40:220–222.

Love RJ, Philbey AW, Kirkland PD et al. 2001. Reproductive diseases and congenital malformations in pigs caused by Menangle virus. Aust Vet J 79:192–198.

Lutz JB, Rampacek GB, Kraeling RR, Pinkert CA. 1984. Serum luteinizing hormone and estrogen profiles before puberty in the gilt. J Anim Sci 58:686–691.

MacLachlan NJ, Dial GD. 1987. An epizootic of endometritis in gilts. Vet Pathol 24:92–94.

Martin PA, Hammitt DG, Strohbehn RS, Keister DM. 1987. Induction of parturition in swine and epostane, a competitive inhibitor of 3b-hydroxysteroid dehydrogenase. J Anim Sci 64:497–506.

Martinat-Botté F, Renaud G, Madec F, Costiou P, Terqui M. 1998. Echographie et Reproduction chez la Truie: Bases et Applications Pratiques. Paris: Institut National de la Recherche Agronomique.

McCaughey WJ, Rea CC. 1979. Pregnancy diagnosis in sows: A comparison of the vaginal biopsy and doppler ultrasound techniques. Vet Rec 104:255–258.

Mengeling WL, Lager KM, Vorwald AC. 2000. The effect of porcine parvovirus and porcine reproductive and respiratory syndrome virus on reproductive performance. Anim Repro Sci 60–61:199–210.

Meredith MJ. 1979. The treatment of anoestrus in the pig: A review. Vet Rec 104:25–27.

Miller H, Foxcroft GR, Aherne FX. 1996. The effects of feed intake in early lactation on sow performance. Swine Research Update, Alberta Agriculture, Food and Rural Development (Electronic Version).

Moeljono MP, Thatcher WW, Bazer FW, Frank M, Owens LJ, Wilcox CJ. 1977. A study of prostaglandin $F_{2\alpha}$ as the luteolysin in swine: II. Characterization and comparison of prostaglandin F, estrogens and progestin concentrations in utero-ovarian vein plasma of nonpregnant and pregnant gilts. Prostaglandins 14: 543–555.

Morbeck DE, Esbenshade KL, Flowers WL, Britt JH. 1992. Kinetics of follicle growth in the prepubertal gilt. Biol Reprod 47:485–491.

Muirhead MR, Alexander TL. 1997. Reproduction: Noninfectious infertility. In Managing Pig Health and the Treatment of Disease: A Reference for the Farm (1st ed). Sheffield, U.K.: 5M Enterprises.

Nelson RE, Robison OW. 1976. Effects of postnatal maternal environment on reproduction in gilts. J Anim Sci 43:71–77.

O'Reilly PJ. 1979. Oestrous cycles and fertility in porcine hermaphrodites. Vet Rec 104:196.

Orr JP, Althouse E, Dulac GC, Durham PJK. 1988. Epizootic infection of a minimal disease swine herd with a herpesvirus. Can Vet J 29:45–50.

Oxender WD, Colenbrander B, van de Wiel DFM, Wensing CJG. 1979. Ovarian development in fetal and prepubertal pigs. Biol Reprod 21:715–721.

Paul PS, Stevenson GW. 1999. Rotavirus and reovirus. In Diseases of Swine (8th ed). BE Straw, S D'Allaire, WL Mengeling, DJ Taylor, eds. Ames: Iowa State University Press, pp. 255–276.

Pearce, GP, Pearce AN. 1992. Contact with a sow in oestrus or a mature boar stimulates the onset of oestrus in weaned sows. Vet Rec 130:5–9.

Polge C. 1978. Fertilization in the pig and horse. J Reprod Fertil 54:461–474.

Polson DD, Dial GD, Marsh WE. 1990a. A biological and financial characterization of nonproductive days. Proc Int Pig Vet Soc Congr 11:372.

Polson DD, Dial GD, Marsh WE et al. 1990b. Relative contributions of commonly used measures of reproductive performance on herd productivity. Proc AD Leman Swine Conf. pp. 74–85.

Preito C, Suarez P, Bautista JM, Sanchez R, Rillo SM, Simarro I, Solana A, Castro JM. 1995. Semen changes in boars after experimental infection with porcine reproductive and respiratory syndrome (PRRS) virus. Theriogenology 45:383–395.

Pressing AL. 1992. Pharmacologic control of swine reproduction. In Swine Reproduction: The Veterinary Clinics of North America. RC Tubbs, AD Leman, eds. Philadelphia: W. B. Saunders, pp. 707–723.

Pressing A, Dial GD, Esbenshade KL, Stroud CM. 1992. Hourly administration of GnRH to prepubertal gilts: Endocrine and ovulatory responses from 70 to 190 days of age. J Anim Sci 70:232–242.

Pressing AL, Dial GD, Stroud CM, Almond GW, Robinson OW. 1987. Prostaglandin-induced abortion in swine: Endocrine changes and influence on subsequent reproductive activity. Am J Vet Res 48:45–50.

Pusateri AE, Smith JM, Smith JW II, Thomford PJ, Diekman MA. 1996. Maternal recognition of pregnancy in swine. I. Minimal requirement for exogenous estradiol-17b to induce either short or long pseudopregnancy in cycling gilts. Biol Reprod 55:582–589.

Quesnel H, Pasquier A, Mounier AM, Prunier A. 1998. Influence of feed restriction during lactation on gonadotropic hormones

and ovarian development in primiparous sows. J Anim Sci 76:856–863.

Rahe CH, Jungst SB, Marple DN, Kuhlers DL. 1987. Effect of animal density on endocrine development of gilts. J Anim Sci 65:439–444.

Reed HCB. 1982. Artificial insemination. In Control of Pig Reproduction. DJA Cole, GR Foxcroft, eds. London: Butterworth, pp. 65–90.

Robertshaw D, Vercoe JE. 1980. Scrotal thermoregulation of the bull and boar. Aust J Agric Res 31:401–407.

Robertson HA, King GJ, Dyck GW. 1978. The appearance of oestrone sulphate in the peripheral plasma of the pig early in pregnancy. J Reprod Fertil 52:337–338.

Robertson HA, Dwyer RJ, King GJ. 1985. Oestrogens in fetal and maternal fluids throughout pregnancy in the pig and comparisons with the ewe and cow. J Endocrinol 106:355–360.

Ryan PL, Raeside JI. 1991. Cystic ovarian degeneration in pigs: A review. Irish Vet J 44:22–36.

Sanders H, Rajamahendran R, Burton B. 1994. The development of a simple fecal immunoreactive progestin assay to monitor reproductive function in swine. Can Vet J 35:355–358.

Seren E, Mattioli M, Gaiani R, Tamanini C. 1983. Direct estimation of urine estrone conjugate for a rapid pregnancy diagnosis in sows. Theriogenology 19:817–822.

Sesti LAC, Britt JH. 1993. Influence of stage of lactation, exogenous luteinizing hormone-releasing hormone, and suckling on estrus, positive feedback of luteinizing hormone, and ovulation in sows treated with estrogen. J Anim Sci 71:989–998.

———. 1994. Secretion of gonadotropins and estimated releasable pools of gonadotropin-releasing hormone and gonadotropins during establishment of suckling-induced inhibition of gonadotropin secretion in the sow. Biol Reprod 50:1078–1086.

Setchell BP, Maddocks S, Brooks DE. 1993. Anatomy, vasculature, innervation and fluids of the male reproductive tract. In The Physiology of Reproduction. E Knobil, JD Neill, eds. New York: Raven Press, pp. 1063–1176.

Sharpe RM. 1994. Regulation of spermatogenesis. In The Physiology of Reproduction. E Knobil, JD Neill, eds. New York: Raven Press, pp. 1363–1434.

Signoret JP, du Mesnil du Buisson F, Mauleon P. 1972. Effect of mating on the onset and duration of ovulation in the sow. J Reprod Fertil 31:327–330.

Singh J, Jamaluddin A. 2002. Nipah virus infection in swine. In Trends in Emerging Viral Infections of Swine. A Morilla, KJ Yoon, JJ Zimmerman JJ (eds). Ames: Iowa State Press, pp. 105–110.

Sisk DB, Cole JR, Pursell AR. 1980. Serologic incidence of eperythrozoonosis in Georgia swine. Proc Am Assoc Vet Lab Diagn 13:91–99.

Smith CA, Almond GW, Esbenshade KL. 1992. Effects of exogenous estradiol-17ß on luteinizing hormone, progesterone and estradiol-17ß concentrations before and after prostaglandin $F_{2\alpha}$-induced termination of pregnancy and pseudopregnancy in gilts. J Anim Sci 70:518–524.

Soede NM, Wetzels C.H, Zondag W, de Koning, MAI, Kemp B. 1995. Effects of time of insemination relative to ovulation, as determined by ultrasonography, on fertilization rate and accessory sperm count in sows. J Reprod Fert 104:99–106.

Stephano HA, Gay GM, Ramirez TC. 1988. Encephalomyelitis, reproductive failure and corneal opacity in pigs, associated with a new paramyxovirus infection (blue eye). Vet Rec 122:6–10.

Swensson T. 1978. Foetus sound detection for control of pregnancy in swine. Svensk Veterin 30:781–783.

Swierstra EE. 1968. Cytology and duration of the cycle of seminiferous epithelium of the boar: Duration of spermatozoan transit through the epididymis. Anat Rec 161:171–185.

Thomford PJ, Sander HK, Kendall JZ, Sherwood OD, Dziuk PJ. 1984. Maintenance of pregnancy and levels of progesterone and relaxin in the serum of gilts following a stepwise reduction in the number of corpora lutea. Biol Reprod 31:494–498.

Tilton SL, Bates RO, Prather RS. 1995. Evaluation of response to hormonal therapy in prepubertal gilts of different genetic lines. J Anim Sci 73:3062–3068.

Tubbs RC, Cox NM, Dyer K. 1996. Effect of PG600 on farrowing rate, litter size, and weaning-to-service intervals in sows with delayed (>7 days) wean-to-estrus interval. Proc Int Pig Vet Soc Congr 14:579.

Ullrey DE, Sprague JI, Becker DE, Miller ER. 1965. Growth in the swine fetus. J Anim Sci 24:711.

van der Steen HAM. 1985. Maternal influence mediated by litter size during the suckling period on reproduction traits in pigs. Livest Prod Sci 13:147–158.

Vannier P. 1999. Infectious causes of abortion in swine. Reprod Dom Anim 34:367–376.

Vanrompay D, Geens T , Desplanques A, Hoang TQT, De Vos L, Van Loock M, Huyck E, Mirry C, Cox E. 2004. Immunoblotting, ELISA and culture evidence for *Chlamydiaceae* in sows on 258 Belgian farms. Vet Microbiol 99:59–66.

Van Til LD, Dohoo IR. 1991. A serological survey of leptospirosis in Prince Edward Island swine herds and its association with infertility. Can J Vet Res 55:352–355.

Varley MA. 1982. The time of weaning and its effect on reproductive function. In Control of Pig Reproduction. DJA Cole, GR Foxcroft, eds. London: Butterworth, pp. 459–478.

——. 1991. Stress and reproduction. Pig News Info 12:567–571.

Waller CM, Bilkei G, Cameron RD. 2002. Effect of periparturient diseases accompanied by excessive vulval discharge and weaning to mating interval on sow reproductive performance. Aust Vet J 80:545–549.

Weitze KF. 1991. Long-term storage of extended boar semen. Reprod Dom Anim (Suppl) 1:231–254.

Weitze KF, Wagner-Rietschel H, Richter L. 1992. Standing heat and ovulation in a sow herd. Proc Int Pig Vet Soc Congr 12:460.

Werdin R, Wold K. 1976. Uterine carcinoma in a sow. Vet Pathol 13:451–452.

West KW, Bystrom J, Wojnarowicz C, et al. 1999. Myocarditis and abortion associated with intrauterine infection of sows with porcine circovirus 2. J Vet Diagn Invest 11:530–532.

Woelders H. 1991. Overview of in vitro methods for evaluation of semen quality. Reprod Dom Anim (Suppl) 1:145–164.

Wrathall AE. 1975. Reproductive Disorders in Pigs. Commonwealth Agricultural Bureaux, Farnham Royal, England.

Xue JL, Dial GD, Marsh WE, Davies PR, Momont HW. 1993. Influence of lactation length on sow productivity. Livest Prod Sci 34:253–265.

Yoon KJ, Janke BH. 2002. Swine influenza: Etiology, epidemiology, and diagnosis. In Morilla A, Yoon KJ, Zimmerman JJ (eds). Trends in Emerging Viral Infections of Swine. Ames: Iowa State Press. pp. 23–28.

Zak LJ, Cosgrove JR, Aherne FX, Foxcroft GR. 1997. Pattern of feed intake and associated metabolic and endocrine changes differentially affect postweaning fertility in primiparous sows. J Anim Sci 75:209–216.

Zannoni A, Bernardini C, Soflai Sohee M, Forni M. 2003. Endonuclease activity in swine ovarian cysts. Vet Res Comm (Suppl 1) 27:635–637.

Zerobin K, Kundig H. 1980. The control of myometrial functions during parturition with a beta 2-mimetic compound, Planipart (clenbuterol). Theriogenology 14:21–35.

Zinn GM, Jesse GW, Dobson AW. 1983. Effect of eperythrozoonosis on sow productivity. J Am Vet Med Assoc 182:369–371.

7 Diseases of the Respiratory System

Vibeke Sørensen, Sven Erik Jorsal, and Jan Mousing

The structure of swine production has changed substantially in most swine-producing areas over several years; large groups of animals are housed under intensive conditions, often in regions with an extremely dense pig population. High stocking density in a closed environment facilitates transmission of airborne pathogens within the herd (Donham 1991; Buddle et al. 1997) and between herds as well (Jorsal and Thomsen 1988; Stark et al. 1992; Christensen et al. 1993). Consequently, respiratory disorders and systemic airborne diseases are today regarded as the most serious disease problems in modern swine production.

STRUCTURE OF THE NORMAL RESPIRATORY SYSTEM

The respiratory tract develops from the anterior part of the embryonic gut as a tree-structured tubular organ. The mature respiratory apparatus comprises the nasal cavity, pharynx, larynx, trachea, and lungs with bronchi, bronchioli, and alveoli. The lungs are embedded in the pleural sac.

There are two separate blood-conducting systems in the lungs. The arteria pulmonalis system vascularizes the capillary plexus surrounding the alveoli with venous blood from the right ventricle. The close structural and functional parallelism between this blood stream and the tubular airway system is important to realize when possible infection routes in the lungs have to be interpreted. The supporting structures around the trachea, bronchi, and bronchioli and even the wall of the arteria pulmonalis are vascularized with blood from the arteria bronchialis tree.

Tubular Tract System

The nasal cavity is divided longitudinally by a wall (septum nasi). Two turbinate bones divide each of the two halves of the cavity into three meatuses: dorsal, middle, and ventral (Figure 7.1). The length of the nasal cavity varies between different breeds. The trachea is relatively short and divides posteriorly into two principal bronchi, one for the left and one for the right lung (Figure 7.2). A special stembronchus branches from the trachea leading to the apical lobe of the right lung. The right principal bronchus sends a stembronchus to the right cardiac lobe and another to the intermediate lobe and then continues until it ramifies into the diaphragmatic lobe. The left principal bronchus gives off a stembronchus that divides into one branch for the apical lobe and one for the cardiac lobe. The principal bronchus then continues posteriorly in the diaphragmatic lobe. The finest branches of the tubular system are the bronchioli, each dividing into alveolar ducts and alveoli.

The vestibular region of the nasal cavity is lined with stratified squamous epithelium. Posteriorly, the epithelium changes from stratified columnar to ciliated pseudostratified epithelium with goblet cells (respiratory epithelium). The respiratory epithelium is covered by mucus produced by the goblet cells and this type of epithelium continues through the respiratory section of the pharynx, larynx, trachea, and bronchi. As the bronchioli approach the alveoli, the epithelium is reduced in height, becoming squamous. Sections of the bronchioli (called *respiratory bronchioli*) and the walls of the alveoli are covered by very flat, single-layered epithelial cells (type I alveolar cells) and by a small percentage of cuboidal epithelial cells (type II alveolar cells). Type II alveolar cells produce pulmonary surfactant and serve as progenitor cells for replacement and turnover of type I alveolar cells. The alveolic wall is very intimately attached to the capillary plexus of the pulmonary blood circulaton.

Gross Appearance of the Lung

In the pig the lungs are divided by deep fissures into seven lobes: the right lung comprises the apical, cardiac, diaphragmatic, and intermediate lobes; the left lung comprises the apical, cardiac, and diaphragmatic lobes (refer to Figure 7.2). The left apical and cardiac lobes are not separated by a fissure but only by the cardiac notch.

149

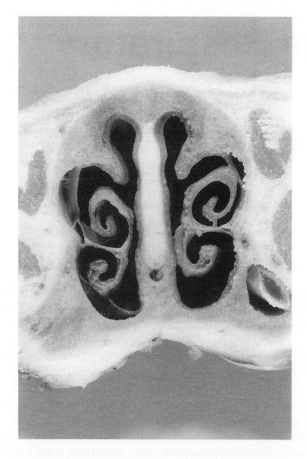

7.1. Transverse section of nasal structures.

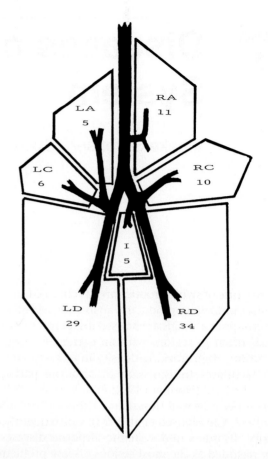

7.2. Schematic outline of lung lobulation and branching of the bronchus tree. LA, RA: left and right apical lobes; LC, RC: left and right cardiac lobes; LD, RD: left and right diaphragmatic lobes; I: intermediate lobe. Numbers = relative lobe weights as percentage of total lung weight based on a study by G. Christensen (unpublished data).

The lobes are subdivided by solid interlobular septa into lobuli. Pathological processes, therefore, often will be retained within lobular structures, typically seen in catarrhal bronchopneumonia as sharp demarcated limits between normal and affected tissue.

When assessing the extent of lung lesions it is necessary to know the relative size or weight of each lobe. Table 7.1 shows the relative weights of the lung lobes as percentages of the total lung weight, as determined in three different studies. The right lung contributes more than half of the total lung weight, with small differences between the investigations. The variations might be caused partly by different average live weights of the animals examined. The animals in study C had a lower average live weight (90 kg) than those in study A (100 kg)

and study B. The difference between the weight of the two lung halves tended to be greater in animals of lower slaughter weight.

FUNCTION OF THE NORMAL RESPIRATORY SYSTEM

The vital gaseous exchange between inhaled air and venous blood from the pulmonary artery takes place at the alveolar level. Each breath renews only a minor part of the total alveolar air volume. In the resting pig, 10–15% of the alveolar air is exchanged per inspiration. The nor-

Table 7.1.   Relative weights of lung lobes as percentages of total lung weight.

| Study | N | Left Lung Lobes | | | Right Lung Lobes | | | |
		Apical	Cardiac	Diaphr.	Apical	Cardiac	Diaphr.	Interm.
A	11	7	7	32	12	8	30	5
B	20	5	7	32	6	9	36	5
C	13	5	6	29	11	10	34	5

Note: A = Morrison et al. (1985) (rounding of numbers caused a total percentage of 101%); B = Heilmann et al. (1988); C = G. Christensen, unpublished data. N = number of pigs examined in each study.

mal respiratory rate (breaths/minute) varies according to age of the animal (piglets and growing pigs, 25–40; finishing pigs, 25–35; sows in gestation, 15–20).

Defense Mechanisms of the Respiratory System

The mucosal surface of the respiratory tract provides a critical interface between the pig and its environment. While the skin is well adapted to prevent invasion of potentially harmful agents and has a limited surface area (about 1.8 m^2 in humans), the epithelial surface of the respiratory tract primarily serves as a diffusion membrane. The gaseous exchange requires a very large surface (in humans more than 100 m^2). Thus, it is understandable that the respiratory tract must be equipped with a potent and specialized defense apparatus. The most important components of the respiratory defense are listed in Table 7.2.

The nasal cavity is designed to remove large particles trapped by hairs in the nostrils and deposited by gravity in the mucus by the eddy currents around the conchal structures. Another function of the nasal cavity with its immense venous sinusoids and wet surfaces is humidification and warming of the air before it reaches the lower airways.

Most inspired particles are trapped in the epithelial mucus of the nasal, pharyngeal, laryngeal, and tracheal cavities. From many experiments it is known that only particles below an aerodynamic diameter of 5 µm (the respirable fraction) are able to reach and settle at the alveolar level. Particles of an aerodynamic diameter greater than 10 µm almost entirely settle before reaching the branches of the bronchial tree (Baskerville 1981).

Mucociliary Defense. Particles trapped in the epithelial mucus are handled by the mucociliary clearance mechanism. The ciliary carpet in the bronchi and bronchioli gives rise to a continuous flow of mucus toward the pharynx. The rhythmic beating of cilia results in a mucus flow of about 4–15 mm/minute (Done 1988). Like the mucus from the nasal cavity, it is delivered to the pharyngeal cavity and subsequently swallowed.

Phagocytes. Alveolar macrophages neutralize foreign material that escapes the mucociliary defense mechanism. Nonpathogenic particles and microbes are handled by simple phagocytic activity and are removed in the mucus flow or by the lymphatic system. Pathogenic microorganisms are neutralized with aid of secretions such as lysozyme, interferons, opsonins, lactoferrins, complement factors, and specific immunoglobulins in the mucus. If the invading agents are not neutralized by the alveolar macrophages, inflammation will occur. Neutrophils from the blood will then invade the alveolus and assist the macrophages in the phagocytic activity. In healthy pigs the normal ratio between the cellular elements in the bronchoalveolar mucus is 70–80%

Table 7.2. Respiratory system defense components.

Physical/Chemical
  Hairs in nostrils
  Structure of the nasal cavity
  Structure of mucosa
  Properties of mucus (physical and chemical—e.g., adhesiveness, nonspecific lysozymes, interferons, opsonins, lactoferrins, complement factors, specific immunoglobulins)
  Humoral components (mucus contents and multiple types of immune modulators—e.g., lymphokines)
Cellular
  Phagocytes (alveolar macrophages, vascular macrophages, histiocytes, monocytes, neutrophils, eosinophils)
  Bone marrow-derived B lymphocytes (plasma cells)
  Thymus-derived T lymphocytes (helper lymphocytes, suppressor lymphocytes, cytotoxic lymphocytes [natural killer cells])

alveolar macrophages, 11–18% lymphocytes, 8–12% neutrophils, and up to 5% eosinophilic granulocytes (Neumann et al. 1985). The phagocytic cell system also comprises intravascular macrophages, which in the pig are particularly numerous (Bertram 1985; Ohgami et al. 1989) in the lung, and histiocytes with phagocytic properties in the connective tissue.

The activity of the phagocytes is highly accelerated if introduced pathogens are not quickly eliminated or if pathogens are recognized from previous infections. A complex immune response is activated by stimulation of the cell-mediated immune system, followed by local and systemic production of specific antibodies (immunoglobulins—Ig).

Immunoglobulins. The production of specific antibodies is of crucial importance in the respiratory immune defense. Their biological function is neutralization of pathogens by generating antigen-antibody complexes.

The predominant antibodies in mucus are of the IgA type and a secretory component takes part in the secretion. IgM antibodies are potent proteins released in the early immune response, particularly in the newborn pig. IgG originating from blood serum form the greater part of the immunoglobulins in mucus of the lower respiratory tract near the alveoli. Immunoglobulins in the mucus carpet act primarily to prevent the initial establishment and penetration of pathogens. IgE are generated in the immune response against parasites, for example, lungworm (*Metastrongylus* sp.) and migrating ascarid larvae.

Cell-Mediated Immune Response. Traditionally, immunity is divided into a humoral immune response, in which the immunoglobulins play an essential role, and a cell-mediated immune response based on antibody-independent components. Today it is realized that immunity cannot be distinctly separated into these two parts, because many mechanisms and elements are closely linked.

Generally, cell-mediated immunity is identified with: cytotoxic T cells, natural killer cells, activated macrophages, and cells mediating antibody-dependent cytotoxicity. The cell-mediated immune response is assumed to be of special importance in viral infections such as influenza, PRRS, PCV2 and Aujeszky's disease, but is also assumed to play an important role in *Mycoplasma hyopneumoiae* infection.

Surface proteins belonging to the swine leukocyte antigen (SLA) gene complex (major histocompatibility gene complex [MHC]) play a significant role in the cellular, as well as the humoral, immune response. Rothschild et al. (1984) demonstrated that the SLA complex was associated with immune response following vaccination with *Bordetella bronchiseptica,* and Mallard et al. (1989) showed differences in serum IgG concentrations in different SLA haplotypes, indicating that selection for increased serum IgG would be possible. Genetic variability of the SLA complex has been demonstrated in different breeds of pigs (Vaiman et al. 1979).

Since placenta of pregnant sows are impermeable to immunoglobulin passage, the neonates are born without antibodies. Although immunocompetent, the piglets are unable to rapidly develop an active immune response to protect them against respiratory diseases. Thus, their survival depends upon the passive acquisition of maternal immunity including at least three components:

- A systemic humoral immunity, transmitted through colostrum
- A local humoral immunity transmitted through milk
- A cellular immunity transmitted via maternal immunocompetent cells present in mammary secretions (Salmon 2000)

Like lambs, piglets are capable of intestinal absorption of intact immunocompetent maternal lymphocytes from colostrum, but only from their own mother (Tuboly et al. 1988; Tuboly and Bernath 2002). Williams (1993) showed the distribution of such cells to liver, lung, lymph nodes, spleen, and gastrointestinal tissue of the piglets by 24 hours postfeeding. Blecha et al. (1983) found that the capability of lymphocytes to undergo blastogenesis was decreased in pigs weaned at 2 and 3 weeks of age and suppressed in pigs weaned at 4 weeks of age. Their data suggested that weaning pigs younger than 5 weeks old causes physiological changes detrimental to cellular immune reactivity, which could alter disease susceptibility in piglets. This information may be useful when managing the farrowing units, where random distribution of piglets between sows and early weaning may contribute to decreased resistance against respiratory infections before as well as after weaning.

Transepithelial passage from the lumen of the respiratory tract into the blood of antigenically intact macromolecules can take place during the first days of life and also to a considerable degree in older pigs (Folkesson et al. 1990). This indicates future possibilities for aerosol-based vaccines against respiratory diseases. Vaccination experiments with Aujeszky's disease in young piglets with passively acquired antibodies indicate that the systemic immune mechanism can be bypassed and a local immune response obtained by application of antigen on the respiratory epithelium (Schlesinger et al. 1990). Nielsen et al. (1990) obtained good immunological protection against *Actinobacillus pleuropneumoniae* with local application of antigens in the respiratory tract.

RESPIRATORY DISORDERS

Under commercial conditions few pigs can be expected to reach slaughter weight without contracting some sort of respiratory lesion. Pathologic alterations can be categorized into three main disease entities: rhinitis, pneumonia, and pleuritis. Detailed characterizations of microscopic and gross pathologies of the individual diseases will be given in other chapters. However, some general features of pathology will be presented here.

Rhinitis

Catarrhal inflammation of the nasal mucosa is common in young animals. The cause is often infectious (Aujeszky's disease virus, cytomegalovirus, *B. bronchiseptica, Mycoplasma hyorhinis*), but ammonia and dust in the air as well as foreign bodies can also provoke mild mucosal inflammation of short duration. However, if toxigenic strains of *Pasteurella multocida* are present, even a slightly damaged mucosa might promote adherence and proliferation of the bacteria and subsequently provoke progressive atrophic rhinitis with permanent alteration of the nasal structure and function. The structural changes in atrophic rhinitis are fundamentally induced by an altered bone metabolic process without inflammation of tissue (Foged et al. 1987).

Pneumonia

Bronchopneumonia. Catarrhal bronchopneumonia, located cranioventrally, is a frequent lesion of the lung in growing pigs. Since M. hyopneumoniae generally is involved, such lesions are often given the term mycoplasmal or mycoplasma-like pneumonia. Noncomplicated mycoplasmal pneumonia typically appears as confluent, purple consolidation, more collapsed than normal lung tissue. Early lesions may be somewhat indistinct, but after 2–3 weeks the lesions are clearly demarcated from adjacent normal tissue by a sharp line following the interlobular septa. When incised, the consistency is "meaty" but not excessively firm. Catarrhal exudate may be expressed from the airway openings of affected tissue. Fissures regularly appear in lobes previously affected with catarrhal bronchopneumonia (Bertschinger et al. 1972).

Lesions with secondary bacterial infections may

change to a more grayish color, and the consistency will be firmer due to formation of fibrous tissue. Further, complicated bronchopneumonia due to secondary bacterial infection usually results in purulent bronchitis or abscess formation. Severe cases may also present pleuritis with adhesion to the thoracic wall.

Fibrinous/Necrotizing Pneumonia. Another common pathological entity of the lung is fibrinous/necrotizing pneumonia, which affects the dorsocaudal portions of the organ in contrast to the cranioventrally located catarrhal or mucopurulent bronchopneumonia. Affected tissue is frequently raised above the adjacent area and crosses interlobular septae, unlike catarrhal bronchopneumonia. Fibrinous/necrotizing pneumonia is often called pleuropneumonia since the pleural surface of affected lung tissue is involved in nearly all cases. In the acute state the inflamed pleural surface is covered with fibrinous exudate. In subacute/chronic cases the associated pleural lesion consists of fibrous tissue, often resulting in firm adherence of the lung to the chest wall.

Interstitial Pneumonia. Interstitial pneumonia is a condition where the inflammatory processes primarily involve the alveolar walls and interstitial tissue, in contrast to bronchopneumonia, where inflammation principally affects the finest branches of bronchioles (the bronchioloalveolar junctions). Also, in contrast to bronchopneumonia, interstitial pneumonia is widely distributed throughout the lung. Interstitial pneumonia is most often caused by viral infections.

Embolic Pneumonia. Embolic pneumonia is caused by hematogenically disseminated agents, mostly pyogenic bacteria from lesions somewhere else in the body. Typically this type of pneumonia starts as minute necrotic foci surrounded by a hemorrhagic zone. Usually suppuration of the centers follows and circumscribed abscesses are formed. A secondary bronchopneumonia or a pleuropneumonia-like inflammation may develop around the primary process. Verminous migration through lung tissue induces small hemorrhagic foci, small abscesses, or firm granulomas. The verminous processes are mainly located dorsocaudally in the lung.

Lesion Distribution Patterns. Cranioventral distribution of mycoplasmal and most other bronchopneumonias might be due to less effective defense mechanisms in this region. This assumption is supported by the fact that *Pasteurella hemolytica* causes pneumonia in this region even if the bacteria reach the lung via the blood (Dungworth 1993). Gravitational influence impeding clearance, leading to pooling or reflux of secretions, is probably a contributing factor.

Experimentally, inhaled aerosolized suspensions of *Bacillus subtilis*, *A. pleuropneumoniae* (Sebunya et al. 1983), and *Staphylococcus aureus* (Kastner and Mehlhorn

1989) are deposited primarily in the caudal lobes. This accords with the fact that *A. pleuropneumoniae*–induced pleuropneumonia is predominantly localized dorsocaudally. In another investigation, inhalation of an aerosolized suspension of radioactively labeled *P. multocida* resulted in a relatively uniform deposition in the lung lobes (Heilmann et al. 1988).

Usually, pneumonic lesions due to hematogenically introduced pyogenic bacteria have a random distribution pattern, which makes them easily distinguishable from lesions due to bronchogenically disseminated bacteria (Buttenschøn 1989). Verminous lung lesions have a caudodorsal location in spite of the assumption that the larvae are introduced via the bloodstream. However, some extravascular migration through the diaphragm might take place (Buttenschøn 1990).

Since chronic pleuritis almost always is associated with a present or, more often, a previous inflammation of lung tissue, the localization of pleuritic lesions is of diagnostic value in determining the type of pneumonia involved.

Healing of Pneumonia. The healing of catarrhal bronchopneumonia is a rather slow process requiring several weeks or months. However, the healing period depends greatly on the agents involved. In specific pathogen free (SPF) pigs inoculated with *M. hyopneumoniae*, induced pneumonic lesions were healed after 2 months, whereas fissuring of the lung persisted for more than 3 months (Bertschinger et al. 1972; Kobisch et al. 1993; Sørensen et al. 1997). By comparing the time of seroconversion with lung lesions at slaughter, Wallgren et al. (1994) estimated the duration of active mycoplasmal lesions to be approximately 12 weeks, and Pattison (1956) still found pneumonic lesions 25 weeks after inoculation with *M. hyopneumoniae*, presumably due to secondary bacterial infection. Unlike catarrhal bronchopneumonia, the interval between appearance and disappearance of *A. pleuropneumoniae*-induced fibrinous/necrotizing pneumonia may be surprisingly short (about 3 weeks) if not complicated with secondary pyogenic infections. This is in accordance with Andreasen et al. (2001) and Wallgren et al. (1994) who found no correlation between seroconversion to *A. pleuropneumonia* and lesions at slaughter. Seroconversion to *M. hyopneumoiae* close to slaughter revealed the largest extent of mycoplasma-like bronchopneumonia and early seroconversion was related to ventrocranial pleuritic lesions. However, infections gained during the early fattening period will generally escape detection at slaughter.

Pleuritis

Fibrotic adherence between the visceral and pleural membranes of the pleural sac (chronic pleuritis, pleural scar) is one of the most frequent pathologic alterations seen in slaughter swine. Fibrous pleuritis affecting larger areas is often associated with similar lesions in the pericardial sac (chronic pericarditis). The repairing of such lesions is a long process, with a duration of at least 1 month, more often 2–3 months (Christensen 1984). The resolving of chronic pleuritis in growing pigs may cause younger fatteners to have a higher frequency of this lesion than older pigs (Mousing 1988). In an investigation of infectious and herd-related factors by logistic regression Enoe et al. (2002) found that seropositivity for *A. pleuropneumoniae* serotype 2 and *M. hyopneumoniae* in conventional herds were associated with 51% and 29% of the occurrence of chronic pleuritis at slaughter, respectively. In SPF herds reinfected with *M. hyopneumoniae*, seropositivity for *M. hyopneumoniae* was associated with 33% of the occurrence of chronic pleuritis detected at slaughter.

CAUSAL FACTORS IN RESPIRATORY DISEASE

General Epidemiologic Considerations

Respiratory disease must be seen as the result of a complexity of events, including infectious, environmental, managemental, and genetic factors. Because the etiology of respiratory disease is multifactorial, one should consider not just specific infectious agent, but other relevant factors as well.

A given pathogen or environmental risk factor will tend to increase the incidence of disease. In quantifying this increase, the ratio between the incidence (or prevalence) among pigs exposed to the factor and the incidence (or prevalence) among pigs that are not exposed can be calculated. This ratio is most often referred to as the relative risk. The higher the relative risk, the stronger the association between the risk factor and disease. When two or more risk factors act simultaneously, the total relative risk will often be greater than the relative risk of the individual factors (Mousing et al. 1990).

Relative risks have to be evaluated with caution, for such associations may be confounded by other factors. Several epidemiologic studies have indicated a positive correlation between herd prevalence of pigs with pneumonia and atrophic rhinitis. This association obviously relies on the fact that the two disease entities are provoked by the same external factors, and not that one disease predisposes to the other. In fact, there was no evidence that animals suffering from one of the diseases were more susceptible to the other when correlation studies included individuals in the same herd (Madec and Kobisch 1984; Straw 1986).

Infection

Respiratory infections occur with a high prevalence in all swine-producing areas (Table 7.3). The spread of respiratory diseases from herd to herd involves two distinct mechanisms. First, like other infections, disease may be disseminated through infectious contacts (purchase of pigs, incoming and outgoing vehicles, birds, rodents, persons, etc.). Second and very important, several respiratory diseases also propagate from herd to herd by means of airborne transmission. The virus causing PRRS can be introduced into a herd with semen (Swenson et al. 1994; Gradil et al. 1996).

Airborne Transmission of Respiratory Diseases Between Herds. Respiratory infections in swine with the capability of airborne transmission over distances up to several kilometers include *M. hyopneumoniae* (Goodwin 1985; Jorsal and Thomsen 1988; Stark et al. 1992;) and porcine respiratory coronavirus (PRCV) (Henningsen et al. 1988). Systemic viral infections such as foot-and-mouth disease (Gloster et al 2003), PRRS (Mortensen et al. 2002) and Aujeszky's disease (Mortensen et al. 1990) follow this pattern. Airborne transmission between small pig units at close range has been induced experimentally with PRRSV, *A. pleuropneumoniae* and *B. bronchiseptica* (Torremorell et al. 1997; Brockmeier and Lager 2002; Kristensen et al. 2004a, b). However, airborne transmission of bacterial infections between herds has still to be documented. The typical pattern of simultaneous influenza outbreaks in many herds is highly suggestive of the airborne transmission of this infection. In Danish epidemics, even though special precautions are taken against introduction of infectious diseases, SPF herds are attacked by influenza just as frequently as conventional neighboring herds. Epidemics in Brittany also seem to follow an airborne transmission (Madec et al. 1982). Table 7.4 lists factors affecting the risk of a herd receiving an airborne infection.

Airborne spread of disease between herds is facilitated by several meteorological factors—most significantly, the direction and velocity of the prevailing winds. Factors such as cloud cover, turbulence, and topography are also important. Overcast skies, night (when the turbulence is often low), and relative humidity of more than 90% (Gloster et al. 1981) facilitate airborne transmission.

Respiratory Infection in Individuals and in Herds. The upper respiratory tract is the natural habitat for myriads of commensal microorganisms, including viruses, mycoplasmas, chlamydias, and other bacteria. The commensal flora may have a favorable competitive effect for their host in outnumbering pathogenic agents. There is no distinct division between commensals and potentially pathogenic microorganisms. Different studies categorize the same microorganism as either commensal or potentially pathogenic. For example, *Mycoplasma flocculare*, *M. hyorhinis*, and *Haemophilus parasuis* belong to a group of microorganisms that can regularly be isolated in the upper respiratory tract and in the bronchial tree of healthy pigs.

Ganter et al. (1990) examined the bacterial flora in live, healthy, 20–30 kg SPF pigs. The bacteria normally found by alveolar lavage belonged to two or three

Table 7.3. The prevalence of some respiratory infections of swine.

Etiologic Agent	Prevalence (%)	Identification	Area
	Positive pigs within affected herds		
Actinobacillus pleuropneumoniae			
Serotype 2	76	se	Denmark[1,9]
Serotype 6	41	se	Denmark[1,9]
Serotype 7	43	se	Denmark[9]
Serotype 12	20	se	Denmark[9]
Swine influenza virus			
H1N1	71–82	se	France[2]
H1N1	75	se	Denmark[9]
H3N2	29–48	se	France[2]
Toxigenic *Pasteurella multocida*	30–50	cu	United Kingdom[3]
	35	se	Germany[4]
Mycoplasma hyopneumoniae	80–90	se	Sweden[5]
	37	cu	Austria[6]
	89	se	Denmark[9]
Haemophilus parasuis	56	se	Denmark[1,9]
	Positive herds		
Actinobacillus pleuropneumoniae			
Serotype 2	24	se	Norway[7]
	84	se	Finland[8]
	41	se	Denmark[1,9]
Serotype 6	29	se	Denmark[9]
Serotypes 1–5	69	se	Iowa[10]
Serotypes 1,3,5,7 or 9	86	se	Minnesota[11]
	23	cl	Ontario[12]
Serotype 7	55	se	Denmark[9]
Serotype 12	36	se	Denmark[9]
Swine influenza virus H1N1	71	se	Denmark[1,9]
Toxigenic *Pasteurella multocida*	11	cl	Missouri[13]
	7	cl	Australia[14]
Mycoplasma hyopneumoniae	85	cl	Australia[14]
	82	se	Denmark[1,9]
	39	se	Finland[15]
Haemophilus parasuis	70	se	Denmark[1,9]

Note: se = serological method; cu = culturing was employed; cl = clinical signs corresponding to the infection were observed.
[1]Mousing et al. (1990).
[2]Madec et al. (1990) (covering 1984, 1985, and 1988).
[3]Goodwin et al. (1990).
[4]Bechmann and Schöss (1990).
[5]Wallgren et al. (1990).
[6]Awad-Masalmeh et al. (1990).
[7]Falk et al. (1990).
[8]Levonen et al. (1994).
[9]Enøe et al. (2002).
[10]Schultz et al. (1982).
[11]Anderson et al. (1990).
[12]Rosendal and Mitchell (1983).
[13]Kliebenstein et al. (1982, 1983).
[14]Mercy and Brennan (1988).
[15]Rautiainen (2001).

species, most often streptococci (nonhemolytic, alpha-hemolytic), staphylococci, *Escherichia coli*, *Klebsiella*, and *Arcanobacterium pyogenes*. *Haemophilus parasuis* and *B. bronchiseptica* were rarely isolated, and *P. multocida* was never isolated in the bronchial tree of healthy pigs. *Haemophilus parasuis* and *M. hyorhinis* were detected in bronchial lavage from about 40% of conventionally reared healthy pigs (Castryck et al. 1990). Møller and Kilian (1990) found that the porcine upper respiratory tract harbors a much wider spectrum of V factor–dependent *pasteurellaceae* species than hitherto recognized, probably with no or low pathogenicity.

Haemophilus parasuis and *M. hyorhinis* behave as commensals only as long as their pathogenicity is neutralized by the respiratory defense. In nonimmune individuals *H. parasuis* (Nielsen and Danielsen 1975) and to some extent *M. hyorhinis* may become pathogenic, resulting in severe systemic disease (polyserositis, polysynovitis, meningitis). Maintenance of the fine balance between animal population and pathogens evidently re-

Table 7.4. Important herd-related factors that increase the risk of airborne disease transmission between herds.

Factor	Disease
Increasing herd size	Porcine respiratory corona virus (PRCV)[1]; Aujeszky's disease[2,3]
Short distance between herds	*Mycoplasma hyopneumoniae*[4,5]; PRCV[1]
Large size of neighboring herd	*Mycoplasma hyopneumoniae*[4,5]; PRCV[1]
High regional pig density	*Mycoplasma hyopneumoniae*[5]
Herd infected with *Actinobacillus pleuropneumoniae*	Aujeszky's disease[3]

[1]Flori et al. (1995).
[2]Mortensen et al. (1990).
[3]Anderson et al. (1990).
[4]Jorsal and Thomsen (1988).
[5]Stark et al. (1992).

quires that all the pigs are exposed to the pathogens in question in early life. Outbreaks appear under circumstances where the normal infection mechanism does not work properly because of restricted contact between individuals—for example, in small herds, in herds with very early weaning or strict separation between animals of different ages, and in SPF herds established originally from cesarean-derived piglets (Nielsen and Danielsen 1975; Smart et al. 1989).

Actinobacillus pleuropneumoniae and *M. hyopneumoniae* can be regarded as representatives of a different type of respiratory microorganisms: they may be common at herd level but are relatively seldom isolated from healthy individuals (Friis 1974; Castryck et al. 1990). Their presence is usually associated with disease, subclinical more often than clinical.

These two groups of microorganisms behave differently, especially in the immunologically weak state between passive and active immunity, for several reasons. First, *A. pleuropneumoniae* and *M. hyopneumoniae* have a higher pathogenicity than *H. parasuis* and *M. hyorhinis*.

Second and very important, it is known that *H. parasuis* and *M. hyorhinis* invade the nasal and tracheobronchial epithelium very early in the piglet's life (Ross 1984). This might facilitate a gradual development of active immunity under the cover of humoral colostral antibodies, a situation beneficial to host as well as to pathogen. A third reason is that the sites (pleural, pericardial, peritoneal, meningeal, articular serotic cavities) where the real pathogenic properties of *H. parasuis* and *M. hyorhinis* predominate are outside the respiratory tract. Here a clear physical barrier exists between the effector site and the residential site of the microorganism. In contrast, *A. pleuropneumoniae* and *M. hyopneumoniae* are easily brought to their point of attack with the inhaled air, directly from the environment or from the nasal and tonsillar epithelium.

Finally, the ability of strains with low pathogenicity to generate protective antibodies against closely related but more pathogenic strains, as demonstrated for *A. pleuropneumoniae* (Nielsen 1988), must be considered.

In conclusion, the constant presence of pathogens that cannot permanently be excluded from the herd

and that behave like *H. parasuis* and *M. hyorhinis* is acceptable for the herd. However, the presence of pathogens that behave like *A. pleuropneumoniae* and *M. hyopneumoniae* cause potential risk of recurrent disease.

The group of acceptable respiratory microorganisms includes species such as *Haemophilus* "minor group," *B. bronchiseptica*, staphylococci, streptococci, most strains of nontoxigenic *P. multocida*, and some strains of *A. pleuropneumoniae*. In contrast, the most pathogenic strains of *A. pleuropneumoniae* and *P. multocida* are highly disadvantageous because herd infections may give rise to episodes of respiratory problems.

Pasteurella multocida probably is the most frequent and damaging invader of the lung. However, this bacterium is a typical secondary invader (Amass et al. 1994). Even the most pathogenic strains are apparently not capable of infecting a healthy lung, unlike *A. pleuropneumoniae Bordetella bronchiseptica* induces only a discrete pneumonia in conventionally reared 7-day-old piglets (Lambotte et al. 1990), but in gnotobiotic piglets the infection causes severe and long-lasting pneumonia (Underdahl et al. 1982). *Bordetella bronchiseptica* is categorized as an acceptable microorganism, because like *P. multocida*, it is not easily kept out of herds due to the fact that several other animal species, including cats and dogs, are reservoirs.

Interaction Between Infectious Agents. Clinically significant disease seldom is the result of an infection with only one pathogen. Several pathogens are very often involved in respiratory disease. One pathogen acts as the key agent, the "door opener," for secondary invaders by lowering the local and sometimes also the systemic defense mechanisms of the host.

Generally, key agents are viruses or mycoplasmas, but secondary invaders are bacteria. For example, susceptibility in swine to *A. pleuropneumoniae* is increased following an influenza infection (Scatozza and Sidoli 1986), PRRS infection (Pol et al. 1997), or Aujeszky's disease (Lai et al. 1986). A similar effect was observed in experiments in mice infected first with influenza virus and subsequently with *A. pleuropneumoniae* (Bröring et al. 1989). Pigs infected with *M. hyopneumoniae* had a decreased resistance against *A. pleuropneumoniae* (Yagihashi et al. 1984), and in another study (Kubo et al. 1995) *M. hyorhinis* increased the severity of pulmonary lesions in piglets infected with PRRS virus. Van Reeth et al. (1994) found higher pathogenicity of a dual infection with influenza virus and PRRS virus than with infection with one of the viruses. Thacker et al. (1999) found that *M. hyopneumoniae* severely potentiated both clinical and pathological manifestations of disease induced by PRRS virus. When disease was induced by swine influenza virus, *M. hyopneumoniae* also potentiated the clinical manifestations, but to a lesser degree the pathological manifestations (Thacker et al. 2001). These findings demonstrate that the relationship between mycoplasmas and viruses varies with the individual agent. In the nasal cavity *B. bronchiseptica* frequently acts as a predisposing key agent facilitating the invasion and replication of toxigenic strains of *P. multocida* (Pedersen and Barfod 1981).

Lesions caused by key agents themselves are often faint and without clinical significance. It is well known from field experiences that influenza and Aujeszky's disease seldom are followed by severe pneumonic complications in herds where *A. pleuropneumoniae* and *M. hyopneumoniae* are absent (e.g., SPF herds), whereas serious respiratory complications regularly follow these viruses in other herds.

As a rule one pathogen intensifies the proliferation of another, but the reverse effect also can be demonstrated. In a cross-sectional seroepidemiological study, Mousing (1991) examined 4800 slaughter pigs for serological evidence of *A. pleuropneumoniae* serotype 2 and serotype 6, *H. parasuis* and swine influenza virus (type H1N1 with American and European variants). The interrelationship between these five respiratory infections is illustrated in Table 7.5, demonstrating the relative risk of confirming a specific infection when a pig also possesses antibodies against another agent.

Most infections appeared to be positively associated with *A. pleuropneumoniae* serotype 2, except for *A. pleuropneumoniae* serotype 6. The probable explanation is that *A. pleuropneumoniae* serotypes share antigens that provoke generation of cross-protecting antibodies (Nielsen 1988). The reverse effect was demonstrated for the two influenza variants.

The effect of an increasing number of infections on prevalence of chronic pleuritis is graphed in Figure 7.3. The prevalence of chronic pleuritis increases from 12.5% in pigs free from all of the five infections to more than 60% in pigs infected with four or all five of them.

Transmission of Infection Between Age Groups. Although the structure of modern pig production is rap-

Table 7.5. Interrelationship between some respiratory infections measured by odds ratio between seroreactions.

Infection A	Infection B			
	AP6	*H.par.*	H1N1(A)	H1N1(B)
AP2	0.4	1.3	1.3	1.5
AP6		(0.9)	(1.0)	0.9
H. par.			1.2	1.3
H1N1(A)				4.0

Source: Mousing (1991).

Note: AP2 = *Actinobacillus pleuropneumoniae* serotype 2; AP6 = *Actinobacillus pleuropneumoniae* serotype 6; *H. par.* = *Haemophilus parasuis*; H1N1(A) = Swine influenza virus A/Swine/New Jersey/8/76 (H1N1); H1N1(B) = Swine influenza virus A/Swine/Belgium/2/79 (H1N1). All infections assessed through individual serological examination of slaughter pigs. Numbers in parentheses are not statistically significant.

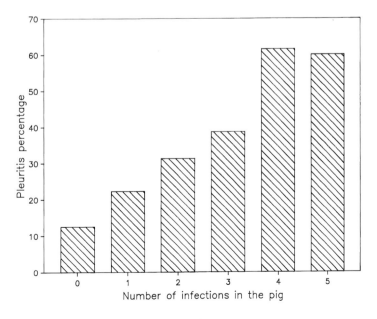

7.3. The prevalence of pleuritis in the presence of an increasing number of infections.

idly changing, preferably toward all-in/all-out and multi-site systems, farrow-to-finish operations still exist. With continuous flow of animals through the system a steady transmission of respiratory pathogens occurs from sows to piglets and, maybe more important, from older to younger pigs. Replication of respiratory pathogens may concentrate in the facilities for growing pigs, which act as "pathogen generators" in the herd. From here the breeding animals are periodically infected. This mechanism explains why it is simpler by far to control respiratory disease in breeding herds marketing all growers and feeders than in herds that also finish the pigs.

Origin of Pigs

The origin of introduced animals significantly influences the risk of the herd contracting respiratory diseases. It is evident that respiratory problems can be expected if pigs with low health status are introduced into a herd. However, there also is a risk when introducing animals with a high health status into herds with a lower health status without taking any precautions to protect the healthy animals against infection. Such animals, insufficiently protected by specific immunity, easily develop clinical disease. Consequently, a sudden rise in infection pressure occurs, and an established herd balance between infection and immunity is jeopardized.

In Danish SPF herds it is clearly illustrated that the risk of a herd contracting respiratory problems increases with the number of animal groups introduced and the number of different sources (Jorsal and Thomsen 1988). Castryck et al. (1990) made the same observation in Belgian conventional pig production systems. Awareness of the herd's status regarding respiratory pathogens and solely buying in breeding animals from a single herd with similar status can contribute to prevent outbreaks of respiratory disease. Establishment of quarantine facilities for introducing breeding animals can often be beneficial for maintaining the herd health status. Furthermore, it is important to keep a good biosecurity in order to prevent unwanted respiratory pathogens to enter the facilities by other routes.

Number of Individuals in Herd or Room

Most empirical epidemiologic studies have revealed that the risk of contracting respiratory disease increases significantly with increasing herd size, and also with the pig density in the vicinity of the herd (Aalund et al. 1976; Bäckström and Bremer 1976; Flesja and Solberg 1981; Mehlhorn and Hoy 1985; Jorsal and Thomsen 1988; Cubero et al. 1992; Stark et al. 1992; Christensen 1995; Goldberg et al. 2000; Maes et al. 2000; Enoe et al. 2002). The theoretical background of the herd size effect has been explained by Willeberg et al. (1994, 1995). Hartley et al. (1988a) and Tielen (1989) found no relationship between respiratory disease at slaughter and herd size, and Martinsson and Lundeheim (1988) found only weak relations. A very large herd might have a somewhat lower level of respiratory disease than one not quite so large (Willeberg et al. 1984/85; Martinsson and Lundeheim 1988). The probable explanation is that very large herd facilities must be subdivided and pigs moved into groups to control infectious diseases.

The number of animals placed in the same airspace significantly affects the incidence of disease. Experience from several investigations (Lindqvist 1974; Tielen et al. 1978; Pointon et al. 1985) indicates that respiratory problems are difficult to control if more than 200–300 animals are housed in the same barn; in the Netherlands housing only 80 fatteners together is advised (Tielen 1989).

Theoretically, for pigs sharing airspace, the risk of exchanging suspended particles increases substantially with increasing number of pigs ($n^2 - n$, where n = number of individuals). The same effect is seen when floor space per pig is decreased (Lindqvist 1974; Bäckström 1978; Mehlhorn and Hoy 1985; Pointon et al. 1985).

Climate

Goodall et al. (1993) combined data from abattoirs with meteorological data from Northern Ireland in 1969–1989 and found significant trends in the occurrence of condemnations due to pleurisy and pneumonia and also significant correlations between the percentage of condemnations and air temperature. In Belgium, Maes et al. (2001) found an increased prevalence of pleuritis at slaughter in January and more severe lesions when pigs were slaughtered in March to April. In Denmark, Bille et al. (1975) found a significantly higher incidence of pneumonia in piglets during the winter season than during the summer months. This indicates that climatic factors are included in the etiology of pneumonia.

A high exchange rate of air often causes local drafts and chilling of animals. As with humans, a sudden chilling by drafts predisposes pigs to respiratory infections. In weaned pigs subjected periodically to drafts, Scheepens (1996) reported a higher frequency of sneezing and coughing than in controls. Subjecting controls and pigs with atrophic rhinitis to similar climatic stress caused an 8-day difference in days to slaughter, compared to a 3-day difference in the two groups of pigs when not exposed to adverse climatic conditions. Flesja et al. (1982) found that solid-sided pens were associated with a reduction in incidence of pneumonia, presumably by preventing drafts and Maes et al. 2001 found that pigs raised in pens with slatted floors were at higher risk of contracting severe pneumonic lesions. According to Kelley (1980) cold drafts and wide temperature differentials stress the immune mechanisms, thus increasing susceptibility to disease. This is confirmed in weaner pigs, where exposure to cold drafts significantly reduced immune response (Scheepens et al. 1988). Prolonged cold stress in suckling piglets experimentally infected with *P. multocida* resulted in lowered levels of serum IgG, lowered phagocytic activity of the polymorphonuclear granulocytes, and delayed local cellular reaction in the lungs of some of the piglets compared with controls. However, the course of infection, the clinical response, and postmortem findings were not influenced by cold stress (Rafai et al. 1987).

Air Pollution

High concentrations of ammonia in the air may be detrimental to respiratory health. Ammonia in concentrations of 50–100 ppm particularly interferes with normal mucociliary function (Curtis et al. 1975a; Johannsen et al. 1987; Neumann et al. 1987). Under normal conditions the ammonia concentration in pig pens does not exceed 20 ppm. Clark et al. (1993) did not find that ammonia concentrations of 18 ppm influenced development of mycoplasmal pneumonia. Nevertheless, epidemiologic studies have revealed the highest incidence of respiratory disease in herds with the highest ammonia concentrations in the air (Pointon et al. 1985). Also, when pigs were given the choice of moving between fresh air and ammoniated air (100 ppm ammonia) they preferred the fresh air (Smith et al. 1996). Donham (1991) found several air contaminants—such as dust, ammonia, and microbes—to be correlated with pneumonia and pleuritis in swine and has proposed maximal safe concentrations on the basis of dose-response correlation to swine health and human health problems: dust 2.4 mg/m^3, ammonia 7 ppm, endotoxin 0.08 mg/m^3, total microbes 10^5 cfu/m^3, and carbon dioxide 1,540 ppm.

However, many investigations have failed to demonstrate significant relation between dust and respiratory disease (Martin and Willoughby 1972; Curtis et al. 1975b; Gilmour 1989; Jansen and Feddes 1995).

Enteritis

A high prevalence of respiratory lesions at slaughter was found in pigs previously experiencing enteritis (Aalund et al. 1976). A highly significant correlation was found between pigs that needed treatment for enteritis and pigs that were treated for pneumonia (Jørgensen 1988). Litters that shed rotavirus during the preweaning period had higher incidence rates of respiratory diseases than virus-free litters (Svensmark et al. 1989). Marois et al. (1989) demonstrated aggravation of experimentally induced mycoplasmal pneumonia in piglets also infected with transmissible gastroenteritis (TGE) virus. Digestive disorders seem to reduce resistance to pneumonia, and also some swine diseases, like postweaning multisystemic wasting syndrome (PMWS) (Allan and Ellis 2000), include both dyspnea and diarrhea in the symptoms.

Gender

From surveillance of slaughter swine at Danish abattoirs it has continuously been revealed that the prevalence of pneumonia and pleuritis in castrated males is 10% higher than in females. Furthermore, Andreasen et al. (2001) found that castrated males have larger pleuritic lesions than females at the time of slaughter. In the Netherlands lesions in lungs, pleura, and pericardium were also more prevalent in castrated males than in females (Kruijf and Welling 1988). Castration may have been responsible for the differences through stress and hormonal changes. Another explanation could be that male pigs grow faster and reach slaughter weight at a younger age than females, which may prevent lung lesions to be healed in males at the time of slaughter.

Heredity

Several investigations indicate that respiratory disorders are to some extent influenced by heredity. In genetically selected obese swine, the phagocytic functions of pulmonary alveolar macrophages were found significantly more effective than those from genetically selected lean swine. The difference was most pronounced during winter and spring months (Caruso and Jeska 1990). Clinical observations in a herd having purebred Hampshires and Yorkshires revealed a much lower level of respiratory diseases in Hampshire than Yorkshire pigs (Lundeheim and Tafvelin 1986). The same investigators examined 45,000 slaughter pigs consisting of Hampshire, Landrace, and Yorkshire crosses. The Hampshire crosses had a significantly lower incidence of pneumonia and pleuritis than the other crosses. The susceptibility to atrophic rhinitis is greater in Yorkshire pigs than in Landrace pigs (Lundeheim 1979; Smith 1983; Straw et al. 1983). Ruiz et al. (2002) provided evidence of different patterns of colonization of *Mycoplasma hyopneumoniae* between pigs sired by three different boars, suggesting a possible genetic effect.

DIAGNOSIS AND DIFFERENTIAL DIAGNOSIS OF RESPIRATORY DISEASE

Definitive diagnoses of respiratory diseases are based upon a combination of history, clinical observations, laboratory tests, and necropsies, including slaughter checks. A clinical diagnosis can only be tentative, since visible signs from the respiratory system may be the result of dysfunction of other organs. Also, pathological disorders of the respiratory system such as acute/subacute pleuropneumonia, chronic pneumonia, and pleuritis will often be without clinical signs or signs typical for respiratory disorders. Acute pleuropneumonia may be widespread in a herd before the disease is revealed at slaughter. Therefore, depression and decreased appetite in fatteners, often misinterpreted and attributed to bad feed, should remind the observer of the possibility of an outbreak of acute pleuropneumonia. Table 7.6 summarizes some principal respiratory disorders. The basic elements in the table are typical pathological-anatomical disease entities. Useful differential diagnostic facts concerning gross pathology, clinical signs, and agents involved are given for each disease entity leading

Table 7.6. Principal respiratory disorders, clinical signs, causative agents, and diagnosis.

Disease Based on Pathology	Important Clinical Signs	Causative Agents	Diagnosis
01 Rhinitis: possibly slight but reversible turbinate atrophy	Sneeze; nasal discharge; conjunctivitis	*Bordetella bronchiseptica*	Nasal swabs; cultivation
02 Progressive atrophic rhinitis: varying turbinate atrophy and nasal wall alteration	Sneeze; nasal discharge; tear tracks below eyes; occasional nasal bleeding; no or varying degree of brachygnathia and snout deviation	Toxigenic *Pasteurella multocida*; predisposing: *Bordetella bronchiseptica*, aerial ammonia, dry air	Necropsy; slaughter checks; nasal swabs; cultivation; ELISA; PCR
03 Catarrhal pneumonia (mycoplasma-like pneumonia): cranioventrally located; lobular; meaty structure	Hard nonproductive cough, particularly when pigs are forced to move; slight fever; slightly decreased appetite	*Mycoplasma hyopneumoniae*; *Mycoplasma hyorhinis*; streptococci, and other bacteria in piglets	Necropsy; slaughter checks; cultivation; immunohistochemistry (IHC); serology
04 Complicated bronchopneumonia (enzootic pneumonia): located as 03; mostly lobular; purulent exudate; eventual formation of abcesses; red to gray; firm fibrous structure; often associated with pleuritis	Productive cough particularly when pigs are forced to move; abdominal "thumping" respiration; periodically high fever; decreased appetite	As 03 + *Pasteurella multocida*, *Bordetella bronchiseptica*, streptococci, staphylococci, *Arcanobacterium pyogenes*, and others; *Salmonella choleraesuis* and viral infections may act as primary agents	As 03; virus detection
05 Disseminated/lobular catarrhal pneumonia: mainly cardiac and apical lobes; red to gray; firm, fibrous structure	Coughing, dyspnea	*Bordetella bronchiseptica*	Cultivation; history: usually in piglets younger than 3 weeks
06 Peracute fibrinous/necrotizing pneumonia (pleuropneumonia): extensive dissemination; associated with blood-tinged fluid in the pleural cavity; extensive fibrinous pleuritis	Depression; prostration; high fever; severe dyspnea, open mouth breathing; occasional blood-tinged foam from nose and mouth; dog-sitting or sternal recumbency	*Actinobacillus pleuropneumoniae*	Necropsy; cultivation; serotyping; PCR
07 Acute/subacute fibrinous/necrotizing pneumonia (pleuropneumonia): predominantly caudodorsal; fibrinous pleuritis	Varying depression; respiration normal to superficial; depressed coughing or no cough; normal to high temperature; decreased appetite	*Actinobacillus pleuropneumoniae*	Necropsy; cultivation; serotyping; PCR
08 Chronic necrotizing pneumonia (pleuropneumonia): located as 07; firm capsulated processes with necrosis and abscesses; local fibrous pleuritis	Slight depression; cough and decreased appetite if secondary infection occurs	*Actinobacillus pleuropneumoniae*; eventually secondary infection with pyogenic bacteria	Necropsy; slaughter checks; cultivation; serotyping; PCR; serology
09 Embolic pneumonia: randomly distributed usually minute abscesses in the lung	Usually no clinical signs from the respiratory system	Pyogenic bacteria; streptococci, staphylococci, *Arcanobacterium pyogenes* and others	Necropsy; slaughter checks; primary conditions causing septicemia
10 Acute disseminated lobular pneumonia: dark purple; bleeding from cuts; lobular emphysema and edema	Varying degree of depression; from no to hard cough; rapid, superficial respiration; fever; prostration; complete anorexia	Swine influenza virus	Virus isolation; PCR; IHC from nasal swabs or affected lung tissue; serology
11 Interstitial pneumonia: variable amount of tan and red mottling; increased amount of clear fluid in thoracic cavity	Varying degree of symptoms from subclinical to inappetence; fever and dyspnea; reproductive failure; suboptimal herd performance	Porcine reproductive and respiratory syndrome virus (PRRS virus); often complicated by other infections	Virus isolation from lung, lymph nodes or serum; PCR; IHC on lung tissue; serology
12 Interstitial pneumonia: often accompanied by other types of pneumonia; lymphadenopathy; enteritis; hepatitis; nephritis	Postweaning multisystemic wasting syndrome (PMWS): wasting; enlarged lymph nodes; dyspnea; diarrhea; pallor; jaundice	Porcine circovirus type 2 (PCV2); often complicated by other infections	Histopathology; detection of PCV2 and characteristic microscopic lesions in lymphatic and other tissues

Table 7.6. *(continued)*

Disease Based on Pathology	Important Clinical Signs	Causative Agents	Diagnosis
13 Verminous pneumonia: small focal areas with hemorrhage, later granulomas or capsulated abscesses	Cough with minimal other signs	*Ascaris suum* and other ascarids	Necropsy; slaughter checks; white spots in the liver
14 Verminous bronchitis: bronchitis, bronchiolitis in caudoventral margins of diaphragmatic lobes; atelectatic areas	Cough with minimal other signs	*Metastrongylus* sp.	Necropsy; history: access to dirt
15 Hemorrhagic pleuritis: associated with 06	As 06; no or depressed cough	As 06	Necropsy
16 Fibrinous pleuritis: associated with 07 or 04, occasionally with 09 and 10; also associated with Glasser's disease	As 07; if associated with Glasser's disease: lameness, central nervous signs	As 07, occasionally other bacteria	Necropsy; cultivation
17 Fibrous pleuritis	None	As 16	Necropsy; slaughter checks

to the diagnosis. Additionally, in Tables 7.7 and 7.8 differential diagnostic information can be found concerning disease entities usually associated with important respiratory signs such as sneezing and coughing.

Monitoring Respiratory Disease

The purpose of monitoring respiratory diseases is to transform observed phenomena in a swine population into numeric values suitable for analysis. Assessment of the level of disease and the effect of therapeutic or preventive measures can be obtained by monitoring disease levels at a point in time (prevalence) or during periods (incidence). Respiratory tract disease data include information collected in the herd, laboratory tests, and slaughter examinations. Large-scale data collection and evaluation on the respiratory health of slaughter swine are routinely carried out in some countries—for example, Finland (Rautiainen et al. 2001), Denmark (Willeberg et al. 1984/85; Mousing 1986), the Netherlands (Van der Valk et al. 1984), and Sweden (Bäckström and Bremer 1976).

Registrations in the Herd. Clinical observations, results of routine slaughter checks, and postmortem examinations of dead or euthanized animals are traditionally the basis for diagnosing and estimating the severity of respiratory disease. The clinical examination is of greatest value in acute outbreaks when fever and specific signs from the respiratory tract are observed. Conditions such as pleuropneumonia, chronic enzootic pneumonia, and pleuritis will often be without clinical signs; thus, a diagnosis based upon clinical observations always will be tentative.

The value of in-herd disease surveillance naturally increases with the quality and amount of objective information. In many situations valuable data can be

Table 7.7. Respiratory disease entities and agents associated with sneezing.

Disease	Agent
Rhinitis (only piglets)	*Bordetella bronchiseptica;* cytomegalovirus; hemagglutinating encephalomyelitis virus
Rhinitis	Dust; ammonia
Atrophic rhinitis	*Bordetella bronchiseptica* and toxigenic *Pasteurella multocida*
Aujeszky's disease	Aujeszky's disease virus

Table 7.8. Respiratory disease entities and agents associated with coughing.

Type of Coughing	Disease	Agent
Hard, nonproductive	Mycoplasmal-like pneumonia	*Mycoplasma hyopneumoniae*
	Acute disseminated lobular pneumonia	Influenza virus
Nonproductive	Disseminated pneumonia (only in piglets)	*Bordetella bronchiseptica*
	Glässer's disease	*Haemophilus parasuisaemophilus parasuis*
	Aujeszky's disease	Aujeszky's disease virus
Productive	Enzootic pneumonia	*Mycoplasma hyopneumoniae* and *Pasteurella multocida* and other species
	Chronic pleuropneumonia	*Actinobacillus pleuropneumoniae* with other infections
Depressed, productive	Cardiac insufficiency	
	Acute pleuropneumonia	*Actinobacillus pleuropneumoniae*

readily obtained by staff recordings, either continuously or during a defined period. Relevant data are number of deaths and treatments associated with respiratory problems, age or weight of affected animals, and performance records—for example, days to market (Pijoan and Leman 1986), daily weight gain or feed efficiency.

Clinical signs are difficult parameters to handle in quantifying a disease problem (Baadsgaard and Jorgensen 2003). Assessment of pneumonia levels through measurement of the amount of coughing has been proposed (Straw et al. 1986). However, in the field such procedures may be too laborious and time consuming.

Laboratory Tests. In recent years tremendous progress in biotechnology has accelerated the development of new, highly specific, and sensitive laboratory tests for respiratory diseases. Useful diagnostic data may be obtained from laboratory examinations made on blood samples, meat juice samples, colostrum or milk samples, nasal swabs, tonsil scrapings, and tissue. It is particularly advantageous to combine data from clinical and pathological examinations with laboratory test results in monitoring the health status of swine herds. For health surveillance, serological analyses are often performed on samples taken from the herds monthly or quarterly, but also samples taken at the abattoirs when the pigs are slaughtered may be used for the analyses. Blood samples are preferable, but often not convenient at the slaughterline, and meat juice samples taken when the carcasses are registered may be a good alternative (Wallgren and Persson 2000). For final verification in the herds, methods like cultivation, PCR, immunohistochemistry or antigen-ELISA, which detect the pathogen directly, may be applied. Here, special attention will be given to diagnostic methods suitable for large-scale monitoring purposes.

When laboratory assays are used for monitoring herd health status or to elucidate the infection dynamic, the sensitivity and specificity of the assays need to be known to interpret the results. These test characteristics are defined and listed for a number of diseases in Chapter 2.

Polymerase chain reaction (PCR) is a relatively new technique for detecting *M. hyopneumoniae* DNA in lungs, tracheobronchiolar washings, nasal swabs, and air (Mattsson et al. 1995; Blanchard et al. 1996; Sørensen et al. 1997; Stark et al. 1998; Verdin et al. 2000). This technique is not as time-consuming as traditional cultivation and can be applied for large-scale use and thereby for surveillance in health programs. Problems with the sensitivity of the PCR technique when using nasal swabs seem to be solved with the nested PCR (Calsamiglia et al. 1999; Kurth et al. 2002; Sibilia et al. 2004). Toxin-producing *P. multocida* can likewise be diagnosed by PCR on nasal and tonsillar swabs (Kamp et al. 1994). Furthermore, an ELISA based on monoclonal antibodies directed against the toxin of *P. multocida* is used on nasal

swabs for health surveillance of progressive atrophic rhinitis in swine herds (Foged et al. 1990).

Much effort has been put into developing PCR tests for direct identification of *A. pleuropneumoniae* in lungs and tonsils (Sirois et al. 1991; Hennessy et al. 1993; Gram et al. 1994, 1996), and in the last years such tests have been implemented for routine identification and serotyping (Fittipaldi et al. 2003; Jessing et al. 2003; Hussy et al. 2004). Three RTX-toxins have been shown to constitute important virulence factors for *A. pleuropneumoniae* infection (Frey 1995). Thus, these toxins might be interesting targets in the development of future diagnostic assays. Already, the hemolytic and cytolytic effects of these toxins form the basis of laboratory assays, and Nielsen et al. (2000) developed ELISAs detecting antibodies against them. However, these assays cannot be expected to be totally specific for *A. pleuropneumoniae* infections, because other bacteria like *Actinobacillus suis* produce similar, but not identical, toxins (Kamp et al. 1994). Schaller et al. (1999) found a fourth toxin, ApxIVA, which is excreted in vivo by all known serotypes of *A. pleuropneumoniae* and this toxin seems to be more species-specific.

A nested PCR for diagnosing PRRS virus in boar semen has proved to have a higher sensitivity than the traditionally used cultivation and is able to distinguish between U.S. and European viruses (Christopher-Hennings et al. 1995).

In the development of new serological assays, biotechnology is introduced in the form of monoclonal antibodies (MABs) against specific epitopes of the agents. MABs are used in blocking ELISAs to detect antibodies against *M. hyopneumoniae* (Feld et al. 1992; Le Potier et al. 1993), toxin-producing *P. multocida* (Foged et al. 1990), and *A. pleuropneumoniae* serotype 2 (Stenbaek and Schirmer 1994) and serotype 5 (Klausen et al. 1996). The *M. hyopneumoniae* ELISA (Feld et al. 1992) has high sensitivity and specificity and can be used on both serum and colostrum (Sørensen et al. 1992, 1993).

The serological *P. multocida* ELISA can also be used on both serum and colostrum. However, serological monitoring of progressive atrophic rhinitis in growing pigs is difficult because only a few of infected pigs seroconvert, and then only in a late stage of infection (Nielsen et al. 1991a). MABs used in serological assays for diagnosing *A. pleuropneumoniae* infections have not been successful so far, probably due to variations in the *A. pleuropneumoniae* strains, giving variable serological response in herds. Serotype-specific blocking ELISAs based on polyclonal antibodies directed against capsular polysaccharides seem more appropriate for *A. pleuropneumoniae* serodiagnosis (Nielsen et al. 1991, 1993; Klausen et al. 1996, 2001; Andresen et al. 2002) Also, serotype specific indirect ELISAs for *A. pleuropneumoniae* based on purified antigen have been used (Gottschalk et al. 1994, 1997; Klausen et al. 2002). For serological herd surveillance it often will be neccesary to analyze the samples for more than one serotype, and ELISAs with mixed antigens (Bosse et al. 1993; Grondahl-Hansen et al. 2003) can facilitate such measurements. Dreyfuss et al. (2004) developed an ELISA based upon recombinant ApxIV toxin for serological screening of all serotypes at one time. Furthermore, this ELISA is expected to give positive results only if the pigs are infected with *A. pleuropneumoniae,* because they do not respond to ApxIV after vaccination with the vaccines available for the time being.

Indirect ELISA (Albina et al. 1992), blocking ELISA (Houben et al. 1995), and immunoperoxidase monolayer assay (Wensvoort et al. 1991) are used for serological monitoring of PRRS infection at the herd level. Combinations of these methods are used in serological profiling of herds to distinguish between chronically and acutely PRRS-infected herds (Bøtner 1997).

For laboratory diagnosis of swine influenza, isolation of the virus in cell culture or embryonated chicken eggs and immunofluorescence on lung tissue are used. Hemagglutination-inhibition tests, which mainly measure antibodies against H-antigens (e.g., H1 and H3), are used for the serological analysis (Palmer et al. 1975).

In countries, where Aujeszky's disease has been eradicated and vaccination is not allowed, serological surveillance of the disease can be carried out using a polyclonal blocking ELISA (Sørensen and Lei 1986) that detects antibodies from both infected and vaccinated pigs. In countries where Aujeszky's disease is common, vaccination programs with vaccines lacking the gene-encoding glycoprotein E (formerly glycoprotein I) can be established, and serological differentiation between infected and vaccinated pigs is possible with an ELISA described by Van Oirschot et al. (1988).

Diagnosis of PMWS is based on a combination of clinical and pathological findings together with evidence of PCV 2 infection. As the etiology of this disease is not yet clearly understood there is no large scale laboratory assays available for the time being.

Examinations on Slaughter Swine. National herd health monitoring programs by means of slaughter inspection are designed for long-term surveillance of herd health. Concurrent and specific examinations on selected groups of swine can be obtained by slaughter checks. Slaughter checks can be a profitable supplementary tool in handling respiratory problems (Pijoan and Leman 1986; Schulz 1986) and are used routinely in the surveillance of the health state of SPF herds (Keller 1988).

Examining the Snout for Atrophic Rhinitis. Slaughter checks for atrophic rhinitis are usually performed by examining a transverse section of the snout. Optimal results are obtained if the cut is placed between premolar 1 and 2 (Martineau-Doizé et al. 1990). Several methods of scoring atrophic rhinitis have been used (Bendixen

1971; Straw et al. 1983; Bäckström et al. 1985). These methods are based on subjective and visual assessment of structures. Results from different slaughter checks should be compared with caution, as demonstrated by D'Allaire et al. (1988). Comparisons should be performed by the same experienced observer using the same scoring system.

A morphometric technique described by Collins et al. (1989) and modified by Gatlin et al. (1996) yielded highly reproducible results. The method is rather time-consuming and therefore of particular interest in experimental work. A rapid method using inspection of longitudinal snout sections may be performed at slaughter (Visser et al. 1988). However, mild cases of atrophic rhinitis can hardly be differentiated from normal cases by this method.

Examining Thoracic Organs (Plucks). Retrospective evaluations of respiratory health by means of slaughter checks are based on the presence of chronic lesions. As demonstrated by Noyes et al. (1988), the progression and regression of pneumonia in growing pigs are highly dependent on the type of pneumonia involved. Generally, infections with *M. hyopneumoniae* gained during the early fattening period cannot be detected macroscopically at slaughter (Wallgren et al. 1994).

Several investigators have described methods of recording enzootic pneumonia in slaughter checks (Morrison et al. 1985), whereas little interest has been given to recording other types of lesions. However, all significant pathological conditions, including cranioventral fissures, pleuritis, and pericarditis should be recorded and categorized according to type and extent.

A reasonable history of respiratory health can be revealed by means of slaughter check, but only if all significant pathologic conditions are included. Also, in estimating the effect of respiratory disease on weight gain, a detailed recording of lesions is important. In a study based on 1700 swine from five herds (Christensen and Mousing 1994) only a weak association was found between uncomplicated catarrhal bronchopneumonia and daily weight gain from weaning to slaughter. However, a significant association was established between daily weight gain and complicated bronchopneumonia, cranioventral fissures, chronic pleuritis, and pericarditis.

Careful slaughter checks of thoracic organs cannot normally be performed at the slaughter line. The material has to be transferred to an appropriate place for a thorough examination. Christensen (unpublished data) devised a method by which 50–100 plucks per hour can be examined per investigator. The extents of all lesions detected are sketched on a special form containing two schematic drawings of the lung (Figure 7.4, left). Lesions affecting lung tissue are marked on the upper drawing, and pleuritis on the lower drawing. The type of lesion is marked by a character indicating lesion category, other than mycoplasmal pneumonia or chronic pleuritis, one

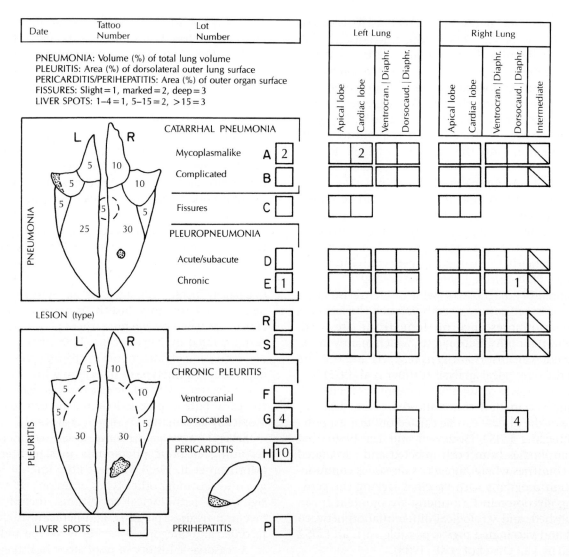

7.4. *Form for recording findings on plucks at slaughter check (left). Form for recording experimental data in slaughter check (right) (Christensen et al. 1999).*

of which occurs in almost 90% of all cases. Following macroscopic examination and sketching, the extent of the lesions is quantified and recorded using the marked lobe measures as guidelines. The recording form illustrated in Figure 7.4, right, is used when experimental studies require detailed data collection.

The result of a slaughter check is presented in Figure 7.5. Specially programmed personal computer software automatically executes the calculations and printing.

The localization of pleuritis is categorized as dorsocaudal or ventrocranial. The border is drawn through the dorsal endpoints of the interlobular fissures. The dorsal areas of the apical and cardiac lobes are regarded as belonging to the dorsocaudal lung surface area. Based on experience with Danish herds we consider dorsocaudally localized pleuritis as nearly pathognomonic for a previous pleuropneumonic lesion.

In most situations slaughter checks should be performed on at least 30 pigs (with similar or known age if possible) to get a sufficient sample and thus a reliable

picture of the herd problem (Morrison et al. 1985; Straw et al. 1989).

The use of a simplified slaughter check procedure based on right-lung examination has been reported by Mousing and Christensen (1993). The procedure interferes much less with normal slaughterhouse routines than a traditional slaughter check and demands fewer people.

CONTROL OF RESPIRATORY DISEASE

Pathogenic microorganisms are involved in all important respiratory disorders, and in practice it can be very difficult to protect pig herds from pathogenic microorganisms. Therefore, the in-herd incidence and prevalence of respiratory disease fundamentally depends on the balance between infection pressure and the pigs' ability to resist this pressure. This balance is fragile and highly affected by numerous factors.

Control of respiratory diseases at the herd level may be based on one of two principles: either to eliminate

```
                          SLAUGHTER CHECK—PLUCKS

Producer:_____                               Slaughter date: 07/03/90


                                                 Tattoo number: 11947

Clinic:   _____
                                                 Number of pigs examined:
                                                            39
```

Type of lesion		Pigs with lesion		Average extension/intensity of lesion
		number	%	
Catarrhal pneumonia, mycoplasmalike	**A**	30	76.9	5.4
Catarrhal pneumonia, complicated	**B**	1	2.6	3.0
Fissures in apical and cardiac lobes	**C**	4	10.3	0.5
Pleuropneumonia, acute/subacute	**D**	1	2.6	3.0
Pleuropneumonia, chronic	**E**	0	0.0	0.0
Chronic pleuritis, ventrocranial	**F**	3	7.7	10.7
Chronic pleuritis, dorsocaudal	**G**	4	10.3	8.7
Embolic pneumonia	**R**	1	2.6	1.0
	S	0	0.0	0.0
Chronic pericarditis	**H**	3	7.7	83.3
Chronic perihepatitis	**P**	0	0.0	0.0
Liver spots	**L**	0	0.0	0.0

```
Average extension of pneumonia: % of total lung vol
Average intensity of fissures: slight=1, marked=2, deep=3
Average extension of pleuritis: area % of outer lung surface
Average extension of pericarditis: area % of heart surface
Average intensity of liverspot: 1–4=1, 5–15=2, >15=3
```

ABC: lesions are often caused by *Mycoplasma hyopneumoniae*
DEG: lesions are often caused by *Actinobacillus pleuropneumoniae*

7.5. *Sample report of results of pluck examination at slaughter check (Christensen et al. 1999).*

pathogens from the herd or to diminish the infection pressure in the herd and simultaneously sustain the animal's defense mechanisms (nonspecific, immunological, and inherited). Elimination of pathogens is by far the most effective remedy in controlling many respiratory disorders. However, understanding of the etiology of respiratory diseases and the transmission route of the pathogens involved is of crucial importance for implementation of succesful reduction/eradication programs. Enzootic pneumonia is a good example of a respiratory disease where intensive research on *M. hyopneumoniae* has made eradication possible (Zimmermann et al. 1989), not only in single herds, but also in geographical areas (Rautiainen et al. 2001). However, in the recent years, the pig industry has struggled with new emerging diseases like PRRS and PMWS, which have increased the significance of respiratory diseases in many pig herds.

Much research has been performed worldwide on PRRS and effective eradication programs have been installed (Dee et al. 1997, 2001). The etiology of PMWS is still not clarified although porcine circovirus type 2 (PCV2) is part of the syndrome, and therefore eradication of this disease is not possible for the time being.

Elimination of Pathogens from the Herd

The United States, Denmark, and Switzerland have implemented specific pathogen free (SPF) pig production many years ago and thereby succesfully controlled respiratory diseases like enzootic pneumonia, pleuropneumonia, and progressive atrophic rhinitis. SPF pig production is principally based on a cesarean-derived and isolator-raised first generation of rather vulnerable breeding animals, which are gradually adapted to a very clean environment. The next generations of SPF pigs are born naturally, but kept and transported with strict biosecurity measures (Barfod 2004). Implementation of such a production system is therefore technically advanced, logistically laborious, and costly, but once established, economical and welfare related benefits from raising healthier pigs may be obtained.

Other methods for eliminating respiratory pathogens from herds include early weaning, strict separation of age groups of pigs, preferably on different geographical sites (multisite systems), removal of certain age groups of pigs, removal of infected individuals, and intensive herd medication. Such elements can be used together in different combinations.

Weaning at 1–3 weeks of age is recommended in segregated early weaning to minimize the risk of infection of piglets from the sow with pathogens like toxigenic *P. multocida*, *M. hyopneumoniae*, and *A. pleuropneumoniae*. Transmission of *M. hyopneumoniae* from sow to offspring was prevented without use of medication by weaning piglets at 7–10 days of age and segregating them off-site (Dritz et al. 1996). However, weaning at such young ages will not be accepted in several countries (Von Borell 1996). *Mycoplasma hyopneumoniae* was successfully eradicated from herds by removing pigs younger than 10 months from the herd and simultaneously stopping farrowings for 2 weeks (Zimmermann et al. 1989). *Actinobacillus pleuropneumoniae* was eliminated from piglets by medicated early weaning (Larsen et al. 1990a) and sometimes from infected herds by means of heavy medication and culling of seropositive animals (Larivière et al. 1990). However, in many countries heavy medication of animals is not accepted anymore in order to prevent problems with antimicrobial resistance. Atrophic rhinitis seems to be impossible to eliminate by medication programs alone (Larsen et al. 1990b), but intensive research and development of effective vaccines within the last decades have minimized the welfare—and economical problems caused by this disease.

PRRS can succesfully be controlled in well-immunized sow herds by nursery depopulation for 14 days (Dee et al. 1996), and Batista et al. (2002) found results indicating that persistence and shedding of PRRS virus are of short duration in breeding-age gilts, which may facilitate maintenance of immunity against PRRS in the sow units. Eradication programs for Aujeszky's disease in geographical areas can be carried out by test and slaughter (Andersen 1991) or by intensive vaccination (Stegeman et al. 1994a, b; Van Oirschot et al. 1996) or by combining the two methods (Leontides 1994).

To prevent reinfection of high-health herds with respiratory pathogens, strict control of brought-in pigs, vehicles, persons, etc., must be maintained. Nielsen and Frederiksen (1990) have demonstrated that human isolates of toxigenic *P. multocida* can induce progressive atrophic rhinitis in pigs, indicating that humans may act as carriers of swine pathogenic *Pasteurella* strains between herds.

Infection Pressure and Sustaining Herd Defense Mechanisms

The influence of several herd factors is decisive in sustaining herd resistance against respiratory pathogens and in reducing the level of such pathogens in the herd. Herd factors influencing the host/pathogen balance are numerous. In Table 7.9, examples of such factors are listed and arbitrarily weighted according to their importance. Short-term control measures against respiratory disease predominantly include correcting managerial factors such as vaccination and antibiotic treatment of sick animals, isolation arrangements, etc. Permanent improvement of respiratory health often requires more radical and expensive changes in production systems and housing. Important long-acting herd factors to take into consideration are stocking rate, flow of animals to

Table 7.9.   Herd factors with detrimental effects on respiratory system.

Factors	Degree of Effect
Production system	
Large herd size	+++
High stocking density	+++
Conventional health system (not SPF or minimal disease production system)	+++
Introduction of animals from herds with unknown or low health status	+++
Continuous flow of animals through facilities (no movement of pigs in batches)	+++
Use of genetically disposed breeds	+
Use of purebreds instead of crosses	+
Housing	
Badly insulated and ventilated facilities (causing improper temperature regulation and air exchange, drafts)	+++
Insufficiently divided facilities combined with housing of differently aged animals in same airspace	+++
Pens divided without solid separations	+++
Large grower or finishing rooms (containing more than 200–300 pigs)	++
Slatted floors	+
Nutrition	
Insufficient caloric intake	+
Improper content of macro- and microelements in feed	+
Feed not supplemented with fat (dust from feed)	+
Presence of nonrespiratory pathogens	
Colibacillosis	++
Dysentery	++
Mange	+
Ascarids	+
Management deficiencies	
Insufficient control of climate	+++
Poor monitoring of signs of disease	++
Lack of or incorrect preventive measures	++
Poor caretaking of sick animals (isolation, treatment)	++
Random distribution of piglets between sows	++
Multiple moving and mingling of pigs during growth period	++
Poor hygiene	++
Poor biosecurity	++

and from the herd and internal flow of animals through the facilities, insulation and ventilation of buildings, separation of large barns, and separation of different age groups in multisite production systems. Also, avoidance of mixing the piglets between sows in the suckling period and weaning the pigs a little older may improve the immunological capacity against respiratory diseases.

Management. Management remains the central factor in controlling respiratory problems. A constant and competent supervising of installations and animal behavior allows immediate and appropriate intervention when problems arise. In this context it has to be recognized that respiratory diseases are not always associated with obvious clinical signs. In fact, most cases of respiratory disease occur subclinically or with only vague symptoms. Even outbreaks of acute pleuropneumonia may occur without clear respiratory symptoms.

Introduction of Genetic Material. The risk of introducing disease through purchase of traditionally reared breeding animals can be avoided if a necessary supply of genetic material is ensured by means of artificial insemination, embryonated eggs, or cesarean-derived piglets. However, under commercial conditions a more practicable alternative will be to introduce breeding animals in batches from a breeding herd with the same health status as the buyer's. Prior to introduction into the herd, the animals could be quarantined for 6 to 12 weeks, blood-tested, and vaccinated if neccesary.

Stocking Density. In spite of the fact that crowding greatly increases the incidence of respiratory diseases, it may be difficult to motivate managers to decrease stocking rate, since calculations do not always reveal a profit by this remedy. In the case of only moderate respiratory problems, the profit due to better health often will be counterbalanced by the loss due to decreased utilization of herd facilities. Nevertheless, lowering stock density remains one of the most effective remedies against serious respiratory problems.

Barriers Between Differently Aged Animals. In herds with an inadequate separation between pigs of different ages microbes are continuously transmitted from older to younger animals, with a subsequently continuous replication of pathogens. Dissimilar climatic needs of different age groups in the same room may be a contributing adverse factor. To limit the multiplication of pathogens, it is of crucial importance in larger herds to build barriers between groups of differently aged animals and to move pigs in batches. The facilities should be adapted to all-in/all-out production, with rooms containing not more than 200–300 individuals. Ideally, the age difference in weaner batches should not exceed 2 weeks.

The potential of age group separation for preventing

transmission of infection increases with the distance between groups. Maximal effect is achieved in multisite production systems with segregated herds for the breeding, nursery, and growing pigs.

Air Pollutants. To prevent massive air pollution and to maintain an acceptable relative humidity, forced ventilation is necessary in confined facilities. The lower the airspace per pig, the higher the air exchange is necessary. However, it is difficult to compensate completely for overcrowding. For example, if the stocking rate is doubled, the ventilation rate should be increased tenfold to maintain the same clearance of air contaminants (Wathes 1983). If a significant effect on the dust concentration is to be achieved, large air-cleaning equipment is necessary (Gustafsson 1989).

Ventilation systems often recirculate room air with fresh air. This mixing of air contributes to the spread of respiratory pathogens. Accordingly, the level of respirable dust is increased in high-speed recirculation systems (Meyer and Manbeck 1986). Hunneman et al. (1986) indicate that respiratory diseases can be controlled better in buildings with negative pressure ventilation, where the polluted air is removed and exchanged for totally fresh air. Nicks et al. (1989) found that the aerial ammonia concentration was 21 ppm and 12 ppm in two compartments of a farrowing house. In the former compartment a larger proportion of the extracted air was recirculated.

Climate. Respiratory problems often arise in cold and humid barns with no artificial heating. Frequently, the choice is between reducing humidity by means of a high air exchange rate, resulting in lower room temperature, or warming up the room by means of a lower air exchange rate. The first alternative is advisable according to experience. Cold, clean, dry air is by far superior to warm, polluted, humid air. Besides, the microclimate in a cold barn can be improved and protected against draft by providing straw bedding or/and some sort of covering for resting places (Feenstra 1985) and by establishing solid separations between pens; pen separations should be solid to a height of 60 cm.

Nutrition. In practice, malnutrition is rarely of importance in creating respiratory problems. Nevertheless, the relevance of vitamin E and selenium for immunity (Hayek et al. 1989) has to be considered. A major part of the dust particles in the air in swine barns arises from the feed. The addition of fat or wet feeding systems significantly reduces the dust problem.

Nonrespiratory Pathogens. There is a well-documented association between enteric disorders and respiratory problems. Therefore, solving respiratory problems is not possible if concurrent enteric problems are neglected. Mange and ascarids also have to be considered. Severe attacks of mange weaken the general resistance, and migrating ascarids cause lung lesions, increasing the susceptibility to respiratory pathogens.

Medication. Due to development of antimicrobial resistance in many bacterial species, restrictions have been put on prophylactic use of antibiotics in livestock production in many countries. However, the ability to quickly combat outbreaks of respiratory disease depends on immediate medication of diseased individuals. Pigs with signs of pneumonia should be treated parenterally with the appropiate antibiotics because their consumption of water and feed might be significantly decreased (Goovaerts et al. 1986; Pijpers et al. 1990). Medication for 2–3 days will be sufficient in most cases. Jørgensen (1988) found that pigs receiving immediate and intensive parenteral treatment against clinical pneumonia had a better weight gain than pigs receiving a less intensive treatment. In outbreaks of pneumonia, it can be necessary that pigs in contact with clinically diseased individuals receive medication in feed or water for 4–7 days.

Vaccination. Vaccines have been developed against progressive atrophic rhinitis, *A. pleuropneumoniae*, *M. hyopneumoniae*, PRRS, and Aujeszky's disease. Vaccines against atrophic rhinitis can be based on a recombinant derivative of the *P. multocida* toxin (Nielsen et al. 1991a) and can be used for vaccination of both sows and pigs. However, some vaccines are still based on *P. multocida* and *B. bronchiseptica* bacterins. *Actinobacillus pleuropneumoniae* vaccines comprise subunit vaccines based on Apx toxins and an outer membrane protein (Bosch 1994), which can be used to vaccinate pigs against all serotypes, and bacterin-based vaccines where it is important to use the homologues serotypes in order to get proper protection (Nielsen, 1982). *Mycoplasma hyopneumoniae* vaccines are based on bacterins and are used for very young pigs (Dayalu et al. 1992; Weiss and Petersen 1992). However, a study by Opriessnig et al. (2003) showed that vaccination with *A. pleuropneumoniae* and *M. hyopneumoniae* bacterins using the approved protocol in the U.S. significantly increased the length of viremia with PCV2. Also, they found a higher copy number of the PCV2 genome in serum, a wider range of tissue distribution of PCV2 antigen, and an increased severity of lymphoid depletion. Thus, veterinarians may need to consider changes in vaccination protocols in herds with recurrent PCV2-associated PMWS. Vaccines against PRRS can be based on live attenuated U.S. or E.U. virus strains or they can be inactivated. The marker vaccines against Aujeszky's disease are gene-deleted (Mettenleiter et al. 1985; Quint et al. 1987; Moormann et al. 1990), which makes it possible to distinguish serologically between vaccinated and naturally infected pigs (Van Oirschot et al. 1986). Vaccines against swine influenza is based on an inactivated whole influenza virus or split-products vaccines prepared from detergent-treated virus. The virus strains used are of human origin and include H1N1 and H3N2, which are the most common types, both in humans and in pigs.

Hygiene. To prevent transmission of respiratory pathogens between herds, particularly in production systems where certain respiratory pathogens are totally prohibited (SPF), it is important to clean, wash, and disinfect possible outside transmitters such as vehicles, delivery rooms, entrance rooms, tools, etc. In all-in/all-out production systems it is also of crucial importance to clean and disinfect the facilities between the batches of animals. However, too much washing in rooms which still are housing pigs can even aggravate a respiratory disease problem by cooling and humidifying the rooms.

ECONOMIC IMPORTANCE OF RESPIRATORY DISEASES

Respiratory disorders cause substantial losses to the swine industry. In a survey of swine health expenditures in Missouri, pneumonia and rhinitis were the two disease categories with the greatest impact on total disease expenses (14% and 10%, respectively) (Kliebenstein et al. 1982/83). Data from the National Animal Health Monitoring System in Ohio, 1986–1987, revealed that pneumonia was by far the most costly disease in swine, accounting for $5.42 U.S. per pig per year out of total costs of $21.34 per pig due to diseases (Miller and Dorn 1987). Respiratory disease expenditures for swine production in the former German Democratic Republic were estimated at DME 700 million per year. This reduction in returns was allocated among damaged lungs, 3%; destroyed and disposed diseased animals, 37%; and reduced growth rate, 60% (Hoy et al. 1987).

Losses associated with respiratory disease vary considerably between herds (Lindqvist 1974; Wilson et al. 1986) but also between seasons. Boessen et al. (1988) reported a seasonal variation of more than 30% in the losses due to pneumonia (from $1.31 per hog in the winter of 1986, to $0.89 in the following summer, and back up to $1.26 in the winter of 1987). Similarly, the variation in losses due to rhinitis was more than 60% (from $0.54 per hog in the winter of 1986, to $1.37 in the following summer, to $0.50 in the winter of 1987). At herd level the total cost of respiratory disease is the sum of output losses—namely, increased mortality, decreased weight gain, increased feed consumption, and decreased meat quality or payment—and of control expenditures—for example, treatments, vaccination programs, hygiene procedures, and extra labor (Schepers 1990). On a national scale, this method of calculation of the costs has been used by Mousing et al. (1996) for PRRS and by Bækbo et al. (1996) for *M. hyopneumoniae*.

In practical situations, the estimated economic impact of respiratory disorders in a herd must be based on slaughterhouse information and data on productivity and disease recordings in the herd: current weight gain or days to slaughter, feed efficiency, incidence of clinical respiratory disease and other diseases, mortality rate, results of necropsies, severity of lesions observed at slaughter, and finally the costs of current treatment and prophylaxis strategy.

The economic effect of each single respiratory disease is difficult to clarify, as reflected in inconsistent results from different studies. It is understandable that disease effects vary between studies: respiratory diseases are always the result of numerous interacting microbial and physical insults, different in type and grade as well. For example, clinical studies on the effect of *M. hyopneumoniae* will show significantly greater losses in areas with a high burden of different pathogens than in areas with few pathogens in the swine population. Thacker et al. (1999) found for example that *M. hyopneumoniae* potentiates the severity and duration of PRRS virus–induced pneumonia. Each disease situation is unique; and data from an investigation can be assessed only by an observer with a detailed knowledge of the situation in question.

Output Losses due to Enzootic Pneumonia

Most investigations on the economic effect of enzootic pneumonia are based on the prevalence of pneumonia at slaughter and the association with daily weight gain. However, in herds where pneumonia predominantly occurs in young pigs, the lesions may be resolved by the time of slaughter (Wallgren et al. 1990). In studies that compare daily weight gain between pigs with pneumonia and control pigs without pneumonia, this could contribute to underestimation of the effect. This may be the main reason for the great variability in reported effects on daily weight gain, varying from positive effect to about 20% decrease (Bäckström et al. 1975; Christensen 1984; Hoy et al. 1985; Love et al. 1985; Wilson et al. 1986; Le Foll et al. 1988; Cowart et al. 1990; Clark et al. 1993). Based on a review and analysis of 27 studies, Straw et al. (1989) concluded that, on the average, mycoplasmal pneumonia caused a 17% decrease in daily weight gain and a 14% decrease in feed efficiency. From different studies on the association between the severity of pneumonia and the decrease in weight gain, Straw et al. (1989) deduced that, on the average, for every 10% of the lung with pneumonic lesions, the mean daily gain is reduced by 37 g.

Lundeheim (1979), Wallgren et al. (1990), and Clark et al. (1993) suggested that pneumonia possesses its greatest influence on total weight gain when it occurs in young pigs. Contrary to this, Dijk et al. (1984), Hartley et al. (1988b), and Jørgensen (1988) proposed that pneumonia in older pigs is more damaging to the average weight gain. The importance of differentiating between uncomplicated and complicated bronchopneumonia in slaughter checks was documented in a study by Christensen and Mousing (1994). The decrease in daily weight gain was 6 g in pigs with uncomplicated bron-

chopneumonia and 38 g in pigs with complicated bronchopneumonia. Maes et al. (1999) made cost benefit analyses on *M. hyopneumoniae* vaccination in multisite herds and found that vaccination significantly improved daily weight gain, feed conversion ratio, medication costs, prevalence of pneumonia, and severity of pneumonic lesions. Vaccination was found economically attractive because it resulted in an increase of the net return to labor with 1.3 ECU per finishing pig sold.

Output Losses due to Pleuropneumonia

As with enzootic pneumonia, results from examinations of the effect of pleuropneumonia on daily weight gain vary over a wide range. Decreases in daily weight gain from none to 20% are reported (Saunders et al. 1981; Christensen 1982; Hunneman 1983; Rosendal and Mitchell 1983; Weibel et al. 1983; Desrosiers 1986; Wilson et al. 1986; Rohrbach et al. 1993). In an *A. pleuropneumoniae*–infected herd, pigs with pleuropneumonic lesions at slaughter had significantly better daily weight gain than pigs without this lesion (Christensen and Mousing 1994). This astonishing observation may indicate that many pigs that did not have lesions at slaughter had nevertheless suffered from pleuropneumonia earlier in the growing period, with high detrimental effect on weight gain. Also, this observation clearly demonstrates the risk of miscalculating the effect of disease from slaughter data for lesions of relatively short duration. Straw et al. (1989) concluded from their review that, on average, pleuropneumonia caused a 34% decrease in daily weight gain and a 26% decrease in feed efficiency.

Occasionally, 10–20% or more of individuals in batches of slaughter swine from newly infected herds are totally condemned at slaughter due to acute pleuropneumonia. The risk of condemnation highly increases if pigs are stored alive at the slaughterhouse for more than 24 hours (Christensen 1986). Slaughter pigs from nonimmune herds, in particular pigs from SPF herds, also are at risk of contracting acute pleuropneumonia if housed for more than 24 hours with infected pigs. The mortality may be as high as 10–20% in acute outbreaks but is usually below 1% in chronically infected herds. Total losses due to pleuropneumonia, including mortality, were assessed at 2% of the value of produced slaughter swine, estimated in three pleuropneumonia-infected herds with high prevalences of pleuritis at slaughter (Christensen 1981).

Output Losses due to Chronic Pleuritis

In Danish pig herds a high frequency of chronic pleuritis at slaughter is closely associated with *A. pleuropneumoniae* infection (Christensen 1981; Mousing et al. 1989). Several studies have been conducted describing the economic implications of pleuritis; in many herds, chronic pleuritis resulted in 7–12 extra days to attain slaughter weight (Christensen 1982, 1984). Following a clinical outbreak of respiratory disease in a large integrated herd, pigs with chronic pleuritis grew slower than pigs without this lesion (requiring 8 extra days to attain market weight), but prior to the outbreak there was no apparent association between chronic pleuritis and days to market (Hartley et al. 1988b). Results from several other studies indicate that pigs with chronic pleuritis have a reduced rate of weight gain (Bäckström et al. 1975; Rasmussen 1984; Hoy et al. 1985; Love et al. 1985). On the other hand, Le Foll et al. (1988) reported no effect of chronic pleuritis on growth rate.

Output Losses due to Atrophic Rhinitis

In experimental studies considerable decrease in daily weight gain has been reported (Nielsen et al. 1991a), but as for pneumonia, the output losses reported for atrophic rhinitis vary from one study to another (Pedersen and Barfod 1977; Love et al. 1985; Straw and Ralston 1986; Le Foll et al. 1988; Lieschke et al. 1989; Cowart et al. 1990; Dumas et al. 1990; Riising et al. 2002). The effect on daily weight gain in these studies varied from no effect to a 13% decrease. Not only have results differed between surveys, but researchers often have found a varying effect between herds in a given survey. In a study of two herds, a decreased rate of weight gain could be attributed to atrophic rhinitis in only one of them (Wilson et al. 1986), and Scheit et al. (1990) could demonstrate a negative effect of atrophic rhinitis in only one out of three herds.

Output Losses due to PRRS

Acute outbreaks of PRRS can give substantial economical losses due to dramatic increase in the mortality rate. In a large breeding farm, Pejsak et al. (1997) observed a mortality rate of nearly 76% during the 5th week of the outbreak when 1,562 out of 2,067 piglets were either born dead or died prior to weaning. Preweaning mortality rates gradually returned to normal values within 16 weeks. However, the incidence of respiratory disease in the weaned and fattening pigs increased during this time. Although prophylactic treatment against respiratory diseases were administered, the mortality rate doubled for the weaned and fattening pigs. Dee et al. (1997) showed that controlling the disease by nursery depopulation reduced the margin over variable costs in 32 out of 34 pig herds. Test and removal of infected animals have also shown to be a way of eliminating PRRS in 5 chronically infected breeding herds (Dee et al. 2001). Garner et al. (2001) estimated that if the disease became established in Australia opportunity losses in gross national income of 5–11% per year would occur.

REFERENCES

Aalund O, Willeberg P, Mandrup M, Riemann HP. 1976. Lung lesions at slaughter: Associations to factors in the pig herd. Nord Vet Med 28:487–495.

Albina E, Leforban Y, Baron T, Plana Duran J, Vannier P. 1992. An enzyme linked immunosorbent assay (ELISA) for the detection of antibodies to the porcine reproductive and respiratory syndrome (PRRS) virus. Ann Rech Vet 23:167–176.

Allan GM, Ellis JA. 2000. Porcine circoviruses: A review. J Vet Invest 12:3–14.

Amass SF, Clark LK, Van Alstine WG, Bowersock TL, Murphy DA, Knox KE, Albregts SR. 1994. Interaction of *Mycoplasma hyopneumoniae* and *Pasteurella multocida* infections in swine. J Am Vet Med Assoc 204:102–107.

Andersen JB. 1991. National programs to eliminate PRV: Eradication in Denmark. In Proc 1st Int Symp on Eradication of Pseudorabies (Aujeszky's) Virus, St. Paul, Minn., pp. 217–223.

Anderson PL, Morrison RB, Molitor TW, Thawley DG. 1990. Factors associated with circulation of pseudorabies virus within swine herds. J Am Vet Med Assoc 196:877–880.

Andreasen M, Mousing J, Krogsgaard Thomasen L. 2001. No simple association between time elapsed from seroconversion until slaughter and the extent of lung lesions in Danish swine. Prev Vet Med 52:147–161.

Andresen LO, Klausen J, Barfod K, Sorensen V. 2002. Detection of antibodies to *Actinobacillus pleuropneumoniae* serotype 12 in pig serum using a blocking enzyme-linked immunosorbent assay. Vet Microbiol 89:61–67.

Awad-Masalmeh M, Köfer J, Schuh M. 1990. On the occurrence of chronic respiratory disease at swine herds in Austria: Bacteriological findings, efficacy of autogenous vaccines. Proc Int Pig Vet Soc 11:107.

Baadsgaard NP, Jorgensen E. 2003. A Bayesian approach to the accuracy of clinical observations. Prev Vet Med 59:189–206.

Bäckström 1978. The relationship between disease incidence of fatteners recorded at slaughter and environmental factors in herds. Nord Vet Med 30:526–533.

Bäckström L, Bremer H. 1976. Sjukdomsregistreringar på Svin vid Slaktbesiktning—Ett Hjälpmedel i Förebyggande Svinhälsovard. Svensk Vet Tidn 28:312–336.

Bäckström L, Bremer H, Dyrendahl I, Olsson H. 1975. Sambandsstudier av produktions- och sjukdomsdata på slaktsvin i en integreret besättning med hög frekvens av atrofisk rhinit, enzootisk pneumoni ock pleurit. Svensk Vet Tidn 27: 1028–1040.

Bäckström L, Hoefling DC, Morkoc AC. 1985. Effect of atrophic rhinitis on growth rate in Illinois swine herds. J Am Vet Med Assoc 187:712–715.

Bækbo P, Kooij D, Mortensen S, Barfod K, Mousing J. 1996. Economic evaluation of national eradication and control strategies for *Mycoplasma hyopneumoniae* in Denmark. Proc Int Pig Vet Soc 14:230.

Barfod K. 2004. Disease control and SPF. In Jensen WK, Devine C, Dikemann M. Encyclopedia of Meat Sciences, 1st edition. Elsevier, Oxford, United Kingdom: Academic Press, pp. 1041–1045.

Baskerville A. 1981. Mechanisms of infection in the respiratory tract. NZ Vet J 29:235–238.

Batista L, Dee SA, Rossow KD, Deen J, Pijoan C. 2002. Assessing the duration of persistence and shedding of porcine reproductive and respiratory syndrome virus in a large population of breeding-age gilts. Can J Vet Res 66:196–200.

Bechmann G, Schöss P. 1990. Neutralizing activity against *Pasteurella multocida* toxin in sera of pigs with atrophic rhinitis. Proc Int Pig Vet Soc 11:50.

Bendixen HC. 1971. Om nysesyge hos svinet. Nord Vet Med (Suppl) 23:1.

Bertram TA. 1985. Quantitative morphology of peracute pulmonary lesions in swine induced by *Haemophilus pleuropneumoniae*. Vet Pathol 22:598–609.

Bertschinger HU, Keller H, Löhrer A, Wegmann W. 1972. Der zeitliche Verlauf der experimentellen enzootischen Pneumonie beim SPF-Schwein. Schweiz Arch Tierheilkd 114:107–118.

Bille N, Larsen JL, Svendsen J, Nielsen NC. 1975. Preweaning mortality in pigs. 6. Incidence and causes of pneumonia. Nord Vet Med 27:482–495.

Blanchard B, Kobisch M, Bové JM, Saillard C. 1996. Polymerase chain reaction for *Mycoplasma hyopneumoniae* detection in tracheobronchiolar washings from pigs. Mol Cell Probes 10:15–22.

Blecha F, Pollmann DS, Nichols DA. 1983. Weaning pigs at an early age decreases cellular immunity. J Anim Sci 56:396–400.

Boessen CR, Kliebenstein JB, Cowart RP, Moore KC, Brurbee CR. 1988. Effective use of slaughter checks to determine economic loss from morbidity in swine. In Proc 5th Int Symp Vet Epidemiol Econ, Acta Vet Scand (Suppl) 84:436–438.

Bosch H. 1994. *Actinobacillus pleuropneumoniae* in swine: Pathogenesis, antigens and vaccination. In Proc *Haemophilus, Actinobacillus* and *Pasteurella* Int Conf, Edinburgh, Scotland.

Bosse JT, Friendship R, Rosendal S, Fenwick BW. 1993. Development and evaluation of a mixed-antigen ELISA for serodiagnosis of *Actinobacillus pleuropneumoniae* serotypes 1, 5, and 7 infections in commercial swine herds. J Vet Diagn Invest 5:359–362.

Bøtner A. 1997. Diagnosis of PRRS. Vet Microbiol 55:295–301.

Brockmeier SL, Lager KM. 2002. Experimental airborne transmission of porcine reproductive and respiratory syndrome virus and *Bordetella bronchiseptica*. Vet Microbiol 89:267–275.

Bröring S, Müller E, Petzoldt K, Schoon HA, Bergmann KC. 1989. Das Zusammenwirken von *Actinobacillus pleuropneumoniae* und influenza A-virus bei experimentell infizirten Mäusen. J Vet Med (B) 36:681–690.

Buddle JR, Mercy AR, Skirrow SZ, Madec F, Nicholls RR. 1997. Epidemiological studies of pig diseases: 1. Use of French protocols for risk factor assessment to predict the health status of Australian herds. Aust Vet J 75:274–281.

Buttenschøn J. 1989. Differentiation between five types of pneumonia distribution pattern in pigs. J Vet Med (A) 36:494–504.

——. 1990. Kvantitativ og kvalitativ karakterisering af pneumonier hos kvæg og svin. Thesis, Institut for Veterinær Mikrobiologi, Den kgl. Veterinær- og Landbohøjskole, Copenhagen.

Calsamiglia M, Pijoan C, Trigo A. 1999. Application of a nested polymerase chain reaction assay to detect *Mycoplasma hyopneumoniae* from nasal swabs. J Vet Diagn Invest 11:246–251.

Caruso JP, Jeska EL. 1990. Phagocytic functions of pulmonary alveolar macrophages in genetically selected lean and obese swine and effects of exogenous linolenic acid upon cell function. Vet Immunol Immunolopathol 24:27–36.

Castryck F, Devriese LA, Hommez J, Cassimon P, Miry C. 1990. Bacterial agents associated with respiratory disease in young feeder pigs. Proc Int Pig Vet Soc 11:112.

Christensen G. 1981. Pleuropneumoni hos svin fremkaldt af *Haemophilus pleuropneumoniae*. II. Undersøgelser vedrørende epidemilogi samt relation til kronisk pleuritis (brysthindear) hos slagtesvin. [Pleuropneumonia in swine due to *Haemophilus pleuropneumoniae*. II. Studies on the epidemiology and the relation to chronic pleuritis (pleural scars) in baconers]. Nord Vet Med 33:236–249.

——. 1982. Pleuropneumoni hos svin fremkaldt af *Haemophilus pleuropneumoniae*. III. Observationer vedrørende klinisk manifestation på besætningsplan samt terapeutiske og immunprofylaktiske muligheder. [Pleuropneumonia in swine due to *Haemophilus pleuropneumoniae*. III. Studies on clinical manifestation in herds, treatment and control by vaccination]. Nord Vet Med 34:113–123.

——. 1984. Brysthindear (kronisk fibrøs pleuritis) hos slagtesvin. En undersøgelse vedrørende brysthindearrenes ætiologi og udviklingsforløb i en lukket, konventionel svinebesætning med høj frekvens af brysthindear. Dansk Vet Tidsskr 67:1067–1075.

——. 1986. Ondartet lungesyge (pleuropneumoni) hos slagtesvin. Betragtninger vedrørende sygdommens natur, udbredelse, kødkontrolmæssige forhold og dens indflydelse på produktionsøkonomi. Hyologisk Tidsskr Svinet 8(6):3–8.

——. 1995. Forekomst af lungebetændelse, lungehindebetændelse, hjertesækbetændelse og ormepletter hos danske slagtesvin (1994-status) [The prevalence of pneumonia, pleuritis, pericarditis, and liver spots in Danish slaughter pigs]. Dansk Vet Tidsskr 78:554–561.

Christensen G, Mousing J. 1994. Udvidet slagtedyrsdiagnostik (USK) på plucks fra svin. II. Daglig tilvækst i relation til forekomst af sygdomsforandringer i pluckset på slagtetidspunktet [Extended postmortem examination on plucks from slaughter pigs. II. Daily weight gain in relation to lesions in the plucks at slaughter]. Dansk Vet Tidsskr 77:753–763.

Christensen G, Sørensen V, Mousing J. 1999. Diseases of the respiratory system. In Straw BE, D'Allaire S, Mengeling WL, Taylor DJ. Diseases of Swine, 8th edition. Ames: Iowa State University Press, pp:927–928.

Christensen LS, Mortensen S, Botner A, Strandbygaard BS, Ronsholt L, Henriksen CA, Andersen JB. 1993. Further evidence of long distance airborne transmission of Aujeszky's disease (pseudorabies) virus. Vet Rec 132:317–321.

Christopher-Hennings J, Nelson EA, Nelson JK, Hines RJ, Swenson SL, Hill HT, Zimmerman JJ, Katz JB, Yaeger MJ, Christopher CLC, Benfield DA. 1995. Detection of porcine reproductive and respiratory syndrome virus in boar semen by PCR. J Clin Microbiol 33:1730–1734.

Clark LK, Armstrong CH, Scheit AB, Van Alstine WG. 1993. The effect of *Mycoplasma hyopneumoniae* infection on growth in pigs with or without environmental constraints. Swine Health Prod 1:10–14.

Collins MT, Bäckström LR, Brim TA. 1989. Turbinate perimeter ratio as an indicator of conchal atrophy for diagnosis of atrophic rhinitis in pigs. Am J Vet Res 50:421–424.

Cowart RP, Lipsey RJ, Hedrick HB. 1990. Measurements of conchal atrophy and their association with growth rate in commingled feeder pigs. J Am Vet Med Assoc 196:1262–1264.

Cubero MJ, Leon L, Contreras A, Lanza I, Zamora E, Caro MR. 1992. Sero-epidemiological survey of porcine respiratory coronavirus (PRCV) infection in breeding herds in southeastern Spain. Zentralbl Veterinarmed B 39:290–298.

Curtis SE, Anderson CR, Simon J, Jensen AH, Day D L, Kelley KW. 1975a. Effects of aerial ammonia, hydrogen sulfide and swinehouse dust on rate of gain and respiratory tract structure in swine. J Anim Sci 41:735–739.

Curtis SE, Drummond JG, Grunloh DJ, Brendan Lynch P, Jensen AH. 1975b. Relative and qualitative aspects of aerial bacteria and dust in swine houses. J Anim Sci 41:1512–1521.

D'Allaire S, Bigras-Poulin M, Paradis MA, Martineau GP. 1988. Evaluation of atrophic rhinitis: Are the results repeatable? Proc Int Pig Vet Soc 10:38.

Dayalu KI, Keich RL, Charlier P, Martinod S. 1992. Evaluation of the beneficial effects of a *Mycoplasma hyopneumoniae* vaccine (Respisure): Results from controlled and field studies. Proc Int Pig Vet Soc 12:302.

Dee SA, Joo HS, Polson DD, Marsh WE, Pijoan C. 1996. An evaluation of nursery depopulation as a strategy for controlling postweaning PRRS: A summary of 34 farms. Proc Int Pig Vet Soc 14:68.

——. 1997. Evaluation of the effects of nursery depopulation of the profitability of 34 pig farms. Vet Rec 140:498–500.

Dee SA, Bierk MD, Deen J, Molitor TW. 2001. An evaluation of test and removal for the elimination of porcine reproductive and respiratory syndrome virus from 5 swine farms. Can J Vet Res 65:22–27.

Desrosiers R. 1986. Therapeutic control and economic aspects of porcine pleuropneumonia in finishing pigs. Vet Rec 119:89–90.

Dijk WPJ van, Klaver J, Verstegen MWA. 1984. Frequentie van enkele aandoeningen bij schlachtvarkens en de effecten op groei en schlachtkwaliteit. Tijdschr Diergeneeskd 109:539–548.

Done SH. 1988. Some aspects of respiratory defence with special reference to immunity. Pig Vet Soc Proc 20:31–60.

Donham KJ. 1991. Association of environmental air contaminants with disease and productivity in swine. Am J Vet Res 52:1723–1730.

Dreyfus A, Schaller A, Nivollet S, Segers RP, Kobisch M, Mieli L, Soerensen V, Hussy D, Miserez R, Zimmermann W, Inderbitzin F, Frey J. 2004. Use of recombinant ApxIV in serodiagnosis of *Actinobacillus pleuropneumoniae* infections, development and prevalidation of the ApxIV ELISA. Vet Microbiol 99:227–238.

Dritz SS, Chengappa MM, Nelssen JL, Tokach MD, Goodband RD, Nietfeld JC, Staats JJ. 1996. Growth and microbial flora of non-medicated segrated, early weaned pigs from a commercial swine operation. J Am Vet Med Assoc 208:711–715.

Dumas G, Denicourt M, D'Allaire S, Bigras-Poulin M, Martineau GP. 1990. Atrophic rhinitis and growth rate: A potential confounding effect related to slaughter weight. Proc Int Pig Vet Soc 11:385.

Dungworth DL. 1993. The respiratory system. In Pathology of Domestic Animals, Vol. 2, 4th ed. KVF Jubb, P C Kennedy, N Palmer, eds. San Diego: Academic Press, p. 592.

Enoe C, Mousing J, Schirmer AL, Willeberg P. 2002. Infectious and rearing-system related risk factors for chronic pleuritis in slaughter pigs. Prev Vet Med 54:337–349.

Falk K, Lium BM, Ødegaard Ø. 1990. Occurrence of lung lesions and antibodies to serotypes 2 and 6 of *Actinobacillus pleuropneumoniae* and to *Haemophilus parasuis* in 5176 slaughter weight pigs from 113 elite herds in Norway. Proc Int Pig Vet Soc 11:31.

Feenstra A. 1985. Effects of air temperatures on weaned piglets. Pig News Inf 6:295–299.

Feld NC, Qvist P, Ahrens P, Friis NF, Meyling A. 1992. A monoclonal blocking ELISA detecting serum antibodies to *Mycoplasma hyopneumoniae*. Vet Microbiol 30:35–46.

Fittipaldi N, Broes A, Harel J, Kobisch M, Gottschalk M. 2003. Evaluation and field validation of PCR tests for detection of *Actinobacillus pleuropneumoniae* in subclinically infected pigs. J Clin Microbiol 41:5085–5093.

Flesja KI, Solberg I. 1981. Pathological lesions in swine at slaughter. Acta Vet Scand 22:272–282.

Flesja KI, Forus IB, Solberg I. 1982. Pathological lesions in swine at slaughter. V. Pathological lesions in relation to some environmental factors in the herds. Acta Vet Scand 23:169–183.

Flori J, Mousing J, Gardner IA, Willeberg P, Have P. 1995. Risk factors associated with seropositivity to porcine respiratory coronavirus in Danish swine herds. Prev Vet Med 25:51–62.

Foged NT, Pedersen KB, Elling F. 1987. Characterization and biological effects of the *Pasteurella multocida* toxin. FEMS Microbiol Lett 43:45–51.

Foged NT, Nielsen JP, Barfod K. 1990. The use of ELISA-determination of *Pasteurella multocida* toxin antibodies in the control of progressive atrophic rhinitis. Proc Int Pig Vet Soc 11:49.

Folkesson HG, Weststrôm BR, Pierzynowski SG, Svendsen J, Lundin S, Karlsson BW. 1990. Lung permeability to different-sized macromolecules in developing pigs. Proc Int Pig Vet Soc 11:430.

Frey J. 1995. Virulence in *Actinobacillus pleuropneumoniae* and RTX toxins. Trends Microbiol 3:257.

Friis NF. 1974. *Mycoplasma suipneumoniae* and *Mycoplasma floculare* in comparative pathogenicity studies. Acta Vet Scand 15:507–518.

Ganter M, Kipper S, Hensel A. 1990. Bronchoscopy and bronchoalveolar lavage of live anaesthetized pigs. Proc Int Pig Vet Soc 11:109.

Garner MG, Whan IF, Gard GP, Philips D. 2001. The expected economic impact of selected exotic diseases on the pig industry of Australia. Rev Sci Tech 20:671–685.

Gatlin CL, Jordan WH, Shryock TR, Smith WC 1996. The quantitation of turbinate atrophy in pigs to measure the severity of induced atrophic rhinitis. Can J Vet Res 60:121–126.

Gilmour MI. 1989. Airborne pollution and respiratory disease in animal houses. Dis Abstr Int (B) 49:2521.

Gloster J, Blackall RM, Sellers RF, Donaldson AI. 1981. Forecasting the airborne spread of foot-and-mouth disease. Vet Rec 108:370–374.

Gloster J, Champion HJ, Sorensen JH, Mikkelsen T, Ryall DB, Astrup P, Alexandersen S, Donaldson AI. 2003. Airborne transmission of foot-and-mouth disease virus from Burnside Farm, Heddon-on-the-Wall, Northumberland, during the 2001 epidemic in the United Kingdom. Vet Rec 152:525–533. Erratum in: Vet Rec, 152:628.

Goldberg TL, Weigel RM, Hahn EC, Scherba G. 2000. Associations between genetics, farm characteristics and clinical disease in field outbreaks of porcine reproductive and respiratory syndrome virus. Prev Vet Med 43:293–302.

Goodall EA, Menzies FD, McLoughlin EM, McIlroy SG. 1993. Prevalence of pleurisy in pigs in Northern Ireland (1969–1989). Vet Rec 132:11–14.

Goodwin RFW. 1985. Apparent reinfection of enzootic pneumonia-free pig herds: Search for possible causes. Vet Rec 116:690–694.

Goodwin RFW, Chanter N, Rutter JM. 1990. Detection and distribution of toxigenic *Pasteurella multocida* in pig herds with different degrees of atrophic rhinitis. Vet Rec 126:452–456.

Goovaerts K, Jansegers L, Lens S. 1986. The effect of the water-consumption of fattening pigs. Proc Int Pig Vet Soc 9:283.

Gottschalk M, De Lasalle F, Radacovici S, Dubreuil JD. 1994. Evaluation of long chain lipopolysaccharides (LC-LPS) of *Actinobacillus pleuropneumoniae* serotype 5 for the serodiagnosis of swine pleuropneumoniae. Vet Microbiol 38:315–327.

Gottschalk M, Altman E, Lacouture S, De Lasalle F, Dubreuil JD. 1997. Serodiagnosis of swine pleuropneumonia due to *Actinobacillus pleuropneumoniae* serotypes 7 and 4 using long-chain lipopolysaccharides. Can J Vet Res 61:62–65.

Gradil C, Dubuc C, Eaglesome MD. 1996. Porcine reproductive and respiratory syndrome virus: Seminal transmission. Vet Rec 138:521–522.

Gram T, Jacobsen MJ, Ahrens P, Nielsen JP. 1994. Evaluation of a PCR detection system of *Actinobacillus pleuropneumoniae* in mixed culture from the respiratory tract of pigs. In Proc *Haemophilus, Actinobacillus* and *Pasteurella* Int Conf, Edinburgh, Scotland, p. 50.

Gram T, Ahrens P, Nielsen JP. 1996. Evaluation of a PCR for detection of *Actinobacillus pleuropneumoniae* in mixed bacterial cultures from tonsils. Vet Microbiol 51:95–104.

Grondahl-Hansen J, Barfod K, Klausen J, Andresen LO, Heegaard PM, Sorensen V. 2003. Development and evaluation of a mixed long-chain lipopolysaccharide based ELISA for serological surveillance of infection with *Actinobacillus pleuropneumoniae* serotypes 2, 6 and 12 in pig herds. Vet Microbiol 96:41–51.

Gustafsson G. 1989. Mass balances of dust in houses for pigs. In Proc 11th Int Cong Agric Eng (CIGR), Dublin, Eire. VA Dod, PM Grace, eds., pp. 1465–1470.

Hartley PE, Wilesmith JW, Bradley R. 1988a. Prevalence of pleurisy in pigs at slaughter. Vet Rec 123:173–175.

———. 1988b. The influence of pleural lesions in the pig at slaughter on the duration of the fattening period: An on-farm study. Vet Rec 123:208.

Hayek MG, Mitchell GE, Harmon RJ, Stahly TS, Cromwell GL, Tucker RE, Barker KB. 1989. Porcine immunoglobulin transfer after prepartum treatment with selenium or vitamin E. J Anim Sci 67:1299–1306.

Heilmann P, Müller G, Finsterbusch L. 1988. Lobäre Deposition radioaktiv markierter *Pasteurella multocida* Aerosole in den Lungen von Ferkeln und Kälbern. Arch Exper Vet Med 42:490–501.

Hennessy KJ, Iandolo JJ, Fenwick BW. 1993. Serotype identification of *Actinobacillus pleuropneumoniae* by arbitrarily primed polymerase chain reaction. J Clin Microbiol 31:1155–1159.

Henningsen D, Mousing J, Aalund O. 1988. Porcint corona virus (PCV) i Danmark. En epidemiologisk tværsnitsanlyse baseret på screening-område spørgeskema data. Dansk Vet Tidsskr 71:1168–1177.

Houben S, Callebaut P, Pensaert MB. 1995. Comparative study of a blocking enzyme-linked-immunosorbent-assay and the immunoperoxidase monolayer assay for the detection of antibodies to the porcine reproductive and respiratory syndrome virus in pigs. J Virol Method 51:125–128.

Hoy S, Mehlhorn G, Eulenberger KH, Erwerth W, Johannsen U, Dorn W, Hörügel K. 1985. Zum Einfluss entzündlicher Lungenveränderungen auf ausgewählte Parameter der Schlachtleistung beim Schwein. Monatsh Veterinarmed 40:584–587.

Hoy S, Mehlhorn G, Liesckhe B. 1987. Zur ökonomischen Bedeutung von Atemwegskrankungen der Schweine. [The economic importance of respiratory diseases of pigs.] Tierzucht 41:334–336.

Hunneman WA. 1983. Vóórkomen, ekonomische betekenis en bestrijding van Haemophilus pleuropneumoniae-infektes bij varkens. Ph.D. diss., Government Univ of Utrecht, Netherlands.

Hunneman WA, Voets MT, School ACM, Verhagen FAP. 1986. *Haemophilus pleuropneumoniae* infections in fattening pigs: Effect of subclinically infected breeding herds and different ventilation systems. Proc Int Pig Vet Soc 9:176.

Hussy D, Schlatter Y, Miserez R, Inzana T, Frey J. 2004. PCR-based identification of serotype 2 isolates of *Actinobacillus pleuropneumoniae* biovars I and II. Vet Microbiol 99:307–310.

Jansen A, Feddes JJR. 1995. Effect of airborne dust on health and performance of growing pigs. Can Agric Eng 37:211–216.

Jessing SG, Angen O, Inzana TJ. 2003. Evaluation of a multiplex PCR test for simultaneous identification and serotyping of *Actinobacillus pleuropneumoniae* serotypes 2, 5, and 6. J Clin Microbiol 41:4095–4100.

Johannsen U, Erwerth W, Menger S, Neumann R, Mehlhorn G, Schimmel D. 1987. Experimentelle Untersuchung zur Wirkung einer chronischen aerogenen Schadgasbelastung des Saugferkels mit Ammoniak unterschiedlicher Konzentrationen. J Vet Med (B) 34:260–273.

Jørgensen B. 1988. Epidemiologiske analyser af sygdomsdata fra svineavlens forsøgsstationer. II. Dansk Vet Tidsskr 71:9–23.

Jorsal SE, Thomsen BL. 1988. A Cox regression analysis of risk factors related to *Mycoplasma suipneumoniae* reinfection in Danish SPF-herds. Acta Vet Scand (Suppl) 84:436–437.

Kamp E, Bokken G, Vermeulen T, de Jong M, Buys H, Reek F, Smits M. 1994. Large scale use of PCR for the detection of toxigenic *Pasteurella multocida* in nasal and tonsillar swabs of pigs. In Proc *Haemophilus*, *Actinobacillus* and *Pasteurella* Int Conf, Edinburgh, Scotland, p. 36.

Kastner P, Mehlhorn G. 1989. Untersuchungen zur Deposition und Clearance inhalierter Bakterien (*Staphylococcus aureus*) in der Lunge von Ferkeln. Arch Exper Vet Med 43:379–389.

Keller H. 1988. The Swiss health service (PHS). Proc Int Pig Vet Soc 10:334.

Kelley KW. 1980. Stress and immune function: A bibliographic review. Ann Vet Res 11:445–478.

Klausen J, Andresen LO, Heegaard P, Nielsen JP, Nielsen R. 1996. Evaluation of blocking ELISAs for serodiagnosis of *Actinobacillus pleuropneumoniae* serotype 5 infections based on monoclonal antibodies against capsular polysaccharides and Lps as well as swine-mouse heterohybridoma-derived monoclonal antibodies. In Proc *Haemophilus, Actinobacillus* and *Pasteurella* Int Conf, Acapulco, Mexico, p. 40.

Klausen J, Andresen LO, Barfod K, Sorensen V. 2001. Blocking enzyme-linked immunosorbent assay for detection of antibodies against *Actinobacillus pleuropneumoniae* serotype 6 in pig serum. Vet Microbiol 79:11–18.

——. 2002. Evaluation of an emzyme-linked immunosorbent assay for serological surveillance of infection with *Actinobacillus pleuropneumoniae* serotype 5 in pig herds. Vet Microbiol 88:223–232.

Kliebenstein JB, Kirtley CL, Selby LA. 1982/83. A survey of swine production health problems and health maintenance expenditures. Prev Vet Med 1:357–369.

Kobisch M, Blanchard B, Le Potier MF. 1993. *Mycoplasma hyopneumoniae* infection in pigs: Duration of the disease and resistance to reinfection. Vet Res 24:67–77.

Kristensen CS, Angen O, Andreasen M, Takai H, Nielsen JP, Jorsal SE. 2004a. Demonstration of airborne transmission of *Actinobacillus pleuropneumoniae* serotype 2 between simulated pig units located at close range. Vet Microbiol 98:243–249.

Kristensen CS, Botner A, Takai H, Nielsen JP, Jorsal SE. 2004b. Experimental airborne transmission of PRRS virus. Vet Microbiol 99:197–202.

Kruijf JM, Welling AAWM. 1988. Het voorkomen van chronische ontstekingen bij gelten en borgen. [Occurrence of chronic inflammatory conditions in gilts and castrated male pigs.] Tijdschr Diergeneeskd 113:415–417.

Kubo M, Kimura K, Kobayashi M, Shimizu M, Yamada S, Morozumi T, Kobayashi H, Mitani K, Ito N, Yamomoto K, Mitura Y, Yamamoto T, Watanabe K. 1995. Pathological studies on natural and experimental porcine pneumonia caused by porcine reproductive and respiratory syndrome (PRRS) virus. Jpn Agric Res Quart 29:201–205.

Kurth KT, Hsu T, Snook ER, Thacker EL, Thacker BJ, Minion FC. 2002. Use of a *Mycoplasma hyopneumoniae* nested polymerase chain reaction test to determine the optimal sampling sites in swine. J Vet Diagn Invest 14:463–469.

Lai SS, Ho WC, Chang WM. 1986. Persistent infection of pseudorabies virus resulted in concurrent infections with *Haemophilus* spp in pigs. Proc Int Pig Vet Soc 9:335.

Lambotte JL, Pecheur M, Charlier, Coignoul F, Deweale A. 1990. Aerosol infection with *Bordetella bronchiseptica*: Morphological alterations in the respiratory tract and in the lung of piglets. Proc Int Pig Vet Soc 11:106.

Larivière S, D'Allaire S, DeLasalle F, Nadeau M, Moore C, Ethier R. 1990. Eradication of *Actinobacillus pleuropneumoniae* serotypes 1 and 5 infections in four herds. Proc Int Pig Vet Soc 11:17.

Larsen S, Jørgensen PH, Nielsen PA. 1990b. Elimination of specific pathogens in 3 to 4 week piglets by use of strategic medication. Proc Int Pig Vet Soc 11:387.

Larsen H, Jørgensen PH, Szancer J. 1990a. Eradication of *Actinobacillus pleuropneumoniae* from a breeding herd. Proc Int Pig Vet Soc 11:18.

Le Foll P, Amara N, Giral B, Solignac T. 1988. Influence de la pathologie sur la croissance des porcs entre le sevrage et l'abattage. Journ Rech Porcine France 20:95–100.

Leontides L. 1994. Evaluation of Vaccination for Controlling the Spread of Aujeszky's Disease Virus in Endemic Regions: An Analytical Approach. Ph.D. diss. Royal Veterinary and Agricultural Univ, Copenhagen, Denmark.

Le Potier MF, Kobisch M, Abiven P, Crevat D, Desmettre P. 1993. Blocking enzyme-linked immunosorbent assay for detection of antibodies to *Mycoplasma hyopneumoniae* in pigs. In Proc World Assoc Vet Lab Diagn Congr, Lyon, France, p. 208.

Levonen K, Veijlanen P, Seppänen J. 1994. *Actinobacillus pleuropneumoniae* serotype 2 antibodies in sow colostrum in Finnish pig-health-scheme herds. J Vet Med (B) 41:567–573.

Lieschke B, Hoy ST, Mehlhorn G, Warnecke HW. 1989. Auswirkungen der Rhinitis atrophicans suum auf die Schlachtleistung gleichaltriger Mastswheine unter Berücksichtung entzündlicher Lungenveränderungen. [Effects of rhinitis atrophicans suum on slaughter yield of equally aged fattening pigs with reference to inflammatory pulmonary alterations.] Monatsh Veterinaermed 44:11–16.

Lindqvist JO. 1974. Animal health and environment in the production of fattening pigs. Acta Vet Scand (Suppl) 51:1–78.

Love RJ, Wilson MR, Tasler G. 1985. Porcine atrophic rhinitis. Austr Vet J 62:377–378.

Lundeheim N. 1979. Genetic analysis of respiratory diseases in pigs. Acta Agric Scand 29:209–215.

Lundeheim N, Tafvelin B. 1986. Pathological lesions at slaughter in Swedish pig production—Hampshire crosses compared with Landrace and Yorkshire crosses. Proc Int Pig Vet Soc 9:380.

Madec F, Kobisch M. 1984. Etat sanitaire du porcelet et évolution des lésions au niveau de l'arbre respiratoire au cours des différentes phases d'élevage. Journ Rech Porcine France 16:215–235.

Madec F, Gourreau JM, Kaizer C. 1982. Epidemiology of swine influenza H^{sw}1N1 on farms in Brittany (first outbreak—1982). Epidemiol Sante Anim 2:56–64.

Madec F, Gourreau JM, Kaizer C, Aymard M. 1990. A retrospective study about influenza infections in the pig in France. Proc Int Pig Vet Soc 11:201.

Maes D, Deluyker H, Verdonck M, Castryck F, Miry C, Vrijens B, Verbeke W, Viane J, de Kruif A. 1999. Effect of vaccination against *Mycoplasma hyopneumoniae* in pig herds with all-in/all-out production system. Vaccine 17:1024–1034.

Maes D, Deluyker H, Verdonck M, Castryck F, Miry C, Vrijens B, de Kruif A. 2000. Herd factors associated with the seroprevalences of four major respiratory pathogens in slaughter pigs from farrow-to-finish herds. Vet Res 31:313–327.

Maes D, Deluyker H, Verdonck M, Castryck F, Miry C, Vrijens B, Ducatelle R, de Kruif A. 2001. Non-infectious factors associated with macroscopic and microscopic lung lesions in slaughter pigs from farrow-to-finish herds. Vet Rec 148:41–46.

Mallard BA, Wilkie BN, Kennedy BW. 1989. The influence of the swine major histocompatibility genes (SLA) on variation in serum immunoglobulin (Ig) concentration. Vet Immunol Immunopathol 21:139–151.

Marois P, DiFranco E, Boulay G, Assaf R. 1989. Enzootic pneumonia in feeder pigs: Association with transmissible gastroenteritis virus infection. Can Vet J 30:328–330.

Martin SW, Willoughby RA. 1972. Organic dusts, sulfur dioxide, and the respiratory tract of swine. Arch Environ Health 25:158–165.

Martineau-Doizé B, Larochelle R, Boutin J, Martineau GP. 1990. Atrophic rhinitis caused by toxigenic *Pasteurella multocida* type D: Morphometric analysis. Proc Int Pig Vet Soc 11:63.

Martinsson K, Lundeheim N. 1988. Effekter av driftsform, besättnings- och stallstorlek. Svensk Vet Tidn 40:313–319.

Mattsson JG, Bergström K, Wallgren P, Johansson KE. 1995. Detection of *Mycoplasma hyopneumoniae* in nose swabs from pigs by in vitro amplification of the 16S rRNA gene. J Clin Microbiol 33:893–897.

Mehlhorn G, Hoy S. 1985. Influence of endogenic and exogenic factors on the prevalence rate of lung lesions of fattening pigs and sows. In Proc 5th Int Congr Anim Hyg, Hannover, pp. 391–396.

Mercy AR, Brennan CM. 1988. The Western Australia pig health monitoring scheme. Proc 5th Int Symp Vet Epidemiol Econ, Acta Vet Scand (Suppl) 84:212–214.

Mettenleiter TC, Lukacs N, Rziha HJ. 1985. Pseudorabies virus avirulent strains fail to express a major glycoprotein. J Virol 56:307–311.

Meyer DJ, Manbeck HB. 1986. Dust levels in mechanically ventilated swine barns. Am Soc Agr Eng Paper 86:4042.

Miller G, Dorn CR. 1987. An economic summary of the National Animal Health Monitoring System data in Ohio, 1986–87. Proc USA Health Assoc 91:154–172.

Møller K, Kilian M. 1990. V factor–dependent *Pasteurellaceae* in the porcine upper respiratory tract. J Clin Microbiol 28:2711–2716.

Moormann RJM, De Rover T, Briarire J, Peeters BPH, Gielkens ALJ, Van Oirschot JT. 1990. Inactivation of the thymidine kinase gene of a gI deletion mutant of pseudorabies virus generates a safe but still highly immunogenic vaccine strain. J Gen Virol 71:1591–1595.

Morrison RB, Hilley HD, Leman AD. 1985. Comparison of methods for assessing the prevalence and extent of pneumonia in market weight swine. Can Vet J 26:381–384.

Mortensen S, Mousing J, Henriksen CA, Andersen JB. 1990. Evidence of long distance transmission of Aujeszky's disease virus. II: Epidemiological and meteorological investigations. Proc Int Pig Vet Soc 11:279.

Mortensen S, Stryhn H, Sogaard R, Boklund A, Stark KD, Christensen J, Willeberg P. 2002. Risk factors for infection of sow herds with porcine reproductive and respiratory syndrome (PRRS) virus. Prev Vet Med 53(1–2):83–101.

Mousing J. 1986. Slagtesvinesundhedstjenesten. En vurdering af omfang og funktion baseret på opgørelser for 1984. Dansk Vet Tidsskr 69:1149–1159.

——. 1988. Chronic pleuritis in pigs: The relationship between weight, age and frequency in 3 conventional herds. Proc 5th Int Symp Vet Epidemiol Econ, Acta Vet Scand (Suppl) 84: 253–255.

Mousing J, Christensen G. 1993. Pathological lesions in the right and left porcine lung: Evaluation of an alternative method for scoring pneumonic lesions based on right lung examination. Acta Vet Scand 34:151–158.

Mousing J, Lybye H, Barfod K, Meyling A, Rønsholt L, Willeberg P. 1989. Brysthindear hos svin. Serologiske reaktioner for luftvejsinfektioner og disses sammenhæng med brysthindearfrekvensen hos slagtesvin. Dansk Vet Tidsskr 72:865–873.

——. 1990. Chronic pleuritis in pigs for slaughter: An epidemiological study of infectious and rearing system-related risk factors. Prev Vet Med 9:107–119.

——. 1991. The relationship between serological reactions to swine respiratory infections and herd related factors. Proc 6th Int Symp Vet Epidemiol Econ, Ottawa, p. 416.

Mousing J, Kooij D, Mortensen S, McInerney J. 1996. Economic analysis of control strategies for porcine reproductive and respiratory syndrome (PRRS) in Danish pork. Proc Int Pig Vet Soc 14:70.

Neumann R, Leonhardt W, Ballin A, Mehlhorn G, Diecke S. 1985. Die Methode der intravitalen Lungenspülen beim Schwein—Gewinnung und Differenzierung von Alveolarzellen. Arch Exp Vet Med 39:525–534.

Neumann R, Mehlhorn G, Buchholz I, Johannsen U, Schimmel D. 1987. Experimentelle Untersuchung zur Wirkung einer chronischen aerogenen Schadgasbelastung des Saugferkels mit Ammoniak unterschiedlicher Konzentrationen. J Vet Med (B) 34:241–253.

Nicks B, Dechamps P, Canart B, Buzitu S, Dewaele A. 1989. Exemple de résultats inattendus lors d'un contrôle de la concentration en ammoniac dans une porcherie. Ann Med Vet 133:613–616.

Nielsen JP, Frederiksen W. 1990. Atrophic rhinitis in pigs caused by a human isolate of toxigenic *Pasteurella multocida*. Proc Int Pig Vet Soc 11:75.

Nielsen JP, Foged NT, Sørensen V, Barfod K, Bording A, Petersen SK. 1991. Vaccination against progressive atrophic rhinitis with a recombinant *Pasteurella multocida* toxin derivative. Can J Vet Res 55:128–138.

Nielsen R. 1982. *Haemophilus pleuropneumoniae* infection in pigs. Thesis. Danish Veterinary Laboratory, Copenhagen, Denmark.

——. 1988. Seroepidemiology of *Actinobacillus pleuropneumoniae*. Can Vet J 29:580–582.

Nielsen R, Danielsen V. 1975. An outbreak of Glässer's disease: Studies of etiology, serology and the effect of vaccination. Nord Vet Med 27:20–25.

Nielsen R, Loftager M, Eriksen L. 1990. Mucosal vaccination against *Actinobacillus pleuropneumoniae* infection. Proc Int Pig Vet Soc 11:13.

Nielsen R, Plambeck T, Foged NT. 1991. Blocking enzyme-linked immunosorbent assay for detection of antibodies to *Actinobacillus pleuropneumoniae* serotype 2. J Clin Microbiol 23:794–797.

——. 1993. Blocking enzyme-linked immunosorbent assay for detection of antibodies against *Actinobacillus pleuropneumoniae* serotype 8. Vet Microbiol 34:131–138.

Nielsen R, van den Bosch JF, Plambeck T, Sorensen V, Nielsen JP. 2000. Evaluation of an indirect enzyme-linked immunosorbent assay (ELISA) for detection of antibodies to the Apx toxins of *Actinobacillus pleuropneumoniae*. Vet Microbiol 71:81–87.

Noyes EP, Feeney D, Pijoan C. 1988. A prospective radiographic study of swine pneumonia. Proc Int Pig Vet Soc 10:67.

Ohgami M, Doershuk CM, English D, Dodek PM, Hogg JC. 1989. Kinetics of radiolabeled neutrophils in swine. J Appl Physiol 66:1881–1885.

Opriessnig T, Yu S, Gallup JM, Evans RB, Fenaux M, Pallares F, Thacker EL, Brockus CW, Ackermann MR, Thomas P, Meng XJ, Halbur PG. 2003. Effect of vaccination with selective bacterins on conventional pigs infected with type 2 porcine circovirus. Vet Pathol 40:521–529.

Palmer DF, Coleman MT, Dowdle WR, Schild GC. 1975. Advanced Laboratory Techniques for Influenza Diagnosis. Washington, D.C.: U.S. Department of Health, Education, and Welfare. Immunology series no. 6.

Pattison IH. 1956. A histological study of transmissible pneumonia of pigs characterized by extensive lymphoid hyperplasia. Vet Rec 68:490–494.

Pedersen KB, Barfod K. 1977. Effect of vaccination of sows with *Bordetella bronchiseptica* on the incidence of atrophic rhinitis in swine. Nord Vet Med 29:369–375.

——. 1981. The aetiological significance of *Bordetella bronchiseptica* and *Pasteurella multocida* in atrophic rhinitis of swine. Nord Vet Med 33:513–522.

Pejsak Z, Stadejek T, Markowska-Daniel I. 1997. Clinical signs and economic losses caused by porcine reproductive and respiratory syndrome virus in a large breeding farm. Vet Microbiol 55:317–322.

Pijoan C, Leman A. D. 1986. Veterinary services to growing and finishing pigs. Proc Int Pig Vet Soc 9:209–213.

Pijpers A, Vernooy JACM, Leengoed LAMG van, Verheijden JHM. 1990. Feed and water consumption in pigs following an *Actinobacillus pleuropneumoniae* challenge. Proc Int Pig Vet Soc 11:39.

Pointon AM, McCloud P, Heap P. 1985. Enzootic pneumonia of pigs in South Australia—Factors relating to incidence of disease. Aust Vet J 62:98–101.

Pol JM, van Leengoed LA, Stockhofe N, Kok G, Wensvoort G. 1997. Dual infections of PRRSV/influenza or PRRS/*Actinobacillus pleuropneumoniae* in the respiratory tract. Vet Microbiol 55:259–264.

Quint W, Gielkens A, Van Oirschot J, Berns J, Cuypers H. 1987. Construction and characterization of deletion mutants of pseudorabies virus: A new generation of "live" vaccines. J Gen Virol 68:523–534.

Rafai P, Neumann R, Leonhardt W, Frenyó L, Rudas P, Fodor L, Boros G. 1987. Effect of environmental temperature on pigs infected with *Pasteurella multocida* type A. Acta Vet Hung 35:211–223.

Rasmussen JF. 1984. The economic importance of chronic pleuritis in slaughter pig production. Proc Int Pig Vet Soc 8:347.

Rautiainen E. 2001. Mycoplasma hyopneumoniae—Aspects of Epidemiology, Protection and Control. Thesis. University of Helsinki, Finland.

Rautiainen E, Oravainen J, Virolainen JV, Tuovinen V. 2001. Regional eradication of *Mycoplasma hyopneumoniae* from pig herds and documentation of freedom of the disease. Acta Vet Scand 42:355–364.

Riising HJ, van Empel P, Witvliet M. 2002. Protection of piglets against atrophic rhinitis by vaccinating the sow with a vaccine against *Pasteurella multocida* and *Bordetella bronchiseptica*. Vet Rec 150:569–571.

Rohrbach BW, Hall RF, Hitchcock JP. 1993. Effect of subclinical infection with *Actinobacillus pleuropneumoniae* in commingled feeder swine. J Am Vet Med Assoc 202:1095–1098.

Rosendal S, Mitchell WR. 1983. Epidemiology of *Haemophilus pleuropneumoniae* infection in pigs: A survey of Ontario pork producers. Can J Comp Med 47:1–5.

Ross RF. 1984. Chronic pneumonia of swine: Emphasis on mycoplasmal pneumonia. In Proc Am Assoc Swine Pract, Kansas City, Mo., pp. 79–95.

Rothschild MF, Chen HL, Christian LL, Lie WR, Venier L, Cooper M, Briggs C, Warner CM. 1984. Breed and swine lymphocyte antigen haplotype differences in agglutination titers following vaccination with *B. bronchiseptica*. J Anim Sci 59:643–649.

Ruiz A, Galina L, Pijoan C. 2002. *Mycoplasma hyopneumoniae* colonization of pigs sired by different boars. Can J Vet Res 66:79–85.

Salmon H. 2000. Mammary gland immunology and neonate protection in pigs homing of lymphocytes into the MG. Adv Exp Med Biol 480:279–286.

Saunders JR, Osborne AD, Sebunya TK. 1981. Pneumonia in Saskatchewan swine: Abattoir incidence of intrathoracic lesions in pigs from a herd infected with *Haemophilus pleuropneumoniae* and from other herds. Can Vet J 22:244–247.

Scatozza F, Sidoli L. 1986. Effects of *Haemophilus pleuropneumonia* infection in piglets recovering from influenza. Proc Int Pig Vet Soc 9:150.

Schaller A, Kuhn R, Kuhnert P, Nicolet J, Anderson TJ, MacInnes JI, Segers RP, Frey J. 1999. Characterization of apxIVA, a new RTX determinant of *Actinobacillus pleuropneumoniae*. Microbiology 145:2105–2116.

Scheepens CJM. 1996. Climatic stress in swine: Hazards for health. Pig J Proc 37:130–136.

Scheepens CJM, Tielen MJM, Hessing MJC. 1988. Influence of climatic stress on health status of weaner pigs. In Proc 6th Int Congr Anim Hyg, (Environment and Animal Health), Skara, Sweden. Vol 2. Ekesbo I, ed., pp. 543–547.

Scheit AB, Mayrose VB, Hill MA, Clark LK, Cline TR, Knox KE, Runnels LJ, Frantz S, Einstein ME. 1990. Relationship of growth performance to pneumonia and atrophic rhinitis detected in pigs at slaughter. J Am Vet Med Assoc 196:881–884.

Schepers JA. 1990. Data requirements and objectives for economic analysis of diseases in farm livestock. In Proc Soc Vet Epidemiol Prev Med, Belfast, pp. 120–132.

Schlesinger KJ, Williams JM, Widel PW. 1990. Intranasal administration of pseudorabies (Bartha K61) vaccine in neonates and grow/finish pigs: Safety and efficacy of vaccination and effects of virulent challenge exposure. Proc Int Pig Vet Soc. 11:260.

Schultz RA. 1986. Swine pneumonia: Assessing the problem in individual herds. Vet Med 81:757–762.

Schultz RA, Young TF, Ross RF, Jeske DR. 1982. Prevalence of antibodies to *Haemophilus pleuropneumoniae* in Iowa swine. Am J Vet Res 43:1848–1851.

Sebunya TNK, Saunders JR, Osborne AD. 1983. A model aerosol exposure system for induction of porcine *Haemophilus pleuropneumoniae*. Can J Comp Med 47:48–53.

Sibilia M, Calsamiglia M, Vidal D, Badiella L, Aldaz A, Jensen JC. 2004. Dynamics of *Mycoplasma hyopneumoniae* infection in 12 farms with different production systems. Can J Vet Res 68:12–18.

Sirois M, Lemire EG, Levesque RC. 1991. Construction of a DNA probe and detection of *Actinobacillus pleuropneumoniae* by using polymerase chain reaction. J Clin Microbiol 29:1183–1187.

Smart NL, Miniats OP, Rosendal S, Friendship RM. 1989. Glasser's disease and prevalence of subclinical infection with *Haemophilus parasuis* in swine in south Ontario. Can Vet J 30:339–434.

Smith JH, Wathes, CM, Baldwin BA. 1996. The preference of pigs for fresh air over ammoniated air. Appl Behav Sci 49:417–424.

Smith WJ. 1983. Infectious atrophic rhinitis: Non-infectious determinants. In Atrophic Rhinitis in Pigs. Copenhagen: CEC Rep Eur En., pp. 149–151.

Sorensen KJ, Lei JC. 1986. Aujeszky's disease: Blocking ELISA for the detection of serum antibodies. J Virol Methods 13:171–181.

Sørensen V, Barfod K, Feld NC. 1992. Evaluation of a monoclonal blocking ELISA and IHA for antibodies to *Mycoplasma hyopneumoniae* in SPF-pig herds. Vet Rec 130:488–490.

Sørensen V, Barfod K, Feld NC, Vraa-Andersen L. 1993. Application of enzyme-linked immunosorbent assay for the surveillance of *Mycoplasma hyopneumoniae* infection in pigs. Rev Sci Tech Off Int Epizoot 12:593–604.

Sørensen V, Ahrens P, Barfod K, Feenstra AA, Feld NC, Friis NF, Bille-Hansen V, Jensen NE, Pedersen MW. 1997. *Mycoplasma hyopneumoniae* infection in pigs: Duration of the disease and evaluation of four diagnostic assays. Vet Microbiol 54:23–34.

Stark KD, Keller H, Eggenberger E. 1992. Risk factors for the reinfection of specific pathogen-free pig breeding herds with enzootic pneumonia. Vet Rec 131:532–535.

Stark KD, Nicolet J, Frey J. 1998. Detection of *Mycoplasma hyopneumoniae* by air sampling with a nested PCR assay. Appl Environ Microbiol 64:543–548.

Stegeman JA, Tielen MJM, Kimman TG, Van Oirschot JT, Hunneman WA, Berndsen FW. 1994. Intensive regional vaccination with a gI-deleted vaccine markedly reduces pseudorabies virus infections. Vaccine 12:527–531.

Stenbæk EI, Schirmer AL. 1994. Detection of *Actinobacillus pleuropneumoniae* serotype 2 antibodies in pig sera by an inhibition enzyme immuno assay (EIA). Vet Microbiol 39:231–244.

Straw BE. 1986. A look at the factors that contribute to development of swine pneumonia. Vet Med 81:747–756.

Straw BE, Ralston N. 1986. Comparative costs and methods for assessing production impact on common swine diseases. In Proc Economics of Animal Diseases, Michigan State Univ, pp. 165–180.

Straw BE, Bürgi EJ, Hilley HP, Leman AD. 1983. Pneumonia and atrophic rhinitis from a test station. J Am Vet Med Assoc 182:607–611.

Straw BE, Henry SC, Schultz RS, Marsteller TA. 1986. Clinical assessment of pneumonia levels in swine through measurement of the amount of coughing. Proc Int Pig Vet Soc 9:275.

Straw BE, Tuovinen VK, Bigras-Poulin M. 1989. Estimation of the cost of pneumonia in swine herds. J Am Vet Med Assoc 195:1702–1706.

Svensmark B, Nielsen K, Dalsgaard K, Willeberg P. 1989. Epidemiological studies of piglet diarrhoea in intensively managed Danish sowherds. III. Rotavirus infection. Acta Vet Scand 30:63–70.

Swenson SL, Hill HT, Zimmermann JJ, Evans LE, Landgraf JG, Wills RW, Sanderson TP, McGinley MJ, Brevik AK, Ciszewski DK, Frey ML. 1994. Excretion of porcine reproductive and respiratory syndrome virus in semen after experimentally induced infection in boars. J Am Vet Med Assoc 204:1943–1948.

Thacker EL, Halbur PG, Ross RF, Thanawongnuwech R, Thacker BJ. 1999. *Mycoplasma hyopneumoniae* potentiation of porcine reproductive and respiratory syndrome virus-induced pneumonia. J Clin Microbiol 37:620–627.

Thacker EL, Thacker BJ, Janke BH. 2001. Interaction between *Mycoplasma hyopneumoniae* and swine influenza virus. J Clin Microbiol 39:2525–2530.

Tielen MJM. 1989. Integrale Qualitätskontrolle: Garantie für Gesundheit? Vortrag am 10. Intensivseminar des steirischer Schweinegesundheitsdienstes vom 2.–9., Nassfeld, Austria.

Tielen MJM, Truijen WT, Van de Groos CAM, Verstegen MAW, Bruin JJM, Conbey RAPH. 1978. De invloed van bedrijfsstructuur en stalbouw op varkensmestbedrijven op het voorkommen van long- en leveraandoeneningen bij slachtvarkens. [Conditions of management and the construction of piggeries on pig-fattening farms as factors in the incidence of disease of the lung and liver of slaughtered pigs.] Tijdschr Diergeneeskd 103:1155–1165.

Torremorell M, Pijoan C, Janni K, Walker R, Joo HS. 1997. Airborne transmission of *Actinobacillus pleuropneumoniae* and porcine re-

productive and respiratory syndrome virus in nursery pigs. Am J Vet Res 58:828–832.

Tuboly S, Bernath S. 2002. Intestinal absorption of colostral lymphoid cells in newborn animals. Adv Exp Med Biol 503:107–114.

Tuboly S, Bernath S, Glavits R, Medveczky I. 1988. Intestinal absorbtion of colostral lymphoid cells in newborn piglets. Vet Immunol Immunopath 20:75–85.

Underdahl NR, Socha TE, Dorster AR. 1982. Long-term effect of *Bordetella bronchiseptica* infection in neonatal pigs. Am J Vet Res 43:622–625.

Vaiman M, Chardon P, Renard C. 1979. Genetic organization of the pig SLA complex: Studies on non recombinants and biochemical lysostrip analysis. Immunogenetics 9:353–361.

Van der Valk PC, Buurman J, Vandenbooren JCMA, Vernoy JCM, Wierda A. 1984. Automatic herd health and production control programs for swine farms. Proc Int Pig Vet Soc 8:342.

Van Oirschot JT, Houwers DJ, Rziha HJ, Moonen PJLM. 1988. Development of an ELISA for detection of antibodies to glycoprotein I of Aujeszky's disease virus: A method for the serological differentiation between infected and vaccinated pigs. J Virol Methods 22:191–206.

Van Oirschot JT, Rhiza HJ, Moonen PJLM, Pol JMA, Van Zaane D. 1986. Differentiation of serum antibodies from pigs vaccinated or infected with Aujeszky's disease virus by a competitive enzyme immunoassay. J Gen Virol 67:1179–1182.

Van Oirschot JT, Kaashoek MJ, Rijsewijk FA, Stegeman JA. 1996. The use of marker vaccines in eradication of herpesviruses. J Biotechnol 44:75–81.

Van Reeth K, Koyen A, Pensaert M. 1994. Clinical effects of dual infections with porcine epidemic abortion and respiratory syndrome virus. Proc Int Pig Vet Soc 13:51.

Verdin E, Saillard C, Labbe A, Bove JM, Kobisch M. 2000. A nested PCR for the detection of *Mycoplasma hyopneumoniae* in tracheobronchiolar washings from pigs. Vet Microbiol 76:31–40.

Visser IJR, Van den Ingh TSGAM, Kruijf JM, Tielen MJM, Urlings HAP, Gruys E. 1988. Atrofische rhinitis: Beoordeling van de lengtedoorsnede van varkenskoppen aan de slachtlijn ter bepaling van voorkomen en mate van concha-atrofie. [Atrophic rhinitis: The use of longitudinal sections of pigs' heads in the diagnosis of atrophy of the turbinate bones at the slaughter line.] Tijdschr Diergeneeskd 113:1345–1355.

Von Borell E. 1996. Current situation on welfare legislation and research within the European Union. Pig News Info 17:105N–107N.

Wallgren P, Persson M. 2000. Relationship between the amounts of antibodies to *Actinobacillus pleuropneumoniae* serotype 2 detected in blood serum and in fluids collected from muscles of pigs. J Vet Med B 47:727–737.

Wallgren P, Mattsson S, Artursson K, Bölske G. 1990. The relationship between *Mycoplasma hyopneumoniae* infection, age at slaughter and lung lesions at slaughter. Proc Int Pig Vet Soc 11:82.

Wallgren P, Beskow P, Fellström C, Renström LHM. 1994. Porcine lung lesions at slaughter and their correlation to the incidence of infections by *Mycoplasma hyopneumoniae* and *Actinobacillus pleuropneumoniae* during the rearing period. J Vet Med (B) 41:441–452.

Wathes CM. 1983. Ventilation, air hygiene and animal health. Vet Rec 113:554–559.

Weibel W, Bühlmann J, Häni H. 1983. Vergleichende Untersuchungen über Mortalität, Morbidität und Mastleistung in konventionellen und dem Schweinegesundheitsdienst angeschlossenen Mastbetrieben. III. Morbidität und Mastleistung. Schweiz Arch Tierheilkd 125:861–869.

Weiss DL, Petersen GR. 1992. *Mycoplasma hyopneumoniae* bacterin field efficacy study. Proc Int Pig Vet Soc 12:305.

Wensvoort G, Terpstra C, Laak EA, Bloemraad M, Kluyver EP, Kragten C, Buiten L, Besten A, Wagenaar F, Broekhuijsen JM, Moonen PJLM, Zetstra T, Boer EA, Tibben HJ, Jong MF, Veld P,

Groenland GJR, Gennep JA, Voets M Th, Verheijden JHM, Braamskamp J. 1991. Mystery swine disease in the Netherlands: The isolation of Lelystad virus. Vet Quart 13:121–130.

Willeberg P, Gerbola MA, Kirkegaard Petersen B, Andersen JB. 1984/85. The Danish pig health scheme: Nation-wide computerbased abattoir surveillance and follow-up at the herd level. Prev Vet Med 3:79–91.

Willeberg P, Gardner IA, Mortensen S, Mousing J. 1994. Model of herd size effects in swine diseases. Proc 7th Int Symp Vet Epidemiol Econ, Kenya 18:189–191.

Willeberg P, Mortensen S, Mousing J. 1995. Effect of herd size on spread of contagious disease. In Proc Animal Health and Related Problems in Densely Populated Livestock Areas of the Community, Brussels, Nov 1994, pp. 53–67.

Williams PP. 1993. Immunomodulating effects of intestinal absorbed maternal colostral leukocytes by neonatal pigs. Can J Vet Res 57:1–8.

Wilson MR, Takov R, Friendship RM, Martin SW, McMillan I, Hacker RR, Swaminathan S. 1986. Prevalence of respiratory diseases and their association with growth rate and space in randomly selected swine herds. Can J Vet Res 50:209–216.

Yagihashi T, Nunoya T, Mitui T, Tajima M. 1984. Effect of *Mycoplasma hyopneumoniae* infection on development of *Haemophilus pleuropneumoniae* pneumonia in pigs. Jpn J Vet Sci 46:705–713.

Zimmermann W, Odermatt W, Tschudi P. 1989. Enzootische Pneumonie (EP): Die Teilsanierung EP-reinfizierter Schweinezuchtbetriebe als Alternative zur Totalsanierung. Schweiz Arch Tierheilkd 131:179–191.

8 Diseases of the Skin

Ranald Cameron

STRUCTURE AND FUNCTION

The skin acts as both a barrier and a communication between the external environment and the internal organs. Its functions include maintenance of body fluids, electrolytes, and macromolecules; protection against chemical, physical, and microbiological damage or invasion; and sensory perception of touch, pressure, pain, itch, and temperature change. Skin also regulates body temperature through support of hair coat, regulation of cutaneous blood supply, and sweat gland function (Scott 1988). Skin has an important function of immunoregulation.

The skin of swine is basically similar in histologic structure to that of other domestic animals and, compared with other species, has many more similarities to human skin (Meyer et al. 1978).

The skin is the largest body organ and can in some animals constitute 12–24% of body weight according to age. In the pig the skin represents between 10% and 12% of body weight at birth and around 7% in adult animals, although in some breeds, such as the Meishan, skin can be 10–12% of adult body weight.

The skin of the pig is divided into two layers, the epidermis and dermis. In most areas the epidermis consists of four layers, since the stratum lucidium is absent except in the snout. The epidermis is relatively thick, the major cells being the keratinocytes in the stratum basale, the polyhedral cells in the stratum spinosum, flattened cells in the stratum granulosum, and cornified cells in the stratum corneum. The thickness of the epidermis varies considerably in different areas of the body (Meyer et al. 1978). Generally the skin of the dorsum is thicker and hairier than the skin of the ventrum. Maximum thickness is between the toes and on the lips, the snout, and the shield, which is unique to the scapular and costal region in older boars. The thinnest layers are found in the axilla, eyelids, and ventral areas of the thorax and abdomen (Marcarian and Calhoun 1966).

The dermis consists of two ill-defined layers beneath which is a prominent layer of adipose tissue (hypodermis). The two layers of the dermis, the stratum papillaris and stratum reticularis, are composed of connective tissue in which are situated blood vessels, nerves, lymphatics, and associated epidermal appendages. Cells found in the dermis include fibroblasts, melanocytes, and mast cells. Origins of hair follicles and sweat glands are found in the hypodermis.

The holocrine sebaceous glands of the pig are branched alveolar and open into the neck of the main hair follicle. The sweat glands are coiled, tubular, and apocrine, and are found in all areas, although there are relatively few (about $25/cm^2$) compared with other species, except on the snout.

In swine the short, stout hair follicles possess arrectores pilorum muscles attached to the outer root sheath; the bristles occur either singly or in groups of two or three. The hair coat consists of 60–70% bristles and 30–40% fine downy hair. Specialized forms of hair are also found—in particular, tactile hairs in the region of the snout (Marcarian and Calhoun 1966; Mowafy and Cassens 1975). Specialized seromucoid glands are found in the carpal glands, located behind the carpus, and in the mental (mandibular) organ, located in the intermandibular space.

CLINICAL EXAMINATION AND DIAGNOSIS

Skin diseases may involve the skin only or be cutaneous manifestations of internal disease (Tables 8.1 and 8.2). Diseases restricted to the skin are, for example, ear necrosis, pityriasis rosea, and swine pox. Examples of skin lesions symptomatic of a more general pathophysiological condition are erysipelas, classical swine fever, and dermatitis/nephropathy syndrome. It is essential therefore that an accurate history be taken, followed by a thorough clinical examination, involving the entire animal first and then the skin itself. Examination of the skin should aim to define the nature of lesions (primary or secondary) or abnormality (vesicles or pustules,

Table 8.1. Causes of diseases of the skin in swine.

A. Infectious			
Bacterial	Viral	Fungal	Parasitic
Exudative epidermitis	Swine pox	Microsporosis	Sarcoptic mange
Streptococcosis	Swine vesicular disease	Trichophytosis	Demodectic mange
Ear necrosis	Vesicular stomatitis	Cutaneous candidiasis	Lice
Spirochetosis	Vesicular exanthema		Fleas
Facial necrosis	Porcine parvovirus		Mosquitoes
Abscesses	Idiopathic vesicular		Flies
Erysipelas	disease		
Salmonellosis	Classical swine fever		
Pasteurellosis	African swine fever		
Mastitis			
Edema disease			
Anthrax			
Malignant edema			

B. Noninfectious				
Environmental	Nutritional	Hereditary	Neoplastic	Miscellaneous
Sunburn	Parakeratosis	Pityriasis rosea	Melanoma	Porcine dermatitis/
Photosensitization	Fatty acid deficiency	Dermatosis vegetans	Rhabdomyoma	nephropathy syndrome
Skin necrosis	Iodine deficiency	Epitheliogenesis imperfecta	Lymphangioma	
Bursitis	Riboflavin deficiency		Papilloma	
Callosities	Pantothenic acid deficiency		Fibroma	
Limb and foot lesions	Biotin deficiency		Hemangioma	
	Vitamin A, C, and E		Sweat gland adenoma	
	deficiencies		Polyp	

Table 8.2. Differential diagnosis of skin diseases.

Location	Lesions and Signs	Diseases
Head and neck	Macules, vesicles, pustules, greasy exudate (seborrhea), crusts in suckling piglets and weaners especially around the eyes	Exudative epidermitis
	Pustules, erosions, crusts, and abscesses	Streptococcosis
	Plaques, pustules, crusts, alopecia with pruritus	Sarcoptic mange
	Pustules, erosions, necrosis, crusts below the eye, cheek, and lips in suckling piglets	Facial necrosis
	Edema around eyes, conjunctiva, and frontal area mainly in weaners and young growers	Edema disease (*E. coli*)
	Edema of head and throat	Malignant edema (*Clostridium* sp.)
	Red to purple discoloration of snout, face, and neck (jowls)	Septicemia
	Discrete ulcer and crust over mandible in sows	Pressure necrosis
	Vesicles, pustules, erosions on snout, lips, mouth, and tongue	Foot-and-mouth disease
		Swine vesicular disease
		Vesicular exanthema
		Vesicular stomatitis
		Porcine parvovirus
		Idiopathic vesicular disease
	Vesicles, erosions, black crusts	Swine pox
Ears	Black necrosis, ulcers on the tips and posterior edge of the pinna in piglets	Ear necrosis
		Salmonellosis
		Erysipelas
	Deep ulcers at the base of the pinna in growers, often bilateral	Ulcerative spirochetosis
	Erythema, red to purple blotchy discoloration	Septicemia
		Classical swine fever
		African swine fever
		Sunburn
	Plaques, brown or gray crusts on the inner ear, ear shaking, pruritus, gray thick crusts on adult animals	Sarcoptic mange
	Macules, pustules, black crusts	Exudative epidermitis
		Streptococcosis
	Circular macules, patches, small scales, pink to red discoloration behind ears and neck	Ringworm (Microsporosis)

Table 8.2.   (*continued*)

Location	Lesions and Signs	Diseases
Dorsum	Hyperkeratosis, dry scales along spine, some alopecia	Essential fatty acid; vitamin A, C, or E; or zinc deficiency Sarcoptic mange
	Complete absence of epithelium (large red shiny areas) in newborn piglets	Epitheliogenesis imperfecta
	Abscesses and pressure necrosis over spine between last ribs and lumbar area in sows	Pressure sores, due to confinement in farrowing crates, pressure from crate bars or prongs
Shoulder	Large deep discrete ulcer, necrosis and crust over spine of scapula in sows often in poor body condition	Pressure sore due to confinement on solid or mesh floors, low energy intake
Ventral abdomen	Erythema, pustules, dark brown crusts, exudate	Exudative epidermitis Streptococcosis Sarcoptic mange Candidiasis Biotin deficiency
	Erythema, round to diamond-shaped red plaques, often with necrotic centers, fever, anorexia, arthritis	Erysipelas
	Papules seen as ringlike lesions, collarettes, flakes and scales (3- to 14-week-old pigs)	Pityriasis rosea
	Circular pink to red macules, scales, or crusts around periphery	Ringworm (Microsporosis, Trichophytosis)
	Papules, thick crusts, fissures, exudate	Zinc deficiency (Parakeratosis) Dermatosis vegetans Exudative epidermitis
	Vesicles, pustules, black scabs, round raised areas with depressed centers	Swine pox
	Erythema, red to purple or black discoloration, skin necrosis in lactating sows	Acute mastitis
	Necrosis of teats, especially pectoral teats in piglets, end of teat appears as red or black (scab) spots	Trauma and infection due to rough floors and poor hygiene in farrowing crates
Lateral abdomen and flank	Erythema, round to diamond-shaped red plaques, often with necrotic centers, fever, anorexia, arthritis	Erysipelas
	Papules, vesicles, pustules, scales, crusts, greasy exudate	Exudative epidermitis Streptococcosis
	Pustules, scales, thick wrinkled skin, alopecia, crusts, with hyperkeratosis	Sarcoptic mange Niacin, pantothenic acid, riboflavin, or vitamin A deficiency
	Erythema, erosion or ulcer on flank	Flank biting
	Papules, plaques seen as ringlike lesions, collarettes, scales (3- to 14-week-old pigs)	Pityriasis rosea
	Circular pink to red macules varying in size, scales or crusts around periphery	Ringworm (Microsporosis, Trichophytosis)
Hindquarters	Erythema of the scrotum, vulva, and perineum	Septicemia Sunburn
	Tail necrosis, ulceration, abscesses (growers)	Tail biting
	Large discrete ulcer, necrosis, scab over hip bone (adult)	Pressure sore
	Erythema, black necrosis, especially scrotum or vulva	Porcine dermatitis/nephropathy syndrome
	Small round raised wheals, urticarial reaction	Insect bites: flies, mosquitoes, fleas
Legs (limbs)	Erythema, red to purple discoloration especially around hocks	Septicemia
	Papules, plaques seen as ringlike lesions, collarettes, scales on medial thighs and legs (3- to 14-week-old pigs)	Pityriasis rosea
	Papules, thick crusts, fissures, papillomas	Parakeratosis (zinc deficiency) Exudative epidermitis
	Complete absence of epithelium (red shiny area) in newborn piglets	Epitheliogenesis imperfecta
	Thick fibrotic areas over joints (hocks, elbows, fetlocks, tuber ischii) often ulcerated	Callosities Bursitis
	Necrosis of carpus, hocks especially, in suckling piglets	Trauma due to rough farrowing-crate floors
Distal limb, coronary band, feet	Thick, dry crusts, deep fissures	Parakeratosis Dermatosis vegetans Exudative epidermitis Sarcoptic mange
	Vesicles, pustules, erosions around coronary band and accessory digits, with lameness	Foot-and-mouth disease Swine vesicular disease Vesicular stomatitis Vesicular exanthema Porcine parvovirus Idiopathic vesicular disease
	Abscesses, discharges, swelling of the coronary band	Bush foot, ascending infections of hoof
	Thickening, ridges and furrows parallel to coronary band	Dermatosis vegetans

edema or erythema). This should be followed by formulation of a differential diagnosis. Tests should then be carried out to confirm a diagnosis (skin scraping, culture, or biopsy) in order to determine the approach to treatment and subsequent prevention.

History

Information obtained should include the following:

Type of Husbandry and Housing System. Extensive or free-range systems may predispose to sunburn or photosensitization. Intensive indoor housing often leads to conditions such as pressure sores in sows or teat necrosis in piglets. Infectious conditions such as exudative epidermitis are more frequently seen in continuous flow through systems than in all-in/all-out systems.

Specific Environmental Conditions. Poor hygiene and high ambient temperatures, relative humidity, and stocking density may predispose to outbreaks of staphylococcal and streptococcal pyoderma. Pityriasis rosea is also more frequently seen with high stocking densities and high humidity. A seasonal pattern may be evident for some skin diseases.

Recent Movement. The mixing of pigs—for example, at weaning—may result in fighting and biting and increase the incidence of exudative epidermitis in the nursery.

Signs of Trauma. Self-inflicted trauma may be due to pruritus associated with sarcoptic mange or lice infestation.

Nutrition. Deficiencies of the B group vitamins, zinc, or essential fatty acids can result in dry, scaly, dandrufflike dermatitis or parakeratosis.

Breed. Breed may indicate a congenital or hereditary condition. Pityriasis rosea has been commonly seen in Landrace pigs and in the progeny of pigs that have had pityriasis rosea as weaners. Other inherited conditions include dermatosis vegetans and epitheliogenesis imperfecta.

Age. A number of diseases are more frequently seen in certain age groups. Exudative epidermitis rarely affects pigs older than 6 weeks of age, and pityriasis rosea is seen only in pigs between 2 and 6 weeks of age. Teat necrosis usually occurs within 24 hours after birth. Nutritional deficiencies are unlikely to occur before weaning.

Chronology of Lesions. Information relating to initial lesions observed and their location may indicate a typical clinical evolution. In swine pox, for example, macules are observed initially, and then vesicles and pustules that rupture to form a dark circumscribed crust before healing. Exudative epidermitis often commences as macules and pustules around the eyes before spreading over the entire body of piglets.

Other Clinical Signs. A history of other signs such as anorexia, depression, loss of body condition, reluctance to move, or diarrhea may indicate the skin lesions are the result of an internal disease.

Incidence. The number of animals affected, the contagious nature, and the history of mortalities may suggest an infectious disease such as exudative epidermitis or erysipelas, which tends to spread rapidly, whereas congenital and hereditary conditions such as pityriasis rosea are seen at a constant rate within a herd.

Response to Therapy. Variation in response to therapy may help to differentiate between viral, bacterial, and fungal infections—for example, swine pox, streptococcal dermatitis, and ringworm. Pityriasis rosea does not respond to any treatment, whereas parakeratosis responds dramatically to the addition of zinc and essential fatty acids to the diet.

Clinical Examination

Before carrying out a detailed examination of the skin a general clinical examination is necessary to determine whether the skin disease is symptomatic of an internal disease.

Internal diseases causing skin lesions or skin abnormalities such as abnormal color changes include erysipelas, salmonellosis, pasteurellosis, mastitis, classical swine and African swine fever, and dermatitis/nephropathy syndrome. Almost any septicemia or toxemia can cause erythema or cyanosis characterized by red to purple discoloration, especially on the extremities and easily seen in the white breeds. Urticaria, seen as multiple pink to purple raised areas of skin, commonly occurs in cases of erysipelas, beta-hemolytic streptococcal infections, food allergy, or insect bites. Blue to black skin discoloration with necrosis can indicate gangrene. Necrosis of the ears and tail of piglets is also black. Pallor is often an indication of blood loss due to conditions such as proliferative enteropathy or gastric ulcerations.

Pruritus causes scratching and should be looked for as a possible sign of sarcoptic mange or lice infestation. Scratching is frequently accompanied by shaking of the head due to the presence of mites in the ears and can result in aural hematomas. Alopecia and excoriation may also be an indicator of intense scratching seen in chronic sarcoptic mange.

Edema of the skin can indicate a systemic disease, for example, hypoproteinemia, vasculitis, increased vascular permeability such as in malignant edema caused by *Clostridium septicum* and in edema disease associated with *Escherichia coli*, the last two conditions producing edema around the head.

Skin lesions are classified as primary, the direct result of the insult or disease, or as secondary, a result of evolutionary changes to the skin dictated by factors such as the cause of the disease, secondary infection, self-trauma, etc.

It is essential for the clinician to differentiate between primary lesions and secondary lesions; however, when the animal is presented, only secondary lesions may be seen. Examination of the entire body of several animals may be necessary to locate primary lesions on recently affected cases.

Primary Lesions. Macules, defined as circumscribed flat discolorations less than 1 cm in diameter, and papules, more solid, raised areas of skin of varying color, are seen in the early stages of exudative epidermitis, erysipelas, and swine pox.

Plaques, elevated superficial lesions more than 0.5 cm in diameter, scattered over the whole body surface of young growing pigs have been associated with erysipelas, pityriasis rosea, and Aujeszky's disease.

Vesicles are well-demarcated, dome-shaped lesions (<1 cm) usually containing serum or inflammatory exudate. They are pale or translucent and are characteristic of a number of the viral skin diseases in swine, such as swine pox, foot-and-mouth disease, swine vesicular disease, and vesicular stomatitis. Similar lesions have been reported in swine with porcine parvovirus infection (Kresse et al. 1985).

Pustules are elevated lesions filled with inflammatory cells (leukocytes) and can be follicular or epidermal. They are white, yellow, or red (hemorrhagic) and, in some cases, are surrounded by erythema. Pustules in swine are commonly associated with streptococcal infections, exudative epidermitis, and swine pox.

Wheals are circumscribed, raised, round or oval areas of skin due to edema. They may be blanched or slightly erythematous. The edema is usually associated with the dermis. Fly and mosquito bites frequently cause wheals.

Secondary Lesions. Scales or flakes can indicate abnormal keratinization and shedding caused by ectoparasites, such as *Sarcoptes scabiei*, or by bacterial skin diseases. Scales are seen on the thinner skin of piglets with exudative epidermitis, on the inner side of the margin of the ringlike lesions of pityriasis rosea, and on the outer periphery of ringworm lesions. Scales may be mixed with sebum and sweat, giving a greasy or oily appearance—seborrhea.

Crusts are a very common secondary skin lesion of swine and are due to a combination of serum, sebum, blood, and cutaneous debris adhering above the normal skin surface. Crusts are seen following bacterial infections and viral vesicular diseases, especially swine pox, and as a result of pruritus associated with sarcoptic mange or lice infestation.

Hyperkeratosis, an increased thickening of the stratum corneum, develops with nutritionally related metabolic disorders such as vitamin A, zinc, and fatty-acid deficiencies or with local callus formation due to trauma associated with pressure and friction. Erythema and intense pruritus with hyperkeratosis and acanthosis have been associated with in-feed tiamulin therapy (Laperle et al. 1988).

Erosions involving the epidermis only and ulcers involving also the dermis are caused by deep bacterial infections (*Staphylococcus* spp., *Streptococcus* spp., *Fusobacterium necrophorum*, and a spirochete referred to as "*Borrelia suis*") or may be due to trauma or pressure.

Severe scratching will result in alopecia, commonly seen over the shoulders and hindquarters in pigs with sarcoptic mange or lice and in pigs irritated by insects such as flies and mosquitoes. The characteristic lesions of pityriasis rosea are typical epidermal collarettes, described as ruptured pustules spreading peripherally with a ring of scales on the inner margins of the ring.

Diagnostic Tests

Diagnosis of skin diseases can be confirmed by a number of relatively simple tests. In swine the most frequently used tests include skin biopsy for histopathological examination, direct smears for identification of bacteria and fungi, and culture for isolation and identification of bacteria and viruses.

Skin Biopsy. Skin biopsy should be used on

- All neoplastic lesions
- Any persistent ulceration
- Skin lesions not responding to treatment

Fully developed primary lesions or early vesicles and pustules are best for biopsy, whereas secondary lesions may be of little value. The technique described by Scott (1988) involves removal of 6–9 mm of skin using a biopsy punch or surgical excision with a scalpel, which may be more suitable for larger lesions, vesicles, and pustules and where the skin is very thick. The skin surface should be cleaned with soap and water but not scrubbed or prepared with antiseptics. Local anesthetic may be indicated. The biopsy should be gently blotted to remove blood and surface material, placed subcutaneous side down on a wooden spatula or cardboard, and gently flattened for 30–60 seconds. The tissue and spatula or cardboard support are immersed within 1–2 minutes in a fixative such as 10% neutral phosphate buffered formalin for at least 24 hours. The volume of fixative should be 10–20 times that of the specimen. Skin biopsies are usually stained with hematoxylin and eosin (H & E).

Skin biopsy, unfixed, can also be used for isolation of bacteria and viruses. For virus isolation, the skin should be cleaned with water or saline only and not with alcohol. Samples should be stored and transported at 4°C in a virus transport medium.

Direct Smear. Direct smear is commonly used for identification of bacteria or fungi. For bacteria, samples of pus or exudate from pustules, macules, or ulcers can be smeared on glass slides, air-dried, and stained with methylene blue, Gram stain, or Diff-Quik for light microscope examination to identify the type of bacteria (cocci or rods, gram-positive or gram-negative) (Scott 1988). Skin scrapings or direct touch impression can be used for suspected fungal diseases. Skin scrapings should be made after defatting the skin with alcohol. Scrapings are warmed in a 20% solution of sodium hydroxide, and spores appear as round highly refractile bodies in chains or mosaics in hair follicles, in epithelial scales, and on the surface of hair fibers.

Culture. Best results are obtained by aspirating samples from intact pustules, vesicles, or abscesses with a needle and syringe. Cultures of open sores (erosions, ulcers, and sinuses) generate confusion (Scott 1988). Bacterial culture is usually done on blood agar or in thioglycolate broth. Virus identification can be done from tissue culture or by electron microscopy. Hair and skin scrapings (surface keratin) can be inoculated onto Sabouraud's dextrose agar or Dermatophyte Test Medium (DTM) for fungal culture (Scott 1988).

BACTERIAL DISEASES

Exudative Epidermitis (Greasy Pig Disease, Impetigo Contagiosa, Seborrhea Contagiosa)

Exudative epidermitis is a generalized dermatitis involving the entire body surface. In the acute form, it usually affects suckling piglets, whereas the chronic form is more commonly seen in older, weaned pigs (Chapter 39).

The disease is caused by *Staphylococcus hyicus*, certain strains of which produce a heat-labile exfoliative toxin (Andresen et al. 1993). Other bacteria frequently isolated from the skin lesions in field cases include *Streptococcus* spp. and *Arcanobacterium pyogenes* (L'Ecuyer and Jericho 1966). Additional factors that may affect the severity and progress of the disease include nutrition, hygiene, immunity, abrasions of the skin, and infection with *Sarcoptes scabiei* var. *suis*. Recent reports have suggested that porcine circovirus type 2 (PCV2) and porcine parvovirus (PPV) could also play an important role in outbreaks of exudative epidermitis (Wattrang et al. 2002; Kim and Chae 2004).

Although pigs develop resistance with age, *S. hyicus* can be recovered from the skin of older pigs, the vagina of sows, and the preputial diverticulum of boars. Piglets can become infected during birth and develop dry scales or flakes over the entire body within 12 hours. These animals are often devoid of hair. Infection usually occurs during the suckling period from sows or in a contaminated farrowing environment. Weaners can be infected after mixing with carrier animals in the nursery.

Suckling piglets, 1–4 weeks old, are the most commonly and often severely affected animals. The morbidity can range from 10% to 90% and mortality from 5% to 90% (average 20%) in suckling piglets. In weaned piglets 3–6 weeks of age, the morbidity can be up to 80% in some groups; however, mortality is usually low. In my experience, lesions may be seen on older animals, especially in immunologically naive gilt herds.

The disease may be acute, subacute, or chronic. In the acute form, the skin lesions are first seen around the eyes, nose, lips, and gums and behind the ears as red-brown spots (macules) that increase in size and develop a vesicular or pustular appearance. The skin soon appears damp and oily as a result of the greasy exudate of sebum, sweat, and serum. Erythema is marked, often over the entire body, and the exudate becomes thick and crusts develop on the skin surface, giving a drier appearance. During this period an obnoxious, rancid odor may be present. When the crusts lift, a raw, highly inflamed skin is left underneath. The feet are frequently affected with erosions on the coronary band and heel. Lesions may develop around the conjunctiva, causing the eyelids to become swollen and matted together. Constipation or, less frequently, diarrhea accompanied by emaciation, dehydration, and often death may be seen 3–5 days after the first signs. The disease has also been associated with lesions of the kidney involving the renal pelvis and tubules (Blood and Jubb 1957). Ulcerative glossitis and stomatitis have been reported by Andrews (1979). Nervous signs were recorded in one outbreak of exudative epidermitis by Blood and Jubb (1957).

The more chronic form (Figure 8.1A) is seen in older pigs 6–10 weeks of age (L'Ecuyer 1966) and up to 5 months of age (Piercy 1966). Occasionally in weaners the disease is seen as only discrete, round, raised lesions (papules), dark red-brown in color, especially on the face and head, with fewer over the body.

The differential diagnosis includes sarcoptic mange, parakeratosis associated with zinc and other nutritional deficiencies, swine pox, pityriasis rosea, and ringworm. Confirmation can be made by biopsy and culture of *S. hyicus*. The biopsy should sample the early typical macules, vesicles, or pustules, before lesions become chronic.

In the early stages of the disease, parenteral antibiotics will greatly reduce the severity and duration as well as mortalities. Antibiotic-resistant *S. hyicus* has frequently been reported but may represent regional differences. The antibiotics of choice include penicillin, ampicillin, amoxicillin, cloxacillin, tetracycline, tylosin, trimethoprim-potentiated sulfonamides, and gentamycin. Resistance to lincomycin, erythromycin, and streptomycin has been reported. Local treatment of the affected areas or the entire body using antibacterial shampoos or skin antiseptics is of value. Preparations used include chlorhexidine, iodophores (providone-iodine), and chloramine. Success when treating large

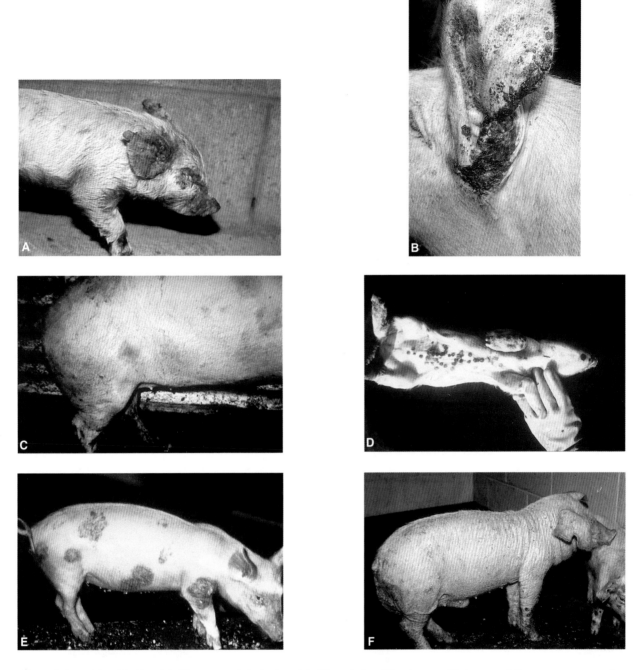

8.1. *(A) Exudative epidermitis (chronic); (B) ear necrosis (spirochetosis); (C) erysipelas; (D) swine pox; (E) ringworm* (Microsporum nanum)*;*
(F) sarcoptic mange. (Color printing courtesy of Pfizer Animal Health Group, New York, N.Y., and MERIAL.)

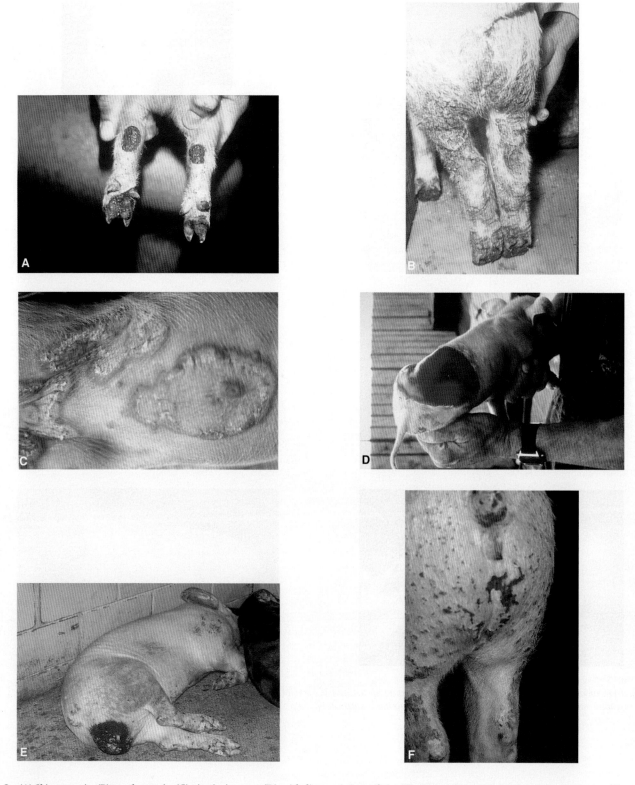

8.2. *(A) Skin necrosis; (B) parakeratosis; (C) pityriasis rosea; (D) epitheliogenesis imperfecta; (E) porcine dermatitis/nephropathy syndrome; (F) porcine dermatitis/nephropathy syndrome. (Color printing courtesy of Pfizer Animal Health Group, New York, N.Y., and MERIAL.)*

numbers of affected animals with in-feed or in-water medication using amoxicillin, oxytetracyclines, or trimethoprim-potentiated sulfonamides has been observed.

During an outbreak, attention should be paid to hygiene, especially in the farrowing and weaner accommodation. Increasing the level of zinc and B group vitamins (especially biotin) in the diet may help in treatment and control. Removal of factors predisposing to skin injury, together with strict hygiene, is important in prevention. Spraying weaner pigs with a skin disinfectant such as chloroxylenol daily for 3 days at the time of weaning and mixing can eliminate outbreaks associated with postweaning fighting. Prevention of sarcoptic mange is also indicated.

Herds derived by hysterectomy or medicated early weaning commonly experience outbreaks of exudative epidermitis soon after being established. Amtsberg (1978) found vaccination to be effective in the prevention of experimentally induced exudative epidermitis. An autogenous vaccine used in commercial herds given to sows twice at 3-week intervals and then every 6 months has also been reported to give good results in eliminating clinical exudative epidermitis (Sieverding 1993).

Pustular Dermatitis (Streptococcosis, Contagious Pyoderma)

Streptococcal infections (Chapter 47) can cause skin necrosis and pustular dermatitis. These conditions are usually caused by the beta-hemolytic streptococci of the Lancefield groups C and L. *Streptococcus zooepidemicus* and *S. equisimilis* have been isolated from abscesses (Miller and Olson 1978, 1980) and porcine ear necrosis (Maddox et al. 1973). Secondary or concurrent infections of the skin frequently involve *S. hyicus*, *Arcanobacterium pyogenes*, and *Borrelia suis* (Penny et al. 1971).

Transmission can be directly from sows to newborn piglets and through skin abrasions and tissue damage associated with tail docking, ear notching, needle teeth clipping, and bite wounds. Abrasions of feet caused by new concrete floors may be associated with streptococcal infections. Outbreaks are usually associated with poor hygiene.

Wounds on any region of the body can become infected, resulting in cellulitis, necrosis, abscess formation, and ulceration. Hare et al. (1942) described the lesions of pustular dermatitis first seen as erythema, occasionally with petechiae over the ventral surface of the abdomen and around the eyes. This is followed by flattened pustules in the inguinal region, on the inner surfaces of the thighs, along the dorsum and tail, and around the eyes, lips, and edge of the ears. On rupture, the pustules heal, forming circular scabs composed of several concentric layers, darker at the center, and resembling large fish scales when peeled. This stage is associated with pruritus. Pustules may form abscesses or

ulcers on the snout, cheeks, tail, legs, and feet. Similar lesions are seen on the udder and teats of sows. The early stages of pustular dermatitis resemble exudative epidermitis and may involve initial infection with *S. hyicus*.

Differential diagnosis includes ulcerative dermatitis, exudative epidermitis, sarcoptic mange, swine pox, and erysipelas. Isolation and identification of streptococci from biopsy material or swabs will confirm a diagnosis.

Treatment with ampicillin, amoxicillin, tetracyclines, or erythromycin can be effective. Local treatment of lesions with disinfectants such as tincture of iodine or iodophores (providone-iodine) is useful. Strict hygiene is essential, especially when carrying out procedures such as clipping needle teeth, ear notching, and tail docking, as well as prevention of injuries by removal of rough, corroded, or splintered surfaces. Regular disinfection in conjunction with all-in/all-out management, especially in the farrowing and nursery accommodation, will help to reduce the buildup of streptococci.

Vaccination with autogenous bacterins has been used as a control measure in herds with contagious pustular dermatitis (Scott 1988).

Ear Necrosis (Necrotic Ear Syndrome, Ulcerative Spirochetosis of the Ear)

Ear necrosis is a syndrome seen in pigs aged from 1 to 10 weeks. It is characterized by bilateral or unilateral necrosis of any part of the ear, but especially in young pigs on the tip and around the posterior edge of the pinna. In growers, necrosis at the base of the ear can occur, with many pigs being affected at any one time. Outbreaks often occur in one pen of pigs, with up to 80% affected.

It is likely that the lesions are the result of a mixed infection following damage to the skin. It has been suggested that infection with *S. hyicus* may take place first, followed by the more invasive streptococci and spirochetes, resulting in necrosis and ulceration (Fraser et al. 1991). Biting following mixing of pigs is a common predisposing factor. In older pigs ear biting can be a vice similar to flank and tail biting, and lead to infection. Self-inflicted trauma resulting from the irritation of *Sarcoptes scabiei* infection in the ears can initiate the early lesions.

The lesions can range from mild, superficial dermatitis (plaques) of the tip, edges, and base of the pinna to more severe inflammation with exudation, ulceration (Figure 8.1B), and necrosis (Harcourt 1973). The areas of necrosis may become dry, crusty, and curled over, with eventual loss of some of the ear or the entire ear. Some pigs may show signs of inappetence, unthriftiness, and fever; death may occur in a few cases.

Bacterial culture and histopathological examination will help to confirm a diagnosis. Injections of penicillin, ampicillin, amoxicillin, or tetracyclines for at least 4–5 days will be of value, especially if combined with local application of a suitable skin disinfectant such as tincture of iodine, iodophore, or chlorhexidine. General hygiene of the environment and elimination of predisposing factors such as ear biting and fighting are essential for control.

Ulcerative Dermatitis (Granulomatous Dermatitis)

Ulcerative dermatitis can occur as ulcerative, necrotic, or tumorlike lesions found on most areas of the body surface and around the buccal cavity of pigs. More specific syndromes such as ear necrosis, facial necrosis, infected bursae, and calluses over joints and bony prominences can be forms of spirochetosis.

The etiology involves initial trauma of the skin, followed by infection, often involving several organisms. Although the typical lesions appear to be caused by a spirochete, which was reported as *Borrelia suis*, early infection with *S. hyicus* and beta-hemolytic *Streptococcus* spp. is most likely. *Arcanobacterium pyogenes* is a common secondary invader (Cameron 1984).

Skin trauma or damage that results in infections can be associated with bite wounds, especially around the face and head and on the flank and tail. Infection following castration, pressure sores, and ulceration of swollen bursae and calluses often leads to spirochetosis. Gum damage following teeth clipping can result in lesions in the buccal cavity.

Lesions are most commonly seen in young pigs or, in the case of pressure sores and bursitis, in older growers and adults. The initial lesions are characterized by erythema and edema followed by necrosis, ulceration, or tumefaction, with fistulae discharging a grayish brown glutinous pus. Lesions may continue to enlarge for several months and involve deeper structures of the body. The central area will often slough.

A differential diagnosis would include foreign-body abscesses, neoplasms, other infectious granulomas, and pressure necrosis. A diagnosis can be made by identification of spirochetes from direct smears, dark-field illumination of wet preparations, or biopsy examination. Culture of secondary invaders will also be of value.

Procaine or benzathine penicillin, ampicillin, or amoxicillin are the drugs of choice. Treatment should continue for at least 5 days. Surgical removal of large granulomas may be indicated. Local treatment may be of value using aerosol preparations of tetracycline or skin disinfectants. Fly repellents are indicated to prevent myiasis. Control of ulcerative dermatitis is by the elimination of factors that result in skin damage and trauma. Improved hygiene at teeth clipping and castration and attention to wounds due to fighting, flank biting, and pressure sores are essential to avoid infection.

Facial Necrosis (Facial Pyemia)

Facial necrosis is a common condition in suckling pigs less than 1 week of age and is characterized by bilateral necrotic ulcers that are often covered by hard brown crusts and that extend from the side of the face to the lower jaw area.

The condition is the result of infection of wounds inflicted by piglets on each other during feeding, often because inexperienced stockpersons have failed to carry out teeth clipping correctly. Lacerations to the side of the face become infected with organisms such as *Fusobacterium necrophorum*, *Streptococcus* spp., and *Borrelia suis*.

Facial necrosis is commonly seen in large litters and especially in the disadvantaged weaker piglets and when milk letdown is slow, that is, when sows suffer from agalactia or hypogalactia.

Facial necrosis occurs during the first few days of life and any number of piglets in a litter can be affected. Initially lesions can be seen as striated lacerations caused by bites from other piglets. The lesions become infected, resulting in shallow ulcerations covered with hard brown crusts. The encrustation may extend over a large area involving the lips and eyelids, making it difficult for the piglet to open its mouth or eyes. These animals have difficulty in feeding and may starve. Facial necrosis can predispose to outbreaks of exudative epidermitis.

The condition is easily diagnosed by the nature and distribution of the lesions on the face of young piglets. Bacteriological examination of the lesions will help identify the organisms involved.

Careful removal of the crusts and application of a mild disinfectant solution of chlorhexidine or iodophores or of an antibiotic cream will help remove the infection as well as soften the lesions. Prevention is by clipping the canine and lateral incisor teeth just above the level of the gum surface during the first 24 hours of life in all piglets in the litter. Instruments used should be thoroughly disinfected. Fostering piglets to eliminate large litters will help reduce competition for teats at feeding. Hygiene in the farrowing accommodation and prevention of milk letdown problems are also important.

Abscesses

Subcutaneous abscesses are common in pigs, usually as a result of fighting, bite wounds, and lacerations from rough floors and housing. Abscesses may also result from injections when using contaminated needles or through dirty skin following castration or tail biting. Tail abscesses can result in infection spreading by lymphatic drainage to the pelvic inlet, sacral region, and vertebral column.

The organisms commonly present in abscesses of the skin in swine include *Arcanobacterium pyogenes*, *Streptococcus* spp., *Bacteroides* spp., and anaerobic gram-positive cocci. *Actinobacillus equuli* and *A. suis* have also been reported as causing subcutaneous abscesses in the neck, withers, and flanks in swine (Mullowney 1984).

The treatment of choice is surgical drainage followed by flushing the open wound with a suitable antiseptic and treatment with antibiotics such as ampicillin, tetracycline, or trimethoprim/sulfonamide.

Erysipelas

Erysipelas is an infectious disease of pigs that manifests in several forms, including septicemia, nonsuppurative arthritis, vegetative endocarditis, and skin lesions (Chapter 37). The disease is seen mainly in pigs between 3 months and 3 years of age. Younger pigs are protected by passive immunity acquired from suckling immune sows. The disease is caused by *Erysipelothrix rhusiopathiae*.

In acute erysipelas, the skin of the extremities—including the snout, ears, lower limbs, tail, and scrotal area, as well as the jowls and ventral surface of the abdomen—is erythematous. The color varies from pink to purple, typical of many systemic infections and not necessarily diagnostic of erysipelas.

The more specific skin lesions associated with erysipelas first appear as small pink or red raised areas (papules) or larger plaques ranging from 3 to 6 cm in diameter. Many of these lesions will develop the characteristic diamond or rhomboidal shape and are raised, firm, and easily palpated (Figure 8.1C). The outer area is pink in color and the center becomes blue to purple (necrosis) as the disease progresses. These discrete lesions are associated with arteritis; the small arterioles show acute cellular infiltration and cellular thrombi with the presence of mainly neutrophils (Jubb et al. 1985). In the chronic stage, skin lesions become more necrotic; appear dark, dry, and firm; and easily peel away from the underlying tissues. Occasionally, sloughing of the ears, tail, or a foot can occur (Scott 1988). Alopecia may be seen in more long-standing cases.

The systemic signs generally associated with the disease, together with the typical skin lesions, usually make the diagnosis of erysipelas on clinical grounds relatively easy. Acute septicemia and erythema have to be differentiated from classical swine fever (hog cholera), African swine fever, salmonellosis, and pasteurellosis. The early, smaller plaques can be confused with insect bites, sarcoptic mange, or exudative epidermitis. Culture of the organism (from the live animal) may be possible in the early stages of the disease from blood and skin biopsy of typical lesions. Several animals should be sampled. Culture is usually more successful at necropsy from a variety of organs: heart, lung, liver, spleen, kidneys, and joints (Wood 1992). A number of serological tests have been used for detecting infection; however, they have limited practical value for clinical diagnosis.

Penicillin is the drug of choice and should be given daily for 3–5 days. In the case of very sick pigs, the first two injections may be given 12 hours apart. At-risk, in-contact animals should also be treated with penicillin. Long-acting preparations can be used.

Prevention is by regular vaccination of sows and boars. Sows should be vaccinated twice at selection and 4 weeks before farrowing, and boars twice yearly. If outbreaks occur in grower stock, a weaner vaccination program may be of value. Reducing contact with effluent and maintaining a good standard of hygiene will help prevent outbreaks.

Salmonellosis

Salmonellosis (Chapter 45) in pigs can cause septicemia and thus skin lesions and changes in skin color. This form of the disease is generally caused by *Salmonella choleraesuis*. All age groups of pigs can be affected, although pigs from weaning to 4 months of age are most frequently affected.

In the acute form associated with septicemia, mortalities can be high, and other pigs may be weak and moribund. Cyanosis of the extremities and abdomen may be seen. The discoloration of the skin is due to intense capillary dilation and congestion in the dermal papillae, followed by thrombosis in the capillaries and venules and, to a lesser extent, arterioles, leading to necrosis and sloughing of the skin. Skin necrosis commonly involves the ears, tail, and feet in young pigs.

Discoloration of the skin is similar to that in other septicemic diseases—that is, swine fever, erysipelas, and pasteurellosis—which therefore have to be considered in a differential diagnosis. Ear necrosis also has to be differentiated from necrosis associated with other infectious agents.

Diagnosis will be made on the basis of clinical signs and isolation and serotyping of the organism—in particular, at necropsy from spleen, liver, lungs, mesenteric lymph nodes, and small intestines.

Acute Mastitis

Some of the acute forms of infectious mastitis in sows immediately following farrowing are accompanied by extensive discoloration of the skin. The affected mammary glands are pink to red and later may become dark purple or black (gangrene).

VIRAL DISEASES

Swine Pox (Contagious Impetigo, Louse-Borne Dermatitis)

Swine pox is a typical poxvirus infection mainly affecting young pigs. There is little or no systemic illness, and lesions are usually confined to the ventrolateral abdomen and thorax (see Chapter 29).

The virus is abundant in the lesions and transmission is by direct contact. Injury to the skin will aid in the infection becoming established. Lice and possibly other blood-sucking insects are an important means of disease transmission in swine herds. Congenital swine pox has been reported (Borst et al. 1990; Thibault et al. 1998a).

The lesions follow the typical pox evolution of erythematous macules becoming papules, and then vesicles progressing to pustules, which rupture and form crusts (Figure 8.1D). Lesions are seen mainly on the side of the body, ventral abdominal wall, and inner thighs. Occasionally lesions are seen on the back, face, and udder. Skin lesions develop within 5 days after experimental intradermal inoculation (Kasza and Griesemer 1962). After first appearance of the lesions, the papules enlarge to 6 mm in diameter. The lesions of the pustular stage become umbilicated, ischemic, and yellow in color. The center of the lesions decreases in height and the peripheral tissue hypertrophies. Within 10 days dark crusts appear, and within 20 days the crusts desquamate, leaving small white discolored spots. The nature and distribution of the lesions may be influenced by secondary bacterial infections. The site of the lesions affects the various stages in the progress of the disease. Vesicles do not form on the thick skin of the back, but proliferative changes with necrosis of the epithelium take place, producing crusts.

Swine pox has to be differentiated from the other vesicular diseases, early cases of sarcoptic mange, and erysipelas. Vesicular diseases such as foot-and-mouth disease and swine vesicular disease are more severe, and lesions are mainly confined to the snout, lips, tongue, palate, coronary band, and feet. Swine pox is relatively mild, and eruptions on mucosal surfaces are rare. Diagnosis can be confirmed by host range studies, serological tests, histological examination, and virus isolation or detection of viral antigens.

Treatment is directed at control of secondary bacterial infections using antibiotics and improving the general health of the animals. No vaccines are available, and prevention of outbreaks is by avoiding the introduction of carrier animals, good sanitation, and control of the pig louse.

Vesicular Diseases

Foot-and-mouth disease, swine vesicular disease, vesicular stomatitis, and vesicular exanthema can all cause vesicular skin lesions in swine. The diseases all produce very similar lesions with similar distribution.

The characteristic lesions of foot-and-mouth disease are vesicles filled with straw-colored fluid that form in the mucosa of the mouth, including the tongue, lips, gums, pharynx, and palate, and in the coronary band. Lesions are also seen between and above the claws and on the snout. Sows may develop lesions on the udder and teats (Mann and Sellers 1989).

Vesicles rupture rapidly, leaving a raw hemorrhagic eroded area with ragged fragments of necrotic epithelium. The lesions heal quickly, beginning with a serofibrinous exudate and a gradual replacement that may or may not be pigmented depending on the cells involved (Callis et al. 1975). With swine vesicular disease, lameness may be severe, as lesions most commonly involve the coronary band, hoof, heel, and supernumerary digits. Separation of the horn of the hoof often occurs, commencing from the coronary band.

The clinician should collect samples for virus isolation and serology, fixed tissue for histopathology, and epithelial and vesicular fluid for complement-fixation and ELISA testing for viral antigens. Animal inoculation studies may also be used.

Porcine Parvovirus

Kresse et al. (1985) reported erosions and vesicles on the snout, mouth, coronet, and interdigital space of swine in the midwestern United States in several herds. The virus was isolated from the skin as well as from serum and other organs.

Idiopathic Vesicular Disease

Several cases of vesicles of unknown or doubtful etiology have been reported in swine. Gibbs et al. (1983) reported vesicles and erosions on only the feet in swine in Florida. Munday and Ryan (1982) and Montgomery et al. (1987) reported vesicles on the snout and feet of swine fed marine products, parsnips, or celery.

Classical Swine Fever (Hog Cholera)

Classical swine fever is caused by a pestivirus of the family Togaviridae. Diffuse erythema followed by purplish discoloration of the skin over the abdomen, snout, ears, and thighs is common in acute cases. Necrosis of the edges of the ears, tail, and vulva may develop. Purple blotching of the ears is characteristic, with generalized hypotrichosis in the chronic form of the disease. Congenital alopecia has been reported in piglets infected in utero (Carbrey et al. 1966).

African Swine Fever

African swine fever is caused by a DNA virus at present unclassified. Besides general signs of fever, depression, anorexia, and incoordination similar to hog cholera, skin changes include cyanotic blotching and purple discoloration of the limbs, snout, abdomen, and ears. Hemorrhages may also occur on the skin of the ears and flanks.

Porcine Reproductive and Respiratory Syndrome (PRRS)

An unusual case of severe cutaneous hemorrhages with dermal and subcutaneous capillary angioplasia has been reported in aborted, stillborn, and live-born weak piglets during an outbreak of PRRS virus abortions (Scruggs and Sorden 2001). The affected full-term stillborn piglets and live-born weak piglets had single or multiple coalescent dark reddish-blue cutaneous hemorrhages on the pinnae, cranium and lateral cervical and shoulder areas. Less severely affected piglets had small (2–10 mm) hemorrhages on the skin of the lateral neck and hind limbs. Because the lesions were seen only during the outbreak of PRRS and disappeared after the abortion storm and localization of PRRS virus antigen within macrophages adjacent to proliferating capillaries was demonstrated, it was suggested the PRRS virus played a role in the development of the lesions.

FUNGAL DISEASES (RINGWORM)

Fungal diseases of swine tend to be superficial mycoses involving the keratinized epithelial cells and hair only. Fungi reported in swine include *Microsporum nanum*, *M. canis*, *M. gypseum*, *Trichophyton mentagrophytes*, *T. rubrum*, *T. tonsurans*, *T. verrucosum*, and *Candida albicans*.

Ringworm is found in both extensively and intensively reared swine. All age groups can be affected and the incidence appears to be higher where sanitation is poor and stocking densities are high with moderate temperatures and high humidity. Bedding may be an important source of infection. Fungal spores can remain viable for many years in a dry and cool environment. Mycelial growth is promoted when the environmental conditions are warm and humid with a slightly alkaline skin pH. Ringworm fungi are strictly aerobic.

Microsporosis

Microsporum nanum is the most common fungal infection in swine; however, *M. canis* produces ringworm in piglets and *M. gypseum* is also found on pigs. Ringworm lesions can be found on almost any part of the body.

Ginther (1965) described the typical lesions as beginning as circumscribed spots, which tend to enlarge in a circle, some to enormous size covering the complete side of the pig (Figure 8.1E). The skin is reddish to light brown in color, roughened but not raised. Dry crusts form around the periphery, the hair is usually not lost, and no pruritus develops. Dirt and dust may obscure the lesions, which often are not noticed until the pigs are washed.

Experimental infection with *M. nanum* (Connole and Baynes 1966) produced lesions that first appeared as pustules or moist brown areas of desquamated tissue 2 cm in diameter. As the lesions extended, fresh pustules were often seen near the periphery. Scales, crusts, and deposits of black material similar to the natural infection appeared. Lesions developed in 2–3 weeks and resolved by 9 weeks. Chronic infections are often seen behind the ears of adult swine and appear as thick, brown crusts that spread over the ear and neck.

Trichophytosis

Trichophyton mentagrophytes is the most common cause of trichophytosis in swine, but *T. rubrum*, *T. tonsurans*, and *T. verrucosum* can also cause ringworm in swine. Lesions are found on the thorax, flank, and neck, behind the ears, and on the legs. The size and shape of lesions vary; some measure up to 12.5 cm across and are roughly circular. Typical lesions are red or covered by a thin brownish dry crust. The disease tends to be self-limiting and lasts about 10 weeks (McPherson 1956). Similar lesions have been described by Pepin and Austwick (1968) in a herd of Wessex pigs. The same authors reported an outbreak of ringworm in a litter of Large White piglets caused by *T. verrucosum*. Arora et al. (1979) described lesions caused by *T. rubrum* as rough and reddish and appearing on several sites; 10% of piglets and 4% of sows in a herd were affected.

Cutaneous Candidiasis

Candidiasis in swine is caused by the yeast *Candida albicans* and appears to cause disease when the host's resistance is lowered. The disease has been reported in grower pigs fed garbage and kept in unsanitary conditions. The morbidity was 40%. The lesions on the most severely affected animals consisted of circular areas approximately 2 cm in diameter coated with moist gray exudate. Lesions were found on all limbs and the lateral and ventral surfaces of the abdomen. The skin was thickened, wrinkled, devoid of hair, and hung loose in folds (Reynolds et al. 1968).

Treatment and Control

Treatment, if indicated, consists of removal of the crusts and local application of products such as a weak solution of iodine, Whitfield's ointment, copper sulfate or copper naphthenate, or thibendazole ointment (2–4%) as a suspension in glycerine. Agriculture Bordeaux mixture (an aqueous solution of copper sulfate and unslaked lime) has been used with good results (Blood and Radostits 1989). Systemic treatment employs oral administration of griseofulvin at a dose rate of 1 g/100 kg body weight daily for up to 40 days.

Control is by maintaining good sanitation. Housing can be disinfected with phenolic disinfectant (2.5–5%), sodium hypochlorite (0.25% solution), or a 2.0% formaldehyde and 1.0% caustic soda solution used as a spray.

PARASITIC DISEASES

Sarcoptic Mange (Scabies)

Sarcoptic mange is the most commonly encountered parasitic skin disease of swine. It is one of the most important skin diseases and of major economic importance (Chapter 53). The disease is caused by the mange mite *Sarcoptes scabiei* var. *suis*.

The disease is more likely to be seen where nutrition, management, and hygiene are of a low standard. The disease affects weight gain (McPherson 1960) and efficiency of feed conversion by as much as 10% in pigs between 18 and 68 kg (Cargill and Dobson 1979b).

The first skin lesions appear about 3 weeks after contact with mites as small encrustations around the ears, eyes, and snout that develop into plaques about 5 mm in diameter. The lesions in the ear may regress and disappear in 12–18 weeks (Cargill and Dobson 1979a). Early pruritus is due to the local irritation from the mites establishing themselves in the skin. As the ear lesions regress, focal erythematous papules associated with hypersensitivity occur on the rump, flank, and abdomen (Cargill and Dobson 1979a). Mites are not usually found in these lesions. The hypersensitivity causes further pruritus, which results in excessive rubbing and the liberation of tissue fluids, giving the animal a greasy or shiny appearance. This is followed by coagulation and drying of the serum, sebum, and sweat to form crusts. In more chronic cases (Figure 8.1F) excessive keratinization and proliferation of the connective tissue occur, with the result that the skin becomes thickened and wrinkled (Dobson and Davies 1992). A common sign seen in grower pigs is shaking of the ears and, in some, the development of large hematomas on the inner surface of the ear.

Chronic cases, usually in adults, develop thick gray-colored, loosely attached scales lining the inner surface of the ears, around the neck, and down the lower limbs, especially over the hock joints. Considerable loss of hair is associated with chronic mange.

Sarcoptic mange needs to be differentiated from exudative epidermitis, parakeratosis associated with zinc and fatty-acid deficiency, B group vitamin deficiency, sunburn, pityriasis rosea, and ringworm. Mange may be present with and predispose to exudative epidermitis. Pruritus may be caused by other parasites such as lice, fleas, and mosquitoes. The clinical signs, together with a range of lesions, will be suggestive of mange. When investigating a herd for evidence of the disease, the ears of adult stock should be examined for chronic lesions.

Demonstration of the mites is best done by examination of the crusts inside the ears. The material can be placed on black paper for a few minutes and then gently tipped or blown off leaving the mites, which will have adhered to the paper. They can be easily examined with a magnifying glass (Brackenridge 1958).

Another method is to place the scales or material from skin scrapings in a 10% solution of sodium or potassium hydroxide for 24 hours, and then concentrate the sediment by centrifugation and examine it for the mites on a glass slide under low power of a microscope. Skin scrapings obtained with a scalpel blade placed on a glass slide and mixed with mineral oil can also be examined in the same way. The movement of live mites allows easy detection.

Sarcoptic mange has been treated with varying success by many remedies and acaricides used in the form of sprays, dusting powders, and pour-ons, in feed medication, and by injection. Insecticides used as sprays or washes (dips) include amitraz, coumaphos, diazinon, lindane, malathion, toxaphene, and trichlorfon. Products that have a systemic action have proved to be more effective, such as the pour-on phosmet and oral or injectable administration of avomectins, such as doramectin, a long-acting endoectocide for use in swine (Cargill et al. 1996). These products are more likely to be successful in eradication of sarcoptic mange, although results have been variable.

For control, monthly treatment of all pigs is effective (Cargill 1981); however, programs are best aimed at sow treatment just before farrowing, followed by weaning

into mite-free accommodations (Cargill and Dobson 1979b). Complete elimination of sarcoptic mange in pig populations can be achieved by the use of hysterectomy-derived piglets and maintained by strict biosecurity. Herds have been kept free of sarcoptic mange for over 20 years in my experience.

Demodectic Mange (Follicular Mange)

Demodectic mange is relatively uncommon and of little economic importance in swine. Clinical signs are seen when pigs are in a poor or debilitated condition. The disease is caused by *Demodex phylloides*, which lives in the hair follicles or sebaceous glands of the skin.

The mites usually invade the soft skin of the snout and around the eyes but can spread over the entire body. Infection is not uncommon on the abdomen between the legs. Lesions start as small red spots which become scaly with a nodular appearance. The nodules contain white caseous material and many mites. Mites can be found on skin scrapings from around the eyes in pigs showing no clinical signs. Treatment is usually not successful and severely affected animals should be culled.

Lice

The pig louse, *Haematopinus suis*, which affects pigs only, causes severe irritation resulting in continual scratching and rubbing against objects.

Lice are easily found around the neck, base of the ears, inner ears, and inside the legs and flank, and the white eggs can also be seen on the bristles, especially in colored pigs. The blood feeding causes considerable irritation; the resultant scratching and rubbing against objects damages the skin, which becomes lacerated and bleeds. Lice tend to congregate around the areas where skin damage has taken place. The continual irritation results in loss of body weight and reduces weight gains. Lice may spread the swine pox virus and erysipelas.

Lice can be controlled by spraying with products such as coumaphos, diazinon, malathion, lindane, or ronnel. Ivermectin in feed or injected also controls lice.

Fleas, Mosquitoes, and Flies

Swine may be affected by fleas (*Ctenocephalides canis, C. felis, Pulex irritans,* and *Echinophaga gallinaceae*), mosquitoes (*Aedes* spp.), flies (*Musca domestica, Stomoxys calcitrans*), and screwworm flies (*Callitroga* spp.).

Clinical signs can include varying degrees of rubbing, scratching resulting in alopecia, excoriations, and bleeding from the skin and circumscribed, raised, rounded (wheal) lesions or edema associated with urticarial reactions.

ENVIRONMENTAL DISEASES

Sunburn

Sunburn is frequently seen in white pigs managed under open-range conditions without adequate protection from sunlight. It is caused by the direct effect of ultraviolet rays upon the skin.

Young pigs and pigs not previously exposed to sunlight are often seriously affected. Erythema occurs within a few hours of exposure and develops most commonly on the back and behind the ears. Edema can develop and affected areas become warm and painful to the touch. Severely affected pigs walk very carefully and are occasionally seen to experience a sudden bout of muscular twitching and jump into the air. The skin becomes dry, scales develop, and the skin peels. In young pigs the tail and ears become necrotic and slough.

A simple and effective treatment is to cover the skin with a bland oil, for example, vegetable oil or light mineral oil. Animals should be removed from direct sunlight and adequate shade provided for prevention.

Photosensitization

Photosensitization is a condition seen in extensive, free-range-managed swine exposed to photodynamic agents and sunlight. Photosensitivity (hypersensitivity to light) results from the ingestion of photodynamic agents such as hypericin found in Saint-John's-wort (*Hypericum perforatum*) and fagopyrin found in buckwheat (*Fagopyrium esculentum* and *Polygonum fagopyrum*). Other plants, including rape (*Brassica* sp.), lucerne (*Medicago sativa*), and *Trifolium* sp., cause photosensitization of unknown etiology. Other substances causing photosensitization in swine are phenothiazine, tetracyclines, sulfonamides (Amstutz 1975), and possibly aphids (McClymont and Wynne 1955).

Lesions are seen in white-skinned breeds and on areas most directly exposed to the sunlight. The severity of the condition depends on the concentration of the photodynamic agent and the length of exposure to light (Jubb and Kennedy 1970).

Erythema and edema develop and serum may exude from the skin and become dry and matted in the hair. Pain causes swine to walk carefully, and severely affected animals may suddenly drop into sternal recumbency and immediately rise again or stagger sideways (Hungerford 1990). The ears become thickened; congestion of the conjunctiva may occur with matting together of the eyelids (Amstutz 1975). Skin becomes dry, hard, and fissured and extremely pruritic. Areas of skin may become necrotic and peel off in strips. Ears and tail may slough.

Sunburn, erysipelas, and sarcoptic mange have to be included in a differential diagnosis. The typical lesions confined to unpigmented or white areas of skin exposed to sunlight and a history of ingestion of a photodynamic agent or plants known to cause photosensitization will suggest a diagnosis.

Affected animals should be placed in darkened housing. Parenteral use of corticosteroids or antihistamines may be of value. Local application of antibiotic creams may also be useful. Control is by preventing access to photodynamic agents, grazing only at night, or keeping pigs indoors.

Skin Necrosis

In piglets, skin necrosis most frequently affects the knees, fetlocks, hocks, elbows, teats, coronets, and soles of the feet. Necrosis of the hocks, vulva, and tail is common in piglets with splayleg. In sows, skin necrosis is common on the shoulder, over the hip region, and on the side of the jaw.

In piglets, necrosis starts as small abraded areas often developing 12–24 hours after birth and reaching maximum severity in 7 days (Penny et al. 1971). Lesions are due to trauma from hard abrasive floors, especially rough concrete in farrowing crates. The alkaline pH of new concrete floors and slats may also affect older pigs. Necrosis of the soles of the feet can be caused by the abrasive surface of rusting wire mesh or metal floors (Figure 8.2A).

Teat necrosis is best looked for at 3 days of age (Stevens 1984). The lesions develop as blackish brown scales or crusts that easily peel off, leaving a new, fresh wound. Teat necrosis usually affects the pectoral (first four) teats, resulting in blind, nonfunctional teats. The highest incidence was found in pigs on heated concrete floors, with decreasing incidence on expanded-metal floors, rubber mats, and plastic-coated wire mesh. A genetic basis for teat necrosis associated with sire lines was demonstrated, but nongenetic causes were more common than genetic causes (Stevens 1984). Females are most commonly affected.

Necrosis of the knees (carpus) is very common in the weaker smaller piglets in large litters and where sows have problems of milk letdown or mastitis. Necrosis of the tail starts at the base, usually encircling the whole tail, which becomes black and may slough. Ear necrosis may be due to fighting or infections.

Skin necrosis in sows is due to a combination of pressure from lying for long periods on hard floors (both concrete and mesh) and poor body condition associated with rapid weight loss during lactation or old age. The condition can occur in young sows after their first litter.

Local application of antibiotic or antiseptic ointments may be of value. Aerosol sprays for wound treatment give good results. Open wounds may require parenteral antibiotic therapy. Control should be aimed at avoiding rough, wet concrete floors and rusting mesh floors and providing bedding or rubber mats in the creep area of farrowing crates. Spreading mash feed over the floors of new pens will help prevent necrosis in young grower pigs. Reducing the incidence of splayleg by selection should be considered.

Stevens (1984) stated that 80% of teat necrosis can be eliminated by replacing concrete floors with raised plastic-coated decks. Resin-reinforced plastic skin has been used to protect teats immediately after birth

(Muirhead 1978). Skin necrosis of sows is best prevented by maintaining good body condition through appropriate feeding before and during lactation, using plastic-coated floors in farrowing crates, and encouraging sows to stand and exercise frequently.

Callosities

Hypertrophy with fibrosis of the skin over joints and bony prominences results in callus formation. Calluses are seen mainly over the fetlocks, elbows, hocks, and tuber ischii. They become very large and hard and contain fluid, which may become infected and result in subcutaneous abscesses. Pigs with leg weakness, foot lesions, or muscular weakness or that spend a lot of time lying down due to illness frequently develop callosities or bursitis.

NUTRITIONAL DISEASES

Swine Parakeratosis

Scott (1988) describes parakeratosis as a nutrition-related metabolic disorder of growing pigs characterized by a generalized nonpruritic, crusting dermatosis. The cause of this condition is now considered to be complex, involving deficiencies of zinc and essential fatty acids or high levels of calcium, phytates, and other chelating agents that affect zinc absorption. Gastrointestinal diseases may also predispose to a more severe zinc deficiency and parakeratosis.

Early lesions (macules and papules) develop on the ventral surface of the abdomen, medial thighs, and distal parts of the legs. The lesions rapidly become covered with scales and then hard dry crusts (Figure 8.2B). The typical keratinous lesions are characterized by crusts and deep fissures. The surface of the skin may be dry and rough, but moist brownish sebum, dirt, and debris accumulate in the fissures. In severe cases animals will have reduced growth rates and reduced appetite, diarrhea, and in some cases vomiting. Testicular development may be affected. Mortalities are rare.

The condition has to be differentiated from chronic sarcoptic mange, exudative epidermitis, and deficiencies of the B group vitamins and iodine.

A history of feeding a diet likely to be deficient in zinc or essential fatty acids or including factors that may interfere with zinc absorption, together with the characteristic lesions and their distribution, will suggest parakeratosis.

Skin biopsy for histopathology will be of value. Serum alkaline phosphatase and zinc levels may be decreased. Response to supplementary zinc and essential fatty acids will support a diagnosis.

Treatment and prevention involve feeding a diet that provides zinc in the form of a zinc salt (zinc sulfate or carbonate) at the rate of 0.02%, or 2 kg per tonne of feed. Fats should provide 1% of the total ration. The calcium levels should not exceed 1% of the ration.

Other Nutritional Deficiencies

Skin changes can result from a number of nutritional deficiencies and excesses. Typical changes are poor hair coat, alopecia, parakeratosis, and eczematous dermatitis.

Essential fatty-acid deficiencies produce a dull, dry hair coat and scaly, dandrufflike dermatitis. Brownish exudate appears on the ears and axillary spaces and under the flanks. This can be followed by necrotic lesions and skin eruptions with loss of hair.

Iodine deficiency is seen as a congenital defect in piglets born to sows fed iodine-deficient diets. Piglets are born full-term but hairless. They have thickened edematous skin over the head, neck, and shoulders.

Riboflavin (vitamin B_2) deficiency in swine produces a dermatitis seen as scales and ulcers with some loss of hair and heavy sebaceous exudate. Conjunctivitis, swollen eyelids, and cataracts may occur. Infertility, weak pigs, and lactation failure are seen in sows.

Pantothenic acid deficiency results in signs of poor growth rate, coughing, diarrhea, and loss of hair. Dermatitis develops as dark brown exudate around the eyes. Incoordination, seen as "goose-stepping," is also characteristic.

Biotin deficiency produces skin changes characterized by dermatitis; dry rough skin with scales, crusts, and brown exudate; generalized alopecia; and ulcerations (Cunha 1977). Lesions of the feet include bruising, erosions, and ulceration of the soles and cracking of the outer wall of the claw (Brooks et al. 1977; Penny et al. 1980).

Vitamin A, C, and E deficiencies have been associated with scurfy (scales) skin lesions. Vitamin E and selenium deficiencies have also been associated with ear necrosis.

CONGENITAL AND HEREDITARY DISEASES

Pityriasis Rosea (Pustular Psoriaform Dermatitis)

Pityriasis rosea in swine is the name used to describe a pustular dermatitis that takes on the appearance of epidermal collarettes, or rings, seen only in young swine, mainly on the ventral abdomen and inner thighs. The disease is self-limiting. The condition, however, does not resemble pityriasis rosea in humans clinically or pathologically; therefore, *pustular psoriaform dermatitis* may be a more suitable name (Scott 1988).

Although the actual cause is unknown, the condition appears to be inherited. Swine that have had the condition are more likely to produce affected progeny. The incidence may be higher in Landrace swine. Attempts to transmit the disease or demonstrate an infectious agent have failed. The condition is seen in piglets derived by hysterectomy and reared in isolation.

The disease is seen in young pigs 3–14 weeks of age. Entire litters or only a few piglets in a litter may be affected. The disease begins as small erythematous papules on the skin of the abdomen and inner thighs. The papules are raised with a central crater and rapidly expand to produce a ring, or collarette, with a raised bright red periphery behind which are scales (Figure 8.2C). As the ring expands, the central area returns to normal. The rings coalesce as they expand to produce mosaic patterns. The hair is usually not lost and little pruritus is seen. The condition usually lasts about 4 weeks, regressing slowly and leaving normal skin as lesions heal.

The extent and severity of the lesions appear to increase when pigs are reared in weaner cages where stocking densities are high with high temperatures and high humidity. Lesions may become infected with bacteria—for example, *S. hyicus*—and resemble an exudative dermatitis.

The condition has to be differentiated from ringworm, dermatosis vegetans, and swine pox. Failure to isolate fungi or microorganisms will help confirm a diagnosis.

Skin biopsy will show psoriaform epidermal hyperplasia and superficial perivascular dermatitis. There is mild to moderate mucinous degeneration of the superficial dermis, and the predominant inflammatory cells are eosinophils and neutrophils. Parakeratotic hyperkeratosis is usually prominent (Scott 1988).

Treatment does not appear to affect the course of the disease. Good hygiene will reduce the chance of secondary infections, whereas overstocking with high humidity and high temperatures appears to increase the incidence. It may be best to cull breeding stock known to produce progeny that develop the condition from the breeding herd.

Dermatosis Vegetans

Dermatosis vegetans is a hereditary and often congenital disease of swine due to a semilethal autosomal recessive factor believed to have originated in the Danish Landrace breed (Done et al. 1967). The condition is seen as an erythematous maculopapular dermatitis with lesions on the coronary band and hoof together with pneumonia.

The main features of the condition are skin lesions, abnormalities of the feet, poor growth, and respiratory dysfunction. The skin lesions may be present at birth or, more commonly, develop within 2–3 weeks of birth. They first develop on the abdomen and inside the thighs as small (0.5–2.0 cm in diameter) raised pink swellings that enlarge rapidly. The lesions spread over the flanks and back of the pigs and become covered with yellowish brown, brittle, papillomatous crusts that are easily removed, leaving a pink granular surface. The lesions become very thick with a hard, horny surface that develops cracks and fissures, giving a characteristic papillomatous appearance. Swine may die after 5–8 weeks, but some will survive and the skin lesions regress.

Lesions of the hoof are usually present at birth and consist of marked swelling and erythema over the coronary band of both the main and the accessory digits and are covered with a yellowish brown greasy exudate. The walls of the hooves are thickened with ridges and furrows parallel to the coronary band. The horn becomes discolored and blackened.

Respiratory dysfunction is due to giant-cell pneumonitis. Respiratory signs of interstitial pneumonia or bronchopneumonia precede death, usually following a course of 4–6 weeks. However, some pigs may survive for 2–3 months but become weak and emaciated. On rare occasions affected pigs have reached maturity and bred.

The condition has to be differentiated from pityriasis rosea, chronic exudative epidermitis, and vitamin deficiencies. The clinical appearance of the skin and hoof lesions seen in young pigs 2–3 weeks of age is, however, characteristic. The very thick papillomatous crusts of the skin lesions are also typical and together with respiratory distress will suggest a diagnosis of dermatosis vegetans.

Skin biopsy reveals intraepidermal pustular dermatitis and microabscesses containing eosinophils and neutrophils, with parakeratotic hyperkeratosis. Older lesions show hyperplastic superficial perivascular dermatitis with multinucleated giant cells in the dermis (Percy and Hulland 1967, 1968). Histopathology of the lungs will help a diagnosis. Done et al. (1967) recommend that lungs should be fixed by filling with, as well as immersing in, 10% neutral formalin, and several samples from each lung should be examined.

There is no treatment for the condition, and prevention is aimed at detection and removal of breeding stock known to have produced affected progeny.

Epitheliogenesis Imperfecta (Aplasia Cutis)

Epitheliogenesis imperfecta is an inherited congenital condition of both white and colored swine and is caused by a simple autosomal recessive trait thought to result in a primary failure of embryonic ectodermal differentiation.

The lesions appear as clearly demarcated discontinuities of the squamous epithelium of varying sizes and shapes but usually on the back, loins, or limbs (Figure 8.2D). The condition may be seen in individual piglets or with a familial incidence in litters. The defect may also affect the dorsal and anterior ventral surface of the tongue with concurrent hydroureter and hydronephrosis (Jubb and Kennedy 1970). Lesions develop as large ulcers and frequently become infected; they may fail to heal or cause septicemia, which may lead to death.

Congenital Swine Pox

Borst et al. (1990) and Thibault et al. (1998a) reported the birth of pigs with pox lesions over the entire body to unrelated sows on different farms. Only one or two pigs in each litter were affected. At the time of the births, no other pigs on the farms had pox lesions, and histological and electron microscopic examination confirmed swine pox in the newborn pigs with lesions. The infections were generally fatal.

NEOPLASTIC DISEASES

Tumors are reported relatively rarely in swine, probably because the majority are slaughtered at 6–8 months of age or around 4–5 years of age for breeding stock. However, a variety of neoplastic conditions have been reported, including lymphangioma, rhabdomyoma, papilloma, sweat gland adenoma, fibroma, and hemangioma.

Melanomas, the result of proliferation of melanoblasts, have been reported most commonly in the Duroc breed and are often found at birth. The tumors are frequently seen on the flank region and have been described as being 1–4 cm in diameter, raised with an irregular black shiny surface. Metastases have been seen in lymph nodes, kidney, liver, lung, heart, brain, and skeletal muscle.

Rhabdomyosarcomas have been reported as solitary or multiple tumors on piglets less than 1 week old in at least 25 piglets in a short period of time in one herd in the Netherlands, indicating a common, possibly genetic cause (Voss et al. 1993).

Small fibrous polyps or wartlike lesions have been seen on sows, especially around the neck, along the back, and on the ears. These lesions frequently bleed and can easily be removed under local anesthetic.

MISCELLANEOUS

Porcine Dermatitis and Nephropathy Syndrome (PDNS)

Porcine Dermatitis and Nephropathy Syndrome (PDNS) has relatively recently been reported in pigs (Smith et al. 1993; White and Higgins 1993; Cameron 1995; Hélie et al. 1995) and is characterized by multifocal skin lesions, weight loss, edema of the limbs, vasculitis, and glomerulonephritis.

The cause is unknown, but histopathological and immunological findings suggest the pathogenesis involves an immune-complex disorder (antibody-antigen complex deposition) possibly due to an infectious agent. Thibault et al. (1998b) suggested that porcine reproductive and respiratory syndrome virus (PRRSV) infection may play a role in the pathogenesis of the disease, because PRRSV antigens were detected by immunochemistry in macrophages located around vessels of skin and kidney tissue examined in acute and chronic cases. Wellenberg et al. (2004) considered that porcine circovirus type 2 (PCV2) was likely to be the primary agent in the development of PDNS. They reported excessively high PCV2 antibody levels in a case-control field study of PDNS and hypothesized that PCV2 plays an important clinical and immuno-pathological role in the development of PDNS. They suggested that the excessive high levels of PCV2 antibodies trigger the develop-

ment of fibrinous deposits (immune complexes) in, for example, kidneys that can initiate an inflammatory process when deposited within the vascular or glomerular capillary wall. They also found an epidemiological association in herds that had experienced postweaning multisystemic wasting syndrome (PMWS) also caused by PCV2. However, their study did not indicate that PRRSV infection was a primary cause of PDNS, nor did they consider *Pasteurella multocida* a primary agent as has previously been suggested (Sierra et al. 1997; Thompson et al. 2001).

Seen mainly in growing swine, 20–65 kg liveweight, the most obvious clinical signs are skin lesions and a rapid loss in body weight with concurrent depression. The skin lesions range from large areas of erythema, macules, and hemorrhagic papules to dark brown to black thick crusts of necrosis on the ears, face, lower limbs, hindquarters, scrotum in boars, and vulva of sows (Figures 8.2E, 8.2F).

Other clinical signs include subcutaneous edema along the ventral abdominal wall and limbs. The lower parts of the legs are obviously swollen, and swelling of the joints is not uncommon. An outbreak in a large specific pathogen free (SPF) herd soon after it had been established by medicated early weaning was investigated. Typical cases were seen in at least 20 growing pigs over a 3-month period. Most pigs had to be destroyed or died within a few weeks (Cameron, unpublished data).

The condition could be confused with erysipelas, with skin necrosis, or, in its early stages, with sarcoptic mange. Of serious concern is that the clinical signs and lesions closely resemble those of classical swine fever and African swine fever. The autopsy findings will reveal enlarged, pale, spotted (petechiation) kidneys, fluid in the body cavities, subcutaneous fluid, and excessive synovial fluid in the joints. Gastric ulceration and hemorrhage are commonly seen. The histopathology of the kidney lesions is consistent with a diffuse necrotizing and proliferating glomerulonephritis. Glomerular spaces contain precipitated protein, necrotic cells (particularly polymorphs), and red blood cells. Secondary renal changes include formation of hyalin/granular casts and distended tubules. Necrotizing vasculitis of arterioles in the dermis and subcutis is associated with skin lesions. Small-vessel vasculitis can be detected in other organs, including lymph nodes, spleen, stomach, liver, bladder, brain, and joints (Higgins 1993). A significant increase in plasma urea and creatinine with a decrease in sodium and chloride and very high levels of protein and red and white blood cells in urine are characteristic. Because the actual causative agent is unknown, control is difficult.

REFERENCES

Amstutz JE. 1975. Heat stroke, sunburn, and photosensitization. In Diseases of Swine, 4th ed. HW Dunne, AD Leman, eds. Ames: Iowa State Univ Press, p. 1014.

Amtsberg G. 1978. Infections versuche mit *Staphylococcus hyicus* an aktiv und passiv immunisierten schweinen. Berl Munch Tierarztl Wochenschr 91:201.

Andresen LO, Wegener HC, Bille-Hansen V. 1993. *Staphylococcus hyicus*: Skin reactions in piglets caused by crude extracellular products and by partially purified exfoliative toxin. Microbial Pathogenesis 15:217–225.

Andrews JJ. 1979. Ulcerative glossitis and stomatitis associated with exudative epidermitis in suckling swine. Vet Pathol 16:432–437.

Arora BM, Das SC, Patgiri GP. 1979. Dermatomycosis in pigs (rubromycosis). Indian Vet J 56:791–793.

Blood DC, Jubb KV. 1957. Exudative epidermitis of pigs. Aust Vet J 33:126–127.

Blood DC, Radostits OM. 1989. Veterinary Medicine, 7th ed. London: Bailliere Tindall, p. 979.

Borst GHA, Kimman TG, Gielkens ALJ, van der Kamp JS. 1990. Four sporadic cases of congenital swinepox. Vet Rec 127:61–63.

Brackenridge DT. 1958. Mange in pigs: A survey. NZ Vet J 6:166–167.

Brooks PH, Smith DA, Irwin VCR. 1977. Biotin-supplementation of diets, the incidence of foot lesions, and the reproductive performance of sows. Vet Rec 101:46–50.

Callis JJ, McKercher PD, Shahan MS. 1975. Foot-and-mouth disease. In Diseases of Swine, 4th ed. HW Dunne, AD Leman, eds. Ames: Iowa State Univ Press, p. 328.

Cameron RDA. 1984. Skin Diseases of the Pig. Univ Sydney Post-Grad Found. Vet Sci Proc Vet Rev 23:9.

——. 1995. Glomerulonephritis: Outbreak of a new disease diagnosed. Pork J, 16(12):28.

Carbrey EA, Stewart WC, Young SH, Richardson GC. 1966. Transmission of hog cholera by pregnant sows. J Am Vet Med Assoc 149:23–30.

Cargill CF. 1981. The treatment and control of sarcoptic mange. Univ Sydney Post-Grad Comm Vet Sci Proc 56:87.

Cargill CF, Dobson KJ. 1979a. Experimental *Sarcoptes scabiei* infection in pigs. I. Pathogenesis. Vet Rec 104:11–14.

——. 1979b. Experimental *Sarcoptes scabiei* infection in pigs. II. Effect on production. Vet Rec 104:33–36.

Cargill C, Davies P, Carmichael I, Hooke F, Moore M. 1996. Treatment of sarcoptic mite infestation and mite hypersensitivity in pigs with injectable doramectin. Vet Rec 138:468–471.

Connole MD, Baynes ID. 1966. Ringworm caused by *Microsporum nanum* in pigs in Queensland. Aust Vet J 42:19–24.

Cunha TJ. 1977. Swine Feeding and Nutrition. New York: Academic Press, p. 101.

Dobson KJ, Davies PR. 1992. External parasites. In Diseases of Swine, 7th ed. AD Leman, BE Straw, WL Mengeling, S D'Allaire, DJ Taylor (eds.). Ames: Iowa State Univ Press, pp. 668–679.

Done JT, Loosmore RM, Saunders CN. 1967. Dermatosis vegetans in pigs. Vet Rec 80:292–297.

Fraser CM, Bergeron JA, Mays A, Aiello SE. 1991. The Merck Veterinary Manual, 7th ed. Rahway, N.J., p. 308.

Gibbs EPJ, Stoddard HL, Yedloutchnig RJ, House JA, Legge M. 1983. A vesicular disease of pigs in Florida of unknown etiology. Florida Vet J 12:25–27.

Ginther OJ. 1965. Clinical aspects of *Microsporum nanum* infection in swine. J Am Vet Med Assoc 146:945–953.

Harcourt RA. 1973. Porcine ulcerative spirochaetosis. Vet Rec 92:647–648.

Hare T, Fry RM, Orr AB. 1942. First impressions of the beta-hemolytic *Streptococcus* infection of swine. Vet Rec 54:267–269.

Hélie P, Drolet R, Germain MC, Bourgault A. 1995. Systemic necrotizing vasculitis in grower pigs in Québec. Can Vet J 36:150–154.

Higgins RJ. 1993. Glomerulo-nephropathy syndrome. Pig Vet J 31:160–163.

Hungerford TG. 1990. Diseases of Livestock, 9th ed. Sydney: McGraw-Hill, p. 678.

Jubb KVF, Kennedy PC. 1970. Pathology of Domestic Animals. Vol. 2. New York: Academic Press, p. 591.

Jubb KVF, Kennedy PC, Palmer N. 1985. Pathology of Domestic Animals, 3rd ed. Vol 1. New York: Academic Press, p. 110.

Kasza L, Griesemer RA. 1962. Experimental swine pox. Am J Vet Res 23:443–450.

Kim J, Chae C. 2004. Concurrent presence of porcine circovirus type 2 and porcine parvovirus in retrospective cases of exudative epidermitis in pigs. Vet. J. 167:104–106.

Kresse JI, Taylor WD, Stewart WW, Eernisse KA. 1985. Parvovirus infection in pigs with necrotic and vesicle-like lesions. Vet Microbiol 10:525–531.

Laperle A, Morin M, Sauvageau R. 1988. Acute dermatitis in feeder pigs administered tiamulin. Proc Int Pig Vet Soc 10:250.

L'Ecuyer C. 1966. Exudative epidermitis in pigs: Clinical studies and preliminary transmission trials. Can J Comp Med 30:9–16.

L'Ecuyer C, Jericho K. 1966. Exudative epidermitis in pigs: Etiological studies and pathology. Can J Comp Med 30:94–101.

Maddox ET, Graham CW, Reynolds WA. 1973. Ampicillin treatment of three cases of streptococcal auricular dermatitis in swine. Vet Med Small Anim Clin 68:1018–1019.

Mann JA, Sellers RF. 1989. Foot-and-mouth disease virus. In Virus Infections of Porcines. MB Pensaert, ed. New York: Elsevier Science Publisher, p. 251–258.

Marcarian NQ, Calhoun ML. 1966. Microscopic anatomy of the integument of adult swine. Am J Vet Res 27:765–772.

McClymont GL, Wynne KN. 1955. Possibility of photosensitization due to ingestion of aphids. Aust Vet J 31:112.

McPherson EA. 1956. *Trichophyton mentagrophytes*: Natural infection in pigs. Vet Rec 68:710–711.

——. 1960. Sarcoptic mange in pigs. Vet Rec 72:869–870.

Meyer W, Schwartz R, Neurand K. 1978. The skin of domestic animals as a model for the human skin, with specific reference to the domestic pig. Curr Probl Dermatol 7:39–52.

Miller RB, Olson LD. 1978. Epizootic of concurrent cutaneous streptococcal abscesses and swine pox in a herd of swine. J Am Vet Med Assoc 172:676–680.

——. 1980. Experimental induction of cutaneous streptococcal abcesses in swine as a sequela to swine pox. Am J Vet Res 41:341–347.

Montgomery JF, Oliver RE, Poole WSH. 1987. A vesiculo-bullous disease in pigs resembling foot-and-mouth disease. I. Field cases. NZ Vet J 35:21–26.

Mowafy M, Cassens RG. 1975. Microscopic structure of pig skin. J Anim Sci 41:1281–1290.

Muirhead MR. 1978. Intensive pig production: Studies in preventive medicine. Fellowship thesis, Royal College of Veterinary Surgeons, London, p. 40.

Mullowney PC. 1984. Skin diseases of swine. Vet Clin North Am: Large Anim Prac 6:107–129.

Munday BL, Ryan FB. 1982. Vesicular lesions in swine—Possible association with feeding of marine products. Aust Vet J 59:193.

Penny RHC, Edwards MJ, Mulley R. 1971. Clinical observations of necrosis of the skin of suckling piglets. Aust Vet J 47:529–537.

Penny RHC, Cameron RDA, Johnson S, Kenyon PJ, Smith HA, Bell AWP, Cole JPI, Taylor J. 1980. Footrot of pigs; the influence of biotin supplementation on foot lesions in sows. Vet Rec 107:350–351.

Pepin GA, Austwick PKC. 1968. Skin diseases of domestic animals. II. Skin diseases, mycological origin. Vet Rec 82:209.

Percy DH, Hulland TJ. 1967. Dermatosis vegetans (vegetative dermatosis) in Canadian swine. Can Vet J 8:3–9.

——. 1968. Evolution of multinucleate giant cells in dermatosis vegetans in swine. Pathol Vet 5:419–428.

Piercy DW. 1966. Greasy pig disease. Vet Rec, 78:477–478.

Reynolds IM, Miner PW, Smith RE. 1968. Cutaneous candidiasis in swine. J Am Vet Med Assoc 152:182–186.

Scott DW. 1988. Large Animal Dermatology. Philadelphia: W. B. Saunders.

Scruggs DW, Sorden SD. 2001. Proliferative vasculopathy and cutaneous hemorrhages in porcine neonates infected with the porcine reproductive and respiratory syndrome virus. Vet Pathol 38:339–342.

Sierra MA, Mulas JM, de las Molenbeek RF, van Maanen C, Vos JH, Quezada M, Gruys E. 1997. Porcine immune complex glomerulonephritis dermatitis (PIGD) syndrome. Eur J Vet Pathol 3:63–70.

Sieverding, E. 1993. Use of an autogenous vaccine against exudative epidermitis in suckled piglets. Pig News Inform, Abstr 135, Mar. 1995.

Smith WJ, Thomson JR, Done S. 1993. Dermatitis/nephropathy syndrome of pigs. Vet Rec 132:42.

Stevens RWC. 1984. Neonatal teat necrosis in pigs. Pig News Info 5:19–22.

Thibault S, Drolet R, Alain R, Dea S. 1998a. Congenital swine pox: A sporadic skin disorder in nursing piglets. Swine Health Prod 6:276–278.

Thibault S, Drolet R, Germain MC, D'Allaire S, Larochelle R, Magar R. 1998b. Cutaneous and systemic necrotizing vasculitis in swine. Vet Pathol 35:108–116.

Thomson JR, MacIntyre N, Henderson LEA, Meikle CS. 2001. Detection of *Pasteurella multocida* in pigs with porcine dermatitis and nephropathy. Vet Rec 149:412–417

Vos JH, Borst GHA, de las Mulas JM, Ramaekers FCS, van Mil FN, Molenbeek RF, Ivanyi D, van den Ingh TSGAM. 1993. Rhabdomyosarcomas in young pigs in a swine breeding farm: A morphologic and immunohistochemical study. Vet Pathol 30:271–279.

Wattrang E, McNeilly F, Allan GM, Greko C, Fossum C, Wallgren P. 2002. Exudative epidermitis and porcine circovirus-2 infection in a Swedish SPF-herd. Vet Microbiol 86:281–293.

Wellenberg GJ, Stockhofe-Zurwieden N, de Jong MF, Boersma WJA, Elbers ARW. 2004. Excessive porcine circovirus type 2 antibody titres may trigger the development of porcine dermatitis and nephropathy syndrome: A case-control study. Vet Microbiol 99:203–214.

White M, Higgins RJ. 1993. Dermatitis nephropathy syndrome of pigs. Vet Rec 132:199.

Wood RL. 1992. Erysipelas. In Diseases of Swine, 7th ed. AD Leman, BE Straw, WL Mengeling, S D'Allaire, DJ Taylor (eds.). Ames: Iowa State Univ Press, p. 483.

9 Diseases of the Urinary System

Richard Drolet and Scott A. Dee

ANATOMY

The kidneys of swine are bean-shaped, generally smooth on the surface, and brown. They are elongated, flattened dorsoventrally, and at least twice as long as wide (Figure 9.1). At the middle of the medial border of each of them is an indentation, the hilus of the kidney, where the vessels, nerves, and ureter communicate with the organ. The kidneys are located ventrally to the psoas muscles at the level of the first four lumbar vertebrae. Their relative location is slightly asymmetrical, but contrary to what is observed in many other species, the left kidney of most individuals is often situated cranially to the right one; the extremity of the cranial pole of the former may reach the last intercostal space. In the adult, the ratio of the combined weight of the kidneys to that of the body is about 0.50–0.66% (Sisson 1975).

The kidneys are enveloped by a rather thin fibrous capsule that can be easily peeled off. In a kidney section, the relative surface occupied by the cortex and the medulla is readily apparent (Figure 9.2). Pigs have multipyramidal or multilobar kidneys but without the external lobation typically found in the bovine species. The medullary portion of each lobe is called a pyramid; some are simple, whereas others are compound, that is, formed by the fusion of two or more primitively separate pyramids. The pale apical portion of a pyramid, called the papilla, projects into the renal pelvis or its ramifications; these latter are referred to as calyces (refer to Figure 9.2). Papillae of simple pyramids are generally narrow and conical, whereas those of compound pyramids, often located in the area of the renal poles, are broad and flattened. There are 8–12 papillae per kidney. Collecting ducts of the kidneys have their openings at the tips of the papillae.

The ureters, which are continuous with the renal pelvis, leave the kidneys in a sharp caudal curve. They ultimately reach the dorsolateral sides of the bladder neck area, penetrating its muscular coat at almost right angles, and pass obliquely through the submucosa, raising the mucosa slightly before ending at the ureteric orifices. In newborn piglets, the length of the portion of the ureter running beneath the bladder mucosa is about 5 mm, whereas it reaches a mean length of about 35 mm in the adult (Carr et al. 1990). The intravesical portion of the ureters acts as a valve that prevents vesico-ureteral reflux of urine.

The urinary bladder of the pig is large and has a long neck. When full, it lies well down into the abdominal cavity. The bladder is supported by one median (ventrally located) and two lateral ligaments. The urethra of the adult female is about 7–8 cm long and its external ostium is located ventrally, at the junction of the vagina and vestibule; beneath it is a small depression, the suburethral diverticulum. In the male, the urethra opens into a slitlike structure at the tip of the penis.

PHYSIOLOGY

Histophysiology

The kidney is involved in many vital functions: the elimination of waste products from the body, the conservation of water, and the regulation of the acid-base balance and electrolyte composition. In addition, it has an endocrine function: it produces a variety of hormones, including erythropoietin, renin, prostaglandins, and vitamin D_3.

Most of these functions are achieved by a multitude of microscopic anatomical structures called nephrons, which, all together, form the bulk of the renal parenchyma. The kidney of a pig contains well over one million nephrons. Newborn piglets have immature kidneys, and nephrogenesis continues during the first 3 months of life (Friis 1980). The nephron, the functional unit of the kidney, consists of a renal corpuscle, proximal tubule, loop of Henle, and distal tubule. The renal corpuscle comprises the glomerulus, a tuft of arterial capillaries, and Bowman's capsule. The first mechanism used to accomplish renal function is glomerular filtra-

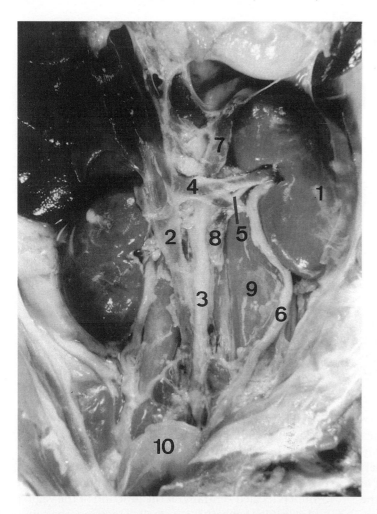

9.1. *Kidneys of pig in situ, ventral view. 1, left kidney; 2, vena cava; 3, aorta; 4, renal vein; 5, renal artery; 6, ureter; 7, adrenal gland; 8, renal lymph node; 9, psoas major; 10, urinary bladder.*

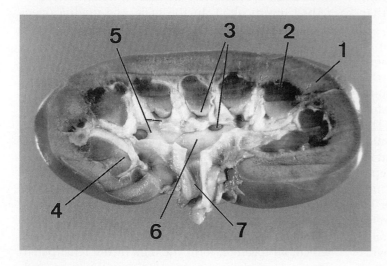

9.2. *Section of kidney from a feeder pig. 1, cortex; 2, medulla; 3, papillae; 4, compound papilla; 5, calyces; 6, pelvis; 7, ureter.*

tion. The volume of plasma filtered depends essentially on the renal perfusion, blood pressure, and integrity of the glomerulus itself. The glomerular filtrate is an ultra-filtrate of blood plasma that contains water, glucose, salts, ions, amino acids, and small amounts of protein of low molecular weight. The glomerular filtrate entering the tubular components of the nephron is profoundly modified by various processes of absorption and secre-

tion that are, at least in part, governed by the needs of the animal. A significant part of these changes takes place in the proximal tubule, a segment of the nephron lined by well-developed and metabolically very active epithelial cells. At that site, for example, 100% of the filtered glucose (in a normoglycemic animal) is reabsorbed by an active transport mechanism, and many other substances, such as water, sodium, amino acids, albumin, and bicarbonate, are also reabsorbed in significant amounts (Banks 1986). Pigs are distinctive in that they reabsorb very few urates from glomerular filtrate compared to most other species. Tubular secretion of various endogenous and exogenous compounds complements the clearance of substances that are filtered at the glomerulus. The filtrate finally enters the collecting ducts, where it may be further concentrated. Under normal conditions, urine expelled into the pelvis is not further modified as it travels through the rest of the lower urinary tract, the mucosa of which is lined with a transitional epithelium often referred to as *urothelium*.

Urine

The volume of urine produced daily depends on several variables, including diet, fluid intake, ambient temperature and humidity, and the size and weight of the animal. Accurate data on the normal ranges of the amount of urine excreted per day in pigs are limited. Salmon-Legagneur et al. (1973) reported a mean urinary output of 9 L and 5.3 L/day in gestating and lactating sows, respectively. Other factors, such as the water distribution system used, may also affect the production of urine if they influence drinking behavior.

The mean specific gravity of urine in adult swine is about 1.020 (plasma >1.010), one of the lowest found in domestic animals (Ruckebusch et al. 1991). Young animals have even lower values. Specific gravity of urine is usually inversely related to urine volume. Urinary pH is usually between 5.5 and 7.5. It is influenced by the metabolism and the composition of the feed; starvation or a high protein intake lowers urinary pH. Urinary infection with urea-splitting bacteria (e.g., *Actinobaculum suis*, formerly *Actinomyces suis*) may result in a significant alkalinization of urine.

As mentioned (see previous section), the small amount of protein that passes through the glomeruli is, for the most part, reabsorbed by the proximal tubules, so normally no protein is detected in urine by usual methods. The presence of proteinuria may be of diagnostic significance and must be interpreted in conjunction with the specific gravity. Significant proteinuria is associated with various renal diseases such as glomerulonephritis (increased permeability to protein), tubular necrosis (decreased reabsorption of protein), and pyelonephritis (inflammation), and with lower urinary tract inflammation. The presence of protein in the urine is, however, not always pathologic, because transient physiological or functional proteinuria also occurs in some instances. Proteinuria is observed in baby pigs in their first few days of life, their glomeruli being permeable to colostral protein found in high levels in the blood. Transient proteinuria may also occur following excessive physical activity (e.g., transport) or intense stress or when excessive amounts of protein are ingested.

The color of urine is usually yellow to amber depending on the concentration of urochromes. Abnormal coloration of urine is observed with some underlying urinary tract diseases. Urine sediment examination is very informative because it may reveal findings of diagnostic significance (e.g., in the case of cystitis-pyelonephritis).

Impaired Renal Function

In some pathological situations, renal function is impaired so much that renal failure ensues. Renal failure may have a prerenal (e.g., any condition that reduces renal blood flow), postrenal (e.g., obstructive uropathy), or primary renal origin (e.g., extensive renal parenchymal disease). Renal failure can cause metabolic acidosis, electrolytic imbalances, and intravascular accumulations of various metabolic waste products, including blood urea nitrogen (BUN) and creatinine. Determination of both BUN and serum creatinine concentration may be used to assess the renal function. The serum creatinine concentration is a more accurate index of the glomerular filtration rate than is the BUN because it is less dependent on nonrenal factors. Concentrations of BUN may rise in animals with high dietary protein intake or in any conditions resulting in increased protein catabolism. Friendship et al. (1984) reported normal-range values for BUN and serum creatinine in weaned and feeder pigs, gilts, and sows. In sows, for example, the mean BUN concentration has been reported as 5.3 mmol/L (n = 102) (Friendship et al. 1984) and 5.0 mmol/L (n = 120) (McLaughlin and McLaughlin 1987), whereas the mean serum creatinine concentrations reported in the same two studies are 160 μmol/L and 186 μmol/L, respectively.

DEVELOPMENTAL ANOMALIES

Anomalies of development occur in all body systems, and the urinary tract is no exception. These anomalies may involve the kidneys as well as the lower urinary tract. Many of these conditions in swine are relatively rare and of little economic significance. Few of these malformations in pigs are common, and only rarely are they associated with clinical signs. In some instances, developmental anomalies have been shown to be inherited.

Malformations of the Kidneys

Most of the well-characterized renal anomalies of development occurring in domestic animals have also been documented in pigs. Depressions of the external surface and partial persistence of fetal lobation of the kidneys have been reported to be relatively common in Norwegian slaughtered pigs (Jansen and Nordstoga 1992). Unilateral renal agenesis (aplasia) occurs sporadically in pigs and is relatively common compared to other domestic animals (Höfliger 1971). Bilateral renal agenesis is obviously incompatible with life and would be encountered in the fetus or stillborn piglet. Cases of bilateral renal agenesis and renal hypoplasia have been described in pigs and linked to a genetic cause (Cordes and Dodd

1965; Mason and Cooper 1985). Malposition of the kidneys (renal ectopia) is not rare and is often characterized by caudal displacement of one kidney, often the left, to the pelvic area (Sisson 1975). Duplication of one kidney has been observed on a number of occasions in pigs (Nieberle and Cohrs 1967). Horseshoe kidney, rarely observed in swine, is a condition in which the kidneys have fused at either the cranial or the caudal poles, resulting in a horseshoe-shaped organ (Nieberle and Cohrs 1967). Renal dysplasia, a disorganized development of renal parenchyma due to anomalous differentiation, also is relatively rare (Maxie 1993).

Congenital renal cysts are not infrequently seen in the kidneys of various species but are more common in swine. The presence of one or a few cysts in the kidney, often referred to as simple renal cysts, is a common incidental finding at abattoirs, and the affected organs are generally condemned. These cystic cavities, filled with serous fluid, vary from a few millimeters in diameter to larger than the organ itself. They are commonly found in the cortex and often protrude from the surface of the organ, where they may appear translucent or opaque depending on the amount of fibrous connective tissue present in their wall (Figure 9.3). Histologically, these cysts are lined with a layer of tubular epithelial cells surrounded by a fibrous capsule.

Polycystic kidney disease represents another form of congenital cysts, occurring far less frequently. This form is characterized by the presence of numerous and generally smaller cysts that occupy a significant proportion of the renal parenchyma. Cystic structures may be found in the liver (cystic bile ducts) as well. Affected piglets usually die from renal failure during the neonatal period (Webster and Summers 1978).

The distinction between simple renal cysts and polycystic kidney disease is not always well demarcated. Wells et al. (1980) reported a prevalence of renal cysts of nearly 50% from a single herd that experienced an abnormally high rate of kidney condemnations at the abattoir. Affected kidneys had variable numbers and sizes of cysts, ranging from one extreme to the other. Further investigation showed that affected animals were the progeny of a Landrace boar. The disease was found to be inherited as an autosomal dominant trait, the number of cysts being determined by polygenic inheritance (Wijeratne and Wells 1980).

Malformations of the Lower Urinary Tract

Developmental anomalies of the lower urinary tract appear to be rare in swine, and like those found in the kidneys, their true prevalence is unknown. Cases of duplication of the ureter (Benko 1969), persistent urachus (Weaver 1966), and congenital ureteral occlusion (Nieberle and Cohrs 1967) have been reported in pigs.

CIRCULATORY DISTURBANCES

Circulatory disturbances may occur in the urinary tract as well as in any other tissues of the body. Some of these disturbances of the circulation produce lesions that may be of diagnostic significance on postmortem inspection.

Hemorrhage

Hemorrhages, in the form of widespread petechiae or less commonly ecchymoses, may be found in any part of the kidney or lower urinary tract in various septicemic illnesses (Figure 9.4). Bacterial infections commonly associated with these lesions include septicemia due to salmonellae, streptococci, *Erysipelothrix rhusiopathiae*, and *Actinobacillus* spp. These lesions are often seen in acute cases of hog cholera and African swine fever and in other viremic diseases such as cytomegalovirus infection (Orr et al. 1988). Petechiation of the renal cortex is also observed occasionally in acute glomerulonephritis, in some acute intoxications, and in electrocuted animals.

Larger intrarenal or subcapsular hemorrhages are usually caused by trauma, necrosis, or clotting defect, including poisoning by anticoagulant rodenticides. They may also occur in some cases of disseminated intravascular coagulation. Widespread hemorrhages in al-

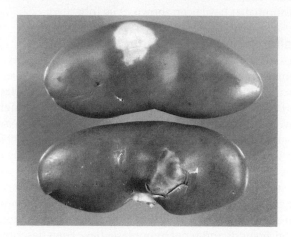

9.3. *Congenital renal cysts in slaughtered sows.*

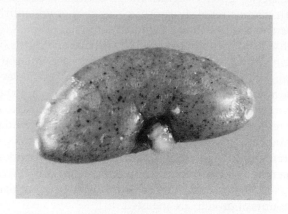

9.4. *Widespread petechiae in the kidney of a piglet with* Staphylococcus hyicus *septicemia.*

most all body systems, including the urinary tract, are a striking pathologic feature in suckling piglets with isoimmune thrombocytopenic purpura due to passively transferred antiplatelet antibody from the dam's colostrum (Andersen and Nielsen 1973; Dimmock et al. 1982). In this relatively common disease, affected piglets appear normal at birth but eventually die between 1 and 3 weeks of age from hemorrhagic diathesis.

Infarction

Renal infarcts, infrequently found in the kidneys of swine, are localized areas of ischemic coagulative necrosis produced by the occlusion of the renal artery or one of its tributaries. The localization and size of the infarct reflect the area vascularized normally by the involved blood vessel. The occlusion is usually due to thrombosis or to aseptic emboli (the consequences of septic emboli are discussed under embolic nephritis). In some instances infarction of the renal parenchyma is primarily associated with renal vasculitis (Jansen and Nordstoga 1992), including polyarteritis nodosa (Nieberle and Cohrs 1967).

Bilateral renal cortical necrosis is seen on rare occasions in pigs and is considered to be the result of an infarct of a major part of the cortex of both kidneys (Häni and Indermühle 1980). The reaction is characterized by disseminated intravascular coagulation with a marked tropism for the small arterial blood vessels of the renal cortex. The etiopathogenesis of these lesions remains unclear but the condition has been associated with septicemia, endotoxemia, and hemorrhagic shock due to bleeding gastric ulcers.

GLOMERULAR DISEASES

Renal diseases that involve primarily the glomeruli include amyloidosis and glomerulonephritis. Renal amyloidosis has been rarely reported in pigs (Jakob 1971; Maxie 1993). Glomerulonephritis represents an important category of renal diseases in animals and in recent years this condition has been recognized with increasing frequency in swine.

Glomerulonephritis

Inflammatory changes in renal glomeruli may take place via a number of mechanisms, including immunologic, thrombotic, toxic, and as yet uncharacterized mechanisms. Most cases of glomerulonephritis (GN) in humans and animals are thought to be immune-mediated.

The main types of glomerular immunologic injury recognized are trapping of circulating immune complexes (antigen-antibody complexes), in situ immune complex formation, activation of the alternate pathway of complement, and cell-mediated processes (Spargo and Taylor 1988). Because immunoglobulins and complement components are frequently found in inflamed glomeruli, antibody-mediated injury has received the

most attention. In veterinary medicine, the commonly used classification for the various morphologic types of immune-mediated GN are membranous, proliferative, and membranoproliferative.

Although the pathogenesis of GN is now reasonably well understood, knowledge of the etiology or triggering event is still unknown in most cases (idiopathic immune-mediated GN). Theoretically GN may be triggered by a variety of factors including drugs, chemicals, food allergens, endogenous antigens, and infectious agents (Drolet et al. 1999).

GN is not often diagnosed in swine but does occur occasionally as a sporadic event (Nieberle and Cohrs 1967; Slauson and Lewis 1979; Maxie 1993; Bourgault and Drolet 1995). It has also been reported as a sequel to chronic infectious diseases such as hog cholera, African swine fever (Maurer et al. 1958; Cheville et al. 1970; Martin-Fernandez et al. 1991; Hervas et al. 1996; Choi and Chae 2003), systemic cytomegalovirus infection (Yoshikawa et al. 1988), and group A streptococcal abscesses (Morales and Guzman 1976). In these cases, the resulting GN appears to be caused by the presence of glomerular immune complexes in which the antigen is related to the agent responsible for the underlying disease (Slauson and Lewis 1979). Nutritionally induced GN has also been reported on a few occasions in pigs. Ingestion of a protein-rich by-product (Elling 1979) and ingestion of "smut fungus" contained in the feedstuff (Müller 1977) have been incriminated.

An inherited renal disease, classified morphologically as membranoproliferative GN type II, has been described in Yorkshire piglets from Norway (Jansen 1993). This familial disease is not associated with the presence of intraglomerular immune complexes but rather is caused by an autosomal recessive deficiency of the complement inhibitory protein "factor H" (Hogasen et al. 1995; Jansen et al. 1995). Deficiency of factor H ultimately provokes activation of the alternate pathway of complement, with subsequent massive deposits of complement in renal glomeruli. This disease in Norwegian Yorkshire pigs represents a promising animal model for the study of membranoproliferative GN type II in humans (Jansen et al. 1998).

In many species, generalized or focal GN is also observed in some cases of systemic vasculitis (mainly immune-mediated vasculitis). In pigs, the best example of this certainly is porcine dermatitis and nephropathy syndrome (PDNS). The condition, first described in the United Kingdom in 1993 (Smith et al. 1993; White and Higgins 1993), was subsequently observed in other parts of Europe, North and South America, Oceania, and Africa, suggesting a worldwide distribution (Segalés et al. 2003). The disease affects nursery and growing pigs and, less commonly, breeding animals (Drolet et al. 1999). Although notable exceptions have been observed, the prevalence of the syndrome in affected herds is usually less than 1%. Affected animals present a sys-

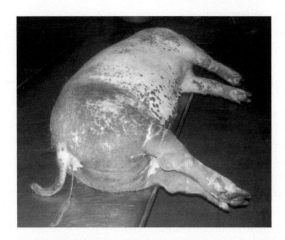

9.5. *Sow affected with PDNS. Note multifocal to coalescent erythematous macules and patches of typical distribution.*

temic necrotizing vasculitis with marked tropism for the skin and kidneys (Smith et al. 1993; Hélie et al. 1995; Thibault et al. 1998). Vascular lesions in the skin provoke a conspicuous dermatopathy (Figure 9.5) (see Chapter 8). Kidney lesions in acute cases may include exudative and occasionally necrotizing GN and vasculitis. Vascular lesions in other tissues vary considerably in frequency and distribution in individual pigs (Thomson et al. 2002). In some atypical cases there may be cutaneous lesions without renal lesions and vice versa. An animal with GN without any other vascular lesions elsewhere should probably not be diagnosed as PDNS since other glomerular diseases not related to this syndrome are known to occur in pigs.

In PDNS, the glomerular and systemic vascular damages are thought to be immune-mediated, possibly through a type III hypersensitivity reaction (Smith et al. 1993; Helie et al. 1995; Sierra et al. 1997; Thibault et al. 1998; Thomson et al. 2002; Wellenberg et al. 2004). The precise etiology of the condition remains unknown at this time. Porcine reproductive and respiratory syndrome (PRRS) virus and porcine circovirus type 2 (PCV2) have been so far the two infectious agents most suspected of being responsible for the development of the disease, either as primary causal agents or as important cofactors (Segalés et al. 1998, 2003; Thibault et al. 1998; Drolet et al. 1999; Rosell et al. 2000; Thomson et al. 2002; Wellenberg et al. 2004). In both of these infections, viremia may coexist with the presence of antibodies, a situation that may facilitate the formation of immune complexes. Also of interest is the fact that these two viruses infect cells of the monocytes/macrophages lineage and may theoretically act indirectly by affecting the efficiency of the mononuclear phagocytic system in removing immune complexes from the circulation (Thomson et al. 2001). Recently it has been shown that animals with PDNS often have relatively low PCV2 loads (Olvera et al. 2004) but very high PCV2 antibody titers (Wellenberg et al. 2004).

Renal fibrosis combined with proliferative glomerular lesions was rather common in Norwegian slaughter pigs (Jansen and Nordstoga 1992, 1994). Further studies are needed to confirm the relationship between this interstitial fibrosis and the mesangioproliferative glomerulopathy observed. Other examples of glomerular disease in swine have been reported in the literature in recent years (Shirota et al. 1984, 1995; Tamura et al. 1986; Yoshie 1991; Pace et al. 1998; Carrasco et al. 2003).

Although several of the previously described glomerulonephropathy types are associated with an underlying disease process (chronic infections, genetic defect, systemic vasculitis, etc.) that gives insight into the likely etiology of the condition, many spontaneous cases of GN, however, remain idiopathic (primary idiopathic GN) (Slauson and Lewis 1979; Shirota et al. 1986; Bourgault and Drolet 1995).

The clinical significance of GN is highly variable, with a spectrum ranging from a subclinical condition to a fulminating and rapidly fatal disease. Shirota and coworkers (1986) found deposition of immune complexes containing IgG and third-complement component (C3) in the glomerular mesangium of most of the 100 normal slaughtered swine they examined. The mesangioproliferative GN, disclosed only upon microscopic examination of the kidneys, was seemingly not associated with clinical disease. On the other end of the spectrum, the proliferative and exudative GN observed in most of the cases of spontaneous GN reported by Bourgault and Drolet (1995) was found to be responsible for the death of at least one-third of the pigs affected. The hereditary GN of Norwegian Yorkshire pigs appears to be invariably fatal; affected piglets die of renal failure within 11 weeks of birth (Jansen et al. 1995). Mortalities are also commonly recorded in pigs affected with PDNS (Smith et al. 1993; White and Higgins 1993; Kavanagh 1994; Hélie et al. 1995; Segalés et al. 1998; Thomson et al. 2002). In this latter condition, the survival of the affected pigs depends on the extent and severity of the vascular lesions in the internal organs, particularly within the kidneys.

Unlike most other domestic animals affected with GN (with the exception of the familial glomerulopathies), pigs appear to be affected at a relatively young age. The condition has been described most commonly in weaned and feeder pigs (1.5–6 months old), occasionally in breeding animals, and rarely in nursing piglets. Clinical signs, when present, may include anorexia, lethargy, unwillingness to move, subcutaneous edema, rapid loss of condition, and death. GN is rarely recognized clinically because most of the signs are nonspecific, and analysis of urine and blood from an individual is rarely considered of practical value in the herd medicine approach applied in our large units of production. Pigs affected with PDNS are often more easy to detect clinically because of the presence of hemorrhagic and necrotizing skin lesions, mainly located on the hindlimbs and perineal area (Segalés et al. 2003). Pigs with GN may show concomitant hypoproteinemia, hypoalbuminemia, and persistent proteinuria which are highly suggestive of a protein-losing glomerulopathy. The urine protein/creatinine ratio may also be increased (Hélie et al. 1995). Proteinuria, hematuria, and pyuria, which are usually compatible with lower urinary tract lesions, may also occur in severe types of GN—namely, in acute proliferative and exudative GN. Blood of affected animals may also reveal elevated urea and creatinine levels suggestive of renal failure (White and Higgins 1993; Hélie et al. 1995; Jansen et al. 1995; Drolet et al. 1999; Thomson et al. 2002).

Gross lesions of GN may be absent, subtle, or very conspicuous. The appearance of the kidneys will depend largely on the severity of the glomerular lesions and the stage (acute vs. chronic) of the disease process. In acute GN, the kidneys may be slightly to markedly enlarged, pale, edematous, often with cortical petechiation (Figure 9.6). The most important differential diagnoses to consider for such acutely affected kidneys are various bacterial septicemia (*Erysipelothrix rhusiopathiae, Actinobacillus suis, Salmonella choleraesuis*), acute viremia (classical swine fever, African swine fever, cytomegalovirus) and intoxications. With time, the surface of the kidneys may become finely granular, and in the chronic phase of the disease, the organs may appear shrunken and contracted due to progressive cortical fibrosis. At this stage, the gross lesions are indistinguishable from chronic interstitial nephritis. They may, however, be differentiated from chronic pyelonephritis, which tends to produce a more irregular pattern of fibrosis, often with intervening areas of normal parenchyma and evidence of lesions upon careful examination of renal calyxes and papillae. Perirenal and subcutaneous edema and serous effusions in body cavities may be observed in some cases of GN. On several occasions a high prevalence of gastric ulcers has been associated with GN (Jansen 1993; White and Higgins 1993; Kavanagh 1994; Bourgault and Drolet 1995).

Treatment of GN, which is usually symptomatic, has received little attention in swine since the disease is not often diagnosed in live animals under normal farm-raising conditions. Pigs affected with PDNS have been tentatively treated with various antimicrobial agents, anti-inflammatory drugs and multivitamin supplements without significantly conclusive results (Segalés et al. 2003).

TUBULAR DISEASES

Renal diseases characterized primarily by degenerative changes affecting the tubular epithelial cells of the nephrons may occur under certain circumstances. In these cases, the epithelial lining cells of the tubules may undergo degeneration, followed by necrosis and sloughing of the cells.

Acute tubular necrosis, often called nephrosis, represents an important cause of acute renal failure in animals. The epithelial cells of the proximal tubules, because of their high metabolic activity, are especially susceptible to damage caused by prolonged ischemia or nephrotoxins, the two main causes of this type of nephropathy.

Ischemic Tubular Necrosis
Ischemic tubular necrosis is generally the result of a severe and prolonged period of hypotension associated with shock of endotoxic, hypovolemic, cardiogenic, or neurogenic origin (Maxie 1993). These renal lesions are potentially life-threatening, and the clinical signs of the resulting renal failure are often hidden by the marked systemic effects of the primary disease responsible for the state of shock.

Nephrotoxic Tubular Necrosis
Nephrotoxic tubular necrosis has been documented in domestic animals in association with a wide variety of exogenous natural and synthetic compounds. These toxic substances may affect tubular function and ultimately cause cellular damage by several mechanisms, including metabolic alterations affecting cellular respiration, interference with the tubular transport system, and damage to specific organelles (Brown and Engelhardt 1987).

Plants, mycotoxins, antimicrobial drugs, heavy metals, ethylene glycol, and some other industrial compounds are potential nephrotoxins in swine. Some of these toxic products are covered in Chapters 56 and 60.

Many plants are nephrotoxic to animals, especially ruminants. Several species of pigweed, particularly redroot pigweed (*Amaranthus retroflexus*) (Figure 9.7), may cause acute renal failure in pigs when ingested. The disease occurs in summer and early fall, corresponding to the months in which animals may have access to the

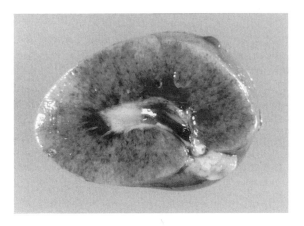

9.6. *Acute glomerulonephritis in a grower pig. Note the edematous and finely petechiated cortical parenchyma (Bourgault and Drolet 1995; reprinted with permission of the American Association of Veterinary Laboratory Diagnosticians).*

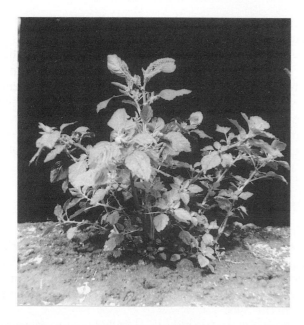

9.7. *Redroot pigweed* (Amaranthus retroflexus). *(Courtesy of the Direction des Services Technologiques, MAPAQ.)*

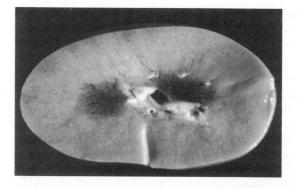

9.8. *Pale and swollen kidney associated with acute tubular necrosis in a sow dead of ethylene glycol poisoning. A leaking valve on the water-heating system was responsible for the poisoning of several animals.*

plants. The onset of clinical signs usually occurs about a week after the ingestion. Characteristic signs include weakness, trembling, and incoordination, rapidly progressing to posterior paralysis and sternal recumbency, and finally to death (Osweiler et al. 1969).

Fungi of some species of *Aspergillus* and *Penicillium* produce nephrotoxins that can contaminate grains used as feedstuff. Ochratoxin A and citrinin are the most common nephrotoxic mycotoxins. Monogastric animals, particularly pigs, may develop significant disease when moldy feed containing ochratoxin A is ingested. Acute clinical signs are relatively rare; a subacute to chronic wasting disease is more commonly associated with this poisoning (Osweiler 1996).

Antibiotic-associated nephropathies are well documented in domestic animals. Classes of antibiotics considered potentially nephrotoxic include the aminoglycosides, tetracyclines (or their degradation products), and sulfonamides. Predisposing factors associated with the toxicity of these agents include the dosage and the route of administration, the duration of the treatment, the solubility of the products, and the general health status (dehydration, shock, preexisting renal disease) of the animal.

Ethylene glycol is another potential cause of poisoning in pigs. This product, found in high concentration in many antifreeze solutions, is not toxic per se, but once it is ingested and absorbed from the gastrointestinal tract, a proportion is enzymatically oxidized in the liver and successively transformed into several nephrotoxic compounds and finally to oxalate. Poisoning occurs in swine with the ingestion of 4–5 ml of ethylene glycol/kg of body weight (Carson 1999). Pigs may be poisoned when they have accidental access to antifreeze so-

lution expelled during engine maintenance or from the plumbing systems in which these products are used to prevent freezing.

Many metallic compounds are nephrotoxic, including inorganic mercury, arsenic, cadmium, lead, thallium, and bismuth. Cases of poisoning with these products are relatively rare in pigs.

Gross renal lesions observed in acute cases of nephrotoxic tubular necrosis are not always conspicuous, but the kidneys may appear slightly swollen, pale, and moist (Figure 9.8). In pigweed (*Amaranthus retroflexus*) poisoning these renal lesions are often accompanied by a marked perirenal edema that may contain blood and possibly by serous effusions elsewhere in the body (Osweiler et al. 1969). In severe acute tubular necrosis, death from acute renal failure may ensue. Animals that survive the acute phase of the disease either recover or develop progressive fibrosis of the kidneys that may or may not lead to chronic renal failure. This chronic evolution appears relatively common in pigs with ochratoxin A toxicosis (Krogh 1977; Rutqvist et al. 1978; Cook et al. 1986).

Histologically, acute tubular necrosis is generally characterized by swelling and necrosis of the lining epithelial cells of the proximal and distal tubules, the presence of granular casts in the tubular lumen, dilated tubules, and mild interstitial edema. The presence of large numbers of calcium oxalate crystals within tubules is a characteristic finding in ethylene glycol poisoning. Kidneys of animals surviving the acute toxic insult show evidence of epithelial regeneration and eventually, at least in some cases, interstitial fibrosis accompanied by focal loss of nephrons and a mild interstitial inflammatory infiltrate.

Since specific therapies for most of these toxicoses is virtually lacking, treatment of affected animals is essentially supportive and symptomatic. When a specific nephrotoxin is suspected, action should be taken to ensure that the offending toxin is rapidly withdrawn or that the pigs are immediately removed from the source of the intoxication. Practical measures can be taken to prevent intoxication by some of these nephrotoxins. Proper drying and storage of grain, for example, is one of the best methods of preventing mycotoxicosis, such as from ochratoxin A.

TUBULOINTERSTITIAL DISEASES

Tubulointerstitial diseases include a relatively large group of conditions characterized primarily by interstitial inflammation and tubular damage: namely, interstitial nephritis (such as that occurring from leptospirosis), embolic nephritis, and pyelonephritis (one of the most significant urinary tract diseases in swine). Immunologically mediated tubulointerstitial disease as occurs in humans has only rarely been documented in domestic animals.

Interstitial Nephritis

Leptospirosis is probably one of the best known causes of interstitial nephritis in pigs. Many serovars of *Leptospira* spp.—those of the serogroups Pomona, Tarassovi, and Australis, for which pigs act as maintenance hosts—cause significant disease in swine, most notably linked with reproductive problems, including infertility, abortion, and birth of weak or dead piglets. The pathogenesis of the disease involves the penetration by the leptospires of mucosal surfaces or skin, a bacteremia of a few days that lasts until the beginning of the humoral immune response, and the preferential localization and persistence of the organisms at sites physically protected from antibodies, such as in the ocular vitreous humor, the cerebrospinal fluid, the genital tract, and the lumen of the renal proximal tubules (Prescott 1993). The passage of the leptospires from the bloodstream to the interstitial tissue of the renal parenchyma and finally to the tubular lumen elicits multifocal lesions of interstitial nephritis (Cheville et al. 1980).

The severity of the interstitial nephritis varies and ranges from grossly undetectable to extensive lesions, particularly when serovars of the Pomona serogroup are involved. The lesions are randomly distributed and appear as poorly circumscribed whitish foci of various shapes and sizes, becoming confluent in severe cases (Figure 9.9). Histologically these foci correspond to the infiltration of lymphocytes, plasma cells, and macrophages in the interstitial tissue, along with some degenerative changes of the surrounding nephrons. In chronic cases, interstitial fibrosis occurs.

In most cases these lesions are not extensive enough to cause renal failure, so the generally asymptomatic animal may shed the leptospires in urine for a relatively long period of time and become an important source of contamination of the premises. With time, the leptospiruria becomes less intense and intermittent, but it has been reported to occur for up to 2 years in some cases (Mitchell et al. 1966).

The association between lesions of interstitial

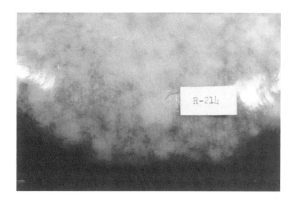

9.9. *Severe interstitial nephritis associated with leptospirosis. (Courtesy of Dr. J.-B. Phaneuf.)*

nephritis in pigs and the detection of leptospires within these kidneys is highly variable among studies (McErlean 1973; Hunter et al. 1987; Jones et al. 1987; Baker et al. 1989; Boqvist et al. 2003). Factors that may influence these results include the serovar of *Leptospira* spp. involved, the methods of leptospiral detection used, the phase of the infection and also the prevalence of leptospirosis and of other infectious causes of interstitial nephritis in swine in a given geographical area. For instance, the prevalence of leptospirosis in fattening pigs and sows in southern Vietnam was found to be high (Boqvist et al. 2002, 2003), whereas similar studies conducted in slaughtered pigs in southwestern Quebec have shown a very low prevalence of this infection (Ribotta et al. 1999; Drolet et al. 2002).

Postweaning multisystemic wasting syndrome (PMWS), a condition affecting nursery and growing pigs, was first described in Canada in 1996 (Clark 1996; Harding 1996). The disease has been linked to PCV2 and is now occurring in many parts of the world. It is characterized by progressive weight loss, respiratory signs, hypertrophic lymphadenopathy, and, in some cases, diarrhea, pallor, or icterus (Allan and Ellis 2000; Segalés and Domingo 2002). Lesions involve several organs and include lymphohistiocytic to granulomatous interstitial pneumonia, nephritis, and hepatitis. The interstitial nephritis is in some cases grossly detectable as whitish foci within renal parenchyma (Figure 9.10). In lymphoid tissues there is lymphocyte depletion and infiltration of histiocytes and multinucleated giant cells that may contain grapelike clusters of basophilic cytoplasmic viral inclusion bodies.

Multifocal lesions of interstitial nephritis also occur in swine with other bacterial (see the section on embolic nephritis) and viral hematogenous infections. Although in most of these cases the lesions do not impair renal function, they are of diagnostic significance because they are suggestive of a systemic disease. Lesions of interstitial nephritis caused by systemic viral infections are often disclosed only upon microscopic examination and are characterized by the presence of foci of nonsup-

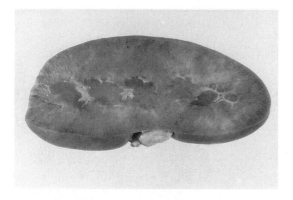

9.10. *Interstitial nephritis in a pig naturally infected with porcine circovirus type 2.*

purative inflammation. Viral infections that may produce these lesions include cytomegalovirus (Kelly 1967), adenovirus (Shadduck et al. 1967; Nietfeld and Leslie-Steen 1993), PRRS virus, and possibly others. Multifocal lesions of nonsuppurative interstitial nephritis have been reproduced experimentally in PRRS virus–infected piglets examined 2–3 weeks postinoculation (Rossow et al. 1995; Cooper et al. 1997). These lesions are found in the renal cortex as well as in the medulla. Similar renal lesions are also frequently found in naturally infected pigs.

Gross lesions of multifocal interstitial nephritis, often called white-spotted or white-dotted kidneys, represent a common cause of kidney condemnation at the slaughterhouse in some areas (Drolet et al. 2002). Lesions generally appear either as few randomly distributed or numerous widely disseminated whitish foci, 1–3 mm in diameter (Figure 9.11). Histologically these foci are composed of mononuclear inflammatory cells that often take up a distinct lymphofollicular pattern (follicular nephritis) (refer to Figure 9.11). This type of interstitial reaction probably represent a nonspecific immunological response to prolonged local antigenic stimulation. In one study it was shown that, although the precise cause of these lesions was uncertain, there was a statistically significant association between the le-

sions and the presence of porcine parvovirus and PCV2 with a stronger association when both viruses were identified in the same kidney (Drolet et al. 2002).

Embolic Nephritis

Embolic nephritis may occur with bacteremia or septic thromboembolism when any of various species of bacteria is seeded within the vasculature of the kidneys. In bacteremia, small aggregates of microorganisms localizing in the renal microcirculation (in particular, in the interstitial and glomerular capillaries) cause the formation of small suppurative foci. Early lesions appear grossly as small hemorrhagic foci bilaterally scattered throughout the renal cortex. They gradually form small (1–3 mm) whitish to yellowish abscesses that may be surrounded by a hyperemic rim (Figure 9.12). These lesions, although more numerous in the cortex, may also be found in the medulla. The finding of such renal lesions, when performing a necropsy, strongly suggests the possibility of a septicemia. In swine, infections with *Streptococcus* spp., *Erysipelothrix rhusiopathiae*, *Actinobacillus suis*, *Escherichia coli*, *Staphylococcus* spp., *Arcanobacterium pyogenes*, and others have to be considered.

Septic thromboembolism occurs when fragments of a septic thrombus enter the bloodstream and occlude the arterial vasculature of the kidneys, resulting in necrosuppurative foci of variable size (Figure 9.13). Such renal lesions, if disclosed during a postmortem examination, should prompt a careful examination of the left cardiac valves (mitral and aortic) for the presence of vegetative endocarditis. In these cases, bacteria most often involved include *Streptococcus* spp., *Erysipelothrix rhusiopathiae*, and *Escherichia coli*.

Cystitis-Pyelonephritis Complex

Urine is formed by the kidneys and stored in the bladder by way of the ureters. The ureteric valves prevent retrograde flow of urine from the bladder to the kidneys. Urine is removed from the bladder via the urethra, which, in females, communicates with the vagina. The distal portion of the urethra and the vaginal tract are not sterile; the composition of the microflora is primarily

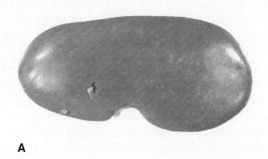

A

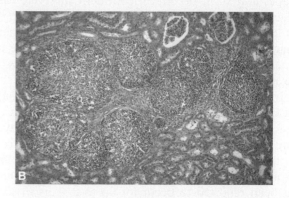

B

9.11. *(A) Kidney from a slaughter pig with multifocal interstitial nephritis. Note the relatively well-demarcated white dots randomly distributed throughout the cortex. (B) Well-demarcated focal area of interstitial nephritis showing a distinct lymphofollicular pattern (follicular nephritis).*

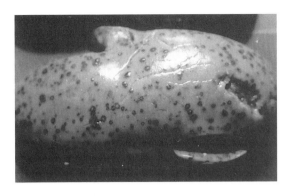

9.12. *Embolic nephritis caused by* Actinobacillus suis. *Scattered suppurative foci are surrounded by a hemorrhagic rim.*

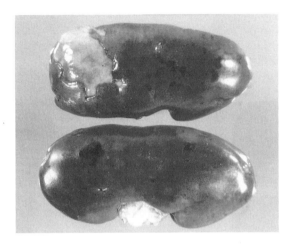

9.13. *Septic thromboembolic nephritis secondary to* Streptococcus suis *endocarditis.*

bacterial. Ascending infection of the sterile portions of the urinary tract may lead to cystitis and pyelonephritis.

The cystitis-pyelonephritis complex has been documented as a leading cause of mortality in sows (D'Allaire and Drolet 1999). Porcine cystitis-pyelonephritis has been reported throughout the world, and the increased incidence appears to be correlated with changes in management, particularly the adoption of confinement housing for gestating sows.

Etiology. A wide variety of bacteria have been isolated from cases of porcine cystitis and pyelonephritis, including *E. coli*, *Arcanobacterium pyogenes*, *Streptococcus* spp., and *Staphylococcus* spp. (Carr and Walton 1993). These endogenous and opportunistic organisms typically inhabit the lower urinary tract and are often referred to as being responsible for "nonspecific" urinary tract infections, which are reviewed in detail in Chapter 38. *Actinobaculum suis*, a specific urinary pathogen, is an important cause of ascending infection in swine. Infection with *A. suis* frequently results in elevated sow mortality, and *A. suis* has been isolated, either alone or

in combination with other bacteria, from nearly half of the reported cases of cystitis and pyelonephritis reviewed by Carr and Walton (1993). Due to the importance of *A. suis* in the pathogenesis of urinary tract infection in swine, the remainder of this section will focus on its role in the disease process.

Formerly classified in the genera *Eubacterium* and *Actinomyces*, *Actinobaculum suis* is a gram-positive rod-shaped bacterium that grows well under anaerobic conditions. *Actinobaculum suis* is urease positive and catalase negative, ferments maltose and xylose, and hydrolyzes starch. Methyl red, Voges-Proskauer, indole, and nitrate reduction tests are negative. A slight alkalinity is produced in litmus milk, but liquification of egg or serum media does not occur. It is nonhemolytic on blood agar, producing pinpoint colonies 2–3 mm in diameter after 2–3 days of incubation under anaerobic conditions at 37°C. During days 4 to 5 postinoculation, colonies flatten and develop a dry, opaque appearance, reaching a diameter of 4–5 mm (Taylor 1999).

Epidemiology. *Actinobaculum suis* is a commensal organism of the porcine urogenital tract. It has been isolated from the preputial cavity of boars at slaughter (Pijoan et al. 1983; Pleschakowa et al. 2004), the vaginal tract of neonatal piglets sampled immediately following parturition, and the vaginal tract of females sampled throughout all stages of production (Dee et al. 1993). *Actinobaculum suis* has been isolated from voided urine, contaminated parturition sleeves of farrowing attendants, pen floors of the farrowing and nursery rooms, and the boots of stockpersons working in the breeding area (Carr and Walton 1990; Dee et al. 1993). The sole route of transmission was believed to be copulation, but it is now understood that the organism is ubiquitous, and colonization of the vaginal tract can take place anytime in the life of the pig.

As the popularity of confinement gestation housing has risen, so has the incidence of *A. suis*–related urinary tract disease. Problems frequently encountered in confinement facilities are the reduced availability of water, increased fecal contamination of the perineal area, excessive weight gain, and leg injuries, all of which result in a reduction in the frequency of urination and enhanced bacterial survival in the urogenital tract. Distinguishing features of endemic cystitis and pyelonephritis within a herd include lack of a temporal relationship between the vulvar discharge and the estrous cycle, minimal effect on herd fertility, low morbidity, high mortality, and an increased frequency in advanced-parity (6+) sows (Pointon et al. 1990).

Pathogenesis. *Actinobaculum suis* is fimbriated, and the short, wide urethra of the sow enhances accessibility to the bladder (Larsen et al. 1986). Once within the bladder lumen, the alkalinity of the environment increases due to the cleavage of urea into ammonia through the use of the urease enzyme. The elevated pH enhances bacterial proliferation and causes an inflammatory reaction of the mucosal surface. The alkaline environment also inhibits the growth of competitive microflora and promotes the precipitation of urinary salts and crystals, particularly struvite. Such precipitates not only further increase inflammatory changes in the bladder mucosa but provide a nidus for bacterial growth and protection from antibiotics and host defense mechanisms. Although the primary means for accessibility to the kidneys is not yet completely understood, it is hypothesized that damage to the ureteric valves secondary to bacterial products (possibly originating from *E. coli*) may predispose the affected animal to pyelonephritis (Carr et al. 1990).

Clinical Signs and Lesions. Clinical signs associated with infections of the urinary tract caused by *A. suis* vary according to the severity and the phase of the disease. In acute and severe cases, affected animals may be found dead, probably from acute renal failure. Symptomatic animals are usually afebrile and may show anorexia, hematuria, and pyuria. The urine is typically reddish brown in color with a strong odor of ammonia. Urinary pH may increase from normal values of 5.5–7.5 up to 8–9. Animals that survive the initial infection frequently experience weight loss and reduced productivity secondary to end-stage renal disease, resulting in premature removal from the breeding herd.

Inflammatory reaction on the mucosal surface of the bladder may be catarrhal, hemorrhagic, purulent, or necrotic, and the bladder wall may be thickened. Struvites can also be found in the lumen. The ureters, often filled with exudate, may increase to as much as 2.5 cm in diameter. Unilateral or bilateral pyelonephritis or pyelitis is the primary lesion detected in the kidneys. The pelvic region, frequently distended with blood, pus, and foul-smelling urine, often shows irregular ulceration and necrosis of the papillae. These suppurative lesions may eventually extend irregularly through the renal medulla and even into the cortex, causing exophytic and discolored deformations of the renal surface (Figure 9.14). These foci of cortical inflammation, when present, seem to occur more frequently at the renal poles. Compound papillae that are mainly located in these latter areas are considered more susceptible to intrarenal reflux of septic urine because of the inability of their papillary ducts to close under intrapelvic pressure (Ransley and Risdon 1974; Carr et al. 1991). In longstanding cases of pyelonephritis, fibrosis ultimately replaces inflammation (Figure 9.15).

Microscopically, necrotizing ureteritis and pyelitis with accumulation of bacterial colonies can be seen, along with epithelial hyperplasia, desquamation of superficial epithelial cells, and goblet cell metaplasia with intraepithelial cyst formation (Woldemeskel et al. 2002). Renal tubules may contain protein casts, bacte-

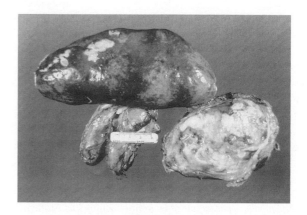

9.14. *Pyelonephritis due to* Actinobaculum suis *in a sow. Note the cortical foci of suppurative inflammation that have extended through the renal capsule (removed on the right).*

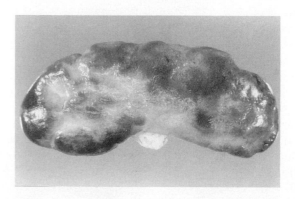

9.15. *Chronic pyelonephritis in a sow.*

ria, and purulent exudate. The interstitium contains mononuclear inflammatory cells, neutrophils, and possibly some fibrosis. Examination of the ureteric valves may reveal inflammation, necrosis, and fibrosis.

Diagnosis. Presumptive diagnosis of cystitis and pyelonephritis in live animals is best achieved when frequent micturition of bloodstained and cloudy urine can be observed. Examination of the urine sediments may also be very informative, because it may reveal the presence of inflammatory cells, erythrocytes, granular renal casts, bacteria, and crystals (Carr and Walton 1992). Due to the striking gross lesions, confirmatory diagnosis of the condition is usually not difficult. In some cases, determination of urea concentration in ocular fluids is a useful aid to postmortem diagnosis of pyelonephritis, especially if it is difficult to ascertain that the lesions found in the urinary tract are responsible for the death of the animal (Drolet et al. 1990; Chagnon et al. 1991). In order to isolate the causative organism properly, care must be taken during sample collection to minimize exposure to oxygen (Dee 1991). In the field, the bladder should remain unopened, and the neck of the bladder should be sealed with umbilical tape. Similar care should be taken with renal tissue. Demonstration of lesions of pyelonephritis can be carried out through the examination of one kidney; however, the other should remain unopened with the ureter sealed as previously described. Upon arrival at the laboratory, a small incision should be made over a portion of the serosal surface of the bladder and kidney, previously seared with a hot iron to reduce surface contamination. A cotton swab should be inserted into the bladder lumen and streaked for isolation on colistin nalidixic acid (CNA) agar and then incubated at 37°C under anaerobic conditions for 5–7 days. If the culture process is to take place at a distant location, swabs can be placed into Kary Blair anaerobic transport media for shipment. Colonial morphology and biochemical characteristics of *A. suis* have been described earlier in the section.

Finally, an indirect fluorescent antibody test for the detection of serum antibodies against *A. suis* has been described (Wendt and Amtsberg 1994). The test appears to be highly specific (100%) but of low sensitivity (79%).

Treatment and Prevention. Treatment of urinary tract infections may be successful if the correct antibiotic is administered early in the course of the disease. Studies have demonstrated consistent susceptibility of *A. suis* to penicillin, cephalosporins, chloramphenicol, tetracyclines, and macrolides, with variable susceptibility to fluoroquinolones, and resistance to aminoglycosides (Biksi et al. 2003). Penicillin and ampicillin are frequently the products of choice, due to their ability to function under alkaline conditions and their propensity for excretion through the urinary tract. Dosages of 2.2 mg/kg are typically administered intramuscularly for 3 consecutive days. Oral administration of penicillin and ampicillin is also possible; however, feed-grade products are of little value, due to the high degree of anorexia in acutely infected sows and a reduced bioavailability, secondary to destruction by gastric enzymes, low pH, and colonic bacteria. Water-soluble ampicillin can be administered at 2.3 mg/kg for 5 consecutive days; however, bioavailability is questionable and cost may become an issue.

Acidification of the urine through oral administration of feed-grade citric acid has been described in the literature (Dee et al. 1994). Results from this study showed a reduction in the incidence of clinical urinary tract disease, as well as highly significant (p <0.0001) differences in urinary pH and bacterial concentration/ml of urine in medicated versus nonmedicated groups. A level of 70 mg of citric acid was administered daily for 14 consecutive days in this study, and palatability problems were not detected in treated animals.

Prevention of urinary tract disease is similar to the steps required to control other diseases of the urogenital system (Dee 1992). The maintenance of a high degree of hygiene during breeding and parturition, as well as throughout the gestation period, is critical. Facilities

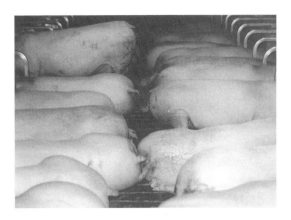

9.16. *Improper facility design enhances the incidence of cystitis-pyelonephritis in gestating sows.*

need to be properly designed to reduce the spread of pathogens within the breeding herd and allow efficient removal of feces from the environment (Figure 9.16).

Restricting water availability through the use of intermittent delivery systems or poor husbandry results in an increase in abnormal urine parameters in gestating sows (Almond et al. 1996). Abnormalities included reduced urine output, elevated specific gravity (≥ 1.026), and increased creatinine concentration. Therefore, it is recommended that free-choice water be available at all times. Finally, because a higher degree of urinary tract disease can be seen in older sows, proper culling procedures are important to ensure that an optimal parity distribution is maintained within the breeding herd.

NEOPLASIA

Neoplasms are infrequent in pigs because of the low average age of the population. However, those most often recorded have been from young animals (Nielsen and Moulton 1990). Tumors of the urinary tract in swine involve mainly the kidneys. Neoplasms of the lower urinary tract, although they have been reported (Nieberle and Cohrs 1967), are generally considered exceedingly rare.

Embryonal nephroma, also named *nephroblastoma,* is one of the most common neoplasms of swine and is certainly the most common primary renal tumor observed in this species, although its relative prevalence varies from one region to another. As its name implies, this neoplasm appears to originate from the embryonic renal blastema. The tumor arises from the kidney or, rarely, from the perirenal tissues (probably from remnants of embryonic renal tissues). Affected animals are typically young, and most of them reach market age without significant clinical signs, the tumor being discovered at postmortem inspection. Embryonal nephroma is most commonly found as a single mass involving one kidney but it may be multiple or bilateral (Nielsen and Moulton 1990). The tumor, which can

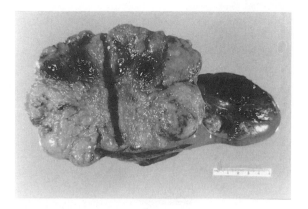

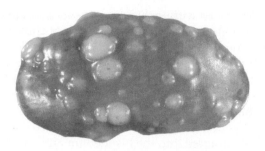

9.18. *Lymphoma in a fattening pig. Multiple tumoral nodules in the kidney.*

9.17. *Large embryonal nephroma at one pole of the kidney of a slaughtered pig. (Courtesy of Dr. Y. Robinson.)*

reach impressive size, often appears firm, pale, and nodular (Figure 9.17). Metastasis infrequently occurs in swine compared to other mammals affected with embryonal nephroma. Histologically, this tumor is very peculiar and resembles disorganized embryonic renal tissue. The primitive tissue from which it arises is pluripotent and accounts for the presence of neoplastic epithelial and mesenchymal elements simultaneously observed within the tumor. Hayashi et al. (1986) classified porcine nephroblastomas into four types according to their contents: nephroblastic, epithelial, mesenchymal, and miscellaneous. Only a few of the nephroblastic tumors described in their case series had metastasized.

Other primary renal tumors are believed to be uncommon in swine. Renal carcinomas have been occasionally reported (Sandison and Anderson 1968; Anderson et al. 1969). Neoplasms originating from the renal pelvis are very rare (Vitovec 1977).

Secondary renal involvement may occur with some multisystemic or generalized cancers such as the malignant lymphoma (lymphosarcoma). In pigs, this relatively common neoplasm occurs predominantly as multicentric and thymic forms. In advanced cases of multicentric and thymic lymphomas, which involve primarily the lymph nodes and the thymus, respectively, infiltration of liver, spleen, kidneys, and other organs may occur. Renal involvement is diffuse or more often nodular so that the organs appear either enlarged and pale or dotted with pale nodules often protruding from the cortical surface (Figure 9.18). In the course of the disease some animals may develop a leukemic phase. Renal lesions in some of these cases appear rather hemorrhagic (Stevenson and DeWitt 1973; Marcato 1987) and may be confused with some systemic infectious diseases (Figure 9.19). The precise pathogenesis of these latter lesions is uncertain but may involve either a coagulation defect or a phenomenon of acute infarction caused by the presence of intravascular neoplastic cells.

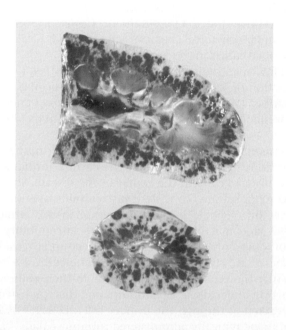

9.19. *Leukemic lymphoma in a gilt showing multiple renal hemorrhagic foci. Histologically these focal interstitial hemorrhages also contain neoplastic lymphoid cells.*

MISCELLANEOUS CONDITIONS

Urolithiasis

Urolithiasis is the presence of calculi, or uroliths, in the urinary passages. Uroliths are macroscopic mineral (polycrystalline) concretions that may contain small quantities of organic material; the term *crystalluria* is used for abnormal microscopic crystalloid precipitates in urine. The mineral composition of calculi found in pigs and their relative importance have not been extensively studied. Nevertheless, various types of calculi can be found, including calcium carbonate, calcium apatite (calcium phosphate), struvite (magnesium ammonium phosphate hexahydrate), and uric acid and urate. Factors known to predispose to the formation of uroliths include the diet, urinary pH, reduced water intake, urinary stasis, and preexisting urinary tract diseases.

Swine are rarely afflicted with urolithiasis in comparison to other domestic animals. The condition is sporadically found in pigs of all ages and is also occasionally observed as incidental findings in slaughtered pigs. Outbreaks of obstructive urolithiasis have been reported on several occasions (Inoue et al. 1977; Sim 1978; Smyth et al. 1986). In these outbreaks, which involved weaned and feeder pigs as well as breeding animals, the predisposing cause for the condition was not elucidated. Animals affected with obstructive urolithiasis may demonstrate decreased appetite, oliguria or anuria, abdominal distension and pain, and death from postrenal uremia. Ruptured bladder may also occur in some cases. Treatment of pigs with obstructive urolithiasis is theoretically feasible but is generally not considered cost-effective.

The bladder of sows sometimes contains yellowish sediments that do not seem to be of clinical significance. On postmortem examination, such sediments, admixed with desquamated epithelial cells, may give the false impression of a cystitis because of the turbidity of the urine. Infection-induced calculi are also observed occasionally in sows with cystitis and pyelonephritis (Figure 9.20).

Uric acid and urate uroliths are frequently found in the kidneys of newborn piglets. These often appear as fine orange precipitates in the medulla and pelvis (Figure 9.21). This peculiar form of urolithiasis is observed mainly in piglets that have no access to the sow's milk (which contains both fluids and nutrients) or are afflicted by a debilitating disease associated with anorexia and diarrhea (e.g., transmissible gastroenteritis), thus contributing to dehydration. Accelerated catabolism of tissue proteins and purines to supply energy needs and decreased kidney function related to dehydration are responsible for the high levels of blood urea and uric acid found in these piglets. The excess solute, poorly reabsorbed from the glomerular filtrate, is ultimately deposited in the inner medulla and pelvis (Maxie 1993).

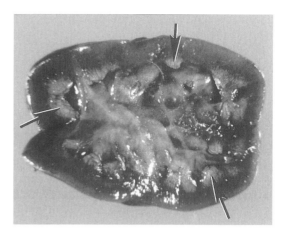

9.21. *Urate calculi in medulla (arrows) of a dehydrated suckling piglet.*

Hydronephrosis

Distension of the renal pelvis and calyces with urine, associated with progressive atrophy of the kidney parenchyma, is the hallmark of hydronephrosis, which is uncommon and sporadic in swine. The pathogenesis of this condition always involves some form of obstructive impediment to the normal passage of urine within the lower urinary tract, anywhere from the pelvis to the distal urethra. The causes of the obstruction include urinary calculi, exudate within urinary passages, ureteral kinking, focal external compression (abcesses, tumors), and posttraumatic or postinflammatory strictures.

Severe unilateral hydronephrosis may develop unnoticed since the remaining kidney, if normal, may compensate adequately. In these cases, the affected kidney shows extensive dilatation of the pelvis and calyces at the expense of the renal parenchyma, which may appear as a thin layer of cortical tissue (Figure 9.22). Depending on the location of the obstruction, hydroureter may also develop. In long-standing cases, the kidney may be virtually transformed into a large fluid-filled sac delimited by a severely distended renal capsule. These extreme lesions may take months to de-

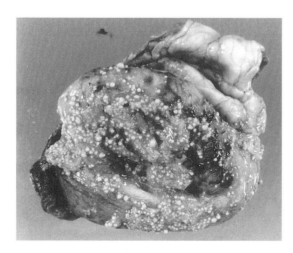

9.20. *Infection-induced calculi in the bladder of a sow with a chronic suppurative cystitis.*

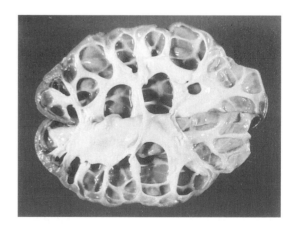

9.22. *Chronic unilateral hydronephrosis.*

velop. Since stagnation of urine predisposes to infection, the urine may be transformed into a purulent exudate in some instances. In cases of bilateral hydronephrosis, affected animals usually die from uremia before renal lesions get fully developed.

Parasitic Infections

The pig is the final or intermediate host of a number of parasitic helminths (see Chapter 55). Compared to some other body systems, the urinary tract is the niche of very few of these parasites. Renal infections with *Dioctophyma renale*, the giant kidney worm, and with larval stages of certain tapeworms may occur on rare occasions. The most significant helminth with tropism for the urinary system of swine is the nematode *Stephanurus dentatus*, the so-called kidney worm of swine.

Stephanurus dentatus is a widely distributed strongyloid worm and is most prevalent in warm climates, including the southern United States. In enzootic areas, this parasitic infection may have significant economical impact since it is associated with deaths, retarded growth, decreased feed efficiency, and condemnations at the abattoir (Batte et al. 1960). Larvae of this nematode need moisture and shade for optimal survival, so pigs raised on soil in this type of environment are the most prone to the disease. Infective larvae penetrate the skin or are ingested by the pigs. Transplacental fetal infection is also possible (Batte et al. 1966).

After being introduced into the host, the larvae molt and migrate to the liver, where they remain for several months, causing severe hepatic damage and inflammation. The presence of the parasite within the hepatic parenchyma is often responsible for extensive liver condemnation in some herds (Hale and Marti 1983). Eventually some larvae escape from the liver and migrate to the abdominal cavity and potentially to various ectopic sites, eliciting a severe inflammatory reaction. To complete the cycle, some adults establish themselves in the perirenal tissues or, more rarely, within the kidney. At that site, the worms, measuring about 3 cm in length, are found in cystic inflammatory nodules that communicate with either the pelvis or the ureter in order to shed their eggs successfully into urine. The prepatent period in most cases is at least 9 months, and adults may shed ova in urine for over 2 years (Batte et al. 1960, 1966). Preventive and curative measures for the control of parasites are addressed in detail in Chapter 55.

Others

Mineralization of the kidneys occurs in swine with acute vitamin D toxicosis. This poisoning is usually observed when excessive amounts of vitamin D_3 are inadvertently added to their feed (Kurtz and Stowe 1979; Long 1984). Affected pigs show lethargy, vomiting, diarrhea, respiratory distress, and death. Salient gross necropsy findings include hemorrhagic gastritis or gastroenteritis, myocardial necrosis, and pulmonary edema and congestion. Histologically, besides the gross lesions described above, there is widespread mineralization accompanied by degenerative changes of varying severity in the kidneys, myocardium, lungs, gastrointestinal tract, and blood vessels.

Mucinous metaplasia of the epithelial cells lining the renal pelvis, ureter, and urinary bladder is occasionally observed in pigs. This rather nonspecific lesion, of uncertain pathogenesis, has been reported in pigs with various conditions, including exudative epidermitis, *E. coli* enteritis, hog cholera, and suppurative arthritis (Brobst et al. 1971), as well as in urinary tract infections.

Ossification of the renal pelvis of unknown etiology has been reported in slaughtered pigs (Bundza 1990).

REFERENCES

Allan GM, Ellis JA. 2000. Porcine circoviruses: A review. J Vet Diagn Invest 12:3–14.

Almond GW, Stevens JB, Routh PA, Feng M, Hevener W, Deen J, Davies PR. 1996. Water deprivation in post-pubertal gilts: Changes in urine and semen constituents. Proc Int Pig Vet Soc 14:734.

Andersen S, Nielsen R. 1973. Pathology of isoimmune purpura thrombocytopenia in piglets. Nord Vet Med 25:211–219.

Anderson LJ, Sandison AT, Jarrett WFH. 1969. A British abattoir survey of tumours in cattle, sheep, and pigs. Vet Rec 84:547–551.

Baker TF, McEwen SA, Prescott JF, Meek AH. 1989. The prevalence of leptospirosis and its association with multifocal interstitial nephritis in swine at slaughter. Can J Vet Res 53:290–294.

Banks WJ. 1986. Urinary system. In Applied Veterinary Histology, 2nd ed. WJ Banks, ed. Baltimore: Williams and Wilkins, pp. 431–446.

Batte EG, Harkema R, Osborne JC. 1960. Observations on the life cycle and pathogenicity of the swine kidney worm (*Stephanurus dentatus*). J Am Vet Med Assoc 136:622–625.

Batte EG, Moncol DJ, Barber CW. 1966. Prenatal infection with the swine kidney worm (*Stephanurus dentatus*) and associated lesions. J Am Vet Med Assoc 149:758–765.

Benko L. 1969. Cases of bilateral and unilateral duplication of ureters in the pig. Vet Rec 84:139–140.

Biksi I, Major A, Fodor L, Szenci O, Vetesi F. 2003. In vitro sensitivity of Hungarian *Actinobaculum suis* strains to selected antimicrobials. Acta Vet Hung 51:53–59.

Boqvist S, Chau BL, Gunnarsson A, Olsson Engvall E, Vagsholm I, Magnusson U. 2002. Animal-and herd-level risk factors for leptospiral seropositivity among sows in the Mekong delta, Vietnam. Prev Vet Med 53:233–245.

Boqvist S, Montgomery JM, Hurst M, Ho Thi Viet Thu, Olsson Engvall E, Gunnarsson A, Magnusson U. 2003. Leptospira in slaughtered fattening pigs in southern Vietnam: Presence of the bacteria in the kidneys and association with morphological findings. Vet Microbiol 93:361–368.

Bourgault A, Drolet R. 1995. Spontaneous glomerulonephritis in swine. J Vet Diagn Invest 7:122–126.

Brobst DF, Cottrell R, Delez A. 1971. Mucinous degeneration of the epithelium of the urinary tract of swine. Vet Pathol 8:485–489.

Brown SA, Engelhardt JA. 1987. Drug-related nephropathies. Part I. Mechanisms, diagnosis, and management. Comp Cont Educ 9:148–159.

Bundza A. 1990. Osseous metaplasia of the renal pelvis in slaughter swine. Can Vet J 31:529.

Carr J, Walton JR. 1990. Investigations of the pathogenic properties of *Eubacterium* (*Corynebacterium*) *suis*. Proc Int Pig Vet Soc 11:178.

———. 1992. Characteristics of plasma and urine from normal adult swine and changes found in sows with either asymptomatic bacteriuria or cystitis and pyelonephritis. Proc Int Pig Vet Soc 12:263.

———. 1993. Bacterial flora of the urinary tract of pigs associated with cystitis and pyelonephritis. Vet Rec 132:575–577.

Carr J, Walton JR, Done SH. 1990. Observations on the intravesicular portion of the ureter from healthy pigs and those with urinary tract disease. Proc Int Pig Vet Soc 11:286.

———. 1991. Cystitis and pyelonephritis in the sow. Pig Vet J 27:122–141.

Carrasco L, Madsen LW, Salguero FJ, Numez A, Sanchez-Cordon P, Bollen P. 2003. Immune complex-associated thrombocytopenic purpura syndrome in sexually mature Göttingen minipigs. J Comp Pathol 128:25–32.

Carson TL. 1999. Toxic minerals, chemicals, plants, and gases. In Diseases of Swine, 8th ed. BE Straw, S D'Allaire, WL Mengeling, DJ Taylor, eds. Ames: Iowa State Univ Press, pp. 783–796.

Chagnon M, D'Allaire S, Drolet R. 1991. A prospective study of sow mortality in breeding herds. Can J Vet Res 55:180–184.

Cheville NF, Mengeling WL, Zinober MR. 1970. Ultrastructural and immunofluorescent studies of glomerulonephritis in chronic hog cholera. Lab Invest 22:458–467.

Cheville NF, Huhn R, Cutlip RC. 1980. Ultrastructure of renal lesions in pigs with acute leptospirosis caused by *Leptospira pomona*. Vet Pathol 17:338–351.

Choi C, Chae C. 2003. Glomerulonephritis associated with classical swine fever virus in pigs. Vet Rec 153:20–22.

Clark EG. 1996. Pathology of the post-weaning multisystemic wasting syndrome of pigs. Proc West Can Assoc Swine Pract, p. 22–25.

Cook WO, Osweiler GD, Anderson TD, Richard JL. 1986. Ochratoxicosis in Iowa swine. J Am Vet Med Assoc 188:1399–1402.

Cooper VL, Heese RA, Doster AR. 1997. Renal lesions associated with experimental porcine reproductive and respiratory syndrome virus (PRRSV) infection. J Vet Diagn Invest 9:198–201.

Cordes DO, Dodd DC. 1965. Bilateral renal hypoplasia of the pig. Pathol Vet 2:37–48.

D'Allaire S, Drolet R. 1999. Culling and mortality in breeding animals. In Diseases of Swine, 8th ed. BE Straw, S D'Allaire, WL Mengeling, DJ Taylor, eds. Ames: Iowa State Univ Press, pp. 1003–1016.

Dee SA. 1991. Diagnosing and controlling urinary tract infections caused by *Eubacterium suis* in swine. Vet Med 86:231–238.

———. 1992. Porcine urogenital disease. In The Veterinary Clinics of North America: Swine Reproduction. RC Tubb, AD Leman, eds. Philadelphia: W. B. Saunders, pp. 641–660.

Dee SA, Carlson AR, Corey MM. 1993. New observations on the epidemiology of *Eubacterium suis*. Comp Cont Ed 15:345–348.

Dee SA, Tracy JD, King V. 1994. Using citric acid to control urinary tract disease in swine. Vet Med 89:473–476.

Dimmock CK, Webster WR, Shiels IA, Edwards CL. 1982. Isoimmune thrombocytopenic purpura in piglets. Aust Vet J 59:157–159.

Drolet R, D'Allaire S, Chagnon M. 1990. The evaluation of postmortem ocular fluid analysis as a diagnostic aid in sows. J Vet Diagn Invest 2:9–13.

Drolet R, Thibault S, D'Allaire S, Thomson JR, Done SH. 1999. Porcine dermatitis and nephropathy syndrome (PDNS): An overview of the disease. Swine Health Prod 7:283–285.

Drolet R, D'Allaire S, Larochelle R, Magar R, Ribotta M, Higgins R. 2002. Infectious agents identified in pigs with multifocal interstitial nephritis at slaughter. Vet Rec 150:139–143.

Elling F. 1979. Nutritionally induced necrotizing glomerulonephritis and polyarteritis nodosa in pigs. Acta Pathol Microbiol Scand 87A:387–392.

Friendship RM, Lumsden JH, McMillan I, Wilson MR. 1984. Hematology and biochemistry reference values for Ontario swine. Can J Comp Med 48:390–393.

Friis C. 1980. Postnatal development of the pig kidney: Ultrastructure of the glomerulus and the proximal tubule. J Anat 130:513–526.

Hale OM, Marti OG. 1983. Influence of an experimental infection of swine kidney worm (*Stephanurus dentatus*) on performance of pigs. J Anim Sci 56:616–620.

Häni H, Indermühle NA. 1980. Bilateral renal cortical necrosis associated with esophagogastric ulcers in pigs. Vet Pathol 17:234–237.

Harding JG. 1996. Post-weaning multisystemic wasting syndrome (PMWS): Preliminary epidemiology and clinical presentation. Proc West Can Assoc Swine Pract p. 21.

Hayashi M, Tsuda H, Okumura M, Hirose M, Ito N. 1986. Histopathological classification of nephroblastomas in slaughtered swine. J Comp Pathol 96:35–46.

Hélie P, Drolet R, Germain MC, Bourgault A. 1995. Systemic necrotizing vasculitis and glomerulonephritis in grower pigs in southwestern Quebec. Can Vet J 36:150–154.

Hervas J, Gomezvillamandos JC, Mendez A, Carrasco L, Sierra MA. 1996. The lesional changes and pathogenesis in the kidney in African swine fever. Vet Res Comm 20:285–299.

Höfliger von H. 1971. Zur kenntnis der kongenitalen unilateralen nierenagenesie bei Haustieren. Schweizer Archiv Tierheilkund 113:330–337.

Hogasen K, Jansen JH, Mollness TE, Hovdenes J, Harboe M. 1995. Hereditary porcine membranoproliferative glomerulonephritis type II is caused by factor H deficiency. J Clin Invest 95:1054–1061.

Hunter P, Van Der Vyver FH, Selmer-Olsen A, Henton MM, Herr S, Delang JF. 1987. Leptospirosis as a cause of "white spot" kidneys in South African pig abattoirs. Onderstepoort J Vet Res 54:59–62.

Inoue I, Baba K, Ogura Y, Konno S. 1977. Pathology of the urinary bladder in urolithiasis in swine. Nat Inst Anim Hlth Quart 17:186.

Jakob W. 1971. Spontaneous amyloidosis of mammals. Vet Pathol 8:292–306.

Jansen JH. 1993. Porcine membranoproliferative glomerulonephritis with intramembranous dense deposits (porcine dense deposit disease). Acta Pathol Microbiol Immunol Scand 101:281–289.

Jansen JH, Nordstoga K. 1992. Renal lesions in Norwegian slaughter pigs: Macroscopic and light microscopic studies. J Vet Med A39:582–592.

———. 1994. Glomerular lesions in fibrotic kidneys of Norwegian slaughter pigs: Light microscopic and immunohistochemical studies. J Vet Med A41:91–101.

Jansen JH, Hogasen K, Grondahl AM. 1995. Porcine membranoproliferative glomerulonephritis type II: An autosomal recessive deficiency of factor H. Vet Rec 137:240–244.

Jansen JH, Hogasen K, Harboe M, Hovig T. 1998. In situ complement activation in porcine membranoproliferative glomerulonephritis type II. Kidney Int 53:331–349.

Jones RT, Millar BD, Chappel RJ, Adler B. 1987. Macroscopic kidney lesions in slaughtered pigs are an inadequate indicator of current leptospiral infection. Aust Vet J 64:258–259.

Kavanagh NT. 1994. Dermatitis/nephropathy syndrome in pigs. Vet Rec 134:311.

Kelly DF. 1967. Pathology of extranasal lesions in experimental inclusion-body rhinitis of pigs. Res Vet Sci 8:472–478.

Krogh P. 1977. Ochratoxin A residues in tissues of slaughter pigs with nephropathy. Nord Vet Med 29:402–405.

Kurtz HJ, Stowe CM. 1979. Acute vitamin-D toxicosis in swine. Proc Am Assoc Vet Lab Diagn 22:61–68.

Larsen JL, Hogh P, Hovind-Hougen J. 1986. Haemagglutinating and hydrophobic properties of *Corynebacterium* (*Eubacterium*) *suis*. Acta Vet Scand 27:520–523.

Long GG. 1984. Acute toxicosis in swine associated with excessive dietary intake of vitamin D. J Am Vet Med Assoc 184:164–170.

Marcato PS. 1987. Swine lymphoid and myeloid neoplasms in Italy. Vet Res Comm 11:325–337.

Martin-Fernandez J, Igual A, Rueda A, Sanchez-Viscaino JM, Alonso-Marti C. 1991. Glomerular pathology in surviving pigs experimentally infected with African swine fever virus. Histol Histopathol 6:115–121.

Mason RW, Cooper R. 1985. Congenital bilateral renal hypoplasia in Large White pigs. Aust Vet J 62:413–414.

Maurer FD, Griesemer RA, Jones TC. 1958. The pathology of African swine fever: A comparison with hog cholera. Am J Vet Res 19:517–539.

Maxie MG. 1993. The urinary system. In Pathology of Domestic Animals, 4th ed. KVH Jubb, PC Kennedy, N Palmer, eds. San Diego: Academic Press, pp. 475–487.

McErlean BA. 1973. The isolation of leptospirae from the kidneys of bacon pigs. Vet J 27:185–186.

McLaughlin PS, McLaughlin BG. 1987. Chemical analysis of bovine and porcine vitreous humors: Correlation of normal values with serum chemical values and changes with time and temperature. Am J Vet Res 48:467–473.

Mitchell DA, Robertson A, Corner AH, Boulanger P. 1966. Some observations on the diagnosis and epidemiology of leptospirosis in swine. Can J Comp Med 30:211–217.

Morales GA, Guzman VH. 1976. Proliferative glomerulonephritis in young pigs. Proc Int Pig Vet Soc 4:R1.

Müller E. 1977. Die Verträglichkeit von Weizensteinbrand beim Schwein. Dtsch Tierarztl Wochenschr 48:43–45.

Nieberle K, Cohrs P. 1967. Urinary organs. In Textbook of the Special Pathological Anatomy of Domestic Animals. Toronto: Pergamon Press, pp. 659–720.

Nielsen SW, Moulton JE. 1990. Tumors of the urinary system. In Tumors in Domestic Animals, 3d ed. JE Moulton, ed. Berkeley: Univ California Press, pp. 458–478.

Nietfeld JC, Leslie-Steen P. 1993. Interstitial nephritis in pigs with adenovirus infection. J Vet Diagn Invest 5:269–273.

Olvera A, Sibila M, Calsamiglia M, Segalés J, Domingo M. 2004. Comparison of porcine circovirus type 2 load in serum quantified by a real time PCR in postweaning multisystemic wasting syndrome and porcine dermatitis and nephropathy syndrome naturally affected pigs. J Virol Methods 117:75–80.

Orr JP, Althouse E, Dulac GC, Durham JK. 1988. Epizootic infection of a minimal disease swine herd with a herpesvirus. Can Vet J 29:45–50.

Osweiler GD. 1996. Mycotoxins. In Toxicology. GD Osweiler, ed. Philadelphia: Williams and Wilkins, pp. 409–436.

Osweiler GD, Buck WB, Bicknell EJ. 1969. Production of perirenal edema in swine with Amaranthus retroflexus. Am J Vet Res 30:557–566.

Pace LW, Schreibman AE, Bouchard G, Luger AM. 1998. Immune-complex mediated glomerulonephritis in miniature swine. Proc Int Pig Vet Soc 15:394.

Pijoan C, Lastra A, Leman AD. 1983. Isolation of Corynebacterium suis from the prepuce of boars. J Am Vet Med Assoc 183:428–429.

Pleschakowa V, Leibold W, Amtsberg G, Konine D, Wendt M. 2004. The prevalence of Actinobaculum suis in boars of breeding herds in the Omsk region (Russian Federation) by indirect immunofluorescence technique. Dtsch Tierarztl Wochenschr 11:67–69.

Pointon AM, Ruen PD, Dial GD. 1990. Vulval discharge syndrome: How to conduct a clinical investigation. Proc Minn Swine Conf Vet 17:280–281.

Prescott JF. 1993. The urinary system. In Pathology of Domestic Animals, 4th ed. JVH Jubb, PC Kennedy, N Palmer, eds. San Diego: Academic Press, pp. 503–511.

Ransley PG, Risdon RA. 1974. Renal papillae and intrarenal reflux in the pig. Lancet 2:1114.

Ribotta M, Higgins R, Perron D. 1999. Swine leptospirosis: Low risk of exposure for humans? Can Vet J 40, 809–810.

Rosell C, Segalés J, Ramos-Vara A, Folch JM, Rodriguez-Arrioja GM, Duran CO, Balash M, Plana-Duran J, Domingo M. 2000. Identification of porcine circovirus in tissues of pigs with porcine dermatitis and nephropathy syndrome. Vet Rec 146:40–43.

Rossow KD, Collins JE, Goyal SM, Nelson EA, Christopher-Hennings J, Benfield DA. 1995. Pathogenesis of porcine reproductive and respiratory syndrome virus infection in gnotobiotic pigs. Vet Pathol 32:361–373.

Ruckebusch Y, Phaneuf LP, Dunlop R. 1991. The urinary collecting and voiding system. In Physiology of Small and Large Animals, 1st ed. Y Ruckebusch, L-P Phaneuf, R Dunlop, eds. Hamilton: B.C. Decker, pp. 184–188.

Rutqvist L, Bjorklund NE, Hult K, Hokby E, Carlsson B. 1978. Ochratoxin A as the cause of spontaneous nephropathy in fattening pigs. Appl Environ Microbiol 36:920–925.

Salmon-Legagneur E, Gayral JP, Leveau JM, Rettagliatti J. 1973. Etude de quelques paramètres de variation de la composition des effluents de porcherie. Journ Rech Porcine France 5:285–291.

Sandison AT, Anderson LJ. 1968. Tumors of the kidney in cattle, sheep, and pigs. Cancer 21:727–742.

Segalés J, Domingo M. 2002. Postweaning multisystemic wasting syndrome (PMWS) in pigs. A review. Vet Quarterly 24:109–124.

Segalés J, Piella J, Marco E, Mateu-de-Antonio EM, Espuna E, Domingo M. 1998. Porcine dermatitis and nephropathy syndrome in Spain. Vet Rec 142:483–486.

Segalés J, Rosell C, Domingo M. 2003. Porcine dermatitis and nephropathy syndrome. In Trends in Emerging Viral Infections of Swine, 1st ed. A Morilla, K-J Yoon, JJ Zimmerman, eds. Ames: Iowa State Press, pp. 313–318.

Shadduck JA, Koestner A, Kasza L. 1967. The lesions of porcine adenoviral infection in germfree and pathogen-free pigs. Pathol Vet 4:537–552.

Shirota K, Nomura Y, Saito Y. 1984. Spontaneous swine glomerulonephritis in littermates from a leukemic sow. Vet Pathol 21:158–163.

Shirota K, Koyama R, Nomura Y. 1986. Glomerulopathy in swine: Microscopic lesions and IgG or C3 deposition in 100 pigs. Jpn J Vet Sci 48:15–22.

Shirota K, Masaki T, Kitada H, Yanagi M, Ikeda Y, Une Y, Nomura Y, Jothy S. 1995. Renal glomerular fibrosis in two pigs. Vet Pathol 32:236–241.

Sierra MA, de las Mulas JM, Molenbeek RF, van Maanen C, Vos JH, Quezada M, Gruys E. 1997. Porcine immune complex glomerulonephritis dermatitis (PIGD) syndrome. Europ J Vet Pathol 3:63–70.

Sim WW. 1978. Urinary obstruction in weaned piglets leading to increased mortality. Proc Pig Vet Soc 4:57–59.

Sisson S. 1975. Porcine urogenital system. In Sisson and Grossman's The Anatomy of Domestic Animals, 5th ed. R Getty, ed. Philadelphia: W. B. Saunders, pp. 1297–1303.

Slauson DO, Lewis RM. 1979. Comparative pathology of glomerulonephritis in animals. Vet Pathol 16:135–164.

Smith WJ, Thomson JR, Done S. 1993. Dermatitis/nephropathy syndrome of pigs. Vet Rec 132:47.

Smyth JA, Rice DA, Kavanagh NT, Collins DS. 1986. Urolithiasis in weaned pigs. Vet Rec 119:158–159.

Spargo BH, Taylor JR. 1988. The kidney. In Pathology, 1st ed. E Rubin, JL Farber, eds. Philadelphia: J. B. Lippincott, pp. 832–889.

Stevenson RG, DeWitt WF. 1973. An unusual case of lymphosarcoma in a pig. Can Vet J 14:139–141.

Tamura T, Shirota K, Une Y, Nomura Y. 1986. Mesangial hyaline droplet formation and mesangiolysis in the renal glomeruli seen in pigs with mastocytosis. Jpn J Vet Sci 48:1183–1189.

Taylor DJ. 1999. Miscellaneous bacterial infections (Actinobaculum suis). In Diseases of Swine, 8th ed., BE Straw, S D'Allaire, WL

Mengeling, DJ Taylor, eds. Ames: Iowa State Univ Press, pp. 635–638.

Thibault S, Drolet R, Germain MC, D'Allaire S, Larochelle R, Magar R. 1998. Cutaneous and systemic necrotizing vasculitis in swine. Vet Pathol 35:108–116.

Thomson JR, MacIntyre N, Henderson LEA, Meikle CS. 2001. Detection of *Pasteurella multocida* in pigs with porcine dermatitis and nephropathy syndrome. Vet Rec 149:412–417.

Thomson JR, Higgins RJ, Smith WJ, Done SH. 2002. Porcine dermatitis and nephropathy syndrome. Clinical and pathological features of cases in the United Kingdom (1993–1998). J Vet Med A49:430–437.

Vitovec J. 1977. Carcinoma of the renal pelvis in slaughter animals. J Comp Pathol 87:129–134.

Weaver ME. 1966. Persistent urachus—An observation in miniature swine. Anat Rec 154:701–704.

Webster WR, Summers PM. 1978. Congenital polycystic kidney and liver syndrome in piglets. Aust Vet J 54:451.

Wellenberg GJ, Stockhofe-Zurwieden N, de Jong MF, Boersma WJA, Elbers ARW. 2004. Excessive porcine circovirus type 2 antibody titres may trigger the development of porcine dermatitis and nephropathy syndrome: A case-control study. Vet Microbiol 99:203–214.

Wells GAH, Hebert CN, Robins BC. 1980. Renal cysts in pigs: Prevalence and pathology in slaughtered pigs from a single herd. Vet Rec 106:532–535.

Wendt M, Amtsberg G. 1994. Serological examinations for detection of antibodies against *Eubacterium suis* in pigs. Proc Int Pig Vet Soc 13:159.

White M, Higgins RJ. 1993. Dermatitis nephropathy syndrome of pigs. Vet Rec 132:199.

Wijeratne WVS, Wells GAH. 1980. Inherited renal cysts in pigs: Results of breeding experiments. Vet Rec 107:484–488.

Woldemeskel M, Drommer W, Wendt M. 2002. Microscopic and ultrastructural lesions of the ureter and renal pelvis in sows with regards to *Actinobaculum suis* infection. J Vet Med A 49:348–352.

Yoshie T. 1991. Study on the swine glomerulopathy resembling human IgA nephropathy. Jpn J Nephrol 33:179–189.

Yoshikawa T, Yoshikawa H, Oyamada T, Saitoh A. 1988. Immune-complex glomerulonephritis associated with porcine cytomegalovirus infection. Proc Int Pig Vet Soc 10:245.

10 Interpretation of Laboratory Results

Ian A. Gardner and Patricia C. Blanchard

Veterinarians use diagnostic tests to assess the health, productivity, and reproductive status of individual pigs and herds. Although tests can take many forms, including history taking, physical examination, and pregnancy testing, the most frequently used tests are those that involve the submission of samples to a laboratory. Laboratory tests are used to

- Detect pathogens or toxins that are responsible for disease outbreaks or suboptimal production.
- Evaluate the infection/exposure status of individual pigs.
- Determine whether a herd was infected with or exposed to a pathogen and, if so, which age or production groups (subpopulations) were affected.
- Estimate the percentage of herds or pigs with antibodies to an infectious agent.
- Monitor a herd's serologic response to vaccination.
- Monitor the progress and success of disease control and eradication programs.

The optimal approach for each of these objectives may differ; a different test, number of samples, and diagnostic strategy may be indicated depending on the information needed. Choice of tests to answer specified objectives is in part determined by the quality and types of sample that are submitted and in part by the availability of tests at the receiving laboratory or at other collaborating laboratories. Additional factors, such as cost, rapidity, ease of performance of the test, and its accuracy (sometimes termed validity) are important considerations. For many tests that are used for swine diseases, estimates of accuracy (commonly measured as sensitivity and specificity) are not published, although it is common for developers to claim that their tests are both highly sensitive and specific. Also, data on the reproducibility (repeatability) of different tests among and within laboratories often are not available.

Although technical modifications to tests (e.g., antigen purification, use of monoclonal vs. polyclonal antibodies, and use of selective culture media) often improve the ability of the test to discriminate infected from noninfected pigs, it is clear that all tests are imperfect.

In this chapter, we describe the principles that are necessary for rational use of tests and interpretation of their results and provide examples of testing strategies and sample sizes that might be appropriate. The increasing availability of rapid serologic, microbiologic, and parasitologic test kits, polymerase chain reaction (PCR)-nucleic acid probes, immunohistochemistry and in situ hybridization, and the continuing expansion of tests offered by laboratories necessitate an understanding of the diagnostic principles of each test and a careful evaluation of its strengths and weaknesses. Most of our examples involve serologic tests for infectious diseases because these tests are commonly used in swine practice. Issues relevant to test interpretation in both a general (Tyler and Cullor 1989) and a food animal setting (Martin 1988) are described elsewhere, but there are few papers that focus specifically on swine disease. Interpretation of surveillance data for swine diseases is described in Chapter 69.

VARIATION IN TEST RESULTS

Some tests yield only a positive or a negative result (e.g., bacterial and viral isolation), and others (including many hematologic, clinical chemistry, and serologic tests) yield a quantitative result that varies among pigs. Results from quantitative serologic tests are of two types:

- Those, such as serum neutralization (SN), for which results are typically reported as a finite number of doubling dilutions or titers
- Those, such as enzyme-linked immunosorbent assays (ELISAs), in which an infinite number of optical density (absorbance) values or sample-to-positive (S/P) ratios theoretically can occur

219

Variability in results of a quantitative serologic test arises from two sources:

- Biologic variation in the response of infected and noninfected pigs
- Variation inherent in the test system or assay

Animal Sources of Variation

For infected pigs, the serologic response depends on the duration of infection, challenge dose of organisms, whether the infection is subclinical or clinical, whether disease is systemic or mild and localized, other concurrent infections, and host factors including age. For acute infectious diseases where the agent is removed by the immune system, pigs that were previously infected might no longer be infected when tested, and therefore, it is often more appropriate to describe infected pigs as "exposed." For noninfected pigs, exposure to cross-reacting organisms, vaccination against the agent, or vaccination against other agents through nonspecific immune stimulation might cause elevated responses in some pigs and lead to false-positive serologic results.

Laboratory Sources of Variation

Sources of variation attributable to the test include variation in the way that different laboratories or technicians perform (e.g., use reagents) or interpret the test (interlaboratory or interobserver variability) and variation in interpretation by the same person at different times (intraobserver variability). As evidenced by a comparison of test variables for the immunoperoxidase monolayer assay (IPMA) for porcine reproductive and respiratory syndrome (PRRS) virus among eight European laboratories, test conditions often are not standardized from laboratory to laboratory (Drew 1995). In addition, laboratory errors (e.g., sample mix-up, error in entry of results, and cross-contamination of samples) might also result in false-positive or false-negative results. Most specialized laboratories, however, have internal and external quality assurance programs that ensure that the internal laboratory sources of test variation are small compared with animal sources. In the following examples, variation attributable to sample quality and handling by the veterinarian and the laboratory is ignored. We describe the effects of these factors later in the chapter.

SENSITIVITY AND SPECIFICITY

Gold Standard Test

We assume that the infection or disease status of each pig can be correctly defined by a so-called gold standard (also known as the diagnostic standard, definitive test, or reference test). A gold standard is a method or combination of methods which determine absolutely and without error whether a pig is infected or diseased. For many diseases the true status might be determined only

at necropsy, and for some diseases, there is no gold standard. In other cases, this perfect diagnostic method is not practical to use in the field due to cost, labor, or invasiveness, so other, less expensive and more practical methods are often used as a compromise. For some diseases such as postweaning multisystemic wasting syndrome (PMWS), definition of a gold standard is difficult, and a working standard such as "compatible histopathology" is used for laboratory diagnosis. For international trade purposes, tests prescribed in the Office International des Epizooties (OIE) *Manual of Standards for Diagnostic Tests and Vaccines* (www.oie.int/eng/normes/mmanual/A_summry.htm) are considered gold standards even though most tests are not perfectly sensitive and specific.

Sometimes, the gold standard is a combined standard where a positive result from one or more perfectly specific tests is considered positive. Bager and Petersen (1991) compared three selective media for isolation of *Salmonella* spp. from pig feces. Because each culture medium detected some *Salmonella* spp. isolates not detected by the other two media, the gold standard for infection was a positive culture by at least one of the methods. The number of positive cultures by each method was expressed as a percentage of the number of samples that tested positive by one or more methods. One hundred and fifteen isolates were detected. Incubation in Rappaport-Vassiliadis broth for 24 hours in combination with plating on brilliant green agar detected 88% (101/115) of the isolates, compared with 51% (59/115) for the selenite broth.

When culture or antigen detection is used as the gold standard for evaluation of a new test, a negative culture result might be viewed with some suspicion depending on the methods used and whether there is other evidence of absence of infection. Confidence in the use of a negative culture result as a standard can usually be increased by inclusion of larger amounts of tissue or material and by culture of more sites from within the same pig. Sometimes, however, the improvements can be negligible. White et al. (1996) compared the sensitivity of serologic tests for detecting latent pseudorabies virus (PRV) infection 2–27 months after experimental infection. Fifty-one pigs were documented as being infected based on a positive PCR assay result of trigeminal nerve and tonsil. Of the 51 positive pigs, 46 were PCR positive on trigeminal nerve and tonsil, 4 were positive on trigeminal nerve and not tonsil, and 1 pig was positive on tonsil and not trigeminal nerve. Therefore, in field investigations where confirmation of PRV infection is necessary, inclusion of tonsillar samples in addition to trigeminal nerve would offer little practical advantage. Confidence in a negative culture result as a standard also might substantially increase if other criteria are incorporated in the definition of negativity. For definition of absence of *Mycoplasma hyopneumoniae* infection, a negative culture result on a pig from a herd without clinical or pathologic evidence of infection would be a more appropriate standard than a negative culture result from a pig from an infected herd or from a herd of unknown status.

For some viral diseases, SN or other serologic tests are used as the standard against which new serological tests are compared. For example, Weigel et al. (1992) compared the performance of two ELISAs with SN for the detection of antibodies to PRV glycoprotein X, and Lanza et al. (1993) compared a monoclonal antibody-capture ELISA with SN for the serodiagnosis of transmissible gastroenteritis (TGE). The problem with use of a serologic test as the standard against which the sensitivity and specificity of a new serologic test are estimated is that if the original serologic test is of poor accuracy and results of the two tests disagree, it may be difficult to determine whether the new test is more accurate. Many authors, including Martin (1988), recommend only measuring the extent of agreement beyond chance between test results using a kappa statistic. If the results of the new test show a sufficiently high level of agreement beyond chance with the standard test, a decision might be made to substitute the new test based on cost and rapidity and ease of use. Questions about the sensitivity and specificity of the new test, however, would remain unanswered.

Statistical approaches that don't require a gold standard (Hui and Walter 1980; Enøe et al. 2000) offer a promising alternative for obtaining sensitivity and specificity estimates for chronic diseases. These methods have been applied to evaluation of serologic tests for *Actinobacillus pleuropneumoniae* serotype 2 (Enøe et al. 2001), evaluation of the accuracy of detection of slaughter lesions in Danish pigs (Enøe et al. 2003), and the detection of classical swine fever virus in tonsillar tissue (Bouma et al. 2001).

Definition of Terms

Results of a quantitative serologic test such as an ELISA used on samples from known infected and noninfected pigs can be displayed graphically as two overlapping frequency distributions (Figure 10.1). Typically, pigs with test results exceeding a predetermined threshold or cutoff value are classed as positive and pigs with values less than the cutoff are considered negative. In contrast, for some tests, such as particle concentration fluorescence immunoassay (PCFIA) and blocking ELISA, a low test value is more indicative of infection.

Because the distributions of test results of infected and noninfected pigs overlap, the designation of a cutoff value results in misclassification of the infection status of some pigs. Four mutually exclusive categories of results are possible: true positives (test-positive and infected), false negatives (test-negative but infected), false positives (test-positive but noninfected), and true negatives (test-negative and noninfected).

Sensitivity, when used with its diagnostic or epidemiologic meaning, is the probability that the test correctly identifies infected pigs: true positives / (true positives + false negatives). For example, a test with 80% sensitivity would correctly identify an average of 80% of infected pigs as test-positive and would incorrectly identify 20% as noninfected because they tested negative (false negatives). The diagnostic definition of sensitivity differs from the use of the term in an analytic context (Saah and Hoover 1997). In the latter context, the term *sensitivity* is often used interchangeably with the minimal or lower detection limit of the test: the smallest number of bacteria or amount of DNA, toxin, antibody, or residue that can be detected. An immunologically more sensitive test (ELISA compared with SN) would be expected to detect antibodies earlier in the course of infection in an individual pig, but for herd diagnosis where prevalence is mod-

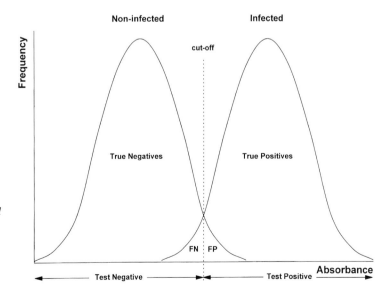

10.1. *Frequency distributions of ELISA results for noninfected (left curve) and infected pigs (right curve). A positive result is an absorbance (optical density) exceeding the cutoff value. (FN = false negatives; FP = false positives.) Although frequencies are depicted as following a normal (Gaussian) distribution, often the distributions are skewed (non-normal).*

erate to high and pigs are at different stages of infection, the need for high sensitivity might not be as great. The contrast in use of the term *sensitivity* is shown in the following example. The PCR for *Mycoplasma hyopneumoniae* is reported by Blanchard et al. (1996) to have a sensitivity (lower detection limit) of between 400 and 5000 organisms per assay. When used on tracheobronchiolar washings, the PCR correctly detected 101/116 experimentally infected pigs (diagnostic sensitivity = 87.1%).

Specificity is the probability that the test correctly identifies noninfected pigs: true negatives / (false positives + true negatives). A test with 90% specificity would correctly classify 90% of noninfected pigs on average as negative and would falsely classify 10% of pigs as infected (false positives). The analogous term in an analytic context is the cross-reaction profile (Saah and Hoover 1997), which indicates the likelihood of cross-reactivity with related pathogens or diseases that present with similar signs. The cross-reaction profile relies substantially on laboratory and clinical experience of the test developers or researchers. For example, a validation study of 8 PCR tests for detection of *Actinobacillus pleuropneumoniae* in tonsillar tissue of chronically infected pigs considered cross-reactions with *A.suis*, *A. minor*, *A.equuli*, *A.lignieresi*, "*A.porcitonsillarum*," and 2 other pathogens often isolated from tonsils, *Streptococcus suis* and *Haemophilus parasuis* (Fittipaldi et al. 2003).

In most field situations, high diagnostic sensitivity and specificity are both desirable although it might be difficult to have both attributes with a single test. Lowering the minimal detection limit of the test will often improve diagnostic sensitivity, depending on the numbers of bacteria, concentration of antibody, etc., typically found in infected pigs, but such a change might lower the specificity of the test. Buyers of pigs and regulatory officials in importing states and countries usually want tests of almost 100% sensitivity to minimize the risk of introducing new pathogens. A similar line of reasoning can also be applied to tests for agents of public health concern—for example, *Salmonella* spp., *Trichinella* spp., and antibiotic residues. Typically, owners of breeding herds want tests of high specificity to maximize their chance of selling replacement boars and gilts. High specificity is also desirable for commercial producers participating in eradication programs based on test and slaughter, where economic losses from false-positive results can be substantial.

One consequence of using multiple imperfectly specific tests is an increased chance of abnormal results in otherwise healthy and nonexposed pigs. The probability of at least one abnormal test result increases as the number of independent tests is increased. For example, suppose that a sow was screened for 10 unrelated bacterial and viral infections. If the sow was never really exposed to any of the agents (unknown to the veterinarian) and each test had a specificity of 95%, the probability that all 10 tests are negative would be 0.95^{10},

or 60%. Hence, the probability that at least one test would yield a positive result is 40%.

Estimation of Sensitivity and Specificity

Diagnostic sensitivity and specificity are determined from experimental and field studies, although it is quite common that an experimental study for an infectious disease will overestimate the sensitivity and specificity of the test when used in the field. One advantage of an experimental study is that it is easier to establish unequivocally a pig's infection status, and the associated serologic response can be followed temporally. From these data, the time to a specified titer value (or time to seroconversion) and duration of titer above the positive cutoff value can be determined. Sørensen et al. (1997) used aerosol challenge of 200 SPF pigs with *Mycoplasma hyopneumoniae* to monitor clinical, serologic, and pathologic responses to the organism and to compare the sensitivity and specificity of culture, immunofluorescence, antigen ELISA, and PCR for detection of the organism in lungs. Because of cost limitations, experimental studies are restricted primarily to infections with short incubation periods but can be very useful for obtaining preliminary data on the sensitivity and specificity of tests and the optimal sampling site. The major limitation of an experimental study is that it may bear little or no resemblance to field situations because the selected experimental conditions are necessarily subjective. In experimental studies, challenge doses are often selected that will ensure clinical disease in most, if not all, pigs, and yet many tests are used in the field to detect subclinical disease in pigs whose immune systems might respond differently because of suboptimal environments and concurrent infections. The control group of noninfected pigs in an experimental study is often comprised of healthy SPF pigs; yet when a test is used for clinical diagnosis, the relevant comparison group of pigs is those with clinical signs caused by pathogens other than the one that the test detects. For example, evaluation of the specificity of an immunochromatographic test for detection of group A rotavirus included samples from pigs with neonatal diarrheas caused by other pathogens (e.g., *Escherichia coli*) as well as samples from healthy rotavirus-free pigs (Klingenberg and Esfandiari 1996).

Even when an experimental infection is used to evaluate a test initially, samples from representative infected and noninfected pigs (age, clinical status, stages of infection, etc.) from commercial herds should be assessed to ensure that test performance is adequate for naturally acquired infections. Test results should be compared with the gold standard (reference test) in a blinded fashion to avoid introducing bias. Sensitivity and specificity and their respective confidence intervals are calculated. As sample sizes to derive these values increase, sensitivity and specificity estimates become more precise, as reflected by narrower confidence intervals. Epidemiologic

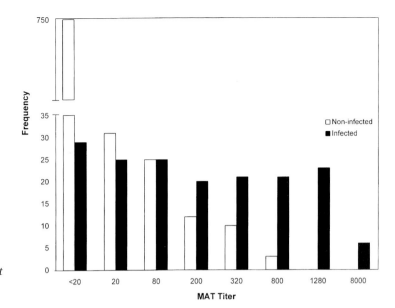

10.2. *Frequency distributions of modified agglutination test titers for* Toxoplasma gondii *for infected and noninfected pigs based on the data from Table 10.1 (Dubey et al. 1995).*

Table 10.1. Modified agglutination test titers for *Toxoplasma gondii* for 170 infected and 830 noninfected sows.

Titer	Infected (n = 170)	Noninfected (n = 830)
<20	29	749
20/40	25	31
80	25	25
200	20	12
320/400	21	10
800	21	3
1280/4000	23	0
≥8000	6	0

Source: Adapted from Dubey et al. (1995).

Table 10.2. 2 × 2 table for hypothetical frequency distributions for modified agglutination test (MAT) results.

		Infection Status	
		+	−
MAT Result	+	141	81
	−	29	749
		170	830

sensitivity = 141/170 = 0.829 (95% confidence interval, 0.764–0.883)
specificity = 749/830 = 0.902 (95% confidence interval, 0.880–0.902)

considerations for test evaluation studies are described in detail elsewhere (Greiner and Gardner 2000a).

Example. Dubey et al. (1995) evaluated the sensitivity and specificity of five diagnostic tests for toxoplasmosis in pigs. The gold standard was isolation of viable *Toxoplasma gondii* by cat or mouse bioassay using heart muscle collected from sows at slaughter. Sows whose samples yielded a positive bioassay result on either bioassay (n = 170) were considered infected, and sows whose samples yielded a negative bioassay result (n = 830) were considered noninfected. Although frequencies of titer values for infected and noninfected sows were not reported in the paper, we generated two hypothetical frequency distributions for modified agglutination test (MAT) results consistent with the published data. Table 10.1 and Figure 10.2 show that results for noninfected and infected pigs overlap over an extensive range of titers (<1:20 to 1:800).

In the study, MAT results were considered positive if titers were ≥1:20, and negative if otherwise. Categor-

ized results were cross-tabulated in a 2 × 2 table, and sensitivity, specificity, and exact binomial confidence intervals were calculated; see Table 10.2.

If a cutoff with 100% specificity is preferred for serologic diagnosis, the cutoff for the MAT would need to be increased to 1:1280. At the cutoff of 1280, however, only 29/170 infected sows (sensitivity = 17.1%) would be correctly identified. These changes in estimates demonstrate the compromise between sensitivity and specificity that is inherent in changing the cutoff value of a quantitative test. Shifting the cutoff point to a lower value will usually increase sensitivity at the expense of specificity and vice versa. In this example, a perfectly sensitive cutoff could not be defined because both infected and noninfected pigs gave negative results at the lowest screening dilution for the test (1:20). The authors discussed the limitations of their gold standard and indicated that false-negative bioassays may have occurred because *T. gondii* were located in tissues other than cardiac muscle or because *T. gondii* were not isolated from inoculated animals even though they were present. Accordingly, if some test-positive pigs that were classed as noninfected by the bioassay were truly infected, the specificity of the MAT might have been underestimated.

Evaluation of a Test at Various Cutoff Values

Sensitivity and specificity values are useful for determining a test's diagnostic limitations and comparing the accuracy of two or more tests. Because many cutoff points are possible for a quantitative test, comparison of tests over a range of cutoff values is often more appropriate than comparison at a single value. The trade-off between sensitivity and specificity as the cutoff value is changed may be represented graphically as a receiver-operating characteristic (ROC) curve (Zweig and Campbell 1993; Greiner et al. 2000). ROC curves, which are graphs of sensitivity (y-axis) versus specificity or 1-specificity (x-axis) for all possible cutoff values of a test, are well accepted in human medicine as a method to quantify test performance. Their acceptance in veterinary medicine and use for swine diseases has been limited. Nodelijk et al. (1996) used an ROC curve to represent the accuracy of a commercial ELISA for PRRS virus, and Elbers et al. (2002; 2003) used ROC analysis to evaluate the use of clinical signs and gross lesions at postmortem to detect outbreaks of classical swine fever in the 1997–1998 epidemic in The Netherlands.

Using the data in Table 10.1 for the *T. gondii* MAT, all sensitivity and specificity pairs at cutoff points from 1:20 to ≥1:8000 were calculated and graphed as an ROC curve (Figure 10.3). The area under the curve (AUC), below and to the right, can be interpreted as the probability that a randomly selected infected pig will have a

MAT result greater than a randomly selected noninfected pig. For these data, the AUC was estimated to be 0.88. The cutoff value closest to the upper-left corner of the figure (≥1:20) is the point that minimizes the number of misclassifications (false positives and false negatives), but as indicated in the following section, other factors are important in selection of a cutoff value.

Selection of Test Cutoff Values

Several factors are considered in selection of test cutoff values, including the purpose of the testing (e.g., screening vs. confirmation), the relative costs (economic, social, or political) of false-positive and false-negative diagnoses, the availability of confirmatory tests of high specificity, and the prevalence of disease (Greiner et al. 2000). Indeed, various cutoffs might be appropriate given different circumstances for testing and consequences of misclassification (costs of a false-positive result compared with costs of a false-negative result). For simplicity, many diagnostic laboratories report results of ELISAs and other tests as positive or negative at a single cutoff. There are two drawbacks to this approach. First, when the cutoff is chosen by the laboratory or test kit manufacturer, and the result is reported only as positive or negative, information is lost to the practitioner. When an S/P ratio for an ELISA or a titer value is well beyond the cutoff value used for test interpretation, a practitioner usually has a stronger belief that a pig is truly infected than if the test result is close to the cutoff value. In the *T. gondii* example, a MAT titer of 1:800 is more likely to come from an infected sow than a titer value of 1:20 (refer to Table 10.1). Likelihood ratios, which range from 0 to infinity, quan-

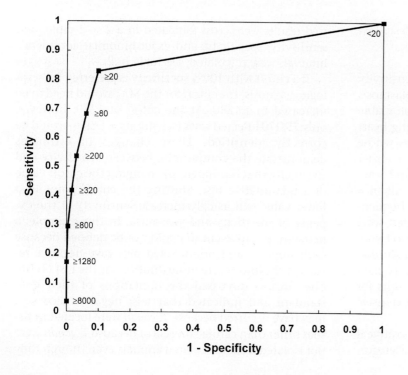

10.3. *Receiver-operating characteristic curve for the modified agglutination test for* Toxoplasma gondii *based on the data from Table 10.1 (Dubey et al. 1995).*

tify how many times more frequently a specific titer value is obtained from infected compared with noninfected pigs. Second, the cutoff chosen by the laboratory may be the one that minimizes the total number of errors, both false positives and false negatives, but it may not take into account the different costs of the two types of misdiagnosis. Depending on the situation, a false-positive diagnosis may be much more damaging than a false negative and vice versa. For example, a veterinarian relying on the results of a test to make a decision about culling a sow probably wants to minimize the chance of a false-positive diagnosis by using a highly specific test, particularly if the sow is asymptomatic and pregnant and there are no other reasons for culling. On the other hand, when screening breeding pigs for purchase into a herd, a false-positive result would be much less harmful to a client than a false-negative, which might allow infected pigs to enter a noninfected herd. Ideally, practitioners need the information to choose the cutoff that best meets their decision requirements at a particular time.

One possible solution to the dilemma of where to set the cutoff value for individual-pig diagnosis is to specify two cutoffs—one value that is 100% sensitive (no false negatives) and another that is 100% specific (no false positives). These cutoffs define an intermediate range of values where false-positive and false-negative results occur. Using this approach, results are reported as negative if they are less than the cutoff value that is 100% sensitive, as positive if they are greater than the cutoff value that is 100% specific, and as suspicious or indeterminate if they are between these values. Suspicious or indeterminate values might be clarified by additional tests, if warranted.

Evaluating Published Sensitivity and Specificity Values

Although sensitivity and specificity estimates might be available on test kit inserts or in industry publications or might be obtained from laboratory diagnosticians, the veterinary medical literature should be consulted, wherever possible, as the most reliable source. Regardless of the source of estimates, practitioners should ask appropriate questions about how the test was validated and how the test will be used:

1. Was the test evaluated under field conditions similar to those in which it will be used?
2. Were test results evaluated with respect to the gold standard in a blinded fashion?
3. Were the positive and negative gold standards appropriate choices given existing technology?
4. Were adequate numbers of representative infected and noninfected pigs included in the study so that sensitivity and specificity estimates are precise? At least 100 infected and 100 noninfected pigs should be used in validation studies, wherever possible.

5. Why was the chosen cutoff value selected, and are estimates of sensitivity and specificity reported at other cutoff values?
6. Will the test be used for individual or herd diagnosis? A test that has low to moderate sensitivity at an individual level might be perfectly appropriate for herd diagnosis if adequate numbers of tests are done and the test has high specificity.
7. Will the test be used by itself or in combination with other tests? If the test is used in combination with other tests, how will multiple test results be interpreted?

If claims are made in publications that one test is more sensitive or more specific than another test, these claims should be based on tests of duplicate samples and appropriate statistical analyses. Often a closer evaluation of the claims shows that the numeric difference in sensitivity or specificity is small and not statistically significant or practically important. If true, other criteria such as cost, ease of use, and rapidity of use become more important in test selection.

PREDICTIVE VALUES

The major advantage of sensitivity and specificity as measures of test accuracy is that they are independent of prevalence and therefore are particularly useful for reporting test performance in the veterinary medical literature. However, these measures have shortcomings in the field, where the diagnostic value of a test varies with the test's inherent accuracy and also with the situation in which the test is used. Because absolute determination of a pig's infection status often is not feasible or economically justified, a veterinarian must estimate the likelihood of infection or absence of infection given test results. These likelihoods are the predictive values of positive and negative test results. Positive predictive value (PPV) is the proportion of the test-positive pigs that are truly infected, and negative predictive value (NPV) is the proportion of test-negative pigs that are truly noninfected.

The distinction between predictive values and sensitivity/specificity might at first seem unclear. Sensitivity and specificity provide estimates of test accuracy given that the disease status is known, whereas predictive values estimate test accuracy given that the test results are known.

Predictive values (also known as posttest or posterior probabilities) are dependent on sensitivity, specificity, and prevalence and can be calculated using Bayes' theorem formulas:

PPV = (sensitivity × prevalence)/[sensitivity × prevalence + (1 − specificity) × (1 − prevalence)]

NPV = [specificity × (1 − prevalence)]/[specificity × (1 − prevalence) + (1 − sensitivity) × prevalence]

Effects of Prevalence on Predictive Values

Clinically, the term *prevalence* means the best estimate of the probability of disease before performing the test. Prevalence is used synonymously with the term *pretest* or *prior probability*. Wherever possible, estimates of prevalence should be based on prior data: for example, frequency of the condition among all cases with similar presenting signs, prior test results for the herd, or test results from herds of similar size in the same geographic area. In the absence of prior data, the following values of prevalence might be reasonable starting values for calculations of predictive values:

1%   Pigs with risk factors for a common disease but without clinical signs, or a herd with no previous history of infection

10%   If a disease is unlikely but possible clinically and a veterinarian wishes to rule it out

50%   If there is substantial uncertainty but the clinical presentation is compatible with the disease

90%   When a disease is very likely clinically or if the herd has a prior history of infection but a practitioner wishes to rule it in using a diagnostic test

To "rule out" disease, a negative result on a highly sensitive test is necessary. This might be done in the initial stage of a diagnostic workup to reduce the number of possibilities on the differential list. To "rule in" or confirm a diagnosis, a positive result is necessary with a nearly perfectly specific test. In general, when a veterinarian does not believe that a disease is present (prevalence ≤10%) or strongly believes that it is (prevalence ≥90%), the test result often does not substantially influence the diagnosis (Martin 1988). Laboratory tests tend to be of greatest value in establishing a diagnosis when a practitioner is most uncertain about infection status (i.e., when presence and absence of infection are equally likely, which is equivalent to a prevalence of 50%).

The effect of prevalence on predictive value can be demonstrated by considering the performance of the MAT test for *T. gondii* (sensitivity = 82.9% and specificity = 90.2%) in two populations, one with a 20% prevalence of infection, which is similar to the prevalence in Dubey et al. (1995), and one where control of *T. gondii* infection is effective and the overall prevalence is 1% (Table 10.3). At 20% prevalence, the positive predictive value of 67.9% indicates that about two in every three pigs with test-positive results is truly infected. At the same prevalence, the negative predictive value is approximately 95%. Hence, the probability that a test-negative pig is truly infected (1 − negative predictive value) is 5%. For the same test at 1% prevalence, the positive predictive value decreases to less than 15% and the negative predictive value becomes almost 100%.

Predictive Value Curves

Prevalence is often not known exactly and a range of values is possible. Predictive value curves can be gener-

Table 10.3. Performance of the MAT test for *T. gondii* (sensitivity = 82.9% and specificity = 90.2%).

prevalence = 20% (assuming a population size of 10,000)

		Infection Status		
		+	−	
MAT Result	+	1658	784	2442
	−	342	7216	7558
		2000	8000	10,000

prevalence = 2000/10,000 = 0.2
positive predictive value = 1658/2442 = 0.679
negative predictive value = 7216/7558 = 0.955

prevalence = 1% (assuming a population size of 10,000)

		Infection Status		
		+	−	
MAT Result	+	97	554	651
	−	3	9346	9349
		100	9900	10,000

prevalence = 100/10,000 = 0.01
positive predictive value = 97/651 = 0.149
negative predictive value = 9346/9349 = 0.999

ated to show how well the test performs in different circumstances. At moderate prevalences (30–70%), most tests, including the MAT (Figure 10.4), perform well regardless of whether results are positive or negative. As prevalence increases above 70%, positive predictive value increases toward 100% with an associated decrease in negative predictive value. As prevalence decreases toward 0%, positive predictive value decreases while negative predictive value increases.

When testing for rare conditions, test specificity is the most important determinant of positive predictive value. As specificity increases at a fixed prevalence value, positive predictive value increases. Only if the test is close to 100% specific will the problem of low positive predictive value be avoided when infection is rare (Figure 10.5).

Practical Implications

The implications of these relationships can be summarized as follows. Given a certain test sensitivity and specificity, a positive finding in a herd without clinical signs or previous history of infection should be interpreted differently from a positive test result in a herd where the infection is endemic and clinical disease is common. However, it is important to note that the clinical usefulness and value of a positive test result are not measured by the positive predictive value (posttest probability) but by the change in probability or diagnostic certainty brought about by use of the test. For example, if a herd had a clinical disease event consistent with either swine influenza or PRRS and the herd had no prior history of either infection but both infections were being commonly diagnosed in other herds at the time of

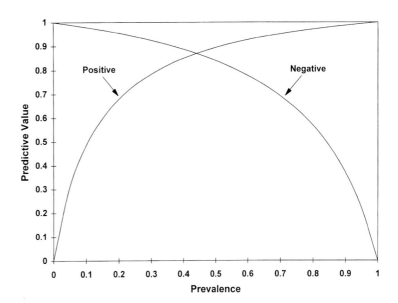

10.4. *Predictive value curves for the modified agglutination test for* Toxoplasma gondii *with sensitivity equal to 82.9% and specificity equal to 90.2%.*

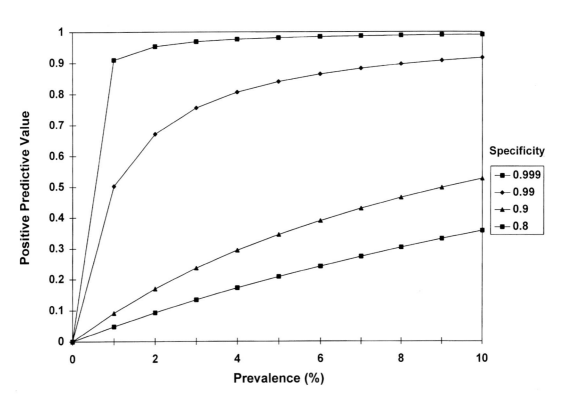

10.5. *Effect of specificity of a laboratory test with a sensitivity equal to 100% on a predictive value of a positive test for prevalence between 0% and 10%.*

the investigation, a practitioner might believe that the pretest probability of each infection was 50%. Isolation of PRRS virus through laboratory testing, assuming perfect specificity, would result in a posttest probability of 100% for PRRS (a 50% gain in probability). If, however, the herd had the same clinical episode and a recent history of PRRS infection, the pretest probability would be higher, perhaps 80%, and even though the posttest probability of PRRS was still 100%, the gain in certainty (20%) would be much smaller. Therefore, the value of

the laboratory test in the second situation would be less than the first, which has more diagnostic uncertainty. Similar reasoning can be used to assess the gain in certainty from negative test results.

USE AND INTERPRETATION OF MULTIPLE TESTS

To improve diagnostic accuracy, tests might be repeated or additional tests might be included in the diagnostic workup. Indeed, most diagnoses are based on the use of multiple tests (e.g., history, physical examination, laboratory tests, etc.). Multiple tests can be used either simultaneously or sequentially and results interpreted in series or parallel. The sensitivity and specificity of a combination of tests differ from the individual sensitivity and specificity values. Interpreting combinations of tests in parallel results in higher sensitivity than any of the individual tests, and interpretation in series results in higher specificity than any of the individual tests. Sometimes, the change in sensitivity and specificity of the combination of tests is less than theoretically predicted because the test results are correlated (also termed *dependent*) for infected or noninfected pigs (Gardner et al. 2000). Correlated results would be expected for serologic tests that measure the same class of antibody but would be far less likely with two tests that measure different biologic responses (e.g., histopathology and serologic testing).

Parallel and Series Interpretation

When two tests are used, one of four results is possible: both tests positive, test 1 positive and test 2 negative, test 1 negative and test 2 positive, and both tests negative. In parallel interpretation, a pig is considered positive if it reacts positively to either test—this increases sensitivity but tends to decrease the specificity of the combined tests. This parallel testing strategy works well when neither test has a particularly high sensitivity but each detects a different type of disease (e.g., early vs. late, rapidly progressing vs. slowly progressing). Culture for a pathogen might be more sensitive than serologic testing early in the course of an infection, but the latter might be more sensitive later in the infection as the pathogen load decreases. Parallel testing with culture and serology should therefore lead to higher sensitivity, although specificity of the combination would be lower than if culture was used alone.

In series interpretation, a pig must be positive on both tests to be considered positive; this increases specificity at the expense of sensitivity. The use of two tests in series might lead to a diagnosis in the following way. The first test might be very sensitive and inexpensive and pigs that test positive are retested with a second test of high specificity to identify false positives. As a cost-saving measure, pigs testing negative on the first test are considered negative and are not tested with the second test. This testing strategy allows veterinarians to rule out disease using fewer tests, although serial testing often takes more time. The probability of disease after both tests are positive is calculated by regarding the predictive value of a positive after the first test as the same as the prevalence of disease before performing the second test. In the example of the MAT for *T. gondii*, the positive predictive value was 67.9% when the test was used in a population with 20% prevalence. If pigs with a positive MAT result were tested with an additional test—for ex-

ample, a latex agglutination test (LAT) with sensitivity of 45.9% and specificity of 96.9% (Dubey et al. 1995)—the value of 67.9% would become the new prevalence before running the LAT test. Substitution of these values in the Bayes' theorem formula would yield a positive predictive value of 96.9% after the second test, assuming that MAT and LAT results were uncorrelated. If the assumption of no correlation was correct, positive results on both the MAT and the LAT would be more indicative of infection than a positive result on the MAT alone.

Choosing Among Testing Strategies

To establish a diagnosis when two tests are available, a veterinarian might decide to use a single test or use both tests. The latter choice incurs additional costs, which need to be passed on to the client. If both tests are used, parallel or series interpretation can be selected depending on the need to emphasize sensitivity or specificity, respectively. As demonstrated in the brucellosis example that follows, the benefits of multiple serologic tests to detect the same pathogen are often less than expected because of correlation between test results. Factors that need to be considered in the final selection of a testing strategy include the sensitivities and specificities of the individual tests, the sensitivities and specificities of the combination of tests when interpreted in series or parallel, costs of false-positive and false-negative diagnoses, prevalence of infection, and the additional costs incurred by adding more tests.

Example. Ferris et al. (1995) estimated the sensitivity and specificity of six serologic tests for brucellosis in 231 swine using bacteriologic culture results from multiple lymph nodes as the gold standard. Sensitivities ranged from 57% (automated complement fixation test) to 85% (particle concentration fluorescence immunoassay [PCFIA] with a cutoff value of 0.81), and specificities ranged from 62% (standard tube test [STT]) to 95% (rivanol test). Sensitivities of the PCFIA and STT were estimated as 85% and 83%, respectively, and specificities were 74% and 62%, respectively. When results of the PCFIA and STT were interpreted in parallel (a positive on any test being considered positive), the sensitivity of the combined tests was 87% and the specificity was 54%. The use of both tests interpreted in parallel yielded a 2% improvement in sensitivity over the higher of the two tests and an 8% loss in specificity compared with the less specific test. Assuming that the two test results were uncorrelated, the sensitivity of the combined tests theoretically should have been 98% and the specificity should have been 46%. The most likely explanation for the difference between the observed and expected values is that the test results were correlated. In this case, use of PCFIA and STT together would increase diagnostic cost for little gain in information. Indeed, even when results of the four additional tests were considered and interpreted in parallel, the sensitivity of the combination did not further increase (40/46 were positive on one or more tests).

Herd-Level Interpretation of Test Results

Assessment of the health status of a population unit (herd, barn, litter, or other grouping of pigs) often is more important than that of an individual pig in the group. A key point that is not widely understood is that herd-level tests must be interpreted differently from individual tests. Interpretation of herd test results often is more complicated, especially when tests are imperfectly specific.

Herd Infection Status

Correct classification of herd status, with respect to one or more pathogens, is important in specific pathogen free (SPF) and other health certification schemes, in assessments of disease introduction risk associated with purchase of pigs, and in studies of risk factors for disease. Similar to the situation for test interpretation for individuals, data are needed on the herd-level sensitivity and specificity of the test being used to determine herd status. The likely performance of a herd test is usually extrapolated from published individual sensitivity and specificity values as described in Martin et al. (1992). With the exception of *Mycoplasma hyopneumoniae* in the Danish SPF scheme (Sørensen et al. 1992; Sørensen et al. 1993), there are few published field studies that have estimated the performance of herd tests used for swine diseases.

Herd Sensitivity and Specificity. Herd-level sensitivity is the probability that an infected herd yields a positive herd-test result, and herd-level specificity is the probability that a noninfected herd yields a negative herd-test result. The respective false-negative and false-positive herd rates can be calculated by subtracting herd sensitivity and herd specificity values from 1. Herd-level sensitivity and specificity depend not only on the respective individual-level sensitivity and specificity values but also on other factors: the number tested, the prevalence of infection within infected herds, and the number of positives (1, 2, 3, etc.) used to classify the herd as positive (Martin et al. 1992; Christensen and Gardner 2000). Usually the individual and herd-level estimates differ. Based on findings from an experimental infection study of 200 SPF pigs (Sørensen et al. 1997), the blocking ELISA for *M. hyopneumoniae* has an individual sensitivity and specificity of 100% and 100%, respectively, at the cutoff of 50% blocking. When samples from 20 pigs are used for herd diagnosis of *M. hyopneumoniae* infection in the SPF scheme, the herd-level sensitivity and specificity were 93% and 96%, respectively, when at least one ELISA positive pig designated a positive herd test (Sørensen et al. 1992). The estimates of herd sensitivity were imprecise because only 15 new infections were detected during the study period. A follow-up study yielded similar estimates (Sørensen et al. 1993).

Some important relationships among factors affecting herd-level sensitivity and specificity warrant comment. First, as the number tested increases, herd-level sensitivity increases. Consequently, the probability of a false-negative herd diagnosis decreases with increasing sample numbers at all values of within-herd prevalence. An increase in sample numbers from 10 to 20 for a perfectly specific test with sensitivity of 50% produces a greater reduction in the probability of a false-negative herd diagnosis if the underlying prevalence is moderate rather than low (30% vs. 1% in Figure 10.6). Second, as the number of pigs used to classify the herd as positive is increased, there is a corresponding increase in herd-level specificity with a decrease in herd-level sensitivity. A change in the number of test-positive pigs in a sample of 20 from at least 1 to at least 2 decreased herd sensitivity for *M. hyopneumoniae* in the Danish SPF system from 100% to 69% but increased herd specificity from 85% to 98% (Sørensen et al. 1993). Third, when testing a fixed number of samples, it is easier to discriminate infected from noninfected herds as within-herd prevalence increases (refer to Figure 10.6). Fourth, as the number of pigs tested with an imperfectly specific test increases, the probability of detecting at least one false-positive pig increases, leading to a lower herd-level specificity (Figure 10.7). This is the same effect that was noted when multiple tests of imperfect specificity were used to evaluate the infection or pathogen exposure status of an individual pig. Testing of pooled rather than individual samples can be used for herd diagnosis (e.g., culture of fecal pools for *Salmonella* spp.; Christensen et al. 2002). Factors affecting the herd sensitivity and specificity of pooled tests are described elsewhere (Christensen and Gardner 2000).

Issues to be considered in the trade-off between herd sensitivity and herd specificity are as described for individual test interpretation. For SPF schemes, herd-level sensitivity is considered more important than herd-level specificity because the costs of failing to detect infection usually outweigh the costs of a false-positive diagnosis in some herds.

Herd-Level Predictive Values. Herd-level predictive values, which are analogous to individual test predictive values, are dependent on herd sensitivity and specificity and the prevalence of infected herds. In this context, prevalence of infected herds means the best guess of the probability that a herd is infected before doing the herd test. Although such estimates might be obtained from state or national surveys, local data based on knowledge of the infection status of herds visited by a veterinarian would be more appropriate. In Denmark, it has been estimated that about 10–15% of SPF herds become reinfected with *M. hyopneumoniae* each year. If 1% is used as the likely prevalence of infected herds as detected by a

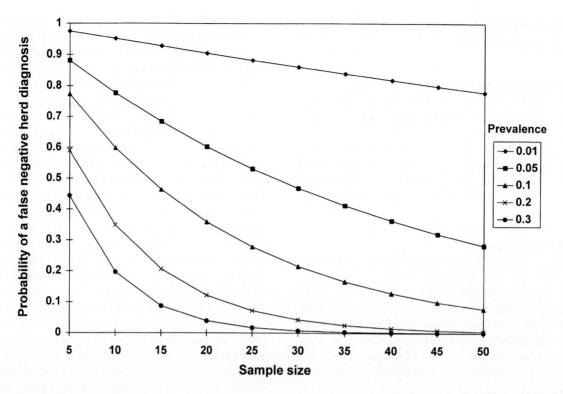

10.6. *Effect of sample size and within-herd prevalence on the probability of a false-negative herd diagnosis (1—herd sensitivity) for a test with an individual-level sensitivity of 50% and individual-level specificity of 100%.*

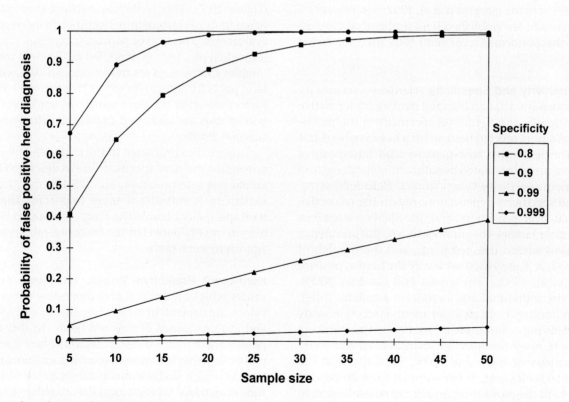

10.7. *Effect of sample size and specificity of a laboratory test on the probability of a false-positive herd diagnosis (1—herd specificity).*

single monthly sampling of 20 pigs, and then using Bayes' theorem and the herd-level sensitivity and specificity estimates of 93% and 96% reported by Sørensen et al. (1992), the positive and negative herd-level predictive values are 19% and 99.9%, respectively. These calculations indicate that only about 1 in 5 test-positive herds is confirmed as infected when followed up by gold standard methods, yet a negative herd test provides strong evidence of freedom from *M. hyopneumoniae* infection.

Because of the lack of sensitivity and specificity data for many individual tests, herd-level sensitivity and specificity and predictive values usually are unknown. Frequently, veterinarians are required to interpret herd results with incomplete knowledge of individual test performance. The number of positive pigs and the apparent prevalence of infection (0–100% test-positive pigs) are both considered in determining the status of the herd. If the seroprevalence is high, the answer to the question about the exposure status of the herd is clear. But what if a low seroprevalence (e.g., <20%) is detected when the herd is tested? In these situations, knowledge of specificity alone would facilitate judgments about the herd's infection status. This question has important practical implications because it is more difficult to use laboratory tests to discriminate herds with a low, rather than a high, prevalence of infection from noninfected herds.

Example. If all sows in a 100-sow nonvaccinated breeding herd were tested by complement fixation test (CFT) for *Actinobacillus pleuropneumoniae* serotype 2 (AP2) and 5 test-positive sows were detected (i.e., seroprevalence is 5%), what can we conclude about the AP2 status of the breeding herd? Without knowing test characteristics, one approach in the absence of a detailed herd history might be to slaughter test-positive sows and culture the upper respiratory tract, including tonsils and nasal cavities, to determine whether AP2 was present. A positive culture would confirm infection, but a negative culture would not rule out infection since culture is imperfectly sensitive. Recently, various PCR assays have been shown to be more sensitive than standard isolation methods on tonsillar tissue (biopsies and whole tonsil collected at slaughter) and would offer an alternative diagnostic strategy for evaluation of the microbiologic status of seropositive sows (Fittipaldi et al. 2003).

If a published estimate of CFT specificity were available, however, a more rational judgment could be made that might avoid unnecessary slaughter and culture of test-positive sows. First, if the CFT had specificity of 95%, the expected number of positives in a noninfected herd of 100 sows would be 5; exactly what was found on the test. Second, if specificity was <95%, the belief that these were false positives would increase since the expected number of false positives even in a noninfected herd would be >5. Third, if the specificity of the test was approximately 99% (as estimated in Enoe et al. 2001),

detection of 5 test-positive pigs would be highly suggestive of infection in the herd.

The conclusions that were made in the example would be less well met in the situation where interpretation was based on a small sample of the herd rather than the whole herd. Even when 30 samples are randomly collected in a large herd, the proportion of positive samples may not always reflect the underlying proportion of positive pigs in the herd (Carpenter and Gardner 1996). Guidelines for selection of an appropriate sample size for evaluation of herd status are described in a following section.

Prevalence Estimation

An estimate of the proportion of infected pigs often is necessary as part of national and regional health-monitoring schemes and for making decisions about vaccination and other disease control and eradication programs. If a random sample of pigs is tested for exposure to an infectious agent, the proportion of positive test results (number positive/number tested) is an estimate of the apparent (test-based) prevalence of infection. If the test is serologic, the term *seroprevalence* is used interchangeably with *apparent prevalence*. The apparent prevalence may over- or underestimate the true prevalence, depending on the sensitivity and specificity of the test that is used. True prevalence can be estimated from apparent prevalence by correcting for the imperfect sensitivity and specificity of the test (Rogan and Gladen 1978):

true prevalence = (apparent prevalence + specificity −1) / (sensitivity + specificity−1)

Confidence intervals for the estimate of true prevalence should be calculated, and for this the reader is referred elsewhere (Greiner and Gardner 2000b). The precision of the estimate or a practitioner's confidence in the accuracy of the estimate is primarily dependent on sample size, with larger samples yielding more precise estimates. Occasionally the calculation yields a negative or zero estimate for true prevalence: such a finding might suggest that the herd is not infected. If sensitivity and specificity are unknown, however, this formula cannot be applied and the true prevalence of infection in the population cannot be calculated directly.

Examples. Assume that a seroprevalence estimate of 15% was obtained when sows in a herd were screened for *T. gondii* using the MAT of sensitivity = 82.9% and specificity = 90.2%. What is the true prevalence of infection in the herd? By substitution of the values in the equation, true prevalence = (0.15 + 0.902 − 1)/(0.829 + 0.902 − 1) = 0.071 (7.1%). This estimated true prevalence is only about one-half of what the test suggests is present, indicating that about 50% of the positive tests are false positives.

Baggesen et al. (1996) found an apparent prevalence of *Salmonella* spp. infection of 6.2% in Danish slaughter pigs based on culture of 5 g of cecal contents. Although the sensitivity of culture can depend on the volume of contents examined and choice of selective medium, the procedure was estimated to be 50% sensitive and 100% specific. Because only 50% of the infected pigs would have been detected by culture, prevalence would have been underestimated twofold. Hence, true prevalence would be 6.2% × 2 = 12.4%.

SAMPLE QUALITY AND OPTIMAL LABORATORY INTERPRETATION

For optimal interpretation of results of animal and tissue submissions to a diagnostic laboratory, a thorough herd history—which includes morbidity and mortality, age of onset, sequence of clinical signs, time from onset to recovery, response to therapy, and recent management and environmental changes—should be obtained. Evidence of differences in incidence or prevalence among different age groups of pigs or those housed under different management conditions could yield important information about the disease agent(s). Valuable insight into a diagnostic investigation often is gained by asking the producers what they suspect is the cause and why they suspect the health or production problem recently occurred. The response to this inquiry also might yield useful information on other issues, which need to be addressed during the farm visit and help focus the laboratory testing.

Goals of Submission and Sample Collection

After completely assessing the problem, the veterinarian and producer should jointly agree on the goals of performing laboratory testing, because this will be critical in selecting appropriate types and numbers of samples from the correct pig groups. The goal of laboratory testing should likewise be communicated to the laboratory performing the testing; laboratory consultation before submission often is valuable to ensure samples are collected, processed, and shipped in a manner which will allow optimal results (i.e., freezing may decrease the recovery of certain bacteria and viruses or may be essential to maintain viability of other agents). Sample collection for detection of toxins may require freezing for labile toxins (i.e., cyanide) or special and individual packaging for toxins which are diffusible or can be contaminated by contact with plastic (i.e., polychlorinated biphenyls) or rubber (i.e., zinc). During consultation with a laboratory diagnostician, the veterinarian should be sure to request information on the various testing methods available and their strengths and weaknesses in detecting the agent(s) of interest, which may vary with the syndrome under investigation and the stage of infection (for PRRS, see Benson et al. 2002, Rossow 1998). The laboratory's ability to detect the agent in the syndrome suspected, quality control procedures used to ensure the test method is working, and, most importantly, whether the laboratory has ever detected this agent before are important issues to be addressed prior to submission.

Selection of Pigs

After the goal is decided and the specimen type and shipping requirements have been determined, it is critical to select pigs for sampling or submission that will provide the information necessary to meet the predetermined goals. For example, if the goal is to determine the initiating cause of a herd outbreak of respiratory disease with high morbidity but low mortality, several agents will be of particular interest to the veterinarian. Diagnosis might require sampling of pigs during the acute phase of illness if the isolation of the agent is desired, whereas sera from acute and convalescent pigs or sera from three groups—nonexposed, acutely infected, and recovered pigs—are more appropriate to confirm the presence of the agent through an immunologic response in infected animals. If, however, the goal is to determine what complicating factors might be leading to the low mortality because most affected pigs recover, pigs late in the disease process will be more appropriate, recognizing that the initiating agent(s) may no longer be present or may be masked by the presence of secondary invaders.

Although gross pathology and histopathology are the diagnostic disciplines that have been the least evaluated in a quantitative manner, this testing is commonly used to diagnose disease problems. Ideally, the veterinarian should be involved in selecting pigs for necropsy to ensure they meet the criteria decided upon. If the veterinarian is unavailable to select the animals, clear communication with the producer on the type of pig required and reasons for the choice will assist the laboratory in providing optimal return for the investment of time and money to perform diagnostic testing. Evaluation of gross lesions and/or histopathology for the early detection of several swine diseases such as classical swine fever and *Lawsonia intracellularis* has shown these methods to be both insensitive and nonspecific (Elbers et al. 2003; Huerta et al. 2003). Therefore, the veterinarian should be cautious when relying on field necropsies alone to either diagnose or exclude various diseases particularly in their early stages.

Additional Considerations

For optimal serologic testing, the quality of serum samples is important. SN tests, for example, are especially susceptible to sample hemolysis and bacterial and chemical contamination of samples. Accordingly, to decrease the risk of samples being toxic to cells in the assay, blood should be collected using sterile equipment, and serum should be separated from the clot and chilled during submission. Toxic samples should not lead to false-positive or false-negative results, but practitioners and owners might be inconvenienced or incur additional costs if pigs need to be resampled (Hill 1988).

Laboratories commonly use PCR-nucleic acid probe assays on fresh tissues or body fluids and immunohistochemistry (IHC) on formalin preserved samples for the detection of infectious agents. Both procedures offer the advantage of not requiring the presence of viable organisms. Both methods have also provided critical information on determination of optimal sampling sites, frequency of repeat sampling, and numbers of samples from one organ to attain a high sensitivity (for PRRS, Benson et al. 2002, Rossow 1998, Yaeger 2002). For example, Yaeger (2002) determined that the likelihood of detecting PRRSV infection in the lung by IHC increased from 48% to >90% when the number of lung sites tested was increased from one to five. PCR has the added advantage of detecting much lower levels of the agent; thus it has a higher sensitivity, but this does not always correlate with a better positive predictive value for the syndrome under investigation as was found with PMWS (Pogranichniy et al. 2002). In fact, increased use of PCR has provided valuable information on the frequency of asymptomatic, subclinical, and carrier states for a number of agents. PCR, because of its much lower detection limit, is more susceptible to problems arising from cross-contamination between sites within the same animal, such as normal nasal flora contaminating lung sites or between animals when using common instruments or gloves during sample collection and processing or when samples are collected in an environment that contains the agent in the air, such as *M. hyopneumoniae* (Kurth et al. 2002). Poorly validated PCR tests may also result in false-positive results through detection of near-neighbor agents, such as bovine viral diarrhea virus with a classical swine fever PCR.

After laboratory testing of samples is completed, interpretation of the results on a herd basis should include evaluation of the agreement of the herd history with the laboratory's gross findings and the individual histories of the pigs submitted. For example, if pigs of appropriate age are submitted to determine the cause of postweaning diarrhea but the gross findings indicate normal feces and significant pneumonia, or if fecal samples are submitted from 10-week-old emaciated pigs, the findings in both cases will be of little or no value in determining the cause of postweaning diarrhea. However, the results in the former case disclose a previously unrecognized respiratory disease. In the latter example, the age and nutritional status indicate pigs are growing poorly, and some agents that initiate postweaning diarrhea (i.e., hemolytic *E. coli*, TGE, or rotavirus) will no longer be present. Another key element in the necropsy report, which complicates interpretation of the results, is the presence of injection sites or medication in the gastrointestinal tract. The use of parasiticides or antibiotics can suppress or kill potential agents under investigation, resulting in false-negative results.

In order to correlate test results with the presence of pathologic lesions or clinical disease, it is important that the samples are labeled with unique animal identifications. The submission paperwork should also indicate the number of pigs sampled. In the absence of identifying information, tissue, swabs, feces, or serum samples from multiple pigs might be assumed to be from the same animal and pooled or only a portion of the samples might be tested.

CAUSE AND EFFECT

Almost all infectious diseases in swine production are multicausal, with environmental and management factors playing a central role in the clinical expression of overt disease and in the determination of a disease's effect on productivity. PMWS is an excellent example of the influence of multiple factors on the expression of clinical disease (Pogranichniy et al. 2002). Although a diagnostic laboratory can help identify agents potentially involved in a disease outbreak or poor-production problem, the importance of infectious agents relative to other host, management, and environmental factors must be determined by the submitting veterinarian.

Considerations if an Agent Is Isolated

Even when an agent is isolated with a 100% specific test and hence there is direct evidence of its presence, questions may arise as to the role of the agent in the disease process. In most investigations that are not done prospectively or that do not include similar testing of healthy cohorts, it is difficult to establish unequivocally that the suspected cause (e.g., agent) preceded the outcome (e.g., morbidity or mortality) or prove that the agent caused disease. Factors that impact a causal interpretation of the agent's role in the disease process need to be considered. Because a certain number of subclinical or normal carriers of an organism occur, it is important to determine whether the goal is to ascertain the presence or absence of a potential disease-causing agent or to determine the role of the agent in causing clinical disease (Huerta et al. 2003, Pogranichniy et al. 2002). The site from which the organism is identified (e.g., nasal vs. lung), the purity of the culture or types of organisms found in mixed cultures, and the quantity of agent present can be important factors in determining the causal relationship of a potential agent to the disease process.

Site of Isolation. The site is important because a number of organisms found in pathologic lesions have also been found in healthy pigs as part of the flora of the skin, respiratory, gastrointestinal, or reproductive tracts (Amass et al. 1996; Dritz et al. 1996; Straw et al. 1996). Therefore, events at the time of death may lead to contamination of deeper organs. For example, the lung may become contaminated with aspirated nasopharyngeal flora, leading to isolation of potential pathogens such as *Haemophilus parasuis* or *Streptococcus suis*, which are reported in the nasal cavities and tonsils of healthy pigs (Amass et al. 1996; Dritz et al. 1996). Most respiratory pathogens are reported more commonly in pneumonic lungs, but they have also been found in a low percentage (2–16%) of normal lungs (Straw et al. 1996). Postmortem contamination can also occur during the organ removal process, such as when nasal flora are found in mixed cultures from a brain that was removed by sawing through the nasal cavity and calvarium.

Pure or Mixed Culture Result. Though uncommon in pigs, finding a single potential pathogen lends greater support to a causal relationship between an agent and a lesion. Co-infections are more common, however; Choi et al. (2003) demonstrated in their findings that 88% of 2872 cases of pneumonia in pigs had two or more pathogens present.

Interpretation of mixed culture results requires knowledge of the flora at the site cultured, as well as the type and relative number of organisms identified. In the absence of inflammation or when potential pathogens are found in mixed culture, determining a causal relationship of any single agent to disease is difficult. Often pigs submitted for evaluation may have been sick and treated with antibiotics for several days, so determining which agents are the primary or secondary pathogens is tricky. The finding of the same pathogens at multiple sites within an affected organ lends support to a causal relationship compared with finding only environmental bacteria, such as coliforms, streptococci and staphylococci. These mixed cultures of environmental bacteria in a parenchymal organ or mixed with rare pathogens suggest aspiration in the lung, postmortem contamination of organs, or poor technique in obtaining cultures. This interpretation is supported by reports that these environmental organisms are found with similar frequency in normal and pneumonic lung cultures (Straw et al. 1996).

Molecular Characterization. In some situations, establishing causality when an agent is identified might require further characterization of the strain found if it is generally of low pathogenicity or if live vaccines, that are detectable by the assay (e.g., PCR), have recently been used. Molecular epidemiologic methods might be required in some instances to determine whether an outbreak is attributable to the introduction of a new, more virulent strain of bacteria or virus or to the reemergence of an endemic strain (e.g., PRRS; Larochelle et al. 2003). Sometimes there is a need to differentiate pathogenic field virus from closely related cross-reacting viruses (e.g., porcine respiratory coronavirus from TGE) or vaccine strains (e.g., PRRS; Wesley et al. 1998), because the first may produce clinical disease whereas cross-reacting viruses and vaccine isolates do not (Mengeling et al. 1996).

Quantity of the Agent. The quantity of an agent present has significance in interpretation of toxicologic and nutritional results. A low level of a toxin might simply reflect a residue rather than clinical toxicosis. However, since toxins are absorbed and metabolized at various rates, a very low level might be significant if clinical signs exist for toxins that are highly volatile (e.g., zinc phosphide) or rapidly broken down (e.g., anticoagulants, ionophores). Some toxins can also result in changes in tissues with a slow turnover, such as hooves, so that lesions persist after the tissue levels have returned to normal (e.g., selenium). The amount of decline below normal levels for minerals in pig sera and tissues is important in determination of clinical or subclinical nutritional deficiencies. In general, antigen and nucleic acid detection assays—such as PCR, IHC, fluorescent antibody (FA), and virus isolation—provide positive or negative results and are not quantitative. Even semi-quantitative testing—such as real-time PCR, bacterial cultures, and fecal parasite counts—will be strongly influenced by the presubmission use of therapeutics, sample handling, nonuniform distribution of the agent in the sample and the stage of infection (e.g., pre-patent). Therefore, quantity of a pathogenic microorganism, though a consideration, should not be a major factor in determining the significance of the agent.

Considerations if No Agent Is Isolated

As described in a previous section, a negative result on laboratory samples should not necessarily rule out an agent as a cause of disease, especially if the negative predictive value of a test is only moderate. False-negative results—such as failure to isolate a viral or bacterial agent or identify a specific pathogen by electron microscopy, FA, histopathology, and other antigen detection or PCR technique—can occur for a variety of reasons. The laboratory performing the test might have little or no experience with isolating some of the fastidious swine pathogens and are not using alternative more sensitive detection methods. For example, a laboratory report stating "*Mycoplasma* cultures were negative" would not exclude the presence of *M. hyopneumoniae*, since most laboratories use a culture technique that is incapable of growing this agent. Nonuniform distribution of the pathogen may be a problem for viral and bacterial respiratory and enteric pathogens when limited sections are taken for laboratory testing (e.g., FA for TGE, IHC for PRRS; see Yaeger 2002) A prolonged time interval since initial onset of disease may lead to a decline in the quantity of the agent to below the detection limit of the assay and would necessitate an alternative assay such as serology or a more sensitive detection method like PCR. The test may detect only specific strains of the pathogen (e.g., commercial ELISA assays detect only group A rotavirus). The combination of transport media, time delay, and shipping and storage temperature may not be conducive to the survival of some pathogens for agent isolation methods, but PCR or antigen detection may still be effective due to greater leeway in their time and temperature requirements. For example, tissue samples maintained at room temperature for 24 hours had less than 50% recovery of PRRS virus by isolation compared with 100% recovery from sequential samples maintained at 4°C (VanAlstine et al. 1993). However, PCR was able to detect PRRSV in 94% of positive samples maintained at room temperature for up to 4 days (Benson et al. 2002). False-negative results on fecal sample PCR for various enteric pathogens may occur within a shorter time frame postcollection and more readily at room temperature or higher temperatures due to the impact of normal flora. In addition, inhibitory substances in feces can result in false-negative PCR results, but new internal control methods have improved the laboratories' ability to detect these substances, thereby rendering the negative results invalid (Jacobson et al. 2003). The incorrect sample (e.g., feces) might be submitted for conditions that many laboratories diagnose on histopathology or IHC (e.g., *Lawsonia intracellularis*, attaching and effacing *E. coli*). For some agents like PRRS, prolonged formalin-fixation can also result in false-negative results by IHC (VanAlstine et al. 2002). In general, problems arising from the inability of the laboratory to identify specific pathogens, nonuniform distribution of lesions, shipping and storage conditions, insensitive assays for the stage of disease, and incorrect samples can be prevented if the laboratory is consulted prior to collection and submission of the samples.

Even when sample selection and shipping conditions are optimal and the laboratory is capable of testing for the agent(s) of interest, a negative result will not rule out the presence of fastidious agents or organisms found in very low numbers. However, in pigs undergoing a thorough pathologic evaluation, the absence of lesions or clinical signs considered specific to that agent is usually adequate evidence to rule out the agent as a cause of disease, although the agent may still be present without causing clinical disease (e.g., *Lawsonia intracellularis,* see Huerta et al. 2003). False-negative results will also occur when pigs are treated prior to sampling. Gram-positive organisms are easily suppressed or killed by the use of penicillin and other antibiotics, substantially reducing the likelihood of isolation of *Erysipelothrix* or beta-hemolytic *Streptococcus* spp. from treated pigs.

Additional Considerations for Serologic Results

Because serologic results often are quantitative and values can vary between laboratories performing the same assay, the relationship of a serologic response to disease can be best interpreted by knowledge of the laboratories' experience with the assay in their submission area. Laboratories should be able to provide information on the common response detected in pigs in their area and in pigs that have been vaccinated. However, for many diseases titers induced by natural infection may not be readily distinguished from vaccinal titers (Hill 1988). An exception is PRV infection for which tests are available for differentiation of field infection from vaccinal responses in pigs vaccinated with gene-deleted PRV vaccines (Weigel et al. 1992). Also of importance is how soon after infection titers become detectable with the assay being used, the time period to reach peak titers, and the duration of detectable antibody after infection or vaccination (Yoon et al. 1995). Lack of a titer on an assay with high sensitivity can be valuable information to rule out the agent in question if the animals sampled have been sick or recovered from the disease within 2–4 weeks prior to sampling.

In young pigs, repeated sampling might help differentiate maternally acquired antibodies from those induced by natural infection. If a veterinarian is interested in using serology to identify TGE as a cause of postweaning diarrhea in a chronically infected herd, a single serum sample taken at weaning might be inadequate because such antibodies could have been passively or actively acquired (Hill 1988). Repeated sampling at 2- to 4-week intervals with evidence of increasing or decreasing titers would provide evidence of active infection or passively acquired antibodies, respectively. However, when interpreting the results of such a sampling strategy, the potential role of porcine respiratory coronavirus maternal antibody or infection, which induces cross-reacting antibody to TGE, would also have to be considered (Sestak et al. 1996; Wesley and Woods 1996).

Although unequivocally establishing a cause-and-effect relationship is difficult, consideration of the above-mentioned factors and testing the diagnosis with an intervention (especially if there is an untreated control group) should provide increased confidence in a causal interpretation of the laboratory findings.

SELECTING APPROPRIATE SAMPLE SIZES

As part of disease investigations and health monitoring of herds, several sample size questions need to be addressed before sample collection. Although collection of too few samples is the most common mistake, the additional cost of submission of more samples must be weighed against the economic cost of the disease and the importance of establishing a correct diagnosis.

Detection of Infection if Present in the Herd

Veterinarians often need to determine whether an infection is or has ever been present in the herd or a subpopulation of the herd. For tests of 100% specificity, a single positive is usually considered sufficient to class the herd as positive, although for serologic tests of imperfect specificity more than one positive might be necessary. To estimate required numbers to detect infection, two values are necessary: the required level of confidence, usually 95%, and the likely prevalence of infection in the herd or in the specific group of pigs being evaluated. The selected prevalence value should be realistic, but if there is doubt, erring toward a lower prevalence is preferable to ensure that adequate numbers of pigs are sampled. If the calculated sample size is large relative to the total population size, these numbers can be adjusted downward.

If a veterinarian's only goal is to detect infection, sampling does not need to be random but can be directed to higher-prevalence groups—for example, different age groups when there is an age-related risk of infection or clinically affected versus otherwise healthy pigs. If there is an age-related risk of exposure—e.g., *Salmonella* spp. in pigs in Denmark (Christensen and Gardner 2000)—this information can be used to target risk-groups for sampling. To detect *T. gondii* in a herd, sows are a better population to sample because prevalence is likely to be higher than in grower-finisher pigs. To detect PRRS virus, samples from older nursery pigs (6–8 weeks old) would be better than samples from sows or finisher pigs. To detect enteric pathogens by fecal culture or antigen detection methods, preference should be given to sampling pigs with diarrhea rather than pigs with normal feces.

A benefit of nonrandom, or targeted, sampling is that a diagnosis can often be established with fewer samples. In an outbreak investigation when samples are selected for culture from typical lesions identified at necropsy (prevalence close to 100%), few samples will be necessary. In other situations, where infection is subclinical and prevalence is lower, more samples should be submitted. For example, a sample size of 30 will give 95% confidence of detecting at least 1 positive in the sample if the prevalence of infection is at least 10% and the test is perfectly sensitive. When sensitivity is less than 100%, numbers should be increased. For example, if culture of feces for *Salmonella* spp. was only 50% sensitive, a sample size of about 60 (double the number needed for a 100% sensitive test) would be needed to satisfy the specified criterion.

Despite adequate planning of sample sizes, laboratory results are sometimes negative. If zero positive test results occur for a sample of pigs from the herd, this should be interpreted differently from negative results based on testing the entire herd. Appropriate interpretation is shown in the example on prevalence estimation that follows.

Prevalence Estimation

Detection of infection and estimation of prevalence can often be done with the same sample of pigs, providing that the sampling is truly random. Usually the random sample for prevalence estimation is collected at a single point in time (cross-sectional sample). Required sample sizes to estimate prevalence with desired accuracy or error limits (usually from 5% to 20%) are presented in Tables 10.2 and 10.3, including corrections for finite population sizes. When prevalence is unknown and a study is planned, we recommend calculating a sample size at 50% prevalence, which represents the maximum number that could be needed. Selection of error limits will be more subjective, although ±10% and ±20% are used more frequently than ±5% because of the substantially increased cost when a more precise estimate is needed.

We emphasize two points with respect to prevalence estimation. First, at moderate prevalences (30–70%), much larger sample sizes are necessary to estimate prevalence accurately than at either low or high prevalences. For a fixed sample size, the precision of the estimate is greater the more the prevalence differs from 50%. Second, small sample sizes can result in sample test results that are very different from the true population values. For example, Gardner et al. (1996) compared samples of 5 and 30 pigs to estimate the prevalence of porcine parvovirus in a large herd and found that sample sizes of 5 frequently failed to reflect herd prevalence, and even a sample size of 30 yielded poor estimates of herd prevalence on some occasions.

Sometimes, even though the sample size is calculated a priori, no positives are found on a random sample of pigs when tested with a perfect test. What conclusions, if any, can be drawn? If there are no positives, the upper 95% confidence limit for prevalence is approximately 3/n where n = number sampled (DiGiacomo and Koepsell 1986). Therefore, if 30 pigs were tested and all were negative, the upper 95% confidence limit would be 3/30, or 10%. Although a veterinarian initially might conclude that a herd was not infected (prevalence = 0%), a more appropriate interpretation would be that the herd has a prevalence of ≤10% with 95% confidence.

This issue of how to interpret negative results correctly extends to health certification schemes. Only if all pigs are tested in a herd with a test of 100% sensitivity and negative results are obtained is there sufficient evidence, based on the test results alone, to certify freedom from a pathogen. In practice, certifications are usually based on a combination of herd history and repeated testing of samples from the herd and are made in the context of knowledge that many herds become infected over time by the spread of pathogens from neighboring herds. Experience from the Danish SPF scheme indicates that the annual reinfection rate of herds with *M. hyopneumoniae* is about 10–15% (Sørensen et al. 1992; Sørensen et al. 1993).

Detection of a Difference in Prevalence or Incidence Between Two Groups

For some investigations a veterinarian might want to determine whether one group of pigs has a higher prevalence or incidence of infection than another group. The grouping factor could be age, reproductive status (preg-

Table 10.4. Sample sizes necessary to detect a significant difference in prevalence or incidence of infection or disease between two groups (one with and one without the risk factor) with 95% confidence and 80% power.

Prevalence in Risk-Factor Positive Group (%)	Prevalence in Risk-Factor Negative Group (%)									
	0	10	20	30	40	50	60	70	80	90
10	93									
20	44	219								
30	27	71	313							
40	19	38	91	376						
50	14	24	45	103	407					
60	11	17	27	48	107	407				
70	9	12	18	28	48	103	376			
80	7	9	13	18	27	45	91	313		
90	5	7	9	12	17	24	38	71	219	
100	4	5	7	9	11	14	19	27	44	93

Note: By convention, the risk-factor positive group is assumed to have a higher prevalence than the risk-factor negative group. Sample sizes assume independence of groups and random sampling. Tabulated numbers are those required in each of the two groups.

nant vs. nonpregnant or aborting vs. nonaborting), production system or husbandry type, or any other comparison factor. If this diagnostic approach was used and a significant association was detected between an infectious agent and an outcome such as clinical disease, reproductive failure, or the prevalence of emaciated pigs, this would provide additional evidence for a causal role of the agent in the syndrome. This comparative approach is often used in serum-profiling schemes where different age groups in the herd are evaluated for exposure to one or more infectious agents.

If a comparison of prevalences is the primary goal of the submission, the required sample size is determined by the level of confidence and the best a priori estimates of prevalence in the groups. As the percentage point difference between the groups decreases, much larger sample sizes become necessary (Table 10.4). For example, to detect a significant difference at the 5% level between 40% and 10% prevalence with 80% power would require 38/group, whereas 91/group would be needed to detect a difference between 40% and 20% prevalence. These calculations indicate that the small sample sizes (5–10 per age group) that are often recommended for serum profiling of herds are typically too small for unequivocal comparisons. Sample sizes necessary to compare prevalences are listed in book tables (Fleiss 1981) or can be calculated with public domain computer software such as Epi Info (available at www.cdc.gov/epiinfo/).

CONCLUSIONS

Laboratories can assist in establishing a diagnosis, but ultimately, practitioners need to assess the laboratory results in the context of other herd information and existing knowledge about the relative importance of infectious agents and other factors in disease occurrence. To maximize the benefits of laboratory testing, veterinarians should do the following:

1. Clearly define the goal of the submission—e.g., confirm a diagnosis, screen for a pathogen, estimate prevalence of a pathogen.
2. Select a laboratory with good internal and external quality control procedures and with experience working with the agent or test of interest.
3. Give the laboratory the maximum chance to achieve the goals desired by
   A. Selecting appropriate sample types—e.g., tissue versus serum;
   B. Using the correct method of submission—e.g., chilled versus frozen versus room temperature;
   C. Ensuring samples are from pigs that are truly representative of the problem under investigation and are collected from pigs at the appropriate stage of disease;
   D. Submitting adequate numbers of samples to meet the specified submission goal, balancing the additional cost of more samples versus the need to establish a diagnosis correctly;
   E. Considering inclusion of a comparison group of samples (controls) if interpretation without them might be equivocal or previous attempts to establish diagnosis have been unproductive.
4. Be knowledgeable about the strengths and limitations of available tests.
5. Interpret results taking into account the predictive values of positive and negative test results, and for quantitative tests, the magnitude of the test result in relationship to the cutoff value.

REFERENCES

Amass SF, Wu CC, Clark LK. 1996. Evaluation of antibiotics for the elimination of the tonsillar carrier state of *Streptococcus suis* in pigs. J Vet Diagn Invest 8:64–67.

Bager F, Petersen J. 1991. Sensitivity and specificity of different methods for the isolation of *Salmonella* from pigs. Acta Vet Scand 32:473–481.

Baggesen DL, Wegener HC, Bager F, Stege H, Christensen, J. 1996. Herd prevalence of *Salmonella enterica* infections in Danish slaughter pigs determined by microbiological testing. Prev Vet Med 26:201–213.

Benson JE, Yaeger MJ, Christopher-Hennings J, Lager K, Yoon KJ. 2002. A comparison of virus isolation, immunohistochemistry, fetal serology, and reverse-transcription polymerase chain reaction assay for the identification of porcine reproductive and respiratory syndrome virus transplacental infection in the fetus. J Vet Diagn Invest 14:8–14.

Bernardo TM, Dohoo IR, Ogilvie T. 1990. A critical assessment of abattoir surveillance as a screening test for swine ascariasis. Can J Vet Res 54:274–277.

Blanchard B, Kobisch M, Bové JM, Saillard C. 1996. Polymerase chain reaction for *Mycoplasma hyopneumoniae* detection in tracheobronchiolar washings from pigs. Molec Cell Probes 10:15–22.

Bøgh HO, Eriksen L, Lawson LG, Lind P. 1994. Evaluation of an enzyme-linked immunosorbent assay and a histamine release test system for the detection of pigs naturally infected with *Ascaris suum*. Prev Vet Med 21:201–214.

Bouma A, Stegeman JA, Engel B, de Kluijver EP, Albers AR, de Jong MC. 2001. Evaluation of diagnostic tests for the detection of classical swine fever in the field without a gold standard. J Vet Diagn Invest 13:383–388.

Cannon RM, Roe RT. 1982. Livestock Disease Surveys: A Field Manual for Veterinarians. Canberra: Australian Government Publishing Service.

Carpenter TE, Gardner IA. 1996. Simulation modeling to determine herd-level predictive values and sensitivity based on individual-animal test sensitivity and specificity and sample size. Prev Vet Med 27:57–66.

Chappel RJ, Prime RW, Millar BD, Mead LJ, Jones RT, Adler B. 1992. Comparison of diagnostic procedures for porcine leptospirosis. Vet Microbiol 30:151–163.

Choi YK, Goyal SM, Joo, HS. 2003. Retrospective analysis of etiologic agents associated with respiratory disease in pigs. Can Vet J 44:735–737.

Christensen J, Bagessen DL, Nielsen B, Stryhn H. 2002. Herd prevalence of *Salmonella* spp. in Danish pig herds after implementation of the Danish Salmonella Control Program with reference to a pre-implementation study. Vet Microbiol 88:175–188.

Christensen J, Gardner IA. 2000. Herd-level interpretation of test results for epidemiologic studies of animal diseases. Prev Vet Med 45:83–106.

Davies PR, Bahnson PB, Grass JJ, Marsh WE, Garcia R, Melancon J, Dial GD. 1996. Evaluation of the monitoring of papular dermatitis lesions in slaughtered swine to assess sarcoptic mite infestation. Vet Parasitol 62:143–153.

DiGiacomo RF, Koepsell TD. 1986. Sampling for detection of infection or disease in animal populations. J Am Vet Med Assoc 189:22–23.

Drew TW. 1995. Comparative serology of porcine reproductive and respiratory syndrome in eight European laboratories, using immunoperoxidase monolayer assay and enzyme-linked immunosorbent assay. Rev Sci Tech Off Int Epiz 14:761–775.

Dritz SS, Chengappa MM, Nelssen JL, Tokach MD, Goodband RD, Nietfeld JC, Staats JJ. 1996. Growth and microbial flora of nonmedicated, segregated, early weaned pigs from a commercial swine operation. J Am Vet Med Assoc 208:711–715.

Dubey JP, Thulliez P, Weigel RM, Andrews CD, Lind P, Powell EC. 1995. Sensitivity and specificity of various serologic tests for detection of *Toxoplasma gondii* infection in naturally infected sows. Am J Vet Res 56:1030–1036.

Elbers ARW, Bouma A, Stegeman A. 2002. Quantitative assessment of the quality of clinical signs for the detection of classical swine fever outbreaks. Vet Microbiol 85:323–332.

Elbers ARW, Vos JH, Bouma A, van Exsel ACA, Stegeman A. 2003. Assessment of the use of gross lesions at post-mortem to detect outbreaks of classical swine fever. Vet Microbiol 96:345–356.

Enøe C, Andersen S, Sorensen V, Willeberg P. 2001. Estimation of sensitivity, specificity and predictive values of two serologic tests for the detection of antibodies to *Actinobacillus pleuropneumoniae* serotype 2 in the absence of a reference test (gold standard). Prev Vet Med 51:227–243.

Enøe C, Christensen G, Andersen S, Willeberg P. 2003. The need for built–in validation of surveillance data so that changes in diagnostic performance of post-mortem inspection can be detected. Prev Vet Med 57:117–225.

Enøe C, Georgiadis MP, Johnson WO. 2000. Estimation of the sensitivity and specificity of diagnostic tests and disease prevalence when the true disease state is unknown. Prev Vet Med 45:61–81.

Ferris RA, Schoenbaum MA, Crawford RP. 1995. Comparison of serologic tests and bacteriologic culture for detection of brucellosis in swine from naturally infected herds. J Am Vet Med Assoc 207:1332–1333.

Fittipaldi N, Broes A, Harel J, Kobisch M, Gottschalk M. 2003. Evaluation and field validation of PCR tests for detection of *Actinobacillus pleuropneumoniae* in subclinically infected pigs. J Clin Microbiol 41:5085–5093.

Fleiss JL. 1981. Statistical Methods for Rates and Proportions. 2d ed. New York: Wiley and Sons, New York.

Gardner IA, Carpenter TE, Leontides L, Parsons TE. 1996. Financial evaluation of vaccination and testing alternatives for control of parvovirus-induced reproductive failure in swine. J Am Vet Med Assoc 208:863–869.

Gardner IA, Stryhn H, Lind P, Collins MT. 2000. Conditional dependence between tests affects the diagnosis and surveillance of animal diseases. Prev Vet Med 45:107–122.

Greiner M, Gardner IA. 2000a. Epidemiologic issues in the validation of veterinary diagnostic tests. Prev Vet Med 45:3–22.

——. 2000b. Application of diagnostic tests in veterinary epidemiologic studies. Prev Vet Med 45:43–59.

Greiner M, Pfeiffer D, Smith RD. 2000. Principles and practical application of the receiver-operating characteristic analysis for diagnostic tests. Prev Vet Med 45:23–41.

Hill, H. 1988. Interpretation of serologic results of some important swine diseases. Compend Contin Educ 10:979–985.

Huerta B, Arenas A, Carrasco L, Maldonado A, Tarradas C, Carbonero A, Perea A. 2003. Comparison of diagnostic techniques in porcine proliferative enteropathy (*Lawsonia intracellularis*) infection. J Comp Path 129:179–185.

Hui SL, Walter SD. 1980. Estimating the error rates of diagnostic tests. Biometrics 36:167–171.

Jacobson M, Englund S, Ballagi-Pordany A. 2003. The use of a mimic to detect polymerase chain reaction-inhibitory substances in feces examined for the presence of *Lawsonia intracellularis*. J Vet Diagn Invest 15:268–273.

Jacobson RH. 1998. Validation of serological assays for diagnosis of infectious diseases. Rev Sci Tech Off Int Epizoot17:469–486.

Klingenberg K, Esfandiari J. 1996. Evaluation of a one-step test for rapid, in practice detection of rotavirus in farm animals. Vet Rec 138:393–395.

Kurth KT, Hsu T, Snook ER, Thacker EL, Thacker BJ, Minion FC. 2002. Use of a *Mycoplasma hyopneumoniae* nested polymerase chain reaction test to determine the optimal sampling sites in swine. J Vet Diagn Invest 14:463–469.

Lanza I, Rubio P, Muñoz M, Carmenes P. 1993. Comparison of a monoclonal antibody capture ELISA (MACELISA) to indirect ELISA and virus neutralization test for the serodiagnosis of transmissible gastroenteritis virus. J Vet Diagn Invest 5:21–25.

Larochelle R, D'Allaire S, Magar R. 2003. Molecular epidemiology of porcine reproductive and respiratory syndrome virus (PRRSV) in Quebec. Virus Res 96:3–15.

Margolis MJ, Hutchinson LJ, Kephart KB, Hattel AL, Whitlock RH, Payeur JB. 1994. Results of using histologic examination and acid-fast staining to confirm a diagnosis of swine mycobacteriosis made on the basis of gross examination. J Am Vet Med Assoc 204:1571–1572.

Martin SW. 1988. The interpretation of laboratory results. Vet Clin N Amer: Food Anim Pract 4:61–78.

Martin SW, Shoukri M, Thorburn MA. 1992. Evaluating the health status of herds based on tests applied to individuals. Prev Vet Med 14:33–43.

Mengeling WL, Vorwald AC, Lager, KM, Brockmeier SL. 1996. Comparison among strains of porcine reproductive and respiratory syndrome virus for their ability to cause reproductive failure. Am J Vet Res 57:834–839.

Murrell KD, Anderson WR, Schad GA, Hanbury RD, Kazacos KR, Gamble HR, Brown J. 1986. Field evaluation of the enzyme-linked immunosorbent assay for swine trichinosis: Efficacy of the excretory-secretory antigen. Am J Vet Res 47:1046–1049.

Nodelijk G, Wensvoort G, Kroese B, Van Leengoed L, Colijn E, Verheijden J. 1996. Comparison of a commercial ELISA and an immunoperoxidase monolayer assay to detect antibodies directed against porcine respiratory and reproductive syndrome virus. Vet Microbiol 49:285–295.

Pogranichniy RM, Yoon KJ, Harms PA, Sorden SD, Daniels M. 2002. Case-control study on the association of porcine circovirus type 2 and other swine viral pathogens with postweaning multisystemic wasting syndrome. J Vet Diagn Invest 14:449–456.

Rogan WJ, Gladen B. 1978. Estimating prevalence from results of a screening test. Am J Epidemiol 107:71–76.

Rossow KD. 1998. Porcine reproductive and respiratory syndrome: Review Article. Vet Pathol 35:1–20.

Saah AJ, Hoover DR. 1997. "Sensitivity" and "specificity" reconsidered: The meaning of these terms in analytical and diagnostic settings. Ann Intern Med 126:91–94.

Sestak K, Lanza I, Park SK, Weilnau PA, Saif LJ. 1996. Contribution of passive immunity to porcine respiratory coronavirus to protection against transmissible gastroenteritis virus challenge exposure in suckling pigs. Am J Vet Res 57:664–671.

Sørensen V, Ahrens P, Barfod K, Feenstra AA, Feld NC, Friis NF, Bille-Hansen V, Jensen NE, Pedersen MW. 1997. *Mycoplasma hyopneumoniae* infection in pigs: Duration of the disease and evaluation of four diagnostic assays. Vet Microbiol 54:23–34.

Sørensen V, Barfod K, Feld NC. 1992. Evaluation of a monoclonal blocking ELISA and IHA for antibodies to *Mycoplasma hyopneumoniae* in SPF-pig herds. Vet Rec 130:488–490.

Sørensen V, Barfod K, Feld NC, Vraa-Andersen L. 1993. Application of enzyme-linked immunosorbent assay for the surveillance of *Mycoplasma hyopneumoniae* in pigs. Rev Sci Tech Off Intl Epizoot 12:593–604.

Straw BE, Dewey CE, Erickson ED. 1996. Interpreting culture reports from swine lungs. Swine Health Prod 4:200–201.

Tyler JW, Cullor JS. 1989. Titers, tests, and truisms: Rational interpretation of diagnostic serology testing. J Am Vet Med Assoc 194:1550–1558.

VanAlstine WG, Kanitz CL, Stevenson GW. 1993. Time and temperature survivability of PRRS virus in serum and tissues. J Vet Diagn Invest 5:621–622.

VanAlstine WG, Popielarczyk M, Albregts SR. 2002. Effect of formalin fixation on the immunohistochemical detection of PRRS virus antigen in experimentally and naturally infected pigs. J Vet Diagn Invest 14:504–507.

Weigel RM, Hall WF, Scherba G, Siegel AM, Hahn EC, Lehman JR. 1992. Evaluation of the sensitivity and specificity of two diagnostic tests for antibodies to pseudorabies virus glycoprotein X. J Vet Diagn Invest 4:238–244.

Wesley RD, Mengeling WL, Lager KM, Clouser DF, Landgraf JG, Frey ML. 1998. Differentiation of porcine reproductive and respiratory virus vaccine strain from North American field strains by restriction fragment length polymorphism analysis of ORF5. J Vet Diagn Invest 10:140–144.

Wesley RD, Woods RD. 1996. Induction of protective immunity against transmissible gastroenteritis virus after exposure of neonatal pigs to porcine respiratory coronavirus. Am J Vet Res 57:157–162.

White AK, Ciacci-Zanella J, Galeota J, Ele S, Osorio, F. 1996. Comparison of the abilities of serologic tests to detect pseudorabies-infected pigs during the latent phase. Am J Vet Res 57:608–611.

Yaeger MJ. 2002. The diagnostic sensitivity of immunohistochemistry for the detection of porcine reproductive and respiratory syndrome virus in the lung of vaccinated and unvaccinated swine. J Vet Diagn Invest 14:15–19.

Yoon K, Zimmerman JJ, Swenson SL, McGinley MJ, Eernisse KA, Brevik A, Rhinehart LL, Frey MI, Hill HT, Platt KB. 1995. Characterization of the humoral immune response to porcine reproductive and respiratory syndrome (PRRS) virus infection. J Vet Diagn Invest 7:305–312.

Zweig MH, Campbell G. 1993. Receiver-operating characteristic (ROC) plots—A fundamental evaluation tool in clinical medicine. Clin Chem 39:561–577.

11 Differential Diagnosis of Disease

Barbara E. Straw, Catherine E. Dewey, and M. R. Wilson

This chapter contains a collection of tables designed to provide assistance in the field diagnosis of swine diseases. These aids do not comprehensively cover all the diseases that could possibly occur in pigs. Diseases that affect only one animal or arise due to unusual circumstances have not been included, since this would greatly lengthen the tables without substantial addition of information useful for diagnosing herd problems that are of real economic importance. In general, diseases have been included that cause herd problems or at least involve a group of animals.

This chapter has been divided into major categories according to the body system affected and subdivided into sections by specific clinical signs. Sometimes pigs will show signs referable to two or more systems. Then the clinician will need to exercise judgment in determining which is the principal one affected or may pursue all signs and look for diseases in common.

Each section begins with a definition of the signs included there and some general remarks about approach to diagnosis. Also included is information about patterns of disease and certain characteristics or signs that are typically associated with specific classes of etiologic agents. When applicable, a table indicates the different ages at which the various diseases are more prominent. Although diseases may be shown to affect pigs in a certain age category, age must not be interpreted to have discrete boundaries. Age categories should be used as a guide to the most common age at which the diseases are seen and should not necessarily be a cause of rejecting a disease as a differential just because the affected pigs are not within the specified category.

The tables list the various possible causes of clinical signs and their differentiating features. Whenever possible, these tables have been designed in a format that leads from clinical signs to the etiologic agents since this most closely parallels the procedure of clinical diagnosis in the field. However, with problems like abortion, there are just not enough differentiating clinical features to proceed from signs to diagnosis and so some charts are in the traditional disease-first format.

GASTROINTESTINAL SYSTEM

Diarrhea

The consistency of feces may vary according to the diet fed, but diarrhea may be considered to occur when there is a change to a more fluid consistency than normal, especially when associated with signs of either large- or small-intestine disease. Signs frequently associated with disease of the small intestine include vomiting, melena, poorly digested feces, bulky voluminous feces, and borborygmus. Vomiting seldom occurs in cases of disease of the large intestine; however, there may be bloody stools, gross mucus on the feces, small frequent defecations, and tenesmus.

Unweaned Pigs (Tables 11.1, 11.3). Many times, a presumptive diagnosis of the cause of baby pig diarrhea can be made on the basis of history, clinical signs, and necropsy findings. Often, however, the clinical picture does not point to a likely etiology because of the variation in clinical signs that can be produced by one disease agent and because of concurrent problems with more than one disease. Therefore, as much information as possible should be collected rather than trying to base a diagnosis on one or two signs.

The most common causes of diarrhea in baby pigs are colibacillosis, hypoglycemia, transmissible gastroenteritis (TGE), clostridial enteritis (CE), coccidiosis, and rotaviral enteritis (RE). These six entities account for the major portion of all preweaning diarrhea. Diseases that occur less frequently or rarely in baby pigs but have diarrhea as their principal sign include *Strongyloides* infestation, swine dysentery (SD), erysipelas, and salmonellosis. Pseudorabies (PR) and toxoplasmosis may cause diarrhea in baby pigs, but generally diarrhea is not their main clinical manifestation.

Table 11.1. Ages at which certain diseases causing diarrhea in pigs are more likely to occur

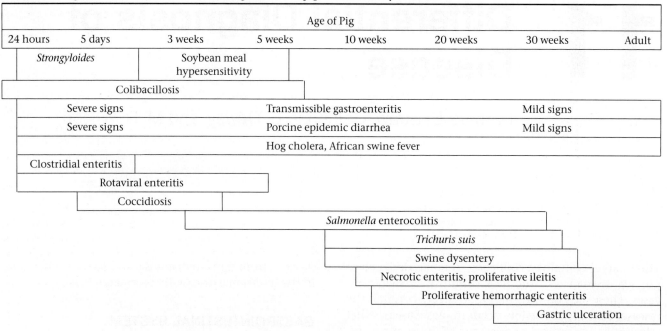

Table 11.2. Change in effective environmental temperature due to various conditions

Condition		Change in Effective Environmental Temperature	
		°C	°F
Airspeed:			
0.2 m/sec	(0.7 ft/sec)	−4	−7
0.5 m/sec	(1.6 ft/sec)	−7	−13
1.5 m/sec	(4.9 ft/sec)	−10	−18
Floor type:			
Straw		+4	+7
Concrete slats		−5	−9
Wet concrete slats		−5 − −10	−9 − −18
Air-to-wall temperature gradient:			
13°C (23°F)		−7	−13
3°C (5°F)		−1.5	−3
1°C (2°F)		−0.5	−1

An explosive onset of diarrhea and rapid spread are usually associated with a viral etiology. An insidious onset, slow spread, and gradual increase in severity over time tend to be seen with bacterial or parasitic disease.

Knowledge of the vaccination status of the herd and previous exposure to infectious disease assists in diagnosis. Diseases such as enzootic TGE, coccidiosis, RE, colibacillosis, and CE are difficult to eliminate once they have become a problem in the herd; and they may still contribute to diarrhea even when control measures are being used. In a herd chronically infected with one of the above diseases, the means of implementing control measures should be reviewed to determine if failure to adequately carry out preventive programs (vaccination or medication) has allowed disease to reoccur.

The age at which pigs are first affected with diarrhea is an indication of the cause (Table 11.1). Diarrhea that occurs on the first or second day after birth is likely to be caused by colibacillosis, hypoglycemia, or CE. Coccidial scours first occur at 5–7 days of age. Diarrhea caused by enzootic TGE, RE, SD, salmonellosis, and erysipelas usually occurs after the first week of life. In addition to appearing during the first few days of life, diarrhea from *Escherichia coli* and agalactia is commonly seen at 3 weeks of age. Sometimes rather than diarrhea that starts at a certain age, there will be a wide range of ages affected simultaneously. An acute onset of severe diarrhea that affects all ages of piglets over 24 hours of age is typical of epizootic TGE and PR. Less severe diarrhea that has no clear time of onset and affects piglets of all ages can be produced by colibacillosis and RE.

Usually when diarrhea occurs in baby pigs, the entire

litter is affected. This occurs because for most infectious diseases either the sow is immune and able to supply sufficient antibodies to the piglets through the milk or the sow is not immune and lacks lactogenic antibodies. CE is an exception since it may affect only a few pigs in the litter and these are usually the biggest and healthiest. Hypoglycemia can also produce disease in only a few pigs in the litter, usually the smallest.

Fecal pH has been used to help differentiate between causes of diarrhea. Fecal materials to be tested should be obtained from several affected piglets by applying pressure to their abdomens, not by collecting fecal material from the floor. Diseases that cause moderate to severe villous atrophy (TGE and RE) produce diarrhea with an acid pH. Other enteric diseases cause diarrhea in which feces are alkaline.

Often, the first sign of diarrhea noticed is dehydration in which the bony prominences are clearly seen and the skin is dry, bluish in color, said to resemble parchment, and remains tented after being pinched between thumb and finger.

Sows tend not to be affected by most disease agents that cause enteritis in their piglets. This general rule is not applicable in cases of piglet hypoglycemia caused by agalactia in the sow and in epizootic TGE and PR, in which sows become sick and may vomit or have diarrhea.

Rare causes of diarrhea in baby pigs include infection with Bacteroides fragilis, Enterococcus durans, and Chlamydia sp.

Noninfectious Contributing Factors (Table 11.2). Two major contributors to baby pig diarrhea are effective environmental temperature (EET) and availability of milk.

The baby pigs' lower critical temperature (LCT)—the temperature below which they must utilize extra energy to maintain their body temperature—is 90°F (33°C). The LCT for recently weaned pigs is about 75°F (28°C). The EET experienced by a pig is a combination of the heat transfer that occurs by radiation through the air, conduction through the floor, evaporation due to wet surfaces and humidity, and convection to walls and windows. The EET may be estimated by measuring the air temperature and adding or subtracting according to the conditions listed in Table 11.2.

Adequate amounts of milk are necessary to provide piglets with lactogenic antibodies and with energy to maintain body temperature. Any factor that limits availability of milk to piglets such as agalactia or impedances of physical access to mammary glands (bars on the farrowing crate that hinder nursing, slippery floors) contributes to the severity of clinical disease.

Baby pig diarrhea is more likely to develop in some environments than in others. Continuous farrowing operations are predisposed to colibacillosis and enzootic TGE. Colibacillosis is found most often where management and sanitation are poor. Within herds affected by colibacillosis, litters of gilts are more often affected than those of sows. In addition to a continuous farrowing schedule, frequent additions of pigs from outside sources is a common practice on farms with enzootic TGE.

Necropsy (Table 11.4). Three areas deserve close attention in the necropsy of pigs with diarrhea. First, examine the lacteals in the mesentery; the presence or absence of fat there reflects the ability of the disease to cause villous atrophy and diminish absorptive capacity of the small intestine. The absence of fat in the lacteals is a prominent finding with TGE and is a variable finding in RE. Colibacillosis does not interfere with the ability of the intestine to absorb fat. Absence of fat in the lacteals also occurs when the pig is not nursing. Milk or a milk curd in the stomach provides evidence that the pig was nursing and makes hypoglycemia unlikely. The second area to examine is the serosal surface of the intestine for reddening (clostridial infection) or transparency (TGE). The mucosal surface is the third area that should be closely examined for signs of petechial or frank hemorrhage (CE, salmonellosis) and a fibrinonecrotic membrane that may be diphtheritic (coccidiosis, chronic CE) or hemorrhagic (acute CE, SD).

Weaned Pigs to Adults (Tables 11.1, 11.5, 11.6). Diarrhea in older pigs may be the only sign of disease or part of a disease syndrome with other signs. The clinician should determine what signs exist, if disease is systemic or confined to the gastrointestinal system, and whether it is likely to involve the large or small intestine or both. Necropsy is similar to that for small pigs.

Loose stools are sometimes seen in pigs a few days to a week after weaning, when pigs have a hypersensitivity to the soybean meal in the diet. *Cryptosporidia* rarely produces diarrhea in weaned pigs.

Vomiting

Vomiting is the ejection of stomach contents through the mouth and should be differentiated from regurgitation, in which food is swallowed, does not reach the stomach, and is ejected through the mouth. If there is any question of whether vomiting or regurgitation is occurring, it may be settled by measuring the pH of the ejected material. Vomitus has an acid pH and regurgitated material is alkaline. In pigs, the act of vomiting may have been observed or the vomitus seen on the floor of the pen.

Unweaned Pigs (Table 11.7). Vomiting is a prominent clinical sign of hemagglutinating encephalomyelitis, porcine epidemic diarrhea, and TGE. Vomiting can also be seen with RE, PR, hog cholera (HC), African swine fever (ASF), and rarely in enteric colibacillosis. Diseases that feature vomiting in baby pigs usually have a viral etiology. Determination of the cause of vomiting in baby pigs is best accomplished by identifying the major system involved and then differentiating between diseases that affect that system.

Table 11.3. Diseases that cause diarrhea in unweaned pigs

Disease	Age When Signs Occur	Morbidity	Mortality	Season	Other Signs in Piglets	Appearance of Diarrhea	Signs in Other Pigs	Onset and Course	Associated Factors
Colibacillosis	Anytime, but see a peak of infection at 1–4 days and 3 weeks of age.	Variable, usually moderate. Typically all of one litter is affected, but nearby litters can be normal.	Variable, moderate.	Any but winter if chilled piglets, summer if agalactia.	Dehydration. Pasty peritoneum. Tail may necrose.	Yellowish white, watery with gas, fetid odor, pH 7.0–8.0.	Sows not affected. Litters of gilts often worse than litters of sows.	Gradual onset and slow spread through the room. Severity worsens toward the end of the farrowing group.	Often associated with poor management, dirty environment, and suboptimal environmental temperatures.
Epizootic transmissible gastroenteritis	Any age over 1 day and all ages at once.	Near 100%.	Near 100% in pigs under 1 week old. Near 0% in pigs over 4 weeks old.	Cold months, November to April.	Vomiting, dehydration.	Yellow-white (possibly greenish), watery, characteristic odor, pH 6.0–7.0	Sows anorexic, may vomit, loose feces, agalactia, rapid spread to other swine.	Explosive, all litters affected at once.	
Enzootic transmissible gastroenteritis	6 days and older.	Moderate, 10–50%.	Low, 0–20%	None.	Vomiting, dehydration.	Yellow-white (possibly greenish), watery, characteristic odor, pH 6.0–7.0	Sows usually not sick. Nursery pigs may have diarrhea.	Litters affected sporadically. Chronic low level.	Frequent additions of pigs and continuous farrowing. Very large farms.
Coccidiosis	Not in pigs under 5 days old. Usually 6–15 (especially at 7) days of age.	Variable, up to 75%.	Usually low.	Peaks in August and September.	Gaunt, rough hair coat. Lower weight at weaning.	Pasty to profuse, watery, yellow-gray, fetid, pH 7.0–8.0. Some pigs with diarrhea, others may have "sheep pellet" feces.	Sows normal.	Slow spread and gradual buildup.	Solid floors.
Rotaviral enteritis	1–5 weeks old.	Variable, up to 75%.	Low, 5–20%.		Occasionally will vomit, gaunt, rough hair coat.	Watery, pasty with yellow curdlike material, pH 6.0–7.0.	Sows rarely sick.	Epizootic: abrupt onset and rapid spread. Enzootic: like TGE.	

(continued)

Table 11.3. Diseases that cause diarrhea in unweaned pigs (*continued*)

Disease	Age When Signs Occur	Morbidity	Mortality	Season	Other Signs in Piglets	Appearance of Diarrhea	Signs in Other Pigs	Onset and Course	Associated Factors
Clostridium perfringens type C or A: PA: Peracute A: Acute SA: Subacute C: Chronic	Typically 1–7 days old. PA: 1 day A: 3 days SA: 5–7 days C:10–14 days	1–4 pigs per litter showing signs. Often the biggest, healthiest piglets are affected.	Nearly 100% of acutely affected pigs. Higher survival if chronic.		PA: Paddling, prostration, occasional vomiting. SA, C: emaciation, rough hair coat.	PA: watery, yellow to bloody; A:reddish brown liquid feces; SA: nonhemorrhagic, watery, yellow-gray; C: yellow-gray, mucoid.	Sows normal.	Slow spread throughout the farrowing room. All four forms may be seen at same time in different litters.	First outbreak often seen after addition of new pigs.
Clostridium difficile	Typically 1–7 days old	10–90%. Often 2/3 of litters and 1/3 of pigs.	Up to 50%. Typically 20%.	None.	Sudden death, with no clinical signs, sometimes dyspnea, mild abdominal distension and scrotal edema.	Pasty yellow to watery.	Sows normal		Treatment at birth with antibiotics
Strongyloides	4–10 days old.		Up to 50%.		Dyspnea, CNS signs.		Sows normal.		Southern states.
Swine dysentery	7 days and older. Especially at 2 weeks of age.	Sporadic by litters.	Low.	Late summer and fall.	No dehydration.	Watery with blood and mucus, yellow-gray.	Sows normal. Older pigs may have diarrhea.		First outbreak often seen after addition of new pigs.
Salmonellosis	3 weeks of age.				Septicemia.	Mucohemorrhagic.			
Erysipelas	Usually over 1 week of age.	Entire litter. Sporadic.	Moderate to High.			Watery.			Sows not vaccinated.
Epizootic pseudorabies	Any age. More severe in younger piglets.	High, up to 100%.	High, 50–100%.	Winter.	Dull, salivate, vomit, dyspnea. ataxia, CNS signs.		CNS signs, abortion.	Explosive outbreak in previously uninfected herd.	
Hypoglycemia (agalactia)	Postpartum agalactia, 1–3 days; inadequate underline, 2–3 weeks.	Variable, 5–15% of litters.	High in affected litters.		Weak, inactive, hypothermia, CNS signs.	Watery.	Sow agalactia, anorexia, mastitis, inverted nipples.		Slick floor, improper crate design or adjustment, failure to remove eyeteeth.
Toxoplasmosis	Any age.	Variable.	Variable.		Dyspnea, CNS signs.	Watery.	Sows normal.		
Porcine epidemic diarrhea	Any age.	Variable, but often high.	Moderate to high.		Vomiting, dehydration.	Watery.	Older pigs may have more severe signs.	Explosive onset and rapid course.	

Table 11.4. Necropsy findings in unweaned pigs with diarrhea

Disease	Gross Necropsy Findings	Microscopic	Diagnosis
Colibacillosis	Stomach is often full, lacteals contain fat, congestion in intestine present or absent, slight edema of intestinal wall, intestine distended with fluid, mucus, and gas.	No lesions.	Demonstration of *E. coli* adhering to the intestinal wall. Culture of 10^4 colonies/mL from the small intestine. Demonstration of the toxin.
Transmissible gastroenteritis	No fat in lacteals, yellow fluid and gas in intestine, congested intestinal vessels, thin-walled small intestine, hemorrhage in stomach wall, stomach contents: first 2–3 days, milk; next 4–5 days, green mucin.	Severe villous atrophy in jejunum and ileum. Possible nephrosis.	Fluorescent antibody test on small intestine. Direct electron microscopic examination of intestinal contents. Isolation of virus.
Coccidiosis	Fibrinonecrotic, diphtheritic membrane, especially in jejunum and ileum. No lesions in large intestine.	Mild to severe villous atrophy, fibrinonecrotic membrane.	Mucosal smear of jejunum or ileum stained with Wright's, Giemsa, or New Methylene Blue for merozoites.
Rotaviral enteritis	Milk or curd in stomach, thin-walled intestines filled with fluid, colon and cecum distended, variable fat in the lacteals.	Moderate villous atrophy in jejunum and ileum.	Fluorescent antibody test on small intestine. Direct electron microscopic examination of gut contents. Virus isolation.
Clostridium perfringens type C or A	Lesions found in the jejunum and ileum. Peracute: hemorrhage in intestinal wall, bloody fluid in lumen, serosanguinous peritoneal fluid, hemorrhagic peritoneal lymph nodes. Acute: jejunal wall, thickening and necrosis of emphysema of mucosa, necrotic membrane. Subacute and chronic: less hemorrhage and thicker membrane.	Hemorrhage throughout wall of gut, mucosal necrosis, presence of gram-positive rods.	Stained mucosal smear and observation of gram-positive rods. Histopathology. Culture of organism and identification of toxin.
Clostridium difficile	Mesocolonic edema	Colon lesions: supporative foci In lamina propria, segmental mecosal erosion, presense of large gram-positive rods.	Isolation of organism. Presence of toxins A and B.
Strongyloides	Petechial hemorrhage in intestinal mucosa. Occasionally hemorrhage in the lungs.		Eggs in feces.
Swine dysentery	Lesions limited to large-intestinal wall are hyperemic and edematous, mild ascites, mucofibrinous, hemorrhagic mucosa, often with pseudomembrane.	Superficial necrosis and hemorrhage.	Culture. Histopathology.
Salmonellosis	Catarrhal to hemorrhagic to necrotic enteritis throughout gastrointestinal tract. Hemorrhage and necrosis in parenchymal organs and lymph nodes. Focal necrotic areas in liver. Diffuse or focal ulcers of gastrointestinal tract.	Intestinal mucosal ulceration. Necrotic foci in liver and spleen.	Culture. Histopathology.
Hypoglycemia	Empty stomach, no fat in lacteals.	No lesions.	Typical signs, absence of disease agents.
Pseudorabies	Necrotic tonsillitis, pharyngitis. Necrotic foci in the liver and spleen. Pulmonary congestion.	Nonsuppurative meningoencephalitis, perivascular cuffing.	Virus isolation from frozen tonsil and brain. Fluorescent antibody of chilled tonsils and brain. Serum antibodies.
Toxoplasmosis	Intestinal ulceration. Necrotic foci in any organ. Lymphadenitis.	Focal necrotic areas.	Histology and demonstration of organism. Serology.

Table 11.5. Diseases of recently weaned and older pigs with diarrhea as the main clinical sign

Blood	Site of Lesions	Possible Causes	Further Differentiation
Diarrhea not bloody	Small intestine.	Transmissible gastroenteritis. Rotaviral diarrhea. Lawsonia-related enteropathies (porcine intestinal adenomatosis [PIA]). Porcine epidemic diarrhea.	Fluorescent antibody test. Direct electron microscopy. Histopathology. Paired serology.
	Large intestine.	*Salmonella enterocolitis. Oesophagostomum* spp.	Bacterial culture. Fecal analysis.
	Both large and small intestine.	Tricothecene toxin.	Feed assay.
	No gross lesions.	Colibacillosis. Lincomycin or tylosin. Soybean meal hypersensitivity. Early sign of edema disease prior to neurologic signs. Acute leptospirosis.	Bacterial culture. History.
Bloody diarrhea, melena	Stomach.	Gastric ulceration.	Blood in feces is black and tarry. Necropsy.
	Large intestine, colon.	Swine dysentery. *Trichuris suis. Salmonella enterocolitis.*	Blood in feces is fresh and red. Histopathology. Fecal assay. Bacterial culture.
	Both large and small intestine.	Proliferative hemorrhagic enteropathy. Tricothecene toxin. Intestinal anthrax.	Histopathology. Feed assay.

Note: Minimal other signs of gastrointestinal tract disease such as vomiting, anorexia, or colic may be present. No signs referable to other systems.

Table 11.6. Diseases of recently weaned and older pigs with diarrhea as part of a clinical syndrome that primarily involves signs referable to systems other than the gastrointestinal tract

Blood	Clinical Signs	Possible Causes	Further Differentiation
Diarrhea not bloody	Reluctance to rise, fever, anorexia, depression, skin discoloration.	Septicemic salmonellosis. Hog cholera. African swine fever.	Bacterial culture. Fluorescent antibody test. Serology.
	Respiratory signs, coughing.	*Ascaris suum.* Just prior to the onset of acute *A. pleuropneumoniae.*	Milk spot liver. Culture of lung.
	Polyuria, polydipsia, dehydration.	Ochratoxin.	Feed assay.
	Increased respiratory rate, dyspnea, ataxia, tremors to convulsions.	Overdose of levamisole, dimetridazole, piperazine. Acute toxoplasmosis.	History of treatment. Histopathology. Mouse inoculation. Serology.
	Wasting, ill-thrift.	Porcine intestinal adenomatosis.	Histopathology.
Bloody diarrhea, melena	Lameness, reluctance to move, anemia.	Warfarin toxicity.	History of access. Stomach contents analysis.
	Wasting, ill-thrift.	Gastric ulceration. Proliferative hemorrhagic enteropathy.	Necropsy. Histopathology.
	Depression, prostrate, fever, anorexia, dyspnea, hyperemia.	Terminal stage of African swine fever.	Fluorescent antibody test. Serology

Table 11.7. Diseases that cause vomiting in unweaned pigs

Disease	Ages Affected	Prominence of Vomition	Primary System Affected[a]	Other Signs	Signs in Sow
Hemagglutinating encephalomyelitis (HEV): encephalitic form	4–14 days old.	Prominent.	Nervous.	Lethargy, huddling, constipation, cyanosis, cough, grinding of teeth, stilted gait, squeal and paddle when handled, posterior paresis, convulsions.	None.
HEV: vomiting and wasting disease	4–14 days old.	Prominent.	Systemic disease.	Thirsty but unable to drink, unthrifty, may have diarrhea, then constipation.	None.
Transmissible gastroenteritis	All ages, younger pigs more severe.	Prominent.	Gastrointestinal.	Profuse, watery diarrhea.	Normal or anorexia, vomit, diarrhea.
Porcine epidemic diarrhea	All ages, younger pigs more severe.	Prominent.	Gastrointestinal.	Profuse, watery diarrhea.	Normal or anorexia, vomit, diarrhea.
Pseudorabies	All ages, younger pigs more severe.	Seen with moderate frequency.	Nervous.	Dyspnea, hypersalivation, diarrhea, trembling, CNS signs, seizures.	Normal or cough, anorexia, constipated, neurologic signs.
Rotaviral enteritis	Uncommon in nursing pigs.	Occasional.	Gastrointestinal.	Watery diarrhea.	None.
Hog cholera	All ages.	Seen with moderate frequency.	Systemic disease.	Lethargy, cyanosis, fever, diarrhea, hemorrhages.	Similar to signs in piglets.
African swine fever	All ages.	Seen with moderate frequency.	Systemic disease.	Lethargy, cyanosis, fever, diarrhea, hemorrhages.	Similar to signs in piglets.

[a]For further differentiation, consult the sections dealing with neurologic, systemic, and gastrointestinal disease.

Weaned Pigs and Adults (Tables 11.8–11.9). Vomiting in older pigs is also frequently associated with viral infection. It also may result from toxins or agents that produce local irritation to the gastrointestinal tract. Usually it is accompanied by other signs that are helpful in making a diagnosis.

Rectal Prolapse
See Table 11.10.

RESPIRATORY SYSTEM

Dyspnea and Cough
Unweaned Pigs (Table 11.11). Labored respiration in baby pigs is generally due to anemia or pneumonia, especially associated with porcine reproductive and respiratory syndrome (PRRS). PR and toxoplasmosis infection can also produce signs of respiratory distress.

In newborns and nursing piglets, PRRS infection produces respiratory distress, thumping, mouth breathing, listlessness, and fading piglet syndrome. Respiratory signs in piglets are more common when the herd is initially infected with PRRS but may also be seen in chronically infected herds experiencing a recurrence of disease.

Anemia causes labored respiration in unweaned pigs. Iron deficiency anemia develops gradually, with signs beginning to be noticeable at about 1.5–2 weeks of age and becoming more severe in older pigs.

Bacterial pneumonias are more rarely seen in baby pigs but when present may cause signs as early as 3 days of age. Coughing is a prominent sign of pneumonia, but it is absent with anemia. Anemic pigs are noticeably pale compared to pneumonic pigs. On necropsy, anemic pigs have an enlarged heart with excess pericardial fluid, an enlarged spleen, and edema in the lung, but no other pulmonary lesions. Bacterial pneumonia in baby pigs may be due to *Actinobacillus, Pasteurella, Bordetella,* or *Streptococci* organisms and these agents should be differentiated in the same way as for older pigs (see Table 11.12). *Bordetella bronchiseptica* can cause a bronchopneumonia in young pigs that has a patchy distribution predominant in the apical and cardiac lobes but also in the dorsal aspects of the lungs.

The respiratory signs caused by PR, toxoplasmosis, HC, and ASF are usually secondary to other signs of systemic or neurologic disease.

Weaned Pigs and Adults (Table 11.12). Most respiratory problems in weaned and growing pigs are due to parasitic, bacterial, or viral invasion of the lungs. In sows, respiratory problems are more commonly caused by anemia or conditions that result in a great increase in

Table 11.8. Diseases that cause vomiting in weaned pigs and adults

Disease	Ages Affected	Prominence of Vomition	Primary System Affected[a]	Nursery Pigs	Other Signs Growing Pigs	Adults
Transmissible gastroenteritis	All ages. More severe in younger pigs.	Moderate in younger pigs and occasional in older pigs.	Gastrointestinal.	Watery diarrhea, dehydration, anorexia lasting up to 1 week.	Inappetence and diarrhea for 1 or a few days.	Brief anorexia, mild diarrhea. Lactating sows may have agalactia, diarrhea.
Porcine epidemic diarrhea	All ages. More severe in younger pigs.	Moderate in younger pigs and occasional in older pigs.	Gastrointestinal.	Watery diarrhea for 4–6 days, dehydration.	Depression and anorexia, watery diarrhea.	Anorexia.
Pseudorabies	All ages. More severe in younger pigs.	Occasionally seen.	Nervous.	CNS signs.	Sneezing, coughing, anorexia, constipation, occasional neurologic signs, pregnant sows may abort.	
Rotaviral enteritis	Nursery pigs, especially after weaning.	Occasionally seen.	Gastrointestinal.	Diarrhea, dehydration.	Not usually a clinical problem at this age.	
Vomitoxin, T-2, diacetoxyscirpenol	All ages.	Moderately frequent.	Gastrointestinal.	Anemia, diarrhea (possibly bloody), ill-thrift, slowed growth rate, occasional feed refusal.		
Hog cholera	All ages.	Moderately frequent.	Systemic disease.	Lethargy, anorexia, ocular discharge, constipation, then diarrhea, weaving, staggering, huddling, posterior paresis, cyanosis, abortion.		
African swine fever	All ages.	Occasionally seen.	Systemic disease.	Lethargy, hyperemia, dyspnea, mucoid to bloody diarrhea, abortion.		
Peracute *Actinobacillus pleuropneumoniae*	All ages, but outbreaks usually in finishing pigs.	Occasionally seen.	Respiratory.	Dyspnea, cough, blood-tinged fluid from the nose and mouth, cyanosis.		
Anthrax: Pharyngeal	All ages.	Moderately frequent.	Systemic disease.	Cervical edema, dyspnea, depression.		
Intestinal	All ages.	Moderately frequent.	Systemic disease.	Anorexia, bloody diarrhea.		
Strongyloides	Weaned to finishing pigs.	Occasionally seen.	Gastrointestinal.	Diarrhea, rapid emaciation, anorexia, anemia.		
Gastric ulcers	Finishing pigs and adults.	Occasionally seen.	Gastrointestinal.	Uncommon.	Anemia, tarry feces, grinding of teeth, weight loss.	
Hairballs, foreign bodies	Finishing pigs and adults.	Occasionally seen.	Gastrointestinal.	Uncommon.	Drop feeding systems that place feed on pigs' backs.	
Thiamin deficiency	Usually only experimental.	Moderately frequent.	Systemic disease.	Anorexia, slow growth, diarrhea, cyanosis.		
Riboflavin deficiency	Usually only experimental.	Moderately frequent.	Systemic disease.	Slow growth; cataracts; stiff gait; scaling, eruption, ulceration, and alopecia of skin.		
Other toxicities (See Table 11.9.)						

[a]For further differentiation, consult the sections dealing with neurologic, systemic, and gastrointestinal disease.

Table 11.9. Toxicities associated with vomiting

Toxin	System Affected	Seen in Pigs with Access to:
Inorganic arsenicals	Gastrointestinal and central nervous.	Ant bait, herbicides, insecticides.
Antimony	Gastrointestinal.	Alloys, paint, tartar emetic.
Cadmium	Gastrointestinal.	Paint, solder, batteries, fungicides.
Fluorine	Gastrointestinal and locomotor.	Water or forage contaminated with industrial waste.
Levamisole	Gastrointestinal and central nervous.	Anthelmintic.
Piperazine	Gastrointestinal.	Anthelmintic.
Organophosphates, carbamates	Neurologic.	Insecticides.
Carbadox	Gastrointestinal.	Swine dysentery treatment.
Ethylene glycol	Neurologic.	Antifreeze.
Solanum nigrum	Gastrointestinal and central nervous.	Nightshade in woods or permanent pastures.

Table 11.10. Causes of rectal prolapse

Cause	Comments
Diarrhea	Abnormally acid stool in the rectum causes irritation, tenesmus, and prolapse. Refer to the section on diarrhea for differentiation between causes of diarrhea.
Cough	Increased abdominal pressure generated during coughing (especially chronic prolonged bouts) causes displacement of the rectum. Refer to the section on cough for differentiation between causes of cough.
Piling	Environmental temperatures too low. Abdominal pressure on the pig at the bottom of the pile produces prolapse.
Zearalenone	Estrogens cause swelling of perineal area, tenesmus, and prolapse.
Floor design	Excessively sloped floors for crated sows causes increased pressure on pelvic structures as pregnancy progresses.
Antibiotics	Rectal prolapse has been reported in pigs in the first few weeks after lincomycin or tylosin has been added to the feed. Prolapses cease later as pigs apparently become accustomed to the antibiotic.
Inherited predisposition	Sporadic reports in the literature of herd outbreaks that occurred in the offspring of certain boars.
Postpartum	Complex etiology surrounding farrowing.
Prepartum	Constipation and pressure of heavily gravid uterus.
Any condition that is associated with tenesmus	Urethritis, vaginitis, rectal or urethral injury postbreeding, urethral calculi. Excess salt in the diet.

Table 11.11. Diseases that cause respiratory distress and cough in unweaned pigs

Disease	Ages Affected	Signs	Necropsy Findings
Iron deficiency anemia	1.5–2 weeks and older.	Pale pigs with normal temperature. Easily exhausted by exertion. Rapid respiratory rate, rough hair coat.	Dilated heart with excess pericardial fluid, lung edema, enlarged spleen.
Porcine reproductive and respiratory syndrome	Any age.	Respiratory distress, open-mouth breathing, fever, palpebral edema. Fading-piglet syndrome.	Mottled-tan, multifocal-to-diffuse pneumonia, enlarged edematous thoracic lymph nodes.
Bordetella bronchiseptica pneumonia	3 days and older.	Coughing, debilitation, rapid respiration, high mortality in affected pigs.	Patchy distribution of pneumonic lesions throughout the lung.
Bacterial pneumonia: *H. parasuis, P. multocida, A. pleuropneumoniae,* or *M. hyopneumoniae, A. suis*	1 week and older.	Dyspnea, cough.	Varies with organism. Often hemorrhage and fibrin.
Pseudorabies	Any age.	Respiratory distress, fever, salivation, vomiting, diarrhea, neurologic signs, high mortality.	Pneumonia, intestinal ulceration, hepatomegaly, white necrotic foci in any organ.
Toxoplasmosis	Any age.	Respiratory distress, fever, diarrhea, neurologic signs.	Pneumonia, intestinal ulceration, hepatomegaly, white necrotic foci in any organ.
Barking-piglet syndrome	Apparent at birth.	Immature domed heads; sparse, erect hair coat; grunting noise produced during attempts to breathe.	Small thyroid, inadequate lung expansion.
Streptococcus spp.	1 week and older.	Dyspnea, cough.	Fibrinous pneumonia.

body temperature. If infectious agents are involved, they tend to be viruses, except in cases where new adult animals have been introduced onto a farm that is infected with a bacteria (especially *A. pleuropneumoniae*) to which they lack previous exposure.

Sneezing

Unweaned Pigs (Table 11.13). Sneezing in piglets can be caused by atrophic rhinitis (AR), porcine cytomegalovirus (PCMV) infection, PRRS, hemagglutinating encephalomyelitis virus infection (encephalitic form), PR infection, or environmental contaminants such as dust, ammonia, or other noxious gases.

AR caused by *Pasteurella multocida, B. bronchiseptica,* and possibly other organisms is by far the most common cause of sneezing in unweaned pigs. AR seldom causes sneezing in pigs that are less than a week old but produces increasing frequencies as pigs approach weaning. Except for nasal discharge and tear staining, AR produces few clinical signs. Piglets are generally in good health otherwise and do not experience higher mortality. On necropsy, lesions are confined to the nose and may include a serous to purulent or blood-tinged exudate, along with turbinate atrophy and nasal septum deviation.

PCMV infection is most severe in newborn pigs. Infection in pigs older than 3 weeks is usually without clinical signs. In addition to sneezing, affected piglets may show edema around the jaw or tarsal joints, shivering, anemia, and respiratory distress. Mortality may reach 25%. In sows, there may be an increase in the numbers of stillbirths and mummies. A mild rhinitis is seen at necropsy. More prominent lesions include subcutaneous edema, generalized petechiation, pericardial and pleural effusion, and enlargement of lymph nodes.

Environmental dust and concentration of ammonia greater than 25 ppm irritate the respiratory mucosa and produce excessive lacrimation, serous nasal discharge, and shallow respiration. Ammonia-induced lesions are differentiated from infectious causes by their complete remission when the pig is removed from the contaminated environment.

PRRS causes a mild rhinitis and associated sneezing which is usually most frequently seen in nursery pigs but can also occur in unweaned pigs or in growing pigs.

Sneezing can be an early sign of PR or part of the clinical picture of hemagglutinating encephalomyelitis. However, in unweaned pigs these infections progress so rapidly to central nervous system involvement that by the time the veterinarian is called, the diagnosis is made from differentials of neurologic disease.

Weaned Pigs to Adults (Table 11.14). Sneezing in older animals is primarily due to AR, PR, or environmental contaminants. Concurrent infections are not uncommon. Rarely, cytomegalovirus affects nursery or growing pigs, in which it produces an acute, severe rhinitis with stenotic breathing that rapidly resolves without treatment in a few days.

EXTERNAL BODY SURFACE

Skin (Tables 11.15–11.18)

If the practitioner is not certain of the appearance of normal pig skin, the neonatal pig should be used as a reference. Mange is so widespread in the swine population that even people who have a long history of association with swine may not recognize how smooth, flat, and unblemished the normal skin is. Changes that are within the skin proper rather than within any of the structures beneath it are covered in Tables 11.16 and 11.17. Lumps or swellings that remain stationary when the skin is moved are covered in Table 11.18. Skin lesions should be examined for color changes, proliferation, distribution, and relation of lesions to normal skin. Pigs should be observed for pruritus. Color changes in the skin without associated lesions are covered in Table 11.17.

NEUROLOGIC SYSTEM

General Signs

Neurologic disorders include diseases that cause behavioral abnormalities, ataxia, abnormal gait, incoordination, paresis, paralysis, muscular tremors, trembling, paddling, dog-sitting, opisthotonos, convulsions, deafness, blindness, nystagmus, coma, or death.

Unweaned Pigs (Table 11.19). One of the major aids in diagnosis of neurologic disease in baby pigs is the distribution of affected piglets. By observing whether disease is occurring sporadically in single pigs, only in certain litters, or across all litters, the range of diagnostic possibilities can be greatly narrowed.

Diseases that occur sporadically and at a low level include middle-ear infection, tetanus, rabies, hypoglycemia, and streptococcal infections. Generally these can be differentiated by clinical signs and necropsy, although streptococcal infections require bacterial culture for confirmation of diagnosis.

Hypoglycemia and streptococcal infections, as well as PR, congenital tremors, vitamin A deficiency, blue eye disease, and iron or organophosphate toxicity may occur in a large number of litters within the farrowing group. History and the presence of signs in the sow are primary aids to differentiating between causes.

HC and ASF cause neurologic signs in baby pigs along with other signs of systemic disease. Inherited or congenital abnormalities that produce neurologic disorders include congenital motor defect in Large White and British Saddleback pigs, Landrace trembles, and Pietrain creeper syndrome. Occasionally Japanese encephalitis causes mild neurologic disease in baby pigs.

Table 11.12. Diseases that cause dyspnea and coughing in weaned and older pigs

	Clinical Signs	Associated Agents
Weaned to growing-finishing pigs	Signs primarily referable to respiratory tract. Dyspnea, cough, anorexia, fever, abdominal respiration, varying severities of clinical signs in an affected group of pigs.	*Mycoplasma hyopneumoniae, Actinobacillus pleuropneumoniae, Salmonella choleraesuis,Bordetella bronchiseptica, pseudorabies,* blue eye disease, *Mycoplasma hyorhinis, Pasteurella multocida, Haemophilus parasuis, Streptococcus suis, Streptococcus* spp., *Staphylococcus* spp., *Klebsiella* spp., *Moraxella* spp., *Corynebacterium* spp., *Fusiformis* spp.
		Porcine reproductive and respiratory syndrome virus. Swine Influenza virus.
	Rapid clinical course, fever, anorexia, depression, severe dyspnea, open-mouth breathing, cyanosis, foamy blood-tinged discharge from nose and mouth.	*Actinobacillus pleuropneumoniae.*
	Coughing with minimal other signs.	*Ascaris suum.*
		Metastrongylus spp.
	No coughing, but dyspnea and cyanosis, depression, fever, anorexia, and reluctance to move, lameness, stiff gait, swollen joints, ataxia, convulsions.	*Haemophilus parasuis, Mycoplasma hyorhinis, Streptococcus suis.*
	Very acute onset, near 100% morbidity, extreme prostration, complete anorexia, labored jerky respiration, hard paroxysmal cough, fever.	Swine influenza.
	Signs of systemic disease, sneezing, coughing, dyspnea, fever, anorexia, vomiting, constipation initially, then diarrhea, possibly tremors, ataxia, and convulsions.	Hog cholera, African swine fever.
		Pseudorabies.
	Rapid or abdominal respiration, moist nonproductive cough if present, pale.	See Table 11.29 on causes of anemia.
	Rapid, panting respiration, no cough, open-mouth breathing, gasping, extremely high temperature.	Porcine stress syndrome, heat prostration, puffer sow syndrome.
Adults	Rapid or abdominal respiration, moist nonproductive cough, subcutaneous edema, enlarged abdomen.	Cardiac insufficiency.
	Dyspnea, abdominal breathing.	Diaphragmatic hernia caused by selenium deficiency, trauma, or genetics.
	Dyspnea.	Fumonisin.

Necropsy	Diagnosis
Usually anterioventral distribution of lesions. Firm areas of tissue with variable intralobular edema. Fibrinous pleuritis suggests involvement with *A. pleuropneumoniae, H. parasuis, P. multocida, M. hyorhinis,* or *S. choleraesuis.*	Culture of organism. Fluorescent antibody test for *M. hyopneumoniae.* Serology for pseudorabies.
Tan to mottled interstitial pneumonia. Enlarged, edematous tan-colored lymph nodes.	Virus isolation. Serology. Immunoperoxidase, polymerase chain reaction.
Acute hemorrhagic necrosis distributed throughout the lungs, especially dorsally in the diaphragmatic lobes. Fibrinous pleurisy, some blood-tinged fluid in the pleural cavity. Bloody foam in the trachea.	Isolation of organism. Serology. Pathology.
Areas of atelectasis, hemorrhage, edema, and emphysema in lungs. Septal and periseptal hemorrhage and necrosis in the liver.	Fecal examination for eggs (may be negative early). Necropsy findings. History of access to soil(absolute requirement for *Metastrongylus*).
Bronchitis, bronchiolitis in posterioventral margins of the diaphragmatic lobes. Areas of atelectasis.	
Fibrinous to serofibrinous pleuritis, pericarditis, arthritis, and meningitis.	Isolation of organism.
Often there is no opportunity to do a necropsy since death due to uncomplicated swine influenza is rare. Tenacious mucus in pharynx, larynx, trachea, and bronchi. Depressed deep purple areas in lung.	Physical examination. Serology. Virus isolation from pharyngeal swab.
Edematous tissue, swollen edematous lymph nodes with mottled hemorrhage, petechial or ecchymotic hemorrhage in bladder and kidneys, enlarged liver and spleen, splenic infarcts.	Hog cholera: fluorescent antibody test. African swine fever: fluorescent antibody test.
Few gross lesions, necrotic tonsillitis and pharyngitis, small white necrotic foci in liver.	Virus isolation or fluorescent antibody test on tonsil. Serology.
Pale musculature, lung edema, dilated heart, excess pericardial fluid, contracted spleen.	Packed-cell volume: 15–20%. Hemoglobin concentration: 6–7 g/dL.
Areas of pale, soft, or exudative muscle. Edema and congestion of lungs. Rapid autolysis.	Creatine kinase. Physical examination.
Enlarged, dilated heart, valvular endocarditis, pulmonary edema, enlarged liver.	Necropsy.
Viscera in thoracic cavity.	Necropsy. Selenium level in liver.
Marked pulmonary edema and serous pleural effusions.	Necropsy. Feed analysis.

Table 11.13. Diseases that cause sneezing in unweaned pigs

Disease	Ages Affected	Associated Signs	Signs in Other Pigs	Necropsy Findings	Diagnosis
Atrophic rhinitis	Signs not usually seen in pigs less than 1 week old. Sneezing occurs more often as pigs near weaning.	Tear stains below the eyes, nasal discharge.	Older pigs may sneeze or have tear-stained eyes and distortion of snout.	Turbinate atrophy, nasal septum deviation, serous to purulent nasal exudate.	Typical necropsy findings. Nasal culture and isolation of toxigenic Pasteurella multocida.
Porcine cytomegalovirus infection	Most severe signs in pigs less than 1 week old. Infection seldom apparent in pigs older than 3 weeks. Occasional outbreak in nursery.	Edema around the jaw and tarsal joints, petechiae, respiratory distress, mortality up to 25%.	Sows: mummification and stillbirths	Mild rhinitis, no turbinate atrophy, petechiae, subcutaneous edema, pericardial and pleural effusion, pulmonary edema, enlarged lymph nodes.	Virus isolation from the nose, lung, or kidney. Indirect fluorescent antibody test on sera of finishing pigs. Histology: inclusion bodies and cytomegaly.
Porcine reproductive and respiratory syndrome	Seen most often in nursery pigs but also in piglets and growers.	Respiratory distress, eyelid edema, poor growth.	Varies.	Mild rhinitis, no turbinate pneumonia, interstitial atrophy, enlarged tan lymph nodes.	Virus isolation. Serology. Immunoperoxidase, polymerase reaction chain.
Environmental contaminants: ammonia, dust	Any age.	Excessive tearing, shallow respiration, serous nasal discharge.	Sow may also have mild signs.	Mild inflammation of respiratory epithelium.	Measurement of dust and ammonia levels in the environment.
Pseudorabies, hemagglutinating encephalomyelitis	Sneezing is a minor sign. In young pigs, neurologic signs predominate and the section on neurologic disease should be consulted to eliminate a diagnosis of pseudorabies or hemagglutinating encephalomyelitis.				

Table 11.14. Diseases that cause sneezing in weaned and older pigs

Disease	Course and Animals Affected	Other Signs	Diagnosis
Atrophic rhinitis	Chronic. Usually see signs in nursery through finishing pigs.	Conjunctivitis, tear-stained areas below eyes, distortion of the snout, occasional epistaxis.	Necropsy: turbinate atrophy, nasal septum deviation. Nasal culture and isolation of toxigenic *Pasteurella multocida*.
Environmental contaminants: ammonia, dust	Chronic. Signs in any age pig but more frequent in younger pigs, especially if on a slatted floor with a pit or a solid floor with urine accumulation.	Excessive tearing, tear-stained areas below eyes, serous nasal discharge, shallow respiration.	Measurement of concentrations of ammonia in the environment greater than 25 ppm. Dust in the environment, especially around feeding time.
Porcine reproductive and respiratory syndrome	Chronic. Other signs of respiratory disease usually more prominent than sneezing.	Coughing, dyspnea, poor growth, mild rhinitis, no turbinate atrophy.	Virus isolation. Serology. Immunoperoxidase, polymerase chain reaction.
Enzootic pseudorabies	Chronic. May see signs to some extent in all age groups but usually worst in one age group.	Cough.	Positive serology from live animals. Necropsy: rhinitis but no turbinate atrophy.
Epizootic pseudorabies	Fairly acute onset of signs. May start in one group of pigs and then spread to others. Signs more severe in younger pigs.	Cough, anorexia, constipation, depression, CNS signs and salivation, vomiting, convulsions.	Necropsy: especially in older pigs may not see any lesions, or may see necrotic tonsillitis, rhinitis, 1–2 mm necrotic foci in liver.
Blue eye paramyxovirus	Transient sneezing and coughing.	Ataxia, swaying, and circling.	Virus isolation.

Table 11.15. Ages at which certain skin diseases are more frequently seen

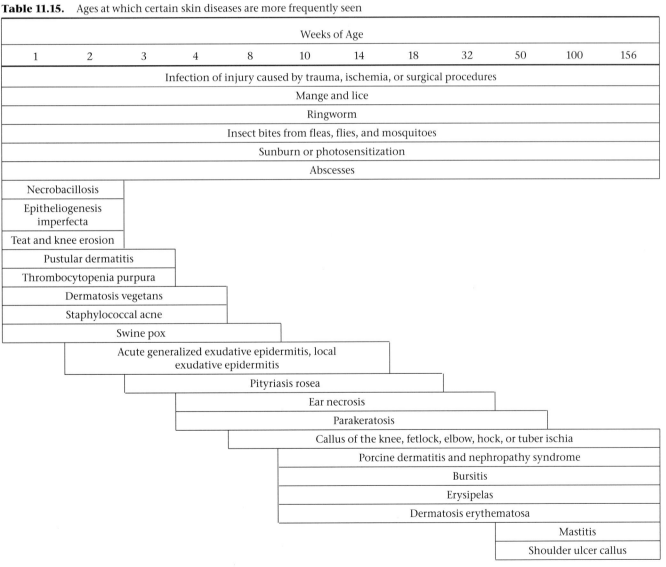

255

Table 11.16. Diseases affecting the skin of pigs

Location	Normal Tissue	Proliferative or Nonproliferative	Demarcation of Lesions	Possible Cause
Face	Elevated		Discrete	Staphylococcal acne
	Flat	Nonproliferative	Discrete	Necrotic stomatitis
Face and feet	Elevated		Discrete	Vesicular diseases[a]
Shoulder	Elevated		Discrete	Hematoma; callus
	Flat	Nonproliferative	Discrete	Ulcer
Knees, elbows, and hocks	Flat	Nonproliferative	Discrete	Knee erosions
	Elevated		Discrete	Callus
	Elevated		Diffuse	Bursitis
Ear	Elevated		Discrete	Hematoma
	Flat	Nonproliferative	Diffuse	Greasy spot behind ear
	Flat	Proliferative	Discrete	Ear necrosis
	Flat	Proliferative	Diffuse	Mange
Ear, eye, and udder	Flat	Nonproliferative	Diffuse	Photosensitization
Extremities	Flat	Nonproliferative	Diffuse	Cyanosis or reddening secondary to disease[b]
Dorsal	Elevated		Discrete	Fleas, flies, mosquitoes
	Elevated	Proliferative	Diffuse	Lumpy skin disease
	Elevated	Proliferative	Diffuse	Hyperkeratinization
	Flat	Nonproliferative	Diffuse	Sunburn
	Flat	Nonproliferative	Discrete	Epitheliogenesis imperfecta
Ventral abdomen	Elevated		Discrete	Pityriasis rosea, eosinophilic dermatitis
	Elevated		Diffuse	Urticarial mange
	Flat	Nonproliferative	Discrete	Transit erythema; teat necrosis
	Flat	Nonproliferative	Diffuse	Mastitis, benign peripartal cyanosis
Ventral cervical area	Elevated		Discrete	Jowl abscess, tuberculosis
	Elevated		Diffuse	Pharyngeal anthrax
Generalized	Elevated		Discrete	Pustular dermatitis, swine pox, infected injuries, neoplasia, abscess
	Elevated		Diffuse	Dermatosis vegetans
	Flat	Proliferative	Diffuse	Parakeratosis, demodectic mange, lice, sarcoptic mange, exudative epidermitis
	Flat	Nonproliferative	Discrete	Ringworm, dermatosis erythematosus, thrombocytopenia purpura, erysipelas
	Flat	Nonproliferative	Diffuse	Carbon monoxide toxicity, porcine stress syndrome, hypotrichosis, cyanosis or reddening secondary to any bacteremia or viremia
	Flat	Nonproliferative	Discrete	Immune complex disorder possibly associated with circovirus

[a]Foot-and-mouth disease, vesicular exanthema, vesicular stomatitis, swine vesicular disease, San Miguel sea lion virus, porcine parvovirus, drug eruption.

[b]Salmonellosis, *H. parasuis, A. pleuropneumoniae,* porcine reproductive and respiratory syndrome, colibacillosis, organophosphate toxicity, hemagglutinating encephalomyelitis.

Weaned Pigs to Adults (Tables 11.20–11.22). As with diagnosis of neurologic disease in baby pigs, a major aid is the distribution of affected animals. Disease occurrence should be identified as to whether it is sporadic or of low, medium, or high prevalence. Since toxicities are seen more frequently in older pigs, recent treatments, changes in the diet, and access to pasture or to chemicals in the pen should be investigated.

EYE AND ADNEXA

Serous Lacrimation

Ammonia in concentrations higher than 25 ppm is the most common cause of lacrimation in swine. Humans can detect ammonia at 10 ppm, so diagnosis can be made by sniffing the environment at pig level and, if ammonia is suspected, removing the pig to an area with clean air, where signs will gradually disappear. Excess tearing is also caused by organophosphate, carbamate, or iodine toxicity. Sources of organophosphates and carbamates include miscalculation of dosage used to treat animals or accidental incorporation of agricultural insecticides into animal feeds. Ethylenediamine dihydroiodide is an expectorant that may cause coughing and increased lacrimation when used in high doses for a prolonged period of time.

Mucopurulent Lacrimation and Conjunctivitis

Conjunctivitis and lacrimation are associated with AR, swine influenza (SI), HC, PR, exudative epidermitis, blue eye disease, and chlamydial and streptococcal infection. The conjunctivitis seen with AR, SI, and PR tends to be

Table 11.17. Cyanosis/hyperemia: discoloration of the skin in the absence of gross skin lesions

	Cause	Pigs Affected and Time of Occurrence	Appearance of Discolored Skin	Associated Conditions
Primary lesion is in the skin	Dermatosis erythematosus	White pigs	Red discoloration over the ears, sides, and abdomen	Possible association with clover pasture but also seen in confinement
	Benign peripartal cyanosis	Sows around the time of farrowing	Generalized cyanosis, especially on the udder and hindquarters	Seen in sows bedded on urine-soaked sawdust
	Sunburn	White pigs	Red discoloration of the dorsum and sides	Recent exposure to the sun
	Transit erythema	Warm months, white pigs	Erythema, especially of ventral areas	Contact with urine, feces, phenolic disinfectants, or lime
	Carbon monoxide toxicity	Perinatal pigs, winter	Uniform, bright red color	Incomplete combustion of fuel in the heater
	Porcine dermatitis and nephropathy syndrome	Weaned and older pigs. Usually finishers.	Multiple flat circular coalescing dark red to purplish, especially over the ham and thighs.	Possible association with circovirus
Primary lesion is in a system other than the skin	Porcine stress syndrome	Heavily muscled pigs, especially Pietrain and Landrace	Blotchy cyanosis becoming coalesced on the dependent side	Triggered by physical exercise, excitement, heat, or halothane anesthesia
	Systemic salmonellosis	Pigs 2–4 months old	Cyanotic ears, tails, ventrum, and extremities	Continuous flow operation, especially after addition of new pigs
	Mastitis	Sows postpartum	Red to purplish udder	
	Haemophilus parasuis	Nursery and grower pigs	Cyanosis of ears, tail, and extremities	Associated with systemic disease
	A. pleuropneumoniae	Growing and finishing pigs	Cyanosis of the nose, ears, and legs progressing to whole body	Associated with peracute respiratory disease
	Organophosphate or carbamate toxicity	Any age pig	Cyanosis of the extremities	Hypoxia develops secondary to increased respiratory tract secretion, bronchoconstriction, erratic slow heart beat and CNS signs
	Porcine reproductive and respiratory syndrome	Sows	Cyanosis of the extremities, blotchy dark red to purple areas over the body	Anorexia, abortion, respiratory signs in younger pigs
	Transitory change prior to onset of typical signs	Has been seen in hog cholera, African swine fever, and *Strep. suis* infections. Transitory hyperemia, especially over the snout, ears, belly, and hindquarters.		
	Terminal sign in disease	Cyanosis of extremities is seen in terminal stages of *E. coli* enteritis and hemagglutinating encephalomyelitis in baby pigs.		
	Porcine dermatitis nephropathy	Nursery to finish	Multiple flat circular coalescing dark red or purplish, especially over the ham and thighs	Possible association with circovirus

Table 11.18.   Diseases that cause lumps or swellings under the skin of pigs

Location of Lumps or Swellings	Possible Causes	Aspirate Appearance
Submandibular region	Jowl abscess (*Streptococcus* group E)	Pus with organisms
	Pharyngeal anthrax	Edema
	Tuberculosis	"Sulfur granules"
Variable distribution	Neoplasia:	Solid tissue, neoplastic cells
	lymphosarcoma	
	malignant melanomatoma	
	cavernous hemangioma	
	others	
	Arcanobacterium pyogenes	Pus with organisms
	Fusiformis necrophorus	Pus with organisms
Over the back, shoulders, thighs	Lumpy skin disease	Solid, dermal cells
Neck caudal to the ear or in the ham	Injection reaction	Pus with or without organisms
Epididymis or testicles	Brucellosis	Pus with organisms
Shoulder, flank, vulva, ear, or over the hindquarters	Hematoma	Blood or serum
Posterior aspect of the hocks, usually bilateral	Adventitious bursitis of the hocks	Synovial fluid (procedure not recommended)
Base of tail, hindquarters	Infection secondary to tail biting	Pus with organisms

fairly mild and to produce a serous to mucopurulent discharge. A more severe conjunctivitis is seen with HC, exudative epidermitis, blue eye disease, and streptococcal and chlamydial infections. In these diseases the discharge is frequently so tenacious as to cause the eyelids to adhere and blind the pig.

Palpebral Edema

Palpebral edema is frequently seen in edema disease and is not uncommon in PRRS, *Haemophilus parasuis,* and blue eye paramyxovirus infection.

Cataracts

Cataract formation has been associated with riboflavin or niacin deficiency and hygromycin toxicity.

Blindness (Table 11.23)

Blindness in pigs is seldom seen in the absence of other signs. The associated signs are usually indicative of the etiology. Two diseases that may cause blindness in the absence of other signs are PR, when blindness occurs in a pig that has recovered from the acute stage of the infection, and arsenilic acid toxicity occurring over a prolonged period of time.

SIGNS NOT REFERABLE TO ANY ONE SYSTEM

Systemic Disease (Tables 11.24, 11.25)

Occasionally pigs become ill or poor-doing without a specific predominant clinical sign. These pigs may be lethargic, depressed, anorexic, febrile, dehydrated, or prostrate with a varying amount of morbidity and mortality. Infectious disease, especially in a subclinical or chronic form, is frequently the cause.

Sudden Death (Table 11.26)

While it might be argued that death is always sudden (i.e., that the transition from living to not living always occurs in a fraction of a second), the term "sudden death" as commonly used in the field refers to the death of an otherwise normal appearing animal.

Wasting and Ill-Thrift (Table 11.27)

Wasting and ill-thrift are signs of chronic disease. Frequently the cause of ill-thrift in one pig cannot be determined even with the aid of a necropsy. This is often the case with diseases that may damage the brain, such as colibacillosis and PR. Because the lesions are microscopic, they are frequently overlooked. When there is a high percentage of poor-doers in a herd, diagnosis should include necropsies of the affected pigs, and in addition the types and levels of acute diseases in the herd should be determined. The combined findings from pigs acutely and chronically affected are most likely to provide a diagnosis.

Anemia

Anemia is the condition of having a blood hemoglobin level that is lower than normal. Minimum normal hemoglobin levels (g/100 mL) for pigs of different ages are as follows: birth, 11; 1 week, 10; 3 weeks, 10; 4 months and older, 12.

Unweaned Pigs (Table 11.28). Anemia in baby pigs is primarily due to iron deficiency. Occasionally eperythrozoonosis, and rarely umbilical hemorrhage, will produce anemic pigs. The primary features that distinguish iron deficiency, eperythrozoonosis, and umbilical hemorrhage are the ages of the affected piglets and the presence of icterus. Icterus is often prominent with eperythrozoonosis and is not seen with iron deficiency or umbilical hemorrhage. Umbilical hemorrhage occurs during the perinatal period, eperythrozoonosis tends to be seen in pigs less than 5 days of age, and iron deficiency is seen in pigs 10 days of age or older. Generally in iron deficiency anemia there is a history of failure to administer an adequate iron preparation. Umbilical hemorrhage is sometimes associated with the use of sawdust for bedding.

Porcine cytomegalovirus infection in utero may cause pigs to be born stunted, anemic, and with edema around the jaw and tarsal joints.

Anemia in baby pigs has also been reported following infestation with *Strongyloides ransomi* and *Balantidium coli*. The primary clinical signs in these pigs are anorexia, diarrhea, and reduced growth rate. Diagnosis is best made at necropsy.

Weaned Pigs to Adults (Table 11.29). Gastric ulceration and parasitism are the most common causes of anemia in weaned to adult pigs. Toxicities that cause anemia other than mycotoxins are rarely encountered clinically. However, anemia has been shown to occur after intoxication with cadmium, cobalt, coal tar, iodine, phenothiazine derivatives, and vitamin D. Nutritional deficiencies are rarely encountered in modern feeding systems, but anemia will result from deficiency of copper, folacin, protein, riboflavin, vitamin B_6, or vitamin K.

MUSCULOSKELETAL SYSTEM

Lameness is the inability to use one or more limbs in a normal fashion while generally displaying a normal degree of alertness and coordination in the other unaffected limbs. Lameness may present as reduced ability or inability to bear weight, alteration or shortening of stride, or recumbency.

Unweaned Pigs (Table 11.30). The major causes of lameness prior to weaning are trauma and infectious polyarthritis. Trauma is more common in pigs that are less than 1 week of age, and infectious polyarthritis is more frequently seen in 1- to 3-week-old pigs. Joint swelling and fever are frequent findings in polyarthritis but are only occasionally seen with trauma.

Splayleg occurs with moderate frequency and is easily recognized by its clinical signs.

Occasionally injections made into the hindleg will produce lameness due to either muscle irritation or nerve damage. In the first case the leg will be swollen and possibly hot, and the pig will tend to carry it. Damage to the sciatic nerve will produce muscle atrophy and the leg will be extended. Injection of iron creates a microenvironment in tissue that favors the growth of *Clostridium perfringens* carried in by a contaminated needle. Diagnosis of improper injection technique is aided by changing the site of the injection to the neck and observing whether lameness continues in the herd.

Arthrogryposis, syndactyly, polydactyly, and thick legs occur rarely and are easily diagnosed by their physical appearance.

Weaned Pigs to Adults (Tables 11.31, 11.32). A major portion of the lameness experienced by young pigs in the age range of 2–4 months is due to infectious polyarthritis. In pigs this age, the clinician should look for multiple sites of infection. Lameness in one leg is easily overlooked because of more severe signs in another leg. Older growing pigs and adults mainly experience lameness that results from injury, especially to the foot. The damage may be limited to the foot or may ascend into one or more joints. Floors that have abrasive, slippery, wet, dirty, or uneven surfaces, protruding sharp edges, exposed aggregate, and uneven or inappropriately sized slats for the size of the pigs predispose to lameness. The amount of competition between pigs should be evaluated when investigating lameness in older pigs. Lameness that occurs in gilts and less so in sows is likely to be due to trauma and secondary infection. Lameness in sows just after weaning may be caused by calcium or phosphorus imbalance in the ration. Osteochondrosis is another common cause of lameness in pigs in the finishing stage or in young adults.

UROGENITAL SYSTEM

Abortion, Stillbirth, and Mummies (Tables 11.33, 11.34)

Diagnosis of the cause of abortion in swine is seldom straightforward and is frequently unsuccessful. Often, the agent that produced death in the fetuses or abortion is no longer present when the problem is recognized clinically. However, there are some characteristic features that are helpful in at least determining the general class of agents likely to be involved. Two major classes exist. First are the agents that cause primary infection of the reproductive tract and that are probably responsible for 30–40% of abortions, mummies, and stillbirths. The second class (including toxins, environmental and nutritional stresses, and systemic disease in the sow) is responsible for the other 60–70%.

A primary aim in diagnosis of abortion is to differentiate between these two major classes by measuring levels of immunoglobulins in aborted fetuses. At 70 days of gestation (17 cm crown-to-rump length) swine fetuses are immunocompetent and will produce antibodies in response to contact with an infectious agent. In the normal pregnancy, the uterine environment is sterile and pigs are born without immunoglobulins. Therefore, the finding of immunoglobulins in fetuses indicates the presence of an infectious agent in the uterus. In abortions that occur in the last third of gestation, fetal serum or thoracic fluid should be collected and submitted for total immunoglobulin determination. If antibodies are present, specific serologic testing against common agents may be done (see Table 11.41).

The age of the fetuses should be determined by crown-to-rump length measurements (Table 11.33) and compared to the stage of gestation. When maternal fail-

Table 11.19. Diseases that cause neurologic signs in unweaned pigs

Disease	Proportion of Litters	Proportion of Affected Piglets within a Litter	Mortality	Age at Onset	Signs in Sow	Signs	Necropsy Findings	Diagnosis
Hypoglycemia	Sporadic.	May be 1 or 2 in a litter if more pigs than teats, or whole litter if sow agalactic.	High, 90–100% of affected pigs.	Usually 2–3 days but can be any age.	May be off feed, not milking, in sternal recumbency.	Ataxia, sternal or lateral recumbency, convulsions, paddling of the forelegs, gasping and chomping of the jaws, bradycardia, subnormal temperature.	No food in the stomach. Absence of body fat, mahogany brown muscles.	Blood glucose less than 50 mg/100 mL, necropsy findings, evidence of lack of milk.
Pseudorabies	High, up to 100%.	High, up to 100% in pigs from nonimmune sows, 20–40% in pigs from immune sows.	High, up to 100%.	Initial outbreak affects all ages of unweaned pigs.	Abortion, vomiting, sneezing, coughing, constipation, CNS signs.	Dyspnea, fever, hypersalivation, vomiting, diarrhea, ataxia, nystagmus, convulsions, coma. Younger pigs are more severely affected.	Few visible gross lesions. Congestion of nasal mucosa and pharynx, edema in lung, necrotic tonsillitis, 1–2 mm white foci in liver and spleen.	Virus isolation and fluorescent antibody on tonsils and brain. Serum antibodies.
Congenital tremors	High.	80% or more.	Low, 0–25%.	Birth.	None.	Severe tremors at birth that gradually diminish within 3 weeks. Tremors disappear when pigs are asleep. Tremors most severe in pigs infected at the beginning of the outbreak.	No gross lesions.	Histological evidence of myelin deficiency.
Streptococcal meningitis	Low to 50%.	Up to 70% of the litter.	High in affected pigs.	A few days up until weaning.	None.	Elevated temperature, hindquarter weakness, stiff gait, stretching movements, tremors, incoordination, paddling, paralysis, opisthotonos, convulsions, blindness, deafness, lameness, sudden death.	Congestion of brain and meninges, suppurative meningitis and polyarthritis, excess turbid cerebrospinal fluid, valvular endocarditis.	Isolation of alpha- and beta-hemolytic streptococci in Lancefield group D, I, and II from lesion of suppurative meningitis.
Teschen	High, up to 100%.	High, up to 100%.	High in affected pigs.	Any.	Similar to piglets.	Fever, anorexia, ataxia, progressing to convulsions, paralysis, opisthotonos, and coma.	No gross lesion. Histological lesions in CNS.	Virus isolation. Fluorescent antibody. Serology.
Talfan	Sporadic.	Low.	Low.	First few weeks.	None.	Fever, anorexia, ataxia, seldom convulsions or paralysis.		
Iron toxicity	As many as were given iron injection.	Usually the entire litter.	High.	Shortly after administration of iron.	None.	Apathy, drowsiness, dyspnea, and coma.	Edema around injection site, pallor of muscles, swollen kidneys, epicardial hemorrhage, hydrothorax, and liver necrosis.	History of iron injection. Necropsy findings.

(continued)

Table 11.19. Diseases that cause neurologic signs in unweaned pigs (*continued*)

Disease	Proportion of Litters	Proportion of Affected Piglets within a Litter	Mortality	Age at Onset	Signs in Sow	Signs	Necropsy Findings	Diagnosis
Organophosphate toxicity	Can be high, depending on how many treated.	High, up to 100%.	High.	Seen at birth.	Usually none.	Salivation, vomiting, stiffness, sawhorse stance, diarrhea, colic, lacrimation, sweating, dyspnea, muscle tremors.	Pulmonary edema.	History of sow being treated prior to farrowing.
Vitamin A deficiency of the sow	High.	High.	High.	At birth.	None.	Incoordination, head tilt, hindleg paralysis, paddling, eye lesions.	Yellow-gray liver, kidney lesions, fluid in body cavities.	Liver biopsy for vitamin A analysis.
Congenital malformation	Sporadic.	Low.	High.	At birth.	None.	Variable: hydrocephalus, cyclops, brain hernia, eyeless, catlin mark, hindleg paralysis, string halt. Cerebellar hypoplasia.	Anomaly of nervous (and other) systems.	Physical exam and necropsy findings. Except for cerebellar hypoplasia, the familial relationships of affected pigs indicate that the trait is heritable.
Blue eye paramyxovirus	High, 20–65%.	High, 20–50%.	High, 80–100%.	Any, especially 2–15 days old.	Mild anorexia, few with corneal opacity.	Depression, ataxia, dilated pupils, nystagmus, ocular discharge, palpebral edema, corneal opacity.		Virus isolation.
Hemagglutinating encephalomyelitis virus	Low to 50%.	Up to 100%.	High.	Usually about 4 days.	None.	Lethargy, vomiting, paddling, squealing.	No gross abnormalities.	Histopathology. Serum antibodies.

Table 11.20. Differential diagnosis of neurologic disease in weaned and older pigs

Condition	Ages Affected	Distribution of Affected Pigs	Clinical Signs	Mortality	Necropsy	Diagnosis
Pseudorabies	All ages. In younger pigs, signs more apt to affect central nervous system and be more severe.	Entire herd affected.	Young to mature swine: sneezing, coughing, constipation, salivation, vomiting, muscle spasms, ataxia, convulsions, paddling, coma. Pregnant swine: resorption, mummification, stillborn piglets.	High, especially in younger pigs.	Few visible gross lesions. Congestion of nasal mucosa and pharynx, pulmonary edema, necrotic tonsillitis, 1–2 mm white necrotic foci in liver and spleen.	Virus isolation from tonsils and brain. Fluorescent antibody test on chilled tonsils and brain. Serum antibodies.
Edema disease	1–2 weeks after weaning.	Up to 15% of pigs in the nursery.	Sudden death in some pigs. Incoordination and staggering gait, ataxia, tremors, paddling, palpebral edema.	High, 50–90%.	Ventral reddening of skin. Edema in subcutaneous tissue, stomach wall, and mesocolon.	Signs, epidemiology. Pure culture of *E. coli* from intestine and colon. Isolation of toxin.
Salt poisoning (water deprivation)	Any age but more commonly seen in nursery to finishing pigs.	Affected by pens.	Blindness, muscle weakness and fasciculations, dullness, anorexia, vomiting, diarrhea, seizures, head tremor, opisthotonos, backing up, falling over, paddling, and chomping. Hemoconcentration, eosinopenia (Na >160 mEq/L).	High.	Gastritis, gastric ulcers, enteritis, constipation.	Histopathology: pathognomonic eosinophilic cuffing of blood vessels in cerebrum.
Brain stem malacia	Nursery pig or occasionally finishing pig.	Sporadic.	Dullness, mild incoordination, unthriftiness, disproportionately large head, failure to grow.	Low.	None.	Histologic evidence of brain stem malacia.
Meningitis due to *Streptococcus suis* (or *Salmonella*)	Usually in nursery pigs. Occasionally in finishing pigs.	A few pigs affected over a few weeks. Occasionally outbreaks.	Elevated temperature, hindquarter weakness, stiff gait, stretching movements, tremors, incoordination, paddling, paralysis, opisthotonos, convulsions, blindness, deafness, lameness.	High.	Congestion of brain and meninges, suppurative meningitis, excess turbid cerebrospinal fluid, suppurative polyarthritis.	Isolation of alpha- and beta-hemolytic streptococci in Lancefield group D, I, and II from lesions or suppurative meningitis (isolation of *Salmonella choleraesuis*).
Middle-ear infection	Any age.	Sporadic.	Abnormal head carriage, tendency to circle.	Low.	Inflammation and/or suppuration in middle ear.	Clinical signs and necropsy findings.

(continued)

Table 11.20. Differential diagnosis of neurologic disease in weaned and older pigs (*continued*)

Condition	Ages Affected	Distribution of Affected Pigs	Clinical Signs	Mortality	Necropsy	Diagnosis
Haemophilus parasuis meningoencephalitis	Usually nursery pigs 5–8 weeks old.	10–50%, especially if recently commingled.	Fever, muscle tremors, incoordination of hindlegs, recumbency, paddling.	Moderate, 20–50%.	Fibrinous meningitis with pleuritis, pericarditis, peritonitis, and arthritis.	Isolation of *Haemophilus parasuis*.
Teschen disease	Any age.	Entire herd may be affected.	Fever, anorexia, ataxia, progressing to convulsions, paralysis, opisthotonos, and coma.	High.	No gross lesions. Histologic lesions in CNS.	Virus isolation. Fluorescent antibody test. Serology.
Organic arsenical toxicity	Any age, but especially in pigs treated for swine dysentery or eperythrozoonosis.	Several to many pigs affected.	Ataxia, posterior paresis, goose-stepping, blindness, paralysis.	Low.	None.	Sciatic nerve demyelination. Kidney and liver arsenic levels >2 ppm.
Brain or spinal cord injury	Any age.	Sporadic.	Tend to show local neurologic deficit.	Low.	Localized damage to brain or spinal cord.	Necropsy reveals trauma, skull or vertebrae fracture, abscesses, parasite migration; *S. dentatus*, fibrocartilaginous emboli.
Tetanus	Any, but most common in recently castrated pigs.	Sporadic.	Stiff gait, erect ears and tail, protrusion of the nictating membrane, progresses to lateral recumbency, opisthotonos, rigid muscles, stiff-legged gait, spasms.	High.	No gross lesions.	Gram-positive bacilli with terminal spores seen at site of injection if found.
Rabies	Usually older than 2 mos.	Sporadic.	Preoccupation with and twitching of nose, prostration, chewing, salivation, generalized clonic muscle spasms.	High, 100%.	No gross lesions.	Fresh brain for animal inoculation. Histopathology. Negri bodies. Fluorescent antibody test.
Listeriosis	Any. Signs more severe in younger pigs.	Sporadic.	Fever, trembling, incoordination, dragging hindlegs while showing stiff gait with forelegs, hyperexcitability.	High in young pigs.	Meningitis, focal hepatic necrosis.	Isolation of *Listeria monocytogenes* from brain, spinal cord, or liver.

Toxicities (See Table 11.21.)
Nutritional deficiencies (See Table 11.22.)

Table 11.21. Toxicities resulting in neurologic disease

Major Signs	Toxic Agent	Other Signs	Neurologic Signs	Source
Clinical signs largely gastrointestinal	Inorganic arsenic	Vomiting, diarrhea	Convulsions	Herbicides, cotton defoliants, insecticides
	Lead (rare)	Vomiting, diarrhea, salivation, anorexia	Muscle tremors, ataxia, clonic seizures, blindness	Motor oil, paint, grease, batteries
Frequently characterized by violent activity	Chlorinated hydrocarbons		Hyperexcitability, hyperesthesia, muscle tremors, tonoclonic seizures	Insecticides
	Strychnine		Tetanic seizures	Rodenticide
	Sodium fluoroacetate		Convulsions, running fits	Rodenticide
	Water intoxication	Anorexia, diarrhea	Depression, blindness, muscle tremors, hyperesthesia, ataxia, convulsions, coma	Unrestricted access to water after deprivation
Signs of cholinesterase inhibition	Dichlorvos	Lacrimation, miosis, cyanosis, reddening of skin, salivation, diarrhea, vomiting	Muscle rigidity, tremors, paralysis, depression	Anthelmintic
	Organophosphates	Lacrimation, miosis, cyanosis, reddening of skin, salivation, diarrhea, vomiting	Muscle rigidity, tremors, paralysis, depression	Insecticides
	Carbamate	Lacrimation, miosis, cyanosis, reddening of skin, salivation, diarrhea, vomiting	Muscle rigidity, tremors, paralysis, depression	Insecticides
Generalized central nervous system signs	Nitrofurans		Hyperirritability, tremors, weakness, convulsions	Antibacterial used to treat swine enteric diseases
	Ammonia salts		Depression, tonoclonic seizures	Cattle feed
	Mercury	Vomiting, diarrhea	Ataxia, blindness, paralysis, coma	Grain treated with mercury as a fungicide, paint, batteries
	Pentachlorophenol	Vomiting	Depression, muscle weakness, posterior paralysis	Wood preservative
	Phenoxy herbicides	Anorexia	Depression, muscle weakness, ataxia	Herbicides
Seen in pigs with access to pasture or fencerows	Pigweed		Weakness, tremors, ataxia, posterior paralysis, coma	Pasture
	Cocklebur	Vomiting	Depression, ataxia, muscle weakness, muscle tremors	Pasture
	Nightshade	Anorexia, vomiting, constipation	Depression, ataxia, muscle tremors, convulsions, coma	Pasture
	Nitrate, nitrite	Salivation, polyuria, miosis	Muscle weakness, ataxia, convulsions	Lamb's-quarter, Canada thistle, simonweed, sweet clover
Deafness	Hygromycin		Deafness, blindness due to cataracts	Anthelmintic
	Streptomycin		Deafness	Antibiotic

Table 11.22. Nutritional imbalances resulting in neurologic disease

Nutrient Imbalance	Signs
Calcium and phosphorus deficiency	Stiff gait, hyperesthesia, posterior paralysis
Magnesium excess	Generalized anesthesia, complete muscular relaxation
Magnesium deficiency	Lameness, bowed legs, hyperirritability, tetany
Sodium chloride deficiency	Ataxia, decreased feed intake and weight gain
Iron toxicity	See Table 11.19
Copper deficiency	May result in demyelinization of nerves, but anemia, cardiac hypertrophy, and crooked hindlegs are more prominent signs
Vitamin A deficiency	Growing pigs: head tilt, incoordination, stiff gait, lordosis, hyperexcitability, muscle spasms, night blindness, paralysis. Pregnant sows: see Table 11.19
Niacin or riboflavin deficiency	May result in demyelinization of nerves, but lameness, skin lesions, cataracts, and poor growth are more prominent signs
Pantothenic acid deficiency	Goose-stepping, incoordination, diarrhea, coughing, hair loss, and poor growth
Vitamin B_6 deficiency	Poor growth, diarrhea, anemia, hyperexcitability, ataxia, epileptiform convulsions

Table 11.23. Diseases that cause blindness in pigs

Cause	Pigs Affected	Other Signs	Associated Factors
Arsenilic acid toxicity	Pigs fed arsenilic acid for swine dysentery or eperythrozoonosis.	Acute: posterior paresis or paralysis. Chronic: blindness, quadriplegia.	History of arsenicals added to the feed in improper dosage.
Salt poisoning (water deprivation)	Usually nursery or finishing pigs but can occur in adults.	CNS signs, ataxia, muscle weakness and fasciculations, convulsions.	Usually a high percentage of affected pigs in one or more pens, associated with disruption in water supply or whey feeding.
Pseudorabies	Usually in 2- to 4- month-old pigs.	Ill-thrift, failure to grow.	Sequelae to pseudorabies infection in an apparently recovered pig.
Lead or mercury toxicity	Nursery to adult.	CNS and gastrointestinal signs.	Access to paint, batteries, motor oil, or seeds treated with organic mercurial fungicides.
Botulism	Grower to adults.	Flaccid paralysis.	Access to a decomposing carcass.
Blue eye disease	Nursery to finishing pigs.	CNS signs. Corneal opacity.	Acute onset of disease in herd with high piglet mortality.
Vitamin A deficiency	Nursery to finishing pigs.	Stiff gait, restlessness, paralysis of rear legs.	Rare. Possible after feeding improperly stored grain.
Hygromycin toxicity	Usually sows.	Cataracts.	Longer feeding period than recommended.
Hemagglutinating encephalitis or *Strep. suis*	Unweaned pigs.	CNS signs, convulsions.	Blindness not apparent until neurologic signs are well advanced.

Table 11.24. Systemic disease in unweaned pigs

Disease	Signs in Sow	Piglet Necropsy	Diagnosis
Streptococci (*S. equisimilis*, *S. suis*)	None.	Congestion of parenchymatous organs, strands of fibrin, meningitis, polyarthritis, enlarged lymph nodes.	Culture of organisms.
Hypoglycemia	Mastitis or nonfunctional mammary glands.	No gross lesions, absence of body fat or food in the stomach.	Necropsy findings.
Iron toxicity	None.	Muscle edema and necrosis around the injection site.	History of recent iron injection and necropsy findings.
Escherichia coli septicemia	None.	Possibly congested organs, enlarged lymph nodes, edema, fibrin tags in abdomen, or minimal changes.	Isolation of *Escherichia coli*.
Porcine reproductive and respiratory syndrome	None or anorexia, agalactia.	Interstitial pneumonia, enlarged tan lymph nodes.	Virus isolation, fluorescent antibody.
Haemophilus parasuis	None.	Fibrinous meningitis, pericarditis, peritonitis, and arthritis.	Isolation of *Haemophilus parasuis*.
Pseudorabies (chronic)	Usually none, may be salivation, constipation, vomiting, abortion.	Usually no gross lesions. Congestion of nasal mucosa, necrotic tonsillitis, focal necrosis in liver and spleen.	Tonsils for fluorescent antibody or virus isolation. Serology.
Erysipelas	Usually none but may show lameness, fever, skin lesions.	Diffuse cutaneous hemostasis, petechial hemorrhage in kidneys.	Isolation of *Erysipelothrix rhusiopathiae*.
Leptospirosis	Possibly abortion, fever, jaundice, or agalactia.	Grayish-white foci in kidneys.	Culture of organism or presence on dark field exam of kidneys.

ure is the cause of pregnancy termination, the fetuses will all be the same age and this age will match the day of gestation. Often when fetal death occurs, fetuses within the litter will have different ages, with the youngest ones having died at some time earlier than the abortion occurred. Viral infection is the major cause of mummified fetuses, but mummies are also seen with a number of other etiologic agents. When there is only one or a few stillborn pigs in an otherwise normal litter, these tend to be caused by events at farrowing such as large litter size, later birth order, prolonged farrowing, or anoxia. When stillbirths are part of a litter that also contains mummies, then an infectious agent is more likely to be involved.

Antibody titers of blood samples taken from the sow must be interpreted carefully. A positive titer only confirms the presence of the organism on the farm; it does not indicate whether that organism was the cause of the reproductive failure. Paired sera and demonstration of a rising titer are more reliable evidence of a recent infection. Positive titers on sera from aborted fetuses are diagnostic for the disease; since there is no transfer of antibodies across the placenta, antibody in the fetus is evidence of infection.

Positive fluorescent antibody tests done on fetal tissue may be diagnostic; however, negative tests in fetuses over 70 days of gestational age do not rule out a diagnosis, since immunocompetent pigs may have produced enough antibody to complex with the infecting agent and interfere with the test.

Polyuria/Polydipsia

Polyuria is not easily recognized in pigs on slatted floors; however, astute stockpersons occasionally observe sows drinking and urinating excessively. In sows, cystitis and nephritis are the most common causes of polyuria. Intoxication with citrinin or ochratoxin may also produce polyuria. Especially during the winter, underfeeding sows causes protein catabolism with increased blood urea nitrogen and subsequent increase in urine volume.

Hematuria

The most common cause of hematuria is cystitis, sometimes associated with pyelonephritis due to organisms such as *Actinobaculum suis*, *Streptococcus spp.*, *Klebsiella spp.*, and *E. coli*. Leptospirosis and *Stephanurus dentatus* infections also may produce hematuria.

Vaginal Prolapse

There is probably a hereditary predisposition to vaginal and uterine prolapse. Sows housed on a floor with an excessive slope, especially if they are kept in a dirty or wet environment, are more prone to developing prolapse. Other causes include zearalenone toxicity, injury from service, and causes of undetermined etiology that occur around the time of farrowing and in gilts following their first estrus.

Vulvar Discharge (Table 11.35)

A purulent or blood-tinged discharge may be due to cystitis, pyelonephritis, vaginitis, or metritis. The first two diseases occur in sows at any stage but are especially noted during gestation, whereas metritis and vaginitis usually occur after farrowing or breeding.

Vulval Enlargement

Unilateral enlargement of one lip of the vulva can be caused by traumatic injury at any time or by hematoma

Table 11.25.   Systemic disease in weaned pigs to adults

Disease	Pigs Affected and Clinical Signs	Necropsy Findings	Diagnosis
Generally Seen in Nursery to Finishing Pigs			
Septicemic salmonellosis	Weaning to 4 months of age. Fever, a few pigs found dead, huddling, low morbidity (10%), high mortality, possibly diarrhea after 3–4 days, depression, anorexia.	Diffuse cutaneous hemostasis, infarcts in gastric mucosa, enlarged liver and spleen, moist swollen lymph nodes, miliary white necrotic foci in liver, serous to necrotic colitis after 3 days.	Isolation of *Salmonella choleraesuis* from liver or spleen.
Haemophilus parasuis	Pigs 1–4 months old. Anorexia, fever, depression, cyanosis, stiff gait, reluctance to move, dog-sitting, eyelid edema, and dyspnea.	Fibrinous or serofibrinous meningitis, pericarditis, pleuritis, peritonitis, and arthritis.	Isolation of *Haemophilus parasuis*.
Mycoplasma hyorhinis infection	Pigs 3–10 weeks old. Moderate fever, depression, reluctance to move, anorexia, possible dyspnea.	Serofibrinous to fibrinopurulent pericarditis, peritonitis, pericarditis, and arthritis.	Isolation of *Mycoplasma hyorhinis*.
Edema disease	Pigs 4–12 weeks old. Usually 1–2 weeks after weaning. Morbidity <15%, mortality 50–90%, often a few pigs found dead. Ataxia, tremors, staggering, eyelid edema, temperature usually normal.	Edema in subcutaneous tissues, submucosa of the stomach, and mesocolon, full stomach, empty small intestine, possibly serous fluid with a few strands of fibrin in the pleural, pericardial, and peritoneal cavities.	Isolation of edema-associated *E. coli* serotypes.
Erysipelas	Pigs 3 months to 3 years old, but also adults. Fever (40–42°C), recumbency, reluctance to rise, anorexia, depression, urticarial skin lesions, cyanosis, often a few pigs found dead.	Diffuse cutaneous hemostasis, congested or edematous lungs, petechial or ecchymotic hemorrhage on epicardium, gastritis, enlarged liver and spleen, excess fluid in joints, and proliferation of synovia.	Isolation of *E. rhusiopathiae* from heart, lungs, spleen, liver, joints, or kidneys.
Postweaning multisytemic wasting syndrome	Usually nursery.	Interstitial pneumonia, enlarged lymph nodes and spleen.	Histopathology.
Any Age from Weaned Pigs to Adults			
Porcine reproductive and respiratory syndrome	Usually nursery to grower pigs. Dyspnea, slow growth, rough hair coat.	Interstitial pneumonia, enlarged tan lymph nodes.	Virus isolation. Fluorescent antibody. Serology.
Porcine dermatitis nephropathy syndrome	Nursery to (especially) finisher pigs.	Reddened and enlarged abdominal lymph nodes, ascites, swollen mottled kidneys.	Histopathology kidneys and skin.
Hog cholera	Any age pigs. Anorexia, fever, depression, conjunctivitis, constipation early, severe watery diarrhea later, huddling, staggering, weaving, cyanosis, possibly convulsions, a few pigs found dead, abortion in pregnant sows.	Edematous tissues, swollen edematous lymph nodes with mottled hemorrhage, petechial to ecchymotic hemorrhage in kidneys, bladder, larynx, and heart, splenic infarcts, button ulcers in the large intestine, bronchopneumonia or lung congestion.	Fluorescent antibody virus determination on tonsil, pharyngeal lymph nodes, or spleen.
African swine fever	Any age pigs. Depression, reluctance to rise, fever, anorexia, hyperemia of skin, dyspnea, possibly diarrhea and vomiting, abortion of pregnant sows.	Edema, ascites, hydrothorax, petechial ecchymotic hemorrhage of epicardium and lungs, swollen edematous lymph nodes, especially gastrohepatic, enlarged spleen with infarcts, edematous noncollapsing lungs, enlarged liver, hemorrhage in kidneys, variable enteritis, ulcers in colon.	Fluorescent antibody test or inoculation of susceptible swine.
Aflatoxin	Any age pigs. Depression, anorexia, anemia, icterus, temperature normal.	Ascites, enlarged fatty liver to liver necrosis or cirrhosis.	Find 200 ppb aflatoxin in the feed.
Citrinin or ochratoxin	Any age pigs. Diarrhea, normal temperature, polyuria, polydipsia, dehydration.	Possibly fibrotic kidney, possibly fatty change and necrosis of liver.	Find 200 ppb mycotoxin in the feed.

Table 11.26. Causes of death without prior clinical signs in weaned pigs to adults

Cause	Pigs Most Commonly Affected and Time
Edema disease	Nursery pigs 1–2 weeks after weaning, especially in the most rapidly growing animals.
Salt poisoning(water deprivation)	Usually nursery or growing and finishing pigs but can be any age.
Vitamin E/selenium deficiency (Mulberry heart disease)	Usually nursery or growing and finishing pigs.
Acute pneumonias due to *A. pleuropneumoniae, Actinobacillus sp., Pasteurella multocida*	Growing and finishing pigs, rarely in adults.
Haemophilus parasuis infection or *Actinobacillus suis* infection	Nursery and growing pigs.
Porcine stress syndrome	Finishing to adult pigs. Heavily muscled animals, especially Pietrain and Landrace breeds.
Gastric ulceration	Finishing pigs to adults.
Hemorrhagic bowel syndrome associated with *Lawsonia intracellularis*	Usually older finishing pigs or young adults.
Hemorrhagic bowel syndrome associated with whey feeding	Usually older finishing pigs or young adults.
Gastric volvulus	Adults, especially sows.
Mesenteric volvulus	Growing and finishing pigs to adults.
Exhaustion	Finishing pigs and adults, especially adults.
Systemic salmonellosis	Growing and finishing pigs and adults.
Electrocution	Any age.
Encephalomyocarditis virus	1–20 weeks of age.
Coal tar toxicity	Usually growing and finishing pigs but also adults.
Clostridium novyi infection	Any age.
Cardiac insufficiency	Any age but more common in heavy finishers or sows.
Asphyxiation from H_2S, CO, CO_2	Any age but more common in finishing pigs.

Necropsy Findings	Associated Factors
Edema in subcutaneous tissue, eyelids, gastric mucosa, and mesocolon, full stomach, empty intestine.	May be associated with ad libitum feeding of highly nutritious and palatable feed.
Usually no gross lesions, may see gastritis or enteritis.	History of recent interruption of the water supply, feeding of whey.
Acute hemorrhagic hepatic necrosis, hemorrhage in the cardiac muscle, excessive pericardial fluid. White, edematous skeletal and cardiac muscle.	Most common in selenium-deficient areas east of the Mississippi River.
Cyanosis, acute necrotizing hemorrhagic pneumonia with fibrin in the pleural cavity, trachea and bronchi filled with foamy blood-tinged mucus.	
Cyanosis, fibrinous peritonitis, pericarditis, pleuritis, arthritis, and meningitis, especially in recently purchased high-health pigs.	
Blotchy cyanosis coalescing on the ventral abdomen, rapid onset of postmortem rigor, areas of pale muscle.	Occurs in pigs that have been moved or were fighting, mating, or farrowing.
Erosion of the pars oesophagea, large amount of blood in the stomach, marked pallor.	Feeding of finely ground feed or whey; interruption of feed availability.
Marked pallor, terminal small intestine and upper spiral colon filled with blood.	Associated with *Lawsonia intracellularis* infections.
Small intestine filled with blood-stained fluid. Bloody fluid in abdomen. Possible volvulus. Gas-distended colon.	Associated with feeding whey, especially acid whey.
Enlarged, gas-filled stomach, splenic engorgement.	Improper crate size that allows the sow to turn around.
Hyperemic segment of the intestine with distinct demarcation between normal and affected areas.	Excessive competition for feed, feeding whey or other large-volume feeds.
Skin abrasions and bruising, pulmonary edema, and froth in the trachea and bronchi.	Fighting, especially in hot, humid environment or after mixing or moving.
Cyanotic extremities, enlarged spleen and liver, enlarged mesenteric lymph nodes, small white, necrotic foci in liver.	Finishing facilities that practice continuous addition of new stock.
Usually no gross lesions, may be petechial hemorrhage in the lungs, singed hair above the coronary band, red streaks on the medial surface of the legs.	Electrical short in the building, lightning during a recent rainstorm.
Cyanotic ventrum, dilated right heart, with areas of pale muscle, fibrin in peritoneal, pericardial, and pleural cavities.	May be more common in rodent-infested buildings, since disease is carried by rodents.
Greatly enlarged and friable liver.	Access to a source such as tar paper, shingles, or clay pigeons.
Rapid postmortem tympany, bloody fluid in pleural, pericardial, and peritoneal cavities, splenomegaly, hepatic necrosis and emphysema, neck swelling.	
Vegetative valvular endocarditis.	*Erysipelas rhusiopathiae, Strep. suis, Actinobacillus pleuropneumoniae*.
	Agitation and pumping of pit, fan failure.

Table 11.27. Ages at which wasting and ill-thrift are seen in baby pigs to adults

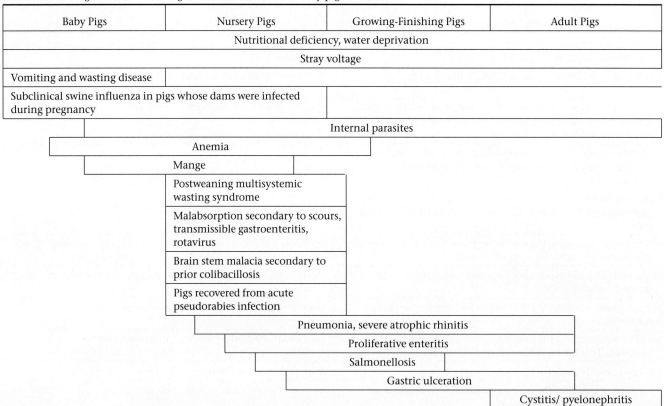

Baby Pigs	Nursery Pigs	Growing-Finishing Pigs	Adult Pigs
Nutritional deficiency, water deprivation			
Stray voltage			
Vomiting and wasting disease			
Subclinical swine influenza in pigs whose dams were infected during pregnancy			
	Internal parasites		
Anemia			
Mange			
	Postweaning multisystemic wasting syndrome		
	Malabsorption secondary to scours, transmissible gastroenteritis, rotavirus		
	Brain stem malacia secondary to prior colibacillosis		
	Pigs recovered from acute pseudorabies infection		
	Pneumonia, severe atrophic rhinitis		
	Proliferative enteritis		
	Salmonellosis		
	Gastric ulceration		
		Cystitis/ pyelonephritis	

Table 11.28. Diseases that cause anemia in unweaned pigs

Disease	Pigs Affected	Signs	Hematologic Findings	Diagnosis
Iron deficiency anemia	Normal at birth; anemia becomes more severe as age increases.	Rough hair coat, pale, rapid respiration, uneven growth.	Microcytic, hypochromic red blood cells.	History that pigs did not receive an appropriate iron injection. Heart dilated, pericardial fluid, pulmonary edema, splenomegaly.
Eperythrozoonosis	Especially pigs under 5 days old but any time from birth to weaning.	Icterus, rough hair coat, uneven growth, listless, swollen yellow-brown liver, splenomegaly.	Organisms seen in red blood cells.	Wright-Giemsa stain of blood from a febrile pig or positive serology from the sow.
Umbilical hemorrhage	Die within a few hours of birth. May be associated with use of wood shavings or vitamin C or zinc deficiency.	Cord remains large and fleshy, fails to shrivel, blood-stained skin.	Normal.	Clinical signs.

Table 11.29. Diseases that cause anemia in weaned pigs to adults

Disease	Ages Affected	Other Signs	Associated Factors	Diagnosis
Gastric ulcer	Older growing pigs and adults.	Inappetence, weight loss, occasional grinding of teeth. Normal feces or firm, dark, and tarry.	Finely ground feed, vitamin E deficiency.	Ulcer observed in the pars oesophagea at necropsy.
Iron deficiency	Nursery pigs.	Reduced growth rate, rough hair coat.	Failure to give sufficient iron before weaning.	Hematology, history, and absence of other lesions.
Sarcoptes scabeii	Nursery pigs to adults. Anemia is more severe in younger pigs.	Scratching and rubbing against walls, rough hair coat, keratinization of skin.	Poor mange control program.	Deep skin scraping from the ear canal to demonstrate mites.
Trichuris suis	Usually in 2- to 6-month-old pigs.	Anorexia, diarrhea with mucus, weight loss. Dark feces, diarrhea with mucus, melena.	Lack of good parasite control program.	Lesions in the large intestine, favorable response to treatment.
Hemorrhagic ileitis	Usually young breeding-age gilts.	Bleeding from the anus, usually with normal body condition.	Seen more often in herds with other *Lawsonia*-associated enteropathies.	Clinical signs and lack of lesions on gross necropsy.
Proliferative enteritis	Nursery to adult pigs, especially 2–5 months old.	Various degrees of weight loss, anorexia. Black, tarry feces to frank blood.	Seen more often in herds with other *Lawsonia*-associated enteropathies.	Necropsy lesions primarily in small intestine. Histopathology: mucosal hyperplasia.
Eperythrozoonosis	Nursery pigs to adults.	Lethargy, reduced growth, occasional icterus, acute episode in sows: mammary and vulvar edema.	Poor mange and lice control program.	Stained blood smear to demonstrate organisms. Indirect hemagglutination titer of 1-80 or higher.
Aflatoxin	All ages. Signs more severe in younger pigs.	Depression, anorexia, ascites, elevated liver enzymes, occasional icterus.	Moldy feed; grains raised, harvested, or stored during wet weather; especially damaged kernels.	Liver lesions of fatty change to necrosis and cirrhosis. Feed analysis for toxin.
Tricothecenes	All ages. Signs more severe in younger pigs.	Gastroenteritis.	Moldy feed; grains raised, harvested, or stored during wet weather; especially damaged kernels.	Feed analysis for toxin.
Zearalenone	All ages. Signs more severe in younger pigs.	Swollen vulvas and mammary glands in prepubertal gilts.	Moldy feed; grains raised, harvested, or stored during wet weather; especially damaged kernels	Feed analysis for toxin.
Warfarin toxicity	Any age.	Lameness, stiff gait, lethargy. Dark, tarry feces.	Access to rodenticides.	Prolonged clotting time. Demonstrate toxin in blood and liver.

Table 11.30. Diseases that cause lameness in unweaned pigs

Condition	Ages Affected	Clinical Signs	Associated Factors	Diagnosis
Infectious polyarthritis: *Streptococcus, Staphylococcus, E. coli*	1–3 weeks old.	Lassitude, rough hair coat, joint swelling, fever.	More frequent in low-parity sows, unsanitary tooth clipping and tail docking.	Necropsy: culture and Gram or Giemsa stain of bacteria in joint fluid.
Trauma	Any, but especially in the first 36–40 hours after birth.	Variable.	Poor crate design, no heat source to draw pigs away from the sow, sows with agalactia.	Presumptive based on lack of heat and poor farrowing crate design.
Splayleg	Birth or within a few hours. 1–4 pigs/litter, occasionally whole litter.	Hindlegs (sometimes forelegs) abducted to the side, pig unable to stand or moves with difficulty.	Birth weight of affected pigs is below average, slippery floors.	Clinical signs. Histology: myofibrillar hypoplasia in semitendinosus or triceps.
Injections	Any time after injection.	Tendency to carry or drag one hindleg.		History of injection.
Arthrogryposis	At birth. 40–50% of a litter affected.	Fixation of the joints in the limbs or vertebral column in various degrees of extension or flexion.	Maternal toxicity (wild black cherry, tobacco stalks, jimsonweed, poison hemlock), deficiency of vitamin A or manganese, or heredity.	Clinical signs in piglets, history of sow access to pasture. Feed analysis.
Syndactyly, polydactyly, thick legs	At birth.	Abnormal number of toes, front legs more likely to be affected.	Genetic.	Clinical signs.
Clostridium perfringens	1–5 days old.	Marked swelling of hindleg, dark reddish-brown discoloration of skin over swelling.	Iron injected within the last 24 hours with contaminated needle.	Necropsy and isolation of the organism.

Table 11.31. Ages at which diseases causing lameness in weaned pigs to adults are more common

Age in Months										
1	1.5	2	3	4	5	6	18	30	42	54

Trauma: muscle bruising, sprains, strains, dislocations, fractures (age 1–54)

Clostridium tetani or septicum infection (age 1–54)

Vesicular diseases: foot-and-mouth, vesicular exanthema, swine vesicular disease, vesicular stomatitis, San Miguel sea lion virus (age 1–54)

Streptococcus suis infection (age 1–1.5)

S. equisimilis infection (age 1–1.5)

Chronic suppurative arthritis due to *S. suis, S. equisimilis, M. hyorhinis, M. hyosynoviae, H. parasuis, Corynebacterium, Staphylococcus* (age 1.5–54)

Acute *Mycoplasma hyorhinis* infection (age 1.5–2)

Haemophilus parasuis infection (age 2–3)

Bursitis (age 3–54)

Rickets (age 3–6)

Acute erysipelas (age 4–18)

Chronic erysipelas (age 18–54)

Asymmetrical hindquarter syndrome (age 4–6)

Foot rot (age 4–54)

Back-muscle necrosis (age 5–54)

Osteochondrosis (age 5–54)

Osteoarthrosis, degenerative joint disease (age 6–54)

Epiphysiolysis (age 6–54)

Brucellosis (age 18–54)

Laminitis (age 18–54)

Apophysiolysis (age 18–30)

Osteomalacia (age 30–54)

Tarsitis (age 30–54)

Arthrosis deformans (age 30–54)

Leg weakness syndrome (age 30–54)

---

at farrowing or mating. Bilateral enlargement is seen with zearalenone toxicity and edema secondary to eperythrozoonosis.

Agalactia (Table 11.36)

Agalactia, the failure to produce milk, becomes apparent because of the behavior of the suckling pigs. They are often noisy and restless and make frequent nursing attempts. With time they become gaunt and emaciated. Agalactic sows should be examined if they show clinical signs, such as pyrexia, depression, or anorexia, which tend to be associated with infectious causes of agalactia; normally bright, alert sows tend to be agalactic due to hormonal or nutritional causes.

POOR REPRODUCTIVE PERFORMANCE
(Tables 11.37–11.41)

Although diseases that deform fetuses or cause abortion attract a great deal of attention when they occur,

greater concern should be directed to the "normal" level of reproductive performance, since when it is suboptimal, a much greater loss of potential profit occurs. Currently, with the advent of computerized record-keeping systems and the use of consultants, requests for assistance in improving poor reproductive performance are common.

Efficiency of reproductive performance is measured by the number of pigs weaned/sow/year (PW/S/Y). Typical North American farms only produce about 14–16 PW/S/Y, although the best farms have demonstrated that 25 PW/S/Y is possible. Three components directly influence PW/S/Y: litters/sow/year (L/S/Y), average live-born litter size, and preweaning mortality. Each of these three major components is in turn influenced by a number of environmental, managemental, genetic, and nutritional factors.

The first step is to determine L/S/Y, average number of live-born per litter, and preweaning mortality. Performance may be suboptimal in one or more areas.

Table 11.32. Diseases that cause lameness in weaned pigs to adults

Clinical Signs	Causes	Diagnosis
Gross swelling of muscles or soft tissue	Trauma.	Physical examination.
	Clostridium septicum infection.	Necropsy, identification of organisms.
	Back-muscle necrosis.	Necropsy, creatine kinase.
	Asymmetric hindquarter syndrome.	Necropsy.
Generalized stiffness, reluctance to move, altered gait, fever, usually also other signs of septicemia	Acute *Mycoplasma hyorhinis infection*, acute *Haemophilus parasuis infection*, acute erysipelas, *Streptococcus suis* infection.	Culture of organisms from heart, liver, spleen, or lesion.
	Tetanus.	Identification of organisms.
Swollen joints	Chronic *Mycoplasma hyorhinis, Haemophilus parasuis,* or erysipelas infection. Infection with *Strep. equisimilis* or *Mycoplasma hyosynoviae.* Suppurative arthritis due to *Staphylococcus, Arcanobacterium pyogenes,* or *Streptococcus.*	Isolation of organisms from the joints.
	Rickets.	Necropsy, bone ash determination, ration analysis.
Posterior paresis or paralysis	Brucellosis.	Necropsy, serology.
	Rickets, osteomalacia.	Necropsy, bone ash determination, ration analysis.
	Apophysiolysis of ischiatic tuberosity; proximal femoral epiphysiolysis; trauma; vertebral, lumbosacral, or pelvic fracture; spondylosis.	Necropsy.
Tail bitten	Abscess in vertebral column.	Necropsy culture.
No external abnormalities	*M. hyosynoviae* infection.	Culture.
	Osteochondrosis, proximal femoral epiphysiolysis, degenerative joint disease, osteoarthrosis, trauma, apophysiolysis of ischiatic tuberosity.	Necropsy.
	Leg weakness syndrome.	Physical examination.
	Fibrocartilaginous embolism. Osteomalacia and fracture.	Necropsy, bone ash determination, ration analysis.
	Selenium toxicity.	Necropsy, selenium levels.
Quarter crack in the hoof wall, pain, heat, swelling	Foot rot (*Arcanobacterium pyogenes* and other opportunist invaders).	Physical examination, culture.
No external deformity, pain, heat, and swelling	Laminitis.	Physical examination, history of postparturient fever.
Hoof abnormalities	Overgrown hooves, bush foot, sand crack, heel separation, trauma.	Physical examination.
Cracks in hoof wall, erosion and bruising of the heel	Rough hooves, wet environment, biotin deficiency.	Physical examination. Ration analysis.
Vesicles and/or hoof separation at coronary band. Shifting lameness.	Foot-and-mouth disease, vesicular stomatitis, vesicular exanthema, swine vesicular disease.	Vesicular fluid for virus isolation.
	Selenium toxicity.	Feed analysis.

Table 11.33. Crown-to-rump length and fetal age

Crown-to-Rump Length (mm)	Approximate Fetal Age (days)
20	25
27	30
46	40
89	50
135	60
170	70
207	85
270	110

Table 11.34. Diseases causing abortion, stillbirth, and mummification in swine

Disease	Signs in Sow	Age of Fetuses	Signs in Fetus and Placenta	Diagnosis
Nutritional Causes				
Overfeeding	None.	Embryonic loss.	None.	Suggestive from history, feed levels after mating.
Underfeeding	Extremely thin sow, possible polyuria, polydipsia.	All the same age, any age.	None.	History, sow condition, competition for feed.
Zinc deficiency	Delayed or prolonged parturition.	At birth.	Low viability, umbilical hemorrhage.	Feed analysis.
Viruses				
Porcine parvovirus	None.	Often fetuses are dead at different stages of development.	Resorption (small litter size), mummies frequent, stillborn or weak pigs, decomposed placenta tightly wrapped around fetus.	Virus isolation.
Japanese B encephalitis	None.	Often fetuses are dead at different stages of development.	Similar to parvovirus with hydrocephalus, subcutaneous edema, hydrothorax, petechial hemorrhage, ascites, necrotic foci in liver and spleen.	Fluorescent antibody test on fetus.
Pseudorabies	Can be mild to severe, sneezing, cough, anorexia, constipation, salivation, vomiting, neurologic signs.	Often fetuses are dead at different stages of development.	Focal necrotic areas in liver, mummies, stillborn pigs, resorption (small litter size). Necrotizing placentitis.	Paired serology from sow.
Swine influenza	Extreme prostration, lethargy, labored respiration, cough.	Often fetuses are dead at different stages of development.	Resorption (small litter size), mummies, stillborn pigs, or pigs born weak.	Paired serology from sow. Virus isolation.
Enterovirus, adenovirus, reovirus, cytomegalovirus	Usually none.	Often fetuses are dead at different stages of development.	Resorption (small litter size), mummies, stillborn pigs, or pigs born weak.	Paired serology from sow.
Hog cholera	Lethargy, anorexia, fever, conjunctivitis, vomiting, dyspnea, erythema, cyanosis, diarrhea, ataxia, convulsions.	Often fetuses are dead at different stages of development.	Mummies, stillbirths, edema, ascites, deformities of head and limbs, petechial hemorrhages, hypoplasia of lungs and cerebellum, liver necrosis.	Fluorescent antibody test on fetal tissue, especially tonsil.
Bovine viral diarrhea virus	None, but sows may be kept in contact with cattle.	Often fetuses are dead at different stages of development.	No lesions.	Virus isolation, serology.
Encephalomyocarditis	None.	Any age, but usually all the same age.	Edema.	Virus isolation.
African swine fever	Lethargy, anorexia, fever, hyperemia, dyspnea, vomiting, diarrhea.	Any age, but usually all the same age.	Petechial and ecchymotic hemorrhages.	Fluorescent antibody test on fetal tissues.
Swine vesicular diseases[a]	Vesicles on snout, mouth, and coronary band.	Any age, but usually all the same age.	No gross lesions.	Vesicular fluid fluorescent antibody or serum neutralization test.
Porcine reproductive and respiratory syndrome	Fever, anorexia, lethargy, blotchy reddening of skin and cyanosis.	Any age, but usually all the same age.	Necrotizing arteritis in the umbilical cord. Edema.	Virus isolation.
Blue eye disease	May be anorexia, fever, depression, rare corneal opacity.	Any age, but usually all the same age.	Stillbirths, mummies, abortions, resorbtion.	Virus isolation.
Bacteria				
Leptospirosis	Few animals showing signs, mild anorexia, fever, diarrhea, abortion.	Usually all near the same age, often mid- to late-term.	Stillbirths or weak neonatal pigs, occasional abortions, diffuse placentitis.	Demonstration of organisms by dark-field examination. Culture or laboratory animal inoculation. Paired sera from sow or single titer >1:800. *(continued)*

Table 11.34. Diseases causing abortion, stillbirth, and mummification in swine (*continued*)

Disease	Signs in Sow	Age of Fetuses	Signs in Fetus and Placenta	Diagnosis
Uterine infection with *E. coli, A. pyogenes, S. aureus, Pasteurella, E. rhusiopathiae, Pseudomonas, Listeria monocytogenes, Strep. equisimilis, Bacillus, Salmonella,* etc.	Generally no clinical signs.	May be any age but usually all are the same age.	May be almost normal or somewhat autolytic with edema, suppurative placentitis.	Culture of organism from fetus.
Brucellosis	Signs seldom recognized, abortion at any time during gestation.	May be any age but usually all are the same age.	May have undergone autolysis or subcutaneous edema. Peritoneal fluid or hemorrhage may be present. Suppurative placentitis.	Culture of organisms from fetus. Positive serology from the herd, paired sera from the sow.
Pyrexia				
Any systemic infection: erysipelas, transmissible gastroenteritis, eperythrozoonosis, *A. pleuropneumoniae,* etc.	Fever. Other signs of disease will vary with the specific agent.	All the same age, any age.	Usually none.	History and clinical signs.
Hostile Environment				
Carbon monoxide	No signs in sows but tends to occur during the coldest weather.	Usually at term, stillborn pigs.	Bright red tissues large amount of serosanguinous pleural effusion.	Suggestive from clinical signs and history. Improvement when fossil fuel replaced.
Carbon dioxide	No signs in sows but tends to occur during the coldest weather.	Usually at term, stillborn pigs.	Muconium on skin and in respiratory tract.	Suggestive from clinical signs and history. Improvement when fossil fuel replaced.
High environmental temperature	High temperature at time of breeding.	Abortion or resorption.	None.	Clinical signs and history.
	High temperature at time of farrowing, sows panting and hyperemia.	Stillborn pigs at term.	None.	Clinical signs and history.
Physical trauma	Sows of different body size and condition penned together, skin abrasions.	All the same age, any age.	None.	Clinical signs and history.
Low environmental temperature	Thin sows and possibly polyuria and polydipsia.	All the same age, any age.	None.	Clinical signs and history.
Seasonal abortion	None.	All the same age, any age.	None.	September–November.
Mold				
Claviceps purpura	Possibly dry gangrene of extremities and tail.	All the same age.	Abortion, stillbirth, weak neonates. No gross lesions.	Feed analysis.
T_2 toxin	Rare but may cause anorexia or lethargy.	Late term.	Abortion, stillbirth, weak neonates. No gross lesions.	Feed analysis.
Zearalenone	Tumescence, edema of the vulva, occasional mammary development in gilts.	Failure of embryo to implant.	Abortion, stillbirth, weak neonates. No gross lesions.	Feed analysis.
Parasite				
Toxoplasma gondii	None.	Any age.	Abortion, stillbirths, weak pigs. Rarely mummies.	Histopathology, serology.
Toxicities				
Organophosphate toxicity	Salivation, defecation, emesis, muscle tremors, paralysis.	All the same age, any age.	None.	Signs, history, whole-blood cholinesterase activity.

Table 11.34. Diseases causing abortion, stillbirth, and mummification in swine (*continued*)

Disease	Signs in Sow	Age of Fetuses	Signs in Fetus and Placenta	Diagnosis
Chlorinated hydrocarbon (CH) toxicity	Hyperexcitability, muscle spasms, seizures.	All the same age, any age.	None.	Signs, history, CH level in liver, kidney, brain.
Pentachlorophenol toxicity	Depression, emesis, muscle weakness, posterior paralysis.	Usually stillborn pigs at term.	None.	Access to pentachlorophenol-treated wood, pentachlorophenol in the blood.
Teratogens				
Vitamin A deficiency	None.	May vary in age or be all the same age.	Stillborn or weak, anophthalmia, cleft palate, microphthalmia, blind, general edema.	History, eye abnormalities.
Methallibure, metrifone, tri chlorfon, iodine deficiency, tobacco stalks	None.	May vary in age or be all the same age.	Mummies, stillbirths, low birth weight, deformed pigs.	History and signs.
Farrowing Complications				
Fatigue: old or fat sow, disturbed or prolonged birth	Prolonged labor, more than 5 hours, especially with large litters or hot weather.	Stillbirths at term.	None.	History, physical exam of sow.
Low maternal hemoglobin level	Pallor, rapid respiration.	Stillbirths at term.	None.	Packed-cell volume or blood hemoglobin too low.

[a]Foot-and-mouth disease, vesicular stomatitis, vesicular exanthema.

Then a systematic investigation can be carried out using the flowchart in Table 11.37.

Maximization of L/S/Y occurs when the proportion of nonpregnant females in the herd is minimized. Unproductive days in the breeding herd are caused by sows that were not bred after weaning, sows that abort or resorb litters, and gilts that remain too long in the gilt pool. About 10% of weaned sows are culled because they fail to show estrus. On the average, unbred weaned sows stay in the herd for 75 days prior to culling, which adds greatly to the number of unproductive herd days. Gilts may spend from 2–20 weeks in the gilt pool and up to one-third of them may never join the breeding herd, again making a major contribution to the total unproductive herd days. When L/S/Y is low (less than 2) then the problem should be characterized as to whether females are anestrus or whether females are returning to heat after breeding. Returns to heat can be further characterized by whether they occur at intervals of 18–21 days postbreeding (failure of conception) or at other intervals (early embryonic loss). Additional observation of management, environment, genetics, and nutrition is used to identify specific contributing factors (Tables 11.39–11.40).

Problems of small litter size are generally due to noninfectious, rather than infectious, causes. Investigation of the cause(s) can be a major undertaking since numerous factors influence litter size, and although each factor may cause only a small reduction by itself, litter size may be considerably reduced when all factors are considered. To investigate small litter size it is necessary to examine information on all farrowings that occur over a 6-month period. Each litter farrowed should be characterized by parity of the sow, number of live-born, number of stillborn, and number of mummies. Data should be recorded and summarized and then analyzed for mean values and trends. When small litter size is due to large numbers of stillborns or mummies, the information in Table 11.34 should be used to assist diagnosis. Other causes of small litter size are given in Table 11.40.

Factors influencing preweaning survival are covered in Chapter 62.

Table 11.35. Causes of vulvar discharges in gilts and sows

| Site of Infection | Characteristics of Discharge | | | Signs and Animals Affected | |
	Amount	Appearance	Frequency and time of occurrence	Parity and stage of reproduction affected	Other clinical manifestations
Vagina	10–50 mL	Purulent, occasionally bloody.	Sporadic with multiple discharges per day. Not related to estrus cycle. Persists days to weeks.	More common in gilts. May be occasional female 10–20% of or herd. Pregnant and open females affected but especially shortly after mating.	Usually no other clinical signs.
Cervix	Less than 20 mL	Purulent.	Not related to estrus. Sporadic over days to weeks.	Usually in cycling females of all parities. Results in delayed return to heat. Also rarely in pregnant females.	Usually no other clinical signs.
Uterus	10–50 mL	Whitish, chalky, odorless.	Normal postpartum discharge.	Any parity after farrowing.	Normal.
	50–100 mL or more	Purulent, occasionally bloody.	Proestrus/estrus: discharge sporadic for 1–2 days near estrus.	Usually in sows after weaning or sows with cystic ovaries. Rarely in pregnant females. More common in higher-parity sows.	Mild fever and inappetence.
	50–100 mL or more	Purulent, occasionally bloody, fetid odor. Decomposing fetal remnants.	Postparturition: somewhat constant discharge for days after farrowing.	More common in older sows after prolonged or assisted farrowing and especially if retained fetuses.	Depression, fever, anorexia, sternal or lateral recumbency.
Urinary bladder	Less than 20 mL	Purulent, mucoid, mucopurulent or mucohemorrhagic.	Seen at urination, especially at end of stream.	Frequent urination of small quantities. Dysuria and straining.	Chronic weight loss and if infection ascends to kidneys may cause uremia and death.

Table 11.36. Causes of agalactia in sows

Condition of Sow	Clinical Findings	Causes	Further Differentiation
Sick sow, elevated temperature, depressed, anorexic	Sternal recumbency. Red, swollen, hot, painful mammary gland(s).	Mastitis due to *E. coli, Klebsiella, Streptococcus, A suis.*	Culture of milk. California mastitis test.
	Hyperemia, cyanosis, anorexia, panting, dyspnea.	Porcine stress syndrome. Heat prostration.	Physical exam. Environmental temperature. DNA test.
	Swollen, edematous, painful mammary glands visible 1–2 weeks prior to farrowing.	Vitamin E/selenium deficiency often with mastitis due to secondary bacterial infection.	Ration analysis. Response to injection of selenium 4–6 weeks prefarrowing.
	Foul-smelling purulent or bloody vaginal discharge, anorexia.	*Metritis due to E. coli, Streptococcus, Klebsiella.*	Uterine culture.
	Anorexia, anemia, possible edema of udder and vulva.	Acute eperythrozoonosis.	Demonstration of organism in blood. Serology.
	Vesicles on snout, mouth, and feet.	Vesicular stomatitis or other vesicular diseases.	Complement fixation or virus neutralization tests.
Normal sow, bright and alert, normal temperature	Abnormal mammary gland conformation.	Blind teats, inverted or damaged nipples.	Physical examination.
	Normal mammary gland conformation with lack of development of underlying glandular tissue.	Undeveloped gilt, asynchrony of hormones (excess 17 beta-estradiol). Feed related: ergot, zearalenone, or deficiency of energy, water, vitamin E, selenium, pantothenic acid, riboflavin.	Ration analysis and observation of feeding practices. Mycotoxin assay.
	Normal mammary gland conformation with excessive firmness of underlying glandular tissue (hard udders).	Excess salt in diet, overfeeding prior to and in first days after farrowing, anything limiting piglets' ability to nurse (splayleg, failure to remove needle teeth, small weak pigs), stray voltage in farrowing pen.	Ration analysis. Observation of feeding. Physical examination. Voltage readings between metal of pens and ground.

Table 11.37. Flowchart for investigation of low numbers of pigs weaned/sow/year (PW/S/Y)

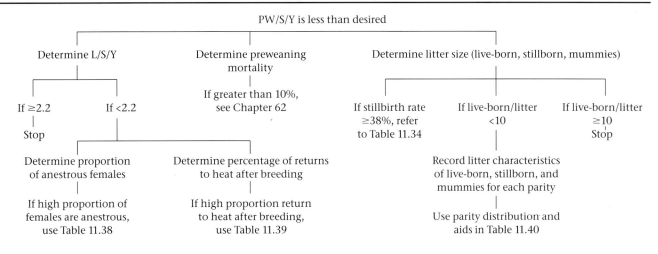

Table 11.38. Causes of anestrus

Factor Contributing to Anestrus	Comments	
	Gilt	Sow Postweaning
Age	The first estrus usually occurs in gilts between 5 and 8 months of age. Gilts raised in outside pens reach puberty earlier than gilts raised in enclosed buildings.	
Breed	There is a large breed variation in age at puberty. Crossbreds reach puberty earlier than purebreds. The percentage of gilts that show estrus by 8.5 months of age in common breeds is Large White, 86%; Landrace, 78%; Duroc, 71%; Hampshire, 71%; and Yorkshire, 56%.	Early weaning (i.e., 10 days). There is a large variation between breeds and lines of sows in percentage of sows returning to heat after weaning at 10 days or less.
Anatomical anomaly	Hermaphrodites, pseudohermaphrodites, intersexuality.	
Exposure to a boar	Gilts raised in contact with a boar reach puberty 20–40 days earlier than gilts raised in isolation.	Sows weaned into an area where they have contact with boars will show earlier and stronger signs of estrus.
Light	Gilts exposed to at least 14 hours of light per day reach puberty earlier than gilts in darker environments.	At least 14 hours of light per day in the farrowing area is associated with a greater percentage of weaned sows returning to estrus within 5 days of weaning.
Season	More fall-born gilts will reach puberty by 8 months of age than spring-born gilts.	Between July and September (in the Northern Hemisphere) a decrease occurs in the number of sows returning to estrus within 7 days after weaning. Primiparous sows are particularly affected.
Length of lactation		Sows weaned earlier than 18 days of lactation show a lower percentage of animals coming into estrus within 7 days.
Nutrition	Undernourished animals are less likely to show estrus.	Animals that were thin prior to entering the farrowing area or lost more than 20 kg because of heavy milk production during lactation are less likely to show estrus within 7 days postweaning.
Management	Many complaints of anestrus or "silent heats" are due to inadequate heat checking by breeding-herd personnel. The boar and sow should be put together in a pen for heat detection. Although the presence of a boar assists the herdsperson to identify females in estrus, the boar should not be relied on to locate estrous sows. Heat checking should be done when there are no distracting influences such as feeding.	
Pregnancy	Usually associated with poor record-keeping and inability to identify animals.	
Pseudopregnancy	May be associated with early pregnancy loss. Corpus luteum maintains pregnant state, even in the absence of fetuses in the uterus. Zearalenone may cause pseudopregnancy.	
Cystic ovaries	Both follicular and luteal cysts develop in swine. Cystic ovarian structures are more common in sows than in gilts.	

Table 11.39. Causes of return to estrus in sows after breeding

	Possible Causes	Diagnosis
		Failures of Ovulation
Regular intervals (18–24 days after breeding)	Zearalenone	Examine prepuberal gilts for vulval redness and enlargement. Test feed samples for presence of zearalenone.
	Seasonal infertility	Between July and September (in the Northern Hemisphere). Problem is more pronounced in gilts and primiparous sows.
	Cystic ovaries	Evaluation of reproductive tracts at slaughter.
		Failures of Conception
	Female anatomical anomaly	Physical examination and evaluation of reproductive tract at slaughter.
	Iatrogenic with artificial insemination	Poor semen handling or insemination technique when using artificial insemination.
		Boar Failure
	Overuse of boar	Examine records of boar usage. Boars should not be used more frequently than four times per week.
	Failure to breed	Physical examination of boar for anatomical defects of reproductive tract and ability to stand and mount. Observation of mating performance for libido and experience. History of recent illness with pyrexia or treatment with corticosteroids.
	Improper timing of mating	Review of mating procedures in the herd. Verification that each female is bred at least twice during estrus. Infections: Early Abortion-Resorption
Irregular intervals (more than 25 days after breeding)	Various diseases: porcine parvovirus, pseudorabies, leptospirosis, brucellosis, eperythrozoonosis, Japanese B encephalitis, cytomegalovirus, and other bacteria, fungi	Serologic demonstration of the presence of the organism in the herd and evidence that there is a susceptible population of animals in the herd.
	Any illness associated with pyrexia	History of illness in the herd. Noninfectious: Early Abortion-Resorption
	High environmental temperatures	History of high environmental temperatures at time sows were mated.
	Trauma	History of excessive fighting among sows. Sows typically kept in large groups of different-sized animals.
	Seasonal	July through September (in the Northern Hemisphere). Most noticeable in gilts and primiparous sows.
	Overfeeding	Consumption of large amounts of feed in the period after mating has been associated with embryonic death.

Table 11.40. Causes of small numbers of pigs per litter at birth

Possible Causes of Small Litters	Diagnosis	Parities Affected
Poor timing and frequency of mating	Observation of estrus detection and mating procedures. Verification that all females are mated twice during estrus.	All
Use of different boars	Double mating with two different boars results in litters 0.4 pigs larger than if the same boar was used twice.	All
Length of previous lactation	Investigation of time of weaning, average, and range. Between 16 and 35 days, for each delay of 5 days, litter size increases by 0.2–0.4 pigs.	2+
Age and weight at first mating (gilts)	History of breeding practices. Waiting to breed a gilt on her second vs. first estrus results in 0.5 more pigs per litter.	1
Split weaning of litters	Split-weaned sows have larger subsequent litters.	2+
Parity	Determination of the parity distribution in the herd. Litter size is smallest in gilts and increases with increasing parities, with the best production in parities 3, 4, 5, and 6.	All
Breed	Analysis of breed composition of herd. White breeds are more prolific than colored breeds.	All
Heterosis	Analysis of breeding program. Determination of heterosis is being appropriately maximized with maternal breeds.	All
Season	Litter size is 0.4 pigs larger in sows bred in January through April than in other months.	All, especially 1
Low lactation feed intake	Examination of sows' condition at the end of gestation and lactation. Evaluation of feeding program for amount and nutrient density. Sows that lose more than 20 kg in weight during a farrowing and lactation have smaller subsequent litters. Too many overweight sows just prior to farrowing.	2+
Low lactation protein	Feed analysis to verify that sows of highly prolific breeds are receiving a ration that contains 1.1% lysine during the lactation period.	2+
Gilt feeding practices	Examine gilt feeding practices. Gilts that are "flushed" (i.e., fed additional amounts 3 weeks prior to mating) produce one more pig per litter.	1
Amount of stress	Examine sow housing for the amount of competition between animals. Large groups of sows, especially when different-sized animals are housed together, or excessive movement or sorting of sows within the first 30 days after mating may result in resorption of embryos.	All
Environmental temperature	History of high environmental temperature just after breeding. Hot environments are associated with resorption.	All
Porcine parvovirus and other viruses	Pattern of titers in breeding herd. Gilts in gilt pool and breeding area negative, bred gilts and older sows positive.	Usually 1

Table 11.41. Interpretation of serology

Disease	Test	Results and Interpretation		
Brucellosis	Standard tube test	If all of the following apply: a. No animals on test with titers greater than 1:1000 b. Not a retest of an infected herd c. Complete herd test or incomplete test of a validated herd. Then use the following:		If one or more of the following apply: a. One or more animals on test with titer greater than 1:1000 b. Retest of an infected herd c. Incomplete test of a herd of unknown status Then use the following:

Brucellosis — Standard tube test detail:

1:25	1:50	1:100		1:25	1:50	1:100	
'	–	–	Negative	'	–	–	Negative
+	–	–	Negative	+	–	–	Reactor
+	'	–	Negative	+	'	–	Reactor
+	+	–	Negative	+	+	–	Reactor
+	+	'	Negative	+	+	'	Reactor
				+	+	+	Reactor

Disease	Test	Results and Interpretation
Eperythrozoonosis	IHA	Results are useful as a herd test; individual titers have not been correlated with clinical signs of disease or production. In herd studies, no consistent correlation was found between disease problems in the herd and the prevalence and magnitude of the titers. Less than 1:40 — Negative 1:40 to 1:80 — Suspect 1:80 and greater — Positive
Circovirus	IFA	Positive at 1:20
Porcine reproductive and respiratory syndrome	IFA	IFA (IgG) is first detected at 9–11 days post infection; the peak titer occurs at 4–5 weeks and gradually declines to undetectable levels at 5–6 months. IFA (IgM) is first detected at 5 days post infection and declines to undetectable levels at 28 days. IgM-positive pigs are likely to be carrier pigs with recent infection. IFA tests do not detect all strains of the virus. A titer of 1:16 is considered low, while 1:256 is high.
	ELISA	Detects both American and European strains of the virus. Antibody is first detected at 9–13 days postinfection; the peak titer occurs at 4–6 weeks and gradually declines to undetectable levels at 4–5 months. An S/P ratio of 0.4 is considered positive.

Disease	Test	Vaccinated Pigs	Nonvaccinated Pigs	
Leptospirosis	MA	2–3 weeks after vaccination, titers may be as high as 1:6400, especially in animals previously vaccinated.	1:100	Of doubtful significance; possibly an old residual titer; however, confirmed cases of leptospiral abortion have resulted in titers no greater than 1:100.
		2–3 weeks after vaccination, titers may be as high as 1:6400, especially in animals previously vaccinated.	1:200 or 1:400	Interpretation difficult; should be checked against another sample 10–20 days later.
		2–3 weeks after vaccination, titers may be as high as 1:6400, especially in animals previously vaccinated.	31:800	Possibly indicates recent infection; sows aborting due to leptospirosis may have titers of 1:12,800.
Actinobacillus pleuropneumoniae	CF	Vaccination may produce titers as high as 1:128, but more typically in the range of 1:8 to1:32. Titers fall to undetectable levels by 2–3 months postvaccination.	Young pigs' (<3 months old) passive immunity: Passively acquired immunity results in titers as high as 1:128. Passive titers usually decline to undetectable levels by 3 months old. Older pigs (34 months): >1:4 = suspect.	
	ESAP-ELISA	2 weeks after a second vaccination, titers are as high as 6.5 on the ESAP scale (0–13).	Because of cross-reaction with *Actinobacillus suis* and other organisms, results should be interpreted with caution, and along with clinical and pathological observation. Early field exposure 10–14 days) gives titers ranging from 2 to 10 on the ESAP scale. The highest titers are seen at 3 weeks postexposure. In late-phase exposure (108–120 days), 87% of the pigs are still seropositive with ESAP titers as high as 13.	

Table 11.41. Interpretation of serology

Disease	Test	Results and Interpretation	
		VACCINATED PIGS	NONVACCINATED PIGS
Porcine parvovirus	HI	At 2 weeks postvaccination, titers generally range from 1:40 to 1:320. Vaccination titers frequently decay to nondetectable levels within 3–4 months.	Young pigs (<6 months old): Passive titers derived from colostral immunity may be up to 1:5120; these titers decline to subdetectable levels by 3–8 months of age. Breeding animals: Within 1 week after exposure to the virus, titers may be as high as 1:10,000. After 2 weeks, the range of values for previously exposed sows in an endemically infected herd is 1:320 to >1:2560.
Pseudorabies	SN	Vaccination may produce titers of 1:32, but more typically at 1:4 to 1:8. Vaccine titers may persist up to 6 months but generally are not detectable after 3 months.	A titer of 1:2 in only one animal of a group generally indicates the need to retest. A 1:4 or greater titer is positive. By 2 weeks after exposure to the virus, titers may reach 1:512.
	ELISA	Results are usually reported as positive or negative and SN tests are run to determine titer. Differential tests are available to detect titers that result from vaccination with gene-deleted vaccines.	
Swine Influenza	HI	At 2 weeks postvaccination, 55% of pigs have titers >1:20. The highest titers are seen 4 weeks postvaccination. Titers are 31:320. Passive immunity of 1:20 interferes with vaccination.	Titers positive 1 week after infection, may be as high as 1:320 by 2 weeks post infection and will persist for 4 weeks before declining. Passive immunity usually declines by 12 wks of age.
	ELISA	At 2 weeks postvaccination, 50% of pigs are seropositive. At 4 weeks postvaccination, 100% have seroconverted.	Specificity 99.7%. Range of values is 0.0–2.5 with the positive cut-off at 0.4. True negative herds have values of 0.05 to 0.2.
Transmissible gastroenteritis	SN	Vaccine titers may reach levels as high as 1:400 but usually are between 1:40 and 1:200. Titers can rise dramatically at farrowing. Cross-reactions occur with porcine corona respiratory virus.	Any titer is considered positive. Titers may range from 1:40 to 1:800. Paired serum samples are the most diagnostic.
	VN	Usually 1:16.	1:4 is positive although recent infection produces titers of 1:32.
Mycoplasma hyopneumoniae	CF	Vaccination usually produces titers in the range of 1:4 to 1:32.	1:8 = positive 1:4 = suspect Titers usually range from 1:4 to 1:128.
	ELISA	2 weeks after a second vaccination, titers are usually 0.4 to 1.6.	Seroconversion starts around 2–3 weeks post exposure. <0.3 is negative, 0.3–0.4 is suspect, and >0.4 is positive. Test may cross-react with *M. hyorhinis* and *M. flocculare*.

Note: CF = complement fixation; ELISA = enzyme-linked immunosorbent assay; IFA = indirect fluorescent antibody; IHA = indirect hemagglutination; HI = hemagglutination inhibition; MA = microtiter agglutination; VN = virus neutralization; SN = serum neutralization; ′ = suspect/borderline.

Viral Diseases

12 Porcine Adenovirus

Steven B. Kleiboeker

An adenovirus was first isolated from a rectal swab of a piglet with diarrhea four decades ago (Haig et al. 1964). A second isolation, made from the brain of a pig with encephalitis, was reported a short time later (Kasza 1966). Since then, porcine adenoviruses have been isolated from a wide variety of samples and associated with pneumonia, diarrhea, and kidney lesions, as well as encephalitis. In swine, however, the virus has been isolated from the feces of normal pigs and the majority of porcine adenovirus infections appear to be asymptomatic. In recent years, porcine adenoviruses have been developed for use as expression vectors and vaccine vectors (Reddy et al. 1999), similar to those based on human adenoviruses.

ETIOLOGY

The three species of porcine adenoviruses (A, B, and C) are classified in family *Adenoviridae*, genus *Mastadenovirus*. Up to six serotypes have been identified by virus-neutralization tests (Clarke et al. 1967; Haig et al. 1964; Hirahara et al. 1990a; Kadoi et al. 1995; Kasza 1966). Serotypes 1, 2, and 3 belong in species porcine adenovirus A, serotype 4 in porcine adenovirus B, and serotype 5 in porcine adenovirus C (Büchen-Osmond 2003).

The structural, chemical, and physical characteristics of porcine adenoviruses are indistinguishable from other members of the *Adenoviridae*. Adenovirus virions are nonenveloped with icosahedral capsid symmetry and are 80–90 nm in diameter. Virions are composed of 240 hexon molecules that form 20 equilateral triangular facets of the icosahedron. A total of 12 pentons per virion are located at the vertices. Fiber proteins, 20–50 nm long with a terminal knob, project from each penton. Adenovirus particles have a precise hexagonal outline when viewed by negative stain electron microscopy (Figure 12.1), and the fiber and terminal knob can occasionally be observed.

Characteristic of family *Adenoviridae*, the porcine adenovirus genome is a single, linear molecule of double-stranded DNA. The genome is approximately 32–34 kilobases in length (Kleiboeker et al. 1993; Reddy et al. 1998; Nagy et al. 2001), based on full-length genome sequencing and restriction fragment length mapping of several porcine adenovirus serotypes. Approximately 40 proteins are encoded by the viral genome and transcribed following complex RNA splicing. About one-third of the genes encode structural proteins. The genome organization is typical of other adenoviruses with early and late gene expression profiles. The ends of the genome form inverted terminal repeats.

Porcine adenoviruses can be isolated and grown in vitro in primary porcine kidney cells using standard virological methods. In addition, continuous porcine kidney cell lines, such as PK-15 cells, and primary porcine cells cultures, such as thyroid cells (Dea and Elazhary 1984a) and testicular cells (Hirahara et al. 1990b), will support productive replication of porcine adenovirus isolates. Viral replication in vitro produces a cytopathic effect characterized by enlargement, clumping, and rounding of cells, followed by detachment. Visible cytopathic effect is typically observed 2–4 days postinoculation and progresses to complete destruction of the cell monolayer. Intranuclear inclusion bodies can be observed in stained cell monolayers. When viewed by thin section electron microscopy, it can be seen that inclusion bodies are formed by crystalline arrays of virus aggregates in the nucleus of the cell.

EPIDEMIOLOGY

Serological studies suggest that porcine adenoviruses are distributed worldwide. Strains of porcine adenovirus B appear to be the most widely distributed, both in North America and Europe.

Swine are the only species known to be susceptible to porcine adenoviruses, although extensive studies on the host range of these viruses have not been performed. Swine appear to be susceptible to infection with human adenoviruses, but in general, the host range of adenoviruses is quite narrow and zoonotic transmission of

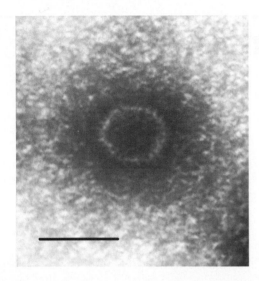

12.1. *Negative stain electron micrograph of porcine adenovirus. A typical adenoviral particle was identified following ultracentrifugation of cell culture supernatant from PK-15 cells showing cytopathic effect. Bar, 100 nm.*

porcine adenoviruses from swine to humans has not been reported.

Transmission of porcine adenoviruses is primarily through the fecal-oral route, although aerosol transmission by inhalation of infectious particles may be possible. Fecal shedding of virus occurs, most commonly after weaning (Derbyshire et al. 1966). The duration of shedding following infection of swine with porcine adenoviruses is unknown, although pathogenesis studies have shown viral antigen in enterocytes up to 45 days postinfection, suggesting that long-term shedding is possible. Adult swine rarely shed virus and frequently have high serum antibody titers, which may prevent productive viral replication in these animals.

Adenoviruses are relatively resistant to heat and are stable at room temperature for up to 10 days, but are readily inactivated by common disinfectants, such as bleach, formaldehyde, alcohol, and phenolic compounds (Derbyshire and Arkell 1971).

PATHOGENESIS

The initial isolation of porcine adenovirus was from the brain of a pig with neurological disease, but porcine adenoviruses are most commonly associated with gastrointestinal disease in swine, although respiratory disease may also be possible. Infection of swine occurs following inhalation or ingestion and the primary sites of replication include the tonsils and distal small intestine (Ducatelle et al. 1982; Shadduck et al. 1967; Sharpe and Jessett 1967). Infection of pregnant swine can result in abortion, and virus will replicate in a number of internal organs of the fetus (Dee 1995). In some disease processes, porcine adenovirus may play a role as a secondary or co-pathogen. For example, research showed that sero-

type 4 and *Mycoplasma hyopneumoniae* produced a more severe pneumonia when inoculated together (Kasza et al. 1969).

CLINICAL SIGNS

The only consistent clinical sign observed following experimental inoculation of piglets with porcine adenovirus was diarrhea (Coussement et al. 1981; Derbyshire et al. 1969; Derbyshire et al. 1975; Sanford and Hoover 1983). Experimental oronasal inoculation of cesarian-derived, colostrum-deprived piglets resulted in diarrhea after an incubation period of 3–4 days. Thus, clinical signs, if present, most often involve generalized gastroenteric disease with watery to pasty diarrhea. Experimental inoculation of pigs with porcine adenovirus did not result in mortality and is considered unlikely to do so in cases of natural infection. Based on pathogenesis studies and clinical reports, clinical signs compatible with respiratory disease are possible, but less likely than gastoenteric disease. Dea and El Azhary (1984b) reported that 15% of adult swine with respiratory disease were seropositive to serotype 4, but did not establish a causal relationship between the two. Porcine adenoviruses have been isolated from aborted fetuses (Dee 1995), although there is little evidence to support a significant etiologic role in swine reproductive failure.

LESIONS

Gross lesions are not likely to be observed in swine with adenovirus infections. Moderate enlargement of lymph nodes has been noted following experimental inoculation. Histological lesions characterized by the presence of intranuclear, basophilic inclusion bodies are suggestive of porcine adenoviral infection. These inclusions can most readily be observed in enterocytes of the distal jejunum and ileum, which is presumably where primary viral replication occurs (Ducatelle et al. 1982). Experimental inoculation has also demonstrated destruction of epithelial cells and blunting of the intestinal villi in the lower jejunum and ileum (Ducatelle et al. 1982). Other lesions attributed to both natural and experimental infection of swine with porcine adenovirus include meningoencephalitis with perivascular infiltration and microglial nodule formation (Edington et al. 1972; Kasza 1966) and kidney lesions involving dystrophy of tubules and capillary dilatation plus severe peritubular infiltration. Pneumonia associated with porcine adenovirus infection is characterized by interstitial pneumonia with alveolar thickening due to proliferation of septal cells and infiltration of inflammatory cells.

DIAGNOSIS

The differential diagnosis for infection of swine with adenoviruses includes other causes of gastroenteric disease, and possibility respiratory disease. Techniques used for diagnosis of porcine adenovirus infection include negative stain electron microscopy (EM) and virus isolation. Electron microscopy is commonly used to detect enteric viral pathogens from diarrheic feces. The relatively large size and characteristic morphology make adenovirus particles straightforward to detect, if present in reasonably high concentrations. In cell culture, the cytopathic effect of porcine adenoviruses is somewhat distinctive, characterized by rounding and the formation of grape-like clusters as cells detach. However, a secondary technique such as EM of cell culture supernatant, neutralization with specific antiserum, or fluorescent antibody (FA) staining with specific antiserum is necessary to confirm the isolation of an adenovirus. For FA staining, an anti-porcine adenovirus fluorescent antibody conjugate is available from the National Veterinary Services Laboratory (United States Department of Agriculture, Animal and Plant Health Inspection Service, Ames, Iowa U.S.A.), although the ability of this conjugate to detect all known species of porcine adenovirus has not been demonstrated. Serologic typing of new isolates by virus neutralizing may be attempted, although reference antiserum may be difficult to obtain.

Serological diagnosis of adenoviral infection may also be attempted using virus neutralization, plaque reduction neutralization assays, or indirect immunofluorescence assays using cells infected with viral stocks in vitro. Demonstration of a rising titer in conjunction with compatible clinical disease is suggestive of a role for porcine adenovirus infection. No commercially available serodiagostic tests specifically for the detection of porcine adenoviruses are available, nor have any been reported in the scientific literature for use in research studies.

In postmortem samples, amphophilic to basophilic adenoviral inclusions that fill the entire nucleus are observed in the early stages of infection. In experimental infections, viral antigen may be detected in enterocytes as early as 24 hours postinoculation. In later stages of infection, inclusions become smaller and are surrounded by a halo. The inclusions are mainly located in enterocytes on the tips and sides of the villi, which may be short and blunt. Viral antigen may persist and can be detected by techniques such as immunoperoxidase staining for up to 45 days following infection (Ducatelle et al. 1982). Specific anti-porcine adenovirus antiserum is available from the same source as the FA conjugate. The presence of intranuclear inclusion bodies is suggestive, but not diagnostic, of porcine adenovirus infection, unless confirmed by positive viral antigen staining by immunofluorescence or immunohistochemistry.

To date, only one report has described a polymerase chain reaction (PCR) assay for detection of porcine adenoviruses (Maluquer de Motes et al. 2004). The assay was validated using fecal samples and a single strain of porcine adenovirus serotype 3. The performance of the assay for other serotypes of porcine adenovirus and other sample matrices is not known.

PREVENTION AND CONTROL

No specific antiviral treatment is available for porcine adenovirus infection of swine. Vaccines have proven useful in control of adenoviruses in other species, but the level of disease caused by porcine adenovirus has not justified the development of vaccines or other control and prevention measures.

REFERENCES

Büchen-Osmond C. 2003. Mastadenovirus. In: ICTVdB—The Universal Virus Database, version 3. ICTVdB Management, The Earth Institute, Biosphere 2 Center, Columbia University, Oracle, AZ, USA.

Clarke MC, Sharpe HB, Derbyshire JB. 1967. Some characteristics of three porcine adenoviruses. Arch Gesamte Virusforsch 21:91–97.

Coussement W, Ducatelle R, Charlier G, Hoorens J. 1981. Adenovirus enteritis in pigs. Am J Vet Res 42:1905–1911.

Dea S, Elazhary MA. 1984a. Cultivation of a porcine adenovirus in porcine thyroid cell cultures. Cornell Veterinarian 74:208–211.

———. 1984b. Prevalence of antibodies to porcine adenovirus in swine by indirect fluorescent antibody test. Am J Vet Res 45:2109–2112.

Dee SA. 1995. Viral causes of porcine reproductive failure—Part I. Compend Contin Educ Vet Pract 17: 962–972.

Derbyshire JB, Arkell S. 1971. The activity of some chemical disinfectants against talfan virus and porcine adenovirus type 2. Br Vet J 127:137–142.

Derbyshire JB, Clarke MC, Collins AP. 1975. Serological and pathogenicity studies with some unclassified porcine adenoviruses. J Comp Pathol 85:437–443.

Derbyshire JB, Clarke MC, Jessett DM. 1966. Observations on the faecal excretion of adenoviruses and enteroviruses in conventional and "minimal disease" pigs. Vet Rec 79:595–599.

———. 1969. The isolation of adenoviruses and enteroviruses from pig tissues. J Comp Pathol 79:97–100.

Ducatelle R, Coussement W, Hoorens J. 1982. Sequential pathological study of experimental porcine adenovirus enteritis. Vet Pathol 19:179–89.

Edington N, Kasza L, Christofinis GJ. 1972. Meningo-encephalitis in gnotobiotic pigs inoculated intranaslly and orally with porcine adenovirus 4. Res Vet Sci 13:289–291.

Haig DA, Clarke MC, Pereira MS. 1964. Isolation of an adenovirus from a pig. J Comp Pathol 74:81–85.

Hirahara T, Yasuhara H, Matsui O, Fukuyama S, Yamanaka M, Izumida A, Yoshiki K, Kodama K, Nakai M, Sasaki N. 1990b. Growth activity of porcine adenoviruses in primary porcine testicular cell cultures. Nippon Juigaku Zasshi 52:1089–1091.

Hirahara T, Yasuhara H, Matsui O, Yamanaka M, Tanaka M, Fukuyama S, Izumida A, Yoshiki K, Kodama K, Nakai M, Sasaki, N. 1990a. Isolation of porcine adenovirus from the respiratory tract of pigs in Japan. Nippon Juigaku Zasshi 52:407–409.

Kadoi K, Inoue Y, Ikeda T, Kamata H, Yukawa M, Iwabuchi M, Inaba Y. 1995. Isolation of porcine adenovirus as a candidate of 5th serotype. J Basic Microbiol 35:195–204.

Kasza L. 1966. Isolation of an adenovirus from the brain of a pig. Am J Vet Res 27:751–758.

Kasza L, Hodges RT, Betts AO, Trexler PC. 1969. Pneumonia in gnotobiotic pigs produced by simultaneous inoculation of a swine adenovirus and Mycoplasma hyopneumoniae. Vet Rec 84:262–267.

Kleiboeker SB, Seal BS, Mengeling WL. 1993. Genomic cloning and restriction site mapping of a porcine adenovirus isolate: Demonstration of genomic stability in a porcine adenovirus. Arch Virol 133:357–368.

Maluquer de Motes C, Clemente-Casares P, Hundesa A, Martin M, Girones R. 2004. Detection of bovine and porcine adenoviruses for tracing the source of fecal contamination. Appl Environ Microbiol 70:1448–1454.

Nagy M, Nagy E, Tuboly T. 2001. The complete nucleotide sequence of porcine adenovirus serotype 5. J Gen Virol 82:525–529.

Reddy PS, Idamakanti N, Hyun BH, Tikoo SK, Babiuk LA. 1999. Development of porcine adenovirus-3 as an expression vector. J Gen Virol 80:563–570.

Reddy PS, Idamakanti N, Song JY, Lee JB, Hyun BH, Park JH, Cha SH, Bae YT, Tikoo SK, Babiuk LA. 1998. Nucleotide sequence and transcription map of porcine adenovirus type 3. Virol 251:414–26.

Sanford SE, Hoover DM. 1983. Enteric adenovirus infection in pigs. Can J Comp Med 47:396–400.

Shadduck JA, Koestner A, Kasza L. 1967. The lesions of porcine adenoviral infection in germfree and pathogen-free pigs. Pathol Vet 4:537–552.

Sharpe HB, Jessett DM. 1967 Experimental infection of pigs with 2 strains of porcine adenovirus. J Comp Pathol 77:45–50.

13 African Swine Fever

José Manuel Sánchez-Vizcaíno

African Swine Fever (ASF) is caused by a DNA virus in family *Asfarviridae,* genus *Asfivirus*. ASF is considered a List A disease by the Office International des Epizooties (OIE) because of its potential for rapid dissemination and significant socioeconomical consequences. ASF is currently endemic in many sub-Saharan countries of Africa and Sardinia (Italy). Under natural conditions, ASF virus (ASFV) infects only porcine species, both wild and domesticated. Inapparent infection with ASFV is common in wart hogs (*Phacochoerus aethiopicus*) and bush pigs (*Potamochoerus porcus*) and both species act as reservoir hosts in Africa (De Tray 1957; Heuschele and Coggins 1965). Soft ticks have been shown to be both reservoirs and vectors of ASFV, especially *Ornithodorus moubata* and *O. erraticus*. ASFV has been introduced into free areas by feeding contaminated pork products collected from international airports and seaports. Once established in domestic herds, infected and carrier pigs become the most important source of virus dissemination. Clinical signs and lesions range from acute to inapparent and can resemble several other hemorrhagic diseases of pigs, especially classical swine fever (hog cholera) and erysipelas. Laboratory tests are required to establish a definitive diagnosis. There is no treatment or effective vaccine available for ASFV. Therefore, control of ASF is based on rapid laboratory diagnosis and the enforcement of strict sanitary measures.

ETIOLOGY

ASFV is the only member of the family *Asfaviridae* genus *Asfivirus* (Murphy et al. 1995). ASFV is a complex, icosahedral, deoxivirus with features common to both the iridovirus and poxvirus families. The virion is composed of several concentric structures and an external hexagonal membrane (Figure 13.1.) acquired by budding through the cell membrane (Carrascosa et al. 1984). By electronic microscopy, the average diameter of ASFV particles is 200 nm (Breese and DeBoer 1966).

ASFV has a double-stranded linear DNA genome 170–190 kilobases in size, depending on the virus strain (Blasco et al. 1989; Tabares et al. 1980), with terminal inverted repeats (Sogo et al. 1984), a conserved central region of about 125 kilobases, and variable ends. The complete DNA sequence of the BA71v strain of ASFV was composed of 170,101 nucleotides, with 151 open reading frames encoding five multigene families (Yañez et al. 1995).

ASFV is a very complex virus. At least 28 structural proteins have been identified in intracellular virus particles (Tabares et al. 1980), and more than 100 virus-induced proteins have been identified in infected porcine macrophages. At least 50 of the latter react with sera from infected or recovered pigs (Alcaraz et al. 1992) and 40 of these polypeptides are incorporated in the viral particle (Carrascosa et al. 1985). Some of these proteins— e.g., p73, p54, p30, and p12—are highly antigenic. Although their role in inducing protective immunity is unresolved (Neilan et al. 2004), they are used in ASF serodiagnosis (Arias and Sánchez-Vizcaíno 1992).

ASFV has been adapted to grow in a large number of stable cell lines, including VERO, MS, and CV, (Hess et al. 1965). In infected pigs, ASFV replicates primarily in monocytes and macrophage cells (Malmquist and Hay 1960; Minguez et al. 1988), but also in endothelial cells (Wilkinson and Wardley 1978), hepatocytes (Sierra et al. 1987), renal tubular epithelial cells (Gomez-Villamandos et al. 1995), and neutrophils (Carrasco et al. 1996). No infection has been observed in T or B lymphocytes (Gomez-Villamandos et al. 1995; Minguez et al. 1988). In nature, ASFV replicates in some soft ticks, principally *Ornithodoros moubata* (Plowright et al. 1970) and *O. erraticus* (Sanchez Botija 1963).

EPIDEMIOLOGY

Montgomery first described ASF in Kenya in 1921. The virus spread from infected warthogs (*Phacochoerus aethiopicus*) to domestic pigs (*Sus scrofa*), causing a disease with a 100% mortality. Since then, ASF has been rec-

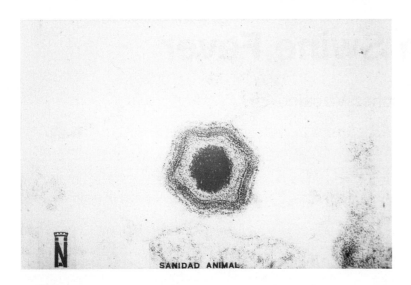

13.1. *Electron micrograph of an ASF virus particle.*

ognized as endemic in many African countries: Angola, Mozambique, Republic of South Africa, São Tomé and Príncipe, Senegal, Sudan, Uganda, and Zimbabwe.

In 1957, ASFV was detected for the first time outside the African continent. It appeared in Lisbon (Portugal) in a peracute form with a mortality of almost 100% (Manso Ribeiro et al. 1963). In 1960, it reappeared near Lisbon, apparently as a new outbreak, spread through the rest of Portugal, and reached Spain the same year (Polo Jover and Sanchez Botija 1961). ASF remained endemic in Portugal and Spain until 1995 when, as a result of an intensive eradication program, both countries were declared ASF-free.

In 1978, ASFV again appeared outside of Africa, this time in Malta, Sardinia (Italy), Brazil, and the Dominican Republic. In 1979, it appeared in Haiti and, in 1980, in Cuba. Today, ASF is present only in Africa, mainly in sub-Saharan countries, and in Sardinia. Elsewhere it has been successfully eradicated

Pigs are the only domesticated animals naturally infected by ASFV. European wild boars are also susceptible to ASFV infection, with clinical signs and mortality rates similar to those observed in naturally infected domesticated pigs in Spain, Portugal, and Sardinia (Italy) (Contini et al. 1983; Sanchez Botija 1982). In contrast, ASFV usually induces an inapparent infection in three African wild suid species: warthogs (*Phacochoerus aethiopicus*), giant forest hog (*Hylochoerus meinertzhageni*) and bushpigs (*Potamochoerus porcus*). Several species of soft ticks have been shown to be ASFV reservoirs and biological vectors, including *Ornithodoros moubata* in Africa (Plowright et al. 1969) and *O. erraticus* in the Iberian Peninsula (Sanchez Botija 1963).

ASFV is maintained in Africa by a cycle of infection between African wild suid species and soft ticks. In some of these wild suids infection is characterized by low levels of virus in tissues and low or undetectable levels of viremia (Plowright 1981). These levels of virus are sufficient for transmission to domestic pigs through tick vec-

tors, but usually not by direct contact between animals. This transmission cycle makes it very difficult to eradicate ASF in Africa.

In contrast to African wild suids, European wild boars are susceptible to ASFV infection and show clinical signs and mortality rates similar to those observed in domestic pigs. In Europe, direct transmission by contact between sick and healthy animals is the most common route of transmission. Indirect transmission by biological vectors, like *O. erraticus*, has also been described in the Iberian Peninsula, especially in outdoor pig productions.

An important difference in the epidemiology of ASFV in Africa vs. Europe is related to ASF virus replication in soft ticks. Transovarial and transtadial transmission of ASFV has been described for *O. moubata* (Plowright et al. 1970), but in Europe only transtadial transmission has been observed in *O. erraticus*. *Ornithodoros savignyi*, also present in Africa, can experimentally transmit ASF virus to domestic pigs (Mellor and Wilkinson 1985). A number of other tick species widely distributed in North and South America are considered capable of harboring and transmitting ASFV (Groocock et al. 1980).

Once ASFV is established in domesticated pigs, carrier pigs become an important source of virus, and their role in the epidemiology of the disease is a major consideration in designing a strategy for ASF eradication. The serological recognition of carrier pigs was an importance facet in the successful eradication of ASF in Spain (Arias and Sánchez-Vizcaíno 2002).

The ASFV is very resistant to inactivation in the environment, particularly by temperature and acid pH. ASFV can be isolated from sera or blood stored at room temperature for 18 months. However, it is inactivated by heat treatment at 60°C for 30 minutes (Plowright and Parker 1967) and by many lipid solvents and commercial disinfectants. In meat products, ASFV may persist for weeks or months in frozen or uncooked meat. In cured or processed products, such as Parma ham, infectious virus was not demonstrated after 300 days of processing and curing (McKercher et al. 1987). Spanish cured pig meat products, such as Serrano hams and Iberian hams and shoulders, were free of viable ASFV by day 140 and Iberian loins by day 112 (Mebus et al. 1993). No infectious ASFV has been found in cooked or canned hams heated to 70°C.

PATHOGENESIS

ASFV is generally spread among domestic pigs via oral or nasal routes of dissemination and exposure (Colgrove et al. 1969; Plowright et al. 1968). Pigs can also be infected by a number of other routes, including tick bite (Plowright et al. 1969), cutaneous scarification, and intramuscular, subcutaneous, intraperitoneal, or intravenous injection (McVicar 1984). The incubation period varies widely (4–19 days), depending on the ASFV isolate and the route of exposure.

The sites of primary replication are the monocytes and macrophages of the lymph nodes nearest to the point of virus entrance. When the exposure is oral, the monocytes and macrophages of the tonsils and mandibular lymph nodes are the first involved. From these sites, the virus spreads through the blood and/or lymphatic system to the main sites of secondary replication—i.e., lymph nodes, bone marrow, spleen, lung, liver, and kidney. Viremia usually begins 4–8 days post infection and, due to the absence of neutralizing antibodies, persists for weeks or months.

ASFV is associated with red blood cell membranes (Quintero et al. 1986) and platelets (Gomez-Villamandos et al. 1996) and causes hemadsorption in affected pigs (Sierra et al. 1991). Recently, the protein involved in hemadsorption was identified (Galindo et al. 2000).

The pathogenesis of the hemorrhage observed in the acute form is believed to be phagocytic activation of endothelial cells aggravated by virus replication in the same cells in the final stages of the disease. In the subacute form, hemorrhages are due mainly to an increase in vascular permeability (Gomez-Villamandos et al. 1995). The pathogenesis of the lymphopenia in the acute form has been related to apoptosis of lymphocytes, mainly on the T area of lymphoid organs (Carrasco et al. 1996). However, there is no evidence of virus replication in T- or B-cells (Gomez-Villamandos et al. 1995; Minguez et al. 1988).

The subacute form is characterized by a transitory thrombocytopenia (Gomez-Villamandos et al. 1996). The alveolar edema observed in the last stages of the acute and subacute form of ASF (and main cause of death) is a consequence of the activation of pulmonary intravascular macrophages (Carrasco et al. 1996; Sierra et al. 1990).

CLINICAL SIGNS

Clinically, ASF can resemble several other diseases of pigs, especially classical swine fever (hog cholera) and erysipelas. Therefore, laboratory tests are required to establish a definitive diagnosis (Sánchez-Vizcaíno 1986). Moreover, ASF can present a range of clinical signs, depending primarily on virus virulence, exposure dose, and exposure route. The clinical forms of ASF range from peracute (i.e., sudden death with few, if any, previous clinical signs) to subclinical or inapparent. In Africa, ASF appears mostly as an acute disease characterized by loss of appetite, high temperature (40–41°C), leukopenia, hemorrhages in internal organs, hemorrhages in the skin (especially the skin of the ears and flanks), and high mortality (Mebus et al. 1983; Moulton and Coggins 1968).

Outside of Africa, it is possible to see acute outbreaks of ASF, but subacute or chronic forms are more common. The subacute form is characterized by transitory thrombocytopenia, leukopenia, and numerous hemorrhagic lesions (Gomez-Villamandos et al. 1997). The chronic form is characterized by respiratory alteration, abortion, and low mortality (Arias et al. 1986).

LESIONS

A wide variety of lesions have been observed in ASF, depending on the virulence of the viral strain. The acute and subacute forms are characterized by extensive hemorrhages and lymphoid tissue destruction. Conversely, lesions may be minimal or absent in the subclinical and chronic forms (Gomez-Villamandos et al. 1995; Mebus et al. 1983).

The principal gross lesions are observed in the spleen, lymph nodes, kidneys, and heart (Sanchez Botija 1982). The spleen may be darkened, enlarged, infarcted, and friable (Figure 13.2). Sometimes lesions are large infarcts with subcapsular haemorrhages. Lymph nodes are hemorrhagic, edematous, and friable (Figure 13.3). They often look like dark-red hematomas. Because of congestion and subcapsular haemorrhage, cut sections of affected lymph nodes sometime have a marbled appearance. Kidneys usually have petechial hemorrhages on the cortical (Figure 13.4) and cut surfaces, as well as in the renal pelvis. An intense hydropericardium with serohemorrhagic fluid is present in some cases. Petechial and echymotic haemorrhages can be observed in epicardium and endocardium. Other lesions can also be observed in acute ASF, such as serohemorrhagic fluid in the abdominal cavity, with edema and hemorrhages throughout the alimentary tract. Congestion of the liver and the gall bladder can be observed, as well as petechial hemorrhages in the mucosa of the urinary bladder. Hydrothorax and petechial hemorrhages of the pleura are frequently found in the thoracic cavity, and lungs are usually edematous. Intense congestion is observed in the meninges, chorioid plexus, and encephalon (Arias et al. 1986).

The most predominant form of ASF outside Africa has been the subacute form, which is similar to the

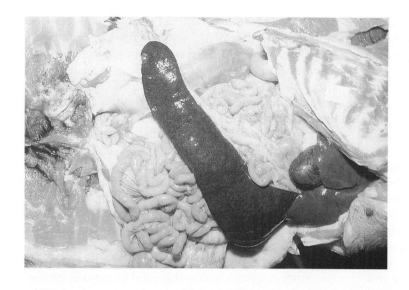

13.2. *Enlarged and darkened spleen from acute ASF.*

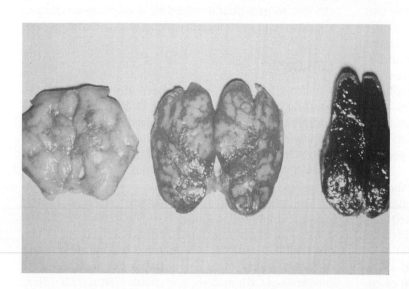

13.3. *Lymph nodes from a normal pig (left), a pig with subacute ASF (center), and a pig with acute ASF (right).*

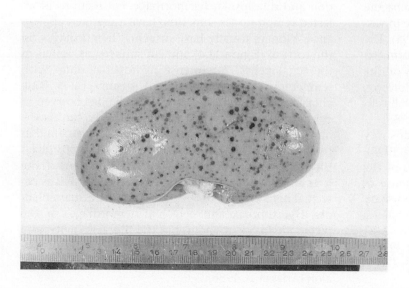

13.4. *Kidney from a pig with acute ASF showing numerous petechiae on the cortical surface.*

acute form except for milder lesions. The subacute form is characterized by large hemorrhages in lymph nodes and kidney. The spleen is enlarged and hemorrhagic. Congestion and edema can be observed in lungs and, in some cases, an interstitial pneumonia has been found (Arias et al. 1986).

In the acute form of ASF, histopathological lesions are present in blood vessels and in lymphoid organs. These lesions are characterized by hemorrhages, microthrombosis, and damage of the endothelial cells with accumulations of dead cells in the subendothelium (Gomez-Villamandos et al. 1995). Hemorrhagic splenomegaly, characteristic of the acute and subacute forms, is a consequence of the loss of splenic architecture caused by viral replication and resulting necrosis of the splenic fixed macrophages (Carrasco et al. 1997). The lymphoid tissue destruction in the acute form is mainly observed on the T area of the lymphoid organs, but no evidence of virus replication in lymphocytes has been observed (Carrasco et al. 1996; Minguez et al. 1988).

The chronic form of ASF is characterized by alterations in the respiratory tract, but lesions in the chronic form may be minimal or absent (Gomez-Villamandos et al. 1995; Mebus et al. 1983). Lesions include fibrinous pleuritis, pleural adhesions, caseous pneumonia, and hyperplasia of the lymphoreticular tissues. Fibrinous pericarditis and necrotic skin lesions are also common (Arias et al. 1986; Moulton and Coggins 1968).

IMMUNITY

The immune mechanisms involved in protection against ASF are poorly understood, and all attempts to develop an effective vaccine have been unsuccessful. The difficulty in inducing effective immunity may be related to the great variability observed among ASFV isolates. It may also be related to the fact that ASFV replicates in some cells typically involved in the immune response. Although there is no evidence for replication of ASFV in either T- and B-cells (Gomez-Villamandos et al. 1995; Minguez et al. 1988), it does replicate in monocytes and macrophages. If immune suppression has a role, however, it is not obvious (Sánchez-Vizcaíno et al. 1981).

ASFV is highly antigenic, and high levels of specific antibodies are produced during ASFV infection. IgM can be detected by 4 days post infection and IgG by 6–8 days post infection (Sánchez-Vizcaíno et al. 1979). Antibodies are detectable for a long time after the initial exposure. Antibodies against ASFV have been shown to delay the onset of the ASF clinical signs, to reduce the levels of viremia, and to protect pigs against the potential fatal consequences of infection (Onisk et al. 1994; Schlafer et al. 1984).

Early experiments demonstrated the absence of neutralizing antibodies against ASFV in sera from naturally or experimental infected pigs. However, recovered pigs produced normal levels of neutralizing antibodies in response to foot and mouth virus vaccine, suggesting that humoral responses are not adversely affected by ASFV (De Boer 1967). Other authors (Ruiz Gonzalvo et al. 1986) have demonstrated that different ASFV isolates are largely neutralized by convalescent porcine sera, but a persistent 10% fraction of nonneutralized virus remained. On the other hand, Gomez-Puertas et al. (1996) reported that ASFV-induced antibodies in serum collected from convalescent pigs effectively neutralized ASFV before and after it was bound to susceptible cells. However, ASFV-specific antibodies have never been demonstrated to entirely fulfill the classic definition of virus neutralization. On the other hand, cytotoxic T lymphocytes from recovered pigs can destroy infected macrophages (Martins and Leitao 1994), suggesting that cell-mediated immunity may be an important component of the protective response. Overall, the relative roles of antibodies and cell-mediated immunity in protecting against ASF are still not well understood.

DIAGNOSIS

Laboratory studies are essential to establish a definitive diagnosis of ASF because of the similarity of ASF clinical signs and lesions to other hemorrhagic pig diseases—e.g., classical swine fever (hog cholera), erysipelas, and septicemic salmonellosis. As in other viral diseases, the laboratory diagnosis of ASF is based on the demonstration of infectious virus, viral antigens, viral DNA, or specific antibodies. A wide variety of laboratory tests are available for detecting either ASFV or homologous antibodies (Arias and Sánchez-Vizcaíno 2002; Sánchez-Vizcaíno 1986).

Several techniques have been adapted for the identification of ASFV. However, at present, the most convenient, safe, and frequently used techniques are direct immunofluorescence (DIF) (Bool et al. 1969), the hemadsorption test (HA) (Malmquist and Hay 1960), and polymerase chain reaction (PCR) (Wilkinson 2000; Aguero et al. 2003).

Direct immunofluorescence (DIF) is based on the demonstration of viral antigen in impression smears or frozen tissues sections from spleen, lung, lymph nodes or kidney reacted with a conjugated immunoglobulin against ASFV. It is a fast, economical test with high diagnostic sensitivity for the acute form of ASF. However, for subacute or chronic forms, DIF has a diagnostic sensitivity of only 40%. This decrease in sensitivity seems to be related to the formation of antigen-antibody complexes in the tissues of infected pigs, which block the reaction between the ASFV antigen and ASF conjugate when such tissues are tested in the laboratory (Sánchez-Vizcaíno 1986).

HA, because of its diagnostic sensitivity and specificity, is useful under the widest range of circumstances.

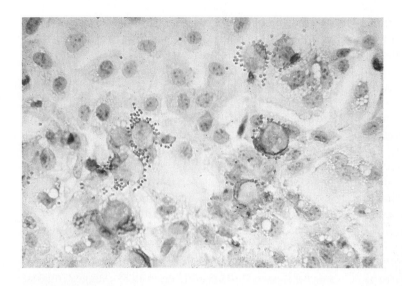

13.5. *Hemadsorption phenomenon: the attachment of erythrocytes to macrophages infected with ASFV.*

It should be performed to confirm any new outbreak, especially when other tests are negative. The HA test is based on the attachment of erythrocytes to the external (cytoplasmic) membrane of ASFV-infected porcine macrophages cultured in vitro. Typically, the erythrocytes form a rosette around the infected macrophages before the appearance of the ASFV-induced cytopathic effects (Figure 13.5) (Malmquist and Hay 1960). However, although HA is the most sensitive test for ASFV detection, it is important to recognize that a few field strains of ASFV have been isolated that induce cytopathic effect in macrophages but do not induce HA (Sanchez Botija 1982). These strains were identified using DIF sediments of these cell cultures.

The detection of a wide range of ASFV isolates by polymerase chain reaction (PCR) was made possible by using primers from a highly conserved region of the viral genome. PCR has been used to identify ASFV isolates from all the known virus genotypes, including both nonhemadsorbing and low virulence viruses (Wilkinson 2000; Aguero et al. 2003). PCR has been particularly useful for identifying viral DNA in tissues unsuitable for other diagnostic tests. It is an excellent and rapid technique that can be used as a routine diagnostic method for ASFV in surveillance, control, and eradication programs (Aguero et al. 2003). A confirmatory method based on restriction endonuclease analysis has been developed recently (Aguero et al. 2003).

The study of antibodies to ASFV is important for two reasons. First, the presence of ASFV antibodies is indicative of infection, since no vaccines are yet available. Second, specific ASFV IgG is detectable in blood from the 6th to 8th day after inoculation and for a long time, even years, thereafter. The early appearance and subsequent persistence of antibodies is the reason they are so useful in studying subacute and chronic forms of the disease. For the same reason, they play an important role in testing strategies implemented as part of eradication programs (Arias and Sánchez-Vizcaíno 2002).

Several techniques have been adapted to ASF antibody detection, but at present indirect immunofluorescense (IIF), indirect enzyme-linked immunosorbent assay (ELISA) (Sánchez-Vizcaíno et al. 1979, 1983) and the immunoblotting assay (IB) (Pastor et al. 1987), are the most frequently used.

The IIF test is a fast technique with high sensitivity and specificity for the detection of ASF antibodies from either sera or tissue exudates (Sanchez Botija et al. 1970). IIF is based on the detection of ASF antibodies that bind to a monolayer of cell lines infected with a cell culture-adapted ASFV. The antibody-antigen reaction is detected by fluorescein-labelled A-protein. Using both tests IIF and DIF, it is possible to detect from 85–95% of ASF cases (acute, subacute, and chronic) in less than 3 hours. (Sánchez-Vizcaíno 1986).

At present, ELISA is the most useful method for large-scale ASF serological studies. It is based on the detection of ASF antibodies bound to the viral proteins by addition of protein A conjugated with an enzyme that produces a visible color reaction when it reacts with the appropriate substrate.

The IB test is a highly specific, sensitive, and easy-to-interpret technique that has been successfully used as an alternative method to IIF for confirmation of questionable ELISA results (Arias and Sánchez-Vizcaíno 1992).

Samples that should be collected for ASF laboratory diagnosis are lymph nodes, kidneys, spleen, lung, blood, and serum. Tissues are used for virus isolation (HA test), viral antigen and DNA detection (DIF, PCR), blood is used for virus isolation (HA, PCR), and tissues exudates and serum for antibodies detection (IIF, ELISA, IB).

PREVENTION AND CONTROL

No treatment or effective vaccine against ASF virus is available. Many attempts have been made to develop a satisfactory vaccine, beginning in 1963, when the first live-attenuated vaccine was used in Portugal (Manso

Ribeiro et al. 1963). Inactivated vaccine does not produce any protection. Live-attenuated vaccine protects some pigs against challenge with the homologous strain of virus, but some of these pigs become carriers and develop chronic lesions, the likelihood of which increases when large numbers of pigs are vaccinated (Manso Ribeiro et al. 1963; Sanchez Botija 1963). Other studies have shown that serum from pigs resistant to homologous and some heterologous strain of ASFV inhibits (in vitro) infection of cells with different, but related, heterologous strains (Ruiz Gonzalvo et al. 1986). However, ASFV-specific antibodies have never been demonstrated to neutralize virus in the classical concept of neutralization. Recently, it has been shown that neutralizing antibodies to ASFV proteins p30, p54, and p72 are not sufficient for antibody-mediated protection (Neilan et al. 2004). The analysis of the complete nucleotide sequence of ASFV (Yañez et al. 1995) has opened new opportunities to explore immune mechanisms of protection and the roles of various ASF virus genes. However, the eradication of ASF from Portugal and Spain, after more than 20 years of endemicity, proved that vaccine is not essential in the eradication of this complex disease.

Because ASF is a costly disease and because there are no effective vaccines for its control, it is especially important that ASF-free areas be maintained free by preventing the introduction of ASFV. Retrospective epidemiological studies have shown that an important source of ASFV has been contaminated garbage from international airports or ports. Therefore, all food leftovers from planes and ships should be incinerated. In infected European areas such as Sardinia, where the disease is endemic and where mild or inapparent clinical signs have been recognized, the most important aspects of prevention are controlling pig movements and implementing extensive serological surveys to detect carriers. In areas of Africa where ASF is endemic, the most important aspects of prevention are controlling natural reservoirs—i.e., soft ticks (*O. moubata*) and warthogs—and preventing their contact with domestic pigs. When ASF is suspected for any reason, pig movement should be restricted and diagnostic evaluations should be performed immediately. Moreover, it is important to remember that low-virulence ASFV strains do not cause signs or lesions that signal their presence.

REFERENCES

Aguero M, Fernández J, Romero L, Sánchez Mascaraque C, Arias M, Sánchez-Vizcaíno JM. 2003. Highly sensitive PCR assay for routine diagnosis of African swine fever virus in clinical samples. J Clin Microbiol 41:4431–4434.

Alcaraz C, Alvarez A, Escribano JM. 1992. Flow cytometric analysis of African swine fever virus-induced plasma membrane proteins and their humoral immune response in infected pigs. Virology 189:266–273.

Arias M, Sánchez-Vizcaíno JM. 1992. Manual de diagnóstico serológico de la peste porcina Africana. Monografias INIA 83:5–44.

——. 2002. African swine fever eradication: The Spanish model. In Trends in Emerging Viral Infections of Swine. A Morilla, K-J Yoon, J Zimmerman, eds. Ames: Iowa State University Press, pp. 133–139.

Arias ML, Escribano JM, Rueda A, Sánchez-Vizcaíno JM. 1986. La Peste Porcina Africana. Med Vet 3:333–350.

Blasco R, Aguero M, Almendral JM, Viñuela E. 1989. Variable and constant regions in African swine fever virus DNA. Virology 168:330–338.

Bool PH, Ordas A, Sanchez Botija C. 1969. The diagnosis of African swine fever by immunofluorescence. Bul Off Int Epizoot 72:819–839.

Breese SS, De Boer CJ. 1966. Electron microscope observation of Africa swine fever virus in tissue culture cells. Virology 28:420–428.

Carrasco L, Bautista MJ, Gomez-Villamandos JC, Martin de las Mulas J, Chacon-M de Lara F, Wilkinson PJ, Sierra MA. 1997. Development of microscopic lesions in splenic cords of pigs infected with African swine fever. Vet Res 28:93–99.

Carrasco L, de Lara FC, Martin de las Mulas J, Gomez-Villamandos JC, Hervas J, Wilkinson PJ, Sierra MA. 1996. Virus association with lymphocytes in acute African swine fever. Vet Res 27:305–312.

Carrascosa AL, del Val M, Santaren JF, Viñuela E. 1985. Purification and properties of African swine fever virus. J Virol 54:337–344.

Carrascosa JL, Carazo JM, Carrascosa AL, Garcia N, Santisteban A, Viñuela E. 1984. General morphology and capsid fine structure of African swine fever virus particles. Virology 132:160–172.

Colgrove G, Haelterman EO, Coggins L. 1969. Pathogenesis of African swine fever virus in young pigs. Am J Vet Res 30:1343–1359.

Contini A, Cossu P, Rutili D, Firinu A. 1983. African swine fever in Sardinia. In African Swine Fever. PJ Wilkinson, ed. Proc CEC/FAO Research Seminar, Sardinia, September, 1981. Commission of the European Communities Publication EUR 8466 EN, pp. 1–6.

De Boer CV. 1967. Studies to determine neutralizing antibody in sera from animals recovered from African swine fever and laboratory animals inoculated with African virus with adjuvants. Arch Gesamte Virusforsch 20:164–179.

De Tray DE. 1957. African swine fever in warthogs (*Phacochoerus aethiopicus*). J Am Vet Med Assoc 130:537–540.

Galindo I, Almazan F, Bustos MJ, Viñuela E, Carrascosa AL. 2000. African swine fever virus EP153R open reading frame encodes a glycoprotein involved in the hemadsorption of infected cells. Virology 266:340–351.

Gomez-Puertas P, Rodriguez F, Oviedo JM, Ramiro-Ibanez F, Ruiz Gonzalvo F, Alonso C, Escribano JM. 1996. Neutralizing antibodies to different proteins of African swine fever virus inhibit both virus attachment and internalization. J Virol 70:5689–5694.

Gomez-Villamandos JC, Bautista MJ, Carrasco L, Caballero MJ, Hervas J, Villeda CJ, Wilkinson PJ, Sierra MA. 1997. African swine fever virus infection of bone marrow: Lesions and pathogenesis. Vet Pathol 34:97–107.

Gomez-Villamandos JC, Bautista MJ, Hervas J, Carrasco L, de Lara FC, Perez J, Wilkinson PJ, Sierra MA. 1996. Subcellular changes in platelets in acute and subacute African swine fever. J Comp Pathol 115:327–341.

Gomez-Villamandos JC, Hervas J, Mendez A, Carrasco L, Martin de las Mulas J, Villeda CJ, Wilkinson PJ, Sierra MA. 1995. Experimental African swine fever: Apoptosis of lymphocytes and virus replication in other cells. J Gen Virol 76:2399–2405.

Groocock CM, Hess WR, Gladney WJ. 1980. Experimental transmission of African swine fever virus by *Ornithodoros coriaceus*, an argasid tick indigenous to United States. Am J Vet Res 41:591–594.

Hess WR, Cox BF, Heuschele WP, Stone SS. 1965. Propagation and modification of African swine fever virus in cell cultures. Am J Vet Res 26:141–146.

Heuschele WP, Coggins L. 1965. Isolation of African swine fever virus from a giant forest hog. Bull Epizoot Dis Afr 13:255–256.

Malmquist WA, Hay D. 1960. Hemadsorption and cytophathic effect produced by African swine fever virus in swine bone marrow and buffy coat cultures. Am J Vet Res 21:104–108.

Manso Ribeiro J, Azevedo R, Teixeira J, Braco M, Rodriguez A, Oliveira E, Noronha F, Grave C, Vigario J. 1963. An atypical strain of swine fever virus in Portugal. Bull Off Int Epizoot 50:516–534.

Martins CL, Leitao AC. 1994. Porcine immune responses to African swine fever virus (ASFV) infection. Vet Immunol Immunopathol 43:99–106.

McKercher PD, Yedloutschnig RJ, Callis JJ, Murphy R, Panina GF, Civardi A, Bugnetti M, Foni E, Laddomada A, Scarano C, Scatozza F. 1987. Survival of viruses in "Prosciutto di Parma" (Parma ham). Can Inst Food Sci Technol J 20:267–272.

McVicar JW. 1984. Quantitative aspects of the transmission of African swine fever virus. Am J Vet Res 45:1535–1541.

Mebus CA, House C, Ruiz Gonzalvo F, Pineda JM, Tapiador J, Pire JJ, Bergada J, Yedlontshning RJ, Sahu S, Becerra V, Sánchez-Vizcaíno JM. 1993. Survival of foot and mouth disease, African swine fever and hog cholera virus in Spanish serrano cured hams and Iberian cured hams, shoulder and loin. Food Microbiol 10:133–143.

Mebus CA, McVicar JW, Dardiri AH. 1983. Comparison of the pathology of high and low virulence African swine fever infections. In African Swine Fever. PJ Wilkinson, ed. Proc CEC/FAO Research seminar, Sardinia, September, 1981. Commission of the European Communities Publication EUR 8466 EN, pp. 183–194.

Mellor PS, Wilkinson PJ. 1985. Experimental transmission of African swine fever virus by Ornithodoros savignyi (Audouin). Res Vet Sci 39:353–356.

Minguez I, Rueda A, Dominguez J, Sánchez-Vizcaíno JM. 1988. Double labeling immunohistological study of African swine fever virus-infected spleen and lymph nodes. Vet Pathol 25:193–198.

Montgomery RE. 1921. On a form of swine fever occurring in British East Africa (Kenya Colony). J Comp Pathol 34:159–191.

Moulton J, Coggins L. 1968. Comparison of lesions in acute and chronic African swine fever. Cornell Vet 58:364–388.

Murphy FA, Fauquet CM, Bishop DHL, Ghabrial SA, Jarvis AW, Martinelli GP, Mayo MA, Summers MD. 1995. Virus taxonomy, 6th report of the International Committee on Taxonomy of Viruses. Arch Virol Supplement 10.

Neilan JC, Zsak L, Lu Z, Burrage TG, Kutish GF, Rock DL. 2004. Neutralizing antibodies to African swine fever virus proteins p30, p54, and p72 are not sufficient for antibody-mediated protection. Virology 319:337–342.

Onisk DV, Borca MV, Kutish G, Kramer E, Irusta P, Rock DL. 1994. Passively transferred African swine fever virus antibodies protect swine against lethal infection. Virology 198:350–354.

Pastor MJ, Laviada MD, Sánchez-Vizcaíno JM, Escribano JM. 1987. Detection of African swine fever virus antibodies by immunoblotting assay. Can J Vet Res 53:105–107.

Plowright W. 1981. African swine fever. In Infectious Diseases of Wild Mammals, 2nd edition. JW Davis, LH Karstand, DO Trainer, eds. Ames: Iowa State University Press, pp. 178–190.

Plowright W, Parker J. 1967. The stability of African swine fever virus with particular reference to heat and pH inactivation. Arch Gesamte Virusforsch 21:383–402.

Plowright W, Parker J, Peirce MA. 1969. The epizootiology of African swine fever in Africa. Vet Rec 85:668–674.

Plowright W, Parker J, Staple RFG. 1968. The growth of a virulent strain of African swine fever virus in domestic pigs. J Hyg 66:117–134.

Plowright W, Perry CT, Peirce MA, Parker J. 1970. Experimental infection of the Argasid tick, Ornithodoros moubata porcinus, with African swine fever virus. Arch Gesamte Virusforsch 31:33–50.

Polo Jover F, Sanchez Botija C. 1961. La peste porcina africana en España. Bull Off Int Epizoot 55:107–147.

Quintero JC, Wesley RD, Whyard TC, Gregg D, Mebus CA. 1986. In vitro and in vivo association of African swine fever virus with swine erythrocytes. Am J Vet Res 47:1125–1131.

Ruiz Gonzalvo F, Carnero ME, Caballero C, Martinez J. 1986. Inhibition of African swine fever infection in the presence of immune sera in vivo and in vitro. Am J Vet Res 47:1249–1252.

Sanchez Botija C. 1963. Reservorios del virus de la peste porcina africana. Investigacion del virus de la PPA en los artropodos mediante la prueba de la hemoadsorcion. Bull Off Int Epizoot 60:895–899.

——. 1982. African swine fever: New developments. Rev Sci Technol Off Int Epizoot 1:1065–1094.

Sanchez Botija C, Ordas A, Gonzalez J. 1970. La inmunofluorescencia indirecta aplicada a la investigacion de anticuerpos de la peste porcina africana: Su valor para el diagnostico. Bull Off Int Epizoot 74:397–417.

Sánchez-Vizcaíno JM. 1986. Africa swine fever diagnosis. In African Swine Fever. J Becker, ed. Boston: Martinus Nijhoff Publishing, pp. 63–71.

Sánchez-Vizcaíno JM, Martin L, Ordas A. 1979. Adaptacion y evaluacion del enzimoinmunoensayo para la deteccion de anticuerpos para la peste porcina africana. Laboratorio 67:311–319.

Sánchez-Vizcaíno JM, Slauson DO, Ruiz Gonzalvo F, Valero F. 1981. Lymphocyte function and cell-mediated immunity in pigs with experimentally induced African swine fever. Am J Vet Res 42:1335–1341.

Sánchez-Vizcaíno JM, Tabares E, Salvador E, Ordas A. 1983. Comparative studies of two antigens for the use in the indirect ELISA test for the detection of ASF antibodies. In: Wilkinson PJ (editor), African swine fever. Proc CEC/FAO Research seminar, Sardinia, September, 1981. Commission of the European Communities Publication EUR 8466 EN, pp. 195–325.

Schlafer DH, Mebus CA, McVicar JW. 1984. African swine fever in neonatal pigs: Passive acquired protection from colostrom or serum from recovered pigs. Am J Vet Res 45:1367–1372.

Sierra MA, Bernabe A, Mozos E, Mendez A, Jover A. 1987. Ultrastructure of the liver in pigs with experimental African swine fever. Vet Pathol 24:460–462.

Sierra MA, Carrasco L, Gomez-Villamandos JC, Martin de las Mulas J, Mendez A, Jover A. 1990. Pulmonary intravascular macrophages in lungs of pigs inoculated with African swine fever virus of differing virulence. J Comp Pathol 102:323–334.

Sierra MA, Gomez-Villamandos JC, Carrasco L, Fernandez A, Mozos E, Jover A. 1991. In vivo study of hemadsorption in African swine fever virus infected cells. Vet Pathol 28:178–181.

Sogo JM, Almendral JM, Talavera A, Viñuela E. 1984. Terminal and internal inverted repetitions in African swine fever virus DNA. Virology 133:271–275.

Tabares E, Marcotegui MA, Fernandez M, Sanchez-Botija C. 1980. Proteins specified by African swine fever virus I. Analysis of viral structural proteins and antigenic properties. Arch Virol 66:107–117.

Wilkinson PJ. 2000. African swine fever. In Manual of Standards for Diagnostic Tests and Vaccines, 4th ed, Office International des Epizooties, World Organisation for Animal Health. Chapter 2.1.12:189–198.

Wilkinson PJ, Wardley RC. 1978. The replication of ASFV in pig endothelial cells. Br Vet J 134:280–282.

Yañez RJ, Rodriguez JM, Nogal ML, Yuste L, Enriquez C, Rodriguez JF, Viñuela E. 1995. Analysis of the complete nucleotide sequence of Africa swine fever virus. Virology 208:249–278.

14 Porcine Circovirus Diseases

Joaquim Segalés, Gordon M. Allan, and Mariano Domingo

In the late 1990s, an apparently novel porcine circovirus (PCV)-like virus was detected worldwide in diseased and nondiseased pigs (Allan and Ellis 2000). This virus was distinct from the known PCV contaminant of PK-15 cell cultures (Tischer et al. 1974, 1982). It was proposed that the original PCV should be designated porcine circovirus type 1 (PCV1), and the new virus associated with clinical disease be designated porcine circovirus type 2 (PCV2) (Allan et al. 1999).

PCV2 infection has been associated with postweaning multisystemic wasting syndrome (PMWS) (Clark 1996; Harding 1996), porcine dermatitis and nephropathy syndrome (PDNS) (Rosell et al. 2000), porcine respiratory disease complex (Allan and Ellis 2000), and reproductive disorders (West et al. 1999). Recently, the terminology "porcine circovirus diseases" (PCVD) has been proposed to group diseases or conditions linked to PCV2 (Allan et al. 2002a). Among PCVD, only PMWS is considered to have a severe impact on swine production, with an estimated cost of approximately 600 million Euros per year to the pig industry in Europe.

ETIOLOGY

PCV2 belongs to the genus *Circovirus* in the family *Circoviridae* (Figure 14.1) (McNulty et al. 2000). The circular, single-stranded DNA genome of PCV2 contains 1767–1768 nucleotides (Hamel et al. 1998; Meehan et al. 1998) and analysis of PCV2 viruses from around the world has shown that they all belong to a phylogenetic cluster with a nucleotide sequence identity greater than 93% (Larochelle et al. 2002).

Little information is available on the biological and physicochemical characteristics of PCV2. However, it is known that PCV1 has a buoyant density of 1.37 g/ml in CsCl, is not able to hemagglutinate erythrocytes from a wide range of species, is resistant to inactivation at pH 3 and by chloroform, and is stable at 70°C for 15 minutes (Allan et al. 1994). It is probable that these properties are also common to PCV2. Exposure of PCV2 for 10 minutes at room temperature to a number of commercial disinfectants based on chlorhexidine, formaldehyde, iodine, and alcohols lead to a reduction in virus titer (Royer et al. 2001).

EPIDEMIOLOGY

PCV2 is considered ubiquitous (Allan and Ellis 2000) and domestic and feral swine appear to be the natural host (Segalés and Domingo 2002; Vicente et al. 2004). Non-suidae species are apparently not susceptible to PCV2 infection (Segalés and Domingo 2002).

Oronasal exposure is considered the most likely and frequent natural route of PCV2 transmission. Attempts to infect fetuses by intranasal inoculation of pregnant sows or artificial insemination have yielded differing, inconclusive results (Cariolet et al. 2001; Nielsen et al. 2004).

PCV2 nucleic acid can be detected by PCR in all excretions and secretions (Bolin et al. 2001; Calsamiglia et al. 2004a; Krakowka et al. 2000; Larochelle et al. 2000) of both PMWS and non-PMWS affected pigs and has also been demonstrated in serum from pigs up to 28 weeks of age under field conditions (Rodríguez-Arrioja et al. 2002).

PMWS is a multifactorial disease of pigs where PCV2 infection is needed for the full expression of the clinical condition. Barrow pigs are considered more prone to develop PMWS than females (Corrégé et al. 2001). Other risk factors for PMWS include litter of origin (Madec et al. 2000), low birth weight, low weaning weight, and low weight at the beginning of the fattening period (Corrégé et al. 2001). PMWS-affected farms commonly have other infections or diseases (Ellis et al. 2004). Field observations from farmers and veterinarians have suggested that certain genetic lines of pigs, specifically in relation to boar lines, are more or less susceptible to PMWS. This observation has been supported by recent experimental studies where Landrace pigs were experimentally shown to be more likely to develop PMWS le-

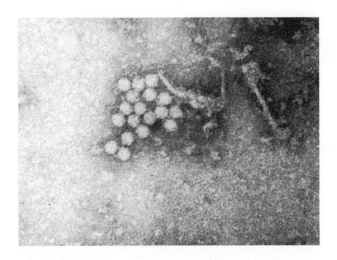

14.1. *Transmission electron photomicrograph of negatively stained PCV2 particles isolated from an affected pig. Virions are 15–20 nm in diameter.*

sions than Duroc and Large White pigs (Opriessnig et al. 2004a). Studies reported contradictory results with the use of the Pietrain boar line. The use of this genetic line did not have an effect on the offspring in one study (Rose et al. 2003a), but another study showed lower general postweaning and PMWS associated mortalities (López-Soria et al. 2004).

PATHOGENESIS

The cells that support PCV2 replication in vivo have not been identified. The large amount of PCV2 virus antigen found in macrophages and dendritic cells of diseased pigs appears to be the result of the accumulation of viral particles (Gilpin et al. 2003, Vincent et al. 2003) and not the result of virus replication in these cells. PCV2 replicates in fetal myocardiocytes in experimentally infected porcine fetuses (Sánchez et al. 2003). PCV2 is also able to replicate in in vivo produced zona pellucida-free morulae and blastocysts (Mateusen et al. 2004), although the importance of this finding in naturally occurring reproductive disease is unknown. To date, studies on tissue sections from pigs with PDNS have failed to consistently demonstrate PCV2 antigen or nucleic acid associated with PDNS lesions.

The effect of PCV2 on the immune system in PMWS-affected and PCV2-subclinically infected pigs may be important in the pathogenesis of the disease. The most repeatable PMWS disease models have been obtained using PCV2 inoculation in combination with infectious and noninfectious cofactors (Allan et al. 2004a). It has been shown experimentally that stimulation and/or activation of the immune system of PCV2-infected pigs by some viruses or noninfectious factors up-regulates PCV2 replication and increases viral loads in tissues and serum (Allan et al. 1999, 2000; Harms et al. 2002; Krakowka et al. 2000, 2001; Rovira et al. 2002), indicating

that PCV2 infection and immunostimulation can be pivotal events in the development of PMWS (Krakowka et al. 2001). The mechanism by which co-infection or immunostimulation may trigger the development of PMWS in PCV2 infected pigs is still unknown (Darwich et al. 2004). Conversely, typical microscopic lymphoid lesions in tissues from PMWS affected pigs (Clark 1997; Rosell et al. 1999), the association of the disease with opportunistic pathogens (Clark 1997; Carrasco et al. 2000; Nuñez et al. 2003; Segalés et al. 2003), and other changes in immune cell subpopulations of lymphoid tissues and peripheral blood mononuclear cells (Chianini et al. 2003; Darwich et al. 2002, 2003b; Nielsen et al. 2003; Segalés et al. 2001) are regular features of PMWS in severely affected pigs, suggesting an immunosuppressive status in diseased pigs (Segalés et al. 2004a).

Recent studies on field cases of PMWS have shown that pigs with clinical disease have an evident and significant alteration of the cytokine mRNA expression patterns of several proinflammatory and regulatory cytokines in different lymphoid tissues (Darwich et al. 2003b). However, it was not clear from these studies whether the altered profiles were related to the development of PMWS or a consequence of the severely altered cell population dynamics in lymphoid tissues of diseased animals. In these studies, a significant overexpression of IL-10 mRNA in the thymus of PMWS-affected pigs, compared to nonaffected pigs, was reported. This was associated with thymic depletion and atrophy (Darwich et al. 2003b). In contrast, Sipos et al. (2004) reported no significant differences in the expression of cytokines in blood and tissue samples from field cases of PMWS-affected pigs when compared to nonaffected pigs and concluded that their results did not support either a Th1 profile response to viral infection or a profile indicative of T cell immunosupression. However, the same authors suggested that animals under investigation were probably at the remitting stage of the disease, potentially ameliorating differences between both groups (Sipos et al. 2004).

Studies on sequential blood samples from pigs experimentally infected with PCV2 have also indicated an increase in IL-10 production in PMWS-affected inoculates, compared to inoculates that remained subclinically infected. This increase was detected only late in the infection and was interpreted by the authors to reflect the effects of clinical PMWS development, rather than contributing to the initiation of the disease (Stevenson et al. 2004). However, in the same study a consistent down-regulation of interferon was noted early in infected pigs that developed PMWS, when compared to infected pigs that remained subclinically infected. It was concluded that the inability of some PCV2-infected pigs to produce interferon early in the infection process may be a key factor in an inappropriate immune response to PCV2 infection that leads to disease (Stevenson et al., 2004). Reduction in interferon production and increase of IL-10 production in PCV2 experimentally infected pigs that develop PMWS have now been confirmed by other workers using a different experimental model (Hasslung et al. 2004). Additionally, it has recently been shown in in vitro studies that PCV2 interaction with porcine natural interferon producing cells (NIPC) results in a down-regulation in the ability of these cells to produce interferon (Vincent et al. 2004).

In vitro studies on peripheral blood mononuclear cells (PBMC) from healthy and PMWS-diseased pigs have revealed substantial and specific effects on functional capabilities of PBMC of PMWS pigs in terms of cytokine release (Darwich et al. 2003a). On the other hand, no specific differences were seen in expression of cell surface markers of PBMC or alveolar macrophages exposed in vitro to PCV2 when compared to mock-infected controls (Gilpin et al. 2001, Vincent et al. 2003)

To date, the results on the interactions of PCV2 with the porcine immune system are controversial and further studies are required. These studies should focus on the interactions following infection and prior to the development of clinical disease in an attempt to elucidate the pathways that determine clinical and/or subclinical infections.

In regard to PDNS, it has been postulated that excessive PCV2 antibody titers may trigger the disease (Wellenberg et al. 2004), but this hypothesis awaits experimental confirmation.

CLINICAL SIGNS AND LESIONS

Postweaning Multisystemic Wasting Syndrome (PMWS)

PMWS most commonly affects pigs at 2–4 months of age. Morbidity in affected farms is commonly 4–30% (occasionally 50–60%), and mortality ranges from 4–20% (Segalés and Domingo 2002). PMWS is characterized clinically by wasting, pallor of the skin, respiratory distress, and occasionally, diarrhea and icterus (Figure 14.2) (Harding and Clark 1997). Enlarged subcutaneous lymph nodes are a common finding in the early clinical phases of PMWS.

PMWS lesions are primarily found in lymphoid tissues and enlargement of lymph nodes is the most prominent feature of the early clinical phases of PMWS (Clark 1997; Rosell et al. 1999). Normal sized, or even atrophied, lymph nodes are usually seen in more advanced phases of PMWS (Segalés et al. 2004b) and the thymus is frequently atrophied in diseased pigs (Darwich et al. 2003b).

The histopathological lymphoid lesions observed in PMWS-affected pigs are characterized by lymphocyte depletion together with infiltration by large histiocytic cells and giant multinucleate cells (Figure 14.3) (Clark 1997; Rosell et al. 1999). In thymus, cortical atrophy is a prominent finding (Darwich et al. 2003b). Cytoplasmic

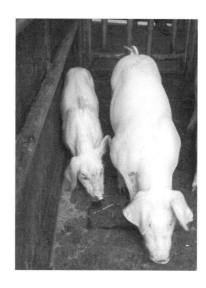

14.2. *PMWS affected pig (left) compared to an age-matched, healthy pig (right). Note the severe growth retardation and the marked spine of the affected animal.*

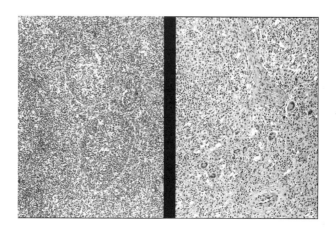

14.3. *Histological appearance of a mesenteric lymph node from a healthy pig (left) versus a PMWS-affected pig (right). Note the lack of follicles in the affected pig together with a marked loss of lymphoid cells and the presence of macrophages and multinucleate giant cells. (Hematoxylin and eosin stain. Original magnification: ×100.)*

viral inclusions may be found in histiocytes or dendritic cells (Figure 14.4).

Lungs may be enlarged, noncollapsed, and rubbery in consistency, in a diffuse or patchy distribution. These findings correspond microscopically to interstitial pneumonia. Peribronchial fibrosis and fibrous bronchiolitis occurs in advanced cases (Clark 1997; Segalés et al. 2004b).

In a few cases of PMWS, the liver is enlarged or atrophied, pale, and firm, with a fine granular surface that corresponds microscopically to widespread cytopathic changes and inflammation (Clark 1997; Segalés et al. 2004b). Pigs may show generalized icterus at this latter stage.

Some pigs show white spots in the kidney cortex

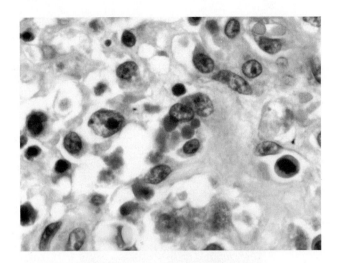

14.4. *Intracytoplasmic, rounded inclusion bodies characteristic of porcine circovirus type 2 infection in a superficial inguinal lymph node from a PMWS-affected pig. (Hematoxylin and eosin stain. Original magnification: ×1000.)*

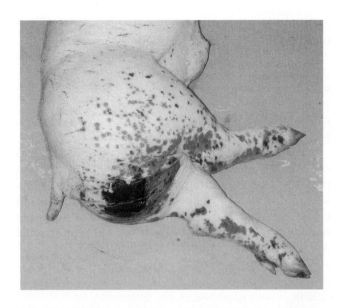

14.5. *PDNS affected pig. Necrotizing cutaneous lesions tend to be more numerous on the hindlimbs.*

(nonpurulent interstitial nephritis). Foci of lymphohistiocytic inflammatory infiltrates may be seen in many tissues of pigs affected by PMWS (Segalés et al. 2004b).

Porcine Dermatitis and Nephropathy Syndrome

PDNS affects nursery, growing, and adult pigs (Drolet et al. 1999). The prevalence of the syndrome is usually below 1% (Segalés et al. 1998), although higher frequency has been described (Gresham et al. 2000). Mortality approaches 100% in pigs older than 3 months of age versus approximately 50% of affected younger pigs. Severe, acutely affected pigs die within a few days after the onset of clinical signs. Surviving pigs tend to recover and gain weight 7–10 days after the beginning of the syndrome (Segalés et al. 1998).

PDNS-affected pigs are anorexic and depressed, with little or no pyrexia (Drolet et al. 1999). They may be prostrate, reluctant to move, and/or stiff-gaited. The most obvious sign of PDNS is the presence of irregular, red-to-purple macules and papules in the skin, primarily on the hind limbs and perineal area (Figure 14.5), but sometimes more generally distributed. With time, the lesions become covered by dark crusts. The lesions gradually fade, sometimes leaving scars (Drolet et al. 1999). Macules and papules are seen microscopically as necrotic and hemorrhagic tissue associated with necrotizing vasculitis (Segalés et al. 2004b). Necrotizing vasculitis is a systemic feature.

Pigs that die acutely with PDNS have bilaterally enlarged kidneys with fine granular cortical surface, small reddish pinpoint cortical lesions, and edema of the renal pelvis (Segalés et al., 2004b). These lesions correspond to a fibrino-necrotizing glomerulitis with nonpurulent interstitial nephritis. Pigs with prolonged disease may show chronic glomerulonephritis (Segalés et al.

1998). Normally, both skin and renal lesions are present in PDNS, but in few occasions, skin or renal lesions may occur alone.

Lymph nodes may be enlarged and red in color. Splenic infarcts may be also present (Segalés et al. 1998). Microscopically, lymphoid lesions similar to PMWS are frequently observed in PDNS affected pigs (Rosell et al. 2000).

Reproductive Disease

PCV2 has been linked to late term abortions and stillbirths (West et al. 1999). However, PCV2-associated reproductive disease under field conditions is rare (Pensaert et al. 2004). This is probably due to the fact that the seroprevalence of PCV2 in adult pigs is high and, therefore, most breeding herds are not susceptible to the clinical disease. In PCV2-associated reproductive disease, stillborn and nonviable neonatal piglets show chronic, passive, hepatic congestion and cardiac hypertrophy with multifocal areas of myocardial discoloration (West et al. 1999). The main microscopic lesion corresponds to a fibrotic and/or necrotic myocarditis (West et al. 1999).

IMMUNITY

In experimentally infected pigs, seroconversion to PCV2 has been demonstrated to occur between 14 and 28 days post infection (PI) (Allan et al. 1999; Balasch et al. 1999; Krakowka et al. 2001; Pogranichniy et al. 2000). Seroconversion has been demonstrated in experimentally infected pigs with and without clinical disease, but some studies have shown that clinically diseased pigs seroconvert at a later stage post infection with PCV2 (Bolin et al. 2001).

Under field conditions, colostral antibodies typically

decline during the lactating and nursery periods, followed by an active seroconversion (Blanchard et al. 2003; Larochelle et al. 2003; Rodríguez-Arrioja et al. 2002; Rose et al. 2002). Seroconversion usually occurs around 7–12 weeks of age, and antibodies may last at least until 28 weeks of age (Rodríguez-Arrioja et al. 2002). PMWS is not usually observed in pigs younger than 4 weeks of age (Segalés and Domingo 2002), which may be associated with maternal immunity against the development of PMWS (Allan et al 2002b; Calsamiglia et al. 2004b). However, other studies have shown no significant protective effect in relation to high levels of colostral-derived serum antibodies to PCV2 in piglets and development of PMWS (Allan et al. 2004b; Hassing et al. 2004). Although a humoral immune response to PCV2 in the field takes place at 2–3 months of age, a variable percentage of growing or finishing pigs may be viremic, suggesting that PCV2 antibodies are not fully protective against the infection (Larochelle et al. 2003; Rodríguez-Arrioja et al. 2002; Sibila et al. 2004). This situation also seems to occur in adult pigs under field conditions, since they can be infected but do not show apparent or detectable clinical signs (Calsamiglia et al. 2002). Whether this is due to humoral immunity to PCV2 or natural age resistance is not known at present.

Only one report has dealt with neutralizing antibodies to PCV2 (Pogranichniy et al. 2000). Virus-neutralizing antibodies were not detected until day 28 post infection. As neutralizing antibodies developed, cross-reactivity with PCV1 also developed using this serological test.

DIAGNOSIS

The respiratory form of porcine reproductive and respiratory syndrome (PRRS) and all diseases and conditions that cause wasting must be differentiated from PMWS (Harding and Clark 1997). For PDNS, differential diagnoses include any condition that causes red to dark discoloration of the skin, as well as conditions that cause petechial hemorrhages in the kidneys (Segalés 2002). Special note should be made of the similarity of gross lesions between PDNS, classical swine fever, and African swine fever. The reproductive form of PCV2 is clinically indistinguishable from other swine diseases that cause late-term abortions and stillbirths.

Postweaning Multisystemic Wasting Syndrome

A pig or group of pigs suffer from PMWS if they fulfill the following criteria (Sorden 2000):

1. Growth retardation and wasting, frequently with dyspnea and enlargement of inguinal lymph nodes and occasionally with jaundice
2. Moderate-to-severe characteristic histopathological lesions in lymphoid tissues

3. Moderate-to-high amounts of PCV2 within the lesions in lymphoid and other tissues of affected pigs

This case definition does not exclude the concomitant presence of other diseases together with PMWS. Neither clinical signs nor gross lesions observed in suspected PMWS affected pigs are sufficient to diagnose the disease.

A herd diagnosis of PMWS is based on the occurrence of a clinical process characterized mainly by wasting and mortality in excess of the expected and/or historical level for the farm and the individual diagnosis of PMWS, as described above, in a number of pigs (Segalés et al. 2003).

Porcine Dermatitis and Nephropathy Syndrome

The diagnosis of PDNS is based on two main criteria (Segalés 2002):

1. The presence of hemorrhagic and necrotizing skin lesions, primarily located on the hind limbs and perineal area, and/or swollen and pale kidneys with generalized cortical petechia
2. Presence of systemic necrotizing vasculitis, and necrotizing and fibrinous glomerulonephritis

Reproductive Disease

The diagnosis of PCV2-associated reproductive disease should include three criteria:

1. Late-term abortions and stillbirths, sometimes with evident hypertrophy of the fetal heart
2. The presence of heart lesions characterized by extensive fibrosing and/or necrotizing myocarditis
3. The presence of high amounts of PCV2 in myocardial lesions and other fetal tissues

Laboratory Confirmation

Several methods have been developed to detect PCV2 in tissues. In situ hybridization (ISH) and immunohistochemistry (IHC) are the most widely used tests (McNeilly et al. 1999; Rosell et al. 1999) for the diagnosis of PCVD. PCV2 nucleic acid or antigen in PMWS and PDNS affected pigs is usually found in the cytoplasm of histiocytes, multinucleate giant cells and other monocyte/macrophage lineage cells (Allan and Ellis 2000), as well as in other cell types (Segalés et al. 2004b). In aborted fetuses, PCV2 is found in the myocardiocyte (Sánchez et al. 2001).

A strong correlation has been observed between the quantity of PCV2 seen in tissues and the severity of microscopic lymphoid lesions in PMWS (Figure 14.6) (Rosell et al. 1999). Since the amount of PCV2 in damaged tissues is the major difference between PMWS affected pigs and PCV2 subclinically infected pigs, techniques that allow PCV2 quantification in tissues and/or

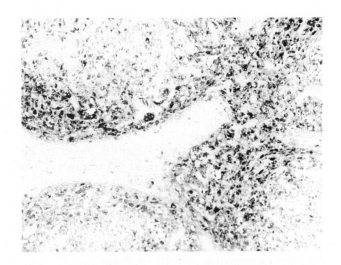

14.6. *Mesenteric lymph node. Marked presence of PCV2 nucleic acid in the cytoplasm of multinucleate giant cells and macrophages (dark-stained cells) in a PMWS-affected pig. (In situ hybridization to detect PCV2; fast green counterstain. Original magnification: ×100.)*

serum could potentially be used to diagnose PMWS (McNeilly et al. 2002, Olvera et al. 2004). Nonquantitative polymerase chain reaction (PCR) techniques should not be used to diagnose PCVD because the virus is ubiquitous and positive results in the absence of clinical disease are common.

Several serological techniques to detect antibodies to PCV2 have been developed (Segalés and Domingo 2002). However, diagnosis of PCVD using serological techniques is problematic because PCV2 is ubiquitous and seroconversion patterns are relatively similar in PMWS affected and nonaffected farms.

PREVENTION AND CONTROL

PMWS is considered a multifactorial disease. In addition to PCV2 infection, environmental conditions are postulated to cause the expression of disease (Madec et al. 2000). Viral and bacterial coinfections with PCV2 are also conjectured to serve as triggers for PMWS (Rose et al. 2003b, Ellis et al. 2004). Consequently, control measures have focused on the control or elimination of postulated cofactors and triggers. The implementation of "Madec's 20-point plan," a list of management practices intended to lower the impact of the disease, significantly decreased the mortality in severely affected farms (Guilmoto and Wessel-Robert 2000). Likewise, the control of concurrent viral and bacterial infections in the postweaning area may decrease the incidence of PMWS.

Some experimental and field studies suggest that immune activation may be an important triggering factor of PMWS in some farms. From a practical point of view, to exclude the use of vaccines from sanitary programs may be inappropriate, since the risk of eliminating effective vaccines may be greater than the risk of inducing

PMWS in a low percentage of pigs in a given pig population. Therefore, producers with PMWS affected herds should consider determining the approximate timing of PCV2 infection, with the final objective of rescheduling the timing of vaccination as a potential plan to minimize the disease (Opriessnig et al. 2004b).

It has been reported that PCV2 infection or low serological titers to PCV2 in sows at farrowing increased the overall mortality of their offspring to PMWS (Allan et al. 2002b, Calsamiglia et al. 2004b). Although these observations were not corroborated in later studies (Hassing et al. 2004, Allan et al. 2004b), measures that increase maternal immunity and decrease sow viremia at farrowing may diminish piglet PMWS mortality in problem herds.

Changes in the diet of affected pigs reportedly led to partial control of PMWS on some farms (Donadeu et al. 2003). Although these results have not been confirmed by other workers, a recent study found that conjugated linoleic acid (CLA) ameliorated PCV2 experimental infection (Bassaganya-Riera et al. 2003). It has been suggested that the addition of vitamin E and/or selenium in the feed may be of benefit in those farms with PMWS (Baebko et al. 2004).

An inactivated, adjuvanted PCV2 vaccine for use in sows and gilts is now commercially available and in use under special license in some countries. In previous studies this vaccine reduced the incidence of PMWS on affected farms (Reynaud et al. 2004). Its efficacy under a wide range of farm conditions still has to be evaluated. Experimental PCV2 vaccines, including inactivated, recombinant, and DNA vaccines, as well as chimeric infectious DNA clones, have shown significant protection when evaluated on the basis of growth rate and rectal temperatures after PCV2 challenge (Blanchard et al. 2003; Fenaux et al. 2004; Pogranichniy et al. 2004).

Subcutaneous injection of suckling or nursery pigs with serum collected from commercial market age pigs (serum therapy) was reportedly successful in reducing mortality in several PMWS affected farms (Ferreira et al. 2001). However, the results of this procedure have been variable and even deleterious in some cases. It is important to note that the use of "serum therapy" presents significant health and biosecurity risks.

REFERENCES

Allan G, Krakowka S, Ellis J. 2002a. PCV2: Ticking time bomb. Pig Progress 18:14–15.

Allan G, McNeilly F, McNair I, Meehan B, Marshall M, Ellis J, Lasagna C, Boriosi G, Krakowka S, Reynaud G, Boeuf-Tedeschi L, Bublot M, Charreyre C. 2002b. Passive transfer of maternal antibodies to PCV2 protects against development of postweaning multisystemic wasting syndrome (PMWS): Experimental infections and a field study. Pig J 50:59–67.

Allan GM, Ellis JA. 2000. Porcine circoviruses: A review. J Vet Diagn Invest 12:3–14.

Allan GM, McNeilly F, Ellis J, Krakowka S, Botner A, McCullough K, Nauwynck H, Kennedy S, Meehan B, Charreyre C. 2004a.

PMWS: Experimental model and co-infections. Vet Microbiol 98:165–168.

Allan GM, McNeilly F, McNair, I, Armstrong D. 2004b. The role of colostrum derived antibodies to PCV2 virus and vertical transmission of PCV2 in PMWS in the United Kingdom. (In preparation).

Allan GM, McNeilly F, Meehan BM, Ellis JA, Connor TJ, McNair I, Krakowka S, Kennedy S. 2000. A sequential study of experimental infection of pigs with porcine circovirus and porcine parvovirus: Immunostaining of cryostat sections and virus isolation. J Vet Med B Infect Dis Vet Public Health Mar 47(2):81–94.

Allan GM, McNeilly F, Meehan BM, Kennedy S, Mackie DP, Ellis JA, Clark EG, Espuña E, Saubi N, Riera P, Botner A, Charreyre CE. 1999. Isolation and characterisation of circoviruses from pigs with wasting syndromes in Spain, Denmark and Northern Ireland. Vet Microbiol 66:115–123.

Allan GM, Phenix K, Todd D and McNulty M. 1994. Some biological and physico-chemical properties of porcine circovirus. J Vet Med B 41:17–26.

Baebko P, Hassing AG, Olsen P, Lorenzen B, Wachmann H, Lauridsen C. 2004. Vitamin E and postweaning mortality in PMWS affected herds. Proc Congr Int Pig Vet Soc, p. 62.

Balasch M, Segalés J, Rosell C, Domingo M, Mankertz A, Urniza A, Plana-Durán J. 1999. Experimental inoculation of conventional pigs with tissue homogenates from pigs with post-weaning multisystemic wasting syndrome. J Comp Pathol 121:139–148.

Bassaganya-Riera J, Pogranichniy RM, Jobgen SC, Halbur PG, Yoon KJ, O'Shea M, Mohede I, Hontecillas R. 2003. Conjugated linoleic acid ameliorates viral infectivity in a pig model of virally induced immunosuppression. J Nutr 133:3204–3214.

Blanchard P, Mahe D, Cariolet R, Keranflec'h A, Baudouard MA, Cordioli P, Albina E, Jestin A. 2003. Protection of swine against post-weaning multisystemic wasting syndrome (PMWS) by porcine circovirus type 2 (PCV2) proteins. Vaccine 21:4565–4575.

Bolin SR, Stoffregen WC, Nayar GP, Hamel AL. 2001. Postweaning multisystemic wasting syndrome induced after experimental inoculation of cesarean-derived, colostrum-deprived piglets with type 2 porcine circovirus. J Vet Diagn Invest 13:185–194.

Calsamiglia M, Olvera A, Segalés J, Domingo M. 2004a. Quantification of PCV2 in different routes of excretion: Possible transmission routes and correlation with presence of PMWS characteristic lesions. Proc Congr Int Pig Vet Soc, p. 11.

Calsamiglia M, Segalés J, Fraile L, Espinal A, Seminati C, Martin M, Mateu E, Domingo M. 2004b. Sow effect on litter mortality in a swine integration system experiencing postweaning multisystemic wasting syndrome (PMWS). Vet J (submitted).

Calsamiglia M, Segales J, Quintana J, Rosell C, Domingo M. 2002. Detection of porcine circovirus types 1 and 2 in serum and tissue samples of pigs with and without postweaning multisystemic wasting syndrome. J Clin Microbiol 40:1848–1850.

Cariolet R, Blanchard P, Le Dimma M, Mahé D, Jolly JP, De Boisseson C, Truong C, Ecobichon P, Madec F, Jestin A. 2001. Experimental infection of pregnant SPF sows with PCV2 through tracheal and muscular routes. Proc ssDNA Viruses Plants, Birds, Pigs and Primates (ESVV), p. 128.

Carrasco L, Segalés J, Bautista MJ, Gómez-Villamandos JC, Rosell C, Ruiz-Villamor E, Sierra MA. 2000. Intestinal chlamydial infection concurrent with postweaning multisystemic wasting syndrome in pigs. Vet Rec 146:21–23.

Chianini F, Majó N, Segalés J, Domínguez J, Domingo M. 2003. Immunohistochemical characterisation of PCV2 associate lesions in lymphoid and non-lymphoid tissues of pigs with natural postweaning multisystemic wasting syndrome (PMWS). Vet Immunol Immunopathol 94:63–75.

Clark E. 1996. Post-weaning multisystemic wasting syndrome. Proc West Can Assoc Swine Pract, pp. 19–20.

——. 1997. Post-weaning multisystemic wasting syndrome. Proc Annu Meet Am Assoc Swine Pract, pp. 499–501.

Corrégé I, Pirouelle D, Gaudré D, LeTiran MH. 2001. La Maladie de l'Amaigrissement du Porcelet (MAP): Influence de différents paramètres zootechniques sur son incidence dans un élevage expérimental. J Rech Porcine France, 33:283–290.

Darwich L, Balasch M, Plana-Duran J, Segales J, Domingo M, Mateu E. 2003a. Cytokine profiles of peripheral blood mononuclear cells from pigs with postweaning multisystemic wasting syndrome in response to mitogen, superantigen or recall viral antigens. J Gen Virol, 84:3453–3457.

Darwich L, Pie S, Rovira A, Segales J, Domingo M, Oswald IP, Mateu E. 2003b. Cytokine mRNA expression profiles in lymphoid tissues of pigs naturally affected by postweaning multisystemic wasting syndrome. J Gen Virol, 84:2117–2125.

Darwich L, Segalés J, Domingo M, Mateu E. 2002. Changes in CD4(+), CD8(+), CD4(+) CD8(+), and immunoglobulin M-positive peripheral blood mononuclear cells of postweaning multisystemic wasting syndrome-affected pigs and age-matched uninfected wasted and healthy pigs correlate with lesions and porcine circovirus type 2 load in lymphoid tissues. Clin Diagn Lab Immunol 9:236–242.

Darwich L, Segales J, Mateu E. 2004. Pathogenesis of postweaning multisystemic wasting syndrome caused by Porcine circovirus 2: An immune riddle. Arch Virol 149:857–874.

Donadeu M, Waddilove J, Marco E. 2003. European management strategies to control postweaning multisystemic wasting syndrome. Proc Allen D. Leman Swine Conf, pp. 136–142.

Drolet R, Thibault S, D'Allaire S, Thomson JR, Done SH. 1999. Porcine dermatitis and nephropathy syndrome (PDNS): An overview of the disease. J Swine Health Prod 7:283–285.

Ellis J, Clark E, Haines D, West K, Krakowka S, Kennedy S, Allan GM. 2004. Porcine circovirus-2 and concurrent infections in the field. Vet Microbiol 98:159–163.

Fenaux M, Opriessnig T, Halbur PG, Elvinger F, Meng XJ. 2004. A chimeric porcine circovirus (PCV) with the immunogenic capsid gene of the pathogenic PCV type 2 (PCV2) cloned into the genomic backbone of the nonpathogenic PCV1 induces protective immunity against PCV2 infection in pigs. J Virol 78:6297–6303.

Ferreira D, Sansot B, Laval A. 2001. Attempt to use serotherapy to control mortality in PMWS. Proc ssDNA Viruses Plants, Birds, Pigs and Primates (ESVV), p. 144.

Gilpin DF, McCullough K, Meehan BM, McNeilly F, McNair I, Stevenson LS, Foster JC, Ellis JA, Krakowka S, Adair BM, Allan GM. 2003. In vitro studies on the infection and replication of porcine circovirus type 2 in cells of the porcine immune system. Vet Immunol Immunopathol 94:149–161.

Gilpin DF, Stevenson LS, McCullough K, Krakowka S, Meehan BM, McNeilly F, Foster C, Adair B, Welsh M, Allan BM. 2001. Studies on the in vitro and in vivo effect of porcine circovirus type 2 infection of porcine monocytic cells. In Proc ssDNA Viruses Plants, Birds, Pigs and Primates (ESVV). p.97.

Gresham A, Giles N, Weaver J. 2000. PMWS and porcine dermatitis nephropathy syndrome in Great Britain. Vet Rec 147:115.

Guilmoto H, Wessel-Robert S. 2000. Control of PMWS in Brittany: a mainly zootechnical approach. In PMWS: A new emerging disease of swine. Melbourne, Australia: Merial Symposium, pp. 45–55.

Hamel AL, Lin LL, Nayar GPS. 1998. Nucleotide sequence of porcine circovirus associated with postweaning multisystemic wasting syndrome in pigs. J Virol 72:5262–5267.

Harding JC. 1996. Postweaning multisystemic wasting syndrome: Preliminary epidemiology and clinical findings. Proc West Can Assoc Swine Pract, p. 21.

Harding JCS, Clark EG. 1997. Recognizing and diagnosing postweaning multisystemic wasting syndrome (PMWS). J Swine Health Prod 5:201–203.

Harms PA, Sorden SD, Halbur PG, Bolin S, Lager K, Morozov I, Paul PS. 2002. Experimental reproduction of severe disease in

CD/CD pigs concurrently infected with type 2 porcine circovirus and PRRSV. Vet Pathol 38:528–539.

Hassing AG, Kristensen CS, Baebko P, Wachmann. 2004. Effect of sow on the mortality of pigs after weaning in PMWS herds. Proc Congr Int Pig Vet Soc, p. 76.

Hasslung F, Wallgren P, Jadekjaer-Mikkelsen AS, Botner A, Nielsen J, Wattrang E, Allan GM, McNeilly F, Ellis J, Timmusk S, Belak K, Segall T, Meilin L, Berg M, Fossum C. 2004. Experimental production of postweaning multisystemic wasting syndrome (PMWS) in Swedish and Danish pigs using a Swedish isolate of porcine circovirus type 2. Vet Microbiol, (submitted).

Krakowka S, Ellis JA, McNeilly F, Ringler S, Rings DM, Allan G. 2001. Activation of the immune system is the pivotal event in the production of wasting disease in pigs infected with porcine circovirus-2 (PCV-2). Vet Pathol 38:31–42.

Krakowka S, Ellis JA, Meehan B, Kennedy S, McNeilly F, Allan G. 2000. Viral wasting syndrome of swine: Experimental reproduction of postweaning multisystemic wasting syndrome in gnotobiotic swine by coinfection with porcine circovirus 2 and porcine parvovirus. Vet Pathol 37:254–263.

Larochelle R, Bielanski A, Muller P, Magar R. 2000. PCR detection and evidence of shedding of porcine circovirus type 2 in boar semen. J Clin Microbiol 38:4629–4632.

Larochelle R, Magar R, D'Allaire S. 2002. Genetic characterization and phylogenetic analysis of porcine circovirus type 2 (PCV2) strains from cases presenting various clinical conditions. Virus Res 90:101–112.

——. Comparative serologic and virologic study of commercial swine herds with and without postweaning multisystemic wasting syndrome. Can J Vet Res 67:114–120.

López-Soria S, Segales J, Nofrarias M, Calsamiglia M, Ramirez H, Minguez A, Serrano IM, Marin O, Callen A. 2004. Genetic influence on the expression of PCV disease. Vet Rec 155:504.

Madec F, Eveno E, Morvan P, Hamon L, Blanchard P, Cariolet R, Amenna N, Morvan H, Truong C, Mahé D, Albina E, Jestin A. 2000. Post-weaning multisystemic wasting syndrome (PMWS) in pigs in France: Clinical observations from follow-up studies on affected farms. Livest Prod Sci 63:223–233.

Mateusen B, Sanchez RE, Van Soom A, Meerts P, Maes DG, Nauwynck HJ. 2004. Susceptibility of pig embryos to porcine circovirus type 2 infection. Theriogenology 61:91–101.

McNeilly F, Kennedy S, Moffett D, Meehan BM, Foster JC, Clarke EG, Ellis JA, Haines DM, Adair BM, Allan GM. 1999. A comparison of in situ hybridization and immunohistochemistry for the detection of a new porcine circovirus in formalin-fixed tissues from pigs with post-weaning multisystemic wasting syndrome (PMWS). J Virol Methods 80:123–128.

McNeilly F, McNair I, O'Connor M, Brockbank S, Gilpin D, Lasagna C, Boriosi G, Meehan B, Ellis J, Krakowka S, Allan GM. 2002. Evaluation of a porcine circovirus type 2-specific antigen-capture enzyme-linked immunosorbent assay for the diagnosis of postweaning multisystemic wasting syndrome in pigs: Comparison with virus isolation, immunohistochemistry, and the polymerase chain reaction. J Vet Diagn Invest 14:106–112.

McNulty M, Dale J, Lukert P, Mankertz A, Randles J, Todd D. 2000. *Circoviridae.* In Virus Taxonomy: Classification and Nomenclature of Viruses The Seventh Report of the International Committee on Taxonomy of Viruses. MHV van Regenmortel, CM Fauquet, DHL Bishop, CH Calisher, EB Carstens, MH Estes, SM Lemon, J Maniloff, MA Mayo, DJ McGeoch, CR Pringle, RB Wickner, eds. San Diego: Academic Press, pp. 299–303.

Meehan BM, McNeilly F, Todd D, Kennedy S, Jewhurst VA, Ellis JA, Hassard LE, Clark EG, Haines DM, Allan GM. 1998. Characterization of novel circovirus DNAs associated with wasting syndromes in pigs. J Gen Virol 79:2171–2179.

Nielsen J, Ladekjaer-Mikkelsen AS, Ville-Hansen V, Lohse L, Botner A. 2004. PCV2-associated disease following intrauterine infection. Proc Congr Int Pig Vet Soc, p. 14.

Nielsen J, Vincent IE, Botner A, Ladekaer-Mikkelsen AS, Allan G, Summerfield A, McCullough KC. 2003. Association of lymphopenia with porcine circovirus type 2 induced postweaning multisystemic wasting syndrome (PMWS). Vet Immunol Immunopathol 92:97–111.

Nuñez A, McNeilly F, Perea A, Sanchez-Cordon PJ, Huerta B, Allan G, Carrasco L. 2003. Coinfection by Cryptosporidium parvum and porcine circovirus type 2 in weaned pigs. J Vet Med B, 50:255–258.

Olvera A, Sibila M, Calsamiglia M, Segales J, Domingo M. 2004. Comparison of porcine circovirus type 2 load in serum quantified by a real time PCR in postweaning multisystemic wasting syndrome and porcine dermatitis and nephropathy syndrome naturally affected pigs. J Virol Methods 117:75–80.

Opriessnig T, Anderson MS, Rothschild MF, Evans RB, Fenaux M, Meng XJ, Halbur PG. 2004a. Evaluation of differences in host susceptibility to PCV2-associated diseases. Proc Congr Int Pig Vet Soc, p. 12.

Opriessnig T, Thacker EL, Yu S, Fenaux M, Meng XJ, Halbur PG. 2004b. Experimental reproduction of postweaning multisystemic wasting syndrome in pigs by dual infection with *Mycoplasma hyopneumoniae* and porcine circovirus type 2. Vet Pathol 41:624–640.

Pensaert MB, Sanchez RE Jr, Ladekjaer-Mikkelsen AS, Allan GM, Nauwynck HJ. 2004. Viremia and effect of fetal infection with porcine viruses with special reference to porcine circovirus 2 infection. Vet Microbiol 98:175–183.

Pogranichniy R, Yoon KJ, Yaeger M, Vaughn E, Stammer R, Roof M. 2004. Efficacy of experimental inactivated PCV2 vaccines for preventing PMWS in CDCD pigs. Proc Annu Meet Am Assoc Swine Vet, pp. 443–444.

Pogranichniy RM, Yoon KJ, Harms PA, Swenson SL, Zimmerman JJ, Sorden SD. 2000. Characterization of immune response of young pigs to porcine circovirus type 2 infection. Viral Immunol 13:143–153.

Reynaud G, Brun A, Charreyre C, Desgouilles S, Jeannin P. 2004. Safety of repeated overdose on an inactivated adjuvanted PCV2 vaccine in conventional pregnant gilts and sows. Proc Congr Int Pig Vet Soc, p. 88.

Rodríguez-Arrioja GM, Segales J, Calsamiglia M, Resendes AR, Balasch M, Plana-Duran J, Casal J, Domingo M. 2002. Dynamics of porcine circovirus type 2 infection in a herd of pigs with postweaning multisystemic wasting syndrome. Am J Vet Res 63:354–357.

Rose N, Abherve-Gueguen A, Le Diguerher G, Eveno E, Jolly JP, Blanchard P, Oger A, Houdayer C, Jestin A, Madec F. 2003a. A cohort study about clinical post-weaning multisystemic wasting síndrome (PMWS) in pigs of different genetic background. Proc Symp Vet Epid Econ, p. 723.

Rose N, Blanchard P, Larour G, Le Diguerher G, Eveno E, Jolly JP, Oler A, Le Dimna M, Jestin A and Madec F. 2002. Post-weaning multisystemic wasting síndrome (PMWS) in France: Serological profiles of affected versus non-affected herds and preliminary analytical epidemiology. Pig J 50:124–134.

Rose N, Larour G, Le Diguerher G, Eveno E, Jolly JP, Blanchard P, Oger A, Le Dimna M, Jestin A, Madec F. 2003b. Risk factors for porcine post-weaning multisystemic wasting syndrome (PMWS) in 149 French farrow-to-finish herds. Prev Vet Med 61:209–225.

Rosell C, Segalés J, Plana-Durán J, Balasch M, Rodríguez-Arrioja GM, Kennedy S, Allan GM, McNeilly F, Latimer KS, Domingo M. 1999. Pathological, immunohistochemical, and in-situ hybridization studies of natural cases of postweaning multisystemic wasting syndrome (PMWS) in pigs. J Comp Pathol 120:59–78.

Rosell C, Segalés J, Ramos-Vara JA, Folch JM, Rodríguez-Arrioja GM, Duran CO, Balasch M, Plana-Durán J, Domingo M. 2000. Identification of porcine circovirus in tissues of pigs with porcine dermatitis and nephropathy syndrome. Vet Rec 146:40–43.

Rovira A, Balasch M, Segalés J, Garcia L, Plana-Duran J, Rosell C, Ellerbrock H, Mankertz A, Domingo M. 2002. Experimental inoculation of conventional pigs with porcine reproductive and respiratory syndrome virus and porcine circovirus 2. J Virol, 76:3232–3239.

Royer RL, Nawagitgul P, Halbur PG, Paul PS. 2001. Susceptibility of porcine circovirus type 2 to commercial and laboratory disinfectants. J Swine Health Prod 9:281–284.

Sánchez RE Jr, Meerts P, Nauwynck HJ, Pensaert MB. 2003. Change of porcine circovirus 2 target cells in pigs during development from fetal to early postnatal life. Vet Microbiol 95:15–25.

Sánchez RE Jr, Nauwynck HJ, McNeilly F, Allan GM, Pensaert MB. 2001. Porcine circovirus 2 infection in swine foetuses inoculated at different stages of gestation. Vet Microbiol 83:169–176.

Segalés J. 2002. Update on postweaning multisystemic wasting syndrome and porcine dermatitis and nephropathy syndrome diagnostics. J Swine Health Prod 10:277–281.

Segalés J, Alonso F, Rosell C, Pastor J, Chianini F, Campos E, López-Fuertes L, Quintana J, Rodríguez-Arrioja G, Calsamiglia M, Pujols J, Domínguez J, Domingo M. 2001. Changes in peripheral blood leukocyte populations in pigs with natural postweaning multisystemic wasting syndrome (PMWS). Vet Immunol Immunopathol 81:37–44.

Segalés J, Calsamiglia M, Domingo M. 2003. How we diagnose postweaning multisystemic wasting syndrome. Proc Emerg Re-Emerg Swine Dis, pp. 149–151.

Segalés J, Domingo M. 2002. Postweaning multisystemic wasting syndrome (PMWS) in pigs. A review. Vet Q 24:109–124.

Segalés J, Domingo M, Chianini F, Majo N, Dominguez J, Darwich L, Mateu E. 2004a. Immunosuppression in postweaning multisystemic wasting syndrome affected pigs. Vet Microbiol 98:151–158.

Segalés J, Piella J, Marco E, Mateu-de-Antonio EM, Espuna E, Domingo M. 1998. Porcine dermatitis and nephropathy syndrome in Spain. Vet Rec 142:483–486.

Segalés J, Rosell C, Domingo M. 2004b. Pathological findings associated with naturally acquired porcine circovirus type 2 associated disease. Vet Microbiol 98:137–149.

Sibila M, Calsamiglia M, Segales J, Blanchard P, Badiella L, Le Dimna M, Jestin A, Domingo M. 2004. Use of a polymerase chain reaction assay and an ELISA to monitor porcine circovirus type 2 infection in pigs from farms with and without postweaning multisystemic wasting syndrome. Am J Vet Res 65:88–92.

Sipos W, Duvigneau JC, Willheim M, Schilcher F, Hartl RT, Hofbauer G, Exel B, Pietschmann P, Schmoll F. 2004. Systemic cytokine profile in feeder pigs suffering from natural postweaning multisystemic wasting syndrome (PMWS) as determined by semiquantitative RT-PCR and flow cytometric intracellular cytokine detection. Vet Immunol Immunopathol 99:63–71.

Sorden SD. 2000. Update on porcine circovirus and postweaning multisystemic wasting syndrome. J Swine Health Prod 8:133–136.

Stevenson LS, McCullough K, Gilpin DF, Vincent I, Summerfield A, Nielsen J, McNeilly F, Adair BM, Allan GM. 2004. Cytokine and C-reactive protein profiles induced by porcine circovirus type 2 experimental infection in 3 week-old pigs. Vet Immunol Immunopathol (submitted).

Tischer I, Gelderblom H, Vettermann W, Koch MA. 1982. A very small porcine virus with circular single-stranded DNA. Nature 295:64–66.

Tischer I, Rasch R, Tochtermann G. 1974. Characterization of papovavirus- and picornavirus-like particles in permanent pig kidney cell lines. Zentralbl Bakteriol [Orig A] 226:153–167.

Vicente J, Segales J, Hofle U, Balasch M, Plana-Duran J, Domingo M, Gortazar C. 2004. Epidemiological study on porcine circovirus type 2 (PCV2) infection in the European wild boar (*Sus scrofa*). Vet Res 35:243–253.

Vincent IE, Carrasco CP, Guzylack-Piriou B, Hermann B, McNeilly F, Allan GM, Summerfield A, McCullough KC. 2004. Circovirus type 2 discriminates plasmocytoid from myeloid dendritic cells by/through selective functional silencing. J Gen Virol (submitted).

Vincent IE, Carrasco CP, Herrmann B, Meehan BM, Allan GM, Summerfield A, McCullough KC. 2003. Dendritic cells harbor infectious porcine circovirus type 2 in the absence of apparent cell modulation or replication of the virus. J Virol 77: 13288–13300.

Wellenberg GJ, Stockhofe-Zurwieden N, de Jong MF, Boersma WJ, Elbers AR. 2004. Excessive porcine circovirus type 2 antibody titres may trigger the development of porcine dermatitis and nephropathy syndrome: A case-control study. Vet Microbiol 99:203–214.

West KH, Bystrom JM, Wojnarowicz C, Shantz N, Jacobson M, Allan GM, Haines DM, Clark EG, Krakowka S, McNeilly F, Konoby C, Martin K, Ellis JA. 1999. Myocarditis and abortion associated with intrauterine infection of sows with porcine circovirus 2. J Vet Diagn Invest 11:530–532.

15 Classical Swine Fever and Other Pestiviruses

Marie-Frédérique Le Potier, Alain Mesplède, Philippe Vannier

Classical swine fever (CSF), formerly known as "hog cholera," is a highly contagious viral disease of worldwide importance and one of the Office International des Epizooties (OIE) List A diseases. Wild and domestic pigs are the only natural reservoirs of classical swine fever virus (CSFV). Clinical outbreaks suggestive of CSF were reported in the early 19th century (Fuchs 1968; Kernkamp 1961; USDA 1889), and CSF was recognized as viral in nature by 1903 (Wise 1981). Historically, peracute, acute, chronic, or prenatal forms of CSF were attributed to distinct levels of virus virulence. However, characterization of strain virulence is difficult since the same isolate can induce different signs depending on pig age, breeding, health status, and immune status.

Pigs are also susceptible to other pestiviruses, including bovine viral diarrhea virus (BVDV) and border disease virus (BDV) (Carbrey et al. 1976; Terpstra and Wensvoort 1988). Bovine viral diarrhea was first described in 1946 as an infectious and contagious disease of cattle; mucosal disease was reported in 1953. Border disease in sheep, characterized by congenital disorders in lambs, was first described in 1959 along the border between England and Wales, but the immunological relationship of BDV with BVDV was only recognized later (Hamilton and Timoney 1973). Cross-species transmission among artiodactyls has been reported for both BVDV and BDV and the terms "bovine viral diarrhea virus" and "border disease virus" are used to indicate that the virus was isolated from either cattle or sheep. In fact, these two viruses cannot be differentiated morphologically or structurally (Laude 1979).

Natural infection of swine with BVDV was first reported in Australia in 1964, but BVDV was not isolated from a naturally infected pig until 1973 (Fernelius et al. 1973). The teratogenic properties of pestiviruses are well established (Terpstra and Wensvoort 1988; Vannier et al. 1988; Wensvoort and Terpstra 1988), and infection of pregnant sows with BVDV or BDV may induce a pathology resembling congenital CSF. Pestivirus isolates from pigs are usually CSFV, but cross-neutralization tests and

tests using monoclonal antibodies (Leforban et al. 1990a; Wensvoort 1989) suggest that BVDV may have been isolated from pigs in the past and misidentified as CSFV by tests based on polyclonal antibodies. Likewise, serum antibodies against BVDV or BDV have the potential to cross-react in assays for the detection of CSFV antibodies. Because of cross-reactions among pestiviruses, it is essential to identify the specific etiologic agent when pestivirus antibodies are detected in CSF eradication programs.

CSFV is endemic in parts of Eastern Europe, Southeast Asia, Central America, and South America. Although eradicated from domestic pigs in Western Europe, CSFV remains endemic in some populations of wild boar, and farms in these areas are at risk of reinfection. At present, the risk of reintroducing CSFV into free areas is high. Producers and veterinarians are in the best position to detect CSF outbreaks in free areas, but early detection will require both vigilance and training in the recognition of clinical signs. A "no vaccination" policy is logical in CSFV-free areas, but emergency vaccination must be included in contingency plans in order to avoid destroying millions of pigs. For this reason, research on efficacious marker vaccines and reliable differential tests should continue. Likewise, the development of simulation models should be encouraged in order to be able to respond to changing epidemiological situations with the most effective control measures.

ETIOLOGY

CSFV, BVDV, and BDV are small, enveloped, positive, single-strand RNA viruses in the genus *Pestivirus* of the family *Flaviviridae* (Becher et al. 1999). Currently the genus *Pestivirus* includes four approved species: CSFV, BVDV-1, BVDV-2, and BDV. A single strain (H138) isolated from a giraffe in Kenya more than 30 years ago represents a tentative fifth species (Becher et al. 1999). Recent phylogenetic and antigenic analysis have led the same authors to propose splitting the BDV group into 3 subgroups: BDV-1 for classical sheep isolates; BDV-2 for isolates, primarily from sheep, related to the previous strain V60 isolated from reindeer; and BDV-3 for the ovine Gifhorn isolate that differs significantly from all previously described pestiviruses, including BDV (Becher et al. 2003).

The majority of pestiviruses are noncytopathogenic in cell culture, but some BVDV isolates from cases of mucosal disease and some CSFV strains are cytopathogenic in vitro. Cytopathogenicity of BVDV is correlated with the expression of the nonstructural protein NS3, which is generated by processing a fusion protein termed NS2-3 (Kummerer and Meyers 2000; Zhang et al. 2003).

The pestivirus genome is 12.5–16.5 kilobases in size and encodes for a single polyprotein (Meyers et al. 1989):

$$NH_2\text{-}(N^{pro}\text{-}C\text{-}E^{rns}\text{-}E1\text{-}E2\text{-}p7\text{-}NS2.3\text{-}NS4A\text{-}NS4B\text{-}NS5A\text{-}NS5B)\text{-}COOH$$

The single polyprotein is co- and posttranslationally converted to mature proteins by a combination of virus and host cell proteases (Rumenapf et al. 1993). The structure and function of some envelope proteins has been studied in some detail, but the nonstructural proteins are not well characterized. Little is known about mechanisms of viral RNA replication, packaging, or how viral particles are assembled. Virions are released from the host cell by exocytosis, usually without morphological cell damage.

CSFV is relatively stable for an RNA virus (Vanderhallen et al. 1999), but is antigenically and genetically diverse, nonetheless. Antigenic variability among CSFV isolates can be characterized using monoclonal antibodies (Edwards et al. 1991) and genetic variability evaluated using genomic sequencing. For example, two panels of monoclonal antibodies, directed against E2 and Erns glycoproteins defined 21 antigenic virus types (Kosmidou et al. 1995). Genetic characterization of new CSFV isolates has become standardized in terms of the genomic fragment sequenced, the algorithms used in constructing phylogenetic trees, and the classification of the genetic groups. Three regions of the viral genome are usually evaluated: the 3' end of the polymerase gene (NS5B), 150 nucleotides of the 5'NTR, and 190 nucleotides of the gene encoding E2. The E2 glycoprotein is most commonly used for genetic typing because abundant sequence data are available.

CSFV is divided into three major genetic groups (Lowings et al. 1996), each with three or four subgroups: 1.1, 1.2, 1.3; 2.1, 2.2, 2.3; 3.1, 3.2, 3.3, 3.4. (Paton et al. 2000c). The phylogenetic analyses of the last decade have demonstrated a link between genotype and geographic origin (Bartak and Greiser-Wilke 2000; Stadejek et al. 1997; Vilcek 1997; Vilcek et al. 1996). Most viruses isolated from outbreaks in Western Europe in the 1990s belonged to Group 2. The situation is more complex in Central and Eastern Europe where isolates usually belong to groups 2.2 or 2.3. Group 1 isolates are present in South America (Frias-Lepoureau and Greiser-Wilke 2002) and Russia (Vlasova et al. 2003); and Group 3 viruses are apparently confined to Asia (Parchariyanon et al. 2000). The Community Reference Laboratory for CSF in Hanover Germany has developed a web-accessible database of sequences from isolates throughout the world (Greiser-Wilke et al. 2000b). This database is a useful tool for identifying possible viral sources for outbreaks occurring in previously uninfected areas (Greiser-Wilke et al. 2000a; Sandvik et al. 2000).

EPIDEMIOLOGY

Classical Swine Fever

Domestic pig populations in Australia, New Zealand, North America, and Western Europe are free of CSF (Paton and Greiser-Wilke 2003). In South America, Chile and Uruguay have been declared CSF-free. Argentina, free of outbreaks since 1999, stopped vaccination in April 2004. CSF remains endemic in Asia (Paton et al. 2000c) and, although the situation in Africa is not well characterized, the disease has been identified in Madagascar. Extensive areas of Central and South America continue using vaccination to control the disease (Morilla and Carvajal 2002; Morilla and Rosales 2002).

The reemergence of CSF is always a risk and several areas previously free of CSF have had incursions in recent years. For example, CSF reemerged in Cuba in 1993 after an absence of more than 20 years. The outbreaks in western Cuba were apparently caused by strain Margarita (group 1.2) used in vaccine potency trials, but outbreaks in eastern Cuba were of uncertain origin, with no demonstrated relationship to Caribbean strains. The outbreaks were exacerbated by the presence of a highly susceptible (unvaccinated) swine population; the result of worsening economics on the island (Frias-Lepoureau 2002). In spite of a campaign of total depopulation carried out in the Caribbean, new infections have occurred, leading the authorities to turn to vaccination as the method of control.

Under natural circumstances, the primary routes of transmission are oronasal by direct or indirect contact with infected wild or domestic pigs, or oral by ingestion of contaminated foodstuffs (Edwards et al. 2000; Fritzemeier et al. 2000; Horst et al. 1997). People should be regarded as the single most important factor in transmission of the virus between herds. In finishing units and in areas with small pig farms, transport and introduction of infected pigs accounts for the majority of outbreaks and for the spread of the disease (Terpstra 1987).

Airborne spread of CSFV has been demonstrated under experimental conditions (Dewulf et al. 2000), although its importance under field conditions is uncertain. However, in a fully susceptible population and in a densely populated region, even a minor route of transmission can have major consequences. A matched case-control study of 135 infected and 99 uninfected pig herds in the 1997 to 1998 CSF epidemic in the Netherlands suggested that airborne transmission did not occur over long distances, but did occur within a holding pen or within a radius of less than 500 meters. In one case, transmission occurred when an aerosol was produced during high-pressure cleaning of the electrocution equipment used to depopulate herds (Elbers et al. 2001).

The possibility of CSFV transmission by semen was raised during the epidemic in the Netherlands. Following infection of two artificial insemination centers, 1680 pig herds were declared CSF-suspect (Elbers et al. 1999; Hennecken et al. 2000). Experimental studies have shown that infected boars could shed CSFV in semen, and it is assumed that the disease might be transmitted by artificial insemination (de Smit et al. 1999; Floegel et al. 2000).

Rodents and pets have been postulated to act as mechanical vectors, but recent work proved that transmission of CSFV by rats, dogs, and cats is unlikely (Dewulf et al. 2001a). Thus, euthanasia of pets during an outbreak cannot be justified, as long as they do not leave the infected farm.

Indirect transmission via people can occur when biosecurity is deficient and, for example, visitors enter the premises without changing into clothing and boots supplied by the farm (Elbers et al. 2001). Vehicles (trucks, trailers, cars) can carry virus-contaminated feces and urine over long distances, but an experiment mimicking the conditions of transport showed that transmission via excretions without direct contact between pigs was unlikely (Dewulf et al. 2002).

A quantitative approach to understanding CSFV spread among animals and herds is an area of active interest, but relatively few studies have been conducted to date. One objective of this approach is to identify the biological and population factors that affect the rate of transmission (Klinkenberg et al. 2002; Laevens et al. 1998). Another objective is to construct mathematical models that predict the course of an epidemic. Ideally, such models could provide insight into the decisions to make to control an outbreak. Such models have been created and tested with data from the epidemic in the Netherlands (Horst et al. 1997; Horst et al. 1999) and in Belgium (Mintiens et al. 2001; Mintiens et al. 2003).

Typical of enveloped viruses, CSFV is inactivated by organic solvents (ether or chloroform) and by detergents. Sodium hydroxide (2%) is still considered the most suitable for disinfection of contaminated premises.

Despite being an enveloped virus, CSFV survives for prolonged periods in favorable environments—i.e., cool, moist, protein-rich conditions, such as those found in meat, but in liquid manure CSFV can survive for 2 weeks at 20°C and more than 6 weeks at 4°C (Haas et al. 1995). CSFV is relatively stable in a range of pH 5–10. The rate of inactivation under pH 5 is dependent on the temperature (Depner et al. 1992).

Thermal and pH stability may vary by strain, but inactivation of the virus is primarily dependent on the medium. For example, CSFV in cell culture loses its infectivity after 10 minutes at 60°C, but survives for up to 30 minutes at 68°C in defibrinated blood. For these reasons, it is difficult to give guidelines for the survival of CSFV in the environment. The survival and inactivation of CSFV was recently reviewed (Edwards 2000).

Bovine Viral Diarrhea Virus and Border Disease Virus

The prevalence of BVDV antibodies in the pig populations of CSFV-free countries (Australia, Ireland, Great Britain, Denmark) have been estimated at 1.6–43.5%, depending on the age of the animals and possibly on the degree of contact with cattle (Jensen 1985). In countries where CSFV is present, the situation with regard to BVDV antibodies seems to be about the same.

Cattle are the most common source of BVDV infection in pigs. In units with dairy farming, one potential source of infection is BVDV-contaminated whey or milk fed to sows (Terpstra and Wensvoort 1988). In some cases, pigs have had contact with cattle recently vaccinated with BVDV 2 (Stewart et al. 1971). In other reports, pigs and cattle were kept in separate lots and buildings, but personnel and equipment moved freely between the different farm units (Carbrey et al. 1976).

The prolonged presence of a persistently infected litter of pigs is the most likely source of BVDV or BDV to susceptible, pregnant sows (Terpstra and Wensvoort 1988; Vannier et al. 1988). Persistent BDV infection of piglets occurs when sows are infected during early pregnancy—i.e., fetuses are transplacentally infected and piglets become immunotolerant and persistently infected (Vannier et al. 1988). The course of the infection is quite similar to that described for BVD infection in pregnant cows (Baker 1987). When a pregnant sow is infected under experimental conditions, the litter may consist of a mixture of virus-positive and antibody-positive piglets. This suggests variability in the time at which individual fetuses became infected (Edwards et al. 1995). Congenitally BDV-infected piglets appear to excrete large amounts of virus, since susceptible young animals kept in contact rapidly seroconvert and produce high antibody titers. Conversely, when piglets are infected after birth, spread of infection to in-contact animals does not occur; suggesting low or perhaps no excretion of virus (Vannier et al. 1988).

Pigs may also become infected through the use of modified live virus vaccines (CSF or Aujeszky's disease) or other biologicals contaminated with virus (Vannier et al. 1988; Wensvoort and Terpstra 1988). In such cases, either ovine or bovine contaminants may be involved.

CLINICAL SIGNS

Classical Swine Fever

In the acute form of the CSF, the initial clinical signs include anorexia, lethargy, conjunctivitis, respiratory signs, and constipation followed by diarrhea. In the chronic form, the same clinical signs are observed, but the pigs survive for a time (2–3 months) before dying. Nonspecific signs—e.g., intermittent hyperthermia, chronic enteritis, and wasting—may also be seen.

Historically, peracute, acute, chronic, or prenatal forms of CSF have been attributed to distinct levels of virus virulence. However, virus strain virulence is difficult to define because clinical signs also depend on pig age, breed, health status, and immune status (Depner et al. 1997; Floegel-Niesmann et al. 2003; Moennig et al. 2003).

Since the early 1980s, the diagnosis of CSF on the basis of clinical signs has been problematic and resulted in the belated recognition of CSF outbreaks, thereby giving time for the virus to spread. CSF is one of several diseases characterized by cutaneous hyperemia or cyanosis and nonspecific clinical signs. Particularly when CSFV strains of low virulence are involved, it may be difficult to differentiate CSF from African swine fever (ASF), porcine reproductive and respiratory syndrome (PRRS), postweaning dermatitis and nephropathy syndrome (PDNS), salmonella, or cumarin poisoning. The one constant sign in CSF is hyperthermia (Davila et al. 2003; Floegel-Niesmann et al. 2003), usually greater than 40°C, and piglets are often seen piled in a corner. Clinical signs are more marked in piglets than adults and hyperthermia may be lower (39.5°C) in adults.

CSFV is able to cross the placenta of pregnant sows and infect fetuses at any stage of pregnancy. Depending on the strain and the time of gestation, infection can cause abortion and stillbirths. However, infection at 50–70 days of gestation can lead to the birth of persistently viremic piglets. Such piglets initially appear clinically normal, but subsequently begin to waste or develop congenital tremors (Vannier et al. 1981). This course of infection has been described as "late onset CSF" (van Oirschot and Terpstra 1977). Similar to BVDV in ruminants, these animals shed high levels of virus for several months and are important reservoirs of CSFV.

Bovine Viral Diarrhea Virus and Border Disease Virus

In the field, infection of pigs with BVDV usually occurs without clinical signs. In some cases, however, natural infection of pig herds with pestiviruses other than CSF has been associated with breeding problems—e.g., poor conception rates, small litters, and a few abortions. Hyperthermia and colic spasms have also been described (Carbrey et al. 1976). In the Netherlands and France, signs compatible with congenital CSF infection were described in piglets born to sows vaccinated 4 months earlier with CSF or Aujeszky's disease vaccines contaminated with a ruminant pestivirus (Vannier et al. 1988; Wensvoort and Terpstra 1988). Clinical signs in piglets included anemia, rough hair coats, growth retardation, wasting, congenital tremors, conjunctivitis, diarrhea, polyarthritis, petechiae in the skin, and blue ear tips (Terpstra and Wensvoort 1988).

Natural infection of sows with BDV has been reported to result in reproductive signs—e.g., repeat breeding, and mummified and stillborn pigs at farrowing (Vannier et al. 1988). A high proportion of piglets from infected sows showed eyelid edema, locomotor disorders, and occasionally, diarrhea and arthritis. The mortality rate in affected litters at 2 days of age ranged from 30–70%.

There are a number of reports of experimental inoculation of pigs, primarily pregnant sows, with BVDV and BDV via oral, intranasal, intramuscular, or intrauterine routes (Leforban et al. 1990b; Stewart et al. 1980; Wrathall et al. 1978). The results are inconsistent, but depend primarily on the strain used and the stage of pregnancy.

Inoculation of pregnant sows with the NADL strain of BVDV between 28 and 54 days of gestation did not produce transplacental infection of the fetuses (Stewart et al. 1980), but eyelid edema was seen in a few piglets (Leforban et al. 1990b). Inoculation of 9–18 kg piglets with the Singer strain of BVDV (Coria and McClurkin 1978) did not produce clinical disease, but the virus could be recovered from blood and tissues of inoculated pigs, and antibodies were detected in their sera after 3 weeks. When later challenged with a virulent CSFV strain, these piglets developed severe disease, but 6 of 7 survived (Stewart et al. 1971). The same strain of BVDV, when administered to fetuses at 41–65 days of gestation by transuterine injection caused death or small-sized fetuses (Mengeling 1988). Dahle et al. (1993) intranasally inoculated weaned pigs with BVDV strain OSLOSS ÷ 2482, and then challenged with decreasing doses of CSFV 4 weeks later. After CSFV challenge, the only clinical sign observed was fever in one animal, although most animals became viremic.

Experimental inoculation of pregnant sows with BDV field strains at 30–32 days of gestation produced transplacental infection of fetuses and newborn piglets with low body weights and short body lengths (Wrathall et al. 1978). Leforban et al. (1990b) reported an increase in perinatal mortality and eyelid edema, hyperthermia, and anemia in survivors during the second week of life. Slow growth rates, respiratory signs, and diarrhea developed in pigs, some of which died by 2 months of age. Pigs without respiratory and enteritic signs survived and had normal growth despite marked snout deformations, including prognathism in one individual. BDV was isolated from blood and organs of all dead piglets, but not from survivors. When 40-day-old specific pathogen free (SPF) pigs were placed in contact with BDV transplacentally infected piglets, they did not show clinical signs, but they developed high levels of antibody to BDV, which was able to protect them completely against challenge with a virulent strain of CSFV.

PATHOGENESIS

Classical Swine Fever

Transmission of CSFV is most commonly oronasal, with primary virus replication in the tonsils. From the tonsils, it spreads to the regional lymph nodes, then via the peripheral blood to bone marrow, visceral lymph nodes, and lymphoid structures associated with the small intestine and spleen. The spread of the virus within the pig is usually complete in less than 6 days.

Within the pig, CSFV replicates in monocyte-macrophage cells and vascular endothelial cells. CSFV is immunosuppressive, and neutralizing antibodies may not appear until 2–3 weeks after infection. Leukopenia, in particular lymphopenia, is a classic early event (Susa et al. 1992). CSF leukopenia impacts leukocyte subpopulations unequally, with B lymphocytes, helper T cells, and cytotoxic T cells the most affected. Depletion of lymphocyte subpopulations occurs 1–4 days before virus can be detected in serum by reverse transcription-polymerase chain reaction (RT-PCR).

The severity of the changes in bone marrow and circulating leukocytes suggest that cytopathic effects in uninfected cells are induced indirectly—e.g., by a soluble factor or by cell-to-cell contact, and are not a direct effect of the virus or viral protein(s). Research has shown that, at high concentration, the glycoprotein Erns induces apoptosis in lymphocytes *in vitro* (Bruschke et al. 1997). However, exposure to supernatant from infected cells did not induce apoptosis in target cells. Although still undescribed, such a mechanism could also account for the delay in cellular and humoral immune responses (Summerfield et al. 2001).

In cell culture, most CSFV strains grow without producing cytopathic effect and without inducing interferon alpha secretion by infected cells. Indeed, CSFV infection causes cells to acquire a greater capacity to resist apoptosis (Ruggli et al. 2003). These observations provide evidence that CSFV interferes with cellular antiviral activity and suggest the possibility that the lesions seen in pigs have an immunopathological basis.

Interactions between CSFV and the monocyte-macrophage system result in the release of mediator molecules that promote the progression of the disease. Changes in hemostatic balance are thought to be caused by proinflammatory and antiviral factors that mediate the thrombocytopenia and hemorrhage characteristic of CSFV infection (Knoetig et al. 1999). The production of inflammatory cytokines by infected endothelial cells could play a role in immunosuppression and facilitate virus dissemination by attracting monocytic cells (Bensaude et al. 2004). It has recently been recognized that CSFV can replicate in dendritic cells. It is possible that these highly mobile cells disseminate CSFV to various sites in the body, especially lymphoid tissues. Of themselves, interactions between CSFV-infected dendritic cells and lymphocytes are not sufficient to induce lymphocyte depletion without other interactions within the environment of the lymphoid follicles (Carrasco et al. 2004).

Understanding the CSFV–host interactions that lead to the evasion of the host's innate immune responses, delay the onset of acquired immunity, and produce the resultant pathogenic effects is currently an active focus of research.

Bovine Viral Diarrhea Virus and Border Disease Virus

BVDV and BDV are pathogenic for fetal pigs, but relatively apathogenic for pigs after birth. The ability of BVDV and BDV to establish intrauterine infections in swine is well established (Stewart et al. 1980; Vannier et al. 1988; Wrathall et al. 1978). The degree of clinical disease depends on the stage of gestation at which the infection occurred. Clinical signs are more serious if sows are infected during the first trimester of pregnancy. The most severe clinical signs and lesions in fetuses or piglets are observed when sows are infected 25–41 days post-breeding (Leforban et al. 1990b; Mengeling 1988). Under experimental conditions, piglets infected in utero with BVDV or BDV became persistently infected and immunotolerant (Leforban et al. 1990b; Vannier et al. 1988). After the disappearance of maternal antibodies, no active humoral response was detected in the majority of piglets. Furthermore, the virus was isolated from piglets and was shed by some, as evidenced by infection in young animals placed in contact.

In some experimental infections of pregnant sows with BDV, the onset of the clinical signs in the piglets was delayed until 13–14 days after birth. The reason for the delayed response is unknown, but colostral antibodies ingested by piglets would presumably block the replication of the virus and/or delay disease in transplacentally infected piglets (Leforban et al. 1990b; Mengeling 1988; Vannier et al. 1988).

The pathogenicity of BVDV or BDV seems to depend on the strain used in the experiment. BDV seems to be more consistently pathogenic for fetuses, whereas variable results are obtained with BVDV viral strains. The Singer strain, adapted to replicate in porcine cells, and BVDV strain 87/6 can infect and cause mortality in porcine fetuses, whereas the NADL strain does not induce clinical disease in piglets (Edwards et al. 1995; Leforban et al. 1990b; Mengeling 1988).

LESIONS

Classical Swine Fever

CSF lesions vary in severity and distribution, depending on the course of the disease. In acute forms, the pathological picture is often hemorrhagic. Leukopenia, thrombocytopenia, petechiae and ecchymoses in the skin, lymph nodes, larynx, bladder, kidney (Figure 15.1), and ileocecal junction are often described. Multifocal infarction of the margin of the spleen is characteristic, but not always present (Figure 15.2). Swollen or hemorrhagic lymph nodes or tonsils are common (Figure 15.3). In chronic forms, button ulcers in the cecum or large intestine may be present (Figure 15.4), as well as a generalized depletion of lymphoid tissues. Hemorrhagic and inflammatory lesions are less common, or even absent, despite the degeneration of endothelial cells. Congenital CSF can result in abortion, fetal mummification, stillbirths, and congenital malformations, such as central dysmyelinogenesis, cerebellar hypoplasia, microen-

cephaly, pulmonary hypoplasia (van der Molen and van Oirschot 1981).

Floegel-Niesmann et al. (2003) compared the clinical signs and lesions produced by four field strains isolated during the 1990s from domestic pigs or wild boars in Europe with the reference Alfort 187 strain. Comparing lesions in skin, subcutis and serosae, tonsil, spleen, kidney, lymph nodes, ileum and rectum, brain, and respiratory system, they found that lymph nodes were the tissues most severely affected by all isolates, followed by necrotic lesions in the ileum and hyperemia of the brain blood vessels (Table 15.1). Thus, these tissues were the most reliable for pathological diagnosis of CSF. Infarction of the spleen and necrotic lesions of the tonsil, although commonly described in the earlier

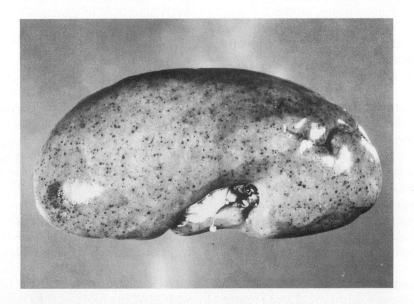

15.1. *Kidney showing numerous petechial hemorrhages (Courtesy W. C. Stewart).*

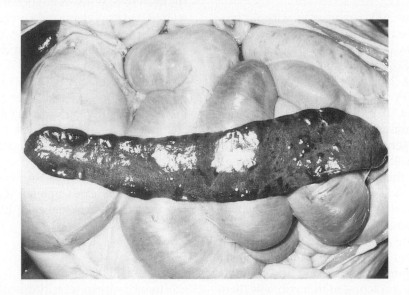

15.2. *Infarction of the spleen (Courtesy L. D. Miller).*

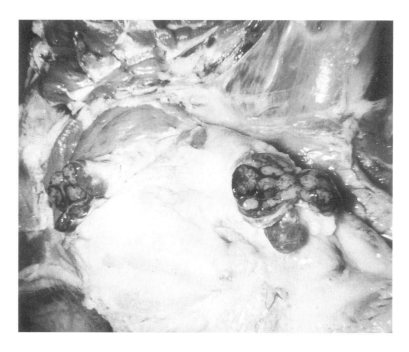

15.3. *Peripheral hemorrhage of the mandibular lymph node (Courtesy W. C. Stewart).*

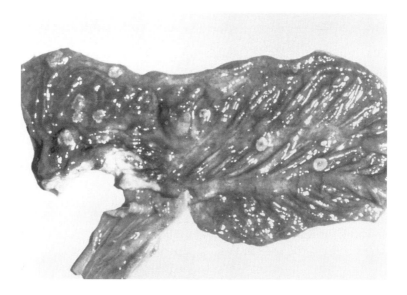

15.4. *Button ulcers in the cecum and colon (Courtesy L. D. Miller).*

literature, were infrequent. Likewise, respiratory signs were absent or mild.

Bovine Viral Diarrhea Virus and Border Disease Virus

When infected postnatally with BVDV or BDV, no or very mild lesions are observed in pigs.

Hyperemia of the small intestine was seen in one pig 11 days after being placed in contact with calves infected with NADL strain BVDV (Stewart et al. 1971). A transient leukopenia was detected during the first week following

experimental infection of pigs with a pig isolate of BVDV (Carbrey et al. 1976). In utero infection of fetuses by transplacental transmission is followed by consistent pathological disorders in fetuses or piglets. In 13 naturally occurring BVDV outbreaks in Holland, chronic gastroenteritis and septicemia with hemorrhages in lymph nodes, epicardium, and kidneys were the most consistent lesions reported. Inflammation of the digestive tract was frequently characterized by catarrh, hypertrophy, or ulceration of the mucosa. Necrotic tonsillitis, icterus, polyserositis, polyarthritis, and atrophy of the thymus were also noted (Terpstra and Wensvoort 1988). A porcine BVDV isolate administered to gilts at 42–46 days of gestation produced significant microscopic lesions in the leptomeninges and the choroid plexus of the fetus, characterized by collections of lymphocytes, histiocytes, and cellular accumulation in the vascular adventitia and perivascular spaces (Stewart et al. 1980).

In the case of BDV, experimental inoculation of sows on day 34 of gestation produced cerebellar hypoplasia in 9 of 19 liveborn piglets, with a small meningocele in one of the nine (Wrathall et al. 1978). The French BDV isolate Aveyron (Chappuis et al. 1984) inoculated into sows at day 30 of gestation produced lesions in lymphoid tissues in some piglets. Marked hemorrhages in lymph nodes and other lymphoid tissues were found in stillborn fetuses or in piglets that died shortly after birth. Histological examination of lymph nodes, spleen, and tonsil revealed marked subacute inflammatory lesions, characterized by accumulations of lymphocytes, plasmocytes, and eosinophilic polymorphonuclear leukocytes, numerous secondary follicles, increased populations of reticulocytes, and lymphoid hypoplasia with pyknosis and karyorrhexis. Thymus, liver and nervous tissues were normal (Leforban 1990).

DIAGNOSIS

Classical Swine Fever

Recent CSF epidemics in Europe have shown that early recognition of CSF and prompt elimination of CSFV-infected animals is the key to control. The longer CSF remains undetected, the greater the opportunity for the virus to spread (Elbers et al. 1999).

It should be recognized that farmers and veterinarians detected 75% of the recent CSFV epidemics on the basis of clinical observations. The need to establish a standardized protocol for evaluating herds for CSF has been recognized (Davila et al. 2003; Elbers et al. 2002; Mittelholzer et al. 2000). However, the list of clinical criteria cannot be overly complex if it is to be used in the field. Average daily gain and feed consumption are two

quantifiable measures that may be of use. Body temperature may also be useful, since hyperthermia is consistently associated with CSF and appears before, or concurrently, with the first clinical signs.

Because there are no pathognomonic clinical signs in CSF, laboratory diagnosis is always required for confirmation. Although it is not a specific diagnostic, leukopenia is an indicator of CSFV infection and a leukocyte count can be used as a screening assay (Dewulf et al. 2004). A variety of specific methods are available for diagnosis of CSFV infection. Since CSFV, BVDV, and BDV share common antigens, it is of the utmost importance to discriminate between these. Clearly, the consequence of a diagnosis of CSF is very distinct from the diagnosis of another pestivirus. Monoclonal antibodies are used in a variety of techniques to specifically identify the virus —e.g., virus isolation (VI), fluorescent antibody test (FAT), or ELISA tests.

Detection of CSFV. Virus isolation (VI) is still the most sensitive and specific method of virus detection. Virus may be isolated from tissue homogenates, serum, plasma, buffy coat, and whole blood collected in heparin or EDTA (Terpstra 2000). The tissues most likely to contain virus are tonsils, spleen, kidney, ileocecal lymph node, and retropharyngeal lymph node (Narita et al. 2000). CSFV can be isolated on porcine kidney cell lines (PK-15 or SK6). It is critical that all cells, media, and reagents have been previously determined to be free of pestiviruses or antibodies against pestiviruses. Although virus isolation is the reference method in most CSFV eradication programs, it is labor intensive, time consuming, and incompatible with the rapid response required to prevent further spread of virus.

The direct fluorescent antibody test (FAT) on frozen sections was the method of choice for detecting viral antigen during the last epidemic in the Netherlands (de Smit et al. 2000). It is rapid and reliable, but requires well-trained technicians. To discriminate between CSFV and other pestiviruses, it is necessary to use monoclonal antibodies. Tonsil tissue, the first site of virus replica-

Table 15.1. Pathological parameters to be evaluated for the diagnosis of CSF during postmortem examination. Scale from 0 points for no alteration up to 3 points for severe alterations, from (Floegel-Niesmann et al., 2003)

Parameter	Points		
	1—Slight Alteration	2—Distinct Lesion	3—Severe CSF Lesion
Skin	Nonspecific erythema	Single CSF-specific hemorrhage	Multiple CSF-specific hemorrhages
Subcutis and serosac	Individual petechiae	Petechiae in several places	Generalized petechiae
Tonsil	Swelling	Erythema	Necrosis
Spleen	Tiny infarction	Obvious infarction	<50% infarction
Kidney	Individual petechiae	Petechiae on surface and interstitium	Multiple petechiae
Lymph nodes	Swelling	Swelling and irregular hemorrhages	Swelling and generalized hemorrhages
Ileum and restum	Erythema	Erythema and small necrosis	Multiple necrosis or "button ulcer"
Brain	Slight hyperemia	Hyperemia	Hyperemia, vessels swollen
Respiratory system	Bronchitis	Bronchopneumonia or pleuritis	Bronchopneumonia and pleuritis

tion, is the most suitable sample. In chronic and subacute cases, ileum is often the only tissue to display fluorescence. FAT is not as sensitive as virus isolation and a negative FAT result is not sufficient to rule out a CSF suspect case.

Antigen-capture enzyme-linked immunosorbent assays (ELISAs) may be used for early diagnosis of CSFV in live pigs. Double-antibody sandwich ELISAs are based on monoclonal and/or polyclonal antibodies directed against a variety of viral proteins. Serum, buffy coat fraction, whole blood in heparin or EDTA, or tissue homogenates can be tested in these assays. The technique is relatively simple to perform, does not require tissue culture facilities, is suitable for automation, and provides results within 36 hours.

It is important to recognize the diagnostic limitations of antigen-capture ELISAs. All currently available commercial ELISAs are less sensitive than virus isolation on cell culture (Dewulf et al. 2004). In addition, their diagnostic sensitivity is significantly better on blood samples from piglets as compared to samples from adult pigs or samples from mild/subclinical cases (Anonymous 2002). To compensate for lack of diagnostic sensitivity, all pigs showing pyrexia in suspect herds should be tested. These tests also have lower diagnostic specificity (Anonymous 2002), and false-positive reactions may occur. For these reasons, the use of antigen-capture ELISAs is recommended only on samples from animals with clinical signs or pathological lesions compatible with CSF and for screening herds suspected to have been recently infected.

A variety of polymerase chain reaction (PCR)–based assays have been described for the detection of CSFV (Hofmann et al. 1994; McGoldrick et al. 1998, 1999; Vilcek et al. 1994), usually targeting the 5' noncoding region. Viral RNA can be detected in blood samples collected from live animals, as well as in tissue samples. Although PCR-based methods have been evaluated in two European ring-tests (Paton et al. 2000a, 2000b), no official PCR protocol has been established. Additional improvement in test performance is required to obtain a rapid, reliable, and automated test for use in routine diagnostics. Theoretically, the use of pooled samples could reduce costs, but the sensitivity of the technique must be validated before implementation on a routine basis.

Detection of Antibodies Against CSFV. ELISAs for the detection of anti-CSFV antibodies are useful for conducting epidemiological surveys and for monitoring CSFV-free areas. Competitive ELISAs are based on competition between anti-CSFV serum antibodies and a CSFV-specific monoclonal antibody directed against the viral glycoprotein gp 55 (E2). Cross-reactions with antibodies against other pestiviruses are reduced in the competitive ELISA format. A baculovirus recombinant E2 protein is often used as the antigen in the system. ELISA-detectable antibodies appear 10–15 days post infection,

similar to the time frame described for the appearance of neutralizing antibodies.

CSFV neutralizing antibody levels are determined by end-point titration of the serum. Briefly, the assay is performed as follows. Serial twofold dilutions of serum are mixed with an equal volume of CSFV (Alfort 187 is usually used as reference strain) prepared to contain around 100 $TCID_{50}$ per ml. After incubation for 1 hour, this is added to plates containing PK-15 cell monolayers. Two to four days later, the cells are stained with CSFV-specific antibodies. The titer of neutralizing antibody is expressed as the reciprocal of the highest serum dilution that prevented virus growth in 50% of two replicate wells.

Because of antibody cross-reactions among pestiviruses, the serum-virus neutralization assay is performed as a double neutralization test. That is, CSFV neutralizing antibody levels are compared to neutralizing antibody titers against BVDV or BDV reference strains. A difference of fourfold or more between the end points of the two titrations is considered conclusive for infection by the virus species yielding the highest neutralizing antibody titer (Terpstra 2000). This method is frequently used to screen neighboring herds around an outbreak prior to lifting control measures.

It is not feasible to perform all available diagnostic assays during an outbreak. Therefore, it is of the utmost importance to perform the assay(s) most appropriate to the situation and intended purpose. Since the key to controlling an outbreak is prevention of virus spread among farms, the assay of choice in terms of diagnostic sensitivity, diagnostic specificity, and speed is reverse transcription-polymerase chain reaction (RT-PCR). However, since the period of viremia is short, antibody detection assays are also useful, especially in herds where clinical signs have been present for more than 2 weeks (Dewulf et al. 2004).

Bovine Viral Diarrhea Virus and Border Disease Virus

BVDV or BDV may be isolated using the same methods previously described for CFSV and from the same tissues submitted for CSFV diagnosis—i.e., tonsils, spleen, kidney, and whole blood collected in heparin or EDTA. In CSF-free countries, BVDV and BDV must be considered in the differential diagnosis of CSFV and all suspect cases of CSF should be tested for BVDV and BDV. If BVDV or BDV is isolated from pigs, it is reported to grow better and to a higher titer in cells of ruminant origin, rather than in porcine cells (Wensvoort et al. 1989).

Pestiviruses share common antigenic structures (or patterns) and serological tests for the detection of antibodies against CSFV may cross-react with antibodies to ruminant pestiviruses. The practical importance of this is that the presence of ruminant pestivirus antibodies in pig sera often cause false positive reactions in serological surveys for CSFV. This presents problems in CSFV eradication campaigns and in epidemiological surveys for CSFV (Jensen 1985).

PREVENTION AND CONTROL

Classical Swine Fever in Domestic Pigs

Classical swine fever remains endemic in many parts of the world and continues to be a disease of worldwide importance. Although some regions are free of the disease, CSFV is still present at the borders between free and endemic areas and in some wild boar populations (Laddomada 2000).

For purposes of international trade, free areas maintain a "no vaccination" policy against CSF, although safe and efficacious live vaccines are available. Thus, control is based on stamping out infected or suspected herds, with the implementation of concomitant quarantine measures. In the last decade, however, the eradication of CSF outbreaks in Europe has raised concerns regarding the "no vaccine" policy. This is especially true in areas of high pig density, where a variety of factors increase the risk of disease spread (Elbers et al. 1999; Koenen et al. 1996; Mintiens et al. 2003). For instance, during the 1997 epidemic in the Netherlands, 9 million pigs were euthanized for reasons linked to movement restriction measures. However, even if emergency vaccination were not prohibited (EU council directive 80/217/EEC), the use of vaccine would have imposed severe economic consequences because vaccinated areas are banned from international trade for at least 1 year. Nevertheless, a more recent council directive (2001/89/EC) (Anonymous 2001) takes recent experiences into account and authorizes emergency vaccination around an outbreak.

Various CSFV vaccines are available, including the well-known live "Chinese" C strain, the Thiverval strain, and the newer marker vaccines that allow differentiation of field virus-infected versus vaccinated animals (for an in-depth review, see van Oirschot 2003). The traditional live vaccines induce a high level of protection against clinical disease, and neutralizing antibodies are detectable at 2 weeks post-challenge (Dahle and Liess 1995; Vandeputte et al. 2001). Duration of immunity is 6–10 months, regardless of the route of administration (intramuscular or oronasal) (Kaden and Lange 2001; Terpstra et al. 1990).

The primary drawback of live vaccines is that it is impossible to differentiate vaccine antibodies from field-virus induced antibodies. Researchers have evaluated a variety of marker vaccines to solve this problem, including nonreplicative Aujeszky's disease (pseudorabies) virus expressing the E2 of CSFV (Peeters et al. 1997), a porcine adenovirus-vectored vaccine (Hammond et al. 1999), and a chimeric pestivirus (Reimann et al. 2004; van Gennip 2001). DNA vaccines have also been developed, but need a prime-boost strategy (DNA-adenovirus) to induce real protection (Hammond et al. 2001).

At present, two differentiable, baculovirus-expressed E2 recombinant protein subunit vaccines are commercially available. The efficacy of the two E2 marker vaccines has been extensively evaluated in vaccination-challenge and transmission trials, but with variable results. A single dose of 32 μg E2 in a water-oil-water adjuvant prevented clinical signs and mortality due to a CSFV challenge 3 weeks after vaccination (Bouma et al. 1999). At least 14 days were needed to obtain clinical protection in growing pigs vaccinated with a single dose (Bouma et al. 2000; Uttenthal et al. 2001). If challenged earlier, no protection against clinical disease and no reduction of virus shedding were observed (Uttenthal et al. 2001).

The ability of the two marker vaccines to prevent transplacental transmission of CSFV has also been evaluated. However, transplacental transmission occurred even when two doses of vaccine (days 25 and 46 of pregnancy) were administered and challenge occurred 14 days after the second dose (Depner et al. 2001). Thus, transplacental infection could not be prevented in most vaccinated animals under the conditions of emergency vaccination. Vaccination could not prevent the "carrier sow syndrome" and, subsequently, the late onset form of CSF (Depner et al. 2001). It was concluded that the two-dose vaccination protocol protected pregnant gilts from clinical disease, but did not prevent horizontal or vertical spread of the CSFV (Dewulf et al. 2001b). Although these results indicated that the efficacy of these vaccines was not ideal, the possible use of these vaccines in an emergency has not been disallowed by the EC.

Differential ELISAs for the E2 marker vaccines are based on the detection of antibodies to the Erns protein (Floegel-Niesmann 2001). Improvement and assessment of these assays has been ongoing. In 2003, the EC conducted a large-scale inter-laboratory assessment of the diagnostic performance of a new version of a companion Erns ELISA test. Although the diagnostic specificity and the sensitivity of the test was improved relative to the kits tested in 1999 (Floegel-Niesmann 2001), it was concluded the need remained for a test that could determine with greater reliability whether a vaccinated pig had been infected and become a CSFV carrier.

Classical Swine Fever in Wild Boars

In Western Europe, vaccination in domestic pigs has been prohibited in EU member states since 1990, but the virus has been periodically reintroduced into domestic pigs via contact with wild boars. In some areas of Germany, an increase in the number of wild boars has promoted the persistence of virus within these populations and created an endemic situation (Fritzemeier et al. 2000; Moennig 2000). CSFV infection is seemingly harmless for wild boars as little mortality has been reported in recent outbreaks. In the presence of natural or manmade barriers, CSFV can be confined to a defined area until it is eliminated (Schnyder et al. 2002), as was done in Moselle (France) (Le Potier et al. 2003) or in Tessin (Switzerland). Classic measures for CSF control in wild boars involve reducing hunting activities to allow the virus to spread within the susceptible population and induce mortality or immunity, followed by targeted hunting of the most susceptible animals—i.e., juveniles and the young sows.

In some areas where it has been difficult to eradicate CSFV using standard methods, oral vaccination using live C strain distributed in bait has been attempted (Kaden et al. 2000). The safety of this vaccine has been demonstrated for other wild animal species (Chenut et al. 1999). In pigs, this oral vaccine can induce strong protective immunity in 10 days (Kaden and Lange 2001). However, recent analysis of the data from oral vaccination field campaigns has shown that three doses were required to induce immunity in the field. Due to poor access to baits, young boars did not acquire sufficient protective immunity in most field studies (Kaden et al. 2002). When vaccine is used, monitoring of the disease becomes very difficult as the only tool to differentiate between infected and vaccinated boars is the detection of the virus. Therefore, there is a real need for the development of an effective marker vaccine delivered by the oral route that would allow for serological monitoring of the spread of the virus among a vaccinated population.

Prevention of BVDV or BDV Infections

To prevent BVDV or BDV infection in pigs, it is necessary to avoid direct or indirect contact with cattle or sheep. Natural infection with BVDV often occurs when pigs are fed with cow's milk or bovine offal and this practice should be avoided.

Inadvertant transmission of these viruses is a risk when live-virus vaccines are used because of contamination of media and/or cells used in production of the vaccine. Cells used for multiplication of master seed virus used to prepare vaccine can be contaminated by BVDV or BDV. Indeed, some batches of CSF and Aujeszky's disease (pseudorabies) vaccines were contaminated by a pestivirus (probably BDV) because secondary lamb kidney cells were used to propagate the vaccine strain virus (Vannier et al. 1988; Wensvoort and Terpstra 1988). Both bovine and non-bovine cell lines can be contaminated with pestiviruses, and all cell cultures need to be monitored carefully for their presence (Potts et al. 1989). The primary source of contamination of cells is bovine serum added to the nutrient medium. BVDV is extremely common and collection from BVDV-infected calves or fetuses results in contaminated bovine serum. Rossi et al. (1980) reported that up to 62% of the lots of nonirradiated bovine fetal sera examined were found positive for BVDV. Therefore, the systematic testing and treatment of bovine serum and of biological products used for the preparation of vaccines is strongly recommended (Makoschey et al. 2003).

REFERENCES

Anonymous. 2001. Council directive 2001/89/EC of 23 October 2001 on community measures for the control of classical swine fever. Official Journal of the European Communities L316, 1.12.2001, pp. 5–35.

——. 2002. Commission decision approving a diagnostic manual establishing diagnostic procedures, sampling methods and criteria for evaluation of the laboratory tests for the confirmation of classical swine fever. Official Journal of the European Communities L39, pp. 71–88.

Baker JC. 1987. Bovine viral diarrhea virus: A review. J Am Vet Med Assoc 190:1449–1458.

Bartak P, Greiser-Wilke I. 2000. Genetic typing of classical swine fever virus isolates from the territory of the Czech Republic. Vet Microbiol 77:59–70.

Becher P, Orlich M, Kosmidou A, Konig M, Baroth M, Thiel HJ. 1999. Genetic diversity of pestiviruses: Identification of novel groups and implications for classification. Virology 262:64–71.

Becher P, Ramirez RA, Orlich M, Rosales SC, Konig M, Schweizer M, Stalder H, Schirrmeier H, Thiel HJ. 2003. Genetic and antigenic characterization of novel pestivirus genotypes: Implications for classification. Virology 311:96–104.

Bensaude E, Turner JL, Wakeley PR, Sweetman DA, Pardieu C, Drew TW, Wileman T, Powell PP. 2004. Classical swine fever virus induces proinflammatory cytokines and tissue factor expression and inhibits apoptosis and interferon synthesis during the establishment of long-term infection of porcine vascular endothelial cells. J Gen Virol 85:1029–1037.

Bouma A, Desmit AJ, Dejong MCM, Dekluijver EP, Moormann RJM. 2000. Determination of the onset of the herd-immunity induced by the E2 sub-unit vaccine against classical swine fever virus. Vaccine 18:1374–1381.

Bouma A, Desmit AJ, Dekluijver EP, Terpstra C, Moormann RJM. 1999. Efficacy and stability of a subunit vaccine based on glycoprotein E2 of classical swine fever virus. Vet Microbiol 66:101–114.

Bruschke CJ, Hulst MM, Moormann RJ, van Rijn PA, van Oirschot JT. 1997. Glycoprotein Erns of pestiviruses induces apoptosis in lymphocytes of several species. J Virol 71:6692–6696.

Carbrey EA, Stewart WC, Kresse JI, Snyder ML. 1976. Natural infection of pigs with bovine viral diarrhea virus and its differential diagnosis from hog cholera. J Am Vet Med Assoc 169:1217–1219.

Carrasco CP, Rigden RC, Vincent IE, Balmelli C, Ceppi M, Bauhofer O, Tache V, Hjertner B, McNeilly F, van Gennip HG, McCullough KC, Summerfield A. 2004. Interaction of classical swine fever virus with dendritic cells. J Gen Virol 85:1633–1641.

Chappuis G, Brun A, Kato F, Dufour R, Durant M. 1984. Isolement et caractérisation d'un pestivirus dans un foyer d'enterocolite leucopenie chez des moutons de l'Aveyron. Epidemiol Santé Anim 6:117–118.

Chenut G, Saintilan AF, Burger C, Rosenthal F, Cruciere C, Picard M, Bruyere V, Albina E. 1999. Oral immunisation of swine with a classical swine fever vaccine (Chinese strain) and transmission studies in rabbits and sheep. Vet Microbiol 64:265–276.

Coria MF, McClurkin AW. 1978. Duration of active and colostrum-derived passive antibodies to bovine viral diarrhoea virus in calves. Can J Comp Med 42:239–243.

Dahle J, Liess B. 1995. Assessment of safety and protective value of a cell culture modified strain "C" vaccine of hog cholera/classical swine fever virus. Berl Munch Tierarztl Wochenschr 108:20–25.

Dahle J, Schagemann G, Moennig V, Liess B. 1993. Clinical, virological and serological findings after intranasal inoculation of pigs with bovine viral diarrhoea virus and subsequent intranasal challenge with hog cholera virus. Zentralbl Veterinarmed B 40:46–54.

Davila S, Cariolet R, Le Potier MF. 2003. Etude de l'influence de la virulence des souches de peste porcine classique sur l'immunopathogénécité du virus chez les suidés et sur la propagation de la maladie en zone de forte densité porcine. Journées de la Recherche Porcine 35:375–382.

de Smit AJ, Bouma A, Terpstra C, van Oirschot JT. 1999. Transmission of classical swine fever virus by artificial insemination. Vet Microbiol 67:239–249.

de Smit AJ, Eble PL, Dekluijver EP, Bloemraad M, Bouma A. 2000. Laboratory experience during the classical swine fever virus epizootic in the Netherlands in 1997–1998. Vet Microbiol 73:197–208.

Depner K, Bauer T, Liess B. 1992. Thermal and pH stability of pestiviruses. Rev Sci Tech 11:885–893.

Depner KR, Bouma A, Koenen F, Klinkenberg D, Lange E, deSmit H, Vanderhallen H. 2001. Classical swine fever (CSF) marker vaccine—Trial II. Challenge study in pregnant sows. Vet Microbiol 83:107–120.

Depner KR, Hinrichs U, Bickhardt K, Greiser-Wilke I, Pohlenz J, Moennig V, Liess B. 1997. Influence of breed-related factors on the course of classical swine fever virus infection. Vet Rec 140:506–507.

Dewulf J, Koenen F, Mintiens K, Denis P, Ribbens S, deKruif A. 2004. Analytical performance of several classical swine fever laboratory diagnostic techniques on live animals for detection of infection. J Virol Methods 119:137–143.

Dewulf J, Laevens H, Koenen F, Mintiens K, deKruif A. 2000. Airborne transmission of classical swine fever virus under experimental conditions. Vet Rec 147:735–738.

——. 2001a. Evaluation of the potential of dogs, cats and rats to spread classical swine fever virus. Vet Rec 149:212–213.

——. 2001b. An E2 sub-unit marker vaccine does not prevent horizontal or vertical transmission of classical swine fever virus. Vaccine 20:86–91.

——. 2002. An experimental infection to investigate the indirect transmission of classical swine fever virus by excretions of infected pigs. J Vet Med B Infect Dis Vet Public Health 49:452–456.

Edwards S. 2000. Survival and inactivation of classical swine fever virus. Vet Microbiol 73:175–181.

Edwards S, Fukusho A, Lefevre PC, Lipowski A, Pejsak Z, Roehe P, Westergaard J. 2000. Classical swine fever: The global situation. Vet Microbiol 73:103–119.

Edwards S, Moennig V, Wensvoort G. 1991. The development of an international reference panel of monoclonal antibodies for the differentiation of hog cholera virus from other pestiviruses. Vet Microbiol 29:101–108.

Edwards S, Roehe PM, Ibata G. 1995. Comparative studies of border disease and closely related virus infections in experimental pigs and sheep. Br Vet J 151:181–187.

Elbers ARW, Bouma A, Stegeman JA. 2002. Quantitative assessment of clinical signs for the detection of classical swine fever outbreaks during an epidemic. Vet Microbiol 85:323–332.

Elbers ARW, Stegeman JA, de Jong MCM. 2001. Factors associated with the introduction of classical swine fever virus into pig herds in the central area of the 1997/98 epidemic in the Netherlands. Vet Rec 149:377–382.

Elbers ARW, Stegeman A, Moser H, Ekker HM, Smak JA, Pluimers FH. 1999. The classical swine fever epidemic 1997–1998 in the Netherlands: Descriptive epidemiology. Prev Vet Med 42:157–184.

Fernelius AL, Amtower WC, Lambert G, McClurkin AW, Matthews PJ. 1973. Bovine viral diarrhea virus in swine: Characteristics of virus recovered from naturally and experimentally infected swine. Can J Comp Med 37:13–20.

Floegel G, Wehrend A, Depner KR, Fritzemeier J, Waberski D, Moennig V. 2000. Detection of classical swine fever virus in semen of infected boars. Vet Microbiol 77:109–116.

Floegel-Niesmann G. 2001. Classical swine fever (CSF) marker vaccine—Trial III. Evaluation of discriminatory ELISAs. Vet Microbiol 83:121–136.

Floegel-Niesmann G, Bunzenthal C, Fischer S, Moennig V. 2003. Virulence of recent and former classical swine fever virus isolates evaluated by their clinical and pathological signs. J Vet Med B Infect Dis Vet Public Health 50:214–220.

Frias-Lepoureau MT. 2002. An update on classical swine fever virus molecular epidemiology. In Trends in Emerging Viral Infections of Swine. A Morilla, K-J Yoon, J Zimmerman, eds. Ames: Iowa State University Press, pp. 165–171.

Frias-Lepoureau MT, Greiser-Wilke I. 2002. Reemergence of Classical Swine Fever in Cuba, 1993 to 1997, In Trends in Emerging Viral Infections of Swine. A Morilla, K-J Yoon, J Zimmerman, eds. Ames: Iowa State University Press, pp. 143–147.

Fritzemeier J, Teuffert J, Greiser-Wilke I, Staubach C, Schluter H, Moennig V. 2000. Epidemiology of classical swine fever in Germany in the 1990s. Vet Microbiol 77:29–41.

Fuchs F. 1968. Schweinepest. In Handbuch der virusinfektionen bei Tieren, Vol 3. H Rohrer, ed. Jena: Gustav Fischer.

Greiser-Wilke I, Fritzemeier J, Koenen F, Vanderhallen H, Rutili D, Demia GM, Romero L, Rosell R, Sánchez-Vizcaíno JM, Sangabriel A. 2000a. Molecular epidemiology of a large classical swine fever epidemic in the European Union in 1997–1998. Vet Microbiol 77:17–27.

Greiser-Wilke I, Zimmermann B, Fritzemeier J, Floegel G, Moennig V. 2000b. Structure and presentation of a World Wide Web database of CSF virus isolates held at the EU Reference Laboratory. Vet Microbiol 73:131–136.

Haas B, Ahl R, Bohm R, Strauch D. 1995. Inactivation of viruses in liquid manure. Rev Sci Tech 14:435–445.

Hamilton AF, Timoney PJ. 1973. Bovine virus diarrhoea-mucosal disease virus and border disease. Res Vet Sci 15:265–267.

Hammond JM, Jansen ES, Morrissy CJ, Goff WV, Meehan GC, Williamson MM, Lenghaus C, Sproat KW, Andrew ME, Coupar BEH, Johnson MA. 2001. A prime-boost vaccination strategy using naked DNA followed by recombinant porcine adenovirus protects pigs from classical swine fever. Vet Microbiol 80:101–119.

Hammond JM, McCoy RJ, Jansen ES, Morrissy CJ, Hodgson AL, Johnson MA. 1999. Vaccination with a single dose of a recombinant porcine adenovirus expressing the classical swine fever virus gp55 (E2) gene protects pigs against classical swine fever. Vaccine 18:1040–1050.

Hennecken M, Stegeman JA, Elbers ARW, Vannes A, Smak JA, Verheijden JHM. 2000. Transmission of classical swine fever virus by artificial insemination during the 1997–1998 epidemic in the Netherlands: A descriptive epidemiological study. Vet Q 22:228–233.

Hofmann MA, Brechtbuhl K, Stauber N. 1994. Rapid characterization of new pestivirus strains by direct sequencing of PCR-amplified cDNA from the 5' noncoding region. Arch Virol 139:217–229.

Horst HS, Dijkhuizen AA, Huirne RBM, Meuwissen MPM. 1999. Monte Carlo simulation of virus introduction into the Netherlands. Prev Vet Med 41:209–229.

Horst HS, Huirne RBM, Dijkhuizen AA. 1997. Risks and economic consequences of introducing classical swine fever into the Netherlands by feeding swill to swine. Rev Sci Tech OIE 16:207–214.

Jensen MH. 1985. Screening for neutralizing antibodies against hog cholera and/or bovine viral diarrhea virus in Danish pigs. Acta Vet Scand 26:72–80.

Kaden V, Heyne H, Kiupel H, Letz W, Kern B, Lemmer U, Gossger K, Rothe A, Bohme H, Tyrpe P. 2002. Oral immunisation of wild boar against classical swine fever: Concluding analysis of the recent field trials in Germany. Berl Munch Tierarztl Wochenschr 115:179–185.

Kaden V, Lange B. 2001. Oral immunisation against classical swine fever (CSF): Onset and duration of immunity. Vet Microbiol 82:301–310.

Kaden V, Lange E, Fischer U, Strebelow G. 2000. Oral immunisation of wild boar against classical swine fever: Evaluation of the first field study in Germany. Vet Microbiol 73:239–252.

Kernkamp HCH. 1961. The natural history of hog cholera. In Symposium on Hog Cholera. GT Mainwaring, DK Sorensen, eds. University of Minnesota, St. Paul, Minnesota, pp. 19–28.

Klinkenberg D, de Bree J, Laevens H, de Jong MC. 2002. Within- and between-pen transmission of classical swine fever virus: A new method to estimate the basic reproduction ratio from transmission experiments. Epidemiol Infect 128:293–299.

Knoetig SM, Summerfield A, Spagnuolo-Weaver M, McCullough KC. 1999. Immunopathogenesis of classical swine fever: Role of monocytic cells. Immunology 97:359–366.

Koenen F, Van Caenegem G, Vermeersch JP, Vandenheede J, Deluyker H. 1996. Epidemiological characteristics of an outbreak of classical swine fever in an area of high pig density. Vet Rec 139:367–371.

Kosmidou A, Ahl R, Thiel HJ, Weiland E. 1995. Differentiation of classical swine fever virus (CSFV) strains using monoclonal antibodies against structural glycoproteins. Vet Microbiol 47:111–118.

Kummerer BM, Meyers G. 2000. Correlation between point mutations in NS2 and the viability and cytopathogenicity of bovine viral diarrhea virus strain Oregon analyzed with an infectious cDNA clone. J Virol 74:390–400.

Laddomada A. 2000. Incidence and control of CSF in wild boar in Europe. Vet Microbiol 73:121–130.

Laevens H, Koenen F, Deluyker H, Berkvens D, deKruif A. 1998. An experimental infection with classical swine fever virus in weaner pigs. I. Transmission of the virus, course of the disease, and antibody response. Vet Q 20:41–45.

Laude H. 1979. Nonarbo-togaviridae: Comparative hydrodynamic properties of the pestivirus genus. Brief report. Arch Virol 62:347–352.

Leforban Y. 1990. Profils epitopiques compares de 18 souches de peste porcine classique: Comparaison des souches isolees de formes chroniques et des autres souches. Rec Med Vet Ec Alfort 166:455–461.

Leforban Y, Edwards S, Ibata G, Vannier P. 1990a. A blocking ELISA to differentiate hog cholera virus antibodies in pig sera from those due to other pestiviruses. Ann Rech Vet 21:119–129.

Leforban Y, Vannier P, Cariolet R. 1990b. Pathogenicity of border disease and bovine viral diarrhoea viruses for pig: Experimental study on the vertical and horizontal transmission of the viruses. Proc Congr Int Pig Vet Soc, p. 204.

Le Potier MF, Kuntz-Simon G, Mesplède A, Boué F, Rossi S, Mazuy D, Hars J, Pacholek X. 2003. Scrological and virological surveillance of a classical swine fever outbreak in wild boar population in Moselle—France. 6th International Congress of the European Society for Veterinary Virology, Saint-Malo, France.

Lowings P, Ibata G, Needham J, Paton D. 1996. Classical swine fever virus diversity and evolution. J Gen Virol 77:1311–1321.

Makoschey B, Keijsers V, Goovaerts D. 2003. Bovine viral diarrhoea virus antigen in foetal calf serum batches and consequences of such contamination for vaccine production. Biologicals 31:203–208.

McGoldrick A, Bensaude E, Ibata G, Sharp G, Paton DJ. 1999. Closed one-tube reverse transcription nested polymerase chain reaction for the detection of pestiviral RNA with fluorescent probes. J Virol Methods 79:85–95.

McGoldrick A, Lowings JP, Ibata G, Sands JJ, Belak S, Paton DJ. 1998. A novel approach to the detection of classical swine fever virus by RT-PCR with a fluorogenic probe (TaqMan). J Virol Methods 72:125–135.

Mengeling WL. 1988. The possible role of bovine viral diarrhoea virus in maternal reproductive failure of swine. Proc Congr Int Pig Vet Soc, p. 228.

Meyers G, Rumenapf T, Thiel HJ. 1989. Molecular cloning and nucleotide sequence of the genome of hog cholera virus. Virology 171:555–567.

Mintiens K, Deluyker H, Laevens H, Koenen F, Dewulf J, deKruif A. 2001. Descriptive epidemiology of a classical swine fever outbreak in the Limburg Province of Belgium in 1997. J Vet Med B Infect Dis Vet Public Health 48:143–149.

Mintiens K, Laevens H, Dewulf J, Boelaert F, Verloo D, Koenen F. 2003. Risk analysis of the spread of classical swine fever virus through 'neighbourhood infections' for different regions in Belgium. Prev Vet Med 60:27–36.

Mittelholzer C, Moser C, Tratschin JD, Hofmann MA. 2000. Analysis of classical swine fever virus replication kinetics allows differentiation of highly virulent from avirulent strains. Vet Microbiol 74:293–308.

Moennig V. 2000. Introduction to classical swine fever: Virus, disease and control policy. Vet Microbiol 73:93–102.

Moennig V, Floegel Niesmann G, Greiser-Wilke I. 2003. Clinical signs and epidemiology of classical swine fever: A review of new knowledge. Vet J 165:11–20.

Morilla A, Carvajal MA. 2002. Experiences with classical swine fever vaccination in Mexico. In Trends in Emerging Viral Infections of Swine. A Morilla, K-J Yoon, J Zimmerman, eds. Ames: Iowa State University Press, pp. 159–164.

Morilla A, Rosales C. 2002. Reemergence of classical swine fever virus in Mexico, In Trends in Emerging Viral Infections of Swine. A Morilla, K-J Yoon, J Zimmerman, eds. Ames: Iowa State University Press, pp. 149–152.

Narita M, Kawashima K, Kimura K, Mikami O, Shibahara T, Yamada S, Sakoda Y. 2000. Comparative immunohistopathology in pigs infected with highly virulent or less virulent strains of hog cholera virus. Vet Pathol 37:402–408.

Parchariyanon S, Inui K, Damrongwatanapokin S, Pinyochon W, Lowings P, Paton D. 2000. Sequence analysis of E2 glycoprotein genes of classical swine fever viruses: Identification of a novel genogroup in Thailand. Dtsch Tierarztl Wochenschr 107:236–238.

Paton DJ, Greiser-Wilke I. 2003. Classical swine fever—An update. Res Vet Sci 75:169–178.

Paton DJ, McGoldrick A, Belak S, Mittelholzer C, Koenen F, Vanderhallen H, Biagetti M, Demia GM, Stadejek T, Hofmann MA, Thuer B. 2000a. Classical swine fever virus: A ring test to evaluate RT-PCR detection methods. Vet Microbiol 73:159–174.

Paton DJ, McGoldrick A, Bensaude E, Belak S, Mittelholzer C, Koenen F, Vanderhallen H, Greiser-Wilke I, Scheibner H, Stadejek T, Hofmann M, Thuer B. 2000b. Classical swine fever virus: A second ring test to evaluate RT-PCR detection methods. Vet Microbiol 77:71–81.

Paton DJ, McGoldrick A, Greiser-Wilke I, Parchariyanon S, Song JY, Liou PP, Stadejek T, Lowings JP, Bjorklund H, Belak S. 2000c. Genetic typing of classical swine fever virus. Vet Microbiol 73:137–157.

Peeters B, Bienkowskaszewczyk K, Hulst M, Gielkens A, Kimman T. 1997. Biologically safe, non-transmissible pseudorabies virus vector vaccine protects pigs against both Aujeszky's disease and classical swine fever. J Gen Virol 78:3311–3315.

Potts BJ, Sawyer M, Shekarchi IC, Wismer T, Huddleston D. 1989. Peroxidase-labeled primary antibody method for detection of pestivirus contamination in cell cultures. J Virol Methods 26:119–124.

Reimann I, Depner K, Trapp S, Beer M. 2004. An avirulent chimeric Pestivirus with altered cell tropism protects pigs against lethal infection with classical swine fever virus. Virology 322:143–157.

Rossi CR, Bridgman CR, Kiesel GK. 1980. Viral contamination of bovine fetal lung cultures and bovine fetal serum. Am J Vet Res 41:1680–1681.

Ruggli N, Tratschin JD, Schweizer M, McCullough KC, Hofmann MA, Summerfield A. 2003. Classical swine fever virus interferes with cellular antiviral defense: Evidence for a novel function of N-pro. J Virol 77:7645–7654.

Rumenapf T, Unger G, Strauss JH, Thiel HJ. 1993. Processing of the envelope glycoproteins of pestiviruses. J Virol 67:3288–3294.

Sandvik T, Drew T, Paton D. 2000. CSF virus in East Anglia: Where from? Vet Rec 147:251.

Schnyder M, Stark KDC, Vanzetti T, Salman MD, Thur B, Schleiss W, Griot C. 2002. Epidemiology and control of an outbreak of classical swine fever in wild boar in Switzerland. Vet Rec 150:102–109.

Stadejek T, Vilcek S, Lowings JP, Ballagi-Pordany A, Paton DJ, Belak S. 1997. Genetic heterogeneity of classical swine fever virus in Central Europe. Virus Res 52:195–204.

Stewart WC, Carbrey EA, Jenney EW, Brown CL, Kresse JI. 1971. Bovine viral diarrhea infection in pigs. J Am Vet Med Assoc 159:1556–1563.

Stewart WC, Miller LD, Kresse JI, Snyder ML. 1980. Bovine viral diarrhea infection in pregnant swine. Am J Vet Res 41:459–462.

Summerfield A, Mcneilly F, Walker I, Allan G, Knoetig SM, Mccullough KC. 2001. Depletion of CD4(+) and CD8(High+) T-cells before the onset of viraemia during classical swine fever. Vet Immunol Immunopathol 78:3–19.

Susa M, Konig M, Saalmuller A, Reddehase MJ, Thiel HJ. 1992. Pathogenesis of classical swine fever: B-lymphocyte deficiency caused by hog cholera virus. J Virol 66:1171–1175.

Terpstra C. 1987. Epizootiology of swine fever. Vet Q 9(Suppl 1):50S–60S.

Terpstra C. 2000. Classical swine fever (hog cholera). In Manual of Standards for Diagnostic Tests and Vaccines, 4th ed, Office International des Epizooties, World Organisation for Animal Health, pp. 202–203.

Terpstra C, Wensvoort G. 1988. Natural infections of pigs with bovine viral diarrhoea virus associated with signs resembling swine fever. Res Vet Sci 45:137–142.

Terpstra C, Woortmeyer R, Barteling SJ. 1990. Development and properties of a cell culture produced vaccine for hog cholera based on the Chinese strain. Dtsch Tierarztl Wochenschr 97:77–79.

USDA. 1889. Hog Cholera: Its history, nature, and treatment as determined by the inquiries and investigations of the Bureau of Animal industry. Washington, Government Printing Office.

Uttenthal A, Le Potier MF, Romero L, De Mia GM, Floegel-Niesmann G. 2001. Classical swine fever (CSF) marker vaccine—Trial I. Challenge studies in weaner pigs. Vet Microbiol 83:85–106.

van der Molen EJ, van Oirschot JT. 1981. Congenital persistent swine fever (hog cholera). II. Further pathomorphological observations with special emphasis on epithelial, vascular and nervous tissues. Zentralbl Veterinarmed B 28:190–204.

van Gennip HG. 2001. Chimeric classical swine fever viruses containing envelope protein Erns or E2 of bovine viral diarrhoea virus protect pigs against challenge with CSFV and induce a distinguishable antibody response. Vaccine 19:447–459.

Vandeputte J, Too HL, Ng FK, Chen C, Chai KK, Liao GA. 2001. Adsorption of colostral antibodies against classical swine fever, persistence of maternal antibodies, and effect on response to vaccination in baby pigs. Am J Vet Res 62:1805–1811.

Vanderhallen H, Mittelholzer C, Hofmann MA, Koenen F, Mittelhozer C. 1999. Classical swine fever virus is genetically stable in vitro and in vivo. Arch Virol 144:1669–1677.

Vannier P, Leforban Y, Carnero R, Cariolet R. 1988. Contamination of a live virus vaccine against pseudorabies (Aujeszky's disease) by an ovine pestivirus pathogen for the pig. Ann Rech Vet 19:283–290.

Vannier P, Plateau E, Tillon JP. 1981. Congenital tremor in pigs farrowed from sows given hog cholera virus during pregnancy. Am J Vet Res 42:135–137.

van Oirschot JT. 2003. Vaccinology of classical swine fever: From lab to field. Vet Microbiol 96:367–384.

van Oirschot JT, Terpstra C. 1977. A congenital persistent swine fever infection I. Clinical and virological observations. Vet Microbiol 2:121–132.

Vilcek S. 1997. Secondary structure of the 5'-noncoding region of border disease virus genome RNAs. Vet Med (Praha) 42:125–128.

Vilcek S, Herring AJ, Herring JA, Nettleton PF, Lowings JP, Paton DJ. 1994. Pestiviruses isolated from pigs, cattle and sheep can be allocated into at least three genogroups using polymerase chain reaction and restriction endonuclease analysis. Arch Virol 136:309–323.

Vilcek S, Stadejek T, Ballagi-Pordany A, Lowings JP, Paton DJ, Belak S. 1996. Genetic variability of classical swine fever virus. Virus Res 43:137–147.

Vlasova A, Grebennikova T, Zaberezhny A, Greiser-Wilke I, Floegel-Niesmann G, Kurinnov V, Aliper T, Nepoklonov E. 2003. Molecular epidemiology of classical swine fever in the Russian Federation. J Vet Med B Infect Dis Vet Public Health 50:363–367.

Wensvoort G. 1989. Topographical and functional mapping of epitopes on hog cholera virus with monoclonal antibodies. J Gen Virol 70:2865–2876.

Wensvoort G, Terpstra C. 1988. Bovine viral diarrhoea virus infections in piglets born to sows vaccinated against swine fever with contaminated vaccine. Res Vet Sci 45:143–148.

Wensvoort G, Terpstra C, de Kluijver EP, Kragten C, Warnaar JC. 1989. Antigenic differentiation of pestivirus strains with monoclonal antibodies against hog cholera virus. Vet Microbiol 21:9–20.

Wise GH. 1981. Hog cholera and its eradication. A review of the U.S. experience. Animal and Plant Health Inspection Service, United States Department of Agriculture, APHIS 91–55.

Wrathall AE, Bailey J, Done JT, Shaw IG, Winkler CE, Gibbons DF, Patterson DS, Sweasey D. 1978. Effects of experimental border disease infection in the pregnant sow. Zentralbl Veterinarmed B 25:62–69.

Zhang G, Flick-Smith H, McCauley JW. 2003. Differences in membrane association and sub-cellular distribution between NS2-3 and NS3 of bovine viral diarrhoea virus. Virus Res 97:89–102.

16 Porcine Cytomegalovirus

Kyoung-Jin Yoon and Neil Edington

Porcine cytomegalovirus (PCMV) infection was originally termed "inclusion body rhinitis" because basophilic intranuclear inclusions were seen in cytomegalic cells in the turbinate mucosa of pigs with rhinitis (Done 1955). Electron microscopy demonstrated herpes virions in turbinate mucous glands, lachrymal glands, salivary glands, and renal tubular epithelium (Duncan et al. 1964). The virus grew slowly in cell culture and produced cytomegaly with intranuclear inclusions (Booth et al. 1967; L'Ecuyer and Corner 1966), placing it in the cytomegalovirus group (Plummer 1973).

PCMV infection is usually subclinical in adults, but often produces a fatal, generalized infection in young swine, particularly piglets infected congenitally or perinatally (Edington et al. 1976a). In susceptible herds, the virus causes fetal and piglet deaths, runting, rhinitis, and pneumonia (Cameron-Stephen 1961; Corner et al. 1964; Duncan et al. 1964; Edington et al. 1977; L'Ecuyer et al. 1972; Orr et al. 1988; Rac 1961; Smith 1997; Yoon et al. 1996). The virus may also cause neurologic disease (Stephano-Hornedo and Edington 1987).

The potential for using live porcine cells, tissues, and organs in humans (xenotransplantation) has heightened interest in PCMV. PCMV is ubiquitous in swine, induces latent infections, and is similar to human and primate CMVs (Garkavenko et al. 2004; Tucker et al. 1999). Cross-species transmission of PCMV was reported in pig-to-primate xenotransplantation (Mueller et al. 2002), but the actual risk of PCMV infection in a human recipient remains unknown.

ETIOLOGY

PCMV (suid herpesvirus 2) is classified in the genus *Cytomegalovirus* in the subfamily *Betaherpesvirinae* of family *Herpesviridae* (Roizman 1982). The PCMV genome is linear, double-stranded, DNA of 130–150 $\times$ 10^6 kilodaltons. Full-length sequences and details of the organization of the viral genome are still lacking. Recent molecular studies of the polymerase, putative glycoprotein B (gB), and major nucleocapsid protein genes indicate that PCMV is genetically closer to human herpesvirus type 6 and 7 (genus *Roseolovirus*) than cytomegaloviruses (Rupasinghe et al. 1999, 2001; Widen et al. 1999, 2001).

The morphology of PCMV is typical of a herpes virion (Duncan et al. 1965; Shirai et al. 1985; Valiček and Smid 1979). The virion is approximately 150–200 nm across. It contains an electron-dense core (30–70 nm) of variable shape surrounded by capsid proteins forming the icosahedral nucleocapsid (80–120 nm). Viral nucleocapsids are present in the nucleus of host cells and acquire an electron-dense coat separated by a translucent halo from the envelope. The envelope is obtained by budding through the membrane of the host cell nucleus or Golgi apparatus. The envelope of extracellular and cytoplasmic virions has 10 nm external projections. The density of the PCMV virion is 1.275 g/ml by CsCl equilibrium-density centrifugation (Shirai et al. 1985).

No distinct PCMV serotypes or genotypes have been identified, although some degree of genetic variation was noted in polymerase and gB genes among PCMV isolates of different geographic origins (Goltz et al. 2000; Widen et al. 2001). Possible antigenic variability has also been reported (Tajima and Kawamura 1998).

The virus is sensitive to chloroform and ether (Booth et al. 1967). Virus infectivity is preserved at subzero temperatures (Booth et al. 1967).

L'Ecuyer and Corner (1966) propagated PCMV in primary pig lung (PL) cells for several passages, and Watt et al. (1973) found that only pig lung macrophages (PLM) were highly sensitive for primary isolation and/or serial propagation. Other culture systems used include primary swine testicle (ST) (Shirai et al. 1985; Kanitz and Woodruff 1976), a porcine fallopian tube (PFT) cell line (Bouillant et al. 1975; Kawamura et al. 1992), PK-15 cell line (Kanitz and Thacker 1974), and porcine turbinate (PT) (Yoon et al. 1996).

Cytomegaly and basophilic intranuclear and, occasionally, small acidophilic intracytoplasmic inclusions

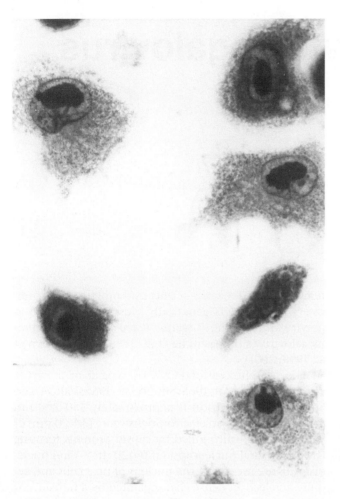

16.1. *Cultured pig macrophages 11 days after infection with PCMV. The basophilic Intranuclear inclusions stand out clearly in the enlarged cells (May-Grünwald-Giemsa; ×720). (Courtesy R.G. Watt.)*

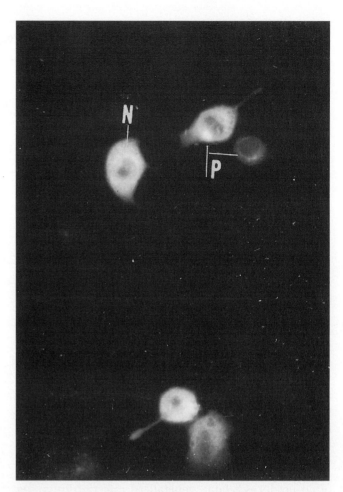

16.2. *Lung macrophage cultures showing fluorescence after IIF, using specific PCMV antiserum. The nuclear staining (N) is most intense at the membrane. Cytoplasmic and discrete paranuclear fluorescence P) can also be seen (×480).*

(Figure 16.1) are generally seen in infected cells at 3–14 days postinoculation (Watt et al. 1973). Infected cells are about six times larger than normal cells, with swelling of the mitochondria, endoplasmic reticulum, and Golgi apparatus (Duncan et al. 1965).

Progeny virus reaches a maximum titer of up to 10^{5-6} $TICD_{50}$ per ml at 10–14 days. Progeny virus yield in cell lines is lower than in primary systems. The absence of lytic cytopathic effect in cell culture requires immuno- or histochemical staining for confirmation of virus growth (Figure 16.2).

EPIDEMIOLOGY

PCMV is found throughout the world (Corner et al. 1964) and infection is ubiquitous, with herd prevalence greater than 90% in Europe, North America, and Japan. Within infected herds, more than 98% of pigs may be seropositive (Goltz et al. 2000; Hamel et al. 1999; Kanitz and Woodruff 1976; Rondhuis et al. 1980; Tajima et al. 1993).

PCMV is transmitted horizontally via the oronasal route, but congenital transmission is well documented (Edington et al. 1977, 1988b; L'Ecuyer et al. 1972). Infection most commonly occurs perinatally or early postnatally in commercial farms (Plowright et al. 1976; Watt 1978).

PCMV can be recovered from nasal and ocular discharge, urine, and cervical fluid (Booth et al. 1967; Edington et al. 1976a–c, 1977). Nasal excretion was demonstrated in gnotobiotic pigs for up to 1 month when exposed at 1 day of age, but for shorter periods (up to 9 days) in older pigs under the same conditions. In the field, the majority of pigs shed PCMV in nasally secretion between 3 and 8 weeks of age (Plowright et al. 1976).

Boars can be infected without apparent clinical signs and Shirai et al. (1985) were able to isolate PCMV from the testis and epididymis. Semen shedding of virus has not been determined.

Typical of herpesviruses, PCMV is able to establish latent infections that can be reactivated and result in virus shedding (Edington et al. 1976c; Narita et al. 1985).

Non-porcine reservoirs and arthropod vectors have not been reported and PCMV infection is considered limited to pigs. The virus does not replicate in mice, rabbits, dogs, cattle, and chicken embryos. However, Mueller et al. (2002) detected virus replication in tissues of baboons that received xenografts of pig origin.

The stability and persistence of PCMV in the environment is unknown. The efficacy of specific disinfectants against PCMV has not been described.

PATHOGENESIS

The primary replication site of PCMV is the nasal mucosa and/or the lachrymal or harderian glands. Cell-associated viremia follows primary replication 14–21 days post infection in animals greater than 3 weeks of age and 5–19 days post infection in neonatal gnotobiotic pigs (Edington et al. 1976c; Edington et al. 1977). Following viremia, virus is shed in nasal, pharyngeal and/or conjunctival secretions, and urine (Booth et al. 1967; Edington et al. 1976c, 1977). Nasal excretion of virus lasts from 10 to over 30 days. Congenitally infected pigs excrete virus until death (Edington et al. 1977).

In sows experimentally infected with PCMV at mid- to late-gestation, the virus was also isolated from cervical fluids, but later than nasal excretion (30–35 days post infection). Neither virus nor inclusions were detected in the cervix or endometrium at this stage, which suggested that cervical shedding was of fetal origin. Excretion in cervical fluids coincided with fetal deaths, implying that the virus required an additional 14–20 days to replicate in the fetus.

The site of secondary viral replication varies with age. In nursery or growing pigs (Edington et al. 1976a, 1977; Kelly 1967; Plowright et al. 1976; Shirai et al. 1985), the virus disseminates predominantly to epithelial sites, particularly the nasal mucosal glands, harderian and lachrymal glands, kidney tubules, and more rarely, the epididymis and mucous glands of the esophagus. Hepatocytes and duodenal epithelium are even more rarely infected.

In the fetus or neonate, there is a predilection for infection of reticuloendothelial cells, particularly capillary endothelium and the sinusoids of lymphoid tissues, thus resulting in generalized lesions (Edington et al. 1977, 1988a). When fetuses were exposed at early gestation, PCMV preferentially replicated in the meninges, Küpffer cells, peritoneal macrophages, and periosteal cells (Edington et al. 1988b). Embryos can be infected shortly after implantation, resulting in embryonic deaths.

Infectious virus persists in lung macrophages, blood monocytes, and CD8+ T cells (Edington et al. 1977; Guedes et al. 2004). Latent infection can be reactivated in vivo by administration of corticosteroids (Edington et al. 1976c; Narita et al. 1985) or in vitro by allogeneic co-cultivation (Guedes et al. 2004).

CLINICAL SIGNS

Uncomplicated infection is usually subclinical in pigs older than 3 weeks, but can be fatal for the fetus or newborn pig. Affected pigs show respiratory signs, e.g., sneezing, nasal discharge, and coughing, and develop rhinitis or neurological disease (Cameron-Stephen 1961; Corner et al. 1964; Done 1955; Duncan et al. 1964; Orr et al. 1988; Rac 1961). PCMV infection does not induce atrophic rhinitis (Rondhuis et al. 1980).

Reproductive problems are another feature of PCMV infection in susceptible herds (Edington et al. 1977, 1988b; L'Ecuyer et al. 1972; Smith 1997; Yoon et al. 1996).

The incubation period of the infection may be 10–20 days (Edington et al. 1977; Goodwin and Whittlestone 1967). During the short viremic phase, animals become lethargic and anorexic, but not febrile. Some congenitally or neonatally infected piglets die without any overt clinical signs. Others often exhibit shivering, sneezing, and respiratory distress, poor weight gain, and rhinitis. The disease is generally self-limiting if uncomplicated. Morbidity is 100%; the average mortality in a naive herd is about 10%, but can rise to 50%.

At farrowing, increased numbers of mummified fetuses and stillbirths are observed, although infected sows may not show any clinical abnormality throughout gestation except lethargy and anorexia. Preweaning mortality also increases. Up to 25% of the litter may be lost and the remainder may show runting. Piglets may be grossly pale and show a variable edema, often around the jaw and tarsal joints.

Although early field observations suggested that the concurrent infection of PCMV and *Bordetella bronchiseptica* might exacerbate the severity of atrophic rhinitis (Cameron-Stephen 1961; Corner et al. 1964), a synergistic effect was not reproducible under experimental conditions (Edington et al. 1976b). Concurrent infection and possible synergism with other agents has not been investigated. However, a field-based, case-control study suggested that PCMV-infected pigs were at a higher risk for respiratory disease than PCMV-uninfected pigs (Yoon et al. 1998).

LESIONS

It is useful to distinguish between disseminated infection of epithelial tissues in the older pigs and generalized infection of reticuloendothelial tissues in the fetus or neonate (Edington et al 1976a).

Epithelial Lesions

No macroscopic changes are seen in epithelial tissues. Microscopically, basophilic intranuclear inclusion bodies and cytomegaly are seen in the nasal mucous glands (Figure 16.3), acinar and duct epithelium of harderian and lachrymal glands, and renal tubular epithelium. In these tissues, the proportion of affected cells may be

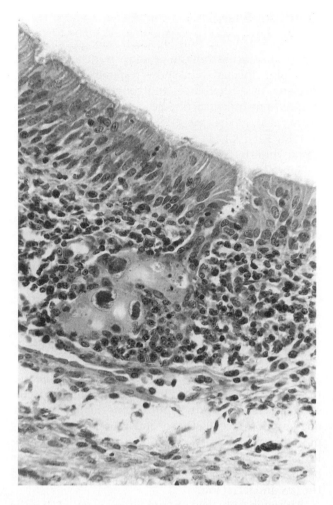

16.3.   *The basophilic intranuclear inclusion, translucent halo, and defined nuclear membrane are prominent in the enlarged superficial mucous gland epithelium of an animal 18 days after experimental intranasal inoculation (H&E; ×480).*

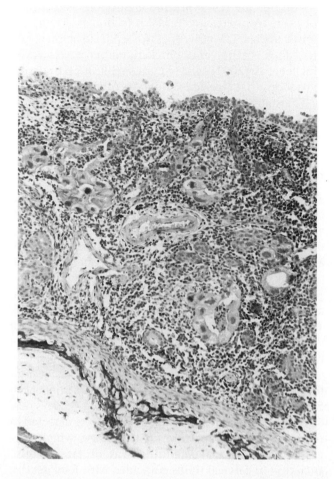

16.4.   *The lamina propria is heavily infiltrated with lymphocytes and plasma cell 24 days after inoculation of PCMV. Many of the acini of the mucous glands still show cytomegaly and prominent inclusion bodies (H&E; ×120).*

high. Isolated inclusions are occasionally seen in the mucous glands of the esophagus, the epithelial lining of the ductus epididymis and the seminiferous epithelium, as well as the epithelial lining of the duodenum and jejunum. The major sites of replication develop focal lymphoid hyperplasia (Figure 16.4). The reparative lesions in the kidney are those of an interstitial nephritis (Kelly 1967). Sparsely distributed focal gliosis is seen in the central nervous system, with inclusions occasionally seen in the glial cells.

Generalized Lesions

In young pigs, petechiae and edema are widespread. Subcutaneous edema is most marked around the throat and tarsal joints. Edema most commonly involves the thoracic cavity and subcutaneous tissues. In the thorax, pericardial and pleural effusions are present. Lungs are edematous, with the interlobular septa becoming distended and the ventral tips of the lobes appearing purple and consolidated (Figure 16.5). The lymph nodes are all

enlarged and edematous, and petechial hemorrhages are observed. Petechiae are most extensive in the kidneys, particularly subcapsular, the appearance varying from speckling to completely purple or black coloration.

In some fetal infections, only reproductive failure, i.e., stillbirths, mummified fetuses, embryonic death, and infertility, is seen. The mummified fetuses are randomly distributed and sometimes of variable age. In the acute fatal syndrome, most inclusions are seen in the capillary endothelial and sinusoidal cells, and thus occur in all lymphoid and parenchymatous tissues. The damaged endothelium is associated with local edema and/or hemorrhage and with macrophages and erythrocytes in the distended extracellular space. Mononuclear cells with inclusions are found in blood vessels and also in the spleen. Infected macrophages are prevalent in alveolar tissues. Replication in hepatocytes results in focal necrosis. In the kidney, inclusions are most common in areas of differentiating renal tissue and in glomerular capillary endothelium (Figure 16.6). Hemor-

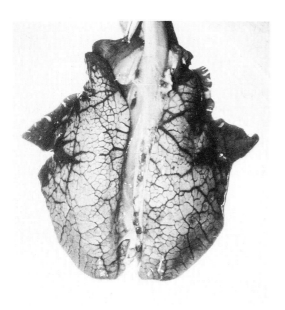

16.5. *This pig was inoculated with PCMV when 1 day old. It died at 16 days of age with widespread petechiae and subcutaneous edema. The interlobular septae of the lungs are distended with transudate, and the tips of the apical, cardiac, and diaphragmatic lobes are also consolidated.*

rhage and gliosis occur throughout the central nervous system, with a predilection for the choroid plexus, cerebellum, and olfactory lobes (Stephano-Horendo and Edington 1987).

IMMUNITY

Experimentally, antibody is detected by the indirect immunofluorescent antibody (IFA) test 2–3 weeks after in-

oculation, peaks at around 6 weeks postinoculation, and remains at high levels for at least 10–11 weeks postinoculation (Edington et al. 1976c, 1977). Development of serum antibody levels detectable by IFA coincides with the disappearance of viremia, but nasal excretion of virus continues for another 2–3 weeks. Longer periods of excretion have been associated with lower levels of antibody (Edington et al. 1988b). A similar pattern of antibody response was seen in commercial farms (Plowright et al. 1976), with antibody persisting until animals were marketed at 23 weeks of age. Neutralizing antibody develops, but very slowly and to very low levels.

Edington et al. (1988a) demonstrated that transplacental infection could be established by superinfection of sows only with low levels of IFA antibody, which suggests that high levels of IFA antibody are indicative of protective immunity.

Piglets with congenital and neonatal infection do not seroconvert, but excrete virus and develop fatal, systemic infections (Edington et al. 1977). Piglets acquire maternal antibodies and these provide some protection, but virus is shed even in the presence of circulating maternal antibody in PCMV-endemic farms (Plowright et al. 1976). Maternal antibody lasts approximately 2 months after birth (Tajima et al. 1994).

No information is available on important aspects of immunity, e.g., cross-protection among isolates or cell-mediated immune responses.

DIAGNOSIS

PCMV-associated respiratory or reproductive diseases must be differentiated from infection with classical swine fever virus, enterovirus, parvovirus, porcine re-

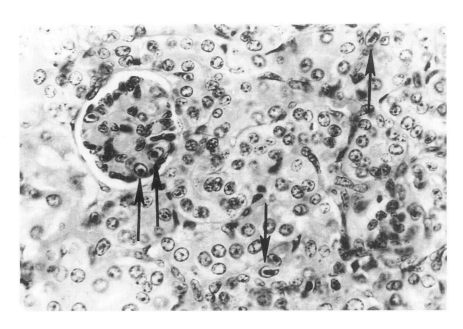

16.6. *Section of kidney from a piglet with viral inclusions (arrows) in capillary endothelium in both the glomerulus and interstitial tissue. Infected cells show enlargement but only reach the size of normal tubular epithelium (H&E; ×240).*

productive and respiratory syndrome (PRRS) virus, and Aujeszky's disease (pseudorabies) virus. Inclusion body rhinitis (IBR) is typically limited to piglets. The initial signs of IBR are sneezing, with nasal discharge in a small number of pigs, which progresses to infrequent coughing. Sometimes a ring of black discoloration can be observed around the eyes due to excessive conjunctival discharge. Clinically affected sows produce smaller litters that may include mummified fetuses and stillborns. Congenitally or perinatally infected piglets present macroscopic lesions of widespread petechiae and edema. No macroscopic changes are seen in older pigs.

Virus isolation or detection must be done to include PCMV as a component of rhinitis. Qualitative or quantitative PCR-based assays for detection of viral DNA can be substituted for virus isolation in clinical cases (Fryer et al. 2001; Hamel et al. 1999; Widen et al. 1999). Antemortem samples of choice are nasal secretion or scrapings and whole blood (Edington et al. 1976a; Watt et al. 1973). Preferred postmortem samples are turbinate mucosa, lung, lung lavage, and kidney (Edington et al. 1976c; Watt 1978). In cases of early reproductive failure, PCMV can occasionally be demonstrated in the brain, liver, and bone marrow of fetuses (Edington et al. 1977, 1988a, 1988b).

Virus isolation can be done on primary or line cells, as previously described. The isolation rate can be increased by incorporating a centrifugal technique into the sample inoculation procedure (Yoon et al. 1998). Kawamura and Matsuzaki (1996) reported that 12-O-tetradecanoylophobol 12-acetate accelerated viral replication in a porcine fallopian tube cell line.

If the carcass is kept chilled, viral antigen can be detected by immunostaining on frozen tissue sections at least 24 hours after virus infectivity has disappeared. Alternatively, pathognomonic inclusions and cytomegaly may be detected in histologic sections.

The presence of PCMV in a herd is most easily confirmed by serology using serum samples from randomly selected grower-finishers. An IFA test on infected PLM, ST, PK-15, or PT cells fixed in acetone has been described (Plowright et al. 1976; Kanitz and Thacker 1974; Kanitz and Woodruff 1976). IFA titers of 1:64 to 1:128 are frequently observed in commercial pigs and occasionally reach titers of 1:1024. Enzyme-linked immunosorbent assays (ELISA) have been described (Assaf et al. 1982; Tajima et al. 1993) and adapted to distinguish IgG and IgM responses (Tajima et al. 1994). It should be noted that no PCMV antibodies are induced by in utero infection. Therefore, antibody is not expected in colostrum-deprived neonatal sera.

PREVENTION AND CONTROL

No PCMV vaccine or specific treatment for PCMV is available. Some antiviral nucleoside analogues, such as ganciclovir, have been shown to inhibit PCMV replica-

tion in vitro in a dose-dependent fashion (Fryer et al 2004; Mueller et al. 2003), but the therapeutic efficacy of these drugs remains to be assessed. No therapeutic efficacy for PCMV was achieved using 6-azauridine and 5-iododeoxyuridine (Steffenhagen et al. 1976). Medication to minimize secondary problems due to concurrent or secondary bacterial infections may be beneficial (Cameron-Stephen 1961; Corner et al. 1964).

Introduction of new stock into herds is a risk since it may stimulate latent infection or give rise to the problems of primary infection in susceptible herds.

A virus-free herd may be established by hysterotomy (Clark et al. 2003). The potential for PCVM transplacental infection should be taken into consideration and monitored.

REFERENCES

Assaf R, Bouillant AM, Di Franco E. 1982. Enzyme-linked immunoassay (ELISA) for the detection of antibodies to porcine cytomegalovirus. Can J Comp Med 46:183–185.
Booth JC, Goodwin REW, Whittlestone P. 1967. Inclusion-body rhinitis of pigs: Attempts to grow the causal agent in tissue cultures. Res Vet Sci 8:338–345.
Bouillant AMP, Dulac G, Willis N, Girard A, Greig AS, Boulanchier P. 1975. Viral susceptibility of a cell line derived from the pig oviduct. Can J Comp Med 39:450–456.
Cameron-Stephen ID. 1961. Inclusion-body rhinitis of swine. Aust Vet J 37:87–91.
Clark DA, Fryer JF, Tucker AW, McArdle PD, Hughes AE, Emery VC, Griffiths PD. 2003. Porcine cytomegalovirus in pigs being bred for xenograft organs: Progress towards control. Xenotransplantation 10:142–148.
Corner AH, Mitchell D, Julian RJ, Meads EB. 1964. A generalized disease in piglets associated with the presence of cytomegalic inclusions. J Comp Path 74:192–199.
Done JT. 1955. An "inclusion body" rhinitis of pigs. Vet Rec 67:525–527.
Duncan JR, Ramsey EK, Switzer WP. 1965. Electron microscopy of cytomegalic inclusion disease of swine (inclusion body rhinitis). Am J Vet Res 29:939–946.
Duncan JR, Ross RF, Switzer WP. 1964. Incidence of inclusion-body rhinitis in Iowa swine. J Am Vet Med Assoc 144:33–37.
Edington N, Broad SC, Wrathall AE, Done JT. 1988a. Superinfection with PCMV initiating transplacental infection. Vet Microbiol 16:189–193.
Edington N, Plowright W, Watt RG. 1976a. Generalised cytomegalic inclusion disease: Distribution of cytomegalic cells and virus. J Comp Pathol 86:191–202.
Edington N, Smith IM, Plowright W, Watt RG. 1976b. Relationship of porcine cytomegalovirus and B. bronchiseptica to atrophic rhinitis in gnotobiotic piglets. Vet Res 98:42–45.
Edington N, Watt RG, Plowright W. 1976c. Cytomegalovirus excretion in gnotobiotic pigs. J Hyg (Camb) 77:283–290.
Edington N, Watt RG, Plowright W, Wrathall AE, Done JT. 1977. Experimental transmission of porcine cytomegalovirus. J Hyg (Camb) 78:243–251.
Edington N, Wrathal AE, Done JT. 1988b. Porcine cytomegalovirus in early gestation. Vet Microbiol 17:117–128.
Fryer JF, Griffiths PD, Emery VC, Clark DA. 2004. Susceptibility of porcine cytomegalovirus to antiviral drugs. J Antimicrob Chemother 53:975–980.
Fryer JF, Griffiths PD, Fishman JA, Emery VC, Clark DA. 2001. Quantitation of porcine cytomegalovirus in pig tissues by PCR. J Clin Microbiol 39:1155–1556.

Garkavenko O, Muzina M, Muzina Z, Powels K, Elliott RB, Croxson MC. 2004. Monitoring for potentially xenozoonotic viruses in New Zealand pigs. J Med Virol 72:338–344.

Goltz M, Widen F, Banks M, Belak S, Ehlers B. 2000. Characterization of the DNA polymerase loci of porcine cytomegaloviruses from diverse geographic origins. Virus Genes 21: 249–255.

Goodwin RF, Whittlestone P. 1967. Inclusion-body rhinitis of pigs: An experimental study of some factors that affect the incidence of inclusion bodies in the nasal mucosa. Res Vet Sci 8:346–352.

Guedes MI, Risdahl JM, Wiseman B, Molitor TW. 2004. Reactivation of porcine cytomegalovirus through allogeneic stimulation. J Clin Microbiol 42:1756–1758.

Hamel AL, Lin L, Sachvie C, Grudeski E, Nayar GP. 1999. PCR assay for detecting porcine cytomegalovirus. J Clin Microbiol 37:3767–3768.

Kanitz CL, Thacker HL. 1974. Tissue culture-indirect fluorescent antibody test for porcine cytomegalalic inclusion disease. Lab Invest 30:399–400.

Kanitz CL, Woodruff ME. 1976. Cell-culture-indirect fluorescent antibody studies of porcine cytomegalovirus. Proc Congr Int Pig Vet Soc, p. 9.

Kawamura H, Matsuzaki S. 1996. Influence of 12-O-tetradecanoyl-phorbol 13-acetate on replication of porcine cytomegalovirus in the 19PFT cell line. J Vet Med Sci 58:263–265.

Kawamura H, Tajima T, Hironao T, Kajikawa T, Kotani T. 1992. Replication of porcine cytomegalovirus in the 19-PFT cell line. Vet Med Sci 54:1209–1211.

Kelly DE. 1967. Pathology of extranasal lesions in experimental inclusion body rhinitis of pigs. Res Vet Sci 8:472–478.

L'Ecuyer C, Corner AH. 1966. Propagation of porcine cytomegalovirus inclusion disease virus in cell cultures: Preliminary report. Can J Comp Med Vet Sci 30:321–326.

L'Ecuyer C, Corner AH, Randall GCB. 1972. Porcine cytomegalic inclusion disease: Transplacental transmission. Proc Congr Int Pig Vet Soc 2:99.

Mueller NJ, Barth RN, Yamamoto S, Kitamura H, Patience C, Yamada K, Cooper DK, Sachs DH, Kaur A, Fishman JA. 2002. Activation of cytomegalovirus in pig-to-primate organ xenotransplantation. J Virol 76:4734–4740.

Mueller NJ, Sulling K, Gollackner B, Yamamoto S, Knosalla C, Wilkinson RA, Kaur A, Sachs DH, Yamada K, Cooper DK, Patience C, Fishman JA. 2003. Reduced efficacy of ganciclovir against porcine and baboon cytomegalovirus in pig-to-baboon xenotransplantation. Am J Transplant 3:1057–1064.

Narita M, Shimizu M, Kawanuru H, Haritari M, Moriwaki M. 1985. Pathologic changes in pigs with prednisolone induced recrudescence of herpesvirus infection. Am J Vet Res 46:1506–1510.

Orr JP, Althouse E, Dulac GC, Durham JPK. 1988. Epizootic infection of a minimal disease swine herd with a herpesvirus. Can Vet J 29:45–50.

Plowright W, Edington N, Watt RG. 1976. The behavior of porcine cytomegalovirus in commercial pig herds. J Hyg (Camb) 75:125–135.

Plummer G. 1973. Cytomegaloviruses of man and animals. Prog Med Virol 15:92–125.

Rac R. 1961. Infectious rhinitis in pigs: Laboratory aspects. Aust Vet J 37:91–93.

Roizman B. 1982. The family Herpesviridae: General description, taxonomy, and classification. In The Herpesviruses (Vol. I). B Roizman,ed. New York: Plenum Press, pp. 1–23.

Rondhuis PR, de Jong MF, Schep J. 1980. Indirect fluorescence antibody studies of porcine cytomegalovirus infections in the Netherlands. Tijdschr Diergeneeskd 105 (suppl 2):56–68.

Rupasinghe V, Iwatsuki-Horimoto K, Sugii S, Horimoto T. 2001. Identification of the porcine cytomegalovirus major capsid protein gene. J Vet Med Sci 63:609–618.

Rupasinghe V, Tajima T, Maeda K, Iwatsuki-Horimoto K, Sugii S, Horimoto T. 1999. Analysis of porcine cytomegalovirus DNA polymerase by consensus primer PCR. J Vet Med Sci 61:1253–1255.

Shirai J, Narita M, Iijima Y. 1985. A cytomegalovirus isolation from swine testicle culture. Jpn J Vet Sci 47:697–703.

Smith KC. 1997. Herpesviral abortion in domestic animals. Vet J 153:253–268.

Steffenhagen KA, Easterday BC, Galasso GJ. 1976. Evaluation of 6-azauridine and 5-iododeoxyuridine in the treatment of experimental viral infections. J Infect Dis 133:603–612.

Stephano-Hornedo A, Edington N. 1987. Encefalitis experimental por cytomegalovirus porcino en credos gnotobioticos: Estudio histopatologica. Vet Mex 18:189–202.

Tajima T, Hironao T, Kajikawa T, Kawamura H. 1993. Application of ELISA for the seroepizootiological survey of antibodies against porcine cytomegalovirus. J Vet Med Sci 55:421–424.

Tajima T, Hironao T, Kajikawa T, Suzuki Y, Kawamura H. 1994. Detection of the antibodies against porcine cytomegalovirus from whole blood collected on the blood sampling paper. J Vet Med Sci 56:189–190.

Tajima T, Kawamura H. 1998. Serological relationship among porcine cytomegalovirus Japanese isolates and a UK isolate. J Vet Med Sci 60:107–109.

Tucker AW, Galbraith D, McEwan P, Onions D. 1999. Evaluation of porcine cytomegalovirus as a potential zoonotic agent in xenotransplantation. Transplant Proc 31:915.

Valiček L, Smid B. 1979. Electron microscopy of porcine cytomegalovirus in pig lung macrophage cultures. Zentralbl Veterinarmed [B] 26:371–381.

Watt RG. 1978. Virological study or two commercial pig herds with respiratory disease. Res Vet Sci 24:147–153.

Watt RG, Plowright W, Sabo A, Edington N. 1973. A sensitive cell culture system for the virus of porcine inclusion body rhinitis (cytomegalic inclusion disease). Res Vet Sci 14:119–121.

Widen F, Goltz M, Wittenbrink N, Ehlers B, Banks M, Belak S. 2001. Identification and sequence analysis of the glycoprotein B gene of porcine cytomegalovirus. Virus Genes 23:339–346.

Widen BF, Lowings JP, Belak S, Banks M. 1999. Development of a PCR system for porcine cytomegalovirus detection and determination of the putative partial sequence of its DNA polymerase gene. Epidemiol Infect 123:177–180.

Yoon K-J, Anderson MS, Zimmerman JJ. 1998. Assessing the significance of porcine cytomegalovirus in respiratory disease of young swine. Proc Congr Int Pig Vet Soc 2:173.

Yoon K-J, Henry SC, Zimmerman JJ, Platt KB. 1996. Isolation of porcine cytomegalovirus (PCMV) from a swine herd with concurrent infection of PRRS virus. Vet Med 91:779–784.

17 Encephalomyocarditis Virus

Frank Koenen

EMCV is noteworthy for its widespread geographic distribution and the large number of species susceptible to EMCV infection. Encephalomyocarditis virus (EMCV) was first isolated from rodents in 1940 (Jungeblut and Sanders 1940). EMCV was later isolated from a chimpanzee in Florida with myocarditis (Helwig and Schmidt 1945). Thereafter, antibodies or virus were detected in a variety of animal species (Tesh and Wallace 1977).

Murnane et al. (1960) isolated EMCV from the lung and spleen of a pig that had abruptly collapsed and died during an outbreak of acute disease in Panama in 1958. This was the first recognition of EMCV as a swine pathogen. In pigs, disease due to the EMCV may take one of two main forms: acute myocarditis, usually causing sudden death in young pigs, and/or reproductive failure in sows.

Even without surveillance mechanisms to track EMCV infections actively, outbreaks in pigs have been reported throughout the world. Several major outbreaks with high mortality have been reported in Australia since 1970 (Acland and Littlejohns 1975; Seaman et al. 1986). Outbreaks have also been reported in South Africa (Williams 1981), New Zealand (Sutherland et al. 1977), Cuba (Ramos et al. 1983), and Canada (Dea et al. 1991). In Europe, clinical disease caused by EMCV was first observed in domestic pigs in 1986 and with greater frequency thereafter. Outbreaks of acute myocarditis have been reported in Italy (Sidoli et al. 1988), Greece (Paschaleri-Papadopoulou et al. 1990), Switzerland (Hani et al. 1992), Belgium (Koenen et al. 1999), and Cyprus (Loukaidis et al. 1996). In Belgium, EMCV has also been frequently isolated from cases of reproductive failure (Koenen et al. 1999).

Infection with EMCV is not uncommon, but clinical disease is infrequent. EMCV outbreaks are often clustered in so-called "endemic areas" (Maurice et al. 2004a). In Italy, 50% of farms without clinical signs in an endemic area had seroprevalence levels similar to farms with clinical EMCV, providing evidence of considerable subclinical infections (Maurice et al. 2004a).

Likewise, in the United Kingdom, antibodies against EMCV were detected, but without isolation of virus (Sangar et al. 1977).

ETIOLOGY

EMCV is an RNA virus in the genus *Cardiovirus* of the family *Picornaviridae*. Several antigenically similar viruses, including Columbia-SK and Mengo viruses, were isolated during the 1940s and are considered to be in the same group as EMCV. Tinsley et al. (1984) reported EMCV to be antigenically related to the cricket paralysis virus.

EMCV virions contain single-stranded RNA of 2.6×10^6 daltons. The viral genome encodes a leader protein that lacks proteolytic activity. The leader protein is cleaved from P1 by the virus-encoded protease 3Cpro. The 1D/2A junction is also cleaved by 3Cpro rather than by 2A. The 2A protein causes cleavage, or polypeptide chain interruption, between P1-2A and downstream sequences at an essential sequence, -NPGP-. EMCV has a poly (C) tract of variable length (usually 80–250 nucleotides) (van Regenmortel et al. 2000).

Although antigenically stabile (Meroni et al. 2000), the D region of EMCV (coding for the capsid protein VP1) displays considerable genetic variability. A single nucleotide mutation can be involved in attenuation or conferring diabetogenicity to a particular EMCV strain (Nelsen-Salz et al. 1996). In particular, isolates from Greece differed from other isolates (Knowles et al. 2000). Limited variability between pig- and rodent-derived EMCV isolates was observed.

EMCV shares many properties with other picornaviruses. It is ether-resistant and stable over a wide pH range. It is inactivated after 30 minutes at 60°C, but some strains have shown a marked thermal stability (Joo 1999).

EMCV replicates well in cell cultures originating from several animal species, including rodents, swine, and primates. Baby hamster kidney (BHK-21) and Vero

331

cells are most commonly used for virus propagation. The virus also replicates in mice and chicken embryos and is pathogenic to many laboratory animals.

The virus hemagglutinates guinea pig, rat, horse, and sheep erythrocytes. Most EMCV strains require KCl-borate (0.12M KCl; 0.05 H_3BO_3) buffered solution for optimal hemagglutination. Some differences in hemagglutinating activity between EMCV strains have been reported (Kim et al. 1991). Serial passage of EMCV in cell culture can alter in vitro growth characteristics, reduce virulence, and affect hemagglutinating activity (Zimmerman 1994).

EPIDEMIOLOGY

EMCV is generally regarded as a virus of rodents, although EMCV has been isolated from over 30 species, including mammals, birds, and insects. In mammals, the host range includes rodents, monkeys (even chimpanzees), elephants, lions, squirrels, mongooses, raccoons, and swine. In some species, EMCV infection may have serious consequences, e.g., lion deaths at a zoo resulted from their feeding on the carcasses of African elephants that had died of EMCV infection (Simpson et al. 1977).

Transmission of EMCV in swine has been poorly described, but rodents are generally believed to serve as a reservoir and as the means of introduction and subsequent spread of the EMCV in pig facilities. The virus usually persists in rodents without causing disease (Acland 1989; Zimmerman 1994) and infected rodents have high levels of EMCV in their tissues and excrete virus in feces and urine. Thus, exposure of swine to EMCV-contaminated feed or water or infected rodent carcasses is considered important in transmission (Acland 1989; Seaman et al. 1986; Spyrou et al. 2004; Tesh and Wallace 1977).

These assumptions were supported by the results of a matched case-control study of an area of Belgium where clinical EMCV outbreaks were regularly reported (Maurice et al. 2005b). At the univariate level, the analyses indicated that rodents, the general farm setup, and general level of hygiene were associated with clinical EMCV. Multivariate relationships between clinical EMCV and potential risk factors were analyzed using conditional logistic regression, and the presence of mice was the most significant risk factor for clinical EMCV infections.

Infected pigs can excrete the virus, at least for a short period of time, and pig-to-pig contacts or contact with infected dead pigs are potential mechanisms of virus spread (Billinis et al. 1999; Foni et al. 1993; Maurice et al. 2002). Transplacental infection has also been described as a potential route of virus spread (Christianson et al. 1992; Koenen and Vanderhallen 1997; Links et al. 1986). Other factors, such as infectious dose, route of infection, and age of the pigs, have been found to be important in the spread of the virus under experimental conditions

(Billinis et al. 2004; Littlejohns and Acland 1975). In certain countries, a seasonal pattern in the outbreaks has been observed, with peaks during the autumn (Maurice et al. 2005a).

CLINICAL SIGNS

Pig age at the time of infection is an important determinate of clinical disease, with particularly severe disease if infected in the first weeks of life. Extremely high mortality, approaching 100%, is limited to pigs of preweaning age (Joo 1999). Infections in pigs from postweaning age to adulthood are usually subclinical, although some mortality may be observed even in adult pigs. Under experimental conditions, Billinis et al. (2004) found no difference in mortality between 20- and 40-day-old pigs, but none of the 105-day-old pigs died.

In young pigs, EMCV infection is most commonly characterized by acute disease with sudden death due to myocardial failure. Other clinical signs may be observed, including anorexia, listlessness, trembling, staggering, paralysis, or dyspnea. Experimentally infected swine (Craighead et al. 1963; Littlejohns and Acland 1975) had body temperatures of up to 41°C and died 2–11 days postinoculation (DPI) (usually 3–5 days) or, occasionally, recovered with chronic myocarditis.

In breeding females, clinical signs may vary from no obvious illness to various forms of reproductive failure, including abortion and increased numbers of mummified and stillborn fetuses (Dea et al. 1991; Koenen and Vanderhallen 1997).

Non-Porcine Species

Among laboratory animals, clinical manifestations and pathogenesis of EMCV are variable. Acute fatal disease is most often produced in mice and hamsters after inoculation by various routes. Neurologic disease due to encephalitis has been reported, but myocarditis is more frequently seen at necropsy. In mice, certain virus strains cause predominantly fatal encephalitis, or widespread myocardial damage, or specific destruction of pancreatic beta cells (Cerutis et al. 1989).

The course of the infection varies in rats, guinea pigs, rabbits, and monkeys, depending on the age of the animals and the virus strain used. In rats experimentally infected with a myocardial EMCV strain, no clinical signs or gross lesions were observed. Regardless, virus was isolated from several tissues from 3 DPI until the end of the observation at 62 DPI. EMCV was most frequently isolated from Peyer's patches and thymus, even in rats killed 60 DPI. The results suggested that these tissues represented a site of persistence after oral infection (Spyrou et al. 2004). Owls, monkeys, and marmosets were reportedly highly susceptible to infection. The virus has seldom been pathogenic for rabbits and rhesus monkeys, causing no apparent infections despite high levels of viremia.

PATHOGENESIS

Divergent reports regarding the clinical picture, in combination with evidence of subclinical infection, suggest that EMCV strains vary in pathogenicity. It is now recognized that some strains cause only reproductive failure or myocarditis, and others can cause both (Koenen and Vanderhallen 1997). Australian strains were shown to be more virulent than New Zealand strains (Littlejohns and Acland 1975; Horner and Hunter 1979), and certain isolates in Florida were found to cause only myocarditis without death (Gainer 1967; Gainer et al. 1968). Thus, the course of EMCV infection in pigs may be influenced by virus strain, virus dose, passage history, level of virus passage, and individual animal factors, e.g., age and pregnancy status.

Natural infection of swine is most likely to occur by the oral route. Following experimental oral inoculation of young pigs, virus was detected as early as 6 hours postinoculation in the intestinal tract. In heart and tonsils, focal positive reactions were found in the cytoplasm of single macrophages and myocardial cells during the first 30 hours postinoculation (acute phase). Thereafter, some animals died with typical postmortem lesions, and clear immunohistochemistry-positive reactions were observed in the tonsils and in the heart. Three days postinoculation, virus was isolated from liver, kidneys, spleen, and lungs. The persistence of virus beyond the viremic period suggests viral replication in the intestine. The highest virus titers were in heart muscle, both in experimental and natural infections. Myocardial lesions were predominant at necropsy. Animals that survived the infection produced EMCV antibodies. Virus detection decreased with the appearance of antibodies (Gelmetti et al. 2006).

The pathogenesis of transplacental EMCV infection in pregnant sows is not well understood. Following intramuscular exposure of pregnant sows with EMCV, transplacental infection and fetal death was observed as early as 2 weeks postinoculation. Early farrowing, abortion, and fetal mummification were observed in sows infected in mid- or late-gestation, and fetal infection in sows during early pregnancy was not conclusive (Koenen and Vanderhallen 1997; Love and Grewal 1986). Antibodies and virus were recovered from the fetuses, but the lesions varied from none to large diffuse patches, depending on the experiment (Kim et al. 1989b; Koenen and Vanderhallen 1997). Little pathogenicity was observed following infection of swine fetuses in utero with laboratory-passaged strains.

LESIONS

Pigs dying during the acute phase of cardiac failure may show only epicardial hemorrhage and no gross lesions. Hydropericardium, hydrothorax, and pulmonary edema are frequently observed at necropsy. The heart is usually enlarged, soft, and pale. The most striking lesions are found in the myocardium (Figures 17.1, 17.2). Multiple foci of various sizes are found, especially in the right ventricle, which may extend to varying depths within the myocardium. These foci are often ill-defined, circular or linear, and an uneven grayish-white in color. These lesions are observed more frequently in fattening pigs than in suckling piglets (Castryck et al. 1996; Littlejohns and Acland 1975).

Infected fetuses are most often apparently normal, but may be hemorrhagic and edematous. With some strains, fetuses may become mummified at various states of development, depending on the stage of infection. Visible myocardial lesions are exceptional.

Histopathologically, the most significant findings in young pigs are seen in the heart. Immunohistochem-

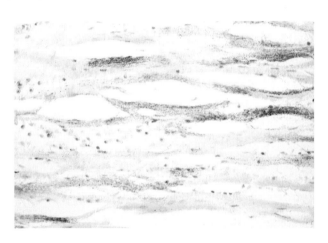

17.1. *Sagittal section of the heart of a pig with EMCV infection showing multiple foci of various sizes (especially in the right ventricle) extending to varying depths (Regional Animal Health Centre Flanders, Torhout, Belgium).*

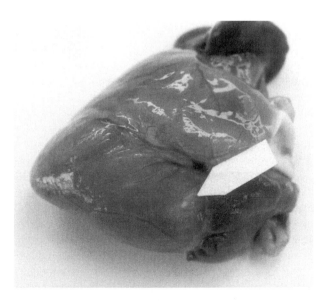

17.2. *Interstitial myocarditis and calcification in heart muscle fibers (Prof. Dr. R. Ducatelle, Faculty of Veterinary Medicine, University of Ghent, Belgium).*

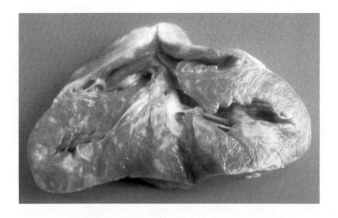

17.3. *Heart of a pig with EMCV infection showing typical white foci in myocardium (Regional Animal Health Centre Flanders, Torhout, Belgium).*

istry (IHC)-positive myocardial cells are seen, with the reaction primarily localized to the cytoplasm of myocardial cells as a fine and granular signal. The intensity and distribution of the reaction correlates with the severity of the lesions. Sometimes, IHC-positive reactions are detected in the Purkinje fibers and in the adjacent endothelial cells. Mineralization of necrotic heart muscle is common, but is not always present (Figure 17.3). In the tonsils, positive reactions are located in the necrotic debris filling the crypts and in the cytoplasm of monocyte-macrophage lineage cells. This last finding has also been reported in lymph nodes (Craighead et al. 1963; Gelmetti et al. 2006; Papaioannou et al. 2003; Psychas et al. 2001). Congestion with meningitis, perivascular infiltration with mononuclear cells, and some neural degeneration may be observed in the brain (Acland and Littlejohns 1975). Nonsuppurative encephalitis and myocarditis have also been described in swine fetuses with natural EMCV infection (Kim et al. 1989a).

DIAGNOSIS

In newborn and suckling piglets, the disease is often characterized by sudden death between 3 days to 5 weeks of age. In most cases, piglets are found dead without any prior clinical signs. In other cases, vomiting and dyspnea, i.e., rapid abdominal breathing due to heart failure, may be observed. Frequently, an entire litter dies in 1 to a few hours, with mortality confined to single, affected litters. Spread of the disease by cross-fostering of piglets has been reported. The most striking lesions, white necrotic areas, are found in the myocardium.

In finishers, sudden death is also the most characteristic sign. All age categories may be affected, but mostly pigs weighing 60–70 kg are involved. The disease is often limited to a single building, and deaths often occur in the late afternoon, when the pigs are most active. In some pigs, squealing can be heard just prior to death. In others, dyspnea can be observed.

A clinical history of reproductive failure and pre-

weaning mortality is suggestive of EMCV infection (Joo 1999). EMCV-induced reproductive problems should be differentiated from other pathogens causing reproductive problems in sows. EMCV causes reproductive failure in sows of all parities, whereas porcine parvovirus infection is manifested as an increase in mummification, primarily in gilt litters, without neonatal mortality. Other infections such as porcine reproductive and respiratory syndrome (PRRS), Aujeszky's disease (pseudorabies), and leptospirosis, should also be considered.

Histopathology may be important in achieving a diagnosis. As described previously, a variable degree of nonsuppurative interstitial myocarditis or encephalitis (infiltration of lymphocytes, histiocytes, and plasma cells) is indicative of EMCV infection. A conclusive diagnosis of EMCV should be demonstrated by virus isolation in mice or cell culture. BHK-21 cell culture is the most sensitive, but HeLa or Vero cell lines are also commonly used. Infected cell monolayers show a rapid and complete cytopathic effect. Identification of the virus can be achieved by cross virus neutralization (VN) using a reference antiserum or by staining with EMCV fluorescent antibody conjugate. Nucleic acid probes and reverse transcription-polymerase chain reaction (RT-PCR) for the detection of EMCV have been reported (Bakkali et al. 2002; Meng et al. 1993; Vanderhallen and Koenen 1997). If available, molecular biotechnological methods may provide sensitive and specific methods of diagnosis, especially when followed by sequencing.

Serologic tests for the detection of serum antibodies against EMCV include the hemagglutination-inhibition (HI) test, ELISA (Brocchi et al. 2000), latex agglutination, immunofluorescent antibody assay (IFA), agar gel immunodiffusion (AGID), and virus neutralization (VN). The VN and ELISA are the most commonly used methods and are considered specific for EMCV. No cross-neutralization was found between EMCV and 62 human enterovirus serotypes or 11 porcine enterovirus serotypes (Zimmerman 1994). For VN, antibody titers of ≥1:16 appear to be significant (Joo 1999). VN antibody reaction starts as soon as 7 DPI and may persist for an extended period (6 months to 1 year).

PREVENTION AND CONTROL

There is no treatment for EMCV infection, but during the acute phase, mortality may be minimized by avoiding situations that stress or excite the pigs at risk.

Rodents are thought to play a role in the introduction and subsequent spread of the EMC virus within pig facilities. Therefore, to prevent clinical outbreaks of EMCV, producers are advised to maintain good hygiene and keep facilities and feed sources as rodent-free as possible, especially in EMCV-endemic areas. The virus can be inactivated by water containing 0.5 ppm residual chlorine. For disinfectants, iodine based preparations or mercuric chloride can also be used.

The direct exposure of pigs to manure has been found to be significantly protective (Maurice et al. 2004b). In pig houses with slatted floors or where manure was moved between "open" manure pits, animals acquired immunity without displaying clinical signs, probably due to infection by exposure to low titers of virus.

An inactivated EMCV-vaccine is commercially available in the United States. The vaccine appears to be effective, since high humoral immunity is detected in vaccinated pigs and vaccinates were protected from clinical disease when challenged with virulent EMCV that killed 60% of unvaccinated controls. Likewise, protection against transplacental infection was demonstrated under experimental conditions.

Public Health

At present, the impact of EMCV on public health is believed to be minimal. Despite the frequency of infection in swine, no association between infection and disease in humans has been recorded (Zimmerman 1994), even in persons at the greatest risk of acquiring the infection (veterinarians, animal caretakers, laboratory staff). In light of the ubiquitous presence of EMCV around the world, secondary EMCV infection in immunocompromised persons can be expected to occur. The outcome of EMCV coinfection under such conditions is not known and there have been no reports of such cases to date. The likelihood of this event is heightened by the current interest in using porcine cells, tissues, and organs in humans (xenotransplantation). Experimental infection of a mouse through the transplantation of pig organs infected with EMCV (Brewer et al. 2003) confirmed this concern.

REFERENCES

Acland HM. 1989. Encephalomyocarditis virus. In Virus Infections of Vertebrates, Vol 2. Virus Infections of Porcines. MB Pesaert, ed. Amsterdam: Elsevier Science Publishers BV, pp. 259–263.

Acland HM, Littlejohns IR. 1975. Encephalomyocarditis virus infection of pigs. I. An outbreak in New South Wales. Aust Vet J 51:409–415.

Bakkali K, Gonzague M, Boutrouille M, Lipobo Mbanda A, Crucière C. 2002. Detection of EMCV in clinical samples by immunomagnetic separation and one step RT-PCR. J Virol Met 101(1-2):197–206.

Billinis C, Leontides S, Psychas V, Spyrou V, Kostoulas P, Koenen F, Papadopoulos O. 2004. Effect of challenge dose and age in experimental infection of pigs with encephalomyocarditis virus. Vet Microbiol 99:187–195.

Billinis C, Paschaleri-Papadopoulou E, Anastasiadis G, Psychas V, Vlemmas J, Leontides S, Koumbati M, Kyriakis SC, Papadopoulos O. 1999. A comparative study of the pathogenic properties and transmissibility of a Greek and a Belgian encephalomyocarditis virus (EMCV) for piglets. Vet Microbiol 70:179–192.

Brewer L, Brown C, Murtaugh MP, Njenga MK. 2003. Transmission of porcine EMCV to mice by transplanting EMCV-infected pig tissues. Xenotransplantation 10:569–576.

Brocchi E, Carra E, Koenen F, De Simone F. 2000. Development of monoclonal antibodies based ELISA's for the detection of EMCV and EMCV-induced antibodies. Proc 1st Congr Soc Ital Diagn Lab Vet, p. 1998.

Castryck F, Miry C, Koenen F, Ducatelle R. 1996. Clinical and pathological aspects of EMCV infections in pigs in Belgium. Proc 14th Congr Int Pig Vet Soc, p. 132.

Cerutis DR, Bruner RH, Thomas DC, Giron DJ. 1989. Tropism and histopathology of the D.B.K and MM variants of encephalomyocarditis virus. J Med Virol 29:63–69.

Christianson WT, Kim HS, Yoon IJ, Joo HS. 1992. Transplacental infection of midgestation sows with encephalomyocarditis virus. Am J Vet Res 53:44–47.

Craighead JE, Peralta PH, Murnane TG, Shelokov A. 1963. Oral infection of swine with the encephalomyocarditis virus. J Infec Dis 112:205–212.

Dea SA, Bilodeau R, Martineau GP. 1991. Isolation of encephalomyocarditis virus among stillborn and post-weaning pigs in Quebec. Arch Virol 117:121–128.

Foni E, Barigazzi G, Sidoli L, Marcato PS, Sarli G, Della Salda L, Spinaci M. 1993. Experimental encephalomyocarditis virus infection in pigs. Zentralbl Veterinarmed B 40:347–352.

Gainer JH. 1967. Encephalomyocarditis virus infection in Florida. 1960–1966. J Am Vet Med Assoc 151:421–425.

Gainer JH, Sauderfur JR, Bigler WJ. 1968. High mortality in a Florida swine herd infected with the encephalomyocarditis virus: An accompanying epizootologic survey. Cornell Vet 58:31–47.

Gelmetti D, Meroni A, Brocchi E, Koenen F, Cammarata G. 2006. EMCV of swine: A pathogenic study under experimental conditions. Vet Res (in press).

Hani H, Zimmermann W, Bestetti GE, Muller HK. 1992. A disease outbreak associated with severe myocarditis resembling encephalomyocarditis virus infection in two Swiss farms: Clinical and pathological characterization of the disease and aetiological studies. Proc 12th Congr Int Pig Vet Soc, p. 105.

Helwig FC, Schmidt ECH. 1945. A filter-passing agent producing interstitial myocarditis in anthropoid apes and small animals. Sciences 102:31–33.

Horner GW, Hunter R. 1979. Experimental infection in pigs with encephalomyocarditis virus. NZ Vet J 27:202–203.

Joo HS. 1999. Encephalomyocarditis virus. In Diseases of Swine, 8th edition. BE Straw, S D'Allaire, WL Mengeling, DJ Taylor, eds. Ames: Iowa State University Press, pp. 139–144.

Jungeblut CW, Sanders M. 1940. Studies of a murine strain of poliomyelitis in cotton rats and white mice. J Exp Med 72:407.

Kim HS, Christianson WT, Joo HS. 1989b. Pathogenic properties of encephalomyocarditis virus isolates in swine fetuses. Arch Virol 109:51–57.

Kim HS, Joo HS, Bergeland ME. 1989a. Serologic, virologic and histopathologic observations of encephalomyocarditis virus infection I, mummified and stillborn pigs. J Vet Diag Invest 1:101–104.

Kim HS, Joo HS, Christianson WT, Morrison RB. 1991. Evaluation of serologic methods for the detection of antibodies to encephalomyocarditis virus in swine fetal thoracic fluids. J Vet Diagn Invest 3:283–286.

Knowles, NJ, Dickinson ND, Wisden G, Carra E, Brocchi E, De Simone F. 2000. Molecular analysis of encephalomyocarditis viruses isolated from pigs and rodents in Italy. Virus Res 57:53–62.

Koenen F, Vanderhallen H. 1997. Comparative study of the pathogenic properties of a Belgian and a Greek EMCV isolate for sows in gestation. Zentralbl Veterinarmed B 44:281–286.

Koenen F, Vanderhallen H, Castryck F, Miry C. 1999. Epidemiologic, pathogenic and molecular analysis of recent encephalomyocarditis outbreaks in Belgium. Zentralbl Veterinarmed B 46:217–231.

Links IJ, Whittington RJ, Kennedy DJ, Grewal A, Sharrock AJ. 1986. An association between encephalomyocarditis virus infection and reproductive failure in pigs. Aust Vet J 63:150–152.

Littlejohns IR, Acland HM. 1975. Encephalomyocarditis virus infection in pigs. II. Experimental diseases. Aust Vet J 51:416–422.

Loukaidis F, Hadjizinonos Z, Hatjisavvas T, Economides P, Paschaleri-Papadopoulou E, Billinis C, Papadopoulos O. 1996. Encephalomyocarditis in Cyprus. Proc 7th Helenic Vet Congr, p. 67.

Love RJ, Grewal AS. 1986. Reproductive failure in pigs caused by encephalomyocarditis virus. Aust Vet J 63:128–129.

Maurice H, Nielen M, Brocchi E, Nowotny N, Bakkali Kassimi L, Billinis C, Loukaides P, O'Harra RS, Koenen F. 2005a. The occurrence of EMCV in European pigs from 1990–2001. Epidemiol Infect 133:547–557.

Maurice H, Nielen M, Stegeman JA, Vanderhallen H, Koenen F. 2002. Transmission of encephalomyocarditis virus (EMCV) among pigs experimentally quantified. Vet Microbiol 88:301–314.

Maurice H, Nielen M, Vyt Ph, Frankema K, Koenen F. 2005b. Factors related to clinical appearance of EMCV at Belgian pig farms. Prev Vet Med (in press).

Meng XJ, Paul, PS, Vaughan EM, Zimmerman JJ. 1993. Development of radiolabeled nucleic acid probe for the detection of EMCV of swine. J Vet Diagn Invest 5:254.

Meroni A, Alborali L, Candotti P, De Simone F, Knowles NJ, O'Hara RS, Brocchi E. 2000. EMC occurrence in Italy and characterisation of EMC virus isolates. Proc 5th Congr ESVV, pp. 201–204.

Murnane TG, Graighead JE, Mondragon H, Shelokov A. 1960. Fatal disease of swine due to encephalomyocarditis virus. Science 131:498–499.

Nelsen-Salz B, Zimmerman A, Wickert S, Arnold G, Botta A, Eggers H, Kruppenbacher P. 1996. Analysis of sequence and pathogenic properties of two variants of encephalomyocarditis differing in a single amino acid in VP1. Virus Res 41:109–122.

Papaioannou N, Billinis C, Psychas V, Papadopoulos O, Vlemmas I. 2003. Pathogenesis of encephalomyocarditis virus (EMCV) infection in piglets during the viraemia phase: A histopathological, immunohistochemical and virological study. J Comp Pathol 129:161–168.

Paschaleri-Papadopoulou E, Axiotis I, Laspidis C, Papadopoulos O. 1990. Encephalomyocarditis virus in Greece: A follow up. Proc 12th Congr Int Pig Vet Soc, p. 106.

Psychas V, Papaioannou N, Billinis C, Paschaleri-papadopoulou E, Leontides S, Papadopoulos O, Tsangaris T, Vlemmas J. 2001. Evaluation of ultrastructural changes associated with encephalomyocarditis virus in the myocardium of experimentally infected piglets. Am J Vet Res 62:1653–1657.

Ramos JR, Gomez L, Mayo M, Sanchez G. 1983. Infection due to encephalomyocarditis virus in swine and other species over the 1975–1981 period. Rev Cub Cienc Vet 14:71–77.

Sangar DV, Rowlands DJ, Brown F. 1977. Encephalomyocarditis virus antibodies in sera from apparently normal pigs. Vet Rec 100:240–241.

Seaman JT, Boulton JG, Carrigan MJ. 1986. Encephalomyocarditis virus disease of pigs associated with a plague of rodents. Aust Vet J 63:292–294.

Sidoli L, Barigazzi G, Foni E, Marcato PS, Barberi G. 1988. Encephalomyocarditis due to cardiovirus in Po Valley swine: Preliminary observations. Proc Italian Soc Swine Pathol, pp. 249–260.

Simpson CF, Lewis AL, Gaskin JM. 1977. Encephalomyocarditis virus infection of captive elephants. J Am Vet Med Assoc 171:902–905.

Spyrou V, Maurice H, Billinis C, Papanastassopoulou M, Nielen M, Koenen F, Papadopoulos O. 2004. Transmission and pathogenicity of encephalomyocarditis virus among rats. Vet Res 35:113–122.

Sutherland RJ, Horner GW, Hunter R, Fyfe BH. 1977. An outbreak of viral encephalomyocarditis in pigs. NZ Vet 25:225.

Tesh RB, Wallace GD. 1977. Observations on the natural history of encephalomyocarditis virus. Am J Trop Med Hyg 27:133–143.

Tinsley TW, MacCallum FO, Robertson JS, Brown F. 1984. Relationship of encephalomyocarditis virus to cricket paralysis virus of insects. Intervirol 21:181–186.

Vanderhallen H, Koenen F. 1997. Rapid diagnosis of EMCV infections in pigs using a reverse transcription-polymerase chain reaction. J Virol Methods 66:83–89.

van Regenmortel MHV, Fauquet CM, Bishop DHL, Carstens EB, Estes MH, Lemon SM, Maniloff J, Mayo MA, McGeoch DJ, Pringle CR, Wickner RB. 2000. Virus Taxonomy: Classification and Nomenclature of Viruses: Seventh report of the International Committee on Taxonomy of Viruses. San Diego, CA: Academic Press, pp. 667–669.

Williams MC. 1981. Encephalomyocarditis virus infection. J S Africa Vet Assoc 52:76.

Zimmerman JJ. 1994. Encephalomyocarditis. In Handbook of Zoonoses, 2nd edition. GW Beran, JH Steele, eds. Boca Raton: CRC Press, Inc., pp. 423–436.

18 Porcine Enteric Picornaviruses

Nick J. Knowles

In previous editions of *Diseases of Swine* this chapter was entitled "Enterovirus." However, complete genome sequences of representatives of all the porcine enterovirus (PEV) serotypes have resulted in the reclassification of the group I serotypes into a new genus, *Teschovirus*, within the family *Picornaviridae* (King et al. 2000). Thus, this chapter will cover the true porcine enteroviruses and the porcine teschoviruses (PTV). Other picornaviruses infecting swine (foot-and-mouth disease virus, swine vesicular disease virus, and encephalomyocarditis virus) are covered in separate chapters.

The first report of porcine teschovirus infection was the occurrence of Teschen disease, a polioencephalomyelitis with high mortality, in Czechoslovakia over 75 years ago. This severe disease has continued to occur sporadically, mainly in Central Europe, but also in Africa. Milder forms of polioencephalomyelitis (Talfan disease, benign enzootic paresis), caused by serologically related but less virulent strains of PTV, have been reported in the last 50 years in Western Europe, North America, and Australia. In France, the encephalomyelitis is intermediate in severity between Teschen and Talfan diseases (Métianu 1986). Porcine enteroviruses and teschoviruses are ubiquitous and no conventional herd of pigs has been shown to be free of infection. Although the majority of infections are asymptomatic, porcine enteroviruses and teschoviruses have been associated with a variety of clinical conditions, including polioencephalomyelitis, female reproductive disorders, enteric disease, and pneumonia. Strains that have not been shown to be pathogenic have been referred to as enteric cytopathogenic swine orphan (ECSO) or enteric cytopathogenic porcine orphan (ECPO) viruses; however, these terms are no longer in general use.

There are no known public health problems associated with any of these viruses.

ETIOLOGY

Taxonomy and Classification

The serotypic classification of porcine enteroviruses and teschoviruses is based upon the virus neutralization (VN) test (Dunne et al. 1971; Knowles et al. 1979). In the 1960s and 1970s there were numerous attempts to achieve a uniform classification. These studies culminated in a classification of eight serotypes proposed by Dunne et al. (1971). This was later extended to 13 serotypes (Auerbach et al. 1994; Knowles et al. 1979) (Table 18.1). A complement-fixation test, suitable for the rapid screening and typing of porcine enteroviruses, has also been described (Knowles and Buckley 1980). Subsequent findings (Knowles 1983) suggested that additional serotypes may exist. Honda et al. (1990a) compared the prototype strains found in Japan with 11 internationally recognized PTV and PEV serotypes by virus neutralization and suggested a further four candidate serotypes. Some limited cross-reactivity among the existing serotypes is evident, and Hazlett and Derbyshire (1978) showed that gastrointestinal antibodies were more broadly specific than serum antibodies.

More recently, the genome sequences of the prototype strains of all the PEV serotypes have been determined, as well as partial genomic data on a number of additional isolates (Doherty et al. 1999; Kaku et al. 1999, 2001; Krumbholz et al. 2002; Peng, Lin, Kitching and Knowles 1998, GenBank accession no. AJ001391; Peng, McCauley, Kitching and Knowles 1997, GenBank accession no. Y14459; Zell et al. 2001). Comparative analyses of these data indicated that PEV types 1 to 7 and 11 to 13 formed a genetic cluster distinct from PEV-8 to 10 and human and bovine enteroviruses. They also possessed a leader polypeptide and a 2A/2B cleavage mechanism similar to the aphthoviruses, cardioviruses, and erboviruses. Thus, these 10 serotypes were renamed porcine teschovirus 1 to 10 and reclassified as a single species, *Porcine teschovirus*, in a new genus, *Teschovirus*. An additional serotype, PTV-11, was also designated, based on

Table 18.1. Classification of porcine enteric picornaviruses

Genus	Species	Serotype	Previous Designation	Reference Strain	Isolated From:	Sequence Accession No.	Reference
Teschovirus	*Porcine teschovirus*	PTV-1	PEV-1	Talfan	Brain	AF231769	Harding et al. 1957
		PTV-2	PEV-2	T80	Tonsils	AF296087	Betts 1960
		PTV-3	PEV-3	O2b	Brain	AF296088	Kasza 1965
		PTV-4	PEV-4	PS36	Fetus	AF296089	Dunne et al. 1965
		PTV-5	PEV-5	F26	Feces	AF296090	Alexander and Betts 1967
		PTV-6	PEV-6	PS37	Fetus	AF296091	Dunne et al. 1965
		PTV-7	PEV-7	F43	Feces	AF296092	Alexander and Betts 1967
		PTV-8	PEV-11	UKG/173/74	Feces	AF296093	Knowles et al. 1979
		PTV-9	PEV-12	Vir 2899/84	CNS	AF296094	Auerbach et al. 1994
		PTV-10	PEV-13	Vir 461/88	CNS	AF296095	Auerbach et al. 1994
		PTV-11	PEV-1	Dresden	CNS	AF296096	Hahnefeld et al. 1965
Enterovirus	*Porcine enterovirus A*	PEV-8	—	V13	Feces	AF406813	Lamont and Betts 1960
Enterovirus	*Porcine enterovirus B*	PEV-9	—	UKG/410/73	Skin lesion	AF363453	Knowles et al. 1979
		PEV-10	—	LP54/UK/75	Skin lesion	AF363455	Knowles et al. 1979

serological and molecular sequence data (Zell et al. 2001).

The remaining porcine enterovirus serotypes are currently classified in two species, *Porcine enterovirus A* (PEV-8) and *Porcine enterovirus B* (PEV-9 and PEV-10), in the genus *Enterovirus*. PEV-9 and PEV-10 are typical enteroviruses most closely related to bovine enteroviruses. However, the taxonomic position of PEV-8 is presently under discussion. Although it clusters genetically with the enteroviruses and rhinoviruses (two genera which may, in the future, be combined), PEV-8 has some distinct genome features that may be the basis for reclassification in a new genus (Krumbholz et al. 2002):

1. The 5' untranslated region (UTR) has an internal ribosome entry site (IRES) that more closely resembles that of hepatitis C virus (a flavivirus) (Kaku et al. 2002; Pisarev et al. 2004).
2. It has a leader polypeptide, absent in all other entero/rhinoviruses.
3. The sequences of the 2A, 2B, and 3A polypeptides are unlike those of the entero/rhinoviruses.

Genetically PEV-8 is most closely related to some simian picornaviruses (Krumbholz et al. 2002; Oberste et al. 2003) and a duck picornavirus (Tseng and Tsai 2004, GenBank accession no. AY563023) that are also in taxonomic limbo (Figure 18-1).

Morphology (Size and Structure)

As with all picornaviruses, the virions of PTVs and PEVs are spherical and nonenveloped with a diameter of 25–30 nm. A single-stranded ribonucleic acid (RNA) genome is surrounded by an icosahedral capsid consisting of 60 copies of four polypeptides. A small basic virus-encoded protein (VPg) is linked to the 5' end of the genome. No three-dimensional structure data is yet available.

Genomic Organization and Gene Expression

The polyproteins of all the porcine enteroviruses and teschoviruses conform to the general picornavirus L-4-3-4 layout (Rueckert and Wimmer 1984) and all processed polypeptides occur in equimolar amounts. A leader polypeptide (absent in PEV-9 and PEV-10) is followed by four structural polypeptides (VP4, VP2, VP3 and VP1, also known as 1A to 1D, respectively) and seven nonstructural polypeptides (2A, 2B, 2C, 3A, 3B^{VPg}, 3C^{pro} and 3D^{pol}). The latter three are a small genome-linked protein, a cysteine proteinase, and an RNA-dependent RNA polymerase, respectively. In the true enteroviruses and rhinoviruses, 2A is also a cysteine proteinase. In the PEVs, primary polyprotein cleavages occur between the precursor polypeptides P1, P2, and P3. However, in the PTVs a self-cleaving mechanism operates between the P1-2A and 2BC polypeptides. Most subsequent processing of PEV and PTV polypeptide precursors is carried out by the 3C protease.

Physicochemical and Biological Properties

The complete PTV virions have a buoyant density of 1.34 g/ml in cesium chloride, which is similar to that of enteroviruses; the PEVs have not been characterized. Lipoprotein is lacking and the viruses are stable when treated with lipid solvents. Porcine teschoviruses are relatively stable to heat, whereas the enteroviruses are more heat labile, unless treated with 1M MgCl$_2$. Heating porcine teschoviruses in the presence of halide ions tends to destabilize the virus. All these viruses are stable at pH values between 2 and 9. Hemagglutination has not been demonstrated for porcine enteroviruses or teschoviruses. Prior to reclassification porcine enteroviruses were divided into three subgroups based on physicochemical properties, type of cytopathic effect (CPE) produced in pig kidney cells, and different cell culture host ranges (Knowles et al. 1979; Zoletto 1965; Zoletto et al. 1974).

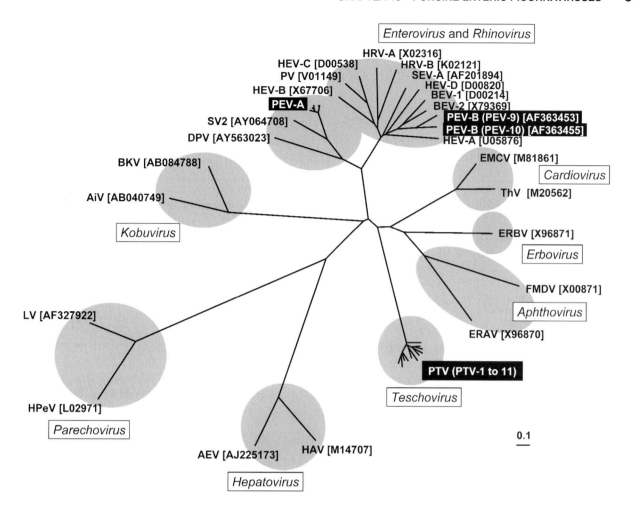

18.1. *Phylogenetic tree showing the relationships between the P1 capsid polypeptides of porcine enteroviruses, porcine teschoviruses, and other members of the Picornaviridae.*

Amino acid sequences were aligned and a neighbor-joining tree constructed using Clustal X. Sequences of the 11 prototype porcine teschoviruses (see Table 18.1) and the following five PEV-A (PEV-8) sequences were included in the tree: V13 [AF406813], 16-S-X [AY392543], 26-T-XII [AY392544], Sek 1562/98 [AY392556], Po 5116 [AY392538].

The following abbreviations are used for the picornavirus species: PV, Poliovirus; HEV-A, Human enterovirus A; HEV-B, Human enterovirus B; HEV-C, Human enterovirus C; HEV-D, Human enterovirus D; SEV-A, Simian enterovirus A; BEV, Bovine enterovirus; PEV-A, Porcine enterovirus A; PEV-B, Porcine enterovirus B; HRV-A, Human rhinovirus A; HRV-B, Human rhinovirus B; EMCV, Encephalomyocarditis virus; ThV, Theilovirus; FMDV, Foot-and-mouth disease virus; ERAV, Equine rhinitis A virus; ERBV, Equine rhinitis B virus; HAV, Hepatitis A virus; AEV, Avian encephalomyelitis-like viruses; HPeV, Human parechovirus; LV, Ljungan virus; AiV, Aichi virus; BKV, Bovine kobuvirus. The following are unclassified entero-like viruses: SV2, Siman virus 2; DPV, Duck picornavirus TW90A. Genus names are enclosed in boxes.

Laboratory Cultivation

Porcine teschoviruses and enteroviruses are readily cultivated in the laboratory in cell cultures of porcine origin. They are normally grown in primary or secondary pig kidney (PK) cell cultures or in established cell lines, such as IB-RS-2. They may also be cultivated in other cells of porcine origin such as the SST cell line or in primary swine testes cells. PEV-8 may additionally be cultivated in monkey kidney (e.g., Vero) and BHK-21 cells (Knowles et al. 1979). Isolates of PEV-9 and PEV-10 are also able to grow in a wide range of established cell lines, including BHK-21, Vero, and HeLa (Knowles et al. 1979).

EPIDEMIOLOGY

The virulent PTV-1 strains associated with classical Teschen disease appear to be restricted to those areas in which the disease occurs and they have not been isolated in North America. Less virulent PTV-1 strains and representatives of the other PTV serotypes appear to be ubiquitous, as is PEV-8 (Odend'hal 1983). However, PEV-9 and PEV-10 have only been identified in Italy, the United Kingdom, and Japan (Caracappa et al. 1985; Honda et al. 1990a; Knowles et al. 1979; Zoletto 1965).

The only known natural host for porcine enteroviruses and teschoviruses is the pig. Experimentally, pregnant guinea pigs infected with PEV-8 developed placental lesions (Lieu 1976).

Transmission of PEV and PTV infection is most frequently by the fecal-oral route. Indirect transmission by fomites is extremely likely to occur since the viruses are relatively resistant.

Endemic infection with several PTV serotypes and PEV-8 can usually be demonstrated in conventional herds and is probably maintained in groups of weaned piglets. Singh and Bohl (1972) demonstrated waves of infection with six different serotypes over a period of 26 months in a long-term study of infection in a single herd. Infection is normally acquired by piglets shortly after weaning, when maternally derived antibodies are withdrawn and pigs from several litters are mixed together, and it persists for at least several weeks. Adults rarely excrete virus, but have high antibody levels. Pigs of any age are, however, fully susceptible to infection with a virus belonging to a serotype to which they have not previously been exposed.

Porcine enteroviruses and teschoviruses are highly resistant to the environment, with Teschen disease virus surviving for more than 168 days at 15°C (Ottis 1976). These viruses survive for long periods in liquid manure, but they are inactivated more rapidly if the manure is aerated (Lund and Nissen 1983). Likewise, they are inactivated in liquid manure by ionizing radiation (Simon et al. 1983) and by anaerobic digestion (Derbyshire et al. 1986).

Porcine enteroviruses and teschoviruses are relatively resistant to many disinfectants. Of 10 commonly used disinfectants tested by Derbyshire and Arkell (1971) against Talfan virus, only sodium hypochlorite or 70% ethanol completely inactivated it.

PATHOGENESIS

Natural infection occurs by ingestion of the virus. It is well established (Long 1985) that initial replication occurs in the tonsil and intestinal tract. The large intestine and ileum are infected more frequently than the upper small intestine, and the former tissues contain higher titers of virus. It has not been clearly established which cells in the intestine support viral replication, but by analogy with experiments on poliovirus (Kanamitsu et al. 1967) it is probable that the reticuloendothelial tissue

of the lamina propria is involved. Epithelial cell destruction is not a feature of these infections. Viremia follows regularly in infections with the virulent PTV-1 strains, but occurs less regularly with the less virulent strains, leading to infection of the central nervous system (CNS) (Holman et al. 1966). It may be assumed that the pregnant uterus is also infected by viremic spread of the virus, since embryonic or fetal infections were demonstrated in gilts following nasal or oral inoculation of PEV-8 or PTV (Huang et al. 1980).

Intranasal inoculation of the virus may lead experimentally to lung infection (Meyer et al. 1966), but the significance of the natural inhalation of viral aerosols is not known. It has also been clearly demonstrated that when piglets are inoculated parenterally with porcine teschoviruses, the virus rapidly infects the intestine. Extraintestinal infections are relatively transient, whereas the virus persists in the large intestine for several weeks.

CLINICAL SIGNS

Although porcine teschovirus and enterovirus infections are most frequently subclinical, various clinical syndromes have been associated with certain serotypes, as indicated in Table 18.2 and outlined below.

Polioencephalomyelitis

The most severe form of polioencephalomyelitis is that produced by the highly virulent PTV-1 strains that cause Teschen disease. This is a disease of high morbidity and high mortality, affecting all ages of swine and associated with major economic losses. The early signs of Teschen disease include fever, anorexia, and listlessness, rapidly followed by locomotor ataxia. In severe cases there may be nystagmus, convulsions, opisthotonus, and coma. Paralysis ensues, and the animal may assume a dog-sitting posture or remain in lateral recumbency. Stimulation by sound or touch may elicit uncoordinated limb movements or opisthotonus. Death is common within 3 or 4 days of the onset of clinical signs. Since the appetite returns after the acute phase, some animals may be kept alive by careful nursing, but these cases show muscle wasting and residual paralysis.

The less virulent PTV-1 strains (Talfan disease, benign enzootic paresis) and strains belonging to other serotypes associated with polioencephalomyelitis pro-

Table 18.2. Natural or experimental clinical syndromes associated with porcine enteric picornavirus infection

Syndrome	PTV Serotypes	PEV Serotypes
Polioencephalomyelitis	PTV-1, PTV-2, PTV-3, PTV-5	—
Reproductive disorders	PTV-1, PTV-3, PTV-6	PEV-8
Diarrhea	PTV-1, PTV-2, PTV-3, PTV-5	PEV-8
Pneumonia	PTV-1, PTV-2, PTV-3	PEV-8
Pericarditis and myocarditis	PTV-2, PTV-3	—
Cutaneous lesions	—	PEV-9, PEV-10

duce a milder disease with relatively low morbidity and mortality. Mainly young pigs are affected, and the disease rarely progresses to complete paralysis.

Recently, encephalomyelitis due to teschovirus infection has been reported in pigs in both the U.S. (Pogranichniy et al. 2003) and Japan (Yamada et al. 2004). No neurological disease has been observed during infection with porcine enteroviruses.

Reproductive Disease

The term SMEDI was initially introduced (Dunne et al. 1965) to designate a group of viruses, subsequently shown to be porcine enteroviruses or teschoviruses, that had been isolated in association with stillbirth (S), mummified fetuses (M), embryonic death (ED), and infertility (I). Subsequent studies by the same group of workers and by others (De Meurichy et al. 1976) indicated that the syndrome could be reproduced experimentally.

However, parvovirus infection may also lead to embryonic death and fetal mummification and this virus may be more frequently associated with these disorders of early and midgestation. Other findings (Cropper et al. 1976) substantiated a role for teschoviruses, as well as parvoviruses, in these disorders, and experimental (Bielanski and Raeside 1977) and field data (Kirkbride and McAdaragh 1978) confirmed an association between teschovirus infection and abortion in swine. These reproductive disorders are not usually accompanied by clinical signs in the sow or gilt. Infection with encephalomyocarditis virus (family *Picornaviridae*, genus *Cardiovirus*) may also result in female reproductive failure.

Porcine teschoviruses have also been isolated from the male genital tract (Philips et al. 1972), although the insemination of gilts with contaminated semen did not influence their fertility (De Meurichy and Pensaert 1977).

Diarrhea

The role of porcine enteroviruses and teschoviruses as enteric pathogens is uncertain. They have frequently been isolated from the feces of piglets with diarrhea, but since they can be readily isolated from normal piglets, particularly postweaning, and since diarrhea can be caused by a variety of other viral and bacterial agents, their presence may be coincidental. However, diarrhea has been produced experimentally by porcine teschoviruses in piglets believed to be free of other pathogens. The diarrhea is mild and relatively transient, and it seems clear that porcine teschoviruses are considerably less important enteric pathogens than rotaviruses or coronaviruses. When piglets were infected with porcine teschoviruses together with rotaviruses, the disease was less severe than in piglets infected only with the rotavirus (Janke et al. 1988). An association between PEV-8 and diarrhea has been suggested based on the relative frequency of isolation of this virus from pigs showing symptoms (Honda et al. 1990b). Conversely, the relative infrequency of isolation of PEV-9/PEV-10 from pig feces would argue against any involvement of these viruses in gastrointestinal disease (Knowles 1988).

Pneumonia, Pericarditis, and Myocarditis

The role of enteroviruses and teschoviruses as respiratory pathogens is also uncertain. It is probable that alone they rarely cause clinical signs of respiratory disease, although Pospisil et al. (1971) noted increased respiration, coughing, snorting, reduced appetite, and depression in piglets exposed to an aerosol of porcine teschovirus. Although pathogenic studies indicate some degree of tropism of these viruses for the lung, the pneumonia produced is usually subclinical. Two serotypes of porcine teschovirus have been shown experimentally to be capable of producing pericarditis, and in one experiment, myocardial involvement occurred (Long et al. 1969). These findings might lead to a suspicion of teschovirus infection in the case of sudden death in piglets, although encephalomyocarditis virus might be more likely candidate.

Possible Association with Cutaneous Lesions

During the course of investigations of swine vesicular disease outbreaks in the United Kingdom, many adventitious agents were isolated from samples of epithelium and feces. Most of these isolates were identified as teschoviruses or enteroviruses (Knowles 1983). Porcine teschoviruses and PEV-8 were evenly distributed in fecal samples (41% and 44%, respectively) and in epithelial samples (21% in each case). However, PEV-9/PEV-10 were rarely found in feces (15%), but were more commonly found in epithelial samples (58%) (Knowles 1988). Examination of another virus collection again revealed an approximately even distribution of PTV and PEV-8 (57% and 43%, respectively), but PEV-9 and PEV-10 were not identified (Knowles 1988). It was assumed that most of the PTV and PEV-8 isolates identified in epithelial samples were incidental contaminants; however, the low level incidence of PEV-9 and PEV-10 in feces could not explain the much higher isolation rate from epithelial tissue collected from atypical skin lesions. This association has yet to be explained.

LESIONS

No specific changes have been associated with intestinal enterovirus or teschovirus infections. They do not appear to cause villous atrophy, which is characteristic of primary intestinal pathogens such as coronaviruses and rotaviruses. Other than muscle atrophy in chronic cases, no gross lesions are found in polioencephalomyelitis. The histological lesions associated with the latter are widely distributed in the CNS but are especially numerous in the ventral columns of the spinal cord, the cerebellar cortex, and the brain stem. The changes are more marked and extensive in Teschen disease than in milder encephalomyelitides, such as Talfan disease. The neurons show progressive diffuse chromatolysis (Koestner et al. 1966) and focal areas of gliosis and perivascular lymphocytes, particularly over the cerebellum, may also occur.

The SMEDI syndrome is remarkable for the lack of specific lesions in stillborn or neonatal piglets, although mild focal gliosis and perivascular cuffing in the brain stem have been found occasionally. Placental changes are restricted to nonspecific degeneration.

Pneumonic lesions have been produced by several investigators. Smith et al. (1973) describes areas of grayish-red consolidation in the ventral anterior lobes of lungs infected with a PTV-2 strain. There were exudates in the alveoli and bronchi, slight perivascular and peribronchiolar cuffing, and some hyperplasia of the bronchiolar epithelium.

A PTV-3 strain consistently produced serofibrinous pericarditis experimentally, and the more severely affected piglets showed focal myocardial necrosis (Long et al. 1969).

IMMUNITY

Infected pigs mount a classical humoral protective immune response (IgM and IgG). Mucosal immunity (IgA) may be produced and have a protective effect in the gastrointestinal tract. In an experimental study of porcine teschovirus infection in piglets, it was shown that cell-mediated responses were weak and localized and not associated with significant antiviral activity (Brundage et al. 1980).

Humoral antibody is thought to be important for protection. In one experiment, immunosuppression (using cyclophosphamide) of pigs infected with a porcine teschovirus led to the lack of a serological response and a persistent infection of the intestinal tract (Derbyshire 1983). This resulted in severe diarrhea and, in one case, signs of encephalomyelitis. Presence of high levels of virus neutralizing IgA antibody in the gastrointestinal tract may protect against oral challenge (Hazlett and Derbyshire 1977).

Since humoral antibody is probably the most important factor in protection, at least in teschoviruses, the relatively large number of serotypes would suggest that cross-protection may not be effective.

It has been reported for both PTV-1 and PEV-8 that maternal antibody has no effect on embryonic or fetal infections after the virus has reached the uterus (Huang et al. 1980). However, possession of preinfection antibody in sows would probably limit infection and prevent the virus from reaching the uterus. Colostral antibody would be expected to protect piglets from infection.

DIAGNOSIS

Teschen disease (Enterovirus Encephalomyelitis) is designated as a List A disease by the World Organisation for Animal Health (OIE) and details of internationally accepted methods for its diagnosis can be found on the World Wide Web as an on-line document (Office International des Epizooties 2004).

The occurrence of clinical signs associated with polioencephalomyelitis is suggestive of viral infection, but the differentiation of teschoviral infection from other neurotropic viruses requires isolation of the virus from the CNS, the demonstration of viral antigen by specific immunofluorescence or presence of viral RNA by RT-PCR. Similarly, with reproductive disorders, diarrhea, pneumonia, pericarditis, and myocarditis, there are no diagnostic clinical signs that would suggest enterovirus or teschovirus involvement and laboratory diagnosis is required.

Virus isolation from the CNS requires the collection of tissues from a piglet showing early nervous signs since animals that have been paralyzed for several days may no longer contain infectious virus in the CNS (Lynch et al. 1984). The virus may be isolated in PK cell cultures from suspensions of the spinal cord, brain stem, or cerebellum. It may subsequently be identified on the basis of its physicochemical characteristics, by immunofluorescence (Watanabe 1971) or immunoperoxidase staining (Sulochana and Derbyshire 1978). Serologic identification of the isolate is desirable. The isolation of a teschovirus or enterovirus from the gastrointestinal tract of a piglet with nervous signs does not establish the etiology of the disease, since the enteric infection may be coincidental. In the SMEDI syndrome, mummified fetuses carried to term rarely contain live virus but may contain viral antigen detectable by immunofluorescence.

Virus isolation in PK cell culture may be attempted from tissues of aborted or stillborn fetuses. Lung tissue appears to be the most reliable source for the isolation of porcine enteroviruses and teschoviruses from fetuses (Huang et al. 1980). VN tests on the body fluids of such fetuses can be carried out against the SMEDI-associated PTV and PEV serotypes. In the investigation of pneumonia or diarrhea, virus isolation from the respiratory or intestinal tract may be attempted, but the virological findings should be interpreted cautiously, especially in relation to diarrhea, since enteric infections with teschoviruses and enteroviruses are common in healthy piglets. In one study porcine enteroviruses and teschoviruses were isolated from 57% of porcine fecal samples submitted for swine vesicular disease diagnosis over a 7-year period (Knowles 1983).

Isolated viruses may be identified by virus neutralization (Knowles et al. 1979), complement fixation (Knowles and Buckley 1980), or immunofluorescence (Auerbach et al. 1994; Dauber 1999) if suitable reference reagents are available. Monoclonal antibodies that are capable of detecting porcine teschoviruses have been described (Dauber 1999).

Now that genomic sequence data is available for all the porcine enteroviruses and teschoviruses, it is possible to use RT-PCR to detect viral RNA in clinical samples or to identify viruses isolated in cell culture. Palmquist et al. (2002) described an RT-PCR using a single set of primers for the simultaneous detection and differentiation (based on amplicon size) of PTVs and PEV-8. Nested RT-PCR assays to specifically detect PTV-1 and to differentiate the PTVs, PEV-8, and PEV-9/10 from each other using virus-specific primer sets have also been described (Zell et al. 2000). More recently, improvements to these assays resulted in the development of a one-step, real-time PCR (Krumbholz et al. 2003).

Serology is of little value for diagnosis, unless paired sera are available and the serotype known. In this case the virus neutralization test would be suitable. An enzyme-linked immunosorbent assay, suitable for mass screening, has been described for the detection of antibodies against Teschen disease virus (Hubschle et al. 1983). However, because these viruses are ubiquitous, serological surveys may not be very helpful.

PREVENTION AND CONTROL

As in most viral infections, control measures for porcine enteroviruses depend on prevention rather than treatment. Potential antiviral chemotherapeutics for porcine enteric picornaviruses have received little attention. Piglets with mild polioencephalomyelitis may recover if nursing care is provided during the period of transient paresis.

Vaccination has been practiced in the field only for the control of Teschen disease. The earlier Teschen disease vaccines, containing inactive virus of pig tissue origin, have been superseded by attenuated or inactivated cell culture vaccines. Mayr and Correns (1959) attenuated Teschen disease virus by cell culture passage and showed that live or formalin-inactivated vaccines prepared from this virus induced similar levels of protection in piglets. Success has been claimed for a Teschen disease eradication program involving ring vaccination and slaughter (Schaupp 1968). Restrictions on the import of swine and pork products from areas in which Teschen disease is endemic seem to be effective in limiting the spread of virulent PTV-1 strains. If such strains were introduced into North America, they would be controlled by a policy of quarantine and slaughter.

Vaccination has not been practiced against the milder forms of polioencephalomyelitis or against the other clinical manifestations of PTV or PEV infection in swine. Only the SMEDI syndrome is of sufficient economic importance to justify specific control measures in the field, but the multiplicity of serotypes that may be involved complicates the development of an effective vaccine.

The best current approach to the prevention of reproductive disorders associated with porcine enteroviruses and teschoviruses would appear to be the application of management practices that ensure that gilts are exposed to the infection with endemic viruses at least 1 month before breeding. This can be achieved naturally if the animals remain in a single building from birth to breeding, with thorough mixing of piglets from different litters at weaning. If breeding stock is segregated at an early age, they should be contaminated with fecal material from recently weaned piglets. This can be readily accomplished by adding fresh feces to the feed of gilts or by dosing gilts with capsules of feces, which should be a pooled sample collected from weaned piglets in several pens to ensure exposure to as wide a range as possible of the virus present in the herd.

The operation of a closed-herd system reduces the risk of introducing extraneous viruses, but it is not possible to eliminate this risk, since the relatively resistant enteric picornaviruses can be transmitted by a variety of fomites. If the introduction of fresh stock is essential for breeding purposes, before the gilts or sows are bred they should be exposed (by fecal contamination as described above) to any virus that may be present or introduced.

Exclusion of porcine enteroviruses or teschoviruses by repopulation of herds with specific pathogen free (SPF) stock seems to be difficult or impossible to achieve over a prolonged period. These viruses have been isolated from commercial SPF herds (Derbyshire et al. 1966) and the accidental introduction of Talfan virus into SPF gilts maintained under strict isolation has been described (Parker et al. 1981). Since transplacental infection of fetuses may occur, even gnotobiotic pigs may be infected.

REFERENCES

Alexander TJ, Betts AO. 1967. Further studies on porcine enteroviruses isolated at Cambridge. II. Serological grouping. Res Vet Sci 8:330–337.

Auerbach J, Prager D, Neuhaus S, Loss U, Witte KH. 1994. Grouping of porcine enteroviruses by indirect immunofluorescence and description of two new serotypes. Zentralbl Veterinarmed B 41:277–282.

Betts AO. 1960. Studies on enteroviruses of the pig—I. The recovery in tissue culture of two related strains of a swine polioencephalomyelitis virus from the tonsils of "normal" pigs. Res Vet Sci 1:57–64.

Bielanski A, Raeside JI. 1977. Plasma concentration of steroid hormones in sows infected experimentally with *Leptospira Pomona* or porcine enterovirus T1 in late gestation. Res Vet Sci 22:28–34.

Brundage LJ, Derbyshire JB, Wilkie BN. 1980. Cell mediated responses in a porcine enterovirus infection in piglets. Can J Comp Med 44:61–69.

Caracappa S, Vesco G, Iannizzotto G, Guercio V, Knowles NJ. 1985. Isolamento ed identificazione di enterovirus suini in Sicilia. Arch Vet Ital 36:167–170.

Cropper M, Dunne HW, Leman AD, Starkey AI, Hoefling DC. 1976. Prevalence of antibodies to porcine enteroviruses and porcine parvovirus in body fluids of fetal pigs from small vs. large litters. J Am Vet Med Assoc 168:233–235.

Dauber M. 1999. Identification of group I porcine enteroviruses by monoclonal antibodies in cell culture. Vet Microbiol 67:1–12.

De Meurichy W, Pensaert M. 1977. Effect of an enterovirus in gilts inseminated with a semen-virus mixture. Zentralbl Veterinarmed B 24:97–103.

De Meurichy W, Pensaert M, Bonte P. 1976. Het SMEDI-syndrome bij het varken: Rol van de enterovirussen en het parvovirus. Vlaams Diergeneeskundig Tijdschrift 45:241–261.

Derbyshire JB. 1983. The effect of immunosuppression with cyclophosphamide on an experimental porcine enterovirus infection in piglets. Can J Comp Med 47:235–237.

Derbyshire JB, Arkell S. 1971. The activity of some chemical disinfectants against Talfan virus and porcine adenovirus type 2. Br Vet J 127:137–142.

Derbyshire JB, Clarke MC, Collins AP. 1966. Observations on the faecal excretion of adenoviruses and enteroviruses in conventional and minimal disease pigs. Vet Rec 79:595–599.

Derbyshire JB, Monteith HD, Shannon EE. 1986. Virological studies on an anaerobic digestion system for liquid manure. Agricultural Wastes 18:309–312.

Doherty M, Todd D, McFerran N, Hoey EM. 1999. Sequence analysis of a porcine enterovirus serotype 1 isolate: Relationships with other picornaviruses. J Gen Virol 80:1929–1941.

Dunne HW, Gobble JL, Hokanson JF, Kradel DC, Bubash GR. 1965. Porcine reproductive failure associated with a newly identified "SMEDI" group of picorna viruses. Am J Vet Res 26:1284–1297.

Dunne HW, Wang JT, Ammerman EH. 1971. Classification of North American porcine enteroviruses: A comparison with European and Japanese strains. Infect Immun 4:619–631.

Hahnefeld H, Hahnefeld E, Wittig W. 1965. Talfan disease der schweine in Deutschland. I. Mitteilung: Isolierung und charakterisierung von Teschenvirus subtyp Talfan bei saugferkeln im bezirk Dresden. Arch Exp Veterinarmed 12:185–218.

Harding JDJ, Done JT, Kershaw GF. 1957. A transmissible polio-encephalomyelitis of pigs (Talfan Disease). Vet Rec 69:824–832.

Hazlett DT, Derbyshire JB. 1977. The protective effect of two porcine enterovirus vaccines in swine. Can J Comp Med 41:264–273.

——. 1978. Broad specificity of gastrointestinal antibodies following vaccination of piglets with a porcine enterovirus. J Comp Pathol 88:467–471.

Holman JE, Koestner A, Kasza L. 1966. Histopathogenesis of porcine polioencephalomyelitis in the germ free pig. Vet Pathol 3:633–651.

Honda E, Hattori I, Oohara Y, Taniguchi T, Ariyama K, Kimata A, Nagamine N, Kumagai T. 1990b. Sero- and CPE-types of porcine enteroviruses isolated from healthy and diarrheal pigs: Possible association of CPE type II with diarrhea. Japanese Journal of Veterinary Science, 52:85–90.

Honda E, Kimata A, Hattori I, Kumagai T, Tsuda T, Tokui T. 1990a. A serological comparison of 4 Japanese isolates of porcine enteroviruses with the international reference strains. Jpn J Vet Sci 52:49–54.

Huang J, Gentry RF, Zarkower A. 1980. Experimental infection of pregnant sows with porcine enteroviruses. Am J Vet Res 41:469–473.

Hubschle OJ, Rajanarison I, Koko M, Rakotondramary E, Rasiofomanana P. 1983. ELISA zur prufung von schweinseren auf antikorper gegen Teschenvirus. Dtsch Tierarztl Wochenschr 90:86–88.

Janke BH, Morehouse LG, Solorzano RF. 1988. Single and mixed infections of neonatal pigs with rotaviruses and enteroviruses: Clinical signs and microscopic lesions. Can J Vet Res 52:364–369.

Kaku Y, Chard LS, Inoue T, Belsham GJ. 2002. Unique characteristics of a picornavirus internal ribosome entry site from the porcine teschovirus-1 Talfan. J Virol 76:11721–11728.

Kaku Y, Sarai A, Murakami Y. 2001. Genetic reclassification of porcine enteroviruses. J Gen Virol 82:417–424.

Kaku Y, Yamada S, Murakami Y. 1999. Sequence determination and phylogenetic analysis of RNA-dependent RNA polymerase (RdRp) of the porcine enterovirus 1 (PEV-1) Talfan strain. Arch Virol 144:1845–1852.

Kanamitsu M, Kasamaki A, Ogawa M, Kasahara S, Inamura M. 1967. Immunofluorescent study on the pathogenesis of oral infection of poliovirus in monkeys. Jpn J Med Sci Biol 20:175–194.

Kasza L. 1965. Swine polioencephalomyelitis viruses isolated from the brains and intestines of pigs. Am J Vet Res 26:131–137.

King AMQ, Brown F, Christian P, Hovi T, Hyypiä T, Knowles NJ, Lemon SM, Minor PD, Palmenberg AC, Skern T, Stanway G. 2000. *Picornaviridae*. In Virus Taxonomy. The Seventh Report of the International Committee on Taxonomy of Viruses. Academic Press, San Diego. MHV van Regenmortel, CM Fauquet, DHL Bishop, CH Calisher, EB Carstens, MH Estes, SM Lemon, J Maniloff, MA Mayo, DJ McGeoch, CR Pringle, RB Wickner, eds. San Diego: Academic Press, pp. 657–673.

Kirkbride CA, McAdaragh JP. 1978. Infectious agents associated with fetal and early neonatal death and abortion in swine. J Am Vet Med Assoc 172:480–483.

Knowles NJ. 1983. Isolation and identification of porcine enteroviruses in Great Britain, 1979 to 1980. Br Vet J 139:19–22.

——. 1988. The association of group III porcine enteroviruses with epithelial tissue. Vet Rec 122:441–442.

Knowles NJ, Buckley LS. 1980. Differentiation of porcine enterovirus serotypes by complement fixation. Res Vet Sci 29:113–115.

Knowles NJ, Buckley LS, Pereira HG. 1979. Classification of porcine enteroviruses by antigenic analysis and cytopathic effects in tissue culture: Description of 3 new serotypes. Arch Virol 62:201–208.

Koestner A, Kasza L, Holman JE. 1966. Electron microscopic evaluation of the pathogenesis of porcine polioencephalomyelitis. Am J Pathol 49:325–337.

Krumbholz A, Dauber M, Henke A, Birch-Hirschfeld E, Knowles NJ, Stelzner A, Zell R. 2002. Sequencing of porcine enterovirus groups II and III reveals unique features of both virus groups. J Virol 76:5813–5821.

Krumbholz A, Wurm R, Scheck O, Birch-Hirschfeld E, Egerer R, Henke A, Wutzler P, Zell R. 2003. Detection of porcine teschoviruses and enteroviruses by LightCycler real-time PCR. J Virol Methods 113:51–63.

Lamont PH, Betts AO. 1960. Studies on enteroviruses of the pig—IV. The isolation in tissue culture of a possible enteric cytopathogenic swine orphan (ECSO) virus (V13) from the faeces of a pig. Res Vet Sci 1:152–159.

Lieu CI. 1976. The experimental infection of pregnant guinea pigs with porcine enterovirus: "SMEDI A" virus. Taiwan Journal of Medicine and Animal Husbandry 28:1–14.

Long JF. 1985. Pathogenesis of porcine polioencephalomyelitis. In Comparative Pathology of Viral Diseases (Volume 1). RA Olsen, S Krakowka, JR Blakeslee, eds. Boca Raton, Florida: CRC Press, Inc., pp. 179–197.

Long JF, Kasza L, Koestner A. 1969. Pericarditis and myocarditis in germfree and colostrum-deprived pigs experimentally infected with a porcine polioencephalomyelitis virus. J Infect Dis 120:245–249.

Lund E, Nissen B. 1983. The survival of enteroviruses in aerated and unaerated cattle and pig slurry. Agricultural Wastes 7:221–223.

Lynch JA, Binnington BD, Hoover DM. 1984. Virus isolation studies in an outbreak of porcine encephalomyelitis. Can J Comp Med 48:233–235.

Mayr A, Correns, H. 1959. Experimentelle Untersuchungen über Lebend- und Totimpfstoffe aus einem modifizierten Gewebekulturstamm des Teschenvirus (poliomyelitis suum). Zentralbl Veterinarmed B 6:416–428.

Métianu T. 1986. La maladie de Teschen-Talfan en France. Bulletin de l'Académie vétérinaire de France 59:291–302.

Meyer RC, Woods GT, Simon J. 1966. Pneumonitis in an enterovirus infection in swine. J Comp Pathol 76:397–405.

Oberste MS, Maher K, Pallansch MA. 2003. Genomic evidence that simian virus 2 and six other simian picornaviruses represent a new genus in *Picornaviridae*. Virology 314:283–293.

Odend'hal S. 1983. The Geographical Distribution of Animal Virus Diseases. Academic Press, New York. p. 415.

Office International des Epizooties. 2004. Enterovirus Encephalomyelitis. Chapter 2.6.3 in Manual of Diagnostic Tests and Vaccines for Terrestrial Animals. http://www.oie.int/eng/normes/mmanual/A_summry.htm.

Ottis K. 1976. Verleichende Untersuchungen über die Tenazitat von Viren in Trink- und Oberflächenwasser. Inaug. diss., Munich.

Palmquist JM, Munir S, Taku A, Kapur V, Goyal SM. 2002. Detection of porcine teschovirus and enterovirus type II by reverse transcription-polymerase chain reaction. J Vet Diagn Invest 14:476–480.

Parker BN, Wrathall AE, Cartwright SF. 1981. Accidental introduction of porcine parvovirus and Talfan virus into a group of minimal disease gilts and their effects on reproduction. Br Vet J 137:262–267.

Phillips RM, Foley CW, Lukert PD. 1972. Isolation and characterization of viruses from semen and the reproductive tract of male swine. J Am Vet Med Assoc 161:1306–1316.

Pisarev AV, Chard LS, Kaku Y, Johns HL, Shatsky IN, Belsham GJ. 2004. Functional and structural similarities between the internal ribosome entry sites of hepatitis C virus and porcine teschovirus, a picornavirus. J Virol 78:4487–4497.

Plagemann PGW. 1996. Lactate dehydrogenase-elevating virus and related viruses. In Fields Virology (3rd edition). BN Fields, DM Knipe, PM Howley, eds. New York: Raven Press, pp. 1105–1120.

Pogranichniy RM, Janke BH, Gillespie TG, Yoon KJ. 2003. A prolonged outbreak of polioencephalomyelitis due to infection with a group I porcine enterovirus. J Vet Diagn Invest 15:191–194.

Pospisil Z, Gois M, Veznikova D, Cerny M. 1971. The pathogenesis of experimental infection of gnotobiotic piglets with enterovirus strain Kr 69TK. Acta Veterinaria Brno 40(Suppl 2):43–46.

Rueckert RR, Wimmer E. 1984. Systematic nomenclature of picornavirus proteins. J Virol 50:957–959.

Schaupp W. 1968. Eradication of contagious paralysis (Teschen disease) in Austria. Wien Tierarztl Monatsschr 55:346–356.

Simon J, Mocsari E, Digleria M, Felkai V. 1983. Effect of radiation on certain animal viruses in liquid swine manure. Int J Appl Radiat Isot 34:793–795.

Singh KV, Bohl EH. 1972. The pattern of enteroviral infections in a herd of swine. Can J Comp Med 36:243–248.

Smith IM, Betts AO, Watt RG, Hayward AH. 1973. Experimental infections with *Pasteurella septica* (sero-group A) and an adeno- or enterovirus in gnotobiotic piglets. J Comp Pathol 83:1–12.

Sulochana S, Derbyshire JB. 1978. Use of indirect immunoperoxidase test for detection of porcine enteroviral antigens in infected PK15 cell cultures. Kerala Journal of Veterinary Science 9:111–119.

Watanabe H, Pospisil Z, Mensik J. 1971. Infection of colostrum-deprived baby pigs with a porcine enterovirus (Kr 69TC strain) isolated from the lung. Jpn J Vet Res 19:107–112.

Yamada M, Kozakura R, Ikegami R, Nakamura K, Kaku Y, Yoshii M, Haritani M. 2004. Enterovirus encephalomyelitis in pigs in Japan caused by porcine teschovirus. Vet Rec 155:304–306.

Zell R, Dauber M, Krumbholz A, Henke A, Birch-Hirschfeld E, Stelzner A, Prager D, Wurm R. 2001. Porcine teschoviruses comprise at least eleven distinct serotypes: Molecular and evolutionary aspects. J Virol 75:1620–1631.

Zell R, Krumbholz A, Henke A, Birch-Hirschfeld E, Stelzner A, Doherty M, Hoey E, Dauber M, Prager D, Wurm R. 2000. Detection of porcine enteroviruses by nRT-PCR: Differentiation of CPE groups I–III with specific primer sets. J Virol Methods 88:205–218.

Zoletto, R. 1965. Caratteristiche differenzialii degli enterovirus suini. Veterinaria Italiana 16:3–20.

Zoletto R, Kadoi K, Turilli C, Cancelloti F, Stilas B. 1974. Cytopathic effect and physico chemical characteristics of swine vesicular disease virus and its relationship with other swine enteroviruses. Proc 3rd Congr Int Pig Vet Soc. Lyon, France, June 12-14, 1974.

19 Porcine Enteric Caliciviruses and Astroviruses

Janice C. Bridger and Nick J. Knowles

Porcine enteric caliciviruses were first recognized when diarrheic feces from postweaning and nursing pigs in the United Kingdom and the United States were examined by electron microscopy (Bridger 1980; Saif et al. 1980). Porcine enteric caliciviruses have not been widely studied and much is unknown concerning their role in naturally occurring swine disease. This is in contrast to the recognized role of caliciviruses in human gastroenteritis (Green et al. 2001). Likewise, research is establishing a role for caliciviruses of the *Norovirus* genus in enteric disease of cattle (Deng et al. 2003; Oliver et al. 2003; Smiley et al. 2003; Wise et al. 2004). Thus, based on their role as disease agents in other species, it may be postulated that caliciviruses play a significant role in porcine enteric disease. Based on the limited data available, there is no evidence that porcine enteric caliciviruses pose a threat to human health.

ETIOLOGY

Human enteric caliciviruses belong to two genera, *Norovirus* (formerly Norwalk-like) and *Sapovirus* (formerly Sapporo-like), in the family *Caliciviridae* (Mayo 2002). Both are common causes of human gastroenteritis. Caliciviruses belonging to both the *Norovirus* and *Sapovirus* genera have also been identified in pigs.

Porcine sapoviruses have been studied the most, but only one isolate (PEC/Cowden) has been studied in any detail (Flynn and Saif 1988; Flynn et al. 1988; Guo et al. 1999; Guo et al. 2001a; Parwani et al. 1990; Saif et al. 1980). PEC/Cowden shows typical calicivirus morphology with clear cup-shaped depressions (Figure 19.1). The virus is approximately 35 nm in diameter and has an RNA genome of 7,320 base pairs organized into two open reading frames, similar to the human sapoviruses and lagoviruses. The highest amino acid identities were with the sapoviruses, with which it grouped phylogenetically, but PEC/Cowden was assigned to genogroup III, a new genogroup distinct from the human sapoviruses (Schuffenecker et al. 2001; Figure 19.2).

Consistent with all other caliciviruses, PEC/Cowden has one major structural capsid protein with a molecular weight of 58 kilodaltons. Antigenic relationships to nonenteric caliciviruses have not been well studied, but PEC/Cowden and a likely porcine sapovirus identified in the United Kingdom were antigenically unrelated to vesicular exanthema of swine virus and feline caliciviruses (Bridger 1980; Saif et al. 1980). Nothing is known about genetic or antigenic variation among porcine sapoviruses because only one isolate has been studied in detail.

The PEC/Cowden sapovirus may be cultured on primary porcine kidney cells and a continuous porcine kidney cell line (LLC-PK), but only by inclusion of intestinal contents in the culture medium (Flynn and Saif 1988; Parwani et al. 1991). It is the only enteric calicivirus to be cultured to date. Bile acids were identified as the active factor that allowed cultivation by affecting the protein kinase A cell signaling pathway (Chang et al. 2002; Chang et al. 2004).

Less is known about porcine noroviruses. A virus with an indistinct morphology was reported in the United Kingdom (Bridger 1980), and six partial gene sequences with close similarity to each other and to human noroviruses have been demonstrated in pigs in the Netherlands and Japan (Sugieda et al. 1998; Sugieda and Nakajima 2002; van Der Poel et al. 2000; Figure 19.2). Phylogenetic analysis grouped the porcine sequences with the genogroup II human noroviruses, but they formed a separate genetic cluster distinct from human noroviruses. Additional data will be required to determine whether human and porcine noroviruses are genetically distinct and whether humans and pigs might share noroviruses. Porcine noroviruses have not been cultured and nothing is known about their physicochemical and other biological properties.

EPIDEMIOLOGY

Porcine enteric caliciviruses have been identified in the United States (Guo et al. 1999; Saif et al. 1980), United

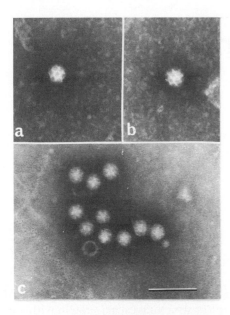

19.1. *Negative stain electron microscopy. Panels A and B: the sapovirus virion has a typical calicivirus morphology with clear cup-shaped depressions and measures approximately 35 nm in diameter. Panel C: the 30 nm diameter, non-enveloped astrovirus particles are distinctive in appearance with some particles showing a 5- or 6-pointed star pattern on their surface. (From Veterinary Record 1980 107:532-533 with permission.)*

Kingdom (Bridger 1980), the Netherlands (van Der Poel et al. 2000), Hungary (Nagy et al. 1996), and Japan (Shirai et al. 1985; Sugieda et al. 1998; Sugieda and Nakajima 2002). The virus identified in the United States was typed as a sapovirus; in the Netherlands and Japan as a norovirus; and in the United Kingdom and Hungary, it was not genetically typed.

The one prevalence study conducted to examine porcine sapoviruses related to PEC/Cowden showed that at least 83% of 30 sow serum samples from Ohio pig herds with PEC-associated postweaning diarrhea had antibodies reactive to PEC/Cowden (Guo et al. 2001b).

Two porcine norovirus prevalence studies have been reported. In Japan, 4 samples were reverse transcription-polymerase chain reaction (RT-PCR) positive among 1,117 cecal content samples collected from healthy pigs on 26 farms in 1997 (Sugieda and Nakajima 2002). In the Netherlands (1998–1999), 2 samples were RT-PCR positive among 100 pooled fecal samples collected from 3–9-month-old pigs on 100 farms (van Der Poel et al. 2000). These studies are likely to have underestimated the prevalence of porcine norovirus infections because PCR primers designed for human noroviruses were used and because investigators did not select for pre- and postweaning diarrheic piglets.

Little is known regarding porcine enteric caliciviruses and natural disease. A study in Hungary found no association with diarrhea when diarrheic and nondi-

arrheic weaned and unweaned pigs were examined for evidence of porcine calicivirus infection by electron microscopy (Nagy et al. 1996).

It is assumed that natural enteric calicivirus transmission is fecal-oral. Whether porcine enteric caliciviruses are species-specific has not been established. It has been postulated that the close genetic similarity of porcine noroviruses and human noroviruses indicates zoonotic potential (Sugieda and Nakajima 2002; van Der Poel et al. 2000).

PATHOGENESIS

Experimental infections with the porcine sapovirus PEC/Cowden produced enteric lesions and disease (Flynn et al. 1988; Guo et al. 2001a). Unusual for a viral enteric pathogen, disease and small intestinal lesions in the duodenum and jejunum resulted from intravenous inoculation of PEC/Cowden, as well as by oral exposure. Viral replication in enterocytes was demonstrated by immunofluorescence with anti-PEC/Cowden antiserum. Calicivirus particles were demonstrated in intestinal contents and in the blood stream, the first time viremia has been associated with an enteric calicivirus. The mechanism by which the virus reached the small intestine and villous enterocytes from the blood stream was not determined. When infected by the oral route, fecal shedding of the sapovirus PEC/Cowden occurred for up to 9 days. When infected by the intravenous route, fecal shedding was observed for at least 8 days.

Experimental infections with porcine noroviruses have not been reported.

CLINICAL SIGNS

With PEC/Cowden, the one strain of porcine sapovirus that has been studied, the incubation period ranged from 2–4 days after oral infection and clinical signs of diarrhea persisted for 3–7 days (Flynn et al. 1988; Guo et al. 2001a). All inoculated pigs became infected and developed clinical signs ranging from mild to severe diarrhea. Control pigs and pigs infected with tissue culture-adapted PEC failed to develop clinical signs, although intestinal lesions were observed in the exposed pigs.

There are no reports of experimental studies with porcine noroviruses.

LESIONS

Infection with PEC/Cowden produced lesions indistinguishable from those produced by other enteric viral pathogens, such as rotaviruses (Flynn et al. 1988; Guo et al. 2001a). Lesions included shortening, blunting, fusion or absence of duodenal and jejunal villi and, by scanning electron microscopy, an irregular microvillous coat on enterocytes. Crypt cell hyperplasia and a reduc-

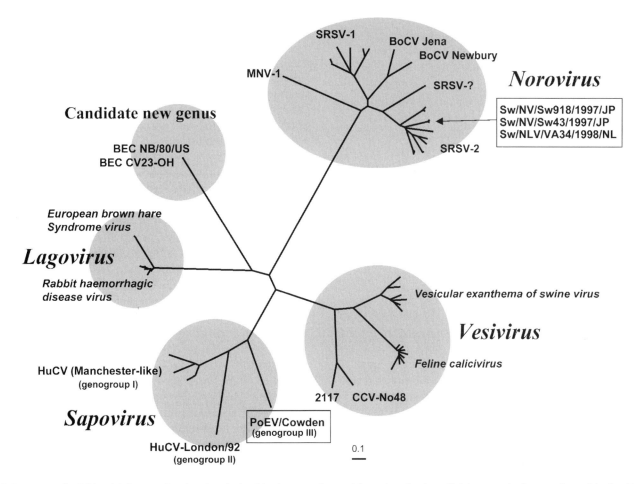

19.2.   *Unrooted neighbor-joining tree showing the relationships between the capsid proteins of swine caliciviruses and other members of the family. Swine caliciviruses are boxed. Members of the four accepted genera (Vesivirus, Lagovirus, Norovirus,* and Sapovirus) *and one candidate genus are within the shaded areas.*

tion of villus/crypt ratios occurred with cytoplasmic vacuolation and infiltration of polymorphonuclear and mononuclear cells into the lamina propria.

IMMUNITY

Immune responses against porcine sapoviruses and noroviruses, protective immunity, and/or the role of maternal antibodies have not been assessed. It may be assumed that protective immune mechanisms are similar to those for other enteric virus pathogens, although the recognition of an extraintestinal phase to the pathogenesis of a porcine sapovirus suggests that other immune strategies might be used in their control. Porcine sapovirus and norovirus infections in pigs may potentially provide useful insights into protective immunity of the equivalent viruses of humans.

DIAGNOSIS

No diagnostic tests for porcine sapoviruses or noroviruses have been developed for use outside the research

laboratory. An antigen and antibody ELISA was developed and used to study PEC/Cowden (Guo et al. 2001b). Porcine noroviruses have been detected using RT-PCR (Sugieda et al. 1998; Sugieda and Nakajima 2002; van Der Poel et al. 2000).

PREVENTION AND CONTROL

Assuming that porcine sapovirus and norovirus epidemiology and immunology are similar to porcine rotaviruses, it is likely that these viruses persist in the environment and that sows pass maternal antibodies in colostrum and milk that limit enteric infection and disease in neonates. Likewise, if these viruses are similar to porcine rotaviruses, it is probably impossible to eliminate infection from pig herds and/or prevent natural infection of piglets. In the case of severely affected pigs, oral rehydration with fluids is likely to be successful.

Porcine Astroviruses

INTRODUCTION

Porcine astroviruses were first recognized when diarrheic feces were examined by electron microscopy (Bridger 1980; Geyer et al. 1994; Shimizu et al. 1990). Their causal role in porcine enteric disease remains undetermined. In some species—for example, humans and sheep—astroviruses have been linked to enteric disease (Matsui and Greenberg 2001), but bovine astroviruses failed to cause clinical disease when inoculated into calves (Woode and Bridger 1978; Woode et al. 1984).

ETIOLOGY

Porcine astroviruses are members of the family *Astroviridae* which is divided into two genera, *Mamastrovirus* (astroviruses of mammals) and *Avastrovirus* (astroviruses of birds). Approximately 30 nm diameter and nonenveloped, astrovirus particles are distinctive in appearance, with some particles showing a 5- or 6-pointed star surface pattern when viewed by negative stain electron microscopy (Figure 19.1; Bridger 1980; Shimizu et al. 1990). Not all particles show this distinctive appearance, and care is needed so as not to confuse them with the indistinct appearance of noroviruses, particularly in the presence of antibody.

The genome is composed of positive sense, single-stranded RNA 6.8 to 7.9 kilobases in length composed of three open reading frames (Matsui and Greenberg 2001). Two porcine astroviruses from Japan have been partially sequenced (Jonassen et al. 2001; Lukashov and Goudsmit 2002; Wang et al. 2001). Phylogenetic analyses grouped human and porcine astroviruses closely together, whereas astroviruses from sheep and avian species were less related to human astroviruses (Figure 19.3). There is evidence that astroviruses from different animal species are antigenically distinct (Matsui and Greenberg 2001). For example, antibodies against porcine astroviruses do not react with bovine astroviruses.

Porcine astroviruses have not been widely studied. In Japan, a cytopathic astrovirus from diarrheic pigs was successfully isolated on a porcine kidney cell line by incorporating trypsin into the medium (Shimizu et al. 1990). Immunofluorescent cells and astrovirus particles were detected. A virus with a buoyant density of 1.35 g/ml was cloned and a serum-virus neutralization test developed. The isolate was stable to treatment with lipid solvents and resisted heating at 56°C for 30 minutes, but showed some lability to acid treatment at pH 3.0. Five structural proteins with molecular masses 13–39 kilodaltons were identified. At present, the number of astrovirus structural proteins is uncertain and has varied in

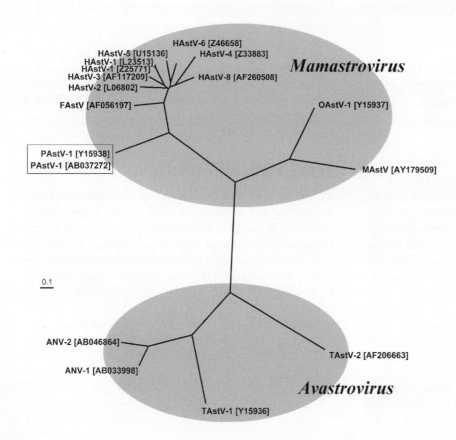

19.3. *Unrooted neighbor-joining tree showing the relationships between the capsid proteins of swine astroviruses and other members of the family. Swine astroviruses are boxed. Members of the two accepted genera (Mamastrovirus and* Avastrovirus) *are within the shaded areas.*

studies with astroviruses from different animal species (Matsui and Greenberg 2001).

EPIDEMIOLOGY

Porcine astroviruses have been identified in feces of pigs in the United Kingdom (Bridger 1980), Japan (Shimizu et al. 1990), and South Africa (Geyer et al. 1994). In a serological survey in Japan, 39% of 128 pigs in 8 herds had serum neutralizing antibodies to porcine astroviruses (Shimizu et al. 1990). All but one herd had antibody and the in-herd prevalence ranged from 7–83%. Transmission is presumed to be fecal-oral.

A study of evolutionary genomic relationships showed that human and animal astroviruses belonged to distinct genomic clusters (Jonassen et al. 2001; Lukashov and Goudsmit 2002; Figure 19.3). However, the genetic data supported the hypothesis that two cross-species transmission events involving pigs, cats, and humans, possibly through intermediate hosts, may have occurred in the past.

Cross-species infectivity of porcine astroviruses has not been demonstrated, and astroviruses are believed to be species-specific.

PATHOGENESIS, CLINICAL SIGNS, LESIONS, IMMUNITY

Porcine astroviruses have been associated with severe diarrhea in natural infections, but only in the presence of other known enteric pathogens (Bridger 1980; Shimizu et al. 1990). Mild diarrhea developed in 4-day-old pigs after oral inoculation with porcine astroviruses grown in cell culture (Shimizu et al. 1990). Diarrhea commenced 1 day after inoculation and continued for 5–6 days. Cytopathic astrovirus was recovered from feces and pigs seroconverted. Intestinal pathology was not studied, but it is reasonable to hypothesize that astroviruses might contribute to the intestinal pathology and clinical signs commonly observed in pre- and postweaning diarrhea. Nothing is known about antigenic differences between porcine astroviruses or the immunity induced by infection with astrovirus.

DIAGNOSIS

Diagnostic assays have not been developed for routine diagnosis, but methods such as isolation on cell culture and identification with immunofluorescence and RT-PCR can be used to diagnose natural porcine astrovirus infection. The serum-virus neutralization and immunofluorescent antibody assays can be used to demonstrate seroconversion (Shimizu et al. 1990).

PREVENTION AND CONTROL

Porcine astroviruses may be just one of several viruses that contribute to pre- and postweaning diarrhea. Elimination of astroviruses from infected farms would be difficult to achieve because of their resistance in the environment. In addition, such an effort would be difficult to justify on the basis of their clinical effects. Assuming that astrovirus pathology is confined to the intestinal tract, oral rehydration would be expected to be effective in affected pigs. There are no commercially available vaccines.

REFERENCES

Bridger JC. 1980. Detection by electron microscopy of caliciviruses, astroviruses and rotavirus-like particles in the faeces of piglets with diarrhoea. Vet Rec 107:532–533.

Chang KO, Kim Y, Green KY, Saif LJ. 2002. Cell-culture propagation of porcine enteric calicivirus mediated by intestinal contents is dependent on the cyclic AMP signaling pathway. Virology 304:302–310.

Chang KO, Sosnovtsev SV, Belliot G, Kim Y, Saif LJ, Green KY. 2004. Bile acids are essential for porcine enteric calicivirus replication in association with down-regulation of signal transducer and activator of transcription 1. Proc Natl Acad Sci USA 101:8733–8738.

Deng Y, Batten CA, Liu BL, Lambden PR, Elschner M, Gunther H, Otto P, Schnurch P, Eichhorn W, Herbst W, Clarke IN. 2003. Studies of epidemiology and seroprevalence of bovine noroviruses in Germany. J Clin Microbiol 41:2300–2305.

Flynn WT, Saif LJ. 1988. Serial propagation of porcine enteric calicivirus-like virus in primary porcine kidney cell cultures. J Clin Microbiol 26:206–212.

Flynn WT, Saif LJ, Moorhead PD. 1988. Pathogenesis of porcine enteric calicivirus-like virus in four-day-old gnotobiotic pigs. Am J Vet Res 49:819–825.

Geyer A, Steele AD, Peenze I, Lecatsas G. 1994. Astrovirus-like particles, adenoviruses and rotaviruses associated with diarrhoea in piglets. J S Afr Vet Med Assoc 65:164–166.

Green KY, Chanock RM, Kapikian AZ. 2001. Human caliciviruses. In Fields Virology (4th edition). DM Knipe, PM Howley, DE Griffin, RA Lamb, MA Martin, B Roizman, SE Straus, eds. Philadelphia: Lippincott Williams and Wilkins, pp. 841–784.

Guo M, Chang KO, Hardy ME, Zhang Q, Parwani AV, Saif LJ. 1999. Molecular characterization of a porcine enteric calicivirus genetically related to Sapporo-like human caliciviruses. J Virol 73:9625–9631.

Guo M, Hayes J, Cho KO, Parwani AV, Lucas LM, Saif LJ. 2001a. Comparative pathogenesis of tissue culture-adapted and wild-type Cowden porcine enteric calicivirus (PEC) in gnotobiotic pigs and induction of diarrhea by intravenous inoculation of wild-type PEC. J Virol 75:9239–9251.

Guo M, Qian Y, Chang KO, Saif LJ. 2001b. Expression and self-assembly in baculovirus of porcine enteric calicivirus capsids into virus-like particles and their use in an enzyme-linked immunosorbent assay for antibody detection in swine. J Clin Microbiol 39:1487–1493.

Jonassen CM, Jonassen TO, Saif YM, Snodgrass DR, Ushijima H, Shimizu M, Grinde B. 2001. Comparison of capsid sequences from human and animal astroviruses. J Gen Virol 82:1061–1067.

Lukashov VV, Goudsmit J. 2002. Evolutionary relationships among Astroviridae. J Gen Virol 83:1397–1405.

Matsui SM, Greenberg HB. 2001. Astroviruses. In Fields Virology. DM Knipe, PM Howley, DE Griffin, RA Lamb, MA Martin, B Roizman, SE Straus, eds. Philadelphia: Lippincott Williams and Wilkins, pp. 875–893.

Mayo MA. 2002. A summary of taxonomic changes recently approved by ICTV. Arch Virol 147:1655–1663.

Nagy B, Nagy G, Meder M, Mocsari E. 1996. Enterotoxigenic Escherichia coli, rotavirus, porcine epidemic diarrhoea virus, adenovirus and calici-like virus in porcine postweaning diarrhoea in Hungary. Acta Vet Hung 44:9–19.

Oliver SL, Dastjerdi AM, Wong S, El-Attar L, Gallimore C, Brown DW, Green J, Bridger JC. 2003. Molecular characterization of bovine enteric caliciviruses: A distinct third genogroup of noróviruses (Norwalk-like viruses) unlikely to be of risk to humans. J Virol 77:2789–2798.

Parwani AV, Flynn WT, Gadfield KL, Saif LJ. 1991. Serial propagation of porcine enteric calicivirus in a continuous cell line. Effect of medium supplementation with intestinal contents or enzymes. Arch Virol 120:115–122.

Parwani AV, Saif LJ, Kang SY. 1990. Biochemical characterization of porcine enteric calicivirus: Analysis of structural and nonstructural viral proteins. Arch Virol 112:41–53.

Saif LJ, Bohl EH, Theil KW, Cross RF, House JA. 1980. Rotavirus-like, calicivirus-like, and 23-nm virus-like particles associated with diarrhea in young pigs. J Clin Microbiol 12:105–111.

Schuffenecker I, Ando T, Thouvenot D, Lina B, Aymard M. 2001. Genetic classification of "Sapporo-like viruses." Arch Virol 146:2115–2132.

Shimizu M, Shirai J, Narita M, Yamane T. 1990. Cytopathic astrovirus isolated from porcine acute gastroenteritis in an established cell line derived from porcine embryonic kidney. J Clin Microbiol 28:201–206.

Shirai J, Shimizu M, Fukusho A. 1985. Coronavirus-, calicivirus-, and astrovirus-like particles associated with acute porcine gastroenteritis. Nippon Juigaku Zasshi 47:1023–1026.

Smiley JR, Hoet AE, Traven M, Tsunemitsu H, Saif LJ. 2003. Reverse transcription-PCR assays for detection of bovine enteric caliciviruses (BEC) and analysis of the genetic relationships among BEC and human caliciviruses. J Clin Microbiol 41:3089–3099.

Sugieda M, Nagaoka H, Kakishima Y, Ohshita T, Nakamura S, Nakajima S. 1998. Detection of Norwalk-like virus genes in the caecum contents of pigs. Arch Virol 143:1215–1221.

Sugieda M, Nakajima S. 2002. Viruses detected in the caecum contents of healthy pigs representing a new genetic cluster in genogroup II of the genus "Norwalk-like viruses." Virus Res 87:165–172.

van Der Poel WH, Vinje J, van Der Heide R, Herrera MI, Vivo A, Koopmans MP. 2000. Norwalk-like calicivirus genes in farm animals. Emerg Infect Dis 6:36–41.

Wang QH, Kakizawa J, Wen LY, Shimizu M, Nishio O, Fang ZY, Ushijima H. 2001. Genetic analysis of the capsid region of astroviruses. J Med Virol 64:245–255.

Wise AG, Monroe SS, Hanson LE, Grooms DL, Sockett D, Maes RK. 2004. Molecular characterization of noroviruses detected in diarrheic stools of Michigan and Wisconsin dairy calves: Circulation of two distinct subgroups. Virus Res 100:165–177.

Woode GN, Bridger JC. 1978. Isolation of small viruses resembling astroviruses and caliciviruses from acute enteritis of calves. J Med Microbiol 11:441–452.

Woode GN, Pohlenz JF, Gourley NE, Fagerland JA. 1984. Astrovirus and Breda virus infections of dome cell epithelium of bovine ileum. J Clin Microbiol 19:623–630.

20 Hemagglutinating Encephalomyelitis Virus

Maurice B. Pensaert

In 1962, a previously unrecognized viral pathogen was isolated in Canada from the brains of suckling pigs with encephalomyelitis (Greig et al. 1962). The virus responsible for this disease was named hemagglutinating encephalomyelitis virus (HEV) and was later classified as a coronavirus (Greig et al. 1971). In 1969, an antigenically identical virus was isolated in England from suckling pigs showing anorexia, depression, and vomiting, but without clear signs of encephalomyelitis (Cartwright et al. 1969). Animals that did not die remained stunted in growth; the condition was therefore called "vomiting and wasting disease" (VWD). Mengeling and Cutlip (1976) were later able to experimentally reproduce both forms of the disease using the same field isolates. Although epidemiologic studies have revealed that infection of swine with HEV is prevalent, naturally occurring disease is uncommon. Neonatal pigs are usually protected by passively acquired colostral antibody, and they subsequently develop an age-related resistance to the potential clinical effects of the virus. Therefore, studies on virus-animal interactions have been scarce in recent years.

ETIOLOGY

HEV belongs to group 2 of the family *Coronaviridae*, a group characterized by the presence of a gene encoding for the hemagglutinin-esterase (HE) protein (Gonzalez et al. 2003). Other members of group 2 include bovine coronavirus (BCV), human respiratory coronavirus OC43 (HCV-OC43), and mouse hepatitis virus (MHV).

Nucleotide sequence analysis of the region covering the S2 probe revealed 92.6% nucleotide sequence homology to BCV and 91.9% to HCV-OC43 (Vieler et al. 1995). An antigenic relationship between HEV and BCV was shown by virus neutralization (VN), hemagglutination-inhibition (HI), immunofluorescence, and immuno-electron microscopy. Moderate cross-reactivity was observed between HEV and turkey enteric coronavirus (Dea and Tijssen 1989). Although HEV is known to be the cause of two distinct clinical syndromes in pigs, only one serotype of the virus is known to exist.

Under electron microscopy, HEV's appearance is similar to other coronaviruses. Negatively stained particles are spherical in shape, with an overall diameter of 120 nm (Greig et al. 1971). Club-shaped surface projections arranged as a solar "corona" protrude from the envelope. Lamontagne et al. (1981) showed that the viral particle contains two concentric membranes—an external envelope and an inner membranous bag—encircling a central core. Virus particles can be seen by electron microscopy in cytoplasmic vesicles of infected cells. Assembly occurs by budding through membranes of the endoplasmic reticulum (Ducatelle et al. 1981).

Studies on the chemical composition of HEV revealed that the virus contains RNA and five polypeptides, four of which are glycosylated, with molecular weights from 31,000–180,000 daltons (Callebaut and Pensaert 1980; Greig and Girard 1969; Pocock and Garwes 1977). The buoyant density was 1.21 g/ml in cesium chloride (Mengeling and Coria 1972) and 1.18 g/ml in potassium tartrate (Greig and Bouillant 1972).

HEV is stable between pH 4 and 10. All viral infectivity is lost after 30 minutes at 56°C, but the titer of infectious virus is reduced by only 0.8 $\log_{10}$ after 7 days at 4°C. HEV was shown by Greig and Girard (1969) to be sensitive to lipid solvents, including sodium desoxycholate.

HEV was first isolated in primary cultures of pig kidney (PK) cells by Greig et al. (1962), who described a cytopathic effect (CPE) characterized by the appearance of syncytia. An immunofluorescence test showed that HEV was also able to propagate in several other porcine cell cultures, including adult thyroid gland, embryonic lung, testicle cell line, PK-15 cell line (Pirtle 1974), IBRS$_2$ cell line (Chappuis et al. 1975), SK cell line (Lucas and Napthine 1971), SK-K cell line (Hirano et al. 1990), and swine embryo kidney cell line KSEK6 (Kadoi et al. 1994). Non-porcine cell cultures have little susceptibility for growth of HEV.

HEV possesses two virion-associated hemagglutinins: the hemagglutinin-esterase (HE) and the S protein (Sasseville et al. 2002; Schultze and Herrler 1993). The virus spontaneously agglutinates erythrocytes of mice, rats, chickens, and several other species of animals (Girard et al. 1964). Elution of HEV from red blood cells has not been observed. These erythrocytes can be used in a hemadsorption test to demonstrate viral growth in inoculated cell cultures.

The natural host of HEV is the pig, but the virus has been adapted experimentally to replicate in mice (Kaye et al. 1977; Yagami et al. 1986) and Wistar rats (Hirano et al. 1993). The virus is neurotropic in mice, but susceptibility was found to be influenced by age and route of inoculation (Yagami et al. 1993). In contrast, 4-week-old Wistar rats died of encephalitis after inoculation of HEV via different routes (Hirano et al. 1993).

EPIDEMIOLOGY

Pigs are the only species known to be naturally susceptible to HEV infection. Most of the infections in this species are subclinical and the economic impact of the disease is low.

The distribution of HEV in the pig population has been studied in several countries. The HI and VN tests proved to be almost equally sensitive for detection of HEV antibodies in swine sera (Mengeling 1975), but the VN test is more specific (Sasaki et al. 2003). Serologic surveys revealed that infection of swine with HEV is very common and probably worldwide. In fattening pigs, 31% of the sera were positive in Canada (Girard et al. 1964), 46% in Northern Ireland (McFerran et al. 1971), 49% in England (Cartwright and Lucas 1970), 52–82% in Japan (Hirai et al. 1974; Hirano and Ono 1998), 75% in Germany (Hess and Bachmann 1978), and 0–89% in the United States, depending on the region surveyed (Mengeling 1975). The percentage of sows with antibodies at slaughter varied from 43% in Northern Ireland to 98% in the United States. A high number of seropositive animals were also found in Denmark (Sorensen 1975), France (Vannier et al. 1981), Australia (Forman et al. 1979), Belgium (Pensaert et al. 1980), and Austria (Mostl 1990). Conversely, Neuvonen et al. (1982) found that 40 Finnish elite breeding pig herds were free of seropositive animals.

HEV was isolated from the respiratory tract of pigs with respiratory illness in Japan in 1984 (Hirahara et al. 1987). The first isolation of HEV in Taiwan was from 30–50-day-old pigs with signs of central nervous disease (Chang et al. 1993).

Under experimental conditions, disease has been reproduced in most instances in which nonimmune pigs were exposed oronasally to HEV during the first few weeks of life (Alexander 1962; Appel et al. 1965). Clinical signs may vary, however. In a study in which the virulence of several HEV field isolates was compared, the severity of signs was related to a difference in host susceptibility (even among littermates), as well as to the apparent virulence of each isolate (Mengeling and Cutlip 1976). In contrast, older pigs and neonatal pigs that had received antibody in colostrum were usually clinically unaffected when exposed to HEV under otherwise similar conditions (Appel et al. 1965).

These observations are believed to explain why naturally occurring disease is relatively uncommon, even though HEV is ubiquitous among swine. That is, in herds where HEV infection is endemic, most pigs receive protective antibody in colostrum, and circulating maternal antibodies persist for 4–18 (mean 10.5) weeks (Paul and Mengeling 1984). By the time maternal antibody wanes, the pigs have already developed an age-related resistance to the disease. Additional support for this concept is provided by a serologic study on two Belgian breeding farms, which showed that passively acquired colostral immunity was replaced by active immunity as a consequence of subclinical infection of pigs between 8 and 16 weeks of age (Pensaert et al. 1980).

Outbreaks of HEV-associated disease are now rarely described in the literature. In a relatively recent outbreak, HEV was isolated from newborn and early-weaned pigs with vomiting and posterior paralysis on a Canadian farm (Sasseville et al. 2001). Remarkably, this recent isolate showed a high degree of genetic and antigenic homology with the 1962 reference strain HEV-67N (Sasseville et al. 2002).

CLINICAL SIGNS

Infection with HEV can produce two clinical syndromes: an acute, clinically apparent encephalomyelitis and vomiting and wasting disease (VWD). Both syndromes are primarily confined to pigs less than 3 weeks of age, although older swine may occasionally vomit and exhibit a brief period of inappetence, listlessness, and nervous signs. Encephalomyelitis caused by HEV was diagnosed in 30–50-day-old pigs in Taiwan (Chang et al. 1993). Prior to the Taiwanese report, the typical encephalomyelitic form had only been described in Canada (Alexander et al. 1959) and the United States (Werdin et al. 1976). Both the nervous and VWD syndromes have many clinical signs in common and varying degrees of severity may be seen, from acute encephalomyelitis to chronic VWD.

Sneezing or coughing may occur at the start of a VWD outbreak. After an incubation period of 4–7 days, the primary sign is repeated retching and vomiting. Pigs under 4 weeks of age start suckling, but soon stop, withdraw from the sow, and vomit the milk they have taken in. Pigs huddle together, appear pale and listless, and often have an arched back. Body temperature may be elevated at the beginning of the outbreak, but returns to normal in 1–2 days. Affected pigs often grind their teeth. They dip their mouths into water bowls, but drink little or nothing, indicating a possible pharyngeal paralysis. Persistent vomiting and decreased food intake result in constipation and a rapid decline in condition.

The youngest pigs become severely dehydrated after a few days, become dyspneic and cyanotic, fall into a coma, and die. Older pigs lose their appetite and rapidly become emaciated. They continue to vomit, although less frequently than in the early stage of the disease. Some animals develop a large distension of the cranial abdomen. This "wasting" state may persist for several weeks until the pigs die of starvation. Mortality approaches 100% within litters and survivors remain permanently stunted.

An outbreak of the encephalomyelitic form may start as a VWD outbreak. Some pigs begin to vomit 4–7 days after birth. The vomiting continues intermittently for 1–2 days, but is rarely severe and does not result in dehydration. In other outbreaks, the first sign is acute depression and a tendency to huddle. Pigs may become sick as soon as 2 days after birth. Occasionally, sneezing, coughing, or upper respiratory compromise is observed. The pigs lose weight rapidly and their hair loses its luster and becomes rough. After 1–3 days, signs of severe encephalomyelitis arise. Younger pigs are most severely affected and exhibit various combinations of nervous signs. Generalized muscle tremors and hyperesthesia are common findings. Pigs that are able to stand usually have a jerky gait and tend to walk backwards, often ending in a dog-sitting position. They soon become very weak, are unable to rise, and paddle their limbs. Their noses and feet become cyanotic. Blindness, opisthotonus, and nystagmus can also occur. Finally, affected animals become prostrate, dyspneic, and lay on their sides. In most cases, coma precedes death.

Mortality in younger pigs is usually 100%. Older pigs usually suffer a mild transient illness in which posterior paralysis may be the most common sign. The paresis in a few cases is accompanied by blindness. The outbreak described in Taiwan (Chang et al. 1993) in 30–to 50-day-old pigs was characterized by fever, constipation, hyperesthesia, muscular tremor, progressive anterior paresis causing pigs to assume a "rabbit-like" posture, posterior paresis, prostration, recumbency, and paddling movements. Morbidity was 4%, but mortality was 100%, with pigs dying 4–5 days after the onset of clinical signs.

The time interval from onset of the disease in the first litter to cessation of the disease or its failure to appear in new litters is usually 2–3 weeks (Werdin et al. 1976). The disappearance of clinical signs coincides with the time it takes sows to develop immunity and to pass this protection on to their offspring. It has been shown that pigs exposed to HEV develop neutralizing and hemagglutination-inhibiting serum antibodies (Pensaert and Callebaut 1974).

PATHOGENESIS

HEV is able to replicate in the upper respiratory tract with or without producing clinical signs. HEV can be isolated from the nasal cavity, trachea, and lungs of diseased or healthy pigs (Hirahara et al. 1989; Mengeling et al. 1972; Pensaert et al. 1980). The virus is excreted for 8–10 days in oronasal secretions (Hirahara et al. 1989; Pensaert and Callebaut 1974), with transmission occurring through exposure to nasal secretions.

Most infections under field circumstances have a subclinical course, but the typical clinical disease can be reproduced by oronasal inoculation of colostrum-deprived piglets. In a series of studies on the pathogenesis of the disease, Andries and Pensaert (1980c) inoculated newborn colostrum-deprived pigs oronasally with an HEV strain from pigs showing the VWD syndrome. Anorexia and vomiting were seen after an incubation period of 4 days. Earlier studies had shown that viremia was probably of little or no importance in the pathogenesis (Andries and Pensaert 1980b). Immunofluorescence studies at different times after inoculation revealed that the epithelial cells of nasal mucosa, tonsils, lungs, and small intestine served as sites of primary viral replication.

After local replication near the sites of entry, the virus spread via the peripheral nervous system to the central nervous system (CNS). At least three pathways appeared to be involved. One pathway led from the nasal mucosa and tonsils to the trigeminal ganglion and the trigeminal sensory nucleus in the brainstem. A second pathway followed along the vagal nerves via the vagal sensory ganglion to the vagal sensory nucleus in the brainstem. A third pathway led from the intestinal plexuses to the spinal cord, also after replication in local sensory ganglia.

In the CNS, the infection started in well-defined nuclei of the medulla oblongata, but later progressed into the entire brainstem, the spinal cord, and sometimes also the cerebrum and cerebellum. Fluorescence in the brain was always restricted to the perikaryon and processes of neurons (Figure 20.1). Vomiting was induced by viral replication in the vagal sensory ganglion (ganglion distale vagi) or by impulses to the vomiting center produced by infected neurons at different sites (Andries 1982).

Experimental inoculation of rats and mice also leads to infection of the central nervous system. In these animals, HEV spreads transsynaptically along the neuronal pathways from the peripheral nerves to the central nervous system (Hirano et al. 2004).

To elucidate the pathogenesis of the wasting in pigs, radiological studies were performed on chronically infected animals, vagotomized animals, and controls (Andries 1982). The stomach of control pigs was always empty within 10 hours, whereas barium was retained in

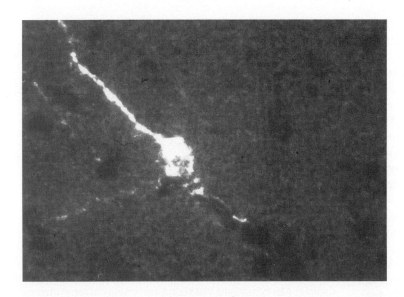

20.1. *Viral multiplication in the brain stem of a pig inoculated with HEV. Fluorescence is seen in the axon and the perikaryon of a neuron (×500).*

the stomachs of pigs with HEV for 2–7 days. In pigs with a bilateral abdominal vagotomy, the stomach emptying was less disturbed. This indicated that the delayed gastric emptying in pigs with HEV was not solely due to earlier viral replication in the vagal ganglion and vagal nuclei in the brain. The virus-induced lesions in the intramural plexi of the stomach were probably also responsible for gastric stasis. The disturbance in normal gastric emptying was considered to play an important role in the pathogenesis of wasting.

LESIONS

The only significant gross lesions reported in natural HEV infections are cachexia and a distension of the abdomen that develops in some chronically affected pigs (Hoorens et al. 1977; Schlenstedt et al. 1969). In these pigs, the stomach is dilated and filled with gas.

Microscopic lesions are found in the tonsils, the nervous system, respiratory system, and stomach of acutely diseased pigs. The lesions tend to disappear in animals surviving acute stages of the disease.

A nonsuppurative encephalomyelitis was reported in 70–100% of pigs with nervous signs and in 20–60% of pigs with the VWD syndrome. The lesions are characterized by perivascular cuffing, gliosis, and neuronal degeneration (Alexander 1962; Chang et al. 1993; Hoorens et al. 1977; Narita et al. 1989b; Richards and Savan 1960). Lesions are most pronounced in the gray matter of the pons Varoli, the medulla oblongata, and the dorsal horns of the upper spinal cord. It has been hypothesized that encephalitic lesions are a specific immune response to HEV following its replication in the CNS (Narita et al. 1989b). Neuritis of peripheral sensory ganglia, particularly the trigeminal ganglia, also occurs.

Changes in the tonsil are characterized by epithelial degeneration and lymphatic cell infiltration into the crypts (Narita et al. 1989a). Degeneration of the epithe-

lial cells of the turbinates, bronchi, and alveoli, as well as interstitial peribronchiolar pneumonia with infiltration of neutrophils and macrophages, were observed in 20% of naturally infected animals (Hoorens et al. 1977) and a much higher proportion of experimentally infected pigs (Cutlip and Mengeling 1972; Hirahara et al. 1989).

Microscopic changes in the stomach wall and the lungs were found only in pigs showing the VWD syndrome. Degeneration of the ganglia of the stomach wall and perivascular cuffing were present in 15–85% of diseased animals. The lesions were most pronounced in the pyloric gland area (Hoorens et al. 1977; Schlenstedt et al. 1969; Steinicke and Nielsen 1959).

DIAGNOSIS

To isolate HEV, the tonsils, brain, and lungs are collected aseptically from young, diseased piglets euthanized shortly after the first signs of infection. It is very difficult to isolate the virus from pigs that have been sick for more than 2 days. Tissue homogenates are inoculated onto primary PK cells, secondary pig thyroid cells, or permissive porcine cell lines. The presence of HEV is shown by the development of syncytia, hemadsorption, and hemagglutination (Andries and Pensaert 1980a). A single blind passage with cells and culture fluid is recommended because clinical specimens from pigs infected with HEV often contain very small amounts of infectious virus.

Antibodies to the virus can be detected by the VN, plaque reduction, or HI tests (Mengeling 1975; Sato et al. 1983). However, since subclinical HEV infections are common, serum antibody titers must be evaluated very carefully. Interpretation of paired serum samples may be difficult. A significant rise in antibody titer will only be observed if acute sera are taken very soon after the appearance of clinical signs. Pigs with clinical signs after an incubation period of 6–7 days may already have produced high serum antibody titers.

The differential diagnoses for HEV include Teschen-Talfan disease and Aujeszky's disease (pseudorabies). In the latter two, clinical signs of encephalomyelitis, including locomotor disorders, are more severe than those associated with HEV infection and may appear in older pigs, as well as in piglets. Aujeszky's disease in unvaccinated animals may also induce respiratory signs in older pigs and abortions in sows. These viruses can be grown in PK and pig thyroid cells; in PK cells they are distinguishable on the basis of cytopathic effect. They can be further differentiated using specific virus identification tests and the production of hemagglutinin by HEV.

PREVENTION AND CONTROL

In most breeding herds, HEV infection is maintained in an endemic cycle through subclinical infection of the respiratory tract. Sows usually come into contact with the virus before their first farrowing and, therefore, provide protective colostral antibodies to their offspring. Infection in such pigs is subclinical. However, if sows are not immune at the time of farrowing, as may occur in newly populated farms or on farms too small to maintain an endemic cycle, infection of pigs within the first weeks after birth will result in clinical signs. Thus, maintaining the virus on farms to obtain immune sows at the time of their first farrowing creates a situation favorable to avoiding disease in piglets.

Once clinical signs are evident, the disease will run its course; spontaneous recoveries are rare. Litters born 2–3 weeks after the onset of disease are usually protected by maternal immunity. Before that time, piglets born to nonimmune sows can be protected by specific hyperimmune serum injected at birth. However, the lapse of time between diagnosis and cessation of the disease is usually too short to gain much benefit from this procedure.

REFERENCES

Alexander TJL. 1962. Viral encephalomyelitis of swine in Ontario. Experimental and natural transmission. Am J Vet Res 32:756–762.

Alexander TJL, Richards WRC, Roe CK. 1959. An encephalomyelitis of suckling pigs in Ontario. Can J Comp Med 23:316–319.

Andries K. 1982. Pathogenese en epizoötiologie van "vomiting and wasting disease," een virale infektie bij het varken. Ph.D. diss., Med Fac Diergeneeskd Rijksuniv, Ghent 24:164.

Andries K, Pensaert M. 1980a. Propagation of hemagglutinating encephalomyelitis virus in porcine cell cultures. Zentralbl Veterinarmed B 27:280–290.

——. 1980b. Virus isolation and immunofluorescence in different organs of pigs infected with hemagglutinating encephalomyelitis virus. Am J Vet Res 41:215–218.

——. 1980c. Immunofluorescence studies on the pathogenesis of hemagglutinating encephalomyelitis virus after oronasal inoculation. Am J Vet Res 41:1372–1378.

Appel M, Greig AS, Corner AH. 1965. Encephalomyelitis of swine caused by a haemagglutinating virus. IV. Transmission studies. Res Vet Sci 6:482–4S9.

Callebaut PE, Pensaert MB. 1980. Characterization and isolation of structural polypeptides in haemagglutinating encephalomyelitis virus. J Gen Virol 48:193–204.

Cartwright SE, Lucas M. 1970. Vomiting and wasting disease in piglets. Vet Rec 86:278–280.

Cartwright SF, Lucas M, Cavill PJ, Gush AF, Blandford TB. 1969. Vomiting and wasting disease of piglets. Vet Rec 84:175–176.

Chang GN, Chang TC, Lin SC, Tsai SS, Chern RS. 1993. Isolation and identification of hemagglutinating encephalomyelitis virus from pigs in Taiwan. J Chin Soc Vet Sci 19:147–158.

Chappuis G, Tektoff J, Leturdu Y. 1975. Isolement en France et identification du virus de la maladie du vomissement et du deperissement des porcelets (coronalike virus). Rec Med Vet 151:557–566.

Cutlip RC, Mengeling WL. 1972. Lesions induced by hemagglutinating encephalomyelitis virus strain 67N in pigs. Am J Vet Res 33:2003–2009.

Dea S, Tijssen P. 1989. Detection of turkey enteric coronavirus by enzyme-linked immunosorbent assay and differentiation from other coronaviruses. Am J Vet Res 50:226–231.

Ducatelle R, Coussement W, Hoorens J. 1981. Morphogenesis of hemagglutinating encephalomyelitis in vivo and in vitro. Vlaams Diergeneeskd Tijdschr 50:326–336.

Forman AJ, Hale CJ, Jones RT, Conaughton ID. 1979. Haemagglutinating encephalomyelitis virus infection of pigs. Aust Vet J 55:503–504.

Girard A, Greig AS, Mitchell D. 1964. Encephalomyelitis of swine caused by a haemagglutinating virus. III. Serological studies. Res Vet Sci 5:294–302.

Gonzalez JM, Gomez-Puertas P, Cavanagh D, Gorbalenya AE, Enjuanes L. 2003. A comparative sequence analysis to revise the current taxonomy of the family Coronaviridae. Arch Virol 148:2207–2235.

Greig AS, Bouillant AMP. 1972. Studies on the hemagglutination phenomenon of hemagglutinating encephalomyelitis Virus (HEV) of pigs. Can J Comp Med 36:366–370.

Greig AS, Girard A. 1969. Encephalomyelitis of swine caused by a haemagglutinating virus. V. Response to metabolic inhibitors and other chemical compounds. Res Vet Sci 10:509.

Greig AS, Johnson CM, Bouillant AMP. 1971. Encephalomyelitis of swine caused by a haemagglutinating virus. VI. Morphology of the virus. Res Vet Sci 12:305–307.

Greig AS, Mitchell D, Corner AH, Bannister GL, Meads EB, Julian RJ. 1962. A hemagglutinating virus producing encephalomyelitis in baby pigs. Can J Comp Med 26:49–56.

Hess RG, Bachmann PA. 1978. Erbrechen und Kummern der Ferkeln. Vorkommen und Verbreitung in Suddeutschland. Tieraertzl Umschau 33:571–574.

Hirahara T, Yamanaka M, Yasuhara H, Matsui O, Kodama K, Nakai M, Sasaki N, Matumoto M. 1989. Experimental infection of pigs with porcine hemagglutinating encephalomyelitis virus. Jpn J Vet Sci 51:827–830.

Hirahara T, Yasuhara H, Kodama K, Nakai M, Sasaki N. 1987. Isolation of hemagglutinating encephalomyelitis virus from respiratory tract of pigs in Japan. Jpn J Vet Sci 49:85–93.

Hirai K, Chang C, Shimakura S. 1974. A serological survey on haemagglutinating encephalomyelitis virus infection in pigs in Japan. Jpn J Vet Sci 36:375–380.

Hirano N, Haga S, Fujiwara K. 1993. The route of transmission of hemagglutinating encephalomyelitis virus (HEV) 67N strain in 4-week-old rats. Adv Exp Med Biol 342:333–338.

Hirano N, Nomura R, Tawara T, Tohyama K. 2004. Neurotropism of swine haemagglutinating encephalomyelitis virus (coronavirus) in mice depending upon host age and route of infection. J Comp Pathol 130:58–65.

Hirano N, Ono K. 1998. A serological survey of human coronavirus in pigs of the Tohoku District of Japan. Adv Exp Med Biol 440:491–494.

Hirano N, Ono K, Takasawa H, Murakami T, Haga S. 1990. Replication and plaque formation of swine haemagglutinating encephalomyelitis virus (67N) in swine cell line, SK-K culture. J Virol Methods 27:91–100.

Hoorens J, Thoonen H, Gheyle M, Van Buyten A. 1977. Braakziekte bij biggen. Vlaams Diergeneeskd Tijdschr 46:209–224.

Kadoi K, Sakai T, Yukawa M, Kamata H, Iwabuchi M. 1994. The propagation of a porcine hemagglutinating encephalomyelitis virus in swine kidney cell cultures. New Microbiol 17:341–344.

Kaye HS, Yarbrouch WB, Reed CJ, Harrison AK. 1977. Antigenic relationship between human coronavirus strain OC43 and hemagglutinating encephalomyelitis virus strain 67N of swine: Antibody responses in human and animal sera. J Infect Dis 135:201–209.

Lamontagne L, Marois P, Marsolais G, Di Franco E, Assaf R. 1981. Inner structure of some coronaviruses. Can J Comp Med 45:177–181.

Lucas MH, Naphtine P. 1971. Fluorescent antibody technique in the study of three porcine viruses. J Comp Pathol 81:111–117.

McFerran JB, Clarke JK, Connor TJ, Knox ER. 1971. Serological evidence of the presence of haemagglutinating encephalomyelitis virus in Northern Ireland. Vet Rec 88:339.

Mengeling WL. 1975. Incidence of antibody for hemagglutinating encephalomyelitis virus in serums from swine in the United States. Am J Vet Res 36:821–823.

Mengeling WL, Boothe AD, Ritchie AE. 1972. Characteristics of a coronavirus (strain 67N) of pigs. Am J Vet Res 33:297–308.

Mengeling WL, Coria MF. 1972. Buoyant density of hemagglutinating encephalomyelitis of swine: Comparison with avian bronchitis virus. Am J Vet Res 33:1359–1363.

Mengeling WL, Cutlip RC. 1976. Pathogenicity of field isolants of hemagglutinating encephalomyelitis virus for neonatal pigs. J Am Vet Med Assoc 168:236–239.

Mostl K. 1990. Erhebungen uber Porcine Coronaviren in Osterreich. III. Teil: Das hemagglutinating Encephalomyelitis Virus (HEV) der Schweine. Wien Tieraerztl Monatsschr 77:117–120.

Narita M, Kawamura H, Haritani M, Kobayashi M. 1989b. Demonstration of viral antigen and immunoglobulin (IgG and IgM) in brain tissue of pigs experimentally infected with haemagglutinating encephalomyelitis virus. J Comp Pathol 100:119–128.

Narita M, Kawamura H, Tsuboi T, Haritani M, Kobayashi M. 1989a. Immunopathological and ultrastructural studies on the tonsil of gnotobiotic pigs infected with strain 67N of haemagglutinating encephalomyelitis virus. J Comp Pathol 100:305–312.

Neuvonen E, Ek-Kommonen C, Veijalainen P, Schulman A. 1982. Absence of hemagglutainaging encephalomyelitis virus in Finnish elite breeding pig herds. Nord Vet Med 34:334–335.

Paul PS, Mengeling WL. 1984. Persistence of passively acquired antibodies to haemagglutinating encephalomyelitis virus in swine. Am J Vet Res 45:932–934.

Pensaert M, Andries K, Callebaut P. 1980. A seroepizootiologic study of vomiting and wasting disease virus in pigs. Vet Q 2:142–148.

Pensaert MB, Callebaut PE. 1974. Characteristics of a coronavirus causing vomiting and wasting in pigs. Arch Gesamte Virusforsch 44:35–50.

Pirtle EC. 1974. Titration of two porcine respiratory viruses in mammalian cell cultures by direct fluorescent antibody staining. Am J Vet Res 35:249–250.

Pocock DH, Garwes FJ. 1977. The polypeptides of haemagglutinating encephalomyelitis virus and isolated subviral particles. J Gen Virol 37:487–199.

Richards WPC, Savan M. 1960. Viral encephalomyelitis of pigs. A preliminary report on the transmissibility and pathology of a disease observed in Ontario. Cornell Vet 50:132–155.

Sasaki I, Kazusa Y, Shirai J, Taniguchi T, Honda E. 2003. Neutralizing test of hemagglutinating encephalomyelitis virus (HEV) in FS-L3 cells cultured without serum. J Vet Med Sci 65:381–383.

Sasseville AM, Boutin M, Gelinas AM, Dea S. 2002. Sequence of the 3'-terminal end (8.1 kb) of the genome of porcine haemagglutinating encephalomyelitis virus: Comparison with other haemagglutinating coronaviruses. J Gen Virol 83 (Pt 10): 2411–2416.

Sasseville AM, Gelinas AM, Sawyer N; Boutin M, Dea S. 2001. Biological and molecular characteristics of an HEV isolate associated with recent acute outbreaks of encephalomyelitis in Quebec pig farms. Adv Exp Med Biol 494:57–62.

Sato K, Inaba Y, Miura Y, Tokuhisa S, Matumoto M. 1983. Inducement of cytopathic changes and plaque formation by porcine haemagglutinating encephalomyelitis virus. Vet Microbiol 8:521–530.

Schlenstedt VD, Barnikol H, Plonait H. 1969. Erbrechen und Kummern bei Saugferkeln. DTW 76:694–695.

Schultze B, Herrler G. 1993. Recognition of N-acetyl-9-O-acetylneuraminic acid by bovine coronavirus and hemagglutinating encephalomyelitis virus. Adv Exp Med Biol 342:299–304.

Sorensen KJ. 1975. [Hemagglutinating encephalomyelitis virus (HEV) infections in swine. Serologic indication for infectional occurrence in Denmark.] Haemagglutinerende encephalomyelitis virus (HEV) infektioner hos grise. Serologisk indikation for infektionens tilstedevaerelse i Denmark. Nord Vet Med 27:208–212.

Steinicke O, Nielsen A. 1959. Histological changes of the mesenteric plexus of the stomach in "baby pig disease." Nord Vet Med 11:399–429.

Vannier P, Chappuis G, Labadie JL, Renault L, Josse J. 1981. A serological survey of the virus of vomiting and wasting disease in piglets. Ann Zootech 30:379.

Vieler E, Schlapp T, Anders C, Herbst W. 1995. Genomic relationship of porcine hemagglutinating encephalomyelitis virus to bovine coronavirus and human coronavirus OC43 as studied by the use of bovine coronavirus S gene-specific probes. Arch Virol 140:1215–1223.

Werdin RE, Sorensen DK, Stewart WC. 1976. Porcine encephalomyelitis caused by haemagglutinating encephalomyelitis virus. J Am Vet Med Assoc 168:240–246.

Yagami K, Hirai K, Hirano N. 1986. Pathogenesis of haemagglutinating encephalomyelitis virus (HEV) in mice experimentally infected by different routes. J Comp Pathol 96:645–657.

Yagami K, Izumi Y, Kajiwara N, Sugiyama F, Sugiyama Y. 1993. Neurotropism of mouse-adapted haemagglutinating encephalomyelitis virus. J Comp Pathol 109:21–27.

21 Japanese Encephalitis and West Nile Viruses

K. B. Platt and Han Soo Joo

Japanese encephalitis virus (JEV) and West Nile virus (WNV) are significant mosquito-borne human and animal pathogens. JEV is considered to be the most important vector-borne virus that causes encephalitis in humans. The rate of apparent to inapparent JEV infection in humans ranges from 1 in 200–300 and the case fatality rate of humans infected with JEV can exceed 40% (Burke and Monath 2001). The virus is also an economically important reproductive pathogen of swine and will cause encephalitis and death in horses. It is widely distributed in Asia, from Southeastern Russia through Japan, Eastern China, Southeastern Asia, to Northern Australia in the south and India in the West.

JEV was first isolated from humans by Fujita (1933) and later by Taniguchi et al. (1936) who concluded that it was the cause of "summer encephalitis" in Japan. A temporal relationship was also recognized between "summer encephalitis" of humans and cases of encephalitis in horses, and abortion and stillbirths in swine (Hosoya et al. 1950). Subsequently Shimizu et al. (1954) demonstrated that JEV was responsible for reproductive failure in swine.

West Nile virus was first isolated in 1937 from a febrile woman in Uganda (Murgue 2002). Prior to 1999 the virus was distributed throughout Africa, the Middle East, and parts of Europe and Asia. WNV first emerged in the U.S. during an outbreak in New York City in 1999. The mechanism of its introduction has not been established. The virus subsequently spread rapidly throughout North America and south through Mexico to Central America and the Caribbean (Gould and Fikrig 2004; Roehrig et al. 2002). The case fatality rate of WNV in humans increases with age and can vary from 2–15% (O'Leary et al. 2004; Tsai et al. 1998). West Nile virus, like JEV, causes fatal disease in horses. Unlike JEV, its role as a swine pathogen has not been thoroughly explored and there are no reports of death or reproductive failure in swine.

ETIOLOGY

JEV and WNV are members of the *Flavivirus* genus of the family *Flaviviridae*. The family contains two other genera, the genus *Pestivirus* represented by viruses causing classical swine fever (hog cholera), bovine viral diarrhea virus, and border disease virus, and genus *Hepacivirus* represented by hepatitis C virus of humans (Lindenbach and Rice 2001). Genus *Flavivirus* is organized into 8 separate antigenic complexes based on serum cross-neutralization assays: Japanese encephalitis (JE), Ntaya, Dengue (DEN), tick-borne encephalitis (TBE), Uganda, Tyuleniy, Rio Bravo, and Modoc serocomplexes. Yellow fever virus, the prototype virus for genus *Flavivirus,* does not fall into any specific serocomplex (Burke and Monath 2001). Notable members of the JE serocomplex include JEV, the prototype of the group, St. Louis encephalitis virus, Murray Valley encephalitis virus, WNV, and Kunjin virus. The latter, which is found in Australia, is currently considered to be a subtype of WNV (Lanciotti et al. 2002).

JEV is classified into 4, and possibly 5, distinct genotypes based on the nucleotide sequences encoding the capsid, prM, and E proteins. Genotype I is the most broadly distributed genotype throughout Asia. Genotypes I and III are most commonly associated with epidemic disease. Genotypes II and IV are found in Southeast Asia and are commonly associated with endemic disease (Solomon et al. 2003). Two major immunotypes of JEV are currently recognized by kinetic neutralization, monoclonal antibody reactivity, and other serological methods. These immunotypes are represented by the Nakayama strain that was isolated from a human brain in 1935 and the JaGAr 01 strain that was isolated from a mosquito in 1959. Antigenic and genetic variation exists among isolates of the same genotype (Burke and Monath 2001). Variations between strains within genotypes and immunotypes can be demonstrated by nucleotide analysis (Holbrook and Barrett 2002).

WNV is represented by 2 genetic lineages based on genomic differences. Lineage 1 viruses are further subdivided into 3 clades: 1a, 1b, and 1c. Lineage 1 viruses are found in Africa, the Middle East, Asia, Europe, and North America. Lineage 2 viruses are found primarily in Africa (Lanciotti et al. 2002). In general, lineage 1 viruses are more virulent than lineage 2 viruses. Serological and molecular techniques can be used to differentiate WNV strains.

Morphology

The JEV and WNV are enveloped, single-stranded, positive polarity RNA viruses approximately 50 nm in diameter. Their genomes are approximately 11 kb in length and surrounded by a polyhedral capsid consisting of a single protein (C) of about 11 kd. The envelope consists of two proteins, E and M, of approximately 50 and 8 kDa, respectively. The E and M protein together form small spikes of approximately 6 nm on the surface of the envelope. The M protein exists as the prM protein before the release of mature virions from infected cells. Nonstructural proteins include NS1, 2A, 2B, 3, 4A, 4B and 5. The E and NS1 proteins are associated with the induction of immunity (Kurane 2002). It is of interest to note that the prM protein of another flavivirus, Dengue, has been reported to induce immunity (Lindenbach and Rice 2001). Neuro-virulence of JEV and WNV strains is associated with common determinants on the E protein (Ni and Barrett 1998; Lee et al. 2004).

The structural proteins of flaviviruses are encoded at the 5' end of the genome and nonstructural proteins are encoded at the 3' end. The flavivirus genome is expressed as a single polyprotein that is cleaved during and after the translation process by both cellular and virus encoded proteases.

Biophysical and Biochemical Properties

Flaviviruses have a buoyant density of 1.22–1.24 g/cm^3 in CsCl. Their sedimentation rates range from 140–200 S20w. In general, flaviviruses are inactivated in whole blood after 30 minutes exposure to 56°C and by low pH, bile, and proteolytic enzymes (Burke and Monath 2001). A study by Remington et al. (2004) demonstrated a loss of WNV infectivity of over 6 orders of magnitude in 5% and 25% albumin solutions after 30 minutes exposure to 60°C. Mayo and Beckwith (2002) demonstrated that WNV maintained in cell culture medium with 10% fetal bovine serum at 28°C lost infectivity at the rate of 1 order of magnitude per 24 hours. In contrast, no infectivity was lost when virus was maintained at 4° over a 4-day period. This point should be considered when submitting clinical specimens for diagnostic evaluation. No information is available on the stability of JEV under dry conditions. However, Johansen et al. (2002) reported that virus activity was lost within 24 hrs when dead JEV-infected mosquitoes were held at 28–32°C in a humidified atmosphere. This suggests that both WNV and JEV virus rapidly lose infectivity outside of their living host.

EPIDEMIOLOGY

A wide range of domestic and wild avian and mammalian species including humans, horses, and swine are susceptible to JEV and WNV infection. These viruses are transmitted almost exclusively by the bite of infected mosquitoes, although experimental tick transmission of WNV has been reported (Lawrie et al. 2004). Rosen (1986) cited two studies, one in which JEV was isolated from midges (*Lasiohelea taiwana*) feeding on humans and the other from the tick *Haemmaphysalis japonica*. There are no reports of contact transmission of either virus between swine. However, contact transmission of WNV between avian species, from which virus can be isolated from throat and cloacal swabs, has been reported (Komar et al. 2003). Contact transmission of WNV between alligators has also been described (Klenk et al. 2004), as has oral infection of cats (Austgen et al. 2004).

Both JEV and WNV are naturally maintained in a mosquito-bird-mosquito cycle. JEV epidemics in human populations typically occur in late summer and early fall in northern temperate climates after JEV amplifies in the fledgling and young bird populations during the nesting season, and subsequently in susceptible pigs and other mammalian species. In endemic tropical areas, JEV infection can occur in swine populations almost immediately after the mosquito season begins. Pigs serve as a significant JEV reservoir for both opportunistic and zoophilic mosquito species that spread the virus to humans which are dead end hosts.

The primary mosquito species involved in transmission of JEV in Asia is *Culex tritaeniorhynchus,* and its role in this capacity has been well documented in reviews by Rosen (1986) and Endy and Nisalak (2002). *Culex tritaeniorhynchus* is opportunistic and feeds on both avian and mammalian species. The titers of blood meals capable of infecting 50% of feeding *Cx. tritaeniorhynchus* vary from $10^{2.9}$–$10^{4.8}$ mouse lethal dose$_{50}$ (LD$_{50}$) per ml of serum depending on the strains of mosquitoes and viruses (Takahashi 1976). These levels of viremia are exceeded in young avian species (Boyle et al. 1983; Buescher et al. 1959) and in young pigs. Maximum serum titers exceeding $10^{6.0}$ LD$_{50}$ per ml were reported by Kodama et al. (1968) in 2-day-old pigs challenged with 10^1 or 10^2 LD$_{50}$. Gresser et al. (1958) observed maximum virus titers in serum of $10^{4.7}$ and $10^{3.9}$ LD$_{50}$ per ml in a 3- and a 5-month-old pig challenged with $10^{5.3}$ LD$_{50}$ and Konishi et al. (1992) reported virus titers in serum that exceeded 10^3 PFU ml in six of ten 25 kg pigs that were challenged with $10^{5.2}$ PFU of JEV. Virus titers exceeded 10^4 PFU per ml of serum in 2 of these pigs. The virus challenge used in these studies was within or near the amounts of JEV that can be delivered by *Cx. tritaeniorhynchus* to a host during feeding (Takahashi 1976).

Several other mosquito species are competent JEV vectors. Examples include; *Cx. pipiens quinquefasciatus*, *Cx. tarsalis* (Endy and Nisalak 2002), *Aedes albopictus* (Weng et al. 1997), and *Ochlerotatus japonicus* (Takashima and Rosen 1989). Each of these species is present in the Western hemisphere. Consequently, if JEV is introduced into this region it will most likely become established.

The mechanisms of interepidemic survival of JEV and WNV have not been fully elucidated. In temperate regions of Asia, outbreaks of JEV are seasonal and occur in late summer after virus has been amplified in fledging bird populations (Buescher and Scherer 1959). Ardeids, such as herons and egrets, are frequently cited as playing a principle role in the epidemiology of JEV. Whether ardeids play a more important role in the epidemiology of JEV than other avian species remains to be determined. Rosen (1986) commented that ardeids have received more attention than other avian species because they are large enough to be bled repeatedly and are found in environments in which the principle *Culex* vectors are present. Virus could be reintroduced into the same general regions by infected mosquitoes that are carried on the wind from warmer endemic regions. However, Takashima et al. (1988) presented a compelling argument that supports the contention that JEV is maintained endemically. Possible mechanisms for interepidemic maintenance include persistence of virus in diapausing adult *Culex* spp., (Nasci et al. 2001), vertical transmission in *Aedes* and *Ochlerotatus* spp., (Rosen et al. 1978; Rosen et al. 1989) and persistent infection in hibernating bats and cold blooded animals (Rosen 1986).

The epidemiology of WNV is similar to that of JEV. In the US, 60 species of mosquitoes from 11 genera are susceptible to WNV (CDC 2005), but the ability to transmit WNV by all of these species has not been established. *Culex* species that feed primarily on birds, such as *Cx. pipiens*, and *Cx. tarsalis,* are considered to be the primary mosquito vectors of WNV. Several other mosquito species that feed primarily on mammals, including humans, can serve as bridge vectors between birds and mammals such as pigs. These species include *Culex quinquefasciatus*, *Aedes albopictus* (a.k.a. Asian tiger mosquito), *Aedes vexans, Ochlerotatus trivittatus, Ochlerotatus triseriatus*, and others (Turell et al. 2005; Tiawsirisup et al. 2004). The general consensus is that the primary reservoir of WNV are birds, especially crows, jays, house sparrows, and grackles (Komar et al. 2003). The role of mammals, including swine, in the epidemiology of WNV has not been fully evaluated.

CLINICAL SIGNS

The primary disease manifestation of JEV infection in sows and gilts is reproductive failure manifested by abortion and abnormal farrowings (Figure 21.1). Litters contain stillborn and mummified fetuses, and weak neonates that may present with hydrocephalus and subcutaneous edema. Live normal piglets can also be present in these litters (Burns 1950). Sexually mature swine do not show any significant clinical signs of infection, but transient anorexia and a mild febrile response have been observed. Reproductive failure occurs in nonimmune sows that become infected before 60–70 days of gestation. Infection after this time does not appear to affect piglets significantly (Sugimori et al. 1974). There have not been any reports of reproductive failure in sows due to WNV infection.

Japanese encephalitis virus has also been associated with infertility in boars. Hashimura et al. (1976) isolated JEV from the testicles of a boar with orchitis. Ogasa et al. (1977) showed that infection of susceptible

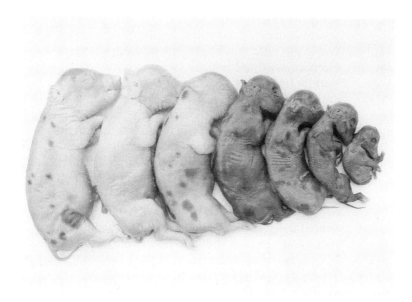

21.1. *Mummified and stillborn fetuses from a gilt following a natural infection with JEV.*

boars resulted in edematous, congested testicles that produced semen with numerous abnormal spermatozoa and significantly depressed total and motile sperm counts. Virus was also excreted in the semen. These changes were usually temporary and most boars recovered completely.

Natural infection of young piglets with JEV resulting in clinical disease has not been recognized as a common occurrence, possibly due to the prevalence of JEV-specific maternal antibody in endemic areas. However, Yamada et al. (2004) reported that JEV was isolated from tonsils of 2 of 4 40-day-old pigs that presented with a wasting syndrome. These pigs did not exhibit neurological signs, but histological examination revealed a nonsuppurative meningoencephalitis. These investigators were able to reproduce nonsuppurative meningoencephalitis in 3-week-old piglets with the isolated viruses. The affected pigs also showed varying degrees of depression and hind limb tremors. Whether or not an association with a wasting syndrome exists was not established, but it is noteworthy that JEV infection in humans can present with wasting of limbs as a result of flaccid paralysis (Solomon and Vaugh 2002). Kodama et al. (1968) also reported that experimental infection of 2-day-old piglets produced tremors and paralysis of the hindlimbs. However, other researchers who infected pigs ranging in age from 10 days to 2–3 months with JEV did not note any significant clinical signs (Gresser et al. 1958; Hale et al. 1957; Ilkal et al. 1994). These differences could have been due to differences in virus strain, virus dose, and the genetic background and age of the piglets.

No clinical signs of infection have been observed in pigs infected with WNV. Ilkal et al. (1994) reported that 4 pigs injected with an Asian isolate of WNV developed viremias that persisted for 1–4 days and reached a maximum titer of $10^{2.2}$ LD_{50} per ml. No mention of adverse clinical effects in the piglets was made. A more recent study by Platt (2004) described experimental infection, by needle and by mosquito bite, of 26 weanling pigs with a New York 1999 WNV isolate. The mean duration of viremia was 4.2 days. The mean daily WNV titer of all pigs was $10^{3.3} \pm 0.5$ $TCID_{50}$ per ml. Some individual pigs had titers in excess of $10^{5.0}$ $TCID_{50}$ per ml. No marked clinical signs of infection were observed. Platt (2004) also reported that nonsuppurative encephalitis and spinal cord lesions were observed in some of these pigs, suggesting that clinical signs, e.g., incoordination, tremors, and paralysis, could occur. A similar study with a NY 1999 WNV strain was reported by Bowen (2003) in which 3 of 6 infected weanling pigs developed maximum WNV titers ranging from $10^{1.9}$–$10^{3.1}$ PFU per ml of serum during an average viremic period of 2.5 days. Only 1 of 6 infected young adult pigs developed a detectable titer that reached 10^1 PFU per ml and persisted for less than a day. None of the pigs developed clinical signs of infection.

PATHOGENESIS

There are no complete studies on the pathogenesis of flaviviruses in swine. However, several studies have been done using the mouse and baby hamster as models (see Burke and Monath 2001). From these studies it can be deduced that virus initially replicates in the skin and regional lymph nodes following injection of virus by mosquito bite. A primary viremia ensues, which is the source of infection for several cell types, including connective tissue, skeletal, cardiac and smooth muscle cells, lymphoreticular cells, and cells of the endocrine and exocrine system. Virus from these tissues constitutes a secondary viremia, which generally occurs within 1–2 days after infection. It is during this period that transplacental infection can occur in pregnant gilts and sows, and virus can reach the fetus by 7 days after infection. The variable mixture of normal piglets, weak neonates, stillborns, and mummified fetuses of different sizes in affected litters indicates that sequential infection of fetuses occurs in utero. These observations suggest that the pathogenesis of JEV in swine is similar to that of porcine parvovirus (Joo et al. 1976).

Whether a causal relationship exists between the level of viremia and transplacental infection remains to be determined. A study by Shimizu et al. (1954) did not find any such relationship among 9 sows that were inoculated with $10^{6.0}$–$10^{9.5}$ LD_{50} with the Fuji or Kanagawa strains of JEV. Viremia persisted for 1–4 days and maximum titers in individual sows ranged from $10^{1.5}$–$10^{5.7}$ LD_{50} per ml of serum. Fetal infection occurred in 4 of the 9 pregnant sows that were infected between 40 and 97 days (mean = 62 days) of gestation. The maximum virus titers in these sows ranged from $10^{1.7}$ to greater than $10^{5.7}$ LD_{50} per ml of serum. Sows in which fetuses were not infected were inoculated with virus between 36 and 92 days (mean = 85 days) of gestation and had maximum virus titers that ranged from $10^{2.1}$ to >$10^{5.7}$ LD_{50} per ml. Fujisaki et al. (1982) concluded from a study using the mouse model that transplacental infection was dependent on the degree of development between placenta and fetal tissue and not on the level of viremia, since the highest rate of transplacental infection by JEV in mice occurred between days 7 and 10 of gestation.

Japanese encephalitis virus can reach the central nervous system as early as 3 days after infection by crossing the blood-brain barrier (Yamada et al. 2004), an event that is more common in neonates and the very young than in older animals. The precise mechanism by which JEV breaches the blood brain barrier has not been definitively established. Liou and Hsu (1998) demonstrated by electron microscopy that JEV could be translocated across endothelial cells in endocytotic vesicles in infected mice. Penetration of the blood brain barrier appears to be enhanced by a JEV-induced cytokine (Mathur et al. 1992).

LESIONS

Significant gross or microscopic lesions caused by JEV in sows have not been reported. The testes of naturally infected boars frequently have a large amount of mucous fluid in the cavity tunica vaginalis. Fibrous thickening along the edge of the epididymis and the visceral layer of the tunica vaginalis is also observed. Microscopically, there are edema and inflammatory changes in the interstitial tissue of the epididymis, tunica vaginalis, and testes. Degenerative changes are often seen in the seminiferous epithelium (Hashimura et al. 1976; Ogasa et al. 1977).

Gross lesions may or may not be seen in stillborn and weak neonatal pigs. When present, they may include hydrocephalus, subcutaneous edema, hydrothorax, ascites, petechial hemorrhages on serosal surfaces, congestion of lymph nodes, necrotic foci in liver and spleen, and congested meninges or spinal cord (Burns 1950). Cerebellar hypoplasia and spinal hypomyelinogenesis have also been described (Morimoto 1969). Microscopic lesions appear to be restricted to the brain and spinal cord. Diffuse nonsuppurative encephalitis and spondylitis may be observed. Yamada et al. (2004) described similar lesions in 3-week-old pigs that were experimentally infected with JEV. These lesions were distributed throughout the cerebrum, midbrain, and cerebellum. Perivascular cuffing, neuronal necrosis, neurophagia, and glial nodules were present. No other macroscopic or microscopic lesions were noted in other organ systems. Similar lesions of the central nervous system were observed in weanling pigs experimentally infected with a New York strain of WNV (Platt 2004).

DIAGNOSIS

Definitive diagnosis of reproductive disease in swine caused by JEV is based on isolating and identifying virus from fetuses, stillborns, neonates, and young piglets. Differential diagnosis must consider porcine parvovirus, porcine reproductive and respiratory syndrome virus, pseudorabies virus, classical swine fever virus, cytomegalovirus, enterovirus, Getah virus (Shibata et al. 1991), toxoplasmosis, and leptospirosis. Seasonal incidence and lack of clinical signs in infected sows and piglets are useful criteria in excluding many diseases.

Tissues from which JEV has been isolated from fetuses and neonates include brain, liver, spleen, lung, and placenta (Shimizu et al. 1954). However, it appears that successful isolation of JEV from pigs of abnormal litters is dependent on the time that pigs were exposed to the virus in utero. Shimizu et al. (1954) isolated JEV from fetuses of 3 litters that were collected 7–22 days after experimental infection of sows with the Kanagawa strain, but not from affected pigs of 2 litters that were collected 62 and 84 days after infection of sows. Susceptible cells for virus isolation include Vero cells, baby hamster kidney cells, pig kidney cells, and the C6/36 cell line derived from *Aedes albopictus*. Virus can also be isolated from infected tissue, such as brain and placenta, by intracerebral inoculation of suckling mice. Neurological signs and death usually occur in mice between 4 and 14 days after inoculation. Final confirmation of the identity of isolated virus can be made serologically using flavivirus-specific monoclonal antibodies (Broom et al. 1998) and/or by the reverse transcription-polymerase chain reaction (RT-PCR) (Huang et al. 2004).

Infection by JEV can also be confirmed by detecting viral antigen in fetal tissue and the placenta by immunohistochemistry (Iwasaki et al. 1986; Kurata et al. 1983; Yamada et al. 2004). The use of flavivirus-specific monoclonal antibodies in these procedures enhances the specificity of the test. Detection of JEV-specific antibody in body fluids of aborted fetuses, weak neonates, and piglets by hemagglutination inhibition, serum virus neutralization, and ELISA is also of diagnostic importance. In older pigs, interpretation of serological results must take vaccination history and maternal antibody into account. Maternal antibody specific for JEV can be detected in some pigs until 8 months of age (Hale et al. 1957). The use of paired serums and tests to detect JEV reactive IgM can facilitate interpretation of serological tests. Burke et al. (1985) demonstrated that porcine IgM antibodies to JEV could be detected within 2–3 days after infection and persist for 2 weeks. Interpretation of serological tests must also take into account whether affected swine could have been exposed to other flaviviruses such as WNV, because there is a high degree of serological cross reactivity between members of the Japanese encephalitis serocomplex (Williams et al. 2001). RT-PCR has also been developed to detect and differentiate JEV and WNV genomic material in clinical specimens (Kleiboeker et al. 2004; Shirato et al. 2003; Yang et al. 2004).

PREVENTION

Japanese encephalitis virus can be controlled by preventing exposure of swine to JEV-infected mosquitoes. However, this method of control is not practical unless pigs are maintained in appropriate confinement facilities. Consequently, vaccination is the method of choice. Monath (2002) reviewed the history of JE vaccine development. The first effective vaccines were formalin inactivated JEV-infected mouse brains. These vaccines were initially developed in Japan during the 1930s. Highly purified inactivated mouse brain vaccines are currently in use throughout the world in humans. Inactivated vaccines derived from infected cell cultures are in various stages of development. A live JE attenuated vaccine based on strain SA-14-2 was licensed in 1988 for human use in the Peoples Republic of China. Live vectored vaccines based on the attenuated vaccinia and canarypox viruses containing the JEV genes for prM, E, and NS1 induce both neutralizing antibodies and cytotoxic T cells.

An effective canarypox recombinant vaccine for WNV has been developed for horses (Siger et al. 2004) and is currently being marketed. A chimeric yellow fever–Japanese encephalitis vaccine virus containing the prM and E genes from the attenuated SA-14-2 strain of JEV induces protective immunity in monkeys and mice (Lai and Monath 2003). Experimental DNA vaccines containing prM and E genes of JEV and WNV have also been developed and induce protective immunity to JEV in swine (Konishi et al. 2000) and to WNV in horses (Davis et al. 2001). Live attenuated and inactivated JEV vaccines are commercially available for swine in Asia. The vaccines are available with porcine parvovirus and Getah virus. It is recommended that boars, gilts, and sows at risk be vaccinated for JEV before the mosquito season.

REFERENCES

Austgen LE, Bowen RA, Bunning ML, Davis BS, Mitchell CJ, Chang GJ. 2004. Experimental infection of cats and dogs with West Nile virus. Emerg Infect Dis 10(1):82–86.

Bowen RA. 2003. Characterization of West Nile virus Infection in Swine. National Pork Board, Final report, project #02-186.

Boyle DB, Marshall ID, Dickerman RW. 1983. Primary antibody responses of herons to experimental infection with Murray Valley encephalitis and Kunjin viruses. Aust J Exp Biol Med Sci 61 (Pt 6):665–674.

Broom AK, Hall RA, Johansen CA, Oliveira N, Howard MA, Lindsay MD, Kay BH, Mackenzie JS. 1998. Identification of Australian arboviruses in inoculated cell cultures using monoclonal antibodies in ELISA. Pathology 30:286–288.

Buescher EL, Scherer WF. 1959. Ecological studies of Japanese encephalitis virus in Japan. IX. Epidemiologic correlations and conclusions. Am J Trop Med Hyg 8:719–722.

Buescher EL, Scherer WF, Rosenberg MZ, McClure HE. 1959. Immunologic studies of Japanese encephalitis virus in Japan III. Infection and antibody responses of birds. J Immunol 83:605–613.

Burke DS, Monath TP. 2001. Flaviviruses. In Fields Virology (4th edition). DM Knipe, PM Howley, DE Griffin, RA Lamb, MA Martin, B Roizman, SE Straus, eds. Philadelphia: Lippincott Williams and Wilkins, pp. 1043–1126.

Burke DS, Tingpalapong M, Elwell MR, Paul PS, Van Deusen RA. 1985. Japanese encephalitis virus immunoglobulin M antibodies in porcine sera. Am J Vet Res 46:2054–2057.

Burns KF. 1950. Congenital Japanese B encephalitis infection of swine. Proc Soc Exp Biol Med 75:621–625.

CDC (Centers for Disease Control and Prevention). 2005. Entomology. http://www.cdc.gov/ncidod/dvbid/westnile/mosquito Species.htm.

Davis BS, Chang GJ, Cropp B, Roehrig JT, Martin DA, Mitchell CJ, Bowen R, Bunning ML. 2001. West Nile virus recombinant DNA vaccine protects mouse and horse from virus challenge and expresses in vitro a noninfectious recombinant antigen that can be used in enzyme-linked immunosorbent assays. J Virol 75:4040–4047.

Endy TP, Nisalak A. 2002. Japanese encephalitis virus: Ecology and epidemiology. Curr Top Microbiol Immunol 267:11–48.

Fujisaki Y, Miura Y, Sugimori T, Murakami Y, Ino T, Miura K. 1982. Experimental studies on vertical infection of mice with Japanese encephalitis virus. III. Effect of gestation days at the time of inoculation on placental and fetal infection. Natl Inst Anim Health Q 22:95–101.

Fujita T. 1933. Studies on the causative agent for epidemic encephalitis. Jpn J Exp Med 17:1441–1501.

Gould LH, Fikrig E. 2004. West Nile virus: A growing concern? J Clin Invest 113:1102–1107.

Gresser JL, Hardy SM, Hu MK, Scherer WF. 1958. Factors influencing transmission of Japanese B encephalitis virus by a colonized strain of Culex tritaeniorhynchus (Giles) from infected pigs and chicks to susceptible pigs and birds. Am J Trop Med Hyg 7:365–373.

Hale JH, Lim KA, Colless DH. 1957. Investigation of domestic pigs as a potential reservoir of Japanese B encephalitis virus on Singapore Island. Am J Trop Med Parasitol 51:374–379.

Hashimura WM, Uemiyada S, Komemura S, Fukumoto S, Okuda G, Miura K, Hayashi S. 1976. Isolation of Japanese encephalitis virus from orchitis in pigs. Summary 81st Meet Jpn Soc Vet Sci, p. 136.

Holbrook MR, Barrett ADT. 2002. Molecular epidemiology of Japanese encephalitis virus. Curr Top Microbiol Immunol 267:75–90.

Hosoya H, Matumoto M, Iwasa S. 1950. Epizootiological studies on stillbirth of swine occurred in Japan during summer months of 1948. Japan J Exp Med 20:587–595.

Huang JL, Lin HT, Wang YM, Weng MH, Ji DD, Kuo MD, Liu HW, Lin CS. 2004. Sensitive and specific detection of strains of Japanese encephalitis virus using a one-step TaqMan RT-PCR technique. J Med Virol 74:589–596.

Ilkal MA, Prasanna Y, Jacob PG, Geevarghese G, Banerjee K. 1994. Experimnental studies on the susceptibility of domestic pigs to West Nile virus followed by Japanese encephalitis virus infection and vice versa. Acta Virol 38:157–161.

Iwasaki Y, Zhao JX, Yamamota T, Konno H. 1986. Immunohistochemical demonstration of viral antigens in Japanese encephalitis. Acta Neuropathol (Berl) 70:79–81.

Johansen CA, Hall RA, van den Hur AF, Ritchie SA, Mackenzie JS. 2002. Detection and stability of Japanese encephalitis virus RNA and virus viability in dead infected mosquitoes under different storage conditions Am J Trop Med Hyg 67(6):656–661.

Joo HS, Donaldson-Wood CR, Johnson RG. 1976. Observations on the pathogenesis of porcine parvovirus infection. Arch Virol 51:123–129.

Kleiboeker SB, Loiacono CM, Rottinghaus A, Pue HL, Johnson GC. 2004. Diagnosis of West Nile virus infection in horses. J Vet Diagn Invest 16:2–10.

Klenk K, Snow J, Morgan K, Bowen R, Stephens M, Foster F, Gordy P, Beckett S, Komar N, Gubler D, Bunning M. 2004. Alligators as West Nile virus amplifiers. Emerg Infect Dis 210:2150–2155.

Kodama K, Sasaki N, Inoue YK. 1968. Studies of live attenuated Japanese encephalitis vaccine in swine. J Immunol 100:194–200.

Komar N, Langevin S, Hinten S, Nemeth N, Edwards E, Hettler D, Davis B, Bowen R, Bunning M. 2003. Experimental infection of North American birds with the New York 1999 strain of West Nile virus. Emerg Infect Dis 9:311–322.

Konishi E, Pincus S, Paoletti E, Laegreid WW, Shope RE, Mason PW. 1992. A highly attenuated host range-restricted vaccinia virus strain, NYVAC, encoding the prM, E, and NS1 genes of Japanese encephalitis virus prevents JEV viremia in swine. Virology 1992 190:454–458.

Konishi E, Yamaoka M, Kurane I, Mason PW. 2000. Japanese encephalitis DNA vaccine candidates expressing premembrane and envelope genes induce virus-specific memory B cells and long-lasting antibodies in swine. Virology 268:49–55.

Kurane I. 2002. Immune responses to Japanese encephalitis virus. Curr Top Microbiol Immunol 267:91–103.

Kurata T, Hondo R, Sato S, Oda A, Aoyama Y, McCormmick JB. 1983. Detection of viral antigens in formalin-fixed specimens by enzyme treatment. Ann NY Acad Sci 420:192–207.

Lai CJ, Monath TP. 2003. Chimeric flaviviruses: Novel vaccines against dengue fever, tick-borne encephalitis, and Japanese encephalitis. Adv Virus Res 61:469–509.

Lanciotti RS, Ebel GD, Deubel V, Kerst AJ, Murri S, Meyer R, Bowen M, McKinney N, Morrill WE, Crabtree MB, Kramer LD, Roehrig JT. 2002. Complete genome sequences and phylogenetic analysis of West Nile virus strains isolated from the United States, Europe, and the Middle East. Virology 298:96–105.

Lawrie CH, Uzcategui NY, Gould EA, Nuttall PA. 2004. Ixodid and argasid tick species and west nile virus. Emerg Infect Dis 10:653–657.

Lee E, Hall RA, Lobigs M. 2004. Common E protein determinants for attenuation of glycosaminoglycan-binding variants of Japanese encephalitis and West Nile viruses. J Virol 78:8271–8280.

Lindenbach BD, Rice CM. 2001. *Flaviviridae*: the viruses and their replication. In Fields Virology (4th edition). DM Knipe, PM Howley, DE Griffin, RA Lamb, MA Martin, B Roizman, SE Straus, eds. Philadelphia: Lippincott Williams and Wilkins, pp. 991–1041.

Liou ML, Hsu CY. 1998. Japanese encephalitis virus is transported across the cerebral blood vessels by endocytosis in mouse brain. Cell Tissue Res 293:389–394.

Mathur A, Khanna M, Chaturvedi UC. 1992. Breakdown of blood-barrier by virus-induced cytokine during Japanese encephalitis virus infection. Int J Exp Pathol 73:603–611.

Mayo DR, Beckwith WH. 2002. Inactivation of West Nile virus during serologic testing and transport. J Clin Microbiol 40:3044–3046.

Monath TP. 2002. Japanese encephalitis vaccines: Current vaccines and future prospects. Curr Top Microbiol Immunol 267:105–138.

Morimoto T. 1969. Epizootic swine stillbirth caused by Japanese encephalitis virus. Proceedings of a symposium on factors producing embryonic and fetal abnormalities, death, and abortion in swine. US ARS 91–73:137–153.

Murgue B, Zeller H, Deubel V. 2002. The ecology and epidemiology of West Nile virus in Africa, Europe and Asia. Curr Top Microbiol Immunol 267:196–221.

Nasci RS, Savage HM, White DJ, Miller JR, Cropp BC, Godsey MS, Kerst AJ, Bennett P, Gottfried K, Lanciotti RS. 2001. West Nile virus in overwintering Culex mosquitoes, New York City, 2000. Emerg Infect Dis 7:742–744.

Ni H, Barrett AD. 1998. Attenuation of Japanese encephalitis virus by selection of its mouse brain membrane receptor preparation escape variants. Virology 241:30–36.

Ogasa A, Yokoki Y, Fujisaki Y, Habu A. 1977. Reproductive disorders in boars infected experimentally with Japanese encephalitis virus. Jpn J Anim Reprod 23:171–175.

O'Leary DR, Marfin AA, Montgomery SP, Kipp AM, Lehman JA, Biggerstaff BJ, Elko VL, Collins PD, Jones JE, Campbell GL. 2004. The epidemic of West Nile virus in the United States, 2002. Vector Borne Zoonotic Dis 4:61–70.

Platt KB. 2004. Characterization of West Nile virus infection in swine. National Pork Board, Clive, Iowa—Final report, project #02-118.

Remington KM, Trejo SR, Buczynski G, Li H, Osheroff WP, Brown JP, Renfrow H, Reynolds R, Pifat DY. 2004. Inactivation of West Nile virus, vaccinia virus and viral surrogates for relevant and emergent viral pathogens in plasma-derived products. Vox Sanguinis 87:10–18.

Roehrig JT, Layton M, Smith P, Campbell GL, Nasci R, Lanciotti RS. 2002. The emergence of West Nile virus in North America: Ecology, epidemiology, and surveillance. Curr Top Microbiol Immunol 267:223–240.

Rosen L. 1986. The natural history of Japanese encephalitis virus. Ann Rev Microbiol 40:395–414.

Rosen L, Lien JC, Shroyer DA, Baker RH, Lu LC. 1989. Experimental vertical transmission of Japanese encephalitis virus by Culex tritaeniorhynchus and other mosquitoes. Am J Trop Med Hyg 40:548–556.

Rosen L, Tesh RB, Lien JC, Cross JH. 1978. Transovarial transmission of Japanese encephalitis virus by mosquitoes. Science 199:909–911.

Shibata I, Hatano Y, Nishimura M, Suzuki G, Inaba Y. 1991. Isolation of Getah virus from dead fetuses extracted from a naturally infected sow in Japan. Vet Microbiol 27:385–391.

Shimizu T, Kawakami Y, Fukuhara S, Matsumoto M. 1954. Experimental stillbirth in pregnant swine infected with Japanese encephalitis virus. Jpn J Exp Med 24:363–375.

Shirato K, Mizutani T, Kariwa H, Takashima I. 2003. Discrimination of West Nile virus and Japanese encephalitis virus strains using RT-PCR RFLP analysis. Microbiol Immunol 47:439–445.

Siger L, Bowen RA, Karaca K, Murray MJ, Gordy PW, Loosmore SM, Audonnet JC, Nordgren RM, Minke JM. 2004. Assessment of the efficacy of a single dose of a recombinant vaccine against West Nile virus in response to natural challenge with West Nile virus-infected mosquitoes in horses. Am J Vet Res 65:1459–1462.

Solomon T, Ni H, Beasley DW, Ekkelenkamp M, Cardosa MJ, Barrett AD. 2003. Origin and evolution of Japanese encephalitis virus in southeast Asia J Virol 77:3091–3098.

Solomon T, Vaugh DW. 2002. Pathogenesis and clinical features of Japanese encephalitis and West Nile virus infections. Curr Top Microbiol Immunol 267:171–194.

Sugimori T, Morimoto T, Fujisaki Y, Sugawara S, Tomishima S, Ogata M. 1974. A status quo survey on stillbirth and abortion in swine. III. Relationship between the day of pregnancy at the time of outbreak of Japanese encephalitis and the occurrence of stillbirth and abortion. J Jpn Vet Med Assoc 27:282–285.

Takahashi M. 1976. The effects of environmental and physiological conditions of *Culex tritaeniorhynchus* on the pattern of transmission of Japanese encephalitis virus. J Med Entomol 13:275–284.

Takashima I, Rosen L. 1989. Horizontal and vertical transmission of Japanese encephalitis virus by *Aedes japonicus* (Diptera: Culicidae). J Med Entomol 1989 26:454–458.

Takashima I, Watanabe T, Ouchi N, Hashimoto N. 1988. Ecological studies of Japanese encephalitis virus in Hokkaido: Interepidemic outbreaks of swine abortion and evidence of the virus to overwinter locally. Am J Trop Med Hyg 38:420–427.

Taniguchi T, Hosokawa M, Kuga S. 1936. A virus isolated in 1935 epidemic of summer encephalitis of Japan. Jpn J Exp Med 14:185–196.

Tiawsirisup S; Platt KB, Evans RB, Rowley WA. 2004. Susceptibility of *Ochlerotatus trivittatus* (Coq.), *Aedes albopictus* (Skuse), and *Culex pipiens* (L.) to West Nile virus infection. J Vector Borne Dis 4:190–197.

Tsai TF, Popovici F, Cernescu C, Campbell GL, Nedelcu NI. 1998. West Nile encephalitis epidemic in southeastern Romania. Lancet 352(9130):767–771.

Turell MJ, Dohm DJ, Sardelis MR, Oguinn ML, Andreadis TG, Blow JA. 2005. An update on the potential of North American mosquitoes (Diptera: Culicidae) to transmit West Nile Virus. J Med Entomol 42:57–62.

Weng MH, Lien JC, Wang YM, Wu HL, Chin C. 1997. Susceptibility of three laboratory strains of *Aedes albopictus* (Diptera: Culicidae) to Japanese encephalitis virus from Taiwan. J Med Entomol 34:745–747.

Williams DT, Daniels PW, Lunt RA, Wang LF, Newberry KM, Mackenzie JS. 2001. Experimental infections of pigs with Japanese encephalitis virus and closely related Australian flaviviruses. Am J Trop Med Hyg 65:379–387.

Yamada M, Nakamura K, Yoshii M, Kaku Y. 2004. Nonsuppurative Encephalitis in piglets after experimental inoculation of Japanese encephalitis flavivirus isolated from pigs. Vet Pathol 41:62–67.

Yang DK, Kweon CH, Kim BH, Lim SI, Kim SH, Kwon JH, Han HR. 2004. TaqMan reverse transcription polymerase chain reaction for the detection of Japanese encephalitis virus. J Vet Sci 5:345–351.

22 Porcine Epidemic Diarrhea

Maurice B. Pensaert and Sang-Geon Yeo

In 1971, previously unrecognized acute outbreaks of diarrhea were observed in feeder pigs and fattening swine in England (Oldham 1972). The clinical appearance was similar to transmissible gastroenteritis virus (TGEV) infection, except for the important difference that suckling pigs did not become sick. TGEV and other known enteropathogenic infectious agents were ruled out. The disease spread to other European countries and the name "epidemic viral diarrhea" (EVD) was adopted.

In 1976, TGE-like outbreaks of acute diarrhea were observed in swine of all ages, including suckling pigs (Wood 1977), but again TGEV and other known enteropathogenic agents were ruled out as the cause. The name "EVD type 2" was used to differentiate these outbreaks from the "type 1" outbreaks observed in 1971, the difference being that baby piglets were involved in type 2 outbreaks.

In 1978, a coronavirus-like agent was associated with the type 2 outbreaks (Chasey and Cartwright 1978; Pensaert and DeBouck 1978). Experimental inoculations with an isolate designated CV777 revealed its enteropathogenic character both for piglets and fattening swine (DeBouck and Pensaert 1980). It appeared that this coronavirus was involved in outbreaks of type 1 as well as of type 2, and the name "porcine epidemic diarrhea" (PED) was proposed (Pensaert et al. 1982) and is still used. The basis for the clinical difference between type 1 and type 2 outbreaks is unknown.

ETIOLOGY

On the basis of genetic and antigenic criteria, PED virus (PEDV) has been categorized in group 1 of the genus *Coronavirus* of the family *Coronaviridae*, together with TGEV, feline coronavirus, canine coronavirus, and human coronavirus 229E (Gónzales et al. 2003; Utiger et al. 1995a). Immunoblotting and immunoprecipitation assays showed that PEDV shares common antigenic determinants with feline coronavirus and that these are located in the N protein (Yaling et al. 1988). The entire genome of CV777 has been sequenced and determined to contain 28,033 nucleotides. Based on the amino acid sequence of the replicase gene, PEDV is considered most closely related to human coronavirus 229E and TGEV (Kocherhans et al. 2001). Sequence determination of the N protein gene confirmed that PEDV holds an intermediate position between 229E and TGEV (Bridgen et al. 1993).

The pattern of the structural proteins of PEDV is similar to that of other coronaviruses. The virus possesses a glycosylated peplomer (spike, S) protein with a molecular weight of 180,000–200,000 daltons, a glycosylated membrane (M) protein of 27,000–32,000 daltons, and an unglycosylated RNA-binding nucleocapsid (N) protein of 57,000 to 58,000 daltons (Duarte and Laude 1994; Egberink et al. 1988; Knuchel et al. 1992; Utiger et al. 1995a, 1995b).

PEDV particles show characteristics of the family *Coronaviridae* (Chasey and Cartwright 1978; Pensaert and DeBouck 1978). The morphogenesis of PEDV in intestinal epithelial cells is identical to that of other coronaviruses. Assembly of the virus occurs by budding through intracytoplasmic membranes (Ducatelle et al. 1981b; Sueyoshi et al. 1995). The particles detected in fecal material are pleomorphic, with a tendency to a spherical shape. Their mean diameter, projections included, is 130 nm, with a range of 95–190 nm. Many particles have an electron-opaque central area. The club-shaped projections measure 18–23 nm and are radially spaced from the core.

Physicochemical characterization has shown that the virus is ether- and chloroform-sensitive. Its density in sucrose is 1.18 g/ml. Cell culture-adapted PEDV loses its infectivity when heated to ≥60°C for 30 minutes, but it is moderately stable at 50°C. The virus is stable between pH 4.0 and 9.0 at 4°C and between pH 6.5 and 7.5 at 37°C (Callebaut and DeBouck 1981; Lee and Yeo 2003a). The virus shows no hemagglutinating activity (Callebaut and DeBouck 1981).

There is no evidence of the existence of more than

one PEDV serotype. Polypeptide bands of a Korean isolate showed molecular weights similar to those of the prototype CV777 strain (Kweon et al. 1993). Genetic comparisons showed 96.5% homology of the N open reading frame (ORF) and 96.8% amino acid identity of the N protein between the Korean (Chinju99) and Belgian (CV777) isolates (Lee and Yeo 2003b). The entire S gene of the Korean strain showed 94.5% homology at the nucleotide level and 92.8% at the amino acid level (Yeo et al. 2003). Likewise, nucleotide sequences of the N gene of a Korean and two Japanese isolates were found to be almost identical (Kubota et al. 1999).

Propagation of PEDV was originally accomplished by orally inoculating piglets (DeBouck and Pensaert 1980). The adaptation of PEDV to laboratory conditions has been difficult. Numerous cell types were tested, but without success. Vero (African green monkey kidney) cells were later found to support the serial propagation of PEDV. Viral growth depends on the presence of trypsin in the cell culture medium. Cytopathic effects consist of vacuolation and formation of syncytia with up to 100 nuclei. Growth kinetics show virus titers peak at about $10^{5.5}$ plaque-forming units per ml 15 hours after inoculation (Hofmann and Wyler 1988, 1989; Lee and Yeo 2003a). PEDV was successfully grown in porcine bladder and kidney cells in Japan (Shibata et al. 2000). A Japanese isolate (P-5V) used as a vaccine strain was cultivated in swine cell lines KSEK6 and IB-RS2 (Kadoi et al. 2002).

EPIDEMIOLOGY

From 1982 to 1990, antibodies to PEDV were detected in swine populations in Belgium, England, Germany, France, the Netherlands, Switzerland, Bulgaria, and Taiwan (DeBouck et al. 1982; Hofmann and Wyler 1987; Möstl et al. 1990). In the northeastern part of India, 21.2% of 528 serum samples from pigs 2–6 months of age were positive for PEDV antibodies (Barman et al. 2003). The virus has been isolated in most swine-raising countries in Europe, as well as China (Qinghua et al. 1992), Korea (Kweon et al. 1993), and Japan (Takahashi et al. 1983). There are no reports of PEDV in North or South America.

In Europe, outbreaks of PED have become rare and there are few recent reports of serologic surveys or diagnostic studies.

In Belgium, a study was performed in 10 groups of multisource feeder pigs entering a fattening unit in September 1991, and none seroconverted. In contrast, the pigs in another 7 groups entering in February 1992 developed diarrhea and seroconverted to PEDV 4 weeks after arrival (Van Reeth and Pensaert 1994). Also in Belgium, a serological study on fattening farms showed 50% positive in 1990 and none in 1997, indicating that virus prevalence has markedly decreased in recent years (Pensaert and Van Reeth 1998).

In Spain, PED was identified as the cause of an epidemic of watery diarrhea in 7 of 15 farms, with the diarrhea becoming persistent in a small number of sows on one farm (Carvajal et al. 1995a). In a Spanish serosurvey conducted in 1992–1993, PEDV-specific antibodies were detected in 1,513 of 5,052 sows and positive animals were found in 55.0% of 803 breeding farms. (Carvajal et al. 1995c).

In the Netherlands, a clinical and virological study of an acute outbreak of PED in a herd with both breeding and finishing pigs was described (Pijpers et al. 1993). Diarrhea was most severe in fattening pigs and pregnant sows, and was mild or absent in suckling pigs and young weaners. The virus became endemic and persisted in 6–10-week-old pigs and in gilts newly introduced to the farm for at least 1.5 years after the original outbreak.

In Britain, a clinical PED outbreak was described in 1998 in 3 consecutive batches of 8–15-week-old pigs in a finishing herd over a 2-month period (Pritchard et al. 1999). In Hungary, 92 diarrhea samples from weaned pigs on 19 farms were examined in 1995 and 5.5% were positive for PEDV, with PED considered the most important cause of postweaning diarrhea (Nagy et al. 1996). In the Czech Republic, 27 of 219 fecal samples from diarrheic pigs less than 21 days old were positive for PEDV, often in combination with other enteric viruses (Rodák et al. 2004).

Distinct from the current situation in Europe, severe outbreaks of diarrhea with high mortality have been reported in Asia. These outbreaks are acute and so severe that they cannot be differentiated clinically from typical acute TGEV outbreaks.

In Japan, outbreaks between September 1993 and June 1994 resulted in 14,000 deaths, with mortality ranging from 30–100% in suckling pigs. During these epidemics, adult pigs showed only a transient inappetence with decreased milk production in sows (Sueyoshi et al. 1995). In the winter of 1996, a PED epidemic occurred in Japan on 108 farms, most of which were farrow-to-finish. Diarrhea was encountered in baby piglets and 39,509 of 56,256 died.

In Korea, PED has caused several outbreaks of diarrhea in swine of all ages. Of 71 viral enteric cases requested for diagnosis at the Veterinary Research Institute between January 1992 and December 1993, 56.3% were identified as PED. Piglets less than 10 days old were involved in 90% of the outbreaks (Hwang et al. 1994). Between August 1997 and July 1999, 50.4% of 1,258 enteric cases in 5 provinces were diagnosed as PED (Chae et al. 2000). A 1994 abattoir serosurvey in Korea of 469 sera from pigs in 7 provinces found seroprevalences of 17.6–79% (mean of 45%), suggesting that the virus had become endemic in some areas (Kweon et al. 1994).

There are suggestions that the PED situation in Asia has recently evolved to reflect a more endemic pattern of disease in a partially immune sow population.

Fecal-oral transmission is probably the primary, if not the only means of transmitting PEDV. Acute outbreaks of PED on susceptible farms often occur 4–5 days after sale or purchase of pigs. The virus probably enters via infected pigs or on virus-contaminated fomites (trucks, boots, etc.). PEDV does not differ markedly from TGEV with regard to modes of transmission, but it appears to persist more easily on a farm once the acute infection has passed. After an outbreak has occurred on a breeding farm, the virus may either be eliminated from the herd or become endemic. An endemic cycle can be established if enough litters of pigs are produced and weaned so as to maintain virus circulation through infection of consecutive litters that have lost their lactogenic immunity at weaning. PEDV may be a cause of persistent postweaning diarrhea on such farms.

CLINICAL SIGNS

The main, and often the only, obvious clinical sign of PED is watery diarrhea. Outbreaks in susceptible breeding herds may show marked variation in morbidity and mortality. On some farms, pigs of all ages become sick, with morbidity approaching 100%. The disease is then very similar to TGE, except for a slower spread and a somewhat lower mortality in baby piglets. Piglets up to 1 week of age may die from dehydration after the diarrhea has lasted 3–4 days. Piglet mortality averages 50%, but may be as high as 100%. Older pigs recover after about 1 week. After the acute outbreak, diarrhea may be seen in pigs 2–3 weeks after weaning, and newly introduced pigs may routinely become sick. In recent years, typical acute outbreaks with high mortality in neonatal pigs are rare in Europe, but have been described in Japan and Korea (Chae et al. 2000; Sueyoshi et al. 1995).

When an acute PED outbreak occurs in multisource feeder pigs or during the fattening period, all the pigs in the unit will show diarrhea within a week. Animals are somewhat anorectic, depressed, and their feces are watery. Clinical PEDV infection towards the end of the fattening period may be more severe than TGEV. The animals appear to have more abdominal pain. As a rule, animals recover in 7–10 days. Mortality of 1–3% may be seen in such fattening pigs and they die acutely, usually in the early stages of diarrhea or even prior to the appearance of diarrhea. A common necropsy finding in these animals is acute necrosis of the back muscle. The highest mortality is found on farms with stress-sensitive pig breeds.

Compared to TGEV, PEDV spreads more slowly between the different units on closed breeding and finishing farms. It may take 4–6 weeks for the virus to infect different groups, and some units may even remain free of infection.

PATHOGENESIS

The pathogenesis of PED has been studied in hysterectomy-derived, colostrum-deprived piglets. Piglets were orally inoculated with the CV777 isolate at the age of 3 days (DeBouck et al. 1981b) and became sick 22–36 hours after inoculation. Viral replication, as demonstrated by immunofluorescence (IF) and transmission electron microscopy (EM), occurred in the cytoplasm of villous epithelial cells throughout the small intestine and also in the colon. Infected epithelial cells were observed as early as 12–18 hours postinoculation, with maximum involvement reached at 24–36 hours. Viral replication in the small intestine resulted in cell degeneration leading to villous shortening. A reduction in the villous height:crypt depth ratio from the normal 7:1 value to 3:1 was observed. No cell degeneration was seen in the infected colonic epithelial cells.

The pathogenic features of PEDV in the small intestine of piglets are very similar to those of TGEV. Since viral replication and progress of the infection in the small intestine with PEDV occurs at a somewhat slower rate, a longer incubation period is observed.

PEDV replication in piglets has not been detected in cells outside the intestinal tract. Shibata et al. (2000) showed that SPF pigs, inoculated with field PEDV between the age of 2 days to 12 weeks, developed age-dependent resistance and deaths occurred only in 2- and 7-day-old pigs.

The pathogenesis of PEDV in older swine has not been studied in detail, but fluorescence was found in the epithelial cells of the small intestinal and colonic villi of conventional fattening swine both after experimental and natural infection (DeBouck and Pensaert 1980). It is not clear how much the colonic infection adds to the severity of clinical signs. Also, no pathogenic explanation can be given for the sudden death with acute back muscle necrosis sometimes observed in finishing pigs and adult pigs.

Pathogenic features described in Korea and Japan are identical to those observed in Europe, except there is no evidence of viral replication in the colon by the Asian strains (Hwang et al. 1994; Kim and Chae 2003; Sueyoshi et al. 1995), and sudden deaths in fatteners have not been reported.

LESIONS

Lesions have been described both in experimentally infected and naturally infected piglets (Ducatelle et al. 1982a,b; Hwang et al. 1994; Pospischil et al. 1981; Sueyoshi et al. 1995).

Lesions are confined to the small intestine, which is distended with yellow fluid. Microscopically, vacuolation and exfoliation of enterocytes occur on the small-intestinal villi starting at 24 hours postinoculation and coinciding with the onset of diarrhea. From that time on, the villi rapidly shorten and enzymatic activity becomes markedly reduced. These findings were confirmed by scanning EM (Ducatelle et al. 1981a). This pathology is very similar to that described for TGEV. No histopathologic changes have been observed in the colon.

Ultrastructural changes were first observed in the cytoplasm of enterocytes in which cell organelles had decreased, leaving electron translucent areas. Later, the microvilli and terminal web disappeared and parts of the cytoplasm protruded into the intestinal lumen. The cells became flattened, the tight junction was lost, and cell release occurred into the gut lumen. Intracellular virus formation was seen by budding through membranes of the endoplasmic reticulum (Ducatelle et al. 1981b; Horvath and Moscari 1981; Pospischil et al. 1981). In the colon, some cellular changes were observed in enterocytes containing virus particles, but no exfoliation was seen.

DIAGNOSIS

A diagnosis of PED cannot be made solely on the basis of clinical signs. Acute PED outbreaks involving pigs of all ages cannot be clinically differentiated from TGE. In Europe, outbreaks may appear as rapidly spreading, watery diarrhea in weaned pigs and older animals on the breeding farm, but without clinical signs in baby piglets.

An etiologic diagnosis can be made by direct demonstration of PEDV and/or its antigens or by detection of antibodies. A direct IF test and an immunohistochemical technique applied on sections of the small intestine of baby pigs are the most sensitive, rapid, and reliable methods. However, they can only be used on the intestines of pigs sacrificed during the acute phase of diarrhea, preferably within 2 days of onset. These techniques are often not reliable on pigs that die naturally, because of loss of enterocytes (Bernasconi et al. 1995; DeBouck et al. 1981a; Guscetti et al. 1998; Sueyoshi et al. 1995).

PEDV particles can be demonstrated in the feces of pigs by direct EM, although the virus particles are not easy to detect if the spikes on the virion are lost or not clearly visible. The highest percentage of positive fecal samples obtained from experimentally inoculated piglets was 73% in feces collected on the first day after the onset of diarrhea. Furthermore, immunoelectron microscopy has to be applied to differentiate PEDV from TGEV, since both viruses have the same morphology.

Isolation of field strains of PEDV in cell cultures from feces may need subpassages before cytopathology appears in Vero cells or in other cell types, but early detection can be done by IF (Hofmann and Wyler 1988; Shibata et al. 2000).

A number of ELISA techniques have been developed for detection of PEDV antigens in feces as well as for demonstration of specific antibodies in serum. They are sensitive and reliable for diagnosis, particularly on a group basis. For the antigen ELISAs, polyclonal and monoclonal antibodies were used with pig-cultivated virus (Callebaut et al. 1982; Carvajal et al. 1995a; van Nieuwstadt and Zetstra 1991). For the antibody ELISA, antigen consists of semipurified virus, either pig- or cell-cultivated (Callebaut et al. 1982; Carvajal et al. 1995b; Kweon et al. 1994), or S and N viral proteins extracted from infected Vero cells (Knuchel et al. 1992). The antibody test has also been used for detection of immunoglobulins in sow's milk (de Arriba et al. 1995).

PEDV antigens can be demonstrated in rectal swabs from 3–11 days after experimental inoculation, with peak excretion being at 4–5 days (Carvajal et al. 1995a). Fecal material should be collected from several pigs, preferably during the acute phase of diarrhea. If proper and sufficient fecal samples are collected, the ELISA antigen test is of reliable sensitivity to detect the virus in pigs with endemic weaning diarrhea on breeding farms.

Other diagnostic tests for detection of PEDV in fecal material include reverse transcription-polymerase chain reaction (RT-PCR) (Ishikawa et al. 1997; Kubota et al. 1999) and in situ hybridization (Kim and Chae 2000). An RT-PCR was established for differential detection of TGEV and PEDV in intestines and stool samples of sick pigs (Kim et al. 2001).

Specific antibodies can be detected in sera from swine after natural or experimental infection with PEDV using ELISA, blocking ELISA, indirect IF, blocking IF, and seroneutralization in Vero cell cultures (Callebaut et al. 1982; Hofmann and Wyler 1989, 1990; Prager and Witte 1981; Shibata et al. 2000; Witte and Prager 1987). Demonstration of PEDV antibodies can be performed using the indirect IF test and the blocking IF test on PEDV-positive cryostat sections of pig intestine or on cell culture. Antibodies detected by blocking ELISA appear at 7 days postinoculation (Carvajal et al. 1995b). With all these tests, paired serum samples should be examined. The convalescent serum sample should be collected no sooner than 2 weeks after the onset of diarrhea.

PREVENTION AND CONTROL

Suckling pigs suffering from PED should have free access to water to diminish dehydration. In fattening swine, it is advisable to withhold feed. Since PEDV does not spread very quickly, preventive measures to temporarily prevent virus entrance into farrowing units with newly born piglets may be of help. Postponing the infection in these piglets until a later age may result in fewer deaths. Concurrently, exposure of pregnant sows to virus-contaminated feces or intestines will stimulate lactogenic immunity and shorten the outbreak on the farm. This approach is similar to that used with TGEV.

If the virus cycles in consecutive litters of weaned piglets, virus elimination can be attempted by removing pigs immediately after weaning to another site for at least 4 weeks. Simultaneously, introduction of new pigs should be stopped temporarily.

Oral administration of chicken egg yolk or cow colostrum containing PEDV immunoglobulins to neonatal pigs showed immunoprophylactic effect by preventing disease or reducing mortality (Kweon et al. 2000; Shibata et al. 2001).

In Europe, the disease is of insufficient economic importance to develop a vaccine. However, outbreaks in Asia have been so severe that attenuated virus vaccines are being developed.

Bernasconi et al. (1995) reported that cell culture adaptation of the CV777 virus made it strikingly different with regard to genomic sequences. Furthermore, the virulence of this cell culture-adapted virus was much lower for newborn cesarean-derived piglets and histopathological changes were decreased in severity. The Korean KPEDV-9 strain, when passaged 93 times in Vero cells, showed a reduction in pathogenicity for neonatal pigs and was found to be safe for pregnant sows. For that reason, the use of a cell culture-adapted virus as a vaccine has been proposed (Kweon et al. 1999), although its efficacy in the field needs to be determined. In Japan, a commercial, attenuated, live virus vaccine of cell-adapted PEDV (P-5V) has been used for prophylaxis in sows since 1997. The vaccine is considered efficacious, but not all sows develop solid lactogenic immunity (Usami et al. 1998).

REFERENCES

Barman NN, Barman B, Sarma K, Pensaert MB. 2003. Prevalence of rotavirus, transmissible gastroenteritis virus and porcine epidemic diarrhoea virus antibodies in pigs of Assam. Indian J Ann Sci 73:576–578.

Bernasconi C, Guscetti F, Utiger A, Van Reeth K, Ackermann M, Pospischil A. 1995. Experimental infection of gnotobiotic piglets with a cell culture adapted porcine epidemic diarrhoea virus: Clinical histopathological and immunohistochemical findings. Proc 3d Congr ESVV, pp. 542–546.

Bridgen A, Duarte M, Tobler K, Laude H, Ackermann M. 1993. Sequence determination of the nucleocapsid protein gene of the porcine epidemic diarrhoea virus confirms that this virus is a coronavirus related to human coronavirus 229E and porcine transmissible gastroenteritis virus. J Gen Virol 74:1795–1804.

Callebaut P, DeBouck P. 1981. Some characteristics of a new porcine coronavirus and detection of antigen and antibody by ELISA. Proc 5th Int Congr Virol, p. 420.

Callebaut P, DeBouck P, Pensaert M. 1982. Enzyme-linked immunosorbent assay for the detection of the coronavirus-like agent and its antibodies in pigs with porcine epidemic diarrhea. Vet Microbiol 7:295–306.

Carvajal A, Diego R, Lanza I, Rubio P, Carmenes P, Schwyzer M. l995a. Evaluation of an ELISA for the detection of porcine epidemic diarrhea virus (PEDV) in feces of naturally infected pigs. Proc 3d Congr ESVV, pp. 516–519.

Carvajal A, Lanza I, Diego R, Rubio P, Carmenes P. 1995b. Evaluation of a blocking ELISA using monoclonal antibodies for the detection of porcine epidemic diarrhea virus and its antibodies. J Vet Diagn Invest 7:60–64.

——. 1995c. Seroprevalence of porcine epidemic diarrhea virus infection among different types of breeding swine farms in Spain. Prev Vet Med 23:33–40.

Chae C, Kim O, Choi C, Min K, Cho WS, Kim J, Tai JH. 2000. Prevalence of porcine epidemic diarrhea virus and transmissible gastroenteritis virus infection in Korean pigs. Vet Rec 18:606–608.

Chasey D, Cartwright SF. 1978. Virus-like particles associated with porcine epidemic diarrhoea. Res Vet Sci 25:255–256.

de Arriba ML, Carvajal A, Lanza I, Rubio P, Carmenes P. 1995. Development of an ELISA for the detection of antibody isotypes against porcine epidemic diarrhoea virus (PEDV) in sow's milk. Proc 3d Congr ESVV, pp. 222–225.

DeBouck P, Callebaut P, Pensaert M. 1981a. The diagnosis of coronavirus-like agent (CVLA) diarrhea in suckling pigs. Curr Top Vet Med Anim Sci 13:59–61.

——. 1982. Prevalence of the porcine epidemic diarrhea (PED) virus in pig population of different countries. Proc Congr Int Pig Vet Soc 7:53.

DeBouck P, Pensaert M. 1980. Experimental infection of pigs with a new porcine enteric coronavirus CV777. Am J Vet Res 41:219–223.

DeBouck P, Pensaert M, Coussement W. 1981b. The pathogenesis of an enteric infection in pigs experimentally induced by the coronavirus-like agent CV777. Vet Microbiol 6:157–165.

Duarte M, Laude H. 1994. Sequence of the spike protein of the porcine epidemic diarrhoea virus. J Gen Virol 75; 1195–1200.

Ducatelle R, Coussement W, Charlier G, DeBouck P, Hoorens J. 1981a. Three-dimensional sequential study of the intestinal surface in experimental porcine CV777 coronavirus enteritis. Zentralbl Veterinärmed B 28:483–493.

——. 1982a. Pathology of experimental CV777 coronavirus enteritis in piglets. II. Electron microscopic study. Vet Pathol 19:57–66.

Ducatelle R, Coussement W, DeBouck P, Hoorens J. 1982b. Pathology of experimental CV777 coronavirus enteritis in piglets. I. Histological and histochemical study. Vet Pathol 19:46–56.

Ducatelle R, Coussement W, Pensaert M, DeBouck P, Hoorens J. 1981b. In vivo morphogenesis of a new porcine enteric coronavirus, CV777. Arch Virol 68:35–44.

Egberink HF, Ederveen J, Callebaut P, Horzinek MC. 1988. Characterization of the structural proteins of porcine epizootic diarrhea virus, strain CV777. Am J Vet Res 49:1320–1324.

Gónzales JM, Gomez-Puertas P, Cavanagh D, Gorbalenya AE, Enjuanes L. 2003. A comparative sequence analysis to revise the current taxonomy of the family *Coronaviridae*. Arch Virol 148:2207–2235.

Guscetti F, Bernasconi C, Tobler K, Van Reeth K, Pospischil A, Ackermann M. 1998. Immunohistochemical detection of porcine epidemic diarrhea virus compared to other methods. Clin Diagn Lab Immunol 5:412–414.

Hofmann M, Wyler R. 1987. Serolgische Untersuchung über das Vorkommen der Epizootischen Virusdiarrhoe der Schweine (EVD) in der Schweiz. Schweiz Arch Tierheilkd 129:437–442.

——. 1988. Propagation of the virus of porcine epidemic diarrhea in cell culture. J Clin Microbiol 26:2235–2239.

——. 1989. Quantitation, biological and physiochemical properties of cell culture-adapted porcine epidemic diarrhea coronavirus (PEDV). Vet Microbiol 20:131–142.

——. 1990. Enzyme-linked immunosorbent assay for the detection of porcine epidemic diarrhea coronavirus antibodies in swine sera. Vet Microbiol 21:263–273.

Horvath I, Moscari E. 1981. Ultrastructural changes in the small intestinal epithelium of suckling pigs affected with a transmissible gastroenteritis (TGE)-like disease. Arch Virol 68: 103–113.

Hwang EK, Kim JH, Jean YH, Bae YC, Yoon SS, Park CK, Kweon CH, Yoon YD, Ackermann M. 1994. Current occurrence of porcine epidemic diarrhea in Korea. RDA J Agri Sci 36:587–596.

Ishikawa K, Sekiguchi H, Ogino T, Suzuki S. 1997. Direct and rapid detection of porcine epidemic diarrhea virus by RT-PCR. J Virol Methods 69:191–195.

Kadoi K, Sugioka H, Satoh T, Kadoi BK. 2002. The propagation of a porcine epidemic diarrhea virus in swine cell lines. New Microbiol 25:285–290.

Kim O, Chae C. 2000. In situ hybridization for the detection and localization of porcine epidemic diarrhea virus in the intestinal tissues from naturally infected piglets. Vet Pathol 37:62–67.

——. 2003. Experimental infection of piglets with a Korean strain of porcine epidemic diarrhoea virus. J Comp Path 129:55–60.

Kim SY, Song DS, Park BK. 2001. Differential detection of transmissible gastroenteritis virus and porcine epidemic diarrhea virus by duplex RT-PCR. J Vet Diagn Invest 13:516–520.

Knuchel M, Ackermann M, Müller HK, Kihm U. 1992. An ELISA for detection of antibodies against porcine epidemic diarrhoea virus (PEDV) based on the specific solubility of the viral surface glycoprotein. Vet Microbiol 32:117–134.

Kocherhans R, Bridgen A, Ackermann M, Tobler K. 2001. Completion of the porcine epidemic diarrhoea Coronavirus (PEDV) genome sequence. Virus Genes 23:137–144.

Kubota S, Sasaki O, Amimoto K, Okada N, Kitazima T, Yasuhara H. 1999. Detection of porcine epidemic diarrhea virus using polymerase chain reaction and comparison of the nucleocapsid protein genes among strains of the virus. J Vet Med Sci 61:827–830.

Kweon CH, Kwon BJ, Jung TS, Kee YJ, Hur DH, Hwang EK, Rhee JC, An SH. 1993. Isolation of porcine epidemic diarrhea virus (PEDV) infection in Korea. Korean J Vet Res 33:249–254.

Kweon CH, Kwon BJ, Kang YB, An SH. 1994. Cell adaptation of KPEDV-9 and serological survey on porcine epidemic diarrhea virus (PEDV) infection in Korea. Korean J Vet Res 34:321–326.

Kweon CH, Kwon BJ, Lee JG, Kwon GO, Kang YB. 1999. Derivation of attenuated porcine epidemic diarrhea virus (PEDV) as vaccine candidate. Vaccine 17:2546–2553.

Kweon CH, Kwon BJ, Woo SR, Kim JM, Woo GH, Son DH, Hur W, Lee YS. 2000. Immunoprophylactic effect of chicken egg yolk immunoglobulin (IgY) against porcine epidemic diarrhea virus (PEDV) in piglets. J Vet Med Sci 62:961–964.

Lee HK, Yeo SG. 2003a. Biological and physicochemical properties of porcine epidemic diarrhea virus Chinju99 strain isolated in Korea. J Vet Clin 20:150–154.

——. 2003b. Cloning and sequence analysis of the nucleocapsid gene of porcine epidemic diarrhea virus Chinju99. Virus Genes 26:207–212.

Möstl K, Horvath E, Bürki F. 1990. Erhebungen über porcine Coronaviren in Osterreich. II. Porcine epidemic diarrhea virus (PEDV) der Schweine. Wien Tierärtztl Monatsschr 77:10–18.

Nagy B, Nagy G, Meder M, Mocsari E. 1996. Enterotoxigenic escherichia coli, rotavirus, porcine epidemic diarrhoea virus, adenovirus and calici-like virus in porcine postweaning diarrhoea in Hungary. Acta Vet Hung 44:9–19.

Oldham J. 1972. Pig Farming (Oct suppl), pp. 72–73.

Pensaert MB, Callebaut P, DeBouck P. 1982. Porcine epidemic diarrhea (PED) caused by a coronavirus: Present knowledge. Proc Congr Int Pig Vet Soc 7:52.

Pensaert MB, DeBouck P. 1978. A new coronavirus-like particle associated with diarrhea in swine. Arch Virol 58:243–247.

Pensaert MB, Van Reeth K. 1998. Porcine epidemic diarrhea and porcine respiratory coronavirus. Am Assoc Swine Pract, pp. 433–436.

Pijpers A, van Nieuwstadt AP, Terpstra C, Verheijden JHM. 1993. Porcine epidemic diarrhoea virus as a cause of persistent diarrhoea in a herd of breeding and finishing pigs. Vet Rec 132:129–131.

Pospischil A, Hess RG, Bachmann PA. 1981. Light microscopy and ultrahistology of intestinal changes in pigs infected with enzootic diarrhoea virus (EVD): Comparison with transmissible gastroenteritis (TGE) virus and porcine rotavirus infections. Zentralbl Veterinärmed B 28:564–577.

Prager D, Witte K. 1981. Die serologische Diagnose der Epizootischen Virusdiarrhoe (EVD) des Schweines mit Hilfe der indirekten Immunofloreszenztechnik (IIFT). II. Antikorper-Antwort nach experimenteller Infektion. Tierärtztl Umsch 36:477–480.

Pritchard GC, Paton DJ, Wibberley G, Ibata G. 1999. Transmissible gastroenteritis and porcine epidemic diarrhoea in Britain. Vet Rec 144:616–618.

Qinghua C, et al. 1992. Investigation on epidemic diarrhea in pigs in Qinghai region. Qinghai Xumu Shaoyi Zazhi 22:22–23.

Rodák L, Smid B, Valíček L, Smítalová R, Nevoránková Z. 2004. Elisa detection of group A rotavirus, transmissible gastroenteritis virus and porcine epidemic diarrhoea virus in faeces of piglets. Proc Congr Int Pig Vet Soc 1:271.

Shibata I, Ono M, Mori M. 2001. Passive protection against porcine epidemic diarrhea (PED) virus in piglets by colostrum from immunized cows. J Vet Med Sci 63:655–658.

Shibata I, Tsuda T, Mori M, Ono M, Sueyoshi M, Uruno K. 2000. Isolation of porcine epidemic diarrhea virus in porcine cell cultures and experimental infection of pigs of different ages. Vet Microbiol 72:173–182.

Sueyoshi M, Tsuda T, Yamazaki K, Yoshida K, Nakazawa M, Sato K, Minami T, Iwashita K, Watanabe M, Suzuki Y. 1995. An immunohistochemical investigation of porcine epidemic diarrhoea. J Comp Path 113:59–67.

Takahashi K, Okada K, Ohshima K. 1983. An outbreak of swine diarrhoea of a new type associated with coronavirus-like particles in Japan. Jpn J Vet Sci 45:829–832.

Usami Y, Yamaguchi O, Kumanomido K, Matsumura Y. 1998. Antibody response of pregnant sows to porcine epidemic diarrhea virus live vaccine and maternally derived antibodies of the piglets. J Jpn Vet Med Assoc 51:652–655.

Utiger A, Tobler K, Brigen A, Ackermann M. 1995a. Identification of the membrane protein of porcine epidemic diarrhea virus. Virus Genes 10:137–148.

Utiger A, Tobler K, Bridgen A, Suter M, Singh M, Ackermann M. 1995b. Identification of proteins specified by porcine epidemic diarrhoea virus. Adv Exp Med Biol 380:287–290.

Van Nieuwstadt AP, Zetstra T. 1991. Use of two enzyme-linked immunosorbent assays to monitor antibody responses in swine with experimentally induced infection with porcine epidemic diarrhea virus. Am J Vet Res 52:1044–1050.

Van Reeth K, Pensaert M. 1994. Prevalence of infections with enzootic respiratory and enteric viruses in feeder pigs entering fattening herds. Vet Rec 135:594–597.

Witte KH, Prager D. 1987. Der Nachweis von Antikorpern gegen das Virus der Epizootischen Virusdiarrhoe (EVD) des Schweines mit dem Immunofluoreszenz-blockadetest (IFBT). Tierärtztl Umsch 42:817–820.

Wood EN. 1977. An apparently new syndrome of porcine epidemic diarrhoea. Vet Rec 100:243–244.

Yaling Z, Ederveen K, Egberink H, Pensaert M, Horzinek MC. 1988. Porcine epidemic diarrhea virus (CV777) and feline infectious peritonitis virus (FIPV) are antigenically related. Arch Virol 102:63–71.

Yeo SG, Hernandez M, Krell PJ, Nagy E. 2003. Cloning and sequence analysis of the spike gene of porcine epidemic diarrhea virus Chinju99. Virus Genes 26:239–246.

23 Porcine Parvovirus

William L. Mengeling

Porcine parvovirus (PPV) causes reproductive failure of swine characterized by embryonic and fetal infection and death, usually in the absence of outward maternal clinical signs. The disease develops mainly when seronegative dams are exposed oronasally to the virus any time during about the first half of gestation, and conceptuses are subsequently infected transplacentally before they become immunocompetent. Porcine parvovirus is ubiquitous among swine throughout the world and is endemic in most herds that have been tested. Diagnostic surveys have indicated that PPV is the major infectious cause of embryonic and fetal death (Cartwright and Huck 1967; Mengeling 1978b; Mengeling et al. 1991; Thacker and Leman 1978; Vannier and Tillon 1979). In addition to its direct causal role in reproductive failure, PPV can potentiate the effects of porcine circovirus type II (PCV2) infection in the clinical course of postweaning multisystemic wasting syndrome (PMWS) (Krakowka et al. 2000; Opriessnig et al. 2004).

ETIOLOGY

PPV is classified in the genus *Parvovirus* (Latin *parvus* = small) of the family *Parvoviridae* (Bachmann et al. 1979; Siegl 1976). All isolates of PPV that have been compared are antigenically similar, if not identical (Cartwright et al. 1969; Johnson and Collings 1969; Johnson et al. 1976; Morimoto et al. 1972a; Ruckerbauer et al. 1978). PPV is also antigenically related to several other members of the genus (Cotmore et al. 1983; Mengeling et al. 1986, 1988). However, its identity can be established by relatively stringent serologic tests such as virus neutralization (VN) and hemagglutination inhibition (HI).

The biophysical and biochemical properties of PPV have been extensively studied (Berns 1984; Molitor et al. 1983; Siegl 1976) and are summarized as follows. A mature virion has cubic symmetry, two or three capsid proteins, a diameter of approximately 20 nm, 32 capsomeres, no envelope or essential lipids, and a weight of 5.3×10^6 daltons. The viral genome is single-stranded deoxyribonucleic acid (DNA) with a molecular weight of 1.4×10^6 (i.e., about 26.5% of the weight of the complete virion). Buoyant densities (g/ml in cesium chloride) of complete infectious virions, incomplete "empty" virions, and extracted virion DNA are 1.38–1.395, 1.30–1.315, and 1.724, respectively. Viral infectivity, hemagglutinating activity, and antigenicity are remarkably resistant to heat, a wide range of hydrogen ion concentrations, and enzymes.

Replication

Replication of PPV in vitro is cytocidal and characterized by "rounding up," pyknosis, and lysis of cells (Figure 23.1A). Many of the cell fragments often remain attached, eventually giving the affected culture a ragged appearance. Intranuclear inclusions develop (Cartwright et al. 1969) but they are often sparsely distributed (Rondhuis and Straver 1972). Infected cultures may hemadsorb slightly (Cartwright et al. 1969) (Figure 23.1B). Cytopathic changes are extensive when cell culture-adapted virus is propagated under appropriate conditions. However, on initial isolation, several serial passages of the virus (Cartwright et al. 1969) or, better, the infected culture may be necessary before the effects are recognized. The use of immunofluorescence (IF) microscopy greatly increases the likelihood of detecting minimally infected cultures (Lucas and Napthine 1971; Mengeling 1975).

Primary and secondary cultures of fetal or neonatal porcine kidney cells are most often used for propagation and titration of PPV, although other kinds of cultures are also susceptible (Pirtle 1974). Replication is enhanced by infection of mitotically active cultures (Bachmann 1972; Cartwright et al. 1969; Hallauer et al. 1972; Mayr et al. 1968). Many cells in such cultures are in the S phase (i.e., the DNA synthesis phase) of their cell cycle, wherein the DNA polymerases of cell origin needed for viral replication are available (Siegl and Gautschi 1973a, b; Tennant 1971).

If either fetal or adult bovine serum is incorporated

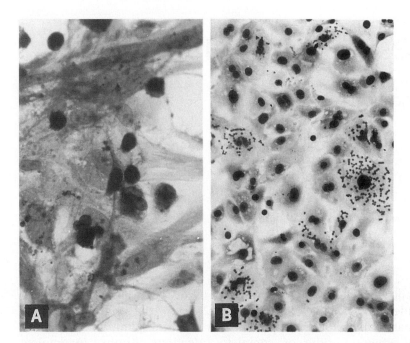

23.1. *Cell cultures infected with PPV. (A) Cytopathic effect, secondary fetal porcine kidney cells, 120 hours after infection (×250) (Mengeling, 1972). (B) Hemadsorption, secondary adult porcine thyroid cells, guinea pig erythrocytes, 22 hours after thyroid cells were infected and then subcultured (May-Grünwald-Giemsa; ×100).*

in the nutrient medium of cell cultures used to propagate PPV, it should be pretested for viral inhibitors (Coackley and Smith 1972; Johnson 1973; Pini 1975). The same may apply to sera of several other species (Joo et al. 1976d). Because replication of PPV is affected by mitotic activity, the effect of the serum on the cells is also especially important. In addition, cultures should be pretested for PPV contamination (Lucas and Napthine 1971; Mengeling 1975). Cultures are sometimes unknowingly prepared from infected tissues of fetal (Mengeling 1975) and postnatal (Bachmann 1969; Cartwright et al. 1969; Hafez and Liess 1979; Huygelen and Peetermans 1967) pigs. Moreover, PPV can be accidentally introduced into cultures in several ways (Hallauer et al. 1971), including the use of contaminated trypsin (Croghan and Matchett 1973; Croghan et al. 1973). If contamination is detected before all cells are infected, the virus can be eliminated by repeatedly subculturing the cells in the presence of nutrient medium containing PPV antiserum (Mengeling 1978a).

Several investigators have used immunofluorescence microscopy to follow the development of PPV in cell culture (Bachmann and Danner 1976; Cartwright et al. 1969; Lucas and Napthine 1971; Mengeling 1972; Siegl et al. 1972). In general, the sequence of events is as follows. Viral antigen is detected in the cytoplasm of cells soon after infection if the inoculum contains a high titer of virus and viral antigen. Most, if not all, of this early cytoplasmic fluorescence is the result of antigen phagocytized from the inoculum (Mengeling 1972; Mengeling and Cutlip 1975). By sequential examinations, such antigen can be demonstrated first on the external surface of the cytoplasmic membrane and later within the cytoplasm, often relatively concentrated in a juxtanuclear location. The first unequivocal evidence of

viral replication is the appearance of nascent viral antigen in the nucleus (Figure 23.2A). In at least some infected cells, nascent antigen next appears in the cytoplasm in sufficient quantity that both cytoplasm and nucleus are brightly fluorescent. The infected cells commonly seen in the lungs of fetuses that develop a high titer of antibody for PPV probably represent this stage of replication (see Figure 23.8C). Affected cells subsequently round up, become pyknotic, and disintegrate with release of virus and viral antigen (Figure 23.2B). Other cells in the culture that are not at the appropriate stage to support viral replication continue to phagocytize and accumulate viral antigen in their cytoplasm (Figure 23.2C). A second wave of viral replication can be induced if these cells are stimulated to enter the S phase of the cell cycle as, for example, by the addition of fresh culture medium.

Hemagglutination

PPV agglutinates human, monkey, guinea pig, cat, chicken, rat, and mouse erythrocytes. Erythrocytes from other animal species that have been tested are relatively or completely insensitive, or the results have been equivocal (Cartwright et al. 1969; Darbyshire and Roberts 1968; Hallauer et al. 1972; Mayr et al. 1968; Mengeling 1972; Morimoto et al. 1972a). Several parameters of the hemagglutination (HA) test—such as the temperature of incubation (Mayr et al. 1968; Mengeling 1972), the species of erythrocyte used, and in the case of chicken erythrocytes the genetic composition (Cartwright et al. 1969; Pini 1975; Ruckerbauer et al. 1978) and age (Morimoto et al. 1972a) of the donor—may quantitatively affect results. The HA test is most commonly conducted at room temperature, at approximately neutral pH, and with guinea pig erythrocytes.

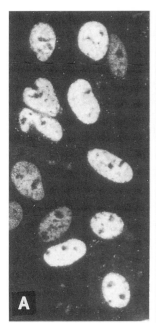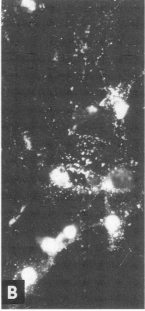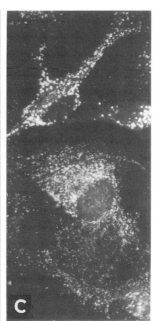

23.2. *Secondary cultures of fetal porcine kidney cells infected with PPV and examined by IF microscopy (×500). (A) 14 hours after infection, culture fixed and then reacted with fluorescent antibodies (FA). (B) 24 hours after infection, culture reacted with FA and then fixed; only extracellular antigen and antigen in cells with disrupted cytoplasmic and nuclear membranes are identified. (C) 48 hours after infection, culture fixed and then reacted with FA.*

Higher HA titers have been recorded when the diluent used in the test was veronal buffer rather than phosphate-buffered saline (Ruckerbauer et al. 1978). Elution of virus (the hemagglutinin is part of the virion) can be induced by suspending erythrocytes in alkaline buffer, pH 9 (Hallauer et al. 1972).

Infectivity Titrations

Infectivity titrations are conducted in a standard manner except that, because cytopathic changes at terminal dilutions are often vague, endpoints of infectivity are often determined either by examining cell cultures for intranuclear inclusions after appropriate staining or by examining cell culture medium for viral hemagglutinin (Cartwright et al. 1969). A titration procedure wherein infected cells are made evident by IF microscopy (Mengeling 1972) and a plaque assay (Kawamura et al. 1988) also have been described.

EPIDEMIOLOGY

Porcine parvovirus is ubiquitous among swine throughout the world. The most common routes of infection for postnatal and prenatal pigs are oronasal and transplacental, respectively.

In major swine-producing areas, infection is endemic in most herds and, with few exceptions, sows are immune. A large proportion of gilts are naturally infected with PPV before they conceive and develop an active immunity that probably persists throughout life. Collectively, the seroepidemiologic data indicate that exposure to PPV is common and that gilts that have not developed immunity before conception are at a high risk of infection and reproductive disease.

Pigs nursing immune dams absorb a high titer of an-

tibody for PPV from colostrum. Passively acquired serum antibody titers decrease progressively with time; both by dilution as pigs grow, as well as by biological degradation. Serum antibody titers usually decline to undetectable levels in 3–6 months, if sera are examined by the HI test (Etoh et al. 1979; Paul et al. 1982), but may persist for a longer interval. Levels of antibody too low to be detected by the HI test may be detected by the VN test (Johnson et al. 1976).

The primary significance of passively acquired antibody is that it interferes with the development of active immunity. High antibody levels can prevent infection and lower levels can minimize dissemination from infected pigs (Paul et al. 1980; Suzuki and Fujisaki 1976). Consequently, some groups of gilts are not fully susceptible to infection and dissemination of virus until either shortly before conception or during early gestation.

Contaminated premises are probably major reservoirs of PPV. The virus is thermostable, resistant to many common disinfectants (Brown 1981), and may remain infectious for months in secretions and excretions from acutely infected pigs. Experimentally, it was shown that pigs transmitted PPV for only about 2 weeks after exposure, but the pens in which they were initially kept remained infectious for at least 4 months (Mengeling and Paul 1986).

The ubiquity of PPV also raises the possibility that some pigs are persistently infected and, at least periodically, shed virus. Shedding beyond the interval of acute infection has not been demonstrated (Johnson et al. 1976), but the possibility of immunotolerant carriers of PPV as a result of early in utero infection has been suggested (Johnson 1973). When gilts were infected with PPV before day 55 of gestation, their pigs were born infected, but without antibody. Virus was isolated from kidneys, testicles, and seminal fluid of such pigs killed at various times after birth up to 8 months of age, at which time the experiment was terminated (Johnson and Collings 1971). Likewise, a study in which dams were infected early in gestation and their pigs were born infected, but without antibody, also suggested immunotolerance (Cartwright et al. 1971). A possible example of an infected, immunotolerant, sexually active boar was reported (Johnson et al. 1976).

Boars may play a significant role in dissemination of PPV at a critical time. During acute infection, the virus is shed by various routes, including semen. The isolation of PPV from semen of naturally infected boars has been reported (Cartwright and Huck 1967; Cartwright et al. 1969; McAdaragh and Anderson 1975). Semen may also become contaminated externally, as for example with feces containing virus, or within the male reproductive tract. For example, PPV was isolated from the testicle of a boar 5 days after it was injected into the boar's prepuce (Lucas et al. 1974) and from testicles of boars killed 5 and 8 days after they were infected oronasally (Mengeling, unpublished data, 1976). Virus was also isolated from scrotal lymph nodes of boars killed 5, 8, 15, 21, and 35 days after oronasal exposure. After day 8, isolation was accomplished by cocultivating lymph node fragments with fetal porcine kidney cells (Mengeling, unpublished data, 1976). Irrespective of their immune status, boars can also function as a vector for mechanical dissemination of PPV among susceptible females.

CLINICAL SIGNS

Acute infection of postnatal pigs, including pregnant dams that subsequently develop reproductive failure, is usually subclinical (Cutlip and Mengeling 1975a; Fujisaki et al. 1975; Johnson and Collings 1969; Johnson et al. 1976; Joo et al. 1976a; Mengeling and Cutlip 1976). However, in young pigs, and probably in older breeding stock as well, the virus replicates extensively and is found in many tissues and organs with a high mitotic index. Viral antigen is especially concentrated in lymphoid tissues (Cutlip and Mengeling 1975a; Fujisaki et al. 1975) (Figure 23.3A, B).

Many pigs, irrespective of age or sex, have a transient, usually mild, leukopenia sometime within 10 days after initial exposure to the virus (Johnson and Collings 1969, 1971; Joo et al. 1976a; Mengeling and Cutlip 1976). PPV and other structurally similar viruses have been identified in the feces of pigs with diarrhea (Dea et al. 1985; Yasuhara et al. 1989). However, there is no experimental evidence to suggest that PPV either replicates extensively in the intestinal crypt epithelium or causes enteric disease, as do parvoviruses of several other species (Brown et al. 1980; Cutlip and Mengeling 1975a). PPV also has been isolated from pigs with lesions described as "vesicle-like." The etiologic role of PPV in such lesions has not been clearly defined (Kresse et al. 1985).

The major and usually only clinical response to infection with PPV is maternal reproductive failure. Pathologic sequelae depend mainly on when exposure occurs during gestation. Dams may return to estrus, fail to farrow despite being anestrus, farrow few pigs per litter, or farrow a large proportion of mummified fetuses. All can reflect embryonic or fetal death or both. The only outward sign in the dam may be a decrease in maternal abdominal girth when fetuses die at midgestation or later and their associated fluids are resorbed. Other manifestations of maternal reproductive failure—e.g., infertility, abortion, stillbirth, neonatal death, and re-

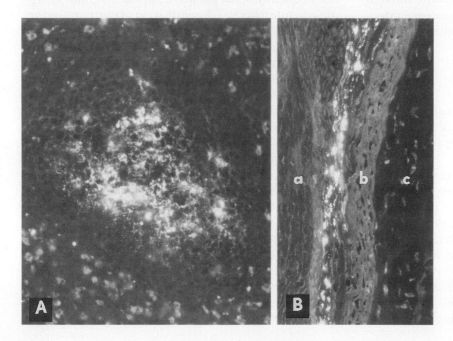

23.3. *Cryostat-microtome sections of tissues from PPV-infected 8-week-old pigs, examined by IF microscopy (×312.5). (A) Viral antigen in germinal center, tonsil. (B) Viral antigen in osteogenic layer of periosteum, rib: a = connective tissue, b = cortical bone, c = marrow cavity.*

duced neonatal vitality, have also been ascribed to infection with PPV (Cartwright and Huck 1967; Forman et al. 1977; Johnson 1969; Morimoto et al. 1972b; Narita et al. 1975). These are normally only a minor component of the disease. The presence of mummified fetuses in a litter can prolong both gestation (Narita et al. 1975) and the farrowing interval (Mengeling et al. 1975). Either may result in stillbirth of apparently normal littermates, whether or not they are infected.

There is no evidence that either fertility or libido of boars is altered by infection with PPV (Biront and Bonte 1983; Thacker et al. 1987).

PATHOGENESIS

Dams are susceptible to PPV-induced reproductive failure if infected anytime during about the first half of gestation. This interval of maternal susceptibility is indicated by the collective results of several experimental studies (Joo et al. 1976a; Mengeling 1979; Mengeling and Cutlip 1976; Mengeling et al. 1980a), by in-depth epidemiological investigations (Donaldson-Wood et al. 1977; Gillick 1977), and by estimates of the time of death of fetuses collected during epidemiological surveys (Mengeling 1978b; Mengeling et al. 1991). Consequences of maternal infection during this interval are embryonic and fetal death followed by resorption and mummification, respectively. Transplacental infection also follows maternal exposure after midgestation, but fetuses usually survive without obvious clinical effects in utero. The likely reason is that transplacental infection often requires 10–14 days (Mengeling et al. 1978, 1980a) or longer (Joo et al. 1976a), and by 70 days of gestation most fetuses are able to develop a protective immunologic response to the virus. In general, fetuses experimentally infected by transuterine inoculation of the virus died if infected before day 70 of gestation, but they have survived and produced antibody when infected later in gestation (Bachmann et al. 1975; Cutlip and Mengeling 1975b; Mengeling and Cutlip 1975; Redman et al. 1974). A strain of PPV of slightly greater virulence also has been reported (Choi et al. 1987). The usual consequences of infection at different stages of gestation are summarized in Table 23.1.

When only part of a litter is infected transplacentally, as is often the case, one or more littermates are fre-

quently infected by subsequent intrauterine spread of virus. The same would apply if initial infection were through contaminated semen. As a result, any combination or all of the sequelae indicated in Table 23.1 can develop in the same litter. Intrauterine dissemination is probably less common when early embryos are infected because they are quickly resorbed after death, effectively removing the intrauterine reservoir of virus (Mengeling et al. 1980a). In such cases there is no evidence at farrowing for the cause of fewer pigs per litter.

The effect, if any, of PPV on the ovum before ovulation is unknown. The virus adheres tenaciously to the external surface of the zona pellucida of the fertilized porcine ovum (Wrathall and Mengeling 1979a,b), and although it apparently cannot penetrate this layer, speculation is that it could pose a threat to the embryo after hatching (Wrathall and Mengeling 1979a).

Despite strong circumstantial evidence (Cartwright et al. 1971), a direct causal role of PPV-contaminated semen in reproductive failure has not been unequivocally established (Lucas et al. 1974). The zona pellucida could protect the early embryo while local immunity is developing. Conversely, the virus may cause uterine changes incompatible with gestation (Wrathall and Mengeling 1979c). In any event, a female infected through semen provides a focus of infection for others.

With the possible exception of the uterine changes alluded to in the preceding paragraph, PPV-induced reproductive failure is caused by the direct effect of the virus on the conceptus. In the absence of an immune response, the virus replicates extensively throughout these tissues. By the time the conceptus dies, most of its cells contain large quantities of intracytoplasmic viral antigen that can be demonstrated by IF microscopy. The relative lack of nuclear fluorescence at the time of death, compared to earlier stages of the disease, indicates that when the conceptus is severely affected, mitotic activity and the associated conditions necessary for viral replication are suppressed more than phagocytic activity.

Death of the conceptus probably results from the collective damage by the virus to a variety of tissues and organs, including the placenta (Cutlip and Mengeling 1975b). However, in the absence of an immune response, changes in almost any vital organ are probably sufficient to eventually cause death. One of the most striking features of viral distribution is the extensive in-

Table 23.1. Consequences of infection with PPV at different intervals of gestation

Interval of Gestation (days)[a]			
Infection of Dam	Infection of Conceptus[b]	Description of Conceptus	Consequences of Infection
≤56	10–30	Embryo	Death and resorption
	30–70	Fetus	Death and mummification
>56	70–term	Fetus	Immune response and usually survival in utero

[a]Intervals are approximations.
[b]Assuming transplacental infection 10–14 days after maternal exposure.

volvement of endothelium. This seems to preclude further development of the vascular network of the conceptus. Preparation for cellular mitosis (i.e., the S phase) results in concomitant viral replication and cell death. Damage to the fetal circulatory system is indicated by edema, hemorrhage, and the accumulation of large amounts of serosanguineous fluids in body cavities. Necrosis of the endothelium is microscopically evident (Lenghaus et al. 1978).

The mechanism of transplacental infection has been investigated by IF microscopy to identify infected cells in maternal and fetal tissues at progressively longer intervals after maternal oronasal exposure (Mengeling et al. 1978). Examination of tissues contiguous with the maternal-fetal junction revealed viral antigen in endothelial and mesenchymal cells of the chorion, with increasing involvement of these tissues at progressively later stages of gestation. Viral antigen was never detected unequivocally in either uterine epithelium or trophectoderm. Consequently, there was no evidence for maternal-fetal transfer of the virus by replicating through these tissues. However, this route cannot be excluded, since only a small part of the total area of contact was examined. Transfer of the virus within macrophages has also been considered (Paul et al. 1979). Whatever the route, maternal viremia seems a likely prerequisite for transplacental infection (Joo et al. 1976a; Mengeling and Cutlip 1976).

LESIONS

Neither macroscopic nor microscopic lesions have been reported for nonpregnant pigs (Brown et al. 1980; Cutlip and Mengeling 1975a). It is possible that cellular infiltrations subsequently described for fetuses could be induced by infection during the perinatal interval.

Macroscopic lesions have not been reported in pregnant dams; however, microscopic lesions have been seen in tissues of gilts killed after their fetuses were infected by transuterine inoculation of virus. Gilts that were seronegative when their fetuses were infected at 70 days of gestation had focal accumulations of mononuclear cells adjacent to the endometrium and in deeper layers of the lamina propria when they were killed 12 and 21 days later. In addition, there were perivascular cuffs of plasma cells and lymphocytes in the brain, spinal cord, and choroid of the eye (Hogg et al. 1977). When fetuses were infected earlier in gestation (35, 50, and 60 days) and their dams were killed 7 and 11 days later, the lesions were similar. However, uterine lesions were more severe and also included extensive cuffing of myometrial and endometrial vessels with mononuclear cells (Lenghaus et al. 1978). Only focal accumulations of lymphocytes were seen in uteruses of gilts that were seropositive when their fetuses were infected (Cutlip and Mengeling 1975b).

Macroscopic changes of embryos are death followed by resorption of fluids (Figure 23.4) and then soft tissues (Figure 23.5). Virus and viral antigen are widely distributed in tissues of infected embryos and their placentas (Mengeling et al. 1980a), and it is probable that microscopic lesions of necrosis and vascular damage, subsequently described for fetuses, also develop in advanced embryos.

There are numerous macroscopic changes in fetuses infected before they become immunocompetent (Figure 23.6). These include a variable degree of stunting and sometimes an obvious loss of condition before other external changes are apparent; occasionally, an increased prominence of blood vessels over the surface of the fetus due to congestion and leakage of blood into contiguous tissues; congestion, edema, and hemorrhage with accumulation of serosanguineous fluids in body cavities; hemorrhagic discoloration becoming progressively darker after death; and dehydration (mummification). Many of these changes also apply to the placenta. Microscopic lesions consist primarily of extensive cellular necrosis in a wide variety of tissues and organs (Joo et al. 1977; Lenghaus et al. 1978) (Figure 23.7A). Inflammation (Joo

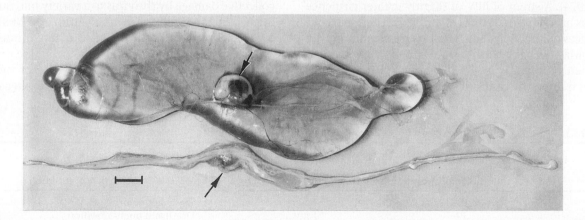

23.4. *Embryos from a gilt experimentally infected oronasally immediately after breeding and killed 22 days later. Bar = 1 cm. (Top) Noninfected, clinically normal embryo (arrow) and associated extraembryonic membranes; (bottom) PPV-infected, dead littermate embryo (arrow) and associated extraembryonic membranes, recent death, no obvious resorption of soft tissues. (Mengeling et al. 1980a.)*

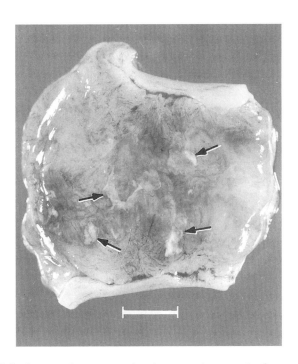

23.5. *Segment of uterus opened to show necrotic remnants of a partially resorbed PPV-infected embryo (arrows) and associated extraembryonic membranes of a gilt experimentally infected oronasally immediately after breeding and killed 22 days later; remnants are laden with virus and viral antigen. Bar = 1 cm. (Mengeling et al. 1980a.)*

et al. 1977) and intranuclear inclusions (Lenghaus et al. 1978) also have been described.

In contrast, macroscopic changes have not been reported for fetuses infected after they become immunocompetent for PPV. Microscopic lesions are primarily endothelial hypertrophy (Hogg et al. 1977) and mononuclear cell infiltrations consistent with an immune response (Hogg et al. 1977; Joo et al. 1977). Meningoencephalitis characterized by perivascular cuffing with proliferating adventitial cells, histiocytes, and a few plasma cells was seen in the gray and white matter of the cerebrum and in the leptomeninges of PPV-infected stillborn pigs. These lesions were believed to be pathognomonic for PPV infection (Narita et al. 1975). Similar lesions have been observed in PPV-infected, live fetuses collected late in gestation (Hogg et al. 1977; Joo et al. 1977) (Figure 23.7B).

Both general types of microscopic lesions (i.e., necrosis and mononuclear cell infiltration) may develop in fetuses infected near midgestation (Lenghaus et al. 1978) when the immune response is insufficient to provide protection.

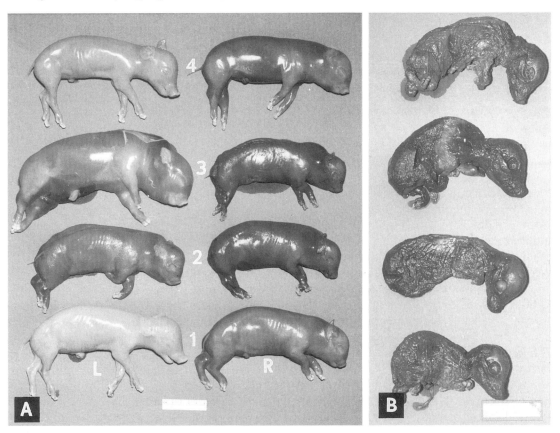

23.6. *PPV-infected fetuses. Bars = −5 cm. (A) Litter of a gilt experimentally infected oronasally on day 47 of gestation and killed 34 days later; fetuses from left (L) and right (R) horn of uterus, numbered 1–4 from cervix toward ovary; fetuses L1 and L4 stunted but alive at necropsy, fetus L3 recently dead, others later stages. (B) Fetuses from litter of a naturally infected gilt, collected at about 114 days of gestation, advanced stage of dehydration (mummification). (Mengeling et al. 1975.)*

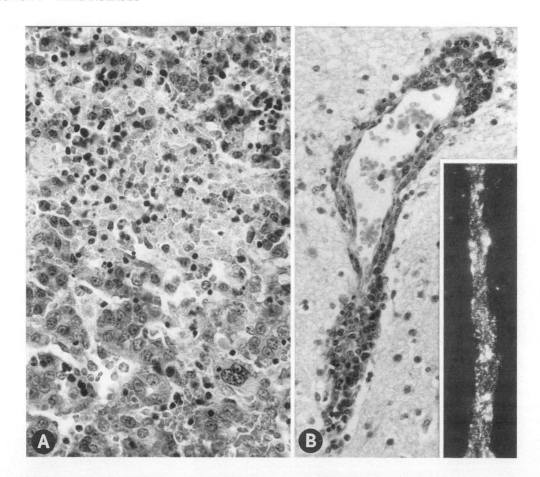

23.7. *Tissues of PPV-infected fetuses of gilts experimentally infected oronasally. (A) Necrotic focus in liver of live fetus of a gilt infected on day 40 of gestation and killed 42 days later; fetus had numerous macroscopic lesions (H&E; ×400). (B) Perivascular cuffing with mononuclear cells in cerebrum of live fetus, littermate of A; fetus had no macroscopic lesions (H&E; ×320). (Insert) Viral antigen associated with endothelium of cerebral vessel of fetus of a gilt infected on day 46 of gestation and killed 25 days later (IF microscopy; ×312.5). All fetuses were probably infected by intrauterine spread of PPV from transplacentally infected littermates. (Photographs A and B courtesy of T. T. Brown, Jr., National Animal Disease Center.)*

DIAGNOSIS

PPV should be considered in a differential diagnosis of reproductive failure of swine whenever there is evidence of embryonic or fetal death or both. A tentative diagnosis of PPV-induced reproductive failure can be made if gilts, but not sows, are affected, maternal illness was not seen during gestation, there are few or no abortions or fetal developmental anomalies, and the evidence suggests an infectious disease. The relative lack of maternal illness, abortions, and fetal developmental anomalies differentiates PPV from most other infectious causes of reproductive failure. However, a definitive diagnosis requires laboratory support.

Several mummified fetuses (<16 cm in length) or lungs from such fetuses, if sufficiently developed, should be submitted to the diagnostic laboratory. Larger mummified fetuses (i.e., more than about 70 days of gestational age) (Marrable and Ashdown 1967), stillborn pigs, and neonatal pigs are not recommended for submission unless they are the only samples available. If infected, their tissues will usually contain antibody that interferes with laboratory tests for either virus or viral antigen.

If females fail to farrow despite being anestrus and are sent to an abattoir, their uteruses should be collected and examined for affected fetuses. Sometimes only remnants of fetal tissues remain when fetuses die early in the middle third of gestation. Nevertheless, these are adequate samples if tested for viral antigen by IF microscopy (Mengeling 1978b; Mengeling and Cutlip 1975). However, the absence of affected fetuses or fetal remnants does not exclude PPV-induced reproductive failure. When all embryos of a litter die and are completely resorbed after the first few weeks of gestation, the dam may remain endocrinologically pregnant and not return to estrus until after the expected time of farrowing (Rodeffer et al. 1975).

Identification of viral antigen by IF microscopy is a reliable and sensitive diagnostic procedure. Sections of fetal tissues are prepared with a cryostat microtome and then reacted with standardized reagents (Mengeling et al. 1975; Mengeling 1978b). The test can be completed

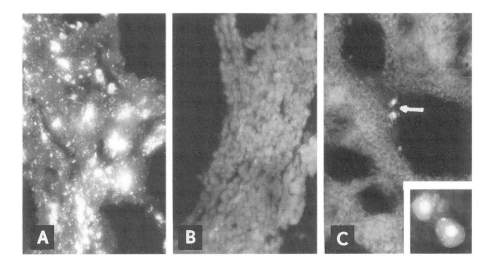

23.8. *Cryostat-microtome sections of lungs of PPV-infected fetuses examined by IF microscopy. (A) Lung of mummified fetus reacted with FA plus nonimmune serum (×312.5). (B) Replicate section reacted with FA plus PPV-immune serum (i.e., blocking control) (×312.5). (C) Lung of live fetus with HI antibody titer of 640 reacted with fluorescent antibodies (FA) plus nonimmune serum, two infected cells (arrow) (×162.5). (Insert) Two similar infected cells in the same section as C (×500). (Mengeling 1978b.)*

within a few hours. In the absence of a fetal antibody response, antigen is seen throughout fetal tissues (Figure 23.8A, B). Even when antibody is present, infected cells usually can be detected in fetal lung (Figure 23.8C).

Detection of viral hemagglutinin also has been recommended as a diagnostic technique (Joo et al. 1976b; Joo and Johnson 1977a). Tissues are triturated in diluent and then sedimented by centrifugation. The supernatant fluid is tested for agglutinating activity for guinea pig erythrocytes. This test requires a minimum of laboratory equipment and is effective in the absence of antibody.

Virus isolation is less suitable as a routine diagnostic procedure than either of the aforementioned tests. Infectivity is slowly but progressively lost after fetal death (Mengeling and Cutlip 1975). As a result, isolation of virus from mummified fetuses that have died as a result of infection is sometimes unsuccessful (Mengeling 1978b). Moreover, the procedure is time-consuming, and contamination is a constant threat because of the stability of PPV in the laboratory (Cartwright et al. 1969) and because cell cultures are sometimes unknowingly prepared from infected tissues (Bachmann 1969; Cartwright et al. 1969; Hafez and Liess 1979; Huygelen and Peetermans 1967; Mengeling 1975). IF microscopy is often used to determine whether PPV has been isolated in cell culture (Cartwright 1970; Johnson 1973; Mengeling 1978b).

In addition to tests that depend on the detection of PPV antigen or antibody, polymerase chain reaction (PCR) assays for PPV been developed (Molitor et al.1991; Prikhod'ko et al. 2003; Soares et al. 1999). In addition, tissues can be directly examined for a portion of the PPV genome by in situ hybridization (Waldvogel et al. 1995).

Serologic Assays

The HI test is frequently used for detection and quantitation of humoral antibody for PPV. Antibody sometimes can be detected as early as 5 days after swine are exposed to live virus, and it may persist for years (Johnson et al. 1976). Sera examined by the HI test are usually pretreated by heat inactivation (56°C, 30 minutes) and by adsorption with erythrocytes (to remove naturally occurring hemagglutinins) and kaolin (to remove or reduce nonantibody inhibitors of HA) (Mengeling 1972; Morimoto et al. 1972a). Trypsin also has been used to remove nonantibody inhibitors of HA (Cartwright et al. 1969). Parameters of the HI test have been studied in detail (Joo et al. 1976c; Kim 1974).

The VN test is occasionally used for detection and quantitation of humoral antibody for PPV. Neutralization of infectivity is usually confirmed by the absence or reduction either of intranuclear inclusions or fluorescent cells in cultures or of viral hemagglutinin in the culture medium (Johnson 1973; Joo et al. 1975; Mengeling 1972). The VN test has been reported to be more sensitive than the HI test (Johnson and Collings 1971; Joo et al. 1975). A microtechnique for application of the VN test has been described (Joo et al. 1975).

Immunodiffusion (Joo et al. 1978), a modified direct complement-fixation test (Ruckerbauer et al. 1978), and enzyme-linked immunosorbent assay (ELISA) (Hohdatsu et al. 1988; Westenbrink et al. 1989) also have been used successfully to detect antibody for PPV.

In general, serologic procedures are recommended for diagnosis only when tissues from mummified fetuses are not available for testing. Results with maternal sera are of value if antibody is not detected, thus excluding PPV as a cause, and if samples collected at intervals reveal seroconversion for PPV coincident with reproductive failure (Mengeling et al. 1975; Morimoto et al. 1972b; Rodeffer et al. 1975). Because PPV is ubiquitous, the presence of antibody in a single sample is otherwise meaningless. However, a determination of relative amounts of antibody present as immunoglobulin M and G can suggest the time frame of infection (Joo et al. 1978; Kim 1974). Detection of antibody in sera of fetuses and stillborn pigs and in sera collected from neonatal pigs before they nurse is evidence of in utero infection, since maternal antibody does not cross the maternal-fetal junction (Cartwright et al. 1971; Chaniago et al. 1978; Johnson and Collings 1969, 1971; Mengeling 1972). When serum is not available, body fluids collected from fetuses or their viscera that have been kept in a plastic bag overnight at 4°C have been used successfully to demonstrate antibody (Cropper et al. 1976; Joo et al. 1976b).

PREVENTION AND CONTROL

There is no treatment for PPV-induced reproductive failure. Gilts should either be naturally infected with PPV or vaccinated for PPV before they are bred. To promote natural infection, a common practice is to arrange contact between seronegative gilts and seropositive sows, with the expectation that one or more of the sows will be shedding virus. Moving gilts to a potentially contaminated area, either currently or recently inhabited by seropositive swine, also can be recommended. Once infection is started, the virus spreads rapidly among fully susceptible swine. Just how effective these procedures are in increasing the incidence of natural infection is unknown. Infection is common, and probably well over one-half of all gilts in areas where PPV is endemic are infected before they are bred for the first time (Mengeling 1972).

The use of vaccine is the only way to ensure that gilts develop active immunity before conception. Both inactivated (Fujisaki 1978; Fujisaki et al. 1978b; Ide et al. 1977; Joo and Johnson 1977b; Mengeling 1977; Mengeling et al. 1979, 1980b; Suzuki and Fujisaki 1976) and modified live-virus (MLV) vaccines (Fujisaki and Murikami 1982; Paul and Mengeling 1980) have been developed. An inactivated vaccine has been tested under field conditions (Fujisaki 1978; Fujisaki et al. 1978a), and both types of vaccines were effective when tested under controlled laboratory conditions (Mengeling et al. 1979, 1980b; Paul and Mengeling 1980).

Vaccines should be administered several weeks before conception with the objective of providing immunity through the susceptible period of gestation. However, vaccines must be administered after the disappearance of passively acquired colostral antibody, which could interfere with the development of active immunity (Paul and Mengeling 1986). These limits may define a very brief interval for effective vaccination of gilts that are bred before 7 months of age. Although inactivated vaccine provides maximum safety, there is experimental

evidence that PPV can be sufficiently attenuated so that it is unlikely to cause reproductive failure, even if inadvertently administered during gestation (Paul and Mengeling 1980). The apparent safety of MLV vaccine may be due to its reduced ability to replicate in tissues of the intact host and cause the level of viremia needed for transplacental infection (Paul and Mengeling 1984). Moreover, it has been shown by transuterine inoculation of both virulent and attenuated virus that a much larger dose of attenuated virus is required to establish infection of fetuses (Mengeling et al. 1984).

Duration of immunity following vaccination is unknown; however, in one study antibody titers were maintained for at least 4 months after administration of an inactivated vaccine (Joo and Johnson 1977b). Low levels of antibody found to be protective allow speculation that, once the immune system has been primed with PPV, subsequent exposure to virulent virus during gestation is unlikely to result in transplacental infection, even if antibody from vaccination is no longer detectable (Mengeling et al. 1979).

Vaccination is also recommended for seronegative sows and boars. Seronegative sows are usually found only in PPV-free herds. In such cases, inactivated vaccine is indicated. Experience has shown that few herds can be expected to remain free of PPV, even if access is carefully controlled. Introduction of PPV into a totally susceptible herd can be disastrous (Donaldson-Wood et al. 1977). Vaccination of boars should reduce their involvement in dissemination of the virus.

Vaccines are used extensively in the United States and in several other countries where PPV has been recognized as an economically important cause of reproductive failure. All federally licensed vaccines marketed in the United States are inactivated.

REFERENCES

Bachmann PA. 1969. Vorkommen und Verbreitung von Picodna (Parvo)-Virus beim Schwein. Zentralbl Veterinarmed B 16:341–345.
——. 1972. Porcine parvovirus infection in vitro: A study model for the replication of parvoviruses. I. Replication at different temperatures. Proc Soc Exp Biol Med 140:1369–1374.
Bachmann PA, Danner K. 1976. Porcine parvovirus infection in vitro: A study model for the replication of parvoviruses. II. Kinetics of virus and antigen production. Zentralbl Veterinarmed B 23:355–363.
Bachmann PA, Hoggan MD, Kurstak E, Melnick JL, Pereira HG, Tattersall P, Vago C. 1979. Parvoviridae: Second report. Intervirology 11:248–254.
Bachmann PA, Sheffy BE, Vaughan JT. 1975. Experimental in utero infection of fetal pigs with a porcine parvovirus. Infect Immun 12:455–460.
Berns KI. 1984. The Parvoviruses. New York: Plenum.
Biront P, Bonte P. 1983. Porcine parvovirus (P.P.V.) infection in boars. I. Possibility of a genital localization in the boar after oronasal infection. Zentralbl Veterinarmed B 30:541–545.
Brown TT Jr. 1981. Laboratory evaluation of selected disinfectants as virucidal agents against porcine parvovirus, pseudorabies

virus, and transmissible gastroenteritis virus. Am J Vet Res 42:1033–1036.

Brown TT Jr, Paul PS, Mengeling WL. 1980. Response of conventionally raised weanling pigs to experimental infection with a virulent strain of porcine parvovirus. Am J Vet Res 41:1221–1224.

Cartwright SF. 1970. Tests available for the detection of some virus infections of pigs and their interpretation. Vet Annu 11:77–82.

Cartwright SF, Huck RA. 1967. Viruses isolated in association with herd infertility, abortions and stillbirths in pigs. Vet Rec 81:196–197.

Cartwright SF, Lucas M, Huck RA. 1969. A small haemagglutinating porcine DNA virus. I. Isolation and properties. J Comp Pathol 79:371–377.

——. 1971. A small haemagglutinating porcine DNA virus. II. Biological and serological studies. J Comp Pathol 81:145–155.

Chaniago TD, Watson DL, Owen RA, Johnson RH. 1978. Immunoglobulins in blood serum of foetal pigs. Aust Vet J 54:30–33.

Choi CS, Molitor TW, Joo HS, Gunther R. 1987. Pathogenicity of a skin isolate of porcine parvovirus in swine fetuses. Vet Microbiol 15:19–29.

Coackley W, Smith VW. 1972. Porcine parvoviruses in Western Australia. Aust Vet J 48:536.

Cotmore SF, Sturzenbecker LJ, Tattersall P. 1983. The autonomous parvovirus MVM encodes two nonstructural proteins in addition to its capsid polypeptides. Virology 129:333–343.

Croghan DL, Matchett A. 1973. Beta-propiolactone sterilization of commercial trypsin. Appl Microbiol 26:832.

Croghan DL, Matchett A, Koski TA. 1973. Isolation of porcine parvovirus from commercial trypsin. Appl Microbiol 26:431–433.

Cropper M, Dunne HW, Leman AD, Starkey AL, Hoefling DC. 1976. Prevalence of antibodies to porcine enteroviruses and porcine parvovirus in body fluids of fetal pigs from small vs. large litters. J Am Vet Med Assoc 168:233–235.

Cutlip RC, Mengeling WL. 1975a. Experimentally induced infection of neonatal swine with porcine parvovirus. Am J Vet Res 36:1179–1182.

——. 1975b. Pathogenesis of in utero infection of eight and ten-week-old porcine fetuses with porcine parvovirus. Am J Vet Res 36:1751–1754.

Darbyshire JH, Roberts DH. 1968. Some respiratory virus and mycoplasma infections of animals. J Clin Pathol 21(Suppl 2):61–92.

Dea S, Elazhary MASY, Martineau GP, Vaillancourt J. 1985. Parvovirus-like particles associated with diarrhea in unweaned piglets. Can J Comp Med 49:343–345.

Donaldson-Wood CR, Joo HS, Johnson RH. 1977. The effect on reproductive performance of porcine parvovirus infection in a susceptible pig herd. Vet Rec 100:237–239.

Etoh M, Morishita E, Watanabe Y. 1979. Transitional antibodies and spontaneous infection in porcine parvovirus infection. Jpn J Swine Husb Res 16:237–239.

Forman AJ, Lenghaus C, Hogg GG, Hale CJ. 1977. Association of a parvovirus with an outbreak of foetal death and mummification in pigs. Aust Vet J 53:326–329.

Fujisaki Y. 1978. Incidence and control of stillbirth caused by porcine parvovirus in Japan. Proc Congr Int Pig Vet Soc 5:KA 14.

Fujisaki Y, Ichihara T, Sasaki N, Shimizu F, Murakami Y, Sugimori T, Sasahara J. 1978a. Field trials on inactivated porcine parvovirus vaccine for prevention of viral stillbirth among swine. Natl Inst Anim Health Q (Tokyo) 18:184–185.

Fujisaki Y, Morimoto T, Sugimori T, Suziki H. 1975. Experimental infection of pigs with porcine parvovirus. Natl Inst Anim Health Q (Tokyo) 22:205–206.

Fujisaki Y, Murikami Y. 1982. Immunity to infection with porcine parvovirus in pigs inoculated with attenuated HT-strain. Natl Inst Anim Health (Tokyo) 22:36–37.

Fujisaki Y, Watanabe Y, Kodama K, Hamada H, Murakami Y, Sugimori T, Sasahara J. 1978b. Protection of swine with inacti-

vated porcine parvovirus vaccine from fetal infection. Natl Inst Anim Health Q (Tokyo) 18:185.

Gillick JC. 1977. An outbreak of swine foetal mummification associated with porcine parvovirus. Aust Vet J 53:105–106.

Hafez SM, Liess B. 1979. Isolation of parvovirus from kidney cell cultures of gnotobiotic piglets. Zentralbl Veterinarmed B 26:820–827.

Hallauer C, Kronauer G, Siegl G. 1971. Parvovirus as contaminants of permanent human cell lines. I. Virus isolations from 1960–1970. Arch Gesamte Virusforsch 35:80–90.

Hallauer C, Siegl G, Kronauer G. 1972. Parvoviruses as contaminants of permanent human cell lines. III. Biological properties of the isolated viruses. Arch Gesamte Virusforsch 38:369–382.

Hogg GG, Lenghaus C, Forman AJ. 1977. Experimental porcine parvovirus infection of foetal pigs resulting in abortion, histological lesions and antibody formation. J Comp Pathol 87:539–549.

Hohdatsu T, Baba K, Ide S, Tsuchimoto M, Nagano H, Yamagami T, Yamagishi H, Fujisaki Y, Matumoto M. 1988. Detection of antibodies against porcine parvovirus in swine sera by enzyme-linked immunosorbent assay. Vet Microbiol 17:11–19.

Huygelen C, Peetermans J. 1967. Isolation of a hemagglutinating picornavirus from a primary swine kidney cell culture. Arch Gesamte Virusforsch 20:260–262.

Ide S, Yamagishi K, Yoshimura M, Maniwa E, Yasuda H, Igarashi J. 1977. Reaction of pigs to injection with a bivalent vaccine of Japanese B encephalitis virus and porcine parvovirus. J Jpn Vet Med Assoc 30:322–325.

Johnson RH. 1969. A search for Parvoviridae (Picornaviridae). Vet Rec 84:19–20.

——. 1973. Isolation of swine parvovirus in Queensland. Aust Vet J 49:257–259.

Johnson RH, Collings DF. 1969. Experimental infection of piglets and pregnant gilts with a parvovirus. Vet Rec 85:446–447.

——. 1971. Transplacental infection of piglets with a porcine parvovirus. Res Vet Sci 12:570–572.

Johnson RH, Donaldson-Wood CR, Joo HS, Allender U. 1976. Observations on the epidemiology of porcine parvovirus. Aust Vet J 52:80–84.

Joo HS, Donaldson-Wood CR, Johnson RH. 1975. A microneutralization test for the assay of porcine parvovirus antibody. Arch Virol 47:337–341.

——. 1976a. Observations on the pathogenesis of porcine parvovirus infection. Arch Virol 51:123–129.

——. 1976b. Rapid diagnostic techniques for detection of porcine parvovirus infection in mummified foetuses. Aust Vet J 52:51.

——. 1976c. A standardised haemagglutination inhibition test for porcine parvovirus antibody. Aust Vet J 52:422–424.

Joo HS, Donaldson-Wood CR, Johnson RH, Campbell RSF. 1977. Pathogenesis of porcine parvovirus infection: Pathology and immunofluorescence in the foetus. J Comp Pathol 87:383–391.

Joo HS, Donaldson-Wood CR, Johnson RH, Watson DL. 1976d. Antibody to porcine, feline and rat parvoviruses in various animal species. Res Vet Sci 21:112–113.

Joo HS, Johnson RH. 1977a. Observations on rapid diagnosis of porcine parvovirus in mummified foetuses. Aust Vet J 53:106–107.

——. 1977b. Serological responses in pigs vaccinated with inactivated porcine parvovirus. Aust Vet J 53:550–552.

Joo HS, Johnson RH, Watson DL. 1978. Serological procedures to determine time of infection of pigs with porcine parvovirus. Aust Vet J 54:125–127.

Kawamura H, Fujita T, Imada T. 1988. Plaque formation and replication of porcine parvovirus in embryonic swine kidney cell line, ESK cells. Jpn J Vet Sci 50:803–808.

Kim YH. 1974. Studies on hemagglutination and hemagglutination-inhibition reaction of porcine parvovirus. Bull AZABU Vet Coll 27:61–65.

Krakowka S, Ellis JA, Meehan B, Kennedy S, McNeilly F, Allan G. 2000. Viral wasting syndrome of swine: Experimental reproduction of postweaning multisystemic wasting syndrome in gnotobiotic swine by coinfection with porcine circovirus 2 and porcine parvovirus. Vet Pathol 37:254–263.

Kresse JI, Taylor WD, Stewart WC, Eernisse KA. 1985. Parvovirus infection in pigs with necrotic and vesicle-like lesions. Vet Microbiol 10:525–531.

Lenghaus C, Forman AJ, Hale CJ. 1978. Experimental infection of 35, 50 and 60 day old pig foetuses with porcine parvovirus. Aust Vet J 54:418–422.

Lucas MH, Cartwright SF, Wrathall AE. 1974. Genital infection of pigs with porcine parvovirus. J Comp Pathol 84:347–350.

Lucas MH, Napthine P. 1971. Fluorescent antibody technique in the study of three porcine viruses: Transmissible gastroenteritis virus, vomiting and wasting disease virus, and the parvovirus 59e/63. J Comp Pathol 81:111–117.

Marrable AW, Ashdown RR. 1967. Quantitative observations on pig embryos of known ages. J Agric Sci 69:443–447.

Mayr A, Bachmann PA, Siegl G, Mahnel H, Sheffy BE. 1968. Characterization of a small porcine DNA virus. Arch Gesamte Virusforsch 25:38–51.

McAdaragh JP, Anderson GA. 1975. Transmission of viruses through boar semen. Proc 18th Annu Meet Am Assoc Vet Lab Diagn, pp. 69–76.

Mengeling WL. 1972. Porcine parvovirus: Properties and prevalence of a strain isolated in the United States. Am J Vet Res 33:2239–2248.

——. 1975. Porcine parvovirus: Frequency of naturally occurring transplacental infection and viral contamination of fetal porcine kidney cell cultures. Am J Vet Res 36:41–44.

——. 1977. Diagnosing porcine parvovirus-induced reproductive failure. Proc 20th Annu Meet Am Assoc Vet Lab Diagn, pp. 237–244.

——. 1978a. Elimination of porcine parvovirus from infected cell cultures by inclusion of homologous antiserum in the nutrient medium. Am J Vet Res 39:323–324.

——. 1978b. Prevalence of porcine parvovirus-induced reproductive failure: An abattoir study. J Am Vet Med Assoc 172:1291–1294.

——. 1979. Prenatal infection following maternal exposure to porcine parvovirus on either the seventh or fourteenth day of gestation. Can J Comp Med 43:106–109.

Mengeling WL, Brown TT Jr, Paul PS, Guntekunst DE. 1979. Efficacy of an inactivated virus vaccine for prevention of porcine parvovirus-induced reproductive failure. Am J Vet Res 40:204–207.

Mengeling WL, Cutlip RC. 1975. Pathogenesis of in utero infection: Experimental infection of 5-week-old porcine fetuses with porcine parvovirus. Am J Vet Res 36:1173–1177.

——. 1976. Reproductive disease experimentally induced by exposing pregnant gilts to porcine parvovirus. Am J Vet Res 37:1393–1400.

Mengeling WL, Cutlip RC, Barnett D. 1978. Porcine parvovirus: Pathogenesis, prevalence, and prophylaxis. Proc Congr Int Pig Vet Soc 5:KA 15.

Mengeling WL, Cutlip RC, Wilson RA, Parks JB, Marshall RF. 1975. Fetal mummification associated with porcine parvovirus infection. J Am Vet Med Assoc 166:993–995.

Mengeling WL, Lager KM, Zimmerman JJ, Samarikermani N, Beran GW. 1991. A current assessment of the relative role of porcine parvovirus as a cause of fetal porcine death. J Vet Diagn Invest 3:33–35.

Mengeling WL, Paul PS. 1986. The relative importance of swine and contaminated premises as reservoirs of porcine parvovirus. J Am Vet Med Assoc 188:1293–1295.

Mengeling WL, Paul PS, Brown TT Jr. 1980a. Transplacental infection and embryonic death following maternal exposure to porcine parvovirus near the time of conception. Arch Virol 65:55–62.

Mengeling WL, Paul PS, Bunn TO, Ridpath JF. 1986. Antigenic relationships among autonomous parvoviruses. J Gen Virol 67:2839–2844.

Mengeling WL, Paul PS, Gutekunst DE, Pirtle EC, Brown TT Jr. 1980b. Vaccination for reproductive failure caused by porcine parvovirus. Proc Congr Int Pig Vet Soc 6:61.

Mengeling WL, Pejsak Z, Paul PS. 1984. Biological assay of attenuated strain NADL-2 and virulent strain NADL-8 of porcine parvovirus. Am J Vet Res 45:2403–2407.

Mengeling WL, Ridpath JF, Vorwald AC. 1988. Size and antigenic comparisons among the structural proteins of selected autonomous parvoviruses. J Gen Virol 69:825–837.

Molitor TW, Joo HS, Collect MS. 1983. Porcine parvovirus: Virus purification and structural and antigenic properties of virion polypeptides. J Virol 45:842–854.

Molitor TW, Oraveerakul K, Zhang QQ, Choi CS, Ludemann LR. 1991. Polymerase chain reaction (PCR) amplification for the detection of porcine parvovirus. J Virol Methods. 32:201–211.

Morimoto T, Fujisaki Y, Ito Y, Tanaka Y. 1972a. Biological and physiochemical properties of porcine parvovirus recovered from stillborn piglets. Natl Inst Anim Health Q (Tokyo) 12:137–144.

Morimoto T, Kurogi H, Miura Y, Sugimori T, Fujisaki Y. 1972b. Isolation of Japanese encephalitis virus and a hemagglutinating DNA virus from the brain of stillborn piglets. Natl Inst Anim Health Q (Tokyo) 12:127–136.

Narita M, Inui S, Kawakami Y, Kitamura K, Maeda A. 1975. Histopathological changes of the brain in swine fetuses naturally infected with porcine parvovirus. Natl Inst Anim Health Q (Tokyo) 15:24–28.

Opriessnig T, Fenaux M, Yu S, Evans RB, Cavanaugh D, Gallup JM, Pallares FJ, Thacker EL, Lager KM, Meng XJ, Halbur PG. 2004. Effect of porcine parvovirus vaccination on the development of PMWS in segregated early weaned pigs coninfected with type 2 porcine circovirus and porcine parvovirus. Vet Microbiol 98:209–220.

Paul PS, Mengeling WL. 1980. Evaluation of a modified live virus vaccine for the prevention of porcine parvovirus–induced reproductive disease in pigs. Am J Vet Res 41:2007–2011.

——. 1984. Oronasal and intramuscular vaccination of swine with a modified live porcine parvovirus vaccine: Multiplication and transmission of vaccine virus. Am J Vet Res 45:2481–2485.

——. 1986. Vaccination of swine with inactivated porcine parvovirus vaccine in the presence of passive immunity. J Am Vet Med Assoc 188:410–413.

Paul PS, Mengeling WL, Brown TT Jr. 1979. Replication of porcine parvovirus in peripheral blood lymphocytes, monocytes, and peritoneal macrophages. Infect Immun 25:1003–1007.

——. 1980. Effect of vaccinal and passive immunity on experimental infection of pigs with porcine parvovirus. Am J Vet Res 41:1368–1371.

Paul PS, Mengeling WL, Pirtle EC. 1982. Duration and biological half-life of passively acquired colostral antibodies to porcine parvovirus. Am J Vet Res 43:1376–1379.

Pini A. 1975. Porcine parvovirus in pig herds in southern Africa. J S Afr Vet Assoc 46:241–244.

Pirtle EC. 1974. Titration of two porcine respiratory viruses in mammalian cell cultures by direct fluorescent antibody staining. Am J Vet Res 35:249–250.

Prikhod'ko GG, Reyes H, Vasilyeva I, Busby TF. 2003. Establishment of a porcine parvovirus (PPV) DNA standard and evaluation of a new lightcycler nested–PCR assay of detection of PPV. J Virol Methods 111:13–19.

Redman DR, Bohl EH, Ferguson LC. 1974. Porcine parvovirus: Natural and experimental infections of the porcine fetus and prevalence in mature swine. Infect Immun 10:718–723.

Rodeffer HE, Leman AD, Dunne HW, Cropper M, Sprecher DJ. 1975. Reproductive failure in swine associated with maternal seroconversion for porcine parvovirus. J Am Vet Med Assoc 166:991–995.

Rondhuis PR, Straver PJ. 1972. Enige kenmerken van een klien, hemagglutinerend DNA-virus, geisoleer uit een verworpen varkensfoetus. Tijdschr Diergeneeskd 97:1257–1267.

Ruckerbauer GM, Dulac GC, Boulanger P. 1978. Demonstration of parvovirus in Canadian swine and antigenic relationships with isolates from other countries. Can J Comp Med 42:278–285.

Siegl G. 1976. The Parvoviruses (1st ed). Vienna, Austria: Springer-Verlag.

Siegl G, Gautschi M. 1973a. The multiplication of parvovirus Lu III in a synchronized culture system. I. Optimum conditions for virus replication. Arch Gesamte Virusforsch 40:105–118.

——. 1973b. The multiplication of parvovirus Lu III in a synchronized culture system. II. Biochemical characteristics of virus replication. Arch Gesamte Virusforsch 40:119–127.

Siegl G, Hallauer C, Novak A. 1972. Parvoviruses as contaminants of permanent human cell lines. IV. Multiplication of KBSH-virus in KB-cells. Arch Gesamte Virusforsch 36:351.

Soares RM, Durigon EL, Bersano JG, Richtzenhain LJ. 1999. Detection of porcine parvovirus DNA by the polymerase chain reaction assay using primers to the highly conserved nonstructural protein gene, NS-1. J Virol Methods. 78:191–198.

Suzuki H, Fujisaki Y. 1976. Immunizing effects of inactivated porcine parvovirus vaccine on piglets. Natl Inst Anim Health Q (Tokyo) 16:81.

Tennant RW. 1971. Inhibition of mitosis and macromolecular synthesis in rat embryo cells by Kilham rat virus. J Virol 8:402–408.

Thacker B, Leman AD. 1978. Evaluation of gravid uteri at slaughter for porcine parvovirus infection. Proc Congr Int Pig Vet Soc 5:M–49.

Thacker BJ, Joo HS, Winkelman NL, Leman AD, Barnes DM. 1987. Clinical, virologic, and histopathologic observations of induced porcine parvovirus infection in boars. Am J Vet Res 48:763–767.

Vannier P, Tillon JP. 1979. Diagnostic de certitude de l'infection a parvovirus dans les trouble de la reproduction de l'espèce porcine. Rec Med Vet 155:151–158.

Waldvogel AS, Broll S, Rosskopf M, Schwyzer M, Pospischil A. 1995. Diagnosis of fetal infection with porcine parvovirus by in situ hybridization. Vet Microbiol 47:377–385.

Westenbrink F, Veldius MA, Brinkhof JMA. 1989. An enzyme-linked assay for detection of antibodies to porcine parvovirus. J Virol Methods 23:169–178.

Wrathall AE, Mengeling WL. 1979a. Effect of porcine parvovirus on development of fertilized pig eggs in vitro. Br Vet J 135:249–254.

——. 1979b. Effect of transferring parvovirus-infected fertilized pig eggs into seronegative gilts. B Vet J 135:255–261.

——. 1979c. Effect of inseminating seropositive gilts with semen containing porcine parvovirus. Br Vet 135:420–425.

Yasuhara H, Matsui O, Hirahara T, Ohgtani T, Tanaka ML, Kodama K, Nakai M, and Sasaki N. 1989. Characterization of parvovirus isolated from diarrheic feces of a pig. Jpn J Vet Sci 51:337–344.

24 Porcine Reproductive and Respiratory Syndrome Virus (Porcine Arterivirus)

J. Zimmerman, D. A. Benfield, M. P. Murtaugh, F. Osorio, G. W. Stevenson, and M. Torremorell

In the late 1980s, catastrophic outbreaks of a previously unrecognized disease were reported in U.S. swine herds (Keffaber 1989; Loula 1991). The clinical picture included severe reproductive losses, extensive postweaning pneumonia, reduction of growth performance, and increased mortality (Hill 1990). Initial efforts to identify the etiology of the outbreaks were unsuccessful and the name "Mystery Swine Disease" (MSD) came into common usage (Hill 1990; Reotutar 1989).

In Europe, outbreaks clinically similar to MSD occurred in Germany in November 1990 (OIE 1992). No common link was found between the outbreaks in Germany and MSD in the U.S. (Anon. 1991). Spreading rapidly, over 3,000 outbreaks were documented in Germany in May 1991 and across Europe in the following 4 years (Baron et al. 1992; Bøtner et al. 1994; Edwards et al. 1992; OIE 1992; Pejsak and Markowska-Daniel 1996; Plana Duran et al. 1992a; Valíček et al. 1997). In Asia, outbreaks occurred in Japan in 1988 (Hirose et al. 1995) and in Taiwan in 1991 (Chang et al. 1993).

The etiology of the disease was resolved in 1991 when Koch's postulates were fulfilled by researchers at the Central Veterinary Institute (Lelystad, the Netherlands) with a previously unrecognized RNA virus (Terpstra et al. 1991a; Wensvoort et al. 1991). Shortly thereafter, the virus was isolated in the U.S. (Collins 1991; Collins et al. 1992) and Canada (Dea et al. 1992a,b). The first virus isolates in the Netherlands and U.S. were designated Lelystad virus and Swine Infertility and Respiratory Syndrome (SIRS) virus (BIAH-001), respectively. European workers introduced the term "porcine reproductive and respiratory syndrome" (PRRS) into the literature in 1991 (Terpstra et al. 1991b). The term "swine arterivirus" is also found in the literature (Albina et al. 1998; Legeay et al. 1997) and is more in keeping with the spirit of the rules of virus nomenclature devised by the International Committee on Taxonomy of Viruses.

ETIOLOGY

PRRS virus (PRRSV) is a small, positive-strand RNA virus. Together with equine arteritis virus, lactate dehydrogenase-elevating virus, and simian hemorrhagic fever virus, PRRSV belongs to family *Arteriviridae*, which together with family *Coronaviridae* form the order *Nidovirales* (Cavanagh 1997). PRRSV is an enveloped virus with a diameter of 50–65 nm, a relatively smooth surface, and a cuboidal, nucleocapsid core with a diameter of 25–35 nm (Benfield et al. 1992) (Figure 24.1).

PRRSV is highly host restricted, growing primarily in porcine alveolar macrophages and in macrophages of other tissues (Pol et al. 1991). PRRSV can also replicate in testicular germ cells (spermatids, spermatocytes, multinucleated giant cells) in infected boars (Sur et al. 1997). In vitro, PRRSV grows in primary cultures of porcine alveolar macrophages, as well as MA-104 African green monkey kidney cells or its derivatives (Benfield et al. 1992, Kim et al. 1993). A cell line derived from cotton rat lung cells has also been reported to be highly susceptible to PRRSV (rat cell line, ATCC PTA-3930).

PRRSV enters the host cell by endocytosis. PRRSV particles have been visualized by electron microscopy at the cell surface or within small vesicles delineated by clathrin-like zones (Kreutz and Ackermann 1996). Meulenberg (2000) concisely described the complete process of morphogenesis: PRRSV is assembled through a process of nucleocapsid budding into the lumen of the smooth endoplasmic reticulum, the Golgi, or both. After budding, virions accumulate in vesicles and then move to the plasma membrane where release takes place through fusion. Under single-step growth conditions, the maximum output of PRRSV particles takes place between 10–20 hours, reaching titers of $10^{6.5}$ to $10^{7.5}$ TCID$_{50}$/ml (Meulenberg 2000).

Genomic Organization

The genomic organization of PRRSV is similar to that of other arteriviruses. The genome is approximately 15 kb

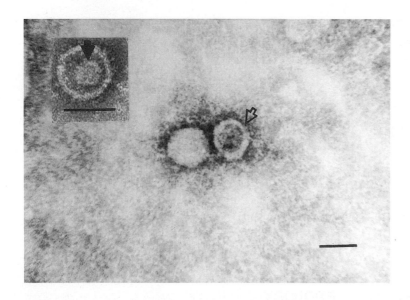

24.1. *A complete PRRSV particle (indicated by the open arrow) and an incomplete (coreless) PRRSV particle. The insert shows a complete PRRSV particle with the 35 nm nucleocapsid core (black arrow) surrounded by an envelope. Bars = 50 nm. (Courtesy of D. Robinson, South Dakota State University.)*

in length with eight open reading frames (ORFs). The complete genome sequence of Lelystad virus and several North American isolates has been published (Allende et al. 1999; Meulenberg et al. 1993; Nelsen et al. 1999; Wootton et al. 2000). A comparison of the amino acid sequences encoded by each PRRSV ORF indicates that PRRSV is more similar to lactate dehydrogenase-elevating virus than to equine arteritis virus.

ORFs 1a and 1b comprise 80% of the genome and encode the RNA replicase required for virus replication. ORFs 1a and 1b are translated as a single poly-protein, which is then processed into smaller nonstructural proteins (nsp). Nsp1-alpha, nsp1-beta, nsp2, and nsp4 are proteases that cleave the entire ORF1 polyprotein into 12 nsps (Snijder and Meulenberg 2001). The nsp10 region of ORF1b encodes a functional helicase (Bautista et al. 2002).

In addition to their functional role in PRRSV replication, the nsps have a potential role in diagnostics and in the host immune response. A significant number of epitopes exist on nsp2 and these are recognized by the immune system of the infected host (Oleksiewicz et al. 2001).

The six ORFs (2, 3, 4, 5, 6, and 7) located at the 3′ end of the genome encode the viral structural proteins. Of these, GP2, GP3, GP4, and GP5, are all N-glycosylated, whereas the nucleocapsid protein N (ORF 7 product) and the integral membrane (or matrix) M protein (ORF 6 product) are not (Dea et al. 2000). Recent evidence also suggests the existence of an additional nonglycosylated, small protein (73 amino acid, 10-kDa) encoded by a small ORF within ORF2 designated ORF2b (Wu et al. 2001).

Structural Proteins

PRRSV possesses a set of six or seven structural proteins. The three major structural proteins are GP5, M, and N.

The N protein is small (15 kDa), highly basic, and in-

teracts with the viral RNA in the assembly of infectious particles. The N protein is expressed at high levels in infected cells and represents 20–40% of the total protein content of the virion. It is active in nuclear shuttling and localization to the nucleolus and may influence nuclear processes during replication (Rowland and Yoo 2003), possibly through rRNA precursor processing and ribosome biogenesis (Yoo et al. 2003). The N protein is not important from an immunogenic or immunoprotective standpoint, but its abundant expression and antigenicity make it an ideal target for diagnostic assays.

The nonglycosylated M (transmembrane) envelope protein is the most genetically conserved of all the structural proteins of PRRSV. As a matrix protein, M is important in virus assembly and budding. It accumulates in the endoplasmic reticulum, forming disulfide-linked heterodimers with the 25 kDa GP5 (Mardassi et al. 1996). These heterodimers are incorporated into the virus particles and are essential for interaction with cellular receptors and are vital for virus infectivity. Evidence for this is supported by the fact that M protein induces PRRSV-neutralizing antibodies (Bastos et al. 2002). The M protein and the M-GP5 complex contribute to PRRSV attachment to a heparin-like receptor on porcine alveolar macrophages (Delputte et al. 2002).

The envelope GP5 contains, after processing, an ectodomain 30 amino acids in length that carries 2 or 3 N-glycans. As the primary envelope protein, GP5 is involved in receptor recognition (Vanderheijden et al. 2003). GP5's role in receptor recognition is supported by the presence of a major neutralization epitope in the N-terminal ectodomain; thus, implying a role for the GP5 ectodomain in the infection process (Ostrowski et al. 2002; Plagemann 2004; Plagemann et al. 2002; Wissink et al. 2003).

The 29–30 kDa GP2 and the 31–35 kDa GP4 envelope proteins are minor constituents of the viral envelope and are typical class I membrane proteins (Meulenberg

2000). It is uncertain whether the 45–50 kDa GP3 protein is present on the structure of the virion, as described for European PRRSV isolates (van Nieuwstadt et al. 1996), or if it is secreted into the medium of infected cells, as reported in studies with a North American isolate (Gonin et al. 1998).

Genomic Diversity

PRRSV strains or isolates are exceptionally variable based on

1. Variation in the clinical presentation of the disease
2. Experimental evidence of differences in pneumovirulence and/or reproductive virulence
3. Antigenic differences as determined by reactivity with polyclonal and monoclonal antibodies
4. Differences in RNA sequences

Concomitant with improvements in the diagnostic assays has been an increased awareness of the genetic/antigenic diversity of PRRSV strains in the field (Meng 2000). In many laboratories, genetic sequencing has become routine in the diagnostic assessment of PRRSV infections.

With the increased use of genetic sequencing has come the realization that genetically diverse PRRSV strains may coexist on the same farm (Dee et al. 2001; Goldberg et al. 2003). Likewise, sequencing has led to the recognition of European genotype (Type 1) strains in areas previously considered to be exclusively populated by U.S. genotype strains (Type 2) (Ropp et al. 2004) and vice versa. Thus, in North America, Europe, and probably elsewhere, two distinct genotypes of PRRSV sharing only partial cross-protection may be found. This has great significance for vaccine strain selection and for the performance of diagnostic assays. Since recombination is likely an important genetic mechanism contributing to PRRSV evolution (Yuan et al. 1999), an additional concern is the possibility that recombination may occur between North American and European viruses coexisting in the same region. However, in vitro (cell culture) conditions indicate that RNA recombination is more likely to occur between two North American (Type 2) strains or two European (Type 1) PRRSV strains than between a Type 1 and Type 2 strain (van Vught et al. 2001).

Systematic application of sequencing has also contributed to concerns about the stability of attenuated vaccine viruses and their possible reversion to virulence. Evidence has suggested the reversion to virulence by attenuated vaccines (Key et al. 2003; Mengeling et al. 1999a; Nielsen et al. 2001; Opriessnig et al. 2002). On the other hand, a significant potential outcome of the study of the genomic structure of attenuated PPRSV strains is a better understanding of the molecular basis for virulence and attenuation in PRRSV. Several genomic pair studies of attenuated strains and their parental wild-type strains have provided an a priori indi-

cation of likely candidate virulence genes (Allende et al. 2000a; Grebennikova et al. 2004; Yuan et al. 2001). These studies are a precursor to studies of gene functions and the molecular basis of PRRSV virulence based on reverse genetics, e.g., infectious cDNA clones (Groot Bramel-Verheije et al. 2000; Meulenberg et al. 1998; Nielsen et al. 2003; Truong et al. 2004; Verheije et al. 2002a; Verheije et al. 2002b; Verheije et al. 2003).

EPIDEMIOLOGY

Geographic Distribution

As diagnostic assays became available during the 1990s, PRRSV was found to have spread nearly everywhere domestic pigs are raised. Retrospective serologic studies found that PRRSV was present in Canada by 1979 (Carman et al. 1995), the U.S. by 1985 (Zimmerman et al. 1997), and the former German Democratic Republic by 1987 (Ohlinger et al. 2000). In Asia, anti-PRRSV antibodies were retrospectively documented in serum from pigs imported into the Republic of Korea (South Korea) in 1985 (Shin et al. 1993), in serum samples collected in 1987 in Taiwan (Chiou 2003), and in samples collected in 1988 in Japan (Hirose et al. 1995). In all cases, the serologic evidence found that PRRSV was in the swine population well before the recognition of clinical PRRS.

Some regions are still free of PRRSV. In Europe, this includes Sweden (Elvander et al. 1997), Norway (OIE 1997), Finland (Bøtner 2003), and Switzerland. Likewise, in Oceania, New Caledonia (OIE 1996), New Zealand (Motha et al. 1997), and Australia (Garner et al. 1996, 1997) are PRRSV-free. In South America, Argentina (Perfumo and Sanguinetti 2003), Brazil (Ciacci-Zanella 2004), Cuba (Alfonso and Frías-Lepoureau 2003), and some areas of the Caribbean may be free of PRRSV.

Accurate estimates of the prevalence of infection with wild-type virus in specific countries or regions are not readily available, but within infected regions, 60–80% of herds are typically infected (Geue 1995; Hirose et al. 1995; Lu et al. 1999; Maes 1997; Mateusen et al. 2002; USDA 1997). The use of modified live virus (MLV) vaccines has made it difficult to estimate prevalence. Antibodies against vaccine virus are not easily differentiated from antibodies against PRRSV field strains. Furthermore, vaccine strain viruses are shed and transmitted in the field, further compounding the problem of identifying infection with wild-type virus (Astrup and Riising 2002; Bøtner et al. 1997; Christopher-Hennings et al. 1996, 1997; Mengeling et al. 1998; Sipos et al. 2002).

Susceptible Species

Presumably, PRRSV entered domestic swine from an as-yet-unidentified wildlife species. A number of species have been determined not to be susceptible to PRRSV, including mice, rats (Hooper et al. 1994), and guinea pigs (J. Zimmerman, unpublished data). Wills et al.

(2000) found no evidence of PRRSV replication in cats, dogs, mice, opossums, raccoons, rats, skunks, house sparrows, or starlings. Zimmerman et al. (1997) reported that mallard ducks (*Anas platyrhynchos*) were susceptible to PRRSV, but subsequent workers have not replicated these results (Trincado et al. 2004b).

Feral swine are susceptible to PRRSV infection, but according to serosurveys, infection in free-ranging feral swine animals is relatively rare (Albina et al. 2000; Lutz and Wurm 1996; Oslage et al. 1994; Saliki et al. 1998).

Even so, in areas where feral swine interact with domestic swine, they could conceivably serve as a source of PRRSV. Within superfamily *Suoidea* (*Sus* spp., peccaries, warthogs, and babirusa), the susceptibility of species, other than *Sus scrofa*, for PRRSV is unknown.

Routes of Shedding

Infected animals shed virus in saliva (Wills et al. 1997a), nasal secretions (Benfield et al. 1994; Christianson et al. 1993; Rossow et al. 1994a), urine (Wills et al. 1997a), semen (Swenson and Zimmerman 1993; Swenson et al. 1994a), and feces (Christianson et al. 1993). Pregnant susceptible females inoculated in late gestation shed virus in mammary secretions (Wagstrom et al. 2001).

Shedding of virus in semen is of particular concern because of the widespread use of artificial insemination. The duration of semen shedding varies widely among boars (Christopher-Hennings et al. 1996). Swenson et al. (1994a) found infectious virus in the semen of experimentally infected boars for up to 43 days following exposure. By PCR, Christopher-Hennings et al. (1995a) detected viral RNA in the semen of experimentally infected boars for up to 92 days postinoculation (DPI) and isolated PRRSV from the bulbourethral gland of a boar euthanized 101 DPI. Semen shedding of MLV vaccine virus occurred for up to 39 days in one study, but prior vaccination eliminated or reduced shedding upon challenge (Christopher-Hennings et al. 1997).

Transmission

Swine are susceptible to PRRSV by several routes of exposure, including intranasal, intramuscular, oral (Magar et al. 1995; Magar and Larochelle 2004; van der Linden et al. 2003b), intrauterine (Christianson et al. 1993), and vaginal (Benfield et al. 2000a; Gradil et al. 1996; Yaeger et al. 1993). Pigs are not equally susceptible to PRRSV by all routes of exposure. That is, the probability that a given dose will result in infection differs by route of exposure. Hermann et al. (2005) estimated the infectious dose$_{50}$ (ID$_{50}$)—i.e., the dose required to infect one-half of the exposed animals—for oral and intranasal routes of exposure to be $10^{5.3}$ TCID$_{50}$ and $10^{4.0}$ TCID$_{50}$, respectively. Based on data from Benfield et al. (2000a), the ID$_{50}$ for exposure via artificial insemination is approximately $10^{4.5}$ TCID$_{50}$. Yoon et al. (1999) reported that exposure to 20 or fewer PRRSV particles by intramuscular exposure resulted in infection.

Overall, the infectivity data indicate that pigs are extremely susceptible to infection via parenteral exposure (breaks in the skin barrier) and much less susceptible by all other routes investigated to date. In the field, potential parenteral exposures include standard husbandry practices, i.e., ear notching, tail docking, teeth clipping, tattooing, and inoculations with medications and biologics. Likewise, because PRRSV is present in saliva for weeks following infection, normal pig behavior commonly results in parenteral exposures, i.e., bites, cuts, scrapes, and/or abrasions that occur during aggressive interactions among pigs. Bierk et al. (2001) associated transmission with aggressive behavior between carrier sows and susceptible contacts. Other behaviors that result in exchange of blood and saliva, i.e., tail-biting and ear-biting, may also function in transmission. The significantly higher ID$_{50}$ estimates for oral and intranasal exposures imply that transmission by these routes is less common and more easily prevented.

Indirect transmission involves transmission by inanimate objects (e.g., equipment, instruments, clothing) or substances (e.g., water, food), living carriers (vectors), or aerosols. Otake et al. (2002b) confirmed needle-borne transmission of PRRSV under experimental conditions. Likewise, Otake et al. (2002a) showed that PRRSV was present on workers' coveralls, boots, and hands following 60 minutes of contact with acutely infected pigs. Importantly, elementary sanitation procedures, e.g., changing coveralls, changing boots, and washing hands, were sufficient to stop transmission (Dee et al. 2004a). Under experimental conditions, Dee et al. (2002, 2003) showed that PRRSV could be moved extensively on fomites in the field under winter conditions, i.e., below 0°C, but to a much lesser degree during warm weather, i.e., 10–16°C, again illustrating the importance of temperature in virus survival.

Preliminary reports suggest a possible role for arthropods in PRRSV transmission. PRRSV has been detected in, or on, wild-caught flies and mosquitoes (Otake et al. 2002c; Pringproa et al. 2004; Schurrer et al. 2004). Under experimental conditions, Otake et al. (2002c) demonstrated mechanical transmission of PRRSV by mosquitoes and house flies (*Musca domestica*) (Otake et al. 2003a). Overall, the current research data suggest that flies and mosquitoes might serve as mechanical vectors of PRRSV. However, the available data have not proven that PRRSV is an arthropod-borne infection. Typically, the ecologic relationships among host, infectious agent, arthropod, and environment in arthropod-borne infections are complex. Additional data are required to connect the current observations into a cohesive understanding of the role of arthropods in the transmission of PRRSV in the field.

Airborne virus was once considered the primary route of PRRS virus transmission. Airborne transmission, along with arthropod-borne transmission, could explain the apparent long-distance transmission (area spread) of PRRSV in the absence of other sources of virus (pigs, inanimate objects, people). However, airborne transmission of PRRSV has been difficult to document. Under experimental conditions, transmission from infected to susceptible pigs over a space of 1.0–2.5 meters has been successful in approximately 50% of the attempts (Lager and Mengeling 2000; Otake et al. 2002d; Torremorell et al. 1997; Wills et al. 1997b). The one exception to this pattern of poor airborne transmissibility is a report by Kristensen et al. (2004). In three trials, approximately 50 acutely infected pigs transmitted PRRSV over a distance of one meter to approximately 50 susceptible pigs when 1%, 10%, or 70% of air was exchanged. In a field setting, airborne transmission did not occur over distances of 15 meters (Trincado et al. 2004a) and 30 meters (Otake et al. 2002d). The role of airborne transmission of PRRSV will not be understood until additional information is available; in particular, the quantity of virus excreted by pigs, the source of the virus, the rate of inactivation of aerosolized virus, and the infectious dose for pigs by aerosol exposure.

Vertical Transmission

PRRSV is transmitted from viremic dams transplacentally to fetuses, resulting in fetal death or birth of infected pigs that are weak or appear normal (Bøtner et al. 1994; Christianson et al. 1992; Terpstra et al. 1991a). Some pigs in affected litters may escape infection with PRRSV. PRRSV can replicate in fetuses 14 days of gestational age or older, but infection of fetuses during the first two-thirds of gestation is uncommon because most strains of PRRSV cross the placenta efficiently only in the last trimester of pregnancy (Christianson et al. 1993; Lager and Mengeling 1995; Mengeling et al. 1994; Prieto et al. 1996a,b). The reason for the difference in efficiency of maternal-placental viral transit at different stages of gestation and the mechanism(s) of viral transit are unknown. Transit is independent of the reproductive virulence of the virus strain. Park et al. (1996) showed that PRRSV strains of low and high virulence for fetuses cross the placenta with equal efficiency when sows are inoculated at 90 days of gestation.

Persistent Infection

PRRSV produces a chronic, persistent infection in pigs. Virus replicates in susceptible cells of clinically inapparent carrier animals for several months. This is the single most significant epidemiological feature of PRRSV infection. Persistent PRRSV infection has been documented through transmission experiments and by detection of virus in animals. Zimmerman et al. (1992) reported transmission of PRRSV from a sow infected 99 days earlier to susceptible sentinels. Following *in utero* exposure at day 90 of gestation, Benfield et al. (2000b) isolated virus from tonsil and lymph nodes from pigs for up to 132 days after farrowing. Wills et al. (1997c) isolated virus from one of 4 pigs at 157 DPI. Horter et al. (2002)

detected infectious PRRSV by virus isolation or swine bioassay in 51 of 59 (84%) animals necropsied between 63 and 105 DPI, including 10 of 11 (91%) of animals euthanized at 105 DPI. Allende et al. (2000b) detected infectious virus by bioassay in 2 of 5 pigs at 150 DPI.

Persistent infection is not a function of pig age at the time of infection. Persistence occurs regardless of whether the pig is exposed in utero (Benfield et al. 1997, 2000b; Rowland et al. 1999), as a young animal, or as an adult (Bierk et al. 2001; Christopher-Hennings et al. 1995a; Fairbanks et al. 2002; Zimmerman et al. 1992). The mechanism(s) by which the virus is able to persevere in the face of an active immune response has not been identified, but probably does not involve evasion of immunity through continual in vivo viral mutation. Chang et al. (2002) found relatively low rates of mutation in persistently infected animals.

Stability in the Environment

Shedding of virus in saliva, urine, and feces results in environmental contamination and creates the potential for transmission via fomites. PRRSV is fragile and quickly inactivated by heat and drying. At 25–27°C, infectious virus was not detected on plastic, stainless steel, rubber, alfalfa, wood shavings, straw, corn, swine starter feed, or denim cloth, beyond day zero (Pirtle and Beran 1996).

PRRSV can remain infectious for an extended time under specific conditions of temperature, moisture, and pH. PRRSV is stable for months to years at temperatures of −70°C and −20°C. Approximately 90% of PRRSV infectivity is lost within 1 week at 4°C, but low titers of infectious virus can still be detected for at least 30 days. In solution, PRRSV infectivity persists for 1–6 days at 20–21°C, 3–24 hours at 37°C, and 6–20 minutes at 56°C. The thermal stability of PRRSV in serum and tissues is similar to that described for virus stored in media. PRRSV was isolated from 47%, 14%, and 7% of porcine serum samples stored at 25°C for 24, 48, and 72 hours, respectively. When serum was stored at 4°C or −20°C, PRRSV was isolated from 85% of the samples after 72 hours (Van Alstine et al. 1993). PRRSV is stable at pH 6.5–7.5, but infectivity is rapidly lost at pH below 6 and above 7.5 (Benfield et al. 1992; Bloemraad et al. 1994).

Disinfection

PRRSV is inactivated by lipid solvents, e.g., chloroform and ether (Benfield et al. 1992). PRRSV is highly unstable in solutions containing low concentrations of detergents, which disrupt the envelope with concomitant release of the noninfectious core particles and loss of infectivity (Snijder and Meulenberg 2001).

Disinfection first requires removal of all organic material. Thereafter, infectious agents are inactivated in a temperature- and contact time–dependent fashion specific to the agent and the disinfectant. PRRSV is relatively labile in the environment and particularly susceptible to drying (Pirtle and Beran 1996). At "room temperature," Shirai et al. (2000) reported complete inactivation of PRRSV with chlorine (0.03%) in 10 minutes, iodine (0.0075%) in 1 minute, and a quarternary ammonium compound (0.0063%) in 1 minute. The effects of temperature or pH were not explored. Dee et al. (2004b, c) reported that protocols involving cleaning, washing, disinfection, and drying were effective at inactivating PRRSV on transport vehicles.

Transmission within Herds

PRRSV tends to circulate within a herd indefinitely. Endemicity appears to be driven by persistent PRRSV infection in carrier animals and the continual availability of susceptible animals either through birth, purchase, or loss of protective immunity. The virus is perpetuated by a cycle of transmission from dams to pigs either in utero or postpartum, or by commingling susceptible animals with infected animals in later stages of production. Under conditions in which susceptible and infectious pigs are mixed, e.g., at weaning, a large proportion of the population may quickly become infected. Dee and Joo (1994a) reported 80–100% of pigs in 3 swine herds were infected by 8–9 weeks of age and Maes (1997) found 96% of market hogs sampled from 50 herds to be positive. However, marked differences in infection rates between groups, pens, or rooms of animals may be observed in endemically infected herds. Houben et al. (1995) even found transmission to vary within litters. Some littermates seroconverted as early as 6–8 weeks of age, but other individuals reached 12 weeks of age, the end of the monitoring period, still free of PRRSV infection. Likewise, Melnichouk et al. (2005) found differences in the pattern of transmission in farms. In 5 farms, approximately 50% of the pigs were infected at 5–7.5 weeks of age and at least 90% were infected by 8.5 weeks of age, but on 2 farms, only 20% to 40% of pigs were infected at 10–12 weeks of age.

Transmission between Herds

The role of infected pigs and virus-contaminated semen in herd-to-herd transmission is firmly established (Dee 1992; Mousing et al. 1997; Weigel et al. 2000). In a regional PRRSV control program in France, Le Potier et al. (1997) estimated that 56% (66 of 118) of herds acquired the infection through the introduction of infected pigs, 20% (23 of 118) through infected semen, 21% (25 of 118) through fomites/slurry, and 3% (4 of 118) through unidentified sources. Mortensen et al. (2002) found that PRRSV entered negative herds through the introduction of animals and semen and through area spread from neighboring farms, which they attributed to aerosol transmission. Dee et al. (2002, 2003) have demonstrated the ease with which PRRSV can be moved between farms on commonplace equipment and objects common to swine farms, e.g., insulated semen coolers, metal toolboxes, plastic lunch pails, and cardboard boxes, es-

pecially when wet and cold. Torremorell et al. (2004) attributed over 80% of new infections in commercial systems to area spread from neighboring units, the movement of pigs in PRRSV infected transports, the lack of compliance of the biosecurity protocols, or possibly, introduction via insects.

Proximity to infected herds is a well-recognized risk factor. The risk of a herd becoming PRRSV-positive increases with the density of PRRSV-positive neighboring herds, but decreased with distances (Zhuang et al. 2002). Le Potier et al. (1997) found that 45% of herds suspected to have become infected through area spread were located within 500 meters (0.3 miles) of the postulated source herd and only 2% were one kilometer from the initial outbreak.

Area spread is a major issue in the control and/or elimination of PRRSV. If area spread is to be prevented, it is essential that the mechanisms by which it occurs be firmly established. Area spread is often attributed to aerosols or insects. However, Goldberg et al. (2000) evaluated the ORF 5 gene sequences from 55 field isolates collected in Illinois (U.S.) and eastern Iowa (U.S.) and found that the genetic similarity of isolates did not correlate with their geographical distance. On that basis, they concluded that PRRSV was most commonly introduced into herds through animals or semen, as opposed to mechanisms associated with spread from neighboring herds.

PATHOGENESIS

The chronology of PRRS viral infection has been described in several key inoculation studies in germ-free, cesarean-derived/colostrum-deprived, or conventional pigs (Duan et al. 1997b; Halbur et al. 1995b, 1996a; Rossow et al. 1994a, 1995, 1996a). Following exposure, viral replication initially occurs primarily in local susceptible macrophages and then rapidly spreads to lymphoid organs, lungs, and, less consistently, to other tissues. Virulent strains of PRRSV cause viremia as early as 12 hours in some pigs, and in all pigs by 24 hours postinoculation along with viral infection of lymphoid tissues and lung. Viral titers increase rapidly and peak in serum, lymph nodes, and lung by day 7–14 with 10^2–10^5 TCID$_{50}$ of virus detected per ml of serum or gram of tissue. The highest viral titers are consistently reported in lung.

PRRSV replicates primarily in well-differentiated subsets of monocyte-derived cells that display a 220 kDa glycoprotein receptor to which PRRSV binds and enters via receptor-mediated endocytosis (Duan et al. 1998; Kreutz and Ackermann 1996; Nauwynck et al. 1999; Wissink 2003a). Differentiated cells known to support replication include pulmonary alveolar macrophages (PAM) and intravascular macrophages (PIM) in the lung (Thanawongnuwech et al. 1997a; Wensvoort et al. 1991) and macrophages in lymphoid tissues (Duan et al.

1997b). Thus, the highest titers of PRRSV and most significant lesions are found in these tissues during acute PRRS.

Maturity and/or activation of PAM, and presumably other macrophages, is required for PRRSV replication (Duan et al. 1997a; Molitor et al. 1996, 1997; Thacker et al. 1998). PRRSV replicates in the subset of differentiated PAM with maximal ability to phagocytose bacteria and produce superoxide anion for bacterial killing in phagolysosomes (Molitor et al. 1996). Both PAM and PIM harvested from younger pigs replicate PRRSV to higher titers compared to older pigs (Mengeling et al. 1995; Thanawongnuwech et al. 1998b).

PRRSV will also replicate in microglia (Molitor et al. 1997), but will not replicate in all monocyte-derived cells, including peripheral blood monocytes, peritoneal macrophages, or bone marrow progenitor cells (Duan et al. 1997a,b).

The largest amount of PRRS viral antigen and/or nucleic acid is observed in lungs and lymph nodes, but is also consistently observed in perivascular and intravascular macrophages in heart, brain, kidney and elsewhere and is inconsistently observed in alveolar, bronchial, and nasal epithelium, endothelium, fibroblasts, spermatids, and spermatocytes (Halbur et al. 1995a,b, 1996a; Magar et al. 1993; Pol et al. 1991; Rossow et al. 1996a; Sirinarumitr et al. 1998; Sur et al. 1997; Thanawongnuwech et al. 1997a).

Generally, clinical disease and consistent lesions correspond to the time and place of highest viral titers, i.e. day 7–14 postinoculation in lung and lymph nodes. In contrast, in stillborn and congenitally infected live born pigs, viral antigen and nucleic acid is in largest amounts in lymphoid organs, but not lung (Cheon and Chae 2001).

After peaking, virus titers in serum decrease rapidly. Most pigs are no longer viremic by 28 DPI, although viral RNA has been detected in serum by rtPCR up to 251 DPI (Duan et al. 1997b; Wills et al. 2003). The duration of viremia may be slightly longer in congenitally infected pigs, being consistently demonstrated by virus isolation for up to 48 days after birth and infrequently by rtPCR for up to 228 days (Rowland et al. 2003).

Following viremia, congenitally- and postnatally infected pigs are persistently infected with virus in tonsil (Wills et al. 1997c) and/or lymph nodes, especially inguinal and sternal (Bierk et al. 2001; Xiao et al. 2004), for extended periods of time. Virus has been detected by virus isolation for as long as 132–157 DPI (Rowland et al. 2003; Wills et al. 1997c). Persistent virus is produced in lymphoid tissues by a low level of continuous replication (Allende et al. 2000b).

Mechanisms of Cell Injury

Replication of PRRS virus in macrophages in lung and lymphoid tissues, and to a lesser extent other tissues, in-

duces lesions and clinical disease by a variety of mechanisms. These include apoptosis of infected cells, apoptotic death of proximate noninfected cells (indirect or bystander apoptosis), induction of inflammatory cytokines, induction of polyclonal B cell activation, and reduction in bacterial phagocytosis and killing by macrophages that results in increased susceptibility to septicemia (also likely due to other forms of immunomodulation by PRRSV).

Direct and indirect (bystander) apoptosis is a major cause of cell death in PRRS. During acute infection when virus titers are high, only a small portion of macrophages in scattered foci are infected with PRRSV (Duan et al. 1997b; Mengeling et al. 1995), but there are large numbers of apoptotic mononuclear cells distributed diffusely (Sirinarumitr et al. 1998; Sur et al. 1998). Apoptotic cells rarely contain PRRSV and are in greatest numbers 10–14 days after PRRSV inoculation. This suggests that PRRSV induces apoptosis in noninfected cells in proximity to infected cells. Most apoptotic cells are morphologically typical of macrophages; fewer are typical of lymphocytes.

The gene product of PRRSV ORF5 (GP5) induces apoptosis when expressed in the simian COS-1 cell line in vitro and may be the cause of apoptosis in PRRSV-infected macrophages in vivo (Suárez et al. 1996). The cause of PRRSV-induced indirect apoptosis is unknown, but is likely due to substances released from, or secreted by, infected macrophages, e.g., p25, apoptogenic cytokines, reactive oxygen species, or nitric oxide (Choi and Chae 2002; Labarque et al. 2003; Suárez 2000).

Secretion of proinflammatory cytokines from PRRSV-infected macrophages likely results in effects that are both positive (recruitment of leukocytes, initiation of immune response, and reduction in viral replication) and negative (increased vascular permeability resulting in pulmonary edema and bronchial constriction). Studies demonstrated variable elevations in cytokine levels in broncho-alveolar lavage from PRRSV-infected vs. uninfected control pigs, including IFN-gamma, TNF-alpha, IL-1, IL-6, IL-10, and IL-12 (Choi et al. 2001; Suradhat and Thanawongnuwech 2003; Thanawongnuwech et al. 2003; van Gucht et al. 2003). Studies using in *situ* hybridization have also shown that production of these cytokines is predominantly by macrophages located in alveolar septa in foci of inflammation and also by lymphocytes positive for IFN-gamma (Choi et al. 2001; Chung and Chae 2003; Thanawongnuwech et al. 2003). Of these cytokines, TNF-alpha, IL-1, and IL-6 are proinflammatory and known to promote influx and activation of leukocytes, increased microvascular permeability (pulmonary edema), and induction of systemic effects such as pyrexia, anorexia, and lethargy. TNF-alpha and IL-1 can also cause bronchial hyper-reactivity and constriction with asthma-like symptoms.

PRRSV replication in lymphoid organs is also associated with polyclonal B cell activation. Grossly, this appears as nodular lymphoid hyperplasia and microscopically as follicular lymphoid hyperplasia (Lamontagne et al. 2001). Inoculation of neonatal gnotobiotic pigs with PRRSV results in lymphoid hyperplasia, extremely elevated levels of all classes of serum immunoglobulins (of which only 1% are specific for PRRSV), circulating immune complexes, immune complex deposition on glomerular basement membranes with associated cellular inflammation, and induction of auto-antibodies to Golgi antigens and dsDNA (Lemke et al. 2004).

CLINICAL SIGNS

Descriptions of the clinical signs of PRRS in swine herds are similar in North America (Bilodeau et al. 1991; Keffaber 1989; Loula 1991; Moore 1990; Sanford 1992), South America (Dewey 2000), Europe (Anon. 1992; Busse et al. 1992; de Jong et al. 1991; Gordon 1992; Hopper et al. 1992; Leyk 1991; Wensvoort et al. 1991; White 1992a,b), and Asia (Chiou 2003; Thanawongnuwech et al. 2003; Tong and Qiu 2003; Yang et al. 2003).

Clinical presentation of PRRS varies greatly between herds, ranging from asymptomatic to devastating. Clinical signs also vary greatly and may be masked or augmented by concurrent infection(s). The only completely consistent clinical feature of PRRS is that there is no consistent feature. For nearly every described clinical sign, there are exceptions. Clinical signs of PRRSV are influenced by virus strain, host immune status, host susceptibility, exposure to lipopolysaccharides (LPS), concurrent infections, and other management factors (Blaha 1992; White 1992a).

Clinical disease in a herd is primarily the consequence of acute viremia in individuals (Collins et al. 1992; Pol et al. 1991; Terpstra et al. 1991a) and transplacental transmission resulting in reproductive failure (Terpstra et al. 1991a). Because PRRSV isolates vary remarkably in virulence, low-virulence isolates can cause completely subclinical epidemic or endemic infections in herds (Morrison et al. 1992), whereas highly virulent isolates can cause severe clinical infections that appear differently, depending on the herd's immune status.

Clinical epidemics occur when PRRSV enters an immunologically naive herd or production site and all ages are affected. Endemic PRRS occurs in herds that have homologous immunity to the infecting strain of PRRSV. In endemic PRRS, clinical disease is observed in susceptible subpopulations, usually in nursery-grower pigs when maternal immunity decays, and/or in replacement gilts or sows that have previously escaped infection, as well as their congenitally infected progeny.

Antigenic variation is great enough among strains of PRRSV that entry of a new, relatively unrelated strain can cause an epidemic in an endemically PRRSV-infected herd.

Epidemic Infection

In PRRS epidemics, the first phase lasts 2 or more weeks and is characterized by anorexia and lethargy in 5–75% of animals of all ages as a result of acute viremia. It begins in one or more stages of production and quickly spreads in 3–7 or more days to all stages of production. Individuals are anorexic for 1–5 days. The spread of the disease through a segregated group of pigs usually requires 7–10 or more days, giving rise to the descriptive term "rolling inappetence." Clinically affected animals may also be lymphopenic, pyretic with rectal temperatures from 39–41°C (102–106°F), hyperpneic and dyspneic, or have transient "blotchy" cutaneous hyperemia or cyanosis on extremities.

The second phase may begin before the first phase of acute illness is completed and continues for 1–4 months, characterized by reproductive failure, primarily in sows that were viremic in their third trimester, and by high preweaning mortality in their live-born progeny. When reproductive performance and preweaning mortality return to near preoutbreak levels, endemic infection of most herds continues.

Sows. During the phase of acute illness, 1–3% of litters may be lost in sows that are from 21–109 days of gestation. This is recognized as overt abortions or, later, as irregular returns to estrus or nonpregnant sows (Hopper et al. 1992; Keffaber 1989; Loula 1991; White 1992a). Also observed inconsistently in acutely ill sows is agalactia (Hopper et al. 1992), incoordination (de Jong et al. 1991), and/or a dramatic exacerbation of endemic diseases, such as sarcoptic mange, atrophic rhinitis, or cystitis/pyelonephritis (White 1992a).

Mortality in sows is typically 1–4% during acute illness and is sometimes associated with pulmonary edema and/or cystitis/nephritis (Hopper et al. 1992; Loula 1991). A few cases of severe acute PRRS in sows have been described with 10–50% abortions, up to 10% mortality, and nervous signs such as ataxia, circling, and paresis (Epperson and Holler 1997; Halbur and Bush 1997).

Late-term reproductive failure begins at approximately 1 week and continues for up to 4 months. Not all affected sows are clinically ill during acute PRRS. Typically, 5–80% of sows farrow on day 100–118 of gestation and have litters composed of any combination of normal pigs, weak variably sized pigs, and dead pigs that are fresh stillborn (intrapartum death), autolytic (brown) partially mummified or completely mummified fetuses. Typically, pigs born dead comprise 0–100% of each affected litter and 7–35% of the total pigs born in a farrowing group. In time, there is a shift from predominantly stillborn pigs and large partially mummified pigs, to smaller more completely mummified pigs, to small weak-born pigs, to pigs of normal size and vigor (Keffaber 1989; Loula 1991; White 1992a). In some herds, the majority of abnormal pigs are born alive, premature, weak, and small, but few are born dead (Gordon 1992). Periparturient mortality in sows may be 1–2% (de Jong et al. 1991; Keffaber 1989). Surviving sows on the subsequent breeding often have delayed return to estrus and low conception rates.

Boars. During acute illness, in addition to anorexia, lethargy, and respiratory clinical signs, boars may lack libido and have variable reduction in semen quality (de Jong et al. 1991; Feitsma et al. 1992; Prieto et al. 1994). Changes in sperm occur 2–10 weeks after infection with virus and include reduced motility and acrosomal defects, but it is unclear whether conception rates are affected (Lager et al. 1996; Prieto et al. 1996a,b; Swenson et al. 1994b; Yaeger et al. 1993). However, of much greater significance is semen shedding of PRRSV that can result in venereal transmission to sows (Swenson et al. 1994b; Yaeger et al. 1993).

Suckling Pigs. During the 1- to 4-month phase of late-term reproductive failure, there is high preweaning mortality (up to 60%) in pigs born prematurely and at term associated most consistently with listlessness, emaciation/starvation, splay-legged posture, hyperpnea, dyspnea ("thumping"), and chemosis. Seen less commonly are tremors or paddling (Keffaber 1989; Loula 1991), slight doming of foreheads (Gordon 1992), anemia and thrombocytopenia with consequent hemorrhage from navels and elsewhere, and an increase in bacterial polyarthritis and meningitis (Hopper et al. 1992; White 1992a). Watery diarrhea was commonly reported in the United Kingdom (Gordon 1992; Hopper et al. 1992; White 1992a) and less commonly elsewhere (Keffaber 1989; Leyk 1991).

Weanling and Grower Pigs. Acute PRRSV infection in nursery or grower-finisher pigs is characterized most consistently by anorexia, lethargy, cutaneous hyperemia, hyperpnea and/or dyspnea without coughing, rough hair coats, and variable reduction in average daily gain creating uneven groups (Moore 1990; White 1992b). Frequently reported is a higher than usual incidence of endemic diseases and elevated mortality of 12–20% (Blaha 1992; Keffaber et al. 1992; Loula 1991; Moore 1990; Stevenson et al. 1993; White 1992a). Diseases most commonly reported include streptococcal meningitis, septicemic salmonellosis, Glasser's disease, exudative dermatitis, sarcoptic mange, and bacterial bronchopneumonia.

Endemic Infection of Herds

Once introduced into a herd, PRRSV becomes endemic in nearly all cases. In endemically infected herds, PRRS is most often seen as regular or occasional outbreaks of typical acute PRRS in susceptible nursery or grower-finisher pigs (Keffaber et al. 1992; Stevenson et al. 1993). Clinical signs are also observed in groups of susceptible gilts or replacement boars exposed to PRRSV after introduction into the herd (Dee et al. 1996; Dee and Joo 1994b; Grosse-Beilage and Grosse-Beilage 1992) but may also be seen in susceptible sows. Acute clinical disease in gilts or boars is as described for epidemics. The reproductive consequences depend on the number of gilts/sows infected and the stage of their reproductive cycle when infected, both of which may vary widely (Torrison et al. 1994). If few gilts are infected on an ongoing basis, there may be scattered abortions, irregular returns to estrus, nonpregnant gilts, and late-term reproductive failure with abnormal litters typical of PRRS. These may be recognized only if records are evaluated on a parity-specific basis (White 1992b). Alternatively, gilts may escape exposure to PRRSV until there is a significant subpopulation of susceptible gilts in various stages of gestation. In this situation, endemic PRRS in the breeding herd manifests as periodic mini-outbreaks of PRRS in gilts and, less commonly, sows, that are identical to those in an epidemic (Dee and Joo 1994b).

Factors Affecting the Severity of Disease

Differences in the expression of clinical disease are incompletely understood and affected by many factors, including virus strain, immune status (discussed elsewhere), host susceptibility, exposure to lipopolysaccharides (LPS), and concurrent infections. Management factors (pig flow, building design, temperature regulation, etc.) likely have impact, but are poorly defined.

PRRS virus strains differ genetically (Murtaugh et al. 1995), antigenically (Nelson et al. 1993; Wensvoort et al. 1992), in severity of induced respiratory disease and lesions (Halbur et al. 1995b, 1996a,b; van der Linden et al. 2003a) and in severity of induced reproductive disease (Mengeling et al. 1996a, 1998; Park et al. 1996). The specific virulence attributes that differ between strains are not known. High virulence strains, as compared to low virulence strains, are known to result in significantly more viral antigen in lung and lymphoid tissues (Halbur et al. 1996a), viremia of higher peak titer and of longer duration (Grebennikova et al. 2004; van der Linden et al. 2003a) and more pulmonary IFN-gamma producing cells (Thanawongnuwech et al. 2003).

A few PRRSV inoculation studies in purebred animals have demonstrated differences in disease between breeds. Halbur et al. (1998) reported significant differences in pulmonary lesions, number of pulmonary PRRSV antigen-positive cells, incidence of myocarditis, and incidence of encephalitis. Christopher-Hennings and others (2001) reported differences in duration of PRRSV shedding in semen of infected boars.

Bacterial LPS, also known as endotoxin, is a major component of bacterial cell walls and is known to be in high levels in dust in poorly ventilated swine buildings (Zejda et al. 1994). Intratracheal administration of LPS in PRRSV-inoculated pigs as compared to pigs given only PRRSV or LPS resulted in consistently more severe clinical respiratory disease that was temporally associated with 10–100-fold elevations of IL-1, IL-6, and TNF-alpha, but not differences in gross and microscopic lung lesions or number of inflammatory -cells in bronchoalveolar lavage fluids (Labarque et al. 2002; van Gucht et al. 2003).

Infection with PRRSV renders pigs more susceptible to some bacterial and viral diseases and has an additive or synergistic effect with some other bacteria or viruses to create more severe disease than either agent alone. Postnatal and congenital infection with PRRSV renders pigs more susceptible to development of septicemia with *Streptococcus suis* (Feng et al. 2001; Galina et al. 1994). Elegant studies have demonstrated that a likely mechanism is replication in and killing of pulmonary intravascular macrophages (PIMS) and alveolar macrophages (PAMS) as well as reduction in ability of virus-infected PIMs and PAMs to phagocytose and kill bacteria (Thanawongnuwech et al. 1997b; 1998a,b; 2000a,b). This mechanism may be operative in rendering pigs with acute PRRS more susceptible to septicemia by other bacteria, but experimental proof is lacking. Infection of weanling pigs with PRRSV also renders them more susceptible to development of bronchopneumonia due to *Bordetella bronchiseptica* (Brockmeier et al. 2000). This might be due to PRRSV infection of PAMs and resulting reduction in ability to kill bacteria (Thanawongnuwech et al. 1997b). Acute PRRS increases incidence and severity of clinical disease following inoculation with *Salmonella choleraesuis* (Wills et al. 2000). Infection with PRRSV also significantly enhances replication of porcine circovirus type 2 (PCV2), resulting in more severe PRRS viral pneumonia as well as lesions of PCV2-associated porcine multisystemic wasting syndrome (Allan et al. 2000; Harms et al. 2001). Attempts to experimentally confirm field observations of increased susceptibility in PRRSV-infected pigs to diseases caused by *A. pleuropneumoniae*, *Pasteurella multocida*, or *Haemophilus parasuis* have been unsuccessful (Cooper et al. 1995; Pol et al. 1997; Segalés et al. 1999). Other studies have demonstrated an additive or potentiating effect between PRRSV and some bacterial and viral agents. That is, dual infection causes more severe disease than either single infection. These include *Mycoplasma hyopneumoniae*, porcine respiratory corona virus, swine influenza virus, and Aujeszky's disease virus (Shibata et al. 2003; Thacker et al. 1999; van Reeth et al. 1996, 2001). No potentiation was observed between PRRSV and classical swine fever virus (Depner et al. 1999).

LESIONS

Postnatal Lesions

Postnatal virulent PRRSV produces consistent gross lesions of interstitial pneumonia and enlarged lymph nodes in all ages of swine. These lesions are suggestive of PRRSV, but are not diagnostic since a variety of other viral and bacterial diseases can cause similar lesions. Typical microscopic lesions of PRRSV sometimes allow a strong presumptive diagnosis. However, a definitive diagnosis always requires demonstration of PRRSV.

Similar lesions are described in all ages of pigs with PRRSV infection. The severity and distribution of lesions varies with the virulence of virus strain (Done and Paton 1995; Halbur et al. 1996b). Most inoculation studies in which lesions have been described were in suckling or weaned pigs 1–70 days of age (Collins et al. 1992; Dea et al. 1992c; Halbur et al. 1995b, 1996a,b; Pol et al. 1991; Rossow et al. 1994a, 1995). Gross and microscopic lesions are consistently observed from 4 to ≥28 DPI in lung and lymph nodes, where most viral replication takes place. Later, only microscopic lesions are inconsistently observed, beginning at approximately 7 to 14 DPI, in kidney, brain, heart, and elsewhere where there is much less virus; mostly in perivascular and intravascular macrophages and endothelial cells. Microscopic lesions are also in the uterus of dams following reproductive failure and in the testicles of boars. Lesions unique to pigs inoculated at ≤13 days of age include periocular edema on days 6–23 postinoculation, scrotal edema on days 11–14 postinoculation, and subcutaneous edema on days 2–7 postinoculation (Rossow et al. 1994a, 1995).

Lungs have interstitial pneumonia from 3 to ≥28 DPI that is most severe 10–14 DPI. Mild lesions are in cranial lungs or diffuse. Affected parenchyma is resilient, slightly firm, noncollapsing, mottled gray-tan, and moist. Severe lesions are diffusely distributed, and parenchyma is mottled or diffusely red-tan, noncollapsing, firm and rubbery, and very moist. Microscopically, alveolar septa are expanded by macrophages, lymphocytes, and plasma cells and may be lined by hyperplastic type II pneumocytes. Alveoli may contain necrotic macrophages, cell debris, and serous fluid. Lymphocytes and plasma cells form cuffs around airways and blood vessels. Rarely, PRRSV antigen is described in few bronchial epithelial cells with cell swelling and loss of cilia (Done and Paton 1995; Pol et al. 1991). In field cases of PRRS, especially in nursery and grower/finisher pigs, PRRS pulmonary lesions are often complicated or obscured by lesions of concurrent bacterial and/or viral diseases.

Lymph nodes have lesions from 4–28 or more DPI (Dea et al. 1992c; Halbur et al. 1995b; Rossow et al. 1994a,b, 1995). Many lymph nodes in most pigs are enlarged from 2–10 times normal. Early postinoculation, enlarged nodes are edematous, tan, and moderately firm. Later, nodes are firm and white or light tan in a nodular or diffuse pattern. Uncommonly, there are multiple fluid-filled 2–5 mm diameter cortical cysts. Microscopic lesions are predominantly in germinal centers. Early in the course of infection, germinal centers are necrotic and depleted. Later, germinal centers are very large and composed of blast-type lymphocytes. The cortices may contain small cystic spaces that are variably lined by endothelium and contain proteinaceous fluid, lymphocytes, and multinucleate prokaryocytes (Rossow et al. 1994b, 1995). Microscopically, there may be mild lymphoid necrosis, depletion, and/or hyperplasia in the thymus, in periarteriolar lymphoid sheaths of the spleen, and in lymphoid follicles in tonsil and Peyer's patches (Halbur et al. 1995b; Pol et al. 1991).

Mild to moderate multifocal lymphohistiocytic vasculitis and perivascular myocarditis may develop in the heart ≥9 DPI (Halbur et al. 1995a, 1996b; Rossow et al. 1994a, 1995). Less commonly, mild myocardial fibrillar necrosis and lymphocytic cuffing of Purkinje fibers is described (Rossow et al. 1995).

Mild lymphohistiocytic leukoencephalitis or encephalitis involving cerebellum, cerebrum, and/or brainstem may develop ≥7 days PI (Collins et al. 1992; Halbur et al. 1996b; Rossow et al. 1995; Thanawongnuwech et al. 1997a). There is segmental cuffing of blood vessels by lymphocytes and macrophages and multifocal gliosis. Necrotizing vasculitis was also described in one field case of PRRS with neurologic clinical disease (Thanawongnuwech et al. 1997a).

Kidneys occasionally have mild periglomerular and peritubular lymphohistiocytic aggregates from 14–42 DPI (Cooper et al. 1997; Rossow et al. 1995). Cooper and others (1997) described mild to severe segmental vasculitis that was most severe in the pelvis and medulla. Affected vessels had swollen endothelium, pooled subendothelial proteinaceous fluid, fibrinoid medial necrosis, and intramural and perivascular aggregates of lymphocytes and macrophages.

By 12 hours postinoculation, the nasal mucosal epithelium may have clumped or absent cilia and epithelial cell swelling, loss or squamous metaplasia (Collins et al. 1992; Halbur et al. 1996b; Pol et al. 1991; Rossow et al. 1995). By 7 DPI, lymphocytes and macrophages are in the epithelium and propria-submucosa.

Microscopic lesions are frequently in the uterus of pregnant sows with natural or experimental PRRS (Christianson et al. 1992; Lager and Halbur 1996; Stockhofe-Zurwieden et al. 1993). The myometrium and/or endometrium is edematous with lymphohistiocytic perivascular cuffs. Less commonly, there is segmental lymphohistiocytic vasculitis in small vessels and microseparations between endometrial epithelium and placental trophoblasts that contain eosinophilic proteinaceous fluid and cell debris.

Atrophy of seminiferous tubules is seen in 5- to 6-month-old boars 7–25 days PI (Sur et al. 1997). Atrophic tubules have PRRSV antigen and nucleic acid in germinal epithelial cells, giant cells with 2–15 nuclei, and apoptosis and depletion of germ cells.

Fetal Lesions

PRRS reproductive failure should be suspected when litters are delivered at ≥100 days of gestation but before term and are composed of variable proportions of clinically normal pigs, small or normal-sized weak pigs, dead variably autolyzed pigs, and mummies. Lesions in fetuses and stillborn pigs are uncommon and rarely contribute to a definitive diagnosis of PRRS. An absence of lesions in fetuses does not rule out PRRS.

PRRSV-infected litters contain variable numbers of normal pigs, small weak pigs, and dead pigs that are either fresh stillborn (intrapartum deaths), autolytic stillborn (prepartum deaths), or partially mummified/completely mummified fetuses. Dead pigs are commonly coated with a thick brown mixture of meconium and amnionic fluid; a nonspecific finding that suggests fetal stress and/or hypoxia (Lager and Halbur 1996; Stockhofe-Zurwieden et al. 1993). Most lesions in fetuses are non-specific and due to sterile in utero autolysis.

PRRSV-specific gross and microscopic lesions are few and inconsistent. These are best observed in fetuses with little or no in utero autolysis (Bøtner et al. 1994; Collins et al. 1992; Done and Paton 1995). Lesions are more commonly seen in live-born PRRSV-infected littermates that die or are sacrificed within a few days after birth. Gross fetal lesions include perirenal edema, edema of the splenic ligament, mesenteric edema, ascities, hydrothorax, and hydroperitoneum (Dea et al. 1992c; Lager and Halbur 1996; Plana Duran et al. 1992b). Microscopic lesions are mild and nonsuppurative and include segmental arteritis and periarteritis in lung, heart, and kidney (Lager and Halbur 1996; Rossow et al. 1996b), multifocal interstitial pneumonia with occasional hyperplasia of type II pneumocytes (Plana Duran et al. 1992b; Sur et al. 1996), mild periportal hepatitis (Lager and Halbur 1996), myocarditis with loss of myocardial fibers (Lager and Halbur 1996; Rossow et al. 1996b), and multifocal leukoencephalitis (Rossow et al. 1996b).

An uncommon, but diagnostically discriminating lesion is segmental hemorrhagic enlargement of the umbilical cord up to three times normal diameter that is caused by segmental necrosuppurative and lymphohistiocytic vasculitis (Lager and Halbur 1996).

IMMUNITY

The difficulty of achieving consistent and reliable control and prevention of PRRS with live, attenuated vaccines emphasizes our incomplete understanding of PRRS immunology. Serious deficits exist in our knowledge of the events initiating immunity at the time of infection, of key immunologic targets for both antibody and cytotoxic T cell-directed protection, of the molecular and cellular mechanisms regulating induction and maturation of the immune response, of the consequences of genetic diversity in PRRSV on immune protection, and of host genetic variation in pig populations on immune resistance to PRRSV.

The immune response to PRRSV begins with an attenuated innate antiviral response in the cytoplasm of an infected macrophage. Interferon (IFN) and inflammatory cytokine responses are weak (Albina et al. 1998; Buddaert et al. 1998; van Reeth et al. 1999). The downregulation of IFN-alpha production facilitates PRRSV replication since IFN-alpha mediates inhibition of PRRSV replication. PRRSV also blocks IFN-alpha production after super-infection with TGEV, a strong inducer of IFN-alpha. This weak innate response may compromise the subsequent initiation and elaboration of antigen-specific adaptive immunity. In addition, suppression of innate antiviral immune mechanisms may increase the risk of secondary infections.

Humoral Immune Response

In serum, PRRSV-specific IgM appears 5–7 days after infection and wanes to undetectable levels after 2–3 weeks. Anti-PRRSV IgG antibodies are detected 7–10 days after infection, peak at about 4 weeks, remain constant for a period of months, and then decline to low levels by 300 days.

The kinetics of anti-PRRSV antibody isotypes in bronchoalveolar lavage (BAL) fluid are similar to those in serum, indicating that these antibodies extravasate from the vasculature. The antibodies in BAL may contribute to the clearance of PRRSV from the lung but are unable to eliminate the virus completely.

Antibodies directed against the nucleocapsid (N) protein are most abundant and are used diagnostically to detect infected animals, but are not neutralizing.

Virus neutralizing (VN) antibodies appear in serum about 3 weeks after infection and are maintained for long periods, but at low levels. There is substantial variation in the VN antibody responses of individual pigs, including lack of response, the kinetics of their appearance, and in the level of titers (Loemba et al. 1996; Nelson et al. 1994; Yoon et al. 1995b). Neutralizing antibodies are produced against glycoproteins GP4 and GP5 and against the matrix (M) protein. A linear epitope on the ectodomain region of GP5 has been identified as the target of neutralizing antibodies, but the characteristics of the specific amino acid sequence involved in neutralization are not fully resolved (Ostrowski et al. 2002; Pirzadeh and Dea 1997; Plagemann et al. 2002; Wissink et al. 2003b).

Antibody responses also are elicited to nonstructural proteins (nsp) of the replicase complex, particularly the nsp2 polypeptide (Oleksiewicz et al. 2001). These antibodies may have diagnostic value and the proteins may be important targets for T cell responses.

The humoral immune response is presumed to play an important role in resistance to reinfection and in prevention or reduction of viral spread from animal to animal since neutralizing antibodies have the potential to clear virus from the circulation. However, the concurrent detection of neutralizing antibodies and infectious PRRSV in blood suggests that the role of neutralizing antibodies in protection against infection may be complex (Loemba et al. 1996; Molitor et al. 1997). Since viremia may occur in the presence of VN antibodies, the level of neutralizing antibodies normally generated against PRRSV may not be sufficient to control the replication of the virus and may even constitute a deleterious, nonprotective response (Yoon et al. 1996).

The kinetics of neutralizing antibody appearance in lung and serum are delayed relative to the changes in viral load in lung and serum. Viral loads peak in the lung at 7–9 days after infection and in serum at 4 days after infection (Labarque et al. 2000; Greiner et al. 2000; Samsom et al. 2000); that is, 2 weeks before VN antibodies first appear. Thus, it appears that neutralizing antibody plays a secondary role in adaptive immune responses to PRRSV.

Cell-Mediated Immune Response

PRRSV titers in the lung peak 7–9 DPI and decline to near zero by day 20, although virus still may be isolated from lung fluids for an extended period. During and subsequent to the decrease in PRRSV, total CD8+ T lymphocyte numbers in the lung may either remain low and constant or increase substantially (Labarque et al. 2000; Samsom et al. 2000). PRRSV-specific T cell responses are transiently induced 2–8 weeks after infection (Bautista and Molitor 1997; Lopez Fuertes et al. 1999; Xiao et al. 2004). T cell responses have been detected against all viral proteins that have been tested, including the products of ORFs 2, 4, 5, 6, and 7 (Bautista et al. 1999). The circulating T cell phenotype is reported as PRRSV-specific CD4+CD8+ memory or CD8+ gamma-delta+, and constitutive CD4+ natural killer (Lopez Fuertes et al. 1999).

The T cell response to PRRSV is highly variable and transient, ranging from insignificant to a high response that occurs after the peak or in the absence of viremia (Xiao et al. 2004). Xiao et al. (2004) found that the abundance of virus-specific T cells in both acutely and persistently infected pigs was highly variable and showed no correlation with the amount of virus. No significant difference in antigen-specific T cell abundance was observed in secondary lymphoid tissues in either acute or persistent infection, except for tonsil, in which the number of responding cells was extremely low. CD4+ and CD8+ T cell frequencies did not change after PRRSV infection, although a decrease in gamma-delta T cells was observed. Macrophages, the permissive cell type for PRRSV, were present in all tissue preparations at various levels that were not in proportion to local virus load. The weak T cell response probably contributes to prolonged PRRSV infection and suggests that PRRSV suppresses T cell recognition of infected macrophages. Meier et al. (2003) also observed that the initial T cell response to PRRSV was weak and transient, but increased steadily for 1–2 years after infection.

Protective Immunity

PRRSV persists for weeks or months in lymphoid tissue (Chang et al. 2002; Horter et al. 2002; Wills et al. 1997c). Persistence in lung and lymph nodes despite the presence of neutralizing antibodies and cell-mediated immunity argues that other factors, such as alteration in macrophage permissiveness to infection and innate immunity, may be important in control of PRRSV infection. The broad genetic and antigenic variation in PRRSV and the presence of multiple viral genotypes circulating on farms or within production systems simultaneously also has an unknown effect on the efficacy of humoral and cell-mediated immune responses.

Nevertheless, pigs infected or vaccinated with live PRRSV are resistant to the reproductive effects of PRRSV upon reexposure to homologous PRRSV (Lager et al. 1997b). Exposure to PRRSV therefore establishes some form of immunological memory that restricts or limits the second infection. The level of protection may be profound; Foss et al. (2002) observed the complete absence of PRRSV following challenge of vaccinated pigs, even though there was no change in specific antibody by two separate measures. Partial-to-high levels of protection may also be achieved against reinfection of immune pigs with heterologous PRRSV strains (Lager et al. 2003; Mengeling et al. 1999b, 2003a, b).

Whether neutralizing antibodies or cytotoxic T cells are essential for protection or even play a key role under natural conditions of reinfection is not known. It is possible that protection against PRRSV is afforded primarily by something other than adaptive immunity, such as a change in the permissiveness of macrophages to infection. Lactate dehydrogenase elevating virus, the arterivirus of mice, elicits ineffective neutralizing antibody and cytotoxic T cell responses, but is controlled primarily by a reduction in macrophages permissive for infection (Plagemann and Moennig 1992). In pigs, the infection in the lung begins to subside before there is evidence of an effective adaptive immune response and more than 98% of macrophages do not become infected (Duan et al. 1997b). Primary prevention and control of PRRSV infection by deletion of permissive macrophages would mean that neutralizing antibody and T cell responses are secondary and are more likely to play a role in the final elimination of virus.

CROSS-PROTECTION

PRRSV is continuously evolving and, therefore, vaccine strains will always be different from current field isolates. Therefore, cross-protection against heterologous field isolates is a key issue in disease prevention strategies that include vaccination.

Experimental studies consistently demonstrate a high level of protection for sows against reproductive losses upon rechallenge with strains homologous to an immunizing virus (Lager et al. 1997a, , 1999; Mengeling et al. 1999b). Attenuated live vaccines also have been effective in reducing disease severity, duration of viremia, virus shedding and the frequency of heterologous PRRSV infection (Christopher-Hennings et al. 1997; Dee and Molitor 1998; Lager et al. 1999, 2003; Mavromatis et al. 1999; Mengeling et al. 1999b, 2003a,b; Nielsen and Bøtner 1997; van Woensel et al. 1998). Still, episodic field observations of chronic and endemic PRRS and of "vaccine failure" suggest that protective immunity may be a variable feature of the immune response to heterologous PRRSV isolates.

MATERNAL IMMUNITY

No specific study has evaluated the effect of maternal immunity on piglet susceptibility to PRRSV infection, but indirect inferences suggest that immune sows provide maternal protection to piglets. Anti-PRRSV antibodies are present in colostrum at the same concentration as in blood (Eichhorn and Frost 1997) and PRRSV infections increase in pigs as maternal antibodies decline (Albina et al. 1994; Chung et al. 1997; Houben et al. 1995; Melnichouk et al. 2005). Maternal immunity appears to be of relatively short duration. In a study of seven commercial herds in Canada, Melnichouk et al. (2005) estimated that 12–44% of pigs had maternal antibodies at 3 weeks of age, but only 2–16% by 5 weeks of age. In the dam, prior immunity does not prevent transplacental infection (Lager et al. 2003) and neutralizing antibodies, particularly at low concentrations, may exacerbate PRRSV infection by antibody-dependent enhancement (ADE) (Yoon et al. 1996). At present, the role of maternal immunity in protection of piglets against PRRS is not known.

DIAGNOSIS

A diagnosis of PRRSV is based on subjective (history, clinical signs, gross and microscopic lesions) and objective (herd production records, detection of virus, and serology) information (Benfield et al. 1999). Table 24.1 summarizes the various diagnostic assays and their recommended use.

A presumptive diagnosis of PRRS is suggested in any herd with reproductive problems in breeding swine and respiratory disease in pigs of any age. Production records in clinically active PRRS herds usually reveal evidence of increased abortions, early farrowings, stillbirths, preweaning mortality, and nonproductive sow days. However, the lack of these signs does not indicate that a herd is free of PRRSV infection. Differential diagnoses include parvovirus, pseudorabies virus, hemagglutinating encephalomyelitis virus, porcine circovirus type 2, enterovirus, swine influenza virus, classical swine fever

Table 24.1. Summary of the use of diagnostic assays for the diagnosis of PRRSV

Assay	Sensitivity	Specificity	Preferred Diagnostic Specimens by Stage of Infection (Days Post Infection (DPI))				Optimum Window of Detection (DPI)
			In Utero Infection	1–28 DPI	30–90 DPI	90–300 DPI	
VI	medium	high	Collect samples from live pigs. Stillborn pigs or mummies are of limited diagnostic value. Refer to list of tissues for acute infection (1–28 DPI). Umbilical cords and umbilical cord blood also appropriate samples.	Serum, lung, tonsil, lymph nodes, lung lavage, heart, kidney, spleen, thymus	Tonsil, oropharyngeal scrapings, serum, lung lavage	Tonsil, oropharyngeal scrapings. Success rate rare to very low.	Serum and most tissues positive through 28–35 DPI. Lymphoid tissues through 157 DPI in limited number of pigs.
FA	medium	Depends on strain of PRRSV used in the test	Lung from live pigs	Lung or macrophages in lung lavage	Lung lavage and direct culture of macrophages from lavage sample.	Not recommended	4–14 DPI
IHC	medium	high	Most tissues from live pigs	See list for VI	Limited success with lymphoid tissues from 30–70 DPI	Not recommended	4–14 DPI
PCR	high	high	Limited success with thoracic fluid and tissues from stillborn fetuses. Most tissues from live pigs.	See list for VI	Good success with tonsil, oropharyngeal scrapings, and lung lavage	Tonsil, oropharyngeal scrapings, and lymph nodes. Success rate low.	Reports of detection by PCR up to 257 DPI.
ELISA	high	high	Can detect antibodies in umbilical cord blood.	serum	serum	serum	Variable from 9–13 DPI to at least 10 months post infection
IFA	high	Depends on strain of PRRSV used in the test	Can detect antibodies in umbilical cord blood.	serum	serum	serum	Variable from 9–14 DPI to 5 months pi
VN	low	Depends on strain of PRRSV used in the test	Not detected in stillborn fetuses or live pigs	serum	serum	serum	Variable from 9–28 DPI, usually 28–46 DPI for appearance and persists up to 12 months

VI=virus isolation; FA=fluorescent antibody on frozen samples; IHC = immunohistochemistry using formalin fixed tissues; PCR=reverse-transcriptase polymerase chain reaction; ELISA= HerdChek 2XR PRRS ELISA, IDEXX Laboratories Inc., Westbrook, Maine; IFA=indirect fluorescent antibody; VN=serum-virus neutralization. Contents of table based on references used in the "Diagnosis" section.

virus, cytomegalovirus, and leptospirosis (Halbur 2003). Co-infections with bacteria and other viruses also complicate the differential diagnosis (Halbur 2003; Zeman 1996). Thus, a definitive diagnosis requires either detection of PRRSV or antibodies in infected pigs.

Pathological Evaluation

There are no pathognomonic gross or microscopic lesions for PRRSV and aborted fetuses and stillborn pigs rarely have lesions of diagnostic value. Gross lesions of interstitial pneumonia and enlarged lymph nodes can be observed in infected pigs of all ages (Lager and Halbur 1996; Stevenson et al. 1993). Microscopically, interstitial pneumonia is the primary lesion. The virus replicates in alveolar macrophages and in macrophages and dendritic cells in germinal centers of lymphoid tissues, vascular endothelial cells, and the intra- and perivascular macrophages of blood vessels in the heart, brain, kidney and other tissues (Halbur et al. 1995; Rossow et al. 1996; Thanawongnuwech et al. 1997b). Lung, lymph nodes, heart, brain, thymus, spleen, and kidney may be fixed in 10% neutral buffered formalin and submitted to the diagnostic laboratory for microscopic evaluation and immunohistochemistry (IHC). The combination of IHC and histopathology allows visualization of cells containing PRRSV antigens in the cytoplasm within or contiguous to microscopic lesions (Halbur et al. 1994; Magar et al. 1993). Tissues should be processed for IHC within 48 hours of fixation to avoid degradation of PRRSV antigens and loss of IHC-positive cells (Van Alstine et al. 2002). Lesions and viral antigens are best observed during acute infection (4–14 DPI), when viral titers in tissues are high and sufficient quantities of viral antigen are present in the cytoplasm of infected cells.

Laboratory Confirmation

Detection of either PRRSV or antibodies is dependent upon proper sample selection and handling. Specimens for virus isolation and detection of viral RNA must be refrigerated (4°C) immediately after collection (freezing may degrade viral RNA for PCR) and shipped to the diagnostic laboratory within 2 days (Yoon et al. 2003). The virus is degraded by heat and has a narrow pH stability. Thus, maintain sterility to avoid pH alterations caused by bacterial contamination and always submit fresh tissues (Benfield et al. 1992, 1999; Bloemraad et al. 1994; Van Alstine et al. 1993). Generally, PRRSV is detected in higher amounts and for longer periods of time in younger, compared to older, pigs. Virus persists longer in tonsil and lymph nodes relative to serum, lung, and other tissues. Virus replicates in most tissues during the acute phase of the disease, reaching peak levels at 4–7 DPI before declining to undetectable levels by 28–35 DPI. Viremia can persist for 28–42 DPI in suckling, weaned, and grower pigs (Mengeling et al. 1996c) and for 7–14 DPI in sows and boars (Christopher-Hennings et al. 1995; Mengeling et al. 1996c). Infectious virus and

viral RNA can be demonstrated in pulmonary lung lavages, tonsil, and lymph nodes for several weeks after cessation of viremia (Benfield et al. 1999; Horter et al. 2002; Mengeling et al. 1995; Rowland et al. 2003; Wills et al. 2003).

Virus Isolation (VI)

Virus isolation is done using either porcine alveolar macrophages (PAMs) or sublines (CL-2621, MARC-145) of the African monkey kidney cell line MA-104 (Benfield et al. 1992; Kim et al. 1993). Isolation of PRRSV on these cell lines followed by fluorescent antibody (FA) or IHC staining of cells to detect viral antigens is the gold standard for detection of infectious virus. Results can be obtained within 1 day after inoculation of cultures, but may take several weeks, depending on the amount of virus in the clinical specimen. PAMs are reported to be more sensitive than MARC-145 cells for VI and the presence of Fc receptors on PAMs enhances the success of isolating PRRSV in the presence of antibodies (Yoon et al. 2003). Use of MARC-145 cells may also bias VI for recovery of modified live vaccine viruses because they are adapted to this cell culture (Benfield et al. 1999; Yoon et al. 2003). Not all PRRSV strains replicate in all cell types (Bautista et al. 1993), suggesting that at least two cell types should be used for VI whenever possible (Yoon et al. 2003). Use of PAMs is required for successful isolation of most European-like strains of PRRSV (Christopher-Hennings et al. 2002; Wensvoort et al. 1991).

Virus can also be detected by VI, FA, and PCR in direct cultures of PAMs from pulmonary lavage collected either from live infected pigs or at necropsy (Mengeling et al. 1995).

The most sensitive assay for detection of PRRSV is the swine bioassay. In this assay, a homogenate of sample suspected to contain PRRSV is injected into a young pig. Presence of PRRSV in the sample is confirmed by seroconversion or detection of replicating virus in the bioassay pig (Horter et al. 2002; Swenson et al. 1994a,b).

Virus isolation is most successful using serum, lung, lymph nodes, and tonsil collected between 4–28 DPI. In late-term abortion and early farrowings, similar tissue samples from liveborn pigs are preferred, because mummies or stillborn fetuses rarely yield positive VI results due to tissue autolysis. For persistent infections, tonsil, oropharyngeal scrapings, and lymph nodes are better samples than serum and lung. Under experimental conditions, virus has been isolated from the tonsil and oropharyngeal scrapings at 130 and 157 DPI, respectively (Rowland et al. 2003; Wills et al. 2003).

Detection of Viral Antigens

Viral antigens are detected by immunohistochemistry (IHC) using formalin fixed tissues (Halbur et al. 1994; Magar et al. 1993; Van Alstine et al. 2002) and fluorescent antibody (FA) using frozen tissue sections (Benfield et al. 1992). Lung, heart, kidney, lymph nodes, spleen, thymus, and tonsil are typically used for IHC, whereas lung is the primary sample for FA (Halbur et al. 1996a; Rossow et al. 1999). Both assays use the SDOW17 or SR30 monoclonal antibodies, either singly or in combination (Nelson et al. 1993; Yoon et al. 1995a), to detect viral nucleocapsid antigen in the cytoplasm of infected cells. The IHC is more sensitive than the FA test and can be done using formalin fixed tissue. The FA test is more rapid and more economical, but requires fresh tissue. Results from both tests are influenced by technician skill, so diagnostic laboratories usually confirm positive IHC and FA tests by VI or PCR. Viral antigens are best detected during peak viral replication (4–7 DPI).

Detection of Viral Nucleic Acid

PCR-based assays detect viral nucleic acid in tissue homogenates, serum, semen, oropharyngeal scrapings, and pulmonary lavage fluids. These assays are highly sensitive and specific (Benson et al. 2002; Horter et al. 2002). While VI amplifies infectious virions, PCR converts viral RNA to DNA using a reverse transcriptase and then exponentially amplifies the DNA to a detectable level. PCR offers several advantages over VI, IHC and FA: (1) Higher sensitivity and specificity; (2) Detection of viral RNA in both acute and persistently infected pigs; (3) Detection of viral RNA in autolyzed fetuses and in samples, such as semen and feces, that are toxic to cell cultures; (4) Rapid turnaround time, with results available in 1–3 days compared to days-to-weeks with other diagnostic assays; and (5) PCR products can be utilized for sequencing, thus expanding the diagnostic utility of this assay. The main disadvantage of PCR is that it does not differentiate between infectious and noninfectious virus. However, under experimental conditions, 94% and 81% correlation was reported between positive PCR results and detection by swine bioassay of infectious virus in semen and oropharyngeal scrapings, respectively (Christopher-Hennings et al. 1995b; Horter et al. 2002).

PCR assays are validated within, and occasionally between, diagnostic laboratories. Results may vary among diagnostic laboratories depending on the PCR assay and the method used to amplify and detect the viral genome (Christopher-Hennings et al. 2002; Kleiboeker et al. 2002). Nested PCR tests are as sensitive as conventional VI techniques, but require stringent controls to avoid false positive results. PCR-based assays are in a period of change and improvement. Several automated PCR methods have recently been developed that are less prone to false positive results, better adapted to screening multiple samples and more economical than nested PCR. These tests target ORF6 and ORF7, i.e., the ORFs with the most consistent nucleotide sequences between different strains of PRRSV. If sequencing is used to monitor viral evolutionary changes within herds, the ORF5 gene is targeted. Recently, a real time PCR assay that uses a primer to the 3'UTR sequence of the PRRSV genome to

detect PRRSV nucleic acid in semen and sera was commercially released. Once licensed for diagnostic use, the industry will have a standardized PRRSV PCR assay (Wasilk et al. 2004).

In acute infections, serum and the tissues recommended for VI are also the preferred diagnostic samples for PCR. During persistence, oropharyngeal scrapings and PCR are the most sensitive combination of sample and assay for detection of PRRSV (Horter et al. 2002). PRRSV nucleic acid has been detected up to 86 DPI in lymph nodes (Bierk et al. 2001), 92 DPI in semen (Christopher-Hennings et al. 1995), 105 DPI in oropharyngeal scrapings (Horter et al. 2002), and 251 DPI in serum and tonsil homogenates (Wills et al. 2003).

Sequencing

Sequencing is commonly done on ORF5 and ORF6 with direct PCR products from diagnostic samples to avoid the potential bias of selection, mutation, or nucleotide changes by passage in cell culture. ORF5 sequences are highly variable and there is an extensive databank of sequences available for comparison. ORF6 is highly conserved and serves as a sequencing control. Sequencing is best used to show the relatedness of strains over time and within a herd. Computer programs compare all possible pairs of sequences and a phylogenetic tree or dendogram is constructed. A phylogenetic tree depicts similarity among genomic sequences like a family lineage. This type of analysis may be used to

1. Determine whether the reappearance of PRRS on a farm is due to the reemergence of a previously existing or a new virus strain.
2. Determine whether PRRS outbreaks on farms are due to a single clone or multiple clones of virus.
3. Track introduction of virus into a swine operation.
4. Monitor spread of PRRSV strains within and between herds.
5. Differentiate vaccine and field viruses (Christopher-Hennings et al. 2002; Roberts 2001, 2003a).

Restriction Fragment Length Polymorphism

Prior to the advent of sequencing, restriction fragment length polymorphism (RFLP) of ORF5 was developed to differentiate a PRRSV modified live vaccine strain from other North American field strains. The ORF5 PCR product is digested using three restriction endonucleases. These enzymes always cleave a nucleic acid chain at a predetermined sequence of nucleotides; thus viruses with the same RFLP pattern contain the same restriction cleavage sites and have similar sequences. Each digest was assigned a three-digit code based on the pattern of digestion (Umthun and Mengeling 1999; Wesley et al. 1998). RFLP patterns are now based on computer-generated digestion patterns from an ORF5 sequence. Experience has shown that RFLP characterizations do not accurately reflect similarity or differences among isolates.

Indeed, many genetically dissimilar PRRSV isolates share the same RFLP pattern. RFLP data were previously used to determine the introduction of a new PRRSV isolate into a herd, monitor spread of an isolate, and differentiate vaccine from field viruses (Christopher-Hennings et al. 2002). Most of the applications of RFLP have been replaced by sequencing and phylogenetic analysis (Roberts 2003a).

Serology

Serological diagnosis is still favored by many practitioners because serum is easily collected in quantities for multiple tests and easily stored for future reference. The demonstration of seroconversion (negative to positive) using acute and convalescent serum samples is the most definitive method to diagnose PRRSV infection serologically. Increasing titers of PRRSV specific antibody demonstrated by FA or rising ELISA S/P ratios in a group of infected animals can also indicate PRRSV infection.

Serology is not a valid approach for diagnosis of PRRSV in previously infected or vaccinated herds, because serologic assays do not differentiate among antibodies resulting from the initial infection, reinfection, or vaccination. Single serum samples are of limited use because of the high prevalence of PRRSV in herds. For that reason, a single positive serologic result does not prove a causal role for PRRSV in a clinical diagnosis. Detection of antibodies in nursing and nursery pigs may be due to the presence of maternal antibodies, which usually persist until pigs reach 3–5 weeks of age (Melnichouk et al. 2005).

Five serological tests to detect antibodies to PRRSV have been described: indirect fluorescent antibody (IFA), ELISA, blocking ELISA, serum-virus neutralization (VN), and immunoperoxidase monolayer assay (IPMA). The proper use of these assays, interpretation, and limitations has been reviewed elsewhere (Christopher-Hennings et al. 2002; Yoon et al. 2003).

The IFA detects IgM and IgG antibodies as early as 5 and 9–14 DPI, respectively (Joo et al. 1997; Zhou et al. 2002). The IgM antibodies persist for 21–28 DPI, whereas IgG antibodies peak at 30–50 DPI and are undetectable 3–5 months after infection. Test sensitivity is impacted by the technical skill of laboratory personnel and antigenic differences between the PRRSV isolate used in the IFA and the field strain that induced antibodies in the pig. Little or no cross reaction between North American and European-like isolates of PRRSV is demonstrated by IFA (Christopher-Hennings et al. 2002). This assay is generally used to confirm a suspicious positive ELISA result.

The commercial ELISA (HerdChek® 2XR PRRS ELISA, IDEXX Laboratories Inc., Westbrook, Maine) is the "gold standard" for detection of antibodies to PRRSV. The assay is sensitive, specific, standardized, and rapid. The test putatively targets antibodies to the nucleocapsid antigens for both North American and European-like strains of PRRSV. Antibodies can be detected as early as 9 DPI, peak at 30–50 DPI and then decline to negative levels 4–12 months after infection. ELISA results are interpreted as positive (S/P ≥0.4) or negative (S/P <0.4). Practitioners have attempted to use ELISA S/P ratios to differentiate animals on the basis of their susceptible, infectious, and resistant immune status. However, this is an overinterpretation of the assay because the response of individual pigs on the ELISA is highly variable (Roberts 2003a).

Interpretation of ELISA negative and positive samples collected at a single point in time can be difficult. Negative ELISA samples have several possible interpretations:

1. Pigs were not infected.
2. Pigs were recently infected and have not yet seroconverted.
3. Pigs are persistently infected, but have become seronegative.
4. Pigs have cleared the infection and reverted to seronegative.
5. Pigs are negative due to low test sensitivity (Roberts 2003a; Yoon et al. 2003).

Pigs negative for antibodies on ELISA can be persistently infected, as demonstrated by recovery of virus or detection of virus or viral RNA in tonsil tissues or oropharyngeal scrapings (Dee et al. 2004a; Horter et al. 2002; Kleiboecker et al. 2002).

False positive (ELISA-positive reactors in expected negative herds) reactions occur at a rate of 0.5–2.0% (Ferrin et al. 2004; Keay et al. 2002; O'Connor et al. 2002; Torremorell et al. 2002a). Both IFA and blocking ELISA are used as confirmatory tests in cases of suspected false positive ELISA results. The blocking ELISA is as sensitive and specific as the commercial ELISA and IFA (Ferrin et al. 2004).

The serum-virus neutralization (VN) assay detects antibodies capable of neutralizing a constant amount of PRRSV in cell culture. The test is highly specific, but antibodies do not develop until 1–2 months after infection; thus the assay is less sensitive than the IFA and ELISA (Benfield et al. 1992). These antibodies typically peak 60–90 DPI and persist up to 1 year after infection. Like IFA, the magnitude of the VN response is highest when homologous virus is used in the assay. Laboratories have not developed standardized VN tests and it is typically used as a research rather than a diagnostic test.

Application of Diagnostic Assays to Herd Monitoring

Herd monitoring is typically done using ELISA and PCR as screening assays and PCR, IFA, and blocking ELISA to confirm suspicious positive results in herds expected to be negative for PRRSV (Dufresne et al. 2003). Issues in herd monitoring are complex and are extensively reviewed elsewhere (Dee 2004; Dufresne et al. 2003; Roberts 2003a,b).

PREVENTION AND CONTROL

Prevention

The objective of PRRSV prevention programs is either to stop the introduction of PRRSV into negative herds or the introduction of new strains into PRRSV-infected herds (Dee et al. 2001). Animals and semen have been considered the primary sources of PRRSV (Le Potier et al. 1997), but the importance of other sources of infection has become evident (Desrosiers 2004). Torremorell et al. (2004) found that over 80% of new infections occurring in commercial systems in the U.S. were not due to pigs or semen, but to area spread from neighboring units, the movement of pigs in PRRSV infected transports, the lack of compliance of the biosecurity protocols, or the possible introduction via insects.

Under ideal conditions, biosecurity starts with the establishment of the production units in isolated areas, but regardless of the herd location, biosecurity efforts should place particular emphasis on all procedures involving the movement of inputs and outputs from the farms, e.g., pigs, supplies and materials, feed, water, personnel, removal of manure, and reclaims. Because PRRSV persists in cold and wet conditions (Dee et al. 2002), all equipment and material used at the farm or for transport of pigs must be cleaned and dried (Dee et al. 2004b,c). All units should also exclude the entry of pests such as rodents, insects, and birds from all buildings.

All replacement breeding stock entering a negative herd should originate from sources known to be PRRSV-negative by a regular schedule of herd testing. In addition, all breeding stock should be properly isolated in isolation/quarantine facilities for a minimum of 30 days and then tested prior to introduction into the herd.

Semen for artificial insemination should come from PRRSV-negative boar studs. Boar studs should be routinely monitored for PRRSV infection. In order to detect early infections, it is recommended that serum or semen from stud boars be tested with a PCR-based assay prior to use in order to detect early infection. Although PCR testing allows for early detection of infections (Christopher-Hennings et al. 1995b; Wasilk et al. 2004), it may not fully prevent infection downstream should an infection in the stud occur (Torremorell and Conroy 2003).

Control

Specific treatments for PRRS are not available. Therefore, the objective of PRRS control is to limit the effects of the virus in the various stages of production. Even so, consistent PRRS control is problematic.

PRRSV cycles in endemically infected herds because, at any given time, animals are in various stages of infection and immunity (Dee et al. 1996). Circulation of the virus in the breeding herd results in PRRSV-infected piglets (Albina et al. 1994). Therefore, the first step in breaking virus circulation in the breeding herd is to use replacement animals that have been exposed to PRRSV and developed immunity prior to their introduction into the herd (Dee 2003). Consistent acclimatization of incoming breeding stock to PRRSV results in the stabilization of clinical signs, improvements in production parameters, and the production of PRRSV negative piglets at weaning.

Gilt introduction is the key to PRRSV control (FitzSimmons and Daniels 2003). This is primarily achieved through management steps involving the gilt pool. Serologically negative replacements are exposed to PRRSV in the acclimatization or isolation unit and are allowed to recover from infection. These animals are then introduced into the breeding herd after they become immune, i.e., when they are no longer viremic and do not constitute a source of infection to herdmates. Different methods for gilt acclimatization have been described (Dee et al. 1994; FitzSimmons and Daniels 2003). It is generally accepted that early exposure (2–4 months of age) will result in protection of the exposed animals and introduction of the replacement animals at a time when shedding has stopped. The exposure methods described in this section utilize PRRSV-negative gilts as the starting point. Regardless of the method of exposure, a major challenge is achieving consistent PRRSV infection.

Continuous-flow gilt development units that rely on contact exposure from previously infected PRRSV positive replacements to newly incoming PRRSV negative animals do not always yield consistent results. In some systems, weaned pigs and culled sows are also used as donor sources for infectious material. However, over time and as the breeding herd becomes immune, virus transmission within the breeding herd stops and the production of PRRSV negative animals at weaning increases. Therefore, incoming gilts may not become exposed to PRRSV when they are commingled with weaned pigs.

Additional exposure methods in replacement gilts may include methods such as feedback with tissues from weak-born piglets and stillbirths in the face of outbreaks, the use of modified live and killed vaccine products, and inoculation of negative replacement animals with serum collected from viremic pigs from the same farm (Batista et al. 2002; Dee 2003; FitzSimmons and Daniels 2003; Thacker et al. 2003).

Modified live virus (MLV) vaccines are used to develop protective immunity and bring consistency to the procedures. The main limitation attributed to PRRSV vaccines is the limited cross-protection that may exist among PRRSV strains. When using MLV vaccine products, the entire population housed in the same air space should be vaccinated at one time. Killed vaccine products may be used in gilt acclimatization protocols as a complement to MLV vaccine products or following exposure with field virus.

The use of planned exposure using serum containing viable field virus has recently increased due to the increased genetic heterogeneity among PRRSV strains and the perception that commercial vaccines do not induce enough protective cross-protection among newly identified PRRSV strains. This method has inherent risks and requires thoughtful application and high quality control standards.

Breeding-Herd Control. The consistent application of acclimatization protocols for incoming replacement animals results in the stabilization of the breeding herd and the production of PRRSV negative animals; therefore, additional procedures directed at breeding/gestating animals may not be required. However, MLV vaccines have also been used in the breeding herd in order to reduce the presence of susceptible animals (Dee 1996; Gillespie 2003), expedite the production of PRRSV-negative pigs (Gillespie 2003; Rajic et al. 2001), and, in the face of outbreaks, to limit field virus replication (although success of the latter measure is still under discussion). Currently, some products are approved for use in nonpregnant females; others are not. Producers and veterinarians should read the product label and understand its application. Vaccination of negative pregnant sows during the third trimester of gestation has been reported to result in fetal infection (Mengeling et al. 1996a).

Planned exposure based on inoculating pigs with serum collected from acutely affected pigs has also been used in the face of acute outbreaks. This procedure should be considered experimental at this time and veterinarians should be cautious in its use. Although it has inherent risks and very little documented information, planned exposure is thought to shorten the duration of the clinical outbreak and speed the recovery of the PRRSV negative weaned pig production. Overall losses expected to be incurred through planned exposure are believed to be similar to a naturally occurring outbreak.

An additional measure to minimize the effects of PRRSV infection in the face of a recent infection or in an effort to accelerate production of PRRSV-negative weaned pigs is the temporal interruption in the introduction of replacement animals (temporal herd closure) (Dee et al. 1994; Torremorell et al. 2003). By discontinuing the introduction of younger, recently infected, replacement animals, a level of herd stabilization is achieved. Periods of 2–4 months may be sufficient to minimize the effects of the virus, but not to eliminate it.

Weaned-Pig Management. Control of chronic PRRS in the weaned-pig population is one of the most frustrating challenges that veterinarians face. The cycle of transmission within the nursery or finishing stage is maintained through transmission of the virus to recently weaned piglets from older, infected pigs. Partial depopulation is a control strategy that consists of a strategic adjustment in the pig flow to prevent the lateral spread of PRRSV within chronically infected populations. Results of partial depopulation have shown highly significant improvements in average daily gain, mortality, and the overall economic performance of the nursery (Dee et al. 1993; Dee et al. 1997). Limitations to this strategy include the logistics involved in depopulating large nurseries and the fact that it may need to be repeated periodically to maintain improvements in performance.

An alternate strategy to eliminate the virus from the infected population is mass MLV vaccination of the growing pig population and unidirectional pig flow (Dee and Phillips 1998). This strategy has been used in commercial settings to displace PRRSV when emptying a site is not a possibility.

Control measures in the weaned pig population should also include the control of concurrent infections aggravated by PRRSV infection, e.g., *Haemophilus parasuis*, *Streptococcus suis*, etc. Appropriate vaccination and medication protocols need to be determined for the individual infections.

If the suckling piglet population is acutely infected, a series of management strategies may be required (Henry 1994; McCaw 2000, 2003). Management practices should limit the movement of piglets between litters to the initial 24 hours of life, humanely destroy chronically infected offspring prior to weaning, and maintain strict all-in/all-out animal flow of the nursery.

Eradication. Spontaneous elimination of PRRSV from a herd has been described (Freese and Joo 1994), but this is considered a rarity for current production systems. Over the last few years major advances have been made to define protocols that can successfully eliminate PRRSV from infected farms (Dee 2004; Torremorell et al. 2003). These include total depopulation/repopulation, partial depopulation, segregated early weaning, test-and-removal, and herd closure.

Successful PRRSV elimination in the breeding herd relies on the introduction of negative nonexposed replacement animals at a time when virus is no longer circulating. Successful control strategies, as described earlier, will prepare the population for eradication since eventually an immune, virus-free, population is developed. A successful elimination plan also requires the implementation of strict biosecurity measures in order to prevent the herds from becoming reinfected (Torremorell et al. 2004).

Total herd depopulation and repopulation is a very successful technique, but it is costly and may be justifiable only if the elimination of other concurrent diseases is desired. This strategy may be the only feasible alternative for farrow-to-finish herds where ongoing replication of PRRSV in the growing population does not allow for the elimination of the virus through other measures.

Partial depopulation, described above, has also been

used for the elimination of PRRSV (Dee et al. 1993; Dee et al. 1997). This measure is indicated for the elimination of the virus from growing pigs when shedding from the breeding population has completely stopped. This technique may be sufficient to eliminate the virus from small-sized farms. However, when used in large units (>500 sows), it requires the application of additional strategies, e.g., herd closure or test-and-removal, to eliminate the virus from the breeding herd prior to attempting elimination in the pig flow.

Segregated early weaning has also been used to produce PRRSV-negative pigs from infected sows. Depending on the level of PRRSV activity in the sow herd, production of PRRSV-negative batches may not be consistent (Donadeu et al. 1999; Gramer et al. 1999). All-in/all-out segregated production of batches of weaned pigs is needed to maximize the success of this technique. In addition, the establishment of PRRSV negative herds from positive sources is possible when negative piglets are produced by the combination of several of these techniques (Torremorell et al. 2002b).

PRRSV elimination through herd closure is based in the fact that PRRSV cannot persist in an immune population (Torremorell et al. 2003). This strategy mimics the principles followed for TGE eradication, whereby all animals are exposed to the virus and no replacement animals are introduced while there is a possibility that they could be exposed to the virus (Harris et al. 1987). In the case of PRRSV, longer periods of herd closure with no introduction of new replacement animals are required. Exposed animals will eventually eliminate the virus from their tissues, although because of the ability of PRRSV to establish persistent infection, this will require a long time. As a rule of thumb, a period of 6 months is recommended, but variations may be needed depending on the status of the farm and pig flow. Introduction of negative replacement animals should be followed by attrition or scheduled culling of the previously infected animals. This strategy will develop a negative population of breeding animals over time. The success rate using this strategy is above 90% for farms with segregated production. Production management practices, such as off-site breeding projects and others, can minimize the economic effects of herd closure.

PRRSV elimination through the test-and-removal technique has also showed promising results (Dee 2004). Elimination of PRRSV by test-and-removal consists of blood-testing the entire breeding herd, identifying PRRSV-infected animals using tests both for antibody and virus, and removing positive animals from the farm. Candidate herds for test-and-removal include herds with segregated production and more than 12 months since the last clinical episode of PRRSV, as well as herds with an estimated prevalence below 25%. Test-and-removal is recommended for herds where there is no indication of virus recirculation in the breeding herd and where the presence of persistently infected animals is considered a potential risk for failure of the program.

Vaccines. Several studies have established that vaccination against PRRSV can result in protective immunity (Gorcyca et al. 1995; Hesse et al. 1996; Mengeling 1996b; Plana Duran et al. 1995). A variety of MLV and inactivated products are available, depending upon the geographic region. In general, it is accepted that MLV vaccines induce a more efficacious immune response, although there are concerns regarding the safety of some of the products. Inactivated vaccines are also available, but in general they are considered less efficacious when used in naive animals. However, when used in combination with attenuated products or in previously infected animals, they may induce a higher production of neutralizing antibodies than when used alone.

When used in the field, vaccines have met with variable degrees of success. These differences may be due to differences in the commercial products available and in how the products are utilized. Likewise, the results may reflect differences in the virus strains circulating in different regions and/or they may relate to the question of cross-protection. In addition, field reports raise the possibility of reversion virulence by attenuated vaccine virus (Nielsen et al. 2001). Vaccine virus behaves very similarly to field PRRSV strains in terms of transmission, persistence, transplacental transmission and congenital infection, shedding in semen, and the length of time required to induce protective immunity. Research to provide safer and more efficacious products is needed in order for practitioners and producers to have a reliable tool to control the devastating effects of PRRSV.

REFERENCES

Albina E, Carrat C, Charley B. 1998. Interferon-alpha response to swine arterivirus (PoAV), the porcine reproductive and respiratory syndrome virus. J Interferon Cytokine Res 18:485–490.

Albina E, Madec F, Cariolet R, Torrison J. 1994. Immune response and persistence of the porcine reproductive and respiratory syndrome virus in infected pigs and farm units. Vet Rec 134:567–573.

Albina E, Mesplede A, Chenut G, Le Potier MF, Bourbao G, Le Gal S, Leforban Y. 2000. A serological survey on classical swine fever (CSF), Aujeszky's disease (AD) and porcine reproductive and respiratory syndrome (PRRS) virus infections in French wild boars from 1991–1998. Vet Microbiol 77:43–57.

Alfonso P, Frías-Lepoureau MT. 2003. PRRS in Central America and the Caribbean region. In The PRRS Compendium (2nd edition). J Zimmerman, K-J Yoon, eds. Des Moines, Iowa: National Pork Board, pp. 217–220.

Allan G, McNeilly F, Ellis J, Krakowka S, Meehan B, McNair I, Walker I, Kennedy S. 2000. Experimental infection of colostrum deprived piglets with porcine circovirus 2 (PCV2) and porcine reproductive and respiratory syndrome virus (PRRSV) potentiates PCV2 replication. Arch Virol 145:2421–2429.

Allende R, Kutish GF, Laegreid W, Lu Z, Lewis TL, Rock DL, Friesen J, Galeota JA, Doster AR, Osorio FA. 2000a. Mutations in the genome of porcine reproductive and respiratory syndrome virus responsible for the attenuation phenotype. Arch Virol 145: 1149–1161.

Allende R, Laegreid WW, Kutish GF, Galeota JA, Wills RW, Osorio FA. 2000b. Porcine reproductive and respiratory syndrome virus: Description of persistence in individual pigs upon experimental infection. J Virol 74:10834–10837.

Allende R, Lewis TL, Lu Z, Rock DL, Kutish GF, Ali A, Doster AR, Osorio FA. 1999. North American and European porcine reproductive and respiratory syndrome viruses differ in nonstructural protein coding regions. J Gen Virol 80(Pt 2):307–315.

Anonymous. 1991. The new pig disease: Conclusions reached at the seminar held. In The New Pig Disease. Porcine Reproductive and Respiratory Syndrome. A report on the seminar/workshop held in Brussels on 29–30 April and organized by the European Commission (Directorate General for Agriculture), pp. 82–86.

——. 1992. Porcine reproductive and respiratory syndrome (PRRS or blue-eared pig disease). Vet Rec 130:87–89.

Astrup P, Riising H-J. 2002. Porcilis PRRS: A laboratory assessment of vaccinal virus spread. Proc Congr Int Pig Vet Soc 2:380.

Baron T, Albina E, Leforban Y, Madec F, Guilmoto H, Plana Duran J, Vannier P. 1992. Report on the first outbreaks of the porcine reproductive and respiratory syndrome (PRRS) in France: Diagnosis and viral isolation. Ann Rech Vet 23:161–166.

Bastos RG, Dellagostin OA, Barletta RG, Doster AR, Nelson E, Osorio FA. 2002. Construction and immunogenicity of recombinant Mycobacterium bovis BCG expressing GP5 and M protein of porcine reproductive respiratory syndrome virus. Vaccine 21:21–29.

Batista L, Pijoan C, Torremorell M. 2002. Experimental injection of gilts with porcine reproductive and respiratory syndrome virus (PRRSV) during acclimatization. J Swine Health Prod 10(4):147–150.

Bautista EM, Faaberg KS, Mickelson D, McGruder ED. 2002. Functional properties of the predicted helicase of porcine reproductive and respiratory syndrome virus. Virology 298:258–270.

Bautista EM, Goyal SM, Yoon I-J, Joo HS, Collins JE. 1993. Comparison of porcine alveolar macrophages and CL2621 for the detection of porcine reproductive and respiratory syndrome (PRRS) virus and anti-PRRS antibody. J Vet Diagn Invest 5:163–165.

Bautista EM, Molitor TW. 1997. Cell-mediated immunity to porcine reproductive and respiratory syndrome virus in swine. Viral Immunol 10:83–94.

Bautista EM, Suárez P, Molitor TW. 1999. T cell responses to the structural polypeptides of porcine reproductive and respiratory syndrome virus. Arch Virol 144:117–134.

Benfield D, Collins JE, Dee SA, Halbur PG, Joo HS, Lager KM, Mengeling WL, Murtaugh MP, Rossow KD, Stevenson GW, Zimmerman JJ. 1999. Porcine reproductive and respiratory syndrome. In Diseases of Swine (8th edition). BE Straw, S D'Allaire, WL Mengeling, DJ Taylor, eds. Ames: Iowa State University Press, pp.201–232.

Benfield D, Nelson J, Rossow K, Nelson C, Steffen M, Rowland R. 2000b. Diagnosis of persistent or prolonged porcine reproductive and respiratory syndrome virus infections. Vet Res 31:71.

Benfield DA, Christopher-Hennings J, Nelson EA, Rowland RRR, Nelson JK, Chase CCL, Rossow KD, Collins JE. 1997. Persistent fetal infection of porcine reproductive and respiratory syndrome (PRRS) virus. Proc Annu Meet Am Assoc Swine Pract, pp. 455–458.

Benfield DA, Nelson C, Steffen M, Rowland RRR. 2000a. Transmission of PRRSV by artificial insemination using extended semen seeded with different concentrations of PRRSV. Proc Annu Meet Am Assoc Swine Pract, pp. 405–408.

Benfield DA, Nelson E, Collins JE, Harris L, Goyal SM, Robison D, Christianson WT, Morrison RB, Goryca D, Chladek D. 1992. Characterization of swine infertility and respiratory syndrome (SIRS) virus (isolate ATCC VR-2332). J Vet Diagn Invest 4:127–133.

Benfield DA, Yaeger MJ, Collins JE. 1994. Experimental studies on the transmission and persistence of swine infertility and respiratory disease virus (Mystery Swine Disease). Research Investment Report. National Pork Producers Council, Des Moines, Iowa, pp. 5–14.

Benson J, Yaeger M, Christopher-Hennings J, Lager K, Yoon K-J. 2002. A comparison of virus isolation, immunohistochemistry, fetal serology and reverse-transcription polymerase chain reaction assay for the identification of porcine reproductive and respiratory syndrome virus transplacental infection in the fetus. J Vet Diagn Invest 14:8–14.

Bierk M, Dee S, Rossow K, Otake S, Collins J, Molitor T. 2001. Transmission of porcine reproductive and respiratory syndrome virus from persistently infected sows to contact controls. Can J Vet Res 65:261–266.

Bierk MD, Dee SA, Rossow KD, Collins JE, Guedes MI, Molitor TW. 2000. Experiences with tonsil biopsy as an antemortem diagnostic test for detecting porcine reproductive and respiratory syndrome virus infection in breeding swine. J Swine Health Prod 8(6):279–282.

Bierk MD, Dee SA, Rossow KD, Otake S, Collins JE, Molitor TW. 2001. Transmission of porcine reproductive and respiratory syndrome virus from persistently infected sows to contact controls. Can J Vet Res 65:261–266.

Bilodeau R, Dea S, Sauvageau RA, Martineau GP. 1991. Porcine reproductive and respiratory syndrome in Quebec [letter]. Vet Rec 129:102–103.

Blaha T. 1992. Epidemiological investigations into PEARS in Germany: Consequences in fattening pigs. Proc Congr Int Pig Vet Soc 12:126.

Bloemraad M, de Kluijver EP, Petersen A, Burkjardt GE, Wensvoort G. 1994. Porcine reproductive and respiratory syndrome: temperature and pH stability of Lelystad virus and its survival in tissue specimens from viraemic pigs. Vet Microbiol 42:361–371.

Bøtner A. 2003. The PRRS situation in Denmark, Norway, Finland, and Sweden. In The PRRS Compendium (2nd edition). J Zimmerman, K-J Yoon, eds. Des Moines, Iowa: National Pork Board, pp. 233–238.

Bøtner A, Nielsen J, Bille-Hansen V. 1994. Isolation of porcine reproductive and respiratory syndrome (PRRS) virus in a Danish swine herd and experimental infection of pregnant gilts with the virus. Vet Microbiol 40:351–360.

Bøtner A, Stradbygaard B, Sorensen KJ, Have P, Madsen KG, Madsen ES, Alexandersen S. 1997. Appearance of acute PRRS-like symptoms in sow herds after vaccination with a modified-live PRRS vaccine. Vet Rec 141:497–499.

Brockmeier S, Palmer M, Bolin S. 2000. Effects of intranasal inoculation of porcine reproductive and respiratory syndrome virus, Bordatella bronchiseptica, or a combination of both organisms in pigs. Am J Vet Res 61:892–899.

Buddaert W, van Reeth K, Pensaert M. 1998. In vivo and in vitro interferon (IFN) studies with the porcine reproductive and respiratory syndrome virus (PRRSV). Adv Exp Med Biol 40:461–467.

Busse FW, Alt M, Janthur I, Neumann W, Schoss AP. 1992. Epidemiologic studies on porcine epidemic abortion and respiratory syndrome (PEARS) in Lower Saxony of Germany. Proc Congr Int Pig Vet Soc 12:115.

Butler JE, Sun J, Weber P, Ford SP, Rehakova Z, Sinkora J. Lager K. 2001. Antibody repertoire development in fetal and neonatal piglets. IV. Switch recombination, primarily in fetal thymus, occurs independent of environmental antigen and is only weakly associated with repertoire diversification. J Immunol 167:3239–3249.

Carman S, Sanford SE, Dea S. 1995. Assessment of seropositivity to porcine reproductive and respiratory syndrome (PRRS) virus in swine herds in Ontario—1978 to 1982. Can Vet J 36:776–777.

Cavanagh, D. 1997. Nidovirales: A new order comprising *Coronaviridae* and *Arteriviridae*. Arch Virol 142:629–633.

Chang CC, Chung WB, Lin MW, Lin MW, Weng CN, Yang PC, Chiu YT, Chang WF, Chu RM. 1993. Porcine reproductive and respiratory syndrome (PRRS) in Taiwan. I. Viral isolation. J Chin Soc Vet Sci 19:268–276.

Chang CC, Yoon K-J, Zimmerman JJ, Harmon KM, Dixon PM, Dvorak CM, Murtaugh MP. 2002. Evolution of porcine reproductive and respiratory syndrome (PRRS) virus during sequential pig passages. J Virol 76:4750–4763.

Cheon D, Chae C. 2001. Distribution of porcine reproductive and respiratory syndrome virus in stillborn and liveborn piglets from experimentally infected sows. J Comp Path 124:231–237.

Chiou M-T. 2003. An overview of PRRS in Taiwan. In The PRRS Compendium (2nd edition). J Zimmerman, K-J Yoon, eds. Des Moines, Iowa: National Pork Board, pp. 281–283.

Choi C, Chae C. 2002. Expression of tumour necrosis factor-alpha is associated with apoptosis in lungs of pigs experimentally infected with porcine reproductive and respiratory syndrome virus. Res Vet Sci 72:45–49.

Choi C, Cho W, Kim B, Chae C. 2001. Expression of interferon-gamma and tumour necrosis factor-alpha in pigs experimentally infected with porcine reproductive and respiratory syndrome virus (PRRSV). J Comp Path 127:106–113.

Christianson WT, Choi CS, Collins JE, Molitor TW, Morrison RB, Joo HS. 1993. Pathogenesis of porcine reproductive and respiratory syndrome virus infection in mid-gestation sows and fetuses. Can J Vet Res 57:262–268.

Christianson WT, Collins JE, Benfield DA, Harris L, Gorcyca DE, Chladek DW, Morrison RB, Joo HS. 1992. Experimental reproduction of swine infertility and respiratory syndrome in pregnant sows. Am J Vet Res 53:485–488.

Christopher-Hennings J. 2000. The pathogenesis of porcine reproductive and respiratory syndrome virus (PRRSV) in the boar. Vet Res 31:57–58.

Christopher-Hennings J, Faaberg KS, Murtaugh MP, Nelson EA, Roof MB, Vaughn EM, Yoon K-J, Zimmerman J. 2002. Porcine reproductive and respiratory syndrome (PRRS) diagnostics: Interpretation and limitations. J Swine Health Prod 10(5): 213–218.

Christopher-Hennings J, Holler L, Benfield D, Nelson E. 2001. Detection and duration of porcine reproductive and respiratory syndrome virus in semen, serum, peripheral blood mononuclear cells, and tissues from Yorkshire, Hampshire, and Landrace boars. J Vet Diagn Invest 13:133–142.

Christopher-Hennings J, Nelson E, Nelson J, Rossow K, Shivers J, Yaeger M, Chase C, Garduno R, Collins J, Benfield D. 1998. Identification of porcine reproductive and respiratory syndrome virus in semen and tissues from vasectomized and non-vasectomized boars. Vet Pathol 35:260–267.

Christopher-Hennings J, Nelson EA, Benfield DA. 1996. Detecting PRRSV in boar semen. Swine Health and Production 4(1):37–39.

Christopher-Hennings J, Nelson EA, Hines RJ, Nelson JK, Swenson SL, Zimmerman JJ, Chase CCL, Yaeger MJ, Benfield DA. 1995a. Persistence of porcine reproductive and respiratory syndrome virus in serum and semen of adult boars. J Vet Diagn Invest 7:456–464.

Christopher-Hennings J, Nelson EA, Nelson JA, Hines RJ, Swenson SL, Hill HT, Zimmermann JJ, Katz JB, Yaeger MJ, Chase CCL, Benfield DA. 1995b. Detection of porcine reproductive and respiratory syndrome virus in boar semen by PCR. J Clin Microbiol 33:1730–1734.

Christopher-Hennings J, Nelson EA, Nelson JK, Benfield DA. 1997. Effects of a modified-live vaccine against porcine reproductive and respiratory syndrome in boars. Am J Vet Res 58:40–45.

Chung H, Chae C. 2003. Expression of interluekin-10 and interleukin-12 in piglets experimentally infected with porcine reproductive and respiratory syndrome virus (PRRSV). J Comp Path 129:205–212.

Chung WB, Lin MW, Chang WF, Yang PC. 1997. Persistence of porcine reproductive and respiratory syndrome virus in intensive farrow-to-finish pig herds. Can J Vet Res 61:292–298.

Ciacci-Zanella JR, Trombetta C, Vargas I, Mariano da Costa DE. 2004. Lack of evidence of porcine reproductive and respiratory syndrome virus (PRRSV) infection in domestic swine in Brazil. Ciçncia Rural 34:449–455.

Collins JE. 1991. Diagnostic note: Newly recognized respiratory syndromes in North American swine herds. American Association of Swine Practitioners Newsletter 3:7–11.

Collins JE, Benfield DA, Christianson WT, Harris L, Hennings JC, Shaw DP, Goyal SM, McCullough S, Morrison RB, Joo HS, Gorcyca D, Chladek D. 1992. Isolation of swine infertility and respiratory syndrome virus (isolate ATCC VR-2332) in North America and experimental reproduction of disease in gnotobiotic pigs. J Vet Diagn Invest 4:117–126.

Cooper V, Doster A, Hesse R, Harris N. 1995. Porcine reproductive and respiratory syndrome: NEB-1 PRRSV infection did not potentiate bacterial pathogens. J Vet Diagn Invest 7:313–320.

Cooper VL, Hesse RA, Doster AR. 1997. Renal lesions associated with experimental porcine reproductive and respiratory syndrome virus (PRRSV) infection. J Vet Diagn Invest 9:198–201.

de Jong MF, Cromwijk W, Van't Veld P. 1991. The new pig disease: Epidemiology and production losses in the Netherlands. In The New Pig Disease. Porcine Reproductive and Respiratory Syndrome. A report on the seminar/workshop held in Brussels on 29–30 April and organized by the European Commission (Directorate General for Agriculture), p. 9–19.

Dea SA, Bilodeau R, Athanassious R, Sauvageau RA, Martineau GP. 1992a. PRRS syndrome in Quebec: Isolation of a virus serologically related to Lelystad virus [letter]. Vet Rec 130:167.

——. 1992b. Swine reproductive and respiratory syndrome in Quebec: Isolation of an enveloped virus serologically-related to Lelystad virus. Can Vet J 33:801–808.

——. 1992c. Isolation of the porcine reproductive and respiratory syndrome virus in Quebec. Can Vet J 33:552–553.

Dea S, Gagnon CA, Mardassi H, Pirzadeh B, Rogan D. 2000. Current knowledge on the structural proteins of porcine reproductive and respiratory syndrome (PRRS) virus: Comparison of the North American and European isolates. Arch Virol 145:659–688.

Dee S, Deen J, Burns D, Douthit G, Pijoan C. 2004c. An assessment of sanitation protocols for commercial transport vehicles contaminated with porcine reproductive and respiratory syndrome virus. Can J Vet Res 68:208–214.

Dee S, Deen J, Rossow K, Weise C, Eliason R, Otake S, Joo HS, Pijoan C. 2003. Mechanical transmission of porcine reproductive and respiratory syndrome virus throughout a coordinated sequence of events during warm weather. Can J Vet Res 67:12–19.

Dee SA. 1992. Investigation of a nationwide outbreak of SIRS using a telephone survey. American Association of Swine Practitioners Newsletter 4:41–44.

——. 1996. The decision of using PRRS vaccine in the breeding herd: When and how to use it. Proc AD Leman Swine Conf, pp. 143–146.

——. 2003. Approaches to prevention, control, and eradication. In The PRRS Compendium (2nd edition). J Zimmerman, K-J Yoon, eds. Des Moines, Iowa: National Pork Board, pp. 119–130.

——. 2004. Elimination of porcine reproductive and respiratory syndrome virus from 30 farms by test and removal. J Swine Health Prod 12(3):129–133.

Dee SA, Deen J, Otake S, Pijoan C. 2004b. An experimental model to evaluate the role of transport vehicles as a source of transmission of porcine reproductive and respiratory syndrome virus to susceptible pigs. Can J Vet Res 68:128–133.

Dee SA, Deen J, Pijoan C. 2004a. Evaluation of four intervention strategies to prevent the mechanical transmission of porcine reproductive and respiratory syndrome virus. Can J Vet Res 68:19–26.

Dee SA, Deen J, Rossow K, Wiese C, Otake S, Joo HS, Pijoan. 2002. Mechanical transmission of porcine and respiratory syndrome virus throughout a coordinated sequence of events during cold weather. Can J Vet Res 66:232–239.

Dee SA, Joo HS. 1994a. Prevention of the spread of porcine reproductive and respiratory syndrome virus in endemically infected pig herds by nursery depopulation. Vet Rec 135:6–9.

——. 1994b. Clinical investigation of recurrent reproductive failure associated with PRRS virus infection in a sow herd. J Am Vet Med Assoc 205:1017–1018.

Dee SA, Joo HS, Henry S, Tokach L, Park BK, Molitor TW, Pijoan C. 1996. Detecting subpopulations after PRRS virus infection in large breeding herds using multiple serologic tests. Swine Health Prod 4(4):181–184.

Dee SA, Joo HS, Pijoan C. 1994. Controlling the spread of PRRS virus in the breeding herd through management of the gilt pool. Swine Health Prod 3(2):64–69.

Dee SA, Joo HS, Polson DD, Park BK, Pijoan C, Molitor TW, Collins JE, King V. 1997. Evaluation of the effects of nursery depopulation on the persistence of porcine reproductive and respiratory syndrome virus and the productivity of 34 farms. Vet Rec 140:247–248

Dee SA, Molitor TW. 1998. Elimination of porcine reproductive and respiratory syndrome virus using a test and removal process. Vet Rec 143:474–476.

Dee SA, Morrison RB, Joo HS. 1993. Eradication of PRRS virus using multi-site production and nursery depopulation. Swine Health Prod 1(5):20–23.

Dee SA, Phillips R. 1998. Using vaccination and unidirectional pig flow to control PRRSV transmission. Swine Health Prod 1(5):21–25.

Dee SA, Torremorell M, Rossow K, Mahlum C, Otake S, Faaberg K. 2001. Identification of genetically diverse sequences (ORF 5) of porcine reproductive and respiratory syndrome virus in a swine herd. Can J Vet Res 65:254–260.

Dee SA, Torremorell M, Thompson R, Deen J, Pijoan C. 2004b. An evaluation of the Thermo-Assisted Drying and Decontamination (TADD) system for the elimination of porcine reproductive and respiratory syndrome virus from contaminated livestock transport vehicles. Can J Vet Res (submitted).

Delputte PL, Vanderheijden N, Nauwynck HJ, Pensaert MB. 2002. Involvement of the matrix protein in attachment of porcine reproductive and respiratory syndrome virus to a heparinlike receptor on porcine alveolar macrophages. J Virol 76:4312–4320.

Depner K, Lange E, Pontrakulpipat S, Fichtner D. 1999. Does porcine reproductive and respiratory syndrome virus potentiate classical swine fever virus infection in weaner pigs? Zentralbl Veterinarmed B 46:485–491.

Desrosiers R. 2004. Transmission of pathogens: We, veterinarians, should change our tune! International Pigletter 2(4):No.2c.

Dewey C. 2000. PRRS in North America, Latin America, and Asia. Vet Res 31:84–85.

Donadeu M, Arias M, Gomez-Tejedor C, Aguero M, Romero LJ, Christianson WT, Sanchez-Vizcaino JM. 1999. Using polymerase chain reaction to obtain PRRSV-free piglets from endemically infected herds. J Swine Health Prod 7(6):255–261.

Done SH, Paton DJ. 1995. Porcine reproductive and respiratory syndrome: Clinical disease, pathology and immunosuppression. Vet Rec 136:32–35.

Duan X, Nauwynxk H, Favoreel H, Pensaert M. 1998. Identification of a putative receptor for porcine reproductive and respiratory syndrome virus on porcine alveolar macrophages. J Virol 72:4520–4523.

Duan X, Nauwynck HJ, Pensaert MB. 1997a. Effects of origin and state of differentiation and activation of monocytes/macrophages on their susceptibility to porcine reproductive

and respiratory syndrome virus (PRRSV). Arch Virol 142:2483–2497.

——. 1997b. Virus quantification and identification of cellular targets in the lungs and lymphoid tissues of pigs at different time intervals after inoculation with porcine reproductive and respiratory syndrome virus (PRRSV). Vet Microbiol 56:9–19.

Dufresne L, Polson DD, Holck JT, Roberts J. 2003. Serological monitoring in negative and low prevalence populations. In The PRRS Compendium (2nd edition). J Zimmerman, K-J Yoon, eds. Des Moines, Iowa: National Pork Board, pp. 87–101.

Edwards S, Robertson IB, Wilesmith JW, Ryan JB, Kilner CG, Paton DJ, Drew TW, Brown I, Sands J. 1992. PRRS ("blue-eared pig disease") in Great Britain. American Association of Swine Practitioners Newsletter 4:32–36.

Eichhorn G, Frost JW. 1997. Study on the suitability of sow colostrum for the serological diagnosis of porcine reproductive and respiratory syndrome (PRRS). Zentralbl Veterinarmed B 44:65–72.

Elvander M, Larsson B, Engvall A, Klingeborn B, Gunnarsson A. 1997. Nation-wide surveys of TGE/PRCV, CSF, PRRS, SVD, *L. pomona,* and *B. suis* in pigs in Sweden. Epidémiol Santé Anim 31–32:07.B.39.

Epperson B and Holler L. 1997. An abortion storm and sow mortality syndrome. Proc Annu Meet Am Assoc Swine Pract, pp. 479–484.

Fairbanks K, Chase C, Benfield DA. 2002. Tonsil biopsies and polymerase chain reaction assay for detection of breeding age gilts persistently infected with porcine reproductive and respiratory syndrome virus. J Swine Health Prod 10(2):87–88.

Feitsma H, Grooten HJ, Schie FW. 1992. The effect of porcine epidemic abortion and respiratory syndrome (PEARS) on sperm production. Proc 12th Int Anim Reprod Congr, pp. 1710–1712.

Feng W, Laster S, Tompkins M, Brown T, Xu J, Altier C, Gomez W, Benfield D, McCaw M. 2001. In utero infection by porcine reproductive and respiratory syndrome virus is sufficient to increase susceptibility of piglets to challenge by *Streptococcus suis* type II. J Virol 75:4889–4895.

Ferrin NH, Fang Y, Johnson CR, Murtaugh MP, Polson DD, Torremorell M, Gramer ML, Nelson EA. 2004. Validation of a blocking enzyme-linked immunosorbent assay for detection of antibodies against porcine reproductive and respiratory syndrome virus. Clin Diagn Lab Immunol 11:503–514.

FitzSimmons MA, Daniels CS. 2003. Control in large systems. In The PRRS Compendium (2nd edition). J Zimmerman, K-J Yoon, eds. Des Moines, Iowa: National Pork Board, pp. 137–142.

Foss DL, Zilliox MJ, Meier W, Zuckermann F, Murtaugh MP. 2002. Adjuvant danger signals increase the immune response to porcine reproductive and respiratory syndrome virus. Viral Immunol 15:557–566.

Freese WR, Joo HS. 1994. Cessation of porcine reproductive and respiratory syndrome (PRRS) virus spread in a commercial swine herd. Swine Health Prod 2(1):13–15.

Galina L, Pijoan C, Sitjar M, Christianson WT, Rossow K, Collins JE. 1994. Interaction between *Streptococcus suis* serotype 2 and porcine reproductive and respiratory syndrome virus in specific pathogen-free piglets. Vet Rec 134:60–64.

Garner MG, Gleeson LJ, Holyoake PK, Cannon RM, Doughty WJ. 1997. A national serological survey to verify Australia's freedom from porcine reproductive and respiratory syndrome. Aust Vet J 75:596–600.

Garner MG, Gleeson LJ, Martin R, Higgins P. 1996. Report on the national serological survey for PRRS in Australia. Pig Research and Development Corporation Project No. BRS 1/1037. Animal and Plant Health Branch, Bureau of Resource Sciences, PO Box E11 Queen Victoria Terrace, Parkes ACT 260.

Geue A. 1995. (Prevalence and incidence of the porcine reproductive and respiratory syndrome in a district of Schleswig-Holstein Germany.) Fachbereich Veterinarmedizin, Freie Universitat, Berlin, Germany.

Gillespie TG. 2003. Control with modified-live virus (MLV) PRRS vaccine. In The PRRS Compendium (2nd edition). J Zimmerman, K-J Yoon, eds. Des Moines, Iowa: National Pork Board, pp. 147–150.

Goldberg TL, Hahn EC, Weigel RM, Scherba G. 2000. Genetic, geographical and temporal variation of porcine reproductive and respiratory syndrome virus in Illinois. J Gen Virol 81:171–179.

Goldberg TL, Lowe JF, Milburn SM, Firkins LD. 2003. Quasispecies variation of porcine reproductive and respiratory syndrome virus during natural infection. Virology 317:193–207.

Gonin P, Mardassi H, Gagnon CA, Massie B, Dea S. 1998. A nonstructural and antigenic glycoprotein is encoded by ORF3 of the IAF-Klop strain of porcine reproductive and respiratory syndrome virus. Arch Virol 143:1927–1940.

Gorcyca D, Schlesinger K, Chladek D, Behan W, Polson D, Roof M, Doitchenoff D. 1995. RespPRRS: A new tool for the prevention and control of PRRS in pigs. Proc Annu Meet Am Assoc Swine Pract, pp. 1–22.

Gordon SC. 1992. Effects of blue-eared pig disease on a breeding and fattening unit. Vet Rec 130:513–514.

Gradil C, Dubuc C, Eaglesome MD. 1996. Porcine reproductive and respiratory syndrome virus: Seminal transmission. Vet Rec 138:521–522.

Gramer ML, Christianson WT, Harris DL. 1999. Producing PRRS negative pigs from PRRS positive sows. Proc Annu Meet Am Assoc Swine Pract, pp. 413–416.

Grebennikova T, Clouser D, Vorwald A, Musienko M, Mengeling W, Lager K, Wesley R, Biketov S, Zaberezhny A, Aliper T, Nepoklonov E. 2004. Genomic characterization of virulent, attenuated, and revertant passages of a North American porcine reproductive and respiratory syndrome virus strain. Virol 321:383–390.

Greiner LL, Stahly TS, Stabel TJ. 2000. Quantitative relationship of systemic virus concentration on growth and immune response in pigs. J Anim Sci 78:2690–2695.

Groot Bramel-Verheije MH, Rottier PJ, Meulenberg JJ. 2000. Expression of a foreign epitope by porcine reproductive and respiratory syndrome virus. Virology 278:380–389.

Grosse-Beilage E, Grosse-Beilage T. 1992. Epidemiological investigations into PEARS in Germany: Influence on reproduction. Proc 12th Congr Int Pig Vet Soc, p. 125.

Halbur PG. 2003. Factors that influence the severity of clinical disease. In The PRRS Compendium (2nd edition). J Zimmerman, K-J Yoon, eds. Des Moines, Iowa: National Pork Board, pp. 17–25.

Halbur PG, Andrews JJ, Huffman EL, Paul PS, Meng X-J, Niyo Y. 1994. Development of a streptavidin-biotin immunoperoxidase procedure for the detection of porcine reproductive and respiratory syndrome virus antigen in porcine lung. J Vet Diagn Invest 6:254–257.

Halbur PG, Bush E. 1997. Update on abortion storms and sow mortality. Swine Health Prod 5(2):73.

Halbur PG, Miller LD, Paul PS, Meng XJ, Huffman EL, Andrews JJ. 1995a. Immunohistochemical identification of porcine reproductive and respiratory syndrome virus (PRRS) antigen in the heart and lymphoid system of three-week-old colostrum-deprived pigs. Vet Pathol 32:200–204.

Halbur PG, Paul PS, Frey ML, Landgraf J, Eernisse K, Meng X-J, Andrews JJ, Lum MA, Rathje JA. 1996a. Comparison of the antigen distribution of two U.S. porcine reproductive and respiratory syndrome virus isolates with that of the Lelystad virus. Vet Pathol 33:159–170.

Halbur PG, Paul PS, Frey ML, Landgraf J, Ernissee K, Meng X-J, Lum MA, Andrews JJ, Rathje JA. 1995b. Comparison of the pathogenicity of two U.S. porcine reproductive and respiratory syndrome virus isolates with that of the Lelystad virus. Vet Pathol 32:648–660.

Halbur PG, Paul PS, Meng XJ, Lum MA, Andrews JJ. Rathje JA. 1996b. Comparative pathogenicity of nine U.S. porcine reproductive and respiratory syndrome virus (PRRSV) isolates in a five-week-old cesarean-derived, colostrum-deprived pig model. J Vet Diagn Invest 8:11–20.

Halbur PG, Rotschild MF, Thacker BJ, Meng XJ, Paul PF, Bruna JD. 1998. Differences in susceptibility of Duroc, Hampshire, and Meishan pigs to infection with a high virulence strain (VR2385) of porcine reproductive and respiratory syndrome virus (PRRSV). J Anim Breed Genet 115:181–189.

Harms P, Sorden S, Halbur P, Bolin S, Lager K, Morozov I, Paul P. 2001. Experimental reproduction of severe disease in CD/CD Pigs concurrently infected with type 2 porcine circovirus and porcine reproductive and respiratory syndrome virus. Vet Pathol 38:528–539.

Harris DL, Bevier GW, Wiseman BS. 1987. Eradication of transmissible gastroenteritis virus without depopulation. Proc Annu Meet Am Assoc Swine Pract, p. 555.

Henry S. 1994. Clinical considerations in "acute" PRRS. Proc Annu Meet Am Assoc Swine Pract, pp. 231–235.

Hermann JR, Muñoz-Zanzi CA, Roof MB, Burkhart K, Zimmerman JJ. 2005. Probability of porcine reproductive and respiratory syndrome (PRRS) virus infection as a function of exposure route and dose. Vet Microbiol (submitted).

Hesse RA, Couture LP, Lau ML, Dimmick SK, Ellsworth SR. 1996. Efficacy of PrimePac PRRS in controlling PRRS reproductive disease: Homologous challenge. Proc Annu Meet Am Assoc Swine Pract, pp. 103–105.

Hill H. 1990. Overview and history of Mystery Swine Disease (Swine infertility/respiratory syndrome). Proceedings of the Mystery Swine Disease Committee Meeting, Livestock Conservation Institute, Denver, Colorado, pp. 29–31.

Hirose O, Kudo H, Yoshizawa S, Hiroike T, Nakane T. 1995. Prevalence of porcine reproductive and respiratory syndrome virus in Chiba prefecture. J Jpn Vet Med Assoc 48:650–653.

Hooper CC, Van Alstine WG, Stevenson GW, Kanitz CL. 1994. Mice and rats (laboratory and feral) are not a reservoir for PRRS virus. J Vet Diagn Invest 6:13–15.

Hopper SA, White ME, Twiddy N. 1992. An outbreak of blue-eared pig disease (porcine reproductive and respiratory syndrome) in four pig herds in Great Britain. Vet Rec 131:140–144.

Horter DC, Pogranichniy RC, Chang CC, Evans RB, Yoon KJ, Zimmerman JJ. 2002. Characterization of the carrier state in porcine reproductive and respiratory syndrome virus infection. Vet Microbiol 86:213–218.

Houben S, van Reeth K, Pensaert MB. 1995. Pattern of infection with the porcine reproductive and respiratory syndrome virus on swine farms in Belgium. Zentralbl Veterinarmed B 42:209–215.

Joo HS, Park BK, Dee SA, Pijoan C. 1997. Indirect fluorescent IgM antibody response of pigs infected with porcine reproductive and respiratory syndrome virus. Vet Microbiol 55:303–307.

Keay S, Moreau IA, Provis P. 2002. A retrospective study of PRRS diagnostic results from routine serologic testing of seven PRRS naïve herds. Proc Annu Meet Am Assoc Swine Vet, pp. 147–148.

Keffaber K, Stevenson G, Van Alstine W, Kanitz C, Harris L, Gorcyca D, Schlesinger K, Schultz R, Chladek D, Morrison R. 1992. SIRS virus infection in nursery/grower pigs. Am Assoc Swine Pract Newsletter 4:38–39.

Keffaber KK. 1989. Reproductive failure of unknown etiology. Am Assoc Swine Pract Newsletter 1:1–10.

Key KF, Guenette DK, Yoon KJ, Halbur PG, Toth TE, Meng XJ. 2003. Development of a heteroduplex mobility assay to identify field isolates of porcine reproductive and respiratory syndrome virus with nucleotide sequences closely related to those of modified live-attenuated vaccines. J Clin Microbiol 41:2433–2439.

Kim HS, Kwang J, Yoon IJ, Joo HS, Frey ML. 1993. Enhanced replication of porcine reproductive and respiratory syndrome (PRRS) virus in a homogeneous subpopulation of MA-104 cell line. Arch Virol 133:477–483.

Kleiboeker SB, Lehman JR, Fangman TJ. 2002. Concurrent use of reverse transcription-polymerase chain reaction testing of oropharyngeal scrapings and paired serological testing for detection of porcine reproductive and respiratory syndrome virus infection in sows. J Swine Health Prod 10(6):251–258.

Kreutz LC, Ackermann MR. 1996. Porcine reproductive and respiratory syndrome virus enters cells through a low pH-dependent endocytic pathway. Virus Res 42:137–147.

Kristensen CS, Bøtner A, Takai H, Nielsen JP, Jorsal SE. 2004. Experimental airborne transmission of PRRS virus. Vet Microbiol 909:197–202.

Labarque G, van Gucht S, Nauwynck H, van Reeth K, Pensaert M. 2003. Apoptosis in the lungs of pigs infected with porcine reproductive and respiratory syndrome virus and associations with the production of apoptogenic cytokines. Vet Res 34:249–260.

Labarque G, van Reeth K, van Gucht S, Nauwynck H, Pensaert M. 2002. Porcine reproductive-respiratory syndrome virus infection predisposes pigs for respiratory signs upon exposure to bacterial lipopolysaccharide. Vet Microbiol 88:1–12.

Labarque GG, Nauwynck HJ, van Reeth K, Pensaert MB. 2000. Effect of cellular changes and onset of humoral immunity on the replication of porcine reproductive and respiratory syndrome virus in the lungs of pigs. J Gen Virol 81:1327–1334.

Lager KM, Halbur PG. 1996. Gross and microscopic lesions in porcine fetuses infected with porcine reproductive and respiratory syndrome virus. J Vet Diagn Invest 8:275–282.

Lager KM, Mengeling WL. 1995. Pathogenesis of in utero infection in porcine fetuses with porcine reproductive and respiratory syndrome virus. Can J Vet Res 59:187–192.

——. 2000. Experimental aerosol transmission of pseudorabies virus and porcine reproductive and respiratory syndrome virus. Proc Annu Meet Am Assoc Swine Pract, pp. 409–410.

Lager KM, Mengeling WL, Brockmeier SL. 1996. Effect of post-coital intrauterine inoculation of porcine reproductive and respiratory syndrome virus on conception in gilts. Vet Rec 138:227–228.

——. 1997a. Homologous challenge of porcine reproductive and respiratory syndrome virus immunity in pregnant swine. Vet Microbiol 58:113–125.

——. 1997b. Duration of homologous porcine reproductive and respiratory syndrome virus immunity in pregnant swine. Vet Microbiol 58:127–133.

——. 1999. Evaluation of protective immunity in gilts inoculated with the NADC-8 isolate of porcine reproductive and respiratory syndrome virus (PRRSV) and challenge-exposed with an antigenically distinct PRRSV isolate. Am J Vet Res 60:1022–1027.

Lager KM, Mengeling WL, Wesley RD. 2003. Strain predominance following exposure of vaccinated and naïve pregnant gilts to multiple strains of porcine reproductive and respiratory syndrome virus. Can J Vet Res 67:121–127.

Lamontagne L, Page C, Larochelle R, Longtin D, Magar R. 2001. Polyclonal activation of B cells occurs in lymphoid organs from porcine reproductive and respiratory syndrome virus (PRRSV)-infected pigs. Vet Immunol Immunopathol 82:165–181.

Le Potier M-F, Blanquefort P, Morvan E, Albina E. 1997. Results of a control programme for the porcine reproductive and respiratory syndrome in the French "Pays de la Loire" region. Vet Microbiol 55:355–360.

Legeay O, Bounaix S, Denis M, Arnauld C, Hutet E, Cariolet R, Albina E, Jestin A. 1997. Development of a RT-PCR test coupled with a microplate colorimetric assay for the detection of a swine arterivirus (PRRSV) in boar semen. J Virol Methods 68:65–80.

Lemke C, Haynes J, Spaete R, Adolphson D, Vorwald A, Lager K, Butler J. 2004. Lymphoid hyperplasia resulting in immune dysregulation is caused by porcine reproductive and respiratory syndrome virus in neonatal pigs. J Immunol 172:1916–1925.

Leyk W. 1991. Observations in three affected herds in North Rhine Westphalia. In The New Pig Disease. Porcine Reproductive and Respiratory Syndrome. A report on the seminar/workshop held in Brussels on 29–30 April and organized by the European Commission (Directorate General for Agriculture), pp. 3–4.

Loemba HD, Mounir S, Mardassi H, Archambault D, Dea S. 1996. Kinetics of humoral immune response to the major structural proteins of the porcine reproductive and respiratory syndrome virus. Arch Virol 141:751–761.

Lopez Fuertes L, Domenech N, Alvarez B, Ezquerra A, Dominguez J, Castro JM, Alonso F. 1999. Analysis of cellular immune response in pigs recovered from porcine reproductive and respiratory syndrome infection. Virus Res 64:33–42.

Loula T. 1991. Mystery pig disease. Agri-practice 12:23–34.

Lu C, Lim K-I, Hahn T-W, Kwon H-M, Han J-H. 1999. Seroprevalence of ELISA antibody to porcine reproductive and respiratory syndrome virus in Korea. Annals of Animal Resources Science 10:127–137.

Lutz W, Wurm R. 1996. [Serological investigations to demonstrate the presence of antibodies to the viruses causing porcine reproductive and respiratory syndrome, Aujeszky's disease, hog cholera, and porcine parvovirus among wild boar (Sus scrofa, L., 1758) in Northrhine-Westfalia.] Zeitschrift fur Jagdwissenschaft 42:123–133.

Maes D. 1997. Descriptive epidemiological aspects of the seroprevalence of five respiratory disease agents in slaughter pigs from fattening herds. Epidémiol Santé Anim 31–32:05.B.19.

Magar R, Larochelle R. 2004. Evaluation of the presence of porcine reproductive and respiratory syndrome virus in pig meat and experimental transmission following oral exposure. Can J Vet Res 68:259–266.

Magar R, Larochelle R, Robinson Y, Dubuc C. 1993. Immunohistochemical detection of porcine reproductive and respiratory syndrome virus using colloidal gold. Can J Vet Res 57:300–304.

Magar R, Robinson Y, Dubuc C, Larochelle R. 1995. Isolation and experimental oral transmission in pigs of a porcine reproductive and respiratory syndrome virus isolate. Adv Exp Med Biol 380:139–144.

Mardassi H, Massie B, Dea S. 1996. Intracellular synthesis, processing, and transport of proteins encoded by ORFs 5 to 7 of porcine reproductive and respiratory syndrome virus. Virology 221:98–112.

Mateusen B, Maes D, Nauwynck H, Balis B, Verdonck M, de Kruif A. 2002. Seroprevalence of porcine reproductive and respiratory syndrome virus (PRRSV) in 20 Belgian farrow-to-finish pig herds. Proc Congr Int Pig Vet Soc 2:240.

Mavromatis I, Kritas SK, Alexopoulos C, Tsinas A, Kyriakis SC. 1999. Field evaluation of a live vaccine against porcine reproductive and respiratory syndrome in fattening pigs. Zentralbl Veterinarmed B 46:603–612.

McCaw MB. 2000. Effect of reducing cross-fostering at birth on piglet mortality and performance during an acute outbreak of porcine reproductive and respiratory syndrome. J Swine Health Prod 8(1):15–21.

——. 2003. McREBEL management. In The PRRS Compendium (2nd edition). J Zimmerman, K-J Yoon, eds. Des Moines, Iowa: National Pork Board, pp. 131–135.

Meier WA, Galeota J, Osorio FA, Husmann RJ, Schnitzlein WM, Zuckermann FA. 2003. Gradual development of the interferon-gamma response of swine to porcine reproductive and respiratory syndrome virus infection or vaccination. Virology 309:18–31.

Melnichouk O, Dewey CE, Friendship RM, Haydon DT. 2005. Seroepidemiological study of porcine reproductive and respiratory syndrome (PRRS) virus infection patterns by age in nursery pigs on seven commercial farms in Ontario, Canada. Prev Vet Med (in press).

Meng XJ. 2000. Heterogeneity of porcine reproductive and respiratory syndrome virus: Implications for current vaccine efficacy and future vaccine development. Vet Microbiol 74:309–329.

Mengeling WL. 1996. An overview on vaccination for porcine reproductive and respiratory syndrome. Proc AD Leman Swine Conf, pp.139–142.

Mengeling WL, Lager KM, Vorwald AC. 1994. Temporal characterization of transplacental infection of porcine fetuses with PRRS virus. Am J Vet Res 55:1391–1398.

——. 1995. Diagnosis of porcine reproductive and respiratory syndrome. J Vet Diagn Invest 7:3–16.

——. 1998. Clinical effects of porcine reproductive and respiratory syndrome virus on pigs during the early postnatal interval. Am J Vet Res 59:52–55.

——. 1999b. Safety and efficacy of vaccination of pregnant gilts against porcine reproductive and respiratory syndrome. Am J Vet Res 60:796–801.

Mengeling WL, Lager KM, Vorwald AD. 1996c. Alveolar macrophages as a diagnostic sample for detecting natural infection of pigs with porcine reproductive and respiratory syndrome virus. J Vet Diagn Invest 8:238–240.

Mengeling WL, Lager KM, Vorwald AC, Clouser DF. 2003a. Comparative safety and efficacy of attenuated single-strain and multi-strain vaccines for porcine reproductive and respiratory syndrome. Vet Microbiol 93:25–38.

Mengeling WL, Lager KM, Vorwald AC, Koehler KJ. 2003b. Strain specificity of the immune response of pigs following vaccination with various strains of porcine reproductive and respiratory syndrome virus. Vet Microbiol 93:13–24.

Mengeling WL, Vorwald AC, Lager KM, Brockmeier SL. 1996a. Comparison among strains of porcine reproductive and respiratory syndrome virus for their ability to cause reproductive failure. Am J Vet Res 57:834–839.

Mengeling WL, Vorwald AC, Lager KM, Clouser DF, Wesley RD. 1999a. Identification and clinical assessment of suspected vaccine-related field strains of porcine reproductive and respiratory syndrome virus. Am J Vet Res 60:334–340.

Meulenberg JJ. 2000. PRRSV, the virus. Vet Res 31:11–21.

Meulenberg JJ, Bos-de Ruijter JN, Wensvoort G, Moormann RJ. 1998. An infectious cDNA clone of porcine reproductive and respiratory syndrome virus. Adv Exp Med Biol 440:199–206.

Meulenberg JJ, Hulst MM, de Meijer EJ, Moonen PL, den Besten A, de Kluyver EP, Wensvoort G, Moormann RJ. 1993. Lelystad virus, the causative agent of porcine epidemic abortion and respiratory syndrome (PEARS), is related to LDV and EAV. Virology 192:62–72.

Molitor TW, Bautista EM, Choi CS. 1997. Immunity to PRRSV: Double-edged sword. Vet Microbiol 55:265–276.

Molitor TW, Xiao J, Choi CS. 1996. PRRS virus infection of macrophages: Regulation by maturation and activation state. Proc Annu Meet Am Assoc Swine Pract, p. 563–569.

Moore C. 1990. Clinical presentation of mystery swine disease in the growing pig. Proceedings of the Mystery Swine Disease Committee Meeting, Livestock Conservation Institute, Denver, Colorado, p. 41–49.

Morrison RB, Collins JE, Harris L, Chladek DW, Gorcyca DE, Joo HS, Christianson W, Benfield DA, Marsh WE, Goyal S, Annelli JF. 1992. Sero-epidemiologic investigation of porcine epidemic abortion and respiratory syndrome (PEARS, PRRS, SIRS). Proc Congr Int Pig Vet Soc 12:114.

Mortensen S, Stryhn H, Sogaard R, Boklund A, Stark KD, Christensen J, Willeberg P. 2002. Risk factors for infection of sow herds with porcine reproductive and respiratory syndrome (PRRS) virus. Prev Vet Med 53:83–101.

Motha J, Stark K, Thompson J. 1997. New Zealand is free from PRRS, TGE, and PRCV. Surveillance 24:10–11.

Mousing J, Permin A, Mortensen S, Bøtner A, Willeberg P. 1997. A case-control questionnaire survey of risk factors for porcine reproductive and respiratory syndrome (PRRS) seropositivity in Danish swine herds. Vet Microbiol 55:323–328.

Murtaugh MP, Elam MR, Kakach LT. 1995. Comparison of the structural protein coding sequences of the VR-2332 and Lelystad virus strains of the PRRS virus. Arch Virol 140:1451–1460.

Nauwynck H, Duan X, Favoreel HW, van Oostveldt P, Pensaert MB. 1999. Entry of porcine reproductive and respiratory syndrome virus into porcine alveolar macrophages via receptor-mediated endocytosis. J Gen Virol 80:297–305.

Nelsen CJ, Murtaugh MP, Faaberg KS. 1999. Porcine reproductive and respiratory syndrome virus comparison: Divergent evolution on two continents. J Virol 73:270–280.

Nelson EA, Christopher-Hennings J, Benfield DA. 1994. Serum immune response to the proteins of porcine reproductive and respiratory syndrome (PRRS) virus. J Vet Diagn Invest 6:410–415.

Nelson EA, Christopher-Hennings J, Drew T, Wensvoort G, Collins JE, Benfield DA. 1993. Differentiation of United States and European isolates of porcine reproductive and respiratory syndrome virus by monoclonal antibodies. J Clin Microbiol 31:3184–3189.

Nielsen HS, Liu G, Nielsen J, Oleksiewicz MB, Bøtner A, Storgaard T, Faaberg KS. 2003. Generation of an infectious clone of VR-2332, a highly virulent North American–type isolate of porcine reproductive and respiratory syndrome virus. J Virol 77:3702–3711.

Nielsen HS, Oleksiewicz MB, Forsberg R, Stadejek T, Bøtner A, Storgaard T. 2001. Reversion of a live porcine reproductive and respiratory syndrome virus vaccine investigated by parallel mutations. J Gen Virol 82:1263–1272.

Nielsen J, Bøtner A. 1997. Hematological and immunological parameters of 4 1/2 month old pigs infected with PRRS virus. Vet Microbiol 55:289–294.

O'Connor M, Fallon M, O'Reilly PJ. 2002. Detection of antibody to porcine reproductive and respiratory syndrome (PRRS) virus: Reduction of cut-off value of an ELISA, with confirmation by immunoperioxidase monolayers assay. Irish Vet J 55:73–75.

Ohlinger VF, Pesch S, Bischoff C. 2000. History, occurrence, dynamics, and current status of PRRS in Europe. Vet Res 31:86–87.

OIE (Office International des Épizooties). 1992. World Animal Health 1991. Volume VII. Number 2. Animal Health Status and Disease Control Methods (Part One: Reports), p. 126.

——. 1996. World Animal Health in 1995. Part 1. Reports on the Animal Health Status and Disease Control Methods and List A Disease Outbreaks—Statistics, p. 211.

——. 1997. World Animal Health in 1996. Part 1. Reports on the Animal Health Status and Disease Control Methods and List A Disease Outbreaks—Statistics, p. 249.

Oleksiewicz MB, Bøtner A, Toft P, Normann P, Storgaard T. 2001. Epitope mapping porcine reproductive and respiratory syndrome virus by phage display: The nsp2 fragment of the replicase polyprotein contains a cluster of B-cell epitopes. J Virol 75:3277–3290.

Opriessnig T, Halbur PG, Yoon KJ, Pogranichniy RM, Harmon KM, Evans R, Key KF, Pallares FJ, Thomas P, Meng XJ. 2002. Comparison of molecular and biological characteristics of a modified live porcine reproductive and respiratory syndrome virus (PRRSV) vaccine (Ingelvac PRRS MLV), the parent strain of the vaccine (ATCC VR2332), ATCC VR2385, and two recent field isolates of PRRSV. J Virol 76:11837–11844.

Oslage U, Dahle J, Muller T, Kramer M, Beier D, Liess B. 1994. [Prevalence of antibodies against hog cholera, Aujeszky's disease, and "porcine reproductive and respiratory syndrome" in feral swine in the federal states Sachsen-Anhalt and Brandenburg.] Dtsch Tierarztl Wochenschr 101:33–38.

Ostrowski M, Galeota JA, Jar AM, Platt KB, Osorio FA, Lopez OJ. 2002. Identification of neutralizing and nonneutralizing epitopes in the porcine reproductive and respiratory syndrome virus GP5 ectodomain. J. Virol 76:4241–4250.

Otake S, Dee SA, Jacobson L, Torremorell M, Pijoan C. 2002d. Evaluation of aerosol transmission of porcine reproductive and respiratory syndrome virus under controlled field conditions. Vet Rec 150:804–808.

Otake S, Dee SA, Moon RD, Rossow KD, Trincado C, Farnham M, and Pijoan C. 2003b. Survival of porcine reproductive and respiratory syndrome virus in houseflies (*Musca domestica* Linnaeus) Can J Vet Res 67:198–203

Otake S, Dee SA, Rossow KD, Deen J, Joo HS, Molitor TW, Pijoan C. 2002a. Transmission of porcine reproductive and respiratory syndrome virus by fomites (boots and coveralls). J Swine Health Prod 10(2):59–65.

Otake S, Dee SA, Rossow KD, Joo HS, Deen J, Molitor TW, Pijoan C. 2002b. Transmission of porcine reproductive and respiratory syndrome virus by needles. Vet Rec 150:114–115.

Otake S, Dee SA, Rossow KD, Moon R, Pijoan C. 2002c. Mechanical transmission of porcine reproductive and respiratory syndrome virus by mosquitoes, *Aedes vexans* (Meigen). Can J Vet Res 66:191–195.

Otake S, Dee SA, Rossow KD, Moon RD, Trincado C, Pijoan C. 2003a. Transmission of porcine reproductive and respiratory syndrome virus by houseflies (*Musca domestica*). Vet Rec 152:73–76.

Park BK, Yoon IJ, Joo HS. 1996. Pathogenesis of plaque variants of porcine reproductive and respiratory syndrome virus in pregnant sows. Am J Vet Res 57:320–323.

Pejsak Z, Markowska-Daniel I. 1996. Viruses as a reason for reproductive failure in pig herds in Poland. Reprod Dom Anim 31:445–447.

Perfumo CJ, Sanguinetti HR. 2003. Argentina: Serological studies on PRRS virus. In The PRRS Compendium (2nd edition). J Zimmerman, K-J Yoon, eds. Des Moines, Iowa: National Pork Board, pp. 209–211.

Pirtle EC, Beran GW. 1996. Stability of porcine reproductive and respiratory syndrome virus in the presence of fomites commonly found on farms. J Am Vet Med Assoc 208:390–392.

Pirzadeh B, Dea S. 1997. Monoclonal antibodies to the ORF5 product of porcine reproductive and respiratory syndrome virus define linear neutralizing determinants. J Gen Virol 78:1867–1873.

Plagemann PG. 2004. GP5 ectodomain epitope of porcine reproductive and respiratory syndrome virus, strain Lelystad virus. Virus Res 102:225–230.

Plagemann PG, Moennig V. 1992. Lactate dehydrogenase-elevating virus, equine arteritis virus, and simian hemorrhagic fever virus: A new group of positive-strand RNA viruses. Adv Virus Res 41:99–192.

Plagemann PG, Rowland RR, Faaberg KS. 2002. The primary neutralization epitope of porcine respiratory and reproductive syndrome virus strain VR-2332 is located in the middle of the GP5 ectodomain. Arch Virol 147:2327–2347.

Plana Duran J, Bastons A, Urniza M, Vayreda M. 1995. Vaccine against porcine reproductive and respiratory syndrome (PRRS). Proceedings of the 2nd International Symposium on Porcine Reproductive and Respiratory syndrome, Copenhagen, Denmark, p. 37.

Plana Duran J, Vayreda M, Vilarrasa J, Bastons M, Porquet L, Urniza A. 1992a. PEARS ("Mystery Swine Disease")—Summary of the work conducted by our group. American Association of Swine Practitioners Newsletter 4:16–18.

Plana Duran J, Vayreda M, Vilarrasa J, Bastons M, Rosell R, Martinez M, San Gabriel A, Pujols J, Badiola JL, Ramos JA, Domingo Mariano. 1992b. Porcine epidemic abortion and respiratory syndrome (mystery swine disease). Isolation in Spain of the causative agent and experimental reproduction of the disease. Vet Microbiol 33:203-211.

Pol JM, van-Dijk JE, Wensvoort G, Terpstra C. 1991. Pathological, ultrastructural, and immunohistochemical changes caused by Lelystad virus in experimentally induced infections of mystery swine disease (synonym: porcine epidemic abortion and respiratory syndrome (PEARS)). Vet Q 13:137–143.

Pol JM, van Leengoed LA, Stockhofe N, Kok G, Wensvoort G. 1997. Dual infections of PRRSV/influenza or PRRSV/Actinobacillus pleuropneumoniae in the respiratory tract. Vet Microbiol 55:259–264.

Prieto C, Sanchez R, Martin-Rillo S, Suárez P, Simarro I, Solana A, Castro JM. 1996a. Exposure of gilts in early gestation to porcine reproductive and respiratory syndrome virus. Vet Rec 138:536–539.

Prieto C, Suárez P, Martin-Rillo S, Simarro I, Solana A, Castro JM. 1996b. Effect of porcine reproductive and respiratory syndrome virus (PRRSV) on development of porcine fertilized ova in vitro. Theriogenology 46:687–693.

Prieto C, Suárez P, Sanchez R, Solana A, Simarro I, Martin-Rillo S, Castro JR. 1994. Semen changes in boars after experimental infection with porcine epidemic abortion and respiratory syndrome (PEARS) virus. Proc 13th Congr Int Pig Vet Soc, p. 98.

Prieto C, Suárez P, Simarro I, García C, Fernández A, Castro JM. 1997b. Transplacental infection following exposure of gilts to porcine reproductive and respiratory syndrome virus at the onset of gestation. Vet Microbiol 57:301–311.

Prieto C, Suárez P, Simarro I, Garcia C, Martin-Rillo S, Castro JM. 1997a. Insemination of susceptible and preimmunized gilts with boar semen containing porcine reproductive and respiratory syndrome virus. Theriogenology 47:647–654.

Pringproa K, Panyathong R, Chungpivat S, Kalpravidh W, Kesdangsakonwut S, Thanawongnuwech R. 2004. Study on potential vectors of PRRSV in mosquitoes captured from a PRRSV-positive pig farm in Thailand. Proc Congr Int Pig Vet Soc 1:70.

Rajic A, Dewey CE, Deckert AE, Friendship RM, Martin SW, Yoo D. 2001. Production of PRRSV-negative pigs commingled from multiple, vaccinated, serologically stable, PRRSV-positive breeding herds. J Swine Health Prod 9(4):179–184.

Reotutar R. 1989. Swine reproductive failure syndrome mystifies scientists. J Am Vet Med Assoc 195:425–428.

Roberts J. 2001. Applying PRRSV sequencing to field cases. Proc Allen D Leman Swine Conf 28:75–78.

——. 2003a. Serological monitoring in infected sow herds. In The PRRS Compendium (2nd edition). J Zimmerman, K-J Yoon, eds. Des Moines, Iowa: National Pork Board, pp. 75–86.

——. 2003b. Monitoring infected sow herds using genomic sequencing. In The PRRS Compendium (2nd edition). J Zimmerman, K-J Yoon, eds. Des Moines, Iowa: National Pork Board, pp. 103–116.

Ropp SL, Wees CE, Fang Y, Nelson EA, Rossow KD, Bien M, Arndt B, Preszler S, Steen P, Christopher-Hennings J, Collins JE, Benfield DA, Faaberg KS. 2004. Characterization of emerging European-like porcine reproductive and respiratory syndrome virus isolates in the United States. J Virol 78:3684–3703.

Rossow KD. 1998. Porcine reproductive and respiratory syndrome. Vet Pathol 35:1–20.

Rossow KD, Bautista EM, Goyal SM, Molitor TW, Murtaugh MP, Morrison RB, Benfield DA, Collins JE. 1994a. Experimental porcine reproductive and respiratory syndrome virus infection in one-, four-, and 10-week-old pigs. J Vet Diagn Invest 6:3–12.

Rossow KD, Benfield DA, Goyal SM, Nelson EA, Christopher-Hennings J, Collins JE. 1996a. Chronological immunohistochemical detection and localization of porcine reproductive and respiratory syndrome virus infection in gnotobiotic pigs. Vet Pathol 33:551–556.

Rossow KD, Collins JE, Goyal SM, Nelson EA, Christopher-Hennings J, Benfield DA. 1995. Pathogenesis of porcine reproductive and respiratory syndrome virus infection in gnotobiotic pigs. Vet Pathol 32:361–373.

Rossow KD, Laube KL, Goyal SM, Collins JE. 1996b. Fetal microscopic lesions in porcine reproductive and respiratory syndrome virus-induced abortion. Vet Pathol 33:95–99.

Rossow KD, Morrison RB, Goyal SM, Singh GS, Collins JE. 1994b. Lymph node lesions in neonatal pigs congenitally exposed to porcine reproductive and respiratory syndrome virus. J Vet Diagn Invest 6:368–371.

Rossow KD, Shivers JL, Yeske PE, Polson DD, Rowland RR, Lawson SR, Murtaugh MP, Nelson EA, Collins JE. 1999. Porcine reproductive and respiratory syndrome virus infection in neonatal pigs characterised by marked neurovirulece. Vet Rec 144(16):444–448.

Rowland R, Lawson S, Rossow K, Benfield D. 2003. Lymphoid tissue tropism of porcine reproductive and respiratory syndrome virus replication during persistent infection of pigs originally exposed to virus in utero. Vet Microbiol 96:219–235.

Rowland RR, Steffen M, Ackerman T, Benfield DA. 1999. The evolution of porcine reproductive and respiratory syndrome virus: Quasispecies and emergence of a virus subpopulation during infection of pigs with VR-2332. Virology 259:262–266.

Rowland RR, Yoo D. 2003. Nucleolar-cytoplasmic shuttling of PRRSV nucleocapsid protein: A simple case of molecular mimicry or the complex regulation by nuclear import, nucleolar localization and nuclear export signal sequences. Virus Res 95:23–33.

Saliki, JT, Rodgers, SJ, Eskew, G. 1998. Serosurvey of selected viral and bacterial diseases in wild swine from Oklahoma. J Wildl Dis 34:834–838.

Samsom JN, Bruin TG, Voermans JJ, Meulenberg JJ, Pol JM, Bianchi AT. 2000. Changes of leukocyte phenotype and function in the broncho-alveolar lavage fluid of pigs infected with porcine reproductive and respiratory syndrome virus: A role for CD8+ cells. J Gen Virol 81:497–505.

Sanford E. 1992. Porcine epidemic abortion and respiratory syndrome (PEARS): Establishment and spread between 1987 and 1992 in Ontario, Canada. Proc 12th Congr Int Pig Vet Soc, p. 117.

Schurrer JA, Dee SA, Moon RD, Rossow KD, Mahlum C, Mondaca E, Otake S, Fano E, Collins JE, Pijoan C. 2004. Spatial dispersal of porcine reproductive and respiratory syndrome virus-contaminated flies after contact with experimentally infected pigs. Am J Vet Res 65:1284–1292.

Segalés J, Domingo M, Solano G, Pijoan C. 1999. Porcine reproductive and respiratory syndrome virus and Haemophilus parasuis antigen distribution in dually infected pigs. Vet Microbiol 64:287–297.

Shibata I, Yazawa S, Ono M, Okuda Y. 2003. Experimental dual infection of specific pathogen-free pigs with porcine respiratory and reproductive syndrome virus and pseudorabies virus. J Vet Med B Infect Dis Vet Public Health 50:14–19.

Shin J, Molitor T. 2002. Localization of porcine reproductive and respiratory syndrome virus infection in boars by in situ riboprobe hybridization. J Vet Sci 3:87–95.

Shin J-H, Kang Y-B, Kim Y-J, Yeom S-H, Kweon C-H, Lee W-Y, Jean Y-H, Hwang E-K, Rhee J-C, An S-H, Cho I-S, Oh J-S, Joo H-S, Choi C-S, Molitor TW. 1993. Sero-epidemiological studies on porcine reproductive and respiratory syndrome in Korea. I. Detection of indirect fluorescent antibodies. RDA J Agri Sci 35:572–576.

Shirai J, Kanno T, Tsuchiya Y, Mitsubayashi S, Seki R. 2000. Effects of chlorine, iodine, and quaternary ammonium compound disinfectants on several exotic disease viruses. J Vet Med Sci 62:85–92.

Sipos W, Indik S, Irgang P, Klein D, Schuh M, Schmoll F. 2002. Transmission of EU-ML-PRRSV (PORCILIS PRRS, INTERVET) from vaccinated to non-vaccinated gilts. Proc Congr Int Pig Vet Soc 2:418.

Sirinarumitr T, Zhang Y, Kluge J, Halbur P, Paul P. 1998. A pneumovirulent United States isolate of porcine reproductive and respiratory syndrome virus induces apoptosis in bystander cells both in vitro and in vivo. J of Gen Virol 79:2989–2995.

Snijder EJ, Meulenberg JM. 2001. Arteriviruses. In Fields Virology (4th edition). DM Knipe, PM Howley, DE Griffin, RA Lamb, MA Martin, B Roizman, SE Straus, eds. Philadelphia: Lippincott Williams and Wilkins, pp. 1205–1220.

Stevenson G. 2003. Pathology. In The PRRS Compendium (2nd edition). J Zimmerman, K-J Yoon, eds. Des Moines, Iowa: National Pork Board, pp. 185–191.

Stevenson GW, Van Alstine WG, Kanitz CL, Keffaber KK. 1993. Endemic porcine reproductive and respiratory syndrome virus infection of nursery pigs in two swine herds without current reproductive failure. J Vet Diagn Invest 5:432–434.

Stockhofe-Zurwieden N, Navarro Camarro JA, Grosse-Beilage E, Chavez J, Pohlenz J. 1993. Uterine and placental alterations in pregnant sows associated with the porcine epidemic abortion and respiratory syndrome (PEARS). Zentralbl Veterinarmed B 40:261–271.

Suárez P. 2000. Ultrastructural pathogenesis of the PRRS virus. Virus Res 31:47–55.

Suárez P, Zardoya R, Martin MJ, Prieto C, Dopazo J, Solana A, Castro JM. 1996. Phylogenetic relationships of European strains of porcine reproductive and respiratory syndrome virus (PRRSV) inferred from DNA sequences of putative ORF-5 and ORF-7 genes. Virus Res 42:159–165.

Sur J, Doster A, Osorio F. 1998. Apoptosis induced in vivo during acute infection by porcine reproductive and respiratory syndrome virus. Vet Pathol 35:506–514.

Sur J-H, Cooper VL, Galeota JA, Hesse RA, Doster AR, Osorio FA. 1996. In vivo detection of porcine reproductive and respiratory syndrome virus RNA by in situ hybridization at different times postinfection. J Clin Microbiol 34:2280–2286.

Sur J-H, Doster AB, Christian JS, Galeota JA, Wills RW, Zimmerman JJ, Osorio FA. 1997. Porcine reproductive and respiratory syndrome virus replicates in testicular germ cells, alters spermatogenesis, and induces germ cell death by apoptosis. J Virol 71:9170–9179.

Suradhat S, Thanawongnuwech R. 2003. Upregulation of interleukin-10 gene expression in the leukocytes of pigs infected with porcine reproductive and respiratory syndrome virus. J Gen Virol 84:2755–2760.

Swenson SL, Hill HT, Zimmerman JJ, Evans LE, Landgraf JG, Wills RW, Sanderson TP, McGinley JM, Brevik AJ, Ciszewski DK, Frey ML. 1994a. Excretion of porcine reproductive and respiratory syndrome virus in semen after experimentally induced infection in boars. J Am Vet Med Assoc 204:1943–1948.

Swenson SL, Hill HT, Zimmerman JJ, Evans LE, Wills RW, Yoon KJ, Schwartz KJ, Althouse GC, McGinley MJ, Brevik AK. 1994b. Artificial insemination of gilts with porcine reproductive and respiratory syndrome (PRRS) virus-contaminated semen. Swine Health Prod 2(6):19–23.

Swenson SL, Zimmerman J. 1993. Porcine reproductive and respiratory syndrome virus in experimentally infected boars: Isolation from semen. Proc Annu Meet Am Assoc Swine Pract, pp. 719–720.

Terpstra C, Wensvoort G, Pol JMA. 1991a. Experimental reproduction of porcine epidemic abortion and respiratory syndrome (mystery swine disease) by infection with Lelystad virus: Koch's postulates fulfilled. Vet Q 13:131–136.

Terpstra C, Wensvoort G, Ter Laak EA. 1991b. The "new" pig disease: laboratory investigations. In: The new pig disease. Porcine reproductive and respiratory syndrome. A report on the seminar/workshop held in Brussels on 29–30 April 1991 and organized by the European Commission Directorate General for Agriculture, pp. 36–45.

Thacker E, Halbur P, Ross R, Thanawognuwech R, Thacker B. 1999. Mycoplasma hyopneumoniae potentiation of porcine reproductive and respiratory syndrome virus-induced pneumonia. J Clin Microbiol 37:620–627.

Thacker E, Thacker B, Wilson W, Ackerman M. 2003. Control with inactivated virus PRRS vaccine. In The PRRS Compendium

(2nd edition). J Zimmerman, K-J Yoon, eds. Des Moines, Iowa: National Pork Board, pp. 151–155.

Thacker EL, Halbur PG, Paul PS, Thacker BJ. 1998. Detection of intracellular porcine reproductive and respiratory syndrome virus nucleocapsid protein in porcine macrophages by flow cytometry. J Vet Diagn Invest 10:308–311.

Thanawongnuwech R, Brown G, Halbur P, Roth J, Royer R, Thacker B. 2000a. Pathogenesis of porcine reproductive and respiratory syndrome virus-induced increase in susceptibility to *Streptococcus suis* infection. Vet Pathol 37:143–152.

Thanawongnuwech R, Damrongwatanapokin S, Horcharoen A. 2003. PRRS in the Republic of Korea. In The PRRS Compendium (2nd edition). J Zimmerman, K-J Yoon, eds. Des Moines, Iowa: National Pork Board, pp. 269–273.

Thanawongnuwech R, Halbur P, Ackermann M, Thacker E, Royer R. 1998a. Effects of low (modified-live virus vaccine) and high (VR2385)-virulence strains of porcine reproductive and respiratory syndrome virus on pulmonary clearance of copper particles in pigs. Vet Pathol 35:398–406.

Thanawongnuwech R, Halbur P, Thacker E. 2000b. The role of pulmonary intravascular macrophages in porcine reproductive and respiratory syndrome virus infection. Anim Health Res Rev 1:95–102.

Thanawongnuwech R, Halbur PG, Andrews JJ. 1997a. Immunohistochemical detection of porcine reproductive and respiratory syndrome virus antigen in neurovascular lesions. J Vet Diagn Invest 9:334–337.

Thanawongnuwech R, Rungsipipat A, Disatian S, Saiyasombat R, Napakanaporn S, Halbur P. 2003. Immunohistochemical staining of IFN-γ positive cells in porcine reproductive and respiratory syndrome virus-infected lungs. Vet Immunol Immunopathol 91:73–77.

Thanawongnuwech R, Thacker E, Halbur P. 1997b. Effect of porcine reproductive and respiratory syndrome virus (PRRSV) (isolate ATCC VR-2385) infection on bactericidal activity of porcine pulmonary intravascular macrophages (PIMs): In vitro comparisons with pulmonary alveolar macrophages (PAMs). Vet Immunol Immunopath 59:323–335.

——. 1998b. Influence of pig age on virus titer and bactericidal activity of porcine reproductive and respiratory syndrome virus (PRRSV)-infected pulmonary intravascular macrophages (PIMs). Vet Microbiol 63:177–187.

Tong G, Qiu H. 2003. PRRS in China. In The PRRS Compendium (2nd edition). J Zimmerman, K-J Yoon, eds. Des Moines, Iowa: National Pork Board, pp. 223–229.

Torremorell M, Conroy P. 2003. Case study: Application of sequencing to investigate an infection in a boar stud and the herds that received semen from it. Proc AD Leman Swine Conf, pp. 44–45.

Torremorell M, Geiger JO, Thompson B, Christianson WT. 2004. Evaluation of PRRSV outbreaks in negative herds. Proc Congr Int Pig Vet Soc 1:103.

Torremorell M, Henry S, Christianson WT. 2003. Eradication using herd closure. In The PRRS Compendium (2nd edition). J Zimmerman, K-J Yoon, eds. Des Moines, Iowa: National Pork Board, pp. 157–161.

Torremorell M, Moore C, Christianson WT. 2002b. Establishment of a herd negative for porcine reproductive and respiratory syndrome (PRRSV) from PRRSV-positive sources. J Swine Health Prod 10(4):153–160.

Torremorell M, Pijoan C, Janni K, Walker J, Joo HS. 1997. Airborne transmission of *Actinobacillus pleuropneumoniae* and porcine reproductive and respiratory syndrome virus in nursery pigs. Am J Vet Res 58:828–832.

Torremorell M, Polson D, Henry SC, Morrison RB. 2002a. Specificity of the PRRSV IDEXX ELISA test in negative farms. Proc Intl Pig Vet Congr 1:209.

Torrison J, Vannier P, Albina E, Madec F, Morrison R. 1994. Incidence and clinical effect of PRRS virus in gilts on commercial swine farms. Proc 13th Congr Int Pig Vet Soc, p. 511.

Trincado C, Dee S, Jacobson L, Otake S, Rossow K, Pijoan C. 2004a. Attempts to transmit porcine reproductive and respiratory syndrome virus by aerosols under controlled field conditions. Vet Rec 154:294–297.

Trincado C, Dee S, Rossow K, Halvorson D, Pijoan C. 2004b. Evaluation of the role of mallard ducks as vectors of porcine reproductive and respiratory syndrome virus. Vet Rec 154:233–237.

Truong HM, Lu Z, Kutish GF, Galeota J, Osorio FA, Pattnaik AK. 2004. A highly pathogenic porcine reproductive and respiratory syndrome virus generated from an infectious cDNA clone retains the in vivo virulence and transmissibility properties of the parental virus. Virology 325:308–319.

Umthun AR, Mengeling WL. 1999. Restriction fragment length polymorphism analysis of strains of porcine reproductive and respiratory syndrome virus by use of a nested set reverse transcription polymerase reaction. Am J Vet Res 60:802–806.

USDA (United States Department of Agriculture). 1997. Prevalence of PRRS virus in the United States. USDA:APHIS:VS NAHMS Info Sheet N225.197.

Valíek L, Pšikal I, Šmid B, Rodak L, Kubalikova R, Kosinova E. 1997. Isolation and identification of porcine reproductive and respiratory syndrome virus in cell cultures. Vet Med (Praha) 42:281–287.

Van Alstine WG, Kanitz CL, Stevenson GW. 1993. Time and temperature survivability of PRRS virus in serum and tissues. J Vet Diagn Invest 5:621–622.

Van Alstine WG, Popielarczyk M, Albergts SR. 2002. Effect of formalin fixation on the immunohistochemical detection of PRRS virus antigen in experimentally and naturally infected pigs. J Vet Diagn Invest 14:504–507.

van der Linden I, Voermans J, van der Linde-Bril E, Bianchi A, Steverink P. 2003a. Virological kinetics and immunological responses to a porcine reproductive and respiratory syndrome virus infection of pigs at different ages. Vaccine 21:1952–1957.

van der Linden IFA, van der Linde-Bril EM, Voermans JJM, van Rijn PA, Pol JMA, Martin R, Steverink PJGM. 2003b. Oral transmission of porcine reproductive and respiratory syndrome virus by muscle of experimentally infected pigs. Vet Microbiol 97:45–54.

van Gucht S, van Reeth K, Pensaert M. 2003. Interaction between porcine reproductive-respiratory syndrome virus and bacterial endotoxin in the lungs of pigs: Potentiation of cytokine production and respiratory disease. J Clin Microbiol 41:960–966.

van Nieuwstadt AP, Meulenberg JJ, van Essen-Zanbergen A, Petersen-den Besten A, Bende RJ, Moormann RJ, Wensvoort G. 1996. Proteins encoded by open reading frames 3 and 4 of the genome of Lelystad virus (Arteriviridae) are structural proteins of the virion. J Virol 70:4767–4772.

van Reeth K, Labarque G, Nauwynck H, Pensaert M. 1999. Differential production of proinflammatory cytokines in the pig lung during different respiratory virus infections: Correlations with pathogenicity. Res Vet Sci 67:47–52.

van Reeth K, Nauwynck H, Pensaert M. 1996. Dual infections of feeder pigs with porcine reproductive and respiratory syndrome virus followed by porcine respiratory coronavirus or swine influenza virus: A clinical and virological study. Vet Microbiol 48:325–335.

——. 2001. Clinical effects of experimental dual infections with porcine reproductive and respiratory syndrome virus followed by swine influenza virus in conventional and colostrum-deprived pigs. J Vet Med 48:283–292.

van Vugt JJ, Storgaard T, Oleksiewicz MB, Bøtner A. 2001. High frequency RNA recombination in porcine reproductive and respiratory syndrome virus occurs preferentially between parental sequences with high similarity. J Gen Virol 82:2615–2620.

van Woensel PA, Liefkens K, Demaret S. 1998. Effect on viremia of an American and a European serotype PRRSV vaccine after challenge with European wild-type strain of the virus. Vet Rec 142:510–512.

Vanderheijden N, Delputte PL, Favoreel HW, Vandekerckhove J, van Damme J, van Woensel PA, Nauwynck HJ. 2003. Involvement of sialoadhesin in entry of porcine reproductive and respiratory syndrome virus into porcine alveolar macrophages. J Virol 77:8207–8215.

Verheije MH, Kroese MV, van der Linden IF, de Boer-Luijtze EA, van Rijn PA, Pol JM, Meulenberg JJ, Steverink PJ. 2003. Safety and protective efficacy of porcine reproductive and respiratory syndrome recombinant virus vaccines in young pigs. Vaccine 21:2556–2563.

Verheije MH, Olsthoorn RC, Kroese MV, Rottier PJ, Meulenberg JJ. 2002a. Kissing interaction between 3' noncoding and coding sequences is essential for porcine arterivirus RNA replication. J Virol 76:1521–1526.

Verheije MH, Welting TJ, Jansen HT, Rottier PJ, Meulenberg J.J. 2002b. Chimeric arteriviruses generated by swapping of the M protein ectodomain rule out a role of this domain in viral targeting. Virology 303:364–373.

Vezina SA, Loemba H, Fournier M, Dea S, Archambault D. 1996. Antibody production and blastogenic response in pigs experimentally infected with porcine reproductive and respiratory syndrome virus. Can J Vet Res 60:94–99.

Wagstrom EA, Chang CC, Yoon KJ, Zimmerman JJ. 2001. Shedding of porcine reproductive and respiratory syndrome virus in mammary gland secretions of sows. Am J Vet Res 62:1876–1880.

Wasilk A, Callahan JD, Christopher-Hennings J, Gay TA, Fang Y, Dammen M, Reos ME, Torremorell M, Polson D, Mellencamp M, Nelson E, Nelson WM. 2004. Detection of U.S. and Lelystad/European-like porcine reproductive and respiratory syndrome virus and relative quantitation in boar semen and serum by real-time PCR. J Clin Microbiol 42:4453–4461.

Weigel RM, Firkins LD, Scherba G. 2000. Prevalence and risk factors for infection with porcine reproductive and respiratory syndrome virus (PRRSV) in swine herds in Illinois (USA). Vet Res 31:87–88.

Wensvoort G, de Kluyver EP, Luijtze EA, den Besten A, Harris L, Collins JE, Christianson WT, Chladek D. 1992. Antigenic comparison of Lelystad virus and swine infertility and respiratory syndrome (SIRS) virus. J Vet Diagn Invest 4:134–138.

Wensvoort G, Terpstra C, Pol JMA, ter Laak EA, Bloemraad M, de Kluyver EP, Kragten C, van Buiten L, den Besten A, Wagenaar F, Broekhuijsen JM, Moonen PLJM, Zetstra T, de Boer EA, Tibben HJ, de Jong MF, van't Veld P, Groenland GJR, van Gennep JA, Voets MTh, Verheijden JHM, Braamskamp J. 1991. Mystery swine disease in the Netherlands: The isolation of Lelystad virus. Vet Q 13:121–130.

Wesley RD, Mengeling WL, Lager KM, Clouser DF, Landgraf JG, Frey ML. 1998. Differentiation of porcine reproductive and respiratory syndrome virus vaccine strain from North American field strains. J Diagn Invest 10:140–144.

White MEC. 1992a. The clinical signs and symptoms of blue-eared pig disease (PRRS). Pig Vet J 28:62–68.

——. 1992b. PRRS: Clinical update. Pig Vet J 29:179–187.

Wills R, Doster A, Galeota J, Sur J, Osorio F. 2003. Duration of infection and proportion of pigs persistently infected with porcine reproductive and respiratory syndrome virus. J Clin Microbiol 41:58–62.

Wills R, Gray J, Fedorka-Cray P, Yoon K, Ladely S, Zimmerman J. 2000. Synergism between porcine reproductive and respiratory syndrome virus (PRRSV) and Salmonella choleraesuis in swine. Vet Microbiol 71:177–192.

Wills RW, Doster AR, Galeota JA, Sur J-H, Osorio FA. 2003. Duration of infection and proportion of pigs persistently infected with porcine reproductive and respiratory syndrome virus. J Clin Microbiol 41:58–62.

Wills RW, Osorio FA, Doster AR. 2000. Susceptibility of selected non-swine species to infection with PRRS virus. Proc Annu Meet Am Assoc Swine Pract, pp. 411–413.

Wills RW, Zimmerman JJ, Swenson SL, Yoon K-J, Hill HT, Bundy DS, McGinley MJ. 1997b. Transmission of porcine reproductive and respiratory syndrome virus by direct close or indirect contact. Swine Health and Production 5:213–218.

Wills RW, Zimmerman JJ, Yoon K-J, Swenson SL, Hoffman LJ, McGinley MJ, Hill HT, Platt KB. 1997a. Porcine reproductive and respiratory syndrome virus: Routes of excretion. Vet Microbiol 57:69–81.

Wills RW, Zimmerman JJ, Yoon KJ, Swenson SL, McGinley MJ, Hill HT, Platt KB, Christopher-Hennings J, Nelson EA. 1997c. Porcine reproductive and respiratory syndrome virus: A persistent infection. Vet Microbiol 55:231–240.

Wissink EH, van Wijk HA, Kroese MV, Weiland E, Meulenberg JJ, Rottier PJ, van Rijn PA. 2003b. The major envelope protein, GP5, of a European porcine reproductive and respiratory syndrome virus contains a neutralization epitope in its N-terminal ectodomain. J Gen Virol 84:1535–1543.

Wissink EHJ, van Wijk HAR, Pol JMA, Godeke GJ, van Rijn PA, Rottier PJM, Meulenberg JJM. 2003a. Identification of porcine alveolar macrophage glycoproteins involved in infection of porcine respiratory and reproductive syndrome virus. Arch Viol 148:177–187.

Wootton S, Yoo D, Rogan D. 2000. Full-length sequence of a Canadian porcine reproductive and respiratory syndrome virus (PRRSV) isolate. Arch Virol 145:2297–2323.

Wu WH, Fang Y, Farwell R, Steffen-Bien M, Rowland RR, Christopher-Hennings J, Nelson EA. 2001. A 10-kDa structural protein of porcine reproductive and respiratory syndrome virus encoded by ORF2b. Virology 287:183–191.

Xiao Z, Batista L, Dee S, Halbur P, Murtaugh MP. 2004. The level of virus-specific T-cell and macrophage recruitment in porcine reproductive and respiratory syndrome virus infection in pigs is independent of the virus load. J Virol 78:5923–5933.

Yaeger MJ, Prieve T, Collins J, Christopher-Hennings J, Nelson E, Benfield D. 1993. Evidence for the transmission of porcine reproductive and respiratory syndrome (PRRS) virus in boar semen. Swine Health Prod 1:7–9.

Yang KS, Park PK, Kim JH. 2003. PRRS in the Republic of Korea. In The PRRS Compendium (2nd edition). J Zimmerman, K-J Yoon, eds. Des Moines, Iowa: National Pork Board, pp. 253–255.

Yoo D, Wootton SK, Li G, Song C, Rowland RR. 2003. Colocalization and interaction of the porcine arterivirus nucleocapsid protein with the small nucleolar RNA-associated protein fibrillarin. J Virol 77:12173–12183.

Yoon KJ, Christopher-Hennings J, Nelson EA. 2003. Diagnosis. In The PRRS Compendium (2nd edition). J Zimmerman, K-J Yoon, eds. Des Moines, Iowa: National Pork Board, pp. 59–74.

Yoon KJ, Wu LL, Zimmerman JJ, Platt KB, 1996. Antibody-dependent enhancement (ADE) of porcine reproductive and respiratory syndrome virus (PRRSV) infection in pigs. Virol Immunol 9:51–63.

Yoon KJ, Zimmerman JJ, Swenson SJ, Landgraf J, Frey ML, Hill HT, Platt KB. 1995a. Failure to consider the antigenic diversity of porcine reproductive and respiratory syndrome (PRRS) virus isolates may lead to misdiagnosis. J Vet Diagn Invest 7:386–387.

Yoon KJ, Zimmerman JJ, Swenson SL, McGinley MJ, Eernisse KA, Brevik A, Rhinehart LL, Frey ML, Hill HT, Platt KB. 1995b. Characterization of the humoral immune response to the porcine reproductive and respiratory syndrome (PRRS) virus infection. J Vet Diagn Invest 7:305–312.

Yoon K-J, Zimmerman JJ, Chang C-C, Cancel-Tirado S, Harmon KM, McGinley MJ. 1999. Effect of challenge dose and route on porcine reproductive and respiratory syndrome virus (PRRSV) infection in young swine. Vet Res 30:629–638.

Yuan S, Mickelson D, Murtaugh MP, Faaberg KS. 2001. Complete genome comparison of porcine reproductive and respiratory syndrome virus parental and attenuated strains. Virus Res 79:189–200.

Yuan S, Nelsen CJ, Murtaugh MP, Schmitt BJ, Faaberg KS. 1999. Recombination between North American strains of porcine reproductive and respiratory syndrome virus. Virus Res 61:87–98.

Zejda JE, Barber E, Dosman JA, Olenchock S A, McDuffie HH, Rhodes C, Hurst T. 1994. Respiratory health status in swine producers relates to endotoxin exposure in the presence of low dust levels. J Occup Med 36:49–56.

Zeman DH. 1996. Concurrent respiratory infections in 221 cases of PRRS virus pneumonia: 1992–1994. J Swine Health and Prod 4:143–145.

Zhou EM, Zimmerman JJ, Zhou KX, Jiang Z, Platt KB. 2002. IgM-capture ELISA as a serodiagnostic test for detection of primary infection of PRRSV in pigs. Proc Annu Meet Am Assoc Swine Vet pp.295–298.

Zhuang Q, Barfod K, Wachmann H, Mortensen S, Willeberg P. 2002. Serological surveillance for PRRS in Danish genetic pig herds and risk factors for PRRS infection. Proc Congr Int Pig Vet Soc 2:231.

Zimmerman J, Sanderson T, Eernisse KA, Hill HT, Frey ML. 1992. Transmission of SIRS virus from convalescent animals to commingled penmates under experimental conditions. Am Assoc Swine Practitioners Newsletter 4(4):25.

Zimmerman JJ, Yoon K-J, Pirtle EC, Wills RW, Sanderson TJ, McGinley MJ. 1997. Studies of porcine reproductive and respiratory syndrome (PRRS) virus infection in avian species. Vet Microbiol 55:329–336.

25 Aujeszky's Disease (Pseudorabies)

Z. K. Pejsak and Marian J. Truszczyński

Pseudorabies (PR) was first described in 1813 in cattle suffering with extreme pruritus. Based on the clinical signs, the disease was called "mad itch" (Baskerville et al. 1973). The term "pseudorabies" was first used in Switzerland in 1849 because the clinical signs in cattle were considered similar to those of rabies. Aladar Aujeszky, the Hungarian for whom the disease is named, determined that the etiologic agent was filterable, i.e., not bacterial, and also conducted research on the disease in the dog and cat. The agent was first recovered from swine in 1909 by Weiss and from sheep in 1910 by Schmiedhoffer (Wittmann and Rziha 1989). Schmiedhoffer also confirmed Aujeszky's findings that the agent was filterable, i.e., that it was viral. In 1934, Sabin and Wright identified the virus as a herpesvirus, later called swine herpes virus 1 (SHV-1) or pseudorabies virus (PRV).

The primary host of PRV is the pig. The pig is the only species able to survive a productive infection and, therefore, serves as the reservoir host (Kretzschmar 1970). Prior to the 1960s, PR was of some importance in pig production, but only in Europe (Wittmann and Jakubik 1979). Beginning in the 1970s, PR achieved global importance (Kluge et al. 1999). The transformation of PR from a sporadic, fatal disease of cattle to a swine disease of major economic significance on a worldwide basis was driven by changes in swine production. Specifically, over a period of 50 years, swine production became concentrated into large farms located relatively close to each other. In addition, intensified international trade led to greater movement of animals, particularly swine and their by-products (Müller et al. 2003; Pensaert and Kluge 1989; Wittmann 1985). At present, PR causes serious losses to swine producers in many parts of the world, both as a result of the disease and because of movement restrictions related to controlling PRV and its impact on trade (Andersson et al. 1997; Bech-Nielsen et al. 1995; Müller et al. 2003; Vannier 1988; Waston 1986).

Significant progress in molecular biology and genetic engineering, most notably by Van Oirschot et al. (1990) and Mettenleiter (1994a, 2000), led to major improvements in diagnostic methods and vaccines and resulted in vast improvements in the prevention and control of the disease in the last 15 years.

ETIOLOGY

PRV belongs to subfamily *Alphaherpesvirinae* of the family *Herpesviridae* (Mettenleiter 2000). Comparison of deduced amino acid sequences of homologous proteins showed PRV to be closely related to bovine herpesvirus 1 (BHV-1), equine herpesvirus 1 (EHV-1), and varicella-zoster virus (McGeoch and Cook 1994). On this basis, it was assigned to the genus *Varicellovirus* of subfamily *Alphaherpesvirinae*.

Alphaherpesviruses are characterized by rapid lytic growth in cell culture, neurotropism, latency in neurons, and a broad host range. All of these features are particularly pronounced in PRV. Numerous strains of PRV have been described, and differences in the severity of clinical signs have shown that strains differ in their infectivity and virulence. Strains also differ in the quantity and duration of virus shedding during infection (Maes et al. 1983). Genomic differences believed to influence virulence have been identified (Gielkens et al. 1985; Lomniczi et al. 1984; Lomniczi and Kaplan 1987).

PRV particles have the typical architecture of a herpes virion. They are quasispherical in shape, with an overall diameter of 150–180 nm (Nauwynck 1997). Mettenleiter (2000) demonstrated that PRV, like all herpesviruses, is composed of a nucleoprotein core that contains the genome, an icosahedral capsid of 162 capsomers, a proteinaceous tegument layer, and a lipid bilayer envelope derived from cellular membranes that contain virus-encoded (glyco) proteins. Figure 25.1 shows an electron micrograph of a PRV virion attached to a bovine kidney cell (Granzow et al. 1997).

Studies on capsid architecture have primarily been done on herpes simplex virus (HSV-1). However, the

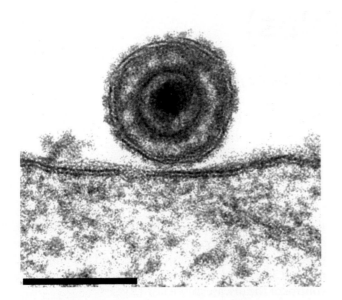

25.1. *Electron micrograph of a PRV virion attached to a bovine kidney cell (MDBK) in culture. Bar: 150 nm (from Mettenleiter 2000).*

morphological similarity of herpesvirus capsids and the homology of capsid components indicate that they share common features.

Little is known about the composition and possible structure of the tegument. In electron micrographs it appears as an electron-dense amorphous structure that lies between capsid and envelope. Several proteins of HSV-1 have been identified as tegument components, and homologues have been found in PRV.

The PRV envelope is derived from intracellular membranes of vesicles in the trans-Golgi area (Granzow et al.

1997). It contains eleven glycoproteins (Table 25.1). All glycoproteins are constituents of the viral envelope, except gG, which is abundantly produced during PRV infection in cell culture and released into the medium. Other putative nonglycosylated membrane proteins are the products of the UL3, UL11, UL20, UL34, and UL43 genes (Mettenleiter 2000).

Genomic Organization and Gene Expression

The PRV genome consists of double-stranded, linear, DNA composed of approximately 150 kilobase pairs (Figure 25.2). Around 90% of the genome has been sequenced. Based on available information from the fully sequenced herpesvirus genomes and partial sequence information from PRV, the only major sequence gap that remains probably contains the homologues of HSV-1 genes UL31 to UL37.

The genome consists of a unique long (UL) region and a unique short (US) region, the latter being bracketed by inverted repeats. So far, three origins of replication which conform to the alphaherpesvirus consensus sequence have been mapped in the repeats (2x) and middle of the unique long region (Klupp and Mettenleiter 1991). Another replication origin with apparently unique features resides at the left end of the genome (Kupershmidt et al. 1991).

Virulence-determining proteins can be divided into viral membrane glycoproteins, virus-encoded enzymes, and nonessential capsid proteins (Mettenleiter 2000). Virus-encoded enzymes involved in nucleic acid metabolism are major determinants of herpesvirus virulence. Their inactivation leads to attenuation of the virus. Deletion of the nonessential envelope glycoprotein gE also leads to a significant decrease in the virulence of some PRV strains. Glycoprotein gE seems to play a prominent role in the spread of PRV within the nervous system, both in the trigeminal and olfactory pathways.

Table 25.1. Properties of PRV glycoproteins (from Mettenleiter 2000; reprinted with permission)

Designation (a)	Gene (b)	Essential	Virion Component	Attachment	Penetration	Cell-to-Cell Spread	Neuronal Spread
gB (gII)	UL27	+	+	-	+ (c)	+	+
gC (gIII)	UL44	-	+	[+] (d)	-	-	-
gD (gp50)	US6	+	+	[+]	+	-	-
gE (gI)	US8	-	+	-	-	[+]	[+]
gG (gX)	US4	-	-	-	-	-	-
gH	UL22	+	+	-	+	+	+
gI (gp63)	US7	-	+	-	-	[+]	[+]
gK	UL53	+	+	-	-	+	? (e)
gL	UL1	+	+	-	+	+	?
gM	UL10	-	+	-	-	[+]	-
gN	UL49.5	-	+	-	[+]	-	-

(a) The old nomenclature of PRV glycoproteins has been added in parentheses.
(b) Gene designation according to the HSV-1 homologue.
(c) + indicates an essential function.
(d) [+] indicates a nonessential or modulating function.
(e) ? indicates no information available.

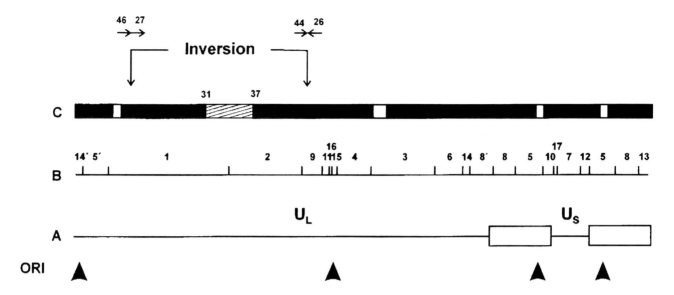

25.2. *The PRV genome. In (A) the division of the genome into a unique long (UL) and unique short (US) region by inverted repeats (open boxes) is shown. Arrows denote identified origins of replication. In (B) the Bam HI restriction fragment map of the PRV strain Ka is depicted. Those areas of the viral genome for which sequence information is available are designated in (C) by closed boxes. Shaded areas denote parts of the genome in which sequence information is present. Only one gap remains, indicated by the hatched area, which contains the open reading frames homologous to the UL31 to UL37 genes of HSV (from Mettenleiter 2000).*

Absence of gE leads to a restricted neural infection (Cheung 1995; Rauh and Mettenleiter 1991; Schang et al. 1994; Van Oirschot et al. 1990).

Replication

The PRV replication cycle is diagrammed in Figure 25.3. Infection of cells is initiated by attachment of free virions to target cells, followed by fusion of the virion envelope and the cellular cytoplasmic membrane (Mettenleiter 1994b). The interaction between viral envelope glycoproteins and cellular surface components that act as virus receptors is critical in both attachment and fusion.

The first contact between PRV and the target cell involves the interaction of glycoprotein gC with heparan sulfate proteoglycans at the cell surface. In addition, gD and two cellular groups of receptors, heparan sulfate proteoglycans and poliovirus-receptor related proteins, are involved in PRV attachment. Entry requires fusion between the cellular cytoplasmic membrane and the viral envelope. The fusion process involves at least four viral glycoproteins: gB, gH/gL, and gD. Absence of any of these glycoproteins in engineered virus mutants renders the virus incapable of fusion. After translocation of the nucleocapsid into the cytoplasm of the cell, it is transported to the nuclear membrane and locates adjacent to nuclear pores. This transport most likely occurs along microtubules. The capsid is invariably oriented toward the nuclear pore so that one vertex is juxtaposed to the pore complex (refer to Figure 25.3). The DNA presumably leaves the virion and enters the nucleus through this vertex. Subsequent intranuclear events and the egress of the virion are described by Mettenleiter (2000).

Laboratory Cultivation

Numerous cell lines or primary cell cultures are permissive to PRV, but porcine cell lines PK-15 or SK-6 are generally used in cultivation (Toma et al. 2004). PRV induces a cytopathic effect (CPE) that usually appears in 24–72 hours, but cell cultures may be incubated for 5–6 days (Figure 25.4). The monolayer develops accumulations of birefringent cells, followed by complete detachment of the cell sheet. Syncytia also develop, the appearance of which is variable. In the absence of obvious CPE, it is advisable to make two blind passages (Granzow et al. 1997).

EPIDEMIOLOGY

PRV is found throughout the world, particularly in regions with dense pig populations, including South America, Europe, and Asia. In Europe, PR has never been reported in Norway, Finland, or Malta. PRV has been eradicated from Germany, Austria, Sweden, Denmark, and the United Kingdom. Canada, New Zealand, and the United States (since 2004) are also free of PR. In these countries, vaccination against PR is prohibited. However, PRV still circulates in wild boar or feral swine populations in the United States, Germany, Poland, France, Italy, and elsewhere (Lipowski and Pejsak 2002).

Pigs are the primary host of the virus, but although a large number of other species can be infected naturally or experimentally. PRV is infectious for cattle, sheep, goats, dogs, cats, foxes in fur farms, rats, and wild mice. PRV in species other than swine causes neurologic disease and death. In cattle, sheep, and goats, clinical pru-

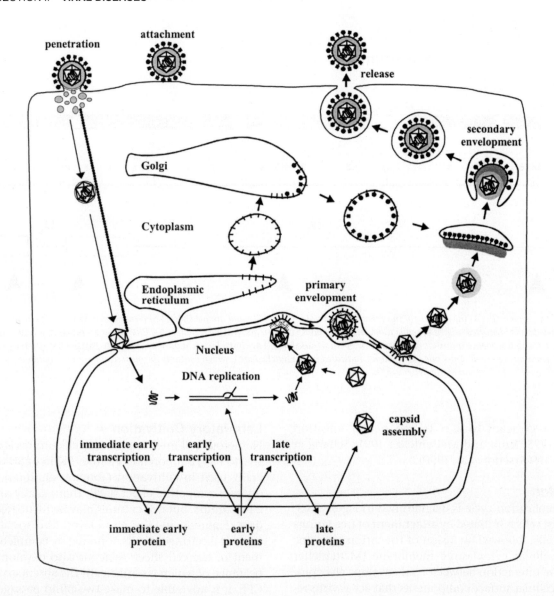

25.3. *The PRV replication cycle (from Mettenleiter 2000).*

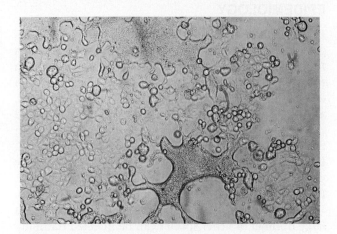

25.4. *Swine kidney cell line SK-6 infected with pseudorabies virus strain NIA-3. Cytopathic effect 24 hours after inoculation (picture courtesy of Dr. Andrzej Lipowski, National Veterinary Research Institute, Pulawy, Poland).*

ritus and encephalitis characterize the uniformly fatal infections. Experimentally infected sheep have transmitted PRV to susceptible swine and to other sheep. Live PRV vaccines are lethal to sheep (Beran 1991). It is very difficult to infect horses and birds; large virus doses are necessary and they must be injected either intracerebrally, subcutaneously, or intramuscularly. Higher primates, including humans, are not susceptible to PRV infection (Wittmann 1985). In non-porcine species, the course of infection is lethal at all ages and recovery is an exception (Wittmann 1985).

The pig is the only species able to survive PRV infection and, therefore, serves as a virus reservoir (Babic et al. 1994; Cheung 1995; Granzow et al. 1997; Enquist et al. 1998). This means that eliminating the virus from the porcine population will ultimately lead to eradication of the disease (Mettenleiter 2000; Wittman 1986). Feral swine are as susceptible to PRV infection as domestic pigs (Lipowski 2003). PRV cycles in the feral swine population independently of the cycle in domestic pigs (Lipowski and Pejsak 2002). Therefore, feral swine should be considered a potential PRV reservoir and source of infection for domestic pigs, especially in those countries where PR eradication programs have been implemented (Lipowski and Pejsak 2002). Naturally occurring PRV also has been identified in peccaries in the southwestern U.S. (Corn et al. 1987).

In pigs, PRV morbidity and mortality are dependent upon the age of the animal. Piglets and young pigs are at the greatest risk. Most risk factors for PR, e.g., swine population density, number of breeders, number of fattening pigs, replacement gilt purchasing, are directly or indirectly linked with the number of susceptible pigs in the population.

Virus is transmitted primarily between swine through nose-to-nose contact. Transmission may occur during breeding either from exposure to contaminated vaginal mucosa or semen, transplacentally during gestation (Beran 1991), or by contact with carcasses of rats, raccoons, swine, and other infected animals (Donaldson 1983). Under favorable circumstances virus may be spread by aerosols (Vannier 1988; Christensen et al. 1990).

Susceptibility to infection is dependent on several factors, including the virulence of the virus strain, the exposure dose, the route of exposure, the age of the pigs (piglets are more susceptible than adult pigs), stress, and the condition of the animal. Larger quantities of virus are necessary for oral infection than for nasal infection (Baskerville 1972a; Jakubik 1977).

PRV is not very contagious. This is supported by the fact that, usually, not all the pigs within a building become infected. The percentage of animals infected varies between 10% and 90%. The spread of infection within a herd is dependent on the opportunity of direct contact between animals. Spread of infection is highest within a pen but lower from pen to pen.

The virus can be isolated from nasal swabs of infected pigs for 8–17 days with maximum virus titers of between $10^{5.8}$ and $10^{8.3}$ TCID$_{50}$ per swab. From oropharyngeal swabs, virus can be isolated for 18–25 days with virus titers of up to 10^6 TCID$_{50}$. At the peak of virus excretion one pig may excrete $10^{5.3}$ TCID$_{50}$ into the air during a 24-hr period. Virus is found in vaginal secretions and foreskin secretions (ejaculate) for up to 12 days and for 2–3 days in milk. The virus is occasionally present in urine, but it has not been isolated from the feces, though it has been detected in rectal swabs for up to 10 days. It is important to note that virus excretion starts before the onset of clinical symptoms (Wittmann 1985).

Persistence in the Environment

PRV is stable under various pH and temperature conditions and is considered resistant in the environment. However, it must be realized that the "environment" is complex and includes both factors favorable and factors unfavorable to virus persistence. Therefore, the data given should be considered only a guide (Wittmann 1985).

The virus survives on hay for 30 days in summer and 46 days in winter. It is stable between pH 4 to 12. Stored in 50% glycerol, it survives for 154 days with little loss of virus titer at refrigerator temperatures. At low temperatures, virus in tissue remains viable for many years. Lyophilized virus survives at least 2 years. Ultraviolet light and drying on glass inactivates the virus (Davies and Beran 1981; Wittmann 1985).

The virus is not inactivated in the course of the maturation of pig meat at 4°C (Weyhe and Benndorf 1970). In urine, the virus retains infectivity for 3 weeks in summer and 8–15 weeks in winter (Atanasowa 1972). In slurry, the virus is thought to remain infectious for about 2 months in winter and about 1 month in summer, in biothermically treated slurry, the virus is inactivated in summer within 5 days and in winter within 12 days. In aerated slurry (pH 9.6, temperature up to 44°C), the virus is inactivated within 50 hrs (Böhm et al. 1980). In packed-down manure the virus is inactivated in 8–15 days. In soil, infectious virus was recovered for 5–6 weeks. Virus dried on sacks and wood persisted for about 10 days in summer and 15 days in winter (Kretzschmar 1970). No data are available on untreated edible waste material, but in material fermented by *Lactobacillus acidophilus* PRV was inactivated at 20°C and 30°C within 24 hrs, but persisted for at least 48 hrs at 10°C and at least for 96 hrs at 5°C (Wooley et al. 1981).

PRV is relatively resistant to heat. It is inactivated at 60°C in 30–60 min, at 70°C in 10–15 min, at 80°C in 3 minutes and at 100°C within 1 minutes (Kunev 1978). The virus is very stable at normal temperatures and in the cold. It stays alive at 25°C about 6 weeks, at 15°C about 9 weeks, at 4°C about 20 weeks and at −40°C for years. However, the virus is relatively unstable at −18°C to −25°C, where inactivation occurs within 12 weeks (Davies and Beran 1981).

Between pH values of 4.0 and 12 the virus is stable and even at pH values of 2.0 and 13.5 it takes 2–4 hours before the virus is completely inactivated (Benndorf and Hantschel 1963). By combining low or high pH levels with elevated temperatures, the inactivation time is significantly reduced (Davies and Beran 1981).

Susceptibility to Disinfectants

Effective disinfectants include orthophenolphenate compounds, 5% phenol, 2% Na hydroxide, trisodium phosphate iodine disinfectants, and chlorhexidine solutions (Beran 1991). Quaternary ammonium compounds, hypochlorites, and in fact, all disinfectants are less effective in the presence of organic matter (Brown 1981). When disinfecting on a large scale, cheaper disinfectants are adopted: calcium chloride milk, calcium chloride preparations that dissolve in water, crude chloramines, and agents containing at least 1% active formaldehyde. For disinfecting slurry, lime (20 kg Ca(OH)2 per cubic meter is recommended (Koch and Euler 1983).

PATHOGENESIS

Following oronasal exposure, primary replication occurs in the epithelia of the upper respiratory tract. Thereafter, infection of tonsils and lungs ensues and the virus is disseminated in the body either in free form or via infected leukocytes. In addition, the virus enters the trigeminal and olfactory nerve endings and invades the central nervous system (Babic et al. 1993; Kritas et al. 1994; Pensaert and Kluge 1989). Replication of PRV in the CNS is characterized by nonsuppurative meningoencephalitis causing severe central nervous disorders (Enquist 1994; Pensaert and Kluge 1989).

The virulence of the infecting strain is, at least in part, determined by viral glycoproteins. According to their relevance for viral replication in cell culture, these have been designated nonessential (gC, gE, gG, gI, gN) and essential (gB, gD, gH, gK, gL). Glycoproteins that mediate attachment of PRV to target cells are of special interest because they may directly determine viral tropism. Primary attachment of PRV to target cells is mediated by binding of the nonessential gC to heparan sulfate proteoglycans (Karger and Mettenleiter 1993; Mettenleiter and Rauh 1990). However, this interaction is not sufficient to trigger fusion between the viral envelope and the cell membrane. The essential glycoprotein gD mediates secondary attachment of PRV (Karger and Mettenleiter 1993) to cellular gD receptors. This gD-gD receptor interaction is thought to be necessary to initiate penetration. Besides gD, gB and the gH-gL complex are required for penetration of free virions into target cells (Mettenleiter 2000). However, in contrast to the situation in herpes simplex virus type 1 (HSV-1) and bovine herpesvirus type 1 (BHV-1), PRV-gD is dispensable for direct viral cell-to-cell spread in vitro (Rauh and Mettenleiter 1991). Thus phenotypically complemented gD-negative PRV (PRV-gD-) is able to infect primary target cells and subsequently spreads via direct cell-to-cell transmission.

Recently, the proteins required for neuroinvasion of PRV were analyzed in detail. Several studies in mice, rats, and pigs have indicated that one of the key proteins in neuroinvasion is glycoprotein E. Deletion of this protein strongly attenuates PRV, but absence of glycoprotein E does not impair primary viral replication in the nasal epithelium after intranasal infection of mice or pigs. It is also not required for the virus to enter primary neurons (Babic et al. 1994, 1996; Enquist 1995). Transsynaptic transfer to second order neurons is, however, severely inhibited, resulting in a dramatic restriction in neuroinvasion. Glycoprotein E, and to a lesser extent glycoprotein I, are the predominant nonessential glycoproteins exhibiting this dramatic phenotype (Enquist et al. 1998).

Latency

Latency is defined as a condition in which viral DNA is present, but infectious virus is not produced. During latency, viral gene expression is restricted to transcription of a distinct part of the viral genome into the so-called latency associated transcripts or LATs (Priola and Stevens 1991).

Latency, with the potential for subsequent reactivation and shedding, is one of the most formidable challenges to the successful control and eradication of PR. A number of studies have suggested that most, if not all, pigs initially exposed to a large quantity of PRV can become latently infected carriers. As a consequence any pig believed to have been previously infected with a field strain of PRV (typically identified by the presence of serum antibody) is assumed to be a latently infected carrier. Despite intensive efforts (Mettenleiter 2000), the molecular basis for alphaherpesvirus latency is still largely unknown. In PRV, latently infected pigs are a constant risk because of the possibility of reactivation, virus shedding (recrudescence), and spread to susceptible individuals.

Major sites of PRV latency are the trigeminal ganglion (TG), the olfactory bulb, and the tonsil. In these organs, viral DNA can be detected in the absence of infectious virus production. LAT transcription can also be demonstrated by highly sensitive methods, such as RT-PCR (Cheung 1995). The most common in vitro method for detecting latency is the examination of the tissue in question via a PCR reaction specific for a portion of the viral genome (Mengeling et al. 1992). The only relatively reliable method for detecting latency in a live pig is to administer large doses of a corticosteroid, with the intent of inducing reactivation followed by virus shedding (Mengeling et al. 1992).

Presumably, after oronasal infection, PRV first replicates in the epithelial tissues and may also directly enter nerve endings of sensory neurons in the nasopharynx. After a first round of replication in the epithelia, progeny virus is abundantly produced, leading to an increased infection of primary neurons. There appears to be a correlation between precolonization of trigeminal ganglia with PRV and failure of a superinfecting strain to become latent itself. This suggests that the number of neurons in which latency can be established is limited and that, probably, a neuron that is already "occupied" resists superinfection. Whether this interference requires a viral function or is dependent on cellular factors is unknown. However, it suggests that attenuated live vaccine strains with a high potential for establishing latency may prevent superinfecting, wild type strains from becoming latent (Schang et al. 1994).

CLINICAL SIGNS

The incubation period for PR ranges from 1–11 days, most frequently 2–6 days. The incubation period in suckling pigs is shorter than in older animals (Wittmann 1986). The clinical severity of PR depends on the age of the pig, the route of infection, and the virulence of the infecting strain, which is at least partially determined by viral glycoproteins (Schmidt et al. 2001), and the immunological status of the animal (Nauwynck 1997). Young piglets are highly susceptible, with mortality rates reaching 100% during the first 2 weeks and decreasing to 50% during the third and fourth week of age. In these animals, severe neurological disorders are observed. The nature of the PRV strain involved determines the degree of the virus invasion within the nervous system of maternally immune neonatal pigs (Kritas et al. 1999).

Differences in the course of the disease are observed between herds. PR may be a rapidly spreading disease affecting swine of all ages, or clinical signs may be absent and infection detected only after serological investigations. The clinical course is more severe in a naive population. In the absence of neonatal pigs, and especially between farrowings, the course of infection is usually inapparent. However, inapparent herd infection does not take place or occurs rarely when PRV is introduced into a herd for the first time and where neonatal pigs are present. This is because these piglets are highly susceptible to PRV infection. In this case, morbidity and mortality may reach 100%.

In breeding herds or separate finishing barns, PRV may cause mild respiratory symptoms, which may be ignored or associated with other etiological agents, e.g., *Streptococcus suis*, *Actinobacillus pleuropneumoniae*, *Pasteurella multocida*, *Mycoplasma hyopneumoniae*, swine influenza virus, or porcine respiratory and reproductive syndrome (PRRS) virus (Zimmerman and Yoon 2003).

According to Kluge et al. (1999), piglets born infected with PRV become listless, anorectic, and within 24 hours, ataxic and convulsive. In such situations, laboratory diagnosis is imperative to establish the role of PRV. The sooner a diagnosis is established, the greater the likelihood of preventing losses by immediate vaccination of the herd against PR.

Piglets that become infected with PRV demonstrate fevers of up to 41°C. Trembling, hypersalivation, incoordination, ataxia, and nystagmus to opistotonos to severe epileptiform-like seizures occur in succession. Pigs may assume the "sitting dog" position because of respiratory distress. Some pigs circle or become recumbent and paddle. Vomiting and diarrhea also occur. In piglets with CNS signs, death occurs within 24–36 hours following the onset of such signs. Mortality of PR in piglets often approaches 100%.

Depending on the dam's level of immunity against PRV, piglets of some litters may not show clinical signs, while piglets in adjacent litters show the clinical signs listed previously. If susceptible sows or gilts are infected with PRV close to parturition, the piglets are born weak, show primarily nervous signs, and die 1–2 days after birth.

In weaned pigs (3–6 weeks), clinical signs are similar to those in neonatal piglets, but less severe, and CNS signs leading to coma and death do not occur as often. Mortality may approach 50%, but it is usually lower. Clinical signs in weaned pigs include listlessness, anorexia, and fever (41–42°C). Respiratory signs are often seen, e.g., sneezing, nasal discharge, dyspnea, and severe cough. Most pigs recover within 5–10 days, with the exception that those demonstrating CNS signs often die. The infection of the respiratory tract with PRV is often complicated by the presence of bacterial infections, e.g., *Pasteurella multocida*, *Actinobacillus pleuropneumoniae*, *Streptococcus suis*, *Haemophilus* spp. or other facultative pathogenic bacteria (Kluge et al. 1999).

In pigs 5–9 weeks of age and in the case of proper veterinary intervention, mortality in pigs 5–9 weeks of age usually does not exceed 10% and is often lower. However, PRV infection in these animals results in a 1- to 8-week delay in reaching market weight compared to uninfected animals.

In grower-finisher pigs, respiratory signs are the most common observation. Morbidity in an infected group often reaches 100%, but in cases uncomplicated by secondary infections, mortality ranges from 1–2%. Complications caused by bacteria, particularly *A. pleuropneumoniae*, increase the losses dramatically. CNS symptoms occur only sporadically. Typically, clinical signs appear in 3–6 days and are characterized by fever (41–42°C), depression, anorexia, and mild-to-severe respiratory signs. Rhinitis with sneezing and nasal discharge may progress to pneumonia. The pigs become gaunt and lose considerable body weight. After 6–10 days, appetite and body temperature return to normal. PRV infection in grower-finisher pigs results in the loss of at least 1 week in the production cycle.

Sows and boars primarily develop respiratory signs. PRV can cross the placenta and infect and kill fetuses in utero. In pregnant females, abortion often occurs and may be the first sign of PR. Sows infected in the first trimester may resorb fetuses and return to estrus. If infection takes place in the second or third trimester of pregnancy, it is usually manifested by abortion or stillborn and/or weak pigs, particularly if the infection occurs close to term. Mortality in adult swine infected with PRV rarely exceeds 2%.

An essential factor affecting the manifestation of clinical signs in a herd is the level of immunization of pregnant sows, weaned pigs, and grower-finisher swine. Likewise, secondary bacterial infections, the age of the animals, and environmental conditions will affect the expression of the disease.

LESIONS

Gross lesions are often absent or minimal, but keratoconjunctivitis, serous-to-fibrinonecrotic rhinitis, laryngitis, tracheitis, and necrotic tonsillitis may be seen.

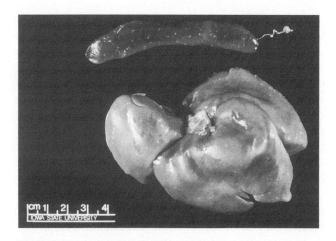

25.5. *Spleen and liver with multiple small focal areas of necrosis (from Kluge et al. 1999).*

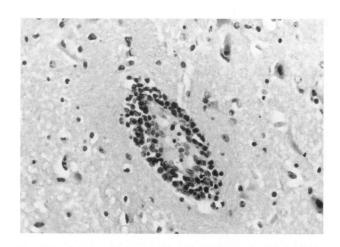

25.6. *Brain with perivascular cuffing (from Kluge et al. 1999).*

Vaccination will reduce both the severity of clinical signs and microscopic lesions (Alva-Valdes et al. 1983). Lesions in the lower respiratory tract range from pulmonary edema to scattered small foci of necrosis, hemorrhage, and/or pneumonia (Becker 1964). Small necrotic white foci (2–3 mm) may be seen on the liver and spleen (Figure 25.5), especially in young pigs that lack passive immunity. In aborted sows, endometritis and a thickened, edematous wall of the uterus are observed (Kluge and Maré 1978). Necrotic placentitis accompanies abortion or parturition. Aborted fetuses may be macerated or, occasionally, mummified. In fetuses or neonatal pigs, necrotic foci in liver and spleen are seen. In addition, hemorrhagic, necrotic foci in lungs and tonsils may be present (Kluge and Maré 1976).

Microscopic lesions most frequently occur in the CNS. These include nonsuppurative meningoencephalitis and ganglioneuritis in the grey and white matter (Baskerville 1972b). Perivascular cuffing (Figure 25.6) consists predominantly of mononuclear cells, with the presence of few granulocytes. Pyknosis and karyorrhexis of the mononuclear cells are often prominent. Neuronal necrosis may be focal, and the neurons surrounded by mononuclear cells or affected neurons may be diffusely scattered. Similar lesions exist in the spinal cord, especially in the cervical and thoracic regions. Meninges over affected areas of brain and cord may be thickened because of infiltrates of mononuclear cells.

Intranuclear inclusion bodies are observed in neurons, astrocytes, and oligodendroglia. According to Kluge et al. (1999) these are much more common in lesions outside the nervous system. They are common in crypt epithelial cells adjacent to necrotic foci. Mucosal epithelial necrosis and submucosal infiltrations of mononuclear cells occur in the upper respiratory tract (Baskerville 1971, 1973). In the lungs, necrotic bronchitis, bronchiolitis, and alveolitis is found. Also, peribronchial mucous gland epithelium may be necrotic.

There is often hemorrhage and fibrin exudation because of the involvement of connective tissue and endothelium. Lesions often are patchy in major airways, and healing by fibrosis is often observed in areas adjacent to acute lesions. Intranuclear inclusion bodies are frequently present in the epithelial lining of the airways, connective tissue cells, and cells sloughed into alveolar spaces.

According to Corner (1965) two types of intranuclear inclusion bodies are observed: a homogenous basophilic body that fills the entire nucleus and an eosinophilic body that has a definite zone between it and the marginated chromatin. In either case, the specificity of the inclusion must be determined by demonstrating PR viral particles or antigen by electron microscopy or immunohistochemistry.

Focal necrotic lesions are similar regardless of the tissue involved. They are most frequently found in spleen, liver, lymph nodes, and adrenal glands. In the uterus, multifocal to diffuse lymphohistiocytic endometritis and vaginitis and necrotic placentitis with coagulative necrosis of chorionic fossae can be found (Bolin et al. 1985; Kluge et al. 1999). Intranuclear inclusion bodies are present in degenerate trophoblasts associated with necrotic lesions (Kluge and Maré 1978; Kluge et al. 1999). In the male reproductive tract there may be degeneration of seminiferous tubules and necrotic foci in the tunica albuginea of the testicles (Hall et al. 1984). Boars with exudative periorchitis have necrotic and inflammatory lesions in the serosa covering the genital organs. Spermatozoa abnormalities are found. Focal necrosis of the mucosal epithelium involving the muscularis mucosa and tunica muscularis develops in the intestines (Narita et al. 1984b). Intranuclear inclusion bodies may be present in degenerative crypt epithelial cells. Necrotizing vasculitis of arterioles, venules, and lymphatic vessels around tonsils and submaxillary lymph nodes is observed (Narita et al. 1984a). Endo-

Table 25.2. Role of PRV proteins in immunity (modified, from Mettenleiter 1996)

Protein	Protection (a)		NT–C (b)	NT+C (c)	Prolif. (d)	CTL (e) (MHC-I restr.)	CTL (f) (LAK)
	Mice	Pigs					
gB	+	+	+	+	+	?	+
gC	+	+	+	+	+	+	+
gD	+	+	+	+	+	?	–
gE	+	?	–	+	–	–	?
gG	–	–	–	–	–	–	?

(a) Protection by administration of purified or genetically engineered antigen, or by administration of antigen-specific monoclonal antibodies.

(b) Neutralization by antigen-specific monoclonal antibodies without complement.

(c) Neutralization by antigen-specific monoclonal antibodies with complement.

(d) Stimulation of proliferation of PBMC derived from immune pigs.

(e) MHC-class I restricted cytotoxic activity.

(f) Non-MHC restricted cytotoxic activity.

thelial nuclei are pyknotic and karyorrhectic, and the vessel walls are infiltrated by neutrophils. Intranuclear inclusion bodies often are present in affected endothelial cells (Kluge et al. 1999).

IMMUNITY

PRV infection evokes antibody production and cell-mediated immunity in pigs. However, immunity is not total and upon reinfection the virus can multiply to a limited degree (Wittmann 1985).

According to Eloit et al. (1988) glycoprotein gp50 is a major target of neutralizing antibodies. However, only a few of the numerous potential PRV antigens has been analyzed, and the relative importance of a single protein to the immune response of the host is difficult, if not impossible to assess (Mettenleiter 1996). An improved understanding of the immune response against PRV is necessary in order to develop vaccines capable of boostering specific effector mechanisms.

Antibodies against PRV and specifically against a number of glycosylated and nonglycosylated viral structural and nonstructural proteins have been detected in infected animals. Monoclonal antibodies have been identified that exhibit virus-neutralizing ability in vitro and in vivo. The role of PRV proteins in immunity is summarized in Table 25.2.

The most potent complement-independent virus-neutralizing antibodies are directed against gC and gD (Mettenleiter 1996). These antibodies work by inhibiting virus attachment (anti-gC) or penetration (anti-gD) and thereby block infection at the first stages. Subunit vaccines consisting of gC or gD, as well as anti-idiotypic anti-gD antibodies have been shown to elicit protective immunity, further emphasizing the important role of these proteins in the humoral immune response (Tsuda et al. 1992). In fact, a large part of the neutralizing activity in convalescent sera of swine appears to be directed against gC (Ben-Porat et al. 1986). The role of the other

Table 25.3. Cell-mediated immunity against PRV (from Mettenleiter 1996)

Cell Type	Antigen Recognized	Negative
CD4+ CD8– (T-helper)	gB, gC	gE, gC, gl
CD4– CD8+ (CTL)	gC	gE, gG, gl
CD4– CD8–/CD4–CD8^low (LAK)	gB, gC	gD, lE
CD4+ CD8+ (T-helper)	gB, gC	?

glycoproteins is less clear. However, vaccination with subunit gB vaccines also induces protective immunity in pigs (Nakamura et al. 1993 in Mettenleiter 1996). Glycoproteins are considered the prime targets for the porcine anti-PRV cell mediated immunity (Table 25.3).

A sow immune to PRV transfers specific antibodies to her offspring via the colostrum. Maternal immunity is able to protect neonatal pigs infected with virulent PRV against clinical disease by limiting virus replication in the CNS (Wittmann and Jakubik 1979). Kritas et al. (1997) showed that high SN titers (272–354) were able to protect neonatal pigs almost completely against neural invasion and spread upon challenge with a virulent strain of PRV. Low SN titers (2–3) did not protect pigs against neural invasion and virus spread, particularly via the olfactory pathway, which is readily accessible to the virus due to the pigs' anatomy. Either low or high SN titers protected pigs against clinical disease. However, the protective role of maternally derived antibodies and maternal immunity against spread of PRV in the nasal mucosa depends on the infecting virus strain.

Maternally derived PRV antibody interferes with immunization of the piglets until it declines to a level that often leaves piglets unprotected. However, Brockmeier et al. (1997) found that certain vaccines—for example, recombinant vaccinia vaccines—were able to circumvent maternally derived antibody and stimulate active immunity.

DIAGNOSIS

Clinical diagnosis of PR disease in individual pigs may be difficult or even impossible. Therefore, a diagnosis of PR should be made on a herd basis. Clinical signs suggestive of PR include numerous deaths of suckling pigs showing nervous signs during the first 3 weeks of life. Nasal discharge, coughing, dullness, somnolence, and nervous disorders may be seen in these and older pigs. In pregnant sows, a high frequency of abortions and stillbirth is observed. It is characteristic of PR that morbidity and mortality decrease as the age of the pigs increases. Signs suggestive of PR may be seen in dogs and cats on the farm. Likewise, the discovery of dead animals of these species is suggestive of PR (Wittmann 1986).

When diarrhea is present in newborn pigs, PR may resemble transmissible gastroenteritis or *E. coli* infection. Similar respiratory signs can be caused by bacteria, e.g., *Pasteurella multocida*, *Actinobacillus pneumoniae*, and *Streptococcus suis*, as well as swine influenza virus. In the latter case, all pigs in all age groups become severely ill without dying. Nervous signs can occasionally occur in classical swine fever (CSF) and, in the absence of gross pathological changes due to CSF, it is difficult to differentiate CSF from PR. Nervous conditions caused by porcine teschovirus infection (previously called Teschen/Talfan disease) are not accompanied by infection of the respiratory tract. NaCl poisoning causes excitement and arsanilic acid and mercurial poisoning causes lethargy of the animals, but these events occur suddenly without fever. Stillbirths and abortion can be induced by parvovirus, *Leptospira*, *Brucella*, and PRRSV infection (Pejsak and Markowska-Daniel 1996; Wittmann 1986; Zimmerman and Yoon 2003).

Classical clinical signs of PR will often lead to a presumptive diagnosis, which is supported if gross lesions—e.g., focal hepatic and splenic necrosis and necrotic tonsillitis—are observed in neonatal pigs. PR is more difficult to diagnose if only grower-finisher pigs or adult swine are involved. A PR outbreak in this age group can easily be misdiagnosed as swine influenza if the disease is manifested only by respiratory signs and lesions. If, however, a few individuals develop CNS signs, it is easier to make a presumptive diagnosis of PR.

In most cases laboratory diagnosis is necessary to confirm the presumptive diagnosis of PR (Toma et al. 2004). The diagnosis of PR can be confirmed by isolation of PRV from the oropharyngeal fluid, nasal fluid (swabs), or tonsil biopsies of living pigs, or from samples from dead pigs. For postmortem isolation of PRV, samples of brain and tonsil are the preferred specimens. In latently infected pigs, the trigeminal ganglion is the most consistent site for virus isolation, although latent virus is usually difficult to culture. Numerous types of cell line or primary cell cultures are sensitive to PRV, but a porcine kidney cell line (PK-15 or SK-6) is generally used. PRV induces a cytopathic effect (CPE, Figure 25.4) that usually appears within 24–72 hours, but cell cultures may be incubated for 5–6 days. The isolation of PRV is confirmation PR, but failure to isolate virus does not guarantee freedom from infection.

In the absence of any obvious CPE, it is advisable to make two blind passages into further cultures. Additional evidence may be obtained by staining infected cover-slip cultures with haematoxylin and eosin to demonstrate the characteristic herpesviral acidophilic intranuclear inclusions with margination of the chromatin. The virus identity should be confirmed by immunofluorescence, immunoperoxidase, or neutralization tests using specific antiserum.

The polymerase chain reaction (PCR) can be used to identify PRV genomes in secretions or organ samples. The primary advantage of PCR over conventional virus isolation techniques is its speed. Preliminary identification can be completed within 1 day, with confirmation of the PCR product on the second day. With the most modern equipment the whole process can be completed in 1 day. Because of the nature of the test, many precautions need to be taken to avoid contamination of samples with extraneous DNA from previous tests or from general environmental contamination in the laboratory. This may limit the value of the test for many laboratories, and therefore this technique cannot be fully recommended for routine diagnosis.

Immunofluorescence (IF) is still of some importance for detection of PRV or its antigen in tissue sections (Wittmann 1986) or in impression smears (Wittmann 1986). IF usually appears in the cytoplasm and only exceptionally in the nucleus.

Virus neutralization (VN) has been recognized as the reference method for serology, but for general diagnostic purposes it has been widely replaced by the enzyme-linked immunosorbent assay (ELISA) because of its suitability for large-scale testing. ELISA can be performed on serum as well as on meat juice (Toma et al. 2004).

The sensitivity of ELISA is generally superior to that of the VN test using 1-hour neutralization without complement. Some weak-positive sera are more readily detected by VN tests using 24-hour neutralization, but others are more readily detectable by ELISA. Commercially available ELISA kits use indirect or competitive techniques for detecting humoral antibody. They differ in their mode of preparation of antigen, conjugate, or substrate, in the period of incubation and in the interpretation of the results. Their general advantage is their capacity for rapid processing of large numbers of samples. Testing can also be automated and the results analyzed by computer. Some of these kits make it possible to differentiate between vaccination and infection with wild-type virus. When using these test systems, it is more appropriate to consider them herd tests rather than individual animal tests.

Interpretation of serological results can be difficult,

especially in young pigs. Maternal antibodies can be present up to 4 months of age. In pigs, the half-life of maternal antibodies is approximately 18 days; for example, it takes 18 days for the antibody titer to decline from 1:16 to 1:8. If pigs from an immune sow are tested too early, they may be identified as infected when the antibody is actually of maternal origin.

Traditional detection methods are complicated by the ability of the PRV to become latent (Gustafson 1986). Several field studies provide circumstantial evidence that pigs can be seronegative to PRV but latently infected (Thawley and Morrison 1988).

PREVENTION AND CONTROL

An essential precondition for effective prevention and control of PR is the obligation for notification. Once a system of notification is in place, the response to the detection of PRV infection in a herd will be largely dictated by local or regional considerations. The primary consideration is whether or not PRV has been, or is in the process of being, eradicated in the area or region and whether vaccination is a control option. Thus, depending on the PRV status of the region, the response may be largely dictated by regional animal health regulations. If permitted, vaccination of the infected herd and neighboring herds should be carried out (Kluge et al. 1999; Wittmann 1985).

Depending on local animal health regulations, control measures imposed on an infected farm could include any of the following: depopulation of the herd; restrictions allowing for movement of pigs to slaughter only; containment and treatment of dead animals, tissues, and offal; decontamination of manure, bedding, waste material, hog lots, and areas of traffic; disinfection of implements, equipment, vehicles, trailers, and buildings; implementation of rat control. Infected herds should refrain from the use of semen for artificial insemination. Unauthorized persons, cats, and dogs should be kept out of the facilities. Persons with access to pigs and facilities should follow strict biosecurity procedures to avoid transporting PRV on their clothing, footwear, or body. Regulations for infected farms may also be adapted to pig markets, pig exhibitions, and to the transport of pigs when a PR outbreak occurs or when animals other than pigs contract PR on a farm.

The most important breakthrough in PR control and eradication has been the development of genetically engineered PR vaccines (Quint et al. 1987) and their accompanying differential ELISA tests (Müller et al. 2003). The use of marker vaccines, i.e., deletion mutants of PRV that do not express glycoprotein gE, has made it possible to identify infected pigs in vaccinated populations. That is, pigs with serum antibodies against gE must necessarily have been infected with wild type virus. Vaccination with marker vaccines increases the virus dose required for infection and reduces, but does not prevent, the shedding of virulent virus and the establishment of latency in pigs infected with virulent PRV. Besides deletion mutant vaccines, there are several conventionally attenuated vaccines containing naturally gE-negative strains (e.g., with Bartha strain).

In general, vaccination prevents or reduces clinical disease and economic losses, but it does not prevent the spread of PRV. Because of the importance of cellular immunity in protection against PRV, live, attenuated vaccines are preferable. In PRV-endemic areas, it is strongly recommended that all animals introduced into the herd be vaccinated. Breeding stock must be vaccinated regularly on breeding or on piglet-producing farms. To reduce circulation of the virus in the herd and to prevent the appearance of subpopulations of susceptible pigs, continuous vaccination of all piglets is recommended. Piglets born to vaccinated sows should be immunized at 10–12 and 14–16 weeks of age. Piglets born to unvaccinated sows should be vaccinated at 6 and 10 weeks of age. Two applications of the vaccine ensure better protection. Unvaccinated animals that stay on the farm should be examined serologically to monitor virus spread. In any case, all such farms remain latently chronically infected and can be sources of virus spread (Kluge et al. 1999; Wittmann 1985). If prophylactic vaccination is practiced, all the fattening herds and all the breeding stock should be vaccinated in the infected geographical area.

As discussed by Mengeling et al. (1992), the most effective method of vaccination is intranasal administration of live, attenuated vaccine. At least part of the advantage of intranasal vaccination can be explained by local replication of virus and by the development of mucosal immunity. Intranasal vaccination is more effective in the presence of passively acquired colostral immunity than intramuscular vaccination (Van Oirschot 1987) and also is most effective at reducing PRV replication and shedding during acute infection. Practical considerations, such as the fact that intranasal vaccination is more labor intensive than intramuscular administration, argues against its wide use. Nevertheless, intranasal vaccination may be recommended for piglets in herds newly infected with PRV.

Eradication

The ultimate objective of PR control is its eradication. Marker vaccines are routinely used for a combined vaccination-eradication program for PR eradication. Such a program generally consists of four elements: a systemic and intensive vaccination campaign; serological screening of pigs for gE-specific antibodies; culling of infected breeding pigs; and in the last stage, abolishment of vaccination (Szweda et al. 2000a, b).

Eradication of PR can be most successfully achieved by the slaughter of all the seropositive animals and by strict control of pig movement. However, such an eradication program is very expensive and time-consuming.

More practical strategies to eliminate PRV include the following:

1. Test-and-removal without vaccination
2. Vaccination followed by test-and-removal
3. Stamping out of infected herds based on serological evidence of PRV in the herd

Test-and-removal is recommended when less than 10% of the breeding herd is PRV-positive and there is no serological evidence of infection in the growing or finishing pens. The entire breeding herd must be tested every 30 days and seropositive swine removed and slaughtered. Following one or two (preferable) negative herd tests, the herd may be considered free of PRV.

Vaccination followed by test-and-removal should be used when a high percentage of the breeding herd is seropositive and/or there is evidence of infection in growing or finishing pigs. The entire herd should be vaccinated with a differential vaccine. Either live or inactivated vaccines can be used in breeding animals, and live vaccines are generally used in weaned pigs. Breeding animals should be vaccinated three times a year (every 4 months). Weaners or/and fattening pigs should be vaccinated twice. Stegeman (1995) showed that the number of finishing pigs showing evidence of infection with wild-type virus (anti-glycoprotein E antibody) at the time of slaughter is higher after a single vaccination than after double vaccination. The first vaccination should be performed at 10–12 weeks of age, followed by revaccination 4 weeks later by either intramuscular, intradermal, or intranasal routes of administration (Visser 1997). If it is only possible to perform a single vaccination, i.e., for economical reasons, immunization should be performed at 14 weeks of age (De Smet et al. 1994). According to Bouma et al. (1997), maternal immunity capable of interfering with vaccine-induced immunity may still be present at 10 weeks of age. On the other hand, a single dose of vaccine at 14 weeks of age may result in transmission of PRV among pigs prior to vaccination.

The vaccination protocol should be followed for at least 3 years. During this period, all sows present on the farm at the start of the program should be rotated out of the herd. Thereafter, a serological survey should be done to determine the level of PRV infection remaining in the herd. If prevalence is sufficiently low, the test-and-removal protocol may be implemented.

Eradication of PR by stamping out should be applied only if the prevalence of PRV-positive farms in a region is very low. Stamping out may be necessary in the last stages of PRV eradication, that is, when only a few PRV-positive farms stand in the way of achieving freedom from PRV.

Inherent to the eradication effort is the control of animal movement and a certification of the health status of herds. All farrowing and farrow-to-finish herds that provide piglets must be free of PR. Likewise, all replacement gilts should be tested for the absence of gE antibodies. Monitoring should be done by the purchaser while the pigs are still at the premises of the supplier. Since transportation is a major stress factor and may lead to reactivation and excretion of latent virus, it is strongly recommended that incoming pigs be kept in quarantine for 2–4 weeks, after which they should again be tested for gE antibodies before joining the breeding herd. It is important to recognize that the use of in-herd replacement breeders is responsible in many cases for maintenance of seropositivity in the holdings (Arias and Sanchez-Vizcaino 2002). A regular systematic census of pig herds in the region and at least a yearly serological screening of each pig herd must be performed.

Serological monitoring of expected-negative herds and populations for PRV creates the problem of singleton reactors. In PR surveillance programs in countries free from PRV—e.g., Sweden and Denmark—and in countries infected with PRV, herds are occasionally observed wherein there is a single seropositive pig (Annelli et al. 1991). Singleton reactors create a major problem because the PR status of such farms is uncertain. According to Bascuñana et al. (1997) and Annelli et al. (1991), singleton reactors may represent one of several possibilities. First, the herd may have been infected at some time in the past and the single reactor is the last seropositive pig in the herd. Second, PRV may have been recently introduced into the herd and the single reactor is the first to seroconvert. Third, the singleton reactor may be a false positive and the pig may never have been exposed to the virus. Fourth, for whatever reason, the single reactor may be the only pig in the herd to be infected. And fifth, virulent PRV is circulating in the herd at a low level.

There is currently no uniform regulatory policy for herds with singleton reactors. In the U.S., such herds are quarantined while the reactor is isolated and retested together with a representative sample of other breeding swine. If only the original positive pig retests positive, the herd owner has the option of remaining under quarantine or submitting the reactor for immunosuppressive treatment and diagnostic testing. If the result is positive, the pig should be culled. If PRV is not detected the quarantine is removed (Annelli et al. 1991).

Several PRV prevention, control, and eradication programs, differing to a larger or smaller degree from those previously described, have been implemented in Europe and the U.S. (Andersson et al. 1997; Bech-Nielsen et al. 1995; Müller et al. 2003; Vannier et al. 1997). The approach differs depending on the epidemiological situation and particular opinions of the representatives of the state veterinary services of the country. It should be noted that PR eradication programs are costly (Bech-Nielsen et al. 1995) and efforts to achieve freedom from PRV by the least expensive means possible should be encouraged. In the U.S., the federal government spent $72 million during the first 10 years of the program. In addition, costs were incurred by the various state governments and private swine producers (Taft 2000). In many areas, the presence of PRV in wild boar and feral pigs poses a challenge to the successful eradication of PRV from domestic swine.

REFERENCES

Alva-Valdes R, Glock RD, Kluge JP, Keune CM. 1983. Effects of vaccination on lesion development in pseudorabies virus-challenged swine. Am J Vet Res 44:588–595.

Andersson HA, Lexmon JA, Robertsson N, Lundeheim N, Wierup M. 1997. Agricultural policy and social returns to eradication programs: The case of Aujeszky's disease in Sweden. Prev Vet Med 29:311–328.

Annelli JF, Morrison RB, Goyal SM, Bergeland ME, Mackey WJ, Thawley DG. 1991. Pig herds having a single reactor to serum antibody tests to Aujeszky's disease virus. Vet Rec 128:49–53.

Arias M, Sánchez-Vizcaino JM. 2002. Aujeszky's disease: The challenge. Pig Progress. Special respiratory diseases. 26–28, June 2002. Elsevier International.

Atanasowa Kh. 1972. Resistance of Aujeszky's disease virus in urine of pigs and sheep. Vet Med Nauki 9:69–74.

Babic N, Klupp B, Brack A, Mettenleiter TC, Ugolini G, Flamand A. 1996. Deletion of glycoprotein gR reduces the propagation of pseudorabies virus in the nervous system of the mouse after intranasal inoculation. Virology 219:279–284.

Babic N, Mettenleiter TC, Flamand A, Ugolini G. 1993. Role of essential glycoproteins gII and gp50 in transneuraltransfer of pseudorabies virus from the hypoglossal nerves of mice. J Virol 67:4421–4426.

Babic N, Mettenleiter TC, Ugolini G. 1994. Propagation of pseudorabies virus in the nervous system of the mouse after intranasal inoculation. Virology 204:616–625.

Bascuñana CR, Björnerot L, Ballagi-Pordány A, Robertsson J-Å, Belák S. 1997. Detection of pseudorabies virus genomic sequences in apparently uninfected "single reactor" pigs. Vet Microb 55:37–47.

Baskerville A. 1971. The histopathology of pneumonia by aerosol infection of pigs with a strain of Aujeszky's disease virus. Res Vet Sci 12:590–592.

——. 1972a. The influence of dose of virus on the clinical signs of experimental Aujeszky's disease in pigs. Brit Vet J 128:394–401.

——. 1972b. Aujeszky's disease encephalitis in pigs produced by different modes of infection. Res Vet Sci 14:223–228.

——. 1973. The histopathology of experimental pneumonia in pigs produced by Aujeszky's disease virus. Res Vet Sci 14:223–228.

Baskerville A, McFerran JB, Dow C. 1973. Aujeszyky's disease in pigs. Vet Bull (London) 43:465–480.

Bech-Nielsen S, Bowman GL, Miller GY, Orloski-Snider KO, Burkholder RH, Dodaro SJ. 1995. Pseudorabies (Aujeszky's disease) eradication progress and program cost in Ohio, USA. Prev Vet Med 22:41–53.

Becker CH. 1964. Zur Bedeutung der Lunge für die pathologisch-anatomische Diagnose der Aujeszkyschen Krankheit des Schweines. Monatsh Veterinärmed. 19:5–11.

Benndorf E, Hantschel H. 1963. Zum Verhalten des Aujeszkyvirus bei veschiedenen Wasserstoffkonzentrationen. Arch Exp Vet Med 17:1357–1362.

Ben-Porat T, DeMarchi JM, Lomniczi B, Kaplan AS. 1986. Role of glycoproteins of pseudorabies virus in eliciting neutralizing antibodies. Virology 154:325.

Beran GW. 1991. Transmission of Aujeszky's disease virus. Proc 1st Int Symp on the Eradication of of Pseudoraies (Aujeszky's) Virus. St. Paul, Minnesota, USA. pp. 93–111.

Böhm HO, Sieber C, Strauch D. 1980. Die Wirkung der Umwätzbelüftung auf das Virus der Aujeszkyschen Krankheit. Berl Münch Tierärztl Wochenschr 93:112–114.

Bolin CA, Bolin SR, Kluge JP, Mengeling WL. 1985. Pathologic effects of intrauterine deposition of pseudorabies virus on the reproductive tract of swine in early pregnancy. Am J Vet Res 46:1039–1042.

Bouma A, De Jong MC, Kimman TG. 1997. The influence of maternal immunity on the transmission of pseudorabies virus and on the effectiveness of vaccination. Vaccine 15:287–294.

Brockmeier SL, Lager KM, Mengeling WL. 1997. Vaccination with recombinant vaccinia virus vaccines expressing glycoprotein genes of pseudorabies virus in the presence of maternal immunity. Vet Microbiol 58:93:103.

Brown TT Jr. 1981. Laboratory evaluation of selected disinfectants as virucidal agents against porcine parvovirus. Am J Vet Res 42:1033–1036.

Cheung AK. 1995. Investigation of pseudorabies virus DNA and RNA in trigeminal ganglia and tonsil tissues of latently infected swine. Am J Vet Res 56:45.

Christensen LS, Mousing J, Mortensen S, Soerensen KJ, Strandbygaard SB, Henriksen CA, Andersen JB. 1990. Evidence of long distance airborne transmission of Aujeszky's disease (pseudorabies) virus. Vet Rec 127:471–474.

Corn JL, Lee RM, Erickson GA, Murphy DC. 1987. Serologic survey for evidence of exposure to vesicular stomatitis virus, pseudorabies virus, brucellosis and leptospirosis in collared peccaries from Arizona. J Wildlife Dis 23:552–557.

Corner AH. 1965. Pathology of experimental Aujeszky's disease in piglets. Res Vet Sci 6:337–343.

Davies EB, Beran GW. 1981. Influence of environmental factors upon the survival of Aujeszky's disease virus. Res Vet Sci 31:32–36.

De Smet K, De Waele K, Pensaert M. 1994. Influence of vaccine medium and vaccination schedules on the induction of active immunity against Aujeszky's disease in maternally immune pigs. Res Vet Sci 56:89–94.

Donaldson AI. 1983. Experimental Aujeszky's disease in pigs: Excretion, survival and transmission of the virus. Vet Rec 113:490–494.

Eloit M, Fargeaud D, L'Haridon RL, Toma B. 1988. Identification of pseudorabies virus glycoprotein gp50 as major target of neutralizing antibodies. Arch Virol 99:45.

Enquist IW. 1994. Infection of the mammalian nervous system by pseudorabies virus (PrV). Semin Virol 5:221–231.

——. 1995. Circuit-specific infection of the mammalian nervous system. ASM News 61:633–638.

Enquist LW, Husak PJ, Banfield BW, Smith GA. 1998. Infection and spread of alphaherpesviruses in the nervous system. Adv Virus Res 51:237–347.

Gielkens ALJ, van Oirschot JT, Berns AJM. 1985. Genome differences among field isolates and vaccine strains of pseudorabies virus. J Gen Virol 66:69–82.

Granzow H, Weiland F, Jons A, Klupp BG, Karger A, Mettenleiter TC. 1997. Ultrastructural analysis of the replication cycle of pseudorabies virus in cell culture: A Reassessment. J Virol 71:2072–2082.

Hall LB, Kluge JP, Evans LE, Hill HT. 1984. The effect of pseudorabies (Aujeszky's) virus infection on young mature boars and boar fertility. Can J Comp Med 48:192–197.

Jakubik J. 1977. Comparative susceptibility of rabbits, rats, mice and pigs to infection with Aujeszky's disease virus (ADV) in the development of an efficacy test to ADV vaccines. Zentralbl Veterinarmed B 24:765–766.

Karger A, Mettenleiter TC. 1993. Glycoproteins gIII and gp50 play dominant roles in the biphasic attachment of pseudorabies virus. Virology 194:654–664.

Kluge JP, Maré CJ. 1976. Gross and microscopic lesions of prenatal pseudorabies (Aujeszky's disease) in swine. Proc Int Congr Pig Vet Soc 4:G3.

——. 1978. Natural and experimental in utero infection of piglets with Aujeszky's disease (pseudorabies) virus. Am Assoc Vet Lab Diagn 21:15–24.

Kluge JP, Beran GW, Hill HT, Platt KB. 1999. Pseudorabies (Aujeszky's Disease). In Diseases of Swine (8th edition). BE Straw, S D'Allaire, WL Mengeling, DJ Taylor, eds. Ames: Iowa State University Press, pp. 233–246.

Klupp BG, Mettenleiter TC. 1991. Sequence and expression of the glycoprotein gH gene of pseudorabies virus, Virology 182:732–741.

Koch KMA, Euler B. 1983. Lime as a disinfectant for Aujeszky's disease virus in slurry. In Hygienic Problems of Animal Manure. D Strauch, ed. Stuttgart: Institut für Tiermedizin, Universität Hohenheim, pp. 107–117.

Kretzschmar C. 1970. Die Aujeszkysche Krankheit: Diagnostik, Epizootiologie und Bekämpfung. Gustav Fischer Verlag, Jena. pp. 131–135.

Kritas SK, Nauwynck HJ, Pensaert MB, Kyriakis SC. 1997. Effect of the concentration of maternal antibodies on the neural invasion of Aujeszky's disease virus in neonatal pigs. Vet Microbiol 55:29–36.

Kritas SK, Pensaert MB, Mettenleiter TC. 1994. Role of envelope glycoproteins gI, gp63 and gIII in the invasion and spread of Aujeszky's disease virus in the olfactory nervous pathway of the pig. J Gen Virol 75:2319–2327.

Kritas SK, Pensaert MB, Nauwynck HJ, Kyriakis SC. 1999. Neural invasion of two virulent suid herpesvirus 1 strains in neonatal pigs with or without maternal immunity. Vet Microb 69:143–156.

Kunev Zh. 1978. Resistance of Aujeszky's disease virus to heat. Vet Med Nauki 15:99–105.

Kupershmidt S, de Marchi, J, Lu Z, Ben-Porat T. 1991. Analysis of an origin of DNA replication located at the L terminus of the genome of pseudorabies virus. J Virol 65:6283–6291.

Lipowski A. 2003. European wild boar (*Sus scrofa* L.) as a reservoir of infectious diseases for domestic pigs. Med Weter 59:861–863.

Lipowski A, Pejsak Z. 2002. Antibody prevalence of pseudorabies virus in feral pigs in Poland. Proc Congr Int Pig Vet Soc 2:223.

Lomniczi B, Kaplan AS. 1987. Multiple defects in the genome of pseudorabies virus can affect virulence without detectably affecting replication in cell culture. Virology 161(1):181–189.

Lomniczi B, Watanabe S, Ben-Porat T, Kaplan AS. 1984. Genetic basis of the neurovirulence of pseudorabies virus. J Virol 52:198–205.

——. 1987. Genone location and identification of functions defective in the Bartha vaccine strain of pseudorabies virus. J Virol 61:796–801.

Maes RK, Kanitz CL, Gustafson DP. 1983. Shedding patterns in swine of virulent and attenuated pseudorabies virus. Am J Vet Res 44:2083–2086.

McGeoch DJ, Cook S. 1994. Molecular phylogeny of the alphaherpesvirinae subfamily and a proposed evolutionary timescale. J Mol Biol 238:9–22.

Mengeling WL, Lager KM, Volz DM, Brockmeier SL. 1992. Effect of various vaccination procedures on shedding, latency, and reactivation of attenuated and virulent pseudorabies virus in swine. Am J Vet Res 53:2164–2173.

Mettenleiter T. 1994a. Pseudorabies (Aujeszky's disease) virus: State of the art. August 1993. Acta Vet Hung 42:153–177.

——. 1994b. Initiation and spread of alpha-herpesvirus infections. Trend Microbiol 2:2–4.

——. 1996. Immunobiology of pseudorabies (Aujeszky's Disease). Vet Immunol Immunopathol 54:221–229.

——. 2000. Aujeszky's disease (pseudorabies) virus: The virus and molecular pathogenesis—State of the art, June 1999. Vet Res 31:99–115.

Mettenleiter TC, Rauh I. 1990. A glycoprotein gX-beta-galactosidase fusion gene as insertional marker for rapid identification of pseudorabies virus mutants. J Virol Methods 30:55–66.

Müller T, Batza HJ, Schluter H, Conraths FJ, Mettenleiter TC. 2003. Eradication of Aujeszky's disease in Germany. J Vet Med B Infect Dis Vet Public Health 50:207–213.

Nakamura T, Ihara T, Nunoya T, Kuwahara H, Ishihama A, Ueda S. 1993. Role of pseudorabies glycoprotein II in protection from lethal infection. Vet Microbiol 36:83–90.

Narita M, Haritani M, Moriwaki M. 1984a. Necrotizing vasculitis in piglets infected orally with the virus of Aujeszky's disease. Nippon Juigaku Zasshi 46:119–122.

Narita M, Kuto M, Fukush OA, Haratani M, Moriwaki M. 1984b. Necrotizing enteritis in piglets associated with the virus of Aujeszky's disease. Vet Pathol 21:450–452,

Nauwynck H. 1997. Functional aspects of Aujeszky's disease (pseudorabies) viral proteins with relation to invasion, virulence and immunogenicity. Vet Microbiol 55:3–11.

Pejsak Z, Markowska-Daniel I. 1996. Virus as a reason for reproductive failure in pig herds in Poland. Reprod Domest Anim 31:445–447.

Pensaert M, Kluge J. 1989. Pseudorabies virus (Aujeszky's disease). In Virus Infections of Vertebrates, Vol 2. Virus Infections of Porcines. MB Pesaert, ed. Amsterdam: Elsevier Science Publishers BV, pp. 39–64.

Priola SA, Stevens JG. 1991. The 5' and 3' limits of transcription in the pseudorabies virus latency associated transcription unit. Virology 182:852–886.

Quint W, Gielkens A, Van Oirschot J, Berns A, Cuypers HT. 1987. Construction and characterization of deletion mutants of pseudorabies virus: A new generation of "live" vaccines. J Gen Virol 68:523–534.

Rauh I, Mettenleiter TC. 1991. Pseudorabies virus glycoproteins gII and gp50 are essential for virus penetration. J Virol 65:5348–5356.

Schang LM, Kutish GF, Osorio FA. 1994. Correlation between precolonisation of trigeminal ganglia by attenuated strains of pseudorabies virus and resistance to wild-type virus latency. J Virol 68:8470–8476.

Schmidt J, Gerdts V, Beyer J, Klupp BG, Mettenleiter TC. 2001. Glycoprotein D-independent infectivity of pseudorabies virus results in an alteration of in vivo host range and correlates with mutations in glycoproteins B and H. J Virol 75(21):10054–10064.

Stegeman A. 1995. Pseudorabies virus eradication by area-wide vaccination is feasible. Ph.D. thesis. University of Utrecht, Utrecht, The Netherlands.

Szweda W, Lipowski A, Bączek W, Dadun M, Platt-Samoraj A, Siemionek J. 2000a. The results of Aujeszky's disease virus elimination from pig farms after 5 years of implementing the "vaccination-eradication programme." Med Weter 56:386–391.

Szweda W, Lipowski A, Bączek W, Platt-Samoraj A, Siemionek J. 2000b. The efficacy of the vaccination-eradication programme in maintaining a pig farm's status as being free from Aujeszky's disease virus. Med Weter 56:447–451.

Taft AC. 2000. The eradication of Aujeszky's disease in the United States. Vet Res 31:157–158.

Tamba W, Calabrese R, Finelli E, Cordioli P. 2002. Risk factors for Aujeszky's disease seropositivity of swine herds of a region of northern Italy. Prev Vet Med 54:203–212.

Thawley DG, Morrison RB. 1988. Programs for the elimination of pseudorabies virus from large herds of swine. J Am Vet Med Assoc 193:184–190.

Toma B, Haddad N, Vannier P. 2004. Aujeszky's disease. In Manual of Diagnostic Tests and Vaccines for Terrestrial Animals (5th edition), Part II. Office International des Epizooties, World Organisation for Animal Health. pp. 295–307.

Tsuda T, Onodera T, Sugimura T, Murakami Y. 1992. Induction of protective immunity and neutralizing antibodies to pseudorabies virus by immunization of anti-idiotypic antibodies. Arch Virol 124:291–300.

Van Oirschot JT. 1987. Intranasal vaccination of pigs against Aujeszky's disease: Comparison with one or two doses of attenuated vaccines in pigs with high maternal antibody titers. Res Vet Sci 42:12–16.

Van Oirschot JT, Gielkens ALJ, Moormann RJM, Berbs AJM. 1990. Marker vaccines, virus protein-specific antibody assays and the control of Aujeszky's disease. Vet Microbiol 23:85–101.

Vannier P. 1988. The control programme of Aujeszky's disease in France: Main results and difficulties. In Vaccination and Control of Aujeszky's Disease. JT Van Oirschot, ed. Boston: Kluwer Academic Publishers, pp. 215–226.

Vannier P, Vedeau F, Allemeersch C. 1997. Eradication and control programmes against Aujeszky's disease (pseudorabies) in France. Vet Microbiol 55:167–173.

Visser N. 1997. Vaccination strategies for improving the efficacy of programs to eradicate Aujeszky's disease virus. Vet Microbiol 55:61–74.

Waston WA. 1986. Epidemiology and control of Aujeszky's disease in Great Britain. Rev Sci Tech OIE 5:363–378.

Weyhe D, Benndorf E. 1970. Zur Haltbarkeit des Aujeszky–Virus in Schlackthausprodukten von infizierten Schweinen unter Kühlhausbedingungen. Arch Exp Vet Med 25:236–239.

Wittmann G. 1985. Aujeszky's disease: Factors important for epizootiology and control. Rev Sci Tech OIE 4:5–20.

——. 1986. Aujeszky's disease. Rev Sci Tech OIE 5:959–977.

——. 1991. Die Beeinträchtigung der Schutzimpfung von Saugferkeln mit inaktivierter Aujeszkyvakzine durch kolostrale Immunität. Tierärztl Umschau 36:523–528.

Wittmann G, Jakubik J. 1979. Colostral immunity in piglets from sows vaccinated with inactivated Aujeszky's disease virus vaccine. Arch Virol 60:33–42.

Wittmann G, Leitzke I. 1985. Die Beeinflussung des Aujeszkyvirus— Neutralisations tests durch verschiedene Testbedingungen. Dtsch Tierärztl Wochenschr 92:262–266.

Wittmann G, Rziha HJ. 1989. Aujeszky's disease (pseudorabies) in pigs. In: Wittmann G (editor), Herpesvirus diseases of cattle, horses, and pigs. Kluwer Academic Publishers, Boston, Massachussets. pp. 230–325.

Wooley RE, Gilbert JP, Whitehead WK, Shotts EB Jr, Dobbins CN. 1981. Survival of viruses in fermented edible waste material. Am J Vet Res 42:87–90.

Zimmerman JJ, Yoon K-J (editors). 2003. The PRRS Compendium (2nd edition). A Comprehensive Reference for Pork Producers, Veterinary Practitioners, and Researchers. National Pork Board, Des Moines Iowa 50306. ISBN 0-9722877-1-X. 294 pages.

26 Rotavirus and Reovirus

Lijuan Yuan, Gregory W. Stevenson, and Linda J. Saif

Porcine Rotavirus

Rotaviruses (RV) are important causes of diarrheal disease in neonates and the young of many species and a common cause of gastroenteritis in sucking and postweaning pigs. Rotaviruses were first discovered in calves (Mebus et al. 1969) and were later detected in humans (Bishop et al. 1973), pigs (Rodger et al. 1975), and other animals (Estes et al. 1983). Porcine RV have been detected in most swine-producing countries and are associated with economic losses caused by diarrheal disease in pigs (Paul and Stevenson 1999).

Porcine rotaviruses are antigenically diverse with four serogroups (A–C, E) and, within serogroup A, 10 G types (VP7 type for glycoprotein) and 7 P types (VP4 type for protease-sensitive protein). Although information pertaining to all porcine RV groups is included, group A RV are most commonly associated with diarrhea in humans and pigs and, therefore, the most extensively studied. In this chapter, if the RV group is not specified, the information pertains to group A RV.

ETIOLOGY
Virus Morphology

Rotaviruses are 65–75 nm, nonenveloped, icosahedral particles. By electron microscopy (EM), the morphology of complete RV particles resembles a wheel (*Rota* in Latin) with short spikes and a smooth outer rim (~75 nm in diameter). The particles are composed of a three-layered viral protein (VP) capsid: the outer layer (VP7 and VP4), the intermediate layer (VP6), and the inner layer (VP2). The viral genome, composed of 11 segments of double-strained (ds) RNA, is enclosed in VP2 along with the RNA-dependent RNA polymerase (VP1). Only the complete triple-layered particles are infectious (Estes 2001). Double-layered particles lacking the outer layer are smaller (~65 nm) with rough edges (Figure 26.1).

Classification

Rotaviruses are classified in the genus *Rotavirus* in the family *Reoviridae*. Based on VP6 antigens, RV are divided serologically into seven distinct groups (A through G) (Estes 2001; Saif and Jiang 1994). Within a group, RVs share cross-reactive antigens on VP6 detectable by serological tests. Groups A–C infect humans and other animals; group E has only been detected in pigs in the UK (Chasey et al. 1986). Groups D, F and G have been detected only in avian species. When subjected to electrophoresis in polyacrylamide gels (PAGE), the RV genome has a characteristic electrophoretic migration pattern referred to as the electropherotype. Each RV serogroup has a unique electropherotype (Pedley et al. 1986; Saif and Jiang 1994). The RNA segments cluster into regions I, II, III, and IV (Figure 26.2). The cluster patterns include 4:2:3:2 (group A), 4:2:2:3 (group B), 4:3:2:2 (group C), and 5:2:2:2 (group D). The group E pattern is similar to group B, except segments 7–11 migrate equidistant from each other. Genome profile analysis using PAGE is a relatively simple technique to identify RV, differentiate them from reoviruses (10 dsRNA segments), and identify RV groups (Janke et al. 1990). However, serologic and nucleic acid-based assays are needed to confirm RV groups and serotypes.

Rotaviruses within serogroup A are further divided into subgroups. In earlier studies, five subgroups (SG) I, II, I+II, and non-I, non-II were defined according to the presence or absence of two distinct epitopes on VP6 reactive with one, both, or neither of the monoclonal antibodies (MAbs) specific for each of the epitopes (Greenberg et al. 1983). Porcine RV strain OSU belongs to SG I and Gottfried strain belongs to SG II. Recent molecular characterization of the subgroup-defining region of VP6 gene suggested two genogroups: genogroup

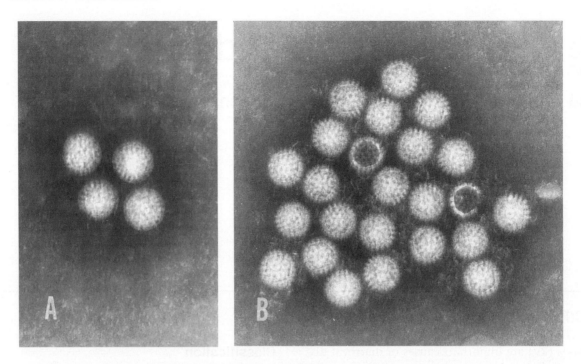

26.1. *Rotavirus particles in feces viewed by negative-staining electron microscopy (×130,000). (A) Triple-layered virus particles with intact outer capsids have characteristic smooth outlines. (B) Double-layered particles lack outer capsids and have spiked outlines.*

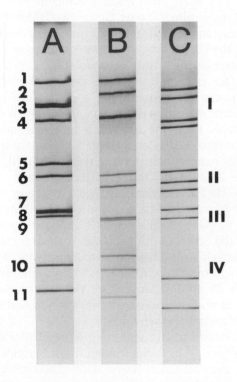

26.2. *Electrophoretic patterns (electropherotypes) of A/OSU, B/IA1146, and C/Cowden strains of groups A, B, and C rotaviruses in polyacrylamide gel stained with silver. Each rotavirus group has a distinct electropherotype. Double-stranded RNA segments cluster in four regions, I–IV. The numbers of bands in the four regions are 4:2:3:2, 4:2:2:3, and 4:3:2:2 for rotavirus groups A, B, and C respectively.*

I (consists of SG I) and genogroup II (includes SG II, I+II, and non-I, non-II) (Iturriza-Gomara et al. 2002).

Within serogroup A, RV are further classified into different G and P serotypes or genotypes (Table 26.1). Serotypes are defined by reactivity of virus in plaque reduction (or fluorescent foci reduction) neutralization assays using polyclonal or MAbs (Estes and Cohen 1989; Hoshino et al. 1984). Genotypes are defined by comparative sequence analysis and/or nucleic acid hybridization data. Strains sharing >89% amino acid sequence identities are considered to belong to the same genotype (Estes 2001; Gorziglia et al. 1990). Serotype is denoted by a number following the letter P or G and genotype is signified by the number in square brackets. For example, porcine RV strain Gottfried is classified as P2B[6]G4 and strain OSU as P9[7]G5. The VP7 serotypes and genotypes are highly consistent; however, a general correlation between P genotypes and P serotypes has not been clearly established due to difficulties in generating type-specific antibodies to VP4 (Estes 2001). Currently, 15 RV G serotypes/genotypes have been identified, whereas, out of 22 different P genotypes reported, only 13 P serotypes have been identified (Hoshino and Kapikian 1996; Hoshino et al. 2002; Liprandi et al. 2003; Martella et al. 2003; Okada et al. 2000). In pigs, at least 10 G types of group A RV (G1–6, 8–10, and 11) and 7 P types (P[5]–[8], [13], [19], and [23]) are associated with diarrhea (Martella et al. 2001). Within serogroup C porcine RV, at least 2 G serotypes have been suggested based on cross-neutralization tests (Tsunemitsu et al. 1992b).

Table 26.1. Serogroup, serotype, and genotype designations of selected porcine rotaviruses[a]

Serogroup	VP7 Serotype/Genotype	Strain	VP4 (P) Serotype (G) [Genotype]	Strain
A	1	C60, C86, C95, S8	1A[8]	S8
	2	C134*b	2B[6]	Gottfried, BEN-144
	3	CRW-8, C176, BEN-307 ISU-65, 4F, MRD-13* LCA843, Clone 8	7[5]	P343 84/52F, 84/106F, 84/158F
	4	Gottfried, SB-1A	9[7]	OSU, EE, TFR-41, C134 CRW-8, BEN-307, SB-1A
	5	OSU, C134*, EE, TFR-41, A34 MDR-13*, A46, S8		C60, C95, YM, A253 LCA843
	6	84/52F, 84/106F, 84/158F	Not tested [13]	MDR-13, A46, Clone 8
	8	field sample	12[19]	4F
	9	ISU-64	14[23]	A34
	10	P343		
	11	YM, A253		
B		Ohio NIAD-1 IA1146		
C		Cowden, HF IA850		
E		DC-9		

Table is adopted and modified from Kapikian et al. 2001; Paul et al. 1999.
*Dual G serotypes were reported.

Other assays used to differentiate RV of different serotypes and/or genotypes include ELISA using serotype-specific MAbs, endonuclease digestion of PCR-amplified VP4 and VP7 gene products (RFLP) (Chang et al. 1996), and reverse transcriptase polymerase chain reaction (RT-PCR) (Barreiros et al. 2003).

Physicochemical and Biological Properties

The RV genome consists of 11 segments of dsRNA that range in size from 0.6–3.3 kilobase pairs (Estes and Cohen 1989). The 11 segments encode six viral structural proteins and six nonstructural proteins (NSP) with segment 12 encoding both NSP5 and 6 (Estes 2001). The six structural proteins are: the core proteins VP1 to 3, the nonglycosylated outer capsid protein VP4 (encoded by gene 4), the major structural component of virions VP6 (encoded by gene 6), and the outer capsid glycoprotein VP7 (encoded by gene 9). Proteolytic cleavage of VP4 into VP5 and VP8 is important for viral infectivity. The VP7 is the second most abundant viral structural protein after VP6. Proteins analogous to VP6 and VP7 have also been described for group C RV (Jiang et al. 1990).

Triple- and double-layered RV particles can be separated by centrifugation in gradients of sucrose or cesium chloride (CsCl). Triple-layered particles have a density of 1.36 g/ml in CsCl and sediment coefficients of 520S to 530S in sucrose, whereas double-layered particles have a density of 1.38 g/cm^3 and sediment at 380S to 400S (Tam et al. 1976). Single-layered core particles have a density of 1.44 g/ml in CsCl and a sedimentation coefficient of 280S (Bican et al. 1982). Treatment of RV particles with calcium-chelating agents (e.g., EDTA) removes the outer capsid and results in loss of infectivity, indicat-

ing that calcium plays a critical role in particle stability by stabilizing the outer capsid VP7 (Ahmadian and Shahrabadi 1999; Bridger and Woode 1976; Estes et al. 1979). The concentration of calcium needed to stabilize the outer capsid varies, depending on the virus strain (Ruiz et al. 1996).

Rotavirus is a nonenveloped virus. Therefore, its infectivity and particle integrity are generally resistant to fluorocarbon extraction and exposure to ether, chloroform, or detergents (deoxycholate) (Estes 2001). Chloroform reduces RV infectivity slightly and destroys hemagglutinating activity. Rotavirus infectivity is relatively stable within the pH range of 3.0–9.0. The hemagglutinating VP4 spikes are removed by treatment at high pH. Repeated freezing and thawing will result in loss of infectivity and hemagglutination activity.

Many RV strains, including some strains of porcine RV, agglutinate human type O, guinea pig, and rat erythrocytes (Eiguchi et al. 1987). Hemagglutination is mediated by the interaction of VP4 with sialic acid on the surface of erythrocytes (Fuentes-Panana et al. 1995). The cell surface molecules employed by RV to initiate infection vary, depending on different strains, and have not been fully identified. The initial contact of RV with the cell surface is mediated by either a neuraminidase-sensitive (requiring sialic acid) or a neuraminidase-resistant cell molecule (Ciarlet et al. 2002). The majority of porcine RV strains are sialic acid-dependent with a few exceptions (OSU, A46 and 4F), whereas most human and animal RV strains are sialic acid-independent. Several cell surface proteins have been implicated as attachment or post-attachment receptors for RV, including gangliosides, integrins and the heat shock protein

70 (Graham et al. 2003; Guerrero et al. 2002; Hewish et al. 2000; Isa et al. 2004; Rolsma et al. 1998). Gangliosides play a major role in recognition of host cells by porcine OSU RV strain (Rolsma et al. 1998).

Laboratory Cultivation

Porcine RV were first adapted to grow in primary porcine kidney cell cultures by pretreatment of viral inoculum with trypsin or pancreatin (Theil et al. 1977). Viruses were later successfully propagated in the African green monkey kidney cell line MA-104 (Bohl et al. 1984) by using roller cultures and addition of trypsin or pancreatin. Roller cultures and proteolytic enzymes are essential for isolation of RV. The enzyme concentrations used for virus activation are 10 µg/ml for trypsin or 2.5 µg/ml for pancreatin before infection. Alternatively, trypsin or pancreatin (0.5–1.0 µg/ml) is added to serum-free culture medium after virus adsorption. Cell culture–adapted RV strains produce a cytopathic effect characterized by rounding of cells followed by cell detachment from the monolayer. Viral antigen can be demonstrated in the cytoplasm of virus-infected cells by IF (Figure 26.3) or immunochemical methods. Rotaviruses form plaques under agarose in the presence of proteolytic enzymes (Ramia and Sattar 1980).

Group C and B porcine RV have been propagated in primary porcine kidney cell cultures using roller cultures and high concentrations of pancreatin (Sanekata et al. 1996; Terrett et al. 1987). The porcine group C RV (Cowden) was subsequently adapted to grow in MA-104 cells (Saif et al. 1988) and a porcine intestinal cell line (Proescholdt 1991). Group E RV, most group B RV, and some group A RV still cannot be serially propagated in cell cultures.

EPIDEMIOLOGY

Rotaviruses are ubiquitous in the environment and in swine herds. It is difficult to raise pigs free of porcine RV under normal husbandry conditions (Bridger and Brown 1985). Multiple RV serogroups (A, B, C, and E) and multiple serotypes within serogroups A and C have been detected in pigs (Atii et al. 1990; Barreiros et al. 2003; Bohl et al. 1984; Geyer et al. 1996; Janke et al. 1990; Kim et al. 1999; Markowska-Daniel et al. 1996; Pongsuwanna et al. 1996; Saif 1999; Saif and Jiang 1994; Theil et al. 1985; Wieler et al. 2001; Will et al. 1994; Winiarczyk et al. 2002). The RV serogroup distributions detected in feces of diarrheic pigs are summarized in Table 26.2.

Group A RV is detected most frequently in pigs under 60 days of age from as early as 1 week to the highest prevalence at 3–5 weeks of age (Bohl 1979). The prevalence of infection increases with age during the sucking period due to the decline in maternal antibody titers. When maternally acquired immunity decreases to unprotective levels, pigs become susceptible to RV diar-

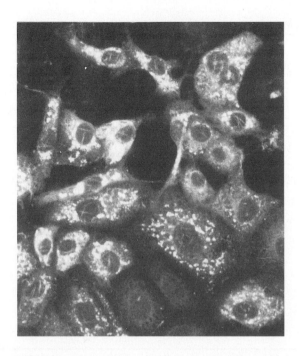

26.3. *Immunofluorescent staining of MA-104 cells infected with group A porcine rotavirus showing cytoplasmic accumulation of rotaviral antigens (×400).*

rhea. Infected pigs shed virus for 1–14 days in feces with an average duration of 7.4 days (Fu and Hampson 1987).

In group B RV infections, lower amounts of RV are shed and for a shorter duration (Bridger 1980; Theil et al. 1985). Group C RV caused diarrhea in 8- to 9-week-old weaned pigs with morbidity ranging from 60 to 80%, but with no mortality in Michigan swine farms (Kim et al. 1999). Group E RV has been reported only in one outbreak of pig diarrhea in the UK (Chasey and Davies 1984), but experimental infection of gnotobiotic pigs with group E RV caused mild diarrhea. A serological survey in the UK indicated a widespread distribution of antibodies to this virus in pigs older than 10 weeks (Chasey et al. 1986).

The serologic prevalence of antibodies to RV varies for each serogroup in different regions of the world and is age-related (Table 26.3) (Bridger and Brown 1985; Brown et al. 1987; Chasey et al. 1986; Hung et al. 1987; Nagesha et al. 1988; Terrett et al. 1987; Theil and Saif 1985; Tsunemitsu et al. 1992a).

Molecular genomic methods, e.g., northern-blot and dot-blot hybridization and reverse transcription-polymerase chain reaction (RT-PCR), have led to a better definition of the distribution of group A RV G and P types in pigs. To date, predominant G types identified in pigs are G3 (CRW-like), G4 (Gottfried-like), G5 (OSU-like), and G11 (YM-like); although human types G1, G2, and G9, and bovine types G6, G8, and G10, have also been detected in pigs. The most common P types in pigs are P2B[6] and P9[7], which are Gottfried-like and OSU-like types, respectively. Other porcine P genotypes P[8]

Table 26.2. Rotavirus prevalence and serogroup distribution

Country	Report	Age	Total No. Samples Tested from Diarrheic Pigs	No. of Rotavirus Positives	% Rotavirus Positive	A	B	C	mixed	Assay Used in the Study
						\multicolumn{4}{c}{% in Each Serogroup Among the Positive Samples}		
Nigeria	Atii et al. (1990)	All ages	96	43	44.8	100				ELISA
		4–6 weeks	41	14	34.2	100				
		1–3 weeks	52	29	55.8	100				
		>6 weeks	3	0	0					
USA	Janke et al. (1990)	All ages	NR[a]	90	NR	68	10	11	11	PAGE
		Suckling pigs	NR	68	NR	76.4	7.4	7.4	8.8	
		Weaned pigs	NR	22	NR	40.9	18.2	22.7	18.2	
USA	Will et al. (1994)	All ages	1048	96	9	89	6	5	1	ELISA, PAGE
Thailand	Pongsuwanna et al. (1996)	Piglets	557	26	4.7	89	4	8	0	PAGE
South Africa	Geyer et al. (1996)	Piglets (<6 weeks)	NR	NR	37.8	84.6	4.6	10.8	ND[b]	PAGE
Poland	Markowska-Daniel et al. (1996)	Piglets	531	169	32	100				ELISA
Germany	Wieler et al. (2001)	1–7 days (suckling)	33	0	0	NR	NR	NR	NR	EM
		8–14 days (suckling)	50	1	2	NR	NR	NR	NR	
		15–21 days (suckling)	19	1	5.3	NR	NR	NR	NR	
		22–28 days (weaned)	16	4	25	NR	NR	NR	NR	
		36–42 days	31	0	0					
Brazil	Barreiros et al. (2003)	All ages	99	53	53.5	100				PAGE
		≤7 days (suckling)	19	10	53	100				
		8–21 days (suckling)	20	12	60	100				
		>21 days (weaned)	60	31	52	100				

[a]NR = not reported.
[b]ND = not determined.

Table 26.3. Prevalence of antibody to serogroup A, B, and C porcine rotaviruses in sera from pigs[a]

Country	Report	Year of Sera Collection	Age	Total No. Sera Tested	A	B	C
					\multicolumn{3}{c}{Rotavirus Serogroup (% Positive)[b]}	
USA	Theil and Saif (1985)	1984–1987	adult	37	100	24	ND[c]
USA	Theil and Saif (1985)	1984–1987	young pigs(3–8 wks)	7	100	17	ND
USA	Terrett et al. (1987)	1984–1987	adult	68	100	ND	100
			young pigs (0–8 wks)	69	100	ND	70
USA	Tsunemitsu et al. (1992)	1988–1992	adult	68	NR[d]	NR	97
Japan	Tsunemitsu et al. (1992)	1988–1992	adult	80	NR	NR	93
UK	Bridger and Brown (1985)	1981	adult	39	97	92	79
UK	Bridger and Brown (1985)	1981	young pigs (3–8 wks)	43	100	70	58
Australia	Nagesha et al. (1988)	1988	adult	12	100	58	100
UK	Brown et al. (1987)	1983	adult	67	ND	97	ND
China	Hung et al. (1987)	NR	adult	202	ND	36	ND

[a]Table is adopted and modified from Saif and Jiang 1994.
[b]Virus antigens used for immunofluorescence, immune electron microscopy, ELISA or counterimmunoelectrophoresis included A/OSU, B/NIRD-1 or B/ADRV, and C/Cowden.
[c]ND = not determined.
[d]NR = not reported.

and P[6] (M37-like) and bovine P genotypes P[1], P[5] and P[11] have also been detected (Table 26.1) (Barreiros et al. 2003; Gouvea et al. 1994a,b; Martella et al. 2001; Pongsuwanna et al. 1996; Rosen et al. 1994; Santos et al. 1999; Winiarczyk and Gradzki 1999; Winiarczyk et al. 2002; Zaberezhny et al. 1994).

Rotavirus is shed in feces and the major route of transmission is thought to be fecal-oral. However, a recent study of gnotobiotic pigs showed that pigs orally or nasally inoculated with a virulent group A human RV (Wa strain) shed similar titers nasally and in feces for 3–4 days (Saif et al. 2003). Whether porcine RV spreads among pigs via the respiratory route needs to be investigated.

Rotavirus can be detected in dust and dried feces in facilities that have been occupied by young pigs (Fu et al. 1989). Rotavirus maintained infectivity in feces for 7–9 months at room temperature (presumably 18–20°C) (Woode 1978) and was still infectious in feces stored at 10°C for 32 months (Ramos et al. 2000). Persistence of RV in the environment provides a mechanism for constant exposure of pigs.

Rotaviruses are resistant to inactivation by many chemical disinfectants and antiseptics (Abad et al. 1997), but can be inactivated by disinfectants such as phenols, formalin, chlorine, and beta-propiolactone. Ethanol (95%), perhaps the most effective disinfectant, exerts its effect by removing the outer capsid (Estes 2001). Disinfectant spray containing ethanol (0.1% o-phenylphenol and 79% ethanol), bleach (6% sodium hypochlorite diluted to give 800 ppm free chlorine), and phenol-based products (14.7% phenol diluted 1:256 in tap water) effectively reduced the RV titer by 95% to 99% after a 10-minute treatment (Sattar et al. 1994).

Many studies have provided evidence for interspecies RV transmission (pigs and cattle, pigs and horses, pigs and humans) and for reassortment of RV. Martella et al. (2001) reported that RV isolated from diarrheic pigs in Italy displayed typical bovine RV G- and P-type specificities, indicating a pathogenic role for bovine RV in piglets. An experimental study of bovine RV strain PP-1 infection in gnotobiotic pigs illustrated that RV circulating in one animal species can pose a risk to another by the emergence of a pathogenic reassortant RV under appropriate conditions (El-Attar et al. 2001). Antigenic and molecular analyses of a horse RV strain H-1 revealed that this virus is closely related to porcine, but not equine RV, suggesting interspecies transmission from pigs to horses (Ciarlet et al. 2001). Molecular characterization of a human RV strain RMC321 from an outbreak of RV diarrhea in India revealed porcine characteristics in most of the genes including VP4, VP6, and NSP1-5 (95–99% amino acid identity) (Varghese et al. 2004). This study provided strong evidence that porcine RV can cross the species barrier and cause severe gastroenteritis in humans. Many studies have also indicated that reassortment occurs between pig and human RV strains (Alfieri et al. 1996; Das et al. 1993; Dunn et al. 1993; Laird et al. 2003; Nakagomi and Nakagomi 2002) and some of the reassortant viruses caused diarrhea in humans (Esona et al. 2004; Gerna et al. 1992; Santos et al. 1999; Timenetsky Mdo et al. 1997). The zoonotic potential of porcine RV requires further investigation and continued surveillance.

PATHOGENESIS

Rotavirus pathogenesis is complex and diarrhea induction involves several mechanisms (Estes et al. 2001). Maladsorption caused by loss of intestinal absorptive cells resulting from villous atrophy is the widely accepted

mechanism of RV-induced diarrhea in pigs and humans (Kapikian et al. 2001). Recent studies have suggested that intestinal inflammatory responses (Zijlstra et al. 1999), activation of the enteric nervous system (Lundgren and Svensson 2001), and the enterotoxin function of RV NSP4 (Ball et al. 1996; Estes et al. 2001) also contribute to a secretory-type diarrhea in RV infection.

Rotavirus replicates predominantly in the cytoplasm of differentiated small intestinal villous epithelial cells (Buller and Moxley 1988) and in cecal or colonic epithelia cells (Collins et al. 1989; Theil et al. 1978; Ward et al. 1996b). Virus replicates most extensively longitudinally in the jejunum and ileum of the small intestine. Vertically, RV antigens were observed in nearly all villous epithelial cells in jejunum and ileum and in a few epithelial cells on villous tips in the duodenum at 12 to 48 hours post inoculation (Figure 26.4) (Collins et al.

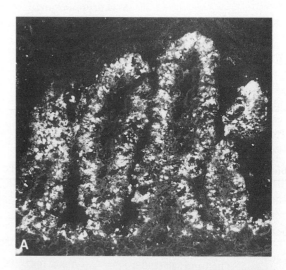

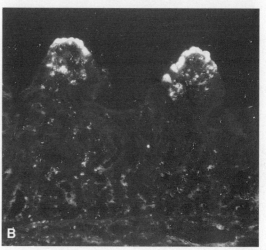

26.4. *Rotavirus antigen in the cytoplasm of villous epithelial cells as viewed by the indirect fluorescent antibody method (×90). (A) Ileum from 1-day-old gnotobiotic pig 16 hours post inoculation with porcine rotavirus. Nearly all villous epithelial cells contain viral antigen. (B) Midjejunum from a 27-day-old weaned conventional pig 3 days postinoculation. Viral antigen is in epithelial cells on villous tips.*

1989; Saif 1999; Shaw et al. 1989; Stevenson 1990; Theil et al. 1978; Ward et al. 1996b).

Rotavirus replication in the villus enterocytes results in cell lysis and attendant villous blunting and atrophy. The degree of villous atrophy and the distribution of atrophic villi in the small intestine vary relative to the RV strain (Collins et al. 1989), serogroup (Saif 1999) and the age of pigs (Shaw et al. 1989). In general, villous atrophy is more severe and extensive in younger pigs. Porcine group A and C RV tend to induce more severe villous atrophy and diarrhea than group B and E in pigs (Saif 1999). Group B RV produces scattered foci of infection in the villous tips of the distal small intestines and mild diarrhea (Saif and Jiang 1994).

Piglets that developed RV diarrhea following administration of porcine or human RV demonstrated functional alterations in small intestinal villous epithelial cells, including impaired glucose-coupled sodium transport (Davidson et al. 1977; Rhoads et al. 1991), decreased disaccharidase activity (Graham and Estes 1991; Zijlstra et al. 1997), and increased thymidine kinase activity (Davidson et al. 1977). These pathophysiological changes all contribute to the maladsorptive diarrhea (Saif 1999). Of importance for swine management, malnutrition increases the severity and duration of RV diarrhea by delaying the restoration of enzymatic and absorptive capacity and hampering the regeneration of damaged intestinal villi (Zijlstra et al. 1997).

In experimentally infected pigs, RV diarrhea precedes the detection of intestinal histopathologic damage, suggesting that other mechanisms, besides villous atrophy, contribute to the RV-induced disease expression (McAdaragh et al. 1980; Theil et al. 1978; Ward et al. 1996b). Intestinal inflammation activates neural reflex pathways in the enteric nervous system. The latter is a critical component in regulating fluid secretion in the normal gut and a key element in the pathophysiology of several important veterinary pathogens such as *Salmonella* sp., *Cryptosporidium parvum*, and RV (Jones and Blikslager 2002; Lundgren et al. 2000). In mice, at least two-thirds of the fluid and electrolyte secretion caused by RV was ascribed to activation of the enteric nervous system (Lundgren and Svensson 2001). Inflammation can also disrupt mucosal integrity and create leaky membranes, further allowing translocation of bacteria and toxins across the intestinal epithelial barrier and initiation of systemic infection (Blikslager and Roberts 1997). Transient increases in macromolecular permeability were observed in piglets infected with RV (Moon 1997), and in vitro studies showed that RV infection led to enhanced toxin uptake into cells (Liprandi et al. 1997). Such findings suggest that RV infections could predispose pigs to more severe bacterial infections via enhanced uptake of toxins or the bacteria, the latter instance leading to septicemia. Mixed infection by RV and enterotoxigenic *E. coli* resulted in more severe diarrhea

than did inoculation of pigs with each agent separately (Benfield et al. 1988).

The RV NSP4 was initially suggested to play a role, along with VP3, VP4, and VP7, in RV pathogenesis in a study using gnotobiotic pigs and reassortant RV (Hoshino et al. 1995). Subsequently, NSP4 was recognized as a viral enterotoxin, contributing to the pathogenesis of RV diarrhea in mice (Ball et al. 1996; Estes et al. 2001). Recombinant baculovirus-expressed NSP4 from simian RV SA11 strain was reported to induce dose- and age-dependent diarrhea in a neonatal mouse model (Ball et al. 1996). It is hypothesized that NSP4 may indirectly participate in the stimulation of the enteric nervous system by causing the release of amines/peptides from villous endocrine cells via its effect on intracellular calcium, which may in turn activate the enteric nervous system in a way similar to that demonstrated for cholera toxin (Lundgren and Svensson 2001). The role of NSP4 in RV diarrhea in pigs and other farm animals has not been confirmed. There are also many other biologically active molecules produced by epithelial cells or immunological cells in RV infection that may participate in activating secretory reflexes in the enteric nervous system and may play a role in RV-induced diarrhea and pathogenesis (Rollo et al. 1999).

Several interrelated factors may be involved in the death of RV-inoculated pigs that could be prevented by effective management strategies. Low environmental temperature (Steel and Torres-Medina 1984), malnutrition (Zijlstra et al. 1997, 1999), and high virus exposure dose (Shaw et al. 1989) are important factors that contribute to more severe diarrhea and higher mortality in RV-infected pigs. Diarrhea causes dehydration and electrolyte imbalances and may lead to exhaustion of extracellular fluid reserves, requiring treatment with oral electrolytes. Malabsorption results in malnutrition and may lead to energy deficiency and hypothermia; which may be countered by providing external heat sources to scouring pigs and rehydration fluids as needed. Observed higher mortality in neonatal pigs is likely related to more severe and extensive villous atrophy, coupled with decreased extracellular fluid and energy reserves, compared to slightly older pigs.

Rotavirus infection was thought to be mostly localized to the intestine. Occasionally, extraintestinal RV infections were reported in humans and animals. Rotavirus was detected in the lung of one of 13 experimentally infected 3-week-old conventional pigs at postinoculation day (PID) two (Shaw et al. 1989). However, recent studies have shown that systemic RV infection (viremia or antigenemia) is not uncommon in animals (calves, mice, rats, and rabbits) and humans (Blutt et al. 2003). A virulent human RV strain (Wa) caused transient viremia in gnotobiotic pigs after oral or intranasal inoculation (Saif et al. 2003). The role of RV viremia in RV pathogenesis and protective immunity to RV is unknown.

CLINICAL SIGNS

Inoculation of naive 1- to 5-day-old gnotobiotic or colostrum-deprived conventional pigs with RV consistently produces severe diarrheal disease (McAdaragh et al. 1980; Pearson and McNulty 1977; Tzipori and Williams 1978; Ward et al. 1996b; Woode et al. 1976). Pigs become listless, anorexic, and occasionally vomit by 12–24 hours after inoculation and then develop profuse watery, yellow-to-white flocculent diarrhea 1–4 hours later. Diarrhea continues for 3–7 days and progressively resolves in 7–14 days. Mortality can reach 50 to 100%. When 7- to 21-day-old pigs are inoculated, diarrhea, and dehydration are less severe and mortality is lower (Crouch and Woode 1978; Shaw et al. 1989; Theil et al. 1978). Conventional pigs inoculated when 28 days old develop mild diarrhea lasting only 1–1.5 days (Lecce et al. 1982; Tzipori et al. 1980c).

Diet influences disease. No clinical disease was observed after RV was inoculated into 21- to 28-day-old pigs that consumed a dry diet for more than 3 days previously (Tzipori et al. 1980c; Paul and Stevenson 1999). In contrast, gnotobiotic pigs fed a liquid diet developed diarrhea when challenged with RV at 7–8 weeks of age (Yuan et al. 1996).

Naturally occurring RV diarrhea is usually less severe than experimental disease due to the impact of maternal lactogenic immunity. Rotavirus infection is endemic in nearly all conventional swine herds. Consequently, a proportion of gilts and sows have immunity to RV, which is passed to their piglets via colostrum and milk (Askaa et al. 1983; Ward et al. 1996a). Levels of RV antibodies in colostrum and milk decline rapidly in the first few days of lactation. Diarrhea occurs in pigs when the oral challenge level of RV exceeds a protective level of lactogenic passive immunity (Saif 1985). Management practices that impact the proportion of dams that are immune (type of housing, sanitation), the level of passive immunity transferred to pigs (factors affecting lactation and suckling), and the level of RV challenge to pigs (crate design, sanitation) differ among swine herds and affect the age of onset and severity of rotaviral diarrhea.

Naturally occurring RV-associated diarrheal disease is reported in 1- to 41-day-old suckling pigs (Askaa et al. 1983; Bohl et al. 1978; Debouck and Pensaert 1983; Roberts et al. 1980; Svensmark et al. 1989; Yaeger et al. 2002) or within 7 days following weaning (Bohl et al. 1978; Lecce and King 1978; Tzipori et al. 1980b; Woode et al. 1976). The age of onset is often consistent in a given herd. Uncomplicated RV diarrhea in suckling pigs usually resolves in 2–3 days. Feces are yellow or white, watery-to-creamy, and variably flocculant. Morbidity is usually less than 20% and mortality due to dehydration is typically less than 15% of diarrheic pigs. Mortality is highest in young pigs. Rotaviral diarrhea in suckling pigs is frequently complicated by infection with *Isospora*

suis (Roberts et al. 1980) or enterotoxigenic *Escherichia coli* (ETEC) (Bohl et al. 1978), which results in more severe disease, higher morbidity, and higher mortality (Lecce et al. 1982; Tzipori et al. 1980a).

The importance of RV in diarrhea in weaned pigs is less clear. Severe diarrhea in weaned pigs has been associated with RV, but usually in combination with TGE virus (Bohl et al. 1978) or β-hemolytic ETEC (Lecce et al. 1982; Tzipori et al. 1980a). Inoculation studies with RV and β-hemolytic ETEC suggest an important role for RV in postweaning diarrhea (Melin et al. 2004). Inoculation of weaned pigs with RV or β-hemolytic ETEC alone resulted in mild transient or no diarrhea, whereas inoculation with RV followed by hemolytic E. coli resulted in enhanced colonization by β-hemolytic ETEC and severe protracted diarrhea.

LESIONS

Lesions caused by RV are only in the small intestines and are due to RV replication within, and destruction of, villous epithelial cells, as well as subsequent adaptive and regenerative responses. Gross lesions appear slightly before, or with, the onset of diarrhea and are most severe in 1- to 14-day-old pigs (Collins et al. 1989; Janke et al. 1988; Pearson and McNulty 1977; Stevenson 1990; Theil et al. 1978). The stomachs usually contain food, and the distal one-half to two-thirds of the small intestine is thin-walled, flaccid, and dilated with watery, flocculant, yellow or gray fluid. The lacteals in the distal two-thirds of the intestine contain no chyle and the associated mesenteric lymph nodes are small and tan. The cecum and colon are dilated with similar contents. Gross lesions are less severe or are absent in pigs that are 21 days of age or older (Shaw et al. 1989; Stevenson 1990).

Light microscopic lesions (Paul and Stevenson 1999) and scanning electron microscopic lesions (Collins et al. 1989; McAdaragh et al. 1980; Stevenson 1990; Torres-Medina and Underdahl 1980) have been described in numerous RV inoculation studies in suckling pigs. Degeneration begins in epithelial cells on the apical portion of villi by 16–18 hours postinoculation and is evidenced by swollen rarified cytoplasm, nuclear swelling, irregular brush borders, and frequent partial detachment from adjacent cells or the basement membrane. By 16–24 hours postinoculation, sloughing of cells results in significant villous atrophy that is most severe by 24–72 hours postinoculation (Figure 26.5). The tips of atrophic villi are eroded or are covered by swollen or attenuated, nearly squamous epithelial cells (Figure 26.6) and there is cellular debris in the lamina propria. Lateral fusion of villi is seen 24–168 hours postinoculation. Hyperplasia of crypt epithelial cells results in significantly deeper crypts beginning 48–72 hours postinoculation. The time required for complete regeneration of normal villi depends on the age of the pig.

Ultrastructural lesions in RV-infected pigs are typical

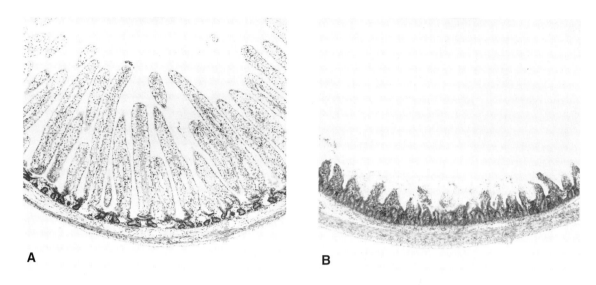

26.5. *Ileum from 3-day-old gnotobiotic pigs (H&E; ×35). (A) Normal villi in an uninoculated control pig. (B) Severe villous atrophy present 18 hours postinoculation.*

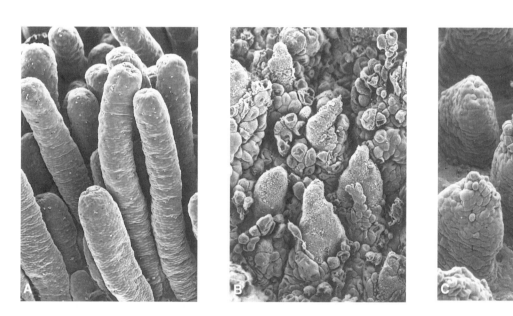

26.6. *Scanning electron micrograph of the ileum of 3-day-old gnotobiotic pigs. (A) Normal villi in an uninoculated control pig (×70). (B) Sloughing, degenerate villous epithelial cells and exposed lamina propria on severely atrophic villi, 18 hours postinoculation (×165). (C) The tips of atrophic villi are covered by a continuous layer of sometimes swollen and degenerate epithelial cells, 24 hours postinoculation (×230).*

of those described for RV in many other mammalian and avian species (Narita et al. 1982; Pearson and McNulty 1979; Saif et al. 1978). The cytoplasm of infected villous epithelial cells contains variably sized, electron-dense granular viroplasms that often have dense subviral cores or double-layered particles on the periphery. Double-layered viral particles obtain the outer capsid by budding through the membranes of the rough endoplasmic reticulum (Figure 26.7). Mature, 75–78 nm triple-layered virus particles accumulate in the cysternae of the endoplasmic reticulum and are released by cell lysis. Other degenerative changes in virus-infected cells include cell swelling, mitochondrial swelling, nuclear swelling, di-

latation of the cytocavity network, and fragmentation of microvilli. Macrophages in the lamina propria contain cellular membrane profiles, virus particles, viroplasm, and other cellular debris in phagosomes.

IMMUNITY

Pigs infected with RV develop intestinal and systemic immune responses. Neonatal gnotobiotic pigs have been used to study immune responses to porcine and human RV infection, correlates of protective immunity, and approaches to improve the immunogenicity and protective efficacy of RV vaccines (Saif et al. 1996, 1997; Yuan and Saif 2002).

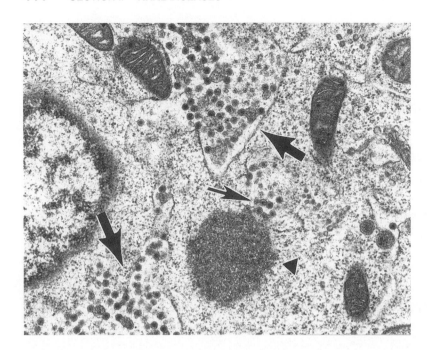

26.7. *Ultrastructure of a swollen and degenerate rotavirus-infected villous epithelial cell containing dense granular viroplasm (arrowhead). Virus particles form and obtain outer capsids through budding into the rough endoplasmic reticulum (small arrow). Many double-shelled virus particles are within the cysternae of the endoplasmic reticulum (large arrows) (×23,800).*

Pigs recovered from virulent RV infection are fully protected from reinfection by homotypic (common P or G type), but not heterotypic, RV (Bohl et al. 1982; Hoshino et al. 1988; Saif et al. 1997).

Rotavirus-specific IgM antibody-secreting cells (ASC) in gnotobiotic pigs orally inoculated with porcine RV (SB1A and Gottfried) occurred by PID 3, and numbers peaked in spleen and mesenteric lymphoid tissues by PID 7 and in intestinal lamina propria by PID 7 to 14 (Chen et al. 1995). Numbers of RV-specific IgA and IgG ASC in these tissues peaked at PID 14 to 21. Rotavirus-specific IgA ASC responses were dominant in the intestine. The B and T cell immune responses to virulent and attenuated human RV Wa strain (P1A[8]G1) were compared in the intestinal lamina propria and systemic lymphoid tissues of neonatal gnotobiotic pigs (Ward et al. 1996c; Yuan et al. 1996, 2001a). Pigs inoculated with one oral dose of virulent human RV developed significantly higher numbers of virus-specific IgA and IgG ASC and memory B cells and higher lymphocyte proliferation responses in the intestinal lamina propria compared to pigs given three oral doses of attenuated human RV. The magnitude of the intestinal IgA ASC and lymphocyte proliferation responses, which reflected the degree of viral replication and lesions within the intestine, was positively correlated with the level of protection induced (Ward et al. 1996c; Yuan and Saif 2002).

After RV infection or oral vaccination, protein-specific antibody responses were predominately against RV inner capsid protein VP6, a nonneutralizing antigen, followed by VP4, NSP2, NSP4, and VP7 (Chang et al. 2001; Yuan et al. 2004). Although VP6 is the most immunogenic protein, VP6 antigen administered in the form of VP2/6 virus-like particles (VLPs) did not protect neonatal pigs (Azevedo et al. 2004; Gonzalez et al. 2004;

Iosef et al. 2002; Nguyen et al. 2003; Yuan et al. 2000, 2001b), or neonatal mice born to 2/6VLP vaccinated dams (Coste et al. 2000). These results indicate that antibodies to VP6 are not sufficient to protect against RV disease (Yuan and Saif 2003). Rotavirus VP4 and VP7 outer capsid proteins both induce virus neutralizing antibodies and independently confer protection in pigs (Hoshino et al. 1988).

Protective Immunity

Protective immunity against RV disease in pigs and humans is most closely related to the presence of neutralizing IgA antibodies in the intestine and serum (Azevedo et al. 2004; Coulsen et al. 1992; Coulsen et al. 1998). The roles of T and B cells in protective immunity to RV infection have been extensively studied, but only in adult mice (reviewed by Franco and Greenberg 2000). Limited studies of presumed CD4+ Th cell responses to RV have been performed in pigs (Ward et al. 1996c), lambs (Bruce et al. 1995), calves (Oldham et al. 1993), and humans (Offit et al. 1993) using lymphocyte proliferation assays. Excluding mice, the role of CD8+ T cells in protective immunity to RV was examined only in calves by injection of MAbs to deplete CD4 or CD8 T cells (Oldham et al. 1993). These investigators suggested that although CD8+ T cells contribute to protection against RV, the major role of CD8+ T cells was in restricting and clearing RV primary infection, whereas CD4+ T cells were important in generation of mucosal antibody responses (Oldham et al. 1993).

Although VP4 and VP7 elicit serotype-specific virus neutralizing antibodies independently from each other (homotypic immunity), they also evoke reduced levels and shorter duration of broad, serotype cross-reactive virus neutralizing antibodies (heterotypic immunity) (reviewed by Hoshino and Kapikian 2000). Among the distinct RV serogroups and serotypes, cross-protection after primary infection or vaccination is minimal or nonexistent, but repeated infection or vaccination (even with the same RV strain) broadens the range of protection against heterotypic RV (Chiba et al. 1993; Gorrell and Bishop 1999). The antigenic divergence among different serotypes/genotypes of RV presents a challenge for design of vaccines capable of inducing heterotypic protection. Reassortant RV containing the VP4 and VP7 genes from different serotypes may be used in multivalent vaccines to induce immunity to each serotype (Hoshino and Kapikian 2000; Hoshino et al. 1988).

Passive Immunity

Pigs are most susceptible to infection with group A RV during the first weeks of life and soon after weaning (Bohl 1979). Outbreaks of diarrhea in animals less than 2 weeks of age are less frequent, presumably because piglets have acquired passive immunity in colostrum/milk from immune dams. Pigs are born agammaglobulinemic and acquire circulating maternal antibodies by consuming colostrum. Piglets are able to uptake antibodies for only a limited time after birth (24–36 hours after birth) before gut closure occurs (Wagstrom et al. 2000). Afterward, maternal antibodies are no longer absorbed from the intestines and only act locally to protect the gut. Piglets born to gilts are more susceptible to RV diarrhea than those born to sows because maternal antibody titers are often lower in gilts (Askaa et al. 1983; Gelberg et al. 1991).

Thus, rotavirus-specific antibodies in the colostrum (mainly IgG) and milk (predominately secretory [S] IgA) provide passive protection against RV to neonatal pigs (Saif 1999). Secretory IgA antibodies are more efficient in mediating protection in the gut of pigs because of their resistance to cleavage by digestive enzymes and higher levels in milk (Saif and Fernandez 1996). High persisting levels of passive IgG RV antibodies transudated from serum back to gut were also protective transiently (Hodgins et al. 1999; Parreno et al. 1999; Parreno et al. 2004; Ward et al. 1996a). Ideally, suckling animals become subclinically infected with RV after receiving adequate passive antibodies to prevent disease and develop active immunity (or are primed) to prevent subsequent diarrhea.

Vaccine Strategies

Current commercially available RV vaccines are used for immunization of sows, as well as nursing pigs. Attenuated RV vaccines are administered orally, orally and intramuscularly (IM), or IM. Inactivated RV vaccines are administered IM in sows and intraperitoneally (IP) in nursing pigs. The efficacy of these vaccines is often uncertain or poor (Saif and Fernandez 1996).

Induction of active immunity in sucking pigs to prevent postweaning diarrhea is problematic because of the

presence of maternal antibodies. Improved vaccines and vaccination approaches are needed. Although oral immunization with replicating vaccines is the simplest and most efficient route for priming SIgA responses in the intestines, maternal antibodies have been shown to interfere with the development of active immunity in neonatal pigs (Hodgins et al. 1999; Parreno et al. 1999). Inactivated vaccines given parenterally may be less affected by maternal antibodies. However, IM immunization of RV seronegative piglets with inactivated RV did not induce SIgA antibody responses in the intestine or confer protection (Yuan et al. 1998).

Besides the traditional vaccines, the immunogenicity and protective efficacy of various alternative RV vaccine formulations (recombinant baculovirus-expressed VLP and DNA vaccines), routes of administration, and adjuvants have been evaluated in RV seronegative gnotobiotic pigs (reviewed by Yuan and Saif 2002). The attenuated human RV as an oral priming dose followed by 2/6-VLPs as intranasal (IN) or oral booster doses (Iosef et al. 2002; Yuan and Saif 2002) or VP6 DNA plasmid as IM booster doses (Yuan et al. 2003) were shown to be highly effective in inducing intestinal IgA antibody responses and protection. However, priming with 2 doses of 2/6-VLPs or VP6 DNA followed by attenuated human RV oral boosting was ineffective.

These results suggest new vaccine approaches that could be developed to prevent enteric viral infections in pigs. The combination of multiple vaccine types, vaccination routes, mucosal adjuvants, and new mucosal delivery systems may lead to optimal stimulation of protective immune responses in the presence or absence of maternal antibodies and improved efficacy of RV vaccines.

DIAGNOSIS

The clinical signs of RV infection in pigs are not unique. Diagnosis requires detection of virus, viral antigen, or viral nucleic acid (RNA). Rotavirus should be considered as a cause of diarrhea in neonatal pigs at 1–8 weeks of age. Fecal samples, intestinal contents, or sections should be collected in the acute phase of disease and submitted for diagnosis. RV is shed at highest concentrations in the first 24 hours after the onset of diarrhea. Sampling during this time frame is especially critical for the detection of certain group RV because the onset, amount, and duration of virus shed is less in pigs infected with group B RV (Bridger 1980; Theil et al. 1985).

A number of methods may be used for the detection of RV, including electron microscopy (EM), immune EM (IEM), immunohistochemistry (IHC), immunofluorescence (IF) on frozen sections or impression smears of small intestines, enzyme-linked immunoassay (ELISA), virus isolation (VI), latex agglutination, dot blot hybridization, RNA electropherotyping, and reverse transcription-polymerase chain reaction (RT-PCR) (Kapikian et al. 2001).

Electron microscopy has been extensively used for detection of RV and used frequently to resolve discrepancies in results from other techniques. It is highly specific because RV have a distinctive morphologic appearance. When only a few samples are to be examined for RV, EM is the most rapid diagnostic method because fecal samples can be stained with phosphotungstic acid and examined directly within a few minutes of collection (Brandt et al. 1981). Use of IEM allows differentiation of RV into serogroups (Saif and Jiang 1994).

ELISA is frequently used for the detection of rotaviral antigens in fecal samples or intestinal contents. Commercial diagnostic kits are available for the detection of porcine group A RV (Benfield et al. 1984; Goyal et al. 1987) and MAb capture ELISAs have also been developed for detection of groups B and C RV (Yolken et al. 1988; Ojeh et al. 1992).

Electropherotyping of viral RNA is used for the detection and differentiation of RV groups. Rotaviruses of different serogroups have distinct electropherotypes (Figure 26.2), which provide a tentative serogroup diagnosis. Electropherotyping results should be confirmed by serologic or nucleic acid–based methods. For electropherotyping, viral RNA is isolated from feces and subjected to polyacrylamide gel electrophoresis and silver staining to visualize the RNA bands (Herring et al. 1982).

Serologic tests are of little value in the diagnosis of RV infection because antibodies are common in most swine herds. However, antibody titers and isotypes are indicators of the immune status of animals. High IgM and IgA antibody titers indicate active or recent infection. There are a variety of techniques for measuring a serologic response to RV infection, including IEM, complement fixation (CF), indirect IF, immune adherence hemagglutination assay, ELISA, VN, hemagglutination inhibition (Eiguchi et al. 1987), inhibition of reverse passive hemagglutination, and immunocytochemical staining (Kapikian et al. 2001).

ELISA using isotype-specific MAbs has been used to detect IgM, IgA, and IgG antibody responses to RV (Azevedo et al. 2004; Parreno et al. 1999; Paul et al. 1989; Coulsen et al. 1998). Antibodies to group C RV have also been detected by blocking ELISA using MAbs (Tsunemitsu et al. 1992a). Plaque reduction and fluorescent focus reduction neutralization assays have been used to detect neutralizing antibodies (Hoshino et al. 1984; Coulsen et al. 1998). Neutralization assays yield the most meaningful information about the identity of the infecting RV and the development of a serotype-specific antibody response. An immunocytochemistry assay using recombinant baculoviruses expressing RV proteins has been developed to measure antibody responses to individual RV proteins (Ishida et al. 1997; Yuan et al. 2004). It is highly sensitive to detect anti-

bodies to both conformation-dependent and independent epitopes on VP4 and VP7.

Nucleic acid probe hybridization assays are highly specific and sensitive for detection of RV RNA and for genotyping (Johnson et al. 1990; Koromyslov et al. 1990; Ojeh et al. 1993; Rosen et al. 1990, 1994; Zaberezhny et al. 1994). The limit of detection for purified viral RNA by the dot hybridization procedure was 8 pg in a homologous reaction. It was ten- to hundredfold more sensitive than ELISA for the detection of RV in various dilutions of fecal samples (Flores et al. 1983).

Currently the most widely used methods for RV detection, genogrouping (A–C, E) and genotyping (group A) is RT-PCR (Barreiros et al. 2003; Elschner et al. 2002; Gouvea et al. 1994a,b; Martella et al. 2001; Pongsuwanna et al. 1996; Winiarczyk and Gradzki 1999; Winiarczyk et al. 2002). Multiplex RT-PCR offers the most sensitive and reliable method for G and P genotyping of group A RV. The RT-PCR method is 100,000 times more sensitive than standard electropherotyping and 5,000 times more sensitive than hybridization assays (Wilde et al. 1991; Xu et al. 1990). The RT-PCR has also been applied for detection of group B and C RV (Eiden et al. 1991; Gouvea et al. 1991).

Newly developed oligonucleotide microarray hybridization technology offers another method for the identification of RV genotypes (Chizhikov et al. 2002). This approach combines the high sensitivity of RT-PCR with the selectivity of DNA-DNA hybridization and was capable of unambiguous identification of the G genotypes of all RV strains.

PREVENTION AND CONTROL

Treatments for diarrhea in animals include antibiotics, antisecretory drugs, adsorbents, and fluid electrolyte therapy (Bywater 1983). However, no known therapeutic agents are available for the specific treatment of porcine RV infections. General supportive therapy, management procedures, and antibiotics are recommended to minimize mortality due to RV and secondary bacterial infections (Paul and Stevenson 1999). Electrolyte solutions containing glucose-glycine minimize dehydration and weight loss induced by RV infection (Bywater and Woode 1980). L-glutamine in oral rehydration solution promotes jejunal sodium and chloride absorption in RV-infected pigs (Rhoads et al. 1991). Oral feeding of transforming growth factor-alpha enhanced jejunal mucosal recovery and electrical resistance in piglets with RV enteritis (Rhoads et al. 1995). Chicken egg powder enriched with Ig specific for RV antigen used as additive to sow's milk reduced the prevalence of diarrhea in 2- to 3-day-old pigs; however, the effect of sow's milk was more pronounced than the effect of the egg powder (Hennig-Pauka et al. 2003).

Optimal ambient temperature (35°C) significantly reduces the nursing piglet mortality caused by RV diarrhea (Steel and Torres-Medina 1984); low temperatures and temperature fluctuations should be avoided. In herds with a persistent problem of postweaning diarrhea with high mortality, a change in weaner diet and weaning procedures should be considered (Paul and Stevenson 1999). Scheduled feeding of a high-energy weaner diet has been successfully used to reduce RV morbidity and mortality (Tzipori et al. 1980b).

The ubiquity of RV in swine herds and its persistence in the environment make it difficult to eradicate RV from swine herds. Rotaviruses persist as subclinical infections and are shed by adult swine (Benfield et al. 1982). Management of farrowing on swine farms is important in controlling diarrhea caused by RV. Management practices should be designed to reduce the level of RV to which susceptible pigs are exposed and to boost levels of passive immunity (Barreiros et al. 2003; Paul and Stevenson 1999; Saif 1985). Exposure levels may be reduced by sanitation. The floors in farrowing and nurs-

ing houses should be constructed for easy cleaning and minimal fecal buildup. Rooms should be cleaned and disinfected between groups. The farrowing interval should be minimized to prevent RV buildup and infection of the litters farrowed latest. A recent study showed that herds using continuous flow in the nurseries had significantly lower rates of RV infection than the herds using all-in/all-out production, suggesting that nursing pigs exposed to RV in the environment may be able to develop an active immune response under the partial protection of maternal antibodies (Dewey et al. 2003). To enhance passive immunity, replacement gilts should be exposed to the feces of older sows to boost RV antibody titers through repeated exposure to RV. Attention to lactation diet, feed intake, sow comfort, and farrowing crate design are important to ensure adequate milk supply and effective suckling necessary to transfer maternal immunity successfully (Paul and Stevenson 1999).

Porcine Reovirus

Although discovered in 1951 (Tyler 2001), the role of reoviruses in the disease process is unclear (Kasza 1970; Kirkbride and McAdaragh 1978; McFerran and Connor 1970). Natural reovirus infection or antibodies to reovirus have been detected in all animal species (Tyler 2001; Yang et al. 1976). Illnesses associated with reovirus infections in animals have involved primarily the respiratory, gastrointestinal, and nervous system (Hirahara et al. 1988; Fukutomi et al. 1996; Tyler 1998). Reoviruses may be detected in pigs with respiratory, enteric, and reproductive diseases, as well as in healthy pigs.

ETIOLOGY

Reovirus was the first genus named in the family *Reoviridae*. The other two genera of importance to animals are genus *Rotavirus* and genus *Orbivirus*. "Reo" is an acronym for "respiratory and enteric orphan." The name was intended to emphasize the fact that these viruses were not associated with any known disease (hence, orphan) (Tyler 2001). Reovirus virions are non-enveloped, icosahedral particles with a rough outer rim. The particles are 75 nm in diameter with the inner capsid measuring 45–50 nm (Figure 26.8).

Reoviruses have a segmented (10 segments) dsRNA genome. The density of a complete (mature) virion in cesium chloride is 1.36 g/ml. Porcine reoviruses are stable at acidic pH and resistant to ether, chloroform, and trypsin, but susceptible to heat at 50°C for 1 hour. They are sensitive to 0.1% sodium deoxycholate (Hirahara et al. 1988). Porcine reoviruses possess a hemagglutinin that agglutinates human group O and porcine erythro-

cytes at 4°C, 22°C, and 37°C. Mammalian reoviruses share a group antigen that can be detected by complement fixation, IF, and immunodiffusion (Sabin 1959). All mammalian reovirus isolates can be divided serologically into three types: 1, 2, and 3. Reoviruses of different types can be distinguished by serum neutralization and hemagglutination inhibition tests.

Reoviruses can be cultivated in a wide variety of cell cultures from many species (Hirahara et al. 1988; Kasza 1970). The most commonly used cell line is mouse L929 fibroblasts for viral growth, purification, and plaque assay (Tyler 2001). Reovirus replicates slowly and the

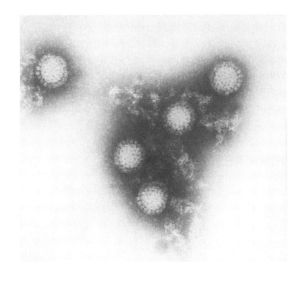

26.8. *Electron micrograph of reovirus particles viewed by negative-staining electron microscopy (×115,000).*

majority (80%) of the nascent virus population remains cell associated. The cytopathic effect of reoviruses varies, depending upon the cell line used. In general, cells round up, become granular, and detach from monolayers. Eosinophilic, intracytoplasmic, inclusion bodies can be seen in cultures stained with May-Greenwald-Giemsa stain (Paul and Stevenson 1999).

EPIDEMIOLOGY

Reoviruses are ubiquitous and porcine reovirus infections are widespread in swine herds. Antibodies to all three types have been detected in pigs (Fukumi et al. 1969; Harkness et al. 1971; Yang et al. 1976). Reoviruses are spread via fecal-oral and respiratory routes. Passively acquired antibodies to reoviruses persist in neonatal pigs for about 11 weeks, at which time pigs become susceptible to infection (Watt 1978).

CLINICAL SIGNS

Reoviruses have been isolated from pigs with respiratory or enteric disease, as well as from clinically healthy pigs (Elazhary et al. 1978; Kasza 1970; McFerran et al. 1971; Robl et al. 1971) and from aborted fetuses (Kirkbride and McAdaragh 1978). Experimental inoculations have not consistently reproduced disease. In most of the studies, intranasal (IN), intraperitoneal, or intracerebral inoculation of conventional and gnotobiotic pigs at 1–6 weeks of age with porcine or human reovirus type 1 did not result in clinical disease, except for a transient febrile reaction (Baskerville et al. 1971; Kasza 1970; McFerran and Connor 1970; McFerran et al. 1971; Watt 1978).

Reovirus is excreted in nasal secretions and feces as early as 24 hours postinoculation and may continue for 6–14 days. Mild respiratory disease characterized by pyrexia, sneezing, inappetence, and listlessness was reproduced in colostrum-deprived pigs and conventional pigs inoculated IN or exposed via aerosol to reovirus type 1 (Hirahara et al. 1988). Intravenous or IM inoculation of seronegative sows between 40 and 85 days of gestation with type 3 reovirus resulted in term litters containing a mixture of mummified, stillborn, weak, and normal pigs. The virus can also be isolated from fecal tissues and the placenta of these sows (Paul and Stevenson 1999).

PATHOGENESIS

Reoviruses replicate mainly in the respiratory and intestinal tracts after natural infection. The pathogenesis and pathology of reoviruses have been studied extensively in mice and the findings have greatly improved our understanding of viruses and virus-host interactions (Tyler 2001). In mice, reoviruses are able to spread from the gastrointestinal tract to extraintestinal organs and the central nervous system after oral inoc-

ulation. Reovirus-induced myocarditis is associated with virus-induced destruction of cardiac myocytes in the absence of a significant inflammatory response (Tyler 2001). The pathogenesis of reoviruses in pigs is unknown.

LESIONS

Reovirus inoculation studies of pigs revealed few gross lesions and only mild microscopic lesions. Oral inoculation of 1-week-old colostrum-deprived pigs with enteric-origin reovirus resulted in focal villous atrophy in the jejunum and ileum (Elazhary et al. 1978). Aerosol exposure of 4-week-old specific pathogen free (SPF) pigs to porcine type 1 reovirus resulted in no gross lesions, but consistent microscopic lesions in the lungs consisting of multifocal aggregates of lymphocytes and macrophages in alveoli and alveolar septae and mild peribronchiolar nodular lymphocytic hyperplasia (Baskerville et al. 1971). Inoculation of 70 kg SPF pigs IN with a respiratory isolate of porcine type 3 reovirus resulted in lobular atalectasis, vesicular emphysema, and peribronchiolar nodular lymphocytic hyperplasia, which varied in intensity between lobules (Paul and Stevenson 1999). Additional studies are needed to characterize the clinical disease and lesions in swine caused by porcine reoviruses.

DIAGNOSIS

Methods similar to those described for RV may be employed for the detection of reoviruses. Virus isolation has commonly been used for diagnosis. Typing of reovirus is achieved by virus neutralization and hemagglutination inhibition tests with reference antisera to the three reovirus types (Paul and Stevenson 1999).

PREVENTION AND CONTROL

No specific methods are available for treatment or prevention of porcine reovirus infections, and possibly none are warranted until the clinical significance of reovirus infections in swine is documented.

REFERENCES

Abad FX, Pinto RM, Bosch A. 1997. Disinfection of human enteric viruses on fomites. FEMS Microbiol Lett 156:107–111.

Ahmadian S, Shahrabadi MS. 1999. Morphological study of the role of calcium in the assembly of the rotavirus outer capsid protein VP7. Biotech Histochem 74:266–273.

Alfieri AA, Leite JP, Nakagomi O, Kaga E, Woods PA, Glass RI, Gentsch JR. 1996. Characterization of human rotavirus genotype P[8]G5 from Brazil by probe-hybridization and sequence. Arch Virol 141:2353–2364.

Askaa J, Bloch B, Bertelsen G, Rasmussen KO. 1983. Rotavirus associated diarrhoea in nursing piglets and detection of antibody against rotavirus in colostrum, milk and serum. Nord Vet Med 35:441–447.

Atii DJ, Ojeh CK, Durojaiye OA. 1990. Detection of rotavirus antigen in diarrhoeic and non-diarrhoeic piglets in Nigeria. Rev Elev Med Vet Pays Trop 42:494–496.

Azevedo MS, Yuan L, Iosef C, Chang KO, Kim Y, Nguyen TV, Saif LJ. 2004. Magnitude of serum and intestinal antibody responses induced by sequential replicating and nonreplicating rotavirus vaccines in gnotobiotic pigs and correlation with protection. Clin Diagn Lab Immunol 11:12–20.

Ball JM, Tian P, Zeng CQ, Morris AP, Estes MK. 1996. Age-dependent diarrhea induced by a rotaviral nonstructural glycoprotein. Science 272:101–104.

Barreiros MA, Alfieri AA, Alfieri AF, Medici KC, Leite JP. 2003. An outbreak of diarrhoea in one-week-old piglets caused by group A rotavirus genotypes P[7],G3 and P[7],G5. Vet Res Commun 27:505–512.

Baskerville A, McFerran JB, Connor T. 1971. The pathology of experimental infection of pigs with type I reovirus of porcine origin. Res Vet Sci 12:172–174.

Benfield DA, Francis DH, McAdaragh JP, Johnson DD, Bergeland ME, Rossow K, Moore R. 1988. Combined rotavirus and K99 *Escherichia coli* infection in gnotobiotic pigs. Am J Vet Res 49:330–337.

Benfield DA, Stotz I, Moore R, McAdaragh JP. 1982. Shedding of rotavirus in feces of sows before and after farrowing. J Clin Microbiol 16:186–190.

Benfield DA, Stotz IJ, Nelson EA, Groon KS. 1984. Comparison of a commercial enzyme-linked immunosorbent assay with electron microscopy, fluorescent antibody, and virus isolation for the detection of bovine and porcine rotavirus. Am J Vet Res 45:1998–2002.

Bican P, Cohen J, Charpilienne A, Scherrer R. 1982. Purification and characterization of bovine rotavirus cores. J Virol 43:1113–1117.

Bishop RF, Davidson GP, Holmes IH, Ruck BJ. 1973. Virus particles in epithelial cells of duodenal mucosa from children with acute non-bacterial gastroenteritis. Lancet 2:1281–1283.

Blikslager AT, Roberts MC. 1997. Mechanisms of intestinal mucosal repair. J Am Vet Med Assoc 211:1437–1441.

Blutt SE, Kirkwood CD, Parreno V, Warfield KL, Ciarlet M, Estes MK, Bok K, Bishop RF, Conner ME. 2003. Rotavirus antigenaemia and viraemia: A common event? Lancet 362:1445–1449.

Bohl EH. 1979. Rotaviral diarrhea in pigs: Brief review. J Am Vet Med Assoc 174:613–615.

Bohl EH, Kohler EM, Saif LJ, Cross RF, Agnes AG, Theil KW. 1978. Rotavirus as a cause of diarrhea in pigs. J Am Vet Med Assoc 172:458–463.

Bohl EH, Saif LJ, Theil KW, Agnes AG, Cross RF. 1982. Porcine pararotavirus: Detection, differentiation from rotavirus, and pathogenesis in gnotobiotic pigs. J Clin Microbiol 15:312–319.

Bohl EH, Theil KW, Saif LJ. 1984. Isolation and serotyping of porcine rotaviruses and antigenic comparison with other rotaviruses. J Clin Microbiol 19:105–111.

Brandt CD, Kim HW, Rodriguez WJ, Thomas L, Yolken RH, Arrobio JO, Kapikian AZ, Parrott RH, Chanock RM. 1981. Comparison of direct electron microscopy, immune electron microscopy, and rotavirus enzyme-linked immunosorbent assay for detection of gastroenteritis viruses in children. J Clin Microbiol 13:976–981.

Bridger JC. 1980. Detection by electron microscopy of caliciviruses, astroviruses and rotavirus-like particles in the faeces of piglets with diarrhoea. Vet Rec 107:532–533.

Bridger JC, Brown JF. 1985. Prevalence of antibody to typical and atypical rotaviruses in pigs. Vet Rec 116:50.

Bridger JC, Woode GN. 1976. Characterization of two particle types of calf rotavirus. J Gen Virol 31:245–250.

Brown DW, Beards GM, Chen GM, Flewett TH. 1987. Prevalence of antibody to group B (atypical) rotavirus in humans and animals. J Clin Microbiol 25:316–319.

Bruce MG, Campbell IC, van Pinxteren L, Snodgrass DR. 1995. Intestinal cellular immunity after primary rotavirus infection. J Comp Pathol 113:155–164.

Buller CR, Moxley RA. 1988. Natural infection of porcine ileal dome M cells with rotavirus and enteric adenovirus. Vet Pathol 25:516–517.

Bywater RJ. 1983. Diarrhoea treatments—Fluid replacement and alternatives. Ann Rech Vet 14:556–560.

Bywater RJ, Woode GN. 1980. Oral fluid replacement by a glucose glycine electrolyte formulation in *E coli* and rotavirus diarrhea in pigs. Vet Rec 106:75–78.

Chang KO, Parwani AV, Saif LJ. 1996. The characterization of VP7 (G type) and VP4 (P type) genes of bovine group A rotaviruses from field samples using RT-PCR and RFLP analysis. Arch Virol 141:1727–1739.

Chang KO, Vandal OH, Yuan L, Hodgins DC, Saif LJ. 2001. Antibody-secreting cell responses to rotavirus proteins in gnotobiotic pigs inoculated with attenuated or virulent human rotavirus. J Clin Microbiol 39:2807–2813.

Chasey D, Bridger JC, McCrae MA. 1986. A new type of atypical rotavirus in pigs. Arch Virol 89:235–243.

Chasey D, Davies P. 1984. Atypical rotaviruses in pigs and cattle. Vet Rec 114:16–17.

Chen WK, Campbell T, VanCott J, Saif LJ. 1995. Enumeration of isotype-specific antibody-secreting cells derived from gnotobiotic piglets inoculated with porcine rotaviruses. Vet Immunol Immunopathol 45:265–284.

Chiba S, Nakata S, Ukae S, Adachi N. 1993. Virological and serological aspects of immune resistance to rotavirus gastroenteritis. Clin Infect Dis 16:S117–121.

Chizhikov V, Wagner M, Ivshina A, Hoshino Y, Kapikian AZ, Chumakov K. 2002. Detection and genotyping of human group A rotaviruses by oligonucleotide microarray hybridization. J Clin Microbiol 40:2398–2407.

Ciarlet M, Ludert JE, Iturriza-Gomara M, Liprandi F, Gray JJ, Desselberger U, Estes MK. 2002. Initial interaction of rotavirus strains with N-acetylneuraminic (sialic) acid residues on the cell surface correlates with VP4 genotype, not species of origin. J Virol 76:4087–4095.

Ciarlet M, Isa P, Conner ME, Liprandi F. 2001. Antigenic and molecular analyses reveal that the equine rotavirus strain H-1 is closely related to porcine, but not equine, rotaviruses: Interspecies transmission from pigs to horses? Virus Genes 22:5–20.

Collins JE, Benfield DA, Duimstra JR. 1989. Comparative virulence of two porcine group—A rotavirus isolates in gnotobiotic pigs. Am J Vet Res 50:827–835.

Coste A, Sirard JC, Johansen K, Cohen J, Kraehenbuhl JP. 2000. Nasal immunization of mice with virus-like particles protects offspring against rotavirus diarrhea. J Virol 74:8966–8971.

Coulsen BS, Grimwood K, Hudson IL, Barnes GL, Bishop RF. 1992. Role of coproantibody in clinical protection of children during reinfection with rotavirus. J Clin Microbiol 30:1678–1684.

Coulsen TL, Ward LA, Yuan L, Saif LJ. 1998. Serum and intestinal isotype antibody responses and correlates of protective immunity to human rotavirus in a gnotobiotic pig model of disease. J Gen Virol 79:2661–2672.

Crouch CF, Woode GN. 1978. Serial studies of virus multiplication and intestinal damage in gnotobiotic piglets infected with rotavirus. J Med Microbiol 11:325–334.

Das BK, Gentsch JR, Hoshino Y, Ishida S, Nakagomi O, Bhan MK, Kumar R, Glass RI. 1993. Characterization of the G serotype and genogroup of New Delhi newborn rotavirus strain 116E. Virology 197:99–107.

Davidson GP, Gall DG, Petric M, Butler DG, Hamilton JR. 1977. Human rotavirus enteritis induced in conventional piglets. Intestinal structure and transport. J Clin Invest 60:1402–1409.

Debouck P, Pensaert M. 1983. Rotavirus excretion in suckling pigs followed under field circumstances. Ann Rech Vet 14: 447–448.

Dewey C, Carman S, Pasma T, Josephson G, McEwen B. 2003. Relationship between group A porcine rotavirus and management practices in swine herds in Ontario. Can Vet J 44:649–653.

Dunn SJ, Greenberg HB, Ward RL, Nakagomi O, Burns JW, Vo PT, Pax KA, Das M, Gowda K, Rao CD. 1993. Serotypic and genotypic characterization of human serotype 10 rotaviruses from asymptomatic neonates. J Clin Microbiol 31:165–169.

Eiden JJ, Wilde J, Firoozmand F, Yolken R. 1991. Detection of animal and human group B rotaviruses in fecal specimens by polymerase chain reaction. J Clin Microbiol 29:539–543.

Eiguchi Y, Yamagishi H, Fukusho A, Shimizu Y, Matumoto M. 1987. Hemagglutination and hemagglutination-inhibition tests with porcine rotavirus. Kitasato Arch Exp Med 60:167–172.

El-Attar L, Dhaliwal W, Howard CR, Bridger JC. 2001. Rotavirus cross-species pathogenicity: Molecular characterization of a bovine rotavirus pathogenic for pigs. Virology 291:172–182.

Elazhary MA, Morin M, Derbyshire JB, Lagace A, Berthiaume L, Corbeil M. 1978. The experimental infection of piglets with a porcine reovirus. Res Vet Sci 25:16–20.

Elschner M, Prudlo J, Hotzel H, Otto P, Sachse K. 2002. Nested reverse transcriptase-polymerase chain reaction for the detection of group A rotaviruses. J Vet Med B Infect Dis Vet Public Health 49:77–81.

Esona MD, Armah GE, Geyer A, Steele AD. 2004. Detection of an unusual human rotavirus strain with G5P[8] specificity in a Cameroonian child with diarrhea. J Clin Microbiol 42:441–444.

Estes MK. 2001. Rotaviruses and their replication. In Fields Virology. DM Knipe, PM Howley, eds. Philadelphia: Lippincott-Raven and Wilkins Publishers, pp. 1747–1786.

Estes MK, Cohen J. 1989. Rotavirus gene structure and function. Microbiol Rev 53:410–449.

Estes MK, Graham DY, Smith EM, Gerba CP. 1979. Rotavirus stability and inactivation. J Gen Virol 43:403–409.

Estes MK, Kang G, Zeng CQ, Crawford SE, Ciarlet M. 2001. Pathogenesis of rotavirus gastroenteritis. Novartis Found Symp 238:82–96.

Estes MK, Palmer EL, Obijeski JF. 1983. Rotaviruses: A review. Curr Top Microbiol Immunol 105:123–184.

Flores J, Boeggeman E, Purcell RH, Sereno M, Perez I, White L, Wyatt RG, Chanock RM, Kapikian AZ. 1983. A dot hybridisation assay for detection of rotavirus. Lancet 1:555–558.

Franco MA, Greenberg HB. 2000. Immunity to homologous rotavirus infection in adult mice. Trends Microbiol 8:50–52.

Fu ZF, Hampson DJ. 1987. Group A rotavirus excretion patterns in naturally infected pigs. Res Vet Sci 43:297–300.

Fu ZF, Hampson DJ, Blackmore DK. 1989. Detection and survival of group A rotavirus in a piggery. Vet Rec 125:576–578.

Fuentes-Panana EM, Lopez S, Gorziglia M, Arias CF. 1995. Mapping the hemagglutination domain of rotaviruses. J Virol 69:2629–2632.

Fukumi H, Takeuchi Y, Ishida M, Saito H. 1969. Serological epidemiology of reovirus infection. 1. Jpn J Med Sci Biol 22:13–21.

Fukutomi T, Sanekata T, Akashi H. 1996. Isolation of reovirus type 2 from diarrheal feces of pigs. J Vet Med Sci 58:555–557.

Gelberg HB, Patterson JS, Woode GN. 1991. A longitudinal study of rotavirus antibody titers in swine in a closed specific pathogen-free herd. Vet Microbiol 28:231–242.

Gerna G, Sarasini A, Parea M, Arista S, Miranda P, Brussow H, Hoshino Y, Flores J. 1992. Isolation and characterization of two distinct human rotavirus strains with G6 specificity. J Clin Microbiol 30:9–16.

Geyer A, Sebata T, Peenze I, Steele AD. 1996. Group B and C porcine rotaviruses identified for the first time in South Africa. J S Afr Vet Assoc 67:115–116.

Gonzalez AM, Nguyen TV, Azevedo MS, Jeong K, Agarib F, Iosef C, Chang K, Lovgren-Bengtsson K, Morein B, Saif LJ. 2004. Antibody responses to human rotavirus (HRV) in gnotobiotic pigs following a new prime/boost vaccine strategy using oral attenuated HRV priming and intranasal VP2/6 rotavirus-like particle (VLP) boosting with ISCOM. Clin Exp Immunol 135:361–372.

Gorrell RJ, Bishop RF. 1999. Homotypic and heterotypic serum neutralizing antibody response to rotavirus proteins following natural primary infection and reinfection in children. J Med Virol 57:204–211.

Gorziglia M, Larralde G, Kapikian AZ, Chanock RM. 1990. Antigenic relationships among human rotaviruses as determined by outer capsid protein VP4. Proc Natl Acad Sci U S A 87:7155–7159.

Gouvea V, Allen JR, Glass RI, Fang ZY, Bremont M, Cohen J, McCrae MA, Saif LJ, Sinarachatanant P, Caul EO. 1991. Detection of group B and C rotaviruses by polymerase chain reaction. J Clin Microbiol 29:519–523.

Gouvea V, Santos N, Timenetsky Mdo C. 1994a. Identification of bovine and porcine rotavirus G types by PCR. J Clin Microbiol 32:1338–1340.

——. 1994b. VP4 typing of bovine and porcine group A rotaviruses by PCR. J Clin Microbiol 32:1333–1337.

Goyal SM, Rademacher RA, Pomeroy KA. 1987. Comparison of electron microscopy with three commercial tests for the detection of rotavirus in animal feces. Diagn Microbiol Infect Dis 6:249–254.

Graham DY, Estes MK. 1991. Pathogenesis and treatment of rotavirus diarrhea. Gastroenterology 101:1140–1141.

Graham KL, Halasz P, Tan Y, Hewish MJ, Takada Y, Mackow ER, Robinson MK, Coulson BS. 2003. Integrin-using rotaviruses bind alpha2beta1 integrin alpha2 I domain via VP4 DGE sequence and recognize alphaXbeta2 and alphaVbeta3 by using VP7 during cell entry. J Virol 77:9969–9978.

Greenberg H, McAuliffe V, Valdesuso J, Wyatt R, Flores J, Kalica A, Hoshino Y, Singh N. 1983. Serological analysis of the subgroup protein of rotavirus, using monoclonal antibodies. Infect Immun 39:91–99.

Guerrero CA, Bouyssounade D, Zarate S, Isa P, Lopez T, Espinosa R, Romero P, Mendez E, Lopez S, Arias CF. 2002. Heat shock cognate protein 70 is involved in rotavirus cell entry. J Virol 76:4096–4102.

Harkness JW, Chapman MS, Darbyshire JH. 1971. A survey of antibodies to some respiratory viruses in the sera of pigs. Vet Rec 88:441–447.

Hennig-Pauka I, Stelljes I, Waldmann KH. 2003. Studies on the effect of specific egg antibodies against Escherichia coli infections in piglets. Dtsch Tierarztl Wochenschr 110:49–54.

Herring AJ, Inglis NF, Ojeh CK, Snodgrass DR, Menzies JD. 1982. Rapid diagnosis of rotavirus infection by direct detection of viral nucleic acid in silver-stained polyacrylamide gels. J Clin Microbiol 16:473–477.

Hewish MJ, Takada Y, Coulson BS. 2000. Integrins alpha2beta1 and alpha4beta1 can mediate SA11 rotavirus attachment and entry into cells. J Virol 74:228–236.

Hirahara T, Yasuhara H, Matsui O, Kodama K, Nakai M, Sasaki N. 1988. Characteristics of reovirus type 1 from the respiratory tract of pigs in Japan. Nippon Juigaku Zasshi 50:353–361.

Hodgins DC, Kang SY, deArriba L, Parreno V, Ward LA, Yuan L, To T, Saif LJ. 1999. Effects of maternal antibodies on protection and development of antibody responses to human rotavirus in gnotobiotic pigs. J Virol 73:186–197.

Hoshino Y, Jones RW, Kapikian AZ. 2002. Characterization of neutralization specificities of outer capsid spike protein VP4 of selected murine, lapine, and human rotavirus strains. Virology 299:64–71.

Hoshino Y, Kapikian AZ. 1996. Classification of rotavirus VP4 and VP7 serotypes. Arch Virol Suppl 12:99–111.

——. 2000. Rotavirus serotypes: Classification and importance in epidemiology, immunity, and vaccine development. J Health Popul Nutr 18:5–14.

Hoshino Y, Saif LJ, Kang SY, Sereno MM, Chen WK, Kapikian AZ. 1995. Identification of group A rotavirus genes associated with virulence of a porcine rotavirus and host range restriction of a human rotavirus in the gnotobiotic piglet model. Virology 209:274–280.

Hoshino Y, Saif LJ, Sereno MM, Chanock RM, Kapikian AZ. 1988. Infection immunity of piglets to either VP3 or VP7 outer capsid protein confers resistance to challenge with a virulent rotavirus bearing the corresponding antigen. J Virol 62:744–748.

Hoshino Y, Wyatt RG, Greenberg HB, Flores J, Kapikian AZ. 1984. Serotypic similarity and diversity of rotaviruses of mammalian and avian origin as studied by plaque-reduction neutralization. J Infect Dis 149:694–702.

Hung T, Chen GM, Wang CG, Fan RL, Yong RJ, Chang JQ, Dan R, Ng MH. 1987. Seroepidemiology and molecular epidemiology of the Chinese rotavirus. Ciba Found Symp 128:49–62.

Iosef C, Nguyen TV, Jeong K, Bengtsson K, Morein B, Kim Y, Chang KO, Azevedo MS, Yuan L, Nielsen P, Saif LJ. 2002. Systemic and intestinal antibody secreting cell responses and protection in gnotobiotic pigs immunized orally with attenuated Wa human rotavirus and Wa 2/6-rotavirus-like-particles associated with immunostimulating complexes. Vaccine 20:1741–1753.

Isa P, Realpe M, Romero P, Lopez S, Arias CF. 2004. Rotavirus RRV associates with lipid membrane microdomains during cell entry. Virology 322:370–381.

Ishida SI, Feng N, Gilbert JM, Tang B, Greenberg HB. 1997. Immune responses to individual rotavirus proteins following heterologous and homologous rotavirus infection in mice. J Infect Dis 175:1317–1323.

Iturriza-Gomara M, Wong C, Blome S, Desselberger U, Gray J. 2002. Molecular characterization of VP6 genes of human rotavirus isolates: Correlation of genogroups with subgroups and evidence of independent segregation. J Virol 76:6596–6601.

Janke BH, Morehouse LG, Solorzano RF. 1988. Single and mixed infections of neonatal pigs with rotaviruses and enteroviruses: Clinical signs and microscopic lesions. Can J Vet Res 52:364–369.

Janke BH, Nelson JK, Benfield DA, Nelson EA. 1990. Relative prevalence of typical and atypical strains among rotaviruses from diarrheic pigs in conventional swine herds. J Vet Diagn Invest 2:308–311.

Jiang BM, Saif LJ, Kang SY, Kim JH. 1990. Biochemical characterization of the structural and nonstructural polypeptides of a porcine group C rotavirus. J Virol 64:3171–3178.

Johnson ME, Paul PS, Gorziglia M, Rosenbusch R. 1990. Development of specific nucleic acid probes for the differentiation of porcine rotavirus serotypes. Vet Microbiol 24:307–326.

Jones SL, Blikslager AT. 2002. Role of the enteric nervous system in the pathophysiology of secretory diarrhea. J Vet Intern Med 16:222–228.

Kapikian AZ, Hoshino Y, Chanock RA. 2001. Rotaviruses, In Fields Virology. DM Kinipe, PM Howley, eds, Philadelphia: Lippincott-Raven and Wilkins Publishers, pp. 1787–1834.

Kasza L. 1970. Isolation and characterisation of a reovirus from pigs. Vet Rec 87:681–686.

Kim Y, Chang KO, Straw B, Saif LJ. 1999. Characterization of group C rotaviruses associated with diarrhea outbreaks in feeder pigs. J Clin Microbiol 37:1484–1488.

Kirkbride CA, McAdaragh JP. 1978. Infectious agents associated with fetal and early neonatal death and abortion in swine. J Am Vet Med Assoc 172:480–483.

Koromyslov GF, Artjushin SK, Zaberezhny AD, Grashuk VN. 1990. Development of hybridization probes on the basis of recombinant DNA to identify porcine parvoviruses and rotaviruses. Arch Exp Veterinarmed 44:897–900.

Laird AR, Ibarra V, Ruiz-Palacios G, Guerrero ML, Glass RI, Gentsch JR. 2003. Unexpected detection of animal VP7 genes among common rotavirus strains isolated from children in Mexico. J Clin Microbiol 41:4400–4403.

Lecce JG, Balsbaugh RK, Clare DA, King MW. 1982. Rotavirus and hemolytic enteropathogenic *Escherichia coli* in weanling diarrhea of pigs. J Clin Microbiol 16:715–723.

Lecce JG, King MW. 1978. Role of rotavirus (reo-like) in weanling diarrhea of pigs. J Clin Microbiol 8:454–458.

Liprandi F, Gerder M, Bastidas Z, Lopez JA, Pujol FH, Ludert JE, Joelsson DB, Ciarlet M. 2003. A novel type of VP4 carried by a porcine rotavirus strain. Virology 315:373–380.

Liprandi F, Moros Z, Gerder M, Ludert JE, Pujol FH, Ruiz MC, Michelangeli F, Charpilienne A, Cohen J. 1997. Productive penetration of rotavirus in cultured cells induces coentry of the translation inhibitor alpha-sarcin. Virology 237:430–438.

Lundgren O, Peregrin AT, Persson K, Kordasti S, Uhnoo I, Svensson L. 2000. Role of the enteric nervous system in the fluid and electrolyte secretion of rotavirus diarrhea. Science 287:491–495.

Lundgren O, Svensson L. 2001. Pathogenesis of rotavirus diarrhea. Microbes Infect 3:1145–1156.

Markowska-Daniel I, Winiarczyk S, Gradzki Z, Pejsak Z. 1996. Evaluation of different methods (ELISA, IF, EM, PAGE) for the diagnosis of rotavirus infection in piglets. Comp Immunol Microbiol Infect Dis 19:219–232.

Martella V, Ciarlet M, Camarda A, Pratelli A, Tempesta M, Greco G, Cavalli A, Elia G, Decaro N, Terio V, Bozzo G, Camero M, Buonavoglia C. 2003. Molecular characterization of the VP4, VP6, VP7, and NSP4 genes of lapine rotaviruses identified in italy: Emergence of a novel VP4 genotype. Virology 314:358–370.

Martella V, Pratelli A, Greco G, Tempesta M, Ferrari M, Losio MN, Buonavoglia C. 2001. Genomic characterization of porcine rotaviruses in Italy. Clin Diagn Lab Immunol 8:129–132.

McAdaragh JP, Bergeland ME, Meyer RC, Johnshoy MW, Stotz IJ, Benfield DA, Hammer R. 1980. Pathogenesis of rotaviral enteritis in gnotobiotic pigs: A microscopic study. Am J Vet Res 41:1572–1581.

McFerran JB, Baskerville A, Connor T. 1971. Experimental infection of pigs with a human strain of type I reovirus. Res Vet Sci 12:174–175.

McFerran JB, Connor T. 1970. A reovirus isolated from a pig. Res Vet Sci 11:388–390.

Mebus CA, Underdahl NR, Rhodes MB, Twiehaus MJ. 1969. Calf diarrhea (scours): Reproduced with a virus from a field outbreak. Univ Nebraska Agri Exp Stn Res Bull 233.

Melin L, Mattsson S, Katouli M, Wallgren P. 2004. Development of post-weaning diarrhoea in piglets. Relation to presence of *Escherichia coli* strains and rotavirus. J Vet Med B Infect Dis Vet Public Health 51:12–22.

Moon HW. 1997. Comparative histopathology of intestinal infections. Adv Exp Med Biol 412:1–19.

Nagesha HS, Hum CP, Bridger JC, Holmes IH. 1988. Atypical rotaviruses in Australian pigs. Arch Virol 102:91–98.

Nakagomi O, Nakagomi T. 2002. Genomic relationships among rotaviruses recovered from various animal species as revealed by RNA-RNA hybridization assays. Res Vet Sci 73:207–214.

Narita M, Fukusho A, Shimizu Y. 1982. Electron microscopy of the intestine of gnotobiotic piglets infected with porcine rotavirus. J Comp Pathol 92:589–597.

Nguyen TV, Iosef C, Jeong K, Kim Y, Chang KO, Lovgren-Bengtsson K, Morein B, Azevedo MS, Lewis P, Nielsen P, Yuan L, Saif LJ. 2003. Protection and antibody responses to oral priming by attenuated human rotavirus followed by oral boosting with 2/6-rotavirus-like particles with immunostimulating complexes in gnotobiotic pigs. Vaccine 21:4059–4070.

Offit PA, Hoffenberg EJ, Santos N, Gouvea V. 1993. Rotavirus-specific humoral and cellular immune response after primary, symptomatic infection. J Infect Dis 167:1436–1440.

Ojeh CK, Parwani AV, Jiang BM, Theil KW, Rosen BI, Saif LJ. 1993. Characterization of field isolates of porcine group C rotaviruses using gene 5 (VP6) and gene 8 (VP7) cDNA probes. J Vet Diagn Invest 5:434–438.

Ojeh CK, Tsunemitsu H, Simkins RA, Saif LJ. 1992. Development of a biotin-streptavidin-enhanced enzyme-linked immunosorbent assay which uses monoclonal antibodies for detection of group C rotaviruses. J Clin Microbiol 30:1667–1673.

Okada J, Urasawa T, Kobayashi N, Taniguchi K, Hasegawa A, Mise K, Urasawa S. 2000. New P serotype of group A human rotavirus closely related to that of a porcine rotavirus. J Med Virol 60:63–69.

Oldham G, Bridger JC, Howard CJ, Parsons KR. 1993. In vivo role of lymphocyte subpopulations in the control of virus excretion and mucosal antibody responses of cattle infected with rotavirus. J Virol 67:5012–5019.

Parreno V, Bejar C, Vagnozzi A, Barrandeguy M, Costantini V, Craig MI, Yuan L, Hodgins D, Saif L, Fernandez F. 2004. Modulation by colostrum-acquired maternal antibodies of systemic and mucosal antibody responses to rotavirus in calves experimentally challenged with bovine rotavirus. Vet Immunol Immunopathol 100:7–24.

Parreno V, Hodgins DC, de Arriba L, Kang SY, Yuan L, Ward LA, To TL, Saif LJ. 1999. Serum and intestinal isotype antibody responses to Wa human rotavirus in gnotobiotic pigs are modulated by maternal antibodies. J Gen Virol 80:1417–1428.

Paul PS, Mengeling WL, Malstrom CE, Van Deusen RA. 1989. Production and characterization of monoclonal antibodies to porcine immunoglobulin gamma, alpha, and light chains. Am J Vet Res 50:471–479.

Paul PS, Stevenson GW. 1999. Rotavirus and Reovirus. In Diseases of Swine (8th edition). B Straw, S D'Allaire, WL Mengeling, D Taylor, eds. Ames: Iowa State University Press, pp. 255–275.

Pearson GR, McNulty MS. 1977. Pathological changes in the small intestine of neonatal pigs infected with a pig reovirus-like agent (rotavirus). J Comp Pathol 87:363–375.

——. 1979. Ultrastructural changes in small intestinal epithelium of neonatal pigs infected with pig rotavirus. Arch Virol 59:127–136.

Pedley S, Bridger JC, Chasey D, McCrae MA. 1986. Definition of two new groups of atypical rotaviruses. J Gen Virol 67:131–137.

Pongsuwanna Y, Taniguchi K, Chiwakul M, Urasawa T, Wakasugi F, Jayavasu C, Urasawa S. 1996. Serological and genomic characterization of porcine rotaviruses in Thailand: Detection of a G10 porcine rotavirus. J Clin Microbiol 34:1050–1057.

Proescholdt T. 1991. Cultivation of porcine group C rotavirus in porcine intestinal cell line. MS thesis, Iowa State University, Ames, Iowa.

Ramia S, Sattar SA. 1980. Proteolytic enzymes and rotavirus SA-11 plaque formation. Can J Comp Med 44:232–235.

Ramos AP, Stefanelli CC, Linhares RE, de Brito BG, Santos N, Gouvea V, de Cassia Lima R, Nozawa C. 2000. The stability of porcine rotavirus in feces. Vet Microbiol 71:1–8.

Rhoads JM, Keku EO, Quinn J, Woosely J, Lecce JG. 1991. L-glutamine stimulates jejunal sodium and chloride absorption in pig rotavirus enteritis. Gastroenterology 100:683–691.

Rhoads JM, Ulshen MH, Keku EO, Chen W, Kandil HM, Woodard JP, Liu SC, Fuller CR, Leary HL Jr, Lecce JG. 1995. Oral transforming growth factor-alpha enhances jejunal mucosal recovery and electrical resistance in piglet rotavirus enteritis. Pediatr Res 38:173–181.

Roberts L, Walker EJ, Snodgrass DR, Angus KW. 1980. Diarrhoea in unweaned piglets associated with rotavirus and coccidial infections. Vet Rec 107:156–157.

Robl MG, McAdaragh JP, Phillips CS, Bicknell EJ. 1971. Experimental swine pneumonia caused by reovirus type 3. Vet Med Small Anim Clin 66:903–909.

Rodger SM, Craven JA, Williams I. 1975. Letter: Demonstration of reovirus-like particles in intestinal contents of piglets with diarrhoea. Aust Vet J 51:536.

Rollo EE, Kumar KP, Reich NC, Cohen J, Angel J, Greenberg HB, Sheth R, Anderson J, Oh B, Hempson SJ, Mackow ER, Shaw RD. 1999. The epithelial cell response to rotavirus infection. J Immunol 163:4442–4452.

Rolsma MD, Kuhlenschmidt TB, Gelberg HB, Kuhlenschmidt MS. 1998. Structure and function of a ganglioside receptor for porcine rotavirus. J Virol 72:9079–9091.

Rosen BI, Parwani AV, Lopez S, Flores J, Saif LJ. 1994. Serotypic differentiation of rotaviruses in field samples from diarrheic pigs by using nucleic acid probes specific for porcine VP4 and human and porcine VP7 genes. J Clin Microbiol 32:311–317.

Rosen BI, Saif LJ, Jackwood DJ, Gorziglia M. 1990. Hybridization probes for the detection and differentiation of two serotypes of porcine rotavirus. Vet Microbiol 24:327–339.

Ruiz MC, Charpilienne A, Liprandi F, Gajardo R, Michelangeli F, Cohen J. 1996. The concentration of Ca2+ that solubilizes outer capsid proteins from rotavirus particles is dependent on the strain. J Virol 70:4877–4883.

Sabin AB. 1959. Reoviruses. A new group of respiratory and enteric viruses formerly classified as ECHO type 10 is described. Science 130:1387–1389.

Saif LJ. 1999. Comparative pathogenesis of enteric viral infections of swine. Adv Exp Med Biol 473:47–59.

Saif L. 1985. Passive immunity to coronavirus and rotavirus infections in swine and cattle: Enhancement by maternal vaccination. In Infectious Diarrhoea in the Young. S Tzipori, ed. New York: Elsevier Science Publishers B.V., pp. 456–467.

Saif LJ, Azevedo MSP, Yuan L, Jeong KI, Nguyen TV, Pouly SM, Gochnauer M. 2003. Nasal and rectal shedding and viremia in gnotobiotic piglets after oral or intranasal inoculation with Wa human rotavirus. 8th International Symposium on ds-RNA Viruses. Abstract W6.3.

Saif LJ, Fernandez FM. 1996. Group A rotavirus veterinary vaccines. J Infect Dis 174:S98–106.

Saif LJ, Jiang B. 1994. Nongroup A rotaviruses of humans and animals. Curr Top Microbiol Immunol 185:339–371.

Saif LJ, Terrett LA, Miller KL, Cross RF. 1988. Serial propagation of porcine group C rotavirus (pararotavirus) in a continuous cell line and characterization of the passaged virus. J Clin Microbiol 26:1277–1282.

Saif LJ, Theil KW, Bohl EH. 1978. Morphogenesis of porcine rotavirus in porcine kidney cell cultures and intestinal epithelial cells. J Gen Virol 39:205–217.

Saif LJ, Ward LA, Yuan L, Rosen BI, To TL. 1996. The gnotobiotic piglet as a model for studies of disease pathogenesis and immunity to human rotaviruses. Arch Virol Suppl 12:153–161.

Saif LJ, Yuan L, Ward L, To T. 1997. Comparative studies of the pathogenesis, antibody immune responses, and homologous protection to porcine and human rotaviruses in gnotobiotic piglets. Adv Exp Med Biol 412:397–403.

Sanekata T, Kuwamoto Y, Akamatsu S, Sakon N, Oseto M, Taniguchi K, Nakata S, Estes MK. 1996. Isolation of group B porcine rotavirus in cell culture. J Clin Microbiol 34:759–761.

Santos N, Lima RC, Nozawa CM, Linhares RE, Gouvea V. 1999. Detection of porcine rotavirus type G9 and of a mixture of types G1 and G5 associated with Wa-like VP4 specificity: Evidence for natural human-porcine genetic reassortment. J Clin Microbiol 37:2734–2736.

Sattar SA, Jacobsen H, Rahman H, Cusack TM, Rubino JR. 1994. Interruption of rotavirus spread through chemical disinfection. Infect Control Hosp Epidemiol 15:751–756.

Shaw DP, Morehouse LG, Solorzano RF. 1989. Experimental rotavirus infection in three-week-old pigs. Am J Vet Res 50:1961–1965.

Steel RB, Torres-Medina A. 1984. Effects of environmental and dietary factors on human rotavirus infection in gnotobiotic piglets. Infect Immun 43:906–911.

Stevenson GW. 1990. Pathogenesis of a new porcine serotype of group A rotavirus in neonatal gnotobiotic and weaned conventional pigs. PhD dissertation, Iowa State University, Ames, Iowa.

Svensmark B, Askaa J, Wolstrup C, Nielsen K. 1989. Epidemiological studies of piglet diarrhoea in intensively managed Danish sow herds. IV. Pathogenicity of porcine rotavirus. Acta Vet Scand 30:71–76.

Tam JS, Szymanski MT, Middleton PJ, Petric M. 1976. Studies on the particles of infantile gastroenteritis virus (orbivirus group). Intervirology 7:181–191.

Terrett LA, Saif LJ, Theil KW, Kohler EM. 1987. Physicochemical characterization of porcine pararotavirus and detection of virus and viral antibodies using cell culture immunofluorescence. J Clin Microbiol 25:268–272.

Theil KW, Saif LJ. 1985. In vitro detection of porcine rotavirus-like virus (group B rotavirus) and its antibody. J Clin Microbiol 21:844–846.Theil KW, Bohl EH, Agnes AG. 1977. Cell culture propagation of porcine rotavirus (reovirus-like agent). Am J Vet Res 38:1765–1768.

Theil KW, Bohl EH, Cross RF, Kohler EM, Agnes AG. 1978. Pathogenesis of porcine rotaviral infection in experimentally inoculated gnotobiotic pigs. Am J Vet Res 39:213–220.

Theil KW, Saif LJ, Moorhead PD, Whitmoyer RE. 1985. Porcine rotavirus-like virus (group B rotavirus): Characterization and pathogenicity for gnotobiotic pigs. J Clin Microbiol 21: 340–345.

Timenetsky Mdo C, Gouvea V, Santos N, Carmona RC, Hoshino Y. 1997. A novel human rotavirus serotype with dual G5-G11 specificity. J Gen Virol 78:1373–1378.

Torres-Medina A, Underdahl NR. 1980. Scanning electron microscopy of intestine of gnotobiotic piglets infected with porcine rotavirus. Can J Comp Med 44:403–411.

Tsunemitsu H, Jiang B, Saif LJ. 1992a. Detection of group C rotavirus antigens and antibodies in animals and humans by enzyme-linked immunosorbent assays. J Clin Microbiol 30:2129–2134.

Tsunemitsu H, Jiang B, Yamashita Y, Oseto M, Ushijima H, Saif LJ. 1992b. Evidence of serologic diversity within group C rotaviruses. J Clin Microbiol 30:3009–3012.

Tyler KL. 1998. Pathogenesis of reovirus infections of the central nervous system. Curr Top Microbiol Immunol 233:93–124.

——. 2001. Mammalian reoviruses. In Fields Virology. DM Kinipe, PM Howley, eds. Philadelphia: Lippincott-William & Wilkins, pp. 1729–1745.

Tzipori S, Chandler D, Makin T, Smith M. 1980a. *Escherichia coli* and rotavirus infections in four-week-old gnotobiotic piglets fed milk or dry food. Aust Vet J 56:279–284.

Tzipori S, Chandler D, Smith M, Makin T, Hennessy D. 1980b. Factors contributing to postweaning diarrhoea in a large intensive piggery. Aust Vet J 56:274–278.

Tzipori S, Williams IH. 1978. Diarrhoea in piglets inoculated with rotavirus. Aust Vet J, 54:188–192.

Tzipori SR, Makin TJ, Smith ML. 1980c. The clinical response of gnotobiotic calves, pigs and lambs to inoculation with human, calf, pig and foal rotavirus isolates. Aust J Exp Biol Med Sci 58:309–318.

Varghese V, Das S, Singh NB, Kojima K, Bhattacharya SK, Krishnan T, Kobayashi N, Naik TN. 2004. Molecular characterization of a human rotavirus reveals porcine characteristics in most of the genes including VP6 and NSP4. Arch Virol 149:155–172.

Wagstrom EA, Yoon KJ, Zimmerman JJ. 2000. Immune components in porcine mammary secretions. Viral Immunol 13:383–397.

Ward LA, Rich ED, Besser TE. 1996a. Role of maternally derived circulating antibodies in protection of neonatal swine against porcine group A rotavirus. J Infect Dis 174:276–282.

Ward LA, Rosen BI, Yuan L, Saif LJ. 1996b. Pathogenesis of an attenuated and a virulent strain of group A human rotavirus in neonatal gnotobiotic pigs. J Gen Virol 77:1431–1441.

Ward LA, Yuan L, Rosen BI, To TL, Saif LJ. 1996c. Development of mucosal and systemic lymphoproliferative responses and protective immunity to human group A rotaviruses in a gnotobiotic pig model. Clin Diagn Lab Immunol 3:342–350.

Watt RG. 1978. Virological study of two commerical pig herds with respiratory disease. Res Vet Sci 24:147–153.

Wieler LH, Ilieff A, Herbst W, Bauer C, Vieler E, Bauerfeind R, Failing K, Klos H, Wengert D, Baljer G, Zahner H. 2001. Prevalence of enteropathogens in suckling and weaned piglets with diarrhoea in southern Germany. J Vet Med B Infect Dis Vet Public Health 48:151–159.

Wilde J, Yolken R, Willoughby R, Eiden J. 1991. Improved detection of rotavirus shedding by polymerase chain reaction. Lancet 337:323–326.

Will LA, Paul PS, Proescholdt TA, Aktar SN, Flaming KP, Janke BH, Sacks J, Lyoo YS, Hill HT, Hoffman LJ. 1994. Evaluation of rotavirus infection and diarrhea in Iowa commercial pigs based on an epidemiologic study of a population represented by diagnostic laboratory cases. J Vet Diagn Invest 6:416–422.

Winiarczyk S, Gradzki Z. 1999. Comparison of polymerase chain reaction and dot hybridization with enzyme-linked immunoassay, virological examination and polyacrylamide gel electrophoresis for the detection of porcine rotavirus in faecal specimens. Zentralbl Veterinarmed B 46:623–634.

Winiarczyk S, Paul PS, Mummidi S, Panek R, Gradzki Z. 2002. Survey of porcine rotavirus G and P genotype in Poland and the United States using RT-PCR. J Vet Med B Infect Dis Vet Public Health 49:373–378.

Woode GN. 1978. Epizootiology of bovine rotavirus infection. Vet Rec 103:44–46.

Woode GN, Bridger J, Hall GA, Jones JM, Jackson G. 1976. The isolation of reovirus-like agents (rota-viruses) from acute gastroenteritis of piglets. J Med Microbiol 9:203–209.

Xu L, Harbour D, McCrae MA. 1990. The application of polymerase chain reaction to the detection of rotaviruses in faeces. J Virol Methods 27:29–37.

Yaeger M, Funk N, Hoffman L. 2002. A survey of agents associated with neonatal diarrhea in Iowa swine including *Clostridium difficile* and porcine reproductive and respiratory syndrome virus. J Vet Diagn Invest 14:281–287.

Yang YF, Yang SC, Tai FH. 1976. Reovirus antibodies among animals in Taiwan. Zhonghua Min Guo Wei Sheng Wu Xue Za Zhi 9:1–4.

Yolken R, Wee SB, Eiden J, Kinney J, Vonderfecht S. 1988. Identification of a group-reactive epitope of group B rotaviruses recognized by monoclonal antibody and application to the development of a sensitive immunoassay for viral characterization. J Clin Microbiol 26:1853–1858.

Yuan L, Azevedo MSP, Jeong K-I, Nguyen TV, Gonzalez AM, Iosef C, Herrmann JE, Saif LJ. 2003. Evaluation of a live attenuated human rotavirus priming and bovine rotavirus VP6 DNA boosting vaccination strategy in a gnotobiotic pig model. Abstract PR.4. 8th International Symposium on ds-RNA Viruses. Abstract PR.4.

Yuan L, Geyer A, Hodgins DC, Fan Z, Qian Y, Chang KO, Crawford SE, Parreno V, Ward LA, Estes MK, Conner ME, Saif LJ. 2000. Intranasal administration of 2/6-rotavirus-like particles with mutant *Escherichia coli* heat-labile toxin (LT-R192G) induces antibody-secreting cell responses but not protective immunity in gnotobiotic pigs. J Virol 74:8843–8853.

Yuan L, Geyer A, Saif LJ. 2001a. Short-term immunoglobulin A B-cell memory resides in intestinal lymphoid tissues but not in bone marrow of gnotobiotic pigs inoculated with Wa human rotavirus. Immunology 103:188–198.

Yuan L, Iosef C, Azevedo MS, Kim Y, Qian Y, Geyer A, Nguyen TV, Chang KO, Saif LJ. 2001b. Protective immunity and antibody-secreting cell responses elicited by combined oral attenuated Wa human rotavirus and intranasal Wa 2/6-VLPs with mutant *Escherichia coli* heat-labile toxin in gnotobiotic pigs. J Virol 75:9229–9238.

Yuan L, Ishida SI, Honma S, Patton JT, Hodgins DC, Kapikian AZ, Hoshino Y. 2004. Homotypic and heterotypic serum isotype-specific antibody responses to rotavirus nonstructural protein 4 and viral protein (VP) 4, VP6, and VP7 in infants who received selected live oral rotavirus vaccines. J Infect Dis 189:1833–1845.

Yuan L, Kang SY, Ward LA, To TL, Saif LJ. 1998. Antibody-secreting cell responses and protective immunity assessed in gnotobiotic pigs inoculated orally or intramuscularly with inactivated human rotavirus. J Virol 72:330–338.

Yuan L, Saif LJ. 2002. Induction of mucosal immune responses and protection against enteric viruses: Rotavirus infection of gnotobiotic pigs as a model. Vet Immunol Immunopathol 87:147–160.

——. 2003. Rotavirus-like particle vaccines evaluated in a pig model of human rotavirus diarrhea and in cattle. In Viral Gastroenteritis. U Desselberger, J Gray, eds. New York: Elsevier Science, B.V., pp. 357–368.

Yuan L, Ward LA, Rosen BI, To TL, Saif LJ. 1996. Systematic and intestinal antibody-secreting cell responses and correlates of protective immunity to human rotavirus in a gnotobiotic pig model of disease. J Virol 70:3075–3083.

Zaberezhny AD, Lyoo YS, Paul PS. 1994. Prevalence of P types among porcine rotaviruses using subgenomic VP4 gene probes. Vet Microbiol 39:97–110.

Zijlstra RT, Donovan SM, Odle J, Gelberg HB, Petschow BW, Gaskins HR. 1997. Protein-energy malnutrition delays small-intestinal recovery in neonatal pigs infected with rotavirus. J Nutr 127:1118–1127.

Zijlstra RT, McCracken BA, Odle J, Donovan SM, Gelberg HB, Petschow BW, Zuckermann FA, Gaskins HR. 1999. Malnutrition modifies pig small intestinal inflammatory responses to rotavirus. J Nutr 129:838–843.

27 Paramyxoviruses: Rubulavirus, Menangle, and Nipah Virus Infections

Peter D. Kirkland and Alberto Stephano

The family *Paramyxoviridae* contains viral pathogens of international significance in most animal species and humans. Until recently, there were no major paramyxovirus pathogens of pigs, the single possible exception being the rubulavirus that causes blue eye (BE) disease (blue eye paramyxovirus, BEP). However, BEP is confined to Mexico, where its economic impact is considered low at present. Then, during a 3-year period commencing in 1997, several new paramyxoviruses were identified, and two (Menangle and Nipah viruses) were found to be serious pathogens of both pigs and humans.

The family *Paramyxoviridae* encompasses a group of large (150–400 nm in diameter) pleomorphic viruses. The genome consists of a long single strand of RNA within a herringbone-like nucleocapsid. The nucleocapsid is surrounded by a lipid envelope that usually contains an outer fringe of surface projections or "spikes."

The paramyxoviruses are currently organized in 2 subfamilies and 7 genera. There are 5 genera in the subfamily *Paramyxovirinae*: *Avulavirus*, *Henipavirus*, *Morbillivirus*, *Respirovirus*, and *Rubulavirus*. There are major pathogens of animals and humans in each of these genera—e.g., Newcastle disease virus of poultry in the genus *Avulavirus*; canine distemper and human measles viruses in the genus *Morbillivirus*; several parainfluenza viruses of animals and humans in the genus *Respirovirus*; and in the genus *Rubulavirus*, human mumps virus, BEP, and Menangle virus. Both of the latter two viruses are infectious for pigs. The genus *Henipavirus* was created for two of the most recently recognized and closely related paramyxoviruses, Hendra and Nipah, reflecting their morphological and genetic differences from other paramyxoviruses.

As a result of their tissue trophisms, there are broad similarities in the diseases caused by paramyxoviruses. Typically, pathogenic paramyxoviruses are associated with diseases of the central nervous system (CNS) (canine distemper and Newcastle disease) and respiratory systems (parainfluenza infections, Hendra, Nipah, and Newcastle disease). Some, especially Menangle virus and BEP, are also important reproductive pathogens.

The only paramyxoviruses that cause significant disease in pigs are BEP, Menangle virus, and Nipah virus. There have been occasional reports of other paramyxoviruses associated with respiratory and CNS disease in pigs in Japan (Sasahara et al. 1954), Canada (Greig et al. 1971), Israel (Lipkind et al. 1986), and the United States (Paul et al. 1994), but none has proven to be of significance. This chapter provides an overview of BEP, Menangle and Nipah viruses, and the diseases they cause.

Rubulavirus (Blue Eye Disease)

As mentioned before, blue eye (BE) is a disease of swine caused by infection with blue eye paramyxovirus (BEP) (Stephano et al. 1988b) or porcine rubulavirus, also known as La Piedad-Michoacan virus (LPMV). The disease was first reported in 1980 in central Mexico, with numerous outbreaks of encephalitis and corneal opacity in piglets (Stephano et al. 1982). A hemagglutinating virus was isolated, characterized, and identified as a serologically distinct member of the family *Paramyxo-* *viridae* (Stephano and Gay 1983, 1984, 1985a; Stephano et al. 1986b).

The first reported outbreak of BE was observed on a commercial farm with 2500 sows located in La Piedad, Michoacán, Mexico (Stephano et al. 1982). Thereafter, BE was recognized as an important pathogen in central Mexico, with serological evidence of BEP in at least 16 states in Mexico (Stephano et al. 1988b). The disease is still recognized in central Mexico, but its economic im-

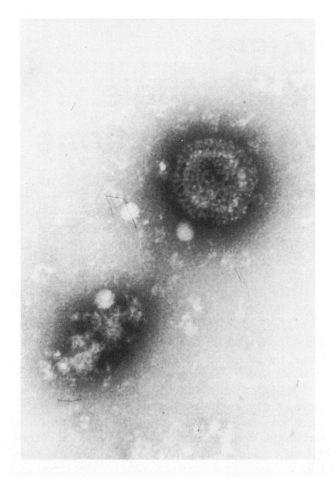

27.1. *Blue eye paramyxovirus particles showing surface projections by negative-stain electron microscopy (×108,200).*

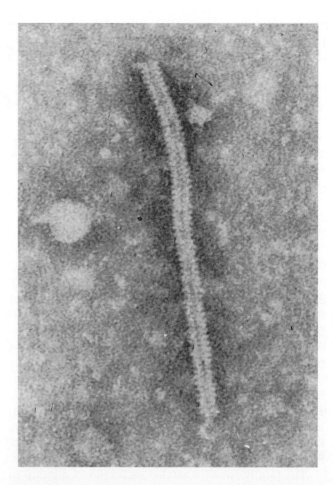

27.2. *Fraction of a nucleocapsid from a disrupted BEP (negative-stain electron microscopy; ×203,000).*

pact has lessened. BE has not been reported outside of Mexico.

ETIOLOGY

Extensive molecular characterization of BEP (Berg et al. 1991, 1992; Sundqvist et al. 1990, 1992), combined with its morphology and biological properties, supports its placement in the rubulavirus genus.

BEP particles are similar to other paramyxoviruses, measuring 135–148 nm by 257–360 nm (Figure 27.1). The virion is pleomorphic, but usually more or less spherical; no filamentous forms have been observed. Nucleocapsids from disrupted virus particles have a diameter of 20 nm and a length of 1000–1630 nm (Figure 27.2) or more (Stephano and Gay 1985a).

In the laboratory, BEP replicates and produces cytopathology in a wide range of cell cultures from many different animal species, including both continuous cell lines and primary cell cultures. Changes consist of individual rounded cells, cytoplasmic vacuoles, and syncytium formation. Some cells also contain viral inclusion bodies (Moreno-Lopez et al. 1986; Stephano and

Gay 1985a; Stephano et al. 1986a). The chick embryo also supports BEP replication.

BEP agglutinates erythrocytes from a wide range of animal species, as well as humans. Spontaneous elution occurs at 37°C after 30–60 minutes. Hemadsorption of chicken erythrocytes has also been described (Stephano and Gay 1985a; Stephano et al. 1986b).

BEP is not known to share any antigens with other paramyxoviruses (Stephano et al. 1986b) and no antigenic differences have been observed between different strains of BEP (Gay and Stephano 1987).

CLINICAL SIGNS

An outbreak of BE may start in any area of a pig farm, but is usually first observed in the farrowing house, with CNS signs and high piglet mortality. At about the same time, corneal opacity may be observed in some weaned or fattening pigs (Stephano and Gay 1985a, 1986a; Stephano et al. 1988a). The mortality rate increases rapidly and then declines within a short time. Once the initial outbreak is over, no new clinical cases appear, unless susceptible pigs are introduced.

Clinical signs are variable and depend primarily on the age of the pig. However, corneal opacity, the sign that gives the disease its name, frequently occurs in pigs of all ages without other signs and resolves spontaneously.

Piglets 2–15 days old are the most susceptible, and the onset of clinical signs is sudden. Healthy piglets may suddenly become prostrate, generally in lateral recumbency, or show nervous signs. However, the disease usually runs a course that starts with fever, a rough hair coat, and an arched back, sometimes accompanied by constipation or diarrhea. These signs are followed by progressive nervous signs, including ataxia, weakness, rigidity (mainly of the hind legs), muscle tremor, and abnormal posture, such as a sitting position. Anorexia does not occur as long as piglets can still walk. Some piglets are hyperexcitable and may squeal and show paddling movements when handled. Other signs include lethargy with some involuntary movements, dilated pupils, apparent blindness, and, occasionally, nystagmus. Some piglets suffer from conjunctivitis, with swollen eyelids and lacrimation. Often the eyelids are closed and adherent with exudate. In up to 10% of affected piglets, either unilateral or bilateral corneal opacity is present.

Of the litters farrowed during an outbreak, about 20% are affected. In these litters, the piglet morbidity is 20–50%, and mortality in affected piglets is about 90%. In the first cases observed, piglets usually died within 48 hours of the appearance of clinical signs, but in later cases, death occurred after 4–6 days. During an initial outbreak, deaths occur for 2–9 weeks, depending on the management system.

Pigs older than 30 days show moderate and transient clinical signs such as anorexia, fever, sneezing, and coughing. Nervous signs are less common and less obvious but, when present, consist of listlessness, ataxia, circling, and, rarely, swaying of the head. Uni- or bilateral corneal opacity and conjunctivitis continue to appear on the farm for another month without other signs. Fewer than 2% of pigs older than 30 days are affected and the mortality is generally low. Outbreaks with 20% mortality and severe CNS manifestations have been observed in 15–45 kg pigs. Corneal opacity was present in up to 30% of these pigs (Stephano and Gay 1985b).

Most of the sows suckling affected litters are clinically normal. Some show moderate anorexia 1 or 2 days before the appearance of clinical signs in piglets. Corneal opacity has also been observed in the farrowing house during outbreaks.

In pregnant sows, reproductive failure lasting 2–11 months (usually 4 months) is observed. Reproductive signs during outbreaks include an increase in the number of animals returning to estrus, a reduction in farrowing rate, and an increase in the weaning-to-service interval and nonproductive sow days. The rate of stillbirths and mummified fetuses also increases and, conse-quently, there is a reduction in the number of pigs born alive. Later, there is also a reduction in the total number of pigs born. Abortion is not a cardinal feature, but has sometimes been observed during an acute outbreak. Gilts and other adult pigs occasionally develop corneal opacity.

Boars, like other adult animals, generally do not show clinical signs, but mild anorexia and corneal opacity have been recorded. Semen evaluation demonstrated that, in herds infected by BEP, about 30% of boars show temporary or permanent infertility, with a decrease in concentration, an increase in abnormalities, and a decrease in motility and viability of spermatozoa. In some boars there is azoospermia, the ejaculate becomes clear and resembles coconut water. Some boars develop swollen testicles. The testis and epididymis become turgid with marked edema. Later, some develop a granular texture and most atrophy (generally unilateral) or become soft and flabby with or without granular epididymitis. Boars with severe lesions lose libido (Campos and Carbajal 1989; Stephano et al. 1990).

Differences in clinical signs became evident a few years after the virus was discovered. In 1980, primarily piglets were affected. Mortality and CNS disorders in pigs older than 30 days were uncommon. In 1983, severe outbreaks of encephalitis with high mortality in pigs weighing 15–45 kg were observed on badly managed farms, always with concomitant viral and bacterial diseases (Stephano and Gay 1985b, 1986a). Also in 1983, reproductive failure in sows and transient infertility in boars were identified (Stephano and Gay 1984, 1985a). In 1988, severe problems of orchitis, epididymitis, and testicular atrophy in boars became evident (Campos and Carbajal 1989; Stephano et al. 1990).

EPIDEMIOLOGY

Pigs are the only species known to be affected clinically by BEP following natural exposure. Experimentally, BEP affects mice, rats, and chick embryos. Rabbits, dogs, cats, and peccaries do not show clinical signs, but rabbits, cats, and peccaries produce antibodies (Stephano and Gay 1985a; Stephano et al. 1988a).

Subclinically infected pigs from affected farms are the primary source of BEP. The virus is apparently disseminated by nose-to-nose contact between infected and susceptible pigs. Transmission through semen has not been proven experimentally, but virus can be recovered from semen, testis, epididymis, prostate, seminal vesicles, and bulbo-urethral glands (M. H. Hernandez, personal communication). The virus may be disseminated by people and vehicles, and possibly by birds and wind. Other sources of infection have not been demonstrated.

The disease is self-limiting in closed herds. Sentinel pigs introduced to a farm 6–12 months after an outbreak remain asymptomatic and do not seroconvert. Although there is evidence of persistence of BEP RNA in the brain and lung of experimentally infected pigs, neither infectious virus nor viral antigen was detected after immunosuppression (Wiman et al. 1998). Further, positive animals moved to seronegative herds did not spread the virus (Stephano and Gay 1986b; Stephano et al. 1986a). However, the disease can recur if a susceptible group of pigs is introduced to a farm. Large farms with a continuous system of production may have cases periodically.

PATHOGENESIS

It has been presumed that BEP infection is acquired by inhalation. Experimentally, intratracheal or intranasal exposures are effective routes of infection. The initial site of BEP replication is thought to be the nasal mucosa and tonsils. The virus has also been observed in the axon of neurons. From the initial site of replication, BEP spreads quickly to the brain and lung. CNS manifestations occur early in the disease. Nervous signs have been induced in 1-day-old piglets 20–66 hours after inoculation, some weaned pigs (21–50 days old) developed a nervous syndrome at 11 days postinoculation, and pregnant sows developed reproductive failure when inoculated during pregnancy. Corneal opacity was occasionally observed in these cases. The disease was also reproduced in susceptible pigs placed in contact with experimentally infected pigs as long as 19 days after experimental infection (Stephano and Gay 1983; Stephano et al. 1988b).

The interstitial pneumonia that is observed suggests dissemination by viremia. In experimentally infected piglets, virus could be isolated from the brain, lung, tonsil, liver, turbinate, spleen, kidney, mesenteric lymph node, heart, and blood.

The cause of the corneal opacity is unknown, but anterior uveitis is commonly observed microscopically in the cornea (Stephano and Gay 1986b). The opacity usually occurs late in the course of the disease and is thought to be due to an immunological reaction similar to that observed in dogs after adenovirus-induced hepatitis.

Infection of pregnant sows in the first one-third of gestation results in reproductive failure due to embryonic mortality. Affected sows usually return to estrus. When infection occurs later in gestation, the result is stillbirths and fetal mummification (Stephano and Gay 1984).

Intranasal infection of young boars results in inflammation and edema of the testis and epididymis by 15 days after inoculation. By 30 days, there is necrosis of the seminiferous tubules and rupture of the epithelial wall of the epididymis with leakage of spermatozoa from the lumen, leading to abscess formation. Boars sacrificed 80 days after infection showed fibrosis and granuloma formation in the epididymis as well as testicular atrophy (Ramirez et al. 1995). BEP was recovered from

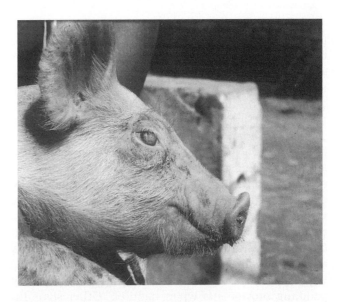

27.3. *Corneal opacity in a 7-day-old piglet.*

testis, epididymis, prostate, seminal vesicles and bulbourethral glands 10–45 days after inoculation.

PATHOLOGY

There are no specific gross changes in cases of BE. In piglets, a mild pneumonia is frequently observed at the ventral tips of the cranial lung lobes. There is mild distension of the stomach with milk, distension of the urinary bladder, and a slight accumulation of peritoneal fluid with fibrin. The brain is often congested and there is an increase in the quantity of cerebrospinal fluid. Conjunctivitis, chemosis, and varying degrees of corneal opacity (Figure 27.3), usually unilateral, are observed. Vesicle formation, ulcers, and keratoconus have been observed in the cornea as well as exudate in the anterior chamber. Pericardial and renal hemorrhages are occasionally observed (Stephano and Gay 1985a, 1986b).

Boars develop swollen testicles and epididymes. These changes are frequently unilateral. There is orchitis, epididymitis, and, later, atrophy of the testicle, with or without granulomatous formation in the epididymis. Hemorrhages are occasionally observed in the tunica albuginia, epididymis, or testis (Campos and Carbajal 1989; Ramirez et al. 1995; Stephano et al. 1990).

The main histological changes are seen in the brain and spinal cord. These reflect a nonsuppurative encephalomyelitis affecting mainly the gray matter of the thalamus, midbrain, and cerebral cortex and include a multifocal and diffuse gliosis, perivascular cuffing with lymphocytes, plasma cells and reticular cells, neuronal necrosis, neuronophagia, meningitis, and choroiditis (Ramirez and Stephano 1982). Intracytoplasmic inclusion bodies are found in neurons (Stephano and Gay 1986b; Stephano et al. 1988a).

The lungs have localized areas of interstitial pneumonia characterized by thickened septa with mononuclear cell infiltration.

Changes in the eye are mainly corneal opacity, characterized by corneal edema and anterior uveitis. Neutrophils, macrophages, or mononuclear cells infiltrate the iridocorneal endothelium, corneo-scleral angle, and cornea (Stephano and Gay 1986b; Stephano et al. 1988a).

In boars, the affected testes show degeneration and necrosis of the germinal epithelium. The interstitial tissue shows Leydig cell hyperplasia, mononuclear cell infiltration, hyalinization of the vascular wall, and fibrosis. The epididymis shows vesicle formation, loss of epithelial cilia, rupture of the epithelial wall, presence of spermatozoa in the intertubular space, and severe infiltration of inflammatory mononuclear cells with macrophage phagocytosis of fragmented sperm. Fibrosis and spermatic granuloma are organized.

DIAGNOSIS

Clinical signs such as encephalitis, corneal opacity, and reproductive failure in the sow and orchitis and epididymitis in the boar are consistent with a diagnosis of BE. Additional diagnostic evidence is provided by histological lesions, such as nonsuppurative encephalitis, anterior uveitis, keratitis, orchitis, and epididymitis. The presence of intracytoplasmic inclusions in neurons and corneal epithelium in conjunction with these clinical signs and histological findings provides strong support for a diagnosis of BE.

Other causes of encephalitis and reproductive disease, especially Aujeszky's disease (pseudorabies) virus and porcine reproductive and respiratory syndrome virus, must be considered. Only BEP produces corneal opacity along with orchitis and epididymitis in boars (Campos and Carbajal 1989; Stephano and Gay 1985b; Stephano et al. 1988a, 1990).

Paired serum samples, 15 days apart, are recommended for serological confirmation. Hemagglutination inhibition (HI), virus neutralization (VN), and enzyme-linked immunosorbent assays (ELISA) have been used for serology. HI is the most frequently used test, but false-positive titers up to 1:16 have been detected when chicken erythrocytes are used or when the

antigen is grown in chicken embryos (Ramirez et al. 1996). Therefore, bovine erythrocytes are recommended. Naturally infected pigs develop antibodies that usually persist for life.

Direct immunofluorescence has been performed to detect antigens in tissue sections and monolayers (Stephano and Gay 1985a; Stephano et al. 1988a).

The brain is the best tissue for virus isolation and antigen detection, but lung and tonsil are also suitable (Stephano et al. 1988a). PK-15 cells or primary pig kidney cells are preferred for virus isolation. Virus replication induces syncytium formation, and the virus is identified by neutralization and immunofluorescence.

PREVENTION AND CONTROL

As with most viral diseases of swine, there is no specific treatment. Pigs with corneal opacity frequently recover spontaneously, whereas pigs with central nervous disease generally die. Antimicrobial therapy is commonly used to treat and prevent secondary infections.

Herd health programs are the most reliable method of preventing the introduction of BEP to a farm. New pigs must be derived from a healthy herd and quarantined prior to introduction. Standard biosecurity measures provide insurance against infection, e.g., perimeter fencing; separate load-out areas; changing rooms and showers; control of birds, rats, and mice; prompt waste removal and disposal of dead pigs; and control of the movement of personnel, visitors, and vehicles. Serological screening of replacement animals is recommended.

Elimination of BEP from infected herds has been accomplished by management practices, e.g., herd closure, cleaning and disinfecting, all-in/all-out production, elimination of clinically affected animals, and disposal of dead pigs. The effectiveness of these procedures should be monitored by serological testing and the introduction of sentinel animals (BEP seronegative pigs) to confirm the elimination of BEP (Stephano et al. 1986b).

At present there are two commercial inactivated virus vaccines approved for use in pregnant sows, gilts, boars, and piglets. Development of a recombinant vaccine is in progress.

Menangle Virus

Menangle virus was first identified during a disease outbreak in New South Wales, Australia, in 1997. This virus causes reproductive disease and congenital defects in pigs, occasionally causes moderately severe disease in humans, and has fruit bats (*Pteropus* sp., flying foxes) as a reservoir host.

ETIOLOGY

Like Blue Eye Paramyxovirus, Menangle virus has been placed in the genus Rubulavirus within the family *Paramyxoviridae*, (Bowden et al. 2001). Other well-known viruses in this genus are human parainfluenza viruses types 2 and 4 and human mumps virus.

Menangle virus has typical paramyxoviruses morphology. Virions are pleomorphic with both spherical and elongated forms that range in size from 100–350 nm. Virions possess a single layer of surface spikes approximately 17 nm in length. Ruptured particles reveal long herringbone shaped nucleocapsids with a diameter of approximately 19 nm (Philbey et al. 1998).

Menangle virus induces pronounced cytopathology in cell culture, including prominent vacuolation of cells and the development of large syncytia. The virus replicates and produces cytopathology in a wide range of cell types from many animal species, including birds and fish. There is no evidence of hemadsorption or hemagglutinating activity (Philbey et al. 1998). Menangle virus is not known to be related antigenically to any other paramyxovirus.

CLINICAL SIGNS

To date, there has been only one known disease outbreak due to Menangle virus in pigs (Love et al. 2001; Philbey et al. 1998). In 1997, over a 5-month period (mid-April to early September), sows in a 3000-sow, intensive farrow-to-finish pig farm near Sydney, New South Wales, Australia experienced severe reproductive failure (Love et al. 2001). There was a marked increase in the incidence of mummified fetuses and stillborn piglets. After a period, some of the stillborn piglets were born with severe malformations. Sows in all four breeding units on the farm were affected. There were some weeks when the farrowing rate decreased from an expected 82% to as low as 38%. Many sows showed delayed returns to estrus at around 28 days after mating, and others remained in a state of pseudopregnancy until more than 60 days post-mating. The disease occurred sequentially in all four breeding units at the pig farm, affecting the progeny of sows of all parities. In the weeks of low farrowing rates, up to 45% of sows farrowed litters with reduced numbers of live piglets and an increase in the proportion of mummified and stillborn piglets, some of which had congenital deformities.

Individual litters contained mummified fetuses of varying size, ranging upward in gestational age from 30 days, together with stillborn piglets (some with malformations) and a few normal piglets (Figure 27.4). Teratogenic defects, including arthrogryposis, brachygnathia, and kyphosis, were frequently seen in stillborn piglets, and there were occasional cases of artiodactyla (Love et al. 2001). The cranium of some piglets was slightly domed.

Although the virus was also detected on two associated growing farms, there were no breeding animals held on these farms and no clinical disease was recognized. Virus had apparently spread to these farms (separated from the main farm and each other by several hundred kilometers) when young growing pigs were moved. There were no clinical signs evident in growing

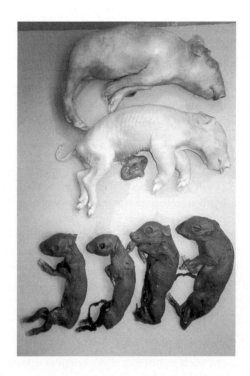

27.4. *Litter of piglets affected by Menangle virus.*

pigs of any age, and the only clinical signs in sows on the main farm were those associated with reproductive failure. It is not known whether Menangle virus can be spread in the semen of acutely infected boars.

Following the isolation of Menangle virus, two seropositive workers were identified (Chant et al. 1998). During subsequent medical investigations, it was found that both had experienced a severe febrile illness with headaches. Extensive testing failed to identify any other possible cause of the illness, and it was concluded that the disease was due to Menangle virus infection (Chant et al. 1998). Both workers recovered fully after a prolonged period of convalescence.

EPIDEMIOLOGY

Studies of archival and newly collected sera suggested that Menangle virus was not highly contagious among the pigs on the affected farm (Kirkland et al. 2001). This was deduced by the relatively slow spread of infection in a building that contained pens of sows, i.e., it took several weeks for all of the sows to become infected. Nevertheless, the virus was widely dispersed through the pig population on the affected farm. About 6 months after the estimated time of entry of the virus to the farm, a high proportion (>90%) of sera collected from pigs of all ages contained high levels of virus-neutralizing (VN) antibody. Positive VN antibody titers ranged from 1:16 to 1:4096 and remained high for at least 2 years after infection. In contrast, all samples collected prior to the estimated time of entry of the virus into the pig population were negative. All serum samples collected at the two grower-fattening farms were positive (Kirkland et al. 2001). Testing of 1114 swine sera from other pig farms throughout Australia indicated that infection was confined to the affected pig farm and the two associated grow-out facilities.

Following the initial spread of the infection through the herd, the virus was maintained by infection of young pigs at about 10–12 weeks of age as they lost the protection provided by maternally derived antibodies. In a large pig population, the constant availability of susceptible animals was sufficient to ensure persistence of the virus. In smaller pig herds, such persistence would be much less likely. Almost all selected replacement breeding pigs on the farm had been exposed to the virus and were seropositive before mating at around 28–30 weeks of age, preventing further reproductive failure.

It appeared that close contact between pigs was required for spread of infection and that the virus did not survive in the environment for long. Susceptible sentinel pigs moved into an uncleaned area occupied 3 days previously by infected pigs did not become infected.

It is believed that Menangle virus has a reservoir in flying foxes (Kirkland et al. 2001; Philbey et al. 1998). During the summer-autumn period, when the virus was thought to have entered the pig farm, there was a large breeding colony of gray-headed fruit bats (*Pteropus poliocephalus*), as well as little red fruit bats (*P. scapulatus*), roosting within 200 meters of the affected pig farm. Sera collected from gray-headed fruit bats in this colony had VN antibodies to Menangle virus. A more extensive study of sera collected from several species of fruit bats in various locations in Australia found that approximately one-third were seropositive, with VN titers ranging from 1:16–1:256. Positive samples were found in gray-headed fruit bats, black fruit bats (*P. alecto*), and spectacled fruit bats (*P. conspicillatus*), but not in little red fruit bats. These results indicated that Menangle virus was endemic in the fruit bat population and preceded the infection in pigs.

Except for spread to humans, there is no evidence that this virus has spread naturally to other animal species. Samples collected from rodents, birds, cattle, sheep, cats, and a dog in the vicinity of the affected pig farm were all seronegative.

PATHOGENESIS

The route of transmission of Menangle virus and the mechanism of spread have not been established, although fecal-oral or urinary-oral transmission is suspected (Love et al. 2001). Infection in pigs appears to be of short duration (10–14 days) and results in strong immunity. Virus was not detected in surviving piglets born during the outbreak, suggesting that persistent infection is unlikely. There is also strong circumstantial evidence that adult pigs do not become persistently infected.

The principal cause of reproductive loss associated with Menangle virus appears to be in utero infection, often resulting in fetal death. In many sows, there was early death of the whole litter, resulting in a delayed return to estrus or sometimes a state of pseudopregnancy.

At parturition, affected litters sometimes contained piglets of varying size and with a range of abnormalities. Some piglets were mummified and were of different gestational ages, some piglets were stillborn and had congenital malformations, and there were a few normal piglets (refer to Figure 27.4). These findings indicated that, as with parvovirus, transplacental infection of a few fetuses can occur early in gestation followed by progressive spread of the virus from fetus to fetus within the uterus. The teratogenic defects observed are the direct result of virus replication and cell destruction in rapidly developing fetal tissues.

PATHOLOGY

Affected litters usually consist of a mixture of mummified fetuses, autolyzed and fresh stillborn piglets, and a few normal live piglets (Love et al. 2001; Philbey et al. 1998). Congenital defects, including arthrogryposis, brachygnathia, kyphosis, and occasionally, artiodactyla are only seen in dead piglets. Affected stillborn piglets frequently have slight-to-severe degeneration of the brain and spinal cord (Figure 27.5). Gross defects ranging from porencephaly to hydranencephaly are most common in the cerebrum. Occasionally, there may be fibrinous body cavity effusions and pulmonary hypoplasia.

Histological changes are most marked in the central nervous system (Love et al. 2001; Philbey et al. 1998). There is extensive degeneration and necrosis of grey and white matter of the brain and spinal cord associated with infiltrations of macrophages and other inflammatory cells. Intranuclear and intracytoplasmic inclusion bodies may be observed in neurones of the cerebrum and spinal cord. These bodies are eosinophilic to amphophilic and consist of aggregates of nucleocapsids. Nonsuppurative

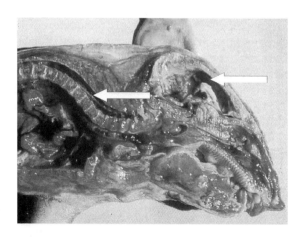

27.5. *CNS abnormalities due to in utero Menangle virus infection.*

multifocal meningitis, myocarditis, and occasionally, hepatitis may also be present in some cases.

DIAGNOSIS

Because Menangle virus is a recently recognized agent that is pathogenic for pigs and only one outbreak has been recorded, most pig populations should be fully susceptible. The birth of litters with a marked reduction of normal live piglets and a number of stillborn piglets with teratogenic defects is suggestive of Menangle virus infection. The most rapid method of excluding Menangle virus infection is to test affected sows for the presence of specific antibody to the virus.

The birth of litters containing mummified fetuses of varying size together with stillborn piglets is indicative of in utero viral infection. By far the most common cause of similar losses is porcine parvovirus, but a variety of other viral infections, e.g., encephalomyocarditis, classical swine fever (hog cholera), Aujeszky's disease (pseudorabies), Japanese encephalitis, porcine reproductive and respiratory syndrome (PRRS), and porcine rubulavirus (blue eye paramyxovirus, BEP) may cause significant fetal death. A feature that distinguishes Menangle virus infection from all but Japanese encephalitis infection is the presence of congenital malformations in piglets. However, it should be noted that these are evident in only approximately one-third of affected litters. In addition, many of these other viral infections cause disease in both piglets and adults. BEP is the only other paramyxovirus to cause significant fetal loss as a presenting sign, but it differs from Menangle virus in that neurological and other signs are usually observed in young piglets and the virus can be readily distinguished as it agglutinates erythrocytes from mammals and birds (Moreno-Lopez et al. 1986). Reproductive disease is not a major feature of infection with Nipah virus.

For laboratory diagnosis, fetal specimens should be collected for virus isolation, serology, and pathology. Virus can be isolated from a number of organs from stillborn piglets, especially brain, lung, and myocardium. A wide range of cell cultures support replication of Menangle virus, but baby hamster kidney cells (BHK-21) have been used for the isolation of the virus from field specimens. Three to five passages may be necessary before suggestive cytopathology is observed. Because the virus does not hemagglutinate, identification will depend on electron microscopy and neutralization of an isolate with specific antiserum. Specific antibodies may be detected in body cavity fluids of some stillborn piglets.

PREVENTION AND CONTROL

There is no specific treatment for Menangle virus. By the time clinical signs are observed, the virus is likely to be widely disseminated in the affected population, negating measures to limit spread.

Fruit bats (Megachiroptera) are considered the primary source of infection for the pig population. Megachiroptera are not found in North America, but are present in Africa, the Middle East, Southern Asia, Australia, and many Pacific Islands. It is not known whether small bats (Microchiroptera) are susceptible to Menangle virus, but it is important to restrict direct and indirect contact between pigs and bats to prevent introduction of this virus to the pig population. Fruit bats do not normally enter pig farm buildings, but they defecate and urinate during flight over and around buildings, and occasionally inadvertently drop their young in flight. All outside areas, e.g., outside walkways, should be covered to prevent contamination and possible infection. Flowering trees and fruiting trees should not be grown in the immediate vicinity of pig farm buildings because these may attract fruit bat activity.

In an outbreak of reproductive disease, the infection will probably have already spread through the entire population of a pig farm by the time the first affected litters are farrowed. In small piggeries, there would be insufficient numbers of susceptible animals available to maintain a cycle of infection because there is no carrier state and, unlike parvovirus, environmental survival of this virus is poor. In large piggeries, infection may become endemic, with the infection being maintained in groups of pigs as they lose their maternally derived protection. In such a situation, it is important to maximize the opportunity for infection of all selected replacement breeding stock prior to mating.

The eradication of Menangle virus from an endemically infected pig population can be achieved by moving all the age groups in which infection is active, e.g., pigs between 10 and 16 weeks of age, to another site (Love et al. 2001). If affected facilities are cleaned, vacated for a few weeks, and then restocked with unexposed pigs or pigs known to be immune to the virus, the cycle of endemic infection in the herd should be broken and the virus eliminated naturally.

PUBLIC HEALTH

In contrast to Nipah virus, Menangle virus does not appear to be highly infectious for humans. However, care should be taken when working with potentially infected pigs or suspect reproductive specimens. Although only 2 out of more than 30 humans directly exposed to infected pigs became infected with the virus, both experienced a severe febrile illness associated with a macular rash followed by prolonged debility (Chant et al. 1998). There was no evidence of infection in a large number of other people, including veterinarians, abattoir workers, and laboratory workers, who had less direct and less protracted contact with potentially infective material. Transmission to humans may require the contamination of cuts and abrasions with infectious body fluids or tissues or possibly splashing of material onto the conjunctivae (Chant et al. 1998).

Nipah Virus

INTRODUCTION

Nipah virus is an important, recently recognized, zoonotic virus that caused a major epidemic in 1998–1999. Although confined to a relatively small geographic area in Southeast Asia, it was associated with significant human mortality. It is believed that this virus jumped from a wildlife reservoir to domestic pigs. From pigs, the virus spread to humans and to other domestic animals, such as cats, dogs, and horses. The virus was not contagious in cats or dogs, but it was associated with a high case fatality rate. In humans, an epidemic occurred in pig farm workers and in others involved in the handling of pigs.

ETIOLOGY

Nipah virus is a novel negative-stranded RNA virus in the family *Paramyxoviridae*. This virus and the related Hendra virus are the sole members of the new genus *Henipavirus* (Chua et al. 2000).

Nipah is a large pleomorphic virus similar to most paramyxoviruses. Virus particles vary in size, but have an average diameter of 500 nm. Surface spikes on the envelope are approximately 10 nm in length. The typical long "herringbone"-shaped nucleocapsids have a diameter of approximately 21 nm and an average length of 1.67 μm.

Nipah virus replicates readily in several continuous cell lines, especially Vero and BHK-21, and produces suggestive cytopathic effects in 3–4 days. In Vero cells, virus replication induces large syncytia in which the cell nuclei are arranged around the periphery of the multinucleated cell. (Daniels et al. 2002). Antigenically, Nipah virus is closely related to Hendra virus and diagnostic reagents for Hendra virus have been utilized to assist Nipah virus investigations.

CLINICAL SIGNS

Nipah virus differs from most paramyxoviruses in that it causes a severe, often fatal disease in a number of species. The clinical signs observed as a consequence of Nipah virus infection in pigs vary in different age groups (Bunning et al. 2000; Nor et al. 2000).

In weaners and grower pigs, an acute febrile illness has been described with temperatures of 40°C and higher. Respiratory signs ranging from increased or forced respiration to a harsh, paroxysmal nonproductive cough (a loud barking cough) or open mouth breathing are prominent, especially if animals are forced to move. There may also be one or more neurological signs, such as muscle fasciculation, rear leg weakness, and varying degrees of spastic paresis and uncoordinated gait when driven and hurried. Illness may progress to lateral recumbency accompanied by thrashing of the limbs or tetanic spasms. Mortality in this age group is low, probably less than 5%. Animals that die may show blood-tinged discharge from the nose. Infection is frequently asymptomatic.

Sows and boars sometimes died suddenly with no overt illness or after a brief period of illness of less than 24 hours' duration. A bloody nasal discharge was frequently apparent after death. Neurological signs were frequently observed and included head pressing, agitation (displayed as biting at the bars of the pen), tetanic spasms or seizures, an apparent pharyngeal muscle paralysis with an apparent inability to swallow, frothy salivation, and drooping of the tongue. Abortions were also reported.

Suckling pigs showed open mouth breathing, leg weakness with muscle tremors, and neurological twitches. Mortality was high in these young animals, but whether from primary disease or as a result of disease in the sow has not been clearly established.

None of the clinical signs described above is pathognomonic, although the barking cough is considered characteristic and the sudden deaths in sows and boars is unusual.

Nipah virus is a dangerous zoonotic agent. Disease and death in people may be the first indication of an outbreak. A full clinical description of Nipah virus–induced disease in humans has been provided by Chua et al. (1999) and Goh et al. (2000). Human Nipah virus infection presents as an encephalitis. Patients may show fever, headache, dizziness, and vomiting. The condition progresses in over 50% of cases to impaired consciousness accompanied by brain stem dysfunction (Goh et al. 2000).

EPIDEMIOLOGY

The disease outbreak observed in Malaysia is presumed to be a result of virus 'jumping' species into farmed domestic pigs (Chua et al. 2000; Daniels 2000; Field et al. 2001; Yob et al. 2001). There is strong evidence for pteropid bats being a reservoir of this virus. A high prevalence of neutralizing antibodies has been detected in both of the species of wild bat (*P. vampirus* and *P. hyomelanus*) present in Malaysia (Yob et al. 2001). Nipah virus has also been isolated from wild *P. hyomelanus* in Malaysia (Chua et al. 2001).

The movement of infected pigs was the main means of spread of Nipah virus in Malaysia, resulting in the spread of the virus between farms, from state to state, and internationally to Singapore where abattoir workers processing Malaysian pigs became infected (Nor 2001; Nor and Ong 2000; Nor et al. 2000; Paton et al. 1999). The outbreak probably originated from a point source

(Lye et al. 2001), implying that the virus moved from its wildlife reservoir on only one occasion.

Human infection was associated with close human-to-pig contact with infected pigs (Parashar et al. 2000). Feeding or handling pigs and assisting with farrowing, treatment, and/or removal of sick or dead pigs were most likely to result in Nipah virus disease in people on infected farms. Living on an infected pig farm was not a significant risk factor.

The major route of excretion of Nipah virus from pigs is via the airways, although the pattern of human infection suggests spread via sputum or large droplets, rather than by fine aerosol. The coughing reported as a frequent clinical sign in infected pigs would facilitate such a mode of transmission.

Domestic animals other than pigs are susceptible to Nipah virus disease and appear to have become infected when there was potential for close contact with infected pigs. Large numbers of dogs died on infected farms, and clinically affected dogs were identified during investigations of the outbreak (Chua et al. 2000; Daniels et al. 2000). There was, however, no evidence of lateral transmission between dogs (Asiah et al. 2001). Cats were reported by farmers to have been affected. Experimentally, they were shown to be susceptible to infection and to excrete Nipah virus in urine (Muniandy 2001). Because virus was also isolated from the kidney of a clinically affected dog in Malaysia (Chua et al. 2000), urinary excretion by domestic carnivores may also be a possible method of spread. There was no evidence of transmission of Nipah virus among horses and serological studies of rodents on infected farms, and various other wildlife species showed no evidence of Nipah virus infection.

PATHOGENESIS

There have been no structured pathogenesis studies with Nipah virus in susceptible species. Therefore, information is limited mainly to observations of naturally occurring clinical cases.

Nipah virus infection in pigs causes an acute febrile infection that may be self-limiting or fatal. Seroconversion occurs at 10–14 days. There is no evidence that persistent infections occur, although the possibility cannot be excluded. Nipah virus primarily infects vascular endothelium. Respiratory epithelium is susceptible to infection in pigs, but infection has not been observed in the nervous system other than the meninges. Immunohistochemical studies of naturally infected pigs have shown large amounts of Nipah viral antigen in the respiratory epithelium at all levels of the lungs, including the minor and major airways and the trachea (Hooper et al. 2001).

PATHOLOGY

The most common syndrome in pigs is respiratory disease characterized by severe coughing. However, there is no pathognomonic gross pathology and concurrent pulmonary disease from other causes may be present. There is mild-to-severe pulmonary consolidation. On the cut surface, the interlobular septae may be distended, The bronchi and trachea are frequently filled with exudate or frothy fluid that is sometimes tinged with blood (Daniels et al. 2000; Hooper et al. 2001; Shahirudin 2001).

Histologically there is pneumonia at all levels, from the alveoli through to the epithelium of the trachea. Syncytial cells are present throughout the respiratory epithelium and in vascular endothelium. Alveolar macrophages are prominent and there appears to be an infiltration of neutrophils into diseased tissue in the absence of intercurrent infections. Viral antigen is readily detectable by immunohistochemistry in syncytia and in respiratory epithelium at all levels of the respiratory tract. In cases where there is neurological disease, there is a nonsuppurative meningitis rather than encephalitis (Hooper et al. 2001; Middleton et al. 2002).

DIAGNOSIS

Nipah virus may be suspected if a clinical syndrome consistent with Nipah virus disease occurs on a pig farm in an area where there is opportunity for contact with pteropid bats. Nipah virus is classified as a Biosafety Level 4 (BSL4) agent and extreme care must be taken in the diagnosis of cases suspected to involve Nipah virus. Some aspects of laboratory diagnosis should be conducted only in a BSL4 laboratory. Ante- and postmortem sampling should be conducted in a manner that will exclude contact of unprotected personnel with body fluids from affected animals. Respiratory protection is advisable (Daniels et al. 2000).

Clinical diagnosis of Nipah virus is difficult because the infection does not produce pathognomonic clinical signs. Furthermore, clinical signs vary by the age and reproductive status of the animals affected. Thus, the differential diagnosis may vary with the age and class of pigs affected. The list of differential diagnoses should include those that cause sudden death in boars and/or sows; reproductive failure characterized by abortion; respiratory disease in any age group characterized by severe coughing; and neurological disease characterized by tremors, muscle fasciculation, and agonal thrashing of the limbs or tetanic spasms in lateral recumbency.

Nipah virus antigens have been demonstrated in formalin- fixed tissues, especially the lung and upper airways, meninges, spleen, and kidney (Daniels 2001). Demonstration of viral antigen in formalin-fixed postmortem samples is a rapid and safe option for confirmation of a diagnosis.

When isolates of virus are required, either for confirmation of a diagnosis or for additional research, it is preferable that virus isolation be conducted in a laboratory with a high level of biosecurity. Nipah virus has been isolated from lung, spleen, kidney, tonsil, meninges, and lymph node collected at postmortem and from throat swabs, cerebrospinal fluid, or urine collected from live animals (Daniels 2001). Vero cells are preferred for virus isolation. Cytopathology may be observed within 2–3 days, but several passages of at least 5 days are usually conducted before declaring an isolation attempt unsuccessful. Cytopathology is characterized by the formation of large syncytia. Polymerase chain reaction (PCR) has been developed as a diagnostic tool and it is likely that a retrospective confirmation could be achieved even with formalin-fixed tissues (Chua et al. 1999; Hooper and Williamson 2000).

For antibody detection, ELISA is the preferred method for routine screening because of the availability of inactivated reagents and the ability to test large numbers of samples quickly (Daniels 2001). However, the possibility that serum samples may contain infectious virus should not be overlooked. Testing of suitable numbers of pig sera by ELISA provides a rapid method for the exclusion of Nipah virus from disease episodes where Nipah virus infection may be considered and is also a valuable approach for confirming that populations are free of infection. Any ELISA reactors should be confirmed by the virus neutralization test (Daniels 2001), but because it employs the use of live virus in cell culture, secure laboratory facilities should be used.

PREVENTION AND CONTROL

As Nipah virus is a dangerous zoonotic agent, treatment of affected animals should not be considered.

In countries where Pteropid bats may be a reservoir of Nipah virus, pig farms should be managed to ensure that infection cannot be introduced (Choo 2001; Daniels 2001). That is, farms should be devoid of fruit trees and other vegetation that may attract the bats to the proximity of the animal housing. Strict biosecurity should be in place to preclude the importation of infected animals. If introductions are necessary for breeding or other purposes, a period of quarantine and isolation separate from the main herd should be enforced.

Control measures in cases of confirmed Nipah virus infection will reflect its extreme hazard as a zoonotic agent. It is essential to prevent spread of infection among domestic animals and to preclude the possibility of infection of humans. Rapid eradication is the recommended response. This was achieved in Malaysia by quarantine of infected premises and the culling of all susceptible animals on those premises. It is essential that quarantine and associated movement controls be enforced during this period of culling (Mangat 2001).

PUBLIC HEALTH

Nipah virus presents a serious threat to public health. In the outbreak in Malaysia, there were numerous human infections and deaths of pig farmers and other people who had close contact with pigs, including abattoir workers in a neighboring country. If there is a risk of an outbreak, it is essential to prevent the movement of all animals and minimize human contact with potentially infected animals.

In the last decade, new viral diseases affecting domestic animals and humans have emerged, with various species of fruit bats as the putative source. Such events would suggest a drastic change in the relationship between fruit bats and domestic animals. This may simply be a further reflection of the worldwide destruction of forest habitat, forcing the wild and domestic species into much closer associations. In Australia, the fruit bat population will remain a potential source of Menangle virus infection for pigs and possibly other species, just as Nipah virus poses a continuing threat in Malaysia. The risk that these viruses pose to pigs in other countries and to other animal species has not been determined, but should not be ignored, especially in countries where Pteropid bats are present.

REFERENCES

Asiah NM, Mills JN, Ong BL, Ksiazek TG. 2001. Epidemiological investigation on Nipah virus infection in peridomestic animals in peninsula Malaysia and future plans. In Report of the regional seminar on Nipah virus infection. Tokyo, Office International des Epizooties Representation for Asia and the Pacific, pp. 47–50.

Berg M, Hjertner B, Moreno-Lopez J, Linne T. 1992. The P gene of porcine paramyxovirus LPMV encodes three possible polypeptides P, V and C: The P protein mRNA is edited. J Gen Virol 73:1195–1200.

Berg M, Sundqvist A, Moreno-Lopez J, Linne T. 1991. Identification of the porcine paramyxovirus LPMV matrix protein gene: Comparative sequence analysis with other paramyxoviruses. J Gen Virol 72:1045–1050.

Bowden TR, Westenberg M, Wang LF, Eaton BT, Boyle DB. 2001. Molecular characterization of Menangle virus, a novel paramyxovirus which infects pigs, fruit bats and humans. Virology 283:358–373.

Bunning M, Jamaluddin A, Cheang H, Kitsutani P, Muhendren, Olson J, Karim N, Field H, Johara, Sharihuddin, Choo Pow Yoon R, Daniels P, Ksiazek T, Nordin M. 2000. Epidemiological traceback studies of the Nipah virus outbreak in pig farms in the Ipoh district of Malaysia, 1997–1999. Proc Congr Int Pig Vet Soc 16:551.

Campos HR, Carbajal SM. 1989. Trastornos reproductivos de los sementales de una granja porcina de ciclo completo ante un brote de ojo azul. Memorias del XXIV Congreso de la Asociación Mexicana de Veterinarios Especialista en Cerdos (AMVEC), pp. 62–64.

Chant K, Chan R, Smith M, Dwyer DE, Kirkland P. 1998. Probable human infection with a newly described virus in the Family Paramyxoviridae. Emerg Infect Dis 4:273–275.

Choo PY. 2001. Pig industry perspectives on herd health monitoring and biosecurity in Malaysia. In Report of the regional seminar on Nipah virus infection. Tokyo, Office International des Epizooties Representation for Asia and the Pacific, pp 90–93.

Chua KB, Bellini WJ, Rota PA, Harcourt BH, Tamin A, Lam SK, Ksiazek TG, Rollin PE, Zaki SR, Shieh W, Goldsmith CS, Gubler DJ, Roehrig JT, Eaton B, Gould AR, Olson J, Field H, Daniels P,

Ling AE, Peters CJ, Anderson LJ, Mahy BW. 2000. Nipah virus: A recently emergent deadly paramyxovirus. Science 288: 1432–1435.

Chua KB, Goh KJ, Wong KT, Kamarulzaman A, Tan PS, Ksiazek TG, Zaki SR, Paul G, Lam SK, Tan CT. 1999. Fatal encephalitis due to Nipah virus among pig-farmers in Malaysia. Lancet 354: 1257–1259.

Chua KB, Koh CL, Cheng SC, Hooi PS, Khong JH, Wee KF, Chua BH, Chan YP, Lim ME, Lam Sai Kit K. 2001. Surveillance of wildlife for source of Nipah virus: Methodologies and outcome II. In Report of the regional seminar on Nipah virus infection. Tokyo, Office International des Epizooties Representation for Asia and the Pacific, pp. 81–83.

Daniels PW. 2000. The Nipah virus outbreak in Malaysia: Overview of the outbreak investigation and the issues that remain. Proc Congr Int Pig Vet Soc 16:553–554.

——. 2001. Nipah virus preparedness—Aspects for a veterinary plan. In Report of the regional seminar on Nipah virus infection. Tokyo, Office International des Epizooties Representation for Asia and the Pacific, pp. 84–89.

Daniels PW, Aziz J, Ksiazek TG, Ong BL, Bunning ML, Yob JM B, Field HE, Olson J, Hoffmann D, Bilou J, Ozawa Y. 2000. Nipah virus: Developing a regional approach. In Comprehensive Reports on Technical Items Presented to the International Committee or Regional Commissions, Edition 1999. Office International des Epizooties, Paris, pp. 207–217.

Daniels PW, Ong BL, Aziz J. 2002. Nipah virus diagnosis and control in swine herds. In Trends in Emerging Viral Infections of Swine. A Morilla, K-J Yoon, J Zimmerman, eds. Ames: Iowa State Press, pp. 111–116.

Field H, Young P, Yob JM, Mills J, Hall L, Mackenzie J. 2001. The natural history of Hendra and Nipah viruses. Microbes Infect 3:307–314.

Gay GM, Stephano AH. 1987. Strain analysis of a new paramyxovirus isolated from 12 outbreaks of encephalitis and corneal opacity in pigs (blue eye syndrome). Proc 23rd World Vet Congr, Montreal, p. 161.

Goh KJ, Tan CT, Chew NK, Tan PS, Kamarulzaman A, Sarji SA, Wong KT, Abdullah BJ, Chua KB, Lam SK. 2000. Clinical features of Nipah virus encephalitis among pig farmers in Malaysia. New Eng J Med 342:1229–1235.

Greig AS, Johnson CM, Bouillant AMP. 1971. Encephalomyelitis of swine caused by a haemagglutinating virus. VI. Morphology of the virus. Res Vet Sci 12:305–307.

Hooper P, Zaki S, Daniels P, Middleton D. 2001. Comparative pathology of the diseases caused by Hendra and Nipah viruses. Microbes Infect 3:315–322.

Hooper PT, Williamson MM. 2000. Hendra and Nipah virus infections. Vet Clin North Am Equine Pract 16:597–603.

Kirkland PD, Love RJ, Philbey AW, Ross AD, Davis RJ, Hart KG. 2001. Epidemiology and control of Menangle virus in pigs. Aust Vet J 79:199–206.

Lipkind M, Shoham D, Shihmanter E. 1986. Isolation of a paramyxovirus from pigs in Israel and its antigenic relationship with avian paramyxoviruses. J Gen Virol 67:427–439.

Love RJ, Philbey AW, Kirkland PD, Ross AD, Davis RJ, Morrissey C, Daniels PW. 2001. Reproductive disease and congenital malformations in pigs caused by Menangle virus. Aust Vet J 79:192–198.

Lye MS, Ong F, Parashar UD, Mounts AW, Mustafa AN, Sahani M, Kamaluddin MA, Premalatha GD, Kitsutani PT. 2001. Report on the epidemiological studies conducted during the Nipah virus outbreak in Malaysia in 1999. In Report of the regional seminar on Nipah virus infection. Tokyo, Office International des Epizooties Representation for Asia and the Pacific, pp. 31–37.

Mangat AA. 2001. Management of Nipah virus outbreaks. In Report on the regional seminar on Nipah virus infection, Tokyo, OIE Representation for Asia and the Pacific, pp. 51–53.

Middleton DJ, Westbury HA, Morrissy CJ, van der Heide BM, Russell GM, Braun MA, Hyatt AD. 2002. Experimental Nipah virus infection in pigs and cats. J Comp Pathol 126:124–126.

Moreno-Lopez J, Correa-Giron P, Martinez A, Ericsson A. 1986. Characterization of a paramyxovirus isolated from the brain of a piglet in Mexico. Arch Virol 91:221–231.

Muniandy N. 2001. Serological screening using ELISA for IgG and IgM. In Report of the regional seminar on Nipah virus infection. Tokyo, Office International des Epizooties Representation for Asia and the Pacific, pp. 73–76.

Nor MN, Ong BL. 2000. Nipah virus infection in animals and control measures implemented in peninsular Malaysia. In Comprehensive Reports on Technical Items Presented to the International Committee or Regional Commissions, Edition 1999. Office International des Epizooties, Paris, pp. 237–251.

Nor MNM. 2001. Overview of Nipah virus infection in peninsular Malaysia. In Report of the regional seminar on Nipah virus infection. Tokyo, Office International des Epizooties Representation for Asia and the Pacific, pp. 24–26.

Nor MNM, Gan CH, Ong, BL. 2000. Nipah virus infection of pigs in peninsular Malaysia. Rev Sci Tech OIE 19:160–165.

Parashar UD, Sunn LM, Ong F, Mounts AW, Arif MT, Ksiazek TG, Kamaluddin MA, Mustafa AN, Kaur H, Ding LM, Othman G, Radzi HM, Kitsutani PT, Stockton PC, Arokiasamy J, Gary HE Jr, Anderson LJ. 2000. Case-control study of risk factors for human infection with a new zoonotic paramyxovirus, Nipah virus, during a 1998–1999 outbreak of severe encephalitis in Malaysia. J Infect Dis 181:1755–1759.

Paton NI, Leo YS, Zaki SR, Auchus AP, Lee KE, Ling AE, Chew SK, Ang B, Rollin PE, Umapathi T, Sng I, Lee CC, Lim E, Ksiazek TG. 1999. Outbreak of Nipah-virus infection among abattoir workers in Singapore. Lancet 354:1253–1256.

Paul PS, Janke BH, Battrell MA, Lyoo YS, Halbur PG, Landgraf J, Huinker C. 1994. Isolation of a paramyxo-like virus from pigs with interstitial pneumonia and encephalitis. Proc Congr Int Pig Vet Soc 13:72.

Philbey AW, Kirkland PD, Ross AD, Davis RJ, Gleeson AB, Love RJ, Daniels PW, Gould AR, Hyatt AD. 1998. An apparently new virus (Family Paramyxoviridae) infectious for pigs, humans and fruit bats. Emerg Infect Dis 4:269–271.

Ramirez MH, Carreon NR, Mercado GC, Rodriguez TJ. 1996. Hemoaglutinacion e inhibicion de la hemoaglutinacion del paramixovirus porcino a traves de la modificacion de algunas variables que participan en la prueba. Veterinaria (México) 27:257–259.

Ramirez MH, Reyes LJ, Kennedy S, Hernandez JP. 1995. Studies on the pathogenesis of the pig paramyxovirus of the blue eye disease on the epididymis and testis. Memorias del XX Reunión de la Academia de la Investigación en Biología y Reproducción (México), pp. 211–214.

Ramirez TCA, Stephano AH. 1982. Histological central nervous system lesions produced by an haemagglutinating virus in naturally infected piglets. Proc Congr Int Pig Vet Soc 7:154.

Sasahara J, Hayashi S, Kumagai T, Yamamoto Y, Hirasawa K, Munekata K, Okaniwa A, Kato K. 1954. On a swine virus disease newly discovered in Japan. 1. Isolation of the virus. 2. Some properties of the virus. Virus 4:131–139.

Shahirudin S. 2001. Clinical and pathological features of the natural Nipah virus infection in pigs. In Report of the regional seminar on Nipah virus infection. Tokyo, Office International des Epizooties Representation for Asia and the Pacific, pp.41–42.

Stephano AH, Doporto JM, Gay, M. 1986a. Estudio epidemiologico en dos granjas afectadas por el ojo azul. Proc Congr Int Pig Vet Soc 9:456.

Stephano AH, Fuentes RM, Hernandez JP, Herradora LM, Carreon R. 1988a. Encefalitis y opacidad de la cornea en cerdos destetados, inoculados experimentalmente con paramyxovirus de ojo azul. Memorias del XXIII Congreso de la Asociación Mexicana de Veterinarios Especialista en Cerdos (AMVEC), pp. 90–92.

Stephano AH, Gay GM. 1983. El syndrome del ojo azul. Estudio experimental. Memorias de la Reunión de Investigación Pecuaria en México, pp. 523–528.

——. 1984. Experimental studies of a new viral syndrome in pigs called "blue eye" characterized by encephalitis and corneal opacity. Proc Congr Int Pig Vet Soc 8:71.

——. 1985a. El syndrome del ojo azul en cerdos I. Síntesis Porcina (México) 4(5):42–49.

——. 1985b. El syndrome del ojo azul en granjas engordadoras. Memorias del IXX Congreso de la Asociación Mexicana de Veterinarios Especialista en Cerdos (AMVEC), pp. 71–74.

——. 1986a. El syndrome del ojo azul. Una nueva enfermedad en cerdos asociada a un paramyxovirus. Veterinaria (México) 17:120–122.

——. 1986b. Encefalitis, falla reproductiva y opacidad de la cornea, ojo azul. Síntesis Porcina (México) 5(12):26–39.

Stephano AH, Gay GM, Ramirez TC. 1988b. Encephalomyelitis, reproductive failure and corneal opacity in pigs, associated with a new paramyxovirus infection (blue eye). Vet Rec 122:6–10.

Stephano AH, Gay GM, Ramirez TC, Maqueda AJJ. 1982. An outbreak of encephalitis in piglets produced by an hemagglutinating virus. Proc Congr Int Pig Vet Soc 7:153.

Stephano AH, Gay M, Kresse J. 1986b. Properties of a paramyxovirus associated to a new syndrome (blue eye) characterized by encephalitis, reproductive failure and corneal opacity. Proc Congr Int Pig Vet Soc 9:455.

Stephano AH, Hernandez D, Perez C, Gonzalez CT, Ramirez MH, Cervantes A. 1990. Boar infertility and testicle atrophy associated with blue eye paramyxovirus infection. Proc Congr Int Pig Vet Soc 11:211.

Sundqvist A, Berg M, Hernandez-Jauregui P, Linne T, Moreno-Lopez J. 1990. The structural proteins of a porcine paramyxovirus (LPMV). J Gen Virol 71:609–613.

Sundqvist A, Berg M, Moreno-Lopez J, Linne T. 1992. The haemagglutinin-neuraminidase glycoprotein of the porcine paramyxovirus LPMV: Comparison with other paramyxoviruses revealed the closest relationship to Simian virus 5 and mumps virus. Arch Virol 122:331–340.

Wiman AC, Hjertner B, Linne T, Herron B, Allan G, McNeilly F, Adair B, Moreno-Lopez J, Berg M. 1998. Porcine rubulavirus LPMV RNA persists in central nervous system of pigs after recovery from acute infection. J Neurovirol 4:545–552.

Yob JM, Field H, Rashdi AM, Morrissy C, van der Heide B, Rota P, bin Adzhar A, White J, Daniels P, Jamaluddin A, Ksiazek T. 2001. Nipah virus infection in bats (order Chiroptera) in peninsular Malaysia. Emerg Infect Dis 7:439–441.

28 Swine Influenza

Christopher W. Olsen, Ian H. Brown, Bernard C. Easterday, and Kristien Van Reeth

Influenza virus infections are a common and important cause of bronchointerstitial pneumonia and respiratory disease in pigs throughout large parts of the world. In any one animal, the disease is typically characterized by an abrupt onset and short course of fever, inappetence, lethargy, coughing, dyspnea, and nasal discharge. However, clinical illness may persist in a herd for several weeks as the virus spreads from pig to pig within the population. Influenza viruses also act synergistically with other viral or bacterial pathogens to cause porcine respiratory disease complex (PRDC). The overall course and severity of an influenza virus infection in a pig may be impacted by these co-infecting agents, the pig's age, overall health and immune status, and, potentially, the strain of influenza virus involved.

Beyond their significance to swine health, influenza virus infections in pigs also pose important human public health concerns, and the histories of influenza in pigs and people are closely linked. In the summer of 1918, an epizootic disease with many clinical and pathologic similarities to influenza in humans appeared among pigs in the north-central U.S., coincident with the 1918 influenza pandemic that killed 20–50 million people around the world. Koen (1919) unapologetically called the disease "flu" because of its similarities to the prevalent clinical disease of flu in human beings. Dorset et al. (1922) also reported on "hog flu" at the annual meeting of the American Veterinary Medical Association in 1922, providing descriptions of the disease that were similar to those given by Koen, and a discussant of the Dorset presentation commented that he believed he had seen a case of "hog flu" in Iowa (U.S.) 5–6 years prior to 1918. Furthermore, McBryde (1927) indicated that it was not uncommon to meet farmers and veterinarians who believed that they had contracted the disease from affected pigs, and he himself suffered an acute febrile disease similar to the hog flu he had been investigating in southeastern Iowa. Finally, Murray (1921) also reported on the nature of influenza in pigs in the U.S. and Beveridge (1977) noted that ". . . in the autumn of 1918

[Aladar Altmann], a Hungarian veterinarian described a disease of pigs which he believed was influenza."

The etiology of swine influenza (SI) was confirmed in 1931 when Shope presented the first reliable experimental evidence that the disease in pigs was caused by a virus (Shope 1931), and 2 years later, Smith et al. (1933) demonstrated that influenza in human beings was also caused by a virus. "When the human pandemic of 1957 . . . first began to spread in Asian countries during the spring of that year, the World Health Organization (WHO) considered it opportune to attempt an animal serum survey in order to throw light on the animal component in the epidemiology of influenza" (Kaplan 1969). That study concluded that the Asian H2N2 strain could infect pigs, and by 1970, there was considerable serologic evidence that people whose occupations brought them into contact with pigs became infected with swine influenza viruses (SIVs). Furthermore, in 1974 and 1975 (Easterday 1986), infections in children were temporally linked to contact with infected pigs, and in 1976, cases of SIV infections occurred among Army recruits at Fort Dix, N.J. (Top and Russell 1977). In the fall of 1976, all speculation about the transmission of SIV from pigs to people came to an end when virus was isolated from pigs and their caretaker on a Wisconsin farm (Easterday et al. unpublished data; Hinshaw et al. 1978).

In more recent times, genetic analyses have confirmed that the early swine viruses and the human viruses of 1918 were closely related to one another, although it remains unclear as to whether a progenitor virus was transmitted from pigs to people or from people to pigs (reviewed in Taubenberger et al. 2001). Currently, more than 85 years since its appearance, SI continues to be an important economic factor in swine production and a public health concern.

ETIOLOGY

Influenza viruses are members of the virus family *Orthomyxoviridae*. They are pleomorphic, enveloped viruses approximately 80–120 nm in diameter. The lipid envelope makes the viruses highly susceptible to detergents and most commonly used antiviral disinfectants. Influenza viruses encode up to 11 viral proteins on 7 to 8 separate segments of negative-sense RNA. The segmented nature of their genomes is a critical structural feature that allows influenza viruses to undergo genetic reassortment.

Influenza viruses are classified by type, subtype, and more recently, genotype. Of the A, B, and C types of influenza viruses (defined by differences in their matrix [M] and nucleoproteins [NP]), only influenza A viruses are of routine clinical significance as swine pathogens. Influenza A viruses are named using the following convention: A/species of origin/location of isolation/isolate number/year of isolation—e.g., A/Swine/Wisconsin/125/98. (If no species is designated, it is, by default, a human isolate.)

Influenza A virus subtypes are defined by the nature of the hemagglutinin (HA or H) and neuraminidase (NA or N) spike-like glycoproteins that project from the surface of the viral envelope. There are 16 different forms of HA and 9 different forms of NA that can be distinguished antigenically and genetically. The combination of HA and NA forms in a virus defines its subtype, e.g., H1N1, H3N2. Functionally, the HA (organized as trimers) binds to sialic acid (SA)-containing receptors and mediates virus infection of host cells. Sialic acid binding is also responsible for the erythrocyte agglutination that underlies virus detection by hemagglutination and hemagglutination-inhibition (HI) serologic assays. The HA protein also contains the major antigenic sites to which neutralizing antibodies (Abs) are directed. The NA protein (organized as tetramers) catalyzes cleavage of sialic acid from adjacent sugar residues, and, thereby, may function to prevent virion aggregation and to enhance the release of budded virus particles. (See Lamb and Krug 2001 and Wright and Webster 2001 for detailed reviews of influenza virus structure and genetics.)

To understand the epidemiology and evolution of influenza A viruses, it is becoming increasingly important to both subtype and genotype viruses. Genotyping is conducted by determining the genetic sequence of each viral RNA segment and then subjecting the sequences to phylogenetic analyses. These analyses define the evolutionary lineages (based on host species and geographic region of the world) from which each gene originated. Genotyping has been extremely important in recent years for understanding the origins of reassortant SIVs isolated in Europe, Asia, and North America.

EPIDEMIOLOGY

Historically, outbreaks of SI in northern climates of the U.S. and western Europe occurred most frequently during the late fall through early winter months, often in association with the onset of colder temperatures and cold autumn rains (Easterday 1980; Easterday and Van Reeth 1999). However, studies have clearly demonstrated that SIVs circulate year-round (Hinshaw et al. 1978; Olsen et al. 2000), and as swine production has increasingly been conducted in total confinement, the seasonal pattern of clinical disease has become less prominent.

Influenza viruses are most commonly introduced into herds with the movement of animals. The primary route of virus transmission is through pig-to-pig contact via the nasopharyngeal route, with virus being shed in nasal secretions at titers of $\geq 10^7$ infectious particles per ml at the peak of shedding (typically 2–5 days after exposure) (Landolt et al. 2003; Van Reeth et al. 2003a). Once the virus has been introduced into a herd, it may continue to circulate as long as susceptible pigs are available. In all-in/all-out systems, the virus should disappear because of the cycle of depopulation and disinfection of facilities. Nonetheless, virus may be reintroduced with new pigs, thus accounting for what appears to be virus persistence on a farm.

The existence of an SI carrier state has been postulated to account for interepidemic persistence of SIVs and, historically, maintenance of influenza viruses on premises was hypothesized to occur via lungworms and earthworms (Shope 1941). However, there is no clear proof of these mechanisms and it appears more likely that virus is maintained through continual availability of susceptible pigs.

Pandemiology and Evolution

Understanding the pandemiology (global epidemiology) and evolution of influenza viruses in pigs requires an understanding of the ecology and epidemiology of influenza viruses in other species.

In horses, marine mammals, poultry, and human beings—as in pigs—influenza viruses may cause clinically and/or economically important disease. In contrast, influenza viruses in waterfowl and shorebirds are generally highly host-adapted, rarely cause disease, and exhibit low evolutionary rates ("evolutionary stasis") (reviewed in Gorman et al. 1990, Webster and Kawaoka 1994, Webster et al. 1992, and Wright and Webster 2001). All 16 HA and 9 NA subtypes of influenza A viruses have been recovered from aquatic birds. In these species, influenza A viruses replicate primarily in enterocytes and, thus, are shed in feces and can contaminate lake water (Hinshaw et al. 1980; Webster et al. 1978). Consequently, aquatic birds provide an omnipresent, global reservoir of influenza viruses. Phylogenetic data indicate that aquatic birds were also the evolutionary progenitors of the lineages of influenza A viruses in mammals (reviewed in Webster et al. 1992 and Wright and Webster 2001). However, only H1, H3, N1, and N2 subtype viruses have established stable lineages and circulated widely among pigs.

Classical H1N1 Swine Influenza Viruses. Viruses of the classical H1N1 lineage were the dominant cause of influenza among pigs in North America from their first isolation by Shope in 1930 through the 1990s (Arora et al. 1997; Chambers et al. 1991; Hinshaw et al. 1978; Morin et al. 1981; Olsen et al. 2000). Classical H1N1 viruses have also been isolated from pigs in South America, Europe, and Asia (reviewed in Brown 2000 and Olsen et al. 2004). Beyond domestic pigs, there is also evidence for infection of wild pigs with classical H1N1 SIVs (Saliki et al. 1998), as well as transmission to domestic turkeys (Hinshaw et al. 1983; Wright et al. 1992).

The classical H1N1 SIVs in the U.S. remained antigenically and genetically highly conserved from 1965 through the 1980s (Luoh et al. 1992; Noble et al. 1993; Sheerar et al. 1989), but antigenic and genetic variants of classical H1N1 viruses were isolated during the 1990s (Dea et al. 1992; Olsen et al. 1993, 2000; Rekik et al. 1994).

Transmission of Human Influenza Viruses to Pigs. There is only limited evidence for maintenance of human H1N1 influenza viruses after natural introduction into swine populations (reviewed in Brown 2000), but human H3N2 viruses have been recovered frequently from pigs in Asia and Europe (reviewed in Brown 2000 and Olsen et al. 2004). There is also evidence for genetic/antigenic drift among the H3N2 viruses that have persistently circulated among pigs in Europe (de Jong et al. 1999), but the drift is relatively minor when compared to that in the human population. In North America, human H3N2 viruses have been recovered from pigs much less frequently (Bikour et al. 1995; Hinshaw et al. 1978; Karasin et al. 2000c), but introduction of a human H3N2 influenza virus into the pig population was likely a critical factor in the emergence of the reassortant viruses that now dominate the swine population in the U.S.

Transmission of Avian Influenza Viruses to Pigs. Experimental infection studies have shown that pigs can be infected with a wide range of avian influenza viruses (AIVs) (Kida et al. 1994) and naturally acquired infections of pigs with AIVs have also been documented from multiple areas of the world. There have been at least three independent introductions of distinct, wholly avian, H1N1 viruses to pigs (Brown 2000; Guan et al. 1996; Karasin et al. 2004; Pensaert et al. 1981). In particular, an avian H1N1 virus introduced into pigs in Europe in the late 1970s spread throughout much of the European continent and United Kingdom and ultimately became a dominant cause of SI in these areas (Brown et al. 1997b; Donatelli et al. 1991; Scholtissek et al. 1983). These avian-like H1N1 viruses have also undergone genetic/antigenic drift (Brown et al. 1997b; de Jong et al. 2001) and have spread from pigs to domestic turkeys (Ludwig et al. 1994; Wood et al. 1997).

Elsewhere in the world, serum antibodies against avian H4, H5, and H9 viruses have been detected in pigs in China (Ninomiya et al. 2002); avian H1N1, H3N2, and H9N2 viruses have been isolated from Asian pigs (Guan et al. 1996; Kida et al. 1988; Peiris et al. 2001a,b); and avian H4N6, H3N3, and H1N1 viruses have been recovered from pigs in Canada (Karasin et al. 2000b, 2004).

Reassortant Influenza Virus Infections in Pigs. The segmented nature of the influenza genome allows two viruses that co-infect a single host to exchange RNA segments during viral replication. Pigs are susceptible to infection with both human and avian influenza A viruses because the cells of their respiratory tract express both the SAα2,6Gal receptors that are preferentially used by human influenza viruses and the SAα2,3Gal receptors preferred by avian influenza viruses (Ito 2000; Ito et al. 1998a, 2000; Suzuki et al. 1997). Several different forms of reassortant viruses have been isolated from pigs in the U.S. and around the world (Olsen 2002a,b).

Reassortant H3N2 Viruses. Reassortant viruses with mixtures of human and classical swine virus genes have been isolated from pigs in Asia and the U.S. (Nerome et al. 1995; Shu et al. 1994; Zhou et al. 1999). In addition, H3N2 viruses with human HA and NA genes and avian internal protein genes have been isolated from pigs in Asia (Peiris et al. 2001a) and are currently the dominant H3N2 virus among pigs in Europe (Campitelli et al. 1997; Castrucci et al. 1993; Lin et al. 2004). Finally, unique "triple reassortant" H3N2 viruses have been isolated frequently from pigs throughout the U.S. since 1998. These viruses contain HA, NA, and PB1 polymerase genes of human influenza virus origin; NP, M, and NS genes of classical swine H1N1 virus origin; and PB2 and PA polymerase genes of North American avian virus origin (Karasin et al. 2000c; Webby et al. 2000; Zhou et al. 1999). Infection with some of the triple reassortant viruses has been associated not only with respiratory disease, but also spontaneous abortion in sows and death of adult pigs (Karasin et al. 2000c; Zhou et al. 1999). These fatal outcomes are uncommon with classical H1N1 swine viruses, and it remains to be determined whether the reassortant virus-associated abortions are due to direct viral effects or simply to high fevers in the affected animals.

Reassortant H1N2 Viruses. Soon after the initial isolations of the triple reassortant H3N2 viruses, influenza-like illness and abortions were associated with infection of pigs in the U.S. with an H1N2 virus. Phylogenetic analyses demonstrated that this virus retained the overall genotype of the triple reassortant H3N2 viruses but had acquired an H1 HA gene through reassortment with a classical H1N1 swine virus (Karasin et al. 2000a). Similar H1N2 viruses subsequently spread throughout the swine population of the U.S. (Choi et al. 2002a,b; Karasin et al. 2002), as well as into domestic turkeys in Missouri (Suarez et al. 2002) and into wild waterfowl in North Carolina (Olsen et al. 2003).

Until 1999, H1N2 viruses had not previously been reported among pigs in North America. However, H1N2 viruses had been recovered from pigs in Japan (Ito et al. 1998b; Nerome et al. 1985; Ouchi et al. 1996; Shimada et al. 2003; Sugimura et al. 1980), France (Gourreau et al. 1994), and Taiwan (Tsai and Pan 2003). These H1N2 viruses were reassortants between human (or human-like swine lineage) H3N2, and classical swine H1N1 viruses. Human-avian reassortant H1N2 viruses were first isolated from pigs in the U.K. in 1994 (Brown et al. 1995, 1998) and subsequently spread to the rest of Europe (Marozin et al. 2002; Schrader and Suss 2003; Van Reeth et al. 2000, 2003a,b). These viruses typically contained human-lineage HA and NA genes and internal protein genes derived from the avian-like European H1N1 swine viruses, although some H1N2 viruses from Italian pigs have contained an avian-like swine H1 HA gene (Marozin et al. 2002).

Reassortant H1N1 Viruses. Since 1998, reassortant H1N1 viruses with classical swine H1N1 HA and NA genes and remaining genes from reassortant H3N2 or H1N2 swine viruses have been isolated in the U.S. This virus genotype was first isolated from a human being with influenza-like illness in Wisconsin who had had direct contact with a pig (Cooper et al. 1999). However, viruses of this genotype have been isolated frequently from pigs in the U.S. since 2001 (Olsen et al. unpublished data; Webby et al. 2002), and current surveillance activities suggest that this has become the predominant genotype of H1N1 virus within the North American swine population (Olsen and Webby, unpublished data).

Reassortant H1N7 and H3N1 Swine Influenza Viruses. These subtypes have been identified among pigs on only a very limited basis. Influenza virus of H1N7 subtype was isolated in 1992 from pigs on a single farm in the U.K.. This virus contained A/Equine/Prague/1/56-like NA and M genes, with the remaining genes being of human influenza virus origin, and was of low pathogenicity in pigs infected experimentally (Brown et al. 1994, 1997a). Reassortant H3N1 viruses (human H3N2 X classical swine H1N1 viruses) have been recovered from pigs in the United Kingdom and Taiwan (Brown unpublished data; Tsai and Pan 2003).

Public Health Aspects

The occurrence of influenza virus infections in pigs poses two important public health issues: zoonotic infections of people with swine influenza viruses and the potential for pigs to serve as hosts for the creation of novel viruses of pandemic potential for the human population.

Zoonotic infections (including fatal infections) with SIVs have been reported in the U.S., Asia, and Europe. Most of these were classical H1N1 SIV infections. However, the wholly avian H1N1 viruses from European pigs, reassortant H3N2 viruses with avian internal protein genes from pigs in Europe and Hong Kong, and a reassortant H1N1 virus from pigs in the U.S. have also been recovered from human beings (reviewed in Alexander and Brown 2000, Olsen 2002a, and Olsen et al. 2002, 2004).

The majority of zoonotic SIV infections have involved individuals in direct contact with pigs, and serologic studies in both Europe and the U.S. have documented increased rates of SIV exposure among persons in contact with pigs (Kluska et al. 1961; Nowotny et al. 1997; Schnurrenberger et al. 1970; Woods et al. 1968, 1981). In addition, a study of swine farm personnel and family members in the U.S. (compared to regional urban control subjects) recently found that SIV seropositivity was statistically associated with being a farm owner or farm family member, living on a farm, or entering a swine barn 4 or more days per week (Olsen et al. 2002). Nonetheless, there are examples of zoonotic SIV infections without apparent animal contact. Although such cases suggest the possibility of human-to-human spread of a virus after initial pig-to-person transmission, with the exception of the Fort Dix incident (Top and Russell 1977), there is little evidence for spread of swine viruses from person to person.

It has also been demonstrated that older lineages of human H3N2 viruses may be maintained by circulation in pigs beyond the time of their active circulation among human beings (reviewed in Brown 2000 and Olsen et al. 2004). Subsequent reintroduction of these viruses into the human population would be a particular concern for young children, because they would be immunologically naive to viruses that circulated prior to their birth.

Finally, because of their susceptibility to infection with influenza viruses of both avian and human origins (reviewed in Ito 2000; Ito et al. 1998a), pigs have also been suggested to be "mixing vessel" hosts in which pandemic human influenza viruses emerge through genetic reassortment (Scholtissek and Naylor 1988; Scholtissek et al. 1985; and reviewed in Brown 2000, Webster et al. 1992, Scholtissek et al. 1998, and Wright and Webster 2001).

PATHOGENESIS

Infection with SIV is generally limited to the respiratory tract, with virus replication demonstrated in epithelial cells of the nasal mucosa, tonsils, trachea, lungs, and tracheobronchial lymph nodes (Brown et al. 1993; Heinen et al. 2000; Lanza et al. 1992). Viremia of low titer and short duration has only rarely been detected (Brown et al. 1993). Similarly, attempts to demonstrate virus replication in extrarespiratory sites have been largely unsuccessful (Choi et al. 2004).

SI is an acute infection and virus clearance is extremely rapid. In most experimental studies, nasal virus shedding begins on day 1 postinoculation (PI) and ceases within 7 days. Likewise, SIV could not be isolated from lungs or other respiratory tract tissues after day 7 (Brown et al. 1993; Choi et al. 2004).

The lungs are clearly the major target organ. Virus titers in the lungs may be >10^8 egg infectious dose 50 (EID$_{50}$) per gram of tissue (Haesebrouck and Pensaert 1986; Van Reeth et al. 1998), and immunofluorescence (IF) and immunohistochemical (IHC) studies demonstrate the virus' highly specific tropism for bronchiolar epithelium (Born et al. 1998; Brown et al. 1993; Haesebrouck and Pensaert 1986; Van Reeth et al. 1998). Up to 100% of the epithelial lining of bronchi/bronchioles and large numbers of alveolar epithelial cells may be positive by IF staining. Typically, bronchi and bronchioli contain exudate with degenerated and detached mucosal cells and neutrophils. However, by 2–3 days after inoculation, lung virus titers and numbers of virus-positive cells begin to decline.

Infection with SIV can be easily reproduced experimentally using intranasal (IN), aerosol, or intratracheal (IT) inoculation routes. However, reproduction of typical SI clinical signs and pathology is most reproducibly accomplished by IT inoculation of high doses of virus ($\geq 10^{7.5}$ EID$_{50}$) (Maes et al. 1984). Less invasive methods, such as IN inoculation, may result in mild or entirely subclinical infections (Larsen et al. 2000; Van Reeth and Pensaert 1994).

Direct cell damage by influenza viruses has been attributed to apoptosis caused by NA and/or PB1F2 proteins (Gibbs et al. 2003; Morris et al. 1999; Schultz-Cherry and Hinshaw 1996). However, proinflammatory cytokines produced by the host during the very acute stage of an infection probably play a critical role in SI disease development. Support for this comes from studies of the lungs of SIV-infected pigs for interferon-α (IFNα), tumor necrosis factor-α (TNFα), interleukin-1 (IL1) and interleukin-6 (IL6) (Van Reeth et al. 1998, 2002). These cytokines are known to induce lung dysfunction and inflammation, fever, malaise, and loss of appetite, and they can enhance each other's effects. In IT infection experiments, excessive levels of all 4 cytokines were found in lung lavage fluids within 18–24 hours PI, when lung virus titers, neutrophil infiltration in the lungs, and clinical signs peaked. In contrast, IN inoculations of SIV produced lower lung virus titers and failed to induce high cytokine levels, and these infections remained clinically mild or subclinical.

Thus, the amount of virus that reaches the deeper airways and the resulting production of infectious virus likely determine the extent of cytokine production in the lungs, which in turn determines the severity of illness. Many cytokines, however, also have antiviral and immunostimulating effects and thus may contribute to clearance of influenza viruses. Therefore, the specific role of individual cytokines during SIV infection merits further study.

CLINICAL SIGNS

Infection with influenza A viruses is typically a herd disease due to rapid spread of virus. Infections with H1N1, H1N2, and H3N2 subtype viruses are clinically similar, and viruses of all subtypes have been associated with acute respiratory episodes in most European countries (reviewed in Brown 2000) and in the U.S. (Karasin et al. 2000a, c, 2002; Zhou et al. 1999). Disease onset is sudden, after an incubation period of 1–3 days. Disease signs typically appear in a large percentage of animals of all ages within a herd or epidemiological unit.

The signs of SI are essentially as they were described in the 1920s (Dorset et al. 1922; McBryde 1927; Shope 1931). Initial signs include pyrexia, anorexia, inactivity, prostration, huddling, and reluctance to rise. Conjunctivitis, rhinitis, nasal discharge, sneezing, coughing, and weight loss may also be observed. The disease may progress to open-mouthed breathing and dyspnea, especially when animals are forced to move. Morbidity is high (near 100%), but mortality typically is low (usually less than 1%) unless there are concurrent infections and/or the pigs are very young. Generally, recovery begins 5–7 days after onset and is as sudden and remarkable as the onset.

Acute outbreaks of clinically typical SI, as described above, are generally limited to fully susceptible, seronegative pigs, including unprotected nursery pigs or older pigs. For instance, in Europe, the sudden reintroduction of influenza viruses into temporarily seronegative breeding-fattening farms has been associated frequently with acute disease in pigs of 50 kg and greater (Loeffen, personal communication). In contrast, breeding animals that have acquired active immunity as a result of previous infections and their maternally immune offspring mostly remain unaffected. Subclinical infections are evidenced by the high seroprevalence of virus subtypes in finishing pigs in the absence of significant respiratory disease during the fattening period and isolation of virus from pigs with no signs of illness (Hinshaw et al. 1978).

However, multiple factors beyond immune status, e.g., age, infection pressure, concurrent infections, climatic conditions, housing, may interact to affect the clinical outcome of SIV infection. For example, it is widely recognized that secondary infections with any of a number of bacterial pathogens, e.g., *Actinobacillus pleuropneumonia*, *Pasteurella multocida*, *Mycoplamsa hyopneumoniae*, *Haemophilus parasuis*, and *Streptococcus suis* type 2, impact the severity and course of infections with SIVs. More recent observations under natural conditions suggest that respiratory viruses can also act as complicating factors. The prevalence of dual or triple infections with influenza virus(es) and either porcine respiratory coronavirus (PRCV) or porcine reproductive and respiratory syndrome virus (PRRSV) is extremely high in intensive fattening units in Europe (Houben et al. 1995; Madec et al. 1987; Van Reeth and Pensaert 1994). The hypothesis that influenza viruses may precipitate disease in combination with other respiratory viruses has been supported by experimental dual infection studies (Van Reeth and Pensaert 1994; Van Reeth et al. 1996, 2001c). In these studies, fever, respiratory disease, and growth retardation were significantly more severe and lasting in dual infections as compared to single virus infected pigs. Nevertheless, unknown factors may impact the development of disease following dual virus infections, because in other studies, clinical signs were not enhanced following simultaneous inoculation of pigs with PRCV and either H1N1 or H3N2 viruses (Lanza et al. 1992; Van Reeth et al. 2001c).

Subsequent to an influenza outbreak in a herd, producers and veterinarians occasionally report reduced reproductive performance through increased infertility, abortion, small weak litters, and stillbirths. However, there is insufficient data to conclude that SI viruses have a specific and direct relationship to the occurrence of reproductive problems and, with rare exceptions (Madec et al. 1989; Woods and Mansfield 1974; Young and Underdahl 1949), influenza viruses are not thought to infect the reproductive tract of pigs.

LESIONS

The gross lesions found in uncomplicated SI are mainly those of a viral pneumonia. Abnormalities are most often limited to the apical and cardiac lobes of the lung. The percent of lung tissue with grossly visible consolidation varies greatly within and between experimental infection studies, but more than 50% of the lung may be affected by 4–5 days PI (Born et al. 1998; Richt et al. 2003). Generally, there is a sharp line of demarcation between the affected and normal lung tissue, and the involved areas will be purple and firm. Some interlobular edema may be evident, airways may be filled with blood-tinged fibrinous exudates, and the associated bronchial and mediastinal lymph nodes are usually enlarged. In naturally occurring SI, however, these lesions may be complicated or masked by concurrent infections, especially bacterial.

Microscopically, the hallmark of an SI infection is necrosis of lung epithelia and desquamation of the bronchial epithelial cell layer (Haesebrouck et al. 1985; Haesebrouck and Pensaert 1986). Within 24 hours after experimental IT inoculation, the airways are plugged with inflammatory and necrotic epithelial cells, mainly neutrophils. In lung lavage fluids collected at this stage of infection, neutrophils may account for up to 50% of the cell population, and macrophages are the dominant

cells in uninfected, healthy pigs (Van Reeth et al. 1998). The neutrophils not only cause obstruction of the airways, but they probably also contribute to lung damage by release of their enzymes. After a few days, there is peribronchial and perivascular infiltration of lymphocytes (Richt et al. 2003). Similar pathologic lesions have been observed in clinically typical SIV outbreaks in the field (Done et al. 1996). Like clinical signs, however, lung lesions can also be mild or unremarkable.

Lastly, a proliferative and necrotizing pneumonia (PNP) characterized by a marked proliferation of type II pneumocytes and coagulates of necrotic cells in the alveoli has been associated with strains of H1N1 and H3N2 SIV (Dea et al. 1992; Girard et al. 1992; Morin et al. 1990). However, recent studies have indicated that PRRSV is the key etiologic agent of this condition (Drolet et al. 2003).

IMMUNITY

The adaptive immune response to SIV infection includes both production of antibodies and cell-mediated immunity (CMI). Antibody responses may develop to the HA, NA, M, and NP proteins. However, only antibodies to the globular head region of the HA can block attachment of the virus to host cell receptors and, thus, neutralize viral infectivity. These antibodies can be measured in virus neutralization (VN) or HI assays. Antibodies to the NA, M, and NP proteins cannot prevent the initiation of infection, but they can mediate killing of infected cells by other antibody-dependent mechanisms. Cytotoxic T lymphocytes (CTLs) are mainly directed to the internal NP and M proteins in mouse models of influenza, and to a lesser degree to the HA and NA. Although CTLs are not capable of preventing infection, they may play a key role in clearing virus from the lungs.

The immune response to SIV infection is remarkably rapid and efficient and results in complete elimination of the virus from the respiratory tract within 1 week PI. T cell responses have been detected from 7 days PI onward (Heinen et al. 2001 a, b; Larsen et al. 2000). HI antibodies in serum can be detected by 7–10 days PI and peak at titers of 1:160 to 1:320 by 2–3 weeks PI (Heinen et al. 2000; Larsen et al. 2000). Antibody titers will remain high for several weeks before beginning to decline by 8–10 weeks PI (Van Reeth et al. 2004, and unpublished data). Using highly sensitive ELISA techniques, HA-specific antibodies have been detected in serum as early as day 3 and in nasal secretions on day 4 after inoculation (Lee et al. 1995). Post infection pig sera also contain antibodies to the NA and NP (Heinen et al. 2000, 2001a; Van Reeth et al. 2003a), and anti-NP Abs have also been found in nasal and lung lavage fluids (Heinen et al. 2000). As would be expected, IgM and later IgG, were the dominant isotypes in serum, whereas IgA was the main isotype in nasal washes (Heinen et al. 2000;

Larsen et al. 2000). Larsen et al. (2000) demonstrated antibody-secreting cells in nasal mucosal tissue, which proved that antibodies were locally produced in the respiratory tract of pigs. Antibodies at the lung level are, at least in part, transudated from serum, as suggested by the dominance of virus-specific IgG in bronchoalveolar lavage samples of pigs (Heinen et al. 2000) and other species (White and Fenner 1994). However, substantial IgA levels were also found in lung lavage fluids of SIV-infected pigs (Larsen et al. 2000), and local antibody production in the lung parenchyma cannot be excluded.

After primary infection with SIV, there is solid protection against reinfection with the same or a similar virus strain. Pigs that had been experimentally infected with H1N1 or H3N2 SIV were completely protected against virus replication in the lungs and nose when rechallenged with homologous virus at 6 and 9 weeks after the initial infection, respectively (Heinen et al. 2001b; Larsen et al. 2000). However, the exact duration of protection is not known. HA-specific VN antibodies are likely the main mediators of this "homologous" immunity. Protection studies to prove the role of other immune mechanisms in the pigs are still lacking.

Because of the concurrent circulation of different subtypes of influenza viruses in Europe and in the U.S., pigs may be exposed to multiple, antigenically different, SIVs during their lifetime. Limited cross-protection (reduced virus shedding and clinical illness severity) between the current European H1N1, H3N2, and H1N2 SIVs was demonstrated in experimental infection studies (Heinen et al. 2001a; Van Reeth et al. 2003a), possibly because these viruses have almost identical NP and M proteins despite very different HA and NA proteins (Van Reeth et al. 2004). The true significance of these data for the field situation is still unknown, as are the immune mechanisms that mediate this "broad" protection. Additionally, protection after vaccination is more subtype-specific (Van Reeth et al. 2003b).

The presence of high titers of VN serum antibodies, reaching the lungs by diffusion, is sufficient to reduce SIV replication in the lungs of vaccinated pigs and protect against disease (Haesebrouck and Pensaert 1986). Protection from nasal virus shedding, on the other hand, appears to be minimal in vaccinated pigs (Macklin et al. 1998; Rapp-Gabrielson et al. 2000). This may be due to a lack of virus-specific IgA antibodies in the nasal mucosa.

Maternally derived antibodies can protect young pigs against SIV, but they will also interfere with the development of an active antibody response to vaccination. Maternal SIV antibody levels in newborn pigs are dependent on antibody levels in the dam, they decline over time, and their precise duration can vary from about 4–14 weeks. In experimental studies, none of the pigs with maternal antibodies were completely protected from nasal virus shedding upon challenge, but some pigs showed complete protection of the lungs (Labarque et al. 2004; Loeffen et al. 2003; Renshaw 1975). Pigs with high passive antibody levels did not develop an immune response to the infection and they remained fully susceptible to reinfection with the same virus; a weak and delayed active immune response was seen in pigs with lower levels of maternal antibodies (Loeffen et al. 2003; Renshaw 1975). Recent studies have also confirmed that maternal immunity does not cross-protect between subtypes (Choi et al. 2004; Labarque et al. 2004).

DIAGNOSIS

A clinical diagnosis of SI is presumptive only because there are no pathognomonic signs and SI must be differentiated from a variety of respiratory diseases of swine. A definite diagnosis is possible only in the laboratory, either through isolation of virus, detection of viral proteins or nucleic acid, or demonstration of virus-specific antibodies.

Isolation of SIV from live animals is typically undertaken on samples of mucus obtained by swabbing the nasal passages or, in the case of very small pigs where it is difficult to swab the nasal passages, the pharynx. Virus is most likely to be found in nasal and pharyngeal secretions during the febrile period of illness. Samples should be collected on polyester (e.g., Dacron), not cotton, swabs. Swabs should be suspended in a suitable transport medium (such as glycerol saline) and kept cold (refrigerator temperature, 4°C) during transport to the laboratory. If the samples for virus isolation can be tested within 48 hours after collection, they should be maintained at 4°C. If the samples must be held longer, storage at −70°C is recommended. SIVs are not stable at −20°C. Filtration of the samples should be avoided to conserve small amounts of virus that might be in the transport medium. Adventitious bacterial and fungal agents may be controlled with the addition of appropriate antimicrobial agents to the transport medium.

Virus may also be isolated from trachea or lung tissues of pigs that die or are euthanized during the acute stage of the disease. The tissue material should be held under the same conditions as swab material until ready for culturing. Before testing, the tissue is homogenized in a sterile saline preparation.

Methods for the isolation of virus have been described in detail (Swenson and Foley 2004). Briefly, the virus can be cultivated in embryonated fowl's eggs, generally by allantoic cavity inoculation of 10- to 11-day-old eggs and subsequent incubation at 35°C for 72 hours. SIVs do not typically kill the embryo, but virus can be detected in allantoic fluid using the hemagglutination assay (generally using chicken or turkey erythrocytes), which provides presumptive evidence for the presence of an influenza virus. Up to two blind passages may be required to confirm the absence of virus. Repeated passages should be done under strictly controlled conditions to avoid cross-contamination in the laboratory.

Increasingly, SIV isolation is being conducted in cell culture. Cell lines of several different origins support the growth of influenza viruses, including bovine, canine, and porcine kidney cells, porcine lung and tracheal epithelial cells, and human diploid cells (Easterday 1975; Ferrari et al. 2003), as well as Vero cells (Govorkova et al. 1995), swine testes cells (Potgeiter et al. 1977), and mink lung cells (Schultz-Cherry et al. 1998). Inoculation of eggs plus cell cultures (Clavijo et al. 2002) or multiple cell lines (Landolt et al. 2005) may enhance recovery of viruses that grow preferentially in different host cells. Furthermore, recent work has demonstrated that Madin-Darby canine kidney and mink lung cells can be co-cultured for SIV isolation (Landolt et al. 2005).

The HA and NA subtypes of influenza viruses have historically been determined in HI and neuraminidase-inhibition (NI) tests (Swenson and Foley 2004). Increasingly, however, molecular-based methods are being used to detect and subtype influenza viruses. The use of reverse transcription-polymerase chain reaction (RT-PCR) assays (both traditional and real-time technologies) offers sensitivity equivalent to virus isolation plus speed and high-volume throughput. These approaches are in their infancy with respect to widespread, commercial diagnostic application for SIV and may have limitations for use in the detection of heterogeneous virus populations. However, such approaches have been used successfully for the detection of the predominant subtypes in pigs and demonstrated good correlation with conventional virus isolation and identification methods (Choi et al. 2002c, 2004; Landolt et al. 2005; Olsen et al. unpublished data; Schorr et al. 1994).

Other methods for detecting virus or viral antigen include direct immunofluorescence techniques applied to lung tissue (Barigazzi et al. 1993), nasal epithelial cells (Onno et al. 1990), or bronchoalveolar lavage contents (Runge et al. 1996); immunohistochemical (IHC) detection in fixed tissues (Haines et al. 1993); ELISA (Lee et al. 1993); rapid cell culture assay using immunoperoxidase staining for typing and subtyping (Ziegler et al. 1995); and a commercially available enzyme immunoassay membrane test (Directigen FLU-A), which rapidly detects influenza A antigen in clinical specimens (Ryan-Poirier et al. 1992).

Serological tests are used to demonstrate the presence of influenza specific antibodies. Diagnosis of acute SIV infection by serology requires the use of paired acute and convalescent (3–4 weeks later) serum samples and appropriate antigens.

Although ELISA assays have become commercially available for SIV, HI remains the most common test for anti-SIV antibody detection. The diagnostician must be aware of the possible presence of nonspecific inhibitors and nonspecific agglutinins in swine serum that may interfere with the HI test. Sera should be treated to reduce or destroy such activity, although some treatments may lower specific antibody levels. The most widely used method is treatment with receptor-destroying enzyme and absorption with chicken erythrocytes (Swenson and Foley 2004). There is considerable antigenic heterogeneity in viruses of the same subtype circulating in pigs because of antigenic drift and lineage variations in different geographical areas of the world. Therefore, the choice of potential viruses for use as antigens in serologic assays should ensure that the strains are well-matched to the current epidemic viruses in a region, country, or continent (Brown et al. 1997b; de Jong et al. 1999; Karasin et al. 2002; Olsen et al. 2000; Richt et al. 2003).

Other assays, such as the VN test (Brown, Olsen, unpublished data) or single radial hemolysis test (Ogawa et al. 1978) have been applied to testing pigs for influenza antibodies. Although these assays do not require pretreatment of sera, they are more appropriate for use in specialized laboratories.

Positive diagnosis of SIV by serological and virological methods among suckling or weanling pigs from dams with antibodies to the virus may be complicated. It has been shown that weanling pigs with maternal antibodies may be infected and may shed virus. The rate of virus recovery and severity of signs of disease are inversely related to levels of maternal antibody (Easterday 1971; Renshaw 1975). In addition, the level of antibody in the convalescent-phase serum will be lower than in the acute-phase serum because of the inhibition of active antibody production by maternal antibody (Easterday 1971; Mensik 1960, 1963, 1966; Renshaw 1975). After maternal antibody is depleted, pigs may be infected again, shed virus, present with signs of disease, and produce a typical primary antibody response.

PREVENTION AND CONTROL

Vaccination and biosecurity remain the primary means of preventing SI in pigs. Commercial inactivated and adjuvanted SIV vaccines for intramuscular administration are available both in Europe and the U.S. Primary vaccination should consist of two injections 2–4 weeks apart. Biannual booster vaccinations are recommended for sows.

SIV vaccine strain composition differs between continents because of the antigenic and genetic differences between SIVs circulating in Europe and the U.S. Vaccines for use in Europe were first licensed during the mid-1980s and contain both subtypes that were prevalent at that time, H1N1 and H3N2. Most of the current vaccines still contain the older human New Jersey/76 (H1N1) and Port Chalmers/73 (H3N2) strains. Whole virus vaccines, as well as "split" vaccines (produced from disrupted highly purified influenza virus) are available. In the U.S., a monovalent H1N1 SIV vaccine was first introduced in 1993. After the emergence of

H3N2 influenza viruses in the U.S. swine population in 1998, monovalent and bivalent (H1N1/H3N2) SIV vaccines became available. The current U.S. vaccines primarily contain a classical H1N1 virus and a triple reassortant H3N2 virus, although a trivalent vaccine also containing reassortant H1N1 virus has recently become available. Autogenous vaccines containing herd-specific strains are also used in the U.S.

Most SIV vaccine efficacy data are from experimental vaccination-challenge studies in which SIV-seronegative pigs are vaccinated twice with commercial vaccine and challenged with virulent SIV 2–6 weeks after the second vaccination. Several studies with European vaccines used a severe IT challenge that results in typical SIV symptoms and high lung virus titers within 24 hours post challenge in unvaccinated controls, but vaccination with New Jersey/76 (H1N1)- and/or Port Chalmers/73 (H3N2)-based commercial vaccines could completely prevent virus replication in the lungs and disease (Haesebrouck and Pensaert 1986; Vandeputte et al. 1986). Based on reports of minor antigenic drift in European H1N1 and H3N2 SIVs during the late 1990s (de Jong et al. 1999, 2001), replacement of the vaccine strains by more recent strains has been considered. In studies in pigs, however, the commercial vaccine still induced high antibody titers to recent H1N1 and H3N2 strains and excellent clinical and virological protection (Heinen et al. 2001b; Van Reeth et al. 2001a,b). Thus, there are no scientific arguments to update H1N1 or H3N2 strains. However, addition of an H1N2 component to these vaccines deserves serious consideration because there is no antigenic cross-reactivity between the European H1N2 virus and the H1N1 and H3N2 strains in the vaccine and because current vaccines failed to protect against H1N2 challenge in experimental infection studies (Van Reeth et al. 2003b).

In studies with U.S. vaccines, challenge has more commonly been by the IN route, and nasal virus shedding was usually the main parameter used to evaluate protection. Complete protection from infection could not be demonstrated, but vaccination could reduce H1N1 challenge virus titers in nasal swabs by 1–2 $\log_{10}$ infectious units. Virus titers in the lungs of vaccinated pigs and macroscopic lung lesion scores were also reduced (Brown and McMillen 1994; Macklin et al. 1998; Rapp-Gabrielson et al. 2000). A bivalent U.S. SIV vaccine was shown to cross-protect against challenge with a 2002 H3N2 isolate that showed genetic drift from the vaccine H3N2 strain (Rapp-Gabrielson et al. 2003).

Though there has to be antigenic overlap between vaccine and challenge strains, antigenic and genetic analyses are not the most accurate predictors of vaccine strain performance. Challenge tests in pigs clearly remain the best measure of vaccine efficacy. Factors other than the nature of the vaccine strains—i.e., the antigenic dose and adjuvant, the health of the pigs at the time of vaccination, proper vaccine administration and timing—all affect vaccine efficacy. Vaccines with higher antigenic doses will generally be more effective, and highly immunostimulatory oil-based adjuvants are used with most commercial vaccines, although the exact adjuvant formulation may differ among vaccines. New generation adjuvants like Quil A and a combination of Quil A, and alhydrogel also induced high antibody titers when administered with an experimental SIV vaccine (Bikour et al. 1994).

HI antibody titers after administration of two doses of vaccine to seronegative pigs generally range from 1:20 to 1:640, but there may be considerable variation between vaccines and different experiments. Vaccine-induced HI antibodies can be short-lived and significant decreases in serum antibody titer have been reported within 10 weeks after vaccination (Erickson et al. 2002). An inverse correlation between prechallenge serum HI antibody titers and lung virus titers after challenge has been reported by several investigators (Bikour et al. 1996; Haesebrouck and Pensaert 1986; Haesebrouck et al. 1987; Van Reeth et al. 2001 a, b). In the studies by Van Reeth et al. (2001 a, b), all vaccinates with HI titers >160 were completely protected against virus replication in the lungs and disease. However, the antibody titer required for complete protection from infection will also depend on the challenge dose, such that antibody titers ≤160 may be effective against challenge with a lower virus dose or under field conditions (Bikour et al. 1996).

Data regarding SIV vaccine efficacy in the field and cost benefit are quite limited. Most SIV vaccine is used for sow vaccination. In sows routinely receiving pre-farrow booster vaccinations, HI serum antibody titers are frequently 1:160 to 1:640 or greater, and this results in higher and longer lasting maternal SIV antibody levels in their piglets. In a study by Thacker (2000), SIV passive antibody levels dropped below 1:40 by 6 weeks of age in nearly all pigs from unvaccinated sows with low residual HI titers. In contrast, in pigs nursing vaccinated sows, antibody titers did not drop below 1:40 until 16 weeks of age. Sow vaccination, therefore, is important in controlling disease in suckling pigs and often protects pigs through the nursery phase.

Vaccination of feeder pigs is less commonly performed, but this strategy may be beneficial in herds where influenza is a problem in growers/finishers. However, vaccination of feeder pigs may be difficult to combine with vaccination of sows because prolonged passive immunity may interfere with effective vaccination of piglets.

So-called new generation vaccines for SIV have also been tested experimentally, but the results have been rather disappointing. DNA vaccines based on the influenza HA or NP reduced the amount and duration of influenza viral shedding (Macklin et al. 1998), but Olsen and coworkers (2000) found no significant protection from challenge infection following HA DNA vaccination. Still, the DNA vaccination primed pigs for a stronger antibody response to infection with virulent virus or to vaccination with a conventional killed SIV vaccine (Larsen et al. 2001; Olsen et al. 2000). Heinen et al. (2002) tested a recombinant vaccine expressing the M2 protein and a DNA vaccine containing NP and M genes. Though both vaccines induced the desired immune responses, there was no protection against infection or disease.

REFERENCES

Alexander DJ, Brown IH. 2000. Recent zoonoses caused by influenza A viruses. Rev Sci Tech Off Int Epiz 19:197–225.

Arora DJS, N'Diaye M, Dea S. 1997. Genomic study of hemagglutinins of swine influenza (H1N1) viruses associated with acute and chronic respiratory diseases in pigs. Arch Virol 142:401–412.

Barigazzi G, Bonardi S, Fibu E, Candotti P, Ferrari B, Bedogni I. 1993. Use of the direct immunofluorescence technique to diagnose swine influenza: A comparison with virus isolation. Atti del XIX Mtg Ann Soc Ital Patol e Allev d Suini, 1992, pp. 309–318.

Beveridge WIB. 1977. Influenza: The Last Great Plague. United Kingdom: Heinemann Educational Books Ltd., p. 124.

Bikour MH, Cornaglia E, Elazhary Y. 1996. Evaluation of a protective immunity induced by an inactivated influenza H3N2 vaccine after an intratracheal challenge of pigs. Can J Vet Res 60:312–314.

Bikour MH, Cornaglia E, Weber JM, Elazhary Y. 1994. Comparative study of the immunostimulatory properties of different adjuvants administered with an inactivated influenza virus vaccine and evaluation of passive immunity in pigs. Immunol Infect Dis 4:166–172.

Bikour MH, Frost EH, Deslandes S, Talbot B, Weber JM, Elazhary Y. 1995. Recent H3N2 swine influenza virus with haemagglutinin and nucleoprotein genes similar to 1975 human strains. J Gen Virol 76:697–703.

Born B, Vincent L, Janke B, Paul P. 1998. Comparative pathogenicity of atypical and typical swine influenza viruses. Proc Annu Meet Am Assoc Swine Pract, pp. 63–66.

Brown GB, McMillen JK. 1994. MaxiVac TM-FLU: Evaluation of the safety and efficacy of a swine influenza vaccine. Proc Annu Meet Am Assoc Swine Pract, pp. 37–39.

Brown IH. 2000. The epidemiology and evolution of influenza viruses in pigs. Vet Microbiol 74:29–46.

Brown IH, Alexander DJ, Chakraverty P, Harris PA, Manvell RJ. 1994. Isolation of an influenza A virus of unusual subtype (H1N7) from pigs in England, and the subsequent experimental transmission from pig to pig. Vet Microbiol 39:125–134.

Brown IH, Chakraverty P, Harris PA, Alexander DJ. 1995. Disease outbreaks in pigs in Great Britain due to an influenza A virus of H1N2 subtype. Vet Rec 136:328–329.

Brown IH, Done SH, Spencer YI, Cooley WA, Harris PA, Alexander DJ. 1993. Pathogenicity of a swine influenza H1N1 virus antigenically distinguishable from classical and European strains. Vet Rec 132:598–602.

Brown IH, Harris PA, McCauley JW, Alexander DJ. 1998. Multiple genetic reassortment of avian and human influenza A viruses in European pigs, resulting in emergence of an H1N2 virus of novel genotype. J Gen Virol 79:2947–2955.

Brown IH, Hill ML, Harris PA, Alexander DJ, McCauley JW. 1997a. Genetic characterisation of an influenza A virus of unusual subtype (H1N7) isolated from pigs in England. Arch Virol 142:1045–1050.

Brown IH, Ludwig S, Olsen CW, Hannoun C, Scholtissek C, Hinshaw VS, Harris PA, McCauley JW, Strong I, Alexander DJ. 1997b. Antigenic and genetic analyses of H1N1 influenza A viruses from European pigs. J Gen Virol 78:553–562.

Campitelli L, Donatelli I, Foni E. 1997. Continued evolution of H1N1 and H3N2 influenza viruses in pigs in Italy. Virology 232:310–318.

Castrucci MR, Donatelli I, Sidoli L, Barigazzi G, Kawaoka Y, Webster RG. 1993. Genetic reassortment between avian and human influenza viruses in Italian pigs. Virology 193:503–506.

Chambers TM, Hinshaw VS, Kawaoka Y, Easterday BC, Webster RG. 1991. Influenza viral infection of swine in the United States 1988–1989. Arch Virol 116:261–265.

Choi YK, Goyal SM, Farnham MW, Joo HS. 2002a. Phylogenetic analysis of H1N2 isolates of influenza A virus from pigs in the United States. Virus Res 87:173–179.

Choi YK, Goyal SM, Joo HS. 2002b. Prevalence of swine influenza virus subtypes on swine farms in the United States. Arch Virol 147:1209–1220.

——. 2004. Evaluation of transmission of swine influenza type A subtype H1N2 virus in seropositive pigs. Am J Vet Res 65:303–306.

Choi YK, Goyal SM, Kang SW, Farnham MW, Joo HS. 2002c. Detection and subtyping of swine influenza H1N1, H1N2 and H3N2 viruses in clinical samples using two multiplex RT-PCR assays. J Virol Methods 102:53–59.

Clavijo A, Tresnan DB, Jolie R, Zhou EM. 2002. Comparison of embryonated chicken eggs with MDCK cell culture for the isolation of swine influenza virus. Can J Vet Res 66:117–121.

Cooper L, Olsen C, Xu X, Klimov A, Cox N, Subbarao K. 1999. Molecular characterization of influenza A viruses bearing swine-like hemagglutinin genes isolated from humans. Proceedings of the Noble Foundation Workshop on Virus Evolution, available at http://www.noble.org/virusevolution/abstracts/Cooperpost.htm.

de Jong JC, Heinen PP, Loeffen WLA, van Nieuwstadt AP, Claas ECJ, Besebroer TM, Bijsma K, Verweji C, Osterhaus ADME, Rimmelzwaan GF, Fouchier RAM, Kimman TG. 2001. Antigenic and molecular heterogeneity in recent swine influenza A (H1N1) virus isolates with possible implications for vaccination policy. Vaccine 19:4452–4464.

de Jong JC, van Nieuwstadt AP, Kimman TG, Loeffen WLA, Bestebroer TM, Bijlsma K, Verwriji C, Osterhaus ADME, Claas ECJ. 1999. Antigenic drift in swine influenza H3 haemagglutinins with implications for vaccination policy. Vaccine 17:1321–1328.

Dea S, Bilodeau R, Sauvageau R, Montpetit C, Martineau GP. 1991. Antigenic variant of swine influenza virus causing proliferative and necrotizing pneumonia in pigs. J Vet Diagn Invest 4:380–392.

Donatelli I, Campitelli L, Castrucci MR, Ruggieri A, Sidoli L, Oxford JS. 1991. Detection of two antigenic subpopulations of A (H1N1) influenza viruses from pigs: Antigenic drift or interspecies transmission. J Med Virol 34:248–257.

Done SH, Brown IH, Harris P, Spencer Y, Cooley W, White MEC. 1996. Swine influenza and interstitial pneumonias in the United Kingdom (1985–1995). Eur J Vet Pathol 2:73–81.

Dorset M, McBryde CN, Niles WB. 1922. Remarks on "hog flu." J Am Vet Med Assoc 62:162–171.

Drolet R, Larochelle R, Morin M, Delisle B, Magar R. 2003. Detection rates of porcine reproductive and respiratory syndrome virus, porcine circovirus type 2, and swine influenza virus in porcine proliferative and necrotizing pneumonia. Vet Pathol 40:143–148.

Easterday BC. 1971. Influenza virus infection of the suckling pig. Acta Vet (Suppl) 2:33–42.

——. 1975. Swine influenza. In Diseases of Swine. HW Dunne, AD Leman, eds. Ames: Iowa State University Press, pp. 141–167.

——. 1980. Animals in the influenza world. Phil Trans Royal Soc (London) B288:433–437.

——. 1986. Swine Influenza. In Diseases of Swine (6th edition). AD Leman, B Straw, RD Glock, WL Mengeling, RHC Penny, E Scholl, eds. Ames: Iowa State University Press, pp. 244–255.

Easterday BC, Van Reeth K. 1999. Swine influenza. In Diseases of Swine (8th edition). BE Straw, S D'Allaire, WL Mengeling, DJ Taylor, eds. Ames: Iowa State University Press, pp. 277–290.

Erickson G, Rapp-Gabrielson V, Jackson T, Eddy B, Gergen L, Bennett K, Velek K. 2002. Duration of HI and ELISA antibodies following vaccination against SIV. Proc Congr Int Pig Vet Soc 1:180.

Ferrari M, Scalvini A, Losio MN, Corradi A, Soncini M, Bignotti E, Milanesi E, Ajmone-Marsan P, Barlati S, Belloti D, Tonelli M. 2003. Establishment and characterization of two new pig cell lines for use in virological diagnostic laboratories. J Virol Methods 107:205–212.

Gibbs JS, Malide D, Hornung F, Bennick JR, Yewdell JW. 2003. The influenza A virus PB1-F2 protein targets the inner mitochondrial membrane via a predicted basic amphipathic helix that disrupts mitochondrial function. J Virol 77:7214–7224.

Girard C, Morin M, Elazhary Y. 1992. Experimentally induced porcine proliferative and necrotising pneumonia with an influenza A virus. Vet Rec 130:206–207.

Gorman OT, Bean WJ, Kawaoka Y, Webster RG. 1990. Evolution of the nucleoprotein gene of influenza A virus. J Virol 64:1487–1497.

Gourreau JM, Kaiser C, Valette M, Douglas AR, Labie J, Aymard M. 1994. Isolation of two H1N2 influenza viruses from swine in France. Arch Virol 135:365–382.

Govorkova EA, Kaverin NV, Gubareva LV, Meignier B, Webster RG. 1995. Replication of influenza A viruses in a green monkey kidney continuous cell line (Vero). J Infect Dis 172:250–253.

Guan Y, Shortridge KF, Krauss S, Li PH, Kawaoka Y, Webster RG. 1996. Emergence of avian H1N1 influenza viruses in pigs in China. J Virol 70:8041–8046.

Haesebrouck F, Biont P, Pensaert MR, Leuven J. 1985. Epizootics of respiratory tract disease in swine in Belgium due to H3N2 influenza virus and experimental reproduction of disease. Am J Vet Res 46:1926–1928.

Haesebrouck F, Pensaert M. 1986. Effect of intratracheal challenge of fattening pigs previously immunized with an inactivated influenza H1N1 vaccine. Vet Microbiol 11:239–249.

Haesebrouck F, Pensaert M, Wyffels R. 1987. Vaccination of swine against H3N2-influenza field isolates using the human Philippines-strain. Vet Q 9:9–14.

Haines DM, Waters EH, Clark EG. 1993. Immunohistochemical detection of swine influenza A virus in formalin-fixed and paraffin-embedded tissues. Can J Vet Res 57:33–36.

Heinen PP, de Boer-Luijtze EA, Bianchi AT. 2001a. Respiratory and systemic humoral and cellular immune responses of pigs to a heterosubtypic influenza A virus infection. J Gen Virol 82:2697–2707.

Heinen PP, Rijsewijk FA, de Boer-Luijtze EA, Bianchi AT. 2002. Vaccination of pigs with a DNA construct expressing an influenza virus M2-nucleoprotein fusion protein exacerbates disease after challenge with influenza A virus. J Gen Virol 83:1851–1859.

Heinen PP, van Nieuwstadt AP, de Boer-Luijtze EA, Bianchi AT. 2001b. Analysis of the quality of protection induced by a porcine influenza A vaccine to challenge with an H3N2 virus. Vet Immunol Immunopathol 82:39–56.

Heinen PP, van Nieuwstadt AP, Pol JM, de Boer-Luijtze EA, van Oirschot JT, Bianchi AT. 2000. Systemic and mucosal isotype-specific antibody responses in pigs to experimental influenza virus infection. Viral Immunol 13:237–247.

Hinshaw VS, Bean WJ, Webster RG, Easterday BC. 1978. The prevalence of influenza viruses in swine and the antigenic and genetic relatedness of influenza viruses from man and swine. Virology 84:51–62.

Hinshaw VS, Webster RG, Bean WJ, Downie J, Senne DA. 1983. Swine influenza viruses in turkeys—A potential source of virus for humans? Science 220:206–208.

Hinshaw VS, Webster RG, Turner B. 1980. The perpetuation of orthomyxoviruses and paramyxoviruses in Canadian waterfowl. Can J Microbiol 26:622–629.

Houben S, Van Reeth K, Pensaert MB. 1995. Pattern of infection with the porcine reproductive and respiratory syndrome virus on swine farms in Belgium. J Vet Med B 42:209–215.

Ito T. 2000. Interspecies transmission and receptor recognition of influenza A viruses. Microbiol Immunol 44:423–430.

Ito T, Couceiro JNSS, Kelm S, Baum LG, Krauss S, Castrucci MR, Donatelli I, Kida H, Paulson JC, Webster RG, Kawaoka Y. 1998a. Molecular basis for the generation in pigs of influenza A viruses with pandemic potential. J Virol 72:7367–7373.

Ito T, Kawaoka Y, Vines A, Ishikawa H, Asai T, Kida, H. 1998b. Continued circulation of reassortant H1N2 influenza viruses in pigs in Japan. Arch Virol 143:1773–1782.

Ito T, Suzuki Y, Suzuki T, Takada A, Horimoto T, Wells K, Kida H, Otsuki K, Kiso M, Ishida H, Kawaoka Y. 2000. Recognition of N-glycolylneuraminic acid linked to galactose by the a2,3 linkage is associated with intestinal replication of influenza A virus in ducks. J Virol 74:9300–9305.

Kaplan MM. 1969. Relationships between animal and human influenza. Bull World Health Org 41:485–486.

Karasin AI, Anderson GA, Olsen CW. 2000a. Genetic characterization of an H1N2 influenza virus isolated from a pig in Indiana. J Clin Microbiol 38:2453–2456.

Karasin AI, Brown IH, Carman S, Olsen CW. 2000b. Isolation and characterization of H4N6 avian influenza viruses from pigs with pneumonia in Canada. J Virol 74:9322–9327.

Karasin AI, Landgraf JG, Swenson SL, Erickson G, Goyal SM, Woodruff M, Scherba G, Anderson GA, Olsen CW. 2002. Genetic characterization of H1N2 influenza A viruses isolated from pigs throughout the United States. J Clin Microbiol 40:1073–1079.

Karasin AI, Schutten MM, Cooper LA, Smith CB, Subbarao K, Anderson GA, Carman S, Olsen CW. 2000c. Genetic characterization of H3N2 influenza viruses isolated from pigs in North America, 1977–1999: Evidence for wholly human and reassortant virus genotypes. Virus Res 68:71–85.

Karasin AI, West K, Carman S, Olsen CW. 2004. Characterization of avian H3N3 and H1N1 influenza A viruses isolated from pigs in Canada. J Clin Microbiol 42:4349–4354.

Kida H, Ito T, Yasuda J, Shimizu Y, Itakura C, Shortridge KF, Kawaoka Y, Webster RG. 1994. Potential for transmission of avian influenza viruses to pigs. J Gen Virol 75:2183–2188.

Kida H, Shortridge KF, Webster RG. 1988. Origin of the hemagglutinin gene of H3N2 influenza viruses from pigs in China. Virology 162:160–166.

Kluska V, Hanson LE, Hatch RD. 1961. Evidence for swine influenza antibodies in human. Cesk Pediat 116:408–414.

Koen JS. 1919. A practical method for field diagnosis of swine diseases. Am J Vet Med 14:468–470.

Labarque G, Barbé F, Pensaert M, Van Reeth K. 2004. Maternal immunity to H1N1 and H3N2 swine influenza viruses fails to protect against the novel H1N2 subtype. Proc Congr Int Pig Vet Soc 1:83.

Lamb RA, Krug RM. 2001. Orthomyxoviridae: The viruses and their replication. In Field's Virology (4th edition). DM Knipe, PM Howley, DE Griffin, RA Lamb, MA Martin, B Roizman, SE Straus, eds. Philadelphia: Lippincott-Raven Publishers, pp. 1487–1531.

Landolt GA, Karasin AI, Hofer C, Mahaney J, Svaren J, Olsen CW. 2005. The use of real-time TaqMAN RT-PCR and cell culture methods to detect swine influenza A viruses. Am J Vet Res 66:119–124.

Landolt GA, Karasin AI, Phillips L, Olsen CW. 2003. Comparison of the pathogenesis of two genetically different H3N2 influenza A viruses in pigs. J Clin Microbiol 41:1936–1941.

Lanza I, Brown IH, Paton DJ. 1992. Pathogenicity of concurrent infection of pigs with porcine respiratory coronavirus and swine influenza virus. Res Vet Sci 53:309–314.

Larsen DL, Karasin A, Olsen CW. 2001. Immunization of pigs against influenza virus infection by DNA vaccine priming followed by killed-virus vaccine boosting. Vaccine 19:2842–2853.

Larsen DL, Karasin A, Zuckermann F, Olsen CW. 2000. Systemic and mucosal immune responses to H1N1 influenza virus infection in pigs. Vet Microbiol 74:117–131.

Lee BW, Bey RF, Baarsch MJ, Larson ME. 1995. Class specific antibody response to influenza A H1N1 infection in swine. Vet Microbiol 43:241–250.

Lee BW, Bey RF, Baarsch MJ, Simonson RR. 1993. ELISA method for detection of influenza A infection in swine. J Vet Diagn Invest 5:510–515.

Lin YP, Bennett M, Gregory V, Grambas S, Ragazzoli V, Lenihan P, Hay A. 2004. Emergence of distinct avian-like influenza A H1N1 viruses in pigs in Ireland and their reassortment with co-circulating H3N2 viruses. In International Conference on Options for the Control of Influenza V. Y Kawaoka, ed. Amsterdam: Elsevier, 1263:209–213.

Loeffen WL, Heinen PP, Bianchi AT, Hunneman WA, Verheijden JH. 2003. Effect of maternally derived antibodies on the clinical signs and immune response in pigs after primary and secondary infection with an influenza H1N1 virus. Vet Immunol Immunopathol 92:23–35.

Ludwig S, Haustein A, Kaleta EF, Scholtissek C. 1994. Recent influenza A (H1N1) infections of pigs and turkeys in northern Europe. Virology 202:281–286.

Luoh SM, McGregor MW, Hinshaw VS. 1992. Hemagglutinin mutations related to antigenic variation in H1 swine influenza viruses. J Virol 66:1066–1073.

Macklin MD, McCabe D, McGregor MW, Neumann V, Meyer T, Callan R, Hinshaw VS, Swain WF. 1998. Immunization of pigs with a particle-mediated DNA vaccine to influenza A virus protects against challenge with homologous virus. J Virol 72:1491–1496.

Madec F, Kaiser C, Gourreau JM, Martinat-Botte F. 1989. Pathologic consequences of a severe influenza outbreak (swine virus A/H1N1) under natural conditions in the non-immune sow at the beginning of gestation. Comp Immunol Microbiol Infect Dis 12:17–27.

Madec F, Kaiser C, Jestin A, Gourreau J-M, Vannier P, Kobisch M, Paboeuf F, Aymard M. 1987. Les syndromes grippaux en porcherie d'engraissement: enquete "flash" realisee en Bretagne. Courte Commun Le Point Veterinaire 19:654–659.

Maes L, Haesebrouck F, Pensaert M. 1984. Experimental reproduction of clinical disease by intratracheal inoculation of fattening pigs with swine influenza virus isolates. Proc Congr Int Pig Vet Soc. p. 60.

Marozin S, Gregory V, Cameron K, Bennett M, Valette M, Aymard M, Foni E, Barigazzi G, Lin Y, Hay A. 2002. Antigenic and genetic diversity among swine influenza A H1N1 and H1N2 viruses in Europe. J Gen Virol 83:735–745.

McBryde CN. 1927. Some observations on "hog flu" and its seasonal prevalence in Iowa. J Am Vet Med Assoc 71:368–377.

Mensik J. 1960. Production and behavior of swine influenza antibodies. 1. Influence of colostral antibodies on immunity in piglets during early life. Sb Cesk Akad Zemed Ved 5:599–619.

——. 1963. Formation of antibodies in swine influenza. Colostral immunity and inhibition of antibody formation. Ved Pr Ustav Vet 3:141–149.

——. 1966. The formation and dynamism of antibodies in swine influenza. V. A long-term depression of the antibody formation in the progeny of hyperimmune mothers. Vet Med (Prague) 11:589–595.

Morin M, Girard C, Elazhary Y, Fajardo R, Drolet R, Lagace A. 1990. Severe proliferative and necrotizing pneumonia in pigs: A newly recognized disease. Can Vet J 31:12.

Morin M, Phaneuf JB, Sauvageau R, Difranco R, Marsolais G, Boudreault A. 1981. An epizootic of swine influenza in Quebec. Can Vet J 22:204–205.

Morris SJ, Price GE, Barnett JM, Hiscox SA, Smith H, Sweet C. 1999. Role of neuraminidase in influenza virus-induced apoptosis. J Gen Virol 80:137–146.

Murray C. 1921. What is "hog flu?" Wallaces' Farmer 46:371

Nerome K, Kanegae Y, Shortridge KF, Sugita S, Ishida M. 1995. Genetic analysis of porcine H3N2 viruses originating in southern China. J Gen Virol 76:613–624.

Nerome K, Yoshioka Y, Sakamoto S, Yasuhara M, Oya A. 1985. Characterization of a 1980—Swine recombinant influenza virus possessing H1 haemagglutinin and N2 neuraminidase similar to that of the earliest Hong Kong (H3N2) virus. Arch Virol 86:197–211.

Ninomiya A, Takada A, Okazaki K, Shortridge KF, Kida H. 2002. Seroepidemiological evidence of avian H4, H5, and H9 influenza A virus transmission to pigs in southeastern China. Vet Microbiol 88:107–114.

Noble S, McGregor MS, Wentworth DE, Hinshaw VS. 1993. Antigenic and genetic conservation of the haemagglutinin in H1N1 swine influenza viruses. J Gen Virol 74:1197–1200.

Nowotny N, Duetz A, Fuchs K, Schuller W, Hinterdorfer F, Auer H, Aspock H. 1997. Prevalence of swine influenza and other viral, bacterial, and parasitic zoonoses in veterinarians. J Infect Dis 176:1414–1415.

Ogawa T, Sugimura T, Tanaka Y, Kumagai T. 1978. A single radial hemolysis technique for the measurement of influenza virus antibody in swine serum. Nat Inst An Health Quart (Japan) 18:58–62.

Olsen CW. 2000. DNA vaccination against influenza viruses: A review with emphasis on equine and swine influenza. Vet Microbiol 74:149–164.

——. 2002a. Emergence of novel strains of swine influenza virus in North America. In Trends in Emerging Viral Infections of Swine. A Morilla, KJ Yoon, JJ Zimmerman, eds. Ames: Iowa State Press, pp. 37–43.

——. 2002b. The emergence of novel swine influenza viruses in North America. Virus Res 85:199–210.

Olsen CW, Brammer L, Easterday BC, Arden N, Belay E, Baker I, Cox NJ. 2002. Serologic evidence of H1 swine influenza virus infection in swine farm residents and employees. Emerg Infect Dis 8:814–819.

Olsen CW, Carey S, Hinshaw L, Karasin AI. 2000. Virologic and serologic surveillance for human, swine and avian influenza virus infections among pigs in the north-central United States. Arch Virol 145:1399–1419.

Olsen CW, Karasin A, Erickson G. 2003. Characterization of a swine-like reassortant H1N2 influenza virus isolated from a wild duck in the United States. Virus Res 93:115–121.

Olsen CW, McGregor MW, Cooley AJ, Schantz B, Hotze B, Hinshaw VS. 1993. Antigenic and genetic analysis of a recently isolated H1N1 swine influenza virus. Am J Vet Res 54:1630–1636.

Olsen CW, Swayne D, Subbarao K. 2004. Epidemiology and control of human and animal influenza. In Contemporary Topics in Influenza Virology. Y Kawaoka, ed. , Norwich: Horizon Scientific Press (in press).

Onno M, Jestin A, Nannier P, Kaiser C. 1990. Diagnosis of swine influenza with an immunofluorescence technique using monoclonal antibodies. Vet Q 12:251–254.

Ouchi A, Nerome K, Kanegae Y, Ishida M, Nerome R, Hayashi K, Hashimoto T, Kaji M, Kaji Y, Inaba Y. 1996. Large outbreak of swine influenza in southern Japan caused by reassortant (H1N2) influenza viruses: Its epizootic background and characterization of the causative viruses. J Gen Virol 77:1751–1759.

Peiris JSM, Guan Y, Ghose P, Markwell D, Krauss S, Webster RG, Shortridge KF. 2001a. Co-circulation of avian H9N2 and human H3N2 viruses in pigs in southern China. In Options for the Control of Influenza IV. Excerpta Medica International Congress Series 1219. A Osterhaus, N Cox, A Hampson, eds. Amsterdam: Excerpta Medica,pp. 195–200.

Peiris JSM, Guan Y. Markwell D, Ghose P, Webster RG, Shortridge KF. 2001b. Cocirculation of avian H9N2 and contemporary "human" H3N2 influenza A viruses in pigs in southeastern China: Potential for genetic reassortment. J Virol 75:9679–9686.

Pensaert M, Ottis K, Vandeputte J, Kaplan MM, Bachmann PA. 1981. Evidence for the natural transmission of influenza A virus from wild ducks to swine and its potential importance for man. Bull World Health Org 59:75–78.

Potgeiter LND, Stair EL, Morton RJ, Whitenack DL. 1977. Isolation of swine influenza virus in Oklahoma. J Am Vet Med Assoc 171:758–760.

Rapp-Gabrielson VJ, Gergen LR, Eddy BA, Junker DE, Weston CQ, Fleck R, Erickson G, Nemechek EC, Wasmoen TL. 2003. Protection of a swine influenza virus vaccine against an H3N2 virus antigenically and genetically distinct from the vaccine virus. In Proceedings of the 4th International Symposium on Emerging and Re-emerging Pig Diseases, pp. 266–267.

Rapp-Gabrielson VJ, Gergen LR, Eddy BA, Wasmoen TL, Lechtenberg KF, Hanna M. 2000. Efficacy and safety of Maxivac-M+, a combination swine influenza vaccine, killed virus—Mycoplasma hyopneumoniae bacterin. Proc Am Assoc Swine Pract. pp. 201–205.

Rekik MR, Arora DJS, Dea S. 1994. Genetic variation in swine influenza virus A isolate associated with proliferative and necrotizing pneumonia in pigs. J Clin Microbiol 32:515–518.

Renshaw HW. 1975. Influence of antibody-mediated immune suppression on clinical, viral, and immune responses to swine influenza infection. Am J Vet Res 36:5–13.

Richt JA, Lager KM, Janke BH, Woods RD, Webster RG, Webby RJ. 2003. Pathogenic and antigenic properties of phylogenetically distinct reassortant H3N2 swine influenza viruses cocirculating in the United States. J Clin Microbiol 41:3198–3205.

Runge M, Ganter M, Delbeck F, Hartwick W, Ruffer A, Franz B, Amtsberg G. 1996. Demonstration of pneumonia in swine as a constant problem: Culture and immunofluorescence microscopic studies of bronchoalveolar lavage (BAL) and serological findings (in German). Berl Munch Tierarztl Wochenschr 109:101–107.

Ryan-Poirier KA, Katz JM, Webster RG, Kawaoka Y. 1992. Application of Directigen FLU A for the detection of influenza A virus in human and nonhuman specimens. J Clin Microbiol 30:1072–1075.

Saliki JT, Rodger SJ, Eskew G. 1998. Serosurvey of selected viral and bacterial diseases in wild swine from Oklahoma. J Wildlife Dis 34:834–838.

Schnurrenberger PR, Woods GT, Martein RJ. 1970. Serologic evidence of human infection with swine influenza virus. Am Rev Resp Dis 102:356–361.

Scholtissek C, Burger H, Bachmann PA, Hannoun C. 1983. Genetic relatedness of hemagglutinins of the H1 subtype of influenza A viruses isolated from swine and birds. Virology 129:521–523.

Scholtissek C, Burger H, Kistner O, Shortridge K. 1985. The nucleoprotein as a possible major factor in determining host specificity of influenza H3N2 viruses. Virology 147:287–294.

Scholtissek C, Hinshaw VS, Olsen CW. 1998. Influenza in pigs and their role as the intermediate host. In Textbook of Influenza. KG Nicholson, RG Webster, A Hay, eds. London: Blackwell Healthcare Communications, pp. 137–145.

Scholtissek C, Naylor E. 1988. Fish farming and influenza pandemics. Nature 331:215.

Schorr E, Wentworth D, Hinshaw VS. 1994. Use of polymerase chain reaction to detect swine influenza virus in nasal swab specimens. Am J Vet Res 55:952–956.

Schrader C, Suss J. 2003. Genetic characterization of a porcine H1N2 influenza virus strain isolated in Germany. Intervirology 46:66–70.

Schultz-Cherry S, Dybdahl-Sissoko N, McGregor M, Hinshaw VS. 1998. Mink lung epithelial cells: Unique cell line that supports influenza A and B virus replication. J Clin Microbiol 36:3718–3720.

Schultz-Cherry S, Hinshaw VS. 1996. Influenza virus neuraminidase activates latent transforming growth factor β. J Virol 70:8624–8629.

Sheerar MG, Easterday BC, Hinshaw VS. 1989. Antigenic conservation of H1N1 swine influenza viruses. J Gen Virol 70:3297–3303.

Shimada S, Ohtsuka T, Tanaka S, Mimura M, Shinohara M, Uchida K, Kimura K. 2003. Existence of reassortant A (H1N2) swine influenza viruses in Saitama Prefecture, Japan. In Conference Program and Abstracts of the Options for the Control of Influenza V Meeting, p. 124.

Shope RE. 1931. Swine influenza. Filtration experiments and etiology. J Exp Med 54:373–385.

——. 1941. The swine lungworm as a reservoir and intermediate host for swine influenza virus. 2. The transmission of swine influenza virus by the swine lungworm. J Exp Med 74:49–68.

Shu LL, Lin YP, Wright SM, Shortridge KF, Webster RG. 1994. Evidence for interspecies transmission and reassortment of influenza A viruses in pigs in Southern China. Virology 202:825–833.

Smith W, Andrewes CH, Laidlaw PP. 1933. A virus obtained from influenza patients. Lancet 2:66–68.

Suarez DL, Woolcock PR, Bermudez AJ, Senne DA. 2002. Isolation from turkey breeder hens of a reassortant H1N2 influenza virus with swine, human, and avian lineage genes. Avian Dis 46:111–121.

Sugimura T, Yonemochi H, Ogawa T, Tanaka Y, Kumagai T. 1980. Isolation of a recombinant influenza virus (Hsw1N2) from swine in Japan. Arch Virol 66:271–274.

Suzuki T, Horiike G, Yamazaki Y, Kawabe K, Masuda H, Miyamoto D, Matsuda M, Nishimura SI, Yamagata T, Ito T, Kida H, Kawaoka Y, Suzuki Y. 1997. Swine influenza virus strains recognize sialylsugar chains containing the molecular species of sialic acid predominantly present in the swine tracheal epithelium. FEBS Letters 404:192–196.

Swenson SL, Foley PL. 2004. Swine influenza. In Manual of Diagnostic Tests and Vaccines for Terrestrial Animals (5th edition), Part II. Office International des Epizooties, World Organisation for Animal Health, pp. 1111–1119.

Taubenberger JK, Reid AH, Janczewski TA, Fanning TG. 2001. Integrating historical, clinical and molecular genetic data in order to explain the origin and virulence of the 1918 Spanish influenza virus. Philos Trans R Soc Lond [Biol] 356:1829–1839.

Thacker B. 2000. Vaccination strategies for swine influenza virus. Proc AD Leman Swine Conf, pp. 21–25.

Top FH, Russell PK. 1977. Swine influenza at Fort Dix, N.J. IV. Summary and speculation. J Infect Dis 136:S376–S380.

Tsai C-P, Pan M-J. 2003. New H1N2 and H3N1 influenza viruses in Taiwanese pig herds. Vet Rec 153:408.

Van Reeth K, Brown I, Essen S, Pensaert M. 2004. Genetic relationships, serological cross-reaction and cross-protection between influenza A virus subtypes endemic in European pigs. Virus Res 103:115–124.

Van Reeth K, Brown IB, Pensaert M. 2000. Isolations of H1N2 influenza A virus from pigs in Belgium. Vet Rec 146:588–589.

Van Reeth K, De Clercq S, Pensaert M. 2001a. The significance of antigenic evolution for vaccine efficacy: Learning from vaccination-challenge studies in pigs. In Proceedings of the Symposium on Emergence and Control of Zoonotic Ortho- and Paramyxovirus Diseases. B Dodet, M Vicari, eds. Paris: John Libbey Eurotext, pp. 99–106.

Van Reeth K, Gregory V, Hay A, Pensaert M. 2003a. Protection against a European H1N2 swine influenza virus in pigs previously infected with H1N1 and/or H3N2 subtypes. Vaccine 21:1375–1381.

Van Reeth K, Labarque G, De Clercq S, Pensaert M. 2001b. Efficacy of vaccination of pigs with different H1N1 swine influenza viruses using a recent challenge strain and different parameters of protection. Vaccine 19:4479–4486.

Van Reeth K, Nauwynck H, Pensaert M. 1996. Dual infections of feeder pigs with porcine reproductive and respiratory syndrome virus followed by porcine respiratory coronavirus or swine influenza virus: a clinical and virological study. Vet Microbiol 48:325–335.

——. 1998. Bronchoalveolar interferon-α, tumor necrosis factor-α, interleukin-1 and inflammation during acute influenza in pigs: A possible model for humans? J Infect Dis 177:1076–1079.

——. 2001c. Clinical effects of experimental dual infections with porcine reproductive and respiratory syndrome virus followed by swine influenza virus in conventional and colostrum-deprived pigs. J Vet Med B 48:283–292.

Van Reeth K, Pensaert MB. 1994. Porcine respiratory coronavirus-mediated interference against influenza virus replication in the respiratory tract of feeder pigs. Am J Vet Res 55:1275–1281.

Van Reeth K, Van Gucht S, Pensaert M. 2002. Correlations between lung proinflammatory cytokine levels, virus replication and disease after swine influenza virus challenge of vaccination-immune pigs. Viral Immunol 15:583–594.

——. 2003b. Investigations of the efficacy of European H1N1- and H3N2-based swine influenza vaccines against the novel H1N2 subtype. Vet Rec 153:9–13.

Vandeputte J, Brun A, Duret C, Haesebrouck F, Devaux B. 1986. Vaccination of swine against H3N2 influenza using a Port Chalmers/1/73 vaccine. Proc Congr Int Pig Vet Soc. p. 219.

Webby RJ, Rossow KD, Goyal SM, Krauss SL, Webster RG. 2002. Proceedings of the American Society for Virology, p. 57.

Webby RJ, Swenson S, Krauss SL, Gerrish PJ, Goyal SM, Webster RG. 2000. Evolution of swine H3N2 influenza viruses in the United States. J Virol 74:8243–8251.

Webster RG, Bean WJ, Gorman OT, Chambers TM, Kawaoka Y. 1992. Evolution and ecology of influenza A viruses. Microbiol Rev 56:152–179.

Webster RG, Kawaoka Y. 1994. Influenza—An emerging and re-emerging disease. Semin Virol 5:103–111.

Webster RG, Yakhno M, Hinshaw VS, Bean WJ, Murti KG. 1978. Intestinal influenza: Replication and characterization of influenza viruses in ducks. Virology 84:268–278.

White DO, Fenner FJ. 1994. Orthomyxoviridae. In Medical Virology. DO White, FJ Fenner, eds. San Diego: Academic Press, pp. 489–499.

Wood GW, Banks J, Brown IH, Strong I, Alexander DJ. 1997. The nucleotide sequence of the HA1 of the haemagglutinin of an H1 avian influenza virus isolate from turkeys in Germany provides additional evidence suggesting recent transmission from pigs. Avian Pathol 26:347–355.

Woods GT, Hanson LE, Hatch RD. 1968. Investigation of four outbreaks of acute respiratory disease in swine and isolation of swine influenza virus. Health Lab Sci 5:218–224.

Woods GT, Mansfield ME. 1974. Transplacental migration of swine influenza virus in gilts exposed experimentally. Res Commun Chem Pathol Pharmacol 7:629–632.

Woods GT, Schurrenberger PR, Martin RJ, Tompkins WAF. 1981. Swine influenza virus in swine and man in Illinois. J Occupat Med 23:263–267.

Wright PF, Webster RG. 2001. Orthomyxoviruses. In Field's Virology (4th edition). DM Knipe, PM Howley, DE Griffin, RA Lamb, MA Martin, B Roizman, SE Straus. eds. Philadelphia: Lippincott-Raven Publishers, pp. 1533–1579.

Wright SM, Kawaoka Y, Sharp GB, Senne DA, Webster RG. 1992. Interspecies transmission and reassortment of influenza A viruses in pigs and turkeys in the United States. Am J Epidemiol 136:488–497.

Young GA, Underdahl NA. 1949. Swine influenza as a possible factor in suckling pig mortalities. I. Seasonal occurrence in adult swine as indicated by hemagglutinin inhibitors in serum. Cornell Vet 39:105–119.

Zhou NN, Senne DA, Landgraf JS, Swenson SL, Erickson G, Rossow K, Liu L, Yoon K-J, Krauss S, Webster RG. 1999. Genetic reassortment of avian, swine, and human influenza A viruses in American pigs. J Virol 73:8851–8856.

Ziegler T, Hall H, Sanchez-Fauquier A, Gamble WC, Cox NJ. 1995. Type and subtype-specific detection of influenza viruses in clinical specimens by rapid culture assay. J Clin Microbiol 33:318–321.

29 Swine Pox

Gustavo Delhon, E. R. Tulman, C. L. Afonso, and Dan L. Rock

Swinepox (SWP) is a mild, acute disease of swine characterized by typical poxviral lesions of the skin. SWP is distributed worldwide and is usually associated with poor sanitation. Morbidity may be high in individual herds where young pigs are most severely affected, but mortality is usually negligible. Clinical signs and epidemiology are usually sufficient for SWP diagnosis.

ETIOLOGY

SWP virus (SWPV) is the sole member of the genus *Suipoxvirus* in the family *Poxviridae* (Moyer 2000). The SWPV virion is morphologically similar to vaccinia virus, exhibiting a brick-like structure approximately 320 x 240 nm in horizontal section (Figure 29.1) (Blakemore and Abdussalam 1956; Cheville 1966a; Teppema and de Boer 1975). The virion is composed of a central biconcave core or nucleoid bordered by two ellipsoid lateral bodies and at least two lipid membranes (Blakemore and Abdussalam 1956; Cheville 1966a; Conroy et al. 1971; Kim and Luong 1975; Smid et al. 1973; Teppema and de Boer 1975). SWPV is ether-sensitive.

The SWPV genome is a double-stranded DNA molecule of 146 kilobase pairs predicted to contain 150 genes. It shares features common with other members of the *Poxviridae*, including a conserved central genomic region containing genes necessary for intracytoplasmic replication and virion structure (Afonso et al. 2002). Although genetically related to viruses of other poxviral genera (*capripoxvirus, leporipoxvirus, yatapoxvirus*), SWPV represents a distinct poxvirus genus and contains in terminal genomic regions a unique complement of genes predicted to affect virus/host interaction and aspects of SWPV virulence and host range (Afonso et al. 2002; Massung et al. 1993).

Despite reports of limited antigenic cross-reactivity, SWPV is antigenically distinct, as evidenced by the failure of SWPV antibodies to cross-protect, cross-neutralize, or efficiently immunoprecipitate viral proteins of other poxviruses (de Boer 1975; Massung and Moyer 1991; Meyer and Conroy 1972; Ouchi et al. 1992; Shope 1940).

Although some isolates have been reported to induce first-passage CPE on swine cells (Afonso et al. 2002; Paton et al. 1990), SWPV generally replicates poorly on initial isolation in swine cell cultures. It requires multiple passages before inducing cytopathic effect (CPE), but maintains pathogenicity for swine (Garg and Meyer 1972; Kasza and Griesemer 1962; Kasza et al. 1960; Meyer and Conroy 1972). CPE, characterized by cytoplasmic vacuoles and inclusion bodies, nuclear "vacuoles," and cell rounding and clumping (Borst et al. 1990; de Boer 1975; Kasza et al. 1960; Meyer and Conroy 1972), is seen 3–5 days postinoculation (PI), and isolated plaques remain relatively small in size (≤1.5 mm)(Kasza et al. 1960; Massung and Moyer 1991; Meyer and Conroy 1972). Infection of cell cultures results in expression of early and late SWPV mRNA by 4 and 8 hours PI, respectively, and viral protein synthesis by 4 hours PI (Massung and Moyer 1991).

Most attempts to grow or adapt SWPV for growth in non-swine cell cultures or on chicken chorioallantoic membranes have failed (Garg and Meyer 1972; Kasza et al. 1960; Meyer and Conroy 1972), indicating a host range restriction for replication at the cellular level. Recently, culture-adapted SWPV has been shown to replicate, albeit to lower titers, in non-swine cell lines (Barcena and Blasco 1998; Hahn et al. 2001).

Due to its restricted host range, SWPV has been proposed as a vaccine expression vector (Foley et al. 1991; Tripathy 1999). Genetically engineered SWPV vectors expressing pseudorabies virus (PRV) and classical swine fever virus antigens have been constructed and, in the case of PRV, shown to induce immune responses in pigs (Hahn et al. 2001; van der Leek et al. 1994). In addition, SWPV is able to express antigens in non-swine cells and may represent a safe, host range-restricted, vaccine vector for non-swine species (Barcena and Blasco 1998; Winslow et al. 2003). Availability of the complete

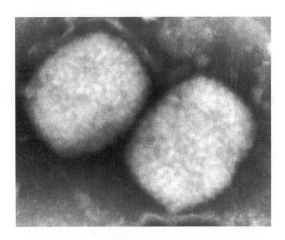

29.1. *Negative stain of swine pox virus particles with characteristic brick-shape and complex woven pattern of external filaments. (Courtesy of D. A. Gregg).*

genome sequence and identification of SWPV virulence and host range genes should enable engineering of live-attenuated, host-range–restricted, SWPV vaccine vectors with enhanced efficacy and greater versatility (Afonso et al. 2002).

EPIDEMIOLOGY

The pig is the only known host of SWPV. Unlike vaccinia virus, SWPV failed to experimentally infect or adapt to several mammalian and avian species (Schwarte and Beiester 1941; Shope 1940), with only a single report of nonproductive SWPV infection following intradermal inoculation of rabbits (Datt 1964). This restricted host range suggests that swine represent the reservoir of SWPV in nature.

SWP is present worldwide. Limited serological survey data from Europe indicated that 8–19% of swine serum samples contained anti-SWPV antibodies (de Boer 1975; Paton et al. 1990). Young swine are most often affected, as adult swine rarely present with clinical disease (McNutt et al. 1929; Kasza et al. 1960). Morbidity rates can be high (up to 100%), but mortality is generally negligible (less than 5%)(de Boer 1975). Overall, SWP is of little economic consequence.

Natural transmission of SWP is not well understood, but is often associated with poor sanitation. SWP has been associated with louse (*Haematopinus suis*) infestation. Lice are able to mechanically transmit SWPV and are thought to affect the extent and distribution of cutaneous lesions, which often occur in less keratinized abdominal and inguinal regions (Kasza et al. 1960; Manninger et al. 1940; Shope 1940). However, SWP without evidence of louse involvement has been described, suggesting a role for other insect vectors or the possibility of horizontal transmission (de Boer 1975; Jubb et al. 1992; Paton et al. 1990; Schwarte and Biester 1941). Vertical SWPV transmission is indicated by sporadic cases of

congenital infection resulting in stillborn fetuses with generalized lesions (Afonso et al. 2002; Borst et al. 1990; Paton et al. 1990).

CLINICAL SIGNS

SWPV causes eruptive dermatitis in pigs. Animals up to 3 months of age are the most susceptible, with adults usually developing a mild, self-limiting form of the disease. Multiple cutaneous lesions are commonly found on the flanks, belly, inner side of the legs, ears, and less frequently, on the face of affected animals (de Boer 1975; Jubb et al. 1992; Kim and Luong 1975; McNutt et al. 1929; Olufemi et al. 1981; Schwarte and Biester 1941). Lesions can also be found in the teats of sows and on the face, lips, and tongue of suckling pigs (Olufemi et al. 1981). In congenital infections, lesions are observed over the entire body and in the oral cavity (Borst et al. 1990; Paton et al. 1990). When virus transmission is associated with mechanical vectors, the distribution of lesions tends to reflect the vector's preferred feeding areas.

The incubation period is thought to be 4–14 days under field conditions (de Boer 1975; McNutt et al. 1929) and 3–5 days after intradermal or intravenous virus inoculation (Kasza and Griesemer 1962; Schwarte and Biester 1941), although longer periods have been described (Shope 1940).

Initial lesions are flat, pale, rounded areas 3–5 mm in diameter (maculae). Over the course of 2 days, these progress to papulae 1–2 mm in height, 1–2 cm in diameter, and occasionally confluent (Figure 29.2). The appearance of papulae may be accompanied by a slight and transient increase in body temperature and loss of appetite (Kasza and Griesemer 1962; Kasza et al. 1960). A true vesicle stage is absent or transient (Borst et al. 1990; Datt 1964; Kasza and Griesemer 1962; Meyer and

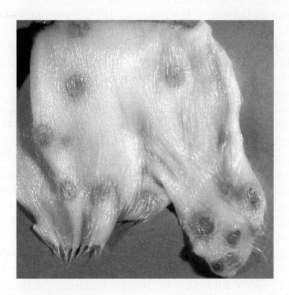

29.2. *Swine pox lesions on the skin of a naturally infected pig (Courtesy of B. Brodersen).*

Conroy 1972). The lesions usually become umbilicated and shrink about a week after appearing. They are replaced by crusts, which are eventually shed, leaving discolored spots (Kasza and Griesemer 1962). Complete recovery is observed 15–30 days post exposure, but it may be delayed if secondary bacterial infection occurs (de Boer 1975; McNutt et al. 1929; Miller and Olson 1980; Schwarte and Biester 1941).

PATHOGENESIS

SWPV may enter the host through preexisting skin abrasions and preferentially replicates in epidermal keratinocytes of the stratum spinosum (Meyer and Conroy 1972). Although mature viral particles have been observed in epidermal basal cells (Teppema and de Boer 1975) and viral antigen has been detected in dermal macrophages (Cheville 1966b), there is no indication that these cell types support virus replication. With the exception of moderate changes in superficial lymph nodes, tissues other than the skin are rarely affected. Infectious virus can be readily isolated from the skin of infected animals as early as 3 days postintradermal inoculation (Kasza and Griesemer 1962), and from regional lymph nodes only if skin lesions are severe (Kasza and Griesemer 1962). A viremic stage has been suggested to account for virus spread from the primary to secondary sites of replication in the skin and for congenital infection; however, virus has not been isolated from blood of infected animals (Borst et al. 1990; Kasza and Griesemer 1962; Paton et al. 1990; Shope 1940).

Functional studies on SWPV pathogenesis are lacking. The complement of virus genes with putative roles in virulence and host range suggests that modulation of host immune responses and inhibition of apoptosis may play a role in the course of the disease (Afonso et al. 2002; Kawagishi-Kobayashi et al. 2000; Massung et al. 1993). SWPV contains genes with sequence similarity to cellular and viral genes encoding CD47 and proteins that bind interferon (IFN) alpha/beta, IFN-gamma, tumor necrosis factor alpha, interleukin-18 (IL-18), and CC chemokines. Products of these genes potentially modulate host immune responses, including NK and T cell responses, and may facilitate SWPV replication and dissemination. SWPV encodes proteins similar to inhibitors of host MHC-I, serine proteases, IL-1/Toll-like receptors, and protein kinase PKR, some of which in other poxviruses are known to interfere with or delay inflammatory responses at the site of virus replication.

Convalescent swine are resistant to SWPV challenge, indicating that infection induces protective immunity (de Boer 1975; Garg and Meyer 1972; Kasza et al. 1960; Schwarte and Biester 1941; Shope 1940). However, the immune mechanisms associated with protection are not known. SWPV neutralizing activity is present in swine sera as early as 7 days PI; however, low neutralizing titers, delayed kinetics of antibody response, and lack of neutralizing antibodies at 50 days PI have been reported (Kasza et al. 1960; Meyer and Conroy 1972; Shope 1940; Williams et al. 1989). Suckling pigs may also be protected by maternal antibody (Manninger et al. 1940), although high neonatal mortality rates have been observed (Olufemi et al. 1981). Decreased mitogen and SWPV-induced proliferative responses have been observed in peripheral blood mononuclear cells from experimentally infected swine (Williams et al. 1989).

LESIONS

The most conspicuous histologic change caused by SWPV infection is hydropic degeneration of stratum spinosum keratinocytes (Figure 29.3A, B) (Borst et al. 1990; Cheville 1966a; Kasza and Griesemer 1962; McNutt et al. 1929; Meyer and Conroy 1972; Olufemi et al. 1981; Paton et al. 1990; Schwarte and Biester 1941; Teppema and de Boer 1975). Hyperplasia of epidermal cells is not as marked as in poxviral infections of other mammals, an observation that might be related to the lack of a SWPV-encoded homologue of the poxviral epidermal growth factor-like gene (Afonso et al. 2002; McNutt et al. 1929; Schwarte and Biester 1941). The cytoplasm of affected cells is brightened and enlarged,

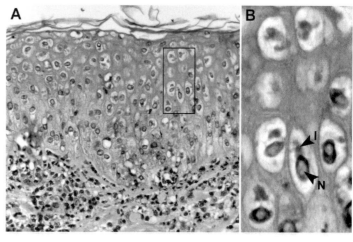

29.3. Histopathological changes caused by SWPV. A. Skin section showing hydropic degeneration in the stratum spinosum of the epidermis and inflammatory cells in the dermis. B. Magnification of the boxed area in A showing ballooned keratinocytes containing cytoplasmic inclusion bodies (I) and central nuclear clearing (N). Hematoxylin and eosin. (Courtesy of D. A. Gregg).

contains eosinophilic inclusion bodies resembling poxviral type B inclusion bodies (Teppema and de Boer 1975) (Figure 29.3B), and reacts strongly with antibodies against viral antigens (Cheville 1966b). Hydropic degeneration and inclusion bodies are also observed in the outer root sheaths of the hair follicles (Kasza and Griesemer 1962; Meyer and Conroy 1972). The nucleus of affected cells exhibits margination of chromatin and a large, central "vacuole" resembling the nuclear clearing observed in sheeppox virus-infected keratinocytes (Figure 29.3B) (Cheville 1966a; Kasza and Griesemer 1962; McNutt et al. 1929; Meyer and Conroy 1972; Plowright and Ferris 1958; Teppema and de Boer 1975). No significant fluid accumulation is observed between keratinocytes. Apical keratinocytes undergo necrosis at later stages of infection. Leukocyte infiltration is observed in the underlying dermis and, to a lesser degree, the affected epidermis (Figure 29.3A), with few viral antigen-containing dermal macrophages (Cheville 1966b). When involved, the inguinal lymph nodes present edema, hyperemia, hyperplasia, and few virus antigen-containing cells (Cheville 1966a; Kasza and Griesemer 1962).

Ultrastructurally, infected cells exhibit a marked decrease in keratin precursors (tonofilaments) and loss of intercellular interdigitations characteristic of the stratum spinosum (Cheville 1966a; Teppema and de Boer 1975). Individual inclusion bodies consist of electrodense central cores surrounded by lamellar bodies and maturing viral particles (viroplasm) (Cheville 1966a; Conroy and Meyer 1971; Kim and Luong 1975; Smid et al 1973; Teppema and de Boer 1975). The large, well-defined nuclear "vacuole" can be more accurately described as a region of low electron density that lacks a surrounding membrane and contains cross-striated fibrils similar to those observed in the cytoplasm.

DIAGNOSIS

Presumptive SWP diagnosis is based on the observation of pox lesions on the skin of affected animals. Differential diagnosis includes vesicular diseases, allergic skin reactions, sunburn, bacterial dermatitis, ringworm, and skin parasitosis (*Tyroglyphus* spp, sarcoptic mange) (Blood and Radostits 1989; Yager and Scott 1985). SWPV involvement can be confirmed by electron microscopy and histopathology and includes pathognomonic epidermal changes: ballooned stratum spinosum keratinocytes containing cytoplasmic eosinophilic inclusion bodies and a "vacuolated" nucleus. SWPV involvement may be definitively confirmed using SWPV-specific antibodies to neutralize virus isolated on swine cell cultures (primary swine kidney cells, PK-15 cell line) (Borst et al. 1990; Meyer and Conroy 1972; Paton et al. 1990) or by performing immunocytochemistry on tissue samples or infected cell cultures (Garg and Meyer 1973; Mohanty et al. 1989; Paton et al. 1990).

Papular/pustular exudate or crusted material are clinical samples of choice for virus isolation. At least seven blind passages should be attempted before considering the sample negative (de Boer 1975).

Serum neutralization and precipitating antibody tests to detect SWPV-specific antibodies in convalescent serum have been described (de Boer 1975; Shope 1940). Since swine do not reliably develop high levels of neutralizing antibodies (Kasza et al. 1960; Shope 1940), negative test results should be interpreted with caution.

The recent availability of the SWPV genome sequence and the identification of unique SWPV gene sequences will permit the development of rapid, sensitive, and specific polymerase chain reaction–based detection and diagnostic assays (Afonso et al. 2002).

Although differential diagnosis of SWP from a vaccinia virus infection in pigs was important when human smallpox vaccination was practiced, this no longer represents a diagnostic concern (Shope 1940).

PREVENTION AND CONTROL

No specific treatment for SWPV exists. Antibiotic regimens are recommended for treatment of secondary bacterial infection. Given that SWP is of relatively low economic impact, no vaccine has been developed. Good animal husbandry, including ectoparasite control, should be practiced.

REFERENCES

Afonso CL, Tulman ER, Lu Z, Zsak L, Osorio FA, Balinsky C, Kutish GF, Rock DL. 2002. The genome of swinepox virus. J Virol 76:783–790.

Barcena J, Blasco R. 1998. Recombinant swinepox virus expressing beta-galactosidase: Investigation of viral host range and gene expression levels in cell culture. Virology 243:396–405.

Blakemore F, Abdussalam M. 1956. Morphology of the elementary bodies and cell inclusions in swine pox. J Comp Pathol 66:373–377.

Blood DC, Radostits OM. 1989. Veterinary Medicine: A Textbook of the Diseases of Cattle, Sheep, Pigs, Goats and Horses (7th edition). Bailliere Tindall, London. pp. 571–958.

Borst GH, Kimman TG, Gielkens AL, van der Kamp JS. 1990. Four sporadic cases of congenital swinepox. Vet Rec 127:61–63.

Cheville NF. 1966a. The cytopathology of swine pox in the skin of swine. Am J Pathol 49:339–352.

——. 1966b. Immunofluorescent and morphologic studies on swinepox. Pathol Vet 3:556–564.

Conroy JD, Meyer RC. 1971. Electron microscopy of swinepox virus in germfree pigs and in cell culture. Am J Vet Res 32: 2021–2032.

Datt NS. 1964. Comparative studies of pigpox and vaccinia viruses. I. Host range pathogenicity. J Comp Pathol 74:62–69.

de Boer GF. 1975. Swinepox, virus isolation, experimental infections and the differentiation from vaccinia virus infections. Arch Virol 49:141–150.

Foley PL, Paul PS, Levings RL, Hanson SK, Middle LA. 1991. Swinepox virus as a vector for the delivery of immunogens. Ann N Y Acad Sci 646:220–222.

Garg SK, Meyer RC. 1972. Adaptation of swinepox virus to an established cell line. Appl Microbiol 23:180–182.

———. 1973. Studies on swinepox virus: Fluorescence and light microscopy of infected cell cultures. Res Vet Sci 14:216–219.

Hahn J, Park S-H, Song J-Y, An S-H, Ahn B-Y. 2001. Construction of recombinant swinepox viruses and expression of the classical swine fever virus E2 protein. J Virol Methods 93:49–56.

Jubb TF, Ellis TM, Peet RL, Parkinson J. 1992. Swinepox in pigs in northern Western Australia. Aust Vet J 69:99.

Kasza L, Bohl EH, Jones DO. 1960. Isolation and cultivation of swine pox virus in primary cell cultures of swine origin. Am J Vet Res 21:269–273.

Kasza L, Griesemer RA. 1962. Experimental swine pox. Am J Vet Res 23:443–450.

Kawagishi-Kobayashi M, Cao C, Lu J, Ozato K, Dever TE. 2000. Pseudosubstrate inhibition of protein kinase PKR by swine pox virus C8L gene product. Virology 276:424–434.

Kim JCS, Luong LC. 1975. Ultrastructure of swine pox. Vet Med Small Anim Clin 70:1043–1045.

Manninger R, Csontos J, Salyi J. 1940. Uber die atiologie des pockenartigen ausschlages der ferkel. Archiv fur Tierheilkunde 75:159–179.

Massung RF, Jayarama V, Moyer RW. 1993. DNA sequence analysis of conserved and unique regions of swinepox virus: Identification of genetic elements supporting phenotypic observations including a novel G protein-coupled receptor homologue. Virology 197:511–528.

Massung RF, Moyer RW. 1991. The molecular biology of swinepox virus. II. The infectious cycle. Virology 180:355–364.

McNutt SH, Murray C, Purwin P. 1929. Swine pox. Am Vet Med Assoc 74:752–761.

Meyer RC, Conroy JD. 1972. Experimental swinepox in gnotobiotic piglets. Res Vet Sci 13:334–338.

Miller RC, Olson LD. 1980. Experimental induction of cutaneous streptococcal abscesses in swine as a sequela to swinepox. Am J Vet Res 41:341–347.

Mohanty PK, Verma PC, Rat A. 1989. Detection of swine pox and buffalo pox viruses in cell culture using a protein A-horseradish peroxidase conjugate. Acta Virol 33:290–296.

Moyer RW, Arif B, Black DN, Boyle DB, Buller RM, Dumbell KR, Esposito JJ, McFadden G, Moss B, Mercer AA, Ropp S, Tripathy DN, Upton C. 2000. Family Poxviridae. In Virus Taxonomy: Classification and Nomenclature of Viruses: Seventh Report of the International Committee on Taxonomy of Viruses. MHV van Regenmortel, CM Fauquet, DHL Bishop, EB Carstens, MH Estes, SM Lemon, J Maniloff, MA Mayo, DJ McGeoch, CR Pringle, RB Wickner, eds. San Diego: Academic Press, pp. 137–157.

Olufemi BE, Ayoade GO, Ikede BO, Akpavie SO, Nwufoh KJ. 1981. Swine pox in Nigeria. Vet Rec 109:278–280.

Ouchi M, Fujiwara M, Hatano Y, Yamada M, Nii S. 1992. Analysis of swinepox virus antigens using monoclonal antibodies. J Vet Med Sci 54:731–737.

Paton DJ, Brown IH, Fitton J, Wrathall AE. 1990. Congenital pig pox: A case report. Vet Rec 127:204.

Plowright W, Ferris RD. 1958. The growth and cytopathogenicity of sheep-pox virus in tissue cultures. Br J Exp Pathol 39:424–435.

Schwarte LH, Biester HE. 1941. Pox in swine. Am J Vet Res 2:136–140.

Shope RE. 1940. Swine pox. Archive fur die Gesamte Virusforschung 1:457–467.

Smid B, Valicek L, Mensik J. 1973. Replication of swinepox virus in the skin of naturally infected pigs. Electron microscopic study. Zentralbl Veterinarmed B 20:603–612.

Teppema JS, De Boer GF. 1975. Ultrastructural aspects of experimental swinepox with special reference to inclusion bodies. Arch Virol 49:151–163.

Tripathy DN. 1999. Swinepox virus as a vaccine vector for swine pathogens. Adv Vet Med 41:463–480.

van der Leek ML, Feller JA, Sorensen G, Isaacson W, Adams CL, Borde DJ, Pfeiffer N, Tran T, Moyer RW, Gibbs EPJ. 1994. Evaluation of swinepox virus as a vaccine vector in pigs using an Aujeszky's disease (pseudorabies) virus gene insert coding for glycoproteins gp50 and gp63. Vet Rec 134:13–18.

Williams PP, Hall MR, McFarland MD. 1989. Immunological responses of cross-bred and in-bred miniature pigs to swine poxvirus. Vet Immunol Immunopathol 23:149–159.

Winslow BJ, Cochran MD, Holzenburg A, Sun J, Junker DE, Collisson EW. 2003. Replication and expression of a swinepox virus vector delivering feline leukemia virus gag and env to cell lines of swine and feline origin. Virus Res 98:1–15.

Yager JA, Scott DW. 1985. The skin and appendages. In KVF Jubb, PC Kennedy, N Palmer, eds. Pathology of Domestic Animals (3rd edition), Volume 1. Orlando: Academic Press, pp. 407–549.

30 Transmissible Gastroenteritis and Porcine Respiratory Coronavirus

Linda J. Saif and Karol Sestak

Transmissible Gastroenteritis

Transmissible gastroenteritis (TGE) is a highly contagious, enteric viral disease of swine characterized by vomiting, severe diarrhea, and a high mortality (often 100%) in TGEV seronegative piglets under 2 weeks of age. Since the 1980s, the appearance and widespread prevalence of a naturally occurring respiratory deletion mutant of TGE virus (TGEV), the porcine respiratory coronavirus (PRCV), has altered the clinical impact of TGE. Although swine of all ages are susceptible to TGEV or PRCV infection, the mortality in TGEV and/or PRCV seropositive herds and in swine over 5 weeks of age generally is low.

TGE was first reported by Doyle and Hutchings (1946) as occurring in the U.S. in 1945, although it undoubtedly had existed earlier. Since then, it has been reported in most countries worldwide, albeit with its clinical impact altered by the prevalence of PRCV. The disease is most easily diagnosed and causes the highest losses when it occurs in TGEV or PRCV seronegative herds at farrowing. In contrast, it often goes undiagnosed when it occurs in growing, finishing, or adult swine because of the mild clinical signs, which usually consist only of inappetence and mild diarrhea.

Because of these undiagnosed infections, serologic surveys were once a more accurate indication of the prevalence of TGEV. However, since the 1980s the prevalence of cross-reactive PRCV antibodies has confounded the serodiagnosis of TGEV based on conventional assays (Laude et al. 1993; Pensaert and Cox 1989). Surveys through the early 1990s indicated that 19–54% of sampled swine herds in North America were seropositive for TGEV antibodies (Egan 1982; USDA APHIS VS 1992). In 1995, 16 of 22 swine herds examined in Iowa were seropositive for TGEV (Wesley et al. 1997). Recent data indicates a decline in the number of TGEV outbreaks diagnosed in the U.S. compared to historical data, pre-sumably due to the spread of PRCV (Yaeger et al. 2002). Currently in many European countries, nearly 100% of swine herds are seropositive for TGEV antibodies. This situation is due to PRCV that appeared in 1984 and rapidly spread in Europe (Brown and Cartwright 1986; Laude et al. 1993; Pensaert 1989; Pensaert and Cox 1989; Pensaert et al. 1986, 1993). Economic losses from TGE can be severe (Mousing et al. 1988; Pritchard 1987); however, with the establishment of endemic PRCV, the economic impact of TGE has decreased (Laude et al. 1993; Pensaert and Cox 1989).

In TGEV/PRCV seronegative herds in North America, TGE remains a cause of sickness and death in piglets. Diagnosis of TGE in PRCV-endemic herds has become problematic because the milder disease in all age groups masks the presence of TGEV infections (Kim et al. 2000b). This poses concerns for maintenance or export of TGEV negative breeding stock.

ETIOLOGY

TGEV is a species in the genus *Coronavirus* of the family *Coronaviridae* (Lai and Cavanagh 1997). TGEV is enveloped and pleomorphic, with an overall diameter of 60–160 nm, as viewed by negative-staining electron microscopy (EM) (Figure 30.1) (Granzow et al. 1981; Okaniwa et al. 1968; Phillip et al. 1971). It has a single layer of club-shaped surface projections or spikes 12–25 nm in length.

TGEV antigen can be demonstrated in the cytoplasm by immunofluorescence (IF) as early as 4–5 hours post infection (Pensaert et al. 1970a). Maturation of virus occurs in the cytoplasm by budding through endoplasmic reticulum, and viral particles (65–90 nm in diameter) are often observed within cytoplasmic vacuoles (Figure 30.2A) (Pensaert et al. 1970a; Thake 1968; Wagner et al.

489

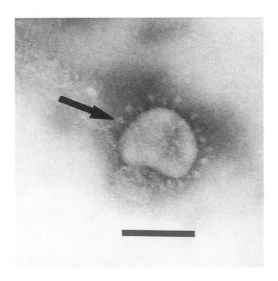

30.1. *Electron micrograph of a TGEV particle showing typical coronavirus morphology. Arrow points to the virus peplomers, or spikes. Bar = 100 nm.*

1973). The virus is frequently seen lining the host cell membranes after exit from infected cells (Figure 30.2B). TGEV glycoproteins have been identified on the surface of infected swine testicular (ST) cells (Laviada et al. 1990).

Biological Properties

TGEV is very stable when stored frozen, but somewhat labile at room temperature or above. No detectable drop in titer occurred when virus of pig intestine origin was stored at −20°C for 6–18 months (Haelterman and Hutchings 1956; Young et al. 1955). In contrast, intestinal virus, when allowed to dry and putrefy at 21°C, was rather labile; after 3 days only two of four inoculated pigs became sick; and after 10 days no viable virus was detected by pig inoculation (Bay et al. 1952). When held at 37°C, there was a log 10 reduction in infectivity titer every 24 hours (Young et al. 1955). Storage of cell culture virus at −20°C, −40°C, or −80°C for 365 days did not result in any significant drop in titer, whereas storage at 37°C for 4 days resulted in total loss of infectivity (Harada et al. 1968). Infectious virus persisted in a liquid manure slurry for more than 8 weeks at 5°C, 2 weeks at 20°C, and 24 hours at 35°C (Haas et al. 1995).

The virus is highly photosensitive. Haelterman (1963) reported that fecal material containing 10^5 pig-infectious doses (PID) was inactivated within 6 hours when exposed to sunlight. Cartwright et al. (1965) reported the photosensitivity of a cytopathic strain when it was exposed to ultraviolet light on a laboratory bench.

In terms of chemical stability, TGEV is inactivated by exposure to 0.03% formalin, 1% Lysovet (phenol and aldehyde), 0.01% beta propiolactone, 1 mM binary ethylenamine, sodium hypochlorite, NaOH, iodines, quaternary ammonium compounds, ether, and chloroform (Brown 1981; Harada et al. 1968; Nakao et al. 1978; VanCott et al. 1993).

As reported for other enteric viruses, TGEV field strains are trypsin resistant, relatively stable in pig bile, and stable at pH 3 (Laude et al. 1981). These properties allow the virus to survive in the stomach and small in-

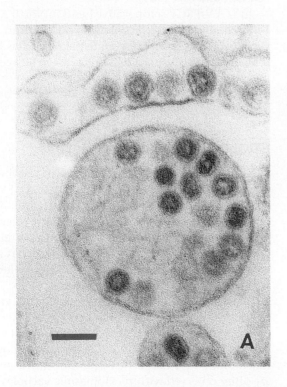

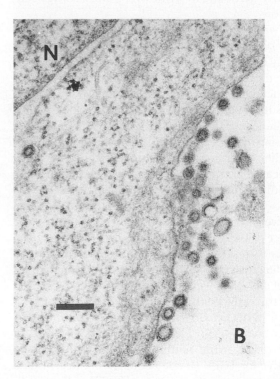

30.2. *(A) TGEV in vesicles of the endoplasmic reticulum of a pig kidney cell (36 hours post infection). Bar = 100 nm. (B) TGEV lining the cell membrane of a pig kidney cell (36 hours post infection). N = nucleus; bar = 200 nm.*

testine. However, attenuated strains, as well as field strains of TGEV vary in these properties, and most studies have failed to show a correlation between susceptibility to these various treatments and cell culture passage level or degree of virulence (Furuuchi et al. 1975; Laude et al. 1981).

Molecular Properties

TGEV and the deletion mutant, PRCV, are enveloped viruses containing one large, polyadenylated, single-stranded, genomic RNA of positive-sense polarity. The genome organization, replication strategy, and expression of viral proteins are similar to those of other coronaviruses (Enjuanes and Van der Zeist 1995; Laude et al. 1993). The genomic RNA of TGEV is infectious (Brian et al. 1980), and the complete sequence of the Purdue-115 strain of TGEV is 28,579 nucleotides long (Eleouet et al. 1995; Kapke and Brian 1986).

TGEV has a buoyant density in sucrose of 1.18–1.20 g/mL (Brian et al. 1980; Jimenez et al. 1986). The phospholipids and glycolipids incorporated into the virus envelope are derived from the host cell, and thus, the envelope composition is host cell dependent (Enjuanes and Van der Zeist 1995; Pike and Garwes 1977).

Intact TGEV contains four structural proteins: a large surface glycoprotein (spike or S); a small membrane protein (E or sM); an integral membrane glycoprotein (M); and a nucleocapsid protein (N) (Garwes and Pocock 1975; Godet et al. 1992).

The N protein (47 kDa) interacts with viral RNA to form a helical ribonucleoprotein complex. This structure, in association with M protein, forms an internal icosahedral core (Risco et al. 1996). The 29–36 kDa M glycoprotein, embedded in the viral envelope by three or four membrane-spanning regions, is present in two topological forms (Risco et al. 1995). In one conformation, the N terminus of the M protein is external to the virus envelope and the C terminus is internal, whereas, in the second conformation, both ends of the molecule are on the outside of the virion. In both conformations, the hydrophilic N terminus with a single accessible glycosylation site is responsible for interferon induction (Charley and Laude et al. 1988). Epitopes on protruding N-terminal and C-terminal ends of M protein molecules bind complement-dependent neutralizing monoclonal antibodies (MAbs) (Laude et al. 1992; Risco et al. 1995; Woods 1988). S glycoproteins, probably as trimer complexes (Delmas and Laude 1990), are visible in electron micrographs as the virus "corona" (Figure 30.1). Functions attributed to the S glycoprotein (170–220 kDa) include virus neutralization (complement-independent), virus-cell attachment, membrane fusion, as well as hemagglutination. Purified S glycoprotein elicited the production of TGEV-neutralizing antibodies, which neutralize at multiple steps in the virus replication cycle (Nguyen et al. 1986; Sune et al. 1990).

Aminopeptidase N and a second 200 kDa surface protein on ST cells and on porcine intestinal enterocytes have been identified as virus receptors (Delmas et al. 1992; Weingartl and Derbyshire 1994). The receptor binding site for aminopeptidase N and the major neutralizing site (site A) on the S protein are located within the same domain (Godet et al. 1994). Moreover, TGEV binds to sialic acid residues on glycoproteins of target cells. This binding was proposed to initiate infection of intestinal enterocytes (Schwegmann-Wessels et al. 2002). Treatment of TGEV with sialidase enhanced hemagglutinating activity (Noda et al. 1987; Schultze et al. 1996). This hemagglutinating activity is located at the N-terminal region of the TGEV S protein, a region that is missing from the PRCV S protein; thus, determining the presence or absence of hemagglutinating activity (Schultze et al. 1996) could be a method to differentiate PRCV and TGEV strains.

Monoclonal antibodies (MAbs) have been produced against attenuated (Correa et al. 1990; Delmas and Laude 1990; Jimenez et al. 1986) and virulent (Simkins et al. 1992, 1993; Welch and Saif 1988; Zhu et al. 1990) strains of TGEV and used to characterize TGEV proteins and map epitopes that elicit antibodies. The major neutralization determinants on the S protein were highly conserved for TGEV and PRCV strains (Garwes et al. 1987; Jimenez et al. 1986; Sanchez et al. 1990; Simkins et al. 1993; Welch et al. 1988). Use of neutralizing MAbs to map epitopes on the S glycoprotein revealed four distinct antigenic sites (A, B, C, D), with site A-B as the highly conserved immunodominant epitope recognized by strongly neutralizing MAbs (Correa et al. 1990; Delmas and Laude 1990; Garwes et al. 1987; Gebauer et al. 1991; Simkins et al. 1992, 1993), although other sites (D, C) also can induce neutralizing antibodies (Laude et al. 1986; Posthumus et al. 1990). The locations of each of the four major antigenic sites were mapped on the primary structure of the S glycoprotein. Starting from the amino terminal end, these sites were designated C, B, D, and A by the Madrid group (Correa et al. 1990) and D, C, and A-B by the Paris group (Delmas and Laude 1990). Paris sites D, C, and A-B (the designation used in this chapter unless specified otherwise) overlap Madrid sites B, D, and A, respectively. Three subsites (Aa, Ab, Ac) for site A were recognized using TGEV-MAb-resistant mutants (Correa et al. 1990).

Antigenic and Genomic Relationships

Only one serotype of TGEV is known (Kemeny 1976). PRCV strains are not distinguished from enteropathogenic strains of TGEV by the virus neutralization (VN) test (Pensaert 1989; Pensaert and Cox 1989), but can be distinguished by a blocking enzyme-linked immunosorbent assay (ELISA) test (see section on diagnosis) or by a large deletion in the S gene of PRCV resulting in a smaller S protein (170–190 kDa) than the S protein of TGEV (220 kDa).

Seven coronaviruses are related antigenically or by

their genomic sequence (Enjuanes and Van der Zeist 1995). These are TGEV, PRCV, canine coronavirus (CCV), feline infectious peritonitis virus (FIPV), feline enteric coronavirus (FECV), porcine epidemic diarrhea virus (PEDV), and human coronavirus (HCV 229E). Within these group I coronavirus, only TGEV, PRCV, CCV, FIPV, and FECV form an antigenically related subset, based on cross-reactivity in VN and IF tests and with MAbs to the S, N, or M protein (Enjuanes and Van der Zeist 1995; Woods 1982). Moreover, all members of this antigenic subset share the antigenic subsite Ac on the S protein (Enjuanes and Van der Zeist 1995). Additional cross-reactivity between the S, M, and N proteins of TGEV, CCV, and FIPV was shown by radioimmunoprecipitation, immunoblotting, and ELISA, and it was suggested that these viruses may actually represent host range mutants of an ancestral virus strain (Horzinek et al. 1982). Similar cross-reactivity among the S, M, and N structural proteins of TGEV and PRCV was observed using polyclonal antisera in immunoblotting assays (Callebaut et al. 1988).

PEDV is another coronavirus of pigs that causes a disease similar to TGEV; this disease has been documented only in swine in Europe and Asia (DeBouck 1982). Antibodies to PEDV have not been detected in a limited survey of adult swine sera from the U.S. (L. J. Saif and M. B. Pensaert, unpublished data, 1990). Some one-way, immunoblotting cross-reactivity with the N protein has been reported for PEDV, FIPV, CCV, TGEV, and a putative mink coronavirus (Have et al. 1992; Zhou et al. 1988). However, no antigenic cross-reactivity between PEDV and TGEV-related coronaviruses has been detected using polyclonal antisera or MAbs in other serologic assays (Callebaut et al. 1988; Enjuanes and Van der Zeist 1995; Pensaert and Debouck 1978). Another coronavirus of pigs, hemagglutinating encephalomyelitis virus, is antigenically and genetically unrelated to the coronaviruses in group I and is a member of coronavirus group II (Enjuanes and Van der Zeist 1995).

Although TGEV, CCV, and FIPV are antigenically closely related, Reynolds et al. (1980) suggested that TGEV and CCV could be distinguished serologically (with sera from naturally infected animals) by employing two-way cross-neutralization tests. Additional in vitro biological differences also have been detected. Whereas both TGEV and CCV will grow in either canine kidney cells (Welter 1965) or an established feline cell line (Woods 1982), neither CCV nor FIPV will grow in ST or porcine thyroid cells, both of which support the growth of TGEV isolates (Reynolds et al. 1980).

In vivo biological differences also exist among TGEV, CCV, and FIPV in their pathogenicity for neonatal pigs (Woods and Pedersen 1979). Whereas virulent FIPV caused diarrhea and intestinal lesions similar to those of virulent TGEV, CCV caused no clinical signs and only slight villous atrophy. IF, using a porcine anti-TGEV serum conjugate, occurred in villous enterocytes of

TGEV- and FIPV-infected pigs but predominated in crypt enterocytes of CCV-infected pigs. CCV shed by acutely infected dogs was shown to infect baby pigs and induced serum neutralizing antibodies for both CCV and TGEV (Woods and Wesley 1992). However, baby pigs and pregnant gilts experimentally infected with FIPV did not produce TGEV-neutralizing antibodies, but did develop some immunity to a TGEV challenge (Woods and Pedersen 1979).

Molecular probes and MAbs are also used to detect and differentiate among these antigenically related coronaviruses. In terms of the S glycoprotein gene that confers host range specificity, the 300 amino acid residues at the N terminus are the most variable. In this domain CCV and FIPV are more similar to each other than to TGEV (Jacobs 1987; Wesseling et al. 1994). Thus, cDNA probes developed from this domain of the TGEV S gene reacted with TGEV RNA but failed to recognize CCV or FIPV RNA under conditions of high stringency. Either cDNA probes or RT-PCR (reverse transcriptase polymerase chain reaction) techniques are used to differentiate U.S. strains of PRCV from prototype strains of TGEV (Bae et al. 1991; Jackwood et al. 1995; Kim et al. 2000a; Vaughn et al. 1994). Similar differentiation of the TGEV-related coronaviruses was possible using certain specific MAbs to the S glycoprotein of TGEV that recognized TGEV strains but failed to react with PRCV, FIPV, or CCV (Callebaut et al. 1988; Laude et al. 1988; Sanchez et al. 1990; Simkins et al. 1992, 1993).

PRCV strains, isolated during the mid-1980s through 2000s, have been characterized and partially sequenced (Britton et al. 1991; Costantini et al. 2004; Kim et al. 2000b; Rasschaert et al. 1990; Vaughn et al. 1995; Wesley et al. 1991b). An overall nucleotide and amino acid sequence homology of 96% between TGEV and PRCV suggests that PRCV evolved from TGEV and that this occurred on a number of independent occasions. Two striking features characterize the PRCV genome: (1) a large deletion (621–681 nucleotides) at a consistent site near the N terminus of the S gene that gives rise to a smaller S protein; and (2) a variable region with deletions that often eliminate the open reading frame (ORF) immediately downstream of the S gene. These genetic changes may account for the altered tissue tropism of PRCV (Ballesteros et al. 1997; Sanchez et al. 1999).

From sequence data, significant homologies occur in the three genes encoding the three main structural proteins within TGEV-related viruses (TGEV, PRCV, CCV, FECV, FIPV) and between TGEV-related viruses and HCV 229E and PEDV (Enjuanes and Van der Zeist 1995). Thus, sequencing data show a genomic relationship between these latter two viruses and TGEV-related viruses that is not demonstrated by serologic analysis (Enjuanes and Van der Zeist 1995).

An altered phenotype was reported for a small plaque (SP) variant of TGEV (Woods 1978; Woods et al. 1981). Although the S gene of the SP variant and the S gene of wild-type TGEV are similar, a large deletion (462 nucleotides) is present in the SP viral genome just downstream from the S gene (Wesley et al. 1990a). This deletion eliminated the ORF of one potential viral encoded protein and eliminated the N-terminal portion of a second potential viral protein. These two ORFs are also missing from the high cell culture–passaged Nouzilly strain, a second attenuated TGEV with an SP phenotype (Britton et al. 1994). Presumably, the altered pathogenicity of SP virus, the Nouzilly virus, and the PRCVs results from these genetic deletions.

The recently emerged severe acute respiratory syndrome (SARS) is a human pneumoenteric disease caused by a novel coronavirus tentatively assigned to coronavirus group IV. Although SARS is believed to be zoonotic, its genetic relationship to TGEV is relatively distant and its exact animal reservoir remains unknown (Drosten et al. 2003; Ksiazek et al. 2003; Marra et al. 2003; Peiris et al. 2003; Rota et al. 2003). However several investigations have reported that SARS coronavirus cross-reacts with antibodies to group I coronaviruses including TGEV and PRCV, mainly through the N-protein (Nagesha et al. 2004; Ksiazek et al. 2003; Sun and Meng 2004). Attempts to transmit SARS coronavirus to 6-week-old pigs (PRCV seropositive) failed, although pigs seroconverted to SARS and shed virus detected by RT-PCR (Weingartl et al. 2004). It is unknown whether the preexisting PRCV antibodies affected susceptibility of the pigs to SARS.

EPIDEMIOLOGY

On a herd basis, two epidemiologic forms of TGE are recognized: epidemic and endemic. In addition, infections with the TGEV deletion mutant PRCV present a different pattern and greatly complicate seroprevalence studies of the epidemiology of TGEV (Pensaert 1989; Pensaert and Cox 1989).

Epidemic TGE

Epidemic TGE refers to the occurrence of TGE in a herd where most, if not all, of the animals are TGEV/PRCV seronegative and susceptible. When TGEV is introduced into such a herd, the disease usually spreads rapidly to swine of all ages, especially during the winter. Some degree of inappetence, vomition, or diarrhea will occur in most animals. Suckling pigs show marked clinical signs and rapidly dehydrate. Mortality is very high in pigs under 2–3 weeks of age, but gradually decreases in older pigs. Lactating sows often show signs, developing anorexia and agalactia, which further contribute to piglet mortality.

The history and severe clinical signs aid in diagnosis of epidemic TGE in the U.S., since diseases with similar signs have not been reported. However, in Europe, PED had similar clinical signs before it became endemic (Pensaert and DeBouck 1978). Likewise, the presence of

PRCV appears to have greatly reduced the incidence and severity of epidemic TGE (Brown and Patton 1991; Laude et al. 1993; Pensaert et al. 1993; Pensaert and Cox 1989).

Endemic TGE

Endemic TGE refers to the persistence of the virus and disease in a herd. This occurs as a result of the continual or frequent influx of susceptible swine which, when infected, tend to perpetuate the disease. Endemic TGE is limited to seropositive herds that have frequent farrowings (Stepanek 1979) or have frequent additions or commingling of susceptible swine.

Endemic TGE represents a common sequel to a primary outbreak in large breeding herds. In endemically infected herds, TGEV spreads slowly among adult swine, particularly herd replacements (Pritchard 1987). Females saved for breeding are frequently immune and will transfer via their colostrum and milk a variable degree of passive immunity to their suckling pigs. Sows usually do not show clinical signs. In these herds, mild TGEV diarrhea occurs in pigs from about 6 days of age until about 2 weeks after weaning. The pig is clinically affected when viral exposure exceeds the pig's passive immunity. The age at which this occurs is related to the management system used in the herd and the degree of immunity of the sow. Mortality is usually less than 10–20%, being determined by the age when infected and by the variable degree of immunity obtained from immune sows. Endemic TGE in suckling or recently weaned pigs can be difficult to diagnose and must be differentiated from other types of endemic diarrheal problems commonly occurring in young pigs, such as rotaviral diarrhea and colibacillosis. Endemic TGE will persist in the herd as long as susceptible or partially immune swine are exposed to TGEV.

The recrudescence or reintroduction of TGEV may occur in herds that contain immune sows, resulting in discrete episodes of disease (Pritchard 1987). This situation commonly occurs in herds in the concentrated swine-rearing areas of the U.S. or other countries. Herds often become reinfected in the winter, and growing and finishing swine are especially affected. Such animals are susceptible because the herd infection from the previous winter has usually terminated during the intervening summer. If the disease enters the farrowing house, the disease in suckling or weaned pigs will resemble that described above since the sows will usually be immune. It is unclear whether the source of virus in these circumstances comes from reactivation of virus shedding in carrier swine or reintroduction of virus into the herd from an external source.

Porcine Respiratory Coronavirus

Evidence that led to the discovery of PRCV was obtained from serologic surveys of slaughterhouse sows or swine tested for international trade in Europe. In 1984, this led to the first isolation of PRCV, a nonenteropathogenic coronavirus, in Belgium (Pensaert et al. 1986). In 1989, two herds in the U.S. unexpectedly were seropositive for TGEV antibodies, although these herds had not been vaccinated for TGE nor had they experienced clinical disease (Hill et al. 1990; Wesley et al. 1990b).

PRCV is a TGEV variant that infects epithelial cells of the respiratory tract and alveolar macrophages (Paul et al. 1994; Pensaert 1989; Pensaert and Cox 1989). After experimental challenge, PRCV infects only a few unidentified cells in the small intestine, and thus, virus shedding in feces is limited or not detected (Brim et al. 1994, 1995; Costantini et al. 2004; Cox et al. 1990a, b; O'Toole et al. 1989; VanCott et al. 1993, 1994). Recently, fecal and nasal isolates of PRCV from the same pigs were compared genetically, and small, but consistent, genetic differences (point mutations) were noted in the S protein (Costantini et al. 2004). However, PRCV-infected pigs produce antibodies that neutralize TGEV.

Swine population density, distances between farms, and season influence the epidemiology of PRCV. PRCV infects pigs of all ages by airborne transmission or by contact. In areas with high swine farm density, the virus can spread to pigs on neighboring farms that are several kilometers away (Pensaert and Cox 1989). In addition, the risk of a farm becoming infected increases as the size of a neighboring herd increases (Henningsen et al. 1989).

PRCV infections are often subclinical and the virus has spread rapidly and extensively in pigs in Europe (Brown and Cartwright 1986; Henningsen et al. 1989; Laude et al. 1993; Martin et al. 1994; Pensaert 1989; van Nieuwstadt et al. 1989) and even into countries that were previously free of TGEV (Pensaert 1989). A limited serologic survey in 1995 in the U.S. suggested that many asymptomatic swine herds in Iowa were seropositive for PRCV (Wesley et al. 1997).

PRCV has become endemic in many European swine herds (Lanza et al. 1993; Laude et al. 1993; Pensaert et al. 1993; Pensaert 1989). The virus circulates in the herd, infecting pigs before the age of 20–26 weeks, after passively acquired maternal antibodies have declined (Pensaert et al. 1993). Introduction of pigs into fattening units and commingling of PRCV-negative and PRCV positive pigs from diverse sources resulted in seroconversion to PRCV in pigs shortly after introduction into most units (Van Reeth and Pensaert 1994a).

Susceptible pigs experimentally infected with PRCV shed virus from nasal secretions for a period of less than 2 weeks (Bourgueil et al. 1992; Brim et al. 1994; Onno et al. 1989; VanCott et al. 1993; Wesley et al. 1990b). There is no evidence for the fecal-oral transmission of PRCV. Pensaert et al. (1993) have shown that pigs on closed breeding farms become infected shortly after weaning— even in the presence of maternal antibodies. Thus, PRCV persists in the herd by regularly infecting newly weaned pigs. PRCV can persist in the herd throughout the entire year or it can disappear temporarily from a herd (mainly in the summer) and reappear in the nursery and fattening units during the colder months of the year (Pensaert et al. 1993). Thus, waves of infection, without clinical disease, coincide with the rainy season in Europe (Laude et al. 1993).

Following the widespread dissemination of PRCV, the seroprevalence of TGEV infections in European swine was examined by blocking ELISA (Brown and Patton 1991; Lanza et al. 1993; Pensaert et al. 1993). The investigators reported low (0.0–7.6%) TGEV seropositives from sows in Spain (Lanza et al. 1993; Pensaert et al. 1993) and from pigs in the U.K. (Brown and Patton 1991). Thus, the seroprevalence of TGEV infections in Europe has decreased coincident with the spread of PRCV.

Transmission and Reservoirs

One of the significant epidemiological features of TGE is its seasonal appearance during the winter months. Haelterman (1962) suggested that this is because the virus is very stable when frozen and more labile when exposed to heat or to sunlight. This would allow virus transmission between herds in winter on fomites or animals. Reduced or fluctuating ambient temperatures also markedly predispose feeder pigs to clinical manifestations of TGE (Shimizu and Shimizu 1979a; Shimizu et al. 1978), thus contributing to transmission in winter.

What is the reservoir of TGEV between seasonal epidemics? Haelterman (1962) proposed at least three possible reservoirs: (1) associated pig farms in which the virus spreads subclinically; (2) hosts other than swine; and (3) carrier pigs.

The most probable explanation for maintenance of the disease is that it exists in an endemic form in feeder-pig operations (Morin et al. 1978) or in herds that are on a continuous farrowing program. These situations could constitute foci for maintenance of the disease during the warmer months and for dissemination during the winter months. This hypothesis is supported by the finding that TGEV infection can spread rather slowly through a group of growing swine under certain conditions, such as during the summer months (Maes and Haelterman 1979).

There is also evidence for the existence of TGEV in non-porcine hosts. Cats, dogs, and foxes have been suggested as possible carriers of TGEV from one herd to another since they can shed virus in their feces for variable periods (Haelterman 1962; McClurkin et al. 1970). Cats and dogs fed TGEV showed no clinical signs, except after repeated passage in dogs and seroconverted to TGEV, but virus excreted by dogs was shown to be infectious for pigs (Haelterman 1962; Reynolds and Garwes 1979).

Massive concentrations of starlings (*Sturnus vulgaris*) in winter in feeding areas of swine may provide a method by which TGEV can be mechanically carried from one farm to another. Pilchard (1965) reported that

TGEV was detected in the droppings of starlings for as long as 32 hours after they were fed TGEV. Houseflies (*Musca domestica*) have also been proposed as possible mechanical vectors for TGEV. TGEV antigen was detected in flies within a swine herd in which TGE was endemic, and experimentally inoculated flies excreted TGEV for 3 days (Gough and Jorgenson 1983).

A third possibility relating to the transmission of TGE is the length of time infected swine shed viable TGEV and the role of the carrier pig. A few reports (Lee et al. 1954; Pensaert 1976; Woods and Wesley 1998) have indicated chronic and/or persistent fecal shedding for periods up to 18 months, rather than the commonly reported 2-week period (Pensaert et al. 1970a). Respiratory shedding of TGEV has been detected in nasal swabs for postexposure periods up to 11 days (Kemeny et al. 1975). However, the virus was detected in lung homogenates for postexposure periods up to 104 days (Underdahl et al. 1975).

TGEV has also been recovered from milk of infected sows during the acute phase of the disease (Kemeny et al. 1975; Kemeny and Woods 1977) and following intramammary infusion or injection of lactating sows with live TGEV (Saif and Bohl 1983). In the latter study, demonstration of TGEV antigen in mammary gland tissue indicated that the virus might replicate in the mammary glands of lactating sows, an event which might contribute to agalactia in sows. Transmission of the virus via milk to suckling piglets, as suggested in the same study, may account, in part, for the rapid spread of the infection among a litter.

Although TGEV has been detected in the intestinal and respiratory tracts for periods of up to 104 days post infection, it is unknown whether such virus is viable and is shed or transmitted in a viable state. Addition of sentinel pigs to a herd at 3, 4, and 5 months after a previous TGE outbreak resulted in no infections in the introduced pigs, as determined by serologic tests (Derbyshire et al. 1969). Nasal shedding of PRCV in experimentally infected pigs occurs through postexposure day 10 (Onno et al. 1989; Wesley et al. 1990b). However, how long pigs recovered from PRCV infection in the field remain infectious is unknown. Thus, a possible role for the long-term carrier hog in transmitting TGEV has been suggested (Woods and Wesley 1998).

CLINICAL SIGNS

Epidemic TGE

The typical clinical signs of TGE in seronegative piglets are transient vomiting and watery, yellowish diarrhea, with rapid loss of weight, dehydration, and high morbidity and mortality in pigs under 2 weeks of age. Diarrhea in young pigs is usually profuse and feces will often contain undigested milk.

The severity of the clinical signs, duration of the disease, and mortality are inversely related to the age of the pig. Most pigs under 7 days of age will die in 2–7 days after first showing clinical signs. Most suckling pigs over 3 weeks of age will survive but are likely to remain stunted. Clinical signs of TGE in growing and finishing swine and in sows are usually limited to inappetence and diarrhea for a few days, with vomiting occasionally observed. The few deaths observed are probably due to complicating factors, such as stress or concurrent infections, which frequently occur after weaning. Some lactating sows become very sick, with an elevated temperature, agalactia, vomiting, inappetence, and diarrhea. These severe signs may be due to a high degree of exposure to the virus from close contact with their affected piglets or to hormonal factors that may influence susceptibility. In contrast, sows in the field having no contact with young infected pigs usually have mild clinical signs or none.

The incubation period is short, usually 18 hours to 3 days. Infection generally spreads rapidly through the entire group of swine so that in 2–3 days most animals are affected, but this is more likely to occur in winter than summer (Maes and Haelterman 1979).

Endemic TGE

Endemic TGE occurs in large herds that have frequent farrowings and in TGEV or PRCV seropositive herds. The clinical signs will usually be less severe than those seen in seronegative pigs of the same age. Death losses are low, especially if pigs are kept warm. The clinical signs in suckling pigs can resemble those caused by rotavirus (Bohl et al. 1978). In some herds, depending on management, endemic TGE is manifested mainly in weaned pigs and may be confused with *Escherichia coli*, coccidia, or rotavirus infections (Pritchard 1987).

Porcine Respiratory Coronavirus

The severity of clinical signs and the degree of pathogenicity appear to be PRCV strain–dependent, and it is speculated that these differences might correlate with slightly different genetic deletions. In addition, infection of swine with PRCV and other respiratory viruses, especially in association with porcine reproductive and respiratory syndrome virus (PRRSV), can alter the severity of disease and clinical signs.

Ultimately, the manifestation of respiratory disease is dependent on a number of variables, including environmental and seasonal factors, management practices, virus load or dose, and presence of other bacterial or viral pathogens in the herd (Van Reeth and Pensaert 1994a, b).

Experimentally infected feeder pigs had only a transient weight loss, whereas 4- and 6-day-old pigs infected with PRCV showed only a reduced rate of weight gain in comparison with control pigs (Lanza et al. 1992; Van Reeth et al. 1996; Vannier 1990; Wesley and Woods 1996).

Many European and American PRCV strains cause subclinical infections, but by histological examination, interstitial pneumonia affecting 5–60% of the lung may be present (Enjuanes and Van der Zeist 1995; Hayes et al. 2000; Laude et al. 1993; Van Reeth and Pensaert 1992). In one study, when American PRCV strains were compared in pigs under the same conditions, differences were observed in pathogenicity among strains (Halbur et al. 1994). Two PRCV isolates, AR310 and LEPP with the same S gene deletion, induced signs of moderate respiratory disease in pigs, while a third strain (1894) produced only mild respiratory disease. However, at a lower dose, even the AR310 strain was asymptomatic in gnotobiotic pigs (Halbur et al. 1993). Likewise, a Canadian PRCV strain (1Q90) isolated in Quebec caused severe pneumonia and 60% mortality in 1-week-old pigs given $10^{8.5}$ TCID$_{50}$ (median tissue culture infectious doses) of virus, but littermates exposed to PRCV by contact, presumably at a lower dose, exhibited mild signs (Jabrane et al. 1994). Inoculation of pigs with a higher dose of PRCV also resulted in longer shedding of PRCV (VanCott et al. 1993).

Thus, clinical signs seen after experimental PRCV exposure may be highly dose related and influenced by the age of the pigs and inoculation techniques. The results of experimental studies were also influenced by the health status of the pigs and their subsequent treatment (Vannier 1990).

Besides a single-virus infection with PRCV, pigs can be exposed concurrently to other respiratory viruses and agents. Often this occurs when pigs from multiple sources are grouped together in nurseries or grower-finisher units (Van Reeth and Pensaert 1994a). The effects of dual-virus inoculations have been investigated and generally found to be more severe than for a single-virus infection. In particular, respiratory signs were enhanced in PRCV-infected pigs when the pigs were inoculated 2 days later with either swine influenza virus or pseudorabies virus (Van Reeth and Pensaert 1994b; Van Reeth et al. 1996). Combined infections with PRRSV followed by PRCV also resulted in a prolonged fever with respiratory disease, a reduced rate of weight gain or longer shedding of PRCV (Hayes et al. 2000; Van Reeth et al. 1996).

Because many respiratory viruses and bacteria are common in swine populations, these combined infections with PRCV may increase the occurrence and severity of respiratory disease (Hayes et al. 2000; Van Reeth et al. 2000). This subject requires additional research including elucidating the mechanism of disease enhancement and shedding in dual infections.

PATHOGENESIS

The pathogenesis of TGE has been reviewed (Hooper and Haelterman 1966; Moon 1978). The early events have been described as follows: TGEV is ingested, infects the mucosa of the small intestine, and causes villous atrophy because of a rapid and extensive loss of functional epithelial cells.

Intestinal Replication

Whether by the oral or the nasal route, the virus is swallowed and, being resistant to low pH and proteolytic enzymes, remains viable until it comes in contact with the highly susceptible villous epithelial cells of the small intestine. Infection and rapid destruction or alteration in function of these cells result in marked reduction in enzymatic activity in the small intestine, which disrupts digestion and cellular transport of nutrients and electrolytes, causing an acute malabsorption syndrome (Moon 1978). Hooper and Haelterman (1966) suggested that the inability of infected pigs to hydrolyze lactose and other nutrients results in the marked deprivation of nutrients critical to the young pig. Furthermore, they suggested that the presence of undigested lactose exerts an osmotic force that causes a retention of fluid in the lumen of the intestine and, thus, contributes to diarrhea and dehydration. Additional mechanisms contributing to diarrhea in TGEV-infected pigs include altered intestinal sodium transport, with accumulation of electrolytes and water in the intestinal lumen (Butler et al. 1974) and loss of extravascular protein (Prochazka et al. 1975). The ultimate cause of death is probably dehydration and metabolic acidosis coupled with abnormal cardiac function resulting from hyperkalemia.

A marked shortening or atrophy of the villi occurs in the jejunum (Figure 30.3) and to a lesser extent in the ileum, but it is often absent in the proximal portion of the duodenum (Hooper and Haelterman 1966). Both virus production and villous atrophy were greater in newborn pigs than in 3-week-old pigs (Moon et al. 1973; Norman et al. 1973), suggesting higher susceptibility of neonates to TGEV infection. Several mechanisms have been proposed to account for this age-dependent resistance to clinical disease. First, the rapidity with which infected villous epithelial cells can be replaced by migration of epithelial cells from crypts of Lieberkühn in older pigs compared to younger may partially account for the higher fatality rate in newborn pigs (Moon 1978). These newly replaced villous enterocytes are reportedly resistant to TGEV infection (Pensaert et al. 1970b), possibly due to onset of innate immunity and presence of intestinal interferon (La Bonnardiere and Laude 1981) or the inability of these regenerating cells to support virus growth. Second, TGEV accumulates and replicates in the apical tubulovascular system of villous absorptive cells in newborn pigs; this system is lacking in pigs older than 3 weeks (Wagner et al. 1973). Third, virus dose may play a major role in infections. Witte and Walther (1976) demonstrated that the infectious dose of TGEV needed to infect a market hog (about 6 months old) was 10^4 times greater than that needed to infect a 2-day-old piglet. However, the severity of clinical signs due to TGE is also increased when pigs are (1) fed a zinc-deficient ration (Whitenack et al. 1978); (2) anemic (Ackerman et al. 1972); (3) exposed to a low temperature or fluctuation in temperature (Shimizu et al. 1978); or (4) injected with a

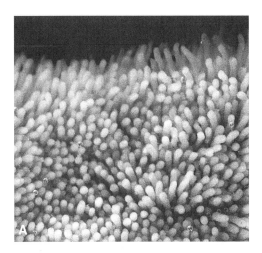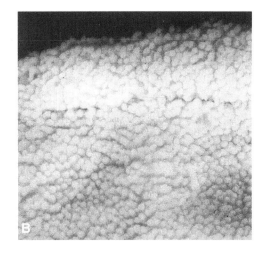

30.3. *Villi of the jejunum from a normal pig (A) and from a TGEV-infected pig (B), as viewed through a dissecting microscope (approximately ×10).*

synthetic corticosteroid, dexamethazone (Shimizu and Shimizu 1979a). In regard to the last two factors, the mechanism is thought to be due to an interference with the early initiation of a local cell-mediated immune response (Shimizu and Shimizu 1979a).

The failure of cell culture-attenuated strains of TGEV to infect large numbers of epithelial cells or those located in the cranial portion of the small intestines of pigs probably explains why such strains cause milder diarrhea than that observed with virulent strains (Frederick et al. 1976; Furuuchi et al. 1979; Hess et al. 1977; Pensaert 1979). Furthermore, there was an inverse correlation between the level of cell culture attenuation of TGEV and the extent of intestinal infection (Hess et al. 1977). Cell-cultured strains of TGEV of reduced virulence in combination with a mildly virulent *E. coli* have been shown to cause a more severe disease in germ-free pigs than when either organism was given alone (Underdahl et al. 1972). Concurrent infections with TGEV and *E. coli* or porcine rotavirus have been reported (Hornich et al. 1977; Theil et al. 1979).

Extraintestinal Replication Sites

TGEV. Although ingestion is undoubtedly the most common portal of entry for the virus, the nasal route, or airborne infection, may be important, but the efficiency of this route of transmission for the spread of TGEV appears much less significant than for PRCV. Only in one study were macroscopic lung lesions observed in gnotobiotic pigs inoculated oronasally with TGEV, but no clinical pneumonia occurred (Underdahl et al. 1975). A preliminary report also indicated that TGEV was present in alveolar macrophages of infected neonatal pigs, suggesting a possible role for these cells in lung infection. However, only cell culture–attenuated, but not virulent TGEV, replicated in cultures of alveolar macrophages in vitro (Laude et al. 1984). Highly attenuated strains of TGEV have also been reported that replicate in the upper respiratory tract and lung but not in the intestine of new-

born pigs, thus, resembling PRCV infections (Furuuchi et al. 1979). Interestingly, 2 amino acid changes (nucleotides 219 and 655) occurred in the S gene between virulent (enteric) and attenuated (respiratory/enteric) TGEV strains that may account for this altered respiratory tropism (Ballesteros et al. 1997; Sanchez et al. 1999). Moreover, nasal shedding of TGEV was detected in infected piglets (VanCott et al. 1993) and in lactating sows exposed to infected piglets (Kemeny et al. 1975). In addition, studies have shown that TGEV is capable of replicating in mammary tissue of lactating sows (Saif and Bohl 1983) and that infected sows shed virus in milk (Kemeny and Woods 1977). The significance of possible mammary gland infection with TGEV under field conditions is unclear, as is whether it plays a role in agalactia, often seen in TGEV-infected sows or rapid spread of infection among piglets. Although natural infection of the porcine fetus with TGEV has not been reported, intrafetal inoculation results in the production of villous atrophy and seroconversion to TGEV (Redman et al. 1978).

Porcine Respiratory Coronavirus. PRCV has a tropism for cells of the respiratory tract. It replicates to high titer in porcine lungs (10^7–10^8 $TCID_{50}$) and also infects epithelial cells of the nares, trachea, bronchi, bronchioles, and alveoli and alveolar macrophages (Hayes et al. 2000; O'Toole et al. 1989; Pensaert et al. 1986). Viremia occurs following primary infection, and virus spreads to parenchymal organs and lymph nodes. Only a few scattered cells containing PRCV antigen are found in the small intestine, even when the virus is directly inoculated into the intestinal lumen. These infected cells are located in, or underneath, the epithelial layer of the intestinal villi and crypts, and the virus does not spread to adjacent cells (Cox et al. 1990a, b). This limited intestinal replication of PRCV explains why no or low titers of virus are detected in feces and most fecal PRCV may reflect swallowed virus (Costantini et al. 2004; VanCott et al. 1993, 1994).

Researchers have used MAb neutralization–resistant mutants and recombinant TGEV strains from infectious TGEV clones to explore the molecular basis for the difference in pathogenicity and tissue tropism between TGEV and PRCV strains (Ballesteros et al. 1997; Bernard and Laude 1995; Sanchez et al. 1999).

Bernard and Laude (1995) reported that most TGEV (Purdue-115 strain) MAb-resistant mutants selected with MAbs to S protein site D (absent on PRCV) exhibited a reduced enteropathogenicity in pigs that correlated with a point mutation or small deletion in the S protein gene encoding the N-terminal subregion of the S protein (similar region deleted in PRCV strains). Using recombinants generated between enteric/respiratory (PUR46) and respiratory (PTV) strains of TGEV, Ballesteros et al. (1997) concluded that a substitution in amino acid 219 of the S protein of the PUR46 recombinants was responsible for the loss of enteric tropism observed after inoculation of pigs with the PUR46 recombinants. The authors speculated that two different domains of the S protein (around amino acid 219) are required to infect intestinal epithelial cells: One domain binds to the cellular receptor, aminopeptidase N, and the other domain may be a binding site for an undefined intestinal coreceptor.

LESIONS

Gross Lesions

Gross lesions with TGE are usually confined to the gastrointestinal tract, with the exception of dehydration. The stomach is often distended with curdled milk and may have small areas of hemorrhage on the diaphragmatic side of the stomach (Hooper and Haelterman 1969). The small intestine is distended with yellow, foamy fluid and usually contains flecks of curdled undigested milk. The wall is thin and transparent, probably due to atrophy of the villi. Although lung lesions have been observed in experimentally infected gnotobiotic pigs (Underdahl et al. 1975), they have not been reported in pigs naturally infected with TGEV.

Subgross Lesions

A highly significant lesion of TGE is the markedly shortened villi of the jejunum and ileum, which Hooper and Haelterman (1969) referred to as villous atrophy (Figure 30.3). This is also seen in rotavirus diarrhea, but is not usually as severe or extensive as in TGE (Bohl et al. 1978). Infections with some strains of E. coli and coccidia have also been reported to produce this lesion (Hornich et al. 1977). However, the pathologic findings and extent of villous atrophy were highly variable in pigs from endemically infected herds (Pritchard 1987).

Microscopic Lesions

The degree of villous atrophy can be judged in histologic sections by comparing the length of the jejunal villi with the depth of the crypts of Lieberkühn. In normal piglets the villi-crypt ratio is about 7:1; in infected piglets the corresponding ratio is about 1:1 (Hooper and Haelterman 1969). Other lesions reported in experimentally challenged 8-week-old pigs include microulceration of the dome epithelium over Peyer's patches (Chu et al. 1982a). By scanning EM, the intestinal lesions of TGE correlate well with those observed by light microscopy (Moxley and Olson 1989b; Waxler 1972). Using scanning EM, Moxley and Olson (1989b) showed that the level of passive immunity in TGEV-infected pigs influenced not only the degree of villous atrophy but also its segmental distribution. Villous atrophy was minimal in pigs nursing sows previously infected with virulent TGEV, compared to pigs nursing seronegative sows or sows given live attenuated vaccines. In partially protected pigs, villous atrophy was seen primarily in the ileum instead of the jejunum. Similar observations were noted in pigs from herds with endemic TGE. Transmission EM of TGEV-infected epithelial cells of the small intestine has revealed alterations in the microvilli, mitochondria, endoplasmic reticulum, and other cytoplasmic components. Virus particles, primarily in cytoplasmic vacuoles, were observed in villous enterocytes and in M cells, lymphocytes, and macrophages in the dome regions of Peyer's patches (Chu et al. 1982a; Thake 1968; Wagner et al. 1973).

PRCV Lesions

In the case of PRCV, villous atrophy is not observed. However, microscopic examination of lungs from asymptomatic pigs reveals that PRCV causes a diffuse interstitial pneumonia in a high percentage of inoculated animals (Cox et al. 1990a; Hayes et al. 2000; O'Toole et al. 1989; van Nieuwstadt and Pol 1989). Others reported more severe respiratory lesions, dependent upon the strain and dose of PRCV used to experimentally infect pigs (Halbur et al. 1993, 1994; Jabrane et al. 1994; Paul et al. 1994).

IMMUNITY

Active Immunity

The duration of active immunity in swine after oral infection with virulent TGEV has not been well characterized. Intestinal infection of breeding-age swine results in detectable serum antibodies that persist for at least 6 months to possibly several years (Stepanek 1979). However, the serum antibody titer, although providing serologic evidence of TGE, provides little indication of the degree of active immunity. Swine that have recovered from TGE are immune to subsequent short-term challenge, presumably due to local immunity within the intestinal mucosa (Brim et al. 1995; Saif et al. 1994; VanCott et al. 1993, 1994). The age and immune status of the animal at initial infection and the severity of the challenge may greatly influence the completeness and duration of this active immunity.

The mechanism of active immunity in the gut probably relates to stimulation of the secretory IgA (sIgA) immune system with production of intestinal sIgA antibodies by lymphoid cells within the lamina propria (Saif et al. 1994; VanCott et al. 1993, 1994). IgA TGEV antibodies and antibody-secreting cells (ASCs) have been detected in the intestine and serum of pigs after oral, but not parenteral, inoculation with TGEV (Kodama et al. 1980; Saif et al. 1994; VanCott et al. 1993, 1994). Kodama et al. (1980) proposed that detection of IgA antibody in the serum, presumably intestinally derived, might serve as an indicator of active immunity to TGE. In another study, oral inoculation of gnotobiotic pigs with TGEV resulted in development of both serum and intestinal TGEV-neutralizing antibodies detectable from 5 to at least 35 days postexposure (DPE) (Saif 1976). IgM (5–15 DPE) and IgA immunocytes (which remained predominant from 7 to 35 DPE) were detected in the intestinal lamina propria of the TGEV-infected gnotobiotic pigs.

More recently, an enzyme-linked immunospot (ELISPOT) technique was used to investigate the kinetics of IgA and IgG TGEV antibody production by the pig's systemic and local gut-associated lymphoid tissues (GALT). High numbers of IgA ASCs were induced in GALT only by virulent TGEV. In contrast, live attenuated (vaccine) TGEV or PRCV strains induced significantly fewer IgA ASCs (Berthon et al. 1990; Saif et al. 1994; VanCott et al. 1993, 1994).

These and other studies (Stone et al. 1982) indicate that the pig is immunocompetent at birth in regard to humoral and mucosal antibody production, but in the intestine, additional maturational time may be required for antibody responses to reach adult levels.

Besides local antibody-mediated immunity, cell-mediated immune responses may also be important in active immunity against TGEV infections. A number of tests have been used to demonstrate cell-mediated immunity (CMI) to TGEV, including macrophage migration inhibition (Frederick et al. 1976), leukocyte migration inhibition (Woods 1977) direct lymphocyte cytotoxicity (Shimizu and Shimizu 1979b), lymphocyte proliferation (Anton et al. 1995, 1996; Brim et al. 1994, 1995; Shimizu and Shimizu 1979c; Welch and Saif 1988), spontaneous cell-mediated cytotoxicity (SCMC), and antibody-dependent cell-mediated cytotoxicity (ADCMC) (Cepica and Derbyshire 1983).

Only indirect evidence exists concerning the role of CMI in resistance to TGEV infection. CMI was demonstrated with lymphocytes obtained from GALT of swine orally infected with virulent TGEV (Brim et al. 1994, 1995; Frederick et al. 1976; Shimizu and Shimizu 1979c; Welch et al. 1988); swine parenterally or oronasally inoculated with attenuated TGEV or PRCV-developed CMI mainly in systemic sites (spleen or peripheral blood lymphocytes). Lymphoproliferative responses to TGEV persisted within GALT, but not systemic lymphocytes, for at least 110 days after oral infection of 6-month-old

swine (Shimizu and Shimizu 1979c) but for only about 14–21 days after infection of younger (7- to 11-day-old) pigs (Brim et al. 1994; Welch et al. 1988). It was confirmed that CD4 T-helper cells are involved in lymphoproliferative responses to TGEV (Anton et al. 1996).

A correlation between lymphoproliferative responses and lactogenic immunity to TGEV was described in sows vaccinated with attenuated or recombinant TGEV vaccines (Park et al. 1998). Although T-cell epitopes were identified by lymphoproliferation studies for each of the three major proteins of TGEV, a dominant functional T-helper epitope was defined on the N protein (N_{321}) (Anton et al. 1995). The N_{321} peptide-induced T cells collaborated in the in vitro synthesis of TGEV-neutralizing antibodies specific for the S protein. These investigators further reported that production of high levels of TGEV-specific antibodies in vitro (from in vivo TGEV-primed mesenteric lymph node cells) required stimulation by at least two TGEV structural proteins, with maximal responses induced by native S protein rosettes in combination with recombinant N protein. Such findings have important implications for the optimal design of TGEV subunit or other recombinant TGEV vaccines.

Because lymphocyte cytotoxicity was absent in newborn piglets and decreased in parturient sows, it was proposed that a lack of K and NK cell activity against TGEV-infected cells may correlate with the increased susceptibility of newborn piglets and parturient sows to TGEV infection (Cepica and Derbyshire 1984). Thus, CMI may play a role in either recovery from TGEV infection or resistance to reinfection via the rapid elimination of TGEV-infected epithelial cells by any one or all of a combination of SCMC, ADCMC, or sensitized T lymphocyte–mediated cytotoxicity.

PRCV

The observation that epidemic outbreaks of TGE in Europe declined dramatically following the widespread dissemination of PRCV among European swine prompted researchers to examine whether a respiratory PRCV infection could induce active intestinal immunity and protection against TGEV. The consensus from several studies was that prior infection of nursing or weaned pigs with PRCV provided partial immunity against TGEV challenge, evident by a reduced duration and level of virus shedding and diarrhea in most (Brim et al. 1995; Cox et al. 1993; VanCott et al. 1994; Wesley and Woods 1996), but not all (van Nieuwstadt et al. 1989), pigs studied.

The mechanism of this partial immunity presumably is related to the rapid increase in TGEV-neutralizing antibody titers (Cox et al. 1993; Wesley and Woods 1996) and numbers of IgG and IgA ASCs observed in the intestines of PRCV-exposed pigs after TGEV challenge (Saif et al. 1994; VanCott et al. 1994). The latter researchers speculated that the migration of PRCV-specific IgG and IgA ASCs from the bronchus-associated lymphoid tissues (BALT) to the gut of the PRCV-exposed pigs after TGEV challenge might explain the rapid anamnestic response and the partial protection induced. However, after PRCV exposure of neonatal pigs, at least 6–8 days were required to develop partial immunity to TGEV challenge (Wesley and Woods 1996), suggesting that induction of active immunity might be too late to protect seronegative newborn piglets from epidemic TGE.

Passive Immunity

Passive immunity is of primary importance in providing newborn piglets with immediate protection against TGEV infection. Swine are born devoid of immunoglobulins (Igs), which they acquire after birth via colostrum. Colostral Igs, consisting primarily of IgG, represent a serum transudate that is transferred from the dam across the piglet's intestinal epithelium to its circulation, thus providing the neonate with the same complement of serum antibodies as in the dam (Bourne 1973; Porter and Allen 1972). These passively acquired humoral antibodies function mainly in protection against systemic infection, but do not protect against intestinal infection (Hooper and Haelterman 1966). The concentration of IgG decreases during the first week of lactation, and IgA becomes the predominant Ig in milk (Porter and Allen 1972). Cells seeded from the intestine produce IgA locally in the mammary tissue (Roux et al. 1977). The piglets do not absorb sIgA milk antibodies, but they play an important role in passive intestinal immunity.

Mechanisms of passive immunity to TGEV infections have been reviewed (Pensaert 1979; Saif and Bohl 1979a, 1981a; Saif and Smith 1985; Saif and Jackwood 1990). Swine that have recovered from TGE can transmit passive immunity to their suckling pigs (Bay et al. 1953). Suckling pigs are protected as a result of the frequent ingestion of colostrum or milk that contains TGEV-neutralizing antibodies. Such antibodies in the lumen of the intestine neutralize any ingested TGEV and thus protect the susceptible epithelial cells of the small intestine. Haelterman (1963) referred to this immunogenic mechanism as *lactogenic immunity*. This is accomplished naturally when piglets suckle immune sows about every 2 hours. Passive protection can also be accomplished artificially by continuous feeding of antiserum to piglets (Haelterman 1963; Noble 1964).

TGEV antibodies in colostrum and milk of sows are primarily associated with IgA or IgG (Abou-Youssef and Ristic 1972; Bohl et al. 1972; Saif et al. 1972). TGEV milk antibodies of the IgA class provide the most effective protection, but IgG antibodies were also protective if high titers could be maintained in milk (Bohl and Saif 1975) or by artificial feeding of colostral IgG (Stone et al. 1977). The greater efficacy of IgA TGEV antibodies is probably because (1) they occur in higher levels in milk (Porter and Allen 1972), (2) they are more resistant to

proteolytic enzymes (Underdown and Dorrington 1974), and (3) they selectively bind to gut enterocytes (Nagura et al. 1978). TGEV antibodies in milk of the IgG class are produced as a result of parenteral or systemic immunization. IgA TGEV antibodies occur in the milk following intestinal infection. To explain their occurrence it was proposed that after antigenic sensitization in the gut, IgA immunocytes migrate to the mammary gland, where they localize and secrete IgA antibodies into the colostrum and milk (Saif and Bohl 1979a; Saif and Smith 1985; Saif et al. 1994; Saif and Bohl 1981a; Saif and Jackwood 1990). This "gut-mammary" immunologic axis, first proposed in relation to TGEV infections in swine (Bohl et al. 1972; Saif et al. 1972), is an important concept that provided the initial description of a common mucosal immune system, and was used for designing optimal vaccination procedures to provide effective lactogenic immunity.

DIAGNOSIS

This subject has been reviewed by Bohl (1981). Collection and preservation of appropriate clinical specimens are necessary for reliable diagnosis. Although villous atrophy is a consistent lesion in severely affected seronegative pigs, it frequently occurs in other enteric infections as well (rotavirus, PED, coccidia, and sometimes *E. coli*). Laboratory diagnosis of TGE may be accomplished by one or more of the following procedures: detection of viral antigen, detection of viral nucleic acids, microscopic detection of virus, isolation and identification of virus, or detection of a significant antibody response.

The serologic assays are complicated by the failure of conventional assays to differentiate between PRCV and TGEV antibodies (discussed under differential blocking ELISA). However, evaluation of clinical signs, histologic lesions, and tissue distribution of viral antigen may provide a presumptive diagnosis because PRCV does not cause diarrhea or villous atrophy and replicates almost exclusively in respiratory tissues (Pensaert 1989; Pensaert and Cox 1989). Thus, PRCV is suspected if there is antigen in lung tissues, seroconversion to TGEV/PRCV by VN test, and no signs of enteric disease.

Detection of Viral Antigen

The detection of TGE viral antigen in epithelial cells of the small intestine is probably the most common method for diagnosing TGE in young pigs. Either IF (Pensaert et al. 1970a) or immunocytochemical (Becker et al. 1974; Chu et al. 1982b; Shoup et al. 1996) techniques may be used, but they require pigs in the early stages of diarrhea. Either mucosal scrapings (these yield a greater sample of the intestinal surface area) (Black 1971) or frozen sections from the jejunum and ileum are prepared and stained by either the direct (Figure 30.4) or indirect IF method.

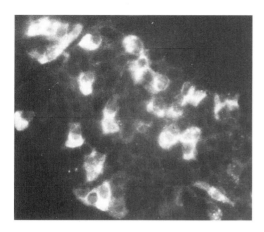

30.4. *Immunofluorescing cells from a TGEV-infected pig. A compression smear was made from a mucosal scraping of the jejunum and stained by the direct fluorescent antibody test (×350).*

Problems that may be encountered in IF tests include (1) lack of sensitivity or specificity of reagents (primary or secondary reagents used must be free of antibodies to other enteric organisms, particularly rotavirus); (2) failure to obtain specimens early after onset of diarrhea before the loss of infected cells (piglets must be euthanized to obtain specimens); and (3) cross-reactions with FIPV, CCV, and PRCV. However, replication of PRCV in villous enterocytes is uncommon, and IF or immunocytochemical staining of villous enterocytes in conjunction with diarrhea almost certainly indicates TGEV.

An immunoperoxidase technique using MAb to the highly conserved N protein of TGEV has been applied to the detection of TGEV (intestinal tissues) or PRCV (lungs) using formalin-fixed paraffin-embedded tissues (Shoup et al. 1996). This permits the diagnosis of TGEV/PRCV on the same tissues as used for histopathology and allows retrospective screening of fixed tissues for TGEV/PRCV. Although polyclonal antibodies will not differentiate between TGEV and PRCV, certain MAbs have been produced that react with TGEV, but not PRCV. These differentiating MAbs have been used in IF and immunocytochemical tests (Garwes et al. 1988; van Nieuwstadt and Pol 1989).

PRCV has been detected in respiratory tissues and nasal epithelial cells by IF and immunocytochemical tests, but use of differentiating MAbs is necessary for confirmation since enteric strains of TGEV may also replicate in these tissues.

A double antibody sandwich ELISA using monoclonal or polyclonal antibodies to TGEV as capture or secondary antibodies is used to detect TGEV antigens in cell culture, feces, and intestinal contents (Bernard et al. 1986; Cornaglia et al. 1994; Lanza et al. 1995; Lu et al. 1991; Sestak et al. 1996, 1999a; van Nieuwstadt et al. 1988) or PRCV antigen in nasal secretions or lung homogenates (Cornaglia et al. 1994; Lanza et al. 1995).

Detection of Viral Nucleic Acids

Nucleic acid hybridization probes have been developed to detect TGEV genome sequences in fecal samples, infected tissues, or infected cell cultures (Benfield et al. 1991; Shockley et al. 1987). Moreover, nucleic acid probes derived from the 5' end of the TGEV spike gene can distinguish between PRCV and TGEV. In a hybridization assay, these probes selectively differentiated enteric TGEV isolates from the U.S., Japan, and England, including live attenuated TGEV vaccine strains from the U.S. and isolates of PRCV, FIPV, and CCV (Bae et al. 1991; Wesley et al. 1990a, 1991a).

RT-PCR and nonradioactive cDNA probes have also been used to detect and differentiate TGEV and PRCV isolates (Costantini et al. 2004; Kim et al. 2000a; Vaughn et al. 1994, 1996). This is accomplished by using PCR primers targeting the region of the S gene spanning the deletion region in PRCV strains.

Electron Microscopy

TGEV has been demonstrated in the intestinal contents and feces of infected pigs by negative-contrast transmission EM (Figure 30.5) (Saif and Bohl 1977). Immune EM (IEM) has advantages over conventional EM in being more sensitive for detecting TGEV and providing serologic identification of the virus from clinical specimens or cell culture harvests. In addition, use of IEM enables one to more readily differentiate TGEV from common enveloped membranous debris and to concurrently detect the presence of other enteric viruses (Saif and Bohl 1977). IEM is at least as sensitive as IF for detection of TGEV. IEM is also ap-

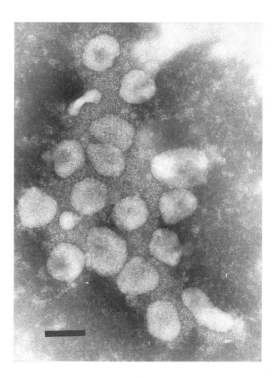

30.5. *Typical virus-antibody aggregates observed by IEM of TGEV and gnotobiotic pig anti-TGEV serum. Bar = 100 nm.*

plicable for detection of PRCV shedding in nasal secretions (L. J. Saif, unpublished). However, this method cannot distinguish between TGEV and PRCV unless MAbs are used, although shedding of large numbers of PRCV in feces would not be expected (VanCott et al. 1993, 1994).

Virus Isolation and Identification

Oral exposure of young, seronegative pigs is probably the most sensitive method for isolating or detecting TGEV (Dulac et al. 1977). However, this procedure is very expensive. Consequently, cell cultures are more frequently used. Primary and secondary pig kidney cells (Bohl and Kumgai 1965) or pig kidney cell lines (Laude et al. 1981), primary porcine salivary gland cells (Stepanek et al. 1971), porcine thyroid cells (Witte 1971), and the McClurkin swine testicle (ST) cell line (McClurkin and Norman 1966) have been successfully used for isolating TGEV from feces or gut contents of infected pigs. However, parvovirus contamination of some cells prepared from porcine thyroid glands may be a disadvantage to the use of these cells (Dulac et al. 1977).

Distinct cytopathogenic effect (CPE) may be negligible upon primary isolation of field strains, and additional passages may be required before CPE is evident. The CPE usually seen in ST and porcine thyroid cells consists of enlarged, rounded, or elongated cells with a balloonlike appearance (Kemeny 1978). The ST cell line has been used for detecting field strains of TGEV by CPE, plaques, or IF (Bohl 1979; Kemeny 1978). For detecting viral CPE or plaques, the sensitivity of ST cells can be further enhanced by adding pancreatin or trypsin to cell culture media (Bohl 1979; Stark et al. 1975; Woods 1982) and using older cells (Stark et al. 1975).

For isolation of PRCV, pig kidney and particularly ST cells have been the cells of choice, but PRCV also grows in a continuous cat fetus cell line (Laude et al. 1993). Nasal swab fluids or lung tissue homogenates from affected swine are used for isolation of PRCV. The CPE resembles that produced by TGEV strains, with syncytia formation frequently observed for PRCV (Pensaert 1989; Pensaert and Cox 1989) similar to that reported for SARS coronavirus grown in Vero cells (Ksiazek et al. 2003; Peiris et al. 2003).

Identification of cell culture virus can be done by VN, IF, or IEM using specific TGEV antiserum. However, MAbs specific for TGEV are required to confirm TGEV and exclude PRCV (Garwes et al. 1988; Laude et al. 1988). Alternatively, isolates can be differentiated using RT-PCR or specific cDNA probes (Enjuanes and Van der Zeist 1995; Kim et al. 2000a; Laude et al. 1993). Confusion with cross-reacting CCV and FIPV should not occur since these viruses do not replicate in ST or pig thyroid cells (Reynolds et al. 1980).

Serology

The detection of TGEV antibodies can assist in diagnosis and control in several different ways. However, the sero-

logic diagnosis of TGEV is complicated by the fact that both TGEV and PRCV induce neutralizing antibodies that are qualitatively and quantitatively similar (Pensaert 1989; Pensaert and Cox 1989). A blocking ELISA test (described later) can differentiate beween these antibodies. Serologic tests can also be used to monitor the TGEV or PRCV infection status of a herd. The entrance of only serologically negative swine will help maintain a herd free of TGEV and PRCV.

A rise in antibody titer between acute and convalescent serum samples provides retrospective evidence for epidemic TGE or infection with PRCV. However, the history of the herd with respect to disease and serologic status is needed to help interpret serologic findings. To determine whether endemic TGE or PRCV is a problem in a herd, serum samples from 2- to 6-month-old swine can be tested for antibodies. At this age, passively acquired antibodies should be absent (Derbyshire et al. 1969); thus, positive results suggest endemic TGEV or PRCV.

TGEV antibodies have been detected by several serologic tests. The VN test has been the most widely used, using cell culture–adapted viruses in cell culture systems by a variety of procedures: inhibition of CPE in microtiter plates (Toma and Benet 1976) and plaque reduction assays (Bohl and Kumgai 1965; Thomas and Dulac 1976) are the most common. Neutralizing antibodies to TGEV can be detected in serum as early as 7–8 days after infection and may persist for at least 18 months. Little is known about the persistence of neutralizing antibodies to PRCV within a herd (Cartwright 1968; Vannier et al. 1982).

Sensitive ELISA tests (Bernard et al. 1989; Berthon et al. 1990; Callebaut et al. 1989; Garwes et al. 1988; Hohdatsu et al. 1987; Nelson and Kelling 1984; Paul et al. 1986; Sestak et al. 1999a, b; van Nieuwstadt et al. 1989) have been described, but require concentrated purified virus or S protein for coating ELISA plates.

Complement-fixing antibodies have not been demonstrated in convalescent swine (Dulac et al. 1977).

Blocking ELISA for Serologic Differentiation of PRCV and TGEV

Studies using MAbs to TGEV have shown that certain antigenic sites on TGEV are not present on the S protein of PRCV because of the deletion from the S protein (Callebaut et al. 1989; Laude et al. 1988; Sanchez et al. 1990; Sestak et al. 1999b; Simkins et al. 1992, 1993). This difference between TGEV and PRCV serves as the basis of serologic tests to determine whether a swine herd is infected with TGEV or PRCV (Bernard et al. 1989; Callebaut et al. 1989; Garwes et al. 1988; Simkins et al. 1993; van Nieuwstadt and Boonstra 1992).

In the blocking ELISA, TGEV antigen or recombinant S protein (Sestak et al. 1999b) coated onto ELISA plates is reacted with either TGEV or PRCV antiserum followed by the distinguishing MAb. TGEV antiserum contains competing antibody that blocks the binding of the

MAb, whereas the PRCV antiserum does not block and allows the MAb to bind. Thus, a negative (no blocking) reaction in ELISA and a positive result in the VN test are evidence of a PRCV infection. The test should be evaluated only on a herd basis because some pigs with low TGEV or PRCV antibody titers, as occurs early in the infection process (7–14 days) or after infection with some TGEV strains, may go undiagnosed (Callebaut et al. 1989; Sestak et al. 1999b; Simkins et al. 1993; van Nieuwstadt and Boonstra 1992). Presently, to export TGE-free swine from countries where PRCV infections occur, only this test provides the differential information required to confirm TGEV seropositive animals. The accuracy of commercial ELISAs for differentiating U.S. strains of PRCV and TGEV is low and therefore appears to be applicable on a herd, but not individual pig, basis (Sestak et al. 1999b).

PREVENTION AND CONTROL

Treatment

Antiviral agents have not yet been developed for the specific treatment of TGE. Some inhibition of TGEV replication in cell culture has been reported for the antiviral compounds amantadine (Dimitrov 1982) and isathiazone (Potopal'skii et al. 1983).

Although high levels of type 1 interferon were detected in the intestine of pigs in the early phase of TGEV infection, the role of this interferon in the recovery or pathogenesis of TGE was undetermined (La Bonnardiere and Laude 1981). Studies suggest that interferon may activate natural killer cells in newborn pigs, thereby contributing a degree of resistance to challenge with TGEV (Lesnick and Derbyshire 1988; Loewen and Derbyshire 1988). In addition, during a field outbreak of TGE, 1- to 12-day-old piglets treated orally for 4 days with 1–20 IU of human interferon-alpha had significantly greater survival rates than placebo-treated piglets (Cummins et al. 1995). However, no increased survival was seen in piglets given human interferon-alpha shortly after birth. Whether such therapy could be cost-effective for treatment of TGEV-infected piglets was not assessed.

The only treatment for TGE presently available is to alleviate starvation, dehydration, and acidosis. Parenteral treatment with fluids, electrolytes, and nutrients would be effective in treating young pigs, but not practical under farm conditions. Oral therapy with balanced electrolyte and glucose solutions is contraindicated in young pigs (Moon 1978). The following measures are suggested: provide a warm (preferably above 32°C), draft-free, dry environment and make water or nutrient solution freely accessible to the thirsty TGEV-infected pigs. Such measures will tend to reduce mortality in pigs that are infected at more than 3–4 days of age. Antibacterial therapy might be beneficial in 2- to 5-week-old pigs, especially if there is concurrent infection with pathogenic strains of *E. coli*. Cross-fostering or put-

ting infected or susceptible litters onto TGE-immune sows was found useful in various field outbreaks (Pritchard 1982; Stepanek 1979).

Management

Preventing Entrance of TGEV into a Herd. Swine in the incubative stage of the disease or those in the viral shedding or carrier state can carry TGEV into a herd. Some precautions to help prevent this possibility are to introduce swine that originate from herds known to be free of TGE, are serologically negative, and/or have been placed in isolation on the farm for 2–4 weeks before being added to the herd proper. A frequent question is, "How soon after a TGE outbreak can pigs be moved to another herd without spreading the disease?" A practical answer to this question is that a period of 4 weeks should elapse from the last sign of disease before introducing such animals into a "clean" herd.

Animal vectors, such as starlings, have been incriminated as a means of spread between herds in winter months because of their tendency to gather in large flocks and feed around swine. Cats, dogs, or foxes might play a role in spreading TGE between herds under certain situations (see section on epidemiology). Feces from TGEV-infected swine can be carried on boots, shoes, clothing, truck beds, feeds, etc., and can be a source of infection to other herds. Especially in winter, this is probably an important means by which TGEV is transmitted during the transport of livestock and feed. Consequently, precautions should be taken to minimize such occurrences.

After Onset of TGE. When TGE has occurred on a farm and pregnant animals have not yet been exposed, two procedures may minimize losses of newborn pigs.

1. If the animals are due to farrow in more than 2 weeks, purposely expose them to virulent virus, such as the minced intestines of infected pigs, so that they will be immune at farrowing.
2. If the animals will farrow in less than 2 weeks, attempt to provide facilities and management procedures that will avoid exposure to TGEV until at least 3 weeks postfarrowing.

To minimize deaths, provide young pigs with a warm, dry, draft-free environment and access to water, nutrient solution, or milk replacer (see section on treatment).

Some success has been achieved in elimination of TGEV from epidemically infected closed breeder herds without depopulation by the following procedures (Harris et al. 1987):

1. Bring in all breeding stock replacements for the next 4–6 months.
2. In the face of an outbreak, feed TGEV-infected minced intestines simultaneously to all pigs in the

herd (including replacement stock) to eliminate susceptible hosts, thereby shortening the time the disease progresses through the herd and ensuring more uniform exposure levels in all pigs.

3. Maintain strict all-in/all-out production in farrowing and nursery units.
4. Add sentinel seronegative pigs about 2 months after clinical signs of TGE disappear and monitor these pigs for seroconversion to TGEV.

Potential hazards associated with feedback control of TGE include possible spread of other pathogens to pregnant sows and throughout the herd.

Endemic TGE. Two approaches can be considered in attempting to control or terminate an endemic TGE herd problem.

First, pregnant seropositive sows can be vaccinated intramuscularly (IM) late in gestation or shortly after farrowing with live attenuated TGEV to boost immunity. Although only limited information is available, this procedure should boost milk antibody levels (Saif and Bohl 1983) and provide longer passive immunity to suckling pigs (Leopoldt and Meyer 1978; Stepanek 1979). Although this procedure may only delay the onset of TGE in exposed pigs, it can be beneficial in reducing mortality.

Second, alterations in management can be made to break the cycle of infection by eliminating reservoirs of susceptible pigs in a unit: prevent the continual influx of susceptible animals into the herd (e.g., by temporarily altering the farrowing schedule), temporarily utilize other facilities, and create smaller farrowing and nursing units to more nearly achieve an all-in/all-out management system.

Immunoprophylaxis

TGE Vaccination of Neonatal or Weaned Pigs. Neonatal pigs have been orally vaccinated with attenuated TGEV in an attempt to induce rapid protection via either interference or local immunity. No early interference has been demonstrated and generally more than 5 days were required before protection due to active immunity could be induced (Pensaert 1979). One study reported a slightly earlier onset of protection, by 3–4 DPI, after maintaining vaccinated pigs at a lowered temperature (18–20°C) to enhance replication of the attenuated virus (Furuuchi et al. 1976). Failure to induce an early interference phenomenon and the delay required for development of active immunity make neonatal vaccination an unlikely method of providing immediate protection against TGEV within the critical first few days of life.

Active immunization of suckling or feeder pigs could be important for control of endemic infections, especially in newly weaned pigs, in which TGEV infections may result in increased mortality. Live attenuated and inactivated TGEV vaccines have been federally licensed for oral or intraperitoneal administration, respectively, shortly after birth. One limited preliminary study reported greater protection in vaccinated, seropositive suckling pigs compared to controls, even though serum antibody levels were not enhanced but were comparable in the two groups (Graham 1980). However, challenge in older piglets usually is much more difficult to standardize, due to age resistance to infection.

Further studies reported that the presence of maternal antibodies in vaccinated pigs decreased (Hess et al. 1982; Lanza et al. 1995; Sestak et al. 1996) or completely suppressed (Furuuchi et al. 1978) active antibody production following oral administration of live TGEV. In the latter study, conducted in suckling piglets nursing naturally infected sows (Furuuchi et al. 1978), high levels of both passive circulating and intestinal antibodies in the suckling piglets probably accounted for the complete interference with active immunization by an attenuated strain of TGEV.

Other approaches have been used in attempts to actively immunize young pigs against TGEV. Woods and Pedersen (1979) noted 33% mortality in challenged pigs vaccinated orally/intraperitoneally with two doses of the antigenically related live virulent FIPV. In comparison, 100% of the challenged pigs died that were orally vaccinated once with an attenuated SP variant of TGEV. Gough and Jorgenson (1983) reported that young weaned pigs inoculated IM with two or three doses of an adjuvanted, soluble, undefined TGEV subunit (23 kDa) vaccine were protected against virus challenge. However, parenteral administration of three doses of a baculovirus-expressed recombinant S protein (containing the four major antigenic sites, A–D) in adjuvant to suckling piglets elicited neutralizing antibodies to TGEV in serum but failed to protect pigs against TGEV challenge (Shoup et al. 1997). When the three major TGEV baculovirus-exressed structural proteins were coadministered intraperitoneally with *E. coli* thermolabile adjuvant to 3-week-old piglets, immune responses associated with virus-specific IgA resulted in markedly reduced rectal virus shedding upon challenge with TGEV (Sestak et al. 1999a). The later study suggests that TGEV-derived baculovirus constructs can be exploited for stimulation of protective mucosal and systemic immune responses.

TGEV Vaccination of the Seronegative Pregnant Dam. A variety of viral vaccines (virulent, attenuated, inactivated, and subunit) and routes of administration (oral, intranasal, intramuscular, subcutaneous, and intramammary) (Bohl and Saif 1975; Kaji and Shimizu 1978; Moxley and Olson 1989a; Pensaert 1979; Saif and Bohl 1979a; Saif et al. 1994; Saif and Jackwood 1990; Voets et al. 1980) have been tested for induction of lactogenic immunity. Oral administration of live virulent virus to pregnant sows generally gave the highest level of immunity, resulting in protective immunity for the sow and consistently producing high titers of persisting IgA TGEV antibodies in milk associated with protective lactogenic immunity for suckling pigs.

Vaccines and Vaccination. There are presently several federally licensed TGEV vaccines. All contain inactivated or live attenuated TGEV and are approved for use in pregnant or neonatal swine. These vaccines and their efficacy will be considered in the following sections according to their respective routes of administration. Many variables complicate the evaluation of both experimental and commercial TGEV vaccines, often resulting in conflicting data. These include the challenge dose and strain of TGEV; the age of the pig at challenge; environmental conditions, especially temperature; the milking efficiency of the vaccinated sow; and the immune status of the dam at vaccination.

Oral and/or Intranasal Vaccination. Based on the observation that sows infected with TGEV during gestation could transmit immunity to their piglets, "planned" infection of pregnant swine with virulent TGEV has been used to mimic this natural immunity. This procedure is accomplished by feeding virulent autogenous virus to pregnant swine at least 2 weeks before farrowing. The virus may consist of minced guts from young pigs acutely infected with TGEV and is administered to sows with food.

Oral vaccination of pregnant swine with attenuated TGEV is a logical route of vaccination for stimulating milk IgA TGEV antibodies aimed at duplicating the natural route of infection and induction of immunity. The intranasal (IN) route alone or with the oral route is used because attenuated strains of TGEV replicate in the respiratory tract (Furuuchi et al. 1979) and upon being swallowed might seed additional virus to the gut. However, results using attenuated strains orally and/or IN have generally been disappointing (Henning and Thomas 1981; Moxley and Olson 1989a; Saif and Bohl 1979a, 1981a; Voets et al. 1980). In previous studies using the high-passaged Purdue strain of TGEV orally, or orally and IM, few IgA TGEV antibodies were evident, and mortality among challenged pigs from vaccinated dams ranged from 25% to 100% (Moxley and Olson 1989a; Saif and Bohl 1979a, b; Saif and Jackwood 1990; Voets et al. 1980).

Concerns that attenuated strains of TGEV might not survive passage through the acidic environment of the stomach prompted studies using lyophilized attenuated virus in enteric-coated gelatin capsules (Hess et al. 1978; Voets et al. 1980). Hess et al. (1978), using the high titered B1 strain of TGEV (300 cell culture passages), reported high levels of IgA TGEV antibodies in milk and only 10% piglet mortality. Voets et al. (1980) used the high-passaged Purdue strain and found that most sows failed to seroconvert after oral vaccination, and even the

sows that seroconverted had a 44% piglet mortality rate. Fichtner et al. (1982) reported 30% mortality in challenged piglets after feeding attenuated Riems TGEV to the dams for 10 days during gestation.

In further efforts to ensure that vaccine virus reached the small intestine, two studies used direct inoculation of attenuated viruses into the intestinal lumen. Again, protection was poor (62% mortality) (Voets et al. 1980) in challenged piglets from dams given a single intralumenal inoculation of attenuated Purdue TGEV during gestation, but greater protection (10% mortality) was achieved when dams received repeated intralumenal inoculations (Fichtner et al. 1982).

Other researchers selected variants of high- and low-passaged TGEV strains resistant to low pH and proteolytic enzymes in vitro and used these strains as vaccines for passive protection studies (Aynaud et al. 1985; Bernard et al. 1989; Chen 1985; Shirai et al. 1988). They reported inconsistent results, with mortality varying from 0–73% among litters challenged with virulent TGEV. In the latter two studies, data interpretation was confounded somewhat by variations in the ages of the pigs at challenge, a factor shown in other studies to dramatically influence piglet survivability (Moxley and Olson 1989a).

A live attenuated SP variant TGEV grown in a persistently infected porcine leukocyte cell line has been used to vaccinate pregnant swine by the oral/IN and/or intramammary routes (Woods 1978, 1984). Challenge of the suckling pigs resulted in mortality of 14–34%. In the latter study the author reported generally high TGEV IgA and IgG antibody titers in 3–4 days postfarrowing (DPF) milk. However, three of eight sows vaccinated with SP TGEV became mildly sick after challenge exposure of their nursing pigs. Although diarrhea was observed in pigs nursing SP-TGEV vaccinates (48% morbidity), it was reportedly mild and delayed in onset (3 DPF). The SP TGEV has been reported to be avirulent for newborn pigs, replicating within the intestinal lamina propria but not epithelial cells (Woods et al. 1981).

Molecular analysis of several attenuated TGEV strains revealed changes in mRNA 2 and 3 affecting the S protein and nonstructural protein 3 (Register and Wesley 1994). Inconsistent results were noted in vaccination studies using a commercial vaccine administered twice orally (in feed) and once IM. Whereas Welter (1980) reported 8% mortality among challenged pigs, others reported higher mortality, similar to that in piglets suckling unvaccinated sows (Bohl et al. 1982; Moxley and Olson 1989a; Saif and Bohl 1981b). The generally poor results obtained with oral or IN vaccination of sows using attenuated TGEV strains may be attributed to the superficial or limited replication of most attenuated strains in the sow's intestine (Frederick et al. 1976; Hess et al. 1977). Consequently, this results in little antigenic stimulation of underlying intestinal IgA plasma cells and correspondingly little IgA antibody secretion in milk.

Attempts to use a low cell culture–passaged TGEV to induce passive immunity led to erratic results in terms of both seroconversion in orally/IN exposed sows and protection in piglets (Saif and Bohl 1979b). The dilemma remains of how to commercially develop a vaccine to prevent epidemic TGEV capable of stimulating IgA in the gut of sows but being sufficiently attenuated or noninfectious so as not to produce disease in newborn pigs.

Parenteral Vaccination. Various experimental and two commercial vaccines composed of live attenuated virus were administered IM about 6 and 2 weeks prefarrowing. Experimental evaluations of this vaccination regime have generally indicated reduced piglet mortality (38–56% in vaccinates compared with 71–92% in controls), but not morbidity (Bohl and Saif 1975; Moxley and Olson 1989a; Voets et al. 1980). However, vaccination results were poor when compared with almost complete protection (0–9% mortality) in litters of naturally infected sows.

Henning and Thomas (1981) and Matisheck et al. (1982) reported more favorable vaccination results, i.e., mortality of 10% and 18%, using two commercial vaccines. The IM vaccination procedure has two major disadvantages. (1) Vaccinated swine develop little or no gut immunity; they usually get sick when exposed to TGEV. If this occurs during lactation, their suckling pigs will be deprived of adequate milk. (2) The TGEV antibodies found in the milk of these vaccinated sows are of the IgG class and of low titer and fail to provide optimal passive protection to suckling pigs.

Intramammary injection of seronegative pregnant swine with TGEV resulted in high titers of primarily IgG TGEV antibodies in milk, whereas similar injections in lactating sows resulted in IgA and IgM TGEV antibodies. Specific antibody activity was found not only in milk from injected glands but also in milk from noninjected glands (Bohl and Saif 1975; Saif and Bohl 1983). Protection was good (14–26% mortality) in litters of intramammarily vaccinated pregnant swine, presumably because exceptionally high levels of IgG antibodies persisted in the milk at the time of challenge, 3 days postfarrowing (Bohl and Saif 1975; Shibley et al. 1973).

A similar, greatly enhanced, predominantly IgG milk antibody titer was noted in two sows vaccinated IM/IN with the high-titered (10^8–$10^{9.3}$ TCID$_{50}$) attenuated TO163 strain of TGEV. No mortality occurred in either of these litters, confirming the protective ability of IgG TGEV antibodies when present in high titers in milk (Kaji and Shimizu 1978).

Heterologous Vaccines. The antigenic relationship between TGEV and FIPV was the basis for studies of the possible efficacy of FIPV as a heterologous coronavirus vaccine in swine. Preliminary studies indicated that some immunity (25% mortality) against TGE was conferred in pigs nursing two sows vaccinated during gestation orally/IN and intramammarily with live virulent FIPV. However, this FIPV was pathogenic in newborn pigs (Woods and Pedersen 1979). Subsequent studies using cell culture–adapted attenuated FIPV in sows by the same routes of inoculation resulted in higher litter mortality (52%) and low TGEV antibody titers of the IgG class in milk (Woods 1984).

Vaccination of TGEV-Infected Swine. Vaccines have been used on two populations of pregnant swine: those that have, and those that have not, previously been naturally infected with TGEV or PRCV. There are significant differences in the immune responses and, consequently, piglet protection in these two groups of animals following vaccination. These differences may account for some of the discrepant results seen in vaccine challenge studies, if previously infected swine were unknowingly used. This possibility can be eliminated only by using a very sensitive test (such as plaque reduction VN) to measure TGEV/PRCV antibodies and by knowing the herd history of test animals in terms of previous TGE outbreaks. Occurrence of PRCV in herds further complicate TGEV vaccine studies.

Limited laboratory research has indicated that parenteral inoculation of previously infected swine during gestation using attenuated TGEV resulted in a boost in TGEV milk antibodies in both the IgA and IgG classes (Saif and Bohl 1981a, b, 1983; Saif and Smith 1985). Others have also reported increased milk TGEV antibody titers (4–7-fold) after intramammary inoculation of previously infected swine with inactivated TGEV (Thorsen and Djurickovic 1971). Currently available parenterally administered TGEV vaccines may be more effective in boosting immunity in previously TGEV or PRCV infected pregnant swine than in initiating immunity in previously uninfected seronegative pregnant swine. These vaccines may be especially useful in herds in which endemic TGE is a problem (Leopoldt and Meyer 1978; Stepanek 1979).

PRCV Maternal Vaccines to Prevent TGE. Since PRCV became widespread in the European swine herds, the incidence and severity of TGE in countries with PRCV have declined (Laude et al. 1993; Pensaert and Cox 1989). This suggests that previous exposure of swine to PRCV imparts partial immunity to TGE (Pensaert 1989; Pensaert and Cox 1989).

A number of researchers have examined the relationship between PRCV infection of sows and passive immunity to TGEV in piglets. Prior natural exposure of sows to PRCV induced a variable degree (44–53% mortality) of passive protection against experimental TGEV challenge of suckling pigs (Bernard et al. 1989; Paton and Brown 1990). Variable protection in the field during TGE outbreaks was also noted among litters of PRCV-exposed sows (Callebaut et al. 1990; Pensaert and Cox

1989). Similar variable levels of protection (30–67% mortality) were reported after TGEV challenge of piglets suckling sows that had been experimentally infected or reinfected with PRCV during pregnancy (Callebaut et al. 1990; De Diego et al. 1992; Lanza et al. 1995; Sestak et al. 1996; Wesley and Woods 1993). Noteworthy in the latter two studies, litter mortality was lowest (range = 0–27%) and IgA and IgG milk antibody titers were highest, in sows multiply exposed to PRCV during two subsequent pregnancies. These experimental findings agree with other reports (Callebaut et al. 1990) that naturally PRCV-exposed sows that are reinfected with PRCV during pregnancy secreted IgA TGEV antibodies in milk and provided a high degree of protection (0–12.5% mortality) to TGEV challenge.

Besides levels of IgA antibodies in milk, a hallmark of protection in these and another study (Wesley and Woods 1993) of passive immunity to TGEV induced by PRCV appeared to be induction of active immunity to TGEV in the sow, preventing illness and/or agalactia. Diarrhea mortality was consistently lower in litters of PRCV-exposed sows that did not become ill or develop agalactia after TGEV challenge of their litters.

The mechanism for the induction of IgA antibodies observed inconsistently in the milk of PRCV-exposed sows is unclear, as is the correlation of such antibodies with passive protection to TGEV challenge (Callebaut et al. 1990; Pensaert and Cox 1989). After a primary exposure to PRCV, IgA antibodies occurred in the milk of only 30% of sows; this percentage increased to 84% in sows reinfected with PRCV. These results concur with a report by Sestak et al. (1996) that the titers of IgA (and IgG) antibodies to TGEV were significantly increased in the milk of sows multiply exposed to PRCV during two sequential pregnancies. The variable IgA antibody responses observed in the milk of sows after primary exposure to PRCV could relate to the low numbers of virus-specific IgA ASCs observed in BALT, GALT, and mesenteric lymph nodes of seronegative pigs exposed to PRCV (VanCott et al. 1993, 1994). Repeated PRCV infections may be necessary to boost numbers of IgA ASCs in BALT and to increase the efficiency of a possible sIgA immunologic link between BALT and the mammary gland. Because IgG antibodies are also prevalent in the milk of sows exposed to other viruses that replicate in the respiratory tract, e.g., attenuated TGEV strains and pseudorabies virus (Saif and Bohl 1977), it is conceivable that an IgG immunologic link may also exist between BALT and the mammary gland in sows, or alternatively, BALT stimulation contributes serum IgG antibodies that are subsequently transudated into the milk.

Besides quantitative differences in the levels of IgA antibodies induced in milk after exposure to TGEV or PRCV, researchers have investigated potential differences in virus epitopes recognized by the IgA milk antibodies induced after TGEV versus PRCV infection of sows (De Diego et al. 1992, 1994). In TGEV-infected sows, antigenic subsite A (Aa, Ab, Ac), followed by antigenic subsite D (Madrid), was the best inducer of IgA antibodies, whereas after PRCV infection, antigenic site D and subsite Ab were immunodominant. These authors concluded that only IgA recognizing at least antigenic sites A and D conferred good protection in vivo, whereas any Ig class recognizing only one antigenic site neutralized virus in cell culture.

Clearly, additional studies are necessary to clarify the levels and mechanisms of active and passive immunity to TGEV established in swine by previous exposure to PRCV. In particular, it is important to elucidate the mechanism by which IgA antibodies are induced after infection with PRCV, whether a BALT-mammary gland immunologic link exists but is less efficient than the gut-mammary link for induction of IgA in milk, why IgA antibodies occur only in some PRCV-exposed sows, and the effectiveness of these IgA antibodies in protecting suckling pigs against intestinal TGEV infections.

New Vaccine Approaches. With existing vaccines being either too attenuated or applied at a dose that is too low, protection is inconsistent (Saif 1996; Saif and Jackwood 1990; Shoup et al. 1997; VanCott et al. 1993) and the search for more reliable vaccines continues. For protection of suckling piglets, research continues to focus on the principle of colostral and lacteal intake of IgA antibodies after immunization of sows with live attenuated vaccines (Park et al. 1998; Saif 1996; Sestak et al. 1999a).

During the last decade, emphasis has been on the construction of TGEV protein subunit vaccines. Among the three major structural proteins of TGEV, the S protein contains immunodominant epitopes that are recognized by virus-neutralizing antibodies (Delmas et al. 1986; Jimenez et al. 1986). Some of these epitopes were shown to be continuous domains (Delmas and Laude 1990; Gebauer et al. 1991; Posthumus et al. 1990), prompting the design of antigenic synthetic peptides derived from the S protein (Posthumus et al. 1991). It was found that the N protein contains the major T helper cell epitopes (Anton et al. 1995). A synthetic 15-mer peptide epitope derived from the N protein was shown to cooperate with the S protein for in vitro induction of TGEV-specific antibody (Anton et al. 1996).

To express the TGEV S, M, or N proteins, several prokaryotic and eukaryotic systems such as *E. coli*, salmonella, adenovirus, vaccinia virus, baculovirus, and plants were used (Britton et al. 1987; Enjuanes et al. 1992; Godet et al. 1991; Gomez et al. 2000; Park et al. 1998; Pulford and Britton 1991; Shoup et al. 1997; Smerdou et al. 1996a; Smerdou et al. 1996b; Torres et al. 1996; Tuboly et al. 1994, 2000). In some studies, protective antibodies were induced in inoculated animals, correlating with partial protection (Torres et al. 1995). In other studies, no induction of protective antibodies was reported (Gomez et al. 1998, 2000; Smerdou et al.

1996a, b; Tuboly et al. 2000) or only serum IgG virus-neutralizing antibodies were induced (Park et al. 1998; Shoup et al. 1997)

When prokaryotic vectors (*E. coli*) including live vectors (attenuated salmonella) were used to express the TGEV S gene or S gene fragments, low or no neutralizing antibodies were induced in mice (Hu et al. 1985), rabbits (Smerdou et al. 1996a), or pigs (Sestak and Schifferli, unpublished, 2004). These failures were attributed to loss or lack of the glycosylation-dependent conformational immunodominant site A in the bacterial expressed S proteins.

Various levels of neutralizing antibodies and protection were induced using eukaryotic vectors to express the TGEV S glycoprotein encoding the glycosylation-dependent antigenic determinants (sites A, B) with or without sites C and D.

The S glycoprotein of TGEV expressed in vaccinia virus induced low titers of neutralizing antibodies, but no protection (Hu et al. 1985). The baculovirus-expressed S protein induced virus neutralizing antibodies to TGEV, detected in the serum of rats and pigs (Shoup et al. 1997; Tuboly et al. 1995). However, the protective ability of these systemic antibodies was low(Godet et al. 1991; Shoup et al. 1997; Tuboly et al. 1995). Only S glycoprotein constructs containing antigenic site A induced high neutralizing antibody titers. S fragments containing sites C and D induced only low titer neutralizing antibodies, but interestingly, they primed pigs for secondary serum antibody responses after challenge (Shoup et al. 1997). When the baculovirus-expressed S glycoprotein with incomplete Freund's adjuvant was administered intramammarily and IM to TGEV seronegative pregnant sows, only low titer IgG antibodies to TGEV were detected in sows' colostrum and milk (Shoup et al. 1997). There was no significant decrease in morbidity or mortality after TGEV challenge exposure of litters from these sows (Shoup et al. 1997).

Similar findings were evident in studies using the same baculovirus-expressed S constructs administered IM to boost antibody responses in sows orally vaccinated with attenuated TGEV vaccines: the S glycoprotein vaccine generated antibody titers in colostrum/milk and partial protection rates (43% mortality) comparable to IM boosting with attenuated TGEV vaccine (57% mortality) (Park et al. 1998). In studies using baculovirus-expressed TGEV structural proteins (S, N, and M) coadministered IP with *E. coli* mutant LT-adjuvant, immune responses associated with IgA antibodies to TGEV were associated with reduced TGEV shedding in the feces of challenged pigs (Sestak et al. 1999a).

Live vectored vaccines expressing TGEV S protein fragments have also been evaluated. A human adenovirus 5 engineered to express the TGEV S protein sites A–D and a smaller fragment expressing sites B+C induced serum neutralizing antibodies in pigs inoculated oronasally and IP (Torres et al. 1996). When newborn

piglets passively fed the immune serum were orally challenged with the immune serum-TGEV mixture, only pigs fed immune serum from swine vaccinated with the S constructs with sites A–D were passively protected against TGE mortality and partially protected against infection.

Other researchers developed a recombinant human adenovirus vector expressing the full length S protein of PRCV (Callebaut et al. 1996). Pigs inoculated oronasally with the recombinant adenovirus S vaccine were not protected against PRCV nasal shedding after PRCV challenge, but they had shorter shedding and a rapid anamnestic neutralizing antibody response to PRCV. In other studies, a porcine adenovirus 5 expressing the TGEV S glycoprotein was used for oral immunization of pigs (Tuboly and Nagy 2001). Although IgA antibodies to TGEV were induced in the intestines of the inoculated pigs, the pigs shed TGEV in feces after challenge (Callebaut et al. 1996).

Recent studies with TGEV infectious cDNA minigenomes indicate that this approach can also be exploited for targeted delivery of immunogens derived from other pathogens to the intestine or respiratory tract (Alonso et al. 2002; Gonzalez et al. 2002; Sola et al. 2003). When nonessential TGEV open reading frames 3a or 3b were replaced by a heterologous green fluorescence gene it was shown that the virus retained immunogenic and also enteropathogenic properties (Sola et al. 2003).

Since the pathology of TGEV remains localized in the intestine, an effective vaccine should primarily elicit an intestinal immune response that can be targeted by oronasal immunizations with adequate doses and forms of attenuated vaccines (Saif and Jackwood 1990; VanCott et al. 1993). Further improvements of TGEV vaccines might be achieved by the use of supplementary mucosal delivery systems such as immunostimulating complexes (ISCOMs), biodegradable microspheres, or infectious recombinant TGEV clones engineered to enhance TGEV immunogenicity and reduce pathogenicity.

REFERENCES

Abou-Youssef MF, Ristic M. 1972. Distribution of antibodies to transmissible gastroenteritis virus in serum and milk of sows: Isolation and identification of the immunoglobulin classes of swine serum and milk. Am J Vet Res 33:975–979.

Ackerman LJ, Morehouse LG, Olson LD. 1972. Transmissible gastroenteritis in three-week-old pigs: Study of anemia and iron absorption. Am J Vet Res 33:115–120.

Alonso S, Sola I, Teifke JP, Reimann I, Izeta A, Balasch M, Plana-Duran J, Moormann RJ, Enjuanes L. 2002. In vitro and in vivo expression of foreign genes by transmissible gastroenteritis coronavirus-derived minigenomes. J Gen Virol 83:567–579.

Anton IM, Gonzalez S, Bullido MJ, Corsin M, Risco C, Langeveld JP, Enjuanes L. 1996. Cooperation between transmissible gastroenteritis coronavirus (TGEV) structural proteins in the in vitro induction of virus-specific antibodies. Virus Res 46:111–124.

Anton IM, Sune C, Meloen RH, Borras-Cuesta F, Enjuanes L. 1995. A transmissible gastroenteritis coronavirus nucleoprotein epitope elicits T helper cells that collaborate in the in vitro antibody synthesis to the three major structural viral proteins. Virology 212:746–751.

Aynaud JM, Nguyen TD, Bottreau E, Brun A, Vannier P. 1985. Transmissible gastroenteritis (TGE) of swine: Survivor selection of TGE virus mutants in stomach juice of adult pigs. J Gen Virol 66:1911–1917.

Bae I, Jackwood DJ, Benfield DA, Saif LJ, Wesley RD, Hill H. 1991. Differentiation of transmissible gastroenteritis virus from porcine respiratory coronavirus and other antigenically related coronaviruses by using cDNA probes specific for the 5' region of the S glycoprotein gene. J Clin Microbiol 29:215–218.

Ballesteros ML, Sanchez CM, Enjuanes L. 1997. Two amino acid changes at the N-terminus of transmissible gastroenteritis coronavirus spike protein result in the loss of enteric tropism. Virol 227:378–388.

Bay WW, Doyle LP, Hutchings LM. 1952. Some properties of the causative agent of transmissible gastroenteritis in swine. Am J Vet Res 13:378–388.

——. 1953. Transmissible gastroenteritis in swine: A study of immunity. J Am Vet Med Assoc 122:200–202.

Becker W, Teufel P, Mields W. 1974. The immunoperoxidase method for detection of viral and chlamydial antigens. III. Demonstration of TGE antigen in pig thyroid cell cultures. Zentralbl Veterinarmed B 21:59–65.

Benfield DA, Jackwood DJ, Bac I, Saif LJ, Wesley RD. 1991. Detection of transmissible gastroenteritis virus using cDNA probes. Arch Virol 116:91–106.

Bernard S, Bottreau E, Aynaud JM, Have P, Szymansky J. 1989. Natural infection with the porcine respiratory coronavirus induces protective lactogenic immunity against transmissible gastroenteritis. Vet Microbiol 21:1–8.

Bernard S, Lantier I, Laude H, Aynaud JM. 1986. Detection of transmissible gastroenteritis coronavirus antigens by a sandwich enzyme-linked immunosorbent assay technique. Am J Vet Res 47:2441–2444.

Bernard S, Laude H. 1995. Site-specific alteration of transmissible gastroenteritis virus spike protein results in markedly reduced pathogenicity. J Gen Virol 76:2235–2241.

Berthon P, Bernard S, Salmon H, Binns RM. 1990. Kinetics of the in vitro antibody response to transmissible gastroenteritis (TGE) virus from pig mesenteric lymph node cells, using the ELISAS-POT and ELISA tests. J Immunol Methods 131:173–182.

Black JW. 1971. Diagnosis of TGE by FA: Evaluation of accuracy on field specimens. Proc US Anim Health Assoc 75:492–498.

Bohl EH. 1979. Diagnosis of diarrhea in pigs due to transmissible gastroenteritis virus or rotavirus. In Viral Enteritis in Humans and Animals. F Bricout, R Scherrer, eds. INSERM (Paris) 90:341–343.

——. 1981. Coronaviruses: Diagnosis of infections. In Comparative Diagnosis of Viral Diseases, Volume 4. E Kurstak, C Kurstak, eds. New York: Academic Press, pp. 301–328.

Bohl EH, Gupta RK, Olquin MV, Saif LJ. 1972. Antibody responses in serum, colostrum, and milk of swine after infection or vaccination with transmissible gastroenteritis virus. Infect Immun 6:289–301.

Bohl EH, Kohler EM, Saif LJ, Cross RF, Agnes AG, Theil KW. 1978. Rotavirus as a cause of diarrhea in pigs. J Am Vet Med Assoc 172:458–463.

Bohl EH, Kumagai T. 1965. The use of cell cultures for the study of swine. Proc US Livest Sanit Assoc 69:343–350.

Bohl EH, Saif LJ. 1975. Passive immunity in transmissible gastroenteritis of swine: Immunoglobulin characteristics of antibodies in milk after inoculating virus by different routes. Infect Immun 11:23–32.

Bohl EH, Saif LJ, Jones JE. 1982. Observations on the occurrence of transmissible gastroenteritis (TGE) in a vaccinated herd. Ohio Swine Res Ind Rep, Anim Sci Ser 82-1, Ohio State Univ., pp. 66–69.

Bourgueil E, Hutet E, Cariolet R, Vannier P. 1992. Experimental infection of pigs with the porcine respiratory coronavirus (PRCV): Measure of viral excretion. Vet Microbiol 31:11–8.

Bourne FJ. 1973. Symposium on nutrition of the young farm animal: The immunoglobulin system of the suckling pig. Proc Nutr Soc 32:205–214.

Brian DA, Dennis DE, Guy JS. 1980. Genome of porcine transmissible gastroenteritis virus. J Virol 34:410–415.

Brim TA, VanCott JL, Lunney JK, Saif LJ. 1994. Lymphocyte proliferation responses of pigs inoculated with transmissible gastroenteritis virus or porcine respiratory coronavirus. Am J Vet Res 55:494–501.

——. 1995. Cellular immune responses of pigs after primary inoculation with porcine respiratory coronavirus or transmissible gastroenteritis virus and challenge with transmissible gastroenteritis virus. Vet Immunol Immunopathol 48:35–54.

Britton P, Garwes DJ, Page K, Walmsley J. 1987. Expression of porcine transmissible gastroenteritis virus genes in E. coli as beta-galactosidase chimaeric proteins. Adv Exp Med Biol 218:55–64.

Britton P, Kottier S, Chen CM, Pocock DH, Salmon H, Aynaud JM. 1994. The use of PCR genome mapping for the characterization of TGEV strains. Adv Exp Med Biol 342:29–34.

Britton P, Mawditt KL, Page KW. 1991. The cloning and sequencing of the virion protein genes from a British isolate of porcine respiratory coronavirus: Comparison with transmissible gastroenteritis virus genes. Virus Res 21:181–198.

Brown I, Cartwright S. 1986. New porcine coronavirus? Vet Rec 119:282–3.

Brown IH, Paton DJ. 1991. Serological studies of transmissible gastroenteritis in Great Britain, using a competitive ELISA. Vet Rec 128:500–503.

Brown TT. 1981. Laboratory evaluation of selected disinfectants as viricidal agents against porcine parvovirus, pseudorabies virus, and transmissible gastroenteritis virus. Am J Vet Res 42:1033–1036.

Butler DG, Gall DG, Kelly MH, Hamilton JR. 1974. Transmissible gastroenteritis. Mechanisms responsible for diarrhea in an acute viral enteritis in piglets. J Clin Invest 53:1335–1342.

Callebaut P, Correa I, Pensaert M, Jimenez G, Enjuanes L. 1988. Antigenic differentiation between transmissible gastroenteritis virus of swine and a related porcine respiratory coronavirus. J Gen Virol 69:1725–1730.

Callebaut P, Cox E, Pensaert M, Van Deun K. 1990. Induction of milk IgA antibodies by porcine respiratory coronavirus infection. Adv Exp Med Biol 276:421–428.

Callebaut P, Enjuanes L, Pensaert M. 1996. An adenovirus recombinant expressing the spike glycoprotein of porcine respiratory coronavirus is immunogenic in swine. J Gen Virol 77:309–313.

Callebaut P, Pensaert MB, Hooyberghs J. 1989. A competitive inhibition ELISA for the differentiation of serum antibodies from pigs infected with transmissible gastroenteritis virus (TGEV) or with the TGEV-related porcine respiratory coronavirus. Vet Microbiol 20:9–19.

Cartwright SF. 1968. Transmissible gastroenteritis of swine (TGE). Br Vet J 124:410–413.

Cartwright SF, Harris HM, Blandfold TB, Fingham I, Glitter M. 1965. A cytopathic virus causing a transmissible gastroenteritis in swine. I. Isolation amd properties. J Comp Pathol 75:386–395.

Cepica A, Derbyshire JB. 1983. Antibody-dependent cell-mediated cytotoxicity and spontaneous cell-mediated cytotoxicity against cells infected with porcine transmissible gastroenteritis virus. Can J Comp Med 47:298–303.

——. 1984. Antibody-dependent and spontaneous cell-mediated cytotoxicity against transmissible gastroenteritis virus infected cells by lymphocytes from sows, fetuses and neonatal piglets. Can J Comp Med 48:258–61.

Charley B, Laude H. 1988. Induction of alpha interferon by transmissible gastroenteritis coronavirus: Role of transmembrane glycoprotein E1. J Virol 62:8–11.

Chen KS. 1985. Enzymatic and acidic sensitivity profiles of selected virulent and attenuated transmissible gastroenteritis viruses of swine. Am J Vet Res 46:632–6.

Chu RM, Glock RD, Ross RF. 1982a. Changes in gut-associated lymphoid tissues of the small intestine of eight-week-old pigs infected with transmissible gastroenteritis virus. Am J Vet Res 43:67–76.

Chu RM, Li NJ, Glock RD, Ross RF. 1982b. Application of peroxidase staining techinique for detection of transmissible gastroenteritis virus in pigs. Am J Vet Res 43:77–81.

Cornaglia E, Chretien N, Charara S, Elazhary Y. 1994. Detection of porcine respiratory coronavirus and transmissible gastroenteritis virus by an enzyme-linked immunosorbent assay. Vet Microbiol 42:349–59.

Correa I, Gebauer F, Bullido MJ, Sune C, Baay MF, Zwaagstra KA, Posthumus WP, Lenstra JA, Enjuanes L. 1990. Localization of antigenic sites of the E2 glycoprotein of transmissible gastroenteritis coronavirus. J Gen Virol 71:271–279.

Costantini V, Lewis P, Alsop J, Templeton C, Saif LJ. 2004. Respiratory and fecal shedding of porcine respiratory coronavirus (PRCV) in sentinel weaned pigs and sequence of the partial S-gene of the PRCV isolates. Arch Virol 149:957–974.

Cox E, Hooyberghs J, Pensaert MB. 1990a. Sites of replication of a porcine respiratory coronavirus related to transmissible gastroenteritis virus. Res Vet Sci 48:165–169.

Cox E, Pensaert MB, Callebaut P. 1993. Intestinal protection against challenge with transmissible gastroenteritis virus of pigs immune after infection with the porcine respiratory coronavirus. Vaccine 11:267–72.

Cox E, Pensaert MB, Callebaut P, van Deun K. 1990b. Intestinal replication of a porcine respiratory coronavirus closely related antigenically to the enteric transmissible gastroenteritis virus. Vet Microbiol 23:237–243.

Cummins JM, Mock RE, Shive BW, Krakowka S, Richards AB, Hutcheson DP. 1995. Oral treatment of transmissible gastroenteritis with natural human interferon alpha: A field study. Vet Immunol Immunopathol 45:355–360.

DeBouck P, Callebaut P, Pensaert M. 1982. Prevalence of the porcine epidemic diarrhea (PED) virus in the pig population of different countries. Proc Int Congr Pig Vet Soc 7:45.

De Diego M, Laviada MD, Enjuanes L, Escribano JM. 1992. Epitope specificity of protective lactogenic immunity against swine transmissible gastroenteritis virus. J Virol 66:6502–6508.

De Diego M, Rodriguez F, Alcaraz C, Gomez N, Alonso C, Escribano JM. 1994. Characterization of the IgA and subclass IgG responses to neutralizing epitopes after infection of pregnant sows with the transmissible gastroenteritis virus or the antigenically related porcine respiratory coronavirus. J Gen Virol 97:2585–2593.

Delmas B, Gelfi J, Laude H. 1986. Antigenic structure of transmissible gastroenteritis virus. II. Domains in the peplomer glycoprotein. J Gen Virol 67:1405–1418.

Delmas B, Gelfi J, L'Haridon R, Vogel LK, Sjostrom H, Noren O, Laude H. 1992. Aminopeptidase N is a major receptor for the entero-pathogenic coronavirus TGEV. Nature 357:417–420.

Delmas B, Laude H. 1990. Assembly of coronavirus spike protein into trimers and its role in epitope expression. J Virol 64:5367–5375.

Derbyshire JB, Jessett DM, Newman G. 1969. An experimental epidemiological study of porcine transmissible gastroenteritis. J Comp Pathol 79:445–452.

Dimitrov P. 1982. Effect of amantadine on different stages of replication of porcine transmissible gastroenteritis virus. Vet Med Nauki 19:90–96.

Doyle LP, Hutchings LM. 1946. A transmissible gastronenteritis in pigs. J Am Vet Med Assoc 108:257–259.

Drosten C, Gunther S, Preiser W, van der Werf S, Brodt HR, Becker S, Rabenau H, Panning M, Kolesnikova L, Fouchier RA, Berger A, Burguiere AM, Cinatl J, Eickmann M, Escriou N, Grywna K, Kramme S, Manuguerra JC, Muller S, Rickerts V, Sturmer M, Vieth S, Klenk HD, Osterhaus AD, Schmitz H, Doerr HW. 2003. Identification of a novel coronavirus in patients with severe acute respiratory syndrome. N Engl J Med 348:1967–1976.

Dulac GC, Ruckerbauer GM, Boulanger P. 1977. Transmissible gastroenteritis: Demonstration of the virus from field specimens by means of cell culture and pig inoculation. Can J Comp Med 41:357–363.

Egan IT, Harris DL, Hill HT. 1982. Prevalence of swine dysentery, transmissible gastroenteritis, and pseudorabies in Iowa, Illinois and Missouri swine. Proc 86th Annu Meet US Anim Health Assoc, pp. 497–502.

Eleouet JF, Rasschaert D, Lambert P, Levy L, Vende P, Laude H. 1995. Complete sequence (20 kilobases) of the polyprotein-encoding gene 1 of transmissible gastroenteritis virus. Virology 206:817–822.

Enjuanes L, Sune C, Gebauer F, Smerdou C, Camacho A, Anton IM, Gonzalez S, Talamillo A, Mendez A, Ballesteros ML, et al. 1992. Antigen selection and presentation to protect against transmissible gastroenteritis coronavirus. Vet Microbiol 33:249–262.

Enjuanes L, Van der Zeist BAM. 1995. Molecular basis of transmissible gastroenteritis virus epidemiology. In The *Coronavidae*. SG Siddell, ed. New York: Plenum Press, pp. 337–376.

Fichtner D, Leopoldt D, Meyer U. 1982. Untersuchungen zur Ermittlung der minimalen Antigenmenge bei der oralen Muttertierimmunisierung gegen die Transmissible Gastroenteritis der Schweine mit Riemser TGE-Vakzine. Arch Exp Veterinarmed 36:577–585.

Frederick GT, Bohl EH, Cross RF. 1976. Pathogenicity of an attenuated strain of transmissible gastroenteritis virus for newborn pigs. Am J Vet Res 37:165–9.

Furuuchi S, Shimizu Y, Kumagai T. 1975. Comparison of properties between virulent and attenuated strains of transmissible gastroenteritis virus. Natl Inst Anim Health Q (Tokyo) 15:159–64.

——. 1976. Vaccination of newborn pigs with an attenuated strain of transmissible gastroenteritis virus. Am J Vet Res 37:1401–4.

——. 1979. Multiplication of low and high cell culture passaged strains of transmissible gastroenteritis virus in organs of newborn piglets. Vet Microbiol 3:169–178.

Furuuchi S, Shimizu M, Shimizu Y. 1978. Field trials on transmissible gastroenteritis live virus vaccine in newborn piglets. Natl Inst Anim Health Q (Tokyo) 18:135–142.

Garwes DJ, Pocock DH. 1975. The polypeptide structure of transmissible gastroenteritis virus. J Gen Virol 29:25–34.

Garwes DJ, Stewart F, Cartwright SF, Brown I. 1988. Differentiation of porcine coronavirus from transmissible gastroenteritis virus. Vet Rec 122:86–87.

Garwes DJ, Stewart F, Elleman CJ. 1987. Identification of epitopes of immunological importance on the peplomer of porcine transmissible gastroenteritis virus. Adv Exp Med Biol 218:509–515.

Gebauer F, Posthumus WP, Correa I, Sune C, Smerdou C, Sanchez CM, Lenstra JA, Meloen RH, Enjuanes L. 1991. Residues involved in the antigenic sites of transmissible gastroenteritis coronavirus S glycoprotein. Virology 183:225–238.

Godet M, Grosclaude J, Delmas B, Laude H. 1994. Major receptor-binding and neutralization determinants are located within the same domain of the transmissible gastroenteritis virus (coronavirus) spike protein. J Virol 68:8008–8016.

Godet M, L'Haridon R, Vautherot JF, Laude H. 1992. TGEV corona virus ORF4 encodes a membrane protein that is incorporated into virions. Virology 188:666–675.

Godet M, Rasschaert D, Laude H. 1991. Processing and antigenicity of entire and anchor-free spike glycoprotein S of coronavirus TGEV expressed by recombinant baculovirus. Virology 185:732–740.

Gomez N, Carrillo C, Salinas J, Parra F, Borca MV, Escribano JM. 1998. Expression of immunogenic glycoprotein S polypeptides from transmissible gastroenteritis coronavirus in transgenic plants. Virology 249:352–358.

Gomez N, Wigdorovitz A, Castanon S, Gil F, Ordas R, Borca MV, Escribano JM. 2000. Oral immunogenicity of the plant derived spike protein from swine-transmissible gastroenteritis coronavirus. Arch Virol 145:1725–1732.

Gonzalez JM, Penzes Z, Almazan F, Calvo E, Enjuanes L. 2002. Stabilization of a full-length infectious cDNA clone of transmissible gastroenteritis coronavirus by insertion of an intron. J Virol 76:4655–4661.

Gough PM, Jorgenson RD. 1983. Identification of porcine transmissible gastroenteritis virus in house flies (Musca domestica Linneaus). Am J Vet Res 44:2078–2082.

Graham JA Jr. 1980. Induction of active immunity to TGE in neonatal pigs nursing seropositive dams. Vet Med Small Anim Clin 75:1618–1619.

Granzow H, Meyer U, Solisch P, Lange E, Fichtner D. 1981. Die Morphologie der Koronaviren—Elektronenmikroskopische Darstellung des Virus der Transmissiblen Gastroenteritis des Schweines im Negativkontrastverfahren. Arch Exp Veterinarmed 35:177–186.

Haas B, Ahl R, Bohm R, Strauch D. 1995. Inactivation of viruses in liquid manure. Rev Sci Tech 14:435–445.

Haelterman EO. 1962. Epidemiological studies of transmissible gastroenteritis of swine. Proc US Livest Sanit Assoc 66:305–315.

——. 1963. Transmissible gastroenteritis of swine. Proc 17th World Vet Congr, Hannover 1:615–618.

Haelterman EO, Huchings LM. 1956. Epidemic diarrheal diseases of viral origin in newborn swine. Ann N Y Acad Sci 66:186–190.

Halbur PG, Paul PS, Vaughn EM. 1994. Virulent porcine respiratory coronavirus isolates exists in the United States. Proc Int Congr Pig Vet Soc 13:70.

Halbur PG, Paul PS, Vaughn EM, Andrews JJ. 1993. Experimental reproduction of pneumonia in gnotobiotic pigs with porcine respiratory coronavirus isolate AR310. J Vet Diag Invest 5:184–188.

Harada K, Kaki T, Kumagai T, Sasahara J. 1968. Studies on transmissible gastroenteritis in pigs. IV. Physicochemical and biological properties of TGE virus. Natl Inst Anim Health Q (Tokyo) 8:140–147.

Harris DLm Bevier GW, Wiseman BS. 1987. Eradication of transmissible gastroenteritis virus without depopulation. Proc Am Assoc Swine Pract, p. 555.

Have P, Moving V, Svansson V, Uttenthal A, Bloch B. 1992. Coronavirus infection in mink (Mustela vison). Serological evidence of infection with a coronavirus related to transmissible gastroenteritis virus and porcine epidemic diarrhea virus. Vet Microbiol 31:1–10.

Hayes J, Sestak K, Myers G, Kim L, Stromberg P, Byrum B, Mohan R, Saif LJ. 2000. Evaluation of dual infection of nursery pigs with U.S. strains of porcine reproductive and respiratory syndrome virus and porcine respiratory coronavirus. Proc VIIth Internat Symp Nidoviruses (Corona and Arteriviruses), Lake Harmony, Pennsylvania, pp. 58-63.

Henning ER, Thomas PC. 1981. Comparison of intramuscular and oral modified-live virus TGE vaccines. Vet Med Small Anim Clin 76:1789–1792.

Henningsen DM, Mousing J, Aalund O. 1989. Porcint corona virus (PCV) i Danmark: En epidemiologisk traersnitsanalyse data. Dansk Vet Tidsskr 71:1168–1177.

Hess RG, Bachmann PA, Hanichen T. 1977. Attempts to establish an immunoprevention of transmissible gastroenteritis (TGE) in

swine. I. Pathogenicity of the B1 strain following serial passages. Zentralbl Veterinarmed B 24:753–763.

Hess RG, Bachmann PA, Mayr A. 1978. Attempts to develop an immunoprevention against transmissible gastroenteritis (TGE) in pigs. III. Passive immunotransfer following oral vaccination of pregnant sows with the attenuated TGE virus strain B1. Zentralbl Veterinarmed B 25:308–318.

Hess RG. Chen YS, Bachmann PA. 1982. Active immunization of feeder pigs against transmissible gastroenteritis (TGE): Influence of maternal antibodies. Proc Int Congr Pig Vet Soc 7:1.

Hill H, Biwer J, Wood R, Wesley R. 1990. Porcine respiratory coronavirus isolated from two U.S. swine herds. Proc Am Assoc Swine Pract, p. 333.

Hohdatsu T, Eiguchi Y, Ide S, Baba K, Yamagishi H, Kume T, Matumoto M. 1987. Evaluation of an enzyme-linked immunosorbent assay for the detection of transmissible gastroenteritis virus antibodies. Vet Microbiol 13:93–97.

Hooper BE, Haelterman EO. 1966. Concepts of pathogenesis and passive immunity in transmissible gastroenteritis of swine. J Am Vet Med Assoc 149:1580–1586.

——. 1969. Lesions of the gastrointestinal tract of pigs infected with transmissible gastroenteritis. Can J Comp Med 33:29–36.

Hornich M, Salajka E, Stepanek J. 1977. Malabsorption in newborn piglets with diarrhoeic Escherichia coli infection and transmissible gastro-enteritis. Zentralbl Veterinarmed B 24:75–86.

Horzinek MC, Lutz H, Pedersen NC. 1982. Antigenic relationships among homologous structural polypeptides of porcine, feline, and canine coronaviruses. Infect Immun 37:1148–1155.

Hu S, Bruszewski J, Smalling R, Browne JK. 1985. Studies of TGEV spike protein gp195 expressed in E. coli and by a TGE-vaccinia virus recombinant. Adv Exp Med Biol 185:63–82. In Viral Enteritis in Humans and Animals. F Bricout, R Scherrer, eds. INSERM (Paris) 90:281–293.

Jabrane A, Girard C, Elazhary Y. 1994. Pathogenicity of porcine respiratory coronavirus isolated in Quebec. Can Vet J 35:86–92.

Jackwood DJ, Kwon HM, Saif LJ. 1995. Molecular differentiation of transmissible gastroenteritis virus and porcine respiratory coronavirus strains. Correlation with antigenicity and pathogenicity. Adv Exp Med Biol 380:35–41.

Jacobs L, de Groot R, van der Zeijst BA, Horzinek MC, Spaan W. 1987. The nucleotide sequence of the peplomer gene of porcine transmissible gastroenteritis (TGEV): Comparison with the sequence of the peplomer protein of feline infectious peritonitis virus (FIPV). Virus Res 8:363–371.

Jimenez G, Correa I, Melgosa MP, Bullido MJ, Enjuanes L. 1986. Critical epitopes in transmissible gastroenteritis virus neutralization. J Virol 60:131–139.

Kaji T, Shimizu Y. 1978. Passive immunization against transmissible gastroenteritis virus in piglets by ingestion of milk of sows inoculated with attenuated virus. Natl Inst Anim Health Q (Tokyo) 18:43–52.

Kapke PA, Brian DA. 1986. Sequence analysis of the porcine transmissible gastroenteritis coronavirus nucleocapsid protein gene. Virology 151:41–49.

Kemeny LJ. 1976. Antibody response in pigs inoculated with transmissible gastroenteritis virus and cross reactions among ten isolates. Can J Comp Med 40:209–214.

——. 1978. Isolation of transmissible gastroenteritis virus from pharyngeal swabs obtained from sows at slaughter. Am J Vet Res 39:703–705.

Kemeny LJ, Wiltsey VL, Riley JL. 1975. Upper respiratory infection of lactating sows with transmissible gastroenteritis virus following contact exposure to infected piglets. Cornell Vet 65:352–62.

Kemeny LJ, Woods RD. 1977. Quantitative transmissible gastroenteritis virus shedding patterns in lactating sows. Am J Vet Res 38:307–310.

Kim L, Chang KO, Sestak K, Parwani A, Saif LJ. 2000a. Development of a reverse transcription-nested polymerase chain reaction assay for differential diagnosis of transmissible gastroenteritis virus and porcine respiratory coronavirus from feces and nasal swabs of infected pigs. J Vet Diag Invest 12:385–388.

Kim L, Hayes J, Lewis P, Parwani AV, Chang KO, Saif LJ. 2000b. Molecular characterization and pathogenesis of transmissible gastroenteritis coronavirus (TGEV) and porcine respiratory coronavirus (PRCV) field isolates co-circulating in a swine herd. Arch Virol 145:1133–1147.

Kodama Y, Ogata M, Simizu Y. 1980. Characterization of immunoglobulin A antibody in serum of swine inoculated with transmissible gastroenteritis virus. Am J Vet Res 41:740–745.

Ksiazek TG, Erdman D, Goldsmith CS, Zaki SR, Peret T, Emery S, Tong S, Urbani C, Comer JA, Lim W, Rollin PE, Dowell SF, Ling AE, Humphrey CD, Shieh WJ, Guarner J, Paddock CD, Rota P, Fields B, DeRisi J, Yang JY, Cox N, Hughes JM, LeDuc JW, Bellini WJ, Anderson LJ. 2003. A novel coronavirus associated with severe acute respiratory syndrome. N Engl J Med 348:1953–1966.

La Bonnardiere C, Laude H. 1981. High interferon titer in newborn pig intestine during experimentally induced viral enteritis. Infect Immun 32:28–31.

Lai MM, Cavanagh D. 1997. The molecular biology of coronaviruses. Adv Virus Res 48:1–100.

Lanza I, Brown IH, Paton DJ. 1992. Pathogenicity of concurrent infection of pigs with porcine respiratory coronavirus and swine influenza virus. Res Vet Sci 53:309–314.

Lanza I, Rubio P, Munoz M, Carmenes P. 1993. Comparison of a monoclonal antibody capture ELISA (MACELISA) to indirect ELISA and virus neutralization test for the serodiagnosis of transmissible gastroenteritis virus. J Vet Diag Invest 5:21–25.

Lanza I, Shoup DI, Saif LJ. 1995. Lactogenic immunity and milk antibody isotypes to transmissible gastroenteritis virus in sows exposed to porcine respiratory coronavirus during pregnancy. Am J Vet Res 56:739–748.

Laude H, Chapsal JM, Gelfi J, Labiau S, Grosclaude J. 1986. Antigenic structure of transmissible gastroenteritis virus. I. Properties of monoclonal antibodies directed against virion proteins. J Gen Virol 67:119–130.

Laude H, Charley B, Gelfi J. 1984. Replication of transmissible gastroenteritis coronavirus (TGEV) in swine alveolar macrophages. J Gen Virol 65:327–332.

Laude H, Gelfi J, Aynaud JM. 1981. In vitro properties of low- and high-passaged strains of transmissible gastroenteritis coronavirus of swine. Am J Vet Res 42:447–449.

Laude H, Gelfi J, Lavenant L, Charley B. 1992. Single amino acid changes in the viral glycoprotein M affect induction of alpha interferon by the coronavirus transmissible gastroenteritis virus. J Virol 66:743–749.

Laude H, Gelfi J, Rasschaert D, Delmas B. 1988. Caracterisation antigenique du coronavirus respiratoireporcin à l'aide d'anticorps monoclonaux diriges contre le virus de la gastro-enterite transmissible. J Rech Porcine Fr 20:89–94.

Laude H, Van Reeth K, Pensaert M. 1993. Porcine respiratory coronavirus: Molecular features and virus-host interactions. Vet Res 24:125–150.

Laviada MD, Videgain SP, Moreno L, Alonso F, Enjuanes L, Escribano JM. 1990. Expression of swine transmissible gastroenteritis virus envelope antigens on the surface of infected cells: Epitopes externally exposed. Virus Res 16:247–254.

Lee KM, Moro M, Baker JA. 1954. Transmissible gastroenteritis in pigs. Am J Vet Res 15:364–372.

Leopoldt D, Meyer U. 1978. Transmissible gastroenteritis of swine as a model for infectious diarrhea. Arch Exp Veterinarmed 32:417–425.

Lesnick CE, Derbyshire JB. 1988. Activation of natural killer cells in newborn piglets by interferon induction. Vet Immunol Immunopathol 18:109–117.

Loewen KG, Derbyshire JB. 1988. The effect of interferon induction in parturient sows and newborn piglets on resistance to transmissible gastroenteritis. Can J Vet Res 52:149–153.

Lu W, Osorio FA, Rhodes MB, Moxley RA. 1991. A capture-enzyme immunoassay for rapid diagnosis of transmissible gastroenteritis virus. J Vet Diag Invest 3:119–123.

Maes RK, Haelterman EO. 1979. A seroepizootiologic study of five viruses in a swine-evaluation station. Am J Vet Res 40:1642–1645.

Marra MA, Jones SJ, Astell CR, Holt RA, Brooks-Wilson A, Butterfield YS, Khattra J, Asano JK, Barber SA, Chan SY, Cloutier A, Coughlin SM, Freeman D, Girn N, Griffith OL, Leach SR, Mayo M, McDonald H, Montgomery SB, Pandoh PK, Petrescu AS, Robertson AG, Schein JE, Siddiqui A, Smailus DE, Stott JM, Yang GS, Plummer F, Andonov A, Artsob H, Bastien N, Bernard K, Booth TF, Bowness D, Czub M, Drebot M, Fernando L, Flick R, Garbutt M, Gray M, Grolla A, Jones S, Feldmann H, Meyers A, Kabani A, Li Y, Normand S, Stroher U, Tipples GA, Tyler S, Vogrig R, Ward D, Watson B, Brunham RC, Krajden M, Petric M, Skowronski DM, Upton C, Roper RL. 2003. The genome sequence of the SARS-associated coronavirus. Science 300:1399–1404.

Martin MC, Casal J, Lanza I, Rubio P, Carmenes P. 1994. Porcine respiratory coronavirus spread in Catalunya, Spain, a previously infection-free area. Prev Vet Med 21:65–74.

Matisheck P, Emerson W, Searl RC. 1982. Results of laboratory and field tests of TGE vaccines. Vet Med Small Anim Clin 77:262–264.

McClurkin AW, Norman JO. 1966. Studies on transmissible gastroenteritis of swine. II. Selected characteristics of a cytopathogenic virus common to five isolates from transmissible gastroenteritis. Can J Comp Med Vet Sci 30:190–198.

McClurkin AW, Stark SL, Norman JO. 1970. Transmissible gastroenteritis (TGE) of swine: The possible role of dogs in the epizootiology of TGE. Can J Comp Med 34:347–349.

Moon HW. 1978. Mechanisms in the pathogenesis of diarrhea: A review. J the Am Vet Med Assoc 172:443–448.

Moon HW, Norman JO, Lambert G. 1973. Age dependent resistance to transmissible gastroenteritis of swine (TGE). I. Clinical signs and some mucosal dimensions in small intestine. Can J Comp Med 37:157–166.

Morin M, Solorzano RF, Morehouse LG, Olson L. 1978. The postulated role of feeder swine in the perpetuation of the transmissible gastroenteritis virus. Can J Comp Med 42:379–384.

Mousing J, Vagsholm I, Carpenter TE, Gardner IA, Herd DW. 1988. Financial impact of transmissible gastroenteritis in pigs. J Am Vet Med Assoc 192:756–759.

Moxley RA, Olson LD. 1989a. Clinical evaluation of transmissible gastroenteritis virus vaccines and vaccination procedures for inducing lactogenic immunity in sows. Am J Vet Res 50:111–118.

Moxley RA, Olson LR. 1989b. Lesions of transmissible gastroenteritis virus infection in experimentally inoculated pigs suckling immunized sows. Am J Vet Res 50:708–716.

Nagesha HS, Han MG, Saif LJ, Ksiasak TG, Anderson LJ, Haynes L. 2004. Antigenic relationships between human severe acute respiratory syndrome (SARS) and animal coronaviruses. Proceedings American Society for Virology, Abstract #7-4.

Nagura H, Nakane PK, Brown WR. 1978. Breast milk IgA binds to jejunal epithelium in suckling rats. J Immunol 120:1333–1339.

Nakao J, Hess RG, Bachmann PA, Mahnel H. 1978. Tenacity and inactivation of transmissible gastroenteritis (TGE) virus of pigs. Berl Munch Tierarztl Wochenschr 91:353–357.

Nelson LD, Kelling CL. 1984. Enzyme-linked immunosorbent assay for detection of transmissible gastroenteritis virus antibody in swine sera. Am J Vet Res 45:1654–1657.

Nguyen TD, Bottreau E, Bernard S, Lantier I, Aynaud JM. 1986. Neutralizing secretory IgA and IgG do not inhibit attachment of transmissible gastroenteritis virus. J Gen Virol 67:939–943.

Noble WA. 1964. Methods used to combat transmissible gastroenteritis. Vet Rec 76:51.

Noda M, Yamashita H, Koide F, Kadoi K, Omori T, Asagi M, Inaba Y. 1987. Hemagglutination with transmissible gastroenteritis virus. Arch Virol 96:109–115.

Norman JO, Lambert G, Moon HW, Stark SL. 1973. Age dependent resistance to transmissible gastroenteritis of swine (TGE). II. Coronavirus titer in tissues of pigs after exposure. Can J Comp Med 37:167–170.

O'Toole D, Brown I, Bridges A, Cartwright SF. 1989. Pathogenicity of experimental infection with 'pneumotropic' porcine coronavirus. Res Vet Sci 47:23–29.

Okaniwa A, Harada K, Park DK. 1968. Structure of swine transmissible gastroenteritis virus examined by negative staining. Natl Inst Anim Health Q (Tokyo) 8:175–181.

Onno M, Jestin A, Cariolet R, Vannier P. 1989. Rapid diagnosis of TGEV-like coronavirus in fattened pigs by indirect immunofluorescence labelling in nasal cells. Zentralbl Veterinarmed B 36:629–634.

Park S, Sestak K, Hodgins DC, Shoup DI, Ward LA, Jackwood DJ, Saif LJ. 1998. Immune response of sows vaccinated with attenuated transmissible gastroenteritis virus (TGEV) and recombinant TGEV spike protein vaccines and protection of their suckling pigs against virulent TGEV challenge exposure. Am J Vet Res 59:1002–1008.

Paton DJ, Brown IH. 1990. Sows infected in pregnancy with porcine respiratory coronavirus show no evidence of protecting their sucking piglets against transmissible gastroenteritis. Vet Res Commun 14:329–37.

Paul PS, Halbur PG, Vaughn EM. 1994. Significance of porcine respiratory coronavirus infection. Compend Contin Educ Pract Vet 16:1223–1234.

Paul PS, Mengeling WL, Saif LJ, Van Deresen RA. 1986. Detection of classes of antibodies to TGE and rotavirus of swine using monoclonal antibodies to porcine immunoglobulins. Proc Int Congr Pig Vet Soc 9:190.

Peiris JS, Lai ST, Poon LL, Guan Y, Yam LY, Lim W, Nicholls J, Yee WK, Yan WW, Cheung MT, Cheng VC, Chan KH, Tsang DN, Yung RW, Ng TK, Yuen KY. 2003. Coronavirus as a possible cause of severe acute respiratory syndrome. Lancet 361:1319–1325.

Pensaert MB. 1976. Transmissible gastroenteritis bij varkens. Tijdschr Diergeneeskd 101:165–177.

———. 1979. Immunity in TGE of swine after infection and vaccination.

———. 1989. Transmissible gastroenteritis virus (respiratory variant). In Virus Infections of Vertebrates, Vol 2. Virus Infections of Porcines. MB Pensaert, ed. Amsterdam: Elsevier Science Publishers BV, pp. 154–165.

Pensaert M, Callebaut P, Vergote J. 1986. Isolation of a porcine respiratory, non-enteric coronavirus related to transmissible gastroenteritis. Vet Quart 8:257–261.

Pensaert MB, Cox E. 1989. Porcine respiratory coronavirus related to transmissible gastroenteritis virus. Agri-Pract 10:17–21.

Pensaert M, Cox E, van Deun K, Callebaut P. 1993. A sero-epizootiological study of porcine respiratory coronavirus in Belgian swine. Vet Quart 15:16–20.

Pensaert MB, Debouck, P. 1978. A new coronaviruslike particle associated with diarrhea in swine. Arch Virol 58:243–247.

Pensaert M, Haelterman EO, Burnstein T. 1970a. Transmissible gastroenteritis of swine: Virus-intestinal cell interactions. I. Immunofluorescence, histopathology and virus production in the small intestine through the course of infection. Arch Gesamte Virusforsch 31:321–334.

Pensaert M, Haelterman EO, Hinsman EJ. 1970b. Transmissible gastroenteritis of swine: Virus-intestinal cell interactions. II. Electron microscopy of the epithelium in isolated jejunal loops. Arch Gesamte Virusforsch 31:335–351.

Phillip JI, Cartwright SF, Scott AC. 1971. The size and morphology of T.G.E. and vomiting and wasting disease viruses of pigs. Vet Rec 88:311–312.

Pike BV, Garwes DJ. 1977. Lipids of transmissible gastroenteritis virus and their relation to those of two different host cells. J Gen Virol 34:531–535.

Pilchard EI. 1965. Experimental transmission of transmissible gastroenteritis virus by starlings. Am J Vet Res 26:1177–9117.

Porter P, Allen WD. 1972. Classes of immunoglobulins related to immunity in the pig. J Am Vet Med Assoc 160:511–518.

Posthumus WP, Lenstra JA, Schaaper WM, van Nieuwstadt AP, Enjuanes L, Meloen RH. 1990. Analysis and simulation of a neutralizing epitope of transmissible gastroenteritis virus. J Virol 64:3304–3309.

Posthumus WP, Lenstra JA, van Nieuwstadt AP, Schaaper WM, van der Zeijst BA, Meloen RH. 1991. Immunogenicity of peptides simulating a neutralization epitope of transmissible gastroenteritis virus. Virology 182:371–375.

Potopal'skii AI, Spivak NIa, Shved AD, Mel'nichenko VS, Krasnova EF. 1983. Activity of certain chemopreparations with respect to the transmissible gastroenteritis virus and pig enterovirus. Mikrobiol Zh 45:75–78.

Pritchard GC. 1982. Observations on clinical aspects of transmissible gastroenteritis of pigs in Norfolk and Suffolk, 1980–81. Vet Rec 110:465–469.

———. 1987. Transmissible gastroenteritis in endemically infected breeding herds of pigs in East Anglia, 1981–85. Vet Rec 120:226–230.

Prochazka Z, Hampl J, Sedlacek M, Masek J, Stepanek J. 1975. Protein loss in piglets infected with transmissible gastroenteritis virus. Zentralbl Veterinarmed B 22:138–146.

Pulford DJ, Britton P. 1991. Intracellular processing of the porcine coronavirus transmissible gastroenteritis virus spike protein expressed by recombinant vaccinia virus. Virology 182:765–773.

Rasschaert D, Duarte M, Laude H. 1990. Porcine respiratory coronavirus differs from transmissible gastroenteritis virus by a few genomic deletions. J Gen Virol 71:2599–2607.

Redman DR, Bohl EH, Cross RF. 1978. Intrafetal inoculation of swine with transmissible gastroenteritis virus. Am J Vet Res 39:907–911.

Register KB, Wesley RD. 1994. Molecular characterization of attenuated vaccine strains of transmissible gastroenteritis virus. J Vet Diag Invest 6:16–22.

Reynolds DJ, Garwes DJ. 1979. Virus isolation and serum antibody responses after infection of cats with transmissible gastroenteritis virus. Brief report. Arch Virol 60:161–166.

Reynolds DJ, Garwes DJ, Lucey S. 1980. Differentiation of canine coronavirus and porcine transmissible gastroenteritis virus by neutralization with canine, porcine and feline sera. Vet Microbiol 5:283–290.

Risco C, Anton IM, Enjuanes L, Carrascosa JL. 1996. The transmissible gastroenteritis coronavirus contains a spherical core shell consisting of M and N proteins. J Virol 70:4773–4777.

Risco C, Anton IM, Sune C, Pedregosa AM, Martin-Alonso JM, Parra F, Carrascosa JL, Enjuanes L. 1995. Membrane protein molecules of transmissible gastroenteritis coronavirus also expose the carboxy-terminal region on the external surface of the virion. J Virol 69:5269–5277.

Rota PA, Oberste MS, Monroe SS, Nix WA, Campagnoli R, Icenogle JP, Penaranda S, Bankamp B, Maher K, Chen MH, Tong S, Tamin A, Lowe L, Frace M, DeRisi JL, Chen Q, Wang D, Erdman DD, Peret TC, Burns C, Ksiazek TG, Rollin PE, Sanchez A, Liffick S, Holloway B, Limor J, McCaustland K, Olsen-Rasmussen M, Fouchier R, Gunther S, Osterhaus AD, Drosten C, Pallansch MA, Anderson LJ, Bellini WJ. 2003. Characterization of a novel coronavirus associated wtih severe acute respiratory syndrome. Science 300:1394–1399.

Roux ME, McWilliams M, Phillips-Quagliata JM, Weisz-Carrington P, Lamm ME. 1977. Origin of IgA-secreting cells in the mammary gland. J Exp Med 146:1311–1322.

Saif LF, Bohl EH. 1977. Immunoglobulin classes of antibodies in milk of swine after intranasal exposure to pseudorabies virus or transmissible gastroenteritis virus. Infect Immun 16:961–966.

——. 1979a. Role of SIgA in passive immunity of swine to enteric viral infections. In Immunology of Breast Milk. PL Ogra, DH Dayton, eds. New York: Raven Press, pp. 237–248.

——. 1979b. Passive immunity in transmissible gastroenteritis of swine: Immunoglobulin classes of milk antibodies after oral-intranasal inoculations of sows with a live low cell culture–passaged virus. Am J Vet Res 10:115–117.

——. 1981a. Passive immunity against enteric viral infections. Proc 3rd Int Symp Neonatal Diarrhea. VIDO, Saskatoon, Canada.

——. 1981b. Experimental studies using TGE vaccines. Ohio Swine Res Ind Rep, Anim Sci Ser, 81-2, Ohio State University, pp. 58–59.

——. 1983. Passive immunity to transmissible gastroenteritis virus: Intramammary viral inoculation of sows. Ann N Y Acad Sci 409:708–723.

Saif LJ. 1976. The Immune Response of Swine to Transmissible Gastroenteritis Virus. Doctoral Thesis, Ohio State University.

——. 1996. Mucosal immunity: An overview and studies of enteric and respiratory coronavirus infections in a swine model of enteric disease. Vet Immunol Immunopathol 54:163–169.

Saif LJ, Bohl EH, Gupta RK. 1972. Isolation of porcine immunoglobulins and determination of the immunoglobulin classes of transmissible gastroenteritis viral antibodies. Infect Immun 6:600–609.

Saif LJ, Jackwood DJ. 1990. Enteric virus vaccines: Theoretical considerations, current status, and future approaches. In Viral Diarrheas of Man and Animals. LJ Saif, KW Theil, eds. Boca Raton, Florida: CRC Press, Inc., pp. 313–329.

Saif LJ, Smith KL. 1985. Enteric viral infections of calves and passive immunity. J Dairy Sci 68:206–28.

Saif LJ, van Cott JL, Brim TA. 1994. Immunity to transmissible gastroenteritis virus and porcine respiratory coronavirus infections in swine. Vet Immunol Immunopathol 43:89–97.

Sanchez CM, Izeta A, Sanchez-Morgado JM, Alonso S, Sola I, Balasch M, Plana-Duran J, Enjuanes L. 1999. Targeted recombination demonstrates that the spike gene of transmissible gastroenteritis coronavirus is a determinant of its enteric tropism and virulence. J Virol 73:7607–7618.

Sanchez CM, Jimenez G, Laviada MD, Correa I, Sune C, Bullido M, Gebauer F, Smerdou C, Callebaut P, Escribano JM, et al. 1990. Antigenic homology among coronaviruses related to transmissible gastroenteritis virus. Virology 174:410–417.

Schultze B, Krempl C, Ballesteros ML, Shaw L, Schauer R, Enjuanes L, Herrler G. 1996. Transmissible gastroenteritis coronavirus, but not the related porcine respiratory coronavirus, has a sialic acid (N-glycolylneuraminic acid) binding activity. J Virol 70:5634–5637.

Schwegmann-Wessels C, Zimmer G, Laude H, Enjuanes L, Herrler G. 2002. Binding of transmissible gastroenteritis coronavirus to cell surface sialoglycoproteins. J Virol 76:6037–6043.

Sestak K, Lanza I, Park SK, Weilnau PA, Saif LJ. 1996. Contribution of passive immunity to porcine respiratory coronavirus to protection against transmissible gastroenteritis virus challenge exposure in suckling pigs. Am J Vet Res 57:664–671.

Sestak K, Meister RK, Hayes JR, Kim L, Lewis PA, Myers G, Saif LJ. 1999a. Active immunity and T-cell populations in pigs intraperitoneally inoculated with baculovirus-expressed transmissible gastroenteritis virus structural proteins. Vet Immunol Immunopathol 70:203–221.

Sestak K, Zhou Z, Shoup DI, Saif LJ. 1999b. Evaluation of the baculovirus-expressed S glycoprotein of transmissible gastroenteritis virus (TGEV) as antigen in a competition ELISA to differentiate porcine respiratory coronavirus from TGEV antibodies in pigs. J Vet Diagn Invest 11:205–214.

Shibley GP, Salsbury DL, Djurickovic SM, Johnson G. 1973. Application of an intramammary route of vaccination against transmissible gastroenteritis in swine. Vet Med Small Anim Clin 68:59–61.

Shimizu M, Shimizu Y. 1979a. Effects of ambient temperatures on clinical and immune responses of pigs infected with transmissible gastroenteritis virus. Vet Microbiol 4:109–116.

——. 1979b. Demonstration of cytotoxic lymphocytes to virus-infected target cells in pigs inoculated with transmissible gastroenteritis virus. Am J Vet Res 40:208–213.

——. 1979c. Lymphocyte proliferative response to viral antigen in pigs infected with transmissible gastroenteritis virus. Infect Immun 23:239–243.

Shimizu M, Shimizu Y, Kodama Y. 1978. Effects of ambient temperatures on induction of transmissible gastroenteritis in feeder pigs. Infect Immun 21:747–752.

Shirai I, Lantier I, Bottreau E, Aynaud JM, Bernard S. 1988. Lactogenic immunity to transmissible gastroenteritis (TGE) of swine induced by the attenuated Nouzilly strain of TGE virus: Neutralizing antibody classes and protection. Ann Rech Vet 19:267–272.

Shockley LJ, Kapke PA, Lapps W, Brian DA, Potgieter LN, Woods R. 1987. Diagnosis of porcine and bovine enteric coronavirus infections using cloned cDNA probes. J Clin Microbiol 25:1591–1596.

Shoup DI, Jackwood DJ, Saif LJ. 1997. Active and passive immune responses to transmissible gastroenteritis virus (TGEV) in swine inoculated with recombinant baculovirus-expressed TGEV spike glycoprotein vaccines. Am J Vet Res 58:242–250.

Shoup DI, Swayne DE, Jackwood DJ, Saif LJ. 1996. Immuno-histochemistry of transmissible gastroenteritis virus antigens in fixed paraffin-embedded tissues. J Vet Diagn Invest 8:161–167.

Simkins RA, Weilnau PA, Bias J, Saif LJ. 1992. Antigenic variation among transmissible gastroenteritis virus (TGEV) and porcine respiratory coronavirus strains detected with monoclonal antibodies to the S protein of TGEV. Am J Vet Res 53:1253–1258.

Simkins RA, Weilnau PA, Van Cott J, Brim TA, Saif LJ. 1993. Competition ELISA, using monoclonal antibodies to the transmissible gastroenteritis virus (TGEV) S protein, for serologic differentiation of pigs infected with TGEV or porcine respiratory coronavirus. Am J Vet Res 54:254–259.

Smerdou C, Anton IM, Plana J, Curtiss R 3rd, Enjuanes L. 1996a. A continuous epitope from transmissible gastroenteritis virus S protein fused to E. coli heat-labile toxin B subunit expressed by attenuated Salmonella induces serum and secretory immunity. Virus Res 41:1–9.

Smerdou C, Urniza A, Curtis R III, Enjuanes L. 1996b. Characterization of transmissible gastroenteritis coronavirus S protein expression products in avirulent S. typhimurium delta cya delta crp: Persistence, stability and immune response in swine. Vet Microbiol 48:87–100.

Sola I, Alonso S, Zuniga S, Balasch M, Plana-Duran J, Enjuanes L. 2003. Engineering the transmissible gastroenteritis virus genome as an expression vector inducing lactogenic immunity. J Virol 77:4357–4369.

Stark SL, Fernelius AL, Booth GD, Lambert G. 1975. Transmissible gastroenteritis (TGE) of swine: Effect of age of swine testes cells culture monolayers on plaque assays of TGE virus. Can J Comp Med 39:466–468.

Stepanek J, Mensik J, Franz J, Hornich M. 1979. Epizootiology, diagnosis and prevention of viral diarrhoea in piglets under intensive husbandry conditions. Proc 21st World Vet Congr, Moscow, 6:43.

Stepanek J, Pospisil Z, Mesaros E. 1971. Growth activity of transmissible gastroenteritis (TGE) virus in primary cultures if pig kidney cells and pig salivary gland cells. Acta Vet Brno 40:235–240.

Stone SS, Kemeny LJ, Jensen MT. 1982. Serum antibody responses of neonatal and young adult pigs to transmissible gastroenteritis coronavirus. Vet Immunol Immunopathol 3:529–533.

Stone SS, Kemeny LJ, Woods RD, Jensen MT. 1977. Efficacy of isolated colostral IgA, IgG, and IgM(A) to protect neonatal pigs against the coronavirus of transmissible gastroenteritis. Am J Vet Res 38:1285–1288.

Sun ZF, Meng XJ. 2004. Antigenic cross-reactivity between the nucleocapsid protein of severe acute respiratory syndrome (SARS) coronavirus and polyclonal antisera of antigenic group I animal coronaviruses: Implication for SARS diagnosis. J Clin Microbiol 42:2351–2352.

Sune C, Jimenez G, Correa I, Bullido MJ, Gebauer F, Smerdou C, Enjuanes L. 1990. Mechanisms of transmissible gastroenteritis coronavirus neutralization. Virology 177:559–569.

Thake DC. 1968. Jejunal epithelium in transmissible gastroenteritis of swine. An electron microscopic and histochemical study. Am J Pathol 53:149–168.

Theil KW, Saif LJ, Bohl EH, Agnes AG, Kohler EM. 1979. Concurrent porcine rotaviral and transmissible gastroenteritis viral infections in a three-day-old conventional pig. Am J Vet Res 40:719–721.

Thomas J, Dulac GC. 1976. Transmissible gastroenteritis virus: Plaques and a plaque neutralization test. Can J Comp Med 40:171–174.

Thorsen J, Djurickovic S. 1971. Experimental immunization of sows with inactivated transmissible gastroenteritis (TGE) virus. Can J Comp Med 35:99–102.

Toma B, Benet JJ. 1976. A technique of research on microplates of the antibodies neutralizing transmissible gastroenteritis virus of swine. Rec Med Vet 152:565–568.

Torres JM, Alonso C, Ortega A, Mittal S, Graham F, Enjuanes L. 1996. Tropism of human adenovirus type 5-based vectors in swine and their ability to protect against transmissible gastroenteritis coronavirus. J Virol 70:3770–3780.

Torres JM, Sanchez C, Sune C, Smerdou C, Prevec L, Graham F, Enjuanes L. 1995. Induction of antibodies protecting against transmissible gastroenteritis coronavirus (TGEV) by recombinant adenovirus expressing TGEV spike protein. Virology 213:503–516.

Tuboly T, Nagy E. 2001. Construction and characterization of recombinant porcine adenovirus serotype 5 expressing the transmissible gastroenteritis virus spike gene. J Gen Virol 82:183–190.

Tuboly T, Nagy E, Dennis JR, Derbyshire JB. 1994. Immunogenicity of the S protein of transmissible gastroenteritis virus expressed in baculovirus. Arch Virol 137:55–67.

——. 1995. Passive protection of piglets by recombinant baculovirus induced transmissible gastroenteritis virus specific antibodies. Can J Vet Res 59:70–72.

Tuboly T, Yu W, Bailey A, Degrandis S, Du S, Erickson L, Nagy E. 2000. Immunogenicity of porcine transmissible gastroenteritis virus spike protein expressed in plants. Vaccine 18:2023–2028.

Underdahl NR, Mebus CA, Stair EL, Twiehaus MJ. 1972. The effect of cytopathogenic transmissible gastroenteritis-like viruses and/or *Escherichia coli* on germfree pigs. Can Vet J 13:9–16.

Underdahl NR, Mebus CA, Torres-Medina A. 1975. Recovery of transmissible gastroenteritis virus from chronically infected experimental pigs. Am J Vet Res 36:1473–1476.

Underdown BJ, Dorrington KJ. 1974. Studies on the structural and conformational basis for the relative resistance of serum and secretory immunoglobulin A to proteolysis. J Immunol 112:949–959.

USDA APHIS VS. 1992. National Animal Health Monitoring System Survey (Data Collection: 1989–1990). Tech Rep USDA APHIS VS.

van Nieuwstadt AP, Boonstra J. 1992. Comparison of the antibody response to transmissible gastroenteritis virus and porcine respiratory coronavirus, using monoclonal antibodies to antigenic sites A and X of the S glycoprotein. Am J Vet Res 53:184–190.

van Nieuwstadt AP, Cornelissen JB, Zetstra T. 1988. Comparison of two methods for detection of transmissible gastroenteritis virus in feces of pigs with experimentally induced infection. Am J Vet Res 49:1836–1843.

van Nieuwstadt AP, Pol JMA. 1989. Isolation of a TGE virus-related respiratory coronavirus causing fatal pneumonia in pigs. Vet Rec 124:43–44.

van Nieuwstadt AP, Zetstra T, Boonstra J. 1989. Infection with porcine respiratory coronavirus does not fully protect pigs against intestinal transmissible gastroenteritis virus. Vet Rec 125:58–60.

Van Reeth K, Nauwynck H, Pensaert M. 1996. Dual infections of feeder pigs with porcine reproductive and respiratory syndrome virus followed by porcine respiratory coronavirus or swine influenza virus: A clinical and virological study. Vet Microbiol 48:325–335.

——. 2000. A potential role for tumour necrosis factor-alpha in synergy between porcine respiratory coronavirus and bacterial lipopolysaccharide in the induction of respiratory disease in pigs. J Med Microbiol 49:613–620.

Van Reeth K, Pensaert M. 1992. Experimental infections with different porcine respiratory coronavirus field isolates: Clinical and virological aspects. Proc Int Congr Pig Vet Soc 12:152.

——. 1994a. Prevalence of infections with enzootic respiratory and enteric viruses in feeder pigs entering fattening herds. Vet Rec 135:594–597.

——. 1994b. Porcine respiratory coronavirus-mediated interference against influenza virus replication in the respiratory tract of feeder pigs. Am J Vet Res 55:1275–1281.

VanCott JL, Brim TA, Lunney JK, Saif LJ. 1994. Contribution of antibody-secreting cells induced in mucosal lymphoid tissues of pigs inoculated with respiratory or enteric strains of coronavirus to immunity against enteric coronavirus challenge. J Immunol 152:3980–3990.

VanCott JL, Brim TA, Simkins RA, Saif LJ. 1993. Isotype-specific antibody-secreting cells to transmissible gastroenteritis virus and porcine respiratory coronavirus in gut-and bronchus–associated lymphoid tissues of suckling pigs. J Immunol 150:3990–4000.

Vannier P. 1990. Disorders induced by the experimental infection of pigs with the porcine respiratory coronavirus (P.R.C.V.). Zentralbl Veterinarmed B 37:177–80.

Vannier P, Toma B, Madec F, Aynaud JM. 1982. Valuation of duration of TGE virus spread among sows of 2 infected herds by means of a serological survey of antibodies persistence. Proc Int Congr Pig Vet Soc 7:3.

Vaughn EM, Halbur PG, Paul PS. 1994. Three new isolates of porcine respiratory coronavirus with various pathogenicities and spike (S) gene deletions. J Clin Microbiol 32:1809–1812.

——. 1995. Sequence comparison of porcine respiratory coronavirus isolates reveals heterogeneity in the S, 3, and 3-1 genes. J Virol 69:3176–3184.

——. 1996. Use of nonradioactive cDNA probes to differentiate porcine respiratory coronavirus and transmissible gastroenteritis virus isolates. J Vet Diag Invest 8:241–244.

Voets MT, Pensaert M, Rondhuis PR. 1980. Vaccination of pregnant sows against transmissible gastroenteritis with two attenuated virus strains and different inoculation routes. Tijdschr Diergeneeskd 105:211–219.

Wagner JE, Beamer PD, Ristic M. 1973. Electron microscopy of intestinal epithelial cells of piglets infected with a transmissible gastroenteritis virus. Can J Comp Med 37:177–188.

Waxler GL. 1972. Lesions of transmissible gastroenteritis in the pig as determined by scanning electron microscopy. Am J Vet Res 33:1323–1328.

Weingartl HM, Copps J, Drebot MA, Marszal P, Smith G, Gren J, Andova M, Pasick J, Kitching P, Czub M. 2004. Susceptiblity of pigs and chickens to SARS coronavirus. Emerg Infect Dis 10:179–184.

Weingartl HM, Derbyshire JB. 1994. Evidence for a putative second receptor for porcine transmissible gastroenteritis virus on the villous enterocytes of newborn pigs. J Virol 68:7253–7259.

Welch SK, Saif LJ. 1988. Monoclonal antibodies to a virulent strain of transmissible gastroenteritis virus: Comparison of reactivity with virulent and attenuated virus. Arch Virol 101:221–35.

Welch SK, Saif LJ, Ram S. 1988. Cell-mediated immune responses of suckling pigs inoculated with attenuated or virulent transmissible gastroenteritis virus. Am J Vet Res 49:1228–1234.

Welter CJ. 1965. TGE of swine. I. Propagation of virus in cell cultures and development of a vaccine. Vet Med Small Anim Clin 60:1054–1058.

——. 1980. Experimental and field evaluation of a new oral vaccine for TGE. Vet Med Small Anim Clin 75:1757–1759.

Wesley RD, Wesley IV, Woods RD. 1991a. Differentiation between transmissible gastroenteritis virus and porcine respiratory coronavirus using a cDNA probe. J Vet Diag Invest 3:29–32.

Wesley RD, Woods RD. 1993. Immunization of pregnant gilts with PRCV induces lactogenic immunity for protection of nursing piglets from challenge with TGEV. Vet Microbiol 38:31–40.

——. 1996. Induction of protective immunity against transmissible gastroenteritis virus after exposure of neonatal pigs to porcine respiratory coronavirus. Am J Vet Res 57:157–162.

Wesley RD, Woods RD, Cheung AK. 1990a. Genetic basis for the pathogenesis of transmissible gastroenteritis virus. J Virol 64:4761–4766.

——. 1991b. Genetic analysis of porcine respiratory coronavirus, an attenuated variant of transmissible gastroenteritis virus. J Virol 65:3369–3373.

Wesley RD, Woods RD, Hill HT, Biwer JD. 1990b. Evidence for a porcine respiratory coronavirus, antigenically similar to transmissible gastroenteritis virus, in the United States. J Vet Diag Invest 2:312–317.

Wesley RD, Woods RD, McKean JD, Senn MK, Elazhary Y. 1997. Prevalence of coronavirus antibodies in Iowa swine. Can J Vet Res 61:305–308.

Wesseling JG, Vennema H, Godeke GJ, Horzinek MC, Rottier PJ. 1994. Nucleotide sequence and expression of the spike (S) gene of canine coronavirus and comparison with the S proteins of feline and porcine coronaviruses. J Gen Virol 75:1789–1794.

Whitenack DL, Whitehair CK, Miller ER. 1978. Influence of enteric infection on zinc utilization and clinical signs and lesions of zinc deficiency in young swine. Am J Vet Res 39:1447–1454.

Witte KH. 1971. Isolation of the virus of transmissible gastroenteritis (TGE) from naturally infected piglets in cell culture. Zentralbl Veterinarmed B 18:770–778.

Witte KH, Walther C. 1976. Age-dependent susceptibility of pigs to infection with the virus of transmissible gastroenteritis. Proc Int Congr Pig Vet Soc 4:K3.

Woods RD. 1977. Leukocyte migration-inhibition procedure for transmissible gastroenteritis viral antigens. Am J Vet Res 38:1267–1269.

——. 1978. Small plaque variant transmissible gastroenteritis virus. J Am Vet Med Assoc 173:643–647.

——. 1982. Studies of enteric coronaviruses in a feline cell line. Vet Microbiol 7:427–435.

——. 1984. Efficacy of vaccination of sows with serologically related coronaviruses for control of transmissible gastroenteritis in nursing pigs. Am J Vet Res 45:1726–1729.

Woods RD, Cheville NF, Gallagher JE. 1981. Lesions in the small intestine of newborn pigs inoculated with porcine, feline, and canine coronaviruses. Am J Vet Res 42:1163–1169.

Woods RD, Pedersen NC. 1979. Cross-protection studies between feline infectious peritonitis and porcine transmissible gastroenteritis viruses. Vet Microbiol 4:11–16.

Woods RD, Wesley RD. 1992. Seroconversion of pigs in contact with dogs exposed to canine coronavirus. Can J Vet Res 56:78–80.

——. 1998. Transmissible gastroenteritis coronavirus carrier sow. Adv Exp Med Biol 440:641–647.

Woods RD, Wesley RD, Kapke PA. 1988. Neutralization of transmissible gastroenteritis virus by complement dependent monoclonal antibodies. Am J Vet Res 49:300–304.

Yaeger M, Funk N, Hoffman L. 2002. A survey of agents associated with neonatal diarrhea in Iowa swine including *Clostridium difficile* and porcine reproductive and respiratory syndrome virus. J Vet Diag Invest 14:281–287.

Young GA, Hinz RW, Underdahl NR. 1955. Some characteristics of transmissible gastroenteritis in disease-free antibody-devoid pigs. Am J Vet Res 16:529–535.

Zhou YL, Ederveen J, Egberink H, Pensaert M, Horzinek MC. 1988. Porcine epidemic diarrhea virus (V777) and feline infections peritonitis virus (FIPV) are antigenically related. Arch Virol 102:63–71.

Zhu XL, Paul PS, Vaughn E, Morales A. 1990. Characterization and reactivity of monoclonal antibodies to the Miller strain of transmissible gastroenteritis virus of swine. Am J Vet Res 51:232–238.

31 Vesicular Diseases

Juan Lubroth, Luis Rodríguez, and Aldo Dekker

The principal vesicular diseases that affect swine are foot-and-mouth disease (FMD), vesicular stomatitis (VS), and swine vesicular disease (SVD). There are other infectious diseases and conditions that can produce signs and pathologies in pigs similar to those seen in these three viral diseases, but they cannot be covered adequately in the scope of this chapter. Salient among the diseases not covered are two caliciviruses (vesicular exanthema of swine virus and San Miguel sea lion virus) and conditions such as caustic agents. It is imperative that practitioners attending a case of a vesicular disease immediately notify and collaborate with the veterinary authorities. The figures included in this chapter are purposely not identified as to which vesicular disease is the causative agent with the objective of emphasizing their identical clinical appearance.

GENERAL CONSIDERATIONS FOR THE OUTBREAK OF A VESICULAR DISEASE (DIFFERENTIAL DIAGNOSIS)

A farm with signs of a vesicular disease should be considered infected with FMD until proven otherwise. This is because of the highly infectious nature of the foot-and-mouth disease virus (FMDV), the fact that lesions caused by agents causing vesicular lesions cannot be differentiated on the basis of gross lesions, and because of the severe consequences for international trade.

When the investigation ensues, it is essential that samples are collected properly and submitted to a laboratory qualified to conduct the appropriate testing. FMDV can be grown on several tissue cell types, but samples for virus isolation recovered from a ruminant species should be assayed on permissive ruminant cells—i.e., bovine thyroid, lamb kidney—and those from swine on permissive swine cells—i.e., swine kidney/IBRS-2. Virus isolation for SVD on IBRS-2 cells is considered one of the most sensitive methods for laboratory diagnosis. In addition to IBRS-2 cells, SK6, PK-15, and primary or secondary porcine kidney cells are also sus-

ceptible to SVDV. Among the cells most commonly used to grow VSV in the laboratory are monkey kidney cells (Vero), hamster cells (BHK, CHO), chick embryo cells, and mouse cells.

As with FMD and VS, RT-PCR techniques have also been developed to detect SVD viral genome (Callahan et al. 2002; Callens and De Clercq 1999; Lin et al. 1997; Niedbalski et al. 2000; Reid et al. 2000). Virus isolation and RT-PCR are the tests of first choice for detection of SVDV in feces or from the principal tissues described earlier. In fresh vesicular material, the amount of virus (FMD, VSV, or SVD) is very high and an ELISA can be used for antigen detection and identification (Hamblin and Crowther 1995).

Other causes of vesicular or erosive lesions, including infectious (swine pox, parvovirus, or mycotic dermatitis), toxic (parsnip or celery contact dermatitis), and chemical burns (Kresse et al. 1985; Montgomery et al. 1987), should also be considered in the diagnostic workup.

THE VETERINARY PRACTITIONER'S RESPONSE

The veterinary practitioner who suspects a vesicular disease, having notified the relevant veterinary authorities, should immediately disinfect their equipment, boots, and vehicle, and should not visit any other premises on which other susceptible animals are kept. Rapid detection and immediate notification of outbreaks are imperative for control of the disease (Geering and Lubroth 2002). The practitioner could provide assistance to the veterinary authorities by beginning a line of epidemiological questioning regarding movements on and off the farm, identification of contacts, e.g., livestock market deliveries, purchases of feed, bedding, or exchanges with other farms. The practitioner's knowledge of the area with regard to producers, auctions and markets, feed distributors, and the activities of other clinicians, can be a valuable asset to the authorities in their attempts to contain and ascertain disease transmission paths.

Foot-and-Mouth Disease

Foot-and-mouth disease virus (FMDV) was recognized over 100 years ago, making it the first animal virus to be discovered. In 1897, Loeffler and Frosch presented their seminal experiments showing that a filterable agent (virus), not a toxin, was responsible for the disease. The disease itself was described in several ancient literary and historical accounts, the first attributed to Aristotle in the third century before the Common Era. Later, a more accurate description appeared in the writings of the Italian poet and physician Girolamo Fracastoro in *De Contagione et Contagiosis Morbis et Curatione* in 1546 (reprinted in part in Casas Olascoaga et al. 1999).

Of all the diseases known to human and animal medicine, foot-and-mouth disease (FMD) is probably the most contagious. Infected animals can shed high titers of virus in excretions, secretions, and from superficial lesions. The virus is found in semen, feces, oropharyngeal fluids, and contaminated food products and waste, and can be carried by aerosols across considerable distances. Importantly, the plethora of virus types makes it difficult to make generalizations based on the characteristics of one virus subtype that apply to all virus types and subtypes. Furthermore, since FMD viruses affect numerous hosts, including both domestic and wild animals, observations based on a certain virus in a specific host may not necessarily be true for another virus in the same or different host species.

All continents have historically been affected by FMD, with the exception of Antarctica. Trade barriers imposed on countries with FMD infection limit their access to international markets. Thus, several regions have either eradicated FMD (i.e., North America and Western Europe) or have undertaken extraordinary regional efforts to control its incidence and eliminate its occurrence altogether (i.e., South America and Oceania). Continued surveillance for vesicular diseases is of the utmost importance to FMDV-free countries and to those that have established control campaigns. Early detection of FMD and early response to its presence are critical to the mission of veterinary services around the world.

Because of its highly infectious nature, FMD has been the leading force behind much of the national and international veterinary service legislation and regulations regarding markets, exports and imports, quarantine, inspection, diagnostic competencies, and the need to establish contingency and emergency response plans.

ETIOLOGY

The viruses of FMD belong to the Genus *Aphthovirus* (*aphtho*—vesicle, blister) in the family *Picornaviridae*. Included in the family are poliovirus, hepatitis A virus, the rhinoviruses, and enteroviruses (such as SVD virus, which is discussed later in this chapter).

Aphthoviruses are small (~25 nm) and composed of ~8.5 kilobases of single-stranded, positive-sense RNA wrapped in a nonenveloped capsid structure comprised of 60 copies each of four viral proteins. The viral RNA encodes for a single polyprotein of some 3000 amino acids. During translation the nascent polyprotein is cleaved into 13 proteins. Proteins, 1A, 1B, 1C, and 1D (historical nomenclature defines these as VP2, VP4, VP3, and VP1, respectively, as reviewed in Grubman and Baxt 2004) form the viral capsid with 3B viral protein linked to the RNA. The nonstructural proteins (2A, 2B, 2C, 3A, 3B [of which there are three copies], 3C, and 3D), are involved in virus replication and host-cell shut off.

Within the FMD viruses, seven distinct serotypes are recognized: serotype A (French for Germany—*Allemagne*); serotype O (for the Oise Region in France, but once referred to as type B); serotype C (the third virus to be recognized as antigenically distinct); serotype Southern African Territories (SAT) 1, SAT 2, and SAT 3; and serotype Asia 1 (Bachrach 1968). Multiple variants or subtypes exist within each serotype (Bachrach 1968; Carrillo et al. 1990; Domingo et al. 1995).

EPIDEMIOLOGY

Geographic Distribution

In Asia, FMDV is endemic in all countries in the region except Brunei, East Timor, Indonesia, Japan, Singapore, and South Korea. The eastern states of Malaysia are also free and the Philippines is well on the way to eradication, with the exception of peri-urban occurrence of FMD around Manila. The most prevalent serotypes are O, A, and Asia 1. The disease causes considerable loss of buffalo draft power for rice cropping and production losses in pigs and cattle, and is a major constraint to trade in cattle, pigs, or their products within the region. The spread of FMD in Asia is closely related to the unofficial movement patterns of cattle and pigs (or their products) for trade purposes. Wildlife reservoirs for FMD in the region are not known, although the possibility exists in wild bovine and porcine species in several countries.

In recent years, the highly contagious Pan-Asian Type O virus has spread through several countries in Asia, including Bangladesh (1996) and Bhutan (1998), Taiwan (1997, 1999), Japan (2000, which had been FMD-free since 1908), the Republic of Korea (2000, which had been FMD-free since 1929), Mongolia (2000, which had been FMD-free for 27 years prior), and the far east of Russia (2000, which had been FMD-free for 36 years prior).

In East Asia, an O virus with a unique tropism for swine emerged in several countries, including Viet Nam, Hong Kong, the Philippines, and Taiwan, producing high mortality in pig populations (Dunn and Donaldson 1997; Knowles et al. 2001). This FMDV has often been erroneously referred to as a "pig-adapted" FMDV. Adaptation, in the ecological sense, connotes cohabitation and symbiosis, which is far from the case for this virulent, porcinophillic virus (Beard and Mason 2000; Mason et al. 2003).

FMDV was introduced to South America in 1870 through the importation of cattle to southern regions (Argentina) from Europe, but only reached northern countries (Colombia and Venezuela, for instance) in the 1950s. Through the *Comisión Sur Americana para la Lucha Contra la Fiebre Aftosa*, the incidence of FMD has declined from several thousand cases in 1980 to a few by early in the 21st century by maintaining effective surveillance, animal control, and vaccination programs in most countries. Critical areas of virus persistence remain in parts of Bolivia, Ecuador, and Venezuela. The only serotypes recorded in South America are A, O, and C. Type C has not been isolated from the field in nearly 10 years and may have disappeared, but its eradication requires confirmation. (Addendum: at the time of publication, Type C has been reported in northern Brazil.)

The situation in Africa is poorly described. This reflects the difficulties for veterinary services of mounting effective disease control initiatives, implementing timely reporting, and garnering sufficient resources to engage villages or incipient private ventures in sustainable healthy livestock development. Six of the seven serotypes of FMDV occur in different African ecosystems. Only Asia 1 has never been reported. South Africa, Namibia, Botswana, and Zimbabwe have been able to control FMD through the production of suitable vaccines, well-designed vaccination campaigns, and the formation of wildlife sanctuaries that separate persistently infected buffalo from domestic operations. Regrettably, land resettlement and civil unrest in Zimbabwe eroded veterinary systems in the early 2000s. Widespread FMD outbreaks have led to the closure of lucrative markets outside Africa and pose a threat to neighboring countries. Although the predominant serotype in the region is SAT-2, others still present a risk. As in South America, type C appears to have disappeared from Africa, but adequate active surveillance is required for confirmation. In southern Africa, the Cape buffalo herds harbor SAT viruses and represent potential sources of infection to domestic livestock.

In the Middle East and Arabian Peninsula, virus types A, O, Asia 1, and occasionally SAT-2 have been identified. Swine are not an important species in these regions and control efforts are focused almost entirely in dairy cattle and small ruminants. However, the needs of the region, in terms of animal protein, necessitate extensive importation from the Horn of Africa or else-where. This situation increases the risk for the entry of FMDV or other transboundary animal diseases. Exclusion of FMDV is, therefore, dependent upon careful pre-embarkation, regulated quarantine, and official laboratory testing undertaken for this purpose. In northern Africa, FMD usually moves in a westerly direction, or as seen in the outbreak in Algeria in the mid-1990s, from western Africa to the north, paralleling the movement of livestock; but again, swine are not part of the disease dynamics in this region either.

Susceptible Species

Natural hosts of FMDV include all artiodactyls (ungulates with a cloven hoof). As such, domestic cattle, buffalo, sheep, goats, camels, South American camelids, deer, antelope, wildebeest, as well as those of the suborder *Suiformes* (domestic swine, feral swine, and wild boar) are susceptible to FMDV infection. FMDV infection has also been reported in other species, including elephants, hedgehogs, and capybara (reviewed in Casas Olascoaga et al. 1999). Of notable epidemiological importance in Africa is the Cape buffalo (*Syncerus caffer*), which serves as a FMDV reservoir host in the region and a potential source of viruses to adjacent livestock production areas (Condy et al. 1985; Dawe et al. 1994). Laboratory models for FMDV include guinea pigs and suckling mice, which historically have been used for virus isolation and studies of vaccine protection determinants (Casas Olascoaga et al. 1999).

Nonhuman primates have also been studied as to their susceptibility to FMD (Schudel et al. 1981). Although there are confirmed cases of FMDV infections in humans, these have been incidental and FMD viruses should not be considered zoonotic (Casas Olascoaga et al. 1999). FMDV is widespread around the world, and the exposure of farmers, veterinarians, and other animal health workers, abattoir personnel, butchers, or researchers is commonplace. However, humans exposed to FMD-infected animals or carcasses have rarely, if ever, developed disease or seroconverted to the virus.

Although equine rhinitis A virus belongs to the aphthovirus genus (King et al. 1999), the FMD viruses do not affect solipeds.

Transmission

FMD viruses can be isolated from exhalations, secretions, urine, feces, milk, and semen during prodromal phases of the infection and during early clinical disease (Casas Olascoaga et al. 1999; Lubroth 2002). Once lesions develop, the virus is easily found in and around the exudations of ruptured vesicles of lesions.

The most common form of transmission is through contact between an infected animal and susceptible cohorts. At the height of clinical manifestation, swine generate more viruses in their exhalations than other species, and thus are often referred to as amplifiers of the virus (Alexandersen and Donaldson 2002). It is estimated that an infected pig can exhale up to 3000 times that of an affected cow. The 1981 FMD outbreak on the Isle of Wight was reported to have come from an infected piggery on France's northern coast, and carried by the prevailing winds and proper humidity from France to England (Donaldson 1986; Gloster and Alexandersen 2004). However, certain FMD viruses isolated from swine actually show the opposite characteristic and are poorly aerosolized, even when pigs are housed in the same room and separated by a double fence meters apart.

As omnivores, pigs ingesting poorly cooked, virus-infected swill or other foodstuffs can acquire FMD. Retrospective epidemiological investigations have shown that ingestion of infected products by swine has been responsible for some important outbreaks of the disease in recent times, such as that in the United Kingdom in 2001 (Gibbens et al. 2001).

Embryo transfer studies in FMD-infected cattle have shown that even at the time of greatest risk—that of peak viremia—proper washing of the collected embryos following protocols established by the International Embryo Transfer Society, will reduce the risk of transmitting the virus to zero, provided that the *zona pellucida* remains intact (Mebus and Singh 1991). FMDV can be recovered from semen from FMD-infected boars, but artificial insemination with contaminated semen failed to transmit the diseases to serviced sows (McVicar et al. 1978).

The persistently infected animal is defined as an animal that harbors the virus in the esophageal-pharyngeal region beyond 28 days post infection (Hedger 1971; Salt 1993). The persistent carrier state has been well described in cattle and buffalo, but less so in sheep and goats, with swine expected not to sustain the virus long term (Salt 1993; Lubroth and Brown 1995). It is likely that persistence is related not only to host factors, but also to those of the specific virus under study.

Salted and processed pork meats can contain viable FMDV under different conditions (Cottral 1969). Studies conducted using Italian and Spanish traditional processes found that by 200 days after post product preparation, no FMDV could be isolated from processed meats (Mebus et al. 1993). During carcass maturation, the lactic acid build up in the skeletal musculature is sufficient to inactivate FMDV, with infectious virus remaining principally in lymph nodes, glands, and bone marrow. It is for this specific reason that export of fresh beef exported from once-endemic areas (South America and southern Africa, primarily) require that it be deboned and deglanded.

FMD viruses are generally subject to rapid inactivation under many physical and chemical environments, but it can survive pasteurization at 72°C for 15 seconds; in cattle stalls after 14 days from urine after 39 days, 28, and 3 days in autumn and summer, respectively; and from contaminated hay after 5 months at 22°C (Cottral

1969; Pirtle and Beran 1991). Thus, under temperate climates characterized by overcast skies and cool temperatures, the virus may survive for a considerable period of time with direct sunlight, dry ambient temperatures destroying the virus. FMD viruses are highly labile to low pH (below 6.7) and high pH (above 10.5). As picornaviruses are nonenveloped, detergents, lipid solvents, and ether-based compounds do not have a primary inactivation effect.

PATHOGENESIS

Great variation exists in susceptibility and clinical presentation of FMD among species and between indigenous and exotic breeds. In addition, variation exists in the virulence of one virus versus another in the same host (Lubroth 2002).

The FMD viruses usually gain entry via the respiratory route, with as few as 10 infectious particles causing infection in cattle (Donaldson et al. 1987). Even if virus-contaminated swill is the source of infection, inhalation of aerosolized virus or entry through breaks in the buccal mucosa leads to viral replication, drainage to local lymph nodes, and subsequent viremia. The lungs, perhaps surprisingly, do not contain as high titers of virus as the upper respiratory tract, particularly the pharyngeal area (Alexandersen et al. 2001). The dissemination of the virus throughout virtually all tissues of the body occurs with remarkable speed, but the classical lesions develop only in the nasal, mucosal, and podal epithelia.

CLINICAL SIGNS

FMD in swine is a crippling disease in adult pigs and often fatal in piglets. The incubation period for FMD may range from 2–10 days following exposure to the virus. In a vaccinated animal, where immunity may vary, the incubation period is often prolonged as the homologous virus replicates (or a closely related one) and eventually overcomes waning immunity.

Infected pigs develop a fever within 24–48 hours and by the third day the fever may surpass 41°C (106°F). Affected pigs are likely prostrate and shivering (Figure 31.1). Blanched areas may be seen at the level of the coronary bands, fringed by congested areas. The feet are warm to the touch. By the fourth to sixth day vesicular lesions, which quickly rupture leaving a raw denuded area and epithelial tags, will have developed along the coronary band; interdigital spaces and bulbs of the heel; and rostral areas of the snout, nares, and chin—all common signs exhibited by affected animals throughout the piggery. Heavy adults often remain prostrate for long periods leading to pressure sores that develop overnight with the epithelia eroding off from carpi and tarsi and much squealing when coaxed to move. Unlike cattle affected by FMD, vesicles rarely develop on the dorsal surface of the tongue in affected pigs. If not humanely

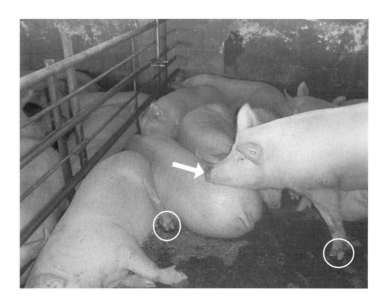

31.1. *Prostration and huddling in swine affected by a vesicular disease. Circle and arrow, foot lesions; arrow, rostral aspect of the snout with ruptured vesicle.*

culled, some pigs will slough off their hooves exposing the raw, underlying, sensitive laminae.

In uncomplicated cases, recovery can be quick and is often complete within 2 weeks, when all mucosal lesions have healed. However, deformation of the claws may be a sequel to the foot lesions. Animals that have lost their claws should be euthanized on humanitarian grounds.

In disease-free areas, the infection can spread quickly and the clinical presentation may become widespread, with a morbidity approaching 100%. In regions where the disease is endemic, or where some degree of vaccination is undertaken, extensive clinical signs may be less pronounced.

The high fevers in sows can lead to abortion storms in the farrowing pens. Piglet mortality can exceed 50% due to virus-induced myocarditis, even before vesicles have developed in these or the adult animals.

By the time the veterinary practitioners or inspectors arrive at the farm, the disease in pigs is characterized by erosions and thick epithelial flaps from ruptured vesicles on the snout, around the nares, under the chin, coronary bands, pads of the heels, bulbs, and interdigital spaces (Figures 31.2–31.5). Some pigs may have sloughed their hooves. Animals in the earliest stages of disease are likely to show turgid or flocculent vesicles on the snout ranging from 4 mm to 2.5 cm and occurring circumferentially around the coronary band. The severity of clinical signs is greatest in heavier pigs. Teat vesicles ranging from a few millimeters to one centimeter may also be apparent (Figure 31.6). The heart muscle from piglets that died due to FMDV should be examined for blanched striations along the epicardium, endocardium, and septum, indicative of myocardial infraction and necrosis.

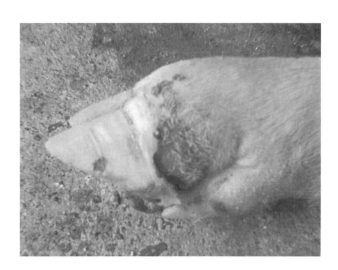

31.2. *Coronary band lesion around the circumference with ruptured vesicle on abaxial surface and intact vesicle on dew claw.*

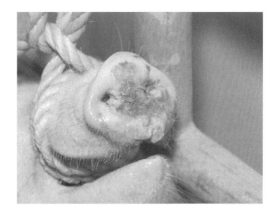

31.3. *Rostral aspect of the snout in an affected pig. Uncomplicated cases can resolve within a few days in individual animals.*

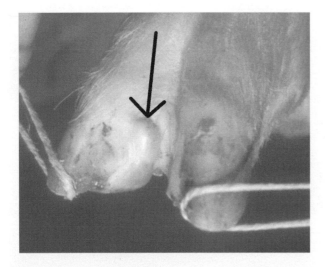

31.4. *Vesicular lesion in the interdigital space. The vesicle on the coronary band extends to the bulb of the heel.*

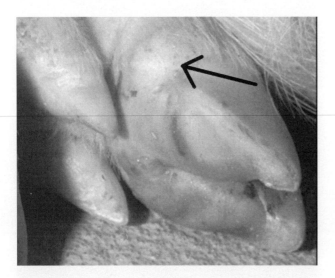

31.5. *Vesicular lesion on the caudal aspect of the coronary band (arrow).*

LESIONS

Histopathologically, early changes can be seen as ballooning degeneration of cells in the midsection of the *stratum spinosum* within the stratified epithelium, with the *stratum germinativum* remaining intact and without neutrophilic infiltrates, unless there are opportunistic pathogens that contaminate the wound. As the cellular pathology progresses, pyknotic nuclei become more salient, and some of the degenerating cells begin to coalesce forming fluid-filled pockets containing large amounts of virus. Subsequently, the multiloculated epithelial changes lead to the formation of a larger blister. This pattern of lesion development is similar in various parts of the body, varying only in the extent of keratinization of the epithelium examined. Histopathological examination of affected myocardial tissues shows

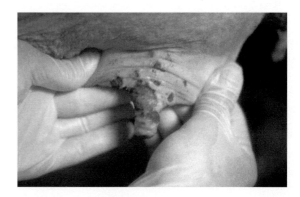

31.6. *Teat lesions in a lactating sow from a field case.*

wide clusters of cells with eosinophilic shrunken cytoplasms and pyknotic nuclei and wide extracellular spaces.

IMMUNITY

Rapid humoral immunity is elicited by the virus, with neutralizing antibodies directed at the three surface capsid proteins: VP1, VP2, and VP3 (Salt 1993). VP1, the immunodominant protein, is also responsible for the serotype classification of the different viruses as well as differentiation between subtypes. As such, vaccine design and certain diagnostic tests, utilize information on the amino acid composition and genomic sequence of VP1 to assess vaccine-virus suitability, molecular epidemiological analysis, and immune response (Doel 1999; Domingo et al. 1995; Knowles and Samuel 1999). However, immune responses to the other viral structural proteins (VP2, VP3, and VP4) and the nonstructural proteins (2C, 3AB, 3ABC, 3D) can also be detected. Reactivity to the nonstructural FMDV proteins is an indication that viral replication has occurred in the host and is the basis for the development of assays that can differentiate between vaccinated, but not infected, animals and those that were infected regardless of their FMD vaccination history (Lubroth 1998; Meyer et al. 1997; Mezencio et al. 1998; Sorensen et al. 1998).

Studies on the duration of protective immunity after recovery from natural infection has been inadequately studied, but in endemic situations where there are at least two viruses in circulation and an ever-changing (replacement) dynamic population, as occurs in flocks of small ruminants, it would appear that protective immunity at the herd level is approximately 2 years in duration (Lubroth, unpublished observations).

No cross-protection is seen across serotypes of FMD viruses (type A to Asia 1, for instance), and only a limited level of protection across virus subtypes (i.e., A5 and A24). There is no cross-protective immunity conferred by infection with other picornaviruses, such as the enteroviruses of domestic animals.

DIAGNOSIS

The veterinary practitioner should take epidemiological considerations into account when trying to determine the causative agent, but must rely on laboratory specialists to confirm the diagnosis using discriminating tests that can quickly differentiate one infectious agent from another (see the section on differential diagnosis).

Laboratory confirmation of FMD depends heavily on the quality of the samples submitted to the diagnostic laboratory. Vesicular fluid or epithelium from oral, nasal, or foot lesions should be fresh, representative of the herd, and collected from several animals. Under field settings, once the veterinary practitioner is called to the farm, intact vesicles may no longer be evident, and the tissues collected for laboratory diagnosis should be from the area of the lesion most apt to contain viral antigens—i.e., at the junction between affected and healthy tissue. If vesicles are seen, fine needle aspirates are an ideal sample for submission, but collection is not easy. Lesions that are 2–3 days old will often have cream-colored coagulated exudate covering the lesion, but these, though easy to sample, are not appropriate diagnostic specimens.

It must be stressed that, when a vesicular disease in swine (or other species) is suspected, the practitioner should immediately contact the official veterinary authorities to conduct a thorough epidemiological evaluation of the incident and collect the appropriate samples for proper laboratory submission.

Antigen-capture enzyme-linked immunoassays (ELISA) using vesicular fluid or well-preserved epithelial tissue samples are used in most countries with endemic FMD or those that have surveillance systems in place as part of their contingency and emergency preparation plans. ELISA has largely replaced the complement fixation test for antigen detection due to its ease in standardization, speed, and high throughput capabilities (Casas Olascoaga et al. 1999).

Penside tests are currently becoming available, but these are limited to subjective interpretation and should be seen as screening tools with a competent laboratory performing the more objective and analytical confirmatory assays.

The inclusion of molecular techniques, such as PCR, into laboratory confirmation can allow rapid identification of group-specific (aphthovirus) or virus-specific (type A24, A96, A22, for instance) gene sequences (Alexandersen et al. 2001; House and Meyer 1993; Reid et al. 2000). Results from ELISA or PCR can be obtained within 3–5 hours after receipt of the samples. Applied research into real-time PCR, in which gene sequences are amplified and visualized on portable computer screens within the hour, has been established for FMD as an ancillary method for diagnosis and is being applied in the field in some countries (Callahan et al. 2002). If the results are negative using these methods,

however, samples should still be processed for virus isolation using sensitive cell culture systems. Most capable laboratories actually begin attempts at virus isolation at the same time as the quicker assays, since virus isolation may take several days to complete and the initial preparation of the specimen is often the same. One of the drawbacks to virus isolation is that it can only be conducted in specially equipped laboratories with trained staff. Once there is evidence that a viral agent has been isolated, the cell culture is tested by ELISA or PCR much the same way as a tissue or vesicular sample.

The more common antibody detection methods for the diagnosis of FMD viruses are ELISA and virus neutralization (VN) assays, both of which have been internationally standardized and included in the *Manual of Standards for Diagnostic Tests and Vaccines,* published by the Office International des Epizooties. ELISA tests can be conducted within a few hours. VN requires 3 days and the use of live virus and cell culture systems, which limit its use to specialized laboratories. VN also requires that the laboratory have antisera and epidemiological knowledge of the circulating viruses to use in the assay system.

The detection of FMDV nonstructural proteins can be accomplished using specific ELISA formats and some rapid penside tests to demonstrate virus persistence or circulation within a herd (Meyer et al. 1997; Shin et al. 2002; Sorensen et al. 1998). The specific detection of the 3D nonstructural FMDV protein (once termed "virus-infection associated antigen" or VIAA) was extensively used as an agar-gel immunodiffusion test. Although still in use today in some laboratories, it has been largely replaced by ELISA methods. ELISA testing has also been developed to detect antibody responses to several other nonstructural proteins and can be used to identify animals in which virus replication has occurred, thereby serving as an indirect method to identify potentially persistently infected animals. Antibodies to VIAA were long used to detect for evidence of virus infection in a population, particularly cattle, but studies have shown that animals receiving multiple doses of vaccine will also develop antibodies to 3D or VIAA, thus limiting its value as an indication of previous infection (Casas Olascoaga et al. 1999; Salt 1993). Countries that do not vaccinate, however, could use a 3D-based assay (or other nonstructural protein), because this protein is highly immunogenic and highly conserved among all FMD viruses, making one test applicable for all serotypes and subtypes. In countries where vaccination is practiced, the use of nonstructural proteins other than 3D could be of great value for determining whether virus circulation and transmission is ongoing in a herd without clinical disease.

PREVENTION AND CONTROL

The only treatment available for pigs infected with FMDV is palliative. The use of antibiotics to prevent secondary bacterial infection could be warranted under endemic situations. FMD is considered a foreign animal disease by many countries and there are ongoing regional and national programs for its progressive control, so treatment is not an option.

The most common method of FMD introduction the world over has been through the movement of clinically ill animals, or those incubating the disease, into a susceptible population (Casas Olascoaga et al. 1999; Geering and Lubroth 2002; Grubman and Baxt 2004; Salt 1993). Contaminated products or by-products of animal origin have also been repeatedly shown as a likely method of spread. Product control restrictions, safety testing of biologicals entering disease-free areas, requirements for health certificates, pre- and post-quarantine testing by government authorities are all attempts to preclude FMD and other diseases from entering into a country or zone.

At the farm level, the application of biosecurity principles has the same basic value as those implemented at an international level. The origin of newly acquired animals should be known and authoritatively certified as healthy. On the farm, recently purchased animals should be quarantined at a distance from the remainder of the herd for a period of 20–40 days to provide added security. Changing outer clothes and footwear when moving between different pens and age groups, with the frequent use of disinfection baths and separate equipment, minimizes the spread of infectious diseases.

The farmer or producer should know the reliability of on-farm contracted services and the origin of all supplies, including feed, veterinary care, equipment, and transport or waste management vehicles. The use of discarded foodstuff as animal feed, even if cooked sufficiently to destroy the virus, should not be allowed. The use of swill for feeding pigs is a high-risk practice and responsible for virus persistence and outbreak occurrence in many parts of the world.

Vaccination

FMD vaccines should contain inactivated antigens representative of the circulating viruses within the region (Doel 2003). Since mutations, antigenic drift, or newly occurring viruses may limit vaccine efficacy, it is critical that laboratory and epidemiological studies be carried out regularly to ensure that vaccine antigens used for the protection of livestock are protective against prevailing viruses.

Two types of vaccines are currently available: aqueous formulations and those emulsified as single or double oil formulations (Black et al. 1984; Casas Olascoaga et al. 1999; Doel 2003). Although ruminants can be vaccinated with either formulation, swine respond to only those prepared with oil adjuvants (Black et al. 1984). Colostral immunity interferes with the induction of protection (Francis and Black 1986a, b).

To obtain herd level protection, all susceptible animals on the premises should be vaccinated in order to ensure that over 80% of the population be adequately immunized. The most successful use of vaccination in FMD-endemic situations has been when quality controlled vaccines are administered twice a year under the supervision of government authorities, with follow-up serological surveys.

The concentration of antigen (referred to as the payload of a vaccine), is one indicator of quality, and those vaccines that have a high payload have been shown to induce some degree of protection 4–5 days after administration (Doel et al. 1994; Doel 2003). Such vaccines can also be used under emergency management of an outbreak if the decision to use vaccine is taken by government authorities.

Some countries, or even continents such as South America, have relied on vaccine coverage in cattle in lieu of swine, sheep and goats, or even wildlife, with much success. In parts of Asia, endemicity differs from the Latin American context in that pig production and marketing are likely to contribute more to the circulation of FMDV. However, vaccination of pigs is haphazard, and progressive control has rarely been achieved.

International and commercial pressure has been placed on vaccine companies to ensure that vaccines are highly purified and do not induce antibodies to FMDV nonstructural proteins. This permits vaccinating countries to demonstrate by serological testing of vaccinates that virus circulation has been halted, thus ensuring access to international markets for their animals and livestock products.

Research into improving vaccines has been undertaken by several government agencies. These include attempts to induce more rapid immunity, vectored vaccines (where FMDV components are incorporated into carrier viruses), and/or the inclusion of antiviral agents or inducers of antiviral properties within vaccine formulations (Moraes et al. 2003). These vaccines have not yet been tested in an endemic or outbreak setting (Grubman and Baxt 2004). In addition, vaccines capable of providing longer duration of protection, able to protect against a wider range of virus subtypes, and without the need for specialized preservation (i.e., refrigeration) are needed.

From the standpoint of an exotic animal disease, the quick and humane elimination of all clinically ill animals and their cohorts to halt further environmental contamination and spread can be warranted (Geering and Lubroth 2002). Burial of the culled animals should be on the affected premises themselves, if an environmentally sound area is available (i.e., away from the water table). When performed correctly, burial is preferable than incineration. Although incineration is suitable for destroying the virus, it falters in that the smoke, smell, and imagery often leads to a strong public outcry regarding animal welfare and it raises environmental concerns that hinder regulatory performance of control operations. In the event that culled animals are to be moved off the farm to burial sites elsewhere or for rendering, it should be done in sealed container trucks and under the escort of regulatory officials, police, or military personnel assisting in the operations.

Biosecurity onto and off farms should be of paramount importance in every instance of FMD occurrence (Geering and Lubroth 2002). Salient in the management of a FMD outbreak are strict standstill orders on animal movement from the outbreak area and restrictions on the movement of people, equipment, and products off affected premises or infected zones, regardless of what other control measures are employed (i.e., emergency vaccination, culling, or allowing the disease to pass its course with the required palliative treatment).

Vesicular Stomatitis

Vesicular stomatitis (VS) is a viral disease affecting swine, cattle, and horses caused by vesicular stomatitis virus (VSV). In cattle and swine, its clinical appearance resembles that of foot-and-mouth disease (FMD) (see the section on differential diagnosis). Economic losses are incurred due to quarantine and trade restrictions and also to decreased production and weight loss. Mortality is rare (Rodriguez and Nichol 1999).

Historical reports dating as far back as 1862 describe vesicular disease in cattle, horses, and swine. The causal agent was first isolated in the United States in 1925 in New Jersey and a year later in Indiana (Cotton 1927). These isolates were determined to be serologically distinguishable and were later classified as serotypes New Jersey (VSNJV) and Indiana (VSIV) (Cartwright and Brown 1972).

VSV is the most common cause of vesicular disease in the Americas, causing thousands of outbreaks every year from southern Mexico to northern South America. VS is considered an exotic animal disease in Europe, Asia, and Australia and is listed by the OIE as a reportable disease. Its report is obligatory within 24 hours of a confirmed diagnosis. In addition to farm animals, VSV can infect humans, resulting in flu-like symptoms and, occasionally, nonfatal encephalitis (Fields and Hawkins 1967; Quiroz et al. 1988). Unlike the other viral agents causing vesicular disease in swine covered in this chapter, which are transmissible by direct contact and fomites, VSV is also transmitted by insects (Stallknecht et al. 1999).

ETIOLOGY

VSV belongs to the Order *Mononegavirales* (nonsegmented, negative-sense RNA viruses), family *Rhabdoviridae*, and genus *Vesiculovirus*. VSV have been classified into two serotypes: New Jersey (VSNJV) and Indiana (VSIV). Two subtypes of VSIV have been found causing livestock disease in South America: Cocal virus or VSIV-2 and Alagoas virus (VSIV-3). A number of vesiculoviruses have been found in nature infecting insects and wild animals. However, only vesicular stomatitis viruses cause outbreaks of vesicular disease in domestic animals (Rodriguez 2002).

VSV has the typical rhabdovirus morphology, with enveloped bullet-shaped virions approximately 70×180 nm in length (Bradish and Kirkham 1966). The core of the virion consists of a helical ribonucleoprotein containing the nucleocapsid (N), polymerase (L), and phosphoprotein (P). The outer shell is made of the matrix protein (M) covered with a lipid membrane containing the glycoprotein (G). Viral entry and exit to and from the infected cell are mediated by the glycoprotein, which also contains the main neutralizing antigenic sites.

The genome consists of a single strand of RNA of negative polarity approximately 1100–1300 nucleotides in length, depending on the virus (Rodriguez et al. 2002). Gene expression is regulated by a simple, yet elegant, mechanism in which level of expression is determined by the distance of each gene from a single promoter near the 3' end of the genome. Gene order is N, P, M, G, L. Therefore, the most frequently expressed gene is N and the least expressed gene is L (Ball et al. 1999). All genes code for a single protein except P, which contains a second open reading frame coding for two additional small basic proteins (C and C') of undetermined function (Kretzschmar et al. 1996; Spiropoulou and Nichol 1993).

In addition to protein and RNA, VS virions contain lipid and carbohydrates associated with the envelope. VSV can persist in the environment for short periods of time. The infectivity of VSV is unstable at pH 3, but stable between pH 5–10. It is rapidly inactivated at 56°C and by UV and x-ray irradiation. Virus infectivity is also sensitive to lipid solvents, detergents, formalin, and various common disinfectants such as sodium hypochlorite (bleach) (Rodriguez and Nichol 1999).

VS viruses are capable of infecting a wide variety of mammalian cell types, as well as insect, amphibian, and fish cells (Seganti et al. 1986). Some studies have implicated phosphatidyl serine, a component of the cell membrane of a wide variety of cells, as a receptor for VSV (Coll 1997; Schlegel et al. 1983). This might explain the wide range of cells that VSV can infect.

Peripheral blood mononuclear cells seem to be resistant to viral infection.

EPIDEMIOLOGY

Outbreaks of vesicular stomatitis are reported every year from southern Mexico to northern South America (Colombia, Venezuela, Ecuador, and Peru). In the United States, VS outbreaks occur in sporadic cycles at approximately 10-year intervals (Rodriguez 2002). The great majority of outbreaks are caused by VSNJV (>80%) and to a lesser extent VSIV-1. In Brazil, two subtypes of VSIV, Cocal (VSIV-2) and Alagoas (VSIV-3), commonly cause outbreaks, and sporadic outbreaks of VSIV-2 have been reported in Argentina (Rodriguez et al. 2000).

VS is not reported to occur outside the Americas, although there was one report of VS in France and other parts of Europe during World War I that was associated with the importation of horses from the United States (Letchworth et al. 1999). There are also reports of "erosive stomatitis" and "acute stomatitis" in cattle in South Africa; however, the causative agent was not identified (Hanson 1950).

Vesicular stomatitis commonly affects cattle, horses, and to a lesser extent swine. However, swine are very susceptible, particularly to VSNJV, and a large number of animals can be affected during outbreaks in swine farms. Sheep and goats seem to be relatively resistant to VSV infection, with clinical cases rarely reported (Hanson 1981). Despite the fact that antibodies to VSV are found in a large number of wild animals, such as peccaries, whitetail deer, several species of rodents, monkeys, and even birds, naturally occurring disease has not been reported in these species.

VSV infects humans causing flu-like symptoms, such as fever, myalgia, and severe headaches. Infections in veterinary and farm personnel during outbreaks of disease in livestock are usually associated with unprotected direct contact with sick animals, particularly when vesicular fluid or contaminated saliva are unintentionally sprayed onto the face. Gloves, goggles, and face masks are recommended to prevent exposure during examination of sick animals (Hanson et al. 1950). Laboratory infections are usually associated with procedures that generate infectious aerosols, such as centrifugation. All laboratory procedures with field viruses should be performed under biological safety level 3. At least one case of encephalitis in a child caused by VSIV-1 has been documented (Quiroz et al. 1988). Symptoms usually resolve within a week and fatalities have never been reported.

Transmission of VSV can occur by direct contact or by insect bites. Strains of VSNJV seem to be more readily transmissible by direct contact than those of VSIV-1 (Stallknecht et al. 1999; Martinez et al. 2003). Swine infected with VSNJV either clinically or subclinically can readily transmit to other swine by direct contact

(Stallknecht 1999). Transmission by fomites is not well documented, but there are anecdotal accounts of transmission by contaminated milking equipment, feed, and rough forage (Hanson 1950; Hansen et al. 1985). Aerosol transmission from animal to animal has never been documented.

At least two groups of biting insects, sand flies (*Lutzomyia* spp.) and black flies (*Simulium* spp.), have been demonstrated to transmit VSV to susceptible hosts (Cupp et al. 1992; Tesh et al. 1972). In addition, virus has been isolated from several groups of wild-caught insects, including gnats and mosquitoes, during VS outbreaks or in the absence of outbreaks in endemic areas (Francy et al. 1988; Sudia et al. 1967). Insect transmission resulting in clinical disease in pigs has been recently demonstrated (Mead et al. 2004).

In infected animals, vesicular stomatitis virus is primarily localized to epithelial surfaces on the snout, mouth, tongue, coronary bands, teats, and lymph nodes draining the affected areas. Virus is not found in blood or urine and only rarely in feces, but saliva, vesicular fluid, and sloughing epithelium can contain large amounts of virus. Virus has been found in epithelial samples and oropharyngeal fluids for up to 10 days after initiation of clinical signs (Martinez et al. 2003).

PATHOGENESIS

Most information on the pathogenesis of VSV is from laboratory inoculation of swine or cattle. VSV pathogenesis is dependent on viral strain, host characteristics, route of inoculation, and virus dose. In swine, clinical disease consistently results when virus is inoculated intradermally by epidermal scarification of the snout or the coronary band with at least 10^6 virus infectious doses. Intradermal inoculation at other sites or intranasal instillation does not result in clinical disease, but virus can be isolated from tonsil swabs, indicating subclinical infection (Howerth et al. 1997).

VSV is a localized infection, with no viremia detected in cattle, horses, or swine. Primary replication seems to occur locally in keratinocytes (Rodriguez, unpublished results). Virus is readily found at the site of lesions or in the tonsil from which virus is shed in saliva or from local draining lymph nodes. Virus is not found in other tissues, including muscle, brain, liver, spleen, mesenteric lymph nodes, kidneys, and spinal cord (Rodriguez, unpublished results). Subclinically infected pigs can shed virus for several days via the saliva and transmit infection to other swine by direct contact (Stallknecht et al. 1999).

Vesicular stomatitis serotype New Jersey seems to cause more severe disease in swine than serotype Indiana. Pigs inoculated with VSNJV by scarification of the snout develop large vesicles at the inoculation site in 2–3 days, followed by coronary band lesions by 5–7 days postinoculation. In contrast, VSINV inoculated swine develop only small lesions at the inoculated site and rarely generalize to the feet or transmit the infection to contact pigs. This difference in virulence between serotypes in swine is likely associated with the glycoprotein gene (Martinez et al. 2003). Host factors also seem to affect outcome of infection; lactating adult animals seem more susceptible to clinical disease than younger animals (Vanleeuwen et al. 1995).

CLINICAL SIGNS

Field studies following animal populations over time in endemic areas or during active outbreaks in areas of sporadic occurrence have demonstrated that the great majority of infections are subclinical (Mumford et al. 1998; Rodriguez et al. 1990; Stallknecht et al. 1985; Webb et al. 1987). The incubation period varies from 2–5 days, depending on the virus, route, and dose of inoculation. Initial signs in swine may include fever of 40–41°C, lethargy, loss of appetite, and increased salivation. Lesions appear 3–4 days after infection. Pigs tend to remain prostrate, because foot lesions can be severe and painful. Snout lesions can be severe and lead to loss of epithelium, leaving a raw reddish surface (refer to Figure 31.3). After vesicles rupture, there is usually crusting of the lesions before healing is complete 2–3 weeks later (Martinez et al. 2003). Morbidity can be high, and in some cases approach 90–100% of individuals in swine herds. But individual cases are also reported, particularly in endemic areas. Mortality is rare.

Factors affecting clinical signs are not clearly defined. Laboratory inoculation models can only partially duplicate the severity of disease. It is hypothesized that environmental factors, such as insect bites, influence the development and severity of disease by modulating the immune response or other host-protective mechanisms (Tabachnick 2000). There is evidence that insect saliva can potentiate virus infection in vitro by decreasing cellular interferon response (Limesand et al. 2000).

LESIONS

Typically, vesicles appear on the snout, tongue, lips, mouth, coronary bands, interdigital space, or foot pads. Multiple lesions at different sites can occur in the same animal. Lesions begin as blanched areas with raised borders that evolve into vesicles or directly into crusted lesions. There may be loss of epithelium, leaving a reddish area covered by clear exudates or dry vesicular fluid. Profuse bleeding is not common. However, in severe cases bleeding may be associated with the loss of claws or epithelium. There are no characteristics unique to VSV gross lesions that differentiate them from other causes of vesicular disease in swine (SVD, FMD, and VES) (Jubb et al. 1985).

Histopathologically, VSV vesicular lesions start at the stratum spinosum with intercellular edema and mi-crovesicles, followed by acantholysis. In early vesicles, epithelial cells remain attached by intercellular desmosomes, giving the tissue a reticular pattern sometimes compared to a stretched Japanese lantern (D. Gregg, personal communication). Later, there are infected and dead keratinocytes and a severe infiltrate of inflammatory cells, mostly neutrophils. Lesions rarely invade the stratum basale. Upper layers above the stratum basale separate, microvesicles coalesce, and vesicular fluid accumulates filling the vesicles (Seibold and Sharp 1960).

IMMUNITY

Immune responses to VSV in livestock species are poorly understood. Neutralizing antibodies are readily detectable as early as 4 days after clinical infection, with antibody titers increasing over time. Interestingly, subclinical infections also result in increasing titers of neutralizing antibodies, but higher titers (2–4 $\log_{10}$) are observed in clinical than in subclinical infections (1–1.5 $\log_{10}$). In endemic regions, neutralizing antibody titers fluctuate among animals without clinical disease, but fourfold increases or greater are usually associated with clinical infections (Rodriguez et al. 1990).

Isotype analyses show a typical IgM response at 4 days post infection, followed by IgG1 and IgG2 responses after 14–21 days, indicating both T-helper-1 and T-helper-2 responses in both clinical and subclinical cases (Rodriguez, unpublished results).

Antibody titers after subclinical infection in livestock do not correlate well with protection. Field evidence suggests that neutralizing antibodies are not protective, even against the homologous serotype, and animals can become clinically ill despite the presence of significant titers of neutralizing antibodies (Rodriguez et al. 1990). Furthermore, viral strains causing disease are fully neutralized by sera obtained from the same animals prior to clinical disease, and there is no evidence of neutralizing escape mutants (Vernon et al. 1990). There is no cross protection between serotypes.

Young animals are less susceptible to clinical disease than adults, but the basis of this resistance is unknown. Maternal neutralizing antibodies are detectable in calves born to seropositive dams, with titers decreasing over time. In most cases, maternal antibodies become undetectable by 6 months of age, but can persist for up to 10 months (Remmers et al. 2000).

DIAGNOSIS

VS lesions are localized in the mouth, tongue, coronary bands, and interdigital space, with occasional lesions in teats of lactating sows. Internal organs are not affected, but virus can also be found in local lymph nodes draining lesion sites (Mebus 1977).

Complement fixation is the traditional laboratory test for detection of viral antigens (Stone and DeLay

1963). The complement fixation test, though still practiced in many countries, has largely been replaced by the antigen-capture ELISA (Ferris and Donaldson 1988). However, the gold standard assay remains virus isolation in green monkey kidney cells (Vero), with subsequent agent characterization. Molecular detection of viral RNA has also been used, including detection by reverse transcription polymerase chain reaction (RT-PCR) individually or in multiplex assays with other vesicular disease (Nuñez et al. 1998; Rodriguez et al. 1993).

The gold standard test for antibody detection is VN using Vero cells as indicators. Nonspecific neutralizing activity of certain sera to VSV can result in false positives, particularly at lower serum dilutions. Paired sera and confirmatory tests, such as complement fixation and ELISA, are recommended (Katz et al. 1997). A competitive ELISA capable of detecting antibodies in various species has also been described (Katz et al. 1995).

PREVENTION AND CONTROL

Treatment of affected animals is not widely recommended, except for palliative measures such as feeding soft feeds and avoiding hard surfaced floors. Topical treatment of lesions with local antiseptics is advised for faster healing and decreasing the risk of secondary opportunistic pathogens. Disinfection of the facilities and separation of affected animals to minimize contact transmission is also recommended. Antibiotic therapy may be implemented to avoid secondary bacterial infections in severe foot or mouth lesions.

Since VSV is transmitted by insects, preventive measures should incorporate insect control with approved insecticides for farm use. Recent studies suggest that permethrin and similar compounds can reduce insect attacks for extended periods (Schmidtmann et al. 2001). In addition, housing animals during times of high insect activity (dawn and dusk) may reduce the attack rate (Hurd et al. 1999). Precautions should be taken to avoid transferring equipment and personnel from affected farms.

Vaccination is available in some endemic countries, where vaccines containing inactivated virus of each serotype are used prior to periods of high vector activity (Arbelaez and Cardona 1982). Vaccination is not recommended or cost-effective in countries with sporadic occurrence of VS. Once an outbreak has occurred, animals should be kept on the premises for at least 30 days after the last clinical case has resolved to avoid spread.

Swine Vesicular Disease

In 1966 a new disease emerged in Italy. The disease was clinically recognized as FMD, but was caused by another enterovirus distinct from FMD (Nardelli et al. 1968). This newly described disease was later called swine vesicular disease (SVD). The virus (SVDV) was subsequently isolated in an FMD vaccine trial in Hong Kong in 1971 (Mowat et al. 1972). In 1972, SVD was diagnosed in Great Britain, Austria, Italy, and Poland. The first case of SVD in the Netherlands occurred in 1975 (Franssen 1975). Recently Portugal (2004) and Italy (2004) have reported outbreaks of SVD (Table 31.1). The last outbreak in Taiwan was reported in 1999, but the virus is probably still present in Asian countries. North and South America are considered free of SVDV, and reports from cases of swine with vesicular conditions in Bolivia and Nicaragua (Table 31.1) are likely considered misdiagnoses.

SVD is currently classified as a list A disease by the Office International des Epizooties (OIE) because the lesions caused by SVD resemble those caused by foot-and-mouth disease. Because of the frequency of subclinical infection, most of the recent outbreaks in Italy were not discovered by clinical inspection, but by serological screening. In the absence of serological screening, the disease would probably be under-reported in Italy. Therefore, it is likely that the virus is present in more countries than those that officially report absence of the disease.

Human infection has been strongly suggested (Brown et al. 1976; Graves 1973), with subsequent need for hospitalization of the infected persons. Sequence homologies to Coxsackie-B5 virus (structural part of the virus) and Echo-virus 9 (nonstructural part of the virus; Zhang et al. 1999) suggest a common ancestor for these viruses. Therefore, SVDV infection in cell lines of human origin would not be surprising. Severe illness in humans, however, has not been reported recently, not even from laboratories working with large quantities of live virus during large-scale screening, so it remains questionable whether the illness leading to hospitalization in earlier reports was actually caused by SVDV.

ETIOLOGY

SVDV is classified as an enterovirus within family *Picornaviridae*. SVD virus is small (30–32 nm), nonenveloped, and contains a single strand of RNA with a positive polarity. Studies with polyclonal antibodies reveal only small antigenic differences among different isolates, and thus SVDV is considered to be a single serotype. Isolates, however, can be divided into four distinct phylogenetic groups by comparing them against panels of monoclonal antibody reaction patterns or nucleotide sequences of the 1D (VP1) gene (Borrego et al. 2002a, b; Brocchi et al. 1997).

The SVDV genome consists of approximately 7400

Table 31.1. Year of last appearance of swine vesicular disease outbreaks in the world. Based on the *FAO-OIE-WHO Animal Health Yearbook (1971–1995)* and information obtained from the European reference laboratory for vesicular diseases in Pirbright (U.K.)

Country	Year of Last Appearance
Europe	
Portugal	2004
Italy	2004
Netherlands	1994
Belgium	1993
Spain	1993
Germany	1985
Romania	1985
France	1983
Great Britain	1982
Austria	1979
Greece	1979
Malta	1978
Ukraine	1977
Russia	1975
Switzerland	1975
Poland	1972
Bulgaria	1971
North and South America	
Bolivia	1991 (See text)
Nicaragua	1986 (See text)
Asia	
Taiwan	1999
Lebanon	1992
Hong Kong	1991
Laos	1991
Macau	1989
Korea	1980
Japan	1975

nucleotides and encodes for a single polyprotein of 2815 amino acids (Inoue et al. 1989). This polyprotein is post-translationally cleaved into 11 proteins. Four of these proteins, 1A, 1B, 1C, and 1D, form the virus capsid (Fry et al. 2003; Jimenez Clavero et al. 2003) and one of these proteins, 3B, is linked to the viral RNA. The nonstructural proteins are involved in virus replication and host-cell shut-off.

SVDV is extremely resistant to adverse environmental conditions and many commonly used disinfectants (Terpstra 1992). The virus remains infectious for months in carcasses and processed meat, e.g., salami or pepperoni sausages (Hedger and Mann 1989; Mebus et al. 1997).

The virus can be grown on primary or secondary porcine kidney cells and a wide range of pig kidney-derived cell lines and secondary lamb kidney cells (Dekker, unpublished data). SVDV can be differentiated from FMDV on the basis of its inability to grow on primary bovine thyroid cells.

SVDV infections in humans have been documented (Brown et al. 1976), and the virus is lethal to newborn mice (Nardelli et al. 1968). It shares with Coxsackie viruses its ability to infect mice, unlike other enteroviruses (Graves 1973). Because of these characteristics (host tropism and antigenic similarity) SVDV is thought to be closely related to Coxsackie B5 virus and likely represents a porcinophillic Coxsackie B5 isolate (Graves 1973). Nucleic acid sequence data show that SVDV has ~75–85% homology with Coxsackie B5 virus (Knowles and McCauley 1997), and phylogenetic analysis indicate that SVDV and recent Coxsackie B5 isolates probably shared a common ancestor in the period between 1945 and 1965 (Zhang et al. 1999).

EPIDEMIOLOGY

Outbreaks of SVD have been limited to a small number of countries (Table 31.1). However, since subclinical infections are common, the disease might have been present or is likely present in other countries and documentation is poor.

Clinical disease is restricted to pigs; not only Euro-Asian pigs, but also American one-toed pigs are susceptible (Wilder et al. 1974). Relatively high titers of SVDV have been detected in the pharynx of sheep kept in close contact with SVD-infected pigs (Burrows et al. 1974). Even neutralizing antibodies were detected in some of these contact sheep, which might indicate that the virus had replicated in this species.

An epidemiological field study in Great Britain revealed that the main source of infection was movement of pigs (48%), either because infected pigs were transported (16%), contaminated transport vehicles were used (21%), or because of contacts at markets (11%). A second source of infection (15%) was feeding of contaminated waste food (Hedger and Mann 1989). The exceptionally high stability of the virus outside the host is the reason why indirect contacts like transporting vehicles or waste food play an essential role in the epidemiology of SVD. Dekker et al. (1995a) showed that contact with a contaminated environment can lead to viremia in 1 day and clinical signs within 2 days. Studies on SVDV transmission within an outbreak farm showed that spread between pens most likely occurs when there is a shared open drainage system or frequent movement of pigs between pens. SVD, therefore, is considered a "pen disease" rather than a farm disease (Hedger and Mann 1989; Dekker et al. 2002).

Because infected herds are culled immediately in countries that maintain heightened surveillance and operational contingency plans, it is not easy to study the transmission of SVD in the field. IgM and IgG ELISAs have been developed to study the time the virus was introduced (Brocchi et al. 1995; Dekker et al. 2002). With these ELISAs, however, the exact time of introduction cannot be fully assessed, and after approximately 50 days the antibody isotype profiles of most infected animals are similar. Therefore, an estimation of the time of introduction beyond 50 days is not possible (Dekker et al. 2002). In contrast to FMDV infections in ruminants, persistence of SVD in infected pigs is not common. There is one report where SVD virus was recovered up to 126 days after infection (Lin et al. 1998), but it has been difficult to reproduce these findings (Lin et al. 2001).

PATHOGENESIS

It has been suggested that SVDV enters the pig through the skin or the mucous membrane of the digestive tract (Chu et al. 1979; Lai et al. 1979; Mann and Hutchings 1980). Experimental SVDV infection can lead to clinical signs within 2 days and SVDV has been isolated from a wide range of tissues (Burrows et al. 1974; Chu et al. 1979; Dekker et al. 1995a; Lai et al. 1979). When pigs are exposed to an SVDV-contaminated environment, viremia can develop within 1 day. This is identical to the time frame when pigs are directly inoculated (Dekker et al. 1995a), which further suggests a mucous or abrasion point of entry.

SVDV has a strong tropism for epithelial tissues, but virus titers in myocardial and brain samples significantly exceed those found in plasma. As such, epithelial tissues, myocardium, and brain are probably the sites of virus replication (Chu et al. 1979; Lai et al. 1979) and excellent samples for analysis. Nevertheless, lymph nodes have also been shown to contain high titers of SVDV after experimental infection, either because of lymphatic drainage or true virus replication (Dekker et al. 1995a).

In vitro studies showed that immunological staining of cells is more efficient than in situ hybridization, with infected cells showing a positive reaction by immunohistochemistry after only 3.5 hours post infection of porcine kidney tissue culture. In situ hybridization, however, seems to be superior when used for staining of SVDV-infected tissue samples (Mulder et al. 1997).

Additional research is required to identify the cells that support SVDV replication, which may help identify the mechanism behind the host tropism of the virus.

CLINICAL SIGNS

Clinical disease is restricted to pigs. In pigs infected with SVDV, vesicles appear principally around the coronary bands (refer to Figures 31.4, 31.5); on the skin of the metacarpus and metatarsus; and to a lesser extent on the snout, tongue, and lips. Lesions are indistinguishable from those induced by an FMD infection. The clinical signs caused by SVD are, however, much milder than those caused by FMD. In the experimental studies performed by the author, fever was always absent and lameness was almost never observed. Sudden death, due to myocardial infarction and necrosis, often observed in young piglets affected with FMD, is not seen in SVD.

Strains of SVDV vary in virulence, and the disease may run a subclinical, mild, or severe course. The latter is usually only seen when pigs are housed on concrete floor structures in humid conditions (Hedger and Mann 1989; Kanno et al. 1996; Kodama et al. 1980).

LESIONS

In typical cases of SVD, lesions are first noticed at the junction of the heel and the coronary band (as can be seen in Figures 31.4 and 31.5). The entire coronary band may eventually be affected with lesions spreading to the metatarsal and metacarpal regions. The horn and sole may be damaged so extensively that the claw(s) slough off. In lactating sows, lesions on the udder and teats can be seen (refer to Figure 31.6). Occasionally, the skin of the thorax and abdomen is also involved, which is not a finding with FMD or VSV infections. Lesions in the mouth, lips, and snout are not too common, but can be seen in approximately 10% of cases. Vesicular snout lesions are usually on the dorsal face of the rostrum and may be hemorrhagic in appearance. Tongue lesions are transient and heal rapidly (Hedger and Mann 1989). In experimentally infected animals, nonsuppurative meningoencephalitis may occur, but this does not result in signs of impaired central nervous system function (Chu et al. 1979).

DIAGNOSIS

The antibody response to SVDV infection is rapid. An IgM-based ELISA can detect a nascent immune response by day 4 post infection in 50% of experimental cases, by day 5 using the VN test, and by day 12 with an IgG-based ELISA (Dekker et al. 2002).

In the aftermath of an outbreak, absence of specific antibodies is essential to prove that no infected farms have been missed, since high titers of neutralizing antibodies are found (Nardelli et al. 1968) and subclinical infection may occur. VN tests, however, are laborious and ELISAs have been developed (Armstrong and Barnett 1989; Brocchi et al. 1995; Chenard et al. 1998; Dekker et al. 1995b; Hamblin and Crowther 1995). Although the ELISA is easier to perform than VN, it produces more false positive results. The specificity of the ELISA can be increased by using specific monoclonal antibodies (Brocchi et al. 1995; Chenard et al. 1998). This protocol has been adopted as the standard assay by the OIE and has been shown to be highly efficient in large-scale serosurveillance (Dekker 2000).

PREVENTION AND CONTROL

When SVD was first recognized, it was not easy to differentiate from FMD, VS, or vesicular exanthema. Therefore, it was generally accepted that SVD would not be tolerated in countries free from the other vesicular diseases. For this reason, SVD was placed on the list A diseases of the OIE and is, therefore, a notifiable disease in most countries. In the case of an outbreak, SVD is strictly controlled by "stamping out" and the imposition of stringent restrictions on livestock movement. Stamping out involves the slaughter and destruction of the infected herds followed by thorough epidemiological tracing and surveillance of pigs on other premises that may have been exposed to infection. After the slaughter and disposal of pigs, the premises are cleaned and disinfected. Adequate disinfection is often difficult, especially in farms with damaged floors and walls. Several cases of recurring infection have been reported after stamping out measures, with infection recurring in the pens where the infected pigs had been previously housed (Hedger and Mann 1989). The costs of control measures and trade restrictions can be very high.

Because clinical signs are not always observed, serosurveillance is required, especially in the aftermath of an outbreak. Serological screening can detect subclinical or previously undetected clinical infections (Hendrie et al. 1978; Larenaudie et al. 1982; Pappous et al. 1980; Tokui et al. 1975). The Netherlands, Italy, and Spain are the only countries in the European Union to have large-scale serosurveillance programs. All other countries in the region rely on detection of SVD on the basis of clinical signs. Because of the large number of sera examined (approximately 500,000 a year in each country), considerable numbers of false-positive reactions are detected, each of which requires an exhaustive and extensive epidemiological study to determine the true status of the result. False-positive reactions, referred to as "singleton reactors," often show cross-reactive antibodies of the IgM isotype (De Clercq 1998). Studies to determine the cause of singleton reactors have identified a sole factor. Moonen et al. (2000) studied the possible role of human Coxsackie B5 as a confounding factor, but all singleton reactor sera reacted more strongly with SVDV than Coxsackie B5 virus. Kadoi et al. (2001), however, reported natural infection of pigs with Coxsackie B5 virus.

Experimental vaccines have been developed to control SVD infection (Delagneau et al. 1974; Gourreau et al. 1975; McKercher and Graves 1976; Mowat et al. 1974). In addition to SVD monovalent vaccines, combinations with FMD (McKercher and Graves 1976; Mitev et al. 1978) and, recently, an SVD subunit vaccine have been described. The latter vaccine was shown not to be efficacious (Jimenez Clavero et al. 1998). Although inactivated virus preparations are efficacious in protecting against clinical signs, these have not been evaluated relative to their ability to reduce wild-type virus transmission. Currently, no SVD vaccine is commercially available and vaccination has not been undertaken in the field.

REFERENCES

Alexandersen S, Donaldson AI. 2002. Further studies to quantify the dose of natural aerosols of foot-and-mouth disease virus for pigs. Epidemiol Infect 128:313–323.

Alexandersen S, Oleksiewicz MB, Donaldson AI. 2001. The early pathogenesis of foot-and-mouth disease in pigs infected by contact: A quantitative time-course study using TaqMan RT-PCR. J Gen Virol 82:747–755.

Arbelaez G, Cardona U. 1982. Vaccine trial against vesicular stomatitis II: Field experimental observations. Rev ACOVEZ 6:27–34.

Armstrong RM, Barnett ITR. 1989. An enzyme linked immunosorbent assay (ELISA) for the detection and quantification of antibodies against swine vesicular disease virus (SVDV). J Virol Methods 25:71–79.

Bachrach HL. 1968. Foot and mouth disease virus. Annu Rev Microbiol 22:201–244.

Ball LA, Pringle CR, Flanagan B, Perepelitsa VP, Wertz GW. 1999. Phenotypic consequences of rearranging the P, M, and G genes of vesicular stomatitis virus. J Virol 73:4705–4712.

Beard CW, Mason PW. 2000. Genetic determinants of altered virulence of Taiwanese foot-and-mouth disease virus. J Virol 74:987–991.

Black L, Francis MJ, Rweyemamu MM, Umebara O, Boge A. 1984. The relationship between serum antibody titers and protection from foot and mouth disease in pigs after oil emulsion vaccination. J Biol Stand 12:379–389.

Borrego B, Carra E, Garcia Ranea JA, Brocchi E. 2002a. Characterization of neutralization sites on the circulating variant of swine vesicular disease virus (SVDV): A new site is shared by SVDV and the related coxsackie B5 virus. J Gen Virol 83:35–44.

Borrego B, Garcia Ranea JA, Douglas A, Brocchi E. 2002b. Mapping of linear epitopes on the capsid proteins of swine vesicular disease virus using monoclonal antibodies. J Gen Virol 83:1387–1395.

Bradish CJ, Kirkham JB. 1966. The morphology of vesicular stomatitis virus (Indiana C) derived from chick embryos or cultures of BHK21/13 cells. J Gen Microbiol 44:359–371.

Brocchi E, Berlinzani A, Gamba D, Desimone F. 1995. Development of two novel monoclonal antibody-based ELISAs for the detection of antibodies and the identification of swine isotypes against swine vesicular disease virus. J Virol Methods 52:155–167.

Brocchi E, Zhang G, Knowles NJ, Wilsden G, McCauley JW, Marquardt O, Ohlinger VF, Desimone F. 1997. Molecular epidemiology of recent outbreaks of swine vesicular disease: Two genetically and antigenically distinct variants in Europe, 1987–94. Epidemiol Infect 118:51–61.

Brown F, Goodridge D, Burrows R. 1976. Infection of man by swine vesicular disease virus. J Comp Pathol 86:409–414.

Burrows R, Mann JA, Goodridge D. 1974. Swine vesicular disease: Virological studies of experimental infections produced by the England/72 virus. J Hyg 72:135–143.

Callahan JD, Brown F, Osorio FA, Sur JH, Kramer E, Long GW, Lubroth J, Ellis SJ, Shoulars KS, Gaffney KL, Rock DL, Nelson WM. 2002. Use of a portable real-time reverse transcriptase-polymerase chain reaction assay for rapid detection of foot-and-mouth disease virus. J Am Vet Med Assoc 220:1636–1642.

Callens M, De Clercq K. 1999. Highly sensitive detection of swine vesicular disease virus based on a single tube RT PCR system and DIG ELISA detection. J Virol Methods 77:87–99.

Carrillo C, Plana J, Mascarella R, Bergada J, Sobrino F. 1990. Genetic and phenotypic variability during replication of foot-and-mouth disease virus in swine. Virology 179:890–892.

Cartwright B, Brown F. 1972. Serological relationships between different strains of vesicular stomatitis virus. J Gen Virol 16:391–398.

Casas Olascoaga R, Gomes I, Rosenberg FJ, Augé de Mello P, Astudillo V, Magallanes N. 1999. Fiebre Aftosa. Organización Panamericana de Salud. Editora Atheneu, São Paulo, Brazil. 458 pp.

Chenard G, Bloemraad M, Kramps JA, Terpstra C, Dekker A. 1998. Validation of a monoclonal antibody based ELISA to detect antibodies directed against swine vesicular disease virus. J Virol Methods 75:105–112.

Chu RM, Moore DM, Conroy JD. 1979. Experimental swine vesicular disease, pathology and immunofluorescence studies. Can J Comp Med 43:29–38.

Coll JM. 1997. Synthetic peptides from the heptad repeats of the glycoproteins of rabies, vesicular stomatitis and fish rhabdoviruses bind phosphatidylserine. Arch Virol 142:2089–2097.

Condy JB, Hedger RS, Hamblin C, Barnett IT. 1985. The duration of the foot-and-mouth disease virus carrier state in African buffalo (i) in the individual animal and (ii) in a free-living herd. Comp Immunol Microbiol Infect Dis 8:259–265.

Cotton WE. 1927. Vesicular stomatitis. Vet Med 22:169–175.

Cottral GE. 1969. Persistence of foot-and-mouth disease virus in animals, their products and the environment. Bull Off Int Epizoot 70:549–568.

Cupp EW, Mare CJ, Cupp MS, Ramberg FB. 1992. Biological transmission of vesicular stomatitis virus (New Jersey) by Simulium vittatum (Diptera: Simuliidae). J Med Entomol 29:137–140.

Dawe PS, Flanagan FO, Madekurozwa RL, Sorensen KJ, Anderson EC, Foggin CM, Ferris NP, Knowles NJ. 1994. Natural transmission of foot-and-mouth disease virus from African buffalo (*Syncerus caffer*) to cattle in a wildlife area of Zimbabwe. Vet Rec 134:230–232.

De Clercq K. 1998. Reduction of singleton reactors against swine vesicular disease virus by a combination of virus neutralisation test, monoclonal antibody based competitive ELISA and isotype specific ELISA. J Virol Methods 70:7–18.

Dekker A. 2000. Pathogenesis, diagnosis and epizootiology of swine vesicular disease (Chapter 7). PhD thesis, Faculty of Veterinary Medice, Utrecht University, Utrecht.

Dekker A, Moonen P, de Boer-Luijtze EA, Terpstra C. 1995a. Pathogenesis of swine vesicular disease after exposure of pigs to an infected environment. Vet Microbiol 45:234–250.

Dekker A, Moonen P, Terpstra C. 1995b. Validation of a screening liquid phase blocking ELISA for swine vesicular disease. J Virol Methods 51:343–348.

Dekker A, Van Hemert Kluitenberg F, Baars C, Terpstra C. 2002. Isotype specific ELISAs to detect antibodies against swine vesicular disease virus and their use in epidemiology. Epidemiol Infect 128:277–284.

Delagneau JF, Guerche J, Adamowicz P, Prunet P. 1974. Swine vesicular disease: Physicochemical and immunogenic properties of the virus strain France 1/73. Ann Microbiol 125B:559–574.

Doel TR. 1999. Optimisation of the immune response to foot-and-mouth disease vaccines. Vaccine 17:1767–1771.

——. 2003. FMD vaccines. Virus Res 91:81–99.

Doel TR, Williams L, Barnett PV. 1994. Emergency vaccination against foot-and-mouth disease: Rate of development of immunity and its implication for the carrier state. Vaccine 12:592–600. (not in text)

Domingo E, Mateu MG, Escarmis C, Martinez-Salas D, Andreu E, Giralt N, Verdaguer, Fita I. 1995. Molecular evolution of aphthoviruses. Virus Genes 11:197–207.

Donaldson AI. 1986. Aerobiology of foot-and-mouth disease (FMD): An outline and recent advances. Rev Sci Tech Epi 5:315–321.

Donaldson AI, Gibson CF, Oliver R, Hamblin C, Kitching RP. 1987. Infection of cattle by airborne FMD: M+inimal doses with O1 and SAT-2 strains. Res Vet Sci 43:555–564.

Dunn CS, Donaldson AI. 1997. Natural adaptation to pigs of a Taiwanese isolate of foot-and-mouth disease virus. Vet Rec 141:174–175.

Ferris NP, Donaldson AI. 1988. An enzyme-linked immunosorbent assay for the detection of vesicular stomatitis virus antigen. Vet Microbiol 18:243–258.

Fields BN, Hawkins K. 1967. Human infection with the virus of vesicular stomatitis during an epizootic. N Engl J Med 277:989–994.

Francis MJ, Black L. 1986a. Humoral response of pregnant sows to foot-and-mouth disease vaccination. J Hyg (Camb) 96:501–511.

——. 1986b. Response of young pigs to foot-and-mouth disease oil emulsion vaccination in the presence and absence of maternally derived neutralizing antibodies. Res Vet Sci 41:33–39.

Francy DB, Moore CG, Smith GC, Jakob WL, Taylor SA, Calisher CH. 1988. Epizootic vesicular stomatitis in Colorado, 1982: Isolation of virus from insects collected along the northern Colorado Rocky Mountain Front Range. J Med Entomol 25:343–347.

Franssen PGJ. 1975. Een geval van vesiculaire varkensziekte (swine vesicular disease—S.V.D.) in Nederland. Tijdschr Diergeneesk 100:1325–1327.

Fry EE, Knowles NJ, Newman JWI, Wilsden G, Rao ZH, King AMQ, Stuart DI. 2003. Crystal structure of swine vesicular disease virus and implications for host adaptation. J Virol 77:5475–5486.

Geering W, Lubroth J. 2002. Foot-and-mouth disease contingency plans. Food and Agriculture Organisation. Animal Production and Health Manual No. 16. Rome, Italy, 100 pp.

Gibbens JC, Sharpe CE, Wilesmith JW, Mansley LM, Michalopoulou E, Ryan JBM, Hudson M. 2001. Descriptive epidemiology of the 2001 foot-and-mouth disease epidemic in Great Britain: The first five months. Vet Rec 149:729–743.

Gloster J, Alexandersen S. 2004. New Directions: Airborne transmission of foot-and-mouth disease virus. Atmos Environ 38:503–505.

Gourreau JM, Dhennin L, Labie J. 1975. Preparation of an inactivated virus vaccine against swine vesicular disease. Rec Med Vet 151:85–89.

Graves JH. 1973. Serological relationship of swine vesicular disease virus and Coxsackie B5 virus. Nature 245:314–315.

Grubman MJ, Baxt B. 2004. Foot-and-mouth disease. Clin Micobiol Rev 17:465–493.

Hamblin C, Crowther JR. 1995. A rapid enzyme linked immunosorbent assay for the serological confirmation of swine vesicular disease. Br Vet J 138:247–252.

Hansen DE, Thurmond MC, Thorburn M. 1985. Factors associated with the spread of clinical vesicular stomatitis in California dairy cattle. Am J Vet Res 46:789–795.

Hanson RP. 1950. The natural history of vesicular stomatitis. Bacteriol Rev 16:179–204.

——. 1981. Vesicular Stomatitis. In Virus Diseases of Food Animals, Vol. II. EP Gibbs, ed. New York: Academic Press, pp. 517–539.

Hanson RP, Rasmussen AF, Brandly CA, Brown JW. 1950. Human Infection with the virus of vesicular stomatitis. J Lab Clin Med 36:754–758.

Hedger RS. 1971. The carrier state in foot-and-mouth disease, and the probang test. Vet J 26:45–50.

Hedger RS, Mann JA. 1989. Swine vesicular disease virus. Virus Infections of Vertebrates, Vol 2. Virus Infections of Porcines. In MB Pesaert, ed. Amsterdam: Elsevier Science Publishers BV, pp. 241–250.

Hendrie EW, Baker K, Hedger R, Davies G, Richards MS. 1978. Swine vesicular disease: Serum surveys 5 and 6. Vet Rec 102:126–127.

House C, Meyer RF. 1993. The detection of foot-and-mouth disease virus in oesophageal-pharyngeal samples by a polymerase chain reaction technique. J Virol Methods 43:1–6.

Howerth EW, Stallknecht DE, Dorminy M, Pisell T, Clarke GR. 1997. Experimental vesicular stomatitis in swine: Effects of route of inoculation and steroid treatment. J Vet Diagn Invest 9:136–142.

Hurd HS, McCluskey BJ, Mumford EL. 1999. Management factors affecting the risk for vesicular stomatitis in livestock operations in the western United States. J Am Vet Med Assoc 215:1263–1268.

Inoue T, Suzuki T, Sekiguchi K. 1989. The complete nucleotide sequence of swine vesicular disease virus. J Gen Virol 70:919–934.

Jimenez Clavero MA, Escribano Romero E, Sanchez Vizcaino JM, Ley V. 1998. Molecular cloning, expression and immunological analysis of the capsid precursor polypeptide (P1) from swine vesicular disease virus. Virus Res 57:163–170.

Jimenez Clavero MA, Ley V, Fita I, Verdaguer N. 2003. Crystallization and preliminary X-ray analysis of swine vesicular disease virus (SVDV). Acta Crystallogr D Biol Crystallogr 59:541–543.

Jubb K, Kennedy PC, Palmer N. 1985. Pathology of Domestic Animals. Vol. 2. New York: Academic Press, pp. 90–110.

Kadoi K, Suzuki H, Nishio O. 2001. Isolation of coxsackievirus B5 from pigs. Microbiologica 24:217–222.

Kanno T, Inoue T, Wang YF, Sarai A, Yamaguchi S. 1996. Identification of the location of antigenic sites of swine vesicular disease virus with neutralization-resistant mutants. J Gen Virol 76:3099–3106.

Katz JB, Eernisse KA, Landgraf JG, Schmitt BJ. 1997. Comparative performance of four serodiagnostic procedures for detecting bovine and equine vesicular stomatitis virus antibodies. J Vet Diagn Invest 9:329–331.

Katz JB, Shafer AL, Eernisse KA. 1995. Construction and insect larval expression of recombinant vesicular stomatitis nucleocapsid protein and its use in competitive ELISA. J Virol Methods 54:145–157.

King AMQ, Brown F, Christian P, Hovi T, Hyypia T, Knowles NJ, Lemon, SM, Minor PD, Palmenberg AC, Skern T, Stanway G. 1999. *Picornaviridae*. In Virus taxonomy: Classification and Nomenclature of Viruses. MHV van Regenmortel, CM Fauquet, DHL Bishop, EB Carstens, MK Estes, SM Lemon, J Maniloff, MA Mayo, DJ McGeoch, CR Pringle, RB Wickner, eds. Seventh report of the International Committee on Taxonomy of Viruses. San Diego: Academic Press, pp. 657–673.

Knowles NJ, Davies PR, Henry T, O'Donnell V, Pacheco JM, Mason PW. 2001. Emergence in Asia of foot-and-mouth disease viruses with altered host range: Characterisation of alterations in the 3A protein. J Virol 75:1551–1556.

Knowles NJ, McCauley JW. 1997. Coxsackievirus B5 and the relationship to swine vesicular disease virus. Cur Top Microbiol Immunol 223:153–167.

Knowles NJ, Samuel AR. 1999. Molecular techniques in foot-and-mouth disease epidemiology. Proc Int Atomic Energy Agency 348:185–201.

Kodama M, Ogawa T, Saito T, Tokuda G, Sasahara J, Kumagai, T. 1980. Swine vesicular disease viruses isolated from healthy pigs in non epizootic period. I. Isolation and identification. Natl Inst Anim Health Q (Tokyo) Nat 20:1–10.

Kresse JI, Taylor WD, Stewart WW, Eernisse KA. 1985. Parvovirus infection in pigs with necrotic and vesicle-like lesions. Vet Microbiol 10:525–531.

Kretzschmar E, Peluso R, Schnell MJ, Whitt MA, Rose JK. 1996. Normal replication of vesicular stomatitis virus without C proteins. Virology 216:309–316.

Lai SS, McKercher PD, Moore DM, Gillespie JH. 1979. Pathogenesis of swine vesicular disease in pigs. Am J Vet Res 40:463–468.

Larenaudie B, Remond M, Gourreau JM. 1982. Swine vesicular disease in France. Results of a serological survey. 10th Conference of the OIE Regional Commission for Europe, 28 September–1 October, London.

Letchworth GJ, Rodriguez LL, Del C, Barrera J. 1999. Vesicular stomatitis. Vet J 157:239–260.

Limesand KH, Higgs S, Pearson LD, Beaty BJ. 2000. Potentiation of vesicular stomatitis New Jersey virus infection in mice by mosquito saliva. Parasite Immunol 22:461–467.

Lin F, Mackay DKJ, Knowles NJ. 1997. Detection of swine vesicular disease virus RNA by reverse transcription polymerase chain reaction. J Virol Methods 65:111–121.

——. 1998. The persistence of swine vesicular disease virus infection in pigs. Epidemiol Infect 121:459–472.

Lin F, Mackay DKJ, Knowles NJ, Kitching, RP. 2001. Persistent infection is a rare sequel following infection of pigs with swine vesicular disease virus. Epidemiol Infect 127:135–145.

Loeffler F, Frosch P. 1897. Summarischer Bericht uber die Ergebnisse der Untersuchungen zur Erforschung der Maul- und-Klauenseuche. Zentbl Backteriol Parasitenkd Abt I 22:257–259.

Lubroth J. 1998. Serological responses to FMDV nonstructural proteins 2C and 3ABC in a vaccinated South American cattle population in the absence of clinical disease. European Commission for the Control of Foot-and-Mouth Disease. Res Group Stand Tech Committee. Aldershot, United Kingdom. Sep 1998. Report FAO, Rome (Italy), pp. 182–190.

——. 2002. Foot-and-mouth disease. A review for the practitioner. Vet Clin North Am Food Anim Pract 18:475–499.

Lubroth J, Brown F. 1995. Identification of native foot-and-mouth disease virus non-structural protein 2C as a serological indicator to differentiate infected from vaccinated livestock. Res Vet Sci 59:70–78.

Mann JA, Hutchings GH. 1980. Swine vesicular disease: Pathways of infection. J Hyg 84:355–363.

Martinez I, Rodriguez LL, Jimenez C, Pauszek SJ, Wertz GW. 2003. Vesicular stomatitis virus glycoprotein is a determinant of pathogenesis in swine, a natural host. J Virol 77:8039–8047.

Mason PW, Grubman MJ, Baxt B. 2003. Molecular basis of pathogenesis of FMDV. Virus Res 91:9–32.

McKercher PD, Graves JH. 1976. A mixed vaccine for swine: An aid for control of foot and mouth and swine vesicular diseases. Bol Centro Panam Fiebre Aftosa 23/24:37–49.

McVicar JW, Eisner RJ, Johnson LA, Pursel VG. 1978. Foot-and-mouth disease and swine vesicular disease in boar semen. Proc Ann Meet US Anim Health Assoc, pp. 221–230.

Mead DG, Gray EW, Noblet R, Murphy MD, Howerth EW, Stallknecht DE. 2004. Biological transmission of vesicular stomatitis virus (New Jersey serotype) by *Simulium vittatum* (Diptera: *Simuliidae*) to domestic swine (*Sus scrofa*). J Med Entomol 41:78–82.

Mebus C. 1977. Ulcerative diseases of animals with an infectious etiology. J Oral Path 7:365–371.

Mebus C, Arias M, Pineda JM, Tapiador J, House C, Sanchez-Vizcaino JM. 1997. Survival of several porcine viruses in different Spanish dry cured meat products. Food Chem 59:555–559.

Mebus CA, House C, Gonzalvo F, Ruiz F, Pineda JM, Tapiador J, Pire JJ, Bergada J, Yedloutschnig RJ, Sahu S, Becerra V, Sanchez-Vizcaino JM. 1993. Survival of foot-and-mouth disease, African swine fever, and hog cholera viruses in Spanish Serrano cured hams and Iberian cured hams, shoulders and loins. Food Microbiol 10:133–143.

Mebus CA, Singh EL. 1991. Embryo transfer as a means of controlling the transmission of viral infections. XIII. Failure to transmit foot-and-mouth disease through the transfer of embryos from viremic donors. Theriogenology 35:435–441.

Meyer RF, Babcock GD, Newman JF, Burrage TG, Toohey K, Lubroth J, Brown F. 1997. Baculovirus expressed 2C of foot-and-mouth disease virus has the potential for differentiating convalescent from vaccinated animals. J Virol Methods 65:33–43.

Mezencio JMS, Babcock GD, Meyer RF, Lubroth J, Salt JS, Newman JFE, Brown F. 1998. Differentiating foot-and-mouth disease virus-infected from vaccinated animals with baculovirus-expressed specific proteins. Vet Quart 20:S11–S13.

Mitev G, Tekerlekov P, Dilovsky M, Ognianov D, Nikolova E. 1978. Experiments on the preparation and testing of associated vaccine against foot and mouth disease and vesicular disease in swine. Arch Exp Veterinarmed 32:29–33.

Montgomery JF, Oliver RE, Poole WSH. 1987. A vesiculo-bullous disease in pigs resembling foot-and-mouth disease. I. Field cases. NZ Vet J 35:21–26.

Moonen P, Van Poelwijk F, Moormann R, Dekker A. 2000. Singleton reactors in the diagnosis of swine vesicular disease: The role of coxsackievirus B5. Vet Microbiol 76:291–297.

Moraes MP, Chinsangaram J, Brum MCS, Grubman MJ. 2003. Immediate protection of swine from foot-and-mouth disease: A combination of adenoviruses expressing interferon alpha and foot-and-mouth disease virus subunit vaccine. Vaccine 22:268–279.

Mowat GN, Darbyshire JH, Huntley JF. 1972. Differentiation of a vesicular disease of pigs in Hong Kong from foot-and-mouth disease. Vet Rec 90:618–621.

Mowat GN, Prince MJ, Spier RE, Staple RF. 1974. Preliminary studies on the development of a swine vesicular disease vaccine. Arch Gesamte Virusforsch 44:350–360.

Mulder WAM, Vanpoelwijk F, Moormann RJM, Reus B, Kok GL, Pol JMA, Dekker A. 1997. Detection of early infection of swine vesicular disease virus in porcine cells and skin sections: A comparison of immunohistochemistry and in situ hybridization. J Virol Methods 68:169–175.

Mumford EL, McCluskey BJ, Traub-Dargatz JL, Schmitt BJ, Salman MD. 1998. Public veterinary medicine: Public health. Serologic evaluation of vesicular stomatitis virus exposure in horses and cattle in 1996. J Am Vet Med Assoc 213:1265–1269.

Nardelli L, Lodetti E, Gualandi GL, Burrows R, Goodridge D, Brown F, Cartwright B. 1968. A foot and mouth disease syndrome in pigs caused by an enterovirus. Nature 219:1275–1276.

Niedbalski W, Kesy A, Fitzner A. 2000. Differential diagnosis of swine vesicular disease virus (SVDV) by DNA amplification in vitro. Med Weter 56:513–516.

Nuñez, JI, Blanco E, Hernandez T, Gomez-Tejedor C, Martin MJ, Dopazo J, Sobrino F. 1998. A RT-PCR assay for the differential diagnosis of vesicular viral diseases of swine. J Virol Methods 72:227–235.

Pappous C, Dimitriadis I, Giannakidis D, Gogos A, Zafiriou G, Zoupidis A, Theodorou E, Iakovidis G, Lyritsis B, Moschovitis S, Tsilios C, Tsironis L. 1980. Serological survey of swine for neutralizing antibodies to swine vesicular disease. Deltion tes Hellenikes Kteniatrikes Hetaireias Bulletin of the Hellenic Veterinary Medical Society 31:244–252.

Pirtle EC, Beran GW. 1991. Virus survival in the environment. Rev Sci Tech 10:733–748.

Quiroz E, Moreno N, Peralta PH, Tesh RB. 1988. A human case of encephalitis associated with vesicular stomatitis virus (Indiana serotype) infection. Am J Trop Med Hyg 39:312–314.

Reid SM, Ferris NP, Hutchings GH, Samuel AR, Knowles NJ. 2000. Primary diagnosis of foot-and-mouth disease by reverse transcription polymerase chain reaction. J Virol Methods 89:167–176.

Remmers L, Perez E, Jimenez A, Vargas F, Frankena K, Romero JJ, Salman M, Herrero MV. 2000. Longitudinal studies in the epidemiology of vesicular stomatitis on Costa Rican dairy farms. Ann NY Acad Sci 916:417–430.

Rodriguez LL. 2002. Emergence and re-emergence of vesicular stomatitis in the United States. Virus Res 85:211–219.

Rodriguez LL, Bunch TA, Fraire M, Llewellyn ZN. 2000. Re-emergence of vesicular stomatitis in the western United States is associated with distinct viral genetic lineages. Virology 271:171–181.

Rodriguez LL, Letchworth GJ, Spiropoulou CF, Nichol ST. 1993. Rapid detection of vesicular stomatitis virus New Jersey serotype in clinical samples by using polymerase chain reaction. J Clin Microbiol 31:2016–2020.

Rodriguez LL, Nichol ST. 1999. Vesicular Stomatitis Viruses. In Encyclopedia of Virology. RG Webster, A Granoff, eds. London: Academic Press,pp. 1910–1919.

Rodriguez LL, Pauszek SJ, Bunch TA, Schumann KR. 2002. Full-length genome analysis of natural isolates of vesicular stomatitis virus (Indiana 1 serotype) from North, Central and South America. J Gen Virol 83:2475–2483.

Rodriguez LL, Vernon S, Morales AI, Letchworth GJ. 1990. Serological monitoring of vesicular stomatitis New Jersey virus in enzootic regions of Costa Rica. Am J Trop Med Hyg 42:272–281.

Salt JS. 1993. The carrier state in foot-and-mouth disease—An immunological review. Br Vet J 149:207–223.

Schlegel R, Tralka TS, Willingham MC, Pastan I. 1983. Inhibition of VSV binding and infectivity by phosphatidylserine: Is phosphatidylserine a VSV-binding site? Cell 32:639–646.

Schmidtmann ET, Lloyd, JE, Bobian RJ, Kumar R, Waggoner JW, Tabachinick WJ, Legg D. 2001. Suppression of mosquito (Diptera: *Culicidae*) and black fly (Diptera: *Simuliidae*) blood feeding from Hereford cattle and ponies treated with permethrin. J Med Entomol 38:728–734.

Schudel AA, Sadir AM, Echeverrigaray ME, Samus S, Colilla O, Rivenson S. 1981. Susceptibility of South American non-human primates to foot-and-mouth disease virus. Bull Off Int Epizoot 93:1345–1350.

Seganti L, Superti F, Girmenia C, Melucci L, Orsi N. 1986. Study of receptors for vesicular stomatitis virus in vertebreate and invertebrate cells. Microbiologica 9:259–267.

Seibold HR, Sharp JB. 1960. A revised concept of the pathological changes of the tongue in cattle with vesicular stomatitis. Am J Vet Res 21:35–51.

Shin N, Yeh MT, Shin H, Jang K, Kang J, Sur JH, An SH, Joo YS, Hyun BH, Lubroth J. 2002. Evaluation of a rapid serological pen-side diagnostic assay for FMD. Proc 17th Congr Int Pig Vet Soc 1:321.

Sorensen KJ, Madsen KG, Madsen ES, Salt JS, Nqindi J, Mackay DKJ. 1998. Differentiation of infection from vaccination in foot-and-mouth disease by the detection of antibodies to the nonstructural proteins 3D, 3AB, and 3ABC in ELISA using antigens expressed in baculovirus. Arch Virol 143:1–16.

Spiropoulou CF, Nichol ST. 1993. A small highly basic protein is encoded in overlapping frame within the P gene of vesicular stomatitis virus. J Virol 67:3103–3110.

Stallknecht DE, Howerth EW, Reeves CL, Seal BS. 1999. Potential for contact and mechanical vector transmission of vesicular stomatitis virus New Jersey in pigs. Am J Vet Res 60:43–48.

Stallknecht DE, Nettles VF, Fletcher WO, Erickson GA. 1985. Enzootic vesicular stomatitis New Jersey type in an insular feral swine population. Am J Epidemiol 122:876–883.

Stone SS and DeLay, PD. 1963. A rapid complement-fixation test for identification of vesicular stomatitis virus in cattle. Am J Vet Res 24:1060–1062.

Sudia WD, Fields BN, Calisher CH. 1967. The isolation of vesicular stomatitis virus (Indiana strain) and other viruses from mosquitoes in New Mexico, 1965. Am J Epidemiol 86:598–602.

Tabachnick WJ. 2000. Pharmacological factors in the saliva of blood-feeding insects. Implications for vesicular stomatitis epidemiology. Ann NY Acad Sci 916:444–452.

Terpstra C. 1992. Swine vesicular disease in the Netherlands. Tijdschr Diergeneeskd 117:623–626

Tesh RB, Chaniotis BN, Johnson KM. 1972. Vesicular stomatitis virus (Indiana Serotype): Transovarial transmission by Phlebotomine sandflies. Science 175:1477–1479.

Tokui T, Kono M, Tokuda G, Kumagai T, Sasahara J. 1975. Outbreaks of swine vesicular disease in Japan: Virus isolation and epizootiological survey. Natl Inst Anim Health Q (Tokyo) 15:165–173.

Vanleeuwen JA, Rodriguez LL, Waltner-Toews D. 1995. Cow, farm, and ecologic risk factors of clinical vesicular stomatitis on Costa Rican dairy farms. Am J Trop Med Hyg 53:342–350.

Vernon SD, Rodriguez LL, Letchworth GJ. 1990. Vesicular stomatitis New Jersey virus glycoprotein gene sequence and neutralizing epitope stability in an enzootic focus. Virology 177: 209–215.

Webb PA, Monath TP, Reif JS, Smith GC, Kemp GE, Lazuick JS, Walton TE. 1987. Epizootic vesicular stomatitis in Colorado, 1982: Epidemiologic studies along the northern Colorado front range. Am J Trop Med Hyg 36:183–188.

Wilder FW, Dardiri AH, Gay JG, Beasley HC, Heflin AA, Acree JA. 1974. Susceptibility of one-toed pigs to certain diseases exotic to the United States. Proc Ann Meet US Anim Health Assoc 78:195–199.

Zhang G, Haydon DT, Knowles NJ, McCauley JW. 1999. Molecular evolution of swine vesicular disease virus. J Gen Virol 80:639–651.

32 Miscellaneous Viral Infections

X. J. Meng, C. A. Baldwin, François Elvinger, Patrick G. Halbur, and Carolyn A. Wilson

This chapter focuses on viruses that are currently important to veterinary and human public health from a zoonotic and xenozoonotic perspective. The clinical significance and economic impact of these viruses on pig health are still uncertain. Swine hepatitis E virus (swine HEV), porcine endogenous retroviruses (PERV), and porcine lymphotropic herpesviruses (PLHV) are all of concern in human xenotransplantation with pig organs, tissues, and cells. Eastern equine encephalomyelitis virus (EEEV), Rabies virus, and swine HEV all pose zoonotic risks.

Swine Hepatitis E Virus
X.J. Meng and P.G. Halbur

Hepatitis E virus (HEV), the causative agent of human hepatitis E, is an important public health problem in many developing countries in Asia and Africa (Emerson and Purcell 2003; Purcell and Emerson 2001). The mortality rate associated with HEV infection is generally low (<1%) but can reach up to 25% during pregnancy (Kumar et al. 2004; Purcell and Emerson 2001). Although only sporadic cases of acute hepatitis E have been diagnosed in patients from industrialized countries, including the United States, a surprisingly high HEV antibody (anti-HEV) prevalence rate has been reported (Drobeniuc et al. 2001; Meng et al. 1999, 2002). The existence of a population of individuals in industrialized countries who are positive for anti-HEV has led to a hypothesis that an animal reservoir for HEV exists and that hepatitis E is a zoonosis (Meng 2003, 2004).

The first experimental evidence of HEV infection of pigs was reported by Balayan et al. (1990) who experimentally infected domestic pigs with a Central Asian strain of human HEV. Clayson et al. (1995) subsequently reported the detection of anti-HEV IgG in 18 of 55 pigs and of HEV RNA from sera and feces in 3 of 47 swine in Nepal. Unfortunately, the identity of the virus infecting swine in those studies was not determined. Meng et al. (1997) isolated and characterized the first animal strain of HEV, swine hepatitis E virus (swine HEV), from pigs in the United States. To isolate swine HEV, a prospective study was conducted in a commercial swine farm in Illinois. Twenty piglets, born to both anti-HEV negative and positive sows, were closely monitored for more than 5 months for evidence of HEV infection. A virus antigenically and genetically related to human HEV, designated swine HEV, was identified from the acute phase sera of the naturally infected piglets. Koch's postulates were subsequently fulfilled, as swine HEV infection was experimentally reproduced in specific-pathogen-free (SPF) pigs, and swine HEV was recovered from experimentally infected SPF pigs (Halbur et al. 2001; Meng et al. 1998a, 1998b).

The discovery of swine HEV and the demonstrated ability of swine HEV to infect across species raised potential concerns relative to food safety, public health, and xenotransplantation with pig organs and cells. However, the clinical implication of this virus in swine health is uncertain.

ETIOLOGY

HEV was initially classified in the family *Caliciviridae* based on the superficial similarity of its genomic organization to the caliciviruses. However, further comparative sequence analyses revealed that the codon usage and genomic organization of HEV are more related to that of rubella virus (a togavirus) than to that of the cali-

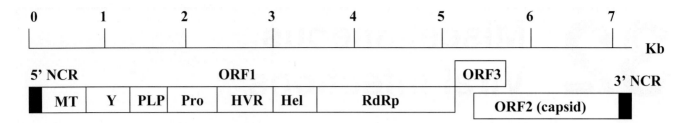

32.1. *Genomic organization of swine HEV. ORF1 encodes for nonstructural proteins, ORF2 for capsid protein and ORF3 for a small protein of unknown function. NCR, nocoding region; MT, methyltransferase; Y, "Y" domain; PLP, a papain-like cysteine protease; Pro, a proline-rich domain that may provide flexibility; HVR, a hypervariable region; Hel, helicase; RdRp, RNA-dependent RNA polymerase.*

civiruses (Koonin et al. 1992). Additionally, HEV possesses a cap structure at its 5′ end of the genome that is absent in calicivirus and does not share significant sequence homology with caliciviruses. Therefore, HEV has recently been reclassified in the new family *Hepeviridae* (Emerson and Purcell 2003). All strains of HEV identified thus far, including swine HEV, belong to the prototype genus *hepevirus* within the family.

HEV is a spherical, nonenveloped, symmetrical virus particle approximately 32–34 nm in diameter, with cup-shaped depressions on the surface similar to caliciviruses (Purcell and Emerson 2001). The morphology of swine HEV is not known, but is expected to be similar to that of human HEV. Like human HEV, swine HEV cannot be efficiently cultivated in cell culture.

The complete genome of swine HEV has been sequenced and shown to be a polyadenylated, single-stranded positive sense RNA molecule of approximately 7.2 kb in size (Meng et al. 1998a). Sequence analyses revealed that the genome of swine HEV contains three open reading frames (ORFs), a short 5′ noncoding region (NCR), and a short 3′ NCR (Figure 32.1).

ORF1, located at the 5′ end of the genome, is predicted to encode the nonstructural proteins. Several putative functional domains and motifs have been identified in the swine HEV ORF1, including the methyltransferase domain, a papain-like cysteine protease (PLP), a proline-rich domain that may provide flexibility, a hypervariable region (HVR), a helicase, and an RNA-dependent RNA polymerase (RdRp) (refer to Figure 32.1).

ORF2 encodes the immunogenic capsid protein. ORF3, encoding a small protein with unknown function, partially overlaps both ORF1 and ORF2. The ORF3 of human HEV is a cytoskeleton-associated phosphoprotein that may be involved in virus replication (Zafrullah et al. 1997).

EPIDEMIOLOGY

Seroepidemiological studies have shown that swine HEV infection is ubiquitous in pigs worldwide, both developing and industrialized countries, regardless of whether HEV is endemic in the respective human population (refer to Table 32.1). Seroprevalence rates vary from herd to herd and from region to region (Table 32.1).

Infected pigs generally have a transit viremia lasting for 1–2 weeks and shed viruses in feces for 3–7 weeks (Huang et al. 2002; Meng et al. 1998b; Takahashi et al. 2003). HEV infection generally occurs at 2–3 months of age (Figure 32.2), shortly after maternal antibodies have waned. This coincides with the time frame when pigs are moved to pens, an environment with increased opportunity for fecal cross-contamination (Huang et al. 2002; Meng et al. 1997). Adult pigs, sows, and boars, although commonly positive for anti-HEV IgG, are generally free of virus shedding.

Sequence analyses of swine HEV isolates identified thus far revealed the existence of at least two genotypes of swine HEV worldwide, i.e., genotypes 3 and 4 (Figure 32.3). In humans, both genotypes 3 and 4 HEV strains are known to cause sporadic cases of hepatitis E, whereas HEV strains of genotypes 1 and 2 are often associated with hepatitis E epidemics in Asia and Mexico (Meng 2004).

Besides domestic pigs, swine HEV also infects wild boars (Chandler et al. 1999). Under experimental conditions, rhesus monkeys and chimpanzees were susceptible to infection by swine HEV (Meng et al. 1998a). Rhesus monkeys experimentally inoculated with swine HEV seroconverted to anti-HEV IgG 4 weeks postinoculation. Viremia and fecal excretion of swine HEV were detected in inoculated rhesus monkeys. Serum liver enzymes, alanine aminotransferase (ALT), and isocitrate dehydrogenase (ICD) were both slightly elevated in the inoculated primates (Figure 32.4). Mild acute viral hepatitis characterized by focal necroinflammatory changes was observed in liver biopsies near the time of serum liver enzyme elevations. A chimpanzee inoculated with swine HEV also became infected, as the chimpanzee seroconverted to anti-HEV and swine HEV RNA was detected in feces.

Infection of nonhuman primates with swine HEV demonstrated the ability of swine HEV to infect across species barriers. Importantly, a genotype 3 human strain of HEV (strain US-2) has been shown to infect SPF pigs (Halbur et al. 2001; Meng et al. 1998a). The inoculated pigs rapidly became viremic and seroconverted to

Table 32.1. Prevalence of IgG anti-HEV in pigs of different countries

Country	Herd	Pig Age	No. Positive/No. Tested (%)	Reference
U.S.	1 herd	6–12 wk	0/16 (0)	Meng et al., 1997
		5 mo–adult	27/41 (66)	
	1 herd	3–8 wk	0/24 (0)	
		3 mo–adult	34/37 (92)	
	1 herd	2 mo	1/8 (13)	
		3 mo–adult	28/32 (88)	
	11 herds	Adult	110/115 (96)	
Japan	25 herds	2 mo	37/500 (7)	Takahashi et al., 2003
		3 mo	301/750 (40)	
		4 mo	433/500 (87)	
		5–6 mo	677/750 (90)	
Spain	6 herds	3 wk–2 mo	2/10 (20)	Pina et al., 2001
		5 mo–adult	13/50 (26)	
Australia	2 herds	Mixed	12/40 (30)	Chandler et al., 1999
	2 herds	16 wk	45 (92-95)	
	Wild pigs	Unknown	15/59 (17)	
Taiwan	10 herds	Mixed	102/275 (37)	Hsieh et al., 1999
Canada (Quebec)	37 herds	Nursery	82/310 (26)	Meng et al., 1999
	16 herds	Adult	34/90 (38)	
Canada (Ontario)	10 herds	Nursery	1/230 (<1)	
	4 herds	Adult	12/82 (15)	
Canada	80 herds	6 mo	594/998 (60)	Yoo et al., 2001
Korea	Multiple	1–2 mo	6/40 (15)	Meng et al., 1999
		3–6 mo	39/80 (49)	
		Adults	12/20 (60)	
	13 herds	1–2 mo	3/90 (3)	Choi et al., 2003
		3 mo	5/50 (10)	
		4–7 mo	28/90 (31)	
		Sows	3/34 (9)	
New Zealand	1 herd	Mixed	54/72 (75)	Garkavenko et al., 2001
Nepal	Multiple	Mixed	18/55 (33)	Clayson et al., 1995
China	3 herds	Mixed	22/72 (31)	Meng et al., 1999
	Multiple	<3 mo	1/10 (10)	Wang et al., 2002
		Adults	329/409 (80)	
Thailand	1 herd	1–2 mo	0/20 (0)	Meng et al., 1999
		3–4 mo	13/20 (65)	
	3 herds	Adults	10/35 (29)	
India	7 herds	2–24 wk	122/284 (43)	Arankalle et al., 2002
	Multiple	3.2–6.4 mo	54/57 (95)	Arankalle et al., 2003

HEV, suggesting that the US-2 strain of human HEV is already competent to replicate in pigs and may be of swine origin.

Cross-species infection of HEV has also been reported in other animal species. Lambs were reportedly infected with human HEV isolates (Usmanov et al. 1994). Similarly, Wistar rats were reportedly infected with a human stool suspension containing infectious HEV (Maneerat et al. 1996). However, attempts to infect laboratory rats and mice experimentally with swine HEV were unsuccessful (Sun and Meng, unpublished data).

Increasing evidence indicates that swine HEV also infects humans. Hsieh et al. (1999) found that about 27% of the Taiwanese pig handlers were positive for anti-HEV compared to only about 8% of control subjects. Recently, Meng et al. (2002) tested a total of 465 swine veterinarians for anti-HEV IgG using recombi-

nant capsid antigens from swine HEV and a Pakistani Sar-55 strain of human HEV. Among the 295 swine veterinarians from 8 U.S. States from which 400 normal U.S. blood donors were available, about 23% (swine HEV antigen) or 27% (Sar-55 antigen) of swine veterinarians were positive for anti-HEV compared to 17% (swine HEV antigen) or 18% (Sar-55 antigen) in normal blood donors. Swine veterinarians in the U.S. were 1.51 times (swine HEV antigen, p = 0.03) and 1.46 times (Sar-55 antigen, p = 0.06) more likely to be anti-HEV positive than normal U.S. blood donors. Veterinarians who reported having needle sticks while performing procedures on pigs were about 1.9 times more likely to be seropositive than those who did not. Also, subjects from traditional major swine states appeared to be more likely seropositive than those from traditionally non-swine States. For example, subjects from Minnesota, a major swine state, were about 5–6 times more likely to be

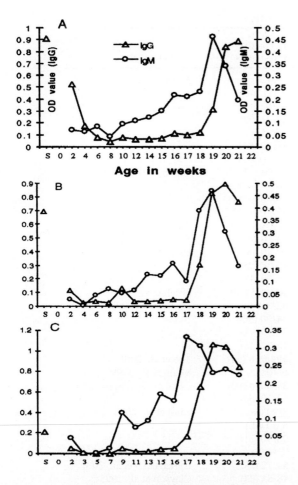

32.2. *Anti-HEV responses of three representative piglets from a prospective study in a commercial swine farm. (A) Piglet born to a seropositive sow with a high titer of IgG anti-HEV. (B) Piglet born to a seropositive sow with a lower titer of IgG anti-HEV. (C) Piglet born to a seronegative sow. The ELISA OD value of IgG anti-HEV in breeder sows is indicated (S). (Reproduced with permission by the National Academy of Science from Meng et al. 1997.)*

seropositive than those from Alabama, which is traditionally not a major swine state.

Drobeniuc et al. (2001) also assessed the anti-HEV prevalence and risk factors to HEV infection in 264 swine farmers and 255 control subjects in Moldova. About 51% of swine farmers were anti-HEV positive whereas only 25% of control subjects with no occupational exposure to swine were seropositive. Withers et al. (2002) reported that swine workers (n = 165) in North Carolina had a 4.5-fold higher anti-HEV prevalence (10.9%) than the control subjects (2.4%, n = 127).

These data provide compelling evidence that hepatitis E is a zoonotic disease and that pigs are reservoirs (Meng 2003, 2004).

The transmission route for swine HEV is presumably fecal-oral. Feces from infected pigs are likely the main source of virus for transmission. It has been shown that an uninoculated sentinel SPF pig housed in the same room with a swine HEV-inoculated pig became infected

about 2 weeks after the experimentally inoculated pig had become infected (Meng et al. 1998a).

It is believed that pigs acquire infection through direct contact with infected pigs or through ingestion of feces-contaminated feed or water. However, experimental reproduction of swine HEV infection in pigs via the oral route of inoculation proved to be difficult (Kasorndorkbua et al. 2002), even though pigs can be readily infected with swine HEV via the intravenous route of inoculation (Halbur et al. 2001; Meng et al. 1998a, b). Other route(s) of transmission cannot be ruled out.

As a fecal-orally transmitted disease, waterborne epidemics are characteristic of hepatitis E outbreaks in humans (Purcell and Emerson 2001). Feces from infected pigs contain large amounts of virus, and thus swine manure and feces could contaminate irrigation water or coastal waters, thereby leading to possible contamination of produce or shellfish (Meng 2004). HEV strains of swine origins have been detected in sewage water (Clemente-Casares et al. 2003; Pina et al. 2000).

Yazaki et al. (2003) recently reported that sporadic cases of acute hepatitis E in Hokkaido, Japan were epidemiologically linked to consumption of grilled or undercooked pig livers about 2–8 weeks prior to the onset of disease. The partial sequences of seven swine HEV isolates recovered from packaged pig livers in local grocery stores are very closely related, or identical in a few cases, to the viruses recovered from human hepatitis E patients, and thus provide more direct evidence of zoonotic transmission between pigs and humans.

PATHOGENESIS

The pathogenesis of swine HEV is largely unknown. It is believed that swine HEV enters the host through the fecal-oral route (Purcell and Emerson 2001; Williams et al. 2001). The primary site of swine HEV replication in pigs is not known. In primates and pigs experimentally infected with swine HEV, virus replication in the liver has been demonstrated (Meng et al. 1998a, b).

It is believed that, after replication in liver, swine HEV is released to the gallbladder from hepatocytes and is then excreted in feces. Williams et al. (2001) showed the existence of extrahepatic sites of HEV replication in pigs experimentally infected with swine HEV and the US-2 strain of human HEV. By using a negative strand-specific RT-PCR, replicative negative-strand HEV RNA, indicative of virus replication, was detected in the liver, as well as in several extrahepatic tissues and organs, including small intestines, colon, and hepatic and mesenteric lymph nodes of infected pigs. Using in situ hybridization, Choi and Chae (2003) also detected swine HEV RNA in hepatocytes and bile duct epithelium as well as in small and large intestines, lymph nodes, tonsil, spleen, and kidney. Although the clinical and pathological significance of these extrahepatic sites of virus

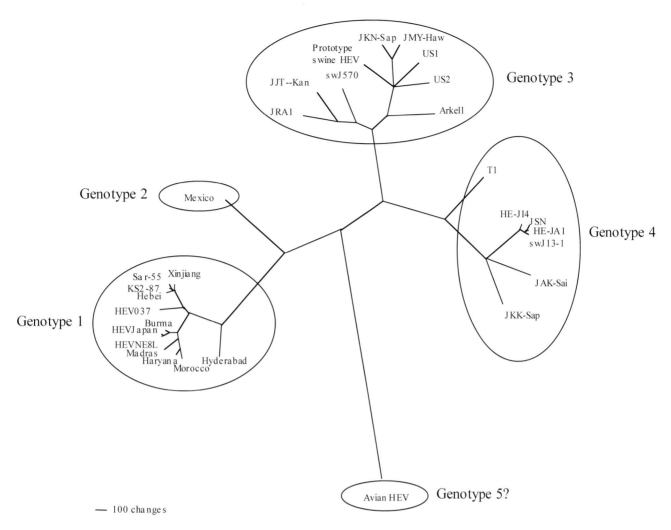

32.3. *A phylogenetic tree based on the complete genomic sequences of 30 human, swine, and avian HEV strains. Swine HEV strains identified thus far belong to either genotype 3 or 4. A scale bar, indicating the number of character state changes, is proportional to the genetic distance. (Reproduced with permission by the Society for General Microbiology from Huang et al. 2004.)*

replication is not known, it is believed that swine HEV may first replicate in the gastrointestinal tract and subsequently spread to its target organ, the liver, via primary viremia.

In humans, it has been reported that pregnancy increased the severity and mortality of the disease. The overall mortality rate caused by HEV in infected pregnant women can reach 25% (Kumar et al. 2004; Purcell and Emerson 2001). However, under experimental conditions, fulminant hepatitis E could not be reproduced in infected pregnant rhesus monkeys, nor was there increased severity of hepatitis in pregnant monkeys when compared to nonpregnant monkeys (Tsarev et al. 1995). Similarly, pregnant gilts experimentally infected with swine HEV did not exhibit any more severe disease than the nonpregnant controls (Kasorndorkbua et al. 2003). Reproductive failure or clinical hepatitis was not observed in HEV-infected gilts. Therefore, the mechanism of fulminant hepatitis E in infected pregnant women is still not known.

CLINICAL SIGNS

Pigs naturally and experimentally infected with swine HEV are asymptomatic. The incubation period, from the time of infection to virus shedding in feces, ranged from 1–4 weeks (Halbur et al. 2001; Meng et al. 1998a, b). The percentage of HEV-infected pigs within a herd is very high (refer to Table 32.1); however, the morbidity and mortality attributable to swine HEV infection is not known.

LESIONS

Four piglets naturally infected with swine HEV in a prospective study were necropsied during the acute stage of infection (Meng et al. 1997). Gross lesions were not detected in the liver or 18 other tissues and organs examined during necropsy. However, all four piglets had microscopic evidence of hepatitis, characterized by mild-to-moderate multifocal and periportal lympho-

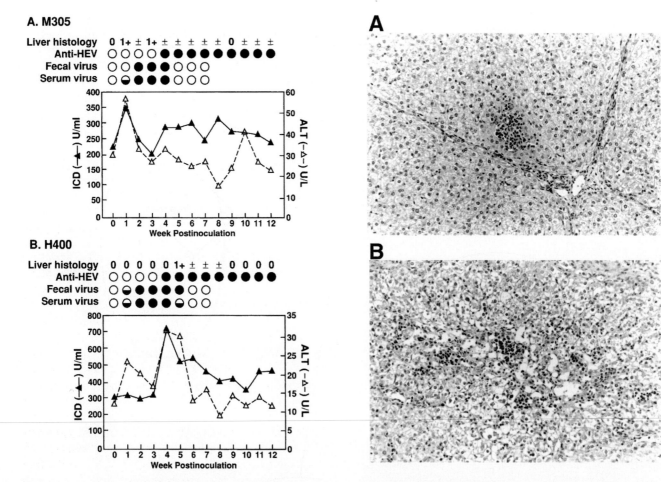

32.4. *Experimental infection of rhesus monkeys with swine HEV. Levels of serum liver enzymes (ALT and ICD) are plotted. Presence (filled circle) or absence (open circle) of anti-HEV and swine HEV RNA in serum and feces is indicated. Half-filled circles indicated detection of swine HEV RNA only by a nested PCR. The degree of liver lesions in liver biopsies is indicated (scale of 0 to 4+). (Modified with permission from Meng et al. 1998.)*

32.5. *Histological liver lesions in pigs experimentally infected with swine HEV or human HEV. (A) Liver of a pig experimentally infected with the swine HEV, showing mild focal infiltration of lymphocytes, plasma cells, and macrophages and mild diffuse inflammation in hepatic sinusoids at 14 days postinoculation (DPI). Hepatocytes are mildly swollen and vacuolated. (B) Liver of a pig experimentally infected with the US-2 strain of human HEV, showing moderate lymphoplasmacytic and histiocytic hepatitis and severe vacuolar degeneration and swelling of hepatocytes at 14 DPI. Hematoxylin and Eosin stain. (Reproduced with permission by the American Society for Microbiology from Halbur et al. 2001.)*

plasmacytic hepatitis with mild focal hepatocellular necrosis. All four piglets also had mild lymphoplasmacytic enteritis and three piglets had mild multifocal lymphoplasmacytic interstitial nephritis.

Under experimental conditions, SPF pigs inoculated with swine HEV and the US2 human HEV remained clinically normal. However, the infected pigs did have mildly to moderately enlarged hepatic and mesenteric lymph nodes from 7–55 days postinoculation (DPI). Microscopic lesions characterized by mild-to-moderate multifocal lymphoplasmacytic hepatitis and focal hepatocellular necrosis were observed in experimentally infected pigs (Figure 32.5). Hepatic inflammation and hepatocellular necrosis peaked in severity at 20 DPI. HEV RNA was detected in feces, liver tissue, and bile of infected pigs from 3–27 DPI (Halbur et al. 2001).

All 12 pregnant gilts experimentally inoculated intravenously with swine HEV at various stages of gestation became infected and shed the virus in feces (Kasorn-

dorkbua et al. 2003). These gilts had no clinical signs of hepatitis or elevation of liver enzymes throughout the 55 days of the study. There was no significant effect of swine HEV on fetal size, fetal viability, or offspring birth weight or weight gain. There were no remarkable gross lesions in the gilts, fetuses, or piglets from gilts that were allowed to farrow. Mild multifocal lymphohistiocytic hepatitis and individual hepatocellular necrosis was observed in 4 of the gilts. There were no remarkable lesions in the fetuses from HEV-infected dams. Evidence that HEV is a reproductive pathogen in pigs is currently lacking.

IMMUNITY

The immune response in pigs to swine HEV infection, characterized by a transient appearance of anti-HEV

IgM followed by long-lasting anti-HEV IgG, appears late during the period of viremia and fecal virus shedding (Meng et al. 1998a, b). Like human HEV, the capsid protein of swine HEV is immunogenic and induces protective immunity. It has been demonstrated that the ORF2 capsid protein of swine HEV shares common antigenic epitopes with that of human HEV and the newly identified avian hepatitis E virus (Haqshenas et al. 2002). All HEV strains identified thus far, including the genotypes 3 and 4 swine HEV, appear to belong to a single serotype. Cross-challenge experiments in primates have demonstrated cross-protection following infection with different genotypes of human HEV strains (Purcell et al. 2003).

Sows with high anti-HEV titers can passively transfer anti-HEV to their offspring, and thus some piglets are seropositive shortly after birth. Piglets born to seropositive sows had maternal antibodies lasting about 7–9 weeks (Meng et al. 1997). It is believed that maternal antibodies confer protective immunity to the piglets against swine HEV infection.

DIAGNOSIS

Swine HEV is a difficult virus to work with because it does not grow in cell culture or cause any clinical disease in pigs. Currently, the diagnosis of swine HEV infection is primarily based on PCR and ELISA (Engle et al. 2002; Huang et al. 2002). However, the sensitivity and specificity of these assays are largely not known. The recombinant human HEV capsid antigen cross-reacted well with antibodies to swine HEV in an ELISA assay and has been used to detect anti-HEV antibody in swine (Engle et al. 2002; Meng et al. 1999, 2002). The capsid protein of a genotype 3 swine HEV has also been expressed and used in an ELISA to detect anti-HEV (Meng et al. 2002). ELISA results based on the recombinant swine HEV antigen correlated well with those obtained with a recombinant antigen from the Sar-55 strain of human HEV. Therefore, both swine HEV and human HEV capsid antigens are suitable for diagnosis of swine HEV infection by ELISA. There is no specific test for differentiating between infections with swine HEV and human HEV.

Serological assays alone are inadequate in screening for acute swine HEV infection since anti-HEV IgG generally occurs in pigs at least 2 weeks after infection. Viremia and fecal virus shedding occur in infected pigs much earlier than the appearance of anti-HEV, and thus seronegative pigs could still be infected with swine HEV (Meng et al. 1998a, b). A sensitive and specific RT-PCR assay has been successfully developed for the detection of swine HEV from infected pigs (Huang et al. 2002). However, the specificity of the current RT-PCR assays in detecting swine HEV in pigs from different geographic regions is not known. Swine HEV strains identified from pigs in different geographic regions vary considerably in their genomic sequences and belong to at least two different genotypes (Meng 2004). Therefore, genetic identification and characterization of additional field strains of swine HEV from different geographic regions will be critical for developing a universal RT-PCR assay that can detect all strains of swine HEV in pigs. Since genotypes 3 and 4 swine and human HEVs are genetically indistinguishable, a differential diagnostic assay for swine HEV is not possible or necessary.

PREVENTION AND CONTROL

Swine HEV is ubiquitous in pigs worldwide and has the ability to infect humans. Therefore, the major concerns for swine HEV are (1) infection in high risk groups, such as swine veterinarians, swine producers, and other pig handlers, and (2) transmission of swine HEV from pig xenografts to human transplant recipients in xenotransplantation and the potential subsequent transmission of the virus to others.

Although swine HEV caused only subclinical infection in pigs, the outcome of exposure of immunosuppressed xenograft recipients is uncertain (Meng 2003). Unlike some other porcine viruses, such as the porcine endogenous retrovirus, xenograft donor pigs free of swine HEV can be derived from infected breeding herds. A recent study showed that piglets negative for swine HEV can be successfully generated through segregated early weaning from pregnant sows experimentally infected with swine HEV (Kasorndorkbua et al. 2003; Brad Thacker, personal communication). Therefore, the potential xenozoonotic risk of infection by swine HEV in xenotransplantation is preventable through adequate screening and strict rearing procedures for donor pigs.

As a zoonotic virus, swine HEV poses a potential public health concern. A vaccine against HEV is not yet available, but experimental recombinant HEV vaccines appear to be effective (Purcell et al. 2003), although their efficacy must be thoroughly evaluated for protection against emerging strains of HEV including genotypes 3 and 4 swine HEV. Vaccination of pig handlers in industrialized countries against HEV, when a vaccine becomes available, appears unnecessary since a high proportion of swine handlers were seropositive for HEV but had no clinical symptoms. However, the occurrence of acute hepatitis E in industrialized countries may be underestimated because sporadic cases of acute hepatitis E may go undiagnosed. Adequate personal and public hygiene can minimize the transmission of the virus. A simple preventive measure for pig handlers is to wash hands thoroughly with soap and water after handling pigs.

Although swine HEV is nonpathogenic in pigs, it is not known whether concurrent infections of swine HEV with other swine pathogens could have any synergistic effects. Therefore, it will be advantageous for the swine industry to produce HEV-free pigs for purposes such as seed stock production, biomedical research, and xenotransplantation. If sporadic cases of hepatitis E continue to occur in people as a result of consumption of under-cooked pork, it may also become important to eliminate swine HEV from commercial production.

REFERENCES

Arankalle VA, Chobe LP, Joshi MV, Chadha MS, Kundu B, Walimbe AM. 2002. Human and swine hepatitis E viruses from Western India belong to different genotypes. J Hepatol 36:417–425.

Arankalle VA, Joshi MV, Kulkarni AM, Gandhe SS, Chobe LP, Rautmare SS, Mishra AC, Padbidri VS. 2001. Prevalence of anti-hepatitis E virus antibodies in different Indian animal species. J Viral Hepat 8:223–227.

Balayan MS, Usmanov RK, Zamyatina NA, Djumalieva DI, Karas FR. 1990. Brief report: Experimental hepatitis E infection in domestic pigs. J Med Virol 32:58–59.

Chandler JD, Riddell MA, Li F, Love RJ, Anderson DA. 1999. Serological evidence for swine hepatitis E virus infection in Australian pig herds. Vet Microbiol 68:95–105.

Choi C, Chae C. 2003. Localization of swine hepatitis E virus in liver and extrahepatic tissues from naturally infected pigs by in situ hybridization. J Hepatol 38:827–832.

Choi IS, Kwon HJ, Shin NR, Yoo HS. 2003. Identification of swine hepatitis E virus (HEV) and prevalence of anti-HEV antibodies in swine and human populations in Korea. J Clin Microbiol 41:3602–3608.

Clayson ET, Innis BL, Myint KS, Narupiti S, Vaughn DW, Giri S, Ranabhat P, Shrestha MP. 1995. Detection of hepatitis E virus infections among domestic swine in the Kathmandu Valley of Nepal. Am J Trop Med Hyg 53:228–232.

Clemente-Casares P, Pina S, Buti M, Jardi R, MartIn M, Bofill-Mas S, Girones R. 2003. Hepatitis E virus epidemiology in industrialized countries. Emerg Infect Dis 9:448–454.

Drobeniuc J, Favorov MO, Shapiro CN, Bell BP, Mast EE, Dadu A, Culver D, Iarovoi P, Robertson BH, Margolis HS. 2001. Hepatitis E virus antibody prevalence among persons who work with swine. J Infect Dis 184:1594–1597.

Emerson SU, Purcell RH. 2003. Hepatitis E virus. Rev Med Virol 13:145–154.

Engle RE, Yu C, Emerson SU, Meng XJ, Purcell RH. 2002. Hepatitis E virus (HEV) capsid antigens derived from viruses of human and swine origin are equally efficient for detecting anti-HEV by enzyme immunoassay. J Clin Microbiol 40:4576–4580.

Garkavenko O, Obriadina A, Meng J, Anderson DA, Benard HJ, Schroeder BA, Khudyakov YE, Fields HA, Croxson MC. 2001. Detection and characterization of swine hepatitis E virus in New Zealand. J Med Virol 65:525–529.

Halbur PG, Kasorndorkbua C, Gilbert C, Guenette D, Potters MB, Purcell RH, Emerson SU, Toth TE, Meng XJ. 2001. Comparative pathogenesis of infection of pigs with hepatitis E viruses recovered from a pig and a human. J Clin Microbiol 9:918–923.

Haqshenas G, Huang FF, Fenaux M, Guenette DK, Pierson FW, Larsen CT, Shivaprasad HL, Toth TE, Meng XJ. 2002. The putative capsid protein of the newly identified avian hepatitis E virus shares antigenic epitopes with that of swine and human hepatitis E viruses and chicken big liver and spleen disease virus. J Gen Virol 83:2201–2209.

Hsieh SY, Meng XJ, Wu YH, Liu ST, Tam AW, Lin DY, Liaw YF. 1999. Identity of a novel swine hepatitis E virus in Taiwan forming a monophyletic group with Taiwan isolates of human hepatitis E virus. J Clin Microbiol 37:3828–3834.

Huang FF, Haqshenas G, Guenette DK, Halbur PG, Schommer SK, Pierson FW, Toth TE, Meng XJ. 2002. Detection by reverse transcription—PCR and genetic characterization of field isolates of swine hepatitis E virus from pigs in different geographic regions of the United States. J Clin Microbiol 40:1326–1332.

Kasorndorkbua C, Halbur PG, Thomas PJ, Guenette DK, Toth TE, Meng XJ. 2002. Use of a swine bioassay and a RT-PCR assay to assess the risk of transmission of swine hepatitis E virus in pigs. J Virol Methods 101:71–78.

Kasorndorkbua C, Thacker BJ, Halbur PG, Guenette DK, Buitenwerf RM, Royer RL, Meng XJ. 2003. Experimental infection of pregnant gilts with swine hepatitis E virus. Can J Vet Res 67:303–306.

Koonin EV, Gorbalenya AE, Purdy MA, Rozanov MN, Reyes GR, Bradley DW. 1992. Computer-assisted assignment of functional domains in the nonstructural polyprotein of hepatitis E virus: Delineation of an additional group of positive-strand RNA plant and animal viruses. Proc Natl Acad Sci USA 89:8259–8263.

Kumar A, Beniwal M, Kar P, Sharma JB, Murthy NS. 2004. Hepatitis E in pregnancy. Int J Gynaecol Obstet 85:240–244.

Maneerat Y, Clayson ET, Myint KS, Young GD, Innis BL. 1996. Experimental infection of the laboratory rat with the hepatitis E virus. J Med Virol 48:121–128.

Meng XJ. 2003. Swine hepatitis E virus: Cross-species infection and risk in xenotransplantation. Curr Top Microbiol Immunol 278:185–216.

——. 2004. Hepatitis E as a zoonosis. In Viral Hepatitis (3rd edition). H Thomas, A Zuckermann, S Lemon, eds. Oxford: Blackwell Publishing Ltd., pp. 611–623.

Meng XJ, Dea S, Engle RE, Friendship R, Lyoo YS, Sirinarumitr T, Urairong K, Wang D, Wong D, Yoo D, Zhang Y, Purcell RH, Emerson SU. 1999. Prevalence of antibodies to the hepatitis E virus in pigs from countries where hepatitis E is common or is rare in the human population. J Med Virol 59:297–302.

Meng XJ, Halbur PG, Haynes JS, Tsareva TS, Bruna JD, Royer RL, Purcell RH, Emerson SU. 1998b. Experimental infection of pigs with the newly identified swine hepatitis E virus (swine HEV), but not with human strains of HEV. Arch Virol 143:1405–1415.

Meng XJ, Halbur PG, Shapiro MS, Govindarajan S, Bruna JD, Mushahwar IK, Purcell RH, Emerson SU. 1998a. Genetic and experimental evidence for cross-species infection by swine hepatitis E virus. J Virol 72:9714–9721.

Meng XJ, Purcell RH, Halbur PG, Lehman JR, Webb DM, Tsareva TS, Haynes JS, Thacker BJ, Emerson SU. 1997. A novel virus in swine is closely related to the human hepatitis E virus. Proc Natl Acad Sci USA 94:9860–9865.

Meng XJ, Wiseman B, Elvinger F, Guenette DK, Toth TE, Engle RE, Emerson SU, Purcell RH. 2002. Prevalence of antibodies to hepatitis E virus in veterinarians working with swine and in normal blood donors in the United States and other countries. J Clin Microbiol 40:117–22.

Pina S, Buti M, Cotrina M, Piella J, Girones R. 2000. HEV identified in serum from humans with acute hepatitis and in sewage of animal origin in Spain. J Hepatol 33:826–833.

Purcell RH, Emerson SU. 2001. Hepatitis E virus. In Fields Virology (4th edition). DM Knipe, PM Howley, DE Griffin, RA Lamb, MA Martin, B Roizman, SE Straus, eds. Philadelphia: Lippincott Williams and Wilkins, pp. 3051–3061.

Purcell RH, Nguyen H, Shapiro M, Engle RE, Govindarajan S, Blackwelder WC, Wong DC, Prieels JP, Emerson SU. 2003. Pre-clinical immunogenicity and efficacy trial of a recombinant hepatitis E vaccine. Vaccine 21:2607–2615.

Takahashi M, Nishizawa T, Miyajima H, Gotanda Y, Iita T, Tsuda F, Okamoto H. 2003. Swine hepatitis E virus strains in Japan form four phylogenetic clusters comparable with those of Japanese isolates of human hepatitis E virus. J Gen Virol 84:851–862.

Tsarev SA, Tsareva TS, Emerson SU, Rippy MK, Zack P, Shapiro M, Purcell RH. 1995. Experimental hepatitis E in pregnant rhesus monkeys: Failure to transmit hepatitis E virus (HEV) to offspring and evidence of naturally acquired antibodies to HEV. J Infect Dis 172:31–37.

Usmanov RK, Balaian MS, Dvoinikova OV, Alymbaeva DB, Zamiatina NA, Kazachkov IuA, Belov VI. 1994. An experimental infection in lambs by the hepatitis E virus. Vopr Virusol 39:165–168.

Wang YC, Zhang HY, Xia NS, Peng G, Lan HY, Zhuang H, Zhu YH, Li SW, Tian KG, Gu WJ, Lin JX, Wu X, Li HM, Harrison TJ. 2002. Prevalence, isolation, and partial sequence analysis of hepatitis E virus from domestic animals in China. J Med Virol 67:516–521.

Williams TP, Kasorndorkbua C, Halbur PG, Haqshenas G, Guenette DK, Toth TE, Meng XJ. 2001. Evidence of extrahepatic sites of replication of the hepatitis E virus in a swine model. J Clin Microbiol 39:3040–3046.

Withers MR, Correa MT, Morrow M, Stebbins ME, Seriwatana J, Webster WD, Boak MB, Vaughn DW. 2002. Antibody levels to hepatitis E virus in North Carolina swine workers, non-swine workers, swine, and murids. Am J Trop Med Hyg 66:384–388.

Yazaki Y, Mizuo H, Takahashi M, Nishizawa T, Sasaki N, Gotanda Y, Okamoto H. 2003. Sporadic acute or fulminant hepatitis E in Hokkaido, Japan, may be food-borne, as suggested by the presence of hepatitis E virus in pig liver as food. J Gen Virol 84:2351–2357.

Yoo D, Willson P, Pei Y, Hayes MA, Deckert A, Dewey CE, Friendship RM, Yoon Y, Gottschalk M, Yason C, Giulivi A. 2001. Prevalence of hepatitis E virus antibodies in Canadian swine herds and identification of a novel variant of swine hepatitis E virus. Clin Diagn Lab Immunol 8:1213–1219.

Zafrullah M, Ozdener MH, Panda SK, Jameel S. 1997. The ORF3 protein of hepatitis E virus is a phosphoprotein that associates with the cytoskeleton. J Virol 71:9045–9053.

Porcine Retroviruses

C. A. Wilson

Retroviruses are defined by the requirement for reverse transcription of their RNA genome into a double-stranded DNA intermediate as a key element to their replication strategy. While there are no known exogenous retrovirus infections of pigs, pigs do carry porcine endogenous retroviruses (PERVs). PERVs comprise a group of heritable viruses that, unlike exogenous viruses, cannot be excluded from pig herds because they are present as genetic elements in the genomes of all pigs.

Although no swine disease has been definitively attributed to PERV, type C retrovirus particles have been detected in porcine cell lines derived from leukemias or lymphomas (Frazier et al. 1969; Moennig et al. 1974) fueling speculation that the endogenous retrovirus of pigs may be tumorigenic. In addition, PERV is related morphologically and genetically to murine retroviruses shown to be the cause of leukemias in mice (Czauderna et al. 2000). However, the association of PERV with leukemic cell lines was not sufficient to assign PERV as the causative agent, since it was impossible to distinguish cause from effect in these studies. As a result, the investigations into whether PERVs may be tumorigenic were ultimately abandoned.

Scientific interest in PERVs was renewed when it was found that co-culture of primary pig cells (Martin et al. 1998; Wilson et al. 1998) or established pig cell lines (Patience et al. 1997) with human cell lines resulted in a productive infection of the human cells. These findings took on particular importance as they coincided with increased interest in developing clinical xenotransplantation, i.e., the transplantation of nonhuman cells or organs into humans. The development of transgenic pigs carrying two human genes that were thought to prevent hyperacute rejection was hoped to spearhead the clinical application of xenotransplantation (Byrne et al. 1997). However, the finding that pig cells harbored endogenous retroviruses capable of infecting human cells underscored the potential public health concerns of xenotransplantation. Many scientists predicted that it would be unlikely that PERV could be removed from the pig genome, given an estimated presence of 50–200 copies of PERV sequences per cell (Akiyoshi et al. 1998; Patience et al. 1997).

While some scientists argued that the pathogenic potential of PERV in humans is low, based on past human exposure to pigs as domesticated animals, others argued that xenotransplantation procedures differed significantly:

1. Xenotransplantation by its nature breaks down the usual boundaries of cross-species transmission of infectious agents, such as skin and mucosal membranes, resulting in essentially a chronic coculture of animal and human cells in vivo.
2. The likelihood that xenotransplant recipients will be immune-suppressed circumvents another natural barrier to transmission of infectious agents.
3. The possibility that transgenic modifications of human complement regulatory proteins could reduce the ability of natural antibodies to protect against PERV transmission.

These considerations were supported by historical examples of naturally occurring cross-species transmission of viruses where the recipient species developed a disease not seen in the host species. For example, HIV is thought to be an outcome of transmission of a nonpathogenic animal virus into humans, resulting in a fatal disease (Hahn et al. 2000). Therefore, efforts to prevent PERV transmission or eliminate PERVs from pig herds are under study because success would enhance the safety profile of xenotransplantation procedures in humans and reduce the potential impact on the public health.

ETIOLOGY

PERVs belong to the family *Retroviridae*, genus *Gammaretrovirus*. Retrovirus particles are characteristically 100 nm in diameter and carry a plasma membrane-derived lipid bilayer envelope and a single-stranded RNA genome in diploid form. The characteristic enzymatic activity of retroviruses is the ability to catalyze the conversion of the retroviral single-stranded RNA genome into a double-stranded DNA intermediate using the virally derived enzyme RNA-dependent DNA polymerase (or reverse transcriptase). A second virally encoded enzyme, integrase, mediates integration into the host genome of the double-stranded viral DNA.

The genomic organization of PERVs is analogous to other gammaretroviruses and has been shown to consist of three open reading frames, gag, pol, and env (Akiyoshi et al. 1998; Czauderna et al. 2000) (Figure 32.6). The genomic RNA also includes elements found at the 5' and 3' ends that are required for poly-adenylation (U5), packaging (Ψ), reverse transcription (primer binding site, PBS), and RNA transcription (U3/R). As an outcome of reverse transcription, the U3/R/U5 elements are repeated at each end of the double-stranded DNA intermediate, and these are termed the Long Terminal Repeats (LTRs). After integration, the promoter and enhancer elements present in the U3 of the 5' LTR mediate RNA transcription of two mRNAs: 1) a full-length genomic RNA that is used for encapsidation into the viral particle as well as for translation of the gag-pol polyprotein, and 2) a spliced mRNA that encodes the envelope precursor. Cellular proteases cleave the envelope precursor into the mature surface envelope glycoproteins (SU) and transmembrane protein (TM). The gag-pol polyprotein is auto-proteolytically cleaved by the virally encoded enzyme, protease, during budding of the viral particle (refer to Figure 32.6). In fact, it is this proteolytic cleavage that results in the change in morphology from an immature particle with an electron dense C-shape into a mature particle bearing the characteristic electron-dense spherical core (Figure 32.7).

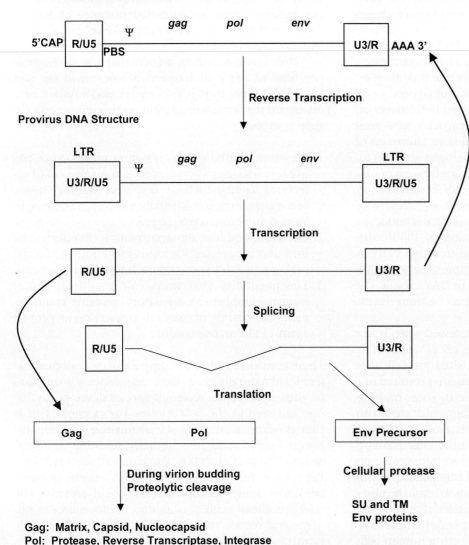

32.6. *Genomic organization and gene expression of porcine endogenous retrovirus. (See text for detailed description.)*

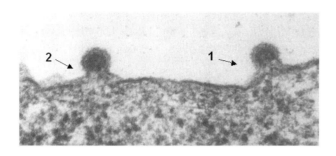

32.7. *Electron micrograph of porcine endogenous retrovirus. Human cells (HeLa) were infected with PERV and then fixed and negatively stained for electron microscopic observation. The micrograph shown is 25,000×. The particle labeled (1) is an immature viral particle demonstrating the hallmark C-shaped electron dense structure within the budding particle. The particle labeled (2) is a particle that has undergone proteolytic cleavage and has the electron-dense spherical structure within the mature virion.*

PERV is somewhat more labile than other gammaretroviruses. It has been shown that PERV infectivity is reduced over hundredfold by storage at −70°C (Wilson, unpublished data), a condition that would typically reduce virus infectivity by only five- to tenfold. Likewise, pelleting virions by ultracentrifugation, a method used to concentrate other gammaretroviruses with moderate impacts on infectivity, will completely abolish PERV infectivity (Wilson, unpublished data).

PERVs have been classified into three receptor classes on the basis of superinfection interference and in vitro cell tropism studies (Takeuchi et al. 1998). PERV-A and PERV-B use distinct receptors, but are both able to infect human cells, while PERV-C essentially only infects porcine cells in vitro. All three receptor classes can be cultured on established cell lines using classic retroviral techniques. PERV-A and PERV-B replicate most efficiently in the human embryonic kidney cell line, HEK293 cells, while viruses representing any of the three receptor classes will also replicate efficiently in the swine testis cell line, ST-IOWA (Takeuchi et al. 1998; Wilson et al. 2000).

EPIDEMIOLOGY

Pigs of all breeds carry in their genome endogenous retrovirus elements. Not all genomic elements will necessarily encode replication competent retrovirus, nor will all replicating retroviruses derived from the pig genome be able to infect human cells (Oldmixon et al. 2002). In fact, molecular analyses of DNA from representative species of the family *Suidae* and *Tayassuidae* have revealed the presence of PERV-like elements in the genomes of these wild relatives to the domesticated pig (Patience et al. 2001; Tonjes and Niebert 2003), indicating that the retroviral sequences were introduced into the germline of the pig long before domestication. Consistent with that observation are reports that PERV

sequences can be identified in all breeds of domesticated pigs examined to date (Edamura et al. 2004; Jin et al. 2000).

Some of the most detailed genetic and phenotypic studies of PERV have been performed in an inbred herd of miniature swine. The results of these studies indicate that genetic heterogeneity of the endogenous retroviral elements in the pig genome give rise to variable results within a herd with respect to whether infectious virus is present and whether that virus may be infectious for human cells in vitro (Oldmixon et al. 2002). In other words, one cannot predict whether a particular herd would express a form of PERV that replicates in human cells, since each individual animal may vary with respect to this characteristic. This finding is promising since it suggests a means to identify and selectively breed those animals that do not express human-tropic PERV.

Although comprehensive examination of PERV expression in different pig tissues and cells has not been reported, there are some data available for certain pig breeds and tissues. While most endogenous retroviruses (for example, those of mice) are maintained in a transcriptionally silent state, where activation of expression may only occur under rare conditions, such as immune activation, PERV may be different. For example, infectious PERV has been directly cultured from pig plasma, indicating that at least some tissue compartments of the pig may constitutively express infectious PERV (Takefman et al. 2001). Likewise, primary cultures of unstimulated pig endothelial cells as well as unstimulated or stimulated porcine bone marrow mononuclear cultures have also been shown to express infectious PERV (Martin et al. 1998; McIntyre et al. 2003). PERV has also been readily isolated from primary cultures of mitogenically activated peripheral blood mononuclear cells (Wilson et al. 1998), as well as cultured porcine islets (van der Laan et al. 2000). Expression of PERV RNA has been shown in a wide variety of other pig tissues (Clemenceau et al. 1999), indicating that perhaps under the right conditions, virus could be isolated from almost any type of pig cell. In general, reports have indicated that tissue-specific expression does not necessarily correspond across different breeds, nor would one animal within a breed necessarily represent all members of the breed with respect to PERV expression (Wilson 2001).

DIAGNOSIS

PERV is not known to cause disease in pigs. Likewise, no disease has been observed in any animals (mice, guinea pigs, nonhuman primates) exposed to PERV to date, although it should be noted that limited or no viral replication has been observed in these studies (Argaw et al. 2004; Martin et al. 1999; van der Laan et al. 2000).

Since PERV is an endogenous retrovirus, all pigs will be positive in laboratory assays used to detect PERV DNA by PCR or Southern blot analysis (Table 32.2). Likewise, detection of PERV RNA expression by RT-PCR, Northern blot analysis, or detection of reverse transcriptase (RT) activity would indicate only that a PERV genetic locus, or loci, is transcriptionally active. However, RNA expression or RT activity may not always correlate with presence of infectious virus because many of the loci encoding PERV are defective due to deletions or point mutations. Therefore, the method recommended by the U.S. Food and Drug Administration (FDA) to qualify a particular porcine tissue or cell type for use in xenotransplantation clinical protocols is to use a culture assay (See *FDA Guidance for Industry: Source Animal, Product, Preclinical, and Clinical Issues Concerning the Use of Xenotransplantation Products in Humans—4/3/2003*). Co-culture of the cells of interest with target cells is used most reliably to detect infectious PERV. FDA has recommended that culture assays include the target cell lines ST-IOWA (to detect PERV-C) and HEK 293 (to detect PERV-A and B). In most cases reported to date, primary pig cells tend to express low levels of PERV, so a culture period of at least 30 days is recommended. At the end of the culture period (or at set time points during the culture), the cells can be examined for evidence of infection by either of these methods: a) detection of the retroviral enzyme, reverse transcriptase by conventional or PCR-enhanced assays (Phan-Thanh et al. 1990; Takefman et al. 2001); or b) detection of PERV DNA or RNA by conventional or quantitative PCR or RT-PCR (Argaw et al. 2002). FDA has recommended that a positive signal be confirmed by serial passage of the virus onto naive indicator cells to show that the signal is indeed due to presence of infectious virus that can replicate in the test system.

In addition to culture methods (refer to Table 32.2), several laboratories have also developed serologic methods for detection of PERV-specific antibody (Galbraith et al. 2000; Matthews et al. 1999; Tacke et al. 2001). These methods would not be of use for screening pigs, since pigs would likely be tolerant to PERV. However, serologic methods have been used to analyze the anti-PERV response in animal models (Argaw et al. 2004;

Specke et al. 2002) or in human subjects of xenotransplantation clinical trials (Heneine et al. 1998; Paradis et al. 1999; Patience et al. 1998; Xu et al. 2003).

PREVENTION AND CONTROL

PERV infection cannot be prevented within a pig, since it is embedded in the genome. However, recent reports indicate that the human-tropic form of PERV may, in some pig breeds, be an exogenous infection (Wood et al. 2004) and that the pig germline may not contain a replication-competent human-tropic PERV (Scobie et al. 2004). These findings suggest that a selective breeding program of individual pigs within a herd that do not contain human-tropic PERV sequences in the germline may allow one to develop a herd of animals that are less likely to express the human-tropic PERV. Use of transgenic knockout technology to eliminate genetic loci that encode infectious PERV has been suggested, but not attempted. Recent reports that the gene encoding the alpha-1,3-galactosyl transferase gene in pigs has been eliminated using this technology (Phelps et al. 2003) demonstrates that a genetic knockout approach is feasible. In addition, newer technologies are being explored. For example, intracellular expression of a heavy-chain variable fragment specific to the PERV matrix protein (part of gag) prevents production of infectious PERV from porcine cells (Dekker et al. 2003). This result could be further developed in the form of transgenic pigs engineered to express this antibody fragment, with the intention that the resulting pigs would not express PERV. Alternatively, transgenic pigs containing PERV-specific siRNAs may prevent expression of infectious PERV, based on studies of siRNA inhibition of replication for a number of other viruses (Joost Haasnoot et al. 2003).

In addition to trying to modulate expression of PERV in the pig, a number of strategies are being explored to determine whether existing antiviral drugs would be useful to treat PERV infection (Qari et al. 2001; Wilhelm et al. 2002). For example, some, but not all inhibitors of RT have been shown to reduce PERV infectivity in vitro, although typically at higher IC50 concentrations than

Table 32.2. Diagnostic methods for PERV detection

Method	Purpose	Specimen	Comments
DNA PCR or Southern blot	Detection of PERV DNA	Pig cells	Will be positive for all tissues
RT-PCR or Northern blot	Detection of PERV RNA	Pig cells	Will likely be positive; may not correlate with presence of infectious virus
Reverse transcriptase assay	Detection of viral enzymatic activity (RT)	Pig cells	Will likely be positive; may not correlate with presence of infectious virus
Culture assay	Detection of infectious virus	Pig cells or fluids cultured with ST-IOWA or HEK-293	Best method to identify infectious virus; detection should include RT assay or RT-PCR or DNA-PCR assays to increase sensitivity
ELISA or Western blot	Detection of immune response to PERV	Human serum	Indicates immune response to PERV in human recipients of xenotransplantation products; possibly indicating transmission of virus.

required for HIV inhibition. In contrast, HIV protease inhibitors have no effect on PERV infectivity.

Naturally preexisting xenoreactive antibody present in human serum against the carbohydrate alpha-1,3-galactosyl epitope present on the PERV envelope (when derived from porcine cells) has been shown to prevent PERV infection of cells both *in vitro* and in vivo (Fujita et al. 2003; McKane et al. 2003). While these data suggest that humans may be naturally protected against PERV infection, recent genetic modifications of pigs (i.e., the functional deletion of alpha-1,3-galactosyl transferase) may circumvent this mechanism of immune protection to PERV infection in humans (Chapman and Wilson 2003).

REFERENCES

Akiyoshi DE, Denaro M, Zhu H, Greenstein JL, Banerjee P, Fishman JA. 1998. Identification of a full-length cDNA for an endogenous retrovirus of miniature swine. J Virol 72:4503–4507.

Argaw T, Colon-Moran W, Wilson CA. 2004. Limited infection without evidence of replication by porcine endogenous retrovirus in guinea pigs. J Gen Virol 85:15–9.

Argaw T, Ritzhaupt A, Wilson CA. 2002. Development of a real time quantitative PCR assay for detection of porcine endogenous retrovirus. J Virol Methods 106:97–106.

Byrne GW, McCurry KR, Martin MJ, McClellan SM, Platt JL, Logan JS. 1997. Transgenic pigs expressing human CD59 and decay-accelerating factor produce an intrinsic barrier to complement-mediated damage. Transplantation 63:149–155.

Chapman LE, Wilson CA. 2003. Commentary: Implications of the advent of homozygous a 1, 3-galactosyltransferase gene deficient pigs on transmission of infectious agents. Xenotransplantation 10:287–288.

Clemenceau B, Lalain S, Martignat L, Sai P. 1999. Porcine endogenous retroviral mRNAs in pancreas and a panel of tissues from specific pathogen-free pigs. Diabetes and Metabolism (Paris) 25:518–525.

Czauderna F, Fischer N, Boller K, Kurth R, Tonjes RR. 2000. Establishment and characterization of molecular clones of porcine endogenous retroviruses replicating on human cells. J Virol 74:4028–4038.

Dekker S, Toussaint W, Panayotou G, de Wit T, Visser P, Grosveld F, Drabek D. 2003. Intracellularly expressed single-domain antibody against p15 matrix protein prevents the production of porcine retroviruses. J Virol 77:12132–9.

Edamura K, Nasu K, Iwami Y, Nishimura R, Ogawa H, Sasaki N, Ohgawara H. 2004. Prevalence of porcine endogenous retrovirus in domestic pigs in Japan and its potential infection in dogs xenotransplanted with porcine pancreatic islet cells. J Vet Med Sci 66:129–135.

Frazier ME, Ushijima RN, Howard EB. 1969. Virus association with 90Sr induced leukemia of miniature swine. In Comparative Leukemia Research. RM Dutcher, ed. Basel: Karger AG, Volume 36, pp. 440–445.

Fujita F, Yamashita-Futsuki I, Eguchi S, Kamohara Y, Fujioka H, Yanaga K, Furui J, Moriuchi R, Kanematsu T, Katamine S. 2003. Inactivation of porcine endogenous retrovirus by human serum as a function of complement activated through the classical pathway. Hepatol Res 26:106–113.

Galbraith DN, Kelly HT, Dyke A, Reid G, Haworth C, Beekman J, Shepherd A, Smith KT. 2000. Design and validation of immunological tests for the detection of porcine endogenous retrovirus in biological materials. J Virol Methods 90:115–124.

Hahn BH, Shaw GM, De Cock KM, Sharp PM. 2000. AIDS as a zoonosis: Scientific and public health implications. Science 287:607–614.

Heneine W, Tibell A, Switzer WM, Sandstrom P, Rosales GV, Mathews A, Korsgren O, Chapman LE, Folks TM, Groth CG. 1998. No evidence of infection with porcine endogenous retrovirus in recipients of porcine islet-cell xenografts. The Lancet 352:695–699.

Jin H, Inoshima Y, Wu D, Morooka A, Sentsui H. 2000. Expression of porcine endogenous retrovirus in peripheral blood leukocytes from ten different breeds. Transpl Infect Dis 2:11–14.

Joost Haasnoot PC, Cupac D, Berkhout B. 2003. Inhibition of virus replication by RNA interference. J Biomed Sci 10:607–616.

Martin U, Kiessig V, Blusch JH, Haverich A, von der Helm K, Herden T, Steinhoff G. 1998. Expression of pig endogenous retrovirus by primary porcine endothelial cells and infection of human cells. The Lancet 352:692–694.

Martin U, Steinhoff G, Kiessig V, Chikobava M, Anssar M, Morschheuser T, Lapin B, Haverich A. 1999. Porcine endogenous retrovirus is transmitted neither in vivo nor in vitro from porcine endothelial cells to baboons. Transplant Proc 31:913–914.

Matthews AL, Brown J, Switzer W, Folks TM, Heneine W, Sandstrom PA. 1999. Development and validation of a western immunoblot assay for detection of antibodies to porcine endogenous retrovirus. Transplantation 67:939–943.

McIntyre MC, Kannan B, Solano-Aguilar GI, Wilson CA, Bloom ET. 2003. Detection of porcine endogenous retrovirus in cultures of freshly isolated porcine bone marrow cells. Xenotransplantation 10:337–342.

McKane BW, Ramachandran S, Yang J, Xu XC, Mohanakumar T. 2003. Xenoreactive anti-Galalpha(1,3)Gal antibodies prevent porcine endogenous retrovirus infection of human in vivo. Hum Immunol 64:708–17.

Moennig V, Frank H, Hunsmann G, Ohms P, Schwarz H, Schafer W. 1974. C-type particles produced by a permanent cell line from a leukemic pig. Virology 57:179–188.

Oldmixon BA, Wood JC, Ericsson TA, Wilson CA, White-Scharf ME, Andersson G, Greenstein JL, Schuurman HJ, Patience C. 2002. Porcine endogenous retrovirus transmission characteristics of an inbred herd of miniature swine. J Virol 76:3045–3048.

Paradis K, Langford G, Long Z, Heneine W, Sandstrom P, Switzer WM, Chapman LE, Lockey C, Onions D, Otto E. 1999. Search for cross-species transmission of porcine endogenous retrovirus in patients treated with living pig tissue. Science 285:1236–1241.

Patience C, Patton GS, Takeuchi Y, Weiss RA, McClure MO, Rydberg L, Breimer ME. 1998. No evidence of pig DNA or retroviral infection in patients with short-term extracorporeal connection to pig kidneys. The Lancet 352:699–701.

Patience C, Switzer WM, Takeuchi Y, Griffiths DJ, Goward ME, Heneine W, Stoye JP, Weiss RA. 2001. Multiple groups of novel retroviral genomes in pigs and related species. J Virol 75:2771–2775.

Patience C, Takeuchi Y, Weiss RA. 1997. Infection of human cells by an endogenous retrovirus of pigs. Nat Med 3:282–286.

Phan-Thanh L, Kaeffer B, Bottreau E. 1990. Porcine retrovirus reverse transcriptase: Optimal conditions for its determination. Develop Biol Standard 72:111–116.

Phelps CJ, Koike C, Vaught TD, Boone J, Wells KD, Chen SH, Ball S, Specht SM, Polejaeva IA, Monahan JA, Jobst PM, Sharma SB, Lamborn AE, Garst AS, Moore M, Demetris AJ, Rudert WA, Bottino R, Bertera S, Trucco M, Starzl TE, Dai Y, Ayares DL. 2003. Production of alpha 1,3-galactosyltransferase-deficient pigs. Science 299:411–414.

Qari SH, Magre S, Garcia-Lerma JG, Hussain AI, Takeuchi Y, Patience C, Weiss RA, Heneine W. 2001. Susceptibility of the porcine endogenous retrovirus to reverse transcriptase and protease inhibitors. J Virol 75:1048–1053.

Scobie L, Taylor S, Wood JC, Suling KM, Quinn G, Meikle S, Patience C, Schuurman HJ, Onions DE. 2004. Absence of replication-competent human-tropic porcine endogenous retroviruses in the germ line DNA of inbred miniature Swine. J Virol 78:2502–2509.

Specke V, Plesker R, Coulibaly C, Boller K, Denner J. 2002. Productive infection of a mink cell line with porcine endogenous retroviruses (PERVs) but lack of transmission to minks in vivo. Arch Virol 147:305–319.

Tacke SJ, Bodusch K, Berg A, Denner J. 2001. Sensitive and specific immunological detection methods for porcine endogenous retroviruses applicable to experimental and clinical xenotransplantation. Xenotransplantation 8:125–135.

Takefman DM, Wong S, Maudru T, Peden K, Wilson CA. 2001. Detection and characterization of porcine endogenous retrovirus in porcine plasma and porcine factor VIII. J Virol 75:4551–4557.

Takeuchi Y, Patience C, Magre S, Weiss RA, Banerjee PT, Le Tissier P, Stoye JP. 1998. Host range and interference studies of three classes of pig endogenous retrovirus. J Virol 72:9986–9991.

Tonjes RR, Niebert M. 2003. Relative age of proviral porcine endogenous retrovirus sequences in *Sus scrofa* based on the molecular clock hypothesis. J Virol 77:12363-12368.

van der Laan LJ, Lockey C, Griffeth BC, Frasier FS, Wilson CA, Onions DE, Hering BJ, Long Z, Otto E, Torbett BE, Salomon DR. 2000. Infection by porcine endogenous retrovirus after islet xenotransplantation in SCID mice. Nature 407:90–94.

Wilhelm M, Fishman JA, Pontikis R, Aubertin AM, Wilhelm FX. 2002. Susceptibility of recombinant porcine endogenous retrovirus reverse transcriptase to nucleoside and non-nucleoside inhibitors. Cell Mol Life Sci 59:2184–2190.

Wilson CA. 2001. Will some pig breeds or tissues be less likely to express infectious PERV? Transplantation 72:1865–1866.

Wilson CA, Wong S, Muller J, Davidson CE, Rose TM, Burd P. 1998. Type C retrovirus released from porcine primary peripheral blood mononuclear cells infects human cells. J Virol 72:3082–3087.

Wilson CA, Wong S, VanBrocklin M, Federspiel MJ. 2000. Extended analysis of the in vitro tropism of porcine endogenous retrovirus. J Virol 74:49–56.

Wood JC, Quinn G, Suling KM, Oldmixon BA, Van Tine BA, Cina R, Arn S, Huang CA, Scobie L, Onions DE, Sachs DH, Schuurman HJ, Fishman JA, Patience C. 2004. Identification of exogenous forms of human-tropic porcine endogenous retrovirus in miniature Swine. J Virol 78:2494–2501.

Xu H, Sharma A, Okabe J, Cui C, Huang L, Wei YY, Wan H, Lei Y, Logan JS, Levy MF, Byrne GW. 2003. Serologic analysis of anti-porcine endogenous retroviruses immune responses in humans after ex vivo transgenic pig liver perfusion. Am Soc Artif Internal Organs J 49:407–416.

Porcine Lymphotropic Herpesviruses
X.J. Meng, P.G. Halbur

Until recently, only two species of herpesviruses have been recognized in swine: pseudorabies virus (PRV) and porcine cytomegalovirus (PCMV) (Chmielewicz et al. 2003a; Murphy et al. 1999). PRV is an alpha-herpesvirus that causes respiratory, reproductive, and central nervous system diseases in pigs. PCMV is a beta-herpesvirus that causes inclusion body rhinitis in swine. Prior to 1999, gamma-herpesvirus was not known to infect pigs. By using a pan-herpesvirus consensus PCR assay, Ehlers et al. (1999a) discovered two closely related gamma-herpesviruses in pigs, designated porcine lymphotropic herpesviruses 1 and 2 (PLHV-1 and PLHV-2). More recently, a third porcine gamma-herpesvirus with considerable sequence differences with PLHV-1 and PLHV-2 was identified and designated PLHV-3 (Chmielewicz et al. 2003b). All three viruses were frequently detected in the blood and lymphoid organs of domestic pigs in different geographic regions. The discoveries of these novel porcine gamma-herpesviruses have raised concerns for the inadvertent transmission of animal pathogens to humans during xenotransplantation with pig cells, tissues, and organs (Chmielewicz et al. 2003b; Tucker et al. 2002, 2003). However, the clinical significance on pig health and the pathogenic potential of these novel viruses alone or in combination with other pathogens in pigs are unknown.

ETIOLOGY

The PLHV group belongs to the subfamily *Gammaherpesvirinae* of the family *Herpesviridae* (Ehlers et al. 1999a). Amino acid sequence analyses based on the partial DNA polymerase gene revealed that PHLV-1 and PHLV-2 displayed the highest (68%) sequence identity to the ruminant gamma-herpesviruses, alcelaphine herpesvirus type 1 (AlHV-1) and ovine herpesvirus type 2 (OvHV-2), about 67% sequence identity to bovine lymphotropic herpesvirus (BLHV), but shared only about 41% sequence identity to porcine alphaherpesvirus PRV and less than 45% identity to porcine betaherpesvirus PCMV (Ehlers et al. 1999a).

The complete DNA polymerase genes of PLHV-1 and PLHV-2 differed by about 7% from each other at the nucleotide sequence level, and 5% from each other at the amino acid sequence level. Since there are 50 amino acid differences between PLHV-1 and PLHV-2 in the DNA polymerase genes, the two viruses belong to two different species rather than strains of the same species (Ulrich et al. 1999).

PLHV-3 was initially detected from the blood sample of a German domestic pig, and was found to share only about 66% amino acid sequence identity in the DNA polymerase gene region with PLHV-1 and PLHV-2 (Chmielewicz et al. 2003b). Phylogenetic analyses showed that all three PLHV viruses clustered together with ruminant gammaherpesviruses BLHV, AlHV-1, OvHV-2, and caprine herpesvirus (CprHV-2) (Figure 32.8); however, PHLV-3 is more distantly related to PLHV-1 and PLHV-2 than the two viruses to each other (Chmielewicz et al. 2003b).

For gammaherpesviruses, the conserved genes are

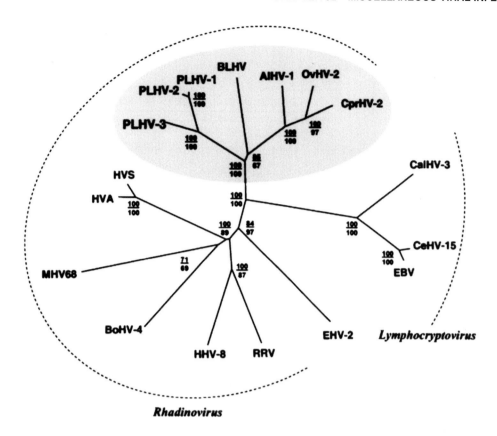

32.8. *A phylogenetic tree based on the concatenated multiple amino acid sequence alignments of conserved regions of gB and DPOL of PLHV-1, -2, and –3 and other related herpesviruses. The bootstrap values derived from 100 replicons are indicated at the branching points of the tree. The upper values were obtained with neighbor/joining analysis, the lower values with parsimonial analysis. Viruses classified to the genus Rhadinovirus and to the genus Lymphocryptovirus are indicated. The PLHVs and several ruminant gammaherpesviruses forming a separate clade are highlighted by gray background. (Reproduced with permission by Academic Press from Chmielewicz et al. 2003b.)*

organized in a common block. Approximately 73 kb genomic sequence of PLHV-1 has been determined and found to encode ORFs 3 to 52 spanning the entire first and second conserved gene blocks and the beginning of the third block (Goltz et al. 2002). In addition, two ORFs not conserved among gammaherpesviruses—E4/BALF1h and A5/BILF1h—three nonconserved ORFs between the second and third conserved gene blocks, and eight unique ORFs outside the conserved gene blocks were also identified in PLHV-1 genome (Goltz et al. 2002). The available 60 kb genomic sequence of PLHV-3 included the first and the majority of the second conserved gene blocks consisting of ORFs 3–46 as well as a putative chemokine receptor and a v-bcl-2 gene (Chmielewicz et al. 2003b). The gene organization of PLHV-3 is identical to that of PLHV-1 and PLHV-2 in the region where sequences are available for all three viruses, including the conserved herpesvirus ORFs; the gammaherpesvirus-specific ORFs 3, 10, 11, 23, and 27; and the nonconserved ORFs E4/BALF1h and A5/BILF1h (Chmielewicz et al. 2003b; Goltz et al. 2002).

Currently, there are no reports of the propagation and isolation of PLHV in cell cultures, and consequently the physicochemical and biological properties of PLHV

are not yet known. However, PLHV-3 has been detected in a persistently infected porcine B cell line L23, which harbors approximately 400 genome copies of PLHV per cell (Chmielewicz et al. 2003b).

EPIDEMIOLOGY

Little is known regarding the epidemiology of PLHV.

Ehlers et al. (1999a) tested peripheral blood mononuclear cells (PBMC) from 42 pigs and spleen samples from 19 pigs in Germany for evidence of PLHV infection, and found that 88% of PBMC and 95% of the spleen samples were positive for PLHV DNA. Three of 8 Spanish pigs tested were also positive. Chmielewicz et al. (2003b) reported that 47 of 92 (51%) peripheral blood leukocyte samples of pigs from 16 different herds in Germany were positive for PLHV-3 DNA. Approximately 88% (14/16) of the swine herds were also positive. Using real-time PCR, PLHV-1 and PLHV-2 DNA were detected in 54% and 16%, respectively, in the same set of samples (Table 32.3). PLHV-1, -2, and –3 DNA were detected in 78%, 41%, and 59% of lung tissue samples and in 59%, 26%, and 62% of the spleen samples, respectively. Of the 20 Italian pigs tested, PLHV-1, -2, and –3 DNA were

Table 32.3. Prevalence of PLHV viral DNA in commercial pigs

Tissue	Farm	Country	Number of Samples Tested	Number of Samples Positive for PLHV-3 DNA by		Number of Samples Positive by gB Real-Time PCR for		
				DPOL PCR	gB PCR	PLHV-3	PLHV-2	PLHV-1
Blood	1	Germany	5	2	2	2	2	4
Blood	2	Germany	6	2	2	2	0	6
Blood	3	Germany	6	3	3	3	1	1
Blood	4	Germany	5	4	5	5	1	4
Blood	5	Germany	7	7	6	6	1	4
Blood	6	Germany	6	2	3	2	0	5
Blood	7	Germany	5	3	3	3	0	3
Blood	8	Germany	5	5	4	4	2	5
Blood	9	Germany	5	1	1	0	0	3
Blood	10	Germany	5	5	5	5	3	2
Blood	11	Germany	5	2	2	2	1	3
Blood	12	Germany	5	3	3	3	0	1
Blood	13	Germany	5	4	3	4	1	3
Blood	14	Germany	8	4	5	3	2	0
Blood	15	Germany	5	0	0	0	1	0
Blood	16	Germany	9	0	0	0	0	6
	Total		92	47 (51%)	47 (51%)	44 (48%)	15 (16%)	50 (54%)
Blood		Italy	20	nd	nd	13 (65%)	4 (20%)	16 (80%)
Lung		Germany	27	nd	nd	16 (59%)	11 (41%)	21 (78%)
Spleen		Germany	34	nd	nd	21 (62%)	9 (26%)	20 (59%)

nd = not done.
Modified with permission by Academic Press from Chielewicz et al. (2003b).

found in 80%, 20%, and 65% of the samples, respectively (Table 32.3). All three PLHV species were also detected from pigs in France, Spain, and the United States (Chmielewicz et al., 2003b).

Analyses of PLHV sequences from pigs in different countries revealed very little variation, indicating that the PLHVs are genetically stable, regardless of their geographic origin. Approximately 21% (9/44) of the miniature swine PBMC were also positive (Tucker et al. 2003). Feral pigs are also found to have a high prevalence of both PLHV-1 and PLHV-2 (Ulrich et al. 1999). Using a pan-herpes consensus PCR assay, Chmielewicz et al. (2003a) analyzed 495 blood and tissue samples collected from 294 pigs, and PLHV sequence was detected in 128 (26%). These molecular epidemiological data suggested that PLHV infection is ubiquitous in commercial swine herds.

The transmission route of PLHV is unknown. Tucker et al. (2003) found that about 80% of the conventional swine spleen samples (15/15) but only 13% (6/47) of cesarean-derived qualified pathogen free (QPF) swine spleen samples were positive for PLHV DNA. The reduced incidence of PLHV infection in cesarean-derived QPF pigs raised in strict biosecurity environment suggested that PLHV transmission may be a combination of both prepartum vertical (transplacental) transfer and postpartum horizontal (piglet-to-piglet, sow-to-piglet). However, the results from a small, transplacental infection study showed that 4 of the 5 sows were positive for PLHV sequences, whereas only one of 33 cesarean-

derived offspring were positive, suggesting that transplacental transfer of PLHV is rare (Tucker et al. 2003).

PATHOGENESIS, CLINICAL SIGNS, AND LESIONS

PLHV infection is not associated with any known disease in pigs under natural conditions. However, due to the close genetic relationship with several pathogenic gammaherpesviruses such as AIHV-1, the cause of malignant catarrhal fever in cattle, it is possible that PLHV might also be pathogenic in pigs. The short lifespan of commercial pigs, generally about 6 months, could make such a disease unrecognizable, especially if it causes a chronic disease. Nevertheless, it has been recently reported that PLHV-1 is associated with posttransplant lymphoproliferative disease (PTLD) in miniature pigs following allogeneic hematopoietic stem cell transplantation (Goltz et al. 2002; Huang et al. 2001). PLHV-1 DNA was abundantly detected in PBMC and lymph node tissues of PTLD pigs (Huang et al. 2001). Most importantly, many PLHV-1 genes such as the immediate-early and late genes, the G-protein coupled receptor (GCR) gene, and the viral homolog of bcl-2 oncogene (v-bcl-2), are actively transcribed in PTLD pigs, but not in healthy pigs (Goltz et al. 2002), supporting the hypothesis that PLHV-1 may be involved in the etiology of porcine PTLD. Since PLHV-2 and PLHV-3 are genetically closely related to PLHV-1, it is reasonable to assume that PLHV-2 and PLHV-3 might also be associated with lym-

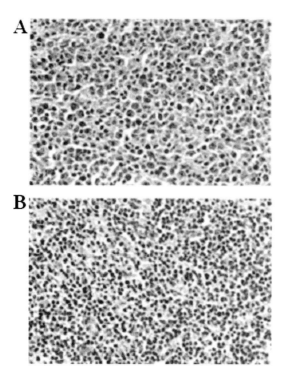

32.9. *Histopathological section from a pig with posttransplantation lymphoproliferative disorder (PTLD) associated with porcine lymphotropic gammaherpesvirus infection. Hematoxylin and eosin staining of mesenteric lymph node tissue taken from a pig during PTLD on day 48 (A) and following complete resolution of PTLD at day 69 (B). Typical polymorphous PTLD with a mixture of immunoblasts, plasmacytoid cells, and plasma cells can be seen in the day 48 but not the day 69 tissue sample (original magnification X 500). (Reproduced with permission from Huang et al. 2001.*

phoproliferative disease in pigs. The clinical symptoms of experimental porcine PTLD, such as fever, lethargy, anorexia, high WBC count, and palpable lymph nodes, are similar to those of human PTLD, which was linked to a human gammaherpesvirus, Epstein-Barr virus (EBV) (Loren et al. 2003; Paya et al. 1999). Characteristic gross pathological lesions in PTLD pigs include enlargement of tonsils and lymph nodes throughout the body with involvement of the gastrointestinal tract and spleen. The enlarged pulmonary lymph nodes and tonsils caused airway obstruction and respiratory failure in these pigs (Huang et al. 2001; Talpe et al. 2001). Microscopically, typical polymorphous PTLD cells with a mixture of immunoblasts, plasmacytoid cells, and plasma cells were seen in the lymph nodes (Figure 32.9).

Several animal gammaherpesviruses, including AlHV-1 and OvHV-2, are genetically closely related to PLHV; however, these viruses are nonpathogenic in their natural hosts, wildebeest and sheep, but cause serious lymphoproliferative and inflammatory diseases in other species such as cattle and deer (Goltz et al. 2002). Therefore, even if PLHV is not associated with any disease in pigs, it could become pathogenic in other animal species, especially in the case of pig-to-human xeno-

transplantation. During xenotransplantation, PLHV could bypass the natural defense barriers such as the mucosal surfaces and be directly introduced into the body of the human recipient via infected organs or cells, thus favoring cross-species infection between pigs and humans. Under immunosuppressive conditions, PLHV could become pathogenic in xenotransplant recipients and cause similar lymphoproliferative diseases in humans (Chmielewicz et al. 2003a; Goltz et al. 2002; Paul et al. 2003; Tucker et al. 2003). The possibility also exists that PLHV from infected xenografts might recombine with known human gammaherpesviruses, which are usually reactivated in the posttransplantation stage. Therefore, donor pigs intended for xenotransplantation should be adequately screened for the presence of PLHV infection.

IMMUNITY

Little is known regarding the immunity of PLHVs or the type of immune response they induce. Several lines of evidence indicated that PLHVs have B cell tropism. PLHV-3 was identified in a continuous porcine B-cell line L23 (Chmielewicz et al. 2003b). In immunosuppressed pigs with PTLD, oligoclonal proliferation of B lineage cells increased by a factor of approximately 10^2, and the amount of PLHV-1 genome copies increased concomitantly by a factor of 10^5 (Huang et al. 2001). In the tissues of PTLD pigs, the transcriptional activity of two ORFs (A7/BZLF2h and A8/BLLF1h) encoding proteins responsible for B cell entry was detected (Goltz et al. 2002). Under field conditions, PLHVs were predominately detected in PBMC in the blood and spleen tissues (Chmielewicz et al. 2003a, b; Ehlers et al. 1999a; Ulrich et al. 1999). Taken together, these data strongly suggested that PLHV infects B-cells. However, it is unclear whether the function of B cells becomes compromised in PLHV-infected pigs.

DIAGNOSIS

PCR is the only diagnostic assay currently available for PLHVs. A pan-herpes consensus PCR assay targeting the conserved regions of herpesvirus DNA polymerase genes has been developed and can detect more than 20 different herpesviruses (Chmielewicz et al. 2003a, b; Ehlers et al. 1999a, b). This pan-herpes consensus PCR assay, when performed in a nested format with degenerate and deoxyinosine-containing primers, can easily detect all three species of PLHV in porcine blood PBMC and spleen tissues. A quantitative real-time PCR assay has also been developed to quantify PLHV-1, -2, and –3 genomic DNA copy numbers in swine samples (Goltz et al. 2003). Ehlers et al. (1999a) developed a differential PCR assay that can differentiate between infections caused by PLHV-1 and PLHV-2. As a group of lymphotropic viruses, PLHV sequences are frequently detected in blood PBMC, spleen, tonsils, and lymph nodes. However, for diagnosis purpose, only blood PBMC is readily available from live pigs. An efficient cell culture for PLHV has not been established, and serological assays are not available.

PREVENTION AND CONTROL

A major concern regarding PLHV is the potential risk of human infection associated with xenotransplantation of pig cells, tissues, and organs (Chmielewicz et al. 2003a; Tucker et al. 2002). PLHV-1 has been shown to be associated with porcine PTLD; thus PLHV–1 is not only potentially pathogenic for pigs, but for human xenograft recipients, as well. Therefore, recipients of xenotransplants from pigs should be carefully monitored for potential PLHV transmission. Adequate screening of donor pigs by PCR assay for PLHV is important to prevent potential infection in xenograft recipients.

Appropriate breeding procedures could eliminate or minimize the risk of PLHV infection. A recent study showed that piglets free of PLHV could be generated through cesarian-derived and barrier-reared breeding procedure (Tucker et al. 2003). Therefore, xenograft donor pigs free of PLHV infection can be produced through a strict breeding and production process.

REFERENCES

Chmielewicz B, Goltz M, Lahrmann KH, Ehlers B. 2003a. Approaching virus safety in xenotransplantation: A search for unrecognized herpesviruses in pigs. Xenotransplantation 10:349–356.

Chmielewicz B, Goltz M, Franz T, Bauer C, Brema S, Ellerbrok H, Beckmann S, Rziha HJ, Lahrmann KH, Romero C, Ehlers B. 2003b. A novel porcine gammaherpesvirus. Virology 308:317–329.

Ehlers B, Borchers K, Grund C, Frölich K, Ludwig H, Buhk HJ. 1999b. Detection of new DNA polymerase genes of known and potentially novel herpesviruses by PCR with degenerate and deoxyinosine-substituted primers. Virus Genes 18:211–220.

Ehlers B, Ulrich S, Goltz M. 1999a. Detection of two novel porcine herpesviruses with high similarity to gammaherpesviruses. J Gen Virol 80:971–978.

Goltz M, Ericsson T, Patience C, Huang CA, Noack S, Sachs DH, Ehlers B. 2002. Sequence analysis of the genome of porcine lymphotropic herpesvirus 1 and gene expression during posttransplant lymphoproliferative disease of pigs. Virology 294:383–393.

Huang CA, Fuchimoto Y, Gleit ZL, Ericsson T, Griesemer A, Scheier-Dolberg R, Melendy E, Kitamura H, Fishman JA, Harris NL, Patience C, Sachs DH. 2001. Posttransplantation lymphoproliferative disease in miniature swine after allogeneic hematopoietic cell transplantation: Similarity to human PTLD and association with a porcine gammaherpesvirus. Blood 97:1467–1473.

Loren AW, Porter DL, Stadtmauer EA, Tsai DE. 2003. Posttransplant lymphoproliferative disorder: A review. Bone Marrow Transplantation 31:145–155.

Murphy FA, Gibbs EPJ, Horzinek MC, Studdert MJ. 1999. *Herpesviridae*. In Veterinary Virology (3rd edition). San Diego, California: Academic Press, Inc., pp. 301–325.

Paul PS, Halbur PG, Janke B, Joo H, Nawagitgul P, Singh J, Sorden S. 2003. Exogenous porcine viruses. Curr Top Microbiol Immunol 278:125–183.

Paya CV, Fung JJ, Nalesnik MA, Kieff E, Green M, Gores G, Habermann TM, Wiesner PH, Swinnen JL, Woodle ES, Bromberg JS. 1999. Epstein-Barr virus-induced posttransplant lymphoproliferative disorders. ASTS/ASTP EBV-PTLD Task Force and The Mayo Clinic Organized International Consensus Development Meeting. Transplantation 68:1517–1525.

Talpe S, Oike F, Dehoux JP, Sempoux C, Rahier J, Otte JB, Gianello P. 2001. Posttransplant lymphoproliferative disorder after liver transplantation in miniature swine. Transplantation 71:1684–1688.

Tucker AW, Belcher C, Moloo B, Bell J, Mazzulli T, Humar A, Hughes A, McArdle PD, Talbot A. 2002. The production of transgenic pigs for potential use in clinical xenotransplantation: Microbiological evaluation. Xenotransplantation 9:191–202.

Tucker AW, McNeilly F, Meehan B, Galbraith D, McArdle PD, Allan G, Patience C. 2003. Methods for the exclusion of circoviruses and gammaherpesviruses from pigs. Xenotransplantation 10:343–348.

Ulrich S, Goltz M, Ehlers B. 1999. Characterization of the DNA polymerase loci of the novel porcine lymphotropic herpesviruses 1 and 2 in domestic and feral pigs. J Gen Virol 80:3199–3205.

Eastern Equine Encephalomyelitis Virus

F. Elvinger, C.A. Baldwin

Eastern equine encephalomyelitis (EEE) is endemic in the eastern United States (Atlantic and Gulf coasts), several Central and South American countries, and Caribbean islands. Naturally occurring EEE in swine was first reported in 1972 (Pursell et al.) when 160 of 200 pigs in one herd died in an outbreak in Georgia, USA. Exposure of domestic and feral swine to the agent had been described earlier in serologic surveys in the states of Georgia, Massachusetts, and Wisconsin (Feemster et al. 1958; Karstad and Hanson 1958, 1959). The disease is diagnosed sporadically in porcine case material at veterinary diagnostic laboratories, but it is likely underrecognized in the field.

The causative agent of EEE, eastern equine encephalomyelitis virus (EEEV), is classified in the United States as a Category B bioterrorism agent because of its moderate ease to disseminate, moderate morbidity, and high case-fatality rates in humans, and its potential impact on the Center for Disease Control and Prevention (CDC)'s diagnostic, surveillance and response capabilities.

ETIOLOGY

EEEV is a single-strand RNA virus in the genus *Alphavirus*, family *Togaviridae*. There are 26 confirmed members in the genus *Alphavirus*, including western equine encephalomyelitis virus (WEEV) and Venezuelan equine encephalomyelitis virus (Hahn et al. 1988). EEEV was described and serologically differentiated from WEEV in 1933 (TenBroeck and Merrill).

Nucleic acid analysis has demonstrated that EEEV has evolved independently into North and South American antigenic varieties (Casals 1964; Weaver et al. 1991), each with distinct virulence characteristics (Walder et al. 1980). Isolates appear to be genetically stable over a discrete time period within a geographic region of transmission (Brault et al. 1999; Roehrig et al. 1990).

EPIDEMIOLOGY

EEEV circulates endemically among many bird species considered to be reservoirs and amplifiers of the virus. EEEV is transmitted from bird-to-bird, mainly by the ornithophilic mosquito vector *Culiseta melanuris*. Other mosquito species from genera such as *Aedes* and *Anopheles* also transmit EEEV. Mosquito species with opportunistic feeding habits on both birds and mammals are responsible for the epidemic virus transmission to mammals. The appearance of EEE in mammals is associated with climatic conditions that influence vector population dynamics and enhance their density (Francy and Wagner 1992; Letson et al. 1993).

Clinical outbreaks have been reported from Georgia and Florida (Elvinger et al. 1994, 1996b; Pursell et al. 1972). Swine on 9 of 45 (20%) farms tested in recent serologic surveys in Georgia had antibodies to EEEV, and 16% of 376 feral swine on a Georgia barrier island had serum virus neutralization antibody titers that ranged from 4 to 128 (Elvinger et al. 1996b).

In general, mammals are considered dead-end hosts due to low virus titers that are insufficient to infect vectors. However, nursing pigs that were experimentally infected developed high titer viremia that lasted up to 168 hours. Virus could be recovered from oropharyngeal and rectal swabs up to 96 hours after virus administration, and virus could be isolated from tonsils of pigs up to 20 days after experimental infection. Contact control pigs, in addition, have seroconverted in experimental infection studies (Baldwin et al. 1993; Karstad and Hanson 1958). Thus, it is conceivable that infected nursing pigs are a source of virus for both vectors and, by direct transmission, for mammals in their close proximity.

CLINICAL SIGNS

EEEV predominantly affects nursing pigs. Clinical signs include depression, anorexia, ataxia, prostration, lateral recumbence, convulsions, and ultimately death. However, clinical disease is not commonly observed following experimental or natural exposure to EEEV. Most nursing pigs exhibit only a transient temperature increase, even when high doses of EEEV are experimentally given by oral, intradermal, or intravenous routes (Baldwin et al. 1993; Elvinger et al. 1996a). Predisposing factors, including adverse environmental conditions or concurrent disease, may contribute to the high mortality observed in natural outbreaks of EEE in swine (Elvinger et al. 1994; Pursell et al. 1972). Experimental infection of older animals did not lead to clinical disease (Karstad and Hanson 1959) and EEE has not been described in adult swine. The oldest pig recorded with clinical EEE was a 2-month-old female (Pursell et al. 1983), however, seroconversion was detected in adult animals following disease outbreaks in piglets (Elvinger et al. 1994).

PATHOGENESIS

Natural infection of pigs likely occurs through transmission of virus by hematophagous vectors, while experimental infection has been achieved by intracranial, intradermal, intravenous, and oral routes of virus administration (Baldwin et al. 1993; Karstad and Hanson 1959; Pursell et al. 1972). Rectal temperature increases within 24 hours of virus administration and is elevated for less than 12 hours in all experimentally infected pigs; however, clinical signs of central nervous system disease are observed in only a few pigs between 18 and 72 hours after virus administration (Baldwin et al. 1993). Circulating virus was isolated 6 hours after experimental infection, regardless of route of infection, and was present in blood for up to 168 hours. Neutralizing antibodies are detectable approximately 120 hours after experimental infection. After the acute viremic phase, EEEV was isolated only from tonsils and central nervous tissues. Virus was isolated or demonstrated by oligonucleotide probe in tonsils up to 20 days after experimental infection. Consequently, tonsil tissues of infected pigs could be a significant source of virus dispersion, especially since contact pigs become infected (Baldwin et al. 1993; Karstad and Hanson 1958). Oligonucleotide probing revealed EEEV in transient liver lesions that appeared early during the viremic phase of the infection, prior to the appearance of lesions in myocardium and central nervous system (Baldwin et al. 1993, 1994a, b). Presence of virus in liver lesions may indicate virus tropism for hepatic tissue and viral replication in the liver.

LESIONS

No gross lesions indicative of EEE have been observed in naturally or experimentally infected pigs (Baldwin et al. 1993; Elvinger et al. 1994, 1996a; Karstad and Hanson 1959; Pursell et al. 1972). Microscopically, necrotizing hepatitis appeared within 12 hours of experimental infection, increasing in size over the next 24 hours, resolving partially by 48 hours, and resolving completely by 72 hours after infection (Baldwin et al. 1993). Central nervous system lesions may not be present in pigs that die in the acute phase of disease. The earliest lesions appeared in brain approximately 48 hours after infection. The appearance of these lesions was concurrent with the appearance of mild lesions in heart and resolution of lesions in liver. Encephalitis was characterized by infiltration of inflammatory cells, disseminated perivascular cuffing, neuronal necrosis and neuronophagia, nodules of glial proliferation, and malacia (Baldwin et al. 1993; Elvinger et al. 1994, 1996a; Pursell et al. 1972). Viral inclusion bodies were not observed. Initially, neutrophils predominated in infiltrates and perivascular cuffs, while lymphocytes were more common at later stages. In addition, histiocytes, adventitial cells, eosinophils, and cellular debris were observed. Hyaline or granular thrombi were found in blood vessels. Lesions occurred primarily in gray matter of brain and spinal cord, but white matter was also affected. Patches of inflammatory cells were noted in the meninges. Multifocal myocardial necrosis had been reported in naturally infected pigs and reproduced in experimental infection (Baldwin et al. 1993; Elvinger et al. 1994, 1996a). Pigs that survived experimental infection with no apparent clinical signs occasionally had lesions of mild encephalitis with lymphocytic perivascular cuffs, focal areas of gliosis and foci of myocardial necrosis that were partially mineralized and surrounded by macrophages (Baldwin et al. 1993).

DIAGNOSIS

Death losses in nursing pigs following clinical signs of central nervous system disease in EEE endemic areas are indicative of virus activity, particularly when climatic conditions are conducive to the development of vector populations. Histopathologic lesions may first appear in liver and myocardium. Lesions in brain consistent with EEE may not have had time to develop in pigs that die during the early viremic phase.

A definitive diagnosis can be supported by virus isolation or detection of virus RNA or antigen. Serologic evidence of exposure in surviving pigs is a good indicator of EEE virus activity, although antibody titers may be due to earlier exposure of sows and transmission of antibodies through colostrum.

A wide spectrum of tests to isolate virus, demonstrate and identify EEEV RNA or antigen, or detect antibodies to EEEV are used to diagnose natural and experimental infections with EEEV (Tsai and Chandler 2003). Fresh and formalin-fixed specimens of brain, spinal cord, liver, heart, and tonsil should be submitted for histopathological examination and virus isolation when EEE is suspected in a swine herd. Virus isolation can be attempted on oropharyngeal swabs from herdmates, since EEEV can persist in tonsil tissue. Precautions should be taken to avoid accidental human infection when collecting the specimens. Serum from affected and nonaffected pigs should be submitted for serologic examination, although disease and death likely will precede the onset of a detectable immune response.

PREVENTION AND CONTROL

Treatment of swine clinically affected with EEE has not been attempted. No treatment of affected horses has been described, and therapeutic efforts in human cases are directed toward management of symptoms (Craven 1991).

Two routes for prevention of EEE can be taken: 1) vaccination of animals at risk, and 2) vector control. Vaccination of sows is an option for protecting swine producers from catastrophic losses due to EEEV infection in pigs. Sows vaccinated experimentally with commercial equine vaccines transferred antibodies to piglets via colostrum that were protective for experimentally infected, early-weaned pigs (Elvinger et al. 1996a). Maternally derived antibodies were measured in pigs for up to 11 weeks after colostrum intake and should be protective until natural susceptibility to clinical disease is outgrown in piglets from vaccinated and naturally infected sows.

The second approach to prevention of EEE is control of exposure to EEEV vectors. Incident cases of EEE in any mammalian or avian species can serve as sentinel cases signaling the need to initiate application of insecticides by local and state governments. Aerial application of insecticides for public health protection benefits swine producers in endemic areas directly by preventing outbreaks and economic losses and, indirectly, by preventing amplification of EEEV in pigs that would put the producers and farm laborers at risk of contracting infection.

REFERENCES

Baldwin CA, Elvinger F, Liggett AD. 1993. Excretion of eastern equine encephalomyelitis virus and oral infection of swine. Proc 74th Conf Res Worker in Anim Dis.

Baldwin CA, Liggett AD, Elvinger F, Tang KN. 1994a. Histopathologic lesions and DNA probing after inoculation of eastern equine encephalomyelitis virus in swine. South East Branch, Annu Meet Am Soc Microbiol, Athens, Georgia.

Baldwin CA, Liggett AD, Niagro F, Elvinger F, Tang KN. 1994b. Porcine liver lesions following inoculation of eastern equine encephalomyelitis virus. Proc 75th Conf Res Worker in Anim Dis.

Brault AC, Powers AM, Chavez CL, Lopez RN, Cachon MF, Gutierrez LF, Kang W, Tesh RB, Shope RE, Weaver SC. 1999. Genetic and antigenic diversity among eastern equine encephalitis viruses from North, Central, and South America. Am J Trop Med Hyg 61:579–586.

Casals J. Antigenic variants of eastern equine encephalitis virus. 1964. J Exp Med 119:547–565.

Craven RB. 1991. Togaviruses. In Textbook of Human Virology (2nd edition). RB Belshe, ed.Littleton, Massachusetts: PSG-Wright, pp. 663–674.

Elvinger F, Baldwin CA, Liggett AD, Tang KN, Dove CR. 1996a. Protection of pigs by vaccination of pregnant sows against eastern equine encephalomyelitis virus. Vet Microbiol 1996:229–239.

Elvinger F, Baldwin CA, Liggett AD, Tang KN, Stallknecht DE. 1996b. Prevalence of exposure to eastern equine encephalomyelitis virus in domestic and feral swine in Georgia. J Vet Diag Invest 8:481–484.

Elvinger F, Liggett AD, Tang KN, Harrison LR, Cole (Jr) JR, Baldwin CA, Nessmith WB. 1994. Eastern equine encephalomyelitis virus infection in swine. J Am Vet Med Assoc 205:1014–1016.

Feemster RF, Wheeler RE, Daniels JB, Rose HD, Schaeffer M, Kissling RE, Hayes RO, Alexander ER, Murray WA. 1958. Field and laboratory studies on equine encephalitis. N Engl J Med 259:107–113.

Francy DB, Wagner BA. 1992. Equine encephalomyelitis in the United States, 1980–1990. Use of weather variables to develop a predictive model for equine cases. In Animal Health Insight. USDA:APHIS:VS Animal Health Information. Spring 1992, pp. 1–8..

Hahn CS, Lustig S, Strauss EG, Strauss JH. 1988. Western equine encephalitis virus is a recombinant virus. Proc Nat Acad Sci USA 85:5997–6001.

Karstad L, Hanson RP. 1959. Natural and experimental infections in swine with the virus of eastern equine encephalitis. J Infect Dis 105:293–296.

Karstad LH, Hanson RP. 1958. Infections in wildlife with the viruses of vesicular stomatitis and eastern equine encephalo-myelitis. In Transactions, 23rd North American Wildlife Conference, pp. 175–185.

Letson GW, Bailey RE, Pearson J, Tsai TF. 1993. Eastern equine encephalitis (EEE): A description of the 1989 outbreak, recent epidemiologic trends, and the association of rainfall with EEE occurrence. Am J Trop Med Hyg 49:677–685.

Pursell AR, Hall RF, Sangster LT, Waller E, Bedell DM. 1983. Eastern encephalomyelitis: The Georgia experience 1982–1983. Proc 26th Annu Meet Am Assoc Vet Lab Diagn, pp. 383–392.

Pursell AR, Peckham JC, Cole (Jr) JC, Stewart WC, Mitchell FE. 1972. Naturally occurring and artificially induced eastern encephalomyelitis in pigs. J Am Vet Med Assoc 161:1143–1147.

Roehrig JT, Hunt AR, Chang GJ, Sheik CB, Bolin RA, Tsai TF, Trent DW. 1990. Identification of monoclonal antibodies capable of differentiating antigenic varieties of eastern equine encephalitis viruses. Am J Trop Med Hyg 42:394–398.

TenBroeck C, Merrill MH. 1933. A serological difference between eastern and western equine encephalomyelitis virus. Proc Soc Exp Biol Med 31:217–220.

Tsai TF, Chandler LJ. 2003. Arboviruses. In Manual of Clinical Microbiology, Volume 2 (8th edition). PR Murray, EJ Baron, JH Jorgensen, MA Pfaller, RH Yolken, eds. Washington, D.C.: ASM Press, pp. 1553–1569.

Walder R, Jahrling PB, Eddy GA. 1980. Differentiation markers of eastern equine encephalitis (EEE) viruses and virulence. Zentralbl Bakteriol Mikrobiol Hyg Suppl 9:237–250.

Weaver SC, Scott TW, Rico-Hesse R. 1991. Molecular evolution of eastern equine encephalomyelitis virus in North America. Virology 182:774–784.

Rabies
F. Elvinger

Rabies is an acute, nearly always lethal, viral, zoonotic disease of the central nervous system (CNS). All mammalian species are believed to be susceptible to rabies virus, although some appear to require higher infectious doses to develop clinical disease, and only a few carnivores/omnivores and bats are important as disease reservoirs.

The geographic distribution of rabies is almost global, with the exception of island nations in the South Pacific (New Zealand and others), where rabies has never been recorded. In Japan, the United Kingdom, Norway, and a few other countries, rabies has been eradicated. The World Health Organization classifies a country as rabies-free if no indigenous cases of rabies have been confirmed in any animal species and humans during the previous 2 years. In some countries, like Australia, rabies-related bat-associated lyssaviruses recently have been described that can cause rabies-like disease and death in humans and terrestrial mammals.

Incidence of rabies is not uniform across regions. The public health and economic impact of the disease varies greatly from highly to less developed regions of the world, from urban to rural environments, and across social strata within countries. Meltzer and Rupprecht (1998a, b) produced a two-part economic assessment in which they estimated costs of a case of human or animal rabies and contrasted those costs to various modalities of control of rabies in dogs and wildlife, and of treatment of exposed human and animal subjects. Costs of rabies are not limited to the economic loss of affected livestock, but also include the costs of regulatory intervention, medical treatment of exposed persons, and the nonfinancial costs of anguish of people who themselves or whose animals have been exposed to the disease.

ETIOLOGY

The bullet-shaped rabies virus of about 180 nm in length and 75 nm in width is a single-stranded, nonsegmented, negative-sense RNA-virus in the *Lyssavirus* genus, family *Rhabdoviridae*, in the order *Mononegavirales*. Another genus in family *Rhabdoviridae* is the genus *Vesiculovirus*, which includes the vesicular stomatitis viruses. Molecular biological analysis and cross-protection assays distinguished 7 genetic lineages in the Lyssavirus genus: rabies virus (classic rabies virus, serotype/genotype 1) and rabies-related viruses including the African viruses Lagos, Mokola, and Duvenhage (serotype/genotypes 2, 3, and 4, respectively); the European bat viruses I and II (genotypes 5 and 6, respectively); and the

Australian bat virus (genotype 7), which, with the exception of Lagos, have all caused disease and death in humans. Additional lyssaviruses that belong to the rabies serogroup, including the Kotonkan and Obodhiang strains from African flies and mosquitoes and the Rochembeau strain from French Guyana mosquitoes currently have been isolated only in invertebrate hosts.

The rabies virion consists of 5 viral proteins of which two are of special interest. The phosphorylated nucleoprotein (N) includes the antibody-binding epitopes that contribute to the differentiation of the various virus groups. Glycoprotein (G) covers the virion, except at the planar end. It is the only one of the 5 proteins that binds virus-neutralizing antibodies, and variation in its amino acid sequence appears to contribute to the variation in pathogenicity of the different strains. Antigenic variation within the sero-type 1 rabies viruses does not appear to affect the efficacy of commonly used vaccines.

EPIDEMIOLOGY

Rabies virus propagates in two epidemiologic cycles. In the *urban cycle,* the street virus circulates in feral and domestic dogs and still puts humans at great risk of exposure and infection in many developing countries. In the developed world there has been a shift from the urban to the *sylvatic cycle,* in which distinctive rabies virus variants circulate in specific wildlife reservoirs within discrete geographic clusters. Reservoirs include different fox species, jackals and coyotes, raccoons, skunks and mongooses, and bats. Wolves and cats can efficiently transmit rabies, but do not serve as reservoirs. Other susceptible animal species in general do not transmit the disease further and are epidemiologically dead-ends. Rabies in humans, companion animals, and livestock in Europe and North America results from spillover from the sylvatic cycle.

The incidence of rabies in swine in North America is low. Two of 2601 rabies cases reported from 1998 through 2003 in Canada (Canadian Food Inspection Agency 2004) and 14 out of 89,011 cases reported from 1991 through 2000 in the United States were in swine (Krebs et al. 2001). Porcine cases, however, are reported to the Office International des Epizooties every year and from all continents (OIE 2003).

PATHOGENESIS

The bite by a rabid animal effectively constitutes a subcutaneous and intramuscular inoculation of large amounts of virus in saliva. Following an eclipse phase, in which virus replication occurs, possibly in myocytes at the bite site, the virus migrates through the axoplasm of the peripheral or cranial nerves to reach the CNS. The lag time between inoculation and neural invasion may be the grace time during which post-exposure prophy-

lactic treatment is most likely to be effective (Acha and Szyfres 2003). Following replication in the CNS, the virus moves centrifugally into non-nervous tissues, including the salivary glands and eyes. Virus may be shed in saliva of infected animals prior to, at, or after onset of clinical disease (Rupprecht et al. 2002).

The incubation period of the disease varies between as little as a few days to several months. The duration of the incubation period depends in part on the virus strain, the site of the bite and the amount of virus transmitted, and the age and immune status of the bitten animal. In a single event in which two of five sows and one boar bitten by a rabid fox developed rabies and died, incubation periods were 39, 56 (boar), and 123 days (Reichel and Möckelmann 1963). Baer and Olson (1972) recorded 32- to 47-day incubation periods in nonlethal infections in feeder pigs. Younger pigs bitten by rabid rats developed rabies 23–42 days after being bitten (Mamatov et al. 1974).

CLINICAL SIGNS

Clinical signs in most species may progress through three phases: the prodromal phase, in which nonspecific respiratory, gastrointestinal or CNS disease signs, including initial behavioral changes may appear; the furious, excitative phase, in which the animal is agitated and aggressive, and which progresses through seizures to coma and death; and the dumb phase, characterized by paralysis, coma, and death.

In swine, as in other species, clinical presentation may be very diverse. Lack of overt clinical signs has been recorded in feeder pigs (Hazlett and Koller 1986). Reported clinical signs include uneasiness, dullness and incoordination, excitement with a tendency to root or attack, drooling/salivation, marked thirst, anorexia, hoarse grunts and vocalizations or lack of squealing, front leg paralysis, twitching of nose and rapid chewing movements with excessive salivation in affected sows, clonic convulsions, fever, and general paralysis proceeding into coma and death (Dhillon and Dhingra 1973; Hazlett and Koller 1986; Merriman 1966; Morehouse et al. 1968; Yates et al. 1983). Duration of the clinical phase in pigs has been reported to be short, lasting from 12 hours to 5 days. Frequently litter- and penmates are affected as well, due to common exposure when attacked by rabid animals. Baer and Olson (1972) described clinical signs of CNS disorder in 4 of 6 pigs bitten by a rabid skunk, including progressive paralysis starting at the forelimbs, and sexual excitement. These signs subsided within 1–2 weeks, and all pigs survived with elevated serum-neutralizing antibody titers to rabies until slaughter 2 months later. Recovery from clinical rabies and survival, including a virus carrier state, have been described in various animal species (Doege and Northrop 1974; Fekadu 1991), and may have occurred in these pigs as well.

LESIONS

Gross lesions due to rabies are not likely to be detected in swine. Swine with rabies may be in good condition, with stomachs full of fresh, normal feed, given the usually short duration of clinical signs (Merriman 1966). Negri bodies, which are eosinophilic inclusions in the cytoplasm of nerve cells and dendrites of infected animals, are frequently absent in rabid swine (Merriman 1966; Morehouse et al. 1968; Reichel and Möckelmann 1963). The most detailed presentation of histopathological changes is given by Morehouse et al. (1968) who examined 5 pigs of 16 that died over a period of 2 months in an outbreak at a Missouri swine farm. Microscopic changes in the CNS varied widely, ranging from mild vasculitis and focal gliosis in the brain to extensive meningoencephalitis and marked neuronal degeneration in brain and spinal cord.

LABORATORY DIAGNOSIS

The direct fluorescent antibody test (FAT) for rabies virus has been, and still is, the most commonly used diagnostic test for rabies in all species. This test, introduced in 1958, is recommended by both the Office International des Epizooties and by the World Health Organization (Aubert et al. 2000). Antigen may be detected in all parts of the CNS of infected animals, in corneal impressions, and in skin biopsies (Fekadu and Smith 1984; Smith 2003). However, the test is the most sensitive (approaches 100%) when examining impression smears from fresh tissues from the medulla oblongata, cerebellum, and hippocampus (Ammon's horn), in which the greatest antigen quantities can be expected. Virus isolation techniques may be slightly more sensitive than the FAT in some tissues; however, the FAT is more likely to detect antigen in specimens in which replication of rabies virus is impaired because of tissue decay or presence of antibodies. The FAT is most sensitive on fresh brain tissue and loses some of its sensitivity when using formalin-fixed specimens following enzymatic treatment of the fixed sample (90–100% relative sensitivity compared to fresh tissue). False-negative FAT have been reported in swine in which rabies was confirmed by mouse inoculation tests (Dhillon and Dhingra 1973; Morehouse et al. 1968; Yates et al. 1983). Mouse inoculation or cell culture tests should be used when the FAT gives an uncertain result or when the FAT is negative, and when there has been human exposure to an animal in which clinical signs strongly suggest rabies. Negri bodies, i.e., intracytoplasmatic acidophilic antigen aggregates, are detected in only 75–80% of specimens found positive by more sensitive diagnostic methods (Fekadu and Smith 1984), and sensitivity of rabies diagnosis by detection of Negri bodies may be even lower in rabid pigs (Merriman 1966; Morehouse et al. 1968; Reichel and Möckelman 1963).

PREVENTION AND CONTROL

Protection of humans and animals from rabies relies on prevention. Control of stray dogs and, later, vaccination of owned dogs had the greatest impact in the reduction of rabies incidence in humans, companion animals, and livestock.

In general, vaccination of swine is not recommended, given the very low number of porcine cases annually in the United States, western Europe, and other countries, which may be due to lower susceptibility of swine to rabies. In the United States there is currently no rabies vaccine licensed for use in swine. Prophylactic vaccination requires the extralabel use of a vaccine product approved for other species.

In case of exposure, unvaccinated livestock should be slaughtered immediately: "If the animal is slaughtered within 7 days of being bitten, its tissues may be eaten without risk of infection, provided that liberal portions of exposed area are discarded" (National Association of State Public Health Veterinarians 2004). Such an animal can be slaughtered for personal consumption in the United States; however, "federal guidelines for meat inspectors require that any animal known to have been exposed to rabies within 8 months be rejected for slaughter."

Prophylactic post-exposure treatment may be indicated to save valuable animals or in countries where culling may impose excessive hardship on the owners of exposed animals. Mitmoonpitak et al. (2002) reported that, following severe rabies exposure involving deep bite wounds on nose, shoulder, vulva, and tail from a rabid dog, 11 pigs received either vaccine alone (inactivated, Rabisin manufactured by Rhone Merieux, France) or vaccine with equine rabies immunoglobulin (ERIG, 40 IU/kg bodyweight; Pasteur Merieux Connaught, France). All treated pigs had detectable antibodies to rabies by 14 days post treatment, and all pigs survived for 1 year following the exposure. Thus, post-exposure rabies treatment of valuable farm animals may be a safe and effective alternative to immediate slaughter. It needs to be pointed out, however, that the lack of licensed rabies vaccine for swine and the potential for the existence of rabies carrier states dictates caution in rabies endemic areas and requires that access of the public to swine in petting zoos or other facilities be restricted (Massachusetts Department of Public Health 2004).

REFERENCES

Acha PN, Szyfres B. 2003. Rabies. In Zoonoses and Communicable Diseases Common to Man and Animals, Volume 2, Chlamydioses, Rickettsioses, and Viroses (3rd edition). Scientific and Technical Publication No. 580. Washington, D.C.: PanAmerican Health Organization, pp. 246–275.

Aubert M, Cliquet F, Barrat J. 2000. Rabies. In Manual of Standards for Diagnostic Tests and Vaccines (4th ed), Office International des Epizooties, World Organisation for Animal Health, pp. 276–291.

Baer GM, Olson HR. 1972. Recovery of pigs from rabies. J Am Vet Med Assoc 160:1127–1128.

Canadian Food Inspection Agency. 2004. Positive Rabies in Canada. accessed June 2, 2004 at http://www.inspection.gc.ca/english/anima/heasan/disemala/rabrag/statse.shtml

Dhillon SS, Dhingra PN. 1973. A note on rabies in swine. Vet Med Small Anim Clin 68:1044.

Doege TC, Northrop RL. 1974. Evidence for inapparent rabies infection. Lancet 7884:825–829.

Fekadu M. 1991. Latency and aborted rabies. In The Natural History of Rabies (2nd edition). GM Baer, ed. Boca Raton, Florida: CRC Press, pp. 191–198.

Fekadu M, Smith JS. 1984. Laboratory diagnosis of rabies. In Rabies Concepts for Medical Professionals. WC Winkler, ed. Miami: Merieux Institute.

Hazlett MJ, Koller MA. 1986. Porcine rabies in a closed feeder barn. Can Vet J 27:116–118.

Hou KC. 1992. Report of suspected cases of rabies in pigs. Chinese Journal of Veterinary Medicine 18:22–28. From CAB Direct, accessed May 31, 2004; Record No: 19932287875.

Krebs JW, Mondul AM, Rupprecht CE, Childs JE. 2001. Rabies surveillance in the United States during 2000. J Am Vet Med Assoc 219:1687–1699.

Mamatov NM, Khushvakov DK, Mamatkudov DM. 1974. Role of rats in outbreaks of rabies among pigs in the Surkhandarin region of Uzbekistan. Trudy Uzbekskogo Naucho-issledovatelskogo Veterinarnogo Instituta 22:136-140. From CAB Direct, accessed June 1, 2004; Record No: 19752286833.

Massachusetts Department of Public Health. 2004. Recommendations for petting zoos, petting farms, animal fairs, and other events and exhibits where contact between animals and people is permitted. accessed May 27, 2004 at http://www.mass.gov/dph/cdc/epii/rabies/petzoo.htm

Meltzer MI, Rupprecht CE. 1998a. A review of the economics of the prevention and control of rabies. Part 1: Global impact and rabies in humans. Pharmacoeconomics 14:365–383.

——. 1998b. A review of the economics of the prevention and control of rabies. Part 2: Rabies in dogs, livestock and wildlife. Pharmacoeconomics 14:481–498.

Merriman GM. 1966. Rabies in Tennessee swine. 1966. J Am Vet Med Assoc 148:809–811.

Mitmoonpitak C, Limusanno S, Khawplod P, Tepsumethanon V, Wilde H. 2002. Post-exposure rabies treatment in pigs. Vaccine 20:2019–2021.

Morehouse LG, Kintner LD, Nelson SL. 1968. Rabies in swine. J Am Vet Med Assoc 153:57–64.

OIE. 2003. World Animal Health in 2002. Part 2. Office International des Epizooties, Paris, France.

Reichel K, Möckelmann. 1963. Rabies in pigs. Tierarztl Umsch 18:445–448, 451. (From Abstracts, Vet Bull 1964 34:143(#891)).

Rupprecht CE, Hanlon CA, Hemachudha T. 2002. Rabies re-examined. Lancet Infect Dis 2:327–343.

Smith JS. 2003. Rabies Virus. In Manual of Clinical Microbiology, Volume 2 (8th edition). PR Murray, EJ Baron, JH Jorgensen, MA Pfaller, RH Yolken, eds. Washington, D.C.: ASM Press, pp. 1545–1552.

National Association of State Public Health Veterinarians Committee. 2004. Compendium of animal rabies prevention and control, 2004. J Am Vet Med Assoc 224:216–222.

Yates WDG, Rehmtulla AJ, McIntosh DW. 1983. Porcine rabies in Western Canada. Can Vet J 24:162–163.

III Bacterial Diseases

33 *Actinobacillus pleuropneumoniae*

Marcelo Gottschalk and David J. Taylor

Actinobacillus pleuropneumoniae is the etiologic agent of pleuropneumonia in pigs. The first observations of this disease were made by Pattison et al. (1957), Matthews and Pattison (1961), and Olander (1963). Shope (1964) later described an acute outbreak of a similar infection on a farm in Argentina. The name *Haemophilus pleuropneumoniae* was given to the causal organism by Shope et al. (1964) and White et al. (1964). The name was confirmed by Kilian et al. (1978). The designation *Haemophilus parahaemolyticus* given to the California strains (Olander 1963) and the Swiss isolates (Nicolet 1968) is considered a synonym.

H. pleuropneumoniae was later transferred to the genus *Actinobacillus* and designated *Actinobacillus pleuropneumoniae* after DNA homology studies had demonstrated the close relationship of *H. pleuropneumoniae* to *A. lignieresii* (Pohl et al. 1983). The *Pasteurella* haemolytica–like organism described by Bertschinger and Seifert (1978) as a causative agent of necrotizing pleuropneumonia is considered to be a nicotinamide adenine dinucleotide (NAD)–independent biotype of *A. pleuropneumoniae* (Pohl et al. 1983) and is known as *A. pleuropneumoniae* biotype II.

Pleuropneumonia is one of the important bacterial diseases of the respiratory tract of the pig and occurs in most pig-keeping countries. The clinical disease is relatively well controlled in the United States and Canada, but it is still a major problem in Latin American and European countries (Gottschalk et al. 2003). Its importance derives from the fact that it can cause pneumonia that results in death, clinical disease that may become chronic, or subclinical disease in successive batches of pigs and causes losses from death, reduced production, and increased costs of medication or vaccination. One of the problems of this disease for the clinician is that animals may be treated with antimicrobials effective against the organism, but they may not respond because of the severity of the initial lesions and their nature. Some herds may be subclinically infected without previous evident episodes of the disease and with the absence of suggestive lesions at the abattoir. This happens often in conventional herds which may be simultaneously infected not only with several serotypes of low pathogenicity (see below) but also with serotypes highly likely to cause disease. In these cases, outbreaks may suddenly appear in the presence of concomitant diseases or as a consequence of changes in management. Hence, early identification of subclinically infected herds is important for the control of the disease because carrier animals are the main source of transmission between herds.

Both the organism and the disease have been studied extensively and in considerable detail, and the knowledge has been used to design new vaccines and diagnostic methods and to propose relatively highly effective eradication programs. However, the best and most economical methods for control of the disease are still a matter for discussion.

ETIOLOGY

The etiologic agent *A. pleuropneumoniae* (formerly *Haemophilus pleuropneumoniae*, *H. parahaemolyticus*) is a small, gram-negative, encapsulated rod with typical coccobacillary morphology. The organism does not grow on blood agar unless it is supplemented with NAD and shows satellitism around colonies of staphylococci (biotype I strains). Staphylococcal streaks are normally required for primary isolation on this medium. The biotype I organism forms colonies 0.5–1 mm after 24h of incubation on blood agar in the presence of staphylococcal colonies and is beta-hemolytic, particularly when sheep red blood cells are used. Biotype I is NAD-dependent, and *A. pleuropneumoniae* produces an increased zone of hemolysis within the zone of partial lysis surrounding a beta-toxinogenic *Staphylococcus aureus* (the CAMP phenomenon) (Nicolet 1970; Kilian 1976), and this CAMP phenomenon has been shown to be related to the possession of the three cytolysins ApxI, ApxII, and ApxIII (Frey et al. 1994; Jansen et al.

1995). Additional detailed morphologic and biochemical characteristics may be found in the original reports (Shope 1964; Nicolet 1968; Kilian et al. 1978). Biotype I strains should differentiate from other actinobacilli normally present in the upper respiratory tract of swine (Kielstein et al. 2001; Gottschalk et al. 2003). Biotype II strains grow easily on blood agar plates without the presence of *Staphylococcus aureus*, and colonies might be similar to those of *Actinobacillus suis*. It is important for diagnostic laboratories to carry out a complete biochemical identification in order to differentiate both species.

A. pleuropneumoniae biotype I has been divided into 13 serotypes and biotype II into 2 serotypes, for a total of 15 serotypes. Serotypes 1–5 were recognized by Kilian et al. (1978), with serotype 5 subdivided into subtypes 5a and 5b (Nielsen 1986a); however, this subdivision has neither epidemiological nor pathological significance, and most laboratories do not perform the subtyping. Subsequently, serotypes 6, 7 (Rosendal and Boyd 1982), 8 (Nielsen and O'Connor 1984), 9 (Nielsen 1985b), 10 (Nielsen 1985c), 11 (Kamp et al. 1987), and 12 (Nielsen 1986b) have been proposed. Serotype 10 was erroneously proposed by Kamp et al. (1987) and was later referred to as serotype 12 (Nielsen 1986b). Nielsen et al. (1997) proposed an integration of the serotyping schemes for biotypes 1 and 2, with two new serotypes, serotypes 13 and 14, belonging to biotype II being added. More recently, Blackall et al. (2002) reported that a new NAD-dependent biotype I serotype (serotype 15) is the predominant serotype in Australia. The association of serotypes and biotypes are not necessarily exclusive, since biotype II strains belonging to serotypes 2, 4, 7, and 9 (normally found among biotype I strains) have been reported (Beck et al. 1994). Two biotype I strains belonging to serotype 13 (a "biotype II serotype") have recently been isolated in Canada and the United States (M. Gottschalk, unpublished observations).

The serologic specificity is given by the capsular polysaccharides (CPS) and the cell wall lipopolysaccharides (LPS). However, some serotypes show structural similarities or have identical LPS O chains, thus explaining the cross-reactions observed between serotypes 1, 9, and 11; serotypes 3, 6, and 8; and serotypes 4 and 7 (Perry et al. 1990; Dubreuil et al. 2000).

Combinations of a given serotype at the capsule and a different serotype at the LPS level have been reported. For example, strains of CPS/LPS of serotype 1/7 and 2/7 have been reported in North America and Europe, respectively (Gottschalk et al. 2000; Nielsen et al. 1996). These strains could complicate the diagnosis, due to the presence of atypical cross-reactions. It has been suggested that serotypes of *A. pleuropneumoniae* would be more rigorously defined by specifying both capsular (K) and LPS (O) antigens (Perry et al. 1990), but this nomenclature has not been widely adopted (Dubreuil et al. 2000).

EPIDEMIOLOGY

Pleuropneumonia of the pig is widely distributed. It has become more important as pig production has become more intensive. Outbreaks have been reported from practically all European countries and from different parts of the United States and Canada, Mexico, South America, Japan, Korea, Taiwan, and Australia. Although some serotypes are prevalent in certain countries (e.g., serotype 2 in Switzerland, Denmark, France and Sweden and serotypes 1 and 5 in the United States, Canada and Mexico), several serotypes often occur in the same country (Dubreuil et al. 2000). Some serotypes (e.g., serotype 3), considered to be of low virulence and of no epidemiologic importance in certain countries, may be epidemic in others (Desrosiers et al. 1984; Brandreth and Smith 1985; Gottschalk et al. 2003). A series of papers provided information on the distribution of serotypes within countries (e.g., Austria, where serotypes 4, 6, and 10 are most common; see Hofer et al. 1996) or within regions of countries (e.g., Catalonia, Spain, where 11 serotypes, principally 1, 2, 4, 7, 9, and 11, have been identified; see Clota et al. 1996; and Quebec, Canada, where serotypes 1, 5, and 7 are predominant; see Mittal et al. 1992). McDowell and Ball (1994) showed that serotypes 1 and 4 were absent from the British Isles, which may reflect the restrictions on imports of live pigs to the U.K. from neighboring countries of the European Union where these serotypes exist. Serotype 4, considered absent from North America in the past, has been isolated from carrier animals in Canada (Lebrun et al. 1999). Different serotypes may also occur within farms. In fact, most conventional herds are infected with more than one serotype of *A. pleuropneumoniae* (Gottschalk et al. 2003). The international relationship of the different serotypes is of special interest, because it points to a transmission through international exchange of animals. For example, serotype 2 is a highly virulent serotype in European countries, but it is infrequently isolated from clinical cases in North America. Recent data showed that European strains produce two toxins, whereas North American strains produce only one (see pathogenesis), which may explain the differences in virulence (M. Kobisch, M. Jacques, and M. Gottschalk, unpublished observations). Biotype II strains are more commonly isolated in Europe than in the United States, where only one report is available (Frank et al. 1992). More recently, an untypable strain of a biotype II *A. pleuropneumoniae* has been reported in the U.S. as an important cause of disease in a commercial herd (Gottschalk et al. 2003). Biotype II strains, considered as low virulence for a long time, seem to be able to cause cases of fatal pleuropneumonia (Gambade and Morvan 2001; Maldonado et al. 2004).

Strains belonging to the same serotype have been genotypically compared. Moeller et al. (1992) analyzed the multilocus enzyme electrophoresis (MEE) types of organisms in one restricted area and found that the electrophoretic type (ET) was unrelated to the severity of the disease. In addition, they concluded that serotype 5 strains possessed a clonal structure. This was confirmed by Chatellier et al. (1999), who used random amplified polymorphic DNA analysis or RAPD to compare Canadian field strains isolated from lungs of diseased animals and from nasal cavities or tonsils of clinically healthy pigs, indicating that these strains have the same potential for virulence. Fussing (1998) reported that serotype 2 field strains were clonally related, using ribotyping, sequence analysis of ribosomal intergenic regions, and pulsed-field gel electrophoresis. On the other hand, Chatellier et al. (1999) showed a relatively high heterogeneity among strains of *A. pleuropneumoniae* serotype 1, especially those recovered from healthy animals, using the RAPD technique.

The economic importance of the disease is principally due to the mortality, production and medical costs in acute outbreaks. In chronically infected herds, results from studies investigating the effect of pneumonia on the average daily gain have been controversial. Hunneman (1986) found that the rate of daily weight gain was not affected, although a study by Hartley et al. (1988) showed that pleurisy at slaughter was associated with an increase of 1 day to slaughter, and clinical disease with an increase of 8 days to slaughter. More recently, Andreasen et al. (2001) explained the lack of significant reduction in the average daily weight gain in *A. pleuropneumoniae* and *Mycoplasma hyopneumoniae* chronically infected herds by either the fact that most pigs included in the study were subclinically infected or because a temporary negative influence of the infection is hidden due to an increased growth in the period following infection.

A. pleuropneumoniae is a parasite of the respiratory tract with high host specificity for pigs. In peracute and acute infections, it can be found not only in pneumonic lesions but also in large numbers in nasal discharges. The incubation period can be quite variable. Experimental infections show that an exposure to large numbers of organisms leads to death within a few hours to a few days. Either exposure to low levels of infection or survival following acute infections may result in subclinical disease, and these animals become carriers. In these cases, the infectious agent is located mainly in necrotic lung lesions and/or in the tonsils, less frequently in the nasal cavity (Kume et al. 1984). Animals that have recovered from acute episodes may remain carriers for several months (Desrosiers 2004).

The main route of spread is by direct contact from pig to pig or by droplets within short distances. In acute outbreaks the infection may not occur in every pen, suggesting the possible role of aerosols and air movement in the transmission of the disease over longer distances within buildings or the indirect transmission of con-

taminated exudates from acutely infected pigs by farm personnel. Transmission between herds occurs through the introduction of carrier animals to naive populations. Different studies showed that *A. pleuropneumoniae* may be transmitted by aerosol over short distances (see Desrosiers 2004), and Kristensen et al. (2004) reported that airborne transmission between closely located pig units is possible but rare. Moving and mixing pigs increases the risk of pleuropneumonia. Introduction of the disease by artificial insemination or embryo transfer is improbable, since the genital tract is not a common site of infection, and antimicrobials in the diluent would prevent survival of the contaminating organism. Transmission by small rodents or birds is doubtful and it is not considered as significant. Survival of the organism in the environment is considered to be of short duration. However, when protected with mucus or other organic matter, it can survive for several days (even weeks) and it can survive in clean water for periods of up to 30 days at 4°C.

Infected sows will transmit the infection to the offspring. It has been suggested that only few piglets get infected by *A. pleuropneumoniae* from their respective sow during the nursing period (when the level of maternal antibodies is usually high), and that these infected pigs spread the bacteria to other pigs after weaning, the age period that corresponds to the age at which the proportion of pigs with detectable levels of colostral antibodies against *A. pleuropneumoniae* is declining (Vigre et al. 2002). These two events (colonization and level of colostral antibodies) are most probably associated. The persistence of colostral antibody in piglets may range from 2 weeks to 2 months postpartum, mainly depending on the initial level of acquired colostral antibodies, and to the serological technique used to measure them (Vigre et al. 2003; M. Gottschalk, unpublished observations).

In the acute phase of the disease, morbidity is generally high. Mortality depends on the virulence of the strain and on the particular environment. Factors such as crowding and adverse climatic conditions, such as rapid changes in temperature and high relative humidity, coupled with insufficient ventilation encourage the development and spread of the disease and, consequently, also affect morbidity and mortality. It is, therefore, not surprising that the highest incidence of outbreaks is observed in growing and finishing pigs, mainly in seasons with adverse weather conditions. As a rule, large herds that mix pigs frequently are more at risk than small herds or herds with separate units. Data from the field seem to indicate that both morbidity and mortality may be exacerbated by the presence of diseases such as Aujeszky's disease and porcine reproductive and respiratory syndrome (PRRS), although experimental studies showed that combined infection with *A. pleuropneumoniae* and PRRS virus may not necessarily result in more severe disease (Pol et al. 1997).

VIRULENCE FACTORS AND PATHOGENESIS OF THE INFECTION

The pathogenesis of swine pleuropneumonia has been studied extensively, both in terms of the development of the lesions and in terms of the relationship of the organism to the tissues at a more molecular level. For a recent complete review, please refer to Bosse et al. (2002). Infection is usually by aerosol or by contact, and experimental studies have shown that the organism can colonize the tonsil and adhere to the alveolar epithelium. In fact, colonization is usually the first step of the infectious process. Chiers et al. (1999) demonstrated that after experimental infection with *A. pleuropneumoniae*, bacteria were mainly associated with the stratified squamous epithelium and detached epithelial cells. Vacuolization and desquamation of the epithelium was observed and many transmigrating neutrophils were present. At later times after inoculation, bacteria were found closely associated with the crypt-walls and with detached cells present in the crypts. A strong neutrophil migration was observed mainly in the deeper parts of the crypts. It was concluded that attachment of *A. pleuropneumoniae* to tonsillar epithelial cells probably constitutes a first step in establishing bacteria at this body site. It seems that this pathogen does not bind well to the cilia or epithelium of the trachea or bronchi (Bosse et al. 2002). However, it seems to significantly adhere to cells of the lower respiratory tract (Bosse et al. 2002; van Overbeke et al. 2002). The presence of fimbriae and fimbrial subunits has been well confirmed (Zhang et al. 2000). It seems that their expression is regulated by growth conditions, which may explain their presence after growth in some media but not in others (Bosse et al. 2002). However, their role in the colonization or any other aspect of the pathogenesis of the infection remains to be elucidated.

Cell adhesion seems to be mediated either by proteins or polysaccharides (van Overbeke et al. 2002). It has been clearly demonstrated that the LPS play an important role in adherence of *A. pleuropneumoniae* to swine cells (Paradis et al. 1999). Recently, glycosphingolipids (gangliotriaosylceramide or GgO$_3$ and gangliotetraosylceramide or GgO$_4$) present in respiratory epithelial cells have been identified as possible receptors for *A. pleuropneumoniae* (Abul-Milh et al. 1999). Originally, high-molecular-mass polysaccharide from the LPS was thought to be involved as adhesin. However, GgO$_3$ and GgO$_4$ were shown to interact with the core oligosaccharide rather than the long chain O polysaccharide (Abul-Milh et al. 1999). Evidence from other pathogen-host cell interactons suggests that adherence to host cells is a complex and multifactorial process (Bosse and Matyunas 1999).

Once in the respiratory tract environment, certain bacterial nutrients are scarce. One of the most important is iron. Mechanisms for overcoming iron-restriction are complex. *A. pleuropneumoniae* expresses a number of factors that are involved in the acquisition and uptake of iron (for a recent review, see Jacques 2004). Among other mechanisms, *A. pleuropneumoniae* is capable of utilizing porcine transferrin and haem compounds including free haem, haemin, haematin, and haemoglobin (Bosse and Matyunas 1999). It also possesses a siderophore (Jacques 2004).

After being able to adhere, resist the clearing function of the normal mucociliary system, and survive in the lower respiratory tract, *A. pleuropneumoniae* may be eliminated by phagocytic cells. Both macrophages and neutrophils phagocytose *A. pleuropneumoniae* in the presence of convalescent pig serum (Cruijsen et al. 1992; Bosse and Matyunas 1999). Production of immunoglobulin proteases, which might interfere with opsonophagocytosis is controversial (Bosse and Matyunas 1999; Negrete-Abascal et al. 1994). Following phagocytosis, *A. pleuropneumoniae* can survive for a certain period of time inside macrophages, but not neutrophils. Different factors produced by this microorganism may contribute to its ability to survive within some phagocytic cells (Bosse and Matyunas 1999). In addition, it appears to be resistant to the action of complement, mainly due to the capsular polysaccharide (CPS) (in the case of serotype 5) and the LPS (in the case of serotype 1) (Ward and Inzana 1994; Rioux et al. 1999, 2000). The presence of the capsule as a protective factor for *A. pleuropneumoniae* serotypes 1 and 5 has been demonstrated by the characterization of nonvirulent isogenic mutants lacking this factor (Bosse and Matyunas 1999; Rioux et al. 2000).

The most important factors involved in impairment of phagocytic function of both macrophages and neutrophils are the RTX-toxins, ApxI, ApxII, and ApxIII, produced by different serotypes of *A. pleuropneumoniae* (Haesebrouck et al. 1997; Frey 2003). In general, strains of serotypes 1, 5, 9, and 11 produce ApxI and ApxII; strains of serotypes 2, 3, 4, 6, 8, and 15 produce ApxII and ApxIII; strains of serotypes 7, 12, and 13 produce only ApxII, and strains of serotypes 10 and 14 produce only ApxI (Gottschalk et al. 2003). It seems that strains of serotype 3 secrete low levels of ApxII. The possible role of the more recently described toxin (ApxIV, produced only in vivo) on macrophages and neutrophils remains to be elucidated (Frey 2003). ApxI and ApxIII are highly toxic for leukocytes, whereas ApxII is moderately toxic for these cells. In fact, most of the pathological consequences of porcine pleuropneumonia can be attributed to these toxins which exert cytotoxic effects on different type of cells (Haesebrouck et al. 1997; Frey et al. 1993; Frey 2003). The production of two toxins by virulent serotypes seems to be important. For example, it has recently been demonstrated that both ApxI and ApxII toxins are necessary for full virulence in serotype 1 strains (Boekema et al. 2004). In addition, highly virulent serotype 2 strains from Europe produce two toxins as expected, but low virulent North American strains produce only ApxII (M. Gottschalk, M. Jacques, and M. Kobisch, unpublished observations). LPS is also considered a cause of toxic effects, due probably to an exacerbation of the inflammatory response (Fenwick 1990). Although several reports indicate an important release of pro-inflammatory mediators (Baarsch et al. 1995), a recent study indicates that pneumonia caused by *A. pleuropneumoniae* infection is not due to the release of systemic inflammatory cytokines (Myers et al. 2004). Other factors include secreted proteases and flagella, but their role in the pathogenesis of the infection remains to be elucidated (Negrete-Abascal et al. 1994, 2000; Negrete-Abascal 2003).

Differences in the virulence between the serotypes or even within the same serotype have often been observed. It is suggested that such differences are due to capsular structure (Jacques et al. 1988), LPS composition (Jensen and Bertram 1986), or type of hemolysin (Frey 2003). In general, strains of serotypes 2, 9, and 11 (in Europe) and 1 and 5 (North America) are found to be more virulent than those of other serotypes. Although it has been previously reported that serotype 10 may be highly virulent (Komal and Mittal 1990), very few clinical cases are reported worldwide. Pigs experimentally infected with this serotype generally present a low level of clinical signs and mortality, but relatively high level of chronic pleuropneumonia and chronic pleuritis (Sorensen 1997; M. Gottschalk, unpublished observations). Interestingly, animals may be carriers of fully virulent strains of serotype 1 or 5 in a herd without the presence of clinical signs. Finally, strains of serotype 1, with no atypical CPS, LPS, or toxin profile have also been shown to be of low virulence after experimental infections (Gottschalk et al. 2003). It is important to note that results obtained after experimental infection may depend on the route of inoculation (intranasal, intratracheal, aerosol, etc.), the dose used, and the immune status of the animals. Conventional animals that might have been in contact with low virulent serotypes of *A. pleuropneumoniae* or with *A. suis* may be more resistant to the infection with a specific strain than specific pathogen-free animals that are negative to all serotypes of *A. pleuropneumoniae* (M. Gottschalk, unpublished observations). Serotypes considered as low pathogenic (such as serotype 3 and 12) can sometimes induce clinical problems, especially in the presence of other pathogens. Concomitant infections with other pathogens of the respiratory tract that aid the development of pleuropneumonia have been described by Caruso and Ross (1990).

Lung lesions resulting from the toxic changes may be seen as early as 3 hours after experimental infection and become progressively more obvious. The alveolar wall becomes edematous and capillary congestion develops. The lymphatics become dilated with edema fluid, fibrin, and inflammatory cells. Platelet aggregation and neutrophil accumulation may also be seen in the damaged alveolar wall, and both arteriolar thrombosis and wall necrosis may develop to produce infarction. Microcolonies of the organism may be seen in infected alveoli, and bacteremia may occur. The edges of the lesions become filled with dead and damaged macrophages or debris and can easily be demarcated from the surrounding lung by 4 days post infection. Purulent exudate containing organisms is present in the bronchi. As the lesions age, their centers become necrotic and healing occurs by fibrosis.

Experimental or natural infections stimulate an immune response, and circulating antibodies can be detected approximately 10–14 days post infection. These antibodies reach a maximum level within 4–6 weeks post infection and may persist for many months (Desrosiers 2004). However, more studies are needed to confirm this fact. Immune sows confer passive immunity on their offspring. Such colostral antibodies may persist for about 5–12 weeks (Vigre et al. 2003), but this may depend on the sensitivity of the test used to detect the antibodies and on the initial level of acquired colostral antibodies. Protection may last for only as little as 3 weeks in some cases (Nielsen 1975), but these data may be due to the use of a very insensitive test such as the complement fixation test. The antibodies are directed against a wide range of bacterial structures and products, including capsule, LPS antigens, toxins (which can be neutralized), outer-membrane proteins, superoxide dismutase, and iron-binding proteins. Both local IgA antibodies and serum IgG antibodies are produced.

CLINICAL SIGNS

Clinical signs vary with the age of the animals, their state of immunity, the environmental conditions, and the degree of exposure to the infectious agent. The clinical course can be peracute, acute, or chronic (Nicolet et al. 1969; Shope 1964; Shope et al. 1964).

In the peracute form, one or more weaned pigs in the same or different pens suddenly becomes very ill with fever to 106.7°F (41.5°C), apathy, and anorexia. There is a short period of slight diarrhea and vomiting. The affected animals lie on the floor without distinct respiratory signs, the pulse rate increases very early, and cardiac and circulatory failure develop. The skin on the nose, ears, legs, and later the whole body becomes cyanotic. In the terminal phase, there is a severe dyspnea with mouth breathing, animals remain in a sitting posture, and rectal temperatures decrease markedly. Shortly before death, there is usually a copious, foamy, blood-tinged discharge through the mouth and nostrils. Death occurs within 24–36 hours of the development of clinical signs. Occasionally an animal may die suddenly without premonitory clinical signs or be found dead in a pen; experimental studies have shown that the course of the disease may be as little as 3 hours from infection to death. In neonatal pigs the disease occurs as a septicemia with fatal results.

In the acute form, many pigs in the same or different pens are affected. Body temperature rises to 105–106°F (40.5–41°C), the skin may be reddened, and the animals are depressed, are reluctant to rise, refuse food, and are reluctant to drink (Pijpers et al. 1990). Severe respiratory symptoms with dyspnea, cough, and sometimes mouth breathing are evident. Cardiac and circulatory failure are usually present, with congestion of the extremities. There is a marked loss of condition, which is apparent within 24 hours of the onset of the disease. The course of the disease differs from animal to animal, depending on the extent of the lung lesions and the time of initiation of therapy. All stages of disease, from intermediate to fatal, subacute, or chronic, may develop within an affected group.

The chronic form develops after the disappearance of acute signs. There is little or no fever, and a spontaneous or intermittent cough of varying intensity develops. Appetite may be reduced, and this may contribute to the decreased rate of gain in body weight. Affected animals can be identified by their intolerance of exercise. When moved, they lag behind the group and struggle only feebly when restrained. In chronically infected herds there are often many subclinically diseased animals. The clinical signs may be exacerbated by other respiratory infections (mycoplasmal, bacterial, or viral). Although a certain synergy between PRRSV and *A. pleuropneumoniae* is often suspected in the field, experimental studies have not shown that previous PRRSV infection of SPF pigs enhanced the severity of a A. pleuropneumoniae infection (Pol et al. 1997). In primary outbreaks abortions may be observed (Wilson and Kierstead 1976), especially in SPF herds. Middle-ear disease has also been associated with *A. pleuropneumoniae* infection (Duff et al. 1996).

It is important to add that some herds are in fact infected by *A. pleuropneumoniae* without the presence of visible clinical signs and with absence of significant lesions at slaughter. These are considered as subclinically infected herds.

LESIONS

The gross pathological lesions are located mainly in the respiratory tract (Nicolet and Köning 1966). The pneumonia is mostly bilateral, with involvement of the cardiac and apical lobes, as well as at least part of the diaphragmatic lobes, where pneumonic lesions are often focal and well demarcated (Figure 33.1). In rapidly fatal cases the trachea and bronchi are filled with a foamy, blood-tinged, mucous exudate and few gross changes may be obvious. In slightly later peracute cases, the pneumonic areas appear dark and solid with little or no fibrinous pleurisy; and the cut surface is friable. Fibrinous pleurisy is very obvious in animals that die in

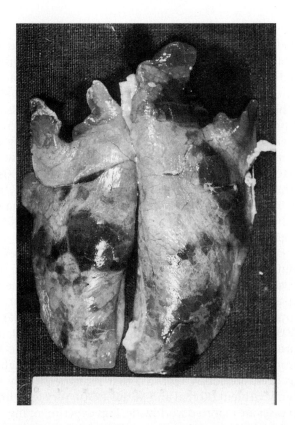

33.1. *Gross lesions of a peracute case of pleuropneumonia showing a well-circumscribed pneumonic area in different lobes with fibrinous pleurisy. (Courtesy Professor H. König, Institute of Animal Pathology, University of Berne.)*

the acute stage of the disease, at least 24 hours after infection, and the thoracic cavity contains a blood-tinged fluid. As the lesions age, the fibrinous pleurisy over the affected areas of lung becomes fibrous and may adhere so strongly to the parietal pleura that lung parenchyma may remain attached to the parietal pleura when the lungs are removed at postmortem examination. The uniform dark red or black of the early lung lesion becomes lighter in color and remains firm only in the worst-affected areas. The lesions shrink in size as resolution progresses, until in more chronic cases nodules of different sizes remain, mostly in the diaphragmatic lobes. These abscess-like nodules are delimited by a thick capsule of connective tissue (Figure 33.2) and may be associated with areas of adhesive fibrous pleurisy. In many cases the lung lesion resolves, and only a residual focus of adhesive fibrous pleurisy remains. A high prevalence of chronic pleuritis at slaughter is very suggestive of pleuropneumonia.

In the early stages of the disease, the histopathologic changes are characterized by necrosis, hemorrhage, neutrophil infiltration, macrophage and platelet activation, vascular thrombosis, widespread edema, and fibrinous exudate (Bertram 1985, 1986, 1990; Liggett and Harrison 1987). Following the acute response, macrophage infiltration, marked fibrosis around areas of

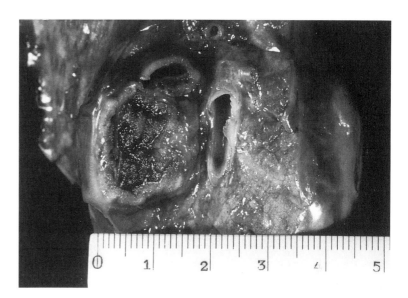

33.2. *Chronic pleuropneumonia. Cross section of a well-capsulated nodule in the diaphragmatic lobe. (Courtesy Professor H. König, Institute of Animal Pathology, University of Berne.)*

necrosis, and fibrous pleuritis are characteristic (Häni et al. 1973).

DIAGNOSIS

Pleuropneumonia may be suspected clinically in acute outbreaks. In such cases the presence of characteristic lung lesions with pleurisy at postmortem examination enhances suspicion, which is enforced by the histological appearance of the lesions. The presence of an acute exudative pneumonia with areas of necrosis surrounded by palisades and whorls of neutrophil debris provides further evidence for pleuropneumonia. In chronic infections the necropsy findings of firm, well-demarcated abscesses associated with pleurisy and pericarditis are very suggestive. In view of the importance of this disease to herd health control programs and the potential for economic loss, bacteriologic confirmation of the diagnosis should be carried out. Hog cholera, erysipelas, and streptococcal infections must be considered in the possible differential diagnosis of peracute and acute cases. Lung lesions caused by other porcine actinobacilli may be indistinguishable from those of pleuropneumonia, and acute pasteurellosis may sometimes resemble pleuropneumonia.

It is relatively easy to demonstrate the etiologic agent in pneumonic lesions from freshly dead animals. Gram-stained smears of lung lesions contain numerous gram-negative coccobacilli. Primary isolation of *A. pleuropneumoniae* from tissues and secretions may be carried out on 5% sheep blood agar with a cross-streak of *Staphylococcus epidermidis* or *S. aureus*. After aerobic incubation overnight, small colonies appear in the neighborhood of the streak (NAD requirement) surrounded by a clear zone of complete hemolysis. This allows a rapid presumptive bacteriologic diagnosis. For some serotypes (such as serotypes 7 and 12), the zone of hemolysis is usually less intense. Altered blood agars ("chocolate agar") allow the

growth of the organism, but it is less distinctive on these media. Presumptive biochemical identification can be carried out by demonstrating the CAMP phenomenon and urease activity. Usually, serotyping will confirm the identity of *A. pleuropneumoniae*. When biochemically atypical isolates are recovered (for example, urease negative isolates) or when the isolates are untypable, it is recommended to carry out a PCR test (see below). Biotype II isolates (NAD-independent) have been recovered more frequently in the last years (Gambade and Morvan 2001; Gottschalk et al. 2003; Maldonado et al. 2004). These isolates might be misidentified as *A. suis*; in these cases, a complete biochemical identification must be done before sending the isolate for serotyping. In fact, *A. suis* isolates present strong cross-reactions with sera against serotypes 3, 6, and 8 of *A. pleuropneumoniae* (unpublished observations). It is strongly recommended to perform a PCR test to confirm the identity of biotype II isolates of *A. pleuropneumoniae*.

The serotyping of isolates is recommended for rapid confirmation of the bacteriologic diagnosis of typical *A. pleuropneumoniae* isolates and is essential when vaccination policy is being considered. It demonstrates the local distribution of serotypes and allows the epidemiologic situation to be evaluated and the performance of specific serologic tests to be monitored. Serotyping can be routinely achieved by slide agglutination from a subculture on a medium enriched with serum (Mittal et al. 1987), unless nonspecific cross-reactions are usually observed (unpublished observations). The coagglutination test (Mittal et al. 1987) is routinely used, but many isolates react with different sera (due to common epitopes) and a confirmatory test, such as agar gel diffusion and indirect hemagglutination (Mittal et al. 1987) is needed. A critical evaluation of the earlier serotyping methods is given by Lida et al. (1990). The use of monoclonal antibodies for serotyping has also been reported (Rodriguez-Barbosa et al. 1995; Lacouture et al. 1997; Lebrun et al.

1999). Finally, toxin typing using a well-described PCR (Frey et al. 1995) could be done in order to anticipate the virulence of the isolated strain.

Bacteriological diagnosis of chronic disease is more complex. It is difficult to culture *A. pleuropneumoniae* from chronic lesions in lungs. Tests for direct detection of *A. pleuropneumoniae* in lung tissues are immunofluorescence, ring precipitation, coagglutination, latex agglutination, ELISA, and counter-immunoelectrophoresis (Dubreuil et al. 2000). Their presence can be confirmed as *A. pleuropneumoniae* either by using a fluorescent or immunoperoxidase antibody test (Gutierrez et al. 1993), or by detection of serotype-specific antigens in lung extracts with a coagglutination test (Mittal et al. 1983). Nucleic acid from bacteria may be detected by a number of methods, including labeled DNA probes in tissue and polymerase chain reaction (PCR). Direct confirmation by PCR of the presence of *A. pleuropneumoniae* in lung tissue is not yet routine.

The detection of *A. pleuropneumoniae* from clinically healthy carrier animals (in subclinically infected herds) is even more complex. Bacteria are usually localized in tonsils and, less frequently, in the nasal cavities. Selective media have been described (Sidibe et al. 1993; Jacobsen and Nielsen 1995), although their sensitivity is very low. In fact, the swine nasal cavities and tonsils are heavily colonized with several NAD-dependent bacterial species, many of them being members of the commensal flora, such as *Actinobacillus minor, Actinobacillus porcinus,* and *Actinobacillus indolicus* (Moeller et al. 1996; Kielstein et al. 2001). Their identity as well as their role as pathogens is controversial (Kielstein et al. 2001; Gottschalk et al. 2003). Although most of these bacterial species probably do not play any significant role as swine pathogens, they may interfere with the culture and identification of *A. pleuropneumoniae*. A bacterial species which is biochemically and antigenically very similar to *A. pleuropneumoniae* has recently been described (Gottschalk et al. 2003). To overcome the presence of a highly contaminating flora, an immunomagnetic separation technique for the selective isolation of a given serotype of *A. pleuropneumoniae* from tonsils has been developed (Gagné et al. 1998). The sensitivity of this technique is a thousandfold higher than direct culture. Molecular techniques can also be used for the detection of *A. pleuropneumoniae* from tonsils. In fact, within the last years, several PCR techniques that amplify well-defined sequences of the *A. pleuropneumoniae* genome have been described as valuable tools for the rapid and affordable detection of the pathogen, and a ready-to-use PCR kit has even been commercialized. Recently, Fittipaldi et al. (2003) have evaluated eight PCR tests for their abilities to detect *A. pleuropneumoniae* from swine tonsils. At first they were compared regarding their specificities by using *A. pleuropneumoniae* and related bacterial species and their analytical sensitivities by using tonsils experimentally infected in vitro. PCRs were carried out both directly with tonsil homogenates (direct PCR) and after culture of the sample (post-culture PCR). Most tests demonstrated good specificities; however, some tests gave false-positive results with some non–*A. pleuropneumoniae* species. High degrees of variation in the analytical sensitivities among the tests were observed for the direct PCRs (10^9 to 10^2 CFU/g of tonsil), whereas those of most of the post-culture PCRs were similar (10^2 CFU/g of tonsil) (Fittipaldi et al. 2003). When some of these techniques were validated in the field, it was shown that the PCR was more sensitive than the standard isolation method with whole tonsils from three infected herds. Post-culture PCR offered the highest degree of sensitivity and the detection rate was higher with whole tonsils than with tonsil biopsy specimens. Most of these tests are specific for the species *A. pleuropneumoniae* and they cannot differentiate among serotypes; since most conventional herds are infected with several low pathogenic serotypes, a positive result is difficult to interpret. To overcome this problem, serotype-specific PCR tests have more recently been described (Jessing et al. 2003; Angen and Jessing 2004; Hussy et al. 2004).

Serological testing has been used widely for the control of swine pleuropneumonia, to replace the fastidious task of detecting individual carrier animals. In fact, serology is the most powerful tool to diagnose subclinical infections due to *A. pleuropneumoniae*. Some countries, such as Canada and Denmark, use serology for the epidemiological surveillance of different herds on a routine basis. Different assays directed to the detection of antibodies against either the toxins or somatic and/or capsular antigens have been developed (for more details, see Dubreuil et al. 2000). Most tests detecting antibodies against ApxI, ApxII, and ApxIII toxins have low specificity, since other microorganisms such as *A. suis* can also produce similar toxins (Dubreuil et al. 2000; Nielsen et al. 2000). An ELISA test detecting antibodies against the ApxIV toxin has recently been reported (Dreyfus et al. 2004). This test would be highly specific for *A. pleuropneumoniae*, but it cannot differentiate among serotypes. Indeed, most conventional herds would probably present high levels of antibodies and its use as a diagnostic tool would be questionable. Although some ELISA tests based on CPS have been reported, some cross-reactions (probably due to antigen contamination during the purification process) were observed (Dubreuil et al. 2000). The tests most commonly used are ELISA tests using O-chain LPS as antigens (Gottschalk et al. 1994; Dubreuil et al. 2000; Klausen et al. 2002; Grondahl-Hansen et al. 2003). These ELISA tests can identify groups of serotypes as follows: 1, 9, and 11; 2; 3, 6, and 8; 4 and 7; 10; and 12. LPS antigens are also used in blocking ELISA tests using polyclonal antibodies (Andresen et al. 2002). Serological tests such as the complement fixation test and the 2-mercaptoethanol test are no longer used due to problems of sensitivity and specificity, respectively (Dubreuil et al. 2000).

TREATMENT

In general, *A. pleuropneumoniae* is susceptible in vitro to penicillin, ampicillin, cephalosporin, chloramphenicol, colistin, sulfonamide, cotrimoxazole (trimethoprim + sulfamethoxazole), and gentamicin, to which it has low minimum inhibitory concentrations (MIC). High MIC values are found for streptomycin, kanamycin, spectinomycin, spiramycin, and lincomycin (Gilbride and Rosendal 1984; Nadeau et al. 1988; Aarestrup and Jensen 1999; Yoshimura et al. 2002). Although antibiotics belonging to the betalactam family (penicillin, ampicillin, amoxycillin) normally show good activity against *A. pleuropneumoniae*, sporadic data from the U.S. and other countries reported a relatively high number of resistant isolates (Nadeau et al. 1988). Resistance seems to be frequent especially in serotypes 1, 3, 5, and 7 (Gilbride and Rosendal 1984; Vaillancourt et al. 1988). The antimicrobial of first choice should be the one with the lowest MIC and with the most satisfactory pharmacokinetic properties. Consequently, the betalactams (principally penicillin and cephalosporin), chloramphenicol, and cotrimoxazole are considered to be most active. Quinolone derivatives (enrofloxacin) (Kobisch et al. 1990) or the semisynthetic cephalosporin ceftiofur sodium (Stephano et al. 1990) have been shown to be particularly effective after experimental challenge. Satisfactory results in the field have been reported with tiamulin (Anderson and Williams 1990) and a combination of lincomycin and spectinomycin (Hsu 1990). Tilmicosin has also been reported as effective (Paradis et al. 2004). The determination of an antibiogram is recommended where problems are being experienced with treatment.

Antibiotic therapy is effective in clinically affected animals only in the initial phase of the disease, when it can reduce mortality. The nature of the lesions means that delay in treatment can result in a degree of infarction and chronic damage which will leave the animal as a respiratory cripple even if it recovers. Antibiotics should be given parenterally (subcutaneously or intramuscularly) and in high dosage, because affected animals may not eat or drink (Pijpers et al. 1990). To ensure effective and durable blood concentrations, repeated injections may be required, depending on the pharmacokinetic properties of the antibiotic used. The success of therapy depends mainly on early detection of clinical signs and on rapid therapeutic intervention. Water treatment may be used to treat members of the affected group that are still able to drink. Feed medicated with any of the above antimicrobials may be used successfully if all pigs have a normal food and water intake. Feed and water medication can be used for the strategic treatment of infected groups on entry to an airspace. A combination of parenteral and peroral medication in a recent outbreak often yields the best results. In spite of apparent clinical success, it must be remembered that antibiotic therapy does not eliminate infection in a herd. Chronic infections in lung abscesses or on the tonsils of carriers persist to form an important source of infection for other animals. Severely affected animals may not recover even after treatment and nursing and should be killed.

PREVENTION

Prevention and control of pleuropneumonia may be accomplished in a number of different ways. Farms free from the disease and infection should maintain a policy of isolation coupled with the use of semen or embryos to introduce new genes. As mentioned, there are good serological tools to monitor herds from where replacement animals are introduced. There are many SPF herds that are free of all serotypes of *A. pleuropneumoniae*. It may be appropriate to hold replacements in quarantine prior to introduction to the herd.

After the infection has been established on a farm, it is difficult to eliminate the infectious agent, although the herd may become clinically normal. Control programs must take account of the epidemiologic features of pleuropneumonia. The first priority must be to control economic loss (mortality, clinical and subclinical disease) and then to consider the control or elimination of infection. Mortality can be controlled by the treatment of cases and of infected groups using the methods and antimicrobials outlined above. Disease may be treated at an early stage by treating groups of animals into clean airspaces and then maintaining them as a group in isolation until slaughter. Where this may not be possible, control of environmental factors such as temperature and ventilation and use of solid partitions between pens may minimize the development and severity of disease. Continuous medication or pulse dosing may be practiced, but neither should be used for long, and the antimicrobial sensitivity of the organism should be monitored continuously. Strategic medication should be targeted at periods of risk, which can be identified by routine postmortem examinations, clinical examinations, and herd antibody profiles. The generalized methods used to control respiratory disease, such as the all-in/all-out system in fattening units, segregated early weaning, and large airspaces with separation, will all considerably reduce the risk of infection. Animals should be brought in only from herds free from infection to avoid introducing new serotypes or new antimicrobial resistances. In chronically infected herds, purchased seronegative animals should be vaccinated before introduction to the herd.

A wide range of vaccines has been developed for this disease. They fall into two main groups: the killed organisms and the subunit vaccines. Vaccination with killed organisms is serotype specific (Nielsen 1984), with possible cross-immunity with cross-reacting serotypes (Nielsen 1984, 1985a). The protection afforded has been extended by including all the serotypes present in an area (e.g., 3, 6, and 8 in the United Kingdom). The type of adjuvant used may affect efficacy, and care may also be necessary before using certain adjuvants in pigs intended for human consumption, because some vaccines can produce undesirable granulomatous lesions at the site of injection (Straw et al. 1985). Recently, a new generation subunit vaccine, composed of the three major RTX exotoxins (ApxI, ApxII, and ApxIII) and a 42 kDa outer membrane protein of *A. pleuropneumoniae*, has been developed and shown to give high protection against all 12 major serotypes (serotypes 1–12) under experimental conditions as well as in field trials (van den Bosch and Frey 2003). Keeping in mind the very complex pathogenesis of porcine pleuropneumonia, inclusion of other bacterial virulence factors in vaccines might also be of value (Haesebrouck et al. 2004). A vaccine containing both Apx toxins and transferrin binding proteins induced better protection against severe challenge than a vaccine solely based on Apx toxins (van Overbeke et al. 2001). A wide range of antigens administered either by parenteral, aerosol, or oral routes have been found to be experimentally protective, but none of them have been used in the field. A live vaccine, based on the use of a nonencapsulated mutant (Inzana et al. 1993), has been commercialized in the United States in the last years.

Vaccines may provide high levels of protection against morbidity in experiments, reduce mortality, reduce the number of treatments required, increase daily liveweight gain, and improve feed conversion efficiency. The quality of the carcass is also improved, with fewer condemnations for pneumonia and lower slaughtering costs through reductions in pleurisy and pericarditis. The decision to vaccinate should be carefully evaluated; the costs of mortality alone should not be the sole consideration, because the other effects on productivity listed above contribute to the benefits of vaccination.

Control of pleuropneumonia on a farm can be accomplished by combining treatment, vaccination, and husbandry practices such as those outlined above. Disinfection should be included in any control program; the organism is sensitive to a wide range of commonly used disinfectants (Gutierrez et al. 1995).

Control of pleuropneumonia in a region or breeding pyramid involves health schemes aimed at pleuropneumonia-free breeding and multiplying herds, serologic monitoring, monitoring at slaughter and postmortem examination of casualties, control of management, and controlled pig traffic (serologic testing, quarantine). For herds infected with *A. pleuropneumoniae* intending to join such a scheme, an eradication program is the method of choice but requires careful evaluation of the economic consequences. Depopulation and restocking with pigs originating from certified pleuropneumonia-free herds can be used; however, this method is expensive and may lead to the loss of important bloodlines. Other methods that have succeeded in the past include an eradication program in the existing herd area but weaning at another farm, at the same time supported by a program of vaccination, medication, and culling and repopulation with disease-free gilts (Larsen et al. 1990). Age of weaning and level of maternal antibodies may have an important influence on the colonization of piglets by *A. pleuropneumoniae* (Vigre et al. 2002). There are several herds that successfully eradicated *A. pleuropneumoniae* using a good medicated early weaning program (M. Gottschalk, unpublished observations). Breeding herds with a relatively low percentage of seropositive animals (up to 30%) have used the "test-and-removal" of seropositive animals under medication (Nielsen et al. 1976). There are different methodologies, but basically the principle is based on the serologic testing of sows shortly before farrowing and by weaning the piglets at 2 weeks of age under strict separation from the potentially infected stock. These piglets, which are seronegative up to the age of 12 weeks, serve to restock the herd. Seropositive sows are systematically eliminated until the entire breeding stock is seronegative. This program can take 6–12 months. During the elimination procedure, the whole herd is protected from reinfection by medicated feed—for example, cotrimoxazole (trimethoprim + sulfamethoxazole 1:20, 250 mg/kg feed). Certain reports suggest that only partial success (Lariviere et al. 1990) or even failure (Hunnemann 1986) has resulted from the application of such eradication programs. In addition, the successful outcome of this method is principally based on the serological test used: a test with low sensitivity will not eliminate all carrier sows, and a test with low specificity will eliminate healthy noncarrier animals, which considerably increases the cost of the program. A successful elimination of certain serotypes *A. pleuropneumoniae* with partial depopulation and tilmicosin has been suggested (Andersen and Gram 2004). However, it has also been demonstrated that tilmicosin treatment cannot completely eliminate the pathogen from carrier animals (Klopfenstein et al. 2004).

REFERENCES

Aarestrup FM, Jensen NE. 1999. Susceptibility testing of *Actinobacillus pleuropneumoniae* in Denmark. Evaluation of three different media of MIC-determinations and tablet diffusion tests. Vet Microbiol 64:299–305.

Abul-Milh M, Paradis SE, Dubreuil JD, Jacques M. 1999. Binding of *Actinobacillus pleuropneumoniae* lipopolysaccharides to glycosphingolipids evaluated by thin-layer chromatography. Infect Immun 67:4983–4987.

Andersen LV, Gram S. 2004. A successful elimination of *Actinobacillus pleuropneumoniae* (serotype 2), *Mycoplasma hyponeumoniae* and PRRS (European and Vaccine-strain) by partial depopulation, early weaning and Tilmicosin (Pulmotil, Elanco) treatment. Proc Int Congr Pig Vet Soc 18:179.

Anderson MD, Williams JA. 1990. Effects of tiamulin base administered intramuscularly to pigs for treatment of pneumonia associated with *Actinobacillus pleuropneumoniae*. Proc Int Congr Pig Vet Soc 11:15.

Andreasen M, Mousing J, Krogsgaard TL. 2001. No overall relationship between average daily weight gain and the serological response to *Mycoplasma hyopneumoniae* and *Actnobacillus pleuropneumoniae* in eight chronically infected Danish swine herds. Prev Vet Med 49:19–28.

Andresen LO, Klausen J, Barfod K, Sorensen V. 2002. Detection of antibodies to *Actinobacillus pleuropneumoniae* serotype 12 in pig serum using a blocking enzyme-lined immunosorbent assay. Vet Microbiol 89:61–67.

Angen O, Jessing S. 2004. PCR tests for serotype specific identification and detection of *Actinobacillus pleuropneumoniae*. Proc Int Congr Pig Vet Soc 18:161.

Baarsch MJ, Scamurra RW, Burger K, Foss DL, Maheswaran SK, Murtaugh MP. 1995. Inflammatory cytokine expression in swine experimentally infected with *Actinobacillus pleuropneumoniae*. Infect Imm 63:3587–3594.

Beck M, van den Bosch J, Jongenelen I, Loeffen P, Nielsen R, Nicolet J, Frey J. 1994. RTX toxin genotypes and phenotypes in *Actinobacillus pleuropneumoniae* field strains. J Clin Microbiol 32:2749–2754.

Bertram TA. 1985. Quantitative morphology of peracute pulmonary lesions in swine induced by *Haemophilus pleuropneumoniae*. Vet Pathol 22:598–609.

——. 1986. Intravascular macrophages in lungs of pigs infected with *Haemophilus pleuropneumoniae*. Vet Pathol 23:681–691.

——. 1990. *Actinobacillus pleuropneumoniae*: Molecular aspects of virulence and pulmonary injury. Can J Vet Res 54:S53–S56.

Bertschinger HU, Seifert P. 1978. Isolation of a Pasteurella haemolytica–like organism from porcine necrotic pleuropneumonia. Proc Int Congr Pig Vet Soc 5:Abstr M19.

Blackall J, Klaasen HL, van den Bosch H, Kuhnert P, Frey J. 2002. Proposal of a new serovar of *Actinobacillus pleuropneumoniae*: Serovar 15. Vet Microbiol 84:47–52.

Boekema BK, Kamp EM, Smits MA, Smith HE, Stockhofe-Zurwieden N. 2004. Both ApxI and ApxII of *Actinobacillus pleuropneumoniae* serotype 1 are necessary for full virulence. Vet Microbiol 100:17–23.

Bosse GM, Matyunas NJ. 1999. Delayed toxidromes. Emerg Med 17(4):679–690.

Bosse JT, Janson H, Sheehan B, Beddek A, Rycroft N, Kroll S, Langford P. 2002. *Actinobacillus pleuropneumoniae*: Pathobiology and pathogenesis of the infection. Micrb Infect 4:225–235.

Brandreth SR, Smith IM. 1985. Prevalence of pig herds affected by pleuropneumonia associated with *Haemophilus pleuropneumoniae* in eastern England. Vet Rec 117:143–147.

Caruso JP, Ross RF. 1990. Effects of *Mycoplasma hyopneumoniae* and *Actinobacillus (Haemophilus) pleuropneumoniae* infections on alveolar macrophage functions in swine. Am J Vet Res 51:227–231.

Chatellier S, Harel J, Dugourd D, Chevallier B, Kobisch M, Gottschalk M. 1999. Genomic relatedness among *Actinobacillus pleuropneumoniae* field strains of serotypes 1 and 5 isolated from healthy and diseased pigs. Can J Vet Res 63:170–176.

Chiers K, Haesebrouck F, van Overbeke I, Charlier G, Ducatelle R. 1999. Early in vivo interactions of *Actinobacillus pleuropneumoniae* with tonsils of pigs. Vet Microbiol 31:301–306.

Clota J, Foix A, March R, Riera P, Costa L. 1996. Caracterizacion serologica de cepas de *Actinobacillus pleuropneumoniae* aisladas en Espana. Med Vet 13:17–22.

Cruijsen TL, Van Leengoed LA, Dekker-Nooren TC, Schoevers EJ, Verheijden JH. 1992. Phagocytosis and killing of *Actinobacillus pleuropneumoniae* by alveolar macrophages and polymorphonuclear leukocytes isolated from pigs. Infect Immun 60:4867–4871.

Desrosiers R. 2004. Epidemiology, diagnosis and control of swine diseases. Howard Dunne Memorial Lecture. Proc Am Ass Swine Vet 9–37.

Desrosiers R, Mittal KR, Malo R. 1984. Porcine pleuropneumonia associated with *Haemophilus pleuropneumoniae* serotype 3 in Quebec. Vet Rec 115:628–629.

Dreyfus A, Schaller A, Nivollet S, Segers RPAM, Kobisch M, Mieli L, Soerensen V, Hüssy D, Miserez R, Zimmermann W, Inderbitzin F, Frey J. 2004. Use of recombinant ApxIV in serodiagnosis of *Actinobacillus pleuropneumoniae* infections, development and prevalidation of the ApxIV ELISA. Vet Microbiol 99:227–238.

Dubreuil D, Jacques M, Mittal K, Gottschalk M. 2000. *Actinobacillus pleuropneumoniae* surface polysaccharides: Their role in diagnosis and immunogenicity. Animal Health Res Rev 2:73–93.

Duff JP, Scott JW, Wilkes MK, Hunt B. 1996. Otitis in a weaned pig: A new pathological role for *Actinobacillus (Haemophilus) pleuropneumoniae*. Vet Rec 139:561–563.

Fenwick BW. 1990. Virulence attributes of the lipopolysaccharides of the HAP group of organisms. Can J Vet Res 54:S28–S32.

Fittipaldi N, Broes A, Harel J, Kobisch M, Gottschalk M. 2003. Evaluation and field validation of PCR tests for detection of *Actinobacillus pleuropneumoniae* in subclinically infected pigs. J Clin Microbiol 41:5085–5093.

Frank RK, Chengappa MM, Oberst RD, Hennessy KJ, Henry SC, Fenwick B. 1992. Pleuropneumonia caused by *Actinobacillus pleuropneumoniae* biotype 2 in growing and finishing pigs. J Vet Diagn Invest 4:270–278.

Frey J. 2003. Detection, identification, and subtyping of *Actinobacillus pleuropneumoniae*. Methods Mol Biol 216:87–95.

Frey J, Beck M, van den Bosch JF, Segers RPAM, Nicolet J. 1995. Development of an efficient PCR method for toxin typing of *Actinobacillus pleuropneumoniae* strains. Mol and Cell Probes 9:277–282.

Frey J, Bosse JT, Chang YF, Cullen JM, Fenwick B, Gerlach GF, Gygi D, Haesebrouck F, Inzana TJ, Jansen R, Kamp EM, Macdonald J, Macinnes JI, Mittal KR, Nicolet J, Rycroft AN, Segers RPAM, Smits MA, Stenbaek E, Struck DK, van den Bosch JF, Wilson PJ, Young R. 1993. *Actinobacillus pleuropneumoniae* RTX toxins: Uniform designation of haemolysins, cytolysins pleurotoxin and their genes. J Gen Microbiol 139:1723–1728.

Frey J, Kuhn R, Nicolet J. 1994. Association of the CAMP phenomenon in *Actinobacillus pleuropneumoniae* with the RTX toxins ApxI, ApxII and Apx III. FEMS Microbiol Lett 124:245–251.

Fussing V. 1998. Genomic relationship of *Actinobacillus pleuropneumoniae* serotype 2 strains evaluated by ribotyping, sequence analysis of ribosomal intergenic regions and pulse-field gel electrophoresis. Lett App Micriobiol 27:211–215.

Gagné A, Lacouture S, Broes A, D'Allaire S, Gottschalk M. 1998. Development of an immunomagnetic method for selective isolation of *Actinobacillus pleuropneumoniae* serotype 1 from tonsils. J Clin Microbiol 36:251–254.

Gambade P, Morvan H. 2001. Episode de mortalités brutales à *Actinobacillus pleuropneumoniae* biovar 2 sur des porcs charcutiers et prophylaxie vaccinale. Bulletin des GTV 12:19–22.

Gilbride KA, Rosendal S. 1984. Antimicrobial susceptibility of 51 strains of *Haemophilus pleuropneumoniae*. Can J Comp Med 48:47–50.

Gottschalk M, Altman E, Charland N, Lasalle F De, Dubreuil JD. 1994. Evaluation of a saline boiled extract, capsular polysaccharides and long-chain lipopolysaccharides of *Actinobacillus pleuropneumoniae* serotype 1 as antigens for the serodiagnosis of swine pleuropneumonia. Vet Micro 42:91–104.

Gottschalk M, Broes A, Fittipaldi N. 2003. Recent developments on *Actinobacillus pleuropneumoniae*. Proc Am Assoc Swine Vet 387–393.

Gottschalk M, Broes A, Mittal K, Kobisch M, Kuhnert P, Lebrun A, Frey J. 2003. Non-pathogenic *Actinobacillus* isolates antigenically and biochemically similar to *Actinobacillus pleuropneumoniae*: A novel species? Vet Microbiol 92:87–101.

Gottschalk M, Lebrun A, Lacouture S, Harel J, Forget C, Mittal KR. 2000. Atypical *Actinobacillus pleuropneumniae* isolates that share antigenic determinants with both serotypes 1 and 7. J Vet Diagn Invest 12(5):444-449.

Grondahl-Hansen J, Barfod K, Klausen J, Andresen LO, Heegaard PM, Sorensen V. 2003. Development and evaluation of a mixed long-chain lipopolysaccharide based ELISA for serological surveillance of infection with *Actinobacillus pleuropneumoniae* serotypes 2, 6 and 12 in pig herds. Vet Microbiol 96:41–51.

Gutierrez CB, Barbosa JIR, Suarez J, Gonzalez OR, Tascon RI, Ferri EFR. 1993. Evaluation of an immunoperoxidase technique using an only biotin-labeled antibody for the demonstration of *Actinobacillus pleuropneumoniae* in tissue sections. Zentralbl Veterinarmed B 40:81–88.

——. 1995. Efficacy of a variety of disinfectants against *Actinobacillus pleuropneumoniae* serotype 1. Am J Vet Res 56:1025–1029.

Haesebrouck F, Chiers K, van Overbeke I, Ducatelle R. 1997. *Actinobacillus pleuropneumoniae* infections in pigs: The role of virulence factors in pathogenesis and protection. Vet Microbiol 58:239–249.

Haesebrouck F, Pasmans F, Chiers K, Maes D, Ducatelle R, Decostere A. 2004. Efficacy of vaccines against bacterial diseases in swine: What can we expect? Vet Microbiol 100:255–268.

Häni H, König H, Nicolet J, Scholl E. 1973. Zur Haemophilus-Pleuropneumonie beim schwein. V. Pathomorphologie. Schweiz Arch Tierheilkd 115:191–203.

Hartley PE, Wilesmith JW, Bradley R. 1988. The influence of pleural lesions in the pig at slaughter on the duration of the fattening period: An on-farm study. Vet Rec 123(8):208.

Hofer J, Schoder J, Buchner A, Vanek E, Lapan G, Fuchs K, Baumgartner W. 1996. Serologischer Querschnittsuntersuchung zu Verbreitung der *Actinobacillus pleuropneumoniae*-Infektion in Österreich unter Berucksichtigung von epidemiologische und betriebspezifischen Einflussfaktoren. Wiener Tierärtzl Monatsschr 83:80–90.

Hsu FS. 1990. Evaluation of lincospectin sterile solution and Linco-Spectin 44 Premix in the treatment of pleuropneumonia. Proc Int Congr Pig Vet Soc 11:15.

Hunneman WA. 1986. Incidence, economic effects, and control of *Haemophilus pleuropneumoniae* infections in pigs. Vet Q 8:83–87.

Hüssy D, Schlatter Y, Miserez R, Inzana T, Frey J. 2004. PCR-based identification of serotype 2 isolates of *Actinobacillus pleuropneumoniae* biovars I and II. Vet Microbiol 99:307–310.

Inzana TJ, Todd J, Veit HP. 1993. Safety, stability and efficacy of non-encapsulated mutants of *Actinobacillus pleuropneumoniae* for use in live vaccines. Infect Immun 61:1682–1686.

Jacobsen MJ, Nielsen JP. 1995. Development and evaluation of a selective and indicator medium for isolation of *Actinobacillus pleuropneumoniae* from tonsils. Vet Micro 47:191–197.

Jacques M. 2004. Surface polysaccharides and iron-uptake systems of *Actinobacillus pleuropneumniae*. Can J Vet Res 68:81–85.

Jacques M, Foiry B, Higgins R, Mittal KR. 1988. Electron microscopic examination of capsular material from various serotypes of *Actinobacillus pleuropneumoniae*. J Bacteriol 170:3314–3318.

Jansen R, Briare J, Kamp EM, Gielkens ALJ, Smits MA. 1995. The CAMP effect of *Actinobacillus pleuropneumoniae* is caused by Apx toxins. FEMS Microbiol Lett 126:139–143.

Jensen AE, Bertram TA. 1986. Morphological and biochemical comparison of virulent and avirulent isolates of *Haemophilus pleuropneumoniae* serotype 5. Infect Immun 51:419–424.

Jessing SG, Angen O, Inzana TJ. 2003. Evaluation of a multiplex PCR test for simultaneous identification and serotyping of *Actinobacillus pleuropneumoniae* serotypes 2, 5, and 6. J Clin Microbiol 41:4095–4100.

Kamp EM, Popma JK, Leengoed LAMG Van. 1987. Serotyping of *Haemophilus pleuropneumoniae* in the Netherlands: With emphasis on heterogeneity within serotype 2 and (proposed) serotype 9. Vet Microbiol 13:249–257.

Kielstein P, Wuthe H, Angen O, Mutters R, Ahrens P. 2001. Phenotypic and genetic characterization of NAD-dependent *Pasteurellaceae* from the respiratory tract of pigs and their possible pathogenetic importance. Vet Microbiol 8:243–55.

Kilian M. 1976. The haemolytic activity of *Haemophilus* species. Acta Pathol Microbiol Scand (B) 84:339–341.

Kilian M, Nicolet J, Biberstein EL. 1978. Biochemical and serological characterization of *Haemophilus pleuropneumoniae* (Matthews and Pattison 1961) Shope 1964 and proposal of a neotype strain. Int J Syst Bacteriol 28:20–26.

Klausen J, Andresen LO, Barfod K, Sorensen V. 2002. Evaluation of an enzyme-linked immunosorbent assay for serological surveillance of infection with *Actinobacillus pleuropneumoniae* serotype 5 in pig herds. Vet Microbiol 88:223–232.

Klopfenstein C, Paradis M-A, Gottschalk M, Fittipaldi N, Broes A, Dick CP. 2004. Evaluation of the efficacy of tilmicosin phosphate premix (Pulmotil) to eliminate *Actinobacillus pleuropneumoniae* from the tonsils of carrier pigs. Proc Int Congr Pig Vet Soc 18:511.

Kobisch M, Vannier P, Delaporte S, Dellac B. 1990. The use of experimental models to study in vivo the antibacterial activity of Enrofloxacin against *Actinobacillus (Haemophilus) pleuropneumoniae* and *Mycoplasma hyopneumoniae* in combination with *Pasteurella multocida*. Proc Int Congr Pig Vet Soc 11:16.

Komal JP, Mittal, KR. 1990. Grouping of *Actinobacillus pleuropneumoniae* strains of serotypes 1 through 12 on the basis of their virulence in mice. Vet Microbiol 25:229–240.

Kristensen CS, Angen O, Andreasen M, Takai H, Nielsen JP, Jorsal SE. 2004. Demonstration of airborne transmission of *Actinobacillus pleuropneumoniae* serotype 2 between simulated pig units located at close range. Vet Microbiol 98:243–249.

Kume K, Nakai T, Sawata A. 1984. Isolation of *Haemophilus pleuropneumoniae* from the nasal cavities of healthy pigs. Jpn J Vet Sci 46:641–647.

Lacouture, S, Mittal, KR, Jacques, M, Gottschalk M. 1997. Serotyping *Actinobacillus pleuropneumoniae* by the use of monoclonal antibodies. J Vet Diagn Invest 9:337–341.

Lariviere S, D'Allaire S, De Lasalle F, Nadeau M, Moore C, Ethier R. 1990. Eradication of *Actinobacillus pleuropneumoniae* serotype 1 and 5 infections in four herds. Proc Int Congr Pig Vet Soc 11:17.

Larsen H, Hogedahl Jorgensen P, Szancer J. 1990. Eradication of *Actinobacillus pleuropneumoniae* from a breeding herd. Proc Int Congr Pig Vet Soc 11:18.

Lebrun A, Lacouture S, Côté D, Mittal K, Gottschalk M. 1999. Identification of *Actinobacillus pleuropneumoniae* strains of serotypes 7 and 4 using monoclonal antibodies: Demonstration of common LPS O-chain epitopes with *Actinobacillus lignieresii*. Vet Microbiol 65:271–282.

Lida J, Smith IM, Nicolet J. Use of monoclonal antibodies for classifying *Actinobacillus (Haemophilus) pleuropneumoniae*. Res Vet Sci 49(1):8–13.

Liggett AD, Harrison LR. 1987. Sequential study of lesion development in experimental *Haemophilus pleuropneumoniae*. Res Vet Sci 42:204–221.

Maldonado J, Riera P, Martinez E, Llopart D, Osorio CR, Artigas C. 2004. NAD-independent *Actinobacillus pleuropneumoniae* implicated in the etiology of fatal swine pleuropneumonia. Proc Int Congr Pig Vet Soc 18:159

Matthews PRJ, Pattison IH. 1961. The identification of a *Haemophilus*-like organism associated with pneumonia and pleurisy in the pig. J Comp Pathol 71:44–52.

McDowell SWJ, Ball HJ. 1994. Serotypes of *Actinobacillus pleuropneumoniae* isolated in the British Isles, 1988–1993. Vet Rec 134:522–523.

Mittal KR, Higgins R, Lariviere S. 1983. Detection of type-specific antigens in the lungs of *Haemophilus pleuropneumoniae*-

infected pigs by coagglutination test. J Clin Microbiol 18:1355–1357.

——. 1987. An evaluation of agglutination and coagglutination techniques for serotyping of *Haemophilus pleuropneumoniae* isolates. Am J Vet Res 48:219–226.

Mittal KR, Higgins R, Lariviere S, Nadeau M. 1992. Serological characterization of *Actinobacillus pleuropneumoniae* strains isolated from pigs in Quebec. Vet Microbiol 32:135–48.

Moeller K, Fussing V, Grimont PAD, Paster BJ, Dewhirst FE, Killian M. 1996. *Actinobacillus minor,* sp.nov.; *Actinobacillus porcinus,* sp.nov. and *Actinobacillus indolicus* sp. nov.; Three new V factor dependent species from the respiratory tract of pigs. Int J Syst Bact 46:951–956.

Moeller K, Nielsen R, Andersen LV, Killian M. 1992. Clonal analysis of the *Actinobacillus pleuropneumoniae* population in a geographically-restricted area by multilocus enzyme electrophoresis. J Clin Micro 30:623–627.

Myers MJ, Farrell DE, Snider TG, Post LO. 2004. Inflammatory cytokines, pleuropneumonia infection and the effect of dexamethasone. 2004. Pathobiology 71:35–42.

Nadeau M, Lariviere S, Higgins R, Martineau GP. 1988. Minimal inhibitory concentrations of antimicrobial agents against Actinobacillus pleuropneumoniae. Can J Vet Res 52:315–318.

Negrete-Abascal E, Garcia R, Reyes ME, Godinez D, de la Garza M. 2000. Membrane vesicles released by *Actinobacillus pleuropneumoniae* contain proteases and Apx toxins. FEMS Microbiol Lett 19:109–113.

Negrete-Abascal E, Reyes ME, Garcia R, Vaca S, Giron J, Garcia O, Zenteno E, de la Garza M. 2003. Flagella and motility in *Actinobacillus pleuropneumoniae.* J Bacteriol 185:664–668.

Negrete-Abascal E, Tenonio VR, Serrano JJ, Garcia CC, Garza M de la. 1994. Secreted proteases from *Actinobacillus pleuropneumoniae* serotype 1 degrade porcine gelatine, haemoglobin and IgA. Can J Vet Res 58:83–86.

Nicolet J. 1968. Sur l'hemophilose du porc. I. Identification d'un agent frequent: *Haemophilus parahaemolyticus.* Pathol Microbiol 31:215–225.

——. 1970. Aspects microbiologiques de la pleuropneumonie contagieuse du porc. These d'habilitation, Berne.

Nicolet J, König H. 1966. Zur Haemophilus-Pleuropneumonie beim Schwein: Bakteriologische, pathologisch-anatomische und histologische Befunde. Pathol Microbiol 29:301–306.

Nicolet J, König H, Scholl E. 1969. Zur Haemophilus-Pleuropneumonie beim schwein. II. Eine kontagiose Krankheit von wirtschaftlicher Bedeutung. Schweiz Arch Tierheilkd 111:166–174.

Nielsen R. 1975. Colostral transfer of immunity to *Haemophilus parahaemolyticus* in pigs. Nord Vet Med 27:319–328.

——. 1984. *Haemophilus pleuropneumoniae* serotypes—Cross protection experiments. Nord Vet Med 36:221–234.

——. 1985a. *Haemophilus pleuropneumoniae (Actinobacillus pleuropneumoniae)* serotypes 8, 3 and 6—Serological response and cross immunity in pigs. Nord Vet Med 37:217–227.

——. 1985b. Serological characterization of *Haemophilus pleuropneumoniae (Actinobacillus pleuropneumoniae)* strains and proposal of a new serotype: Serotype 9. Acta Vet Scand 26:501–512.

——. 1985c. Serological characterization of *Haemophilus pleuropneumoniae (Actinobacillus pleuropneumoniae)* strains and proposal of a new serotype: Serotype 10. Acta Vet Scand 26:581–585.

——. 1986a. Serology of *Haemophilus (Actinobacillus) pleuropneumoniae* serotype 5 strains: Establishment of subtypes A and B. Acta Vet Scand 27:49–58.

——. 1986b. Serological characterization of *Actinobacillus pleuropneumoniae* strains and proposal of a new serotype: Serotype 12. Acta Vet Scand 27:453–455.

Nielsen R, Andresen LO, Plambeck P. 1996. Serological characterization of *Actinobacillus pleuropneumoniae* biotype 1 strains antigenically related to both serotypes 2 and 7. Acta Vet Scand 37:327–336.

Nielsen R, Andresen LO, Plambeck T, Nielsen JP, Krarup LT, Jorsal SE. 1997. Serological characterization of *Actinobacillus pleuropneumoniae* biotype 2 strains isolated from pigs in two Danish herds. Vet Microbiol 54:35–46.

Nielsen R, O'Connor PJ. 1984. Serological characterization of 8 *Haemophilus pleuropneumoniae* strains and proposal of a new serotype: Serotype 8. Acta Vet Scand 25:96–106.

Nielsen R, Thomsen AD, Vesterlund SD. 1976. Pleuropneumonia caused by *Haemophilus parahaemolyticus*: An attempt to control the disease at two progeny testing stations by serological blood testing followed by removal of the seropositive animals and their litter mates. Nord Vet Med 28:349–352.

Nielsen R, van den Bosch JF, Plambeck T, Sorensen V, Nielsen JP. 2000. Evaluation of an indirect enzyme-linked immunosorbent assay (ELISA) for detection of antibodies to the Apx toxins of *Actinobacillus pleuropneumoniae.* Vet Microbiol 71:81–87.

Olander HJ. 1963. A Septicaemic Disease of Swine and Its Causative Agent *Haemophilus parahaemolyticus.* Ph.D. diss. Univ California.

Paradis MA, Vessie GH, Merrill JK, Dick CP, Moore C, Charbonneau G, Gottschalk M, MacInnes JI, Higgins R, Mittal KR, Girard C, Aramini JJ, Wilson JB. 2004. Efficacy of tilmicosin in the control of experimentally induced *Actinobacillus pleuropneumoniae* infection in swine. Can J Vet Res 68:7–11.

Paradis SE, Dubreuil JD, Gottschalk M, Archambault M, Jacques M. 1999. Inhibition of adherence of *Actinobacillus pleuropneumoniae* to porcine respiratory tract cells by monoclonal antibodies directed against LPS and partial characterization of the LPS receptors. Curr Microbiol 39:313–320.

Pattison IH, Howell DG, Elliott J. 1957. A Haemophilus-like organism isolated from pig lung and the associated pneumonic lesions. J Comp Pathol 67:320–329.

Perry MB, Altman E, Brisson JR, Beynon LM, Richards JC. 1990. Structural characteristics of the antigenic capsular polysaccharides and lipopolysaccharides involved in the serological classification of *Actinobacillus (Haemophilus) pleuropneumoniae* strains. Serodiagnosis and Immunotherapy in Inf Dis 4:299–308.

Pijpers A, Vernooy JACM, Leengoed LAMG Van, Verheijden JHM. 1990. Feed and water consumption in pigs following an *Actinobacillus pleuropneumoniae* challenge. Proc Int Congr Pig Vet Soc 11:39.

Pohl S, Bertschinger HU, Frederiksen W, Manheim W. 1983. Transfer of *Haemophilus pleuropneumoniae* and the *Pasteurella haemolytica*-like organism causing porcine necrotic pleuropneumonia to the genus *Actinobacillus (Actinobacillus pleuropneumoniae* comb. Nov.) on the basis of phenotypic and deoxyribonucleic acid relatedness. Inst J Syst Bacteriol 33:510–514.

Pol JMA, Leengoed LAMG Van, Stockhofe N, Kok G, Wensvoort G. 1997. Dual infections of PRRS/influenza or PRRSV/ *Actinobacillus pleuropneumoniae* in the respiratory tract. Vet Micro 55:259–264.

Rioux S, Galarneau C, Harel J, Frey J, Nicolet J, Kobisch M, Dubreuil D, Jacques M. 1999. Isolation and characterization of mini-Tn10 lipopolysaccharide mutants of *Actinobacillus pleuropneumoniae* serotype 1. Can J Microbiol 45:1017–1026.

Rioux S, Galarneau C, Harel J, Kobisch M, Frey J, Gottschalk M, Jacques M. 2000. Isolation and characterization of a capsule-deficient mutant of *Actinobacillus pleuropneumoniae* serotype 1. Microb Pathog 28:279–89.

Rodriguez-Barbosa JI, Gutierrez CB, Tascon RI, Suarez J, Noronia F de, Rodriguez-Ferri EF. 1995. Characterisation of monoclonal antibodies to O antigen of lipopolysaccharide of *Actinobacillus pleuropneumoniae* serotype 2 and their use in the classification of field isolates. FEMS Immunol and Med Micro 11:35–44.

Rosendal S, Boyd DA. 1982. Serotyping of *Haemophilus pleuropneumoniae.* J Clin Microbiol 16:840–843.

Shope RE. 1964. Porcine contagious pleuropneumonia. I. Experiment transmission, etiology and pathology. J Exp Med 119:357–368.

Shope RE, White DC, Leidy G. 1964. Porcine contagious pleuropneumonia. II. Studies of the pathogenicity of the etiological agent *Haemophilus pleuropneumoniae*. J Exp Med 119:369–375.

Sidibe M, Messier S, Lariviere S, Gottschalk M, Mittal KR. 1993. Detection of *Actinobacillus pleuropneumoniae* in the porcine upper respiratory tract as a complement to serological tests. Can J Vet Res 57:204–208.

Sorensen V. 1997. Evaluation of Laboratory Diagnostic Assays for Monitoring Respiratory Infections in pigs. Ph.D. thesis. Frederiksberg, Denmark: The Royal Veterinary and Agricultural University.

Stephano A, Navarro R, Rayo CD, Osorio M. 1990. Effect of the use of ceftiofur sodium injectable (Excenel sterile powder) for the treatment of induced *Actinobacillus pleuropneumoniae*: Multiple dose titration study. Proc Int Congr Pig Vet Soc 11:41.

Straw BE, MacLachlan NJ, Corbett WT, Carter PB, Schey HM. 1985. Comparison of tissue reactions produced by *Haemophilus pleuropneumoniae* vaccines made with six different adjuvants in swine. Can J Comp Med 49:149–151.

Vaillancourt JP, Higgins R, Martineau GP, Mittal KR, Lariviere S. 1988. Changes in the susceptibility of *Actinobacillus pleuropneumoniae* to antimicrobial agents in Quebec (1981–1986). J Am Vet Med Assoc 193:470–473.

van den Bosch H, Frey J. 2003. Interference of outer membrane protein PalA with protective immunity against *Actinobacillus pleuropneumoniae* infections in vaccinated pigs. Vaccine 21:3601–3607.

van Overbeke I, Chiers K, Charlier G, Vandernberghe I, Van Beeumen J, Ducatelle R, Haesebrouck F. 2002. Characterization of the in vitro adhesion of *Actinobacillus pleuropneumniae* to swine alveolar epithelial cells. Vet Microbiol 88:59–74.

van Overbeke I, Chiers K, Ducatelle R, Haesebrouck F. 2001.Effect of endobronchial challenge with *Actinobacillus pleuropneumoniae* serotype 9 of pigs vaccinated with a vaccine containing Apx toxins and transferrin-binding proteins. J Vet Med B Infect Dis Vet Public Health 48:15–20.

Vigre H, Angen O, Barfod K, Thanning Lavristsen D, Sorensen V. 2002. Transmission of *Actinobacillus pleuropneumoniae* in pigs under field-like conditions: Emphasis on tonsillar colonisation and passively acquired colostral antibodies. Vet Microbiol 89:151–159.

Vigre H, Ersboll AK, Sorensen V. 2003. Decay of acquired colostral antibodies to *Actinobacillus pleuropneumoniae* in pigs. J Vet Med B Infect Dis Vet Public Health 50:430–435.

Ward CK, Inzana TJ. 1994. Resistance of *Actinobacillus pleuropneumoniae* to bactericidal antibody and complement is mediated by capsular polysaccharide and blocking antibody specific for lipopolysaccharide. J Immunol 153:2110–2121.

White DC, Leidy G, Jamieson JD, Shope RE. 1964. Porcine contagious pleuropneumonia. III. Interrelationship of *Haemophilus pleuropneumoniae* to other species of Haemophilus: Nutritional, metabolic, transformation and electron microscopy studies. J Exp Med 120:1–12.

Wilson PJ, Deneer HG, Potter A, Albritton W. 1989. Characterization of a streptomycin-sulfonamide resistance plasmid from *Actinobacillus pleuropneumoniae*. Antimicrob Agents Chemother 33:235–238.

Wilson RW, Kierstead M. 1976. Haemophilus parahemolyticus associated with abortion in swine. Can Vet J 17(8):222.

Yoshimura H, Takagi M, Ishimura M, Endoh YS. 2002. Comparative in vitro activity of 16 antimicrobial agents against *Actinobacillus pleuropneumoniae*. Vet Res Commun 26:11–19.

Zhang Y, Tennent JM, Ingham A, Beddome G, Prideaux C, Michalski WP. 2000. Identification of type 4 fimbriae in *Actinobacillus pleuropneumoniae*. FEMS Microbiol Lett 189:15–18.

34 Progressive and Nonprogressive Atrophic Rhinitis

M. F. de Jong

A disease condition in pigs referred to as "atrophic rhinitis" (or "infectious atrophic rhinitis") and "chronic atrophic rhinitis" has been recognized for nearly two centuries. A disease of the pig characterized by stunted development or total disappearance of the nasal turbinates (called "turbinate atrophy") has been recognized for over 160 years and was first described as "*Schnüffelkrankheit*" in Germany (Franque 1830), where it became prevalent in several areas.

These conditions are now classified as either nonprogressive atrophic rhinitis (NPAR), caused by toxigenic *Bordetella bronchiseptica,* or progressive atrophic rhinitis (PAR), caused by toxigenic *Pasteurella multocida,* alone or in combination with other agents (e.g., *B. bronchiseptica*). The characteristic lesion caused by both agents is a hypoplasia of the nasal turbinate bones (conchal atrophy); in moderate to severe outbreaks this is accompanied by degrees of facial distortion (including brachygnathia superior, lateral deviation of the snout, and septum deviation) and nasal hemorrhage as a result of frequent sneezing. Nasal hemorrhage is rare in NPAR but characteristic in PAR.

In contrast to NPAR, PAR is of global economic significance to swine production, since in PAR, these signs are accompanied by poor growth of fattening pigs (Pedersen and Barfod 1981). Toxigenic *P. multocida* is still spreading in the pig population, especially where disease control measurements are carried out ineffectively (Glattleider et al. 1996; Frymus et al. 1996). The PAR toxigenic *P. multocida* is also able to cause disease in other species, such as rabbits, goats, sheep, cattle, poultry, and turkeys. Even humans can become infected, and lesions somewhat comparable to those in swine can result. Poultry, sheep, and cattle, along with rats, cats, and dogs, are described as carriers (Avril et al. 1990; Donnio et al. 1991; Nielsen and Frederiksen 1990). Toxigenic *P. multocida* should therefore be considered a zoonosis and should be of concern to governmental and human and veterinary health organizations.

Toxigenic *B. bronchiseptica* is widespread in swine production and considered to cause a minor or insignificant growth depression in diseased pigs and is therefore called nonprogressive atrophic rhinitis.

The individual and combined importance of both agents will be discussed in this chapter.

The precise etiology of the "condition" atrophic rhinitis (AR) has been actively debated, with intermittent attempts at definition, for well over a century. Since the 1930s, observations by Ratke (1938), Thunberg and Carlstrom (1940), and Philips (1946) have implied that the disease was contagious. Shortly thereafter it was demonstrated experimentally that turbinate atrophy was transmissible between pigs; when young pigs were inoculated intranasally with crude material from atrophic turbinates, they frequently developed turbinate atrophy (Jones 1947; MacNabb 1948; Philips et al. 1948; Gwatkin et al. 1949, 1951; Terpstra and Akkermans 1960). Much research has since been directed toward defining the precise microbiological agent(s) responsible. While several management and husbandry factors can influence the severity and clinical expression of PAR, this disease is now established primarily as an infectious disease despite attempts at one time to redefine it as a disorder fundamentally of nutritional origin (Brown et al. 1966).

In 1956 Switzer suggested that turbinate atrophy may be caused by several agents, including trichomonads (Switzer 1951), filter-passing agents (Switzer 1953), viruses (Switzer and L'Ecuyer 1960; Edington et al. 1976), and mycoplasmas (Switzer 1955; Edington et al. 1976; Gois et al. 1977). Only special AR-toxigenic strains of *B. bronchiseptica* and AR-toxigenic strains of *P. multocida* have consistently produced "turbinate atrophy" when sufficient quantities of pure (broth) cultures have been inoculated intranasally into young susceptible (e.g., colostrum-deprived specific pathogen free [SPF]) pigs. Despite these observations, however, clinical (and pathological) disease cannot be attributed solely to infection with either one or both agents, since these infections can occur in the field in the (temporary) absence of clinical disease (the so-called subclinical stage of PAR). Interruptions between periods of clinical disease that can vary in duration from approximately 2 months to about 2 years can occur in infected herds. Herd monitoring based on clinical (and/or pathological) features, therefore, cannot guarantee the absence of infectious PAR in a pig herd. Complementary monitoring of a herd or connected (breeding) herds for over 1 year, based on bacteriologic and/or serologic detection of the PAR-toxigenic *P. multocida*, may be necessary to obtain sufficient information concerning the PAR-infected or PAR-free status of the herd.

DEFINITION

At this point it is important to define carefully the conditions described in this chapter. All diseases that cause turbinate atrophy in swine are called infectious atrophic rhinitis by farmers. The term "infectious progressive atrophic rhinitis" should be reserved for the disease produced by one etiologic agent, *P. multocida*. Pedersen and Nielsen (1983) first recommended the use of this term as a result of the deliberations of a European Economic Community commission of specialists on PAR. To obtain a consensus in a worldwide forum, the proposal was repeated by Pedersen and coworkers in 1988. The first agreement among specialists in swine diseases from Europe, North and South America, and Asia was achieved in 1988 (de Jong and Nielsen 1990). It was agreed to define PAR as a disease caused by infection with toxigenic *P. multocida*. In herds where suspicious manifestations such as sneezing, nose bleeding, snout deformation, growth retardation, turbinate atrophy, and septum deviation are observed and where toxigenic *P. multocida* is detected (bacteriologically or serologically), the diagnosis of PAR can be confirmed. However, the disease may also develop in or be transmitted by pigs from herds harboring toxigenic *P. multocida* even though only slight or subclinical disease is present. The advantage of an etiologic definition of PAR rests on the possibility of identifying, independently of actual clinical status, those herds that are able to transmit or develop the severe clinical disease (Bollwahn 1988).

Estimates of the economic impact of PAR in swine have varied, but in moderate to severe outbreaks it can be of considerable economic importance (Pedersen and Nielsen 1983; Glattleider et al. 1996). From the clinical and pathological points of view, it is probably no longer useful to employ the term "atrophic rhinitis" as denoting a single disease complex. Rather, bordetellosis and toxigenic pasteurellosis should be distinguished as NPAR and PAR. The infectious agents have completely different economic impacts in swine production and require different methods and strategies for prevention and treatment.

ETIOLOGY

Research suggests that toxigenic strains of both *B. bronchiseptica* and *P. multocida* are the primary infectious eti-

ologic factors in NPAR and PAR, respectively. The severity of the disease that develops in a pig is related to the amount of one or of both toxins absorbed by the animal (Van Diemen et al. 1994a). The susceptibility of pigs to a certain amount of toxin that causes turbinate bone reduction has been shown to be age related. Toxigenic strains of *P. multocida* have been shown to produce severe PAR, including extreme growth retardation, even in pigs older than 3 months of age; toxigenic strains of *B. bronchiseptica* produce turbinate hypoplasia only in pigs until about the age of 6 weeks.

The conditions for the growth and/or colonization of *P. multocida* or *B. bronchiseptica* necessary to produce sufficient amounts of toxin are influenced by bacteriologic and/or virologic damage to the mucosa and by certain environmental, management, and husbandry factors that create the (multifactorial) disease complex. When these factors are all present, very severe clinical PAR can result. Since growth retardation and clinical PAR also occur after parenteral dosing with the toxin of *P. multocida*, colonization of toxigenic *P. multocida* in the nose may not be necessary for the development of the disease. Tonsils and lungs also have to be considered as locations for toxin production (Ackermann et al. 1994).

Infectious Agents

Bordetella Bronchiseptica. *B. bronchiseptica* is a small, motile, gram-negative rod or coccobacillus measuring approximately 1.0×0.3 µm in size. The bacterium is aerobic, does not ferment carbohydrates, utilizes citrate, and splits urea.

B. bronchiseptica has been isolated widely from young pigs with rhinitis and from pigs with pneumonia and also from animals in herds showing no clinical signs of respiratory disease. It is also a pathogen or potential pathogen of many other mammals, including dogs, cats, and rats.

In the United States during the 1960s, *B. bronchiseptica* was said to be the principal cause of atrophic rhinitis (Switzer and Farrington 1975). After intranasal instillation of pure cultures of *B. bronchiseptica* in colostrum-deprived pigs a few days old, Cross and Claflin (1962) were able to produce typical experimental turbinate atrophy. This work was repeated by Ross et al. (1967), who were able to reproduce turbinate atrophy with pure cultures of AR-toxigenic *B. bronchiseptica* in 95% of pigs inoculated at 1–3 days of age but in only 66% of 4-week-old pigs. Brassinne et al. (1976) reported that only high numbers of AR-toxigenic *B. bronchiseptica* caused turbinate lesions. A toxigenic strain that caused 100% turbinate atrophy in 3-week-old colostrum-deprived SPF pigs did not cause typical atrophy when intranasally instilled during 4 successive days in 6-week-old pigs (de Jong and Akkermans 1986). This indicated that between 3 and 6 weeks of age, the sensitivity to a heavy infection with an AR-toxigenic *B. bronchiseptica* strain dropped drastically. Duncan et al. (1966a) had already stated that experimental infections with *B. bronchiseptica* did not cause severe progressive lesions. Pearce and Roe (1966) were unsuccessful in producing turbinate atrophy with cultures of *B. bronchiseptica* in naturally farrowed pigs but were able to produce the lesions when the culture was inoculated into colostrum-deprived pigs. This indicated protection against AR lesions by colostral immunity.

Bacteriologic data from nasal swabs taken from pigs at different ages suggested that *B. bronchiseptica* infection starts to build up in conventional herds with and without clinical signs of PAR in the third week of age, when the nasal sensitivity for toxigenic *B. bronchiseptica* has already started to decrease (Pedersen and Nielsen 1983; de Jong 1985). This meant that, under natural (conventional) conditions, the influence of *B. bronchiseptica* as a primary cause of PAR has been overestimated. Turbinate atrophy can occur in 2- to 3-month-old piglets in exceptional circumstances, such as after a primary *B. bronchiseptica* infection in SPF herds (Schöss 1982) and after experimental infections in piglets free from antibodies. Partial or total regeneration of such atrophy has been described and such infections seem to result in only a limited and low percentage of transient clinical snout deviations; animals with lesions caused by *B. bronchiseptica* did not develop significant growth depression (Pedersen and Barfod 1982).

Nearly all *B. bronchiseptica* strains from pigs produced the thermolabile AR toxin. *B. bronchiseptica* can also affect the lower respiratory system, and toxin production from such regions may have some influence on clinical symptoms of NPAR.

Variations in virulence among porcine *B. bronchiseptica* strains are known to exist. Collings and Rutter (1985) determined that only those strains in phase 1 and isolated from pigs caused turbinate atrophy, and they established that the ability to both colonize the nasal cavity in large numbers and produce a cytotoxin were important virulence determinants. The role of the cytotoxin was clearly established by Magyar et al. (1988), who also examined the role of several other putative virulence determinants, including a hemolysin, adenylate cyclase, and an adhesin. By comparing the pathogenic effects of a porcine cytotoxic phase 1 strain with a noncytotoxic phase 1 strain also of porcine origin, they established that it is the cytotoxin (which is probably the same as the mouse lethal factor and dermonecrotic toxin) that is the key virulence determinant in the production of turbinate hypoplasia.

In a comparison of three biological assays for the detection of toxigenic properties of *B. bronchiseptica*, discrepancies were found between the guinea pig skin test, the mouse spleen atrophy assay, and the suckling mice mortality assay (Mendoza 1993), suggesting that differences exist between these toxigenic properties.

Discrepancies in the results of studies obtained in different countries could arise from variation in virulence or the amount of toxin produced by the organism concerned. This has been reported for isolates of *B. bronchiseptica* in the United States (Ross et al. 1967; Skelly et al. 1980), Canada (Miniats and Johnson 1980), the United Kingdom (Collings 1983), and Hungary (Elias et al. 1982). However, even the most virulent of 10 U.K. isolates did not cause progressive turbinate atrophy or significant snout deformation in experimental infections (Rutter and Rojas 1982). More important, strains isolated from herds with or without progressive disease in the United Kingdom all caused nonprogressive lesions of similar severity (Rutter and Rojas 1982; Giles and Smith 1983). From observations in this laboratory, it appeared that strains isolated in PAR-diseased herds and in herds not suspected of PAR produced roughly the same amount of toxin. Only a few strains differed from this pattern (de Jong and Akkermans 1986). Thus, there is strong evidence, contrary to the opinions of Kielstein (1983) and Nakai et al. (1986), that although there are differences in the virulence of isolates of *B. bronchiseptica*, the severe lesions of clinical PAR cannot be attributed only to this organism. Pigs infected with *B. bronchiseptica* in the deeper respiratory system may be more sensitive to other pulmonary infections. This means that *B. bronchiseptica* infections should not be neglected as a respiratory pathogen.

Pasteurella Multocida. *P. multocida* is a nonmotile, gram-negative rod or coccobacillus approximately 0.3 × 0.6 μm in size. The bacterium is aerobic, ferments glucose without gas, and produces indole. In fresh smears the organism shows distinct bipolar staining. The colonies of *P. multocida* type A are larger and more mucoid than those of type D. On blood agar plates a characteristic odor is generally produced.

P. multocida and its subspecies have been isolated widely from pigs with and without clinical symptoms of rhinitis or pneumonia. Early studies (reviewed by Gwatkin 1959) established that *P. multocida* could experimentally produce turbinate atrophy in pigs and rabbits and that it was frequently but not always isolated from field outbreaks.

Several workers subsequently examined the ability of this organism to produce turbinate atrophy under controlled experimental conditions. Some strains studied produced a mild rhinitis but were unable to induce marked turbinate hypoplasia (Harris and Switzer 1968; Smith 1971; Koshimizu et al. 1973; Nakagawa et al. 1974; Edington et al. 1976), whereas in other studies, particularly from Europe, cultures of *P. multocida* produced nasal deformity and turbinate atrophy (Dirks et al. 1973) and even severe PAR (Nielsen et al. 1976). In Germany and in the Netherlands particularly, *P. multocida* was considered to be an important primary pathogen in PAR (Dirks et al. 1973). Medication and vaccination with bordetella vaccines in PAR herds reduced *B. bronchiseptica* successfully but failed to affect PAR. In these herds *P. multocida* was found to be the major pathogen. Reducing *P. multocida* in these herds decreased PAR (de Jong 1976–1979, 1980).

A major step in resolving these conflicting opinions began in the Netherlands when de Jong (1976–1979) and de Jong et al. (1980) began to test different *P. multocida* strains isolated from herds with and without PAR in colostrum-deprived SPF piglets, as described earlier by Ross et al. (1967) for *B. bronchiseptica*.

P. multocida grows in a semifluid mucus on the mucosal membrane of the nose rather than on the nasal epithelium itself, so studies were redirected from cultures washed off solid medium and resuspended to broth cultures. These broth cultures contained substances excreted by the bacteria. After this change it was easy to reproduce AR lesions with the same strain in 3-week-old pigs (or older) instead of in 3-day-old pigs.

Martineau et al. (1982) showed the importance of using broth cultures instead of cultures washed from solid media, and explained that this could be a possible reason for the different findings of investigators (Nakai et al. 1986). Pure cultures of both dermonecrotic and nondermonecrotic type D and type A isolates of *P. multocida* establish themselves poorly in the nasal cavity of healthy conventional (Voets 1990), SPF (de Jong 1985), and gnotobiotic piglets (Rutter and Rojas 1982; Rutter 1983). Nasal instillations of pure broth cultures of toxigenic *P. multocida* needed to be repeated for approximately 4 days to produce a severe *P. multocida* nasal infection that resulted in PAR. Uninoculated pigs kept in contact with inoculated pigs became infected, but only mild lesions were noticed 4 weeks later. Sneezing was sporadic in these experiments with gnotobiotic and SPF pigs. In contrast, experimental infection with toxigenic *P. multocida* in conventional pigs pretreated with chemical irritants or with *B. bronchiseptica* resulted in sneezing, and PAR lesions also occurred in pigs in contact. The strains that caused PAR lesions were called AR pathogenic. This characteristic correlated with the ability to produce a thermolabile toxin. PAR could be reproduced completely with bacteria-free filtrates of these unheated toxins.

Nasal infection by aerosol with 0.5 mL 5 and 13 µg toxin/mL per nostril in 4-week-old piglets induced subclinical ventral turbinate hypoplasia (atrophy). Amounts of 40 µg/mL induced severe lesions. During the 5-week period after challenge, depression of weight gain started in week 3 after challenge. In the 5, 13, 20, and 40 µg/mL groups, the growth depressions during this period were 32, 54, 52, and 96 grams/day/pig, respectively (Van Diemen et al. 1994a). The severity of atrophy depended on the amount of toxin administered into the nose of the pig.

The first publication explaining the role of toxigenic *P. multocida* in AR was by Ilina and Zasukhin (1975) in Russia and it encouraged the development of tests for selecting toxigenic *P. multocida* isolates. Instead of using a rabbit test, the guinea pig skin test was chosen because it also selected AR-pathogenic *B. bronchiseptica* strains (de Jong 1980; Blobel and Schliesser 1981; de Jong and Akkermans 1986). Differences between infections with toxigenic *B. bronchiseptica* and toxigenic *P. multocida* strains were revealed when pure broth cultures were instilled intranasally in groups of colostrum-deprived SPF pigs aged 3, 6, 9, 12, and 16 weeks. In pigs infected with *B. bronchiseptica*, macroscopic turbinate lesions were noticed only in 3- and 6-week-old pigs, not in pigs of 9 weeks and older. Toxigenic *P. multocida* still induced typical snout and turbinate alterations, including septal deviation, in pigs infected at 12 and at 16 weeks of age. The severity of nose lesions decreased with increasing age with the same dose of toxigenic *P. multocida*.

Other Factors

Despite the major role of infectious agents, other factors contribute to the cause or at least the clinical expression of AR, but they have proved difficult to evaluate and have been inadequately defined quantitatively. Most experienced clinicians have concluded that the severity of the disease is markedly influenced by extrinsic factors (Penny 1977; Goodwin 1980). Smith (1983) provided a useful review of these noninfectious determinants.

Nutrition. Although the role of the dietary calcium: phosphorus imbalance is now discounted as a primary cause (Brown et al. 1966), nutritional deficiency of any kind may enhance the severity of infectious disease. Feed consumption may be influenced by AR, since piglets with an acute rhinitis may accept feed less readily and become stunted and weak. Growing pigs with conchal damage may also have reduced feed intake, thus contributing to the reduced daily gain associated with the condition.

Genetic Influences. In the past it has been suggested that heredity played a major role, but heritability estimates have varied greatly, and attempts to control the disease solely by genetic selection have failed. There is probably a measure of genetically linked predisposition to AR, since breeds and strains that vary in susceptibility to the disease and are susceptible to genetic pressure do occur. In the United Kingdom, for example, Large White pigs are now generally considered more vulnerable than Landrace pigs, although 30 years ago the reverse could have been the case. The subject has been reviewed by Smith (1983), Voets et al. (1986a), and Martineau et al. (1988).

Management, Housing, and Environment. Severe growth-retarding AR is closely associated with intensive methods of production; it is undoubtedly most severe when successive batches of pigs are housed in densely stocked, continuously occupied, poorly ventilated

Table 34.1. Management factors influencing the severity of atrophic rhinitis

Increase	Decrease
Large herds, open herds	Small herds, closed herds
Expanding herds	Static herd size
High proportion of gilts	Mainly old sows
Large farrowing unit	Small or single farrowing unit (all-in/all-out)
Multiple suckling—piglets fostered between litters	Single suckling
Large weaner pools	More isolation, modular systems (all-in/all-out)
Large number in one airspace	Small number in one airspace
Frequent moving and mixing	Little movement and mixing
Intensive systems indoors	Outdoor rearing
High stocking density	Low stocking density
Poor ventilation and no temperature control	Good ventilation and temperature control
Poor hygiene, little disinfection	Good hygiene and disinfection
Continual pig throughput	Buildings rested
Dry-feeding, dusty atmosphere	Wet-feeding, clean atmosphere
Mechanical food handling	Hand delivery

Source: After Penny 1977.

buildings (Smith and Giles 1980). Penny (1977) has identified several management factors that tend to predispose to an increased severity of AR (Table 34.1).

Instances have been observed where the disease was controlled, or at least reduced to economically acceptable levels, solely by the manipulation of housing and environment and improved management. It is also a common belief that the disease may be more severe in a dusty atmosphere, particularly where dry and dusty feed is delivered by automatic equipment. The influences of housing and feed, including the feed delivery system, on respiratory diseases of the pig have been reviewed by Owen (1982) and Strang (1982), respectively.

EPIDEMIOLOGY

Bordetella bronchiseptica

B. bronchiseptica is widely prevalent in the pig population in countries with major swine-producing industries. The prevalence of *B. bronchiseptica* infection greatly exceeds that of clinical AR or marked turbinate atrophy at slaughter (Cameron et al. 1980), and although *B. bronchiseptica* is frequently isolated from young pigs in outbreaks of AR, the infection also occurs widely in herds without the condition (Tornoe et al. 1976; Giles et al. 1980; Rutter 1981; Whittlestone 1982).

The dam has been considered a possible source of the important nasal infections for her suckling piglets, and she has been reliably incriminated as a source of *B. bronchiseptica* and *P. multocida*. Transmission also occurs between sows and boars. Although traditionally viewed as important, some observers have concluded that the sow's role might be minor, since clinically NPAR-free progeny resulted when sows from an affected herd were reared under improved conditions (Bercovich 1978).

The degree of resistance to natural *B. bronchiseptica* infection among sows does not appear to be marked, but younger sows are more likely to be active shedders of the organism. Although infection from the dam is probably the chief method of initiating the infection among populations of suckling piglets, infection in weaner houses may often be endemic because of infection passing laterally between different batches, particularly in systems where an all-in/all-out approach is not practiced.

B. bronchiseptica is primarily introduced by the introduction of carrier pigs (in SPF herds); recently purchased breeding stock are often held responsible.

Whether or not the sow is important in transmission, the recognized infectious agents pass readily between populations of young weaned pigs. Infection of pigs at an early age may be vital, even when the clinical signs appear late in the fattening period.

The chief mode of transmission of *B. bronchiseptica* from pig to pig is by aerosol droplet infection. The high prevalence of infection among growing pigs suggests that transmission may occur at any age, but it is probably more common and more readily accomplished in susceptible young pigs, in which an active rhinitis with sneezing develops. The infection can certainly spread rapidly among populations of susceptible (nonimmune) piglets (Smith et al. 1982).

B. bronchiseptica colonizes the ciliated mucosa of the porcine respiratory tract very effectively; it is frequently isolated from the tonsils, and large numbers have been found in the intestinal contents of infected gnotobiotic pigs (Rutter 1985). Thus, direct-contact droplet infection, and perhaps ingestion of fecal material, are likely to be the main routes of transmission. The cycle of infection appears to be maintained by a small proportion of breeding females. Litters within the farrowing house become infected at an early age, but in the United Kingdom as well as in the Netherlands, the major spread seems to occur after 2–3 weeks of age or after weaning, especially in large groups on flat decks, when 70–80% of a group can become infected. The infection persists for several months, with a gradual reduction in the intensity and rate of infection. The age at which animals first become infected with *B. bronchiseptica* has an important effect on the development of lesions. The most severe lesions occur in nonimmune animals infected during the first week of life (Duncan et al. 1966a). Animals infected at 4 weeks show less-severe lesions, while those infected at 9 weeks show virtually no lesions (de Jong and Akkermans 1986).

The amount and type of immunity also influence the epidemiology of bordetella infection. The presence of passive antibody in the sera of piglets born to naturally infected dams (with toxigenic bordetellae) appeared to provide protection against the development of turbinate lesions (Rutter 1981) but not against infection (Kobisch and Pennings 1989; Voets 1990). However, vaccination of sows appeared to delay infection in their piglets until 12–16 weeks of age compared to nonvaccinated herds, in which litters became infected by 2 weeks of age (Rutter et al. 1984).

B. bronchiseptica shedding from vaccinated sows seems to be reduced in herds in which the sow population has been vaccinated for some years.

B. bronchiseptica has been isolated from most domestic and wild animal species (Goodnow 1980), and because it is a ubiquitous pathogen, there is always the risk that infection could be introduced by nonporcine vectors. Most isolates from other species appear to be of low virulence in pigs, but it is possible that rodents might become infected with pig strains and transmit them. Virtually every pig herd is infected with *B. bronchiseptica*, and variable amounts of brachygnathia superior (BS), moderately severe turbinate atrophy, and moderate signs of septum deviation can be expected in all herds. For this to occur, pigs from nonimmune dams must become infected within the first 4 weeks of life and develop lesions that persist to slaughter, but in most, regeneration of turbinates begins approximately 4 weeks after the start of infection, when the scrolls are not totally damaged. Lesions such as septal deviation, turbinate bone hyperplasia, and BS may be apparent at slaughter. The percentage of pigs with a twisted snout generally does not reach 1%.

In the field, however, the picture is likely to be more complicated. For example, there are reports that *Haemophilus parasuis* in combined infections with type A strains of *P. multocida* can produce mild turbinate lesions (Gois et al. 1983a). Others could not repeat these results.

B. bronchiseptica is killed in 30 minutes at 56°C. It survives outside the body in dried droplets for up to 5 days on glass, 3 days on cloth, and a few hours on paper. The survival time of *B. bronchiseptica* in soil is about 6 weeks. Low humidity and raised temperatures rapidly reduce numbers of live bacteria. In liquid media *B. bronchiseptica* survived for more than 8 weeks at 21°C. In lake water

and in phosphate buffered saline solution (PBS), *B. bronchiseptica* remained viable for at least 3 weeks (Porter et al. 1991). In a rotating aerosol chamber, the mean half-life at 21°C and 76% relative humidity was 118.8 minutes (Stehmann et al. 1992), and at 23°C and 75% relative humidity, it was 56.7 minutes (Müller et al. 1992). The organism is sensitive to common disinfectants (Stehmann et al. 1990).

Pasteurella multocida

The introduction of a disease and its subsequent spread within a population depend on numerous factors, including the nature of the etiologic agent, the host, and the structure of the population. In intensive pig rearing, many animals are in close contact and there is often widespread movement of breeding and replacement stock between herds. The main risks of introducing infection are associated with purchased pigs, and disease may then spread rapidly within a seronegative herd. Early reports that did not distinguish between PAR and NPAR clearly recognized that (P)AR was introduced by carrier pigs. The disease appeared in many Norwegian herds that had imported pigs, several of which eventually developed severe clinical signs. This led Braend and Flatla (1954) to conclude that "atrophic rhinitis was practically unknown in Norway prior to [World War II,] after which it has been rather common, most certainly because of importation of pigs from Sweden where the disease is common." It was, therefore, assumed that a new infectious organism had been imported. The disease was declared notifiable, and a slaughter policy was carried out. This strategy was also followed in other European countries, such as in the United Kingdom until 1959 and in the Netherlands until 1980. Similarly, the introduction of AR into the United Kingdom was attributed to the importation of Swedish stock (Anon. 1954). There are at least two possible explanations for these observations: either *B. bronchiseptica* was introduced in uninfected animals and exacerbated existing infections with toxigenic *P. multocida* or, more likely, toxigenic *P. multocida* was introduced with the imported stock.

Estimates of the prevalence of PAR, whether from an individual farm or larger population, are usually conducted by an examination of the heads of pigs after slaughter. Such surveys have indicated that macroscopic nasal turbinate atrophy is widespread in pig populations. It occurred in about 40% of Danish and British herds (Nielsen 1983) in the late 1970s, although a later estimate from England showed a decline to 25% (Cameron et al. 1980). Such a high level of turbinate atrophy, however, does not reflect an equivalent level of clinical disease, since mild lesions are common in commercial fattening pigs, and mild or even moderate atrophy in individuals may occur in herds without obvious clinical disease or adverse economic effects. Today it is believed that these lesions are caused by *B. bronchiseptica*

(NPAR); growth retardation associated with more severe outbreaks has proved difficult to quantify, and some observers (Straw et al. 1983) have found no correlation between the degree of turbinate atrophy and production parameters and, in these herds, now consider atrophy to result from infection with *B. bronchiseptica* (NPAR). Nevertheless, where clinically apparent disease occurs, there is frequently a reduction in average daily gain; this has been conservatively estimated as 5–8% for pigs with severe atrophy (Nielsen 1983). In combination with pleurisy and pneumonia this reduction can double.

The epidemiology of *P. multocida* infection in pigs is less well understood than that of *B. bronchiseptica*. The organism colonizes the tonsils, but some factor or factors, the mechanisms of which are not understood, are needed to assist colonization of the nasal mucosa. Nontoxigenic and toxigenic type A strains can be isolated from the lungs of pigs with pneumonia (Baekbo 1988), but *P. multocida* is much less effective than *B. bronchiseptica* in colonizing the trachea. In contrast to type A strains, toxigenic and nontoxigenic type D strains are isolated less frequently in the lungs but more frequently in the nose. *P. multocida* has also been isolated from most animal species and is well recognized as an important pathogen in cattle, rabbits, poultry, and turkeys (Carter 1967). In some studies its distribution in pig herds was limited; only 9% were infected in one report (Harris and Switzer 1969), but such results may be attributable to the presence of the commensal flora in the nasal cavity (Chanter and Rutter 1989). Today in most laboratories, selective media and the technique of mouse passage can be used for primary isolation of the organism. Material from herds examined in this way (Rutter 1985) has yielded toxigenic and nontoxigenic isolates of type A or D, and mixed infections with these two types in the same pig can occur.

In contrast, the distribution of toxigenic isolates of *P. multocida* appears to be limited to those herds with PAR or a history of the disease (Rutter 1985). In Germany, the Netherlands, and Denmark (Pedersen 1983), the picture is similar, indicating that the majority of herds infected with toxigenic *P. multocida* exhibit clinical signs of progressive disease. In the Netherlands, however, toxigenic *P. multocida* has been isolated from 15% of breeding herds with no history or clinical signs of progressive disease at the moment of the first detection of the toxigenic *P. multocida*. Most of these breeding herds were monitored and became clinically diseased within 2 years after this detection. Only 5% of pigs 4–12 weeks of age were infected in these herds. A few herds remain clinically unaffected for some years (de Jong 1983a; Goodwin et al. 1990), which indicates that toxigenic strains may be present in some clinically unaffected herds, and these could transmit progressive disease if infected stock were purchased from them.

The main source of *P. multocida* infection for young pigs appears to be pharyngeal transport of the organism among breeding stock; 10–15% of sows in farrowing houses were infected with toxigenic isolates (de Jong 1983b), and some piglets were already infected with these strains within a week after birth. Toxigenic *P. multocida* was also isolated from the vaginas of a few sows. The age at which piglets first become infected with *P. multocida* affects the severity of the lesions produced, but unlike *B. bronchiseptica* infection, older pigs may still develop lesions. Significant turbinate atrophy occurred in pigs infected with toxigenic *P. multocida* up to 16 weeks of age; Rutter et al. (1984) found that pigs that became naturally infected between 12 and 16 weeks of age had turbinate lesions. It has been shown that apparently healthy 3-month-old pigs can develop PAR when introduced into a commercial production unit where severe disease is occurring (Nielsen et al. 1976). Injection of *P. multocida* toxin (125 µg/kg) produced significant atrophy in conventional pigs of 10 weeks of age (Rutter 1985). With 13 µg/mL instilled nasally, a subclinical PAR could be achieved in 4-week-old piglets necropsied 5 weeks later. With 40 µg/mL, severe lesions were obtained in the trials (Van Diemen et al. 1994a).

The prevalence of toxigenic *P. multocida* may be related to the extent of clinical disease. The organism was isolated from 50% to 60% of young pigs sampled in a herd in which almost 30% of fattening pigs had twisted snouts. In less severely affected herds, larger numbers of young pigs had to be sampled before toxigenic strains were isolated (Rutter 1985; de Jong et al. 1988).

The distribution of toxigenic *P. multocida* in other species has still to be determined. Pedersen (1983), de Jong (1985), Rutter (1985), Baalsrud (1987), Ohkubo et al. (1987), Kamp et al. (1990), and Frymus et al. (1996) reported that dermonecrotic strains occurred in cattle, rabbits, dogs, cats, rats, poultry, goats, and sheep. A toxigenic strain from pasteurellosis in turkeys produced severe turbinate atrophy in gnotobiotic pigs, but a toxigenic strain thought to have been isolated from ovine pneumonia colonized the nasal cavity of pigs poorly and did not produce significant lesions in combined infection with *B. bronchiseptica* (Rutter 1983, 1985). Toxigenic strains were isolated from humans suffering from tonsilitis, rhinitis, sinusitis, pleuritis, appendicitis, and septicemia and were pathogenic for pigs (Nielsen and Frederiksen 1990; Donnio et al. 1991). This implies special risks for all persons who have contact with herds or animals infected with toxigenic *P. multocida*: farmers and their families, farmhands, drivers, merchants, vets, consultants, butchers, and employees of slaughterhouses. Wearing face masks will reduce the risk of becoming infected and spreading the infection.

The infectious agents are usually introduced into a previously unaffected herd by carrier pigs. Recently purchased breeding stock, gilts or boars, are commonly held responsible, although the evidence for their involvement is often circumstantial. The introduction of toxigenic strains of *P. multocida* is the principal event preceding an outbreak. Poorly colonizing strains with a low toxin production may represent an exception (Kavanagh 1994). Infection from other sources is rare but seems to become more important if the spread of toxigenic *P. multocida* in pigs is not stopped.

P. multocida is easily destroyed by 60°C in 10 minutes, by 0.5% phenol in 15 minutes, and by a 3.5% solution of cresol in a few minutes. In manure *P. multocida* remains infective for a month and in decomposing or frozen carcasses for 3 months. In a rotating aerosol chamber, the mean half-life was 20.85 minutes at 23°C and 75% relative humidity.

The organism is susceptible to commonly used disinfectants, including those of the following general categories: quaternary ammonium compounds, phenolics, sodium hypochlorite, iodophores, glutaraldehyde, and chlorhexidine.

Formalin at a concentration of 0.2% or greater and phenol at 0.5% will kill in less than 18 hours at 3°C. On stock culture agar *P. multocida* often survives for months or even years if kept at room temperature, but if stored in the refrigerator, the bacteria may die in several days. Their viability can be maintained for many years in blood or tissues in the frozen state at −20°C or lower (Blobel and Schliesser 1981).

PATHOGENESIS

Bordetella bronchiseptica

It is believed that *B. bronchiseptica* colonizes the nasal cavity by adhering to the nasal mucosa, where it probably preferentially attaches to the ciliated epithelial cells (Yokomizo and Shimizu 1979). This is followed by multiplication at the mucosal surface and toxin production, leading to inflammatory, proliferative, and degenerative changes in the nasal epithelium, including the loss of cilia (Duncan et al. 1966a; Edington et al. 1976). The organism is not believed to invade the deeper tissues.

It is assumed that the organism at the mucosal surface elaborates a toxin that diffuses into the osseous core of the nasal turbinate and is responsible for the osteopathy. The nature of this toxic factor has received much attention. Cell-free sonicated extracts from phase 1 *B. bronchiseptica* were originally shown to contain a heat-labile and dermonecrotic toxin, and it was assumed that this was probably an important factor in the pathogenesis. Since then, such bacteria-free extracts containing high levels of this toxin have been repeatedly inoculated intranasally into piglets, where they produce nasal lesions similar to those seen in naturally occurring AR (Hanada et al. 1979; Nakase et al. 1980; Magyar et al. 1988).

The degree of severity of the hypoplastic lesions seen in young pigs varies, and only rarely does severe hypoplasia result (Figs. 34.1–34.3). The ventral scroll of the ventral turbinate is the area most commonly and consistently affected; grossly it varies in appearance from a slightly shrunken and distorted scroll to virtually complete absence. In the more severe cases the dorsal scrolls of the ventral turbinate and the dorsal turbinate are also usually affected. The important factors that affect the severity of the hypoplasia are the degree of resistance of the pig to the infection (Smith et al. 1982) and the age when it was first acquired, since susceptibility to the damage the infection can produce declines as the pig gets older.

The histologic changes in bordetella-induced hypoplastic rhinitis have been reported by Duncan et al. (1966a) and are detailed in Switzer and Farrington (1975). Briefly, there is a hyperplasia of the epithelium and, in places, a metaplasia, the epithelium becoming more stratified in structure with polyhedral cells devoid of cilia. There is a degree of cellular infiltration (principally with neutrophils and mononuclear cells), a fibroblastic proliferation in the lamina propria, and a reduction in size and replacement fibrosis of the osseous core. In more chronic stages there are increased numbers of osteoblasts around the trabeculae, but osteoclasts are rarely found.

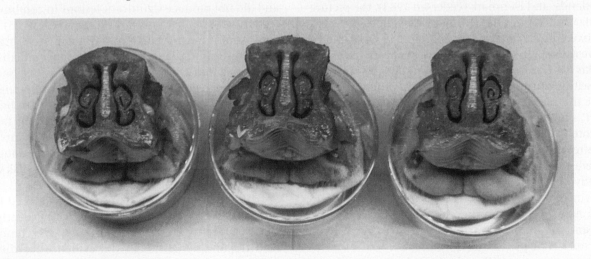

34.1. *Cross section of the snouts of three uninfected 6-week-old pigs showing normal anatomy of the turbinate scrolls (conchae Kontr. 1-2-3). (Courtesy P. Schöss.)*

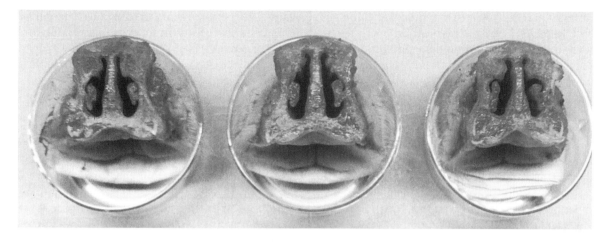

34.2. *Turbinate hypoplasia in three pigs experimentally infected at 5 and 10 days old with* B. bronchiseptica *and necropsied 40 days postinfection (Va 6-7-8). (Courtesy P. Schöss.)*

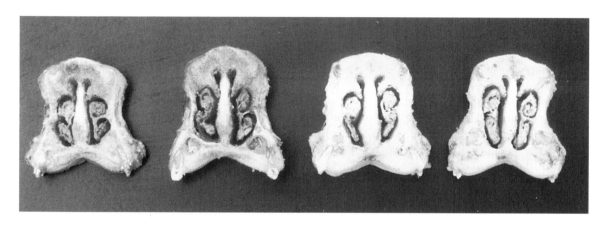

34.3. *Cross section of the snouts of four pigs infected at 5 and 10 days old with + and slaughtered at 6 months of age. Presumed turbinate regeneration and deformations of the ventral turbinates and nasal bones (os vomer) (Va 9-10-11-12). (Courtesy P. Schöss.)*

There is some variation in the toxigenicity of different strains of *B. bronchiseptica*; porcine phase 1 strains are more toxigenic than phase 3 or nonporcine isolates (Collings and Rutter 1985).

Turbinate Regeneration. There is considerable field and experimental evidence that the hypoplasia of the turbinates produced by the uncomplicated infection of young pigs (up to about 8 weeks old) is capable of regeneration, which may sometimes be almost complete (Duncan et al. 1966a; Tornoe and Nielsen 1976; Rutter 1981; Smith et al. 1982).

A degree of turbinate hypoplasia in young pigs (Fig. 34.2), with a variable amount of subsequent regeneration as the pig grows to slaughter weight (Fig. 34.3), may thus occur in most herds infected with *B. bronchiseptica*. This probably accounts for the high prevalence of mild lesions of turbinate atrophy seen at slaughter in the many bordetella-infected herds free from obvious clinical AR, especially in cases where the nasal cavity remains

infected with other species, particularly with nontoxigenic *P. multocida* or *Haemophilus spp.*

A reaction in the regeneration of the scrolls is the irregular increased ("hyperplastic") bone structures in the turbinate bones and other nose bones as well. Once induced, the BS does not seem to regenerate and is difficult to separate from breed-associated BS. Only after elimination of *B. bronchiseptica* in such pig populations can the breed-associated BS be studied properly.

Pasteurella multocida

The mechanisms of colonization by *P. multocida* and the subsequent processes affecting the turbinate bone cells and leading to progressive atrophy and clinical PAR have been partially clarified. Furthermore, the mechanisms by which these chronic nasal changes and their associated malfunctions cause growth retardation have been clarified to a large extent (Becker et al. 1986; Williams et al. 1986; Doster et al. 1990; Dugal and Jacques 1990).

P. multocida apparently colonizes the nasal cavity

poorly unless there is preexisting mucosal damage (Elling and Pedersen 1983). Chemical irritants (e.g., acetic acid and *B. bronchiseptica*) induce different modifications of the nasal epithelium, but both actions cause the production of nasal mucus, which results in a nasal environment favorable to colonization by *P. multocida* (Gagne and Martineau-Doize 1993). The different types of mucins produced by the piglets' nasal mucosa at different ages may contribute to an understanding of *P. multocida* and *B. bronchiseptica* colonization (Martineau-Doize et al. 1991a, b).

Given this preconditioning, the organism will set up a nasal infection and, if toxigenic, the toxin will be elaborated. The nasal cavity, however, is not necessarily the only possible site of toxin production. The toxin appears to be of crucial significance in the pathogenesis of PAR, since only toxigenic strains of *P. multocida* produce PAR lesions; furthermore, the toxin will produce progressive snout shortening and turbinate atrophy when given to pigs intranasally (Ilina and Zasukhin 1975) and by a variety of parenteral routes (Rutter and Mackenzie 1984).

The precise mechanism of action of the *P. multocida* toxin has not been clearly defined; but it will produce a variety of changes in the ventral turbinates, consisting of epithelial hyperplasia, atrophy of mucosal glands, increasing volume of blood vessels, osteolysis, and a proliferation of mesenchymal cells. These eventually will replace the bone trabeculae and osteogenic and osteoclastic tissues (Rutter and Mackenzie 1984). PAR therefore seems to result from a combination of early osteoblastic damage followed by a series of toxin-induced chronic changes that result in osteolysis and subsequent replacement fibrosis. The toxins of *B. bronchiseptica* and *P. multocida* are different. Also, the ways in which the turbinates are destroyed differ. The combination of both toxins has detrimental effects on the turbinates and skull bones (Martineau-Doize et al. 1990).

CLINICAL SIGNS

Bordetella bronchiseptica

Rhinitis. The principal signs seen in bordetellosis are sneezing and snuffling in young pigs. This can occur in piglets as young as 1 week but is frequently seen at 3–4 weeks of age or about the time of weaning, which may be related to both maternal colostral protection and the mixing of pigs at this stage.

Affected piglets sneeze, snuffle, and snort with a variable degree of catarrhal rhinitis producing a variable amount of serous or frequently mucopurulent nasal discharge, which may be observed by swabbing the nasal cavity. Generally, the younger the piglet when initially affected, the more severe the clinical signs. The appetite is usually only moderately to slightly impaired. The clinical signs increase in severity for a time, then tend to abate after a few weeks, except in herds with clinical PAR, where continued progressive turbinate damage

causes frequent sneezing to continue. Uncomplicated *B. bronchiseptica* infections in older pigs produce only mild signs or remain clinically inapparent.

Not all sneezing in young pigs is attributable solely to *B. bronchiseptica*, since infection with porcine cytomegalovirus or other agents may also produce or exacerbate these signs.

Bronchopneumonia. A more severe manifestation of infection is bronchopneumonia, which is usually seen as a primary condition in very young piglets (3–4 days). Although this type of disease is relatively uncommon compared with the wide prevalence of nasal infection, *B. bronchiseptica* is an important pathogen in those cases of pneumonia with bronchitis that occur in young pigs. The condition only affects young pigs and is most common in winter (Whittlestone 1982). The major clinical sign is coughing, perhaps with whooping and dyspnea. Pyrexia is not usually marked (Switzer and Farrington 1975). Morbidity is high within litters, and mortality may be so in untreated cases.

B. bronchiseptica is not infrequently isolated from pneumonic lesions in older fattening pigs, but it is considered to be a secondary opportunist pathogen, and the clinical significance of its presence remains largely unknown.

Pasteurella multocida

Clinical signs of PAR are not usually seen in pigs until about 4–12 weeks of age or later, depending on the severity of the outbreak, but sneezing and snuffling in baby pigs are commonly recorded as the first signs. They are not, however, specific to or diagnostic of the condition, since they frequently occur in the absence of subsequent clinical PAR. Sneezing and snuffling in baby pigs is merely a reflection of an acute catarrhal rhinitis, which may be due to bordetellosis and/or infection with porcine cytomegalovirus; other agents may possibly be involved, for example, *Mycoplasma* sp., *Actinobacillus* sp., and Aujeszky's disease, influenza, and porcine reproductive and respiratory syndrome (PRRS) viruses. In herds where subsequent infectious and other factors combine to cause progression to clinical AR, affected pigs will continue to sneeze, snuffle, and snort throughout the growing period; this is accompanied by a variable amount of serous to mucopurulent nasal discharge. In severely affected animals, sneezing may be pronounced and occasionally nasal bleeding may occur. Hemorrhage is usually unilateral and varies in severity. Blood may be seen on the walls of the pen or on the backs of the pigs; mucopurulent material and even pieces of turbinate debris may be expelled from the nose following episodes of forceful, violent sneezing. In gilts and sows the hemorrhage in late gestation and farrowing can be life threatening to the dam and her piglets.

The most characteristic clinical signs of PAR are due to disturbances of normal bone development of the

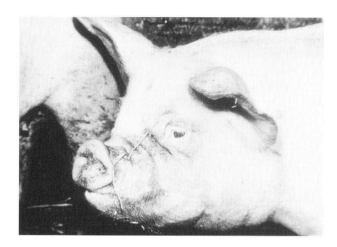

34.4. *A 17-week-old pig with clinical PAR showing marked brachygnathia superior, wrinkling of the skin on the dorsum of the nose, and tear staining.*

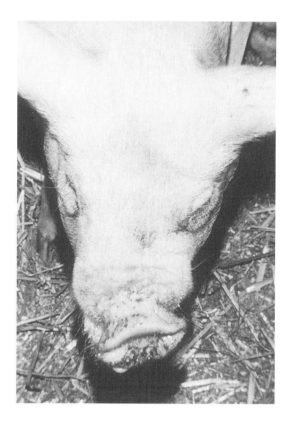

34.5. *The head of a 15-week-old pig with clinical PAR showing severe lateral deviation of the snout. The anatomy of the skull is distinctly abnormal due to a failure of normal bone development.*

nose; conspicuous deformities of the face may occur. The most common is BS, in which the upper jaw is shortened in relation to the lower, as a result of growth depression of the ossa nasales and maxillares, giving the face a "pushed-up" appearance. The skin and subcutis over the dorsum of the shortened snout are thrown into folds; when the disturbance of bone growth affects one side of the face more than the other, lateral deviation of the snout occurs (Figs. 34.4 and 34.5). This may vary in severity from a barely perceptible misalignment to severe twisting (possibly by as much as 50°). These facial deformities reflect an underlying turbinate atrophy; in the case of lateral deviation the atrophy is more pronounced on the side of the deviation. The prevalence of facial distortion varies among outbreaks, and not all pigs with significant turbinate atrophy develop marked facial distortion.

Dirty streaks on the face radiating from the medial canthus of the eye, caused by tear staining and the entrapment of dust following occlusion of the nasolachrymal duct, are common in PAR outbreaks (Fig. 34.4). However, they are not diagnostic and may occur in the absence of PAR.

In moderate to severe herd outbreaks of PAR, the clinical signs are frequently accompanied by growth retardation and reduction in the efficiency of feed utilization. Feed utilization is particularly reduced in severely diseased pigs. The amount of *P. multocida* toxin may influence growth performance (Doster et al. 1990; Van Diemen et al. 1994a).

Some clinical parameters have been used in an attempt to monitor and quantify disease levels. The prevalence of gross distortion among growing pigs is a crude measure of disease level but is not a sensitive index of turbinate atrophy. The prevalence and degree of BS in weaned pigs can provide useful information (Bercovich and de Jong 1976) but is not always diagnostic (Schöss 1983), and confusion can arise with breeds that are nat-

urally brachygnathic (e.g., Large White) (Van Groenland 1984). Sneeze counts have been used successfully in an attempt to assess the effects of treatment (Douglas and Ripley 1984; Kobisch and Pennings 1989).

LESIONS OF NPAR AND PAR

Gross Lesions

The gross lesions of PAR are restricted to the nasal cavity and adjacent structures of the skull, although in severe cases the pig may also be stunted. At necropsy both BS and facial distortion are observed in the intact head. The dominant lesion is an atrophy of the ventral and dorsal turbinates, and this can vary greatly in severity. The atrophy is assessed by a cross section of the snout at the level of the first/second upper premolar, at which point the conchae, dorsal and ventral, are symmetrically and maximally developed in the normal pig (Fig. 34.6). In mild to moderate cases the ventral scrolls of the turbinates are by far the most consistently and severely affected area; they vary from slightly shrunken to complete atrophy (Figs. 34.7 and 34.8).

In more severe cases, atrophy of the dorsal scrolls of the ventral turbinate and the dorsal and ethmoidal turbinates may occur (Figs. 34.9 and 34.10); in the most severe form there is a complete absence of all turbinate structures (Fig. 34.11). In between these mild and severe

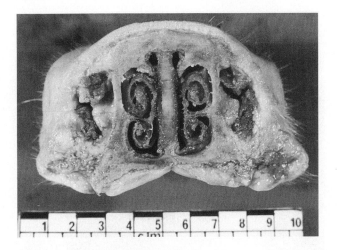

34.6. *Cross section of the snout of an 18-week-old pig showing normal anatomy of the turbinates.*

forms, a whole spectrum of atrophic changes may be observed; occasionally the turbinates are bizarrely shaped (Fig. 34.10), which may represent some degree of regrowth of the conchae (Done 1985). Another gross change that may be observed is bowing or buckling of the nasal septum (Fig. 34.11); this is not uncommon and is often associated with BS, facial distortion, and/or asymmetrical atrophy. Irregular formation of the ossa nasales and maxillares also occurs in PAR (de Jong 1985) and should not be neglected (Figs. 34.10 and 34.11).

Exudate may be found in the nasal cavity but is not a constant finding. The amount and character depend on the age of the lesion and the type of infection. The exudate consists of variable amounts of mucopurulent to purulent material, possibly flecked with blood. The mucosa lining the frontal sinus is sometimes inflamed, and the sinus itself may contain mucopurulent material. The bones surrounding the nasal cavity may have undergone thinning or may be irregularly shaped to some

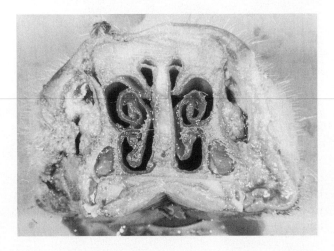

34.7. *Cross section of the snout of an 18-week-old pig. Slight distortion of the ventral scrolls of the turbinates is present, a common finding.*

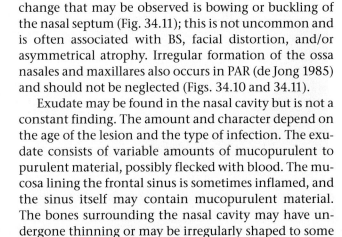

34.9. *Cross section of the snout of an 18-week-old pig showing severe bilateral turbinate atrophy.*

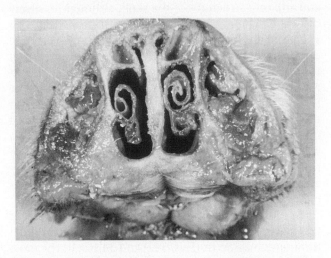

34.8. *Cross section of the snout of an 18-week-old pig showing modest but definite turbinate atrophy.*

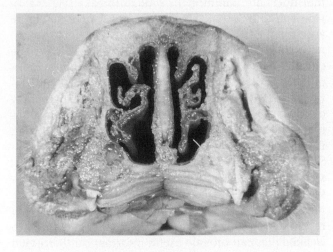

34.10. *Cross section of the snout of an 18-week-old pig; the atrophic turbinates have developed into bizarre shapes.*

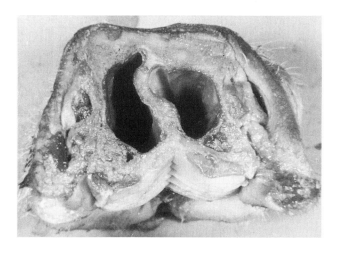

34.11. *Cross section of the snout of a 22-week-old pig showing total atrophy of all turbinate structures, with severe bending of the nasal septum.*

extent. Hyperplasia/hyperostosis can be observed in older pigs (de Jong 1985).

Assessment of Turbinate Atrophy. The varying severity of the atrophic changes has led to the development of methods of quantitative assessment, but unfortunately, no one system has gained universal acceptance. Subjective scoring of snouts (e.g., on a 0–5 scale as in the British system; Anon. 1978) has proved very useful in evaluating treatment and monitoring schemes. As well as wide variation between systems, there is also considerable interobserver variation within a system (D'Allaire et al. 1988). At least one reason for this is probably the clinicians' unwillingness to score a herd as having PAR, despite a degree of mild atrophy, when there has never been any clinical evidence of disease. Today, bacteriologic or serologic tests are necessary to confirm downgrading of the health status of a herd (e.g., when toxigenic *P. multocida* is present). The cutoff point between normality and being affected is imprecise, and the condition should not be regarded as a simple all-or-nothing phenomenon (Done 1985). The situation in many herds with only mild atrophy probably represents only the effects of a normally transient and often-resolving hypoplastic rhinitis without the progression characteristic of clinical PAR (see Definition above).

Objective measures of assessing atrophy on a continuous scale have also been developed, including a morphometric index (area of free space as a percentage of total cross-sectional area of snout section) (Done et al. 1984). Such systems provide parametric data suitable for analysis, but as diagnostic tools they offer few advantages over subjective snout scoring (Collins et al. 1988, 1989).

Histologic Changes

Depending on the type of process active at the time of necropsy, acute, subacute, or chronic histologic changes may be observed.

The pathognomonic lesion of PAR by toxigenic *P. multocida* is a fibrous replacement of the bony plates of the ventral conchae (Done 1983a; Elling and Pedersen 1983; Martineau-Doize et al. 1990). Additionally, there may be a variable metaplasia of the respiratory epithelium and inflammation of the mucosal lamina propria; subacute cases of rhinitis in conventional pigs will show various mixtures of degenerative, inflammatory, dystrophic, and reparative processes. In SPF pigs infection with toxigenic *P. multocida* does not induce a typical inflammatory reaction but does induce toxic alterations. The histologic changes in pigs with PAR that show retarded growth have been described by Yoshikawa and Hanada (1981).

Lesions in parenchymatous organs may also be present in cases of severe infection with toxigenic *P. multocida* (de Jong 1983a; Rutter 1983). Parenteral injections with *P. multocida* toxin induced liver cirrhosis, renal failure, marked decrease of peripheral blood lymphocytes without lysis, and growth retardation (Becker et al. 1986; Williams et al. 1986; Cheville et al. 1988).

Bronchopneumonia. Pneumonic lesions occur principally in young pigs and have a characteristic scattered monolobular or bilobular distribution, mainly in the apical and cardiac lobes. Affected areas are initially dark red, become brown, then yellowish brown after a time and develop a contracted appearance. The lesions are associated with the *B. bronchiseptica* element of the complex.

Histologically, the pneumonic lesions in bordetellosis are characteristic. Detailed descriptions of the histopathology of experimental *B. bronchiseptica* bronchopneumonia are given by Duncan et al. (1966b) and Meyer and Beamer (1973) in conventional and germfree swine, respectively. The lesions from these experimental cases are similar to those of field cases. Briefly, the most severe cases affect the pneumonic vasculature, and there are areas of extensive alveolar hemorrhage with necrosis and interlobular edema. In areas where hemorrhagic changes are less extensive, there is an acute inflammatory reaction with cellular infiltration, principally with neutrophils. There is an accompanying bronchiolitis with neutrophilic exudate. As the lesions age, vascular changes become less prominent and epithelialization of the alveoli, fibroblastic activity, and deposition of collagen occur. Large alveolar macrophages are present in some alveoli.

DIAGNOSIS

Bordetella bronchiseptica

Although the clinical signs are suggestive of infection, a definitive diagnosis of bordetellosis in pigs is only possible by the bacteriologic examination of lung washings, lungs at postmortem, or nasal secretions. Nasal secretions are best collected on cotton-tipped swabs with either metal or elastic plastic stems. Wooden-stemmed swabs and swabs with quick-breaking plastic stems should be avoided, since sudden movement of the pig may break the shaft. The live pig should be adequately restrained and the external nares cleaned. Swabs are carefully inserted in a naris with a gentle rotating motion and pushed carefully along the ventral meatus so as to avoid trauma to the delicate turbinates. The swabs are then submitted for laboratory examination, preferably in a bacteriologic transport medium or a phosphate buffered saline solution (PBS) under cool conditions (±4°C).

The organism grows well on blood agar or MacConkey agar plus 1% glucose, but its isolation from field specimens is often complicated by the overgrowth of other organisms (Smith and Baskerville 1979); hence, culture on more selective media is recommended. Procedures for isolating and identifying the organism from field specimens from pigs are given by Farrington and Switzer (1977), Smith and Baskerville (1979), and Rutter (1981). Selective media to isolate both *B. bronchiseptica* and *P. multocida* on the same plate are discussed below under the detection of *P. multocida*.

The serologic diagnosis of bordetella infection by the detection of agglutinating antibodies in the serum has been described. The various methods of antigen preparation, details of some of the tests employed, and their interpretation have been reviewed by Giles and Smith (1983). Agglutinating antibodies to *B. bronchiseptica* are widespread in the pig population, but although their detection by serologic tests can be useful in making a herd diagnosis of bordetellosis, these are not commonly employed for routine diagnostic purposes, since, practically, serologic tests offer few advantages over the culture of nasal swabs.

Pasteurella multocida

Clinical Diagnosis. When the full range of clinical signs is present, a preliminary diagnosis of PAR on clinical signs alone is possible, but none of the snout deformations by themselves are pathognomonic for PAR. Animals showing lateral deviation of the snout and/or marked BS, especially at an age of 10–12 weeks, almost always have pronounced turbinate atrophy (Bercovich and de Jong 1976; de Jong 1985; Kobisch and Pennings 1989). However, when these signs are not apparent or are of decreasing prevalence (e.g., following treatment), it is not possible for even experienced observers to assess the extent of turbinate atrophy in the live animal. The presence of a few twisted snouts or sneezing alone is not sufficient evidence to justify a diagnosis of PAR (see Definition).

Radiographic Diagnosis. Radiographic examination of the snout has been developed to facilitate improved diagnosis of turbinate atrophy in the live animal; a suitable procedure is described by Done (1976). In some countries this method has enjoyed widespread popularity, but it is beset with technical difficulties and problems in interpretation of the radiographs. The method may not detect mild lesions reliably, and its value has been questioned (Eikelenboom et al. 1978; Webbon et al. 1978); furthermore, pigs must be sedated, anesthetized, or physically immobilized, and the procedure is costly and time-consuming. With experience, however, some observers consider radiographic examination a useful aid (Schöss 1983). The same disadvantages apply to rhinoscopy (Plonait et al. 1980). Modern methods such as computerized tomography, used as a diagnostic tool for PAR, facilitate the macroscopic grading of the nasal structures in live pigs of any age (Jolie et al. 1990).

Postmortem Diagnosis. The prevalence and severity of turbinate atrophy are best estimated by examination of snouts after slaughter. Snouts should be transversely sectioned at the level of the first/second upper premolar; sectioning cranial to this should be avoided, since this will reveal a different pattern of turbinate development. Pigs of 4 weeks old or older that died during weaning or prefattening can present turbinate atrophy at an early stage, and cross-sectioning can be carried out with a simple iron saw by qualified local veterinarians during regular herd inspections. Material from tonsils, lungs, and the nose can be sent to laboratories to ensure a proper diagnosis. To make a preliminary herd diagnosis, pigs have to be examined at slaughter at regular intervals. As many pigs as practical should be examined; between 20 and 30 per time is suggested by Goodwin (1988). Atrophy is scored on subjective grading systems (Bendixen 1971; Anon. 1978; Done 1983a, b; de Jong 1985). With low levels it is not possible to define a single cutoff point as representing freedom from PAR. An acceptable level for an individual (toxigenic *P. multocida*–infected) herd is a matter of reasoned clinical judgment but must be one in which the economic effects of the disease are minimal (Goodwin 1988). A monitoring scheme that could serve as a useful model with a diagrammatic representation of snout grading is described by Goodwin (1980). Computerized versions have been developed by Collins et al. (1988), Barfod et al. (1990), and Jolie and Thacker (1990).

Cultural and Serologic Diagnosis. Today, a definite diagnosis of PAR cannot be based solely on clinical and pathomorphologic observations but requires laboratory tests (Pedersen 1983). Detection of the two most significant bacterial pathogens is possible by the culture of nasal and tonsillar swabs or tonsillar biopsies. The live pig should be adequately restrained and the external nares cleaned; slender cotton-tipped swabs with plastic or metal shafts should be inserted with slight rotation deep into both sides of the nasal cavity. Swabbing the tonsillar surface or tonsillar biopsies can aid the isolation and differentiation of *P. multocida* and toxigenic *P. multocida* (Van Leengoed et al. 1986; de Jong et al. 1988; Ackermann et al. 1994). Swabs should be transported to the laboratory within 24 hours, preferably in a transport medium under cooled conditions (4–8°C). Nutrient transport media that support the growth of fast-growing contaminants are best avoided, but sterile phosphate-buffered saline is suitable (Pedersen 1983).

Detection of *P. multocida* (and *B. bronchiseptica*). Special selective media are described on which both *B. bronchiseptica* and *P. multocida* can grow (de Jong and Borst 1985; de Jong 1994; Moore 1994).

The cultural isolation of *P. multocida* from nasal swabs and the testing of their toxigenicity are detailed by Pedersen (1983). When the nasal cavity is heavily infected with *P. multocida*, the organism can be recovered on simple blood agars (Smith and Baskerville 1983). However, field specimens frequently contain low numbers of organisms, and the other nasal flora may mask the presence of *P. multocida* on nonselective media. Mouse inoculation greatly improves the recovery rate from field specimens, but a good in vitro method would be preferable. Some selective media are described by Smith and Baskerville (1983), Rutter and Luther (1984), de Jong and Borst (1985), Leblanc et al. (1986a, b), Chanter and Rutter (1989), Avril et al. (1990), and de Jong (1994). Evidence suggests that the tonsil is the preferred habitat for *P. multocida* in the pig, and improved detection rates may be achieved by the collection of tonsillar swabs or biopsies in combination with nasal swabs (de Jong et al. 1988). Tonsils and lungs can also be collected in the slaughterhouse and examined in the laboratory. Swabs from noses of pigs sampled after immersion in the hot-water tank are unsatisfactory for the detection of toxigenic *P. multocida* (Chanter and Rutter 1989).

When clinical severe PAR is first detected in pigs, infection by toxigenic *P. multocida* actually occurred weeks or months earlier. The detection of the toxigenic *P. multocida* from these pigs can be difficult. Therefore, it is recommended to also examine clinically less severely affected pigs in such groups or pens.

Detection of *P. multocida* Toxin. The central etiologic importance of toxigenic strains of *P. multocida* is that classification of field isolates into PAR toxin-positive or toxin-negative strains is necessary in understanding the epidemiology of the disease. The toxin is thermolabile, dermonecrotic in the guinea pig and lethal for the mouse when administered intraperitoneally. All three tests give broadly comparable results; the methods are described by de Jong (1980, 1985), Pedersen (1983), and Rutter (1983), respectively. An in vitro system of detection by assessing the cytopathogenic effect in monolayers of Vero cells or embryonic bovine lung cells has been developed (Pennings and Storm 1984; Rutter and Luther

1984). Today, enzyme-linked immunosorbent assays (ELISAs) are replacing the earlier tests (Foged et al. 1988). DNA probes have been developed to detect the gene responsible for toxin production in toxigenic *P. multocida* (Andresen et al. 1990; Kamps et al. 1990; Lax and Chanter 1990). The use of polymerase chain reaction (PCR) tests is becoming of interest in diagnosis and in proposals for eradication of toxigenic *P. multocida* in PAR-diseased herds (Nagai et al. 1994; de Jong 1994; de Jong et al. 1996).

P. multocida Serotypes. Determination of the capsular serotype of *P. multocida* is also often useful for epidemiological purposes; most toxin-positive strains are type D, although toxin-positive type A strains also occur. In some regions the toxigenic type D is prevalent, in others it seems to be type A (Cowart and Backstrom 1984; Iwamatsu and Sawada 1988; Pijoan et al. 1988). The usual method of capsular serotyping is the indirect hemagglutination test with rabbit antisera (Carter 1955). The hyaluronidase test (Carter and Rundell 1975) and acriflavine test (Carter and Subronto 1973) are simpler methods for the detection of type A and D strains, respectively, but not all porcine isolates are typeable by these methods (Pedersen 1983). Piliation, hemagglutination, and capsular serotypes did not show a correlation with toxin production (Trigo and Pijoan 1988). An atypical *P. multocida* strain producing a toxin similar to the dermonecrotic toxin of *P. multocida* subsp. *multocida* has been described in cattle (Kamp et al. 1990). Not only the capsule and somatic structure are of epidemiological interest; the phage types and plasmid types are also interesting tools with which to follow the distribution pattern of the different toxigenic strains (Lugtenberg et al. 1984; Nielsen and Rosdahl 1988, 1990; Hoje et al. 1990; Rubies et al. 1996).

Serologic Tests. Although agglutinating antibodies to *B. bronchiseptica* can be detected in pig serum (Giles and Smith 1983), this is of little diagnostic value. Serologic tests to detect antibodies against toxigenic *P. multocida* resulting from vaccination or infection have been described (de Jong and Akkermans 1986; Bechmann and Schöss 1990; Foged et al. 1990; Schimmelpfennig 1990). The toxin in natural infection is a weak immunogen, and antibodies to it take 3 months or longer to detect and only then in some pigs (Bording et al. 1990; Van Diemen et al. 1994b). This means that serology may only be of importance in detecting antibodies in the sow population. A skin test has been described to detect antibodies in sow herds that have been infected (Schimmelpfennig and Jahn 1988; Breuer and Schimmelpfennig 1990).

In the skin test the purified concentrated toxin is applied intradermally in one or different concentrations. Neutralization of the toxin indicates the presence of antibodies as a response to the infection or vaccination with toxigenic *P. multocida*. Difficulties in application and in the identification of the correct amount of toxin per dose have limited the use of the skin test in practice.

Differential Diagnosis. Sneezing in young pigs occurs in herds with active PAR, but it is not diagnostic itself, since it regularly occurs due to uncomplicated bordetellosis or porcine cytomegalovirus infection (Rondhuis et al. 1980). Both agents are widely spread in the pig industry and can cause severe mucous membrane damage, which is necessary for colonization by toxigenic *P. multocida*. The frequency of severe sneezing can be used in clinical monitoring of PAR (Kobisch and Pennings 1989). Influenza, PRRS, and pseudorabies are other viruses causing damage to the nasal mucosa.

A variety of other conditions (reviewed by Done 1977) may cause facial deformity in pigs; these are likely to cause confusion in clinical and postmortem diagnosis, since malformations of the turbinates can be observed. A localized bacterial infection entering via wounds may produce a paranasal abscess (bull nose) in young pigs.

Problems with Diagnosis. Should pigs from a herd with no clinically apparent disease that have no obvious growth retardation but show mild turbinate atrophy at slaughter be considered to be suffering from PAR or NPAR? It is suggested that when BS, lateral deviation, and poor growth are obvious within the herd and atrophy at slaughter is marked, the herd should be suspected of having clinical PAR. Conversely, where no turbinate atrophy is seen in slaughtered pigs, the herd must be regarded as clinically free from PAR. However, defining the status of herds where mild atrophy occurs in the absence of clinical disease presents problems, since there is no satisfactory single cutoff point between affected and unaffected herds (Goodwin 1988). These low levels of atrophy have been regarded as representing degrees of subclinical PAR but are probably better viewed as indicating risk of developing clinical PAR. The level of atrophy deemed satisfactory or acceptable for a given enterprise is often a matter of reasoned clinical judgment. With the help of bacteriologic and serologic investigations this problem can be avoided (see Definition).

BS can occur as a breed-associated characteristic in certain lines of the Large White/Yorkshire breed. Breed-associated BS increases with age and cannot be influenced by a medication program intended to combat the influence of a bordetella and/or a pasteurella infection in these pigs. The breed-associated level of BS can easily be assessed by such a medication method. All BS grading higher than this lower genetic level may be a result of PAR or NPAR. A warning limit can be chosen (e.g., at an age of 8–12 weeks) to allow early selection of clinically diseased animals and to limit further damage in grower or fattening pigs as well as in the younger pigs that will follow such groups.

Breed-associated BS is easily distinguished from PAR by the absence of turbinate atrophy, except where regeneration of the turbinates has occurred.

Sows and gilts kept in stalls often bite, chew, or play with bars or drinkers, and this can give rise to asymmetric bone development causing protrusion of the lower jaw or mandibular misalignment. These conditions can be confused with the facial deformity of AR, especially in the older pig, but careful inspection should reveal that the lower jaw is abnormally placed rather than that the snout is shortened or laterally deviated. A useful technique is to draw an imaginary line between the center of the ears and eyes and project it forward onto the snout. Some sows keep their snouts more to one side. This can cause misinterpretation. By pressing the molar teeth on top of each other and comparing the diastema between the incisor teeth in the upper and lower jaw, distortion can be noticed clinically at an early stage. This method can be carried out in combination with the BS-grading method. With thin nasal swabs an increase in internasal space can be observed clinically, but some experience is necessary for the interpretation.

TREATMENT

The effective treatment of an outbreak of NPAR or PAR requires a selected combination of management, environmental, chemotherapeutic, and vaccination procedures. No one combination is equally applicable to all affected herds. The overall aims of treatment are (1) to reduce the prevalence and load of the important specific bacterial infections (bordetellosis and pasteurellosis) in young pigs by sow vaccination, medication of feed, and antibiotic treatment of piglets; (2) to treat growing pigs with an acute rhinitis to reduce the weight of bacterial infection and severity of the hypoplastic changes and maintain efficient growth and feed utilization; and (3) to manipulate housing, ventilation, and management to improve the overall environment for the pigs (de Jong and Bartelse 1980; Smith 1983).

Management and therapeutic measures to control bordetellosis in commercial pig herds are required or usually deemed necessary by experienced clinicians only in herds where this infection is associated with clinically significant disease, whether rhinitis, bronchopneumonia, or infectious PAR. The mere presence of the infection within an ordinary commercial herd is not, on its own, sufficient ground for initiating therapeutic measures against it.

The sulfonamides were the first drugs to be used successfully in this respect (Switzer 1963) and are still widely employed, either alone or in combination with antibiotics, or potentiated with trimethoprim. Bronchopneumonia in piglets should be treated with parenteral injections of sulfadoxine or sulfadiazine at 12.5 mg/kg with trimethoprim at 2.5 mg/kg daily for 3–5 days.

Alternatives to the sulfonamide drugs have been examined. Most porcine isolates of *B. bronchiseptica* appear to be sensitive to the tetracyclines (Sisak et al. 1978; Smith et al. 1980; Pijpers et al. 1989), and these drugs, particularly a long-acting formulation of oxytetracycline given by parenteral injection to young pigs, appear to be suitable for the control of bordetellosis.

The new fluoroquinolones are also active against porcine *B. bronchiseptica* (Hannan et al. 1989).

Antibiotic Resistance

The in vitro activity of 12 sulfonamide drugs against *B. bronchiseptica* was compared by Mengelers et al. (1989), who showed that the minimum inhibitory concentration (MIC)50 ranged from 0.5 to 8 μg/mL. Against a selection of the pathogenic respiratory bacteria of swine, sulfamethoxazole had the highest antimicrobial activity, and sulfamezathine had an overall low activity. Isolates of *B. bronchiseptica* from pigs have been shown to have transmissible R factors that carry antibiotic resistance (Terakado et al. 1974).

Medication

Sows and Piglets. To reduce the prevalence and severity of nasal infection acquired from dams, the feed of the sow can be medicated during the final month of gestation. Sulfadimidine (sulfamethazine) (400–2000 g/ton) and oxytetracycline (400–1000 g/ton) are the products most widely used.

Suckling piglets are best medicated by strategic injections of antibacterial agents in therapeutic dosages four to eight times during the first 3–4 weeks of life. The most useful are potentiated sulfonamides, oxytetracycline, and penicillin/streptomycin.

If bordetellosis is the major infection in suckling piglets, potentiated sulfonamides are the drugs of choice (12.5 mg/kg sulfadiazine or sulfadoxine + 2.5 mg/kg trimethoprim). Injections of oxytetracycline (20–80 mg/kg) once or twice a week are also clinically effective for PAR (de Jong and Oosterwoud 1977; Mefford et al. 1983). The long-acting formulation (20–80 mg/kg) may be the preferred product and is best given once or twice a week during each of the first 3 or 4 weeks of life. If the organism is not resistant, the drug is effective against pasteurellosis, since, experimentally, long-acting oxytetracycline has reduced the prevalence of nasal infection and the severity of turbinate atrophy induced by *P. multocida* (Gois et al. 1983b); although other researchers prefer doxycycline (Pijpers et al. 1988). In the Netherlands, intranasal spraying of oxytetracycline in a 5% solution is used in piglets twice a week, when starting the treatment. If effective after 2–3 months, a reduction from twice to once a week can be recommended (de Jong 1983b). This withdrawal of medication also depends on the average antibody titer against the toxin of *P. multocida* in the dams resulting from the vaccination program.

Other antibiotics to which *P. multocida* may be sensitive and that are frequently used in therapeutic concentrations against pneumonia caused by pasteurellosis include penicillin/streptomycin (20,000 IU/10–25 mg/kg), tylosin (10–25 mg/kg), lincomycin/spectinomycin (50/100 mg/kg), ampicillin (10–20 mg/kg), amoxycillin (10–20 mg/kg), spiramycin (25 mg/kg), quinolone derivatives (0.5–5 mg/kg), cephalosporins (1–5 mg/kg), and tiamulin (10–20 mg/kg) (Plonait and Bickhardt 1988). The benefits of the treatments have not been critically evaluated as far as nasal and pulmonary protection and/or elimination of the toxigenic *P. multocida* are concerned.

Weaners and Growers. The PAR in weaned pigs that leads eventually to marked turbinate atrophy at slaughter can be controlled to some extent by medication of weaner and/or grower rations or by the addition of antibiotics to the drinking water. Such medication also assists in the maintenance of growth and efficiency of feed utilization in the face of active PAR, but as might be expected, medication is always much more effective when the pigs' environment is improved. Various antibacterial agents alone or in combination are effective. The sulfonamides are frequently included in rations because of their known efficacy against bordetellosis. Their use and the problems of the development of drug resistance are of great concern.

Well-established drugs or combinations suitable for the control of PAR are (1) sulfadimidine (sulfamethazine) (400–2000 g/ton) in feed or sulfathiazole (0.08–0.13 g/L) in the drinking water; (2) chlortetracycline (165 g/ton), sulfadimidine (sulfamethazine) (165 g/ton), and penicillin G (83 g/ton) in feed; (3) tylosin (100 g/ton) and sulfadimidine (sulfamethazine) (100 g/ton) in feed; (4) carbadox (50 g/ton) and sulfadimidine (sulfamethazine) (100 g/ton) in feed; (5) oxytetracycline in feed (400 g/ton) or in drinking water (0.18 g/L) (Giles 1986). Various other antibacterial agents, alone or in combination, also have broadly similar beneficial effects on PAR lesions and help to maintain growth. For example, the following have been demonstrated as clinically effective in feed: lincomycin (220 g/ton); lincomycin (220 g/ton) and sulfamethazine (550 g/ton); lincomycin, spectinomycin, and amoxicillin trihydrate (10–20 g/ton).

When a number of drugs are used in feed, a decrease of bioavailability can occur, which may result from the amount of calcium, the feed processing, and the water ration given to the treated pigs (Counotte et al. 1984; Froe 1990; Sutter and Wanner 1990). The availability of some of these drugs and the regulations regarding their use in food-producing animals vary between countries.

Selection of an appropriate antibiotic or combination depends partly on cost, legislation, and clinical experience but should also be related to the antibiotic sensitivity patterns of *B. bronchiseptica* and *P. multocida* isolates and the established MICs (Pijpers et al. 1988; Fales et al. 1990; Awad-Masalmeh et al. 1994). Differences in MIC between *P. multocida* type D and type A strains may occur in the same herd (Schimmelpfennig 1990). In a severe outbreak, treatment should be directed at pigs of all age groups other than those immediately destined for slaughter; as the severity declines, reducing antibiotic use for the older fatteners should be the first priority. The appropriate withdrawal times before slaughter must always be adhered to. It is usually necessary for pigs at risk to receive medicated feed for a minimum of 4–5 weeks and frequently for longer periods, depending on the results of the vaccination program and the improvement in housing, ventilation, and management.

Vaccination

Sows. Vaccination of the sow induces a significant degree of passive colostral protection against *B. bronchiseptica* in the serum of her suckling piglets (Koshimizu et al. 1973; Smith et al. 1982); in the field, this protection will often persist until about the time of weaning. The colostral protection afforded by sow vaccination is thus an effective aid in controlling *B. bronchiseptica* infections among populations of young suckling piglets; in herds where early piglet infection occurs and rhinitis and/or bronchopneumonia develop in young pigs, sow vaccination should be recommended. Initially two doses should be given 6 and 2 weeks before farrowing, followed by revaccination at 2 weeks before each subsequent farrowing. Bordetella vaccines which induce toxin-neutralizing antibodies and pilus antibodies are of interest.

In a prolonged vaccination scheme for gilts and the sow and boar population, the number of *B. bronchiseptica* carriers is reduced. This in combination with the increased colostrum protection and all-in/all-out procedures in the farrowing and weaner sections may be helpful in producing *B. bronchiseptica*–free offspring or in reducing the *B. bronchiseptica* colonization in such populations. These procedures also reduced bordetella pneumonia. In NPAR herds the use of combined bordetella and pasteurella vaccines is not recommended, because the antibodies against the pasteurella toxin lead to suspicion of PAR in such herds. Downgrading the health status could be the result.

Vaccination of the sow with a potent *B. bronchiseptica* vaccine is an effective way to reduce the prevalence and severity of nasal bordetellosis in suckling and weaned piglets (de Jong 1985) but exerts only a limited effect on clinical PAR (Giles and Smith 1983). Pathogenic determinants important in vaccines include the toxigenic characters, the pilus-producing factor, and outer-membrane proteins. Lack of antibody to some of these properties seems to influence the reduction of *B. bronchiseptica* in sows and piglets.

B. bronchiseptica/P. multocida vaccines have been evaluated experimentally and in the field. In some countries combined vaccines are available commercially. Such vaccines have reduced the prevalence of clinical PAR (Schuller et al. 1980; Baars et al. 1982; de Jong et al. 1984) but do not eliminate the condition. As might be expected, the thermolabile toxin for *P. multocida* appears to be an important determinant in eliciting protection, because experimental vaccination of sows with crude toxin significantly protected their offspring against PAR (Baars et al. 1982, 1986; Pedersen and Barfod 1982). The specific importance of the toxoid fraction has been elucidated (Nagy et al. 1986; Foged et al. 1989; Frymus et al. 1989; Chanter and Rutter 1990).

The antigens and mechanisms of protection against toxigenic *P. multocida* infection and associated disease have yet to be fully defined; reports show that toxoid preparations of *P. multocida* produce an antitoxin response, with an effect on colonization (Chanter and Rutter 1990). Claims made for *B. bronchiseptica* vaccines in the control of AR were not fully substantiated in field use (Giles and Smith 1983); thus, a rush to develop further combined vaccines without full appraisal of the required antigens is undesirable.

Some of the currently available combined *B. bronchiseptica/P. multocida* vaccines may be of benefit in controlling bordetellosis and toxigenic pasteurellosis and in reducing the prevalence and severity of PAR when combined with housing and management changes (de Jong et al. 1984). The marked reduction in toxigenic *P. multocida* in the nose following vaccination with a potent toxoid vaccine requires further evaluation to determine whether the expression of high antibody levels can eradicate toxigenic *P. multocida*. Vaccination of sows with combined vaccines can be as effective as piglet medication. However, neither procedure constitutes a means of protection against the condition nor necessarily obviates the need for medication. Such a vaccination program, once started in an infected herd, has to be maintained, at least for many years.

Piglets. Vaccination of older pigs undoubtedly produces an active humoral response but its value is debatable, since the main effects of the infection occur in younger animals. Specific measures against *B. bronchiseptica* infection should be directed toward preventing the infection from arising in suckling pigs (by management, sow vaccination, or chemotherapy) or mitigating its effects in young pigs (by management and/or chemotherapy).

B. bronchiseptica vaccine has been widely employed. Although some observers have concluded that it has little benefit against clinical PAR and is generally less effective than sow vaccination (Giles and Smith 1982, 1983), in some countries (notably the United States) the procedure nevertheless still enjoys fairly widespread use. *B. bronchiseptica/P. multocida* bacterin vaccines are also widely employed, but the composition of many of them means that they may be of little benefit in the field. In a study in which both sows and piglets were inoculated with a combined vaccine, Mefford et al. (1983) demonstrated that vaccination alone did not influence turbinate atrophy and only marginally improved profitability.

Only vaccination of the piglets born of inadequately vaccinated or unvaccinated dams is of value in the case of *P. multocida* toxoid vaccines. When sows are properly vaccinated and produce good levels of antitoxic antibodies, piglets may not respond to vaccination. If the dams show good titers, the colostral protection in pigs can last for 3–4 months. Vaccinations of the young breeding stock can be started after this age. A high antitoxin titer seems to reduce colonization by toxigenic *P. multocida*.

The additional use of therapeutics (e.g., long-acting oxytetracycline) in piglets significantly reduced turbinate atrophy at slaughter and markedly improved profitability (Pejsak et al. 1990). Furthermore, some commercially available vaccines contain neither toxigenic strains nor *P. multocida* toxoid, the manufacturers only claiming efficacy against pneumonic pasteurellosis.

Housing and Husbandry

Medication and vaccination procedures should never be introduced without concurrent attempts to improve swine management and husbandry. Although the noninfectious factors that contribute to the severity of PAR are inadequately defined quantitatively, steps should always be taken to reduce their influence. All-in/all-out systems are favored for farrowing, weaner, and preferably fattener management; the age of the sow herd can be allowed to rise and the introduction of large numbers of infected new gilts can be avoided; stocking density can be reduced; strict hygiene measures should be implemented; and correct ventilation rates should be maintained to reduce the airborne concentration of bacterial pathogens, noxious gases, and dust. Steps should also be taken to reduce factors that stress young pigs, including large temperature variations, chilling, and drafts. Replacement breeding stock should not only be free from clinical signs of disease but also be raised in herds free from infections with toxigenic *P. multocida*; introduced weaners should be free from active rhinitis and the associated sneezing and typical BS. Newly purchased stock should originate from herds free from toxigenic *P. multocida*, be isolated (quarantined), be tested bacteriologically or serologically for freedom from toxigenic *P. multocida*, and be integrated slowly. Severely affected pigs with obvious and severe growth retardation should be culled. Vaccination programs should be started if breeding stock free from toxigenic *P. multocida* infection is brought into infected herds. Vaccination can reduce colonization by toxigenic *P. multocida* when infection cannot be avoided. Such an AR vaccination program needs to be carried out continuously in the

whole sow population of the infected herd. Effective vaccination with potent vaccines in sows alone can also limit the economic damage in weaners. The risk to breeders, multipliers, and fatteners of becoming infected by toxigenic *P. multocida* can be limited by asking for or giving guarantees that the pigs bought or sold originate directly from herds certified free from the organism. This certification can be carried out under governmental legislation. Only by means of such a system of enforced restrictions can the spread of toxigenic *P. multocida* via sales or auctions be prevented.

Depopulation

Depopulation and restocking with swine from a source known to be free from toxigenic *P. multocida* are often the only viable solution. Buildings should be thoroughly cleaned and disinfected, then fumigated and left empty for 2 weeks to 2 months, depending on the efficacy and quality of the hygiene program. Eradication of rats, mice, and birds must be carried out properly and continually. Replacement pigs should be bought from sources known to be free from PAR and toxigenic *P. multocida* infection, based on clinical, abattoir, bacteriologic, and/or serologic monitoring.

PREVENTION

Since *B. bronchiseptica* is widely prevalent in the pig population, its total exclusion from a herd is only possible by the development of an SPF system or by medicated and segregated early-weaning methods and the strict maintenance of an effective barrier. *B. bronchiseptica* is often one of the first agents to infect an SPF herd.

Vaccination

B. bronchiseptica vaccines have been developed and used in several countries in an attempt to control both the infection and the clinical condition AR by immunologic methods. Killed whole-culture vaccines with aluminum salt adjuvants were the first to be available commercially and have been licensed for use in several countries since the 1970s. Other types of vaccine have also been investigated, including live avirulent strains (Krüger and Horsch 1992) and subunit vaccines, but generally have not been used widely in practice. Killed whole-culture adjuvanted vaccines were at one time widely employed in pig herds because several reports, mainly from the United States and Japan (e.g., Nakase et al. 1976; Goodnow 1977; Goodnow et al. 1979), indicated that such products were highly effective in the control of field outbreaks of clinical PAR. In Europe, however, these benefits were much less obvious (Bercovich and Oosterwoud 1977; Pedersen and Barfod 1977; Giles and Smith 1982). Later, further studies from the United States also concluded that such bordetella vaccines are of limited efficacy in the overall control of PAR. A critical review of bordetella vaccines (Giles and Smith 1983) concluded that, as single antigens, their beneficial effects in the control of PAR are indeed limited and the previous claims for their usefulness overstated. In the light of new knowledge, combined vaccines have been developed consisting of *B. bronchiseptica/P. multocida* bacterins or *B. bronchiseptica* bacterin combined with *P. multocida* toxoid. Such vaccines are of use in the field, provided their limitations are fully realized by the clinician.

Single bordetella vaccines should be used to limit the influence of bordetellosis or NPAR but not in PAR-diseased herds.

PAR can be prevented effectively only by rearing swine free from the specific infections required for disease to develop. The adoption of an SPF system of production and the maintenance of an effective microbiologic barrier are the only sure ways of achieving this. Medicated early weaning (Alexander et al. 1980) may well be a viable alternative to the established methods of producing SPF stock free from toxigenic *P. multocida* (James 1989; Blaha et al. 1990; Larsen et al. 1990). Traditional vaccination or medication regimes applied to infected herds are not likely to create herds free from the infections; thus, the infected herds pose a serious threat to free herds in their neighborhood and also pose risks to other branches of animal production, such as poultry, rabbits, goats, sheep, and cattle (Nielsen et al. 1986; Frymus et al. 1996). In a preventive disease control program, eradication schemes have to be carried out in all types of herds and in all kinds of animals infected with toxigenic *P. multocida*. *B. bronchiseptica* appears to be very widespread in the pig population, but the prevalence of infection with toxigenic strains of *P. multocida* is less well defined. A positive correlation exists between the prevalence of toxigenic strains of *P. multocida* in a herd and the known occurrence of PAR (de Jong 1983b; Nielsen 1983; Pedersen 1983; Cowart and Backstrom 1984; Leblanc et al. 1986b; Bechmann and Schöss 1988; Cowart et al. 1989), although the mere presence of this infection does not always mean clinical disease. The potential risk of clinical PAR developing in a herd could be eliminated simply by ensuring that pigs are free from toxigenic *P. multocida* infection. Therefore, it is desirable to monitor breeding herds for this pathogen and to take steps to reduce its dissemination and introduction into unaffected herds. It is definitely beneficial to maintain herds with no history of PAR and low scores of atrophy at slaughter behind effective barriers or to bring in pigs only from sources known to be free from the condition. Breeding companies that sell and export pigs from infected herds, inadequately monitored for infectious diseases like PAR, are involved more and more in financial claims by new clients who will not accept the cost of medication and vaccination and the degradation of the health status of their own breeding herds. Because aerogenic spread has been described (Baekbo and Nielsen 1988; Stehmann et al. 1989) and spread of infection may be possible from surrounding herds, special attention to

air filtration and decontamination systems (Rutter et al. 1986; Voets et al. 1986b) could be necessary if distances become too small (probably within 200–2000 m, depending on the size of the surrounding herds). PAR has also been found in outdoor systems. Prevention of toxigenic *P. multocida* infection in outdoor systems can be difficult. Prevention by artificial insemination seems possible, but some risks exist when the antibiotics used in the semen diluter do not eliminate the toxigenic pasteurellae (Overby 1990).

Monitoring

Commercial producers should be aware of the current disease status of their herds. This applies to herds that have past or present evidence for the clinical condition, as well as to producers who need to monitor the effects of control measures or whose herds have remained free from the condition and who appreciate early warning of any change in herd status. Hence, ideally, herds need monitoring systems that can quantify not only the presence but also the effects of PAR (Done 1983b), especially in the case of an infected herd. Since this disease is not a simple all-or-nothing condition, merely relying on the presence of clinical disease disguises moderate to low levels of infection and recognizes it too late for the introduction of prophylactic measures.

Parameters that can be usefully measured are indirect production or economic data, such as liveweight gain or efficiency of feed utilization, and clinical/pathological data related to PAR, including the amount of sneezing, the incidence of facial distortion, and the two most useful criteria, the prevalence and extent of BS in weaned pigs and the prevalence and severity of turbinate atrophy at slaughter. The latter is the most popular in some countries. In large, modern slaughterhouses the gathering of snouts and cross sections is difficult; in such situations a scoring system on longitudinally opened snouts can be useful (Visser et al. 1988). Sophisticated methods of monitoring have been developed, one of which is the plotting of cumulative-sum charts with decision boundaries, since it gives early signals of deterioration or improvement. Done (1983b) has reviewed the methods of monitoring PAR. Use of computer technology in slaughterhouses and on pig farms means that important disease-monitoring systems may be effectively employed without laborious clerical work (Collins et al. 1988). Because the antibody titer against the toxin of *P. multocida* correlates with increased protection against turbinate atrophy (Sorensen et al. 1990), serologic monitoring becomes of interest in determining a possible increase in PAR risk when a decrease in the titers occurs in herds with a sow vaccination program. A program in which only sows are vaccinated can also protect the pigs during the fattening period. Recent investigations have shown a relationship between antitoxin titers and some protection against colonization by toxigenic pasteurellae (Chanter and Rutter 1990). Modern methods for the detection of toxigenic *P. multocida* by DNA probes from samples of noses, tonsils, or lungs may soon become useful in monitoring systems (Kamps et al. 1990). Positive results have already been achieved by bacteriologic (Schöss 1982; Schöss and Thiel 1984; de Jong et al. 1988) or serologic monitoring (de Jong et al. 1988; Bechmann and Schöss 1990; Foged et al. 1990; Schimmelpfennig 1990).

Toxigenic *P. multocida* can be eliminated from infected breeding farms after intensive vaccination for a period of more than 5 years. These regularly vaccinated sows produce high anti–*P. multocida* toxin titers. During this period the replacement gilts and boars must be bought from herds free from toxigenic *P. multocida*. The replacements should be introduced into the infected sow population only after being vaccinated several times with an atrophic rhinitis toxoid (ART) vaccine. The herd vaccination program needs to be continued until the last sow from the infected population has left the farm, which generally takes about 5 years. Methods to shorten such periods by selecting and slaughtering the toxigenic *P. multocida* carriers are being developed with the help of the new PCR techniques. First attempts have been partially successful (de Jong 1994; de Jong et al. 1994, 1996; de Jong and Braamskamp 1994).

Selecting carrier sows in nonvaccinating herds by bacteriological procedures and by the (DAKO) ELISA test or the PCR test and removing them have been described as successful in creating infection-free sow herds (Alt et al. 1996).

REFERENCES

Ackermann MR, De Bey MC, Register KB, Larson D J, Kinyon J M. 1994. Tonsil and turbinate colonization by toxigenic and nontoxigenic strains of *Pasteurella multocida* in conventionally raised Iowa swine. Proc Int Congr Pig Vet Soc 13:162.

Alexander TJL, Thornton K, Boon G, Lysons RJ, Gush AF. 1980. Medicated early weaning to obtain pigs free from pathogens endemic in the herd of origin. Vet Rec 106:114.

Alt M, Meyer K, Schöss P. 1996. Eradication of progressive atrophic rhinitis by bacteriological and serological examination. Proc Int Congr Pig Vet Soc 14:246.

Andresen LO, Petersen SK, Christiansen C, Nielsen JP. 1990. Studies on the location of the *Pasteurella multocida* toxin gene, tox A. Proc Int Congr Pig Vet Soc 11:60.

Anon. 1954. New pig disease in Britain. Vet Rec 66:316.

———. 1978. Atrophic Rhinitis: A System of Snout Grading. Ministry of Agriculture, Fisheries and Food Booklet LPD 51. Pinner, UK.

Avril JL, Donnio PY, Pouedras P. 1990. Selective medium for *Pasteurella multocida* and its use to detect oropharyngeal carriage in pig-breeders. J Clin Microbiol 28:1438–1440.

Awad-Masalmeh M, Kourouma G, Köfer J, and Schuh M. 1994. Investigation on *Pasteurella multocida* lesions of slaughter swine suffering from chronic respiratory disorders. Proc Int Congr Pig Vet Soc 13:172.

Baalsrud KJ. 1987. Atrophic rhinitis in goats in Norway. Vet Rec 121:350–353.

Baars JC, de Jong MF, Storm PK, Willems H, Pennings A. 1982. Atrophic rhinitis and its control with an adjuvant vaccine consisting of *B. bronchiseptica* and *P. multocida* strains. Proc Int Congr Pig Vet Soc 7:121.

Baars JC, Pennings A, Storm PK. 1986. Challenge and field experiments with an experimental atrophic rhinitis vaccine, containing *Pasteurella multocida* DNT-toxoid and *Bordetella bronchiseptica*. Proc Int Congr Pig Vet Soc 9:247.

Baekbo P. 1988. Pathogenic properties of *Pasteurella multocida* in the lung of pigs. Proc Int Congr Pig Vet Soc 10:58.

Baekbo P, Nielsen JP. 1988. Airborne *Pasteurella multocida* in pig fattening units. Proc Int Congr Pig Vet Soc 10:51.

Barfod K, Sorensen V, Nielsen JP. 1990. Methods of evaluation of the degree of atrophic rhinitis. Proc Int Congr Pig Vet Soc 11:70.

Bechmann G, Schöss P. 1988. Untersuchungen über das Vorkommen toxinbildener Pasteurella-multocida-Stamme in Tonsillen und Nasen von Ferkeln aus Rhinitis-atrophicans-unverdächtigen Zuchtbeständen. Dtsch Tierärztl Wochenschr 95:257–312.

———. 1990. Neutralizing activity against *Pasteurella multocida* toxin in sera of pigs with atrophic rhinitis. Proc Int Congr Pig Vet Soc 11:50.

Becker HN, Reed P, Woodard JC, White EC. 1986. The effects of *P. multocida* type D toxin on turbinates, body weight gains, and liver weight in piglets when injected intramuscularly. Proc Int Congr Pig Vet Soc 9:249.

Bendixen HC. 1971. Om nysesyge hos svinet. Chronic dystrophic s. Atrophic s. Infectious rhinitis in pigs. Vet Med (Suppl 1) 23:177.

Bercovich Z. 1978. Contamination and age as factors in the pathogenesis of atrophic rhinitis. Tijdschr Diergeneeskd 103:833.

Bercovich Z, de Jong MF. 1976. Shortening of the upper jaw (Brachygnathia superior) as a clinical feature of atrophic rhinitis in approximately 8-week-old piglets. Tijdschr Diergeneeskd 101:1011–1022.

Bercovich Z, Oosterwoud RA. 1977. Vaccination with *Bordetella bronchiseptica* vaccine on a farm with atrophic rhinitis: An evaluation of a field experiment. Tijdschr Diergeneeskd 102:485.

Blaha T, Schimmel D, Erler W, Burch DGS. 1990. Use of tiamulin for the production of pigs with healthy lungs, suitable for research into respiratory diseases. Proc Int Congr Pig Vet Soc 11:110.

Blobel H, Schliesser T. 1981. Handbuch der bakteriellen Infektionen bei Tieren. Band III V.E.B. Jena: Gustav Fischer Verlag.

Bollwahn W. 1988. Forensische Aspekte der Rhinitis atrophicans der Schweine. Tierärztl Prax (Suppl) 3:59–61.

Bording A, Petersen S, Foged NT. 1990. Immunological and pathological characterization of the *Pasteurella multocida* toxin and its derivates. Proc Int Congr Pig Vet Soc 11:62.

Braend M, Flatla JL. 1954. Rhinitis infectiosa atroficans hos gris. Nord Vet Med 6:81–122.

Brassinne M, Dewaele A, Gouffaux M. 1976. Intranasal infection with *Bordetella bronchiseptica* in gnotobiotic piglets. Res Vet Sci 20:162–166.

Breuer J, Schimmelpfennig H. 1990. Skin testing for *P. multocida* antitoxic antibodies in breeding herds. Proc Int Congr Pig Vet Soc 11:51.

Brown WR, Krook L, Pond WG. 1966. Atrophic rhinitis in swine: Etiology, pathogenesis and prophylaxis. Cornell Vet (Suppl 1) 56:1–107.

Cameron RDA, Giles CJ, Smith IM. 1980. The prevalence of *Bordetella bronchiseptica* and turbinate (conchal) atrophy in English pig herds in 1978–1979. Vet Rec 107:146.

Carter GR. 1955. Studies on *Pasteurella multocida*. I. A hemagglutination test for the identification of serological types. Am J Vet Res 16:481–484.

———. 1967. Pasteurellosis: *Pasteurella multocida* and Pasteurella hemolytica. Adv Vet Sci Comp Med 11:321–379.

Carter GR, Rundell SW. 1975. Identification of type A strains of *P. multocida* using staphylococcal hyaluronidase. Vet Rec 96:343.

Carter GR, Subronto P. 1973. Identification of type D strains of *Pasteurella multocida* with acriflavine. Am J Vet Res 34:293.

Chanter N, Rutter JM. 1989. Comparison of methods for the sampling and isolation of toxigenic *Pasteurella multocida* from the nasal cavity of pigs. Res Vet Sci 47:355–358.

——. 1990. The role of osteolytic toxin in colonisation by toxigenic *P. multocida*. Proc Int Congr Pig Vet Soc 11:67.

Cheville NF, Rimler RB, Thurston JR. 1988. A toxin from *Pasteurella multocida* type D causes acute hepatic necrosis in pigs. Vet Pathol 25:518–520.

Collings LA. 1983. The Pathogenicity of *Bordetella bronchiseptica* in Porcine Atrophic Rhinitis. Ph.D. diss, Univ Reading, U.K.

Collings LA, Rutter JM. 1985. Virulence of *Bordetella bronchiseptica* in the porcine respiratory tract. J Med Microbiol 19:247.

Collins MT, Backstrom L, Brim A. 1989. Turbinate perimeter ratio as an indicator of conchal atrophy for diagnosis of atrophic rhinitis in pigs. Am J Vet Res 50:421–424.

Collins MT, Backstrom LR, Conrad TA. 1988. Evaluation of semi-automatic digitizertablet snout morphometry technique. Proc Int Congr Vet Soc 10:37.

Counotte GHM, Eefting T, Bosch A. 1984. Stability and distribution of oxytetracycline hydrochloride during the manufacture and storage of pig-rearing pellets under field conditions. Tijdschr Diergeneeskd 109(9):339–344.

Cowart RP, Backstrom L. 1984. Prevalence of dermonecrotic, toxin-producing *Pasteurella multocida* strains in Illinois swine herds with varying levels of atrophic rhinitis and pneumonia. Proc Int Congr Pig Vet Soc 8:159.

Cowart RP, Backstrom L, Brim TA. 1989. *Pasteurella multocida* and *Bordetella bronchiseptica* in atrophic rhinitis and pneumonia in swine. Can J Vet Res 53(3):295–300.

Cross RF, Claflin RM. 1962. *Bordetella bronchiseptica* induced porcine atrophic rhinitis. J Am Vet Med Assoc 141:1467–1468.

D'Allaire S, Bigras-Poulin M, Paradis MA, Martineau GP. 1988. Evaluation of AR: Are the results repeatable? Proc Int Congr Pig Vet Soc 10:38.

de Jong MF. 1976–1979. Atrofische Rhinitis onderzoek. Annual Report Central Veterinary Institute, C.D.I. Postbus 65, Lelystad, Netherlands.

——. 1980. Some aspects of the study of atrophic rhinitis in pigs. Tijdschr Diergeneesk 105:711–714.

——. 1983a. Atrophic rhinitis caused by intranasal or intramuscular administration of broth-culture and broth-culture filtrates containing AR toxin of *Pasteurella multocida*. In Atrophic Rhinitis of Pigs. KB Pedersen, JC Nielsen, eds. Comm Eur Communities Rep EUR 8643 EN. Luxembourg, p. 136.

——. 1983b. Atrophic Rhinitis of Pigs. KB Pedersen, JC Nielsen, eds. Comm Eur Communities Rep EUR 8643 EN. Luxembourg.

——. 1985. Atrophic Rhinitis in Pigs. Thesis, Univ Utrecht. Elinkwijk B.V. Utrecht.

——. 1994. [Atrophic rhinitis: Problems of diagnosis.] Rhinitis atrophicans: Problematik der Diagnostik. Praktische Tierarzt 75 (Sondemummer): 82–83.

de Jong MF, Akkermans JPWM. 1986. I. Atrophic rhinitis caused by *Bordetella bronchiseptica* and *Pasteurella multocida* and the meaning of a thermolabile toxin of *P. multocida*. Vet Q 8(3):204–214.

de Jong MF, Bartelse A. 1980. The influence of management and housing on the isolation frequency of *Bordetella bronchiseptica* in piglet populations. Proc Int Congr Pig Vet Soc 6:212.

de Jong MF, Borst GHA. 1985. Selective medium for the isolation of *P. multocida* and *B. bronchiseptica*. Vet Rec 9:167.

de Jong MF, Braamskamp J. 1994. Atrophic rhinitis–herd monitoring: The investigation of toxigenic *Pasteurella multocida* from tonsils of culled sows collected in the slaughterhouse. Proc Int Congr Pig Vet Soc 13:161.

de Jong MF, Kamp E., Bokken G. 1994. Selecting sows harbouring AR toxigenic *Pasteurella multocida* by a PCR-test to eliminate progressive AR in a breeding herd. Proc Int Congr Pig Vet Soc 13:167.

de Jong MF, Kamp E, Van Der Schoot A., Von Banniseth T. 1996. Elimination of AR toxinogenic pasteurella from infected sow herds by a combination of ART vaccination and testing sows with a PCR and Elisa test. Proc Int Congr Pig Vet Soc 13:245.

de Jong MF, Nielsen JP. 1990. Definition of progressive atrophic rhinitis. Vet Rec 27:93.

de Jong MF, Oei HL, Tetenburg GJ. 1980. AR pathogenicity tests for *Pasteurella multocida* isolates. Proc Int Congr Pig Vet Soc 6:211.

de Jong MF, Oosterwoud RA. 1977. Treatment with oxytetracycline hydrochloride in the prevention of atrophic rhinitis in baby pigs. Tijdschr Diergeneeskd 102:266.

de Jong MF, Oosterwoud RA, Bouwkamp FR. 1984. A field evaluation of the Nobi-Vac AR vaccine. Proc Int Congr Pig Vet Soc 8:174.

de Jong MF, Wellenberg G, Schaake J, Frik K. 1988. Selection of pig breeding herds free from atrophic rhinitis by means of a bacteriological screening of pigs on DNT producing *Pasteurella multocida*: A field evaluation from 1981 until 1987. Proc Int Congr Pig Vet Soc 10:49.

Dirks C, Schöss P, Schimmelpfennig H. 1973. Aetiology of atrophic rhinitis of swine. Dtsch Tierärztl Wochenschr 80:342.

Done JT. 1976. Porcine atrophic rhinitis: Snout radiography as an aid to the diagnosis and detection of the disease. Vet Rec 98:23.

——. 1977. Facial deformity in pigs. Vet Annu 17:96.

——. 1983a. Atrophic rhinitis: Pathomorphological diagnosis. In Atrophic Rhinitis of Pigs. K B Pedersen, JC Nielsen, eds. Comm Eur Communities Rep EUR 8643 EN. Luxembourg, p. 3.

——. 1983b. Monitoring of atrophic rhinitis. In Atrophic Rhinitis of Pigs. KB Pedersen, NC Nielsen, eds. Comm Eur Communities Rep EUR 8643 EN. Luxembourg, p. 193.

——. 1985. Porcine atrophic rhinitis—An update. Vet Annu 25:180–191.

Done JT, Upcott DH, Frewin DC, Hebert CN. 1984. Atrophic rhinitis: Snout morphometry for quantitative assessment of conchal atrophy. Vet Rec 113:33.

Donnio PY, Avril JL, Andre PM, Vaucel J. 1991. Dermonecrotic toxin production by strains of *Pasteurella multocida* isolated from man. J Med Microbiol 34:333–337.

Doster AR, Frantz JC, Brown AL, Huseman BR, Hogg A. 1990. Effects of *Pasteurella multocida* serotype D dermonecrotic toxin in swine. Proc Int Congr Pig Vet Soc 11:72.

Douglas RGA, Ripley PH. 1984. Sneeze counts as a diagnostic aid in pig production. Vet Rec 114:321.

Dugal F, Jacques M. 1990. Enhanced adherence of *Pasteurella multocida* to porcine tracheal rings pre-infected with *Bordetella bronchiseptica*. Proc Int Congr Pig Vet Soc 11:73.

Duncan JR, Ramsey RK, Switzer WP. 1966b. Pathology of experimental *Bordetella bronchiseptica* infection in swine: Pneumonia. Am J Vet Res 27:467.

Duncan JR, Ross RK, Switzer WP, Ramsey RK. 1966a. Pathology of experimental *Bordetella bronchiseptica* infection in swine: Atrophic rhinitis. Am J Vet Res 27:457–466.

Edington N, Smith IM, Plowright W, Watt RG. 1976. Relationship of porcine cytomegalovirus and *Bordetella bronchiseptica* to atrophic rhinitis in gnotobiotic piglets. Vet Rec 98:42.

Eikelenboom G, Dik KJ, de Jong MF. 1978. De waarde van het röntgenologisch onderzoek voor de diagnostiek van Atrofische Rhinitis. Tijdschr Diergeneeskd 103:1002–1008.

Elias B, Kruger M, Ratz F. 1982. Epizootiologische Untersuchung der Rhinitis Atrophicans des Schweines. II. Biologische Eigenschaften der von Schweinen isolierten *Bordetella bronchiseptica* Stämme. Zentralbl Veterinärmed (B) 29:619–635.

Elling E, Pedersen KB. 1983. Atrophic rhinitis in pigs induced by a dermonecrotic type A strain of *Pasteurella multocida*. In Atrophic Rhinitis of Pigs. KB Pedersen, NC, eds. Nielsen. Comm Eur Communities Rep EUR 8643 EN. Luxembourg, p. 123.

FalesWH, Turk JR, Miller MA, Bean-Knudsen C, Nelson SL, Morehouse GL, Gossen HS. 1990. Antimicrobial susceptibility of *Pasteurella multocida* type D from Missouri swine. J Vet Diagn Invest 2:80–81.

Farrington DO, Switzer WP. 1977. Evaluation of nasal culturing procedures for the control of atrophic rhinitis caused by *Bordetella bronchiseptica* in swine. J Am Vet Med Assoc 170:34.

Foged NT, Nielsen JP, Barfod K. 1990. The use of ELISA determination of *Pasteurella multocida* toxin antibodies in the control of progressive atrophic rhinitis. Proc Int Congr Pig Vet Soc 11:49.

Foged NT, Nielsen JP, Jorsal SE. 1989. Protection against progressive atrophic rhinitis by vaccination with *Pasteurella multocida* toxin purified by monoclonal antibodies. Vet Rec 125:7–11.

Foged NT, Nielsen JP, Schrimer AL. 1988. Use of monoclonal antibodies in the diagnosis of atrophic rhinitis. Proc Int Congr Pig Vet Soc 10:33.

Franque. 1830. Was ist die Schnüffelkrankheit der Schweine? Dtsch Z Gesammte Tierheilkd 1:75.

FroeDL II. 1990. Oral tetracyclines: Factors affecting serum levels and efficacy. Proc Int Congr Pig Vet Soc 11:353.

Frymus T, Lésniewsky SF, Zurawski A. 1996. Possible sources of progressive atrophic rhinitis: Toxigenic pasteurella strains in species other than the pig. Proc Int Congr Pig Vet Soc 14:247.

Frymus T, Muller E, Franz BA, Petzold K. 1989. Protection by toxoid-induced antibody of gnotobiotic piglets challenged with dermonecrotic toxin of *Pasteurella multocida*. J Vet Med (B) 36:674–680.

Gagne S, Martineau-Doize B. 1993. Nasal epithelial changes induced in piglets by acetic acid and by *B. bronchiseptica*. J Comp Pathol 109:71–81.

Giles CJ. 1986. Atrophic rhinitis. In Diseases of Swine, 6th ed.AD Leman, B Straw, RD Glock, WL Mengeling, RHC Penny, E Scholl, eds. Ames: Iowa State Univ Press, pp. 455–469.

Giles CJ, Smith IM. 1982. The value of vaccinating pigs with *Bordetella bronchiseptica*. Pig Vet Soc Proc 9:61.

——. 1983. Vaccination of pigs with *Bordetella bronchiseptica*. Vet Bull 53:327.

Giles CJ, Smith IM, Baskerville AJ, Brothwell E. 1980. Clinical, bacteriological and epidemiological observations on infectious atrophic rhinitis of pigs in southern England. Vet Rec 106:25.

Glattleider L, Laval A, Espeisse O. 1996. Horizontal transmission of atrophic rhinitis. Proc Int Congr Pig Vet Soc 14:251.

Gois M, Barnes HJ, Ross RF. 1983a. Potentiation of turbinate atrophy in pigs by long-term nasal colonization with *Pasteurella multocida*. Am J Vet Res 44:372.

Gois M, Farrington DO, Barnes HJ, Ross RF. 1983b. Long acting oxytetracycline for control of induced *Pasteurella multocida* rhinitis in swine. J Am Vet Med Assoc 183:445.

Gois M, Kuksa F, Sisak F. 1977. Experimental infection of gnotobiotic piglets with *Mycoplasma hyorhinis* and *Bordetella bronchiseptica*. Zentralbl Veterinärmed 34:89.

Goodnow RA. 1977. Control of atrophic rhinitis with *Bordetella bronchiseptica* bacterin. Vet Med Small Anim Clin 72:1210.

——. 1980. Biology of *Bordetella bronchiseptica*. Microbiol Rev 44:722–738.

Goodnow RA, Shade FJ, Switzer WP. 1979. Efficacy of *Bordetella bronchiseptica* bacterin in controlling enzootic atrophic rhinitis in swine. Am J Vet Res 40:58.

Goodwin RFW. 1980. Atrophic rhinitis of pigs. Vet Rec (Pract Suppl) 2:5.

——. 1988. Monitoring for atrophic rhinitis: The problem of higher snout scores. Vet Rec 123:566–568.

Goodwin RFW, Chanter N, Rutter JM. 1990. Detection and distribution of toxigenic *Pasteurella multocida* in pig herds with different degrees of atrophic rhinitis. Vet Rec 126:452–456.

Gwatkin R. 1959. Rhinitis of swine. XII. Some practical aspects of the rhinitis complex. Can J Comp Med Vet Sci 23:338.

Gwatkin R, Plummer PJG, Byrne JL, Walker RVL. 1949. Rhinitis of swine. III. Transmission to baby pigs. Can J Comp Med Vet Sci 13:15.

——. 1951. Rhinitis of swine. V. Further studies on the aetiology of infectious atrophic rhinitis. Can J Comp Med Vet Sci 15:32.

Hanada M, Shimoda K, Tomita S, Nakase Y, Nishiyama Y. 1979. Production of lesions similar to naturally occurring atrophic rhinitis by cell-free sonicated extract of *Bordetella bronchiseptica*. Jpn J Vet Sci 41:1.

Hannan PCT, O'Hanlon PJ, Rogers NH. 1989. In vitro evaluation of various quinolone antibacterial agents against veterinary mycoplasmas and porcine respiratory bacterial pathogens. Res Vet Sci 46:202.

Harris DL, Switzer WP. 1968. Turbinate atrophy in young pigs exposed to *Bordetella bronchiseptica*, *Pasteurella multocida* and combined inoculum. Am J Vet Res 29:777.

——. 1969. Nasal and tracheal resistance of swine against reinfection by *Bordetella bronchiseptica*. Am J Vet Res 30:1161–1166.

Hoje S, Norby K, Falk K. 1990. Plasmid profiles of selected strains of *Pasteurella multocida* from pneumonic lesions of slaughter weight swine. Proc Int Congr Pig Vet Soc 11:104.

Ilina ZM, Zasukhin MI. 1975. Sib Nauch Rab, Sib Zonal' Nauchno-Issled Vet Inst, Omsk 25:76 (cited in Vet Bull 1977).

Iwamatsu S, Sawada T. 1988. Relationship between serotypes, dermonecrotic toxin production of *Pasteurella multocida* isolates and pneumonic lesions of porcine lung. Jpn J Vet Sci 50(6):1200–1206.

James A. 1989. The manifestation and attempted eradication of atrophic rhinitis in a newly established Duroc herd. Pig Vet J 23:113–121.

Jolie R, De Roose P, Tuyttens N. 1990. Diagnosis of atrophic rhinitis by computerized tomography: A preliminary report. Vet Rec 126:591–594.

Jolie R, Thacker B. 1990. Comparison of atrophic rhinitis morphometric measurements and macroscopic grades of nasal cross sections on computerized tomography scans in pigs. Proc Int Congr Pig Vet Soc 11:53.

Jones TL. 1947. Rhinitis in swine. Agric Inst Rev 2:274.

Kamp, E. M., Ter Laak, E. A., de Jong, M. F. 1990. Atypical pasteurella strains producing a toxin similar to the dermonecrotic toxin of *Pasteurella multocida* subs*p. multocida*. Vet Rec 126:434–437.

Kamps AMIE, Buys WECM, Kamp EM., Smits MA. 1990. Specificity of DNA probes for the detection of toxigenic *Pasteurella multocida* subs*p. multocida* strains. J Clin Microbiol 28:1858–1861.

Kavanagh NT. 1994. Isolation of toxigenic *P. multocida* type D from pigs in a herd free from progressive atrophic rhinitis in Ireland. Proc Int Congr Pig Vet Soc 13:121.

Kielstein P. 1983. Zur Bordetelleninfektion des Schweines und die Bedeutung von Tiermodellen zum Nachweis protektiver Eigenschaften von *Bordetella bronchiseptica*. Monatsh Vet Med 38:504–509.

Kobisch M, Pennings A. 1989. An evaluation in pigs of Nobi-Vac AR and an experimental atrophic rhinitis vaccine containing *Pasteurella multocida* DNT-toxoid and *Bordetella bronchiseptica*. Vet Rec 124:57–61.

Koshimizu K, Kodama Y, Ogata M, Sanbyakuda S, Otake Y, Mimura M. 1973. Studies on the etiology of infectious atrophic rhinitis of swine. V. Experimental *Bordetella bronchiseptica* infection in conventional piglets. Jpn J Vet Sci 35:223.

Krüger M, Horsch F. 1992. Spezifische Stimulation des Respirationstraktes von Ferkeln mit *Bordetella bronchiseptica*-Lebendimpfstoffen. Mh Vet Med 47:75–78.

Larsen S, Hogedal Jorgensen P, Nielsen PA. 1990. Elimination of specific pathogens in 3 to 4 week old piglets by use of strategic medication. Proc Int Congr Pig Vet Soc 11:387.

Lax AJ, Chanter N. 1990. Cloning of the toxin gene from *Pasteurella multocida* and its role in atrophic rhinitis. Proc Int Congr Pig Vet Soc 11:61.

Leblanc R, Denicourt M, Lariviera S, Martineau GP. 1986a. Comparison of isolation methods for the recovery of *Bordetella bronchiseptica* and *Pasteurella multocida* from the nasal cavities of piglets. Proc Int Congr Pig Vet Soc 9:226.

Leblanc R, Lariviera S, Martineau GP, Mittal KR. 1986b. Characterization of *Pasteurella multocida* isolated from the nasal cavities of piglets from farms with or without atrophic rhinitis. Proc Int Congr Pig Vet Soc 9:225.

Lugtenberg B, Boxtel RV, de Jong MF. 1984. Atrophic rhinitis in swine, correlation of *Pasteurella multocida* pathogenicity with membrane protein and lipopolysaccharide patterns. Infect Immun 46:48–54.

MacNabb AL. 1948. Rhinitis. Ont Vet Col Rep.

Magyar T, Chanter N, Lax AJ, Rutter JM, Hall GA. 1988. The pathogenesis of turbinate atrophy in pigs caused by *Bordetella bronchiseptica*. Vet Microbiol 18:135.

Martineau GP, Broes A, de Jong MF, Martineau-Doize B. 1982. Experimental reproduction of atrophic rhinitis with *Pasteurella multocida* in gnotobiotic and conventional piglets. Proc Int Congr Pig Vet Soc 7:88.

Martineau GP, Denicourt M, Charette P, Lambert J, Desilets A, Sauvageau R, Cousineau G. 1988. Retrospective study on atrophic rhinitis and enzootic pneumonia found in pigs at Quebec central testing station. Pt 2. Breed effect. Med Vet Quebec 18(4):175–179.

Martineau-Doize B, Frantz JC, Martineau GP. 1990. Cartilage and bone lesions: An explanation of the severity of conchal atrophy induced by *Pasteurella multocida* type D dermonecrotic toxin. Proc Int Congr Vet Soc 11:68.

Martineau-Doize B, Larochelle R, Martineau GP. 1991a. Nasal mucosa of the piglet: Risk factor for atrophic rhinitis. 23 Journées de la Recherche Porcine en France, Paris, 5, 6, 7, febr. Instituut Technique Porc. MNE, pp. 175–178.

Martineau-Doize B, Trepanier H, Martineau GP. 1991b. Histological changes in the nasal ventral conchae of piglets infected with *Bordetella bronchiseptica*. Can J Vet Res 55:42–49.

Mefford DE, Vinson RA, Swafford WS, Pinkston ML. 1983. The efficacy of long-acting oxytetracycline and/or Bordetella/Pasteurella bacterin in a swine herd with enzootic atrophic rhinitis. Vet Med Small Anim Clin 78:1911.

Mendoza S. 1993. Comparison of three biological assays for the detection of toxigenic properties of *Bordetella bronchiseptica* associated with atrophic rhinitis. Vet Microbiol 36:215–219.

Mengelers MJB, Van Klingeren B, Van Miert ASPPAM. 1989. In vitro antimicrobial activity of sulfonamides against some porcine pathogens. Am J Vet Res 50:1022.

Meyer RC, Beamer PD. 1973. *Bordetella bronchiseptica* infections in germ-free swine: An experimental pneumonia. Vet Pathol 10:550.

Miniats OP, Johnson JA. 1980. Experimental atrophic rhinitis in gnotobiotic pigs. Can J Comp Med 44:358.

Moore MK. 1994. A new selective enrichment procedure for isolating *Pasteurella multocida* from avian and environmental samples. Avian Dis 38:317–324.

Müller W, Schneider J, Von Dossow A. 1992. Survival times of *Pasteurella multocida* (subsp. *multocida*) and *Bordetella bronchiseptica* strains in a rotating aerosol chamber—A contribution to the epidemiology of atrophic rhinitis. Monatsh Vet Med 47(5):253–256.

Nagai S, Someno S, Yagihashi T. 1994. Differentiation of toxigenic from nontoxigenic isolates of *Pasteurella multocida* by polymerase chain reaction. Proc Int Congr Pig Vet Soc 13:163.

Nagy LK, Mackenzie T, Scarnell J. 1986. Serum antibody values to *Pasteurella multocida* type D toxin and susceptibility of piglets to experimental challenge with toxigenic type D of *P. multocida*. Proc Int Congr Pig Vet Soc 9:224.

Nakagawa M, Shimizu T, Motoi Y. 1974. Pathology of experimental atrophic rhinitis in swine infected with *Alcaligenes bronchisepticus* or *Pasteurella multocida*. Natl Inst Anim Health Q (Tokyo) 14:61.

Nakai T, Kume K, Yoshikawa H, Oyamada T, Yoshikaw T. 1986. Changes in the nasal mucosa of specific-pathogen-free neonatal pigs infected with *Pasteurella multocida* or *Bordetella bronchiseptica*. Jpn J Vet Sci 48:693–701.

Nakase Y, Kimiura M, Shimoda K. 1976. Efficacy of inactivated *Bordetella bronchiseptica* vaccine for atrophic rhinitis under field conditions. Proc Int Congr Pig Vet Soc 4:8.

Nakase Y, Kume K, Shimoda K, Sawata A. 1980. Experimental atrophic rhinitis produced by cell-free extract of *Bordetella bronchiseptica*. Proc Int Congr Pig Vet Soc 6:202.

Nielsen JP, Frederiksen W. 1990. Atrophic rhinitis in pigs caused by a human isolate of toxigenic *Pasteurella multocida*. Proc Int Congr Pig Vet Soc 11:75.

Nielsen JP, Rosdahl VT. 1988. Phage-typing of toxigenic *Pasteurella multocida*. Proc Int Congr Pig Vet Soc 10:34.

——. 1990. Development and epidemiological application of a bacteriophage system for typing *Pasteurella multocida*. J Clin Microbiol 28:103–107.

Nielsen NC. 1983. Prevalence and economic significance of atrophic rhinitis. In Atrophic Rhinitis of Pigs. KB Pedersen, NC Nielsen, eds. Comm Eur Communities Rep EUR 8643 EN. Luxembourg, p. 35.

Nielsen NC, Bisgaard M, Pedersen KB. 1986. Occurrence of toxin producing strains of *Pasteurella multocida* in different mammalian and avian species. Proc Int Congr Pig Vet Soc 9:232.

Nielsen NC, Riising HJ, Bille N. 1976. Experimental reproduction of atrophic rhinitis in pigs reared to slaughter weight. Proc Int Congr Pig Vet Soc 4:202.

Ohkubo Y, Hiramune T, Kikuchi N. 1987. Sero-types and dermonecrotic activity of *Pasteurella multocida* isolates from nares of rabbits. J College Dairying, Jpn, Nat Sci 12(1):279–285.

Overby E. 1990. Determination of a possible survival rate of *Actinobacillus pleuropneumoniae* bacteria in an EDTA semen dilution experimentally infected. Proc Int Congr Pig Vet Soc 11:45.

Owen JE. 1982. The influence of buildings on respiratory disease. Pig Vet Soc Proc 9:24.

Pearce HG, Roe CK. 1966. Infectious atrophic rhinitis: A review. Can Vet J 7:243.

Pedersen KB. 1983. Cultural and serological diagnosis of atrophic rhinitis in pigs. In Atrophic Rhinitis of Pigs. KB Pedersen, JC Nielsen, eds. Comm Eur Communities Rep EUR 8643 EN. Luxembourg, p. 22.

Pedersen KB, Barfod K. 1977. Effect of vaccination of sows with *Bordetella bronchiseptica* on the incidence of atrophic rhinitis in swine. Nord Vet Med 29:369.

——. 1981. The aetiological significance of *Bordetella bronchiseptica* and *Pasteurella multocida* in atrophic rhinitis of swine. Nord Vet Med 33:513–522.

——. 1982. Effect on the incidence of atrophic rhinitis of vaccination of sows with a vaccine containing *Pasteurella multocida* toxin. Nord Vet Med 34:293.

Pedersen KB, Nielsen JP, Foged NT, Elling F, Nielsen NC, Willeberg P. 1988. Atrophic rhinitis in pigs: Proposal for a revised definition. Vet Rec 20:190.

Pedersen KB, Nielsen NC., eds. 1983. Atrophic Rhinitis of Pigs. Comm Eur Communities Rep EUR 8643 EN. Luxembourg, p. 205.

Pejsak Z, Hogg A, Foreman K, Wasinska B. 1990. The effect of terramycin LA in combination with a Bordetella/Pasteurella vaccine in controlling atrophic rhinitis in swine. Proc Int Congr Pig Vet Soc 11:76.

Pennings AMMA, Storm PK. 1984. A test in Vero-cell monolayers for toxin production by strains of *Pasteurella multocida* isolated from pigs suspected of having atrophic rhinitis. Vet Microbiol 9:503–508.

Penny RHC. 1977. The influence of management changes on the disease picture in pigs. Vet Annu 17:111.

Philips CE. 1946. Infectious rhinitis in swine (bull nose). Can J Comp Med Vet Sci 10:33.

Philips CE., Longfield HF, Miltimore JE. 1948. Porcine infectious atrophic rhinitis experiments. Can J Comp Med Vet Sci 12:268.

Pijoan C, Trigo E, Hogg A. 1988. Atrophic rhinitis in pigs associated with a toxigenic strain of *Pasteurella multocida* serotype A. Proc Int Congr Pig Vet Soc 10:32.

Pijpers A, Van Klingeren B, Schoevers EJ, Verheyden JHM, Van Miert ASP. 1988. The in vitro activity of some antimicrobial agents against 4 porcine respiratory tract pathogens. Proc Int Congr Pig Vet Soc 10:98.

Pijpers A, Van Klingeren B, Schoevers EJ, Verheijden JHM, Van Miert ASJPAM. 1989. In vitro activity of five tetracyclines and some other antimicrobial agents against four porcine respiratory tract pathogens. J Vet Pharmacol Therap 12:267–276.

Plonait H, Bickhardt K. 1988. Lehrbuch der Schweinekrankheiten. Berlin: Verlag Paul Parey.

Plonait H, Heinel KG, Bollwahn W. 1980. Vergleich von Endoskopie und Rontgenaufnahmen als Hilfsmittel zur Diagnose der Rhinitis atrophicans am lebenden Schwein. Prakt Tierärztl 61:1056–1064.

Porter JF, Parton R, Wardlaw AC. 1991. Growth and survival of *Bordetella bronchiseptica* in natural waters and in buffered saline without added nutrients. Appl Environ Microbiol 57:1202–1206.

Ratke G. 1938. Untersuchungen über die Ursache und das Wesen der Schuffelkrankheit des Schweines. Archiv Wiss Prakt Tierheild 72:371.

Rondhuis PR, de Jong MF, Schep J. 1980. Indirect fluorescence antibody studies in porcine cytomegalovirus infections in the Netherlands. Vet Q 2:65–68.

Ross RF, Switzer WP, Duncan JR. 1967. Comparison of pathogenicity of various isolates of *Bordetella bronchiseptica* in young pigs. Can J Comp Med Vet Sci 31:53–57.

Rubies X, Casal J, Fernandez J, Pijoan C. 1996. Transmission of *Pasteurella multocida* clones in a swine pyramid structure. Proc Int Congr Pig Vet Soc 14:243.

Rutter JM. 1981. Quantitative observations on *Bordetella bronchiseptica* infection in atrophic rhinitis of pigs. Vet Rec 108:451–454.

——. 1983. Virulence of *Pasteurella multocida* in atrophic rhinitis of gnotobiotic pigs infected with *Bordetella bronchiseptica*. Res Vet Sci 34:287.

——. 1985. Atrophic rhinitis in swine. Adv Vet Sci Comp Med 29:239–279.

Rutter JM, Beard M, Carpenter GA, Fryer JT. 1986. The effect of air filtration on the performance and health of pigs. Proc Int Congr Pig Vet Soc 9:400.

Rutter JM, Luther PD. 1984. Cell culture assay for toxigenic *Pasteurella multocida* from atrophic rhinitis of pigs. Vet Rec 114:393–396.

Rutter JM, Mackenzie A. 1984. Pathogenesis of atrophic rhinitis in pigs: A new perspective. Vet Rec 114:89.

Rutter JM, Rojas X. 1982. Atrophic rhinitis in gnotobiotic piglets: Differences in the pathogenicity of *Pasteurella multocida* in combined infection with *Bordetella bronchiseptica*. Vet Rec 110:531.

Rutter JM, Taylor RJ, Crighton WG, Robertson IB, Bentson AJ. 1984. Epidemiological study of *Pasteurella multocida* and *Bordetella bronchiseptica* in atrophic rhinitis. Vet Rec 115:615–619.

Schimmelpfennig H. 1990. Rhinitis atrophicans (Ra) des Schweines: Zur Neutralisation des Toxins von *Pasteurella multocida*. Dtsch Tierärztl Wochenschr 97:195–196.

Schimmelpfennig H, Jahn B. 1988. Rhinitis atrophicans (R.a.) des Schweines: Ein Hauttest zum Nachweis antitoxischer *Pasteurella multocida* Antikorper. Dtsch Tierärztl Wochenschr 95:285–286.

Schöss P. 1982. *Bordetella bronchiseptica* Infektionen in einem SPF Schweinebestand: Ein Beitrag zur Atiologie der Rhinitis atrophicans. Dtsch Tierärztl Wochenschr 89:177–181.

——. 1983. Clinical diagnosis of atrophic rhinitis. In Atrophic Rhinitis of Pigs. KB Pedersen, NC Nielsen, eds. Comm Eur Communities Rep EUR 8643 EN. Luxembourg, p. 13.

Schöss P, Thiel CP. 1984. Occurrence of toxin-producing strains of *Pasteurella multocida* and *Bordetella bronchiseptica* in pig herds with atrophic rhinitis and in unaffected herds. Proc Int Congr Pig Vet Soc 8:94.

Schuller W, Trubrich H, Kosztolich O, Flatscher J, Jahn J. 1980. Vaccination against atrophic rhinitis in swine with a combined *Bordetella bronchiseptica*, *Pasteurella multocida* vaccine. Zentralbl Veterinärmed 27:125.

Sisak F, Gois M, Kuksa F. 1978. The sensitivity of the strains of *Bordetella bronchiseptica*, *Pasteurella multocida* and *Mycoplasma hyorhinis*, isolated from pigs, to antibiotics and chemotherapeutics. Vet Med (Praha) 23:531.

Skelly BJ, Pruss M, Pellegrino R, Andersen D., Abruzzo G. 1980. Variation in degree of atrophic rhinitis with field isolants of *Bordetella bronchiseptica*. Proc Int Congr Pig Vet Soc 6:210.

Smith IM. 1971. Studies on the Role of Some Microorganisms in Respiratory Infections of the Pig with Special Reference to the Involvement of Pasteurella septica. Ph.D. diss., Univ London.

Smith IM., Baskerville, A. J. 1979. A selective medium facilitating the isolation and recognition of *Bordetella bronchiseptica* in pigs. Res Vet Sci 27:187.

——. 1983. A selective medium for the isolation of *Pasteurella multocida* in nasal specimens from pigs. Br Vet J 139:476.

Smith IM, Giles CJ. 1980. Vaccines for atrophic rhinitis. Pig Farming Suppl (Oct.):83.

Smith IM, Giles CJ, Baskerville AJ. 1982. The immunisation of pigs against experimental infection with *Bordetella bronchiseptica*. Vet Rec 110:488.

Smith IM, Oliphant J, Baskerville AJ, Giles CJ. 1980. High prevalence of strains of *Bordetella bronchiseptica* resistant to potentiated sulphonamide in English pig herds in 1978–1979. Vet Rec 106:462.

Smith WJ. 1983. Infectious atrophic rhinitis: Noninfectious determinants. In Atrophic Rhinitis of Pigs. KB Pedersen, JC Nielsen, eds. Comm Eur Communities Rep EUR 8643 EN. Luxembourg, p. 151.

Sorensen V, Barfod K, Nielsen JP, Foged NT. 1990. Effect of degree of atrophy and serum antitoxin titer on the daily weight gain and feed conversion. Proc Int Congr Pig Vet Soc 11:57.

Stehmann R, Huster A, Mehlhorn G, Neuparth V. 1990. Survival and sensitivity to disinfectants of *Bordetella bronchiseptica*, *Haemophilus parasuis*, and *Actinobacillus pleuropneumoniae*. Dtsch Vet Med Gesellschaft, pp. 315–320.

Stehmann R, Mehlhorn G, Neuparth V. 1989. Detection of *Bordetella bronchiseptica* in the air of farrowing and weaned piglet pens. Monatsh Vet Med 44:307–311.

Stehmann R, Rottmayer J, Zschaubitz K, Mehlhorn G. 1992. Investigations on the survival of *Bordetella bronchiseptica* in the air. Zentralbl Veterinärmed (B) 39:546–552.

Strang MM. 1982. The influence of feed and feed delivery systems on respiratory disease. Pig Vet Soc Proc 9:36.

Straw BE, Burgi EJ, Hilley HD, Leman AD. 1983. Pneumonia and atrophic rhinitis in pigs from a test station. J Am Vet Med Assoc 182:607.

Sutter MT, Wanner M. 1990. Higher bioavailability of tetracyclines given with liquid feed in weaned pigs. Proc Int Congr Pig Vet Soc 11:353.

Switzer WP. 1951. Atrophic rhinitis and trichomonads. Vet Med 46:478.

——. 1953. Studies on infectious atrophic rhinitis of swine. I. Isolation of a filterable agent from the nasal cavity of swine with infectious atrophic rhinitis. J Am Vet Med Assoc 123:45.

——. 1955. Studies on infectious atrophic rhinitis. IV. Characterization of a pleuropneumonia-like organism isolated from the nasal cavities of swine. Am J Vet Res 16:540.

——. 1956. Studies on infectious atrophic rhinitis. V. Concept that several agents may cause turbinate atrophy. Am J Vet Res 17:478.

——. 1963. Elimination of *Bordetella bronchiseptica* from the nasal cavity of swine by sulphonamide therapy. Vet Med 58:571.

Switzer WP, Farrington DO. 1975. Infectious atrophic rhinitis. In Diseases of Swine, 4th ed. HW Dunne, AD Leman, eds. Ames: Iowa State Univ Press, p. 687.

Switzer WP, L'Ecuyer C. 1960. Detection of swine nasal viruses in cell culture. Am J Vet Res 21:967.

Terakado N, Azechi H, Ninomiya K, Fukuyasu T, Shimizu T. 1974. Incidence of R. factors in *Bordetella bronchiseptica* isolated from pigs. Jpn J Microbiol 18:45.

Terpstra JI, Akkermans JPWM. 1960. Enkele aantekeningen over Atrofische Rhinitis. Tijdschr Diergeneeskd 85:1222–1233.

Thunberg E., Carlstrom B. 1940. Om nyssjuka hos svin fran epizootisynpunkt. Skand Vet 30:711. Can J Comp Med Vet Sci 10:169.

Tornoe N, Nielsen NC. 1976. Inoculation experiments with *Bordetella bronchiseptica* strains in SPF pigs. Nord Vet Med 28:233.

Tornoe N, Nielsen NC, Svendsen J. 1976. *Bordetella bronchiseptica* isolations from the nasal cavity of pigs in relation to atrophic rhinitis. Nord Vet Med 28:1.

Trigo E, Pijoan C. 1988. Effect of piliation, hemagglutination and capsular serotype of *Pasteurella multocida* on the production of atrophic rhinitis in swine. Proc Int Congr Pig Vet Soc 10:31.

Van Diemen PM, de Jong MF, De Vries Reilingh G, Van Der Hel W, Schrama JW. 1994a. Intranasal administration of *Pasteurella multocida* toxin in a challenge-exposure model used to induce subclinical signs of atrophic rhinitis in pigs. Am J Vet Res 55:49–54.

Van Diemen PM, De Vries Reilingh G, Noordhuizen JPTM, Parmentier HK. 1994b. Effect of *Pasteurella multocida*-toxin on the immune system of piglets. Proc Int Congr Pig Vet Soc 13:120.

Van Groenland GJ. 1984. Measuring the distance between tooth edges in piglets as a way to monitor breeding farms for atrophic rhinitis. Proc Int Congr Vet Soc 8.

Van Leengoed LA, Kamp E, Vecht U. 1986. Tonsil biopsy: A tool in epidemiological studies of atrophic rhinitis and streptococcal meningitis in pigs. Proc Int Congr Pig Vet Soc 9:227.

Visser IJR, Van den Ingh TSGAM, De Kruijf JM, Tielen MJM, Urlings HAP, Gruys E. 1988. Atrofische rhinitis: The use of longitudinal sections of pigs' heads in the diagnosis of atrophy of the turbinate bones at the slaughter line. Tijdschr Diergeneeskd 113:1345–1355.

Voets MT. 1990. Evaluation of the challenge model to test AR vaccine. Proc Int Congr Pig Vet Soc 11:56.

Voets MT, Tielen MJM, Hunneman W. 1986a. The heritability of conchal atrophy in a slight AR-infection. Proc Int Congr Pig Vet Soc 9:391.

——. 1986b. UV-ray treatment of air to prevent atrophic rhinitis. Proc Int Congr Pig Vet Soc 9:404.

Webbon PM, Penny RHC, Gray J. 1978. Atrophic rhinitis. The value of radiography for diagnosis in piglets. Br Vet J 134:193.

Whittlestone P. 1982. Infectious agents associated with porcine respiratory diseases. Pig Vet Soc Proc 9:71.

Williams PR, Hall RM, Rimler RB. 1986. Effect of purified *Pasteurella multocida* turbinate atrophy toxin on porcine peripheral blood lymphocytes in vivo and in vitro. Proc Int Congr Pig Vet Soc 9:234.

Yokomizo Y, Shimizu T. 1979. Adherence of *Bordetella bronchiseptica* to swine nasal epithelial cells and its possible role in virulence. Res Vet Sci 27:15.

Yoshikawa T, Hanada T. 1981. Histological studies on pigs with atrophic rhinitis showing retarded growth. Jpn J Vet Sci 43:221.

35 Brucellosis

A. P. MacMillan, Heidi Schleicher, John Korslund,
and William Stoffregen

Brucellosis of pigs is an infectious disease that has been recognized as a specific entity since 1914, when Traum (1914) isolated the organism from aborted porcine fetuses in Indiana, but for many years it was thought to be caused by an exceptionally pathogenic form of *Brucella abortus* until Huddleston (1929) named the infectious agent, *B. suis*, as a separate species. Brucellosis occurs in most countries throughout the world where pigs exist in the wild or domesticated state.

In the United States porcine brucellosis was recognized as a major disease, causing considerable economic loss during the 1920s–1950s. Since that time, changes in management combined with regulatory programs to eradicate the disease have gradually eliminated brucellosis as a major disease problem from large areas of the country. As of late 2004 all states except Texas were in Stage III (Free) status of the Swine Brucellosis Control/ Eradication Program. All outbreaks of infection in domestic herds have been attributed to feral swine exposure for several years, including those in Texas. In fiscal year 2004, there were only 2 small-herd isolated outbreaks reported in the U.S. swine population, both feral-related (Holland and Barton 2004). The disease is essentially eradicated in the commercial production swine herd in the United States.

Swine brucellosis appears to be widespread in South America, where it is predominantly caused by biovar 1. In Europe (apart from Britain and Scandinavia, which are brucellosis free), there is a general low prevalence of porcine brucellosis. In Africa, the disease is reported by some countries, but the number of pigs on the continent is not large, and the true position is not entirely clear. Asia, particularly Southeast Asia, seems to have a generally high prevalence of the disease, predominantly caused by biovar 3 in south China and Singapore and by biovar 1 elsewhere. In Australia the disease is confined to feral pigs in Queensland (Alton 1990).

Porcine brucellosis also has noteworthy public health implications. Until recently the source of the majority of human brucellosis has been *Brucella suis*–infected pigs (Fox and Kaufmann 1977). The public health hazard caused by porcine brucellosis is of proportionately greater significance than the risk from bovine brucellosis primarily because *B. suis* (biovars 1 and 3) appears to have a much higher degree of pathogenicity for humans than *B. abortus*. There also tend to be higher numbers of *B. suis* organisms in the tissues, providing a greater exposure to persons who come in contact with infected pigs. As pigs do not produce dairy products, the incidence of *B. suis* in humans is almost entirely occupational: in farmers, veterinarians, abattoir workers, and individuals, such as hunters, having direct contact with feral swine. Interestingly, although the infection of cattle with *B. suis* is rare, Cook and Noble (1984), working in Australia, reported several cases, probably contracted following contact with feral pigs. Persistent excretion in the milk may give rise to human epidemics (Borts et al. 1943). *B. suis* infection of a ram has been reported by Paolicchi et al. (1993), who suggest that this may represent a public health hazard.

ETIOLOGY

The genus *Brucella* comprises six nomen species: *B. abortus*, *B. melitensis*, *B. suis*, *B. neotomae*, *B. ovis*, and *B. canis* (Brinley-Morgan and McCullough 1974; Alton et al. 1975). In addition to the traditional six species, recent identifications of *Brucella* organisms in marine mammal species have led to the provisional speciation of *B. cetaceae* and *B. pinnipediae* (Cloeckaert et al. 2001). The genus appears to be genetically very homogeneous (Verger et al. 1985) but does not appear to be closely related to any other animal pathogens (de Ley et al. 1987). The first three nomen species are further divided into 8, 3, and 5 biovars, respectively. The principal hosts for *B. melitensis* are goats and sheep; for *B. abortus*, cattle, bison, and elk; for *B. neotomae*, desert wood rats; for *B. ovis*, sheep; for *B. canis*, dogs; for provisionally named *B. cetaceae*, dolphins, porpoises, and minke whale; and for provisionally named *B. pinnipediae*, seals. The most common host for *B. suis* biovars 1 and 3 is the pig, and these biovars are worldwide in distribution. *B. suis* biovar 2 occurs in Europe, where the hosts are pigs and the European hare (*Lepus capinensis*), which can form a reservoir for occasional outbreaks in both wild and domestic pigs. The disease in pigs caused by biovar 2 differs slightly from that caused by biovars 1 and 3 in that miliary brucellosis of the uterus is a feature, and unlike them, it does not appear to be pathogenic for humans. *B. suis* biovar 4 is enzootic in reindeer and caribou (*Rangifer* spp.) in Siberia, Alaska, and Canada and is apparently not pathogenic for pigs although it causes many cases of human brucellosis. *B. suis* biovar 5 causes murine brucellosis.

B. suis is the only recognized *Brucella* species that causes systemic or generalized infection leading to reproductive failure in pigs. Pigs can be infected naturally or experimentally with other *Brucella* species, but a characteristic of the infection is almost invariably a symptomless, self-limiting localized infection of lymph nodes regional to the point of entry. It should be noted, however, that the differentiation of biovars of *Brucella* must be accomplished using methods only available in large reference centers, and this probably accounts for the frequent reports before the early 1960s of the isolation of *B. melitensis* from pigs (Alton 1990).

Bacteriological examination is often of great assistance in aiding a diagnosis, but it must be remembered that handling *B. suis* in the laboratory is extremely hazardous unless appropriate precautions are taken. The genus *Brucella* belongs to Hazard Group III and should be handled in a Class I/III safety cabinet within Containment Level III accommodation by staff with adequate training and experience.

Primary isolations of *B. suis*, like the other species in the genus, appear as small, convex, translucent, honey-colored colonies on the surface of clear agar media after incubation at 37°C for 2–7 days. Colonies grown on more opaque agar media types may appear pearl-colored. All *Brucella* species and biovars, except *B. ovis* and *B. canis*, occur naturally with smooth colonial morphology. *B. ovis* and *B. canis* always occur as rough forms, even on primary isolation. All smooth forms of

brucellae may dissociate into intermediate, rough, or mucoid forms under certain artificially induced environmental conditions. This dissociation frequently occurs if cultures are left for a long period without being subcultured, and it renders them incapable of being assigned to species or biovar. Microscopically, *Brucella* organisms are small, gram-negative bacilli or coccobacilli and are nonmotile and arranged singly. *B. suis* organisms from different sources may vary considerably in size but are generally 0.4–0.8 by 0.6–3.0 μm.

Several commercially available agar media are suitable for isolation and propagation of *B. suis*; those more commonly used include tryptose, trypticase-soy, Albimi, serum dextrose, Farrell's, and potato infusion. The addition of serum to the media to a final concentration of 5% frequently enhances the growth of brucellae, particularly on primary isolation. Increased carbon dioxide tension is not required for growth of *B. suis*. A more complete discussion of biotyping procedures, biovars, and formulation of growth media, as well as descriptive characteristics of the entire genus, can be obtained from Alton et al. 1988.

In general, all biovars of *B. suis* have a noticeably greater urease and catalase activity than other species of *Brucella*. Classification of *B. suis* into biovars is based on the combined findings of a variety of conventional and specialized tests. Briefly, *B. suis* biovar 1 produces large amounts of hydrogen sulfide, whereas biovars 2, 3, 4, and 5 produce little or none; growth of biovars 1, 2, and 5 is inhibited to a greater degree by basic fuchsin than growth of biovars 3 and 4; *B. suis* is not lysed by routine test dilutions (RTD) of Tbilisi *Brucella* phage but may be partially lysed by 10,000 × RTD; using monospecific antisera for the dominant A and M antigens, *B. suis* biovars 1, 2, and 3 are A dominant, while biovar 4 is AM (the only distinguishing feature separating biovars 3 and 4), and biovar 5 is M dominant (Table 35.1).

As the oxidative metabolic characteristics of all *B. suis* biovars are very similar, there are insufficient differences for differentiation.

Among the *B. suis*, only biovars 1 and 3 are known to occur in pig-raising areas of the United States. Until 1946 the only recognized cause of pig brucellosis in the

Table 35.1. Characteristics used for the differentiation of *Brucella suis*

	H$_2$S Production	Growth on Thionin	Growth on Fuchsin	Dominant Antigen[a]	Lysis by Tb Phage at RTD	Lysis by Tb Phage at 10^4 RTD
Biovar 1	+	+	–	A	NL[b]	L[c]
Biovar 2	–	+	–	A	NL	L
Biovar 3	–	+	+	A	NL	L
Biovar 4	–	+	–[d]	AM	NL	L
Biovar 5	–	+	–	M	NL	L

[a]Agglutination with A and M monospecific serum.
[b]No lysis.
[c]Lysis.
[d]Some strains may grow.

United States was the organism now known as *B. suis* biovar 1. At that time, *B. suis* biovar 3 (originally classified as American *B. melitensis*) was first isolated from tissues of infected pigs by S. H. MacNutt (Borts et al. 1946). For a period of time, reported isolations of *B. suis* biovar 1 had become comparatively less frequent, while isolations of *B. suis* biovar 3 had become more frequent. However, recent isolations of *B. suis* from feral swine have been identified as biovar 1, and both *B. suis* biovars 1 and 3 are most likely still present within the United States.

EPIDEMIOLOGY

Most evidence indicates that most *B. suis* infection is transmitted to susceptible animals through direct association with infected pigs. In this species, the most important routes of infection are through the alimentary and genital tracts. The habits of pigs and usual character of the disease strongly suggest that the alimentary tract is the most common portal of entry. Pigs of all ages may eat food or drink fluid contaminated with discharges from infected pigs. Piglets are frequently infected by nursing infected dams, and when breeding pigs are confined together, aborted fetuses and fetal membranes are readily consumed. Brucellosis is a venereal disease in pigs, and sows are readily infected when mated with infected boars or when artificially inseminated with semen containing *B. suis*. Experimentally, pigs are readily infected by conjunctival or intranasal exposure with suspensions of *B. suis*. It is possible that organisms could also enter through scarified or, possibly, intact skin.

The survival of brucellae under environmental conditions is a relatively important factor in transmission of the disease. The survival rate of brucellae is similar to that of other nonsporing gram-negative bacteria and as such is extremely variable depending on prevailing conditions. Experimental evidence indicates that *B. suis* is readily killed by pasteurization, 2–4 hours of direct sunlight, and the most commonly used disinfectants. *Brucellae* can survive in organic matter at freezing or near-freezing temperatures in excess of 2 years. Consequently, efforts to eliminate brucellosis from pig-raising premises must include an effective sanitation program (Luchsinger et al. 1965). The most suitable methods for preserving *Brucella* organisms for long periods are lyophilization and/or storage at subfreezing temperatures.

There are few known reservoirs of *B. suis* infection other than infected domestic pigs. Only the European hare and feral pigs have been established as significant potential reservoirs. The European hare was incriminated as a natural host for *B. suis* biovar 2 as early as 1954 (Bendtsen et al. 1954) and is apparently responsible for periodic outbreaks of brucellosis of pigs in Europe. Feral pigs in the southeastern United States, and to a much lesser extent elsewhere (Drew et al. 1992), have been discovered to have a high rate of serologic reactors, with isolation of *B. suis* biovar 1 from some animals (Wood et al. 1976; Becker et al. 1978). Extensive studies conducted in Florida showed that although only some populations are infected, the incidence within these groups is usually high (Leek et al. 1993). The epidemiological importance of feral pigs in the maintenance of porcine brucellosis depends largely on the degree of contact between wild and domestic pigs (Nettles 1991). If pig management systems in regions where feral pigs exist prevent contact, *B. suis* infection in feral pigs may be of greater public health importance than a threat to the pig industry. There have been numerous instances of *B. suis* infection or seropositivity in rodents or carnivorous species trapped near areas where brucellosis in domesticated pigs has occurred. However, general indications are that these species acquired infection from the pigs and are terminal hosts of the infection. With few or no exceptions, epidemiological investigation of newly infected pig herds has revealed the source as another herd of domesticated pigs.

Experimental studies have shown that pigs can be infected with *B. suis* biovar 4, *B. abortus*, *B. melitensis*, *B. canis*, and *B. neotomae*. However, there has been no evidence that these organisms invade the genital tract, are transmissible between pigs, or localize in any tissues other than lymph nodes draining the site of infection. All available evidence indicates that these biovars or species are not highly pathogenic for pigs, pigs are not likely to show clinical evidence of disease, and the infection is self-limiting and usually persists less than 60 days. Nevertheless, these infections do have importance for public health. In particular, pigs are associated with *B. abortus* infection in packinghouse workers.

Pigs infected with *B. suis* biovars 1, 2, or 3 can serve as a source of infection for other domesticated animal species. *B. suis* infection can occur naturally in horses, cattle, and dogs. Although the most common brucella infection in horses is *B. abortus*, fistulous withers and other syndromes have been recorded as caused by *B. suis* when horses were associated with infected pigs. Cattle are rarely infected with *B. suis*; when infection does occur, the characteristic infection is mastitis, with *B. suis* organisms excreted in the milk representing a public health risk. It can cause an acute infection in dogs, with pregnant bitches frequently aborting. There is some evidence that *B. canis*, a significant pathogen in dogs, evolved from *B. suis* biovar 3.

PATHOGENESIS

Available literature and comparative studies indicate that the pathogenesis of *B. suis* biovars 1, 2, and 3 is very similar (Thomsen 1934; Hutchings 1950; Hoerlein et al. 1954; Deyoe 1967). Differences are generally related to factors such as method of exposure, infecting dose, age and breed of pigs, and possibly minor differences between strains of the same biovar. However, the characteristics of the disease produced are usually indistinguishable.

Regardless of the route of infection, the organism must be able to attach to and penetrate the mucosal epithelium, although the mechanisms for this have not yet been fully elucidated. Following the initial penetration, submucosal aggregations of lymphocytes and plasma cells form in response. Invading organisms are carried to local lymph nodes, although it is not known whether they travel as free organisms or within phagocytes, and infected nodes become enlarged due to lymphoid and reticuloendothelial hyperplasia and infiltration. *Brucella* organisms surviving regional node colonization enter a phase of bacteremia, now protected from humoral immune mechanisms by their intracellular location within neutrophils and macrophages.

In *B. suis* infection of pigs, bacteremia is an invariable finding in acute stages of the disease if frequent blood samples are collected and examined bacteriologically. In general, the onset of bacteremia ranges from 1–7 weeks after exposure, with a mean of about 2 weeks post exposure. Bacteremia persists an average of about 5 weeks and is generally continuous during that time. Intermittent bacteremia in individual pigs has been observed to be as brief as 1 week to as long as 34 months. It is this bacteremia that is probably responsible for the wide range of tissues secondarily infected during the course of the disease.

Within a short time after the bacteremia stage, *B. suis* can be isolated from a large number of sites in the body (Deyoe and Manthei 1967). The entire lymphatic system is often affected for a period of time. With increasing time after exposure, the sites of localization of the organism tend to be reduced in number. Among lymph nodes, the most frequent sources of *B. suis* are mandibular, gastrohepatic, internal iliac, and suprapharyngeal, in that order, depending essentially on the route of infection. Organs of the genital system containing high levels of erythritol, a sugar promoting the growth of brucellae, become involved in many pigs and may remain persistently infected. The placenta is a privileged site, and brucellae localize in the rough endoplasmic reticulum of the chorionic trophoblasts. Despite severe placental infection, only mild inflammation of the endometrium is observed. The spleen, liver, kidney, bladder, mammary gland, and brain may be involved (Jubb et al. 1985), although not as regularly as lymph nodes. Other significant sources of *B. suis*, particularly in chronically infected pigs, are joint fluids and bone marrow.

The response to invasion of *B. suis* becomes evident with the appearance of humoral antibody, activation of the cell-mediated immune system, and development of microscopic lesions. These manifestations may occur simultaneously but usually are subsequent to the appearance of detectable bacteremia; bacteremia may precede detectable antibody levels possibly by as much as 6–8 weeks. As pigs recover from *B. suis* infection (i.e., when viable organisms are no longer present in their tissues), other manifestations, such as antibody levels, cellular hypersensitivity, and microscopic lesions, recede and disappear also. Unfortunately, many pigs remain permanently infected.

In a series of experiments, infection was established in 248 sexually mature pigs (Deyoe 1972a). They were killed at various intervals after exposure to *B. suis* and their tissues subjected to thorough bacteriological examination. Three-fourths of the pigs in each group of females had recovered from infection by 4–6 months or longer after exposure, whereas the recovery rate in males never exceeded 50%. In contrast, Goode et al. (1952) and Manthei et al. (1952) isolated *B. suis* from only 12 of 474 adult pigs exposed as suckling pigs. This information demonstrates beyond doubt that the majority of pigs infected with *B. suis* will eventually recover spontaneously. Nevertheless, sufficient numbers of permanently infected animals will remain to serve as a continual source of infection.

CLINICAL SIGNS

Clinical evidence of *B. suis* infection varies considerably in different herds. The majority of affected herds may have no signs of brucellosis recognizable by the herd owner. The classic manifestations of pig brucellosis are abortion, infertility, orchitis, posterior paralysis, and lameness. Infected pigs fail to show any persisting or undulating pyrexia. Clinical signs may be transient and death is a rare occurrence.

Abortions may occur at any time during gestation and are influenced more by the time of exposure than by the time of gestation. The rate of abortion is highest in sows or gilts exposed via the genital tract at the time of breeding (Deyoe and Manthei 1969). Abortions have been observed as early as 17 days following natural insemination by boars disseminating *B. suis* in the semen. Early abortions are usually overlooked under field conditions, and the first indication is a large percentage of sows or gilts showing signs of estrus 30–45 days after the service that resulted in conception. Little or no vaginal discharge is observed with early abortions. Abortions that occur during the middle or late stages of gestation are usually associated with females that acquire infection after pregnancy has advanced past 35 or 40 days. The persistence of genital infection in females varies considerably.

A small percentage of sows have been shown to shed *B. suis* in vaginal discharges for as long as 30 months. However, the majority ceased shedding organisms within 30 days. A clinically apparent abnormal vaginal exudate is seldom observed in sows that have uterine infection except just prior to and for a short time after abortion. The majority of female pigs eventually recover from genital infection.

When genital infection in sows persists only a short

time after abortion, parturition, or breeding to an infected boar and the sows are permitted two or three estrous cycles of sexual rest, subsequent conception rates and reproductive capacity are usually very good.

Genital infection tends to be more persistent in boars than in sows. Some infected boars do not develop a localized genital infection. However, boars that do develop genital infection seldom recover from it. Pathologic changes in the male accessory glands or testes are generally more extensive and irreversible than in the uterus. Infertility and lack of sexual drive may occur in infected boars and are frequently associated with testicular involvement. More commonly, however, boars have infection in accessory genital glands and as a result disseminate large numbers of *B. suis* in their semen. These boars do not necessarily have reduced fertility (Vandeplassche et al. 1967). In most circumstances, clinically apparent lesions of *B. suis* biovar 1, 2, or 3 infection in boars are seldom encountered.

Clinical brucellosis in suckling and weaning pigs may appear as diskospondylitis associated with posterior paralysis or arthritis. These clinical signs are occasionally observed in any age of pigs.

LESIONS

Macroscopic pathologic changes produced by *B. suis* in pigs are quite variable. Enough abscess formation may occur in affected organs to result in necrosis and desquamation of a significant proportion of the mucous membrane. Generally, the histopathological changes consist of uterine glands filled with leukocytes, cellular infiltration of the endometrial stroma, and hyperplasia of periglandular connective tissue. Diffuse suppurative inflammation is usually present in affected placentas, resulting in purulent, necrotizing placentitis with fibrinous polyserositis. There also may be considerable necrosis of epithelium and diffuse hyperplasia of fibrous connective tissue.

Focal microscopic granulomatous lesions frequently can be observed in livers of pigs with brucellosis, particularly during bacteremic phases of the disease. These foci frequently are necrotic areas infiltrated with lymphocytes, macrophages, neutrophils, and giant cells, with sheets of histocytic and epithelioid cells with a central zone of caseous or coagulative necrosis. The lesions are usually partially or completely enclosed by a fibrous capsule. The necrotic portions of the granulomas are heavily infiltrated with neutrophils, and liquefaction and mineralization may occur (Enright 1990). Aborted fetuses may exhibit purulent hepatitis as well.

These lesions are not specific for brucellosis, since similar hepatic lesions are associated with other bacterial infections.

Microscopic lesions of bones are sometimes caused by *B. suis* infection. These occur both in vertebrae and in long bones. The lesions are most frequently located ad-

jacent to the epiphyseal cartilage and usually consist of caseous centers surrounded by a zone of macrophages and leukocytes and often by an outer zone of fibrous connective tissue.

Focal areas of chronic lymphocytic and macrocytic inflammation or focal abscesses are found infrequently in kidneys, spleen, brain, ovaries, adrenal glands, lungs, and other tissues of infected pigs (Deyoe 1968).

DIAGNOSIS

The most accurate and possibly the most sensitive method of diagnosis of porcine brucellosis is isolation of *Brucella* organisms by direct culture methods. It has been shown that routine culture of a small sample of lymph nodes from carcasses will reveal as many positives as serologic diagnosis (Alton 1990; Rogers et al. 1989). This is a very practical survey strategy, as virtually all the produce of the industry passes through abattoirs and the material can be removed without damage to the carcass. Culture of other material that becomes available is often fruitful, such as vaginal swabs or products of abortion, semen samples or castrated testicles, the contents of swollen joints, and blood samples. However, culture is often not feasible because of inadequate or unavailable laboratory facilities and trained personnel (Deyoe 1969). *B. suis* can readily be grown on all the normal *Brucella* media in the absence of added CO_2, the techniques being fully described by Alton et al. (1988).

Detection of *B. suis* antigen in tissues of infected pigs has been investigated, primarily using fluorescent antibody (FA) techniques. The general conclusion has been that brucellae are seldom detectable in lymph node impression smears with FA procedures because of the relatively low numbers of organisms typically present (Deyoe 1972b). Nevertheless, FA tests could probably be useful for examining aborted materials, since large numbers of *B. suis* are typical in such specimens. More recently, potentially sensitive methods for the detection of the presence of brucellae, such as the polymerase chain reaction (PCR), are gradually being introduced into routine use and may, in the future, prove a valuable method of diagnosis in certain situations (Lealklevezas et al. 1995).

Serologic procedures to detect antibodies against brucellae in infected pigs are generally the most practical and most common means of diagnosis, but the results obtained are far from perfect. Market pig surveys have shown that as many as 18% of normal pigs may react at the 1:25 level when plate agglutination tests are used (Deyoe 1969). On the other hand, some pigs produce little or no antibody against brucellae. Because of variation in the stage of disease, an infected herd of pigs will nearly always contain some infected animals that have no detectable brucella antibody. Some strains of *B. suis* apparently do not stimulate antibody production as well as others (Deyoe 1967). Pigs exposed to a minimal infective dose of *B. suis* generally have a prolonged incubation period before significant quantities of antibody are produced.

Because of the foregoing factors, current serologic tests are much less effective for the diagnosis of individual pigs than they are in cattle. However, most serologic tests are entirely adequate as herd tests. Characteristically, infected herds include a majority or large numbers of infected individuals. Because of close contact between animals and the tendency of brucellosis to spread rapidly through a herd, 50–80% is a common morbidity range (Spencer and Mattison 1975). When large herds have only a single serologic reactor disclosed during a herd test, it can generally be concluded that *B. suis* infection is not present.

Numerous serologic tests are available or have been investigated for use in diagnosis of porcine brucellosis (Alton et al. 1988). Many of these were developed for diagnosis of bovine brucellosis and have been adapted for testing pig sera. Most tests utilize *B. abortus* whole-cell antigens. Since the commonly used antigen strains *B. abortus* 1119-3 and S99 have the same or very similar surface lipopolysaccharide complexes as smooth *B. suis*, the standardized antigens produced and distributed by the Animal and Plant Health Inspection Service (APHIS) of the USDA and by the Central Veterinary Laboratory, Weybridge, United Kingdom, are equally useful for diagnosis of both bovine and porcine brucellosis. This has been confirmed by extensive laboratory testing of pig sera with both *B. abortus* and *B. suis* antigens.

The original test methods for the diagnosis of porcine brucellosis were tube and plate agglutination procedures. Interpretation of results was based on the finding that most infected pig herds contained one or more animals with more than 100 international units (IU) of agglutination. It is now known that serum agglutination tests (SAT), although sensitive, are not sufficiently specific to be reliable diagnostic tools when used alone. Some of the inaccuracies can be overcome in situations where frequent and repeated testing is practicable and the trend of antibody titers can be determined.

Reducing the pH of antigen-serum mixtures to 3–4 was also found to reduce nonspecific agglutination while not affecting agglutination caused by serum from infected animals. This led to the development of methods classified as buffered brucella antigen tests, in which stained brucella antigen is buffered at pH 3.65. The buffered brucella antigen became the basis of the brucellosis card test and similar procedures such as buffered plate antigen and Rose-Bengal tests (RBT). These tests are the most practical method of diagnosis for porcine brucellosis at present, are possibly still the preferred method for large-scale surveillance testing, and are "prescribed tests for international trade" (Office International des Epizooties 1997). They have a distinct advantage over standard agglutination tests because they are relatively unaffected by nonspecific agglutinins and are

generally as sensitive as any other serologic test for diagnosis of porcine brucellosis.

Other tests, such as the Rivanol precipitation–serum agglutination, 2-mercaptoethanol, and complement fixation tests (CFT), are frequently used for the diagnosis of brucellosis in pigs and are very useful in confirming results of card tests. The above tests very seldom or never detect IgM brucella antibodies in pig serum; therefore, they are highly specific. However, the relative sensitivity of these methods is usually low in early stages of brucellosis. By the time the antibody response peaks and thereafter in chronic stages, the Rivanol, mercaptoethanol, and CFT methods are generally as sensitive as the card test. An evaluation of a range of serologic tests on culture-positive pigs was reported by Rogers et al. (1989). The sensitivity of the RBT was 79%; of the CFT, 49%; and of the SAT, 51%. The specificity of the RBT was reported to be 98% based on the results of testing over 30,000 serum samples. Other studies generally confirm the low levels of diagnostic sensitivity achievable (Ferris et al. 1995; Payeur et al. 1990).

The Particle Concentration Fluorescence Immunoassay (PCFIA) is a competitive immunoassay for IgG1, IgG2, and IgM antibodies which has been reported to have a sensitivity of 80% and specificity of 89% (Ferris et al. 1995). The PCFIA interpretation ranges for swine have been established as a ratio of Sample to Negative Control signal (S/N) of 0.0 to 0.5 for reactors, 0.51 to 0.70 for suspects, and greater than 0.70 for negatives.

Recently, the Fluorescence Polarization Assay (FPA) has also been evaluated for the detection of Brucellosis in swine (Nielsen and Gall 2001). The FPA test is based on the size and rotation rate of molecules in solution and the depolarization of light by these molecules (see Nielsen and Gall 2001 for a complete description.) One study in swine has shown the FPA to have a sensitivity of 94% and a specificity of 97% (Nielsen et al. 1999). The FPA test is currently being incorporated as an official test into the USDA Swine Brucellosis Control/Eradication program.

Limited investigation of the enzyme-linked immunosorbent assay (ELISA) has been conducted, and it appears that this method may be equal or slightly superior to other serologic procedures for diagnosis of porcine brucellosis in the future (Office International des Epizooties 1997). Further investigation of this test for use in eradication campaigns is warranted.

Regardless of the serologic test used for diagnosis, detection of 80–90% of infected pigs must be regarded as the best that can be achieved at present.

Experimental studies reviewed by Corbel (1985) have shown that infection with organisms of several other genera can produce antibodies reactive in brucellosis diagnostic tests. These organisms include *Escherichia coli* serogroup O:157, Salmonella serobiovars of Kaufman-White group N, and most importantly *Yersinia enterocolitica* serogroup O:9. Infection of pigs with this latter organism has often been confirmed, and the cross-reaction that results (the dominant O polysaccharide antigen is chemically identical to the A antigen present on the surface of all smooth brucellae) is highly significant. In some situations, yersiniosis poses a greater threat to the agricultural industry than does brucellosis itself, due to the confusion with brucellosis in diagnosis and the consequent effect on the export trade. Great Britain has always been free from *B. suis* infection and enjoys a thriving export trade as a result of the generally high health status of its stock. During the 7 years prior to 1988, the number of pigs tested for export certification giving a CFT reaction of greater than 20 international complement-fixation test units (icftu) never exceeded 0.004%, whereas the figures for 1988, 1989, and 1990 were 0.42%, 0.70%, and 1.5%, respectively. Since 1988, at least 4% of exporting herds have had more than 5% CFT positive reactions, with some herds reaching levels of more than 50% of animals tested failing at this level. *Y. enterocolitica* O:9 has been isolated from many herds involved, and despite extensive investigation, *B. suis* has not been recovered (Wrathall et al. 1991).

Lymphocyte transformation tests have been used to measure cell-mediated immune responses in infected pigs on a limited scale (Kaneene et al. 1978). There was high correlation between recovery of *B. suis* from tissues and detectable lymphocyte stimulation responses. However, the complexity of the method probably eliminates it from consideration as a diagnostic tool except in special cases.

Tests for delayed hypersensitivity, using intradermal injection of brucella allergens, have been studied, but results have not stimulated much enthusiasm in the United States. However, they are of similar accuracy to serologic tests and would be more appropriate for farm testing in some circumstances, although they are more difficult to apply and read and would not be applicable in testing programs for market pigs. In the face of cross-reactions caused by *Y. enterocolitica* O:9, the use of such tests is perhaps the most specific method of diagnosis. Skin tests are used frequently for diagnosis of porcine brucellosis in many countries, particularly in Eastern Europe.

One of the most important aids to diagnosis is an adequate herd history. Good records of clinical manifestations, movement of animals, additions to the herd, breeding records, and illnesses in persons working with the pigs provide invaluable information necessary to arrive at a diagnosis of brucellosis. Accurate epidemiological information is an essential supplement to laboratory tests.

TREATMENT

No treatments, such as antibiotic therapy, dietary supplements, or other chemotherapy, have been proven effective and economically feasible in curing pigs of brucellosis. Large doses of tetracyclines, streptomycin, or sulfonamides given over relatively long periods have been investigated. In some trials these antibiotics alone or in combination appeared promising. In general, however, antibiotic therapy was effective in limiting the bacteremic stage of the disease, but after therapy was discontinued, viable *B. suis* was still present in tissues. Although treatments have not been effective in eliminating all organisms from the host, chemotherapy in carefully selected circumstances could probably suppress multiplication of *B. suis* in vivo sufficiently to alleviate clinical manifestations and shedding of organisms. Even though such an approach may have limited practicability, it could have beneficial effects in an infected herd and should not be dismissed as useless.

PREVENTION

Immunity

Safe and reliable vaccines that produce serviceable immunity against brucellosis in pigs have not been developed. Significant resistance can be stimulated, but persistence of immunity has been a limiting factor (Deyoe 1972a). Interest in vaccination of pigs in the United States has declined along with the decline in incidence of the disease. With the present incidence of porcine brucellosis in the United States, the cost of developing and applying vaccination cannot be justified.

There have been no basic studies specifically directed toward the mechanism of immunity against *B. suis* infection in pigs. Nevertheless, one must assume from the overwhelming evidence accumulated in research on brucellosis in other species that the fundamental mechanism is a cell-mediated immunity, with humoral immunity having only a minor or nonexistent role.

Investigations into antibrucella immunity in pigs can be summarized as follows:

1. Some pigs are naturally resistant to brucella infection, and this resistance could be enhanced markedly by selective breeding programs (Cameron et al. 1941) if all other genetic factors could be ignored.
2. Some pigs infected with virulent *B. suis* will recover from the disease, but subsequent resistance induced by the virulent infection may be transient, as most will be susceptible to reexposure probably within 6–12 months after the initial infection. Commonly, many pigs, especially boars, become persistently infected with *B. suis*.
3. Trials with attenuated *B. suis* or *B. abortus* strain 19 have been unsuccessful in producing a persistent immunity with products considered to be safe for use.
4. Bacterins or extracts of killed *B. suis* have generally been ineffective in stimulating immunity or else there has been no conclusive evidence that the persistence of immunity is adequate.

Control Measures

Experiences in control of porcine brucellosis indicate that eradication of the disease from pigs in the United States is desirable and feasible. Marked reduction in the incidence of the disease has occurred since 1950. One significant factor in this reduction has been the tendency for pig production to become more specialized and less a part of diversified farming operations. Consequently, the occurrence of reproductive disease in pigs has become proportionately more important, confinement systems and closed herds have eliminated many opportunities for interfarm spread of disease, and larger units have eliminated the "community boar" in most instances. Another important instrument in control of porcine brucellosis has been the establishment and maintenance of validated brucellosis-free herds, particularly purebred herds or those selling breeding stock. Implementation of effective surveillance programs such as identification and testing of market pigs (sows and boars) has been instrumental in locating and eliminating large numbers of infected herds. Finally, it has been found that whenever recommended procedures to eradicate brucellosis from an individual herd or an enzootic area are conscientiously followed, there is very seldom any recurrence of the disease in that locality (e.g., Spencer and Mattison 1975).

The current brucellosis eradication program in the United States is a joint state-federal and livestock industry program. The program is administered, supervised, and funded by cooperative efforts between state and federal animal health regulatory agencies. This program is now nearing successful completion, with all states and U.S. territories, except Texas, in Stage III (Free) status. Texas will likely gain equal status once Uniform Methods and Rules are revised to reflect federal-state-industry consensus to remove loosely managed feral-exposed domestic herds from commercial herd classification.

The swine brucellosis eradication program has evolved to recognize that the organism will continue to exist indefinitely in the feral swine reservoir and associated transitional swine population. Transitional swine are defined as those feral swine that are captive or swine that have reasonable opportunities to be exposed to feral swine (USDA 2003). Efforts are now concentrated on effective separation of commercial production swine from transitional and feral swine, with adequate surveillance and testing of at-risk populations to assure compliance. The Pseudorabies Eradication Program now requires each state to file a Feral-Transitional Swine Management Plan, outlining its plans for dealing with feral swine pseudorabies virus threats. This plan will address swine brucellosis infection threats from feral swine populations as well. Swine brucellosis will be considered but one of many swine pathogens to be controlled by effective management and biosecurity measures against potential feral-transitional swine infections.

REFERENCES

Alton GG. 1990. *Brucella suis*. In Animal Brucellosis. Boca Raton: CRC Press.

Alton GG, Jones LM, Angus RD, Verger JM. 1988. Techniques for the brucellosis laboratory. Paris: INRA.

Alton GG, Jones LM, Pietz DE. 1975. Laboratory Techniques in Brucellosis, 2d ed. Geneva: World Health Organisation.

Becker HN, Belden RC, Breault T, Burridge MJ, Frankenberger WB, Nicoletti P. 1978. Brucellosis in feral swine in Florida. J Am Vet Med Assoc 173:1181–1182.

Bendtsen H, Christiansen M, Thomsen A. 1954. *Brucella* enzootics in swine herds in Denmark—Presumably with hare as a source of infection. Nord Vet Med 6:11–21.

Borts IH, Harris DM, Joynt MF, Jennings JR, Jordan CF. 1943. A milk borne epidemic of brucellosis caused by the porcine biotype of *Brucella* (*Brucella suis*) in a raw milk supply. J Am Vet Med Assoc 121:319.

Borts IH, McNutt SH, Jordan CF. 1946. *Brucella melitensis* isolated from swine tissues in Iowa. J Am Vet Med Assoc 130:966.

Brinley-Morgan WJ, McCullough NB. 1974. Genus *Brucella*. In Bergey's Manual of Determinative Bacteriology, 8th ed. Baltimore: Williams and Wilkins, pp. 278–282.

Cameron HS, Gregory PW, Hughes EH. 1941. Studies on genetic resistance in swine to *Brucella* infection. II. A bacteriological examination of resistant stock. Cornell Vet 31:21–24.

Cloeckaert A, Verger JM, Grayon M, Paquet JY, Garin-Bastuji B, Foster G, Godfroid J. 2001. Classification of *Brucella* spp. isolated from marine mammals by DNA polymorphism at the omp2 locus. Microbes and Infection 3:729–738.

Cook DR, Noble JW. 1984. Isolation of *B. suis* from cattle. Aust Vet J 61:263–264.

Corbel MJ. 1985. Effect of atrophic rhinitis vaccines on the reaction of pigs to serological tests for brucellosis. Vet Rec 117:150.

de Ley J, Mannheim W, Segers P, Lievens A, Denijin M, Vanhouke M, Gillis M. 1987. Ribonucleic acid cistron similarities and taxonomic neighbourhood of *Brucella* and CDC group Vd. Int J Syst Bacteriol 37:35–42.

Deyoe BL. 1967. Pathogenesis of three strains of *Brucella suis* in swine. Am J Vet Res 28:951–957.

——. 1968. Histopathologic changes in male swine with experimental brucellosis. Am J Vet Res 29:1215–1220.

——. 1969. Diagnostic tests for swine brucellosis. Proc Annu Meet Livest Conserv 53:20–22.

——. 1972a. Immunology and public health significance of swine brucellosis. J Am Vet Med Assoc 160:640–643.

——. 1972b. Research findings applicable to eradication of swine brucellosis. Proc Annu Meet US Anim Health Assoc 76:108–114.

Deyoe BL., Manthei CA. 1967. Sites of localization of *Brucella suis* in swine. Proc Annu Meet US Livest Sanit Assoc 71:102–108.

——. 1969. Swine brucellosis. In Proc 1967 Symp on Factors Producing Embryonic and Fetal Abnormalities, Death, and Abortion in Swine. ARS 91–73, pp. 54–60.

Drew ML, Jessup DA, Burr AA, Franti CE. 1992. Serological survey for brucellosis in feral swine, wild ruminants, and black bear of California. J Wildl Dis 28:355–363.

Enright FM. 1990. The pathogenesis and pathobiology of *Brucella* infection in domestic animals. In Animal Brucellosis. Boca Raton: CRC Press.

——. 1995. Update on research with RB51 strain of *Brucella abortus*. Proc Annu Meet US Anim Health Assoc 99:647–648.

Ferris RA, Schoenbaum MA, Crawford RP. 1995. Comparison of serological tests and bacteriologic culture for detection of brucellosis in swine from naturally infected herds. J Am Vet Med Assoc 207:1332–1333.

Fletcher WO, Chreekmore TE, Smith MS, Nettles VF. 1990. A field trial to determine the feasibility of delivering oral vaccines to wild swine. J Wildl Dis 26:503–510.

Fox MD., Kaufmann AF. 1977. Brucellosis in the United States, 1965–1974. J Infect Dis 136:312–316.

Frye GH, Gilsdorf MJ, Lenard D. 1993. Status report—Fiscal year 1993. Cooperative State-Federal Brucellosis Eradication Program. Proc Annu Meet US Anim Health Assoc 97:138–154.

Goode ER, Jr, Manthei CA, Blake GE, Amerault TE. 1952. *Brucella suis* infection in suckling and weanling pigs. II. J Am Vet Med Assoc 121:456–464.

Hoerlein AB, Hubbard ED, Leith TS, Biester HE. 1954. Swine Brucellosis. Vet Med Res Inst, Iowa State Coll.

Holland SD, Barton CE. 2004. Report of the Committee on Brucellosis. Proc Annu Meet US Anim Health Assoc. http://www.usaha.org/committees/bru/bru.shtml.

Huddleston IF. 1929. The Differentiation of the Species of the Genus *Brucella*. Bull Mich Agric Exp Stn no. 100.

Hutchings LM. 1950. Swine brucellosis. In Brucellosis: American Association for the Advancement of Science Symposium. Washington, D.C.: Waverly Press, pp. 188–198.

Jubb KVF, Kennedy PC, Palmer N. 1985. Pathology of Domestic Animals, vol. 3. Orlando: Academic Press, p. 349.

Kaneene JM, Anderson RK, Johnson DW, Angus RD, Muscoplate CC, Pietz DE, Vanderwagon LC, Sloane EE. 1978. Cell-mediated immune responses in swine from a herd infected with *Brucella suis*. Am J Vet Res 39:1607–1611.

Lealklevezas DS, Martinez-Vazquez IO, Lopez-Merino A, Martinez-Soriano JP. 1995. Single-step PCR for detection of *Brucella* spp. from blood and milk of infected animals. J Clin Microbiol 33:3087–3090.

Leek ML van der, Becker HN, Humphrey P, Adams CL, Belden RC, Frankenberger WB, Nicoletti PL. 1993. Prevalence of *Brucella* sp. antibodies in feral swine in Florida. J Wildl Dis 29:410–415.

Luchsinger DW, Anderson RK, Werring DF. 1965. A swine brucellosis epizootic. J Am Vet Med Assoc 147:632–636.

Manthei CA, Mingle CK, Carter RW. 1952. *Brucella suis* infection in suckling and weaning pigs. 1. J Am Vet Med Assoc 121:373–382.

Nettles VF. 1991. Short- and long-term strategies for resolving problems of pseudorabies and swine brucellosis in feral swine. Proc Annu Meet US Anim Health Assoc 95:551–556.

Nielsen K, Gall N. 2001. Fluorescence Polarization Assay for the Diagnosis of Brucellosis: A Review. J. Immunoassay & Immunochemistry 22(3):183–201.

Nielsen K, Gall N, Smith P, Vigliocco A. et al. 1999. Validation of the fluorescence polarization assay as a serologic test for the presumptive diagnosis of porcine brucellosis. Veterinary Microbiology 68:245–253.

Office International des Epizooties. 1997. Manual of Standards for Diagnostic Tests and Vaccines. 3rd Edition. Paris.

Paolicchi FA, Terzolo HR, Campero CM. 1993. Isolation of *Brucella suis* from the semen of a ram. Vet Rec 132:67.

Payeur JB, Miller CD, Hennager SG, Ewalt DR. 1990. Comparison of five serologic tests and culture for brucellosis in swine experimentally infected with *Brucella suis* biovar 1. Proc Annu Meet US Anim Health Assoc 94:147–152.

Rogers RJ, Cook DR, Kettlerer PJ, Baldock FC, Blackall PJ, Stewart RW. 1989. An evaluation of three serological tests for antibody to *Brucella suis* in pigs. Aust Vet J 66:77–80.

Spencer PL, Mattison JR. 1975. Pike County, Illinois, swine brucellosis project. Proc Annu Meet US Anim Health Assoc 79:86–91.

Thomsen A. 1934. *Brucella* infection in swine. Acta Pathol Microbiol Scand (Suppl) 21.

Traum J. 1914. Report to the Chief. Bureau of Animal Industry, USDA, p. 30.

United States Department of Agriculture, Animal and Plant Health Inspection Service. 2003. Pseudorabies Eradication, State-Federal-Industry, Program Standards (APHIS 91-55-071). Effective November 1, 2003. http://www.aphis.usda.gov/vs/nahps/pseudorabies/prv-prgm-std.pdf.

Vandeplassche M, Herman J, Spincemaille J, Bouters R, Dekeyser P, Brone E. 1967. *Brucella suis* infection and infertility in swine. Meded Veeartsenijsch Rijksuniv Gent 11:1–40.

Verger JM, Greymont F, Gremont PAD, Grayon M. 1985. *Brucella*, a monospecific genus as shown by deoxyribonucleic acid hybridisation. Int J Syst Bacteriol 35:292–295.

Wood GW, Hendricks JB, Goodman DE. 1976. Brucellosis in feral swine. J Wildl Dis 12:579–582.

Wrathall AE, Broughton ES, Gill KPW, Goldsmith GP. 1991. Serological reactions to *Brucella* in British pigs. Vet Rec 132:449–454.

36 Clostridial Infections

J. Glenn Songer and David J. Taylor

Clostridia are large, gram-positive, spore-forming rods, and are strict–to–oxygen-tolerant anaerobes. *Clostridium perfringens* types A and C, *C. difficile, C. tetani, C. novyi, C. botulinum,* and occasionally *C. chauvoei* and *C. septicum*, are primary pathogens of swine, but may also invade existing wounds or lesions (Table 36.1). Many maintain a residence in the intestinal tract, and postmortem invasion of other tissues can confuse diagnosis.

ENTERIC INFECTIONS

Clostridium perfringens
Production of the so-called major toxins [alpha (CPA), beta (CPB), epsilon (ETX), and iota (ITX)] divides *C. perfringens* into five toxinotypes (Table 36.2). Strains of type A are widespread in the intestines of warm-blooded animals and in the environment, and others tend to be present in lower numbers in normal animals.

Type C Enteritis. *Clostridium perfringens* type C infection occurs in all swine-producing areas of the world (Field and Gibson 1955; Szent-Ivanyi and Szabo 1955; Barnes and Moon 1964; Hogh 1965; Matthias et al. 1968; Plaisier 1971; Morin et al. 1983; Azuma et al. 1983). Type C causes frequently hemorrhagic, often-fatal, necrotic enteritis in young piglets. Hallmark lesions are profound mucosal necrosis and emphysema in small intestine, sometimes extending into cecum and proximal colon.

Etiology and Epidemiology. Type C is a primary pathogen but can apparently colonize lesions of other diseases, such as transmissible gastroenteritis (TGE). Types B (Bakhtin 1956) and D (Harbola and Khera 1990) have apparently been isolated from type C-like syndromes, but given the vagaries of the in vivo typing system, it may be prudent to confirm these reports before accepting types B and D as even rare causes of severe enteritis in neonatal pigs.

Infection can be transmitted piglet-to-piglet, but the ultimate source is likely the intestine of the sow. Prevent-ing introduction of disease by screening of replacement stock is likely not a viable option. Type C in normal sow feces accounts for only a tiny percentage of the total population of *C. perfringens*; it nearly always goes undetected by any but highly specialized methods, which are impractical for screening large numbers of animals. Piglets may act as enrichment vessels, in which small numbers of type C outcompete other bacteria and multiply to large numbers, with resulting disease production.

The organism persists in the environment as vegetative cells or spores, and the latter are resistant to heat, disinfectants, and ultraviolet light. Environmental organisms cycle through nonvaccinated piglets over long periods.

Disease is most common in 3-day-old piglets, but may appear as early as 12 hours after birth and is rarely seen in pigs older than one week (Bergeland et al. 1966; Meszaros and Pesti 1965; Matthias et al. 1968). Type C enteritis occurs epizootically in nonvaccinated populations (Bergeland et al. 1966) and prevalence of affected litters can reach 100%. The case fatality rate varies with the form of the disease, but 100% mortality in litters of nonimmune sows is not unusual, and total herd mortality may be as high as 50–60% (Bergeland et al. 1966; Hogh 1967b). When herd immunity rises, due to exposure of sows to infected piglets, disease may become enzootic. Milder cases occur over a period of months in individual herds, but continued appearance of acute disease usually indicates a deficiency in herd immunity (e.g., repeated introduction of naive gilts or sows) or failure of piglets to receive adequate levels of specific antibody in colostrum.

Clinical Signs and Lesions. Clinical signs vary according to immune status and age of affected piglets. Most *peracutely affected piglets* develop hemorrhagic diarrhea, accompanied by staining of the perineum. Piglets become weak, move with reluctance, and rapidly become moribund, risking crushing by the sow. Rectal temperature falls to 35°C and abdominal skin may blacken be-

Table 36.1.   Major clostridia and associated syndromes affecting swine

Clostridium species	Syndrome
C. perfringens type A	Neonatal necrotizing enteritis, myonecrosis
C. perfringens type C	Neonatal hemorrhagic, necrotic enteritis
C. difficile	Neonatal enteritis
C. tetani	Tetanus
C. botulinum	Botulism
C. novyi	Sudden death in sows
C. septicum	Blackleg
C. chauvoei	Blackleg

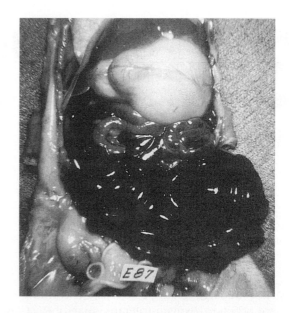

36.1.   *Necrohemorrhagic jejunitis in a 1-day-old piglet with peracute* C. perfringens *type C enteritis.*

fore death. Many are found dead within 12–36 hours of birth. Death occurs in some animals without diarrhea being seen. The abdominal wall is often edematous when cut, but the most immediate and striking findings are intensely hemorrhagic small intestines (Figure 36.1) and bloodstained fluid in the abdominal cavity. Lesions are typically in jejunum and ileum; they may extend anterior to within a few centimeters of the pylorus and posterior to the proximal colon, or may affect only a few centimeters of jejunum. Gross mucosal lesions are reddish or black in color, with intense hemorrhage and gas bubbles in the intestinal wall. Mesenteric lymph nodes may be reddened. Contents of the affected area contain blood and may be found as far distal as the rectum. Microscopic examination reveals necrotic jejunal villi and a surface covered by a carpet of large gram-positive bacilli. Crypt epithelium may be necrotic, and there is profuse hemorrhage throughout the mucosa and submucosa (Figures 36.2 and 36.3).

Acutely affected piglets may survive for 1–2 days after onset of clinical signs, but usually die shortly thereafter. They have reddish-brown diarrhea containing gray shreds of tissue debris, may be dehydrated, with loss of body condition, and there may be scalding of the perineum and adherent reddish feces. Nursing is minimal, and these piglets rapidly lose condition and become gaunt and weak. Gross lesions (refer to Figure 36.1) are usually localized, and emphysema may be observed in a sharply demarcated portion of jejunum. This portion of intestine may be loosely adherent to adjacent segments by acute fibrinous peritonitis (Figure 36.4), and intes-

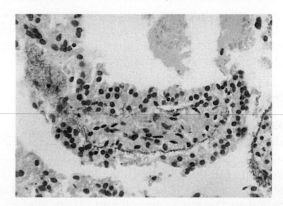

36.2.   *Villus of the jejunum early in the course of* C. perfringens *type C infection in a 12-hour-old piglet. Numerous bacilli are present beneath the desquamated epithelium in the area of the epithelial basement membrane (H&E).*

tinal wall is usually thickened and yellow or grayish; contents may be bloodstained and contain necrotic debris. Deposition of urate crystals in kidney is common. Microscopic examination reveals loss of most villi, and those surviving are necrotic and covered with bacteria. The exposed submucosa is also carpeted by bacteria,

Table 36.2.   Production of so-called major toxins by types of *Clostridium perfringens* and associated diseases

Toxin Type	Major Diseases	Major Toxins
A	Food poisoning, poultry necrotic enteritis, lamb enterotoxemia, porcine neonatal necrotizing enterocolitis, bovine neonatal hemorrhagic enteritis	alpha
B	Lamb dysentery, ovine chronic enteritis, bovine/equine hemorrhagic enteritis	alpha, beta, epsilon
C	Fowl necrotic enteritis, hemorrhagic or necrotic enterotoxemia in piglets, lambs, calves, goats, foals, acute enterotoxemia ("struck") in adult sheep	alpha, beta
D	Ovine enterotoxemia, caprine enterocolitis, bovine enterotoxemia (calves, possibly adults)	alpha, epsilon
E	Bovine (possibly ovine) neonatal enterotoxemia	alpha, iota

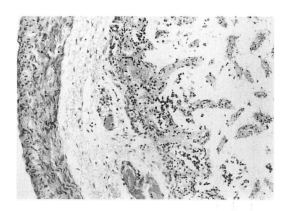

36.3. *Jejunum of a piglet with peracute* C. perfringens *type C enteritis. There is acute necrosis of the mucosa and massive hemorrhage in the submucosa (H&E).*

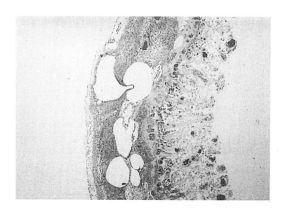

36.5. *Jejunum of a piglet with acute* C. perfringens *type C enteritis. The mucosa is completely necrotic, and there is emphysema of the submucosa and tunica muscularis (H&E).*

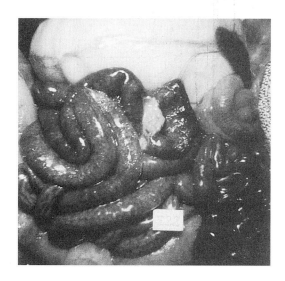

36.4. *Acute* C. perfringens *type C enteritis in a 3-day-old piglet. An emphysematous segment of upper jejunum (left) is held together by acute peritonitis. Mucosal necrosis of the lower jejunum (right) is seen from the serosal surface.*

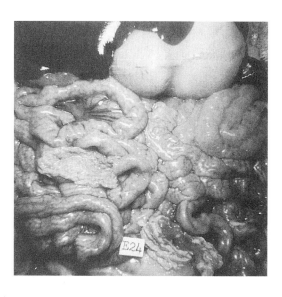

36.6. *Subacute form of* C. perfringens *type C enteritis in a 6-day-old piglet. The entire jejunum is lined with a necrotic membrane.*

shed epithelial cells, fibrin, and degenerating inflammatory cells. Submucosal vessels are necrotic and many contain thrombi and emphysema may be evident in submucosa, tunica muscularis, and under the serosa (Figure 36.5). Large gram-positive bacteria may be present in deeper layers of intestinal wall.

Diarrhea in *pigs with subacute disease* is nonhemorrhagic. These animals remain active, alert, and appetant, but become progressively emaciated; they may be thin and dehydrated at the time of death, usually at about 5–7 days of age. Stools are often yellow initially, but then become clear, with flecks of necrotic debris. There may be adhesions between affected areas of small intestine, and intestinal wall is thickened and friable. The mucosal surface is covered by a tightly adherent necrotic membrane which may be seen from the serosal surface as longitudinal grayish-yellow bands (Figure 36.6).

Chronic cases usually have intermittent diarrhea for

more than a week. Feces are yellow-gray and mucoid, and tail and perineum may be fecal-stained, and although these piglets remain alert and vigorous, they may die after several weeks or be euthanized because of unthriftiness. Lesions may resemble those in subacute disease, but may not be obvious from the serosa. There may be local thickening of intestinal wall and well-defined areas (in many cases only 1–2 cm in length) to which necrotic membrane is adherent. Deeper layers of the intestinal wall show evidence of chronic inflammation (Figure 36.7).

Pathogenesis. *Clostridium perfringens* has a very short generation time, and type C organisms can multiply to numbers approaching 10^8–10^9 per gram of contents in only a few hours (Ohnuna et al. 1992). Attachment to jejunal epithelial cells at villous apices (Arbuckle 1972; Walker et al. 1980) is followed by desquamation of these

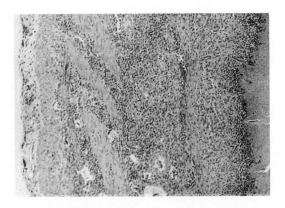

36.7. *Ileum of a piglet with chronic* C. perfringens *type C enteritis. The mucosa is replaced by a necrotic membrane containing a variety of bacterial species. The submucosa, tunica muscularis, and serosa are infiltrated by chronic inflammatory cells (H&E).*

cells and proliferation of the organism along the basement membrane. Necrosis of the villous lamina propria is extensive, and hemorrhage accompanies necrosis. The necrotic zone advances to involve crypts, muscularis mucosa and submucosa, and occasionally the muscular layers. Perforation of intestinal wall leads to emphysema (sometimes with thrombosis) in muscle layers, beneath the peritoneum, and in mesenteric lymph nodes. Bacteria remain adhered to necrotic villi or are shed into intestinal lumen with cell debris and blood, and sporulation may be observed (Kubo and Watase 1985).

The lethal and necrotizing beta toxin (CPB) is the key factor in pathogenesis of type C infections (Warrack 1963; Hogh 1967a). Toxoid vaccines protect against infection, but it is worth noting that these are crude, containing many clostridial antigens other than beta toxoid. Experimental evidence for the primacy of CPB in pathogenesis is equivocal. Disease was reproduced by oral administration of toxin, but in pigs subsequently found to be infected with the organism (Field and Goodwin 1959). Typical lesions appeared in gut loops inoculated with broth cultures of type C (Bergeland 1972), but necrosis was not produced by inoculation with CPB alone. There are numerous potentially confounding factors in much of the published literature, including use of older pigs as experimental animals; trypsin secretion deficiencies and colostral protease inhibitors probably account for susceptibility of piglets less than 4 days old.

Death is primarily due to effects of intestinal damage and toxemia. CPB has been detected in both intestinal contents and peritoneal fluid of affected pigs. Toxin-containing preparations administered IV in high doses cause sudden death, and lower doses cause polioencephalomalacia, adrenal cortical necrosis, nephrosis, and pulmonary edema. Hypoglycemia and secondary bacteremia due to *C. perfringens* or *E. coli* may raise the mortality rate (Field and Goodwin 1959; Hogh 1967b).

Beta2 toxin (CPB2), produced by most or all porcine type C isolates, may also play a role in pathogenesis (see below, under "Type A Enteritis").

Diagnosis. Compatible clinical signs, pattern of mortality, and nature of gross and microscopic lesions are sufficient basis for a presumptive diagnosis of type C enteritis. Diagnosis of chronic disease may depend upon a more-detailed history of infection in the herd, elimination of other causes of necrotic enteritis, and detection of type C organisms in lesions. Coccidiosis *(Isospora suis)* and other causes of villous atrophy, such as rotavirus infection, TGE, and porcine epidemic diarrhea, may cause lesions which become colonized by *C. perfringens* type C. It is especially important in subacute and chronic cases to distinguish type C infections from those caused by *C. perfringens* type A, and this can be done only by bacteriologic culture and toxin detection or genotyping.

Laboratory aspects of diagnosis include bacteriologic culture and examination of smears of intestinal contents and mucosal lesions and histological sections of intestine for large, gram-positive rods. *Clostridium perfringens* is not an efficient sporulator, but ovoid-to-eccentric spores are sometimes observed. Colonies after 24 hours' incubation on horse or bovine blood agar are usually 3–5 mm in diameter, grayish, and circular; on primary isolation, these may be mixed with smaller colonies, which are smoother and have a gumdrop-like morphology. The organism usually produces an inner, complete zone of hemolysis, caused by theta toxin (perfringolysin O, PFO), and a less-complete outer zone caused by CPA. Identification to species is based in addition upon biochemical characteristics and production of toxins.

Microscopic lesions are almost pathognomonic. Diagnosis can be confirmed by demonstration of CPB in eluates of hemorrhagic intestinal contents or in peritoneal fluid. Mouse protection tests are seldom used today, having been replaced by enzyme immunoassays (Havard et al. 1992). PCR methods to detect genes for the major toxins are an acceptable substitute for toxin detection in typing of isolates, and can provide useful supportive findings in diagnosis (Buogo et al. 1995; Songer and Meer 1996; Meer and Songer 1997).

In the absence of methodology to detect toxins in pathologic specimens, bacterial isolation and genotyping are useful aids in establishing a diagnosis. In most cases, type C is isolated in large numbers and in pure culture from scrapings of the intestinal mucosa. Results may be misleading in rare situations, in that type C can be found as a secondary agent, colonizing lesions of TGE and other viral diseases. Cultures may be negative in chronic cases, and when positive usually yield a mixture of type C and type A organisms. Thus, it is important to determine genotype or phenotype of multiple primary isolates. Diagnosis must, in some cases, be based upon findings in the herd as a whole, rather than from examination of individual diseased animals.

Treatment and Prevention. Treatment is of little use in animals with clinical signs (Szabo and Szent-Ivanyi 1957; Hogh 1967b), and prophylaxis is the preferred approach. Passive immunization with equine antitoxin can be useful for protection of litters of nonimmune sows in an outbreak, and protection may last as long as 3 weeks (Ripley and Gush 1983). Antitoxin should be injected parenterally as soon after birth as possible. Oral antimicrobials, such as ampicillin or amoxicillin, may also be given prophylactically, beginning immediately after birth and continuing daily for 3 days. There are reports of antimicrobial resistance in *C. perfringens*, and tetracycline resistance plasmids have been identified (Rood et al. 1985). However, the organism remains uniformly susceptible to penicillins. Ceftiofur may be an alternative for treatment of piglets, and bacitracin methylene disalicylate can be administered to sows before and after farrowing to prevent infection of piglets.

Prevention is best achieved by vaccination of sows with type C toxoid, at breeding or midgestation and 2–3 weeks before farrowing (Kennedy et al. 1977). Commercial toxoid vaccines are quite effective, and instituting a vaccination program usually eliminates the disease within one farrowing cycle. Tenfold reductions in mortality are common (Ripley and Gush 1983), assuming normal responses of the sow to vaccination (Matishek and McGrinley 1986) and ingestion of adequate colostrum. Booster injections should be given about 3 weeks before subsequent farrowings. Toxoid may also be of value in protecting weaned pigs (Meszaros and Pesti 1965).

Type A Enteritis. *Clostridium perfringens* type A is part of the normal flora of the swine intestine (Mansson and Smith 1962), but is also a cause of enteric disease, both in neonatal piglets and, occasionally, in weaned pigs (Jestin et al. 1985). Disease has been reported worldwide (Amtsberg et al. 1976; Ramisse et al. 1979; Nabuurs et al. 1983; Secasiu 1984; Collins et al. 1989). There is a continuing association of type A with hemorrhagic bowel syndrome, but this etiologic link is not supported by experimental evidence.

Etiology and Epidemiology. *Clostridium perfringens* type A resembles type C in culture, but it produces CPA as its sole major toxin (refer to Table 36.2). Recent information (Bueschel et al. 2003; Waters et al. 2003) suggests a role for beta2 toxin (CPB2) in porcine clostridial enteritis, and nearly all type A strains from this condition produce this protein (Bueschel et al. 2003; Waters et al. 2003; see below). Clinical signs have been reproduced experimentally (Johannsen et al. 1993a).

Human clostridial food poisoning usually occurs when enterotoxigenic (CPE-producing) strains grow in slowly cooling meats following cooking. Involvement of

CPE-producing strains in animal disease is apparently uncommon (Estrada Correa and Taylor 1989; Damme-Jongsten et al. 1990; Miwa et al. 1997; Collins et al. 1989). Food poisoning strains probably originate most commonly in poultry; porcine strains can also be fully enterotoxigenic, so pigs may also be a source. In general, *cpe* is chromosomal in human strains and plasmid-borne in animal strains.

Disease occurs usually during the first week, and it is assumed that sows are the source of infection for piglets. Antibody is widespread in finishing pigs and in sows (Estrada Correa and Taylor 1989). However, it should be understood that it is not possible to differentiate between normal flora type A strains and those which cause disease, with the possible exception of *cpb2* positivity. Furthermore, it may be that, under the right conditions, *any* strain of type A can cause disease. Type A is ubiquitous in gut contents and in soil, although most of these strains are *cpb2* negative. Thus, discussion of the epidemiology of type A enteric infections amounts to little (or nothing) more than speculation.

As noted previously, *C. perfringens* is an inefficient sporulator, but spores are nonetheless likely to be important in maintaining the organism in the environment. The organism can also be isolated from pig feed.

Clinical Signs and Lesions. Piglets develop creamy or pasty diarrhea within 48 hours of birth, displaying rough hair coat and fecal staining of the perineum (Johannsen et al. 1993a). Diarrhea lasts for up to 5 days, and feces become mucoid and sometimes pink. Most piglets recover, but are stunted, sometimes through the entire growing and finishing period. Disease has been reproduced in gnotobiotic colostrum-deprived and conventional pigs (Johannsen et al. 1993).

On postmortem, small intestine is flaccid, thin-walled, and gas-filled, with watery contents and no blood. Mucosal inflammation is mild, occasionally with adherent necrotic material. Large intestine may be distended, with whitish, pasty contents, but without lesions. Microscopic lesions in piglets may include superficial villous tip necrosis and accumulation of fibrin, but villi may also be completely normal in appearance (Figure 36.8). Jejunal and ileal lesions may be heavily colonized with *C. perfringens* (Nabuurs et al. 1983), although it is common to find masses of organisms in the lumen (Johannsen et al. 1993c). Capillaries may be dilated, but there is no hemorrhage.

Mucosal necrosis and villous atrophy are superficial in infections by enterotoxigenic *C. perfringens* (Nabuurs et al. 1983; Estrada-Correa and Taylor 1989; Collins et al. 1989). Signs in experimental infections range from creamy diarrhea and emaciation with low mortality to profuse, bloodstained diarrhea, enteritis, and death (Olubunmi and Taylor 1985). Morphology of small intestinal villi and enterocytes are normal, and there are no colonic or cecal lesions, but numerous spore-

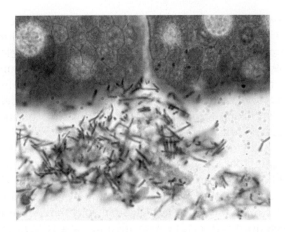

36.8. *Association of* C. perfringens-*like organisms with villus tips and accumulation of large numbers of organisms in jejunal lumen in* C. perfringens *type A infection in a 3-day-old piglet (Jane Christopher-Hennings).*

bearing, gram-positive rods are found in the lumen or apposed to epithelial cells at tips of villi.

Enterotoxigenic strains have been linked to diarrheal disease in growing pigs, and in these cases onset and the severity of diarrhea correlate with presence of CPE in feces. Affected pigs develop serum antibodies to CPE (Jestin et al. 1985).

Pathogenesis. Type A can be isolated from any normal piglet's first feces, and although pathogenesis of infections is poorly understood, it is likely multifactorial. Numbers in ileum and jejunum reach 10^8–10^9 per gram of contents, producing CPA, CPB2, and possibly other toxins. Attachment and invasion do not occur in experimental infections (Johannsen et al. 1993c). Intestinal epithelial necrosis occurs in experimental infections, but may not be apparent in natural cases; absence of gross and microscopic lesions suggests that type A enteritis is mainly a secretory diarrhea.

There is no direct information on the role of specific toxins in pathogenesis. There are no consistent changes in gut loops inoculated with purified CPA, but slight edema of villi occurs when 6-hour-old piglets are given 80–800 mouse lethal doses (Johannsen et al. 1993b). The specific role of CPB2 in pathogenesis is unknown, but its strong association with enteric disease in pigs suggests that it is at least a marker of virulence (Gibert et al. 1997; Herholz et al. 1999; Bueschel et al. 2003). Few isolates from normal pigs contain *cpb2*, but >90% from porcine neonatal enteritis strains are positive, and the gene is rarely silent (Bueschel et al. 2003). CPE causes villous necrosis and fluid secretion into intestinal lumen. Anti-CPE antibody is present in colostrum, and disease associated with CPE commonly occurs in weaned pigs after maternal antibody disappears (Estrada Correa and Taylor 1989).

Diagnosis. Diagnosis of type A enteritis is seldom unequivocal. The most useful findings are compatible clinical signs and isolation of large numbers of *C. perfringens* from affected jejunum or ileum. Genotyping almost invariably reveals type A organisms with *cpb2*. Microscopic examination may reveal organisms intimately associated with the mucosa, or they may be massed in the lumen. Detection of CPA in gut contents is also supportive, but tests are not widely available. Commercial assays for CPE are prone to false positives, but diarrhea has been associated with fecal CPE titers >1:32 (Popoff and Jestin 1985). Failure to demonstrate other agents is also supportive.

Treatment and Prevention. Treatment with antimicrobials is more likely to be successful than in cases of type C infection. Vaccination against type A is possible via custom biologics, and products available in some countries for immunization of other species are used off-label in pigs. Commercial vaccines do not include CPE toxoid. Growth promoters, such as avoparcin (Taylor and Estrada Correa 1988) and salinomycin (Kyriakis et al. 1995), have been used in feed, and bacitracin methylene disalicylate can be used prophylactically in sows or for treatment of piglets (Madsen 1995).

Clostridium difficile-Associated Disease (CDAD)

Etiology and Epidemiology. Human *C. difficile*-associated disease (CDAD) accounts for one-fourth of all cases of antibiotic-associated diarrhea (Bartlett 1992; Bartlett et al. 1978; Borriello and Wilcox 1998; Johnson et al. 1999). Spores germinate in ileum, cecum, and colon (Kelly et al. 1984), and vegetative cells fill empty niches and produce toxins. Disease presents as diarrhea, colitis, pseudomembranous colitis, or fulminant colitis (Kelly et al. 1984).

CDAD also occurs in antibiotic-treated hamsters (Libby et al. 1982) and guinea pigs and neonatal foals (Jones et al. 1988), and is emerging as a cause of enteritis in neonatal pigs. More than one-third of piglets submitted for diagnosis of enteritis in major swine-producing areas of the U.S. have uncomplicated CDAD and mixed infections occur in a further 20–25% (Songer et al. 2000). Prevalence in a production system was 47.6% on a per litter basis, and 90% of herds were infected (J.G. Songer and K.W. Post, unpublished observations).

Clinical Signs, Lesions, and Pathogenesis. Typical CDAD affects piglets 1–7 days of age born to gilts or multiparous sows. They present with a history of early-onset scours, occasionally with respiratory distress and sudden death (with hydrothorax and/or ascites). Gross lesions usually include mesocolonic edema (Figure 36.9), and large intestines may be filled with pasty-to-watery yellowish feces. Extensive sampling in CDAD-affected herds has revealed that two-thirds of litters and more

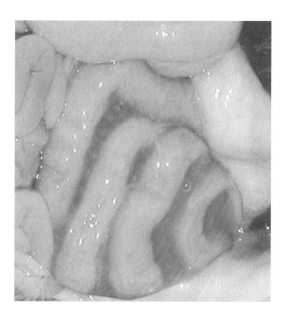

36.9. *Mesocolonic edema in a 4-day-old piglet with* C. difficile *infection (J. Glenn Songer).*

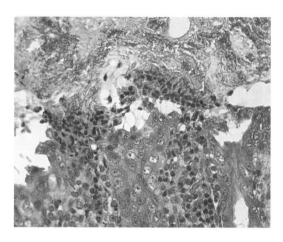

36.10. *Colitis in neonatal* C. difficile *infection. Neutrophils entering the colonic lumen form the so-called "volcano" lesion (J. Glenn Songer).*

than one-third of individual pigs are toxin positive in an infected barn. Piglets without enteric signs may be toxin positive (Yaeger et al. 2002; Waters et al. 1998). Focal suppuration in colonic lamina propria is the hallmark lesion, and colonic serosal and mesenteric edema and infiltration of mononuclear inflammatory cells and neutrophils into the edematous areas is common. Segmental erosion of colonic mucosal epithelium and volcano lesions (exudation of neutrophils and fibrin into lumen) may occur (Figure 36.10) (Songer et al. 2000). Pathogenesis of CDAD in domestic animals is likely mediated by the monomeric toxins A (TcdA, 308 kDa, an enterotoxin) and B (TcdB, 270 kDa, a cytotoxin).

Diagnosis. The gold standard for diagnosis of porcine CDAD is detection of TcdA and TcdB in feces or colonic contents. The reference method is measurement of neutralizable cytotoxicity in monolayers of Chinese hamster ovary cells, but most laboratories now use commercially available enzyme immunoassays. Culture for *C. difficile* can be somewhat challenging, in that this organism is more strictly anaerobic than some clostridia (Songer et al. 2000; Post et al. 2002). Most isolates are fully toxigenic, but some produce only TcdB or no toxins at all. Gross lesions are minimal, but careful microscopic examination of colon and cecum reveals suppurative foci, as described above. Colitis due to other causes is relatively rare.

Treatment and Prevention. Immunoprophylaxis of CDAD in domestic animals has not been studied, but precedent in other species suggests that immunity will be antitoxic. Antibodies against TcdA prevent toxin binding in mouse and hamster models, eliminating secretion, inflammation, and clinical disease (Allo et al. 1979). AntiTcdB antibodies also participate (Kink and Williams 1998; Viscidi et al. 1983). No commercial product is available, but some have attempted to prevent CDAD by use of custom biologics. Results of in vitro antimicrobial susceptibility testing suggest that virginiamycin administered to sows before and after farrowing might be useful for prophylaxis, and tylosin may be effective in treatment of piglets.

CELLULITIS AND GAS GANGRENE

Clostridial wound infections are characterized by acute inflammation, edema, and extensive tissue emphysema and local tissue necrosis. Inflammation spreads rapidly from the primary site, often with terminal generalized sepsis. *Clostridium septicum, C. perfringens* type A, *C. novyi,* and *C. chauvoei* are most likely to cause porcine clostridial cellulitis and gas gangrene.

Clostridium septicum Infection (Malignant Edema)

Etiology and Epidemiology. *Clostridium septicum* appears to be the most common etiologic agent of clostridial cellulitis and gas gangrene of swine. It is an anaerobic gram-positive rod, which forms oval subterminal spores, is found in soil and feces (Finegold et al. 1983; Kahn 1924; Princewill 1985; Princewill and Oakley 1976), and is a frequent postmortem invader (MacLennan 1962). Incidence of malignant edema is particularly high on certain premises that have had large populations of livestock for many years, suggesting that there is a buildup of spore numbers in the environment of these farms.

Clinical Signs and Lesions. *Clostridium septicum* causes malignant edema, which has an acute course and is often fatal in less than 24 hours. Hemorrhage, edema, and necrosis develop as the infection spreads along muscular fascial planes. Common sites include the inguinal and ventral abdominal region, the head and ventral cervical area, and the shoulder. There is reluctance to bear weight on affected limbs, and skin overlying the swollen area has a blotchy reddish-purple discoloration. Tissues that are initially painful and warm, with pitting edema, become rapidly crepitant and cold. In the terminal stage, affected swine lie in lateral recumbency and commonly make a groaning noise during forced expiration.

Swelling at the primary infection site (Figure 36.11) overlies subcutaneous edema that is colorless with focal hemorrhages or uniformly sanguinous. Adjacent skeletal muscle may be edematous, with essentially normal color, or may be black, dry, and crepitant (Figure 36.12). Affected muscle may have a butyric odor comparable to that in ruminant blackleg (*C. chauvoei* infection). Regional lymph nodes are enlarged and hemorrhagic, and may be emphysematous. Acute fibrohemorrhagic

peritonitis is common, the spleen is slightly enlarged, and there is moderate pulmonary edema and congestion. Varying amounts of blood-tinged fluid and fibrin may be found in the pleural cavity and pericardial sac.

Postmortem accumulation of subcutaneous gas progresses until the subcutis of the entire carcass is emphysematous. Focal postmortem lysis of the liver, evidenced by grayish-tan foci, are evident within several hours after death. These foci become confluent, giving the liver a uniform tan color with numerous gas bubbles. Microscopically, edematous subcutis contains large numbers of degenerating acute inflammatory cells and bacteria. Septic thrombi in subcutaneous veins and lymphatics are commonly found (Figure 36.13). Affected skeletal muscle fibers undergo coagulation necrosis with fragmentation and lysis, and bacteria are readily found between degenerating muscle fibers (Figure 36.14).

Pathogenesis. Most cases result from wounds, and tissue damage at the site of inoculation favors initial establishment of the infection. Lesions are largely the result of the necrotizing effect of alpha toxin. Hyaluronidase

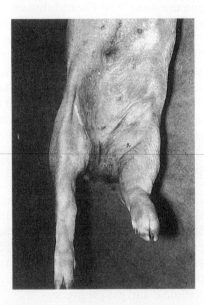

36.11. C. septicum *infection. The grossly swollen area involves the entire left rear leg and extends cranially to the umbilicus. The overlying skin has a blotchy reddish-purple discoloration.*

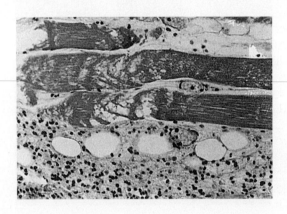

36.13. *Acute septic thrombophlebitis involving the subcutaneous vein of a pig with* C. septicum *infection. The thrombus contains many long slender rods and degenerating leukocytes (H&E).*

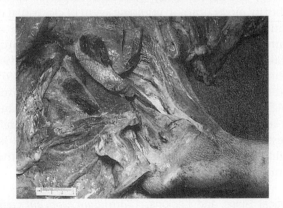

36.12. *Rear leg of a pig with* C. septicum *infection. There is prominent subcutaneous edema. The infection extends into the ham, which has foci of black, dry necrotic muscle.*

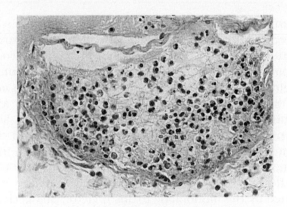

36.14. C. septicum *infection of the rear leg of a pig. Skeletal muscle fibers are undergoing fragmentation and lysis. The adjacent connective tissues are edematous and emphysematous and contain bacteria and degenerating inflammatory cells (H&E).*

may cause disappearance of the endomysium (Aikat and Dible 1960), which may aid spread of the infection through muscle. Toxemia is probably the ultimate cause of death. Alpha toxin is a pore-former (Ballard et al. 1993) and intravenous infusion specifically affects coronary and pulmonary circulation and causes pulmonary edema (Kellaway et al. 1941).

Diagnosis. Presumptive diagnosis is based upon gross lesions. Laboratory confirmation is based on pathologic findings, exclusion of other diseases, and identification of the organism. Bacteria are seen in direct smears of affected subcutis or muscle, and fluorescent-labeled antibody staining is a rapid and accurate method to positively identify *C. septicum* (Batty and Walker 1963). Bacteriologic culture is an alternative method, but is time-consuming and often less reliable than immunofluorescence (Martig 1966). Swarming of *C. septicum* may cause small numbers of the organism to appear predominant, resulting in a false-positive diagnosis.

Treatment and Prevention. Prevention is preferred to treatment, given the fulminant clinical course. It is important to practice good sanitation and prevent injuries. Infection may be iatrogenic, and adequate sanitary procedures should be followed when making injections or performing surgery. On premises where the disease recurs, immunization could be considered, although this is uncommon in swine. Antibodies to somatic and toxin antigens provide lifelong immunity, although there are differences in immunogenicity by vaccine and host species (Green et al. 1987). Treatment with antibiotics may be successful if given early (Zeller 1956). Experimental prophylactic use of tetracyclines, penicillin, or chloramphenicol prevents disease in mice, although their effectiveness was greater when administered at the inoculation site than when given systemically (Taylor and Novak 1952).

Clostridium perfringens Type A Infection (Gas Gangrene)

Etiology and Epidemiology. Most cases of *C. perfringens*-associated myonecrosis are apparently caused by type A strains. The source is usually endogenous, and few cases are nontraumatic. High intraherd incidence in young piglets is often a complication of injection of iron-containing preparations for prevention of nutritional anemia. Anecdotal evidence supports a view that such injections create a tissue microenvironment that favors growth of *C. perfringens* (Jaartsveld et al. 1962; Taylor and Bergeland 1992) in pure or mixed culture. The case fatality rate approaches 50%.

Clinical Signs and Lesions. Affected animals have marked swelling of the entire affected limb, and in the case of piglets with iatrogenic infections, the swelling extends cranially to the umbilical area. The skin overly-

ing the swollen area has a dark reddish-brown discoloration. There is extensive edema, and a copious quantity of gas may be found in muscle and subcutis. The inflammatory exudate is stained by the injected iron preparation and the lesion usually has a putrid odor. Postmortem decomposition is rapid, and livers of pigs dead more than a few hours may have conspicuous gray foci of lysis that surround minute gas bubbles. Acute thrombophlebitis may be evident microscopically, and muscle fibers undergo fragmentation and liquefaction necrosis.

Uterine gangrene and decomposition of its contents may follow dystocia and bungled attempts to assist in delivery. Foul-smelling, reddish, watery vulval discharge may be seen, and death ensues in 12–24 hours. The uterus and its contents are usually dark green or black, malodorous, and contain gas bubbles. There may be foul-smelling reddish fluid in the peritoneal cavity. Decomposition of the remainder of the carcass is rapid, and lesions in other sites are rarely identified.

Pathogenesis. Spores germinate and vegetative cells multiply in ischemic tissue and infection spreads to healthy muscle. CPA and PFO toxins play local and systemic synergistic roles in myonecrosis (Awad et al. 2000), although the entirety of our knowledge in this area comes from studies in mice. The protective effect of CPA-containing toxoids against gas gangrene has been long known, and antibodies against native CPA and its C-terminus protect mice against challenge with toxin or multiple LD_{50} of spores (Titball et al. 1993; Williamson and Titball 1993).

Diagnosis. Diagnosis is based on clinical and pathologic findings, together with isolation and identification of *C. perfringens*. Gram-stained smears of the lesion are helpful in estimating the relative numbers of bacteria. Isolation of the organism is easily accomplished by anaerobic incubation for 18–24 hours on blood agar or egg yolk agar.

Prevention and Treatment. Prevention of gas gangrene requires prevention of deep, contaminated wounds and prompt treatment of any such wounds with systemic penicillins. Treatment may be successful if instituted early in the course of the disease. Infection of mice was prevented by administration of penicillin coincident with *C. perfringens*, but if the antimicrobial was delayed by as little as 3 hours, the survival rate was appreciably lowered (Hac and Habert 1943). Clinically ill pigs may recover following penicillin injection (Jaartsveld et al. 1962).

Specific immunization of domestic animals against infection by type A in North America is focused at present upon anti-CPA immunity, and both toxoids and bacterin:toxoids are widely available elsewhere in the world.

Clostridium chauvoei Infection (Blackleg)

Etiology and Epidemiology. *Clostridium chauvoei* is a pleomorphic, anaerobic, gram-positive rod that readily forms central to subterminal spores. It causes blackleg (Burke and Opeskin 1999; Kuhnert et al. 1996), an emphysematous, necrotizing myositis of ruminants and other domestic species (refer to Table 36.1), which resembles malignant edema.

Clinical Signs and Lesions. Pigs are generally quite resistant to *C. chauvoei* infection, and there have been very few substantiated reports of disease in swine. Blackleg has occurred in swine kept under poor hygienic conditions on premises with previous losses of cattle from blackleg (Sterne and Edwards 1955; Gualandi 1955), although *C. septicum* may also be involved in these cases. Disease may follow consumption by swine of meat from blackleg-affected calves (Eggleston 1950), and in these cases, swelling of the face and throat were prominent. Lesions are perhaps more common in limbs (Mavenyengwa and Matope 1995). Signs include high fever, anorexia, depression, and lameness, with crepitant lesions and sudden death. Lesions are often dry and emphysematous at the center, but edematous, hemorrhagic, and necrotic at the periphery, with little leukocytic infiltration.

Pathogenesis. Pathogenesis of *C. chauvoei* infection in pigs is poorly understood. Infection may be by the oral route, rather than beginning as a wound infection. The organisms may lie dormant in various tissues until a microenvironment favorable for their growth is generated, such as by tissue damage from bruising. The roles of alpha toxin, which is necrotizing, hemolytic, and lethal, and beta toxin, a DNase (Ramachandran 1969), remain undefined. Flagellar expression is associated with virulence, and phase variation occurs in motility and flagellation (Tamura et al. 1995); flagella are apparently protective antigens (Kojima et al. 2000; Verpoort et al. 1966).

Diagnosis. A diagnosis of blackleg can be made only by bacterial identification, due to similarities in the clinical presentation and pathology of *C. septicum* and *C. chauvoei* infections. The fluorescent antibody test, applied to direct impression smears of infected tissue, is a rapid and practical method of identification (Batty and Walker 1963). Bacterial isolation may be difficult in decomposing specimens, since *C. chauvoei* is easily overgrown by other bacteria, including *C. septicum*.

Treatment and Prevention. Prevention of *C. chauvoei* infection involves minimizing exposure to the organism. *Clostridium chauvoei* is not a common soil organism, but anecdotal evidence suggests that keeping swine on known contaminated premises or allowing them to eat carcasses of ruminants dead of blackleg are risk factors.

Clostridium novyi Infection (Sudden Death)

Etiology and Epidemiology. *Clostridium novyi* is an anaerobic, spore-forming, gram-positive rod that is generally the largest of the clostridia encountered in swine. Types A and B are involved in swine infections (Itoh et al. 1987; Duran and Walton 1997).

Clinical Signs and Lesions. *Clostridium novyi* has been associated with sudden death in swine (Batty et al. 1964), with unusually rapid postmortem decomposition. Necropsy findings include rapid postmortem tympany, submandibular swellings, bloodstained fluid in pleural, pericardial, and peritoneal cavities, serosal hemorrhages, and splenic enlargement. The hallmark is perhaps marked hepatic degeneration and emphysema, often referred to as "aerochocolate liver." Its bronze color and the presence of large numbers of small gas bubbles are common (Duran and Walton 1997). The organism can be demonstrated in various tissues, including liver, heart, and blood.

The disease affects large finishing pigs and breeding stock, principally sows, and was recorded more frequently in spring, in older, periparturient sows of parity greater than 4 in moderate to good condition (Duran and Walton 1997).

Pathogenesis. Livers of normal sows often yield *C. novyi* when subjected to bacteriologic culture, although the route by which the organism reaches the liver has not been documented. The conditions under which dormant spores germinate are also unknown. Pathogenesis is likely mediated by the lethal, necrotizing alpha toxin. A so-called large clostridial cytotoxin (Busch et al. 2001; Selzer et al. 1996), it is produced by strains of types A and B. Beta toxin, a phospholipase related to CPA of *C. perfringens*, is produced in small quantities by type B strains. Systemic effects, with acute or peracute death, follow dissemination of alpha toxin (Elder and Miles 1957). Cardio-, neuro-, histo-, and hepatotoxic effects result in edema, serosal effusion, and hepatic necrosis (Elder and Miles 1957; Cotran 1979; Rutter and Collee 1967).

Treatment and Prevention. The disease can be controlled by reducing the incidence of pneumonias, metritis, and enteritis in affected groups of pigs, coupled with vaccination of finishing pigs and sows against the disease using alum-adjuvanted vaccines such as those readily available for sheep. Zinc bacitracin (200 ppm in feed twice daily) may reduce mortality in sows (Marco 1995). Prompt carcass disposal by incineration or deep burial may reduce spore contamination of the environment.

Diagnosis. Diagnosis of *C. novyi* infection in swine is difficult, since suspect cases are usually found dead, and the interval between death and necropsy introduces the possibility of postmortem invasion. Other possible causes of death should be excluded, but disease should be suspected when there is a history of sudden death and typical necropsy findings. Subcutaneous edema is particularly notable in cervical and inguinal regions. Pulmonary edema and tracheal froth, serofibrinous or serosanguinous exudates in pericardial and pleural cavities, and unusually rapid decomposition with accumulation of gas in the liver are all common. Gas bubbles in the liver in an otherwise fresh carcass are particularly significant (Duran and Walton 1997).

The organism is rapidly identified by fluorescent antibody staining of direct smears of infected tissue. It is the most fastidious of the clostridia commonly encountered in swine, but it can be isolated (Itoh et al. 1987; Duran and Walton 1997; J.G. Songer and K.W. Post, unpublished observations).

Treatment and Prevention. Given that definition of the syndrome is sudden death, treatment is not a factor in management of the disease. It may be possible to prevent disease by feeding bacitracin methylene disalicylate in the periparturient period. Prevention may also be achievable by use of bacterin:toxoids or toxoids, and second-generation vaccines may be based upon native or recombinant alpha (Amimoto et al. 1998) or beta toxoids.

NEUROTOXIGENIC CLOSTRIDIA

Tetanus

Tetanus is caused by *C. tetani* and is characterized by toxin-mediated, uncontrollable spasms of voluntary muscles. Swine of all ages may be affected, but most cases involve young pigs and originate with castration wounds or umbilical infection.

Etiology and Epidemiology. *Clostridium tetani* is a slender, anaerobic, gram-positive rod. It forms terminal spores, which are ubiquitous in the environment. Spores often enter via traumatic wounds, including those from tail-docking. Castration is a risk factor for infection, and sows may be infected by contamination of uterine prolapses.

Clinical Signs and Lesions. Tetanus is characterized by generalized skeletal muscle spasms. The incubation period ranges from several days to several weeks. In general, cases with a short incubation period run a more acute and fulminating course with a higher fatality rate than cases with a long incubation period.

The earliest sign is a stiffened gait, but the disease progresses rapidly over 1–2 days. Ears become erect, the tail extends straight out posteriorly, the head is slightly elevated, and there may be protrusion of the nictitating membrane. The pig becomes incapable of walking, and the skeletal muscles are very firm on palpation. Ultimately, the pig lies in lateral recumbency in opisthotonus, with both thoracic and pelvic limbs extended

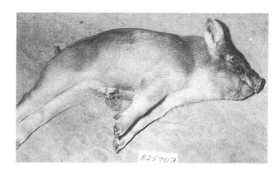

36.15. *Generalized tetanus in a 10-day-old pig that apparently resulted from umbilical infection. The ears are erect and the limbs are rigidly extended.*

and directed posteriorly (Figure 36.15). Tetanic spasms proceed from periodic to continuous and are noticeably heightened by sudden sensory stimuli, such as noise, touch, or movement. Tachycardia and increased respiration rate are common terminal signs, and white froth may be present around the mouth and external nares.

Many factors may contribute to the eventual death of the affected pig. In acute cases, respiratory failure resulting from severe skeletal muscle spasms is likely to be the single most important factor. Prolonged recumbency and nutrient deprivation may be factors in animals with a relatively long survival time. No lesions specific for tetanus are found at necropsy. Conspicuous abrasions of the skin over pressure points may be seen, and there may be pulmonary congestion and edema.

Pathogenesis. Development of tetanus depends upon the presence of *C. tetani* in a tissue environment that will support spore germination, vegetative cell growth, and toxin production. Spores usually gain entrance via a deep penetrating wound. Spore germination is facilitated by the presence of foreign bodies or facultative anaerobes which reduce Redox potential (Eh) in tissue. Bacterial multiplication and tetanospasmin (TeNT) production is enhanced by tetanolysin, a cholesterol-binding toxin, which inhibits neutrophil and macrophage chemotaxis and causes local tissue necrosis. Spores may remain latent in healed wounds for 10 years or more. *Clostridium tetani* is not invasive and remains localized at the primary site of infection. The most commonly reported location of tetanus infection in swine is castration wounds (Kaplan 1943).

Toxin-containing vesicles pass by retrograde axonal transport along the motor nerve fibers from neuromuscular junctions at the site of the infection, acting eventually on the inhibitory neurons in the ventral horn of the spinal cord. The toxin consists of a light chain that is enzymatic (a zinc-dependent endopeptidase) and a heavy chain that binds to receptors. The L chain cleaves synaptobrevin, a protein involved in the exocytosis of neurotransmitters by neurons, resulting in tetany.

Diagnosis. Diagnosis is based upon typical clinical signs. An obvious area of infection (e.g., a castration wound or umbilical abscess) may be apparent. The organism may be isolated by bacteriologic culture or identified by immunofluorescence (Batty and Walker 1963), but this is usually not necessary if there is adequate antemortem clinical observation of the affected animals.

Treatment and Prevention. There is no practical way to eliminate spores from soil, so control is directed toward prevention of wound contamination by soil or feces. Good sanitation in the farrowing house, treatment of the umbilical cord with antiseptics soon after birth, and prompt clipping of the canine incisors are recommended preventive measures against neonatal tetanus. Sharp objects that may cause skin wounds should be removed from the environment. Because most tetanus in swine follows castration, particular emphasis should be placed on proper surgical technique, with the provision of clean quarters for the pigs after castration to prevent undue contamination of the castration wound by soil or feces.

Passive immunization with tetanus antitoxin, prophylactic use of antibiotics, and/or active immunization with tetanus toxoid may be indicated. Prophylactic use of large doses of long-acting penicillin or tetracycline may be superior to antitoxin in preventing experimental tetanus in mice, if treatment is instituted within a few hours after infection (Veronesi 1966). Active immunity may be obtained from a single injection of alum-precipitated tetanus toxoid, and excellent protection for a year or more can be expected if three doses are given several weeks apart.

Prognosis is poor, and there is little evidence that treatment by currently practical methods is of real benefit (Mihaljevic 1966; Kaplan 1943). Various suggested treatments include reopening castration wounds and flushing them with hydrogen peroxide, administration of antitoxin in an attempt to neutralize toxin not already fixed by nervous tissue, administration of antibiotics, and the use of tranquilizers or barbiturates as muscle relaxants.

Botulism

Clostridium botulinum produces eight types of botulinum neurotoxin (BoNT) (Smith 1979; Linial 1995; Smith 1977) which have unique geographic distribution and species susceptibility patterns (Smith 1977; Shapiro et al. 1998; Smith and Milligan 1979; CDC 1998; Hatheway 1990, 1995). Thus, botulism is a toxicosis characterized by rapidly progressive flaccid paralysis. Swine are highly resistant to botulism, and there are few authentic reports of naturally occurring botulism in this species.

Etiology and Epidemiology. Botulism spores are ubiquitous in soil throughout the U.S. (Smith 1979; Whitlock and Williams 1999; Kelch et al. 2000). Disease in other species is associated with forage (Kinde et al. 1991; Whitlock 1997; Wichtel and Whitlock 1991; Ricketts et al. 1984; Franzen et al. 1992; Kelly et al. 1994), contamination of grain by decomposing animal carcasses (Whitlock and Williams 1999; Divers et al. 1986; Enfors et al. 1975; Galey et al. 2000), or transport of BoNT by ravens or crows feeding on a decomposing carcass (Schoenbaum et al. 2000). Type D botulism has been linked to pica, in which phosphorous-deficient animals consume bones of confederates dead of botulism (Dobereiner et al. 1992). Prevalence may be associated with the quantity of organic matter in the soil, and factors such as fertilization with manure may increase bacterial numbers. Botulism in swine is rare, so there are few recorded toxin sources, but type C disease due to consumption of dead fish (Beiers and Simmons 1967) and swill and decomposing brewers waste (Doiurtre 1967) have been reported.

The organism is a strictly anaerobic, gram-positive bacillus (Smith and Holdeman 1968), which forms oval, usually subterminal, spores. Growth is perhaps optimal at about 30°C.

Eating habits of nonconfined pigs should make them likely candidates for botulism, but there appears to be innate resistance when toxin is administered by the oral route. The swine intestine may have a low permeability for botulinum toxin (Dack and Gibbard 1926b; Scheibner 1955; Smith et al. 1971).

Clinical Signs and Lesions. The latent period between consumption of toxic material and onset of signs ranges from 8 hours to 3 days or more, largely determined by the amount of toxin consumed (Beiers and Simmons 1967; Smintzis and Dunn 1950). Initial signs are weakness, incoordination, and staggering, with weakness appearing first in the forelegs, followed by involvement of the hindlegs and general motor paralysis and dilation of the pupils of the eyes (Smith et al. 1971). The clinical effect is progressive flaccid paralysis of voluntary muscles, which manifests in the end as lateral recumbency with complete flaccidity. Other clinical signs include anorexia, reduced vision or complete blindness, aphonia, excessive salivation, involuntary urination, and deep labored breathing (Smintzis and Dunn 1950; Beiers and Simmons 1967).

No specific lesions are found at necropsy. Significant findings might include presence in the stomach of the material suspected as the toxin source and the occurrence of aspiration pneumonia as a result of paralysis of the muscles of deglutition (Beiers and Simmons 1967).

Pathogenesis. Botulinum toxin relative potency varies among toxin types, and amounts of toxin produced varies with strain. Botulism occurs after ingestion of preformed BoNT or by dissemination of toxin from a wound or focus of clostridial multiplication in the gastrointestinal tract (Hatheway 1995; Swerczek 1980;

Bernard et al. 1987). Absorption varies among species and with different areas of the intestine (May and Whaler 1958).

Botulinum toxin is composed of an enzymatic light chain (a zinc-dependent endopeptidase) and a heavy chain that binds to receptors and facilitates internalization. The light chain cleaves proteins involved in exocytosis of neurotransmitters by neurons. Toxin types B, D, and F cleave synaptobrevin, types A and E act on SNAP-25, and type C toxin acts on syntaxin, at the myoneural junction, preventing muscular contraction. Death is generally ascribed to asphyxia resulting from paralysis of the muscles of respiration.

Diagnosis. Toxin is detected inconsistently in serum or plasma of acutely affected animals, and this may be a manifestation of relative sensitivity of various species. Gross or histological lesions are usually absent, although inhalation pneumonia may occur due to an abnormal deglutition reflex. Affected animals are dysphagic and will usually have relatively empty gastrointestinal tracts. A diagnosis of botulism should be considered in afebrile, alert animals with progressive weakness and recumbency. Because the pig apparently is quite highly resistant to botulism, a diagnosis should be made only after thorough investigation and exclusion of other possible diagnoses (Beiers and Simmons 1967).

Isolation and identification of *C. botulinum* may also be of some value in establishing the diagnosis (Narayan 1967; Muller 1967; Yamakawa et al. 1992).

Treatment and Prevention. If botulism is suspected, an effort should be made to find the toxin source and prevent further consumption of any remaining suspect material by the herd.

Antitoxin is the only specific treatment for botulism, and it has been effective in reducing mortality in humans when given after consumption of food suspected to contain toxin (Lamanna and Carr 1967; Burgen et al. 1949). Therapy in animals demands use of polyvalent antitoxins that incorporate the types most commonly present in a geographic area. Therapy aimed at reducing continued absorption of toxin from the intestine (administration of magnesium sulfate) may be helpful.

Prevention requires eliminating opportunities to consume potentially toxic material, such as spoiled garbage and decomposing animal tissue. Prophylactic immunization with toxoids is not practical in swine because of the infrequent occurrence of the disease.

REFERENCES

Aikat BK, Dible JH. 1960. The local and general effects of cultures and culture filtrates of *Clostridium oedematiens, Cl. septicum, Cl. sporogenes,* and *Cl. histolyticum.* J Pathol 79:277.

Allo M, Silva J Jr, Fekety R, Rifkin GD, Waskin H. 1979. Prevention of clindamycin-induced colitis in hamsters by *Clostridium sordellii* antitoxin. Gastroenterol 76:351.

Amimoto K, Sasaki O, Isogai M, Kitajima T, Oishi E, Okada N, Yasuhara H. 1998. The protective effect of *Clostridium novyi* type B alpha-toxoid against challenge with spores in guinea pigs. J Vet Med Sci 60:681.

Amtsberg GW, Bisping W, el-Sulkhon SN, Matthiesen I, Krobischi P. 1976. *Clostridium perfringens* type A infection. Berl Munch Tierarztl Wochenschr 21:409–414.

Arbuckle JBR. 1972. The attachment of *Clostridium welchii (Cl. perfringens)* type C to intestinal villi of pigs. Pathol 106:65.

Awad MM, Ellemor DM, Bryant AE, Matsushita O, Boyd RL, Stevens DL, Emmins JJ, Rood JI. 2000. Construction and virulence testing of a collagenase mutant of *Clostridium perfringens.* Microb Pathog 28:107.

Azuma R, Hamacka T, Shioi H, Tanji T, Yamaguchi H, Shiga K. 1983. Case report of necrotic enteritis in neonatal pigs caused by *Clostridium perfringens* type C. Nippon Juigaku Zasshi 45:135.

Bakhtin AG. 1956. Dysentery of newborn piglets. Veterinariya (Moscow) 33:30.

Ballard J, Sokolov Y, Yuan WL, Kagan BL, Tweten RK. 1993. Activation and mechanism of *Clostridium septicum* alpha toxin. Mol Microbiol 10:627–634.

Barnes DM, Moon HW. 1964. Enterotoxemia in pigs due to *Clostridium perfringens* type C. J Am Vet Med Assoc 144:1391.

Bartlett JG. 1992. Antibiotic-associated diarrhea. Clin Infect Dis 15:573.

Bartlett JG, Chang TW, Gurwith M, Gorbach SL, Onderdonk AB. 1978. Antibiotic-associated pseudomembranous colitis due to toxin-producing clostridia. N Engl J Med 298:531.

Batty I, Buntain D, Walker PD. 1964. *Clostridium oedematiens:* A cause of sudden death in sheep, cattle and pigs. Vet Rec 76:1115.

Batty I, Walker PD. 1963. Differentiation of *Clostridium septicum* and *Clostridium chauvoei* by the use of fluorescent-labelled antibodies. J Pathol 85:517.

Beiers PR, Simmons GC. 1967. Botulism in pigs. Aust Vet J 43:270.

Bergeland ME. 1972. Pathogenesis and immunity of *Clostridium perftingens* type C enteritis in swine. J Am Vet Med Assoc 160:658.

Bergeland ME, Dermody TA, Sorensen DK. 1966. Porcine enteritis due to *Clostridium perfringens* type C. I. Epizootiology and diagnosis. Proc US Livest Sanit Assoc 70:601.

Bernard W, Divers TJ, Whitlock RH, Messick J, Tulleners E. 1987. Botulism as a sequel to open castration in a horse. J Am Vet Med Assoc 191:73.

Borriello SP, Wilcox MH. 1998. *Clostridium difficile* infections of the gut: The unanswered questions. J Antimicrobial Chemotherapy 41 Suppl C:67–69.

Bueschel DM, Jost BH, Billington SJ, Trinh HT, Songer JG. 2003. Prevalence of *cpb2*, encoding beta2 toxin, in *Clostridium perfringens* field isolates: Correlation of genotype with phenotype. Vet Microbiol 94:121.

Buogo C, Capaul S, Haeni H, Frey J, Nicolet J. 1995. Diagnosis of *Clostridium perfringens* type C enteritis in pigs using a DNA amplification technique (PCR). Vet Med Ser B 42:51–58.

Burke MP. Opeskin K. 1999. Nontraumatic clostridial myonecrosis. Am J Forensic Med Pathol 20:158.

Burgen AS, Dickens F, Zatman LJ. 1949. The action of botulinum toxin on the neuro-muscular junction. J Physiol 109(1–2):10–24.

Busch C, Schomig K, Hofmann F, Aktories K. 2001. Characterization of the catalytic domain of *Clostridium novyi* alpha-toxin. Infect Immun 68:6378.

Centers for Disease Control and Prevention. 1998. Botulism in the United States, 1899–1996. Handbook for Epidemiologists, Clinicians, and Laboratory Workers, Atlanta, GA. Centers for Disease Control and Prevention.

Collins JE, Bergeland ME, Bouley D, Ducommun AL, Francis DH, Yeske P. 1989. Diarrhea associated with *Clostridium perfringens* type A enterotoxin in neonatal pigs. J Vet Diagn Invest 1:351–353.

Cotran RS. 1979. Studies on inflammation. Ultrastructure of the prolonged vascular response induced by *Clostridium oedematiens* toxin. Lab Invest 17:39.

Dack GM, Gibbard J. 1926b. Permeability of the small intestine of rabbits and hogs to botulinum toxin. J Infect Dis 39:181.

Damme-Jongsten M van, Haagsma J, Notermans S. 1990. Enterotoxin gene not found in *Clostridium perfringens* isolates from pigs. Vet Rec 126:191–192.

Divers TJ, Bartholomew RC, Messick JB, Whitlock RH, Sweeney RW. 1986. *Clostridium botulinum* Type B toxicosis in a herd of cattle and a group of mules. J Am Vet Med Assoc 188:382.

Dobereiner J, Tokarnia CH, Langenegger J, Dutra IS. 1992. Epizootic botulism of cattle in Brazil. Dtsch Tierarztl Wschr 99:188.

Doiurtre MP. 1967. Botulism in animals in Senegal. Bull Off Int Epizoot 67:1497.

Duran CO, Walton JR. 1997. *Clostridium novyi* sudden death in sows: Toxaemia or postmortem invader? Pig J 39:37–53.

Eggleston EL. 1950. Blackleg in swine. Vet Med 45:253.

Elder JM, Miles AA. 1957. The action of the lethal toxins of gas gangrene clostridia on capillary permeability. J Pathol Bacteriol 74:133.

Enfors E, Gunnarsson A, Hurvell B, Ringarp N. 1975. Outbreak of botulism caused by *Clostridium botulinum* Type C in cattle. Svensk Vet 27:333–339.

Estrada Correa AE, Taylor DJ. 1989. *Clostridium perfringens* type A spores, enterotoxin and antibody to enterotoxin. Vet Rec 124:606–611.

Field HL, Gibson EA. 1955. Studies on piglet mortality. II. *Cl. welchii* infection. Vet Rec 67:31.

Field HL, Goodwin RFW. 1959. The experimental reproduction of enterotoxaemia in piglets. J Hyg (Camb) 57:81.

Finegold SM, Sutter VL, Mathisen GL. 1983. Normal indigenous intestinal flora. In Human Intestinal Microflora in Health and Disease. D. Hentges, ed. New York: Academic Press, pp. 3–31.

Franzen P, Gustafsson A, Gunnardsson A. 1992. Botulism in horses associated with feeding big bale silage. Svensk Veterinar tidning 44:555–559.

Galey FD, Terra R, Walker R, Adaska J, Etchebarne MA, Puschner B, Fisher E, Whitlock RH, Rocke T, Willoughby D, Tor E. 2000. Type C botulism in dairy cattle from feed contaminated with a dead cat. J Vet Diagn Invest 12:204–209.

Gibert M., Jolivet-Renaud C, Popoff MR. 1997. Beta2 toxin, a novel toxin produced by *Clostridium perfringens*. Gene 203:65–73.

Green DS, Green MJ, Hillyer MH, Morgan KL. 1987. Injection site reactions and antibody responses in sheep and goats after the use of multivalent clostridial vaccines. Vet Rec 120:435–439.

Gualandi GL. 1955. L'infezione da *"Clost chauvoei"* nel suino. Arch Vet Ital 6:57.

Hac LR, Habert AC. 1943. Penicillin in treatment of experimental *Clostridium welchii* infection. Proc Soc Exp Biol Med 53:61.

Harbola PC, Khera SS. 1990. Porcine enteritis due to *Clostridium perfringens* and its immunoprophylaxis. Proc Int Congr Pig Vet Soc 11:164.

Hatheway CL. 1990. Toxigenic clostridia. Clin Microbiol Rev 3:66–98.

——. 1995. Botulism: The present status of the disease. Curr Topics Microbio Immun 195:55–75.

Havard HL, Hunter SEC, Titball RW. 1992. Comparison of the nucleotide sequence and development of a PCR test for the epsilon toxin gene of *Clostridium perfringens* type B and type D. FEMS Microbiol Lett 97:77–81.

Herholz C, Miserez R, Nicolet J, Frey J, Popoff M, Gibert M, Gerber H, Straub R. 1999. Prevalence of beta2-toxigenic *Clostridium perfringens* in horses with intestinal disorders. J Clin Microbiol 37:358–61.

Hogh P. 1965. Enterotoksaemi hos pattegrise forarsaget of *Clostridium perfringens* type C. Nord Vet Med 17:1.

Hogh P. 1967a. Necrotizing infectious enteritis in piglets caused by *Clostridium perfringens* type C. I. Biochemical and toxigenic properties of the Clostridium. Acta Vet Scand 8:26.

Hogh P. 1967b. Necrotizing infectious enteritis in piglets caused by *Clostridium perfringens* type C. II. Incidence and clinical features. Acta Vet Scand 8:301.

Itoh H, Uchida M, Sugiura H, Oguso S, Yamakawa K. 1987. Outbreak of *Clostridium novyi* infection in swine and its rapid diagnosis. J Jpn Vet Med Assoc 40:365–369.

Jaartsveld FHJ, Janssens FTM, Jobse CJ. 1962. *Clostridium* infectie bij biggen. Tijdschr Diergeneeskd 87:768.

Jestin A, Popoff MR, Mahe S. 1985. Epizootiologic investigations of a diarrheic syndrome in fattening pigs. Am J Vet Res 46:2149–2151.

Johannsen U, Arnold P, Köhler B, Selbitz HJ. 1993. Studies into experimental *Clostridium perfringens* type A enterotoxaemia of suckled piglets: Experimental provocation of the disease by *Clostridium perfringens* type A intoxication and infection. Monatsh für Veterinaermed 48:129–136.

——. 1993a. Untersuchungen zur experimentellen *Clostridium perfringens* typ A enterotoxaemie der Saugferkel. Monatsh fur Veterinaermed 48:129–136.

Johannsen U, Menger S, Arnold P, Kohler B, Selbitz HJ. 1993b. Untersuchungen zur experimentellen *Clostridium perftingens* typ A enterotoxaemie der Saugferkel. Monatsh fur Veterinaermed 48:267–273.

——. 1993c. Untersuchungen zur experimentellen *Clostridium perfringens* typ A enterotoxaemie der Saugferkel: Licht un elektronmikroskopischen Untersuchungen zur Pathologie und Pathogenesis der experimentellen *Clostridium perfringens* typ A Infektion. Monatsh fur Veterinaermed 48:299–306.

Johnson S, Samore MH, Farrow KA. 1999. Epidemics of diarrhea caused by a clindamycin-resistant strain of *Clostridium difficile* in four hospitals. N Engl J Med 341:1645–1651.

Jones RL, Adney WS, Alexander AF, Shideler RK, Traub-Dargatz JL. 1988. Hemorrhagic necrotizing enterocolitis associated with *Clostridium difficile* infection in four foals. J Am Vet Med Assoc 193:76–79.

Kahn CM. 1924. Anaerobic spore-bearing bacteria of the human intestine in health and in certain diseases. J Infect Dis 35:423–478.

Kaplan MM. 1943. An unusual epizootic of tetanus in young pigs. Middx Vet 3:8.

Kelch WJ, Kerr LA, Pringle JK, Rohrbach BW, Whitlock RH. 2000. Fatal *Clostridium botulinum* toxicosis in eleven Holstein cattle fed round bale barley haylage. J Vet Diagn Invest 12:453–455.

Kellaway CH, Reid G, Trethewie ER. 1941. Circulatory and other effects of the toxin of *Cl. septicum*. Aust Exp Biol Med Sci 19:277.

Kelly AR, Jones RJ, Gillick JC, Sims LD. 1984. Outbreak of botulism in horses. Eq Vet J 16:519–521.

Kennedy KK, Norris SJ, Beckenhauer WH, White RG. 1977. Vaccination of cattle and sheep with combined *Clostridium perfringens* type C and type D toxoid. Am J Vet Res 38:1515–1518.

Kinde H, Betty RL, Ardans A, Galey FD, Daft BM, Walker RL, Eklund MW, Byrd JW. 1991. *Clostridium botulinum* type C intoxication associated with consumption of processed hay cubes in horses. J Am Vet Med Assoc 199:742–746.

Kink JA, Williams JA. 1998. Antibodies to recombinant *Clostridium difficile* toxins A and B are an effective treatment and prevent relapse of *C. difficile*-associated disease in a hamster model of infection. Infect Immun 66:2018–2025.

Kojima A, Uchida I, Sekizaki T, Sasaki Y, Ogikubo Y, Kijima M, Tamura Y. 2000. Cloning and expression of a gene encoding the flagellin of *Clostridium chauvoei*. Vet Microbiol 76:359–372.

Kubo M, Watase H. 1985. Electron microscopy of *Clostridium perfringens* in the intestine of pigs with necrotic enteritis. Jap J Vet Sci 47:497–501.

Kuhnert P, Capaul SE, Nicolet J, Frey J. 1996. Phylogenetic positions of *Clostridium chauvoei* and *Clostridium septicum* based on 16S rRNA gene sequences. Int J Syst Bacteriol 46:1174–1176.

Kyriakis SC, Sarris K, Kritas SK, Saolidis K, Tsinas AC, Tsioyannis VK. 1995. The effect of salinomycin on the control of *Clostridium perfringens* type A infection in growing pigs. J Vet Med Ser B 42:355–359.

Lamanna C, Carr CJ. 1967. The botulinal, tetanal, and enterostaphylococcal toxins: A review. Clin Pharmacol Ther 8:286–332.

Libby JM, Jortner BS, Wilkins TD. 1982. Effects of the two toxins of *Clostridium difficile* in antibiotic-associated cecitis in hamsters. Infect Immun 36:822–829.

Linial M. 1995. Bacterial neurotoxins—A thousand years later. Isr J Med Sci 31:591–595.

MacLennan JD. 1962. Histotoxic clostridial infections of man. Bacteriol Rev 26:177.

Madsen DP. 1995. Managing management induced *Clostridium perfringens* type A enteric infection in sucking pigs: A case study. Swine Health Prod 3:207–208.

Mansson I, Smith LDS. 1962. Atypical strains of *Clostridium perfringens* from swine. Acta Path Microbiol Scand 55:342–348.

Marco E. 1995. Sudden deaths in sows. Pig J 35:157–163.

Martig J. 1966. Zur Differentialdiagnose zwischen Rauschbrand und Pararauschbrand mit Hilfe der Immunofluoreszenz. Schweiz Arch Tierheilkd 108:303.

Matishek PH, McGrinley M. 1986. Colostral transfer of *Clostridium perfringens* type C beta antitoxin in swine. Am J Vet Res 46:2147–2148.

Matthias D, Illner F, Bauman G. 1968. Untersuchungen zur Pathogenese der Magen-Darm-Veranderungen bei der infektiosen Gastroenteritis der Schweine. Arch Exp Veterinarmed 22:417.

Mavenyengwa M, Matope G. 1995. An outbreak of quarter evil in weaner pigs in Zimbabwe. Zimbabwe Vet J 26:135–138.

May AJ, Whaler BC. 1958. The absorption of *Clostridium botulinum* type A toxin from the alimentary canal. Br J Exp Pathol 39:307.

Meer RR, Songer JG. 1997. Multiplex PCR method for genotyping *Clostridium perfringens*. Am J Vet Res 58:702–705.

Meszaros J, Pesti L. 1965. Studies on the pathogenesis of gastroenteritis in swine. Acta Vet Acad Sd Hung 15:465.

Mihaljevic K. 1966. A contribution to the study of lockjaw in animals. Vet Arh 36:152.

Miwa N, Nishima T, Kubo S, Atsumi M. 1997. Most probable number method combined with nested polymerase chain reaction and enumeration of enterotoxigenic *C. perfringens* in cattle, pigs and chickens. J Vet Med Sci 59:89–92.

Morin M, Turgeon D, Jolette J, Robinson Y, Phaneuf JB, Sauvageau R, Beauregard M, Teuscher E, Higgins R, Lariviere S. 1983. Neonatal diarrhea of pigs in Quebec: Infectious causes of significant outbreaks. Can J Comp Med 47:11.

Muller J. 1967. On the occurrence of *Clostridium botulinum* type C beta in the livers of slaughter animals in Denmark. Bull Off Int Epizoot 67:1473–1478.

Nabuurs MJA, Haagsma J, van der Molen EJ, van der Heijden PJ. 1983. Diarrhea in one to three week-old piglets associated with *Clostridium perfringens* type A. Annales de Recherches Veterinaires 14:408–411.

Narayan KG. 1967. Culture isolation and identification of clostridia. Zentralbl Bakteriol [Orig] 202:212–220.

Ohnuna Y, Kondo H, Saino H, Taguchi M, Ohno A, Matsuda T. 1992. Necrotic enteritis due to *Clostridium perfringens* type C in newborn piglets. J Jpn Vet Med Assoc 45:738–741.

Olubunmi PA, Taylor DJ. 1985. *Clostridium perfringens* type A in enteric diseases of pigs. Trop Vet 3:28–33.

Plaisier AJ. 1971. Enterotoxemia in piglets caused by *Clostridium perfringens* type C. Tijdschr Diergeneesk 96:324.

Popoff MR, Jestin A. 1985. Enteropathogenicity of purified *Clostridium perfringens* enterotoxin in the pig. Am J Vet Res 47:1132–1133.

Post KW, Jost BH, Songer JG. 2002. Evaluation of a test for *Clostridium difficile* toxins A and B for the diagnosis of neonatal swine enteritis. J Vet Diagn Invest 14:258–259.

Princewill TJ, Oakley CL. 1976. Deoxyribonucleases and hyaluronidases of *Clostridium septicum* and *Clostridium chauvoei*. III. Relationship between the two organisms. Med Lab Sci 33:110–118.

Princewill TJT. 1985. Sources of clostridial infections in Nigerian livestock and poultry. Bull Anim Hlth Produc Africa 33:323–326.

Ramachandran S. 1969. Haemolytic activities of *Cl. chauvoei*. Indian Vet J 46:754–768.

Ramisse J, Brement A, Poirier J, Rabreaud C, Simonnet P. 1979. Flore microbienne isolae au cours de diarrhees neonatales mortelles chez le veau, l'agneau et le porcelet. Rev Vet Med 130:111–122.

Ricketts SW, Greet TRC, Glyn PJ, Ginnett CDR, McAllister EP, McCaig J, Skinner PH, Webbon PM, Frape DL, Smith GR, Murray LG. 1984. Thirteen cases of botulism in horses fed big bale silage. Eq Vet J 16:515–518.

Ripley PH, Gush AF. 1983. Immunisation schedule for the prevention of infectious necrotic enteritis caused by *Clostridium perfringens* type C in piglets. Vet Rec 112:201.

Rood JI, Buddle JR, Wales AJ, Sidhu R. 1985. The occurrence of antibiotic resistance in *Clostridium perfringens* from pigs. Aust Vet J 62:276–279.

Rutter JM, Collee JG. 1967. Studies on the soluble antigens of *Clostridium oedematiens* (*Cl. novyi*). J Med Microbiol 2:395–417.

Scheibner G von. 1955. Die Emfanglichkeit des Schweines fur Botulinus toxin der Typen A–E. Dtsch Tierarztl Wochenschr 62:355.

Schoenbaum MA, Hall SM, Glock RD, Grant K, Jenny AL, Schiefer TJ, Sciglibaglio PS, Whitlock RH. 2000. An outbreak of type C botulism in 12 horses and a mule. J Am Vet Med Assoc 217:365–368.

Secasiu V. 1984. Diagnosticul bacteriologic welchiozel porcine (enterotoxiema anaeroba). Rev crestarea animalelor 2:38–45.

Selzer J, Hofmann F, Rex G, Wilm M, Mann M, Just I, Aktories K. 1996. *Clostridium novyi* alpha-toxin-catalyzed incorporation of GlcNAc into Rho subfamily proteins. J Biol Chem 271:25173–25177.

Shapiro RL, Hatheway C, Swerdlow DL. 1998. Botulism in the United States: A clinical and epidemiologic review. Ann Int Med 129:221–228.

Smintzis G, Dunn D. 1950. Epizootie de botulisme chez le porc. Bull Soc Sci Vet (Lyon), p. 71.

Smith GR, Milligan RA. 1979. *Clostridium botulinum* in soil on the site of the former metropolitan (Caledonian) cattle market, London. J Hyg Camb 83:237–241.

Smith LDS. 1977. Botulism in animals. In Botulism: The Organism, Its Toxins, the Disease. CC Thomas, ed. Springfield, Ill: Charles C. Thomas, p. 236.

———. 1979. *Clostridium botulinum*: Characteristics and occurrence. Rev Inf Dis 1:637–641.

Smith LDS, Davis JW, Libke KG. 1971. Experimentally induced botulism in weanling pigs. Am J Vet Res 32:1327.

Smith LDS, Holdeman LV. 1968. The Pathogenic Anaerobic Bacteria. Springfield, IL: Charles C. Thomas.

Songer JG, Meer RR. 1996. Genotyping of *Clostridium perfringens* by polymerase chain reaction is a useful adjunct to diagnosis of clostridial enteric disease in animals. Anaerobe 2:197–203.

Songer JG, Post KW, Larson DJ, Jost BH, Glock RD. 2000. Enteric infection of neonatal swine with *Clostridium difficile*. Swine Health Produc 8:185–189.

Sterne M, Edwards JB. 1955. Blackleg in pigs caused by *Clostridium chauvoei*. Vet Rec 67:314.

Swerczek TW. 1980. Toxicoinfectious botulism foals and adult horses. J Am Vet Med Assoc 176:348–350.

Szabo S, Szent-Ivanyi T. 1957. Infectious necrotic enteritis in sucking pigs. II. Incidence and control of the disease in Hungary. Acta Vet Acad Sci Hung 7:413.

Szent-Ivanyi T, Szabo S. 1955. 1. *Clostridium welchii* type C causing infectious necrotic enteritis in newborn piglets. Magy Allatorv Lapja 10:403.

Tamura Y, Kijima-Tanaka M, Aoki A, Ogikubo Y, Takahashi T. 1995. Reversible expression of motility and flagella in *Clostridium chauvoei* and their relationship to virulence. Microbiology 141:605–610.

Taylor DJ, Bergeland ME. 1992. Clostridial infections. In Diseases of Swine, 7th ed. AD Leman, BE Straw, WL Mengeling, S DAllaire, DJ Taylor, eds. Ames: Iowa State Univ Press, pp. 454–469.

Taylor DJ, Estrada Correa AE. 1988. Avoparcin in the prevention of enterotoxigenic *C perfringens* type A infections and diarrhoea in pigs. Proc Int Congr Pig Vet Soc 10:140.

Taylor WI, Novak M. 1952. Antibiotic prophylaxis of experimental clostridial infections. Antibiot Chemother 2:639.

Titball RW, Fearn AM, Williamson ED. 1993. Biological and immunological properties of the C-terminal domain of the alpha-toxin of *Clostridium perfringens*. FEMS Microbiol Lett 110:45–50.

Veronesi R. 1966. Antibiotics versus antitetanic serum in the prevention of human tetanus. Principles on Tetanus. Proc 2d Int Conf Tetanus, p. 417.

Verpoort JA, Joubert FJ, Jansen BC. 1966. Studies on the soluble antigen and haemolysin of *Clostridium chauvoei* strain 64. S Afr J Agric Sci 9:153–172.

Viscidi R, Laughon BE, Yolken R. 1983. Serum antibody response to toxins A and B of *Clostridium difficile*. J Infect Dis 148:93–100.

Walker PD, Murrell TGC, Nagy LK. 1980. Scanning electron microscopy of the jejunum in enteritis necroticans. J Med Microbial 13:445.

Warrack GH. 1963. Some observations on the typing of *Clostridium perftingens*. Bull Off Int Epizoot 59:1393.

Waters EH, Orr JP, Clark EG, Schaufele CM. 1998. Typhlocolitis caused by *Clostridium difficile* in suckling piglets. J Vet Diagn Invest 10:104–108.

Waters M, Savoie A, Garmory HS, Bueschel D, Popoff MR, Songer JG, Titball RW, McClane BA, Sarker MR. 2003. Genotyping and phenotyping of beta2-toxigenic *Clostridium perfringens* fecal isolates associated with gastrointestinal diseases in piglets. J Clin Microbiol 41:3584–3591.

Whitlock RH. 1997. Botulism. Vet Clin North Am Equine Pract 13:107–128.

Whitlock RH, Williams JM. 1999. Botulism toxicosis of cattle. Proc Bovine Practitioner 32:45–53.

Wichtel JJ, Whitlock RH. 1991. Botulism associated with feeding alfalfa hay to horses. J Am Vet Med Assoc 199:471–472.

Williamson ED, Titball RW. 1993. A genetically engineered vaccine against the alpha-toxin of *Clostridium perfringens* protects mice against experimental gas gangrene. Vaccine 11:1253–1258.

Yaeger M, Funk N, Hoffman L. 2002. A survey of agents associated with neonatal diarrhea in Iowa swine including *Clostridium difficile* and porcine reproductive and respiratory syndrome virus. J Vet Diagn Invest 14:281–287.

Yamakawa K, Kamiya S, Yoshimura K, Nakamura S. 1992. *Clostridium botulinum* type C in healthy swine in Japan. Microbiol Immunol 36:29–34.

Zeller M. 1956. Enzootischer Pararauschbrand in einer Schweinmastanastalt. Tierarztl Umsch 11:406.

37 Erysipelas

Richard L. Wood and Louise M. Henderson

The bacterium *Erysipelothrix rhusiopathiae*, a small gram-positive rod, is a primary pathogen of swine and turkeys as well as a sporadic cause of disease in humans and other species. It is the causative agent of swine erysipelas (SE) (Sneath et al. 1986), which is manifested most commonly by acute or subacute septicemia and chronic proliferative lesions. The disease is worldwide in distribution and of economic importance throughout Europe, Asia, and the Australian and American continents.

The identification of SE as a disease entity began in 1878 when Koch isolated from an experimental mouse an organism that he called "the bacillus of mouse septicemia." In 1882–1883 Pasteur and Thuillier briefly described the organism isolated from pigs with *rouget*. In 1886 Löffler published the first accurate description of the causative agent of *Schweinerotlauf* and described the infection in swine. In the United States the recorded history of SE began when Smith (1885) isolated the causative organism from a pig. Serious outbreaks were reported in South Dakota in 1928; by 1959 acute SE had been reported in 44 states. Since that time the prevalence of SE apparently had decreased overall (Wood 1984); but in 2001, SE reemerged in the midwestern U.S. (Opriessnig et al. 2004).

E. rhusiopathiae also causes polyarthritis of sheep and lambs and serious death losses in turkeys and marine mammals, including dolphins. It has been isolated from body organs of many species of wild and domestic mammals and birds as well as reptiles, amphibians, and the surface slime of fish. In humans *E. rhusiopathiae* causes erysipeloid, a local skin lesion that occurs chiefly as an occupational disease of persons engaged in handling and processing meat, poultry, fish, and lobsters as well as of rendering-plant workers, veterinarians, game handlers, leather workers, and laboratory workers. The organism occasionally is isolated from cases of endocarditis in humans and rarely causes acute septicemic disease.

ETIOLOGY

E. rhusiopathiae is a gram-positive bacillus with a tendency to form elongated filaments. Plasmid DNA has been detected in some strains of *E. rhusiopathiae*, but the functions of the plasmid are unknown (Noguchi et al. 1993). The morphology of *E. rhusiopathiae* is variable. In smears made directly from tissues in cases of acute infection, the organism appears as slender, straight or slightly curved rods, 0.2–0.4 by 0.8–2.5 μm, occurring singly or in short chains (Figure 37.1). An occasional coccoid or clubbed form may be seen. Palisades and angular formations ("snapping division") are common. The organism is nonmotile, non–spore-forming, non-acid-fast, and produces no flagella. It stains readily with ordinary dyes and is gram-positive but is easily decolorized. After several subcultures on an artificial medium, filamentous forms of the organism begin to appear and may predominate in old cultures or in chronic lesions. Filamentous forms are somewhat thickened, are greatly elongated (4–60 μm), and may form a mass resembling mycelia, especially in a liquid medium (refer to Figure 37.1). The filamentous forms sometimes have a beaded appearance when Gram's stain is used. Growth of *E. rhusiopathiae* at 37°C in a nutrient broth appears at 24 hours as a faint turbidity with no pellicle. Growth is much heavier in broth enriched with serum. In gelatin stabs incubated at 22°C for 4–8 days, growth produces a test-tube brush appearance.

Colonies of *E. rhusiopathiae* on agar media at 48 hours are tiny (less than 1 mm), transparent, and vary from smooth to rough, (refer to Figure 37.1). Colonies of most strains have entire edges, but some strains form colonies that are slightly larger and have somewhat undulate edges. Granulelike structures usually appear under a colony just below the surface of the agar. Dissociation from smooth to rough form may occur during the development of a colony, producing a sector (refer to Figure 37.1); the morphology of cells from these

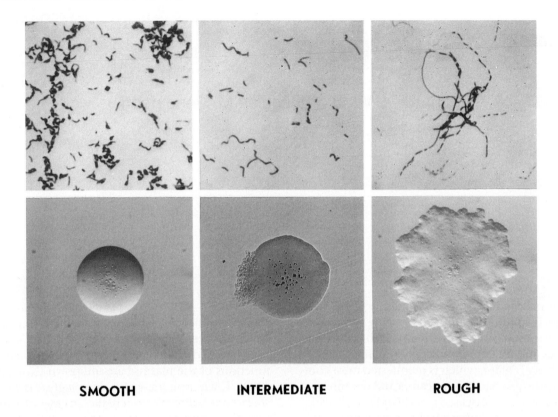

SMOOTH   **INTERMEDIATE**   **ROUGH**

37.1. *Cellular and colonial morphology of* Erysipelothrix rhusiopathiae. *Upper row: ×1200, crystal violet; lower row: ×32. (Courtesy National Animal Disease Center, Ames, Iowa.)*

intermediate forms will include a variety of shapes from short, curved rods to short filaments. Most strains of *E. rhusiopathiae* produce a narrow zone of partial hemolysis on blood agar, usually with a greenish color. Rough colonies do not induce hemolysis. *E. rhusiopathiae* produces acid but no gas from certain fermentable carbon compounds and produces hydrogen sulfide along the stab in triple-sugar iron agar (Vickers and Bierer 1958; White and Shuman 1961). Most, if not all, strains have one or more common heat-labile antigens, which are proteins or protein-saccharide-lipid complexes. Heat-stable antigens consisting of peptidoglycan fragments from the cell wall form the basis for identification of various serovars within the species. The serovars are identified by precipitin reactions with specific hyperimmune rabbit sera, usually in a gel double-diffusion system. Most isolates of the organism (75–80%) from swine fall into two major serovars designated 1 and 2 (Wood and Harrington 1978; Takahashi et al. 1996). About 20% of isolates make up a group of less-common serovars. Under a numerical system introduced by Kucsera (1973), a total of 26 serovars have been described so far (Kucsera 1973; Wood et al. 1978; Nørrung 1979; Xu et al. 1984, 1986; Nørrung et al. 1987; Nørrung and Molin 1991). Strains that do not possess the specific antigen are referred to as serovar N. Pulsed-field gel electrophoresis (PFGE) has been used to characterize field isolates and vaccine strains, with 23 PFGE patterns identified from

20 characterized strains (Opriessnig et al. 2004). Using PGFE to genotype is easy to perform and allows characterization without the need to rely on difficult-to-obtain antisera.

E. rhusiopathiae is a facultative anaerobe; some strains grow better in an atmosphere of reduced oxygen containing 5–10% carbon dioxide. It will grow at temperatures of 5–42°C. Optimum growth occurs at 30–37°C and at a pH range of 7.4–7.8. Growth is enhanced by serum, glucose, protein hydrolysates, or surfactants such as Tween-80. The organism is fastidious, requiring a complex medium, but no specific nutrient requirements are known. It is relatively resistant to adverse conditions and somewhat resistant to drying and can remain viable for several months in animal tissues under a variety of conditions. It can persist in frozen or chilled meat, decaying carcasses, dried blood, or fish meal. It is remarkably resistant to salting, pickling, and smoking and can survive several months in cured and smoked hams. The organism can survive in swine feces or fish slime for 1–6 months if temperatures remain below 12°C. It is sensitive to penicillin and usually to the tetracyclines; it is quite resistant to polymyxin B, neomycin, and kanamycin and is relatively resistant to streptomycin and the sulfonamides (see the section on treatment). It is killed readily by common disinfectants, heat (15 minutes at 60°C), and gamma irradiation.

Another species, *E. tonsillarum*, has been identified

(Takahashi et al. 1987a). This species is distinguished from *E. rhusiopathiae* by DNA homology. Protein profiles using sodium dodecyl sulphate-polyacrylamide gel electrophoresis (SDS-PAGE) demonstrated differences between the strains but were unable to establish sufficient differences to support identification to a species (Bernath et al. 2001). Phenotypic characteristics of the two species are indistinguishable by the usual diagnostic bacteriologic methods. *E. tonsillarum* has been isolated from a variety of sources, including the tonsils of healthy swine. Reported isolates have little or no virulence for swine and are not considered significant in the etiology of SE.

EPIDEMIOLOGY

The most important reservoir of *E. rhusiopathiae* is the domestic pig. Carriers can discharge the organism in their feces or oronasal secretions, and swine affected with acute erysipelas shed profusely in feces, urine, saliva, and nasal secretions. The large variety of wild mammals and birds known to harbor *E. rhusiopathiae* provides an extensive reservoir (Wood and Shuman 1981; Shuman 1971). Various species of domestic animals from which the organism has been isolated provide an additional potential reservoir. The agent can be found in the soil; however, Wood (1973) and others have found no evidence of maintenance of the organism in test soils, and current evidence indicates that soil provides only a temporary medium for transmission of *E. rhusiopathiae*. Swine between 3 months and 3 years of age are generally most predisposed to SE, most likely due to naturally acquired passive immunity in the young and active immunity following subclinical infection or vaccination in older animals. Suckling pigs of immune sows are immune to infection up to several weeks of age. There is no experimental evidence that susceptibility to SE is related to genetics of the animal; however, naturally acquired active immunity induced by previous infection, often with organisms of low virulence, is not uncommon. The role of parasites in transmission of disease has not been well defined, but the poultry red mite has been shown to carry the agent (Chirico et al. 2003).

SE can occur with other swine diseases, but the significance of preexisting infectious disease as a predisposing factor is uncertain. Parasitic infestations have been reported to increase the severity of clinical SE. In addition, Cysewski et al. (1978) showed that the susceptibility of swine to acute SE can be enhanced by subclinical toxicity from aflatoxin in the feed. This treatment also interfered with vaccination efficacy. Environmental and stress factors such as nutrition, ambient temperature, and fatigue, particularly sudden changes in these conditions, have long been linked to the appearance of SE. A number of molecular techniques may provide useful tools for epidemiological investigations. SDS-PAGE can be utilized for such purposes (Bernath et al. 1998).

PATHOGENESIS

Investigations using germfree pigs have demonstrated that *E. rhusiopathiae is* the sole causative agent of SE and does not require the presence of any other infectious agent for its disease-producing ability. The organism can gain entry to the body by a variety of routes. Infection through ingestion of contaminated feed and water is considered a common mode. The organism can readily gain access to the body through the palatine tonsils or other lymphoid tissue but entrance is probably not limited to these areas. Natural infection can result from infected skin wounds, and experimental infection can be easily accomplished by inoculation of scarified skin (Shuman 1951).

Acute systemic SE begins with bacteremia, which quickly results in clinical signs of generalized infection (septicemia). A nonsystemic infection consisting only of a local skin lesion may occur upon cutaneous exposure to a strain of low virulence or with partial immunity. In such cases the organism is eliminated without inducing septicemia and the lesion disappears. In the more typical systemic infection caused by virulent organisms, bacteremia usually develops within 24 hours after exposure. The organism usually can no longer be cultured from blood or most body organs after a few days but may persist in the joints and in lymphoid tissue such as tonsils, Peyer's patches, and spleen.

According to Schulz et al. (1975b, 1977), pathogenesis of the early septicemic phase consists of changes involving capillaries and venules of most body organs, including synovial tissues. As early as 36 hours after subcutaneous exposure, swelling of endothelium, with adherence of monocytes to vascular walls and evidence of widespread hyaline thrombosis was observed. This process was referred to as a shocklike generalized coagulopathy leading, within 4 days, to fibrinous thrombosis, diapedesis, invasion of vascular endothelium, and deposition of fibrin in perivascular tissues leading to connective-tissue activation in joints, heart valves, and blood vessels.

In severe acute SE, hemolysis is commonly observed. Ischemic necrosis of perivascular tissues may occur, caused by interference with microcirculation. Drommer et al. (1970) observed a high incidence of encephalomalacia in acute experimental SE and theorized that certain strains of the organism are endotheliotropic and damage the endothelial cell barrier in the central nervous system (CNS). Mild, delayed hypersensitivity responses to *E. rhusiopathiae* can be elicited and transferred by lymphoid cells. It is doubtful, however, that delayed hypersensitivity has a significant part in the pathogenesis of acute SE.

Information on the pathogenesis of chronic SE is derived primarily from studies on development of the arthritic lesion, which has stimulated interest because of its apparent similarity to the lesion of rheumatoid arthritis of humans. According to observations by Schulz et al. (1975a, 1977), the joint lesion in chronic SE begins with acute synovitis that may occur as early as 4–10 days after exposure. Within 3 months, fibrinous exudation, proliferation, and pannus formation occur, developing further into severe fibrosis and destruction of articular cartilage in 5–8 months. During this time, the organism can be found sequestered within chondrocytes in addition to its presence in synovial tissue and fluid (Franz et al. 1995). The earliest changes in the synovial tissue are described as consisting of coagulopathy and fibrinous exudate into perivascular tissues. Fibrin deposited during the vascular phase, not bacterial colonization, is believed to act as mediator of the subsequent connective-tissue proliferation. Affected joints are culture-negative after 3–6 months; yet the arthritic lesions usually undergo a progressive development that can continue at least 2 years. Hypersensitivity may be a significant factor in the chronic proliferative and destructive changes but probably not in initiation of the lesion. The porcine homologues of intracellular adhesion molecule-1 (ICAM-1)F and MHC class II, which are not constitutively expressed on porcine chondrocytes, appear to be induced as a result of arthritis and support the use of the model for immunopathological studies (Davies et al. 1994).

There is evidence that the bacteria do not entirely disappear from chronically affected joints, and the long-term progressive lesion may occur in response to the continued presence of either whole bacterial cells or their antigens. Schulz et al. (1977) reported that living *E. rhusiopathiae* was occasionally isolated from such joints for up to 2 years. Furthermore, they stated that *E. rhusiopathiae* antigen could be detected by immunofluorescence, and whole or fragmented bacteria could be seen with the electron microscope in culturally negative joints. Denecke and Trautwein (1986) reported detection of *E. rhusiopathiae* in arthritic joints microbiologically and immunohistologically for up to 3 years. Specific antibodies to the organism have been detected in synovial fluid of chronically arthritic joints and apparently are produced locally by plasma cells in the synovial tissue, which can assume a lymphoid function. It is not known whether the chronicity of the joint lesion is maintained entirely by specific immune reactions against *E. rhusiopathiae* antigen or whether superimposed autoimmune reactions are involved.

A preponderance of evidence exists to indicate that erysipelatous arthritis is initiated by active infection of the joint. Mild synovitis and arthritis have been induced in rabbits and rats by massive intravenous or intra-articular injections with nonliving whole cells or fractions of the organism (White et al. 1975; Hermanns et al. 1982), but the lesions were not as severe as those typically caused by infection. White et al. (1975) suggested that the mild response induced by such antigens may predispose the joint to infection during a subsequent transient septicemia. Studies on the pathogenesis of endocarditis indicate that the valvular lesions begin with vascular inflammation and myocardial infarcts, possibly resulting from bacterial emboli. These processes, together with exudation of fibrin, lead to destruction of valvular endocardium.

The mechanism by which *E. rhusiopathiae* incites disease processes is not clearly understood, but considerable evidence indicates that neuraminidase, an enzyme that specifically cleaves alpha-glycosidic linkages in neuraminic acid (sialic acid), a reactive mucopolysaccharide on surfaces of body cells, is a factor. The amount of enzyme produced by the strain seems to increase as virulence increases (Müller 1981). Specific antibody activity against *E. rhusiopathiae* neuraminidase has been demonstrated in sera of swine with chronic SE and commercial equine antierysipelas antibody. Neuraminidase activity could be a major factor mediating the widespread vascular damage, thrombosis, and hemolysis described (see the section on pathogenesis of acute SE). The ability to adhere to cell surfaces may also play a role in the pathogenicity of *E. rhusiopathiae*, and there is evidence that the process involves neuraminidase. Takahashi et al. (1987b) reported that virulent strains of the organism adhered better to porcine kidney cells in vitro than did avirulent strains. Nakato et al. (1987) reported that neuraminidase was essential for adherence of *E. rhusiopathiae* bacteria to vascular endothelial cells.

Although neuraminidase activity may be largely responsible for the pathogenicity of *E. rhusiopathiae* and may be a virulence factor, other virulence factors play an important role in disease processes. The virulence of *E. rhusiopathiae* is related to the organism's ability to resist the action of phagocytes, and resistance to phagocytosis is correlated with the presence of a protective capsulelike structure on the surface of virulent strains but not on avirulent mutants (Shimoji et al. 1994).

In the U.S., reports of field cases frequently have described serovar 1 (usually subserovar 1a) as the predominant isolate from acute septicemic disease and serovar 2 as the most common isolate from subacute and chronic cases of SE. However, experimentally, all clinical forms of SE can be induced readily in susceptible swine by strains of serovar 1 or 2. The less-common serovars (3 through 26; N) tend to have low virulence for swine.

CLINICAL SIGNS

The clinical signs of SE can be divided into three general classifications: acute, subacute, and chronic. In addition, subclinical infection can occur in which no visible signs of acute disease are evident but which can lead to chronic SE.

Acute SE is characterized by sudden onset, sometimes with sudden death. Other animals in the herd may have temperatures of 104–108°F (40–42°C) and over, and those with the higher temperatures may show signs of chilling. Some pigs may appear normal and yet have temperatures of 106°F (41°C). In surviving pigs, temperatures usually return to normal within 5–7 days. Affected animals withdraw from the herd and will be found lying down. When approached, they resent being disturbed but usually will get up and move away. This usually is accompanied by squealing; when walking, they show a stiff, stilted gait. Upon stopping, they may be seen to shift their weight in an apparent effort to ease the pain in their legs. If left alone, they will soon lie down carefully. Pigs showing severe depression are nevertheless usually aware of activities around them. They may show some resentment at being disturbed but will make little or no effort to rise. Upon being forced to get up, they may stand for only a few moments before lying down again. While standing, the feet are carried well under them and the head is hung dejectedly, giving the back line a marked arched appearance. Others will not be able to stand even when assisted. Most affected animals will show partial or complete inappetence. Bowel movements are usually retarded and the feces firm and dry in pigs of market age and older, although as the disease progresses, a diarrhea may appear in younger animals. Abortion may occur in sows that contract acute or subacute SE during pregnancy.

Characteristic cutaneous lesions (urticarial, or "diamond-skin" lesions) appear as early as the second, and usually by the third, day after exposure to *E. rhusiopathiae* (Figure 37.2). On the light-skinned pig they can be seen as small, light pink to dark purple areas that usually become raised, are firm to the touch, and in most instances are easily palpated. In animals with dark-pigmented skin, one must rely mainly on palpation, although the weltlike lesions may be detected by observing raised areas in the hair coat. The lesions may be few in number and easily overlooked or so numerous it would be difficult to count them all. An animal also may die before recognizable urticarial lesions are evident. Individual lesions, by extension of the borders, assume a characteristic square or rhomboid shape. In acute nonfatal erysipelas, these lesions may spread considerably but will gradually disappear within 4–7 days after their first appearance, with no subsequent effect other than a superficial desquamation to mark the site. The intensity of skin lesions has a direct relationship to the outcome of the disease. Light pink to light purplish-red lesions are characteristic of acute nonfatal SE, whereas angry dark purplish-red lesions usually precede death of the animal. In acute fatal disease, extensive dark purplish discoloration often occurs over the belly, ears, tail, posterior aspect of the thighs, and jowls. Infrequently, severely affected pigs do not die, and skin necrosis may follow the severe cutaneous lesions. The areas of necrotic skin are dark, dry, and firm and eventually become separated from the healing underlying tissue. Affected areas, particularly the ears and tail, will eventually slough, and secondary infection may occur.

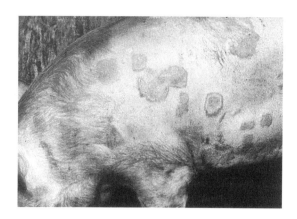

37.2. *Typical rhomboid urticarial lesions ("diamond-skin" lesions) of SE. (Courtesy National Animal Disease Center, Ames, Iowa.)*

Subacute SE includes signs that are less severe in their manifestations than the acute form. The animals do not appear as sick; temperatures may not be as high and may not persist as long; appetite may be unaffected; a few skin lesions may appear that may be easily overlooked; and, if visibly sick, the animals will not remain so for as long as those acutely ill. Some cases of subacute SE are so mild as to remain unnoticed.

Chronic SE may follow acute or subacute disease or subclinical infection and is characterized most commonly by signs of arthritis, or, occasionally, signs of cardiac insufficiency that are most noticeable following exertion, sometimes causing sudden death. Chronic arthritis results in joints that show various degrees of stiffness and enlargement, sometimes as early as 3 weeks after infection. Interference with locomotion ranges from a slight limp to complete refusal to put weight on the limb, depending upon the extent of damage. Arthritis is the most important clinical manifestation of SE from an economic standpoint. The condition not only affects growth rate but is responsible for significant losses of prime cuts at slaughter.

LESIONS

Rhomboid urticarial lesions ("diamond-skin" lesions) are characteristic of acute SE, and when generalized (refer to Figure 37.2), they are a reliable indicator of septicemia. This observation is important in meat inspection as well as in field diagnosis. Most lesions of acute SE are similar to those of septicemia caused by a variety of organisms.

In acute SE, macroscopic lesions include evidence of diffuse cutaneous hemostasis, which is often prominent, particularly in the skin of the snout, ears, jowls, throat, abdomen, and thighs. The lungs may be congested and edematous. Petechial and ecchymotic hemorrhages may be seen on the epicardium and in the musculature of the atria, particularly the left atrium. Catarrhal to hemorrhagic gastritis is common, and hemorrhage of the serosa of the stomach may be present. The liver usually is congested. The appearance of the spleen is of particular note, for it may be congested and markedly enlarged, particularly in animals affected for several days. Petechial hemorrhages may be present in the cortex of the kidneys. The appearance of the lymph nodes will depend upon the degree of involvement in the area they drain. There is some degree of enlargement with moderate to marked congestion; subcapsular hemorrhage of peripheral nodes may be seen after several days of illness. The mucosa of the urinary bladder usually appears normal but may present areas of congestion. A histologic examination of skin lesions reveals damage to the capillaries and venules, with perivascular infiltration by lymphoid cells and fibroblasts. The pathologic changes occur in the papillae and upper layers of the derma. Blood vessels of the papillae are congested and may contain microthrombi and bacteria. The papillae may also present focal necrotic areas as a result of circulatory stasis. Vascular lesions can be seen in the heart, kidney, lung, liver, nervous system, skeletal muscle, and synovial membranes. Cellular response consists predominantly of mononuclear leukocytes and macrophages. Neutrophils may appear but do not predominate. Purulent lesions are not characteristic.

Affected lymph nodes usually show acute hyperplastic lymphadenitis, with hyperemia and hemorrhage. In some nodes there may be evidence of thrombosis and necrosis of small blood vessels and capillaries. Hemorrhagic nephritis with inflammatory changes in glomeruli may be seen occasionally. In addition, necrosis of renal tubules with hyaline and granular casts has been reported. Focal accumulations of mononuclear cells may be seen in subcapsular sinuses of the adrenal cortex. Lesions of skeletal muscle may occur, associated with vascular lesions. These consist of a segmented hyaline and granular necrosis of muscle fibers, which may be followed by fibrosis, calcification, and regeneration. Lesions of the CNS have been described, consisting of angiopathies with disturbances in permeability, degeneration of neurons, swelling of endothelial cells, and malacic foci in the cerebrum, brain stem, and spinal cord.

Leukocytosis may occur in field cases of SE that last for several days or possibly from mixed bacterial infection, but in uncomplicated acute SE a leukopenia accompanied by a relative lymphocytosis is characteristic during the first 3–5 days. There may be a relative increase in the number of eosinophils. Hemoglobin and hematocrit values decrease during acute disease, followed later by the appearance of nucleated erythrocytes. The sedimentation rate increases. Changes during acute SE include a decrease in glucose and increases in glutamic oxaloacetic transaminase activity, blood creatinine, and blood urea nitrogen.

The predominant lesion of chronic SE is a proliferative, nonsuppurative arthritis, occurring most commonly in hock, stifle, elbow, and carpal joints with occasional spondylitis. Vegetative proliferation on heart valves is less common. Animals affected with chronic arthritis have an enlargement of one or more joints, most readily visible in hock and carpal joints. The joint capsule is thickened with fibrous connective tissue. The joint cavity contains an excessive amount of serosanguinous synovial fluid, which may be slightly cloudy, indicating a small amount of purulent material. The presence of frank pus, however, is not characteristic of the lesion. The synovial membrane presents varying degrees of hyperemia and proliferation (Figure 37.3), which gives the tissue a swollen, somewhat granular appearance, and often takes irregular forms, producing fringes ("tags") that project into the joint cavity. These fringes may be caught between the articulating surfaces and produce severe pain. The proliferating tissue also may extend across the surface of articular cartilage, forming a pannus that leads to destruction of the articular surface and eventually to fibrosis and ankylosis of the joint. Lymph nodes associated with arthritic joints are usually enlarged and edematous. Vegetative endocarditis consists of proliferative granular growths on the

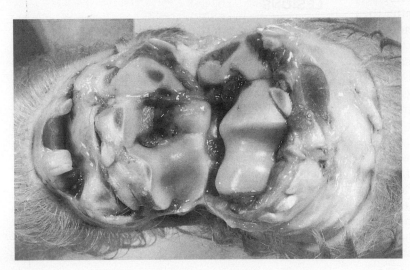

37.3. *Synovitis and arthritis of chronic SE in a hock joint 8 weeks after exposure to* E. rhusiopathiae. *Note hyperemia and proliferation of synovial tissue. (Courtesy National Animal Disease Center, Ames, Iowa.)*

heart valves and may be accompanied by lesions resulting from cardiac insufficiency. Other internal organs may show chronic inflammatory changes such as infarcts of kidneys and spleen. Enlargement of the adrenal gland has been reported.

Lesions of the synovial tissue may vary in severity, from slight perivascular accumulation of mononuclear cells to an extensive proliferative process. The typical synovial lesion in chronic SE is characterized by pronounced hyperplasia of the synovial intima and subintimal connective tissue, with vascularization and accumulation of lymphoid cells and macrophages, forming a villous pad of inflammatory tissue. Deposition and organization of fibrin may be seen. As the lesion progresses, proliferation of fibrous connective tissue becomes more prominent, and long fronds of hyperplastic synovium may be seen. The surface lining may become necrotic, with deposition of a fibrinous to fibrinopurulent exudate. Some tendency to follicle formation may be evident in the heavy accumulations of lymphoid cells. There may be erosion of the articular cartilages along with periostitis and osteitis. In old lesions ankylosis of the involved joint by fibrous adhesion may be accompanied by calcification. Vegetative growths on the heart valves are composed of granulation tissue and superimposed masses of fibrin. Connective tissue proliferation occurs with additional fibrin formation, which can be the source of emboli.

DIAGNOSIS

Clinical and bacteriologic examinations are useful to diagnose acute SE, which often cannot readily be differentiated clinically from other septicemic diseases (Miniats et al. 1989). Nevertheless, certain clinical features of an outbreak in a herd are more characteristic of SE than of other diseases if viewed in combination. For example, the following are presumptive of SE: a history of a few sudden deaths with no prior evidence of illness; several others sick with high temperatures and apparent stiffness in legs; reluctance of sick pigs to move but unexpected vitality when aroused; and clear, alert eyes. Other characteristic signs include a fair appetite in some visibly sick animals; normal to dry feces; death or recovery of sick animals within a few days; and, when present, the characteristic rhomboid skin lesions. Marked improvement within 24 hours after treatment with penicillin supports the diagnosis. At necropsy the presence of an enlarged spleen is suggestive.

Isolation of *E. rhusiopathiae* from the acutely affected animal provides a definitive laboratory diagnosis of SE. Hemoculture is a useful diagnostic aid in living animals, but specimens should be taken from several affected animals in the herd, because the presence of the organism in the blood may vary. At necropsy of a pig that has died in the acute phase, the organism is easily cultured from a variety of body organs (heart, lungs, liver, spleen, kidneys, joints). If the illness has persisted for several days, however, the organism often can no longer be cultured from internal organs but may still be found in the joints. Under these conditions it is important to take several specimens of fluid and synovial tissue from as many synovial sacs of a joint as possible, because the organisms may be present in small numbers and limited to certain areas.

Culture of *E. rhusiopathiae* from tissue specimens is relatively simple. In addition to use of blood agar, selective culture methods for isolation of the organism from contaminated specimens are described elsewhere (Cottral 1978). The use of immunofluorescence for rapid identification of *E. rhusiopathiae* has been reported; however, the method is not in widespread use for routine diagnostic purposes (Harrington et al. 1974).

A variety of serologic tests have been used in attempts to diagnose SE. These include plate, tube, and microtitration agglutination; passive hemagglutination; hemagglutination inhibition; complement fixation; enzyme-linked immunosorbent assay (ELISA); and indirect immunofluorescence. An agglutination test involving the use of growing culture as antigen was developed by Wellmann (1955). Most recently, a serological assay using nitrocellulose impregnated with a 65 kDa antigen has been developed (Chin et al. 1992). No serologic test has proved useful for routine diagnosis of acute infection or to determine immune status but may have some value in detection of chronic infection, primarily on a herd basis. Microtitration agglutination, growth agglutination, and ELISA are probably the most reliable for this purpose. It can be concluded that serologic testing has limited practical application in clinical diagnosis of SE in the field. The chief value of serologic procedures resides in research. Polymerase chain reaction (PCR) methods have improved the detection of *E. rhusiopathiae* in clinical and environmental samples. The use of these techniques for routine diagnosis is growing.

TREATMENT

The treatment of SE with hyperimmune serum, usually obtained from horses, was introduced in 1899, several years after it had been developed for use in conjunction with live-culture vaccination. Until the introduction of antibiotics nearly 50 years later, the administration of antiserum was the only effective treatment available. Polyclonal and monoclonal antiserum directed against protective antigens have been shown to protect animals from challenge with virulent strains of *E. rhusiopathiae* if administered early.

It is generally accepted that the treatment of choice for acute erysipelas is administration of penicillin; treatment early in an acute outbreak usually results in dramatic response within 24–36 hours. Specific treatment regimens generally involve giving penicillin alone or in combination with other antibiotics or antiserum (occasionally both) to provide a longer action. For example, long-acting penicillin (available under various proprietary names), consisting of a combination of 150,000 units procaine penicillin G and 150,000 units benzathine penicillin G/cm^3, may be given intramuscularly at a single dose of 5000–10,000 units/pound (454 g) to visibly sick pigs. The entire herd may be treated with tetracycline in the drinking water: 500 mg/gallon, 132 mg/l until 5 days after no sick pigs are observed or given antiserum if the outbreak is very severe. As an alternative, long-acting penicillin may be given in severe outbreaks, and procaine penicillin G in less severe cases. The use of antiserum for treatment of suckling pigs is a fairly common practice. Although penicillin has been consistently found to be the most effective antibiotic for treatment of acute SE, satisfactory results have been reported also with tetracyclines (including chlortetracycline and oxytetracycline), lincomycin, and tylosin. The organism is sensitive in vitro to erythromycin, but this antibiotic has been reported to be relatively ineffective in vivo. Streptomycin, dihydrostreptomycin, chloramphenicol, bacitracin, polymyxin B, neomycin, and sulfonamides are not effective against SE. Some isolates of the organism from swine have been found to be resistant to tetracyclines. There is no practical treatment for chronic SE. Experimentally, the administration of antiinflammatory agents has provided some alleviation of the effects of chronic arthritis, and they may be used in treatment of especially valuable individual animals. Initiation of a vaccination program in herds where outbreaks occur is strongly recommended.

PREVENTION

Prevention of SE is best accomplished by sound practices of herd health management, including a program of immunization. Swine should be raised according to sound husbandry practice relative to nutrition, housing, and condition of lots and pastures, and they should be observed regularly for deviations from their usual attitude. Replacements should be obtained from clean sources. The recent introduction of a new boar is a relatively common historical finding preceding acute outbreaks of SE in a herd. Newly purchased animals should be isolated for at least 30 days. It is advisable to eliminate chronically affected swine from the herd, as they can remain carriers of the organism indefinitely. Good sanitation is important in general herd management and is essential following the cessation of an outbreak. Walls and floors should be cleaned and disinfected. Phenolic, alkali, hypochlorite, or quaternary ammonium disinfectants are effective against the organism but must be applied to clean surfaces.

A variety of veterinary biologics developed for the purpose of inducing immunity to SE are licensed for use in the U.S. Active immunization can be induced using either live attenuated vaccines or killed bacterins. Bacterins are inactivated whole-cell or subunit preparations and have been used in the U.S. since 1953. Many licensed bacterins are made from selected strains of serovar 2 that produce a soluble immunogenic product when grown in a complex liquid medium containing serum. This substance, most of which is released into the medium, has been described as a glyco-lipoprotein (White and Verwey 1970). The most active component of the immunogenic substance has been identified as a protein fraction with a molecular weight of 64–66 kDa (Timoney and Groschup 1993; Sato et al. 1995; Goodman 1996; Zarkasie et al. 1996). The properties of the 64–66 kDa immunogenic substance have been the subject of a number of studies. A monoclonal antibody recognizing the 64–66 kDa (and a 43 kDa degradation product) immunogen was developed in 1992 and shown to provide passive protection to mice and swine challenged with virulent *E. rhusiopathiae* (Henderson et al. 1993b). An affinity purified protein, shown to be 99% pure by HPLC, that was derived using the monoclonal antibody was also shown to protect pigs from challenge. The 64 kDa immunogen has since been identified as Spa A.1, a cell surface protein, and the protective immunogenic region has been shown to reside within the N-terminal two-thirds of the SpaA.1. region (Shimoji et al. 1999).

Conventionally attenuated live vaccines, developed by passage through rabbits or chicken embryos, by air-drying, or by growth in media containing acridine dyes resulting in low virulence for swine, were first licensed in the U.S. in 1955. They stimulate immunity in swine by limited multiplication in the body, with very few or no clinical disease. Passive protection or antiserum given concomitantly may interfere with development of immunity following vaccination. Manufacturers generally do not recommend use of serum with their attenuated products except when immediate protection is necessary, as in the case of suckling pigs being given both vaccine and serum during a herd outbreak. In this case, repeated vaccination at weaning is recommended. Treatment with antibiotics that affect replication of *E. rhusiopathiae* should be discontinued at least 8–10 days before vaccination with attenuated vaccines. Attenuated vaccines are usually given by injection or administered orally in drinking water. In some parts of Europe and the former Soviet Union, vaccination by aerosol has been practiced. Acapsular mutants of *E. rhusiopathiae* may be useful for the development of live vaccines (Shimoji et al. 1998).

Lysate bacterin, first reported in 1953, has been used in the U.S. since 1955. It is similar to whole-culture bacterin except that the bacterial cells have been lysed. Bacterins are given by subcutaneous or intramuscular injection; a second (booster) injection in 3–5 weeks is generally recommended. Some studies have demonstrated that the immunity induced by bacterins may not protect animals for sufficient periods of time to reach market weight from challenge (Henderson et al. 1992). Subsequently, some manufacturers have demonstrated longer duration of immunity for their bacterins; this information is available on the label of the product. An enzyme-linked immunosorbent assay (ELISA) has been developed for use in potency testing of bacterins. The assay uses a monoclonal antibody to the protective 64–66 kDa protein and reduces the use of animals in testing bacterin potency (Henderson et al. 1993b). An alternative ELISA has been developed for detection of a protective antibody response in mice to replace the mouse challenge model for potency testing of erysipelas bacterins (Imada 2003).

Temporary passive immunity can be induced by administration of commercially available polyclonal antiserum as well as monoclonal antibody to the 64–66 kDa protein fraction. Pigs given antiserum by subcutaneous or intravenous administration receive immediate passive protection, which persists for about 2 weeks. Antiserum may be useful during a herd outbreak for temporary protection of suckling pigs until they are old enough to be vaccinated.

The mechanism of immunity to *E. rhusiopathiae* infection is not clearly defined, but serologic responses play a key role in immunity. Studies have shown that virulent *E. rhusiopathiae* bacteria opsonized with immune serum were readily eliminated by polymorphonuclear leukocytes (Sawada et al. 1988) and by macrophages (Shimoji et al. 1996). Nonopsonized virulent organisms were resistant to phagocytosis. Immunity induced by vaccination may not always prevent chronic SE. Many investigators agree that vaccination has little effect on the incidence of arthritis caused by *E. rhusiopathiae*, although this observation is difficult to evaluate in the field, since SE vaccination is not universally practiced in the U.S. Some believe vaccination actually causes an increase in arthritic lesions by initiating a state of hypersensitivity to subsequent contact with the organism. An alternative explanation for the failure of vaccination to prevent arthritis may exist, however. The organism may be carried to synovial tissues by loaded macrophages soon after exposure, thereby escaping the opsonic effects of humoral immunity (Drommer et al. 1970). Sequestration of the bacteria in chondrocytes (Franz et al. 1995) might provide similar protection from immune mechanisms. It is possible that certain uncommon serovars of *E. rhusiopathiae* may be refractory to the immunity induced in swine by standard SE vaccines. However, such serovars are usually isolated from healthy carrier pigs or nonporcine sources, and none have been directly associated with cases of acute SE in the field.

Vaccination provides a worthwhile means of control when used with other good management practices. A regular vaccination program for both breeding and market animals is recommended. Because of the ubiquity of *E. rhusiopathiae*, together with its poorly understood ability to exist in nature, the possibility of eradication of the organism seems remote.

REFERENCES

Bernath S, Nemet L, Toth K, Morovjan G. 2001. Computerized comparison of the protein compositions of *Erysipelothrix rhusiopathiae* and *Erysipelothrix tonsillarum* strains. J Vet Med B Infect Dis Vet Public Health 48(1):73–79.

Bernath S, Morovian G. 1998. Computerized evaluation procedure for comparing the electrophoretic protein patterns of bacterial strains. Lett Appl Microbiol 27(4):235–238.

Cottral GE. 1978. Manual of Standardized Methods for Veterinary Microbiology. Ithaca, N.Y.: Cornell Univ Press, pp. 429–436, 671, 672, 679, 687.

Chin JC, Turner B, Eamens GJ. 1992. Serological assay for swine erysipelas using nitrocellulose particles impregnated with an immunodominant 65 kDa antigen from *Erysipelothrix rhusiopathiae*. Vet Microbiol 31(2–3):169–180.

Chirico J, Eriksson H, Fossum O, Jansson D. 2003. The poultry red mite, *Dermanyssus gallinae*, a potential vector of causing erysipelas in hens. Med Vet Entomol 17(2):232–234.

Cysewski SJ, Wood RL, Pier AC., Baetz AL. 1978. Effects of aflatoxin on the development of acquired immunity to swine erysipelas. Am J Vet Res 39:445–448.

Davies ME, Horner A, Franz B. 1994. Intercellular adhesion molecule-1 (ICAM-1) and MHC class II on chondrocytes in arthritic joints from pigs experimentally infected with *Erysipelothrix rhusiopathiae*. FEMS Immunol Med Microbiol 9(4):265–272.

Denecke R, Trautwein G. 1986. Lokale Antigenpersistenz und Chronizität der experimentellen Rotlauf-Polyarthritis. Berl Münch Tierärztl Wochenschr 99:200–208.

Drommer W, Schultz LC, Pohlenz J. 1970. Experimenteller Rotlauf beim Schwein: Permeabilitatsstorungen und Malazien im zentralen Nervensystem. Pathol Vet 7:455–473.

Franz B, Davies ME, Horner A. 1995. Localization of viable bacterial antigens in arthritic joints of *Erysipelothrix rhusiopathiae*-infected pigs. FEMS Immunol Med Microbiol 12:137–142.

Goodman SA. 1996. USDA: Progress toward in vitro tests and other trends. Dev Biol Stand 86:41–47.

Harrington R, Jr., Wood RL, Hulse DC. 1974. Comparison of a fluorescent antibody technique and cultural method for the detection of *Erysipelothrix rhusiopathiae* in primary broth cultures. Am J Vet Res 35:461–462.

Henderson LM, Coe NE, Scheevel KF, Egemo CL, Wood RL. 1992. Duration of Immunity Elicited in Swine Vaccinated with *Erysipelothrix rhusiopathiae* Bacterins. Fourth Annual Veterinary Biologics Public Meeting, Ames, Iowa.

Henderson LM, Jenkins PS, Scheevel KF, Walden DM. 1993a. A Monoclonal Antibody Specific for a Putative Protective Immunogen of *Erysipelothrix rhusiopathiae*. Iowa State University doctoral thesis.

Henderson LM, Scheevel KF, Walden DM. 1993b. An Enzyme-Linked Immunosorbent Assay (ELISA) for Potency Testing of Erysipelothrix rhusiopathiae Bacterins Based on a Protective Monoclonal Antibody. Iowa State University doctoral thesis.

Hermanns W, Jessen H, Schulz LC, Kerlen G, Böhm KH. 1982. Über die Induktion einer chronischen Polyarthritis mit Bestandteilen von Rotlaufbakterien (*Erysipelothrix rhusiopathiae*). II. Mitteilung: Versuche zur Arthritis-Induktion bei Ratten. Zentralbl Veterinärmed (B) 29:85–98.

Imada Y, Mori Y, Daizoh M, Kudoh K, Sakano T. 2003. J Clin Microbiol 41(11):5015–5021.

Kucsera G. 1973. Proposal for standardization of the designations used for serotypes of *Erysipelothrix rhusiopathiae* (Migula) Buchanan. Int J Syst Bacteriol 23:184–188.

Miniats OP, Spinato MT, Sanford SE. 1989. *Actinobacillus suis* septicemia in mature swine: Two outbreaks resembling erysipelas. Can Vet J 30:943–947.

Müller HE. 1981. Neuraminidase and other enzymes of *Erysipelothrix rhusiopathiae* as possible pathogenic factors. In Arthritis: Models and Mechanisms. H Deicher, ed. Berlin: Springer-Verlag, p. 58.

Nakato H, Shinomiya K, Mikawa H. 1987. Adhesion of *Erysipelothrix rhusiopathiae* to cultured rat aortic endothelial cells: Role of bacterial neuraminidase in the induction of arteritis. Path Res Pract 182:255–260.

Noguchi N, Sasatsu M, Takahashi T, Ohmae K, Terakado N, Kono M. 1993. Detection of plasmid DNA in *Erysipelothrix rhusiopathiae* isolated from pigs with chronic swine eryipelas. J Vet Med Sci 55(2):349–350.

Nørrung V. 1979. Two new serotypes of *Erysipelothrix rhusiopathiae*. Nord Vet Med 31:462–465.

Nørrung V, Molin G. 1991. A new serotype of *Erysipelothrix rhusiopathiae* isolated from pig slurry. Acta Vet Hung 39:137–138.

Nørrung V, Munch B, Larsen HE. 1987. Occurrence, isolation and serotyping of *Erysipelothrix rhusiopathiae* in cattle and pig slurry. Acta Vet Scand 28:9–14.

Opriessnig T, Hoffman LJ, Harris DJ, Gaul SB, Halbur PG. 2004. *Erysipelothrix rhusiopathiae*: Genetic characterization of Midwest US isolates and live commercial vaccines using pulsed-field gel electrophoresis. J Vet Diagn Invest 16(2):101–107.

Sato H, Hirose K, Saito H. 1995. Protective activity and antigenic analysis of fractions of culture filtrates of *Erysipelothrix rhusiopathiae*. Vet Microbiol 43:173–182.

Sawada T, Tamura Y, Takahashi T. 1988. Mechanism of protection induced in mice against *Erysipelothrix rhusiopathiae* infection by treatment with porcine antiserum to the culture filtrate of an attenuated strain. Vet Microbiol 17:65–74.

Schulz LC, Drommer W, Ehard H, Hertrampf B, Leibold W, Messow C, Mumme J, Trautwein G, Überschär S, Weiss R, Winklemann J. 1977. Pathogenetische Bedeutung von *Erysipelothrix rhusiopathiae* in der akuten und chronischen Verlaufsform der Rotlaufarthritis. Dtsch Tierärzt Wochenschr 84:107–111.

Schulz LC, Drommer W, Seidler D, Ehard H, Leimbeck R, Weiss R. 1975a. Experimenteller Rotlauf bei verschiedenen Spezies als Modell einer systemischen Bindegewebskrankheit. II. Chronische Phase mit besonderer Berucksichtigung der Polyarthritis. Beitr Pathol 154:27–51.

Schulz LC, Drommer W, Seidler D, Ehard H, Von Mickwitz G, Hertrampf B, Böhm KH. 1975b. Experimenteller Rotlauf bei verschiedenen Spezies als Modell einer systemischen Bindegewebskrankheit. I. Systemische vaskulare Prozesse bei der Organmanifestation. Beitr Pathol 154:1–26.

Shimoji Y, Mori Y, Fischetti VA. 1999. Immunological characterization of a protective antigen of *Erysipelothrix rhusiopathiae*: Identification of the region responsible for passive immunity. Infect Immuno 67(4):1646–1651.

Shimoji Y, Mori Y, Sekizaki T, Shibahara T, Yokomizo Y. 1998. Infect Innum. 1998. 66(7):3250–3254.

Shimoji Y, Yokomizo Y, Mori Y. 1996. Intracellular survival and replication of *Erysipelothrix rhusiopathiae* within murine macrophages: Failure of induction of the oxidative burst of macrophages. Infect Immun 64:1789–1793.

Shimoji Y, Yokomizo Y, Sekizaki T, Mori Y, Kubo M. 1994. Presence of a capsule in *Erysipelothrix rhusiopathiae* and its relationship to virulence for mice. Infect Immun 62:2806–2810.

Shuman RD. 1951. Swine erysipelas induced by skin scarification. Proc Am Vet Med Assoc, p. 153.

——. 1959. Comparative experimental evaluation of swine erysipelas bacterins and vaccines in weanling pigs, with particular reference to the status of their dams. Am J Vet Res 20:1002–1009.

——. 1971. *Erysipelothrix*. In Infectious and Parasitic Diseases of Wild Birds. JW Davis, RC Anderson, LH Karstad, DO Trainer, eds. Ames: Iowa State Univ Press, p. 141.

Smith T. 1885. Second Annual Report of the Bureau of Animal Industry. Washington, D.C.: U.S. Department of Agriculture, p. 187.

Sneath PHA, Mair NS, Sharpe ME, Holt JG. 1986. Bergey's Manual of Systematic Bacteriology. Vol. 2. Baltimore: Williams & Wilkins, pp. 1245–1249.

Takahashi T, Fujisawa T, Benno Y, Tamura Y, Sawada T, Suzuki S, Muramatsu M, Mitsuoka T. 1987a. *Erysipelothrix tonsillarum* sp. nov. isolated from tonsils of apparently healthy pigs. Int J Syst Bact 37:166–168.

Takahashi T, Hirayama N, Sawada T, Tamura Y, Muramatsu M. 1987b. Correlation between adherence of *Erysipelothrix rhusiopathiae* strains of serovar 1a to tissue culture cells originated from porcine kidney and their pathogenicity in mice and swine. Vet Microbiol 13:57–64.

Takahashi T, Nagamine N, Kijima M, Suzuki S, Takagi M, Tamura Y, Nakamura M, Muramatsu M, Sawada T. 1996. Serovars of *Erysipelothrix* strains isolated from pigs affected with erysipelas in Japan. J Vet Med Sci 58:587–589.

Timoney JF, Groschup MM. 1993. Properties of a protective protein antigen of *Erysipelothrix rhusiopathiae*. Vet Microbiol 37:381–387.

Vickers CL, Bierer BW. 1958. Triple sugar iron agar as an aid in the diagnosis of erysipelas. J Am Vet Med Assoc 133:543–544.

Wellmann G. 1955. Die subklinische Rotlaufinfektion und ihre Bedeutung für die Epidemiologie des Schweinerotlaufs. Zentralbl Bakteriol (Orig A) 162:265–274.

White RR, Verwey WF. 1970. Solubilization and characterization of a protective antigen of *Erysipelothrix rhusiopathiae*. Infect Immun 1:387–393.

White TG, Puls JL, Hargrave P. 1975. Production of synovitis in rabbits by fractions of a cell-free extract of *Erysipelothrix rhusiopathiae*. Clin Immunol Immunopathol 3:531–540.

White TG, Shuman RD. 1961. Fermentation reactions of *Erysipelothrix rhusiopathiae*. J Bacteriol 82:595–599.

Wood RL. 1973. Survival of *Erysipelothrix rhusiopathiae* in soil under various environmental conditions. Cornell Vet 63:390–410.

——. 1984. Swine erysipelas: A review of prevalence and research. J Am Vet Med Assoc 184:944–949.

Wood RL, Harrington R, Jr. 1978. Serotypes of *Erysipelothrix rhusiopathiae* isolated from swine and from soil and manure of swine pens in the United States. Am J Vet Res 39:1833–1840.

Wood RL, Haubrich DR, Harrington R, Jr. 1978. Isolation of previously unreported serotypes of *Erysipelothrix rhusiopathiae* from swine. Am J Vet Res 39:1958–1961.

Wood RL, Shuman RD. 1981. *Erysipelothrix* infection. In Infectious Diseases of Wild Mammals, 2d ed. JW Davis, LH Karstad, D O Trainer, eds. pp. 297–305. Ames: Iowa State Univ Press.

Xu K, Gao C, Hu X. 1986. Study on a new serotype of *Erysipelothrix rhusiopathiae* isolated from marine fishes. Anim Infect Dis 3:6–7, 48.

Xu K, Hu X, Gao C, Lu Q. 1984. A new serotype of *Erysipelothrix rhusiopathiae*. Anim Infect Dis 4:11–14.

Zarkasie K, Sawada T, Yoshida T, Takahashi I, Takahashi T. 1996. Growth ability and immunological properties of *Erysipelothrix rhusiopathiae* serotype 2. J Vet Med Sci 58:87–90.

38 *Escherichia coli* Infections

John M. Fairbrother and Carlton L. Gyles

Introduction
J. M. Fairbrother

The genus *Escherichia* is named after the German pediatrician Theodor Escherich (1857–1911). It is classified with the family *Enterobacteriaceae*, which belongs to the gram-negative facultatively anaerobic rods. The species *Escherichia* (*E.*) *coli* includes normal inhabitants of the gastrointestinal tract and strains causing a broad variety of intestinal and extraintestinal diseases in swine.

BACTERIOLOGY

E. coli are gram-negative, peritrichous flagellated rods of variable length and with a diameter of about 1 μm. Colonies on solid media reach their full size within 1 day of incubation. Their appearance may vary from smooth to rough or mucoid. A wide range of selective media is available for growth of *E. coli*. Some strains produce hemolysins. Species identification relies mainly on biochemical characters, bearing in mind that there are exceptions with every single biochemical character. Commercially available identification kits therefore make use of up to 50 characters to achieve a high level of accuracy. The interpretation may be facilitated by computer-assisted processing of the data. The determination of DNA relatedness, the scientific base of discrimination between species, is restricted to research laboratories.

SEROTYPING

There are several ways to subdivide the species into types. So far, serotypes have shown the best association with certain virulence traits. Complete serotyping includes determination of O (somatic), K (capsular or microcapsular), H (flagellar), and F (fimbrial) antigens. Unlike salmonellae, only a small percentage of *E. coli* isolates are typeable with available antisera, since sero-typing has been limited to isolates of proven or suspected pathogenicity. Presently, at least 175 O, 80 K, 56 H, and over 20 F antigens are officially recognized.

In diagnostic laboratories serotyping is often reduced to one or two classes of antigens and to a limited spectrum of antisera. This may be quite suitable, since in a given region, animal species, and organ, pathogenic serotypes maintain their characteristic antigenic makeup. Thus one may deduce the complete serotype from a simple slide agglutination with a living culture. Serotyping is diagnostically helpful in communicable types of disease caused by a limited number of serotypes, such as postweaning *E. coli* diarrhea and edema disease.

VIRULENCE FACTORS

Bacterial traits involved in pathogenesis are called virulence factors. The nomenclature for pathogenic *E. coli* has evolved over the last few years. The term "pathotype" is now used to identify types of *E. coli* on the basis of their virulence mechanism, as indicated by the presence of virulence factors that characterize the method by which disease is caused. This system identifies broad classes of pathogenic *E. coli*, such as enterotoxigenic *E. coli* (ETEC), edema disease *E. coli* (EDEC), and attaching and effacing *E. coli* (AEEC) and these classes are referred to as pathotypes (Gyles and Fairbrother 2004). Potent exotoxins trigger the secretion of fluid into the gut lumen in ETEC infections and are responsible for systemic pathology caused by EDEC strains. Endotoxin is present in the outer membrane of most *E. coli* strains. Its significance is well documented only in extraintestinal infections, such as septicemia, mastitis, and urinary tract infections.

Many *E. coli* infections require the colonization of

mucous membranes. With ETEC and EDEC, adhesion to the small intestine is mediated by extracellular proteinaceous appendages, which are called fimbriae, fimbrial adhesins (F antigens), or pili and are highly host-specific. In some strains capsular polysaccharide has been shown to enhance the ability to colonize. AEEC colonizing the lower gastrointestinal tract adhere by an attaching and effacing mechanism. In the pig, colonization of the urinary tract has received little attention to date.

In extraintestinal sites, *E. coli* have to resist the natural bactericidal activity of serum, a characteristic called serum resistance. Some *E. coli* utilize high-affinity iron-uptake systems to compete with the host for available iron. A given pathogenic strain may exhibit a whole set of virulence factors, that is, more than one toxin and even more than three adhesins. Detection of more virulence factors can be expected.

GENETICS OF VIRULENCE

Very specific sets of virulence factors are needed to cause a particular disease. Thus, strains causing enteric diseases are usually not associated with extraintestinal infections and vice versa. Detection of virulence factors is important for the identification of pathogenic *E. coli* and the term virotype is now used to refer to the combination of these factors for a particular isolate. Many virulence factors examined so far are plasmid determined. This applies in particular to hemolysins, toxins, and adhesins of ETEC. In strains from most extraintestinal infections, however, the genes encoding for fimbriae, cytotoxins, and hemolysin are chromosomally located. In the laboratory, plasmids can easily be transmitted from donor to recipient strains. However, such exchanges of genetic material do not appear to play a major role in the field. The genetic makeup of pathogenic *E. coli* strains is remarkably stable. This may be because a whole set of virulence factors is involved in the virulence of a particular strain, and certain recipient strains may not express transmitted plasmid-determined functions. The clinically important development of antimicrobial resistance is an exception to this observation.

The time-consuming and sometimes cumbersome assays for detection of virulence factors are increasingly being replaced by hybridization and polymerase chain reaction (PCR) techniques for the detection of the genes encoding these factors.

ECOLOGY

The particular ecology of pathogenic *E. coli* strains has been somewhat neglected. Intestinal infections caused by ETEC and EDEC are often contagious. The same strain is usually found in many sick pigs and often in consecutive batches of pigs. When edema disease spread through Denmark, 63% of the outbreaks were con-

nected by trade of pigs to one single infected breeding herd (Jorsal et al. 1996). On the other hand, clinical edema disease occurred in no more than 5% of the herds with trading contacts. These strains may sometimes appear in healthy pigs without overt disease. They are usually shed in high numbers for only a few days. The ensuing dramatic decrease seems to be due to the development of local immunity.

Extraintestinal infections, however, do not behave like communicable diseases. Individual pigs in a given herd are affected most often by different strains. Mixed infections by more than one strain are frequent. In humans, the fecal flora is obviously the reservoir of such pathogenic strains. Most extraintestinal infections in the pig are also endogenous. For example, in 18 out of 67 sows with mastitis, *E. coli* of the same O types present in samples of mammary secretion were isolated from the feces (Awad-Masalmeh et al. 1990).

The primary habitat of *E. coli* in the pig is the gastrointestinal tract. The *E. coli* flora of individual pigs is extremely complex. When strains were distinguished by the combined application of O serogrouping, biotyping, and resistance pattern, up to 25 strains were identified in the gastrointestinal tract of one individual (Hinton et al. 1985). Numerically dominant strains change at intervals from 1 day to several weeks, leading to successive waves of dominant strains (Katouli et al. 1995). Proliferation of *E. coli* takes place mainly during the passage through the small intestine. Subsequent increases in bacterial numbers from the ileum to the rectum is minimal or absent (McAllister et al. 1979). Numbers in the large intestine fluctuate around 107 colony-forming units/g. However, *E. coli* contribute less than 1% to the total bacterial count. When found elsewhere (feed, water, soil, etc.), *E. coli* are derived from this habitat, usually by fecal contamination. Long survival times in the environment are promoted by low temperature and sufficient available water, among other factors. In an experiment with five slurry samples, a porcine *E. coli* O139:K82(B) strain remained viable for between 5 and more than 11 weeks (Burrows and Rankin 1970).

REFERENCES

Awad-Masalmeh M, Baumgartner W, Passernig A, Silber R, Hinterdorfer F. 1990. Bakteriologische Untersuchungen bei an puerperaler Mastitis (MMA-Syndrom) erkrankten Sauen verschiedener Tierbestände Österreichs. Tierärztl Umschau 45:526–535.

Burrows MR, Rankin JD. 1970. A further examination of the survival of pathogenic bacteria in cattle slurry. Br Vet J 126:32–34.

Gyles CL, Fairbrother JM. 2004. *Escherichia coli*. In Pathogenesis of Bacterial Infections in Animals (3rd edition). CL Gyles, JF Prescott, JG Songer, CO Thoen, eds. Ames, Iowa: Blackwell Publishing, p. 193–223.

Hinton M, Hampson DJ, Hampson E, Linton AH. 1985. A comparison of the ecology of *Escherichia coli* in the intestine of healthy unweaned pigs and pigs after weaning. Journal of Applied Bacteriology 58:471–478.

Jorsal SE, Aarestrup FM, Ahrens P, Johansen M, Baekbo P. 1996. Oedema disease in Danish pig herds: Transmission by trade of breeding animals. Proc Int Congr Pig Vet Soc 14:265.

Katouli M, Lund A, Wallgren P, Kühn I, Söderlind O, Möllby R. 1995. Phenotypic characterization of intestinal *Escherichia coli* of pigs during suckling, postweaning and fattening periods. Applied and Environmental Microbiology 61:778–783.

McAllister JS, Kurtz HJ, Short ECJr. 1979. Changes in the intestinal flora of young pigs with postweaning diarrhea or edema disease. J Anim Sci 49:868–879.

Neonatal *Escherichia coli* Diarrhea

J. M. Fairbrother

Diarrhea has become an economically important disease in pigs as a result of increasing intensification of farrowing management. It may be classified into three main entities: neonatal diarrhea (within the first few days of birth), young piglet diarrhea (from the first week of birth to weaning), and postweaning diarrhea. *Escherichia coli* is the most important etiologic agent of neonatal and postweaning diarrhea. Etiologic agents of diarrhea in young piglets are more numerous and include transmissible gastroenteritis virus, rotavirus, coccidia, and *E. coli* (Biehl and Hoefling 1986). A less frequently encountered manifestation of enteric *E. coli* infection is an acute shock syndrome which provokes gross lesions of hemorrhagic gastroenteritis. Neonatal diarrhea in pigs has been reviewed by Alexander (1994).

ETIOLOGY

Neonatal diarrhea associated with *E. coli* is observed most commonly in pigs aged from 0–4 days. Causative strains produce one or more enterotoxins and are referred to as ETEC. ETEC adhere to the small intestinal mucosa in neonatal pigs by means of one or more of the fimbrial adhesins F4 (K88), F5 (K99), F6 (987P), or F41 (Table 38.1). They may also produce an adhesin involved in diffuse adherence (AIDA). They colonize the small intestine and produce one or more of the enterotoxins STa (STI), STb (STII), EAST1, or LT. Until recently, the most commonly observed ETEC in cases of neonatal diarrhea belonged to the classic serogroups O149, O8, O147, and O157, were F4-positive, and produced the enterotoxins LT and STb (Harel et al. 1991; Soderlind et al. 1988; Wilson and Francis 1986). An increasing number of ETEC of serogroups such as O8, O9, O64, and O101 which are F5-, F6-, and/or F41-positive and mainly produce the enterotoxin STa, or less often STb, are now being isolated. These ETEC cause diarrhea mainly in pigs aged from 0–6 days, and to a lesser extent in older pigs, whereas F4-positive ETEC may be isolated in diarrheic pigs from birth to the postweaning period. F4-positive ETEC now predominantly belong to the serogroup O149, also the main cause of postweaning diarrhea.

Table 38.1. Predominant *E. coli* pathotypes, virotypes, and O serogroups associated with neonatal diarrhea

Pathotype	Virotypes	O Serogroups
ETEC	STa:F5:F41, STa:F41, STa:F6, LT:STb:EAST1:F4, LT:STb:STa:EAST1:F4, STb:EAST1:AIDA	8,9,20,45,64, 101,138,141, 147,149,157

Source: The *Escherichia coli* Laboratory, Université de Montréal.

Enteric colibacillosis complicated with shock also occurs in young pigs before and after weaning. *E. coli* associated with this disease either (1) are ETEC and commonly belong to serogroups O149, O157, and O8, which are F4-positive, produce STb and LT, but only occasionally produce Shiga toxin (Stx2e) (Faubert and Drolet 1992), or (2) produce Stx2e and are associated with edema disease. The latter will be discussed in a later section.

EPIDEMIOLOGY

The occurrence of *E. coli* diarrhea depends on an interaction between the causative bacteria, environmental conditions, and certain host factors. Only *E. coli* that carry virulence factors as described in the previous section and that are ingested in large numbers are able to cause diarrhea. The newborn pig, on leaving the uterus and before reaching the teats of the sow, encounters the heavily contaminated environment of the farrowing crate and the skin of the dam, resulting in ingestion of microbes from the intestinal flora of the sow. Thus, in conditions of poor hygiene or in a continuous-farrowing system, a buildup of pathogenic *E. coli* in the environment could lead to an outbreak of neonatal *E. coli* diarrhea. The colostrum contains nonspecific bactericidal factors and specific antibody (IgG and IgA) that inhibit the adherence of pathogenic *E. coli* in the intestine. If the dam has not been exposed to the pathogenic *E. coli* present in the environment of the piglets, specific antibodies are not present in the colostrum, and the piglets are susceptible to infection. Similarly, when individual piglets do not have access to colostrum, due to injury or inability to compete or due to agalactia or insufficient teats of the sow, they are more susceptible to infection. Ambient temperature in the farrowing house is also very important. In pigs kept at temperatures of less than 25°C, intestinal peristaltic activity is greatly reduced, and passage of bacteria and protective antibodies through the intestine is delayed (Sarmiento 1983). Increased numbers of pathogenic *E. coli* in the intestinal tract of these pigs result in a more severe diarrhea than in pigs kept at 30°C.

PATHOGENESIS

In the presence of the appropriate predisposing environmental conditions and host factors, pathogenic *E. coli* proliferate in the intestine and cause diarrhea by means of specific virulence factors. Pathogenesis will be discussed with respect to the *E. coli* pathotypes defined by the production of these factors.

Enterotoxigenic *E. coli*

Most pathogenic *E. coli* produce one or more fimbrial adhesins that mediate their attachment to specific receptors on mucosal epithelial cells and in the adjacent mucous layer. These fimbriae (or pili) are hairlike appendages extending from the bacterial cell and consist of structural protein subunits that, in many cases, act as a support for a separate adhesive protein found at the tips of the fimbriae. Fimbriae are classified by serologic reactivity or by receptor specificity, the latter being manifested by agglutination of red blood cells from different animal species. The nomenclature for fimbriae has been very diverse. For example, the first fimbrial adhesins demonstrated on porcine ETEC were thought to be capsular antigens and were named K88 and K99. A more standardized nomenclature based on serologic activity in crossed immunoelectrophoresis and using an F designation has been proposed (Orskov and Orskov 1983) and is now widely accepted. Hence, K88 and K99 are now called F4 and F5, respectively. The latter nomenclature will be used in this chapter.

Although an increasing number of fimbrial adhesins have been described (more than 30), most fimbrial adhesins, with the exception of F1 (type 1) common fimbriae, are associated with *E. coli* of particular serogroups isolated from specific animal species. F1 fimbriae are found on most *E. coli* isolates and cause an agglutination of guinea pig red cells which is inhibited by D-mannose. Their role in attachment of porcine ETEC to the intestinal mucosa is still unclear (Jayappa et al. 1985; To et al. 1984).

F1 has been found in the absence of any other known fimbrial adhesins on certain diarrheagenic ETEC strains (Broes et al. 1988). The four important fimbrial adhesins of neonatal porcine ETEC are F4 (K88), F5 (K99), F6

(987P), and F41. F4 (K88) fimbriae have been divided into three variants, F4ab, F4ac, and F4ad, based on serologic cross-reactions (Guinée and Jansen 1979). Many ETEC isolates produce more than one fimbrial adhesin, and common combinations are F5 and F6, F5 and F41, and F4 and F6. Production of fimbriae is controlled by genes on the bacterial chromosome (F1, F41) or on plasmids (F4, F5, F6). Many fimbriae, such as F1 and F6, undergo phase variation and may be very poorly expressed after several passages in culture conditions. Other fimbriae (F5 and F41) undergo quantitative variation and are only well expressed in culture media low in glucose or alanine, such as Minca medium (Guinée et al. 1977).

The adhesin involved in diffuse adherence (AIDA), an autotransported 100-kDa mature protein, was originally detected in *E coli* isolates from humans with diarrhea, and has been detected recently in *E. coli* strains from pigs with diarrhea (Mainil et al. 2002; Niewerth et al. 2001). ETEC isolates of the STb or STb:EAST-1 virotypes from neonatal or weaned pigs may be AIDA-positive and induce diarrhea in neonatal pigs (Ngeleka et al. 2003).

Fimbriae adhere to specific receptors on the cell membrane of intestinal epithelial cells and to specific receptors or nonspecifically in the mucus coating the epithelium. ETEC producing fimbriae F5, F6, and F41 mostly colonize the posterior jejunum and ileum, whereas F4-positive ETEC tend to colonize the length of the jejunum and the ileum. Certain pigs do not have receptors for the F4 adhesin on intestinal epithelial cells and are thus resistant to infection by F4-positive ETEC (Sellwood et al. 1975). This genetic resistance to infection is inherited in a simple Mendelian way, and the allele for the receptor is dominant. Subsequent studies have demonstrated at least five pig phenotypes, based on susceptibility of brush borders of different pigs to adherence of isolates producing the different variants F4ab, F4ac, and F4ad (Bijlsma et al. 1982; Hu et al. 1993). The loci encoding porcine intestinal receptors for F4ab and F4ac are closely linked on chromosome 13 (Edfors-Lilja et al. 1995). A similar genetic resistance has not been observed for the other fimbriae of neonatal porcine ETEC. On the other hand, there appears to be an age resistance to infection by F5-and F6-positive isolates, which is not observed for F4-positive isolates. Piglets are most susceptible to infection with F5- and F6-positive ETEC during the first several days of life and subsequently become more resistant. This susceptibility could be related to a reduction of the number of receptors present on intestinal epithelial cells with age in the case of F5 (Runnels et al. 1980). F6-mediated intestinal colonization in older pigs is thought to be inhibited by preferential binding of bacteria to F6 receptors present in the mucus rather than to those on the intestinal epithelium (Dean-Nystrom and Samuel 1994).

ETEC adhering to the intestinal mucosa produce enterotoxins that change the water and electrolyte flux of the small intestine and may lead to diarrhea if the excess fluid from the small intestine is not absorbed in the large intestine. Two major classes of enterotoxin are produced by porcine ETEC: heat-stable toxin (ST), which is resistant to heat treatment at 100°C for 15 minutes, and heat-labile toxin (LT), which is inactivated at 60°C for 15 minutes (Guerrant et al. 1985). ST has been further divided into STa and STb based on solubility in methanol and biological activity (Burgess et al. 1978). The gene for EAST1, which is related to STa, has been recently reported in ETEC isolates from pigs. The *E. coli* enterotoxins have been reviewed in detail elsewhere (Gyles and Fairbrother 2004).

LT is a high–molecular-weight toxin complex that consists of five B subunits able to bind to ganglioside receptors on the intestinal epithelial cell surface and a biologically active A subunit (Gill et al. 1981). After binding, the latter activates adenylate cyclase, which stimulates the production of cyclic AMP. High levels of cyclic AMP in the cell result in increased secretion of Cl, Na, HCO$_3$, and water into the intestinal lumen. Excessive secretion will lead to dehydration, metabolic acidosis, and eventually death. Two subgroups of LT, LTI and LTII, have been described (Holmes et al. 1986). Only LTI is neutralized by anticholera toxin. LT produced by porcine isolates belongs to the LTI subgroup. The LT produced by human and porcine ETEC has been designated LTh and LTp, respectively, based on slight differences in the genes coding for the toxin.

STa (STI, ST1, and ST mouse) is a small, nonimmunogenic protein with a molecular weight (MW) of 2000 (Lallier et al. 1982). STa binds to a guanylyl cyclase intestinal epithelial receptor (De-Sauvage et al. 1991) and activates guanylate cyclase, which stimulates production of cyclic GMP. High levels of cyclic GMP in the cell inhibit the Na/Cl cotransport system and reduce the absorption of electrolytes and water from the intestine (Dreyfus et al. 1984). STa is active in infant mice and young piglets of less than 2 weeks of age but is less active in older pigs. This could be due to differences in the concentration of intestinal receptors with age (Cohen et al. 1988). As with LT, STa produced by human and porcine ETEC has been designated STah and STap, respectively, based on differences in the genes coding for the toxin.

STb (STII, ST2, ST pig) is a small, 5000 MW protein that is antigenically and genetically unrelated to STa and is poorly immunogenic (Dubreuil 1997). STb stimulates cyclic-nucleotide-independent fluid secretion in the gut (Kennedy et al. 1984), which is independent of the cyclic nucleotides but appears to be mediated by prostaglandin E$_2$ and possibly other secretagogues (Harville and Dreyfus 1995; Peterson and Whipp 1995). STb is inactivated by trypsin and, in the presence of trypsin-inactivator, is active in intestines of mice, rats, and calves (Whipp 1990). STb is found in 74% of all porcine ETEC isolates (Moon et al. 1986). The role of STb in the development of diarrhea has been questioned

(Casey et al. 1998), although ETEC producing only STb can induce diarrhea in experimentally infected newborn pigs (Fairbrother et al. 1989), and STb induces some villous atrophy in pig intestinal gut loops (Rose et al. 1987).

EAST1 was first identified in enteroaggregative *E. coli* isolated from humans and was subsequently reported in ETEC from pigs with diarrhea (Yamamoto and Nakazawa 1997). It is commonly found in F4-positive ETEC strains from pigs with diarrhea and in F18:Stx2e strains from pigs with edema disease (Choi et al. 2001). EAST1 is a 38 amino acid peptide of 4100 Da that is different from STa and STb, although it shares 50% homology with the enterotoxic domain of STa (Savarino et al. 1993) and appears to interact with the STa receptor guanylate cyclase C to elicit an increase in cGMP. Hence, the mechanism of action of EAST1 is proposed to be identical to that of STa. However, the role of EAST1 in the development of diarrhea has not yet been defined.

Attaching and Effacing *E. coli*

Porcine AEEC attach to the intestinal mucosa and cause lesions similar to those observed for enteropathogenic *E. coli* (EPEC) isolated from human infantile diarrhea (Hélie et al. 1990). They attach intimately to the intestinal epithelial cell membrane by means of a bacterial outer-membrane protein termed "intimin" or "EPEC attaching and effacing factor" (Eae), efface the microvilli, and invade the epithelial cells (Zhu et al. 1994).

CLINICAL SIGNS

Enteric *E. coli* infection is usually manifested by diarrhea, the severity of which depends on the virulence factors of the *E. coli* and the age and immune status of the piglets. In severe cases, clinical signs of dehydration, metabolic acidosis, and death are observed. In certain cases, particularly in young animals, the infection may be so rapid that death occurs before the development of diarrhea.

Neonatal diarrhea may first be observed 2–3 hours after birth and may affect single pigs or whole litters. Gilt litters are more often affected than sow litters. A large number of piglets in a farrowing house may be affected and mortality may be very high in the first few days of life. Diarrhea may be very mild with no evidence of dehydration or may be clear and watery. The feces vary in color from clear to whitish or various shades of brown. The fecal material may just dribble from the anus down the perineum and be detected only by close examination of the perineal area. In very severe outbreaks, a small proportion of affected animals may vomit. In severe cases, 30–40% of total body weight may be lost as fluid into the intestinal lumen and result in signs of dehydration. The abdominal musculature is flaccid and atonic, the pigs are depressed and sluggish, the eyes may be sunken, and the skin may be bluish-gray in color and resemble parchment in texture. The loss of fluid and weight results in the exaggerated appearance of the bony prominences. These animals usually die. In more chronic or less severely affected cases, the anus and perineum may be inflamed from contact with the alkaline fecal material. Pigs with less severe dehydration may continue to drink and, if treated appropriately, may recover with only minimal long-term effects.

Diarrhea in pigs from the neonatal to the postweaning period is similar to that observed in neonatal piglets but tends to be less severe. Morbidity may be the same as in the neonatal period but mortality is invariably lower. The feces vary from grayish to whitish in unweaned piglets to brownish in recently weaned piglets. Enteric colibacillosis complicated by shock, when associated with ETEC strains, occurs both in unweaned pigs from a few days of age and in recently weaned pigs (Faubert and Drolet 1992). Apparently healthy pigs die suddenly or decline rapidly with cyanosis of the extremities. A yellowish to brownish diarrhea is sometimes observed.

LESIONS

Few specific pathological changes may be attributed to enteric *E. coli* infection. Gross lesions that may be observed include dehydration, dilation of the stomach (which may contain undigested milk curd or feed in the case of postweaning diarrhea), venous infarcts on the greater curvature of the stomach, and dilation of the small intestine with some congestion of the small-intestinal wall. In cases of ETEC infection complicated by shock, characteristic lesions include marked congestion of the small-intestinal and stomach walls and blood-tinged intestinal contents.

Histologic lesions depend on the category of *E. coli* involved. In ETEC infections, layers of *E. coli* are observed adhering to the mucosal epithelial cells of most of the jejunum and ileum in the case of F4-positive ETEC isolates, and of the posterior jejunum and/or the ileum in the case of other ETEC isolates. Adhering bacteria may be found only in the crypts of Lieberkühn, or more often covering the crypts and the tips of the villi. On transmission electronmicroscopy, bacteria are usually located approximately half a bacterial width away from the microvilli, and fimbriae may sometimes be visualized between the bacteria and the microvilli (Figure 38.1). Histological lesions, if observed, may include vascular congestion in the lamina propria with some hemorrhages into the intestinal lumen, increased numbers of neutrophils and macrophages in the lamina propria and migrating into the lumen, and some villous atrophy. In cases of ETEC enteric infection complicated by shock, *E. coli* are found adhering to the mucosal epithelial cells of the small intestine. Congestion, some hemorrhages, and in severe cases villous necrosis and microvascular fibrinous thrombi are observed in the lamina propria of the stomach, small intestine, and colon.

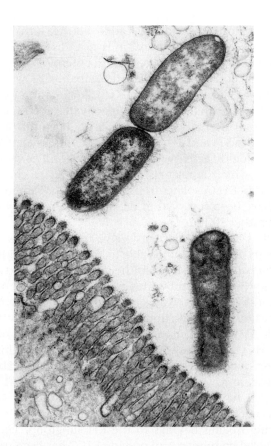

38.1. *Electron micrograph of attachment of E. coli 987P positive strain in the intestine.*

In pigs infected with AEEC isolates, a multifocal colonization of the brush border of mature enterocytes by *E. coli* arranged in palisades with enterocyte degeneration and light to moderate inflammation of the lamina propria is observed, mostly in the ileum (Hélie et al. 1990). Colonization is most intense in the duodenum and cecum, bacteria are sometimes observed in intracytoplasmic vacuoles in enterocytes, and there is a light to moderate villous atrophy in the small intestine. On transmission electronmicroscopy, bacteria are intimately attached to the cytoplasmic membrane of mature enterocytes and arranged in regular palisades, parallel to the microvilli, with effacement of adjacent villi (Figure 38.2). The bacterial cell wall and the apical cell membrane of the enterocyte are separated by a narrow, regular gap of 10 nm at the cupping pedestal, and apical dense regions are seen at attachment sites.

DIAGNOSIS

Enteric *E. coli* infection in young, unweaned pigs must be differentiated from other common infectious causes of diarrhea in pigs of this age group. These include *Clostridium perfringens*, transmissible gastroenteritis virus, rotavirus, and coccidia. More than one etiologic agent may be associated with a particular animal or outbreak. A presumptive diagnosis may be made by determination

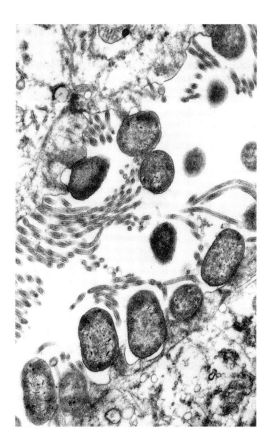

38.2. *Electron micrograph of AEEC lesions.*

of the fecal pH. Secretory diarrheic fluid as a result of enteric ETEC infection has an alkaline pH, whereas that from diarrhea associated with malabsorption as a result of transmissible gastroenteritis virus or rotavirus infection is acid.

Diagnosis of enteric *E. coli* infection is based on clinical signs, histopathological lesions, and the presence of gram-negative organisms usually closely adhering to the small-intestinal mucosa (Wilson and Francis 1986). This diagnosis is strengthened by the isolation of *E. coli* of the appropriate serogroup or, more important, possessing one or more of the above-mentioned virulence factors. Production of enterotoxins and cytotoxins may be ascertained by detection of toxin biological activity. STa activity is determined in the infant mouse test, STb activity in pig and rat ligated gut loops, and LT and Stx in cell culture assays. Fimbrial adhesins may be detected by serologic assays such as slide agglutination, immunofluorescence, and ELISA, using rabbit polyclonal antisera. However, F5 and F41 are only produced when *E. coli* are grown on special minimal media, and F6 is often poorly produced in in vitro conditions. Alternatively, *E. coli* adhering to the intestinal mucosa may be demonstrated directly in infected pigs by examination of frozen sections using indirect immunofluorescence or by examination of formalin-fixed, paraffin-embedded tissues using the immunoperoxidase technique.

Recent technological advances have greatly improved the detection of *E. coli* virulence factors (Wray and Woodward 1994). Use of monoclonal antibodies has led to more specific, sensitive, and reproducible assays for the detection of STa, F4, F5, F6, and F41. Such antibodies may be used in diagnostic kits for the rapid detection and identification of pathogenic *E. coli* directly in the feces or intestinal contents of affected piglets. Currently, genotypic analysis is more commonly used to define the virotypes involved in an infection. Colony hybridization probes and the multiplex polymerase chain reaction (PCR) have been developed for the detection of the genes coding for the fimbrial adhesins and enterotoxins of swine ETEC isolates (Francis 2002; Frydendahl 2002; Osek 2001; Wray and Woodward 1994). There is a high correlation between the results of the standard serologic and biological assays and those of gene probes for the detection of fimbrial adhesins and enterotoxins of swine ETEC isolates (Harel et al. 1991). Gene probe techniques often involve the use of radioactivity and thus must be performed in controlled laboratory conditions. Multiplex PCR amplification may be used to rapidly detect the genes encoding for the virulence factors of pathogenic *E. coli* associated with diarrhea in pigs, either following enrichment culture or directly in the feces or intestinal contents (Tsen et al. 1998). The latter approach is more rapid and indicates the presence of pathogenic *E. coli,* but it does not permit the identification of specific virotypes, as is possible when isolates are tested. However, the traditional approach for identification of pathogenic *E. coli* by serotyping will still be necessary, at least in reference laboratories, in order to monitor changing trends and to identify new, emerging *E. coli* virulence determinants that could gain importance due to the pressure of vaccination of sows against the currently predominant determinants.

TREATMENT

Treatment of enteric *E. coli* infection should be aimed at removal of the pathogenic *E. coli*, correction of their harmful effects, and provision of optimal environmental conditions. Therapy should be rapidly instituted to be as effective as possible. It is important to confirm the diagnosis of *E. coli* infection by culture and to perform antibiotic sensitivity tests, because antibiotic sensitivity varies greatly among *E. coli* isolates (Table 38.2). A broad-spectrum antibiotic treatment could be used initially until the results of antibiotic sensitivity are known. In vitro resistance of *E. coli* isolates to a wide range of antimicrobial agents has dramatically increased over the last several years. In newborn piglets, treatment with antibiotics may be on an individual or litter basis, by mouth or parenteral injection. Commonly used antibiotics are ampicillin, apramycin, ceftifur, gentamycin, neomycin, spectinomycin, furizoli-

Table 38.2. Sensitivity to antimicrobial agents of *E. coli* isolates from pigs aged from 0 to 7 days with diarrhea in Quebec

Antimicrobial Agent	*n* = 38 % Sensitive Isolates
Amikacin	100
Ampicillin	46
Apramycin	79
Ceftiofur	92
Cephalothin	70
Enrofloxacin	100
Gentamycin	63
Neomycin	56
Spectinomycin	41
Tetracycline	7
Tiamulin	5
Trimethoprim-sulfamethoxazole	71

Source: The *Escherichia coli* Laboratory, Université de Montréal 1994–1996.

done, and potentiated sulfa drugs. An alternative approach to the treatment of enteric *E. coli* infection is the use of bacteriophages, an approach that has been successful experimentally but has not been extensively applied in the field.

Fluid therapy, consisting of electrolyte replacement solutions containing glucose given orally, is useful for the treatment of dehydration and acidosis. Drugs which inhibit the secretory effects of enterotoxin, such as chlorpromazine and berberine sulfate, may be useful for the treatment of diarrhea, although many of these drugs have undesirable side effects. The use of such antisecretory drugs as bencetimide and loperamide, alone or in combination with antibacterial agents, has also been suggested (Solis et al. 1993).

It is important to ensure that younger piglets are maintained at a constant temperature of 30–34°C and that recently weaned pigs are held in a draft-free environment at a constant temperature of about 29.5°C.

PREVENTION

A program for prevention of enteric *E. coli* infection should be aimed at reduction of numbers of pathogenic *E. coli* in the environment by good hygiene, maintenance of suitable environmental conditions, and provision of a high level of immunity. Because most pathogenic *E. coli* belong to a limited number of serogroups, enteric *E. coli* infection could be eliminated from some herds.

Husbandry

One of the most important factors in prevention of enteric *E. coli* infection is the maintenance of piglets at an adequate environmental temperature (30–34°C for unweaned pigs), free of drafts, and on a low–heat-conducting floor. This is particularly true for piglets of below-average weight, who lose heat more rapidly because they have a greater skin surface area per unit body weight.

Good hygiene in the farrowing area leads to a reduction in the numbers of *E. coli* being presented to the piglet to a level that it is able to control through its own defense mechanisms.

Farrowing-crate design is important because it affects the position at which feces are deposited by the sow. In crates that are too long, the feces are deposited over a large area of the available floor space, thereby increasing the heavily contaminated area. Ideally, the crate should be adjustable, allowing for a shorter crate for gilts than for sows. Crates on raised, perforated floors allow fecal material to drop through and away from the piglets, and litters farrowed onto such floors have a noticeably lower incidence of diarrhea than those on solid concrete floors.

A dry, warm environment reduces the moisture available to enhance the survival of *E. coli*. This is largely affected by ventilation rates, although if room temperature is too high, sows tend to try and spread water over their lying area to cool themselves, thereby defeating other hygienic procedures. The sow should be at a temperature of approximately 22°C, necessitating a warmer creep area for the piglets.

Quarantine should be used to control the introduction of different *E. coli* virotypes or other infectious agents into the herd. Animals in the herd will have little immunity to *E. coli* fimbrial antigens with which they have not had contact. Farrowing crates should be thoroughly cleaned and disinfected between litters. An all-in/all-out farrowing system with thorough disinfection of the farrowing room between batches will reduce the *E. coli* population in the environment.

Diet may be modified in order to reduce colonization of the intestine by *E. coli* (Thomlinson and Lawrence 1981). Feeding of cultures of *Streptococcus faecium* to young pigs may reduce the incidence of diarrhea (Morkoc et al. 1984).

Immunity

Immunity to enteric *E. coli* infections is humoral and is initially provided through the maternal colostrum, lactogenic antibodies in the milk of the sow, and subsequently by a local intestinal immune response. Specific antibodies inhibit bacterial adherence to receptors on the intestinal epithelial cells and neutralize the activity of the enterotoxins or cytotoxins produced by *E. coli*.

Colostrum from the sow contains high levels of immunoglobulin G (IgG), which rapidly decrease during lactation and IgA becomes the main immunoglobulin class (Bourne 1976). The latter protects the gut against *E. coli* infection. It appears that most IgA, IgM, and IgG in the milk of the sow is produced within the mammary gland. During pregnancy, a proportion of the lymphocytes stimulated by antigens in the intestine migrate to the mammary gland and produce specific antibody against enteric pathogens. These antibodies are actively transported to the colostrum and then the milk during lactation.

The newborn piglet begins to synthesize specific immunoglobulin and develop intestinal immunity during the first week of life (Butler 1973). At first, IgM predominates, but after 12 weeks, it is replaced by IgA as the most important immunoglobulin class in the intestine (Bianchi et al. 1999). Thus, during the first weeks of life, colostrum is the main source of immunologic protection for the piglet.

Breakdown in the protection provided by colostrum may occur for several reasons. If the dam has not been exposed to ETEC present in the environment of the piglets, her colostrum will not contain the specific antibodies necessary for protection against adherence and proliferation of ETEC. Also, any disease process causing agalactia in the sow will diminish transfer of colostrum. Generalized systemic infection may cause a total reduction in colostrum production, whereas mastitis or injured teats may affect production in one or several glands. Piglets failing to receive colostrum due to deformities, infection, small size, or damage at birth will also be more susceptible to ETEC infection.

Maternal vaccination has been one of the most effective ways of controlling neonatal ETEC diarrhea in piglets. Identification of virulence factors important in the pathogenesis of ETEC diarrhea and application of recombinant DNA technology have resulted in the production of more efficient vaccines over the last several years. One of the earliest vaccination techniques consisted of taking the small-intestinal contents from a piglet with diarrhea, culturing it in milk, and feeding the culture to pregnant sows, usually about a month before parturition (Kohler 1974). This technique is effective, conferring an immunity lasting throughout the suckling period, and is still used, particularly in the United States.

Commonly used commercially available vaccines are given parenterally and may be killed whole-cell bacterins or purified fimbrial vaccines. Both of the latter types of vaccines appear to work equally well (Fahy 1987). Bacterins usually contain strains representing the most important serogroups and producing the fimbrial antigens F4, F5, F6, and F41 (Nagy 1986). They are usually given parenterally at about 6 weeks and 2 weeks prior to parturition. Addition of the common fimbrial antigen F1 to a fimbrial bacterin appeared to have been protective in one study (Jayappa et al. 1985) but was not protective in another study (To et al. 1984). Recombinant DNA technology has enabled the production of large quantities of purified fimbrial antigens for use in parenteral vaccines for immunization of the dam (Clarke et al. 1985).

In cases where vaccination is ineffective, it is important to identify the serotypes involved for possible inclusion into an autogenous bacterin. Further characterization of these isolates may identify new or variant fimbrial adhesins important in the pathogenesis of ETEC diarrhea. An alternative approach to the problem of emerging ETEC negative for the known fimbriae has been the use of vaccines containing the nontoxic form of the enterotoxin LT-B conjugated to the nonimmunogenic STa (Klipstein 1986). Following conjugation, STa becomes immunogenic, and this vaccine has given protection in experimental animals. Addition of these components to fimbrial vaccines will provide protection against emerging ETEC with new fimbrial antigens in neonates and against ETEC negative for the known fimbrial antigens and commonly found in older pigs. Isaacson (1994) has recently reviewed the use of vaccines for the prevention of *E. coli* diseases.

Finally, a novel approach to the prevention of ETEC diarrhea in piglets could be the oral administration of exogenous proteases such as bromelain (Mynott et al. 1996). Such proteases can inhibit attachment of F4-positive ETEC to the intestinal mucosa due to modification of the receptor attachment sites.

REFERENCES

Alexander TJL. 1994. Neonatal diarrhea in pigs. In *Escherichia coli in Domestic Animals and Humans*. CL Gyles, ed. Wallingford, U.K.: CAB International, pp. 151–170.

Bianchi AT, Scholten JW, Moonen Leusen BH, Boersma WJ. 1999. Development of the natural response of immunoglobulin secreting cells in the pig as a function of organ, age and housing. Developmental and Comparative Immunology 23:511–520.

Biehl LG, Hoefling DC. 1986. Diagnosis and treatment of diarrhea in 7- to 14-day-old pigs. J Am Vet Med Assoc 188:1144–1146.

Bijlsma IGW, De Nijs A, Van Der Meer C, Frik JF. 1982. Different pig phenotypes affect adherence of *Escherichia coli* to jejunal brush borders by K88ab, K88ac, or K88ad antigen. Infect Immun 37:891–894.

Bourne FJ. 1976. Humoral immunity in the pig. Vet Rec 98:499–501.

Broes A, Fairbrother JM, Larivière S, Jacques M, Johnson WM. 1988. Virulence properties of enterotoxigenic *Escherichia coli* O8:KX105 strains isolated from diarrheic piglets. Infect Immun 56:241–246.

Burgess MN, Bywater RJ, Cowley CM, Mullan NA, Newsome PM. 1978. Biological evaluation of a methanol-soluble, heat-stable *Escherichia coli* STb enterotoxin in infant mice, pigs, rabbits, and calves. Infect Immun 21:526–531.

Butler JE. 1973. Synthesis and distribution of immunoglobulins. J Am Vet Med Assoc 163:795–800.

Casey TA, Herring CJ, Schneider RA, Bosworth BT, Whipp SC. 1998. Expression of heat-stable enterotoxin STb by adherent *Escherichia coli* is not sufficient to cause severe diarrhea in neonatal pigs. Infect Immun 66:1270–1272.

Choi C, Cho W, Chung H, Jung T, Kim J, Chae C. 2001. *Escherichia coli* heat-stable enterotoxin 1 (EAST1) gene in isolates in weaned pigs with diarrhea and/or edema disease. Vet Microbiol 81:65–71.

Clarke S, Cahill A, Stirzaker C, Greenwood P, Gregson R. 1985. Prevention by vaccination-animal bacteria. In Infectious Diarrhea in the Young. Amsterdam: Elsevier Science Publishers, p. 481.

Cohen MB, Guarino A, Shukla R, Giannella RA. 1988. Age-related differences in receptors for *Escherichia coli* heat-stable enterotoxin in the small and large intestine of children. Gastroenterology 94:367–373.

Dean-Nystrom EA, Samuel JE. 1994. Age-related resistance to 987P fimbria-mediated colonization correlates with specific glycolipid receptors in intestinal mucus in swine. Infect Immun 61:4789–4794.

De-Sauvage FJ, Camerato TR, Goeddel DV. 1991. Primary structure and functional expression of receptor for *Escherichia coli* heat-stable enterotoxin. J Biol Chem 266:17912–17918.

Dreyfus LA, Jaso-Friedmann L, Robertson DC. 1984. Characterization of the mechanism of action of *Escherichia coli* heat stable enterotoxin. Infect Immun 44:493–501.

Dubreuil JD. 1997. *Escherichia coli* STb enterotoxin: Review. Microbiology 143:1783–1795.

Edfors-Lilja I, Gustafsson U, Duval-Iflah Y, Ellergren H, Johansson M, Juneja RK, Marklund L, Andersson L. 1995. The porcine intestinal receptor for *Escherichia coli* K88ab, K88ac: Regional localization on chromosome 13 and influence of IgG response to the K88 antigen. Animal Genetics 26:237–242.

Fahy VA. 1987. Preweaning colibacillosis. In Proceedings of Conference Australasian Pig Science Association, p. 177.

Fairbrother JM. 1999. *Escherichia coli* infection in farm animals. In Current Veterinary Therapy—Food Animal Practice. Florida: W. B. Saunders, p. 328–330.

Fairbrother JM, Broes A, Jacques M, Larivière S. 1989. Pathogenicity of *Escherichia coli* O115:K"V165" strains isolated from pigs with diarrhea. Am J Vet Res 50:1029–1036.

Faubert C, Drolet R. 1992. *Escherichia coli* hemorrhagic gastroenteritis in the piglet: Clinical, pathological and microbiological findings. Can Vet J 33:251.

Francis DH. 2002. Enterotoxigenic *Escherichia coli* infection in pigs and its diagnosis. J Swine Health Prod 10:171–175.

Frydendahl K. 2002. Prevalence of serogroups and virulence genes in *Escherichia coli* associated with postweaning diarrhoea and oedema disease in pigs and a comparison of diagnostic approaches. Vet Microbiol 85:169–182.

Gill DM, Clements JD, Robertson DC, Finkelstein RA. 1981. Subunit number and arrangement in *Escherichia coli* heat-labile enterotoxin. Infect Immun 33:677–682.

Guerrant RL, Holmes RK, Robertson CC, Greenberg RN. 1985. Roles of enterotoxins in the pathogenesis of *Escherichia coli* diarrhea. In Microbiology—1985. L Leive, PF Bonventre, JA Morello, S Schlesinger, SD Silver, HC Wu, eds. Washington: American Society for Microbiology, USA. pp. 68–73.

Guinée PAM, Jansen WH. 1979. Behavior of *Escherichia coli* K antigens K88ab, K88ac, and K88ad in immuno-electrophoresis, double diffusion, and hemagglutination. Infect Immun 23:700–705.

Guinée PAM, Veldkamp J, Jansen J. 1977. Improved minca medium for the detection of K99 antigen in calf enterotoxigenic strains of *Escherichia coli*. Infect Immun 15:676–678.

Gyles CL, Fairbrother JM. 2004. *Escherichia coli*. In Pathogenesis of Bacterial Infections in Animals (3rd edition). CL Gyles, JF Prescott, JG Songer, CO Thoen, eds. Ames, Iowa: Blackwell Publishing, p. 193–223.

Harel J, Lapointe H, Fallara A, Lortie LA, Bigras-Poulin M, Larivière S, Fairbrother JM. 1991. Detection of genes for fimbrial antigens and enterotoxins associated with *Escherichia coli* serogroups from pigs with diarrhea. J Clin Microbiol 29:745–752.

Harville BA, Dreyfus LA. 1995. Involvement of 5-hydroxytryptamine and prostaglandin E_2 in intestinal secretory action of *Escherichia coli* heat-stable enterotoxin B. Infect Immun 63:745–750.

Hélie P, Morin M, Jacques M, Fairbrother JM. 1990. Experimental infection of newborn pigs with an attaching and effacing *Escherichia coli* O45: K"E65" strain. Proc Int Congr Pig Vet Soc p. 143.

Holmes RK, Twiddy EM, Pickett CL. 1986. Purification and characterization of type II heat-labile enterotoxin of *Escherichia coli*. Infect Immun 53:464–473.

Hu ZL, Hasler-Rapacz J, Huang SC, Rapacz J. 1993. Studies in swine on inheritance and variation in expression of small intestinal receptors mediating adhesion of the K88 enteropathogenic *Escherichia coli* variants. J Hered 84:157–165.

Isaacson RE. 1994. Vaccines against *Escherichia coli* diseases. In *Escherichia coli* in Domestic Animals and Humans. CL Gyles, ed. Wallingford, U.K.: CAB International, pp. 629–647.

Jayappa HG, Goodnow RA, Geary SJ. 1985. Role of *Escherichia coli* type 1 pilus in colonization of porcine ileum and its protective nature as a vaccine antigen in controlling colibacillosis. Infect Immun 48:350–354.

Kennedy DJ, Greenberg RN, Dunn JA, Abernathy R, Ryerse JS, Guerrant RL. 1984. Effects of *Escherichia coli* heat stable enterotoxin STb on intestines of mice, rabbits, and piglets. Infect Immun 46:639–643.

Klipstein FA. 1986. Development of *Escherichia coli* vaccines against diarrheal disease in humans. In Development of Drugs and Vaccines against Diarrhea. 11th Nobel Conf Stockholm 1985. Lund: Stdentlitteratur, p. 53.

Kohler EM. 1974. Protection of pigs against neonatal enteric colibacillosis with colostrum and milk from orally infected sows. Am Vet J 35:331–338.

Lallier R, Bernard F, Gendreau M, Lazure C, Seidah NG, Chretien M, St-Pierre S. 1982. Isolation, purification, and structure of *Escherichia coli* heat stable enterotoxin of porcine origin. Anal Biochem 127:267–275.

Mainil JG, Jacquemin E, Pohl P, Kaeckenbeeck A, Benz I. 2002. DNA sequences coding for the F18 fimbriae and AIDA adhesion are localized on the same plasmid in *Escherichia coli* isolates from piglets. Vet Microbiol 86:303–311.

Moon HW, Schneider RA, Mosely SL. 1986. Comparative prevalence of four enterotoxin genes among *Escherichia coli* isolated from swine. Am J Vet Res 47:210–212.

Morkoc A, Backstrom L. Savage D. 1984. Streptococcus faecium in prevention of neonatal colibacillosis in piglets. Proc Int Congr Pig Vet Soc 8:76.

Mynott TL, Luke RK, Chandler DS. 1996. Oral administration of protease inhibits enterotoxigenic *Escherichia coli* receptor activity in piglet small intestine. Gut 38:28–32.

Nagy B. 1986. Vaccines against toxigenic *Escherichia coli* disease in animals. In Development of Drugs and Vaccines against Diarrhea. 11th Nobel Conf Stockholm 1985. Lund: Stdentlitteratur, p. 53.

Ngeleka M, Pritchard J, Appleyard G, Middleton DM, Fairbrother JM. 2003. Isolation and association of E. coli AIDA-I/STb, rather than EAST1 pathotype with diarrhea in piglets and antibiotic sensitivity of isolates. J Vet Diagn Invest 15:242–252.

Niewerth U, Frey A, Voss T, Le Bouguenec C, Baljer G, Franke S, Schmidt MA. 2001. The AIDA autotransporter system is associated with F18 and stx2e in *Escherichia coli* isolates from pigs diagnosed with edema disease and postweaning diarrhea. Clinical and Diagnostic Laboratory Immunology 8:143–149.

Orskov I, Orskov F. 1983. Serology of *Escherichia coli* fimbriae. Progress in Allergy 33:80–105.

Osek J. 2001. Multiplex polymerase chain reaction assay for identification of enterotoxigenic *Escherichia coli* strains. J Vet Diagn Invest 13:308–311.

Peterson JW, Whipp SC. 1995. Comparison of the mechanisms of action of cholera toxin and the heat-stable enterotoxins of *Escherichia coli*. Infect Immun 63:1452–1461.

Rose R, Whipp SC, Moon HW. 1987. Effects of *Escherichia coli* heat stable enterotoxin on small intestinal villi in pigs, rabbits, and lambs. Vet Pathol 24:71–79.

Runnels PL, Moon HW, Schneider RA. 1980. Development of resistance with host age to adhesion of K99+ *Escherichia coli* to isolated intestinal epithelial cells. Infect Immun 28:298–300.

Sarmiento JI. 1983. Environmental temperature: A predisposing factor in the enterotoxigenic *Escherichia coli*–induced diarrhea of the newborn pig. M.S. thesis, Univ Guelph, Ont.

Savarino SJ, Fasano A, Watson J., Martin BM, Levine MM, Guandalini S, Guerry P. 1993. Enteroaggregative *Escherichia coli* heat-stable enterotoxin 1 represents another subfamily of E. coli heat-stable toxin. In Proceedings of National Academy of Sciences, USA. 90:3093–3097.

Sellwood R, Gibbons RA, Jones GW, Rutter JM. 1975. Adhesion of enteropathogenic *Escherichia coli* to pig intestinal brush borders: The existence of two pig phenotypes. Journal of Medical Microbiology 8:405–411.

Soderlind O, Thafvelin B, Mollby R. 1988. Virulence factors in *Escherichia coli* strains isolated from Swedish pigs with diarrhea. J Clin Microbiol 26:879–884.

Solis CA, Sumano LH, Marin HJA. 1993. Treatment of *Escherichia coli* induced diarrhoea in piglets with antisecretory drugs alone or combined with antibacterials. Pig Vet J 30:83–88.

Thomlinson JR, Lawrence TJL. 1981. Dietary manipulation of gastric pH in the prophylaxis of enteric disease in weaned pigs: Some field observations. Vet Rec 109:120–122.

To SCM, Moon HW, Runnels PL. 1984. Type 1 pili (F1) of porcine enterotoxigenic *Escherichia coli*: Vaccine trial and tests for production in the small intestine during disease. Infect Immun 43:1–5.

Tsen HY, Jian LZ, Chi WR. 1998. Use of a multiplex PCR system for the simultaneous detection of heat labile toxin I and heat stable toxin II genes of enterotoxigenic *Escherichia coli* in skim milk and porcine stool. Journal of Food Protection 61:141–145.

Whipp SC. 1990. Assay of enterotoxigenic *Escherichia coli* heat-stable toxin b in rats and mice. Infect Immun 58:930–934.

Wilson RA, Francis DH. 1986. Fimbriae and enterotoxins associated with *Escherichia coli* serogroups isolated from pigs with colibacillosis. Am J Vet Res 47:213–217.

Wray C, Woodward MJ. 1994. Laboratory diagnosis of *Escherichia coli* infections. In *Escherichia coli* in Domestic Animals and Humans. CL Gyles, ed. Wallingford, U.K.: CAB International, pp. 595–628.

Yamamoto T, Nakazawa M. 1997. Detection and sequences of the enteroaggregative *Escherichia coli* heat-stable enterotoxin 1 gene in enterotoxigenic *E. coli* strains isolated from piglets and calves with diarrhea. J Clin Microbiol 35:223–227.

Zhu C, Harel J, Jacques M, Desautels C, Donnenberg MS, Beaudry M, Fairbrother JM. 1994. Virulence properties and attaching-effacing activity of *Escherichia coli* O45 from swine postweaning diarrhea. Infect Immun 62:4153–4159.

Postweaning *Escherichia coli* Diarrhea and Edema Disease

J. M. Fairbrother and C. L. Gyles

Postweaning *Escherichia coli* diarrhea and edema disease are treated in one section because they often both occur in the same age group of pigs, the causative bacteria share certain virulence factors, and some strains of *E. coli* can cause both diseases. There are also important differences in the two diseases.

E. coli postweaning diarrhea (PWD) is a communicable diarrhea mediated by enterotoxins and observed mainly after weaning. It is also called "postweaning enteric colibacillosis."

Edema disease (ED) is a communicable enterotoxemia caused by certain *E. coli* that colonize the small intestine and produce a protein toxin that enters the bloodstream and damages vessel walls in certain tissues. The names "edema disease," "bowel edema", and "gut edema" were coined because edema of the submucosa of the stomach and the mesocolon is often a prominent feature of the disease.

E. coli PWD and ED may occur independently, but they may also occur in a single outbreak or in the same pig. The early history of the two diseases has been extensively reviewed by Sojka (1965).

E. coli is an important cause of death in weaned pigs. Losses due to PWD are reported worldwide, whereas mortality due to ED does not appear to be as great in North America as is observed in Europe.

ED bears some similarity to the human diseases caused by enterohemorrhagic strains of *E. coli* (EHEC), which produce closely related, but not identical, Shiga toxins. However, the human EHEC strains colonize the intestine by a mechanism distinct from edema disease *E. coli* (EDEC) (Tzipori et al. 1986). Serotypes associated with ED are different from those of EHEC that cause disease in humans.

ETIOLOGY

PWD and ED are caused by strains of *E. coli* that possess certain adhesion factors enabling the bacteria to colonize the small intestine and that produce one or several exotoxins. Nearly all of these *E. coli* are alpha-hemolytic. Most of them belong to a very limited number of serotypes. In a given area, the serotypes are closely associated with a rather constant set of fimbrial adhesins and toxins. Thus, the serogroup O139 has been found worldwide to produce the fimbrial variant F18ab. Strains of this serogroup from Australia always cause PWD, whereas those from Europe typically induce ED. The serogroup O149 has been found worldwide to produce the fimbrial variant F4ac and to induce PWD.

At present, by far the most predominant serogroup of *E. coli* associated with PWD in pigs is O149. The most important virotypes and O serogroups of *E. coli* associated with PWD throughout the world are found in Table 38.3. These virotypes usually have either F4 or F18 as fimbrial adhesin. Some F4- and F18-negative virotypes have been identified by The *Escherichia coli* Laboratory in Quebec and by others (Frydendahl 2002) in *E. coli* from pigs with PWD. The role of these virotypes in the development of diarrhea has not yet been established. Some differences in the predominant virotypes have been observed from country to country. For example, the fimbrial adhesins F4 and F18 were detected in 45% and 39%, respectively, of isolates from pigs with PWD or

Table 38.3. Important pathotypes, virotypes, and O serogroups of *E. coli* causing disease in postweaning pigs

Disease	Pathotype	Virotypes	O Serogroups
Postweaning diarrhea	ETEC	LT:STb:EAST1:F4, LT:STb:STa:EAST1:F4, STa:STb, STa:STb:Stx2e[1]:F18ac, STa:F18ac, LT:STb, STb:EAST1:AIDA, LT:STb:STa[1]:EAST1:F4[1]: AIDA[1]:Stx2e[1]:F18ac, AIDA:F18ac	8, 38, 139, 141, 147, 149, 157
Postweaning diarrhea	EPEC	Eae:EAST1[1]	45, 103
Edema disease	EDEC	Stx2e:F18ab:AIDA[1]	138, 139, 141

Source: The *Escherichia coli* Laboratory, Université de Montréal; Francis 2002; Frydendahl 2002; and Mainil et al. 2002.
[1]Not always present.

ED in Denmark during 1999–2000 (Frydendahl 2002). Of the F4-positive isolates, all were O149: two-thirds were of virotype LT:STb:EAST1:F4 and one-third were of virotype LT:STa:STb:EAST1:F4. The F18 isolates were much more heterogeneous, the most common serotype/virotype profiles being O149:LT:STb:EAST1:F18, O138:STa:STb:F18, O138:LT:STb:EAST1:Stx2e:F18, and O139:Stx2e:F18. More than half of the ETEC isolated from pigs with diarrhea in South Dakota, U.S., in 2001–2002 were of virotypes LT:STb:F4, STa:STb:F18, or STa:STb:Stx2e:F18, F4 isolates being slightly more prevalent than F18 isolates (Francis 2002). On the other hand, the predominant fimbrial adhesin found in ETEC isolated from pigs with diarrhea in Quebec, Canada, both in diagnostic cases from 1994 to 1998 (Fairbrother et al. 2000) and in a study of 17 farms with at least 15% diarrhea in pigs in the first 3 weeks postweaning (personal observations 2002), was F4. In both studies, about half of ETEC isolates produced F4. All F4-positive isolates were O149, half being of virotype LT:STb:EAST1:F4, half being of virotype LT:STa:STb:EAST1:F4. Only 2% of isolates were F18-positive and were mostly of virotype STa:STb. All other ETEC produced neither F4 nor F18, the most common virotypes being STa:STb and STb:EAST1:AIDA. AIDA has been detected recently in *E. coli* strains from pigs with edema disease or postweaning diarrhea, particularly in strains of the virotypes Stx:F18 and F18 alone (Mainil et al. 2002). AIDA is encoded by genes present on a plasmid, possibly the same as that containing the *fed* genes that encode F18 fimbriae. ETEC isolates of the STb or STb:EAST-1 virotypes from weaned pigs may also be AIDA-positive (Ngeleka et al. 2003).

The antigenic variants of F18 fimbriae were serologically determined using 380 isolates from fatal cases of PWD and ED in Germany (Wittig et al. 1995). Variants F18ab and F18ac were found in 40% and 35%, and F4 in 14%, of the isolates. The remaining isolates were negative for F18 and F4.

An interesting evolution in the virotype of O149 isolates has been observed. In retrospective studies in Canada, it has been observed that O149 strains isolated

before 1990 were predominantly of virotype LT:STb:EAST1 (Fontaine et al. 2002; Noamani et al. 2003). Since 1990, a new virotype, LT:STa:STb:EAST1, has appeared and is now either as prevalent as (Fontaine et al. 2002; Frydendahl 2002) or has almost replaced (Noamani et al. 2003) the old virotype. This trend may not be universal, because most O149 strains isolated from 4- to 6-week-old weaned pigs with diarrhea in Poland (Osek 2003) were of the LT:STb:EAST1 virotype, and the new virotype did not appear to be prevalent in the 2001–2002 South Dakota study (Francis 2002).

PWD and ED are mediated by toxins—enterotoxins in the case of *E. coli* PWD, and Shiga toxin in the case of ED. It is noteworthy that ETEC and EDEC strains may occur in pigs in the absence of PWD or ED. In these cases, the pathogenic *E. coli* constitute a low percentage of the fecal *E. coli*. In contrast, in disease, they constitute most or all of the *E. coli* in the feces.

A more detailed description of the enterotoxins is given in the preceding subchapter. The term "Shiga toxin" (Stx2e) is a synonym of Shiga-like toxin, verotoxin, edema disease principle, neurotoxin, and vasotoxin. MacLeod and Gyles (1990) developed a purification scheme resulting in a homogeneous preparation of Stx2e free of endotoxin. As little as 3 ng of pure Stx2e per kilogram of body weight administered intravenously to young pigs induces disease. Clinical signs and gross and microscopic lesions are characteristic of ED, thus confirming that Stx2e and EDP (edema disease principle) are identical. Incubation time and severity of disease are directly related to the toxin dose.

Enteropathogenic *E. coli*

An enteric syndrome distinct from classic PWD was described by several investigators. It is characterized by attaching and effacing lesions caused by *E. coli* (AEEC). The clinical outcome of the infection is difficult to evaluate, because mixed infection, such as with F4-positive ETEC, often occurs. The AEEC do not possess any virulence factors of classic PWD or ED strains (Zhu et al. 1994). Their virulence attributes are dealt with in the subchapter on neonatal *E. coli* diarrhea. Experimental infection of gnotobiotic pigs allows reproduction of the lesions (Figure 38.2). Several predisposing factors, such as a weaner diet containing soya and field peas or Porcine Reproductive and Respiratory Syndrome (PRRS) virus infection, may enhance bacterial colonization and development of attaching and effacing lesions (Neef et al. 1994, personal observations). AEEC will not be further dealt with in this chapter.

Comprehensive overviews of *E. coli* and its role in animal disease may be found elsewhere (Gyles 1994; Gyles and Fairbrother 2004).

EPIDEMIOLOGY

The epidemiologies of PWD and ED have many features in common. The age group primarily affected by PWD and/or ED depends on the weaning age. There are some differences between *E. coli* with F4 and those with F18. The former can cause neonatal, preweaning, and postweaning diarrhea, most often in the very first days after weaning. In farms where husbandry measures at weaning, such as addition of higher levels of protein of animal source, plasma, acidifying agents, and zinc oxide are being used, peaks of diarrhea and enteric colibacillosis complicated by shock may be observed often at 3 weeks after weaning, or even at 6–8 weeks after weaning, at the time when the pigs enter the growing barns (Fairbrother, unpublished observations). The latter, however, more often cause disease between 5 and 14 days after weaning (Svendsen et al. 1974) or after introduction to fattening herds. Unweaned piglets can also be affected by *E. coli* diarrhea and ED. In suckling pigs, the severity of the disease depends on antibody titers in the milk of the sow (Sarmiento et al. 1988b).

The morbidity in an affected herd is extremely variable. Within a particular litter it may be up to 80% or more, but the average is 30–40%. With ED, the case fatality rate ranges from 50% to over 90%. The course of the disease in the herd varies from 4–14 days, the average being slightly under a week. The disease disappears as abruptly as it appears. Recurrence on premises is common (Kurtz et al. 1969). With PWD the case fatality rate and the mortality tend to be lower. In untreated herds, the latter may attain 26% (Svendsen et al. 1974).

The environment of the weaner unit appears to be the most likely source of pathogenic *E. coli* strains. Unweaned pigs may acquire infection in the farrowing house, presumably from the same source, and carry it into the weaning unit. Routine cleaning and disinfection are usually insufficient to break the cycle of infection (Hampson et al. 1987). Under experimental conditions, however, transmission can be prevented by strict hygienic measures (Smith and Halls 1968; Kausche et al. 1992). The minimal infectious dose is not known. In transmission experiments with a F4-positive ETEC strain, airborne transmission between pigs in wire cages

1.5 m apart was repeatedly observed (Wathes et al. 1989). Outbreaks tend to involve only one strain of F4-positive *E. coli* at any one time. Occasionally, two potential pathogens are isolated, but one usually predominates. Multiple infections of herds involving more than one serogroup were detected in 47% of 84 herds (Awad-Masalmeh et al. 1988).

The spread of pathogenic *E. coli* is presumed to occur via aerosols, feed, other vehicles, pigs, and possibly other animals. Introduction of new pathogenic strains of *E. coli* into closed primary specific pathogen free (SPF) herds with a high isolation standard was observed at intervals of 1–2 years. Once a site is contaminated with a particular strain, it can remain so for an extended period. The serotypes associated with postweaning diseases tend to be similar in broad geographic areas. When ED entered Denmark in 1994, it spread from one SPF breeding herd by trade of pigs to at least 37 other herds. The close clonal relationship of the causal strains was confirmed (Aarestrup et al. 1997; Jorsal et al. 1996). Another 22 herds became infected without known trading contact.

PATHOGENESIS

For the sake of clarity, intestinal colonization and toxemia will be presented separately. However, there may be mutual interactions.

Colonization of the Small Intestine

E. coli causing PWD and/or ED enter the animal by ingestion and, when present in sufficient numbers, colonize the small intestine following bacterial attachment to receptors on the small intestinal epithelium or in the mucus coating the epithelium, by means of specific fimbrial adhesins. These bacteria then proliferate rapidly to attain massive numbers to the order of 10^9 in the midjejunum to the ileum. The degree of colonization determines whether disease results from infection. Adhering microcolonies or layers of bacteria were observed on the small-intestinal mucosae of pigs experimentally infected with two strains of O group 139 (Figure 38.3) (Bertschinger and Pohlenz 1983; Methiyapun et al. 1984; Bertschinger et al. 1990). EDEC adhere to the brush border similarly to ETEC. Some of the known factors influencing colonization by pathogenic *E. coli* are discussed here.

Brush border receptors for pathogenic *E. coli* are not present in every pig. Genetic resistance resulting from lack of receptors for F4 was first described by Sellwood et al. (1975) (see section on neonatal colibacillosis). The receptor for F18 fimbriae is also controlled in a single locus, and the presence of a receptor is dominant over absence (Bertschinger et al. 1993). The receptor for F18 is distinct from the receptor for F4. The genes for the F4 receptor were determined on chromosome 13 (Guérin et al. 1993), whereas the genes for the F18 receptor were lo-

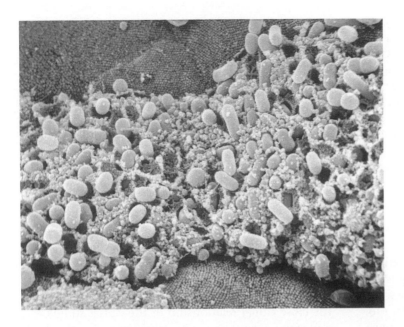

38.3. *Bacteria adhering patch-wise to microvilli of small-intestinal epithelium of a weaner 6 days after oral inoculation with a culture of E. coli O139:K12:H1.*

cated on chromosome 6 close to the locus for stress susceptibility. In a high proportion of the Swiss pig population, resistance against stress is linked to susceptibility to adhesion of *E. coli* with F18 fimbriae (Vögeli et al. 1996). In view of the low prevalence of stress-susceptible pigs, the frequency of pigs with the F18 receptor would be predicted to be high. This has been confirmed in a number of studies.

Fimbrial receptors are thought to be glycoconjugates that are subject to modulation by feed lectins such as constituents of leguminous plants (Kelly et al. 1994). It may be speculated that feed-induced changes of the receptor are involved in the reduced susceptibility to colonization by F18-positive *E. coli* in the first days after weaning (Bertschinger et al. 1993). Endogenous as well as orally administered proteases may reduce the receptor activity for F4 fimbriae (Mynott et al. 1996). Receptors for F4 are fully expressed from birth to adult age, whereas the F18 receptor is not yet fully expressed by piglets under about 20 days of age (Nagy et al. 1992). Hence, *E. coli* with F18 fimbriae do not cause disease in neonatal pigs. Constant expression of receptors may underlie the earlier appearance after weaning of *E. coli* strains with F4 in herds where F4- and F18-positive strains are endemic.

Loss of milk antibodies appears to contribute significantly to susceptibility of pigs to *E. coli* enteric infections in the postweaning period (Deprez et al. 1986, Sarmiento et al. 1988b).

A variety of viruses infect the porcine intestine and may thereby change the bacterial environment. Dual infection of pigs with rotavirus and with an ETEC strain without F4 results in a more severe diarrhea than inoculation with either agent alone (Lecce et al. 1982). The investigators concluded that viral damage of the epithelium favors colonization by *E. coli*. Infection by the PRRS virus results in a decreased efficacy of the immune system, permitting ETEC to cause a septicemia leading to death (Nakamine et al. 1998).

An acid environment has an inhibitory effect on *E. coli*. The pH of the stomach contents falls after weaning (Risley et al. 1992). Several investigators found that the pH of the jejunum cannot be reduced by acidification of the feed. The pH close to the jejunal brush border is slightly acid and highly regulated. It is not influenced by the pH of the chyme (McEwan et al. 1990).

Veterinary practitioners and farmers were convinced many years ago that nutritious feed would play an important role in development of disease. Thus ED was named "protein intoxication." Smith and Halls (1968) inoculated pigs on various feed regimens with an O141:K85ac EDEC strain. They found that severe feed restriction resulted in much lower fecal numbers of the bacteria and absence of disease. A similar effect was achieved by feeding pigs ad libitum on a diet extremely rich in fiber and low in nutrients. The authors concluded that the physiological state of the intestinal epithelium might influence bacterial adhesion. These experiments were extended by Bertschinger et al. (1978) using an O139:K12 EDEC strain. The findings of Smith and Halls (1968) were confirmed. However, the poor diets inhibited growth of the pigs. When these diets were replaced by a conventional type of feed, colonization and clinical disease developed. The inhibitory effect of the poor diet was abolished by supplementation with fish meal but not with starch or fat. The precise mechanism behind these phenomena remains to be elucidated.

Low room temperature in the weaner rooms was proposed as being responsible for a more severe course of PWD (Wathes et al. 1989). Under experimental conditions, ED was not aggravated by cold stress (Kausche et al. 1992).

Diarrhea

The mechanisms by which enterotoxins induce diarrhea are described in the preceding section (neonatal *E. coli* diarrhea). Almost all *E. coli* involved in fatal cases of PWD produce LT (Imberechts et al. 1994). Pigs colonized about 12 days after weaning with ETEC producing one or both heat-stable enterotoxins develop diarrhea only exceptionally (Sarrazin and Bertschinger 1997). This difference between neonates and weaned pigs may be explained at least in part by the marked increase of antisecretory factor beginning a few days after weaning (Lange et al. 1993).

Enterotoxemia

Highly purified Stx2e induces a disease indistinguishable from ED when administered intravenously to pigs (MacLeod and Gyles 1990). Stx2e produced by EDEC in the intestine is absorbed into the circulation and can bind to globotetraosyl ceramide on red blood cells. Thus, vessels are subjected to prolonged toxin exposure (Boyd et al. 1993). By immunological methods the toxin can be detected in endothelial cells of small blood vessels of the intestine and in microvillous membranes of enterocytes at the base of the villi (Waddell et al. 1996).

The most consistent injury observed in natural cases, after injection of partially purified toxin (Clugston et al. 1974b; Gannon et al. 1989) and in pigs inoculated orally with live cultures (Methiyapun et al. 1984; Kausche et al. 1992) is a degenerative angiopathy of small arteries and arterioles. The edema fluid found in various tissues is low in protein and could be the result of a mild increase in vascular permeability. Information on pathophysiology of ED is scarce. Clugston et al. (1974a) observed an increase of blood pressure after intravenous administration of EDP. Hypertension developed later than clinical edema and was therefore thought to be the result of vascular injury rather than its cause. Hypertension might exacerbate the lesions in the already damaged vessels. The development of injuries in the nervous system may be due to hypoxia resulting from impaired blood flow (Clugston et al. 1974b).

A distinct type of ED is characterized by terminal bloody diarrhea and hemorrhagic lesions in the cardiac region of the stomach, the ileum, and the large intestine (Figure 38.4) (Bertschinger and Pohlenz 1983). According to Gannon et al. (1989) and MacLeod and Gyles (1990), acute hemorrhagic gastroenteritis occurs in some of the pigs to which a high dose of Stx2e is administered. Epithelial necrosis secondary to necrosis of small arteries and arterioles may be responsible for luminal hemorrhage.

CLINICAL SIGNS

Postweaning Diarrhea

In the spontaneous outbreaks caused by an *E. coli* strain of O149 without F4 investigated by Svendsen et al.

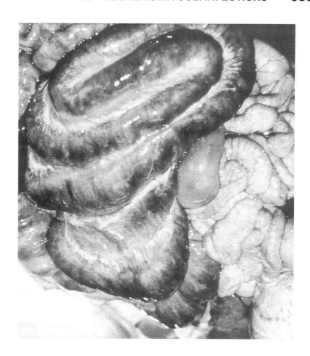

38.4. *Extended hemorrhages and minor mesenteric edema in the colon of a pig that developed bloody diarrhea 5 days after inoculation with a culture of E. coli O139:K12:H1.*

(1974), the first manifestation of PWD was sudden death of one or several pigs as early as 2 days after weaning. At the same time, feed consumption of the affected batch of pigs dropped markedly, and a watery diarrhea developed. At the onset, some pigs exhibited a characteristic quivering of the tail. The rectal temperature was normal. Affected pigs became dehydrated and depressed. They ate irregularly, but even in the terminal stage of the disease, they tried to drink. Many pigs showed cyanotic discoloration of the tip of the nose, the ears, and the abdomen. Even severely affected pigs tried to move around with staggering, uncoordinated movements. The peak of mortality occurred 6–10 days after weaning. Surviving pigs recovered well. Some pigs were completely spared from the disease.

In pigs experimentally infected with a strain with virulence factors F4, LT, and STb, diarrhea started 1–2 days after inoculation and was fulminating and fatal in some of the pigs, whereas others survived after diarrhea of 3–4 days' duration (Sarmiento et al. 1988a). The pigs lost some weight in the first 2 days after inoculation. From the fifth day on, the growth curve of susceptible pigs resumed a course parallel to that of genetically resistant pigs. The latter were not colonized and remained free from any symptoms.

Postweaning Diarrhea Combined with Edema Disease

Smith and Halls (1968) described the disease experimentally induced with a strain of serogroup O141:K85a,c, obviously a producer of Stx2e and of enterotoxin(s). The first sign was anorexia, which started at the onset of shedding bacterial numbers above 10^9 colony-forming units (CFU)/g of feces 3 (2–5) days postinoculation (PI) and was observed in most pigs. Anorexia lasted for several days in the pigs that recovered and until euthanasia in the pigs killed when death was imminent. Diarrhea appeared on day 4 (1–8) PI. Usually it was severe but of short duration. It was rarely fatal. In most pigs diarrhea was no longer present when signs of nervous involvement became apparent, that is, on day 6 (5–13) PI. Swollen eyelids were seen at about the same time. Ataxia was accompanied with varying degrees of mental confusion and was usually progressive. Affected pigs soon became completely recumbent. Severe dyspnea was usually present at this final stage. Most of the pigs with ataxia had to be killed on the day the signs of impairment of the nervous system appeared. Pigs were moribund 7 (5–13) days PI. The rectal temperature always remained within the normal range.

Edema Disease

A similar disease was seen in pigs inoculated with a nonenterotoxigenic ED strain of serotype O139:K12:H1 (Bertschinger et al. 1978). However, diarrhea was not associated with colonization and a more pronounced edema developed in some cases. In such cases ears, subcutaneous tissue over the frontal bones, nose, and lips were swollen (Figure 38.5). In mild cases, subcutaneous edema was accompanied by pruritus, which disappeared after recovery. In some pigs with or without dyspnea, respiration was accompanied by a snoring sound.

Watery diarrhea with clots of fresh blood became apparent in a few pigs at the terminal stage (Bertschinger and Pohlenz 1983). Hemorrhagic colitis developed also

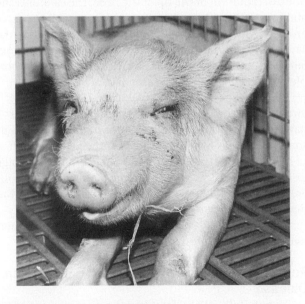

38.5. *Edematous swelling of eyelids, forehead, and lips, breathing through open mouth, and inability to rise in a weaner 4 days after oral inoculation with a culture of E. coli O139:K12:H1.*

in pigs to which high doses of toxin Stx2e were administered (MacLeod et al. 1991).

Chronic ED occurred in a variable, but mostly low, proportion of pigs recovering from acute attacks of ED or *E. coli* PWD (Bertschinger and Pohlenz 1974; Nakamura et al. 1982). The condition was called cerebrospinal angiopathy before its association with ED became apparent. For periods varying from days to several weeks after intestinal infection, growth stops, and sick pigs often show unilateral nervous disturbances such as circling movements, twisting of the head, or atrophy of limb muscles with progressive weakness. Subcutaneous edema is rare. Affected pigs should be destroyed. Subclinical ED was observed in most pigs surviving for 2 weeks after inoculation with a strain of *E. coli* O139 positive for Stx2e and STb. The pigs were clinically normal but developed vascular lesions. No pigs were allowed to survive beyond the 2 weeks (Kausche et al. 1992).

LESIONS

Postweaning Diarrhea

Gross Lesions. Pigs dead from *E. coli* PWD are generally in good condition but severely dehydrated with sunken eyes and some cyanosis. Lungs look pale and dry, as observed in well-bled pigs (Svendsen et al. 1974). The stomach is often distended with dry feed. Variable hyperemia of the gastric mucosa is often noted in the fundic region. The small intestine is dilated, slightly edematous, and hyperemic. The contents vary from watery to mucoid, with a characteristic smell. The mesentery is heavily congested. Contents of the large intestine most often look light greenish or yellowish and are mucoid to watery. Pigs dying late in an outbreak look emaciated and exhibit a strong smell of ammonia. There are irregularly shaped superficial ulcerations in the fundic region of the stomach and similar lesions of smaller size in the large intestine. The feces look yellow and pasty. The fluid from the anterior chamber of the eye may give a positive reaction for urea.

Some authors use the terms "hemorrhagic gastroenteritis" or "enteric colibacillosis complicated by shock" to describe a form of *E. coli* diarrhea characterized by severe congestion of the gastric fundus and the small intestine with or without blood-tinged contents of the small intestine and sometimes the upper large intestine, but only exceptionally with bloody feces (Faubert and Drolet 1992). This type of lesion was always caused by *E. coli* with F4 fimbriae. The syndrome of enteric colibacillosis complicated by septicemia was recently reproduced in gnotobiotic pigs and deletion of the gene for LT resulted in reduction of F4-mediated colonization, reduced dehydration, and less frequent septicemia (Berberov et al. 2004).

Microscopic Lesions. Bacteria adhering to the ileal and less consistently to the jejunal surface are always seen. The bacterial layers are restricted to villi and look patchy (Sarmiento et al. 1988a; Casey et al. 1992; Faubert and Drolet 1992). The mucosa and the epithelium appear intact. Some investigators have reported increased numbers of neutrophils in the superficial lamina propria. In pigs with enteric colibacillosis complicated by shock, severe congestion of the gastric and small-intestinal mucosae is commonly associated with microvascular fibrinous thrombi. Necrosis of villi with marked infiltration of neutrophils occurs in severe cases. There is only occasional hemorrhage in the lamina propria of the jejunum and the ileum (Svendsen et al. 1974; Faubert and Drolet 1992).

Edema Disease

Gross Lesions. Pigs dead of ED are mostly in good condition, somewhat pale, and the bodies retain a fresh appearance. Edema at specific sites is variable and may be absent in some animals. Subcutaneous edema may occur. Edema in the submucosa of the stomach is characteristic when present and is located in the region of the glandular cardia (Figure 38.6). It may vary from being barely detectable to 2 cm or more in thickness. The edema fluid is usually serogelatinous and occasionally may be bloodstained adjacent to the mucosa. If severe, the edema may extend into the fundic submucosa. Inflammatory edema associated with acute ulceration of the esophageal cardia must not be confused with that of ED.

Edema of the gallbladder is sometimes seen. The mesocolon is a common site for edema. Careful inspection of the pericardial, pleural, and peritoneal cavities may reveal occasional whitish fibrin strands and a slight increase in serous fluid. The mesenteric and colic nodes vary in appearance from normal to being swollen, edematous, and congested. Typically, the stomach is full of

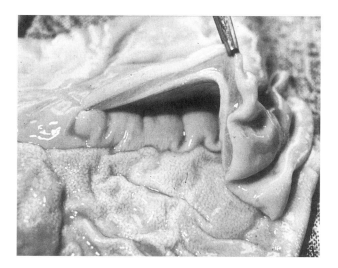

38.6. *Edematous swelling of glandular mucosa of the cardiac region and gelatinous submucosal edema of the cut stomach wall from a field case from which E. coli O139:K12:H1 was isolated.*

dry, fresh-looking feed, and the small intestine is relatively empty. Colonic contents may be diminished in amount. It may be inferred that this is a manifestation of delayed gastric emptying, since some animals have a period of anorexia before death. Also, it has been shown experimentally that pigs with ED may eat very little for 48 hours before death and at necropsy have full stomachs (Smith and Halls 1968). The suggestion that some pigs with ED are affected by constipation also agrees with these observations.

The lungs may display varying degrees of edema and a characteristic, patchy, sublobular congestion. In some cases this may be the only observable lesion. Cases with laryngeal edema have also been observed. A few epicardial and endocardial petechiae may occur. This lesion must not be confused with mulberry heart disease.

In some pigs with spontaneous or experimental ED, a form of hemorrhagic gastroenteritis occurs, which is quite different from that described with *E. coli* PWD. In addition to marked edema, the edematous submucosa of the cardiac region of the stomach and the mucosa of the lower small and upper large intestine show extensive hemorrhage. Watery diarrhea with clots of coagulated blood occurs shortly before death in some of these pigs (Bertschinger and Pohlenz 1983). Endothelial swelling, vacuolation and proliferation, microthrombus formation, subendothelial fibrin, medial necrosis, and perivascular edema were detected in such cases (Methiyapun et al. 1984). The similarity to human hemorrhagic colitis is striking.

If the causative strain of *E. coli* is also capable of producing enterotoxin, lesions of postweaning diarrhea may be added, and edema may be mild or absent.

Microscopic Lesions. Patchy layers of adhering bacteria are present throughout the small intestine early in the course of ED (Bertschinger and Pohlenz 1983; Methiyapun et al. 1984; Bertschinger et al. 1990). Contrasting with *E. coli* PWD, the colonization has often disappeared when pigs with ED become moribund (Smith and Halls 1968).

The most important microscopic lesions are those of a degenerative angiopathy affecting small arteries and arterioles (Clugston et al. 1974b; Kausche et al. 1992). The lesions may occur in many organs and tissues. The dense arterial network in the mesocolon adjacent to the colic lymph nodes is frequently affected. The early acute lesion is one of necrosis of smooth muscle cells in the tunica media characterized by pyknosis and karyorrhexis of nuclei and hyaline change in cytoplasmic elements. In the walls of some affected vessels, fibrinoid material is deposited (Figure 38.7). Swelling of endothelial cells has also been observed. In acute experimental cases, edema of the leptomeninges and perivascular spaces has been demonstrated. In older lesions, there may be proliferation of adventitial and medial cells (Figure 38.8).

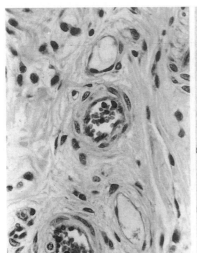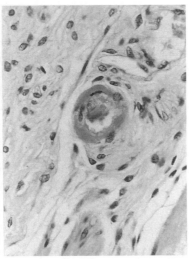

38.7. Arterioles in submucosa of the urinary bladder: (left) normal; (right) fibrinoid or hyaline change, acute experimental ED (Clugston et al. 1974b).

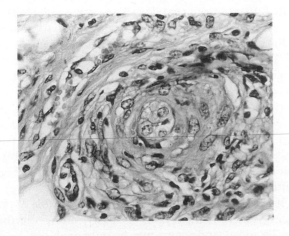

38.8. Submucosa of cardial gland region of the stomach 17 days after inoculation with EDP (edema disease principle containing STL-IIe); arteriole with proliferative arteriopathy (Clugston et al. 1974b).

Vascular lesions may be difficult to detect in acute cases, but in surviving pigs or those affected subclinically, they are more readily apparent (Kausche et al. 1992). Thrombosis is not usually a feature of uncomplicated naturally occurring ED.

In pigs that have recovered from natural outbreaks or survived for several days following acute signs, there are lesions of focal encephalomalacia in the brain stem together with lesions in the small arteries and arterioles (Kurtz et al. 1969; Kausche et al. 1992). These are thought to be the result of vascular injury leading to edema and ischemia. A cerebrospinal angiopathy of pigs has been recognized as a clinicopathologic entity for some years. Its microscopic features are those described above as well as the occurrence of eosinophilic, Periodic Acid Schiff (PAS)–positive droplets around affected vessels. This angiopathy is most likely a manifestation of edema disease (Bertschinger and Pohlenz 1974).

DIAGNOSIS

Postweaning Diarrhea

Postweaning diarrhea is a very complex disease with multiple etiologies (see Chapter 3). Occurrence of diarrhea early after weaning, marked dehydration, and at least some mortality are characteristics in the field allowing a preliminary diagnosis of ETEC. The gross lesions, including the characteristic smell, are also helpful. The final diagnosis requires detection of ETEC (see neonatal *E. coli* diarrhea), which are shed in high numbers. Hemolysis is not a valid criterion for identification of ETEC. Laboratories not equipped for the determination of virulence factors should at least use serotyping of living cultures with OK-antisera against serotypes most prevalent in a given region.

Edema Disease

The diagnosis of acute ED is based on sudden appearance and on clinical signs of neurologic disease in thriving pigs 1–2 weeks after weaning. In the live pig the most important and constant diagnostic sign is partial ataxia or a staggering gait. Subcutaneous edema in the palpebrae and over the frontal bones is also a cardinal sign when present. At necropsy the characteristic lesions of edema, when present, are helpful in confirming the diagnosis but may be absent in a significant number of cases, especially when severe diarrhea has preceded ED. Diagnosis of ED in adult pigs (Imberechts et al. 1996) may require additional efforts, such as histopathology and postmortem examination of more than one pig.

Bacteriologic examination of the small intestine and colon usually yields pure or nearly pure cultures of hemolytic *E. coli*. However, bacterial numbers may have declined in more protracted cases (Bertschinger and Pohlenz 1983). In contrast to ETEC infections, a negative bacteriologic result therefore does not exclude the diagnosis of ED. Serologic identification of the common serotypes associated with ED is additional evidence. Serotyping is essential, because hemolytic *E. coli* not associated with other virulence factors are frequently encountered in the intestinal flora and may be present in high numbers. Polymerase chain reaction (PCR) amplification of the genes for Stx2e and F18 fimbriae may be used to obtain a rapid and definitive identification of EDEC.

Subacute or chronic ED is diagnosed by the demonstration of arteriopathy and eventually lesions of focal encephalomalacia.

In cases of sudden death, differential diagnosis includes microangiopathia dietetica and circulatory failure, as seen after severe fighting. When pigs show signs of neurological disease, viral encephalitis (enteroviral polioencephalomyelitis, pseudorabies) and bacterial meningoencephalitis (*Streptococcus suis*, *Haemophilus parasuis*) as well as water deprivation should be considered.

TREATMENT

Much less is known about the treatment of these diseases than about pathogenesis and about treatment of neonatal colibacillosis.

Antimicrobial Therapy

Chemotherapeutic control of bacterial proliferation is therapeutically much more effective in *E. coli* PWD than in ED, because in the latter, toxin has already been absorbed into the circulation and become bound to its receptor when clinical signs become visible. The development of bacterial resistance against a wide range of antimicrobial drugs (Table 38.4) renders this approach uncertain. It is not possible to give universal data on resistance, because the situation varies in different pig populations depending on the antimicrobials preferentially used.

Sick pigs must be treated parenterally. They eat and drink very little, even if they stand close to the creep and to the drinking nipple. Substances must be selected that reach the intestinal lumen, such as amoxicillin/clavulanic acid, fluoroquinolones, cephalosporins, apramycin, ceftiofur, neomycin, or trimethoprim. Testing bacterial resistance is indispensable if there is a herd problem.

Supportive Therapy for PWD

The supportive therapy has to counteract dehydration and acidosis. Attractive rehydration fluid should be offered for spontaneous intake or injected intraperitoneally if the pig is anorectic. Such fluids may contain glucose, glycine, citric acid, and potassium dihydrogen phosphate in an isotonic solution (Bywater and Woode 1980). Uptake should be equal to the loss (i.e., up to 25% of the body weight).

Table 38.4. Sensitivity to antimicrobial agents of *E. coli* O149 isolates from pigs with PWD or ED in Switzerland and PWD in Quebec

	% Sensitive O149 Isolates	
Antimicrobial Agent	Switzerland[1] $n = 59$	Quebec[2] $n = 52$
Ampicillin	73	36
Amoxicillin/clavulanic acid	100	NT[3]
Cefoxitin	100	NT
Streptomycin	37	NT
Spectinomycin	19	NT
Neomycin	81	73
Apramycin	93	58
Gentamicin	91	81
Tetracycline	47	0
Chloramphenicol	81	NT
Enrofloxacin	100	98
Colistin[4]	100	NT
Ceftiofur	NT	100
Sulfonamide	15	NT
Trimethoprim	73	NT
Trimethoprim-sulfamethoxazole	NT	30
Furazolidone	100	NT

[1]Bertschinger et al. 1996.
[2]The *Escherichia coli* Laboratory, Université de Montréal 1996–2000.
[3]Not tested.
[4]Modified agar dilution technique (Bertschinger et al. 1996).

Edema Disease

There is little likelihood of saving the lives of pigs with advanced signs such as severe subcutaneous edema, respiratory distress, or inability to rise. Evaluation of therapy is difficult because the severity of the illness cannot be quantified. Numerous remedies have been recommended in the past and have then been abandoned.

PREVENTION

Breeding of Resistant Pigs

This is the approach to prevention that may be most effective and economical in the long term. Work in this direction is in progress. It will be important to avoid co-selection of unwanted traits closely linked with loci coding for the F4 and the F18 receptors. It cannot be predicted whether additional types of adhesive fimbriae or new variants of known types will emerge that could bind to yet unidentified receptors.

Eradication of EDEC

The transmissible character of *E. coli* PWD and ED is evident. In Denmark most of the recent spread of ED followed the routes of the pig trade (Jorsal et al. 1996). It was logical to start an eradication program involving depopulation of affected farms and disinfection of the buildings (Johansen et al. 1996b). With one exception, the 15 farms participating in this program remained free of clinical disease for a minimum of 4–7 months. They are under continuing surveillance. Some problems render this approach risky. The tools to prove the absence of pathogenic *E. coli* from a given herd are not yet adequate. Also, *E. coli* has a high tenacity in the environment.

Immunoprophylaxis

Acquired immunity may result in protection against intestinal colonization and/or against effects of the toxins. Weaned pigs can be protected passively or actively.

Passive Immunity. A daily dose of 525 mL, but not of 270 mL, milk obtained from sows in late lactation fed to weaned pigs completely inhibited colonization, whereas pigs fed the same amount of cow's milk shed high numbers of the EDEC bacteria (Deprez et al. 1986). Spray-dried porcine blood plasma fed at a dose of 90 g per pig/day had a similar inhibitory effect that lasted only as long as the plasma was fed, and the inhibitory effect could be improved by vaccination of the donor pigs (Deprez et al. 1990, 1996). Immune protection against colonization with F4- and F18-positive *E. coli* may be attained by feeding eggs produced by vaccinated hens (Imberechts et al. 1997; Marquardt et al. 1999). It remains to be shown whether the antibody-containing egg powder can be produced at an acceptable price.

Active Immunity. Few commercial vaccines are available for the prevention of postweaning *E. coli* PWD and ED. Injectable vaccines, such as those administered to sows for the prevention of neonatal diarrhea, stimulate mostly the systemic rather than mucosal immunity, giving rise to circulating antibodies which do not reach intestinal bacteria in high enough levels to be very effective (Van den Broeck et al. 1999). Such vaccines may even suppress the mucosal immune response upon subsequent oral infection with a pathogenic *E. coli* (Bianchi et al. 1996). Several approaches for the control of postweaning *E. coli*–associated diarrhea are currently being investigated. Most of these control strategies are specific for the adhesin or O serogroup of the causative *E. coli*. Hence, an accurate diagnosis and identification of the adhesin type is essential to assure a more effective control of the diarrhea. New vaccination strategies include the oral immunization of piglets with live attenuated avirulent *E. coli* strains carrying the fimbrial adhesins. Such vaccine strains may be administered to weaned piglets in the drinking water or to unweaned piglets by oral dosing at least 1 week prior to the expected onset of diarrhea, to allow the intestinal colonization by these bacteria and induction of local intestinal antibodies which will block the adherence of the pathogenic *E. coli* and hence prevent the development of diarrhea. This approach appears to be effective for the control of both F4 and F18 *E. coli*–associated diarrhea, using a vaccine strain carrying the appropriate adhesin. A large scale on-farm study in the United States has demonstrated a decreased mortality and reduced use of antimicrobials fol-

lowing oral administration of a live nonenterotoxigenic F4 *E. coli* strain to pigs immediately following weaning (Fuentes et al. 2004). Pigs that have been colonized by an F18 ETEC producing STI and STb are protected against recolonization by a heterologous ETEC sharing no other antigens with the immunizing strain except F18 fimbriae. However, the cross-protection between strains with fimbrial variants F18ab and F18ac may not be very high (Bertschinger et al. 2000). Current research is aimed at the oral administration of purified F4 fimbriae, instead of the whole bacteria, as a vaccine for the control of outbreaks of *E. coli*–associated diarrhea in weaned pigs (Van den Broeck et al. 1999). Use of such a subunit vaccine results in a specific mucosal immune response in the intestines and a significant reduction in fecal excretion of the pathogenic F4.

In the pig, the small intestine is the major site of IgA and IgM production. IgM is more a mucosal isotype than in other animal species and probably has an important role in mucosal immunity (Bianchi et al. 1999). In the porcine lamina propria, the frequency of IgM secreting cells is similar to that of IgA secreting cells at 4 weeks of age and increases thereafter. The shift from IgM to IgA as predominant mucosal isotype is at about 12 weeks of age. Vaccines for preventing PWD should activate the mucosal immune system and evoke antigen-specific IgA or IgM responses in order to induce a protective mucosal immunity (Van den Broeck et al. 1999).

Gannon et al. (1988) did not detect neutralizing antibody against Stx2e in the sera of neonatal pigs and weaned pigs from herds with and without ED. However, pigs do mount an antibody response; Wieler et al. (1995) showed that pigs that had survived an outbreak of ED had antibodies reacting in an ELISA to the B subunit of Stx2e.

Active immunity against intravenous challenge with Stx2e was induced in young pigs by a toxoid vaccine prepared from an ultrasonic lysate of an EDEC by treatment with glutaraldehyde (Dobrescu 1982). A similar toxoid was used for vaccination of pigs 1 week before weaning (Awad-Masalmeh et al. 1989). The vaccine conferred highly significant protection against ED after the pigs were orally challenged with EDEC serogroup O139:K12. Vaccinated principals shed lower numbers of the inoculated bacteria and had better weight gains than placebo-vaccinated littermates.

A toxoid prepared by treatment of Stx2e with formaldehyde was not completely free of toxic activity. Therefore, the toxin was modified by site-directed mutagenesis of the *stx2e* gene. The genetically modified toxin was found to have no deleterious effect on the growth of vaccinated pigs, and it prevented overt and subclinical ED when vaccinated pigs were challenged with an *E. coli* O139:F18 positive for Stx2e and STb (Bosworth et al. 1996). A different approach was chosen by MacLeod and Gyles (1991), who detoxified purified Stx2e with glutaraldehyde. An adjuvanted experimental vaccine was evaluated in two herds infected by a strain of *E. coli*

O139:F18, Stx2e. Mortality due to ED was significantly reduced, and daily gain in the nursery was significantly improved. Deaths caused by ETEC in one of the herds were not prevented (Johansen et al. 1996a). These toxoid vaccines are not yet commercially available.

Chemoprophylaxis

At present, preventive feed medication is practiced in a majority of the affected herds in most countries despite serious drawbacks such as nonacceptance by the consumer, impaired buildup of immunity, and selection of resistant bacteria. Resistance is often induced within days or a few weeks. Isolates from *E. coli* PWD and ED show the highest rate of resistance within porcine *E. coli*. Besides the classes of antimicrobials mentioned above for parenteral therapy, the aminoglycosides and colistin are widely used. The latter has the advantages of high stability, low toxicity, absence of infectious resistance, and slow development of resistance. With colistin, resistance cannot reliably be detected by the agar diffusion technique (Bertschinger et al. 1996). Investigators have reported that oxytetracycline reduces the adhesion of *E. coli* at concentrations below the minimum inhibitory concentration. Sarmiento and Moon (1988) reported that *E. coli* PWD induced by a tetracycline-resistant strain takes an identical course in pigs eating feed with and without tetracycline.

Zinc oxide offers an alternative to antimicrobials. Feeds with contents between 2400 and 3000 ppm of zinc reduce diarrhea and mortality and improve growth. The activity is explained by an antibacterial effect (Holm and Poulsen 1996). However, environmental considerations should be included in discussions of zinc oxide at such high levels.

Dietary Measures

Restriction of feed intake, high-fiber diets, or ad libitum feeding of fiber have been reported as effective deterrents to the development of ED and postweaning diarrhea (Smith and Halls 1968; Bertschinger et al. 1978; Rantzer et al. 1996). The nutritive value of the feed may be reduced by increasing fiber content to 15–20% and reducing crude protein and digestible energy to one-half of the normal values (Bertschinger et al. 1978). The addition of fiber to normal diets may be beneficial. Dunne (1975) advocated feeding high-quality alfalfa coupled with restriction of daily feed intake. To be effective, nutrient intake has to be low enough to maintain daily gain below 1% of body weight in the 2 weeks after weaning. Such diets prevent colonization and impair the development of immunity in the same way as antimicrobials. Later outbreaks are frequently seen.

A lower mortality due to *E. coli* enterotoxemia and improved weight gains were reported after introduction of rations with a reduced acid-binding capacity. A similar effect is ascribed to organic acids. Others were unable to reduce the mortality due to ED by the inclusion of a mixture of organic and inorganic acids in the feed (Johansen et al. 1996b). This result is not surprising in view of the highly regulated pH close to the mucosal surface (McEwan et al. 1990).

An improved weight gain and lower frequency of scours was observed in early weaned (10 days of age) pigs fed a spray-dried porcine plasma (SDPP)–based diet (Owusu-Asiedu A et al. 2002). This was partly attributed to the presence of specific anti-ETEC antibodies in the SDPP. In another study, addition of SDPP to the ration of weaned pigs did not prevent losses due to experimental challenge with an ETEC strain, although improved weight gain was observed (Van Dijk et al. 2002). However, the lack of effect on losses could be due to the severity of the experimental model.

Exogenous as well as endogenous proteases lower the activity of intestinal F4 receptors. Bromelain, a protease from pineapple stems, applied orally to pigs reduced the binding of F4-positive ETEC to brush borders in a dose-dependent manner (Mynott et al. 1996). The efficacy in a clinical situation remains to be demonstrated.

Scandinavian workers have shown that antisecretory factor reverses secretory diarrhea induced by heat-labile enterotoxin. The levels of antisecretory factor in the blood plasma can be increased by addition of glucose and of some amino acids to the feed. Treated weaner pigs were reported to have a lower incidence of diarrhea and a greater weight gain (Göransson et al. 1993). Antisecretory factor probably exerts its effects on the enteric nervous system (Hansen and Skadhauge 1995).

Bacterial Probiotics

In recent investigations *Enterococcus faecium*, *Lactobacillus* sp., and *Bacillus cereus* strain "toyoi" were fed to experimentally infected (De Cupere et al. 1992) and to naturally infected (Johansen et al. 1996b) pigs. No preventive effect was recorded. Schulze (1977) confirmed earlier comparative quantitative studies of the gastrointestinal flora in weaned and in unweaned pigs, where no evidence was found for an interdependence between *E. coli* and the other components of the flora.

General Management

Management of the weanling pig should minimize environmental and other forms of stress such as unnecessary mixing of litters, chilling, transportation, and assignment to new pens. Wathes et al. (1989) observed a higher incidence of scours and greater mortality due to *E. coli* PWD in experimentally infected pigs kept at 15°C than in controls at higher temperatures. The experiment was not perfectly conclusive because genetic resistance was neglected.

REFERENCES

Aarestrup MF, Jorsal SE, Ahrens P, Jensen NE, Meyling A. 1997. Molecular characterization of *Escherichia coli* strains isolated from pigs with edema disease. J Clin Microbiol 35:20–24.

Awad-Masalmeh M, Reitinger H, Quakyi E, Hinterdorfer H, Silber R, Willinger H. 1988. Observations on the isolation and characterization of *E. coli* derived from edema disease cases. Proc Int Congr Pig Vet Soc 10:114.

Awad-Masalmeh M, Schuh M, Köfer J, Quakyi E. 1989. Überprüfung der Schutzwirkung eines Toxoidimpfstoffes gegen die Ödemkrankheit des Absetzferkels im Infektionsmodell. Dtsch Tierärztl Wochenschr 96:397–432.

Berberov EM, Zhou Y, Francis DH, Scott MA, Kachman SD, Moxley RA. 2004. Relative importance of heat-labile enterotoxin in the causation of severe diarrheal disease in the gnotobiotic piglet model by a strain of enterotoxigenic *Escherichia coli* that produces multiple enterotoxins. Infect Immun 72:3914–3924.

Bertschinger HU, Bachmann M, Mettler C, Pospischil A, Schraner EM, Stamm M, Sydler T, Wild P. 1990. Adhesive fimbriae produced in vivo by *Escherichia coli* O139:K12(B):H1 associated with enterotoxaemia in pigs. Vet Microbiol 25:267–281.

Bertschinger HU, Eggenberger U, Jucker H, Pfirter HP. 1978. Evaluation of low nutrient, high fibre diets for the prevention of porcine *Escherichia coli* enterotoxaemia. Vet Microbiol 3:281–290.

Bertschinger HU, Mettler C, Blaser C, Fritzsche C. 1996. Colistin resistance of *E. coli* isolated from pigs with oedema disease and postweaning diarrhoea detected by a modified agar dilution method. Proc Int Congr Pig Vet Soc 14:271.

Bertschinger HU, Nief V, Tschape H. 2000. Active oral immunization of suckling piglets to prevent colonization after weaning by enterotoxigenic *Escherichia coli* with fimbriae F18. Vet Microbiol 71:255–67.

Bertschinger HU, Pohlenz J. 1974. Cerebrospinale Angiopathie bei Ferkeln mit experimenteller Coli-Enterotoxämie. Schweiz Arch Tierheilk 116:543–554.

——. 1983. Bacterial colonization and morphology of the intestine in porcine *Escherichia coli* enterotoxemia (edema disease). Vet Pathol 20:99–110.

Bertschinger HU, Stamm M, Vögeli P. 1993. Inheritance of resistance to oedema disease in the pig: Experiments with an *Echerichia coli* strain expressing fimbriae 107. Vet Microbiol 35:79–89.

Bianchi AT, Scholten JW, Moonen Leusen BH, Boersma WJ. 1999. Development of the natural response of immunoglobulin secreting cells in the pig as a function of organ, age and housing. Developmental and Comparative Immunology 23:511–520.

Bianchi ATJ, Scholten J-W, van Zijderveld AM, van Zijderveld FG, Bokhout BA. 1996. Parenteral vaccination of mice and piglets with F4' *Escherichia coli* suppresses the enteric anti-F4 response upon oral infection. Vaccine. 14:199–206.

Bosworth BT, Samuel JE, Moon HW, O'Brien AD, Gordon VM, Whipp SC. 1996. Vaccination with genetically modified Shiga-like toxin IIe prevents edema disease in swine. Infect Immun 64:55–60.

Boyd B, Tyrrell G, Maloney M, Gyles C, Brunton J, Lingwood C. 1993. Alteration of the glycolipid binding specificity of the pig edema toxin from globotetraosyl to globotriaosyl ceramide alters in vivo tissue targetting and results in a verotoxin 1–like disease in pigs. J Exp Med 177:1745–1753.

Bywater RJ, Woode GN. 1980. Oral fluid replacement by a glucose glycine electrolyte formulation in *E. coli* and rotavirus diarrhoea in pigs. Vet Rec 106:75–78.

Casey TA, Nagy B, Moon HW. 1992. Pathogenicity of porcine enterotoxigenic *Escherichia coli* that do not express K88, K99, F41, or 987P adhesins. Am J Vet Res 53:1488–1492.

Clugston RE, Nielsen NO, Roe WE. 1974a. Experimental edema disease of swine (*E. coli* enterotoxemia). II. The development of hypertension after the intravenous administration of edema disease principle. Canadian Journal of Comparative Medicine 38:29–33.

Clugston RE, Nielsen NO, Smith DLT. 1974b. Experimental edema disease of swine (*E. coli* enterotoxemia). III. Pathology and pathogenesis. Canadian Journal of Comparative Medicine 38:34–43.

De Cupere F, Deprez P, Demeulenaere D, Muylle E. 1992. Evaluation of the effect of 3 probiotics on experimental *Escherichia coli* enterotoxaemia in weaned piglets. Journal of Veterinary Medicine Series B: Infectious Diseases and Veterinary Public Health 39:277–284.

Deprez P, Van den Hende C, Muylle E, Oyaert W. 1986. The influence of the administration of sow's milk on the post-weaning excretion of hemolytic *E. coli* in the pig. Veterinary Research Communications 10:469–478.

Deprez P, De Cupere F, Muylle E. 1990. The effect of feeding dried plasma on experimental *Escherichia coli* enterotoxemia in piglets. Proc Int Congr Pig Vet Soc 11:149.

Deprez P, Nollet H, Van Driessche E, Muylle E. 1996. The use of swine plasma components as adhesin inhibitors in the protection of piglets against *Escherichia coli* enterotoxemia. Proc Int Congr Pig Vet Soc 14:276.

Dobrescu L. 1982. Immunological studies in pigs using edema disease principle (*E. coli* neurotoxin). Proc Int Congr Pig Vet Soc 7:19.

Dunne HW. 1975. Colibacillosis and edema disease. In Diseases of Swine (4th edition). HW Dunne, AD Leman, eds. Ames: Iowa State Univ Press, p. 674.

Fairbrother JM, Higgins R, Desautels C. 2000. Trends in pathotypes and antimicrobial resistance of *E. coli* isolates from weaned pigs. Proc Int Congr Pig Vet Soc 16:17.

Fontaine F, Pérès S, Gyles CL, Fairbrother JM. 2002. Trends in O149:K91 Enterotoxigenic *E. coli* from pigs in Québec. Proc Int Congr Pig Vet Soc 17:70.

Faubert C, Drolet R. 1992. Hemorrhagic gastroenteritis caused by *Escherichia coli* in piglets: Clinical, pathological and microbiological findings. Can Vet J 33:251–256.

Francis DH. 2002. Enterotoxigenic *Escherichia coli* infection in pigs and its diagnosis. J Swine Health Prod 10:171–175.

Frydendahl K. 2002. Prevalence of serogroups and virulence genes in *Escherichia coli* associated with postweaning diarrhoea and oedema disease in pigs and a comparison of diagnostic approaches. Vet Microbiol 85:169–182.

Fuentes M, Pijoan C, Becton L, Morrison B, Pieters M. 2004. Inoculation of non pathogenic *Escherichia coli* to control disease and reduce antibiotic usage. Proc Int Congr Pig Vet Soc 18:258.

Gannon VPJ, Gyles CL, Friendship W. 1988. Characteristics of verotoxigenic *Escherichia coli* from pigs. Can J Vet Res 52:331–337.

Gannon VPJ, Gyles CL, Wilcock BP. 1989. Effects of *Escherichia coli* Shiga-like toxins (verotoxins) in pigs. Can J Vet Res 53:306–312.

Göransson L, Martinsson K, Lange S, Lönnroth I. 1993. Feed-induced lectins in piglets: Feed-induced lectins and their effect on post-weaning diarrhoea, daily weight gain and mortality. Journal of Veterinary Medicine Series B: Infectious Diseases and Veterinary Public Health 40:478–484.

Guérin G, Duval-Iflah Y, Bonneau M, Bertaud M, Guillaume P, Ollivier L. 1993. Evidence for linkage between K88ab, K88ac intestinal receptors to *Escherichia coli* and transferrin loci in pigs. Animal Genetics 24:393–396.

Gyles CL. 1994. *Escherichia coli* in Domestic Animals and Humans. Wallingford, U.K.: CAB International.

Hampson DJ, Fu ZF, Robertson ID. 1987. Investigation of the source of haemolytic *Escherichia coli* infecting weaned pigs. Epidemiology and Infection 99:149–153.

Gyles CL, Fairbrother JM. 2004. *Escherichia coli*. In Pathogenesis of Bacterial Infections in Animals (3rd edition). CL Gyles, JF Prescott, JG Songer, CO Thoen, eds. Ames, Iowa: Blackwell Publishing, p.193–223.

Hansen MB, Skadhauge E. 1995. New aspects of the pathophysiology and treatment of secretory diarrhoea. Physiological Research 44:61–78.

Holm A, Poulsen HD. 1996. Swine nutrition management update: Zinc oxide in treating *E. coli* diarrhea in pigs after weaning. Compend Contin Educ Vet Pract 18:S26–S48.

Imberechts H, Bertschinger HU, Stamm M, Sydler P, Pohl P, De Greve H, Hernalsteens J-P, Van Montagu M, Lintermans P. 1994. Prevalence of F107 fimbriae on *Escherichia coli* isolated from pigs with oedema disease or postweaning diarrhoea. Vet Microbiol 40:219–230.

Imberechts H, Deprez P, Van Driessche E, Pohl P. 1997. Chicken egg yolk antibodies against F18ab fimbriae of *Escherichia coli* inhibit shedding of F18 positive *E. coli* by experimentally infected pigs. Vet Microbiol 54:329–41.

Johansen M, Andresen LO, Jorsal SE, Thomsen LK, Waddell T, Gyles CL. 1996a. Vaccination against oedema disease. Proc Int Congr Pig Vet Soc 14:378.

Johansen M, Baekbo P, Thomsen LK. 1996b. Control of edema disease in Danish pig herds. Proc Int Congr Pig Vet Soc 14:256.

Jorsal SE, Aarestrup FM, Ahrens P, Johansen M, Baekbo P. 1996. Oedema disease in Danish pig herds: Transmission by trade of breeding animals. Proc Int Congr Pig Vet Soc 14:265.

Kausche M, Dean EA, Arp LH, Samuel JE, Moon HW. 1992. An experimental model for subclinical edema disease (*Escherichia coli* enterotoxemia) manifested as vascular necrosis in pigs. Am J Vet Res 53:281–287.

Kelly D, Begbie R, King TP. 1994. Nutritional influences on interactions between bacteria and the small intestinal mucosa. Nutrition Research Reviews 7:233–257.

Kurtz HJ, Bergeland ME, Barnes DM. 1969. Pathologic changes in edema disease of swine. Am J Vet Res 30:791–806.

Lange S, Martinsson K, Lönnroth I, Göransson L. 1993. Plasma level of antisecretory factor (ASF) and its relation to postweaning diarrhoea in piglets. Journal of Veterinary Medicine Series B: Infectious Diseases and Veterinary Public 40:113–118.

Lecce JG, Balsbaugh RK, Clare DA, King MW. 1982. Rotavirus and hemolytic enteropathogenic *Escherichia coli* in weanling diarrhea of pigs. J Clin Microbiol 16:715–723.

MacLeod DL, Gyles CL. 1990. Purification and characterization of an *Escherichia coli* Shiga-like toxin II variant. Infect Immun 58:1232–1239.

——. 1991. Immunization of pigs with a purified Shiga-like toxin II variant toxoid. Vet Microbiol 29:309–318.

MacLeod DL, Gyles CL, Wilcock BP. 1991. Reproduction of edema disease of swine with purified Shiga-like toxin-II variant. Vet Pathol 28:66–73.

Mainil JG, Jacquemin E, Pohl P, Kaeckenbeeck A, Benz I. 2002. DNA sequences coding for the F18 fimbriae and AIDA adhesion are localized on the same plasmid in *Escherichia coli* isolates from piglets. Vet Microbiol 86:303–311.

Marquardt RR, Jin LZ, Kim JW, Fang L, Frohlich AA, Baidoo SK. 1999. Passive protective effect of egg-yolk antibodies against enterotoxigenic *Escherichia coli* K88+ infection in neonatal and early-weaned piglets. FEMS Immunology and Medical Microbiology 23:283–288.

McEwan GTA, Schousboe B, Skadhauge E. 1990. Direct measurement of mucosal surface pH of pig jejunum in vivo. Journal of Veterinary Medicine Series A: Physiology Pathology Clinical Medicine 37:439–444.

Methiyapun S, Pohlenz JFL, Bertschinger HU. 1984. Ultrastructure of the intestinal mucosa in pigs experimentally inoculated with an edema disease–producing strain of *Escherichia coli* (O139:K12:H1). Vet Pathol 21:516–520.

Mynott TL, Luke RKJ, Chandler DS. 1996. Oral administration of protease inhibits enterotoxigenic *Escherichia coli* receptor activity in piglet small intestine. Gut 38:28–32.

Nagy B, Casey TA, Whipp SC, Moon HW. 1992. Susceptibility of porcine intestine to pilus-mediated adhesion by some isolates of piliated enterotoxigenic *Escherichia coli* increases with age. Infect Immun 60:1285–1294.

Nakamine M, Kono Y, Abe S, Hoshino C, Shirai J, Ezaki T. 1998. Dual infection with enterotoxigenic *Escherichia coli* and porcine reproductive and respiratory syndrome virus observed in weaning pigs that died suddenly. J Vet Med Sci 60:555–561.

Nakamura K, Kubo M, Shoya S, Kashiwazaki M, Koizumi S, Onai M. 1982. Swine cerebrospinal angiopathy with demyelination and malacia. Vet Pathol 19:140–149.

Neef NA, McOrist S, Lysons RJ, Bland AP, Miller BG. 1994. Development of large intestinal attaching and effacing lesions in pigs in association with the feeding of a particular diet. Infect Immun 62:4325–4332.

Ngeleka M, Pritchard J, Appleyard G, Middleton DM, Fairbrother JM. 2003. Isolation and association of *E. coli* AIDA-I/STb, rather than EAST1 pathotype with diarrhea in piglets and antibiotic sensitivity of isolates. J Vet Diagn Invest 15:242–252.

Noamani B, Fairbrother JM, Gyles CL. 2003. Virulence genes of O149 enterotoxigenic *Escherichia coli* of postweaning diarrhea in pigs. Vet Microbiol 97:87–101.

Osek J. 2003. Detection of the enteroaggregative *Escherichia coli* heat-stable enterotoxin 1 (EAST1) gene and its relationship with fimbrial and enterotoxin markers in *E. coli* isolates from pigs with diarrhoea. Vet Microbiol 91:65–72.

Owusu-Asiedu A, Baidoo SK, Nyachoti CM, Marquardt RR. 2002. Response of early-weaned pigs to spray-dried porcine or animal plasma-based diets supplemented with egg-yolk antibodies against enterotoxigenic *Escherichia coli*. .J Anim Sci 80: 2895–2903.

Rantzer D, Svendsen J, Weström B. 1996. Effects of strategic feed restriction on pig performance and health during the postweaning period. Acta Agriculturae Scandinavica Section A: Animal Science 46:219–226.

Risley CR, Kornegay ET, Lindenmann MD, Wood CM, Eigel WN. 1992. Effect of feeding organic acids on selected intestinal content measurements of varying times postweaning in pigs. J Anim Sci 70:196–206.

Sarmiento JI, Casey TA, Moon HW. 1988a. Postweaning diarrhea in swine: Experimental model of enterotoxigenic *Escherichia coli* infection. Am J Vet Res 49:1154–1159.

Sarmiento JI, Dean EA, Moon HW. 1988b. Effects of weaning on diarrhea caused by enterotoxigenic *Escherichia coli* in three-week-old pigs. Am J Vet Res 49:2030–2033.

Sarmiento JI, Moon HW. 1988. Postweaning diarrhea in swine: Effects of oxytetracycline on enterotoxigenic *Escherichia coli* infection. Am J Vet Res 49:1160–1163.

Sarrazin E, Bertschinger HU. 1997. Role of fimbriae F18 for actively acquired immunity against porcine enterotoxigenic *Escherichia coli*. Vet Microbiol 54:133–144.

Schulze F. 1977. Quantitative Magen-Darm-Flora-Analysen beim Ferkel vor und nach dem Absetzen unter Berücksichtigung der Pathogenese der Kolienterotoxämie. Archiv Experimentelle Veterinarmedizin 31:299–316.

Sellwood R, Gibbons RA, Jones GW, Rutter JM. 1975. Adhesion of enteropathogenic *Escherichia coli* to pig intestinal brush borders: The existence of two pig phenotypes. Journal of Medical Microbiology 8:405–411.

Smith HW, Halls S. 1968. The production of oedema disease and diarrhoea in weaned pigs by the oral administration of *Escherichia coli*: Factors that influence the course of the experimental disease. Journal of Medical Microbiology 1:45–59.

Sojka WJ. 1965. *Escherichia coli* in Domestic Animals and Poultry. Bucks, England: Commonw Agric Bur, Farnham Royal, pp. 104–156.

Svendsen J, Larsen J, Bille N. 1974. Outbreaks of post weaning *Escherichia coli* diarrhoea in pigs. Nord Vet Med 26:314–322.

Tzipori S, Wachsmuth IK, Chapman C, Birner R, Brittingham J, Jackson C, Hogg J. 1986. The pathogenesis of hemorrhagic colitis caused by *Escherichia coli* O157:H7 in gnotobiotic piglets. Journal of Infectious Diseases 154:712–716.

Van den Broeck W, Coxa E, Goddeeris BM. 1999. Induction of immune responses in pigs following oral administration of purified F4 Fimbriae. Vaccine 17:2020–2029.

Van Dijk AJ, Enthoven PM, Van den Hoven SG, Van Laarhoven MM, Niewold TA, Nabuurs MJ, Beynen AC. 2002. The effect of dietary spray-dried porcine plasma on clinical response in weaned piglets challenged with a pathogenic *Escherichia coli*. Vet Microbiol 84:207–218.

Vögeli P, Bertschinger HU, Stamm M, Stricker C, Hagger C, Fries R, Rapacz J, Stranzinger G. 1996. Genes specifying receptors for F18 fimbriated *Escherichia coli*, causing oedema disease and postweaning diarrhoea in pigs, map to chromosome 6. Animal Genetics 27:321–328.

Waddell TE, Lingwood CA, Gyles CL. 1996. Interaction of verotoxin 2e with pig intestine. Infect Immun 64:1714–1719.

Wathes CM, Miller BG, Bourne FJ. 1989. Cold stress and postweaning diarrhoea in piglets inoculated orally or by aerosol. Anim Prod 49:483–496.

Wieler LH, Franke S, Menge C, Rose M, Bauerfeind R, Karch H, Baljer G. 1995. Investigations on the immunoresponse during edema disease of piglets after weaning by using a recombinant B subunit of Shiga-like toxin IIe. Dtsch Tierärztl Wochenschr 102:40–43.

Wittig W, Klie H, Gallien P, Lehmann S, Timm M, Tschäpe H. 1995. Prevalence of the fimbrial antigens F18 and K88 and of enterotoxins and verotoxins among *Escherichia coli* isolated from weaned pigs. Zbl Bakt 283:95–104.

Zhu C, Harel J, Jacques M, Desautels C, Donnenberg MS, Beaudry M, Fairbrother JM. 1994. Virulence properties and attaching-effacing activity of *Escherichia coli* O45 from swine postweaning diarrhea. Infect Immun 62:4153–4159.

Systemic Infection
J. M. Fairbrother

Escherichia coli may induce systemic infections, such as septicemia, or localized extraintestinal infections, such as meningitis or arthritis, resulting from bacteremia (Fairbrother and Ngeleka 1994; Fairbrother et al. 1989; Morris and Sojka 1985). Septicemia due to *E. coli* may be primary, occurring predominantly in newborn to 4-day-old pigs, or secondary, when associated with diarrhea or other compromising diseases in young pigs.

ETIOLOGY

Only a relatively small number of *E. coli* serogroups have been reported in natural cases of septicemia. Serogroups O6, O8, O9, O11, O15, O17, O18, O20, O45, O60, O78, O83, O93, O101, O112, O115, and O116 have most commonly been identified in isolates associated with septicemia (Morris and Sojka 1985; Nielsen et al. 1975a; Fairbrother et al. 1989). Other gram-negative bacteria such as *Klebsiella* spp. and *Pseudomonas* spp. have been reported to be associated with systemic infections in pigs (Nielsen et al. 1975b). In a 4-year study at the *Escherichia coli* Laboratory from 1989 to 1992, the most commonly observed serogroups in isolates from cases of primary septicemia were O9 (10%) and O20 (18%) (Fairbrother and Ngeleka 1994). Serogroups O1, O18, O60, O78, O101, O141, and O147 were isolated in rela-

tively lower numbers (2–4% each), but 49% of isolates were nontypeable. Not all *E. coli* isolates are able to cause septicemia in colostrum-deprived piglets (Meyer et al. 1971; Murata et al. 1979).

The characteristics of *E. coli* involved in porcine septicemia have not been greatly studied. However, septicemia-inducing strains may express virulence determinants, which include fimbriae, polysaccharide capsule and O-antigen capsule, lipopolysaccharide (LPS), the aerobactin system, hemolysin, and other cytotoxins (Table 38.5). Fimbrial adhesins associated with *E. coli* isolates from piglets with septicemia include the $F165_1$, $F165_2$ (Contrepois et al. 1989; Fairbrother et al. 1986), and other fimbriae of the P, S, and F1C fimbrial families (Dozois et al. 1997).

ETEC may be associated with secondary septicemia, particularly in older piglets. These isolates most frequently belong to the virotypes listed in Table 38.3.

The virulence determinants most frequently associated with isolates from primary septicemia in pigs or isolates inducing septicemia in newborn colostrum-deprived pigs are $F165_1$, $F165_2$, or other fimbriae of the P, S, and F1C fimbrial families, production of colicin V, production of the siderophore aerobactin, and resistance to the bactericidal effects of serum (Fairbrother and Ngeleka 1994). Isolates from cases of primary septicemia

Table 38.5. Important pathotypes, virulence factors, and O serogroups of *E. coli* causing extraintestinal disease in pigs

Disease	Pathotype	Virulence Factors	O Serogroups
Septicemia	SEPEC	Aerobactin, F165-1 (P fimbrial family), F165-2 (S fimbrial family), CNF1 or CNF2, CDT	6,8,9,11,15, 17,18,20,45, 60,78,83,93, 101,112,115, 116
Urogenital tract infection	UPEC	P, S, aerobactin, CNF1	1,4,6,18

Source: The *Escherichia coli* Laboratory, Université de Montréal.

may occasionally produce cytotoxic necrotizing factor (CNF1).

EPIDEMIOLOGY

Primary septicemia is most often seen as sporadic cases and rarely in the form of a small outbreak (Nielsen et al. 1975a). The disease may occur throughout the suckling period, with exceptional cases in pigs up to 80 days old. Epidemiology of the secondary systemic infection is determined by the underlying disease.

PATHOGENESIS

Primary neonatal septicemia occurs in piglets lacking immunity, due either to an absence of ingested colostrum or to ingestion of colostrum lacking specific antibody. The disease may develop after bacterial invasion of the respiratory or the gastrointestinal tract in the nonimmune host. Contamination of the umbilicus after birth may also lead to colisepticemia. However, the intestine is considered as a major route of *E. coli* invasion since the disease can be experimentally induced by oral or intragastric administration of the organisms (Ngeleka et al. 1993).

Secondary septicemia may develop after invasion of the host by ETEC, but in most cases development of primary neonatal septicemia is associated with intestinal permeability to macromolecules, to some defect of the immune system (e.g., low levels of maternal colostrum), to low birth weight, and to sublethal malformations (Gyles and Fairbrother 2004; Murata et al. 1979).

Bacteria may pass through the mucosa of the alimentary tract, probably by endocytic uptake into intestinal epithelial cells or through the intercellular spaces formed by lateral plasma membranes of adjacent epithelial cells, to locate in the mesenteric lymph nodes before entering the bloodstream. This bacterial invasion may result in a generalized infection (septicemia, polyserositis) with bacteria disseminated in different extraintestinal organs such as lung, liver, spleen, kidney, brain, and heart blood, or in a localized infection (meningitis or arthritis) (Morris and Sojka 1985). In the sow, a puerperal sepsis may be induced by an enteric *E. coli* soon after farrowing (Sojka 1965).

Septicemia may be produced experimentally in colostrum-deprived piglets by intragastric inoculation with isolates of porcine origin (Fairbrother and Ngeleka 1994; Ngeleka et al. 1993). However, the disease can also be reproduced in piglets with isolates from other sources, such as calves, cats, and poultry (Fairbrother et al. 1993; Murata et al. 1979; Meyer et al. 1971). Animals may develop fever, anorexia, diarrhea, dyspnea, or nervous signs, due in part to the effect of bacterial endotoxin or cytotoxins or to the effects of inflammatory cytokines induced by these bacterial products (Nakajima et al. 1991; Jesmok et al. 1992).

The role of some of the virulence determinants associated with *E. coli*–inducing septicemia is only partially understood. LPS, K capsule and O-antigen capsule, and production of siderophores such as aerobactin are thought to allow the bacteria to invade the host and escape its defense mechanisms. These determinants increase bacterial resistance to the bactericidal effect of complement and to phagocytosis and allow bacterial growth in body fluids with low concentrations of free iron (Crosa 1989; Ngeleka et al. 1992, 1993).

Fimbriae appear to be important for the survival and spread of bacteria within the host and subsequent bacterial pathogenicity, in part by promoting bacterial resistance to the bactericidal effects of phagocytosis (Ngeleka et al. 1992, 1993, 1994). One mechanism for this resistance appears to be an inhibition of the oxidative response (Ngeleka and Fairbrother 1999).

CLINICAL SIGNS

Clinical signs of infection include depression, lameness, reluctance to move, anorexia, rough hair coat, and labored respiration (Nielsen et al. 1975a). The affected piglets may show sternal recumbency and the abdomen may be somewhat distended. Sometimes piglets become unconscious, with convulsions and paddling movements; they may be in good bodily condition but cyanosis of the extremities may be observed. Some piglets are found dead whereas others are comatose without any sign of diarrhea. These clinical signs may develop within 12 hours after birth and piglets can die within 48 hours (Taylor 1989). In older piglets, the clinical signs may include periodic scouring or other ailments that precede the onset of acute septicemia with clinical signs resembling those in the newborn pigs.

LESIONS

In acute primary septicemia, there may be no gross lesions other than congestion of the intestine, the mesenteric lymph nodes, and the extraintestinal organs. In subacute cases, subserous or submucosal hemorrhages and fibrinous polyserositis with gross signs of pneumonia are usually observed, often accompanied by fibrinopurulent arthritis and meningitis (Morris and Sojka 1985; Waxler and Britt 1972). Histological examination of the lung reveals interalveolar interstitial pneumonia with edema and neutrophilic infiltration, but alveoli are free of exudates. In secondary septicemia resulting from enteric colibacillosis, icterus, petechial hemorrhages in the serosal membranes, and splenomegaly accompanied by severe diarrhea and dehydration can be observed in some cases (Svendsen et al. 1975). In many cases of secondary systemic *E. coli* infection, presumably occurring at a very late stage in the underlying disease, the changes are slight or no lesions at all are recorded.

DIAGNOSIS

Systemic colibacillosis is generally suspected with the appearance of the clinical signs described above. However, in the case of polyserositis, a differential diagnosis between *Mycoplasma hyorhinis* and *Haemophilus parasuis* has to be made. In the former infection, gross lesions can be detected more than 6 days after infection. Mortality is lower than in *E. coli* infection. In polyserositis due to *E. coli*, the exudates encountered in piglets are serofibrinous or fibrinopurulent, whereas in *H. parasuis* infections they tend to be serofibrinous. In the central nervous system and joints, these exudates are fibrinopurulent to purulent (Waxler and Britt 1972). Infection due to *H. parasuis* is rarely seen in the early suckling period but is more common in piglets of 2–3 months of age. However, differential diagnosis can be established after a careful microbiological examination. In most of the cases, postmortem examination and bacteriology are useful for identifying the infection. Diagnosis of primary systemic colibacillosis is strengthened by the isolation in pure culture or by the predominance of *E. coli* in extraintestinal tissues, particularly *E. coli* of one of the above-mentioned serogroups or, more important, possessing one or more of the virulence factors, such as adhesins of the P or S families, serum resistance, or production of aerobactin (Table 38.5). The genes for these virulence factors may be detected by hybridization probes and the multiplex polymerase chain reaction (PCR), as described in the section on neonatal diarrhea. Diagnosis of secondary systemic colibacillosis is strengthened by the isolation in pure culture or by the predominance in extraintestinal tissues of *E. coli* possessing the genes for one or more of the enterotoxins LT, STa, or STb and possibly one of the fimbrial adhesins associated with ETEC, particularly F4.

PREVENTION AND TREATMENT

Inadequate hygiene and poor environmental temperature control increase the likelihood of infection. Thus, prevention of infection should focus on reduction or elimination of significant pathogenic *E. coli* populations in the environment of the piglets and in providing a plentiful supply of colostrum at birth. Hygiene, especially washing and disinfection of the farrowing pens, will efficiently contribute to reduction of the infection. Young piglets should be maintained at an even temperature of 35°C for the first week of life. They must be kept dry and warm in clean surroundings. Affected piglets should be treated if necessary, and other litters of susceptible age watched. However, in the case of small outbreaks, careful monitoring of the causative serogroup(s) and autovaccination of the pregnant sows might be beneficial.

Treatment may be attempted after diagnostic confirmation of *E. coli* infection and antibiotic sensitivity testing. Meanwhile, parenteral or oral administration of broad-spectrum antimicrobials to affected piglets is recommended while waiting for results of diagnostic tests. This treatment may be useful in subacute cases of infection but is mostly ineffective after the appearance of clinical signs. However, the remaining piglets in the litter and affected piglets and littermates in adjacent litters should be treated.

REFERENCES

Contrepois M, Fairbrother JM, Kaura YK, Girardeau JP. 1989. Prevalence of CS31A and F165 surface antigens in *Escherichia coli* isolates from animals in France, Canada, and India. FEMS Microbiology Letters 59:319–324.

Crosa JH. 1989. Genetics and molecular biology of siderophore-mediated iron transport in bacteria. Microbiological Reviews 53:517–530.

Dozois CM, Clement S, Desautels C, Fairbrother JM. 1997. Expression of P, S, and F1C adhesins by cytotoxic necrotizing factor I (CNF1)–producing *Escherichia coli* from septicaemic and diarrheic pigs. FEMS Microbiology Letters 152:307–312.

Fairbrother JM, Broes A, Jacques M, Larivière S. 1989. Pathogenicity of *Escherichia coli* O115:K"V165" strains isolated from pigs with diarrhea. Am J Vet Res 50:1029–1036.

Fairbrother JM, Harel J, Forget C, Desautels C, Moore J. 1993. Receptor binding specificity and pathogenicity of *Escherichia coli* F165-positive strains isolated from piglets and calves and possessing pap related sequences. Can J Vet Res 57:53–55.

Fairbrother JM, Larivière S, Lallier R. 1986. New fimbrial antigen F165 on *Escherichia coli* serogroup O115 strains isolated from piglets with diarrhea. Infect Immun 51:10–15.

Fairbrother JM, Ngeleka M. 1994. Extraintestinal *Escherichia coli* infections in pigs. In *Escherichia coli* in Domestic Animals and Humans. CL Gyles, ed. Wallingford, U.K.: CAB International, pp. 221–236.

Gyles CL, Fairbrother JM. 2004. *Escherichia coli*. In Pathogenesis of Bacterial Infections in Animals (3rd edition). CL Gyles, JF Prescott, JG Songer, CO Thoen, eds. Ames, Iowa: Blackwell Publishing, p.193–223.

Jesmok G, Lindsey C, Duerr M, Fournel M, Emerson TJr. 1992. Efficacy of monoclonal antibody against human recombinant tumor necrosis factor in *E. coli*–challenged swine. American Journal of Pathology 141:1197–1207.

Meyer RC, Saxena SP, Rhoades HE. 1971. Polyserositis induced by *Escherichia coli* in gnotobiotic swine. Infect Immun 3:41–44.

Morris JA, Sojka WJ. 1985. *Escherichia coli* as a pathogen in animals. In The Virulence of *Escherichia coli*: Reviews and Methods. M Sussman, ed. London: Academic Press, pp. 47–77.

Murata H, Yaguchi H, Namioka S. 1979. Relationship between the intestinal permeability to macromolecules and invasion of septicemia-inducing *Escherichia coli* in neonatal piglets. Infect Immun 26:339–347.

Nakajima Y, Ishikawa Y, Momotani E, Takahashi K, Madarame H, Ito A, Ueda H, Wada M, Takahashi H. 1991. A comparison of central nervous lesions directly induced by *Escherichia coli* lipopolysaccharide in piglets, calves, rabbits and mice. Journal of Comparative Pathology 104:57–64.

Ngeleka M, Fairbrother JM. 1999. F1651 fimbriae of the P fimbrial family inhibit the oxidative response of porcine neutrophils. FEMS Immunology and Medical Microbiology 25:265–274.

Ngeleka M, Harel J, Jacques M, Fairbrother JM. 1992. Characterization of a nonacidic polysaccharide capsular antigen of septicemic *Escherichia coli* O115:K"V165":F165 and evaluation of its role in pathogenicity. Infect Immun 60:5048–5056.

Ngeleka M, Jacques M, Martineau-Doizé B, Harel J, Fairbrother JM. 1993. Pathogenicity of an *Escherichia coli* O115:K"V165" mutant negative for $F165_1$ fimbriae in septicemia of gnotobiotic pigs. Infect Immun 61:836–843.

Ngeleka M, Martineau-Doizé B, Fairbrother JM. 1994. Septicemia-inducing *Escherichia coli* O115:K"V165" resist killing by porcine polymorphonuclear leukocytes in vitro: Role of F165$_1$ fimbriae and K "V165" O-antigen capsule. Infect Immun 62:398–404.

Nielsen NC, Bille N, Riising HJ, Dam A. 1975a. Polyserositis in pigs due to generalized *Escherichia coli* infection. Canadian Journal of Comparative Medicine 39:421–426.

Nielsen NC, Riising HJ, Larsen JL, Bille N, Svendsen J. 1975b. Preweaning mortality in pigs: Acute septicaemias. Nord Vet Med 27:129–139.

Sojka WJ. 1965. *Escherichia coli* in Domestic Animals and Poultry. Commonw Agric Bur, Farnham Royal, Bucks, England.

Svendsen J, Bille N, Nielsen NC, Larsen JL, Riising H-J. 1975. Preweaning mortality in pigs. 4. Diseases of the gastrointestinal tract in pigs. Nord Vet Med 27:85–101.

Taylor DJ. 1989. Bacterial Diseases. In Pig Diseases (5th ed.). Cambridge: Book Production Consultants, pp. 171–172.

Waxler GL, Britt AL. 1972. Polyserositis and arthritis due to *Escherichia coli* in gnotobiotic pigs. Canadian Journal of Comparative Medicine 36:226–233.

Coliform Mastitis

J. M. Fairbrother

The term "coliform mastitis" (CM) is used to refer to puerperal mastitis in the pig, underlining the parallel of this disease with CM in the cow (Bertschinger 1999). Other terms used to denominate CM and related conditions are discussed in Chapter 4 of this book. In one study, it was found that 59 of 72 agalactic sows (82%) had gross lesions of mastitis (Ross et al. 1981).

CM has a worldwide distribution. Hermansson et al. (1978) reported an average incidence of postpartum agalactia of 12.8%, individual herds varying from 0.5–50%. In a Danish study, on farms with a high management level, an incidence of 9.5% of mastitis-metritis-agalactia (MMA) among 72,000 farrowings was observed (Jorsal 1986). In these studies, the precise incidence of CM was not determined. In another study, *E. coli* or *Klebsiella pneumoniae* was isolated from 79% of the 131 mammary complexes with mastitis examined in herds with an MMA problem (Wegmann et al. (1986).

Economic loss due to CM is difficult to estimate, being multifactorial. In the affected sows, mortality is low, and it is difficult to assess the cost of extra care and of treatment. On the other hand, the mortality in piglets nursing multiparous sows with MMA has been reported to be as high as 55.8%, compared to 17.2% in piglets nursing healthy sows (Bäckström et al. 1984) and 21% compared to 17% in another study (Madec et al. 1992). Mortality of piglets may result from lengthened farrowing time, crushing by the sow, starvation, and impaired immunity to infectious agents because of insufficient uptake of colostral immunoglobulins. The average milk yield of three sows affected with CM on the first 2 days after farrowing was about half the yield of healthy sows, and the piglets of the sick sows lost some weight (Ross et al. 1975). Piglets sucking glands with mastitis of sows with subclinical CM had smaller weight gains only for days 1–4 postpartum (Bertschinger et al. 1990).

ETIOLOGY

The term "coliform," when used in the context of mastitis, refers to the bacterial genera *Escherichia*, *Klebsiella*, *Enterobacter*, and *Citrobacter*. However, the methods used for identification in several studies were not adequate to determine the genera and even less the species of the bacterial isolates. *E. coli* was the organism most often identified in either milk samples or affected mammary tissue (Ringarp 1960; Armstrong et al. 1968; Bertschinger et al. 1977a; Ross et al. 1981; Wegmann et al. 1986). No one serotype has been associated with *E. coli* isolated from the milk of sows with CM (Morner et al. 1998). The virulence factors of *E.coli* from CM are not well known, although serum resistance and ability to bind to fibronectin have been associated with these isolates. Nevertheless, *E. coli* isolates from sows with mastitis are very heterogeneous, as shown by random amplified polymorphic DNA genotyping (Ramasoota et al 2000). *Klebsiella*, mostly *K. pneumoniae*, was prevalent in the cases investigated by Ross et al. (1975) and Jones (1976). *Staphylococcus epidermidis* and a variety of streptococci have also been found in the mammary glands of sows with signs of mastitis, either mixed with coliforms or as pure cultures. Nevertheless, noncoliform organisms were rarely associated with microscopic lesions of mastitis (Bertschinger et al. 1977a; Ross et al. 1981).

EPIDEMIOLOGY

CM of the sow appears to be noncontagious. Multiple serological types of isolate from cases of mastitis may be found within a herd and even within distinct glands of one sow. A significant proportion of subcomplexes harbor more than one type (Bertschinger et al. 1977a; Awad-Masalmeh et al. 1990). The great variety of coliform bacteria associated with CM indicates an abundant reservoir of potentially pathogenic bacteria. The coliforms causing mastitis may originate from the flora of the sow as well as from the environment. In about one-third of the sows with mastitis, identical isolates were found in mastitic glands, the uterine contents, and the urinary bladder (Bertschinger et al. 1977a). The intestinal flora of the sow, the oral flora of the neonatal piglet, and environmental bacteria may significantly contribute to contamination of the nipples. Awad-Masalmeh et al. (1990) found identical O serogroups of *E. coli* in mammary secretion and in feces of about one-fourth of 67 sows with CM. Muirhead (1976) considered the bedding of the sow of paramount importance. Dung and urine contaminate the udder. *Klebsiella* spp. may also originate from wood shavings used for bedding. Bertschinger et al. (1990) compared 12 farrowings each in conventional farrowing crates and in an experimental pen where the sows could lie down in a clean resting area. Sows in the experimental pen had much lower counts of coliform bacteria on their teat ends and an incidence of intramammary *E. coli* infections 10 times lower than that of the sows in the crates.

PATHOGENESIS

Invasion of the Mammary Gland

Mastitis was reproduced in the sow by intramammary instillation of not more than 120 organisms of a strain of *K. pneumoniae*. Following massive external contamination of the nipples with the same strain, the bacteria were recovered from 60 out of 142 subcomplexes examined. External contamination of the nipples was as successful on gestation day 111 as 2 hours after completion of farrowing (Bertschinger et al. 1977b). It is largely unknown at what time spontaneous invasion of the cistern takes place. McDonald and McDonald (1975) found significant numbers of coliform bacteria in about one-fourth of mammary glands cultured immediately prior to parturition. In a sequential examination of the mammary secretions, *E. coli* was isolated from 30 glands. In 17 of these glands, the bacteria were detected before the first piglet was born (Bertschinger et al. 1990). New infections appeared not later than day 2 postpartum.

The bacteria are located in the ductular and alveolar lumina, either free or within phagocytic cells. Little adhesion to surfaces is observed. At postmortem examination the causative bacteria are frequently isolated from regional lymph nodes, whereas isolations from the liver, spleen, or kidney are rare (Armstrong et al. 1968; Bertschinger et al. 1977a, b; Ross et al. 1981).

Multiplication of bacteria in the mammary secretion is controlled by antimicrobial mechanisms. The antimicrobial activity of cow's milk is due to a variety of inhibitors acting in concert and conferring on the dry udder a nearly total resistance to coliform proliferation (Bramley 1976). A lower opsonic activity observed in mammary secretions of sows at parturition (Osterlundh et al. 1998), as well as a lower phagocytic capacity of polymorphonuclear (PMN) cells in colostrum as compared to in milk (Osterlundh et al. 2001) may explain the increased susceptibility to the development of CM at parturition. CM is a self-curing disease. The bacteria generally disappear between 1 and 6 days after parturition (Wegmann and Bertschinger 1984; Bertschinger et al. 1990). In severe cases, however, they persist in necrotic foci throughout lactation (Löpfe 1993).

Mammary Inflammation

CM in the sow is associated with massive accumulation of neutrophils in the lumina of affected glands. Simultaneous induction of CM in several mammary subcomplexes of sows from which the piglets had been removed resulted in severe leukopenia within 24 hours (Bertschinger et al. 1977b). Intracisternal instillation of identical bacterial inocula following a highly standardized protocol led to a spectrum of reactions ranging from very severe local and general signs to subclinical mastitis (Löpfe 1993; Mossi 1995). Severe reaction is the consequence of massive and persistent multiplication of inoculated bacteria. In the experiments of Löfstedt et al. (1983) susceptibility to experimental infection was associated with impaired function of circulating neutrophils. The cause of the impaired neutrophil function is still a mystery. Magnusson et al. (2001) showed that sows were more susceptible to experimental infection immediately prior to parturition than at 4 days before parturition, the number of neutrophils in the blood being greater in the former. This suggests a role for the number of circulating neutrophils at the time of infection in the development of clinical CM in the sow. Nevertheless, Osterlundh et al. (2002) have shown in experimental inoculation studies that impaired chemotactic or phagoctyic capacity of blood granulocytes does not appear to be involved in susceptibility of sows to develop clinical CM at parturition. Cytological findings in the secretion must be interpreted with caution. Mammary glands not chosen by a piglet undergo involution soon after parturition. Involution is accompanied by an increase in the total somatic cell count as well as in the proportion of PMN cells (Wegmann and Bertschinger 1984). In some sows many glands show increases of total somatic and of PMN cells in the absence of cultivable bacteria (Bertschinger et al. 1990).

Systemic Reaction

The systemic signs of CM are brought about by the bacterial endotoxin. An outline of the systemic changes is given in Chapter 4. CM in the absence of systemic reaction is often revealed by methodical examination of mammary secretion (Wegmann 1985; Bertschinger et al. 1990; Persson et al. 1996b).

Immunity

CM apparently does not result in protection against homologous reinfection (Bertschinger and Bühlmann 1990). Ringarp (1960) reported a higher incidence in sows than in gilts, as well as repeated occurrence, up to 10 times, in individual sows.

CLINICAL SIGNS

Ross et al. (1975) described the clinical findings in sows with proven CM and demonstrated changes quite similar to those described earlier in sows with lactational failure. Interpretation of clinical parameters is rendered difficult by the presence of subclinical CM in apparently healthy sows (Nachreiner and Ginther 1972; Middleton-Williams et al. 1977; Persson et al. 1996b).

The initial signs are most often detected on the first or second day and more rarely on the third day after farrowing. However, they may be observed as early as during parturition (Martin et al. 1967). The first symptoms are body temperature response, listlessness, weakness, and loss of interest in the piglets. Affected sows prefer sternal recumbency. In severe cases they become stiff, do not stand up, and may even become comatose. Consumption of feed and water is either reduced or absent. Body temperature is moderately elevated and only rarely exceeds 42° C. Afebrile cases have been reported; although the temperature was not taken continuously and temperature peaks may have been missed. On the other hand, many normal sows will have rectal temperatures that exceed the 39.7°C limit on the day of parturition and for 2 days thereafter (King et al. 1972). In affected sows, respiratory and heart rates are increased. In general, symptoms do not last for more than 2–3 days.

The behavior of the piglets is very helpful in the early detection of lactational failure. Undernourished piglets look gaunt. They frequently try to suck, move from nipple to nipple, nibble at litter, and lick urine from the floor. If access to the nipples is given by the sow, the periods of suckling are shortened. After suckling, the piglets wander instead of resting in close contact with their littermates.

Precise localization of mammary lesions is often not possible because reddening and heat of the skin extend over several subcomplexes. The reliable clinical assessment of the state of the actual mammary tissue is rendered difficult by subcutaneous fat and considerable subcutaneous edema. If palpable, the mastitic tissue is firmer and palpation may cause pain. The red color of the skin is blanched by finger pressure, which causes a depression of the tissue lasting for some time. Mere clinical examination will at best detect some of the affected subcomplexes (Persson et al. 1996b). The inguinal lymph nodes may be swollen.

The fluid expressed from a nipple originates from more than one subcomplex, because two or, rarely, three teat canals end in each nipple. Therefore, in samples taken from a nipple, secretion from the unaffected, productive subcomplex dominates. The exudate from inflamed subcomplexes looks serous to creamy, like pus. It may contain clots of fibrin or blood. The pH is of limited diagnostic value (Ross et al. 1981; Persson et al. 1996b), but cytological examination allows differentiation between healthy and mastitic complexes at least during the first 48 hours after parturition (Wegmann and Bertschinger 1984). Because mastitis is a local process, samples must be taken from individual complexes and not pooled. The threshold value of the total cell count varies depending on the investigator. Bertschinger et al. (1990)

suggested 5×10^6 cells per mL and fewer than 70% PMN. In a recent study, Persson et al. (1996a) proposed 10×10^6 cells per mL. However, these authors did not distinguish between sucked and unsucked glands. Involution of some glands starts as early as 1 day after parturition (Wegmann and Bertschinger 1984). It leads to a significant increase of the total cell count accompanied by a transient increase of up to 60% of the proportion of PMN cells. As a consequence, cytological distinction between involution and mastitis may be difficult or impossible between 2 and 7 days postpartum (Wegmann 1985). Bacteriological examination of the secretion may be necessary in unclear cases. Infection persisting for several days is limited to severely affected complexes (Löpfe 1993).

LESIONS

Despite the high incidence of CM, there are not many reports of necropsy findings (Martin et al. 1967; Jones 1976; Middleton-Williams et al. 1977; Ross et al. 1981). In general, lesions are confined to the mammary glands and regional lymph nodes. The subcutaneous tissue may be edematous over affected parts of the udder. For reliable demonstration of mastitis, Middleton-Williams et al. (1977) recommended a longitudinal section at the level of the nipples through each row of glands. Using this technique, irregularly scattered foci of mastitis were detected in 1–23 subcomplexes (Figure 38.9). The appearance of affected mammary tissue varied from slightly increased firmness and grayish discoloration to sharply demarcated, red-mottled, hard, and dry areas

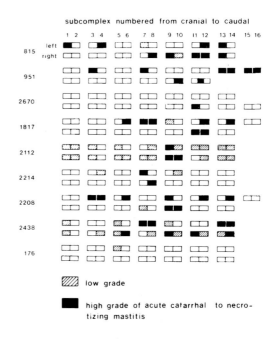

38.9. *Distribution and intensity of histologic lesions on nine field cases of CM (modified from Middleton-Williams et al. 1977).*

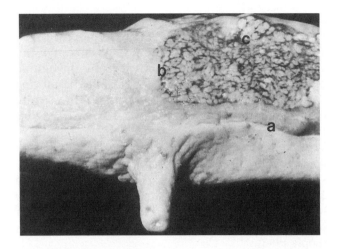

38.10. *Acute CM of one subcomplex adjacent to unaltered glandular tissue in longitudinal cut surface: (a) subcutaneous edema, (b) demarcation from adjacent subcomplex, (c) mottled appearance of affected tissue.*

(Figure 38.10). The secretion was sparse and sometimes mixed with clots.

Histological examination permitted the detection of additional lesions that had not been recognized at gross examination. In every case there was an acute purulent exudative mastitis with congestion. An extreme variability in severity ranging from a small number of neu-trophils in the alveolar lumina to severe purulent infiltration with necrosis was obvious (Figure 38.11). The severity of the lesions varied not only between but also within subcomplexes, where unaffected tissue was found adjacent to severely inflamed areas. Acute purulent lymphadenitis was present in the inguinal and iliac lymph nodes (Middleton-Williams et al. 1977). A sequential study of the microscopic lesions following experimental intracisternal inoculation revealed in severe cases the persistence throughout lactation of abscesslike large necrotic foci surrounded by granulomatous connective tissue (Löpfe 1993). A predilection of microscopic lesions for certain areas within a given complex was not evident. The mucosa lining the cisternae was not affected.

DIAGNOSIS

Any hypogalactia at the beginning of lactation arouses suspicion of CM. The diagnosis may be supported by fever, anorexia, reluctance to stand up, lying on the gland, and disinterest in the piglets. In severe cases some affected glands may be reddened, swollen, and firm, and the secretion may look abnormal. A reliable rapid test for use on the farm is not available. Due to the higher cell content of sow milk, tests developed for use with the cow cannot be recommended. Bacteriological and cytologi-

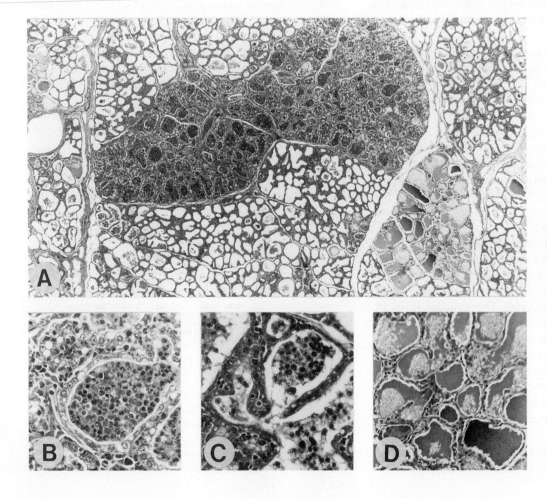

38.11. *Histopathology of a mammary gland 24 hours after experimental inoculation with a culture of Klebsiella pneumoniae. (A) Low-power magnification within a single subcomplex showing different types of mastitis next to secreting alveoli. (B) Dark area filled with densely packed polymorphonuclear leukocytes and local destruction of epithelium. (C) Nearly empty-looking alveoli containing low numbers of polymorphonuclear leukocytes. (D) Alveoli with normal-looking secretion. (Institute of Veterinary Pathology, University of Zurich.)*

cal examinations of the secretion are valuable only if all glands are sampled or if affected glands are known. The differential diagnosis of CM is reviewed in Chapter 4.

TREATMENT

Therapeutic measures are usually not taken before the sow shows signs of dysgalactia. Thus, treatment may at best shorten the period of underfeeding of the piglets.

Chemotherapy is complicated by the heterogeneous pattern of antimicrobial susceptibility of individual isolates, not only within a herd but also within a sow. Therefore, sensitivity testing is of little value in individual cases.

The pharmacokinetics of antimicrobials has received only limited attention. One injection of 20 mg/kg body weight of a slow-release formulation of oxytetracycline results in milk levels not surpassing 2 µg/mL, that is, just above the minimum inhibitory concentration (MIC) of susceptible *E. coli* (Schoneweis et al. 1982). Enrofloxacin, a quinolone antibiotic, given at 2.5 mg/kg body weight orally twice daily, is concentrated in colostrum and milk to mean levels of 1.2 µg/mL, which is 20 times higher than the MIC (Oliel and Bertschinger 1990). Awad-Masalmeh et al. (1990) tested 107 strains of *E. coli* isolated from sows with CM from 43 herds and found no resistance to enrofloxacin (Table 38.6). Therapeutic trials are generally difficult to evaluate because the curative effect is not quantified and is often difficult to distinguish from spontaneous improvement. Options for supportive therapy are discussed in Chapter 4.

Much attention should be given to the piglets. They may either be fostered by other sows or remain with their mother and receive a milk substitute. Sweetened condensed milk diluted with water 1:1 can be used instead of commercial products. A sterile 5% glucose solution at a dose of approximately 15 mL can be repeatedly injected intraperitoneally every several hours, or a more concen-

trated solution may be administered intragastrically. When the pig obtains insufficient amounts of milk, protection against chilling is particularly important.

PREVENTION

Hygiene Measures

Muirhead (1976) and Jones (1979) suggested that protection of the teats from bacterial contamination might be an effective prophylaxis of CM. Bertschinger et al. (1990) performed a prospective study of farrowing in two types of pens. They concluded that the density of the coliform flora on the teat apex reflects the degree of contamination of the lying area. Optimal prophylaxis is achieved by designing farrowing accommodation in such a manner that the sow is prevented from lying down in her own excreta. On the other hand, washing and disinfection of the pen and of the newly housed sow contribute much less to efficient prophylaxis. If cases of CM accumulate, the bedding materials should be checked.

Nutrition of the Sow

Drastic reduction of the sow's ration shortly before parturition is a widespread practice. In a carefully designed long-term study using pairs of full siblings, the reduction of the daily feed allowance from 3.2 to 1.0 kg of a commercial-type feed lowered the incidence of agalactia from 26.6% to 14.4% (Persson et al. 1989). Udder changes were observed in a high percentage of the agalactic sows, and significant numbers of bacteria were found in more than 80% of the agalactic sows. The two feed regimens did not influence the total cell count, the PMN levels, or the pH of the secretion (Persson et al. 1996b). Plonait et al. (1986) reported a corresponding observation. Experimentally induced CM takes a similar course with sows on high and low rations (H. U. Bertschinger and A. Bühlmann, unpublished data). This finding led to the suggestion that feed reduction might act through reduced exposure of the teats to microbial infection due to the much smaller amounts of feces and urine contaminating the lying area.

Immunoprophylaxis

Vaccination is not a promising method for control of mastitis. Induction of specific immunity is hampered by the wide range of antigenic types of coliforms isolated from sows with CM. Use of an *E. coli* bacterin induced poor protection in sows against intramammary challenge with the same strain used to prepare the bacterin (R. Ross, Ames, Iowa, unpublished data, 1982).

In the cow, there is considerable evidence that vaccination with an R-mutant of *E. coli* results in a dramatically reduced incidence of CM (Tyler et al. 1993). Vaccination has little impact on the frequency of new infections but decreases the incidence of overt disease. No reports have appeared to date on the efficacy of such vaccines in the sow.

Table 38.6. Sensitivity to antimicrobial agents of coliform isolates from mammary glands in Switzerland and Austria

Antimicrobial agent	% Sensitive Isolates		
	Switzerland		Austria
	$n = 80$[1]	$n = 107$[2]	$n = 107$[3]
Ampicillin	90	86	74
Tetracycline	19	42	16
Chloramphenicol	95	81	64
Streptomycin	21	21	21
Neomycin	96	92	86
Gentamicin	100	100	100
Trimethoprim-sulfamethoxazole	100	84	51
Enrofloxacin	NT[4]	NT	100

[1]Bertschinger et al. 1977a.
[2]Wegmann et al. 1986.
[3]Awad-Masalmeh et al. 1990.
[4]Not tested.

Hormones

Some investigators found an extended period of gestation in sows developing lactational failure. The length of gestation can be controlled by use of prostaglandins. However, the prophylactic application led to conflicting results. Studies focusing on CM are not known.

Chemoprophylaxis

At present, chemoprophylaxis appears to be the most promising method of control where accommodation cannot be improved. The prevalence of drug resistance (Table 38.6) and the wide variety of bacteria associated with the disease in a given herd must be considered when the drug is selected. Feed medication should be replaced by individual application of the drug in a small amount of feed because the feed consumption of the sow in the periparturient period is quite variable. Minimizing the period of treatment helps postpone the emergence of drug resistance. In field trials, the morbidity from MMA was reduced from 30% to 12% by giving 0.4 g trimethoprim, 1 g sulfadimidine, and 1 g sulfathiazole/150 kg body weight twice a day. The treatment began on gestation day 112 and lasted for 4 days regardless of the day of farrowing (Bollwahn 1978). Six intramuscular injections of apramycin (6.25 mg/kg) at 12-hour intervals reduced the severity of experimentally induced mastitis (Ross and Zimmermann 1982).

Oliel and Bertschinger (1990) evaluated the effect of oral chemoprophylaxis with enrofloxacin on experimentally induced CM. Three glands of each sow were inoculated with *E. coli* and three glands with *K. pneumoniae*. Eight sows were not treated (treatment I), eight sows received 2.5 mg (treatment II), and eight sows received 5.0 mg/kg body weight twice a day (treatment III). The inoculated bacteria were reisolated in treatment I from 100%, in treatment II from 10%, and in treatment III from 2% of the inoculated glands. A beneficial effect on milk productivity would be expected but could not be demonstrated because the control sows did not develop systemic signs.

REFERENCES

Armstrong CH, Hooper BE, Martin CE. 1968. Microflora associated with agalactia syndrome of sows. Am J Vet Res 29:1401–1407.

Awad-Masalmeh M, Baumgartner W, Passernig A, Silber R, Hinterdorfer F. 1990. Bakteriologische Untersuchungen bei an puerperaler Mastitis (MMA-Syndrom) erkrankten Sauen verschiedener Tierbestände Österreichs. Tierärztl Umschau 45:526–535.

Bäckström L, Morkoc AC, Connor J, Larson R, Price W. 1984. Clinical study of mastitis-metritis-agalactia in sows in Illinois. J Am Vet Med Assoc 185:70–73.

Bertschinger HU. 1999. *Escherichia coli* Infections: Coliform Mastitis. In Diseases of Swine (8th edition). BE Straw, S D'Allaire, WL Mengeling, DJ Taylor, eds. Ames: Iowa State University Press, pp. 457–464.

Bertschinger HU, Bühlmann A. 1990. Absence of protective immunity in mammary glands after experimentally induced coliform mastitis. Proc Int Congr Pig Vet Soc 11:175.

Bertschinger HU, Pohlenz J, Hemlep I. 1977a. Untersuchungen über das Mastitis-Metritis-Agalaktie-Syndrom (Milchfieber) der Sau. II. Bakteriologische Befunde bei Spontanfaellen. Schweiz Arch Tierheilkd 119:223–233.

Bertschinger HU, Pohlenz J, Middleton-Williams DM. 1977b. Untersuchungen über das Mastitis-Metritis-Agalaktie-Syndrom (Milchfieber) der Sau. III. Galaktogene Erzeugung von Klebsiellen-Mastitis. Schweiz Arch Tierheilkd 119:265–275.

Bertschinger HU, Bürgi E, Eng V, Wegmann P. 1990. Senkung der Inzidenz von puerperaler Mastitis bei der Sau durch Schutz des Gesäuges vor Verschmutzung. Schweiz Arch Tierheilkd 132:557–566.

Bollwahn W. 1978. Effect of strategic TMP/S treatment on puerperium and conception in sows. Proc Int Congr Pig Vet Soc 5:KA16.

Bramley AJ. 1976. Variations in the susceptibility of lactating and non-lactating bovine udders to infection when infused with *Escherichia coli*. Journal of Dairy Research 43:205–211.

Hermansson I, Einarsson S, Larsson K, Bäckström L. 1978. On the agalactia postpartum in the sow: A clinical study. Nord Vet Med 30:465–473.

Jones JET. 1976. Bacterial mastitis and endometritis in sows. Proc Int Congr Pig Vet Soc 4:E6.

———. 1979. Acute coliform mastitis in the sow. Veterinary Annual 19:97–101.

Jorsal SE. 1986. Epidemiology of the MMA-syndrome, a field survey in Danish sow herds. Proc Int Congr Pig Vet Soc 9:93.

King GJ, Willoughby RA, Hacker RR. 1972. Fluctuations in rectal temperature of swine at parturition. Can Vet J 13:72–74.

Löpfe PJ. 1993. Experimentelle Mastitis bei der Sau: Korrelation der pathologisch-anatomischen und histologischen Befunde mit den klinischen Befunden 4–30 Tage nach der Ansteckung mit *E. coli* und Klebsiella pneumoniae. DVM thesis, Zurich.

Löfstedt J, Roth JA, Ross RF, Wagner WC. 1983. Depression of polymorphonuclear leukocyte function associated with experimentally induced *Escherichia coli* mastitis in sows. Am J Vet Res 44:1224–1228.

Madec F, Miquet JM, Léon E. 1992. La pathologie de la parturition chez la truie: Étude épidémiologique dans cinq élevages. Recueil de Médecine Vétérinaire 168:341–349.

Magnusson U, Pedersen Morner A, Persson A, Karlstam E, Sternberg S, Kindahl H. 2001. Sows intramammarily inoculated with *Escherichia coli* influence of time of infection, hormone concentrations and leucocyte numbers on development of disease. Journal of Veterinary Medicine Series B: Infectious Diseases and Veterinary Public Health 48:501–512.

Martin CE, Hooper BE, Armstrong CH, Amstutz HE. 1967. A clinical and pathologic study of the mastitis-metritis-agalactia syndrome of sows. J Am Vet Med Assoc 151:1629–1634.

McDonald TJ, McDonald JS. 1975. Intramammary infections in the sow during the peripartum period. Cornell Veterinarian 65:73–83.

Middleton-Williams DM, Pohlenz J, Lott-Stolz G, Bertschinger HU. 1977. Untersuchungen über das Mastitis-Metritis-Agalaktie-Syndrom (Milchfieber) der Sau. I. Pathologische Befunde bei Spontanfaellen. Schweiz Arch Tierheilkd 119:213–222.

Morner AP, Faris A, Krovacek K. 1998. Virulence determinants of *Escherichia coli* isolated from milk of sows with coliform mastitis. Zentralbl Veterinarmed B 5:287–295.

Mossi R. 1995. Experimentelle Kolimastitis bei der Sau: Korrelation der pathologisch-anatomischen und histologischen mit den klinischen Befunden 6–72 Stunden nach der Inokulation. DVM thesis, Zurich.

Muirhead MR. 1976. Veterinary problems of intensive pig husbandry. Vet Rec 99:288–292.

Nachreiner RF, Ginther OJ. 1972. Porcine agalactia: Hematologic, serum chemical and clinical changes during the preceding gestation. Am J Vet Res 33:799–809.

Oliel N, Bertschinger HU. 1990. Prophylaxis of experimentally induced coliform mastitis in the sow with enrofloxacin (BAYTRIL). Proc Int Congr Pig Vet Soc 11:186.

Osterlundh I, Holst H, Magnusson U. 1998. Hormonal and immunological changes in blood and mammary secretion in the sow at parturition. Theriogenology 50:465–477.

——. 2001. Effect of mammary secretions on functions of polymorphonuclear leukocytes in pigs. Am J Vet Res 62:1250–1254.

Osterlundh I, Hulten F, Johannisson A, Magnusson U. 2002. Sows intramammarily inoculated with *Escherichia coli* at parturition: I. Functional capacity of granulocytes in sows affected or non-affected by clinical mastitis. Vet Immunol Immunopathol 90:35–44.

Persson A, Pedersen AE, Göransson L, Kuhl W. 1989. A long term study on the health status and performance of sows on different feed allowances during late pregnancy. I. Clinical observations, with special reference to agalactia post partum. Acta Vet Scand 30:9–17.

Persson A, Pedersen, Mörner A, Kuhl W. 1996a. A long term study on the health status and performance of sows on different feed allowances during late pregnancy. II. The total cell content and its percentage of polymorphonuclear leucocytes in pathogen-free colostrum and milk collected from clinically healthy sows. Acta Vet Scand 37:279–291.

——. 1996b. A long term study on the health status and performance of sows on different feed allowances during late pregnancy. III. *Escherichia coli* and other bacteria, total cell content, polymorphonuclear leucocytes and pH in colostrum and milk during the first 3 weeks of lactation. Acta Vet Scand 37:293–313.

Plonait H, Kump AW-S, Schöning G. 1986. Prophylaxis of the MMA-syndrome by antibacterial medication and restricted feeding. Proc Int Congr Pig Vet Soc 9:96.

Ramasoota P, Krovacek K, Chansiripornchai N, Mornerm AP, Svenson SB. 2000. Identification of *Escherichia coli* recovered from milk of sows with coliform mastitis by random amplified polymorphic DNA (RAPD) using standardized reagents. Acta Vet Scand 41:249–259.

Ringarp N. 1960. Clinical and experimental investigation into a post-parturient syndrome with agalactia in sows. Acta Agriculturae Scandinavica, Suppl 7.

Ross RF, Zimmermann BJ. 1982. Control of *Escherichia coli*–induced mastitis in sows with apramycin. Proc Int Congr Pig Vet Soc 7:14.

Ross RF, Zimmermann BJ, Wagner WC, Cox D. 1975. A field study of coliform mastitis in sows. J Am Vet Med Assoc 167:231–235.

Ross RF, Orning AP, Woods RD, Zimmermann BJ, Cox DF, Harris DL. 1981. Bacteriologic study of sow agalactia. Am J Vet Res 42:949–955.

Schoneweis DA, Hummels S, Schulteis L. 1982. Levels of oxytetracycline in plasma and milk in pig. Proc Int Congr Pig Vet Soc 7:291.

Tyler JW, Cullor JS, Ruffin DC. 1993. Immunization and immunotherapy for mastitis. Veterinary Clinics of North America: Food Animal Practice 9:537–549.

Wegmann P. 1985. Zur Pathogenese der Colimastitis beim Mutterschwein. DVM thesis, Zurich.

Wegmann P, Bertschinger HU. 1984. Sequential cytological and bacteriological examination of the secretions from sucked and unsucked mammary glands with and without mastitis. Proc Int Congr Pig Vet Soc 8:287.

Wegmann P, Bertschinger HU, Jecklin H. 1986. A field study on the prevalence of coliform mastitis (MMA) in Switzerland and the antimicrobial susceptibility of the coliform bacteria isolated from the milk. Proc Int Congr Pig Vet Soc 9:92.

Urinary Tract Infection

J. M. Fairbrother

Urinary tract infection (UTI) is present whenever any of the typically sterile sections of the urinary tract are colonized by microbes. UTI may or may not be accompanied by clinically manifest or subclinical disease. In the pig, specific UTI caused by *Actinobaculum suis* (Chapter 9) is distinguished from nonspecific UTI caused by a variety of microbes, the subject of this chapter. According to Liebhold et al. (1995), a nonspecific UTI often predisposes for *A. suis* infection.

UTI is the predominant cause of death in pigs over 1 year of age (Häni et al. 1976). In a survey of culled sows, significant bladder colonization was detected in 17% of the sows, and 80% of the colonized bladders exhibited histological lesions of cystitis (Colman et al. 1988).

Many authors have suggested a relationship between bacteriuria and reproductive disorders, including MMA. Sows developing MMA have a much higher prevalence of UTI in the preceding gestation period than sows with a normal puerperium (Miquet et al. 1990). According to Petersen (1983), examination of urine in late pregnancy allows recognition of sows at risk to develop MMA at a subsequent farrowing. However, similar prevalences of UTI in herds with and without MMA were reported by Becker et al. (1985). Potential pathogenetic relations between UTI and MMA were discussed in detail by Berner (1988).

ETIOLOGY

A. suis is often associated with severe cases of urinary tract disease. Nonspecific UTI may be caused by one or more of a number of bacterial species, often including *E. coli*. In one study of sows with acute urinary tract disease, *A. suis* was the bacterial species most commonly detected, mostly together with two or three other bacterial species, such as *E. coli*, *Streptococcus* sp., *Staphylococcus epidermidis*, *Klebsiella* sp., *Pseudomonas* sp., *Aeromonas* sp., and *Bacteroides* sp. (Stirnimann and Tschudi 1985). *A. suis* was also the bacterial species most commonly detected, mostly in mixed infections, in cases of pyelonephritis (Carr and Walton 1993). In this study, the isolation of large numbers of *E. coli* in the upper urinary tract was associated with linear renal scarring.

In a study of sows with severe acute urinary tract disease, mostly cystitis and often with pyelonephritis, *A. suis* was detected in fewer cases and *E. coli* was the principal pathogen, followed by streptococci and *Pseudomonas* (Stirnimann 1984). In another study, half of the sows with a significant bacteriuria but no pyelonephritis were infected with enterobacteria and streptococci but were free from *A. suis* (Liebhold et al. 1995).

In a study of aspirates taken at a slaughterhouse from sow bladders, *E. coli* was the most commonly isolated bacterial species, mostly in pure culture (Colman et al. 1988). *S. aureus, S. hyicus, E. faecalis, E. faecium, S. dysgalactiae,* and diverse gram-positive bacteria were also isolated, but to much lesser extent. Cystitis was present in most of the examined bacteriologically positive sows. *A. suis* was not detected in this study.

The urinary tract is a dynamic microbiological ecosystem. Dominant bacterial species change spontaneously in a significant proportion of sows surveyed over prolonged periods (Berner 1990). These changes become more frequent when sows are treated with antimicrobials.

EPIDEMIOLOGY

Nonspecific UTI behaves like a noncontagious infectious disease of endogenous origin. In dogs, *E. coli* isolates from urine and from rectal samples of the same individual show identity in phenotypic and genotypic tests (Low et al. 1988). Corresponding studies with the pig are lacking. The fecal flora may achieve access to the urinary tract more efficiently in females than in males. Under intensive confinement conditions, sows' vulvas are often placed in direct contact with feces (Smith 1983). The dog-sitting position helps to force fecal material into the vagina. Sows resting for long periods void urine at longer intervals. However, housing conditions have not yet been studied with respect to UTI.

The age distribution of UTI favors the concept of continuous exposure to fecal contamination. The prevalence of UTI increases from 18% in young sows with 1–3 litters to 38% in older sows with 7 and more litters (Becker et al. 1985).

PATHOGENESIS

In humans and in dogs colonization of the lower genital tract and of the urinary tract by uropathogenic *E. coli* is greatly facilitated by fimbrial adhesins, particularly Type 1 and P fimbriae (Gyles and Fairbrother 2004). Similarly, P fimbriae and mannose-sensitive hemagglutination indicative of type 1 pili, were found in *E. coli* isolates from the urine of pigs with bacteriuria (de Brito et al. 1999). It is assumed that most agents ascend through the urethra (Smith 1983). Invasion is favored by the short, wide urethra of the female pig, the relaxation of the sphincter muscle in late pregnancy and puerperium, trauma to the urethra and bladder at coitus and parturition, abnormal bacterial colonization of the sinus urogenitalis and the genital organs, incomplete closure of the vulva, and catheterization of the bladder

(Berner 1988). Repeated examination of individual sows led to the conclusion that asymptomatic bacteriuria may temporarily deteriorate to cystitis with spontaneous remission (Berner 1988). Liebhold et al. (1995) assumed that nonspecific infection promotes colonization of the bladder by *A. suis*. Carr et al. (1990) postulate that bacterial colonization leads to shortening and deformation of the ureteric valve and thereby promotes vesicoureteric reflux. The latter could be easily demonstrated postmortem in cases of acute pyelonephritis.

Serum antibody against the infecting *E. coli* strain can regularly be detected in sows with pyelonephritis, less often in sows with cystitis, and rather rarely in sows with asymptomatic bacteriuria (Wagner 1990). *E. coli* strains may persist in the urinary tract despite high antibody concentrations in the urine.

UTI predisposes to MMA in one of several ways (Berner 1988). Ascending invasion of the uterus at parturition and of the mammary glands from contamination of the lying area appears most likely. However, other routes cannot be ruled out. Identical OK serotypes of *E. coli* were found in the urinary bladders and in the uteri of 3 sows and in the bladder and mammary gland of 1 out of 9 sows with MMA killed for postmortem examination (Bertschinger et al. 1977).

CLINICAL SIGNS

In the vast majority of nonspecific UTI cases there are no clinical signs (Berner 1988). Akkermans and Pomper (1980) concluded from an extended field study that sows with a significant bacteriuria tend to wean small litters, have increased intervals between litters, show a lower fertility rate, and exhibit an inferior body condition. In many sows with cystitis, careful observation reveals abnormal urination (Becker et al. 1988). The sows stand in one place before they void urine in small quantities with straining. They are more often seen in a dog-sitting position. Proteinuria, macrohemoturia, and pH increases are more prevalent in sows infected with *A. suis* than with *E. coli* (Liebhold et al. 1995).

Vulval discharge may appear as dried deposits around the vulva, on the underside of the tail, or more often as a pool on the floor underneath the sows (Dial and MacLachlan 1988a). The discharge may be mucoid, mucohemorrhagic, or purulent and is observed most often during the final phase of urination. However, discharge may result from inflammation of any part of the urogenital tract. Significant discharge is more often the consequence of endometritis than of UTI.

Severe pyelonephritis becomes clinically manifest during the first 2 weeks postpartum in 40% of the cases (Stirnimann 1984). Typical cases exhibit a rectal temperature below 38.0°C, a heart rate over 120, polypnoea, cyanosis, ataxia, and more rarely generalized tremor (Stirnimann and Tschudi 1985). The blood concentrations of urea and creatinine are higher than normal.

LESIONS

Berner (1981) examined 118 culled sows for bacteria and lesions. Twenty-six out of 29 sows with a UTI presented a cystitis, and 12 sows presented an additional pyelonephritis.

The gross lesions of cystitis begin as focal or diffuse mucosal hyperemia (Dial and MacLachlan 1988b). Subsequently, there may be mucosal ulceration with fibrinopurulent exudate over affected areas. The bladder wall becomes thickened. Similar lesions occur in the ureters and the renal pelvis if infection ascends the urinary tract. In pyelonephritis the inflammatory process extends into the renal parenchyma. Wedge-shaped foci extend from the distorted pelvis to the cortex. Fibrosis of the kidneys may occur with time.

Microscopic bladder lesions can be found even in sows with nonspecific UTI and no proteinuria. They consist of a prominent goblet cell proliferation and of intraepithelial cysts containing a few granulocytes. The epithelial layer is infiltrated with neutrophils, whereas mononuclear cells dominate in the lamina propria (Liebhold et al. 1995).

DIAGNOSIS

Mere clinical examination of the animal is of little value in the diagnosis of UTI (Stirnimann 1984); urine must be examined in most cases. Bacteriology of the urinary tract is complicated by the presence of the normal flora colonizing the vagina and the distal part of the urethra. Therefore, distinction between contamination and infection is based on the number of bacteria in the urine. A viable count of 10^5 CFU/mL is interpreted as indicative of infection and 10^4 CFU/mL as suspicious. Dip slides (i.e., commercially available slides covered by bacterial culture media) give satisfactory quantitative results (Akkermans and Pomper 1980). Nevertheless, dip slides have the shortcoming that anaerobes such as *A. suis* and slow growers will be missed.

Catheterization of the sow is possible (Stirnimann 1984) but does not circumvent contamination and involves the risk of setting up a new UTI. Voiding can be induced by rousing the sows in the morning before feeding time (Becker et al. 1985). When collecting midstream urine, the attendant should avoid contact with the urine, which may contain zoonotic agents such as leptospires.

Diagnostic test strips are applicable to the urine of pigs, except for nitrite. The sensitivity of the latter test is too low due to the low nitrite concentration in porcine urine (Becker et al. 1985). The most useful parameters are protein, hemoglobin, and pH. In cases due to *A. suis*, the pH is strongly alkaline (greater than 8.5) (Carr et al. 1995). Cytological examination may allow discrimination between bacteriuria, cystitis, and pyelonephritis. The presence and concentrations of antibodies in the

urine are not well correlated with the severity of the condition (Wagner 1990). Test strips permit the rapid determination of blood urea (Liebhold et al. 1995). Concentrations greater than 10 mmol/L indicate uremia.

TREATMENT

Nearly all the treatments recommended in the literature are aimed at elimination of the bacteria by antimicrobials. The variable susceptibilities of the diverse bacteria involved and the frequent acquisition of R factors pose considerable problems (Table 38.7). With regard to the observed changes of infecting bacterial species or types in the course of antimicrobial treatments, Berner (1990) recommended the use of either broad-spectrum or combined antimicrobials and suggested intensifying the search for alternative strategies.

Becker et al. (1988) treated 9 sows twice daily for 2 weeks via feed with sulfadimidine 1.0 g, sulfathiazole 1.0 g, and trimethoprim 0.4 g/sow. Significant bacteriuria was present in 2 sows 1 week after the treatment and in 3 sows 7 weeks later. The same substances applied over 4 days gave greatly inferior results. Gentamicin, 2.5 mg/kg body weight, was injected intramuscularly to 15 sows on the first day, followed by 2.0 mg on the next 3 days. One week after this treatment, 10 sows were free of significant bacteriuria. The authors concluded that prolonged treatment should be preferred. Antimicrobial resistance was not checked.

Treatment of severely affected sows was reported by Stirnimann (1988). Injection of ampicillin 3 g/sow daily

Table 38.7. Sensitivity to antimicrobial agents of significant isolates from porcine UTI in Belgium and Switzerland

| | % Sensitive Isolates | | |
| | Belgium[1] | | Switzerland[2] |
Antimicrobial Agent	Gram-Negative $n = 62$	Gram-Positive $n = 18$	E. coli $n = 21$
Penicillin G	NT[3]	44	NT
Penicillinase-stable Penicillins	NT	72	NT
Ampicillin	68	44	71
Amoxycillin/clavulanic acid	100	72	NT
Streptomycin	40	44	NT
Neomycin	98	61	86
Spectinomycin	85	72	NT
Gentamicin	100	61	100
Tetracycline	47	61	33
Chloramphenicol	82	83	67
Nitrofurane	95	94	14
Sulfonamide	37	50	52
Trimethoprim	76	61	NT
Trimethoprim and sulfonamide	NT	NT	76
Macrolide	NT	61	NT
Lincomycin	NT	72	NT

[1]Colman et al. 1988.
[2]Stirnimann 1988.
[3]Not tested.

for 4 days or of the same antibiotic combined with no-vaminsulfon 10 g/sow was compared. The combined treatment led to a smaller number of emergency slaughters. Subclinical UTI persisted in about half of the successfully treated sows.

Dial and MacLachlan (1988b) concluded that treatment of urogenital infections of swine generally is frustrating.

PREVENTION

Results of long-term prospective studies are not available. Berner (1988) recommended that all pregnant sows be checked repeatedly for UTI and that positive sows be treated with antimicrobials shortly before parturition. Smith (1983) suggested medicating all dry sows on problem farms for 7–10 days at 6-week intervals. The interval between treatments can be increased gradually as experience dictates. Antibiotics such as tetracyclines or a suitable form of penicillin have been successfully used in the diet. In view of the disappointing results reported by Berner (1990), these recommendations should be viewed with caution.

According to Wagner (1990), immunoprophylaxis holds little promise. Thus, Smith (1983) and Carr et al. (1995) recommended the reduction of environmental exposure by improving fecal drainage and housing conditions. These factors as well as the role of water intake should be further investigated. Frequency of urination was increased by giving access to an exercise yard and by increasing water intake, which was achieved by a salt content of 1% in the diet (Smith 1983).

REFERENCES

Akkermans JPWM, Pomper W. 1980. The significance of a bacteriuria with reference to disturbances in fertility. Proc Int Congr Pig Vet Soc 6:44.

Becker H-A, Kurtz R, Von Mickwitz G. 1985. Chronische Harnwegsinfektionen beim Schwein, Diagnose und Therapie (I). Prakt Tierarztl 66:1006–1011.

Becker W, Kurtz R, Von Mickwitz G. 1988. Chronische Harnwegsinfektionen beim Schwein, Diagnose und Therapie (III). Prakt Tierarztl 69:41–45.

Berner H. 1981. Untersuchungen zum Vorkommen von Harnwegsinfektionen bei Muttersauen. 2. Mitteilung: Harnwegsinfektionen bei Schlachtschweinen. Tierärztl Umsch 36:250–255.

——. 1988. Cystitis in der MMA-Diagnostik. Prakt Tierarztl 69:124–131.

——. 1990. Erregerwechsel als Ursache von Misserfolgen bei der Therapie bakteriell bedingter Krankheiten der Urogenitalorgane des Schweines. Dtsch Tierärztl Wochenschr 97:20–24.

Bertschinger HU, Pohlenz J, Hemlep I. 1977. Untersuchungen über das Mastitis-Metritis-Agalaktie-Syndrom (Milchfieber) der Sau. Schweiz Arch Tierheilkd 119:223–233.

Carr J, Walton JR. 1992. The characterization of *Escherichia coli* isolates from the porcine urogenital tract. Proc Int Congr Pig Vet Soc 12:262.

——. 1993. Bacterial flora of the urinary tract of pigs associated with cystitis and pyelonephritis. Vet Rec 132:575–577.

Carr J, Walton JR, Done SH. 1990. Observations on the intravesicular portion of the ureter from healthy pigs and those with urinary tract disease. Proc Int Congr Pig Vet Soc 11:286.

——. 1995. Cystitis and ascending pyelonephritis in the sow. Practice 17:71–79.

Colman J, Devriese L, Verdonck M. 1988. Bacteriuria and urinary tract infection in sows. Vlaams Diergeneesk Tijdschr 57:192–198.

de Brito BG, Leite DS, Linhares RE, Vidotto MC. 1999. Virulence-associated factors of uropathogenic *Escherichia coli* strains isolated from pigs. Vet Microbiol 65:123–132.

Dial G, MacLachlan NJ. 1988a. Urogenital infections of swine. Part I. Clinical manifestations and pathogenesis. Compendium on Continuing Education for the Practicing Veterinarian 10:63–71.

——. 1988b. Urogenital infections of swine. Part II. Pathology and medical management. Compendium on Continuing Education for the Practicing Veterinarian 10:529–540.

Gyles CL, Fairbrother JM. 2004. *Escherichia coli*. In Pathogenesis of Bacterial Infections in Animals (3rd edition). CL Gyles, JF Prescott, JG Songer, CO Thoen, eds. Ames, Iowa: Blackwell Publishing, pp. 193–223.

Häni H, Brändli A, Luginbühl H, König H. 1976. Vorkommen und Bedeutung von Schweinekrankheiten: Analyse eines Sektionsgutes (1971–1973). Schweiz Arch Tierheilkd 118:1–11.

Imberechts H, Bertschinger HU, Stamm M, Sydler T, Pohl P. De Greve H, Hernalsteens JP, Van-Montagu M, Lintermans P. 1994. Prevalence of F107 fimbriae on *Escherichia coli* isolated from pigs with oedema disease or postweaning diarrhoea. Vet Microbiol 40(3–4):219–230.

Liebhold M, Wendt M, Kaup F-J, Drommer W. 1995. Clinical and light and electron microscopical findings in sows with cystitis. Vet Rec 137:141–144.

Low DA, Braaten BA, Ling GV, Johnson DL, Ruby AL. 1988. Isolation and comparison of *Escherichia coli* strains from canine and human patients with urinary tract infections. Infect Immun 56:2601–2609.

Miquet JM, Madec F, Paboeuf F. 1990. Epidemiology of farrowing disorders in the sow: Preliminary results of a prospective inquiry in 2 farms. Proc Int Congr Pig Vet Soc 11:472.

Petersen B. 1983. Methods of early recognition of puerperal and fertility disorders in the sow. Livest Prod Sci 10:253–264.

Smith WJ. 1983. Cystitis in sows. Pig News Info 4:279–281.

Stirnimann J. 1984. Akute Harnwegsentzündung bei der Muttersau. Schweiz Arch Tierheilkd 126:597–605.

——. 1988. Zur Behandlung der akuten Harnwegsentzündung bei der Muttersau. Schweiz Arch Tierheilkd 130:605–611.

Stirnimann J, Tschudi PR. 1985. Beurteilung der Nierenfunktion bei Muttersauen mit akuter Harnwegsentzündung. Schweiz Arch Tierheilkd 127:575–582.

Wagner S. 1990. Die Immunreaktion bei der durch *Escherichia coli* bedingten chronischen Harnwegsinfektion des weiblichen Schweines. DVM thesis, Univ München.

39 Exudative Epidermitis

H. C. Wegener and E. W. Skov-Jensen

Exudative epidermitis (EE) has been known by its clinical signs for over 160 years (Spinola 1842). The classic disease occurs as an acute or peracute infection in suckling and newly weaned piglets in which a generalized epidermitis may lead to dehydration and death. Early occurrence and distribution have been comprehensively reviewed by Jones (1956), who provided a good description of the disease and its effects on production. It has been recorded in most pig-rearing countries in both piglets and weaners. Major studies have been carried out by Sompolinsky (1953), Jones (1956), Underdahl et al. (1963, 1965), L'Ecuyer (1966), L'Ecuyer and Jericho (1966), Hunter et al. (1970), and Wegener and Skov-Jensen (1992). The condition is of sporadic occurrence in all countries but may be of great importance in individual herds, especially in newly established or repopulated herds (Pepper and Taylor 1977).

ETIOLOGY

Staphylococcus hyicus is the causal agent of the generalized form of the disease seen in piglets. Although it is present in profuse culture in lesions in adult pigs, the disease has not been reproduced in that age group. Strains of *S. hyicus* can be divided into virulent and avirulent types with regard to the ability to reproduce EE experimentally in piglets (Wegener et al. 1993). Both types can be present simultaneously on the skin of diseased, as well as healthy, piglets (Park and Kang 1986; Wegener et al. 1993). The production of an exfoliative toxin appears to be the single most important virulence determinant of *S. hyicus* (Amtsberg 1979; Sato et al. 1991; Wegener et al. 1993; Andresen et al. 1993; Andresen et al. 1997). However, a range of other factors may also be necessary, but not sufficient, to render *S. hyicus* capable of causing EE in piglets.

S. hyicus was first described by Sompolinsky (1953) as *Micrococcus hyicus;* it was then defined as a staphylococcus by Baird-Parker (1965). *S. hyicus* was separated into *S. hyicus* subsp. *hyicus* and *S. hyicus* subsp. *chromogenes,* a nonpathogen, by Devriese et al. (1978). *S. hyicus* subsp. *chromogenes* was subsequently elevated to species *S. chromogenes* by Hajek et al. (1986), making *S. hyicus* the taxonomically correct designation for the causal agent of EE. The organism is a gram-positive coccus that forms 3–4 mm porcelain-white nonhemolytic colonies on sheep blood agar after 24 hours' incubation. It is coagulase negative using the slide test and is heat-stable DNase, lipase, and hyaluronidase positive, and mannitol and acetoin negative. These biochemical characteristics are of value in distinguishing the organism by conventional means from other staphylococci found in pigs (Devriese 1977). A selective indicator medium described by Devriese (1977) which utilizes the lipase activity as the indicative principle can be very useful for isolation of *S. hyicus* from pathological samples.

S. hyicus may be isolated from a range of other animals, including ruminants and fowl (Devriese et al. 1978). Phenotypic and genotypic differences from porcine isolates suggest that *S. hyicus* from other animals may belong to separate ecovars (Devriese et al. 1978; Schleifer 1986; Takeuchi et al. 1988). Their virulence with regard to EE is not known.

EPIDEMIOLOGY

EE has been described from all major pig-producing countries, and the incidence has been reported to be increasing in some regions (Anon. 1991; Wegener 1992). This increase may reflect changes in pig production toward larger units, earlier weaning, and higher animal densities. The disease may occur sporadically and with low morbidity among litters in some pig herds, whereas in others it reaches epidemic proportions affecting all litters. This suggests that immunity plays an important part in the cause of the disease in the individual animal as well as in the herd. The significance of immunity in relation to EE has, however, not been thoroughly investigated.

The disease occurs most commonly following the

introduction of carrier animals to a nonimmune herd and affects successive litters of piglets, usually those born to nonimmune sows. All litters in an affected herd may be affected, and up to 70% of affected piglets may die. Outbreaks are usually self-limiting and last for 2–3 months but may persist or recur if nonimmune sows are brought into infected buildings or exposed to infected animals. Outbreaks may start among the weaned piglets, possibly as a result of mixing nonimmune litters and litters of immune carriers, and then spread to the farrowing section of the herd.

S. hyicus can frequently be recovered from the nasal mucosa of healthy pigs, from the conjunctiva, the skin of the snout or ear, and from the vagina in gilts and sows (Hajsig et al. 1985; Wegener and Skov-Jensen 1992). *S. hyicus* strains indistinguishable from those present in the vaginas of sows have been recovered from the skin of their offspring, suggesting that colonization takes place during passage through the birth canal (Wegener and Skov-Jensen 1992).

S. hyicus is very resistant to adverse conditions (as most staphylococci are) and can persist in the environment for long periods. The organism can persist for weeks on fittings and surfaces, and it has been recovered from the air of infected units at levels up to $2.5 \times 10^4/m^3$, suggesting that airborne transmission is possible (Wegener 1992). Other species such as horses, dogs, cattle, goats, and chickens may be of little importance as sources of infection for pigs.

PATHOGENESIS

Application of pure cultures of virulent *S. hyicus* to the scarified skin of a nonimmune pig is sufficient to reproduce the disease (Underdahl et al. 1965; L'Ecuyer and Jericho 1966), but it can also be produced by subcutaneous injection in specific pathogen free (SPF) piglets (Underdahl et al. 1965; Wegener et al. 1993). Conventional animals may be resistant to such applications, suggesting that immunity may be an important protective factor. Studies indicate that other elements of the skin flora, especially other staphylococci, may contribute to this resistance to colonization (Allaker et al. 1988). Trauma from fighting, unclipped teeth, rough bedding, or pen walls leading to exposure of dermis may allow the organism to establish infection, although *S. hyicus* may also be able to penetrate the epidermis directly.

The earliest changes are seen as skin reddening accompanying the multiplication of the organism on the skin surface and its growth between the corneocytes of the epidermis, where microcolonies develop. Inflammation, marked hyperplasia of the stratum corneum, and invasion by neutrophils occur, with an increase in thickness of the epidermis, followed by its erosion. The stratum germinativum becomes disorganized and penetrates deeply into the dermis. Clinical signs develop in gnotobiotic piglets when the number of organisms on the skin ex-

ceeds $10^5/cm^2$ (Allaker et al. 1988). *S. hyicus* may adhere to fibronectin in the dermis by fibronectin-binding proteins on the bacterial surface (Lämmler et al. 1985).

The phagocyte-opsonin system is the pig's first active line of defense against the infection. Many *S. hyicus* strains harbor determinants that may protect them from phagocytosis: protein A, present in the cell wall of most porcine *S. hyicus* strains, reduces opsonization by binding immunoglobulins at the Fc terminal (Takeuchi et al. 1990), and a capsule present in all virulent but not all avirulent strains of *S. hyicus* inhibits phagocytosis by neutrophils and macrophages (Wegener 1990). All porcine *S. hyicus* strains coagulate pig plasma, suggesting a potential for forming aggregates which may increase protection of the bacterium against phagocytosis. In addition, the production of catalase may protect the bacterium from being killed by the phagocytic cells. All of these properties may contribute to overcoming the initial immune response of the piglet.

The most important factor in the pathogenesis is probably the production of an exfoliative toxin of approximately 30 kDa. Crude or purified exfoliative toxin, which is demonstrable in culture supernates of the organism, can reproduce the skin alterations seen in clinical EE when injected subcutaneously in piglet skin locally (Wegener et al. 1993; Andresen et al. 1993; Sato et al. 1991). There are different antigenic variants of the toxin; however, they all seem to exert the same activity in pig skin (Andresen et al. 1997). The effect of the purified toxin is separation of the cells in the epidermis, notably separation of cells in the upper stratum spinosum, allowing for rapid intraepidermal spread of the bacteria (Andresen et al. 1993). Exfoliation of the skin is accompanied by excess sebaceous secretion and serous exudate. *S. hyicus* is present in large numbers in the skin and may be isolated from the draining lymph nodes and blood. The mortality associated with this disease results from dehydration and possibly also septicemia.

Exudative epidermitis shares many similarities with the human infection called the staphylococcal scalded skin syndrome, which is a *Staphylococcus aureus* infection of the skin of neonates. The infection leads to a local or a generalized exfoliation of the epidermis and excessive sebaceous secretion and is caused by strains of *S. aureus* capable of producing exfoliative toxins. Two variants of the toxin are known: ET-A, which is encoded by a gene located on the chromosome, and ET-B, which is plasmid encoded. The exfoliative toxins of *S. aureus* and *S. hyicus* have different species specificity. ET-A and ET-B affect the skin of humans and mice but not pigs, whereas the exfoliative toxin of *S. hyicus* affects pigs and chickens but not mice.

CLINICAL SIGNS

Piglets usually develop the disease between 4–6 days and 5–6 weeks of age. Clinical signs begin with dejection

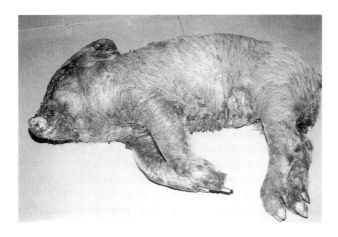

39.1. *Generalized exudative epidermitis in a 3-week-old piglet.*

and a reddish or coppery skin color. Thin, pale brown scales of exudate develop in the axillae and groin and within 3–5 days spread to all parts of the body and rapidly become dark in color and greasy in texture (Fig. 39.1). The skin of affected piglets often feels hot, the hair coat is matted, and exudate may extend to the eyelashes. Ulcers may occur in the mouth, and separation of horn may occur at the bulbs of the heels. Anorexia and dehydration are features of this disease. Severely affected piglets lose weight rapidly and may die within 24 hours; death usually occurs within 3–10 days. There is no pruritis, and fever is not common.

Not all piglets in a litter are affected to the same extent, and some individuals will suffer from chronic disease in which smaller areas of the body are involved (Fig. 39.2). Mildly affected piglets may have a yellowish skin,

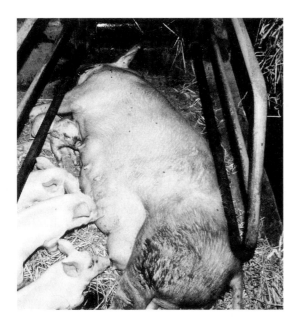

39.2. *A single piglet with generalized exudative epidermitis among only mildly affected or unaffected littermates.*

appear hairy, and have only a few flakes of exudate in the axillae or groin or near facial scratches or damage on the knees or adjacent to badly clipped teeth. Growth depression is marked in survivors, and productivity of the herd may be depressed by up to 35% during an outbreak and up to 9% in the year following infection (Pepper and Taylor 1977). Disease in adults varies in severity but occurs as localized lesions on the back or flanks. Mild forms may appear as brownish areas of EE, but in some cases, there may be ulceration (Smith et al. 1990).

LESIONS

Gross Lesions
Early lesions of the infection include reddening of skin and the presence of a clear exudate. The abdominal skin can be peeled off by slight rubbing. Early lesions are usually present around the mouth, eyes, and ears as well as on the abdomen. Later cases are covered by a thick brownish, greasy, and odorous layer due to dirt and feces sticking to the affected skin. During the recovery phase, the skin is dry and crusted for a period of several days to weeks. The carcasses of pigs that have died from EE are dehydrated and emaciated. The superficial lymph nodes are usually edematous and swollen. Most animals have empty stomachs, and urate crystals may be seen in the medulla of the kidney on section. There is often an accumulation of mucoid or crystalline material in the pelvis of the kidney, and pyelonephritis may be present.

Microscopic Lesions
Early changes of the epidermis are exfoliation, exocytosis, crust formation, and formation of vesicles and pustules classified as an "intraepidermal vesicular and pustular dermatitis." In the later stages, acanthosis (hyperplasia of the epidermis) is observed (Fig. 39.3). In the dermis, perivascular inflammation occurs (Andresen et al. 1993). In histological sections of the skin, bacterial microcolonies may occur in the keratinized layer of the epidermis.

Bacteriology
S. hyicus can usually be isolated from the lesions, from the superficial lymph nodes, and frequently also from the liver and spleen of untreated cases but may be difficult to demonstrate on nonselective culture media if treatment has been given or if secondary infection by *Proteus* sp. and *Pseudomonas aeruginosa* has occurred. The use of a selective indicative agar facilitates isolation of *S. hyicus* from pathological samples (Devriese 1977). Both virulent and avirulent strains of *S. hyicus* can be isolated as mixed cultures from the skin, lymph nodes, and organs of diseased piglets (Wegener 1992). Whether the avirulent strains take any active part in the establishment or course of the infection remains unknown.

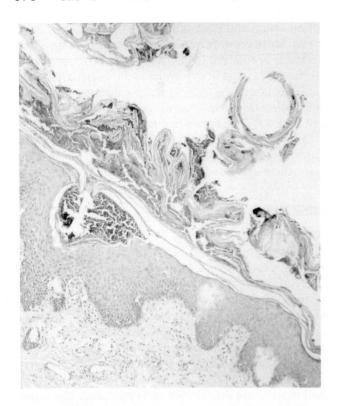

39.3. *Histological section of skin of pig with generalized exudative epidermitis (original magnification ×1200). Changes present in the epidermis are exfoliation, exocytosis, crust formation, formation of vesicles and pustules classified as an "intraepidermal vesicular and pustular dermatitis," and acanthosis (hyperplasia of the epidermis). In the dermis, perivascular inflammation can be seen.*

DIAGNOSIS

The clinical signs are generally sufficient to reach a diagnosis in young piglets. The lack of fever or of pruritis and the generalized nature of the lesions, their appearance, and the variation in severity within an affected litter are all features suggestive of the disease. Confirmation may be obtained by histological and bacteriological means. It may be necessary to confirm the identity of the staphylococci isolated as *S. hyicus* by conventional bacteriological means (Devriese 1977) or by use of strip tests such as the Staph-Zym test (Lämmler 1989). These have the advantage of revealing the identity of non–*S. hyicus* staphylococci.

S. hyicus from pigs are very heterogeneous with regard to phago-, sero-, and DNA fingerprinting types (Wegener 1993a; Park and Kang 1987). Diagnosis is complicated by the simultaneous presence of up to 8 different types of *S. hyicus* on diseased piglets. Wegener (1993b) found that each diseased piglet on average harbored 1.9 different phage types and 2.3 different antibiotic resistance patterns among 10 randomly selected isolates of *S. hyicus* recovered from the skin. Only a slightly lower diversity was observed for strains recovered from the liver or the spleen of the animals. In the absence of simple methods to differentiate virulent from avirulent strains in the diagnostic laboratory, all types of *S. hyicus* should be regarded as potentially virulent. Thus, antimicrobials for therapy which affect all types present should be chosen. Similarly, autogenous vaccines should be prepared from all types present on the diseased animals.

Diagnosis is less easy when the lesions are mild, localized around predisposing lesions such as fight wounds, or have been treated. The demonstration of *S. hyicus* and response to antimicrobials may help confirm uncomplicated disease of this type, but the organism may be present in lesions caused by a number of initiating agents.

Other skin conditions that may be confused with EE include swine pox (localized lesions, rarely fatal), mange (pruritis, demonstration of mites), ringworm (expanding superficial lesions, isolation of fungus), pityriasis rosea (expanding circles, nonfatal, lesions not greasy), zinc deficiency (weaners, symmetrical dry lesions), dermatosis vegetans (inherited in Landrace, fatal pneumonitis), and local wounds such as facial fight wounds and abraded knees in piglets and crate injuries in adults. The organism may be isolated from other pathologic conditions such as arthritis in piglets (Noda and Fukui 1986) and cystitis in sows as well as from the skin of healthy pigs.

TREATMENT AND PREVENTION

Treatment is most successful if carried out early in the disease; severely affected animals may not respond. The effect of systemic treatment is reduction in the severity of the skin lesions, development of only superficial lesions, and promotion of the healing process. *S. hyicus* is frequently resistant to antibiotics. This resistance has been shown to be predominantly mediated by plasmids (Wegener and Schwarz 1993). Combinations of trimethoprim and sulfonamides or lincomycin and spectinomycin have been shown to have good in vitro activity against *S. hyicus* (Wegener et al. 1994). Antimicrobial treatment should be accompanied by the provision of a fluid replacer or at least clean water for affected piglets and by local treatment with antibiotics or skin disinfectants such as cetrimide, hexocil, or Virkon X in order to speed recovery and prevent spread of the infection. Treatment may have to be continued for at least 5 days, and clinically affected piglets may make a slow recovery or remain stunted.

Vaccination of sows with autogenous bacterins made from strains isolated on the affected farm may be of value in protecting the litters of newly purchased sows when given before farrowing. Antibodies can effectively neutralize the effect of the exfoliative toxin in the skin. It is possible that the toxin may be able to serve as a single protective antigen; however, this has not yet been shown under field conditions. Therefore, autogenous vaccines should be prepared from both the bacterial cells and the culture supernatant, which contains the exfoliative toxin.

The incidence of the disease may be reduced by clipping the teeth of litters at risk, by ensuring that pen surfaces are not abrasive, and by providing soft and dry bedding, such as softwood sawdusts or chaffed straw. Sows entering farrowing accommodation should be washed and disinfected and placed in clean, disinfected, or fumigated pens. Prompt treatment of local lesions on both sows and piglets may also help.

REFERENCES

Allaker RP, Lloyd DH, Smith LM. 1988. Prevention of exudative epidermitis in gnotobiotic piglets by bacterial interference. Vet Rec 123:287–288.

Amtsberg G. 1979. Nachweis von Exfoliation auslösenden Substanzen in Kulturen von *Staphylococcus hyicus* des Schweines und *Staphylococcus epidermidis* Biotyp 2 des Rindes. Zentralbl Veterinärmed (B) 26:257–272.

Andresen LO, Bille-Hansen V, Wegener HC. 1997. *Staphylococcus hyicus* exfoliative toxin: Purification and demonstration of antigenic diversity among toxins from virulent strains. Microbial Pathogenesis (in press).

Andresen LO, Wegener HC, Bille-Hansen V. 1993. *Staphylococcus hyicus*–skin reactions in piglets caused by extracellular products and by partially purified exfoliative toxin. Microbial Pathogen 15:217–225.

Anon. 1991. Greasy pig (disease review). Int Pigletter 11:30–32.

Baird-Parker AC. 1965. The classification of staphylococci and micrococci from world-wide sources. J Gen Microbiol 38:363–387.

Devriese LA. 1977. Isolation and identification of *Staphylococcus hyicus*. Am J Vet Res 38:787–792.

Devriese LA, Hajek V, Oeding P, Meyer SA, Schleifer KH. 1978. *Staphylococcus hyicus* (Sompolinsky 1953) comb. nov. and *Staphylococcus hyicus* subsp. *chromogenes* subsp. nov. Int J Syst Bacteriol 28:482–490.

Hajek V, Devriese LA, Mordarski M, Goodfellow M, Pulverer G, Varaldo PE. 1986. Elevation of *Staphylococcus hyicus* subsp. *chromogenes* (Devriese et al. 1978) to species status: *Staphylococcus chromogenes* (Devriese et al. 1978) comb. nov. System Appl Microbiol 8:169–173.

Hajsig D, Babic T, Madic J. 1985. Exudative epidermitis in piglets. II. Distribution of *Staphylococcus hyicus* subsp. *hyicus*: Findings in healthy piglets. Vet Arh 55:45–51.

Hunter D, Todd JN, Larkin M. 1970. Exudative epidermitis of pigs. Br Vet J 126:225–229.

Jones LD. 1956. Exudative epidermitis of pigs. Am J Vet Res 17:179–193.

Lämmler C. 1989. Evaluation of the Staph-Zym system for identification of *Staphylococcus hyicus* and *Staphylococcus intermedius*. J Vet Med (B) 36:180–184.

Lämmler C, De Freitas JC, Chatwal GS, Blobel H. 1985. Interaction of immunoglobulin G, fibrinogen, fibronectin with *Staphylococcus hyicus* and *Staphylococcus intermedius*. Zbl Bakt Hyg (A) 260:232–237.

L'Ecuyer C. 1966. Exudative epidermitis in pigs: Clinical studies and preliminary transmission trials. Can J Comp Med 30:9–16.

L'Ecuyer C, Jericho K. 1966. Exudative epidermitis in pigs: Etiological studies and pathology. Can J Comp Med 30:94–101.

Noda K, Fukui T. 1986. Outbreaks of pyogenic arthritis in newborn piglets and stillbirth caused by *S. hyicus* subsp. *hyicus*. Jpn J Vet Med Assoc 39:305–310.

Park CK, Kang BK. 1986. Studies on exudative epidermitis in pigs. I. Isolation and some properties of *Staphylococcus hyicus* subsp. *hyicus* from diseased and healthy pigs. Korean J Vet Res 26:251–257.

——. 1987. Studies on exudative epidermitis in pigs. II. Serological typing of Staphylococcus hyicus subsp. hyicus isolated from pigs. Korean J Vet Res 27:47–52.

Pepper TA, Taylor DJ. 1977. The effect of exudative epidermitis on weaner production in a small pig herd. Vet Rec 101:204–205.

Sato H, Tanabe T, Kuramoto M, Tanaka K, Hashimoto T, Saito H. 1991. Isolation of exfoliative toxin from *Staphylococcus hyicus* subsp. *hyicus* and its exfoliative activity in the piglet. Vet Microbiol 27:263–275.

Schleifer KH. 1986. *Micrococcaceae*. In Bergey's Manual for Determinative Bacteriology, 9th ed. Ed. PHA. Sneath. Baltimore: William & Wilkins, pp. 1003–1035.

Smith WJ, Taylor DJ, Penny RHC. 1990. A Colour Atlas of Diseases and Disorders of the Pig. London: Wolfe Publishing, pp. 113–114.

Sompolinsky D. 1953. De l'impetigo contagiosa suis. Schweiz Arch Tierheilkd 95:302–309.

Spinola J. 1842. Die Krankheiten der Schweine. Berlin: Verlag Hirschwald, pp. 146–148.

Takeuchi S, Kobayashi Y, Mori Y. 1990. Assay of protein A in *Staphylococcus hyicus* subsp. *hyicus* by ELISA and immunoelectron microscopy. Vet Microbiol 25:297–302.

Takeuchi S, Kobayashi Y, Morosumi T, Mori Y. 1988. Protein A in *Staphylococcus hyicus* subsp. *hyicus* isolated from pigs, chickens and cows. Jpn J Vet Sci 50:153–157.

Underdahl NR, Grace PD, Twiehaus MJ. 1965. Porcine exudative epidermitis: Characterisation of bacterial agent. Am J Vet Res 26:617–624.

Underdahl NR, Grace PD, Young GA. 1963. Experimental transmission of exudative epidermitis of pigs. J Am Vet Med Assoc 142:754–762.

Wegener HC. 1990. Studies on *Staphylococcus hyicus* virulence in relation to exudative epidermitis in piglets. Proc Int Congr Pig Vet Soc 11:197.

——. 1992. *Staphylococcus hyicus* Epidemiology and Virulence in Relation to Exudative Epidermitis in Pigs. Ph.D. diss. Nat Vet Lab and Royal Vet Agric Univ, Copenhagen, Denmark.

——. 1993a. Development of a phage typing system for *Staphylococcus hyicus*. Res Microbiol 144:237–244.

——. 1993b. Diagnostic value of phage typing, antibiogram typing and plasmid profiling of *Staphylococcus hyicus* from piglets with exudative epidermitis. J Vet Med (B) 40:13–20.

Wegener HC, Andresen LO, Bille-Hansen V. 1993. *Staphylococcus hyicus* virulence in relation to exudative epidermitis in the piglet. Can J Vet Res 57:119–125.

Wegener HC, Schwarz, S. 1993. Antibiotic resistance and plasmids in *Staphylococcus hyicus* isolated from pigs with exudative epidermitis and from healthy pigs. Vet Microbiol 35:363–372.

Wegener HC, Skov-Jensen EW. 1992. A longitudinal study of *Staphylococcus hyicus* colonization of vagina of gilts and transmission to piglets. Epidemiol Infect 109:433–444.

Wegener HC, Watts L, Salmon SA, Yancey RJ., Jr. 1994. Antimicrobial susceptibility of *Staphylococcus hyicus* isolated from exudative epidermitis in pigs. J Clin Microbiol 32:793–795.

40 *Haemophilus parasuis*

Vicki J. Rapp-Gabrielson, Simone R. Oliveira, and Carlos Pijoan

Once considered a sporadic disease of young pigs compromised by stress, porcine polyserositis and arthritis (Glässer's disease), caused by *Haemophilus parasuis*, has emerged as one of the significant bacterial diseases affecting swine throughout the world. Adoption of new production technologies resulting in high-health-status herds and the emergence of new respiratory syndromes have contributed to an increase in prevalence and severity of the disease. Disease management with antibiotics, vaccination, and other strategies is not always successful in countering production losses due to *H. parasuis* infection. It has long been known that the immune status of a herd is a determinant of pathogenic outcome of infection (Nielsen and Danielsen 1975). However, the heterogeneity among *H. parasuis* strains is striking, and a better understanding of the association of these phenotypic and genotypic differences with virulence potential and protective immunity has emerged in recent years.

ETIOLOGY

Glässer (1910) first reported the association of a small gram-negative rod with fibrinous serositis and polyarthritis of swine. Initially, the causative agent was identified as *Haemophilus suis* by Hjärre and Wramby (1943) and as *Haemophilus influenza suis* by Lecce (1960). The name was changed to *H. parasuis* based on demonstration that the organism did not require X factor (haemin or other porphyrins) for growth (Biberstein and White 1969; Kilian 1976). The taxonomic position of *H. parasuis* within the Pasteurellaceae is still uncertain, due to a lack of nucleic acid homology with other *Haemophilus* species (De Ley et al. 1990; Dewhirst et al. 1992). Taxonomic studies on the NAD-dependent swine Pasteurellaceae based on nucleic acid hybridization or 16s rRNA gene sequencing have led to the classification of 6 bacterial species (Møller at al. 1996). However, considerable genetic, biochemical, serological, and virulence differences exist among strains provisionally clas-

sified as *Actinobacillus minor, Actinobacillus porcinus,* and *Actinobacilus indolicus*, indicating that these may represent groups of similar organisms rather than clearly defined species (Kielstein et al. 2001). Considerable genotypic heterogeneity has also been demonstrated among *H. parasuis* strains (Smart et al. 1988; Rapp-Gabrielson et al. 1992a; Blackall et al. 1997; Rafiee et al. 2000; Ruiz et al. 2001; Oliveira et al. 2001b; De la Puente Redondo et al. 2003; Oliveira et al. 2003a). It has been proposed that more than one bacterial species may be represented by strains identified as *H. parasuis* (Morozumi et al. 1986; Dewhirst et al. 1992).

Microscopically, *H. parasuis* cells are small, non-motile, pleomorphic rods, varying from single coccobacilli to long, thin, filamentous chains. A capsule can usually be demonstrated, but expression is influenced by in vitro culture (Rapp-Gabrielson et al. 1992b). Thus, the significance of reports associating lack of capsule with virulence needs further investigation (Kobisch and Desmettre 1980; Morozumi and Nicolet 1986a; Kielstein 1991). Nicotinamide adenine dinucleotide (NAD, or V factor) is required for growth and can be supplied by heated blood (chocolate agar) or by satellitic growth in the vicinity of a streak of a staphylococcus strain. After 24–48 hours' growth, colonies are small, translucent, and nonhemolytic on blood agar.

The existence of serovars was first reported by Bakos et al. (1952). In subsequent years, expansion of this serotyping scheme by other investigators led to several proposals for new serovars (Schimmel et al. 1985; Morozumi and Nicolet 1986b; Nicolet et al. 1986; Kielstein 1991; Rapp-Gabrielson and Gabrielson 1992). Presently, 15 serovars based on immunodiffusion (ID) are recognized (Kielstein and Rapp-Gabrielson 1992). The type-specific antigen is heat-stable polysaccharide (Morozumi and Nicolet 1986b) presumed to be capsule or lipopolysaccharide (LPS). Although some geographic differences are apparent, serotyping of isolates from Japan, Germany, Australia, the United States, Canada, Spain, and Denmark shows serovars 4, 5, and 13 to be

Table 40.1.   Prevalence of *Haemophilus parasuis* serovars

	Percent Frequency									
H. parasuis serovar	Japan 1990[b]	Canada & USA1992	Germany 1992	Germany 1998	USA 2003	Canada & USA 2004[c]	Australia 1996,2000	Spain 1999	Spain 2003[c]	Denmark 2004
1	3	2	4	7	7	3	1	3	9	1
2	6	8	6	11	4	8	6	9	6	2
4	9	16	17	11	39	27	7	16	20	13
5	14	23	24	9	2	15	36	18	23	36
7 or 10[a]	—	5	5	4	2	11	5	5	11	3
12	—	7	3	6	7	8	4	3	9	3
13	—	11	5	4	1	13	13	8	3	21
14	—	9	2	0	3	3	0	3	2	1
3,6,8,9,11 or 15	—	4	10	17	8	2	3	6	11	6
Nontypeable	68	14	26	31	27	10	28	29	8	15

Sources: Morikoshi et al. 1990; Rapp-Gabrielson and Gabrielson 1992; Kielstein and Rapp-Gabrielson 1992; Blackall et al. 1996; Kielstein and Wuthe 1998; Rúbies et al. 1999; Rafiee and Blackall 2000; del Rio et al. 2003; Oliveira et al. 2003; Tadjine et al. 2004a; Angen et al. 2004.

[a]Differences between the type strains and field isolates for serovars 7 and 10 have been reported and these serovars cannot always be distinguished by ID (Rapp-Gabrielson 1995, unpublished; Blackall et al. 1996; Rafiee and Blackall 2000; Tadjine et al. 2004).

[b]Only tested for *H. parasuis* serovars 1–7.

[c]Typed by Indirect Hemagglutination (IHA).

most prevalent (Table 40.1). Serovar 15, which is of low prevalence in most countries, was identified in 65% of outdoor units in Hungary/Romania/Serbia (Docic and Bilkei 2004). A large percentage of isolates are nontypeable, indicating that some isolates may not express sufficient type-specific antigen, the presence of antigenic diversity within serovars, or the existence of additional serovars. More recently, indirect hemaglutination (IHA) may also be used to serotype *H. parasuis* (del Rio et al. 2003; Tadjine et al. 2004a; Angen et al. 2004). Initial reports indicated that the IHA technique reduced the percentage of nontypeable isolates from 30% to less than 10% compared to ID. However, Turni and Blackall (2005) reported that a similar high percentage of field isolates were nontypeable by ID and IHA. Discordant results were evident for almost 36% of the isolates they examined, and the IHA test did not identify some serovar 4, 5, 13, and 14 field isolates. They recommend that ID be used as the primary typing method, with IHA as a secondary test.

The heterogeneity of *H. parasuis* isolates can also be demonstrated based on genomic fingerprints by Enterobacterial Repetitive Intergenic Consensus polymerase chain reaction (ERIC-PCR) testing (Figure 40.1) (Rafiee et al. 2000; Ruiz et al. 2001; Oliveira et al. 2003a). With this technique, extensive strain variation within serovar groups has been demonstrated. Analysis of strains from the United States identified at least 12 different strains among serovar 4 isolates. The remaining serovar groups contained either 1 (serovar 5), 2 (serovars 1, 3, and 7), 3 (serovars 12 and 14), or 4 (serovar 2) different strains. There was also high genetic diversity among nontypeable isolates, and at least 18 different strains were identified (Oliveira et al. 2003a).

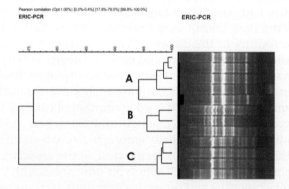

40.1.   Haemophilus parasuis *genotyping by means of ERIC-PCR. Three clusters of genetically related strains are shown in the dendrogram (A, B, and C). The scale represents the percent of similarity between strains.*

EPIDEMIOLOGY

The pig is the natural host for *H. parasuis*. This organism is commonly isolated from nasal secretions and tracheal swabs of healthy swine (Bertschinger and Nicod 1970; Harris et al. 1969; Smart et al. 1989; Cu et al. 1998) and from the lungs of pigs with pneumonia, but not generally from normal lungs (Little 1970; Møller et al. 1993). In conventional herds, *H. parasuis* is one of the earliest and most prevalent bacterial isolates from nasal swabs of pigs at 1 week of age (Kott 1983).

Historically, Glässer's disease has been considered a sporadic disease of young swine compromised by stress. However, the epizootiologic picture in specific pathogen free (SPF) or high-health-status herds that represent an immunologically naive population is much different (Nielsen and Danielsen 1975; Baehler et al. 1974; Menard and Moore 1990). Introduction of *H. parasuis* may result in systemic disease of high morbidity and mortality, affecting swine at any stage of production. In conventional herds that use segregated early weaning (three-site production), late infection with a virulent *H. parasuis* strain can have severe consequences if it occurs when maternal immunity is no longer present. Presently, *H. parasuis* is one of the most serious problems associated with mixing swine from different herds or introduction of new breeding stock into a herd (Smart et al. 1989; Menard and Moore 1990).

There is support for *H. parasuis* as a contributor in the swine respiratory disease complex as a predisposing agent, a secondary invader, or a primary pathogen involved in pneumonia. Demonstration of purulent rhinitis associated with *H. parasuis* colonization supports a possible role as a predisposing factor for other viral and bacterial pathogens (Gois et al. 1983; Vahle et al. 1995, 1997). In pneumonia, *H. parasuis* has often been assumed to be an opportunistic secondary invader, causing disease only in association with other viral or bacterial agents. Such a relationship was evident after accidental infection of pigs experimentally inoculated with pseudorabies virus with *H. parasuis* serovar 4 (Narita et al. 1994). Isolation of *H. parasuis* from pneumonia has increased substantially in recent years and is believed to be associated with the increased prevalence of mycoplasma pneumonia as well as viral respiratory pathogens such as porcine reproductive and respiratory syndrome (PRRS) virus, swine influenza virus, and porcine respiratory coronavirus. *H. parasuis*, in combination with *Mycoplasma hyorhinis*, was isolated from 51.2% of lungs from PRRS-infected swine (Kobayashi et al. 1996). Although an association between PRRS virus and *H. parasuis* appear to be evident in the field, the potential interaction between these two agents has not been substantiated in experimental in vitro or in vivo models (Solano et al. 1997; Cooper et al. 1995; Segalés et al. 1998, 1999). However, Solano et al. (1998) reported that in later stages of infection, pulmonary alveolar macrophages from PRRS virus–infected pigs had a decrease in ability to kill *H. parasuis*. A recent study indicated that pigs harboring a virulent *H. parasuis* strain may develop pneumonia by this agent following PRRS virus challenge (Oliveira et al. 2004d). Several reports support field observations that *H. parasuis* may be a primary agent in pneumonia without the involvement of other pathogens (Pöhle et al. 1992; Barigazzi et al. 1994; Solano et al. 1997; Brockmeier 2004; Müller et al. 2003).

The pathogenic potential of *H. parasuis* strain(s) occurring in a herd is also a factor in the severity and progression of systemic disease. Serovars and strains commonly isolated from upper respiratory sites in swine are not commonly isolated from systemic sites (Bloch 1985; Rapp-Gabrielson 1993; Oliveira et al. 2003a). There may be a subpopulation of *H. parasuis* strains occurring in the respiratory tract that is capable of invading systemi-

Table 40.2. Virulence of strains representing *H. parasuis* serovars for SPF swine

H. parasuis Serovar	No. of Strains Evaluated	Virulence[a]
1, 5, 10, 12, 13, 14	10	Death within 96 hours
2, 4, 15	10	Severe polyserositis and arthritis at necropsy
8	1	Mild clinical signs and gross lesions
3, 6, 7, 9, 11	8	No clinical signs or gross lesions

Source: Kielstein and Rapp-Gabrielson 1992.
[a]Swine inoculated intraperitoneally with 5×10^8 colony-forming units.

cally and causing disease (Rapp et al. 1986; Rapp-Gabrielson 1993).

An association between serovar and isolation from polyserositis was apparent in several studies (Bakos et al. 1952; Morozumi and Nicolet 1986b; Kielstein 1991; Oliveira et al. 2003a; Docic and Bilkei 2004). Differences in virulence among serovars were demonstrated by inoculation of SPF or cesarean-derived, colostrum-deprived (CDCD) swine and guinea pigs with strains representing the 15 serovars (Rapp-Gabrielson et al. 1992b, 1995; Kielstein and Rapp-Gabrielson 1992; Nielsen 1993; Amano et al. 1994, 1996). In these studies, strains representing some serovars were highly virulent and strains representing other serovars were of lesser virulence or avirulent. Virulence of field isolates was consistent with that of the reference strain, indicating a causal relationship between serovar and virulence (Table 40.2). However, the demonstration that two serovar 14 strains differed in virulence for CDCD pigs indicates that factors other than serovar contribute to the virulence potential of a strain (Rapp-Gabrielson et al. 1995).

Sodium dodecyl sulfate-polyacrylamide gel electrophoresis (SDS-PAGE) of whole-cell and outer-membrane (OM) proteins also demonstrates phenotypic heterogeneity among strains (Morozumi and Nicolet 1986a; Rapp et al. 1986; Morikoshi et al. 1990; Rosner et al. 1991; Rapp-Gabrielson et al. 1992a; Ruiz et al. 2001; Oliveira and Pijoan 2004a). These reports indicate a possible association of virulence potential with specific protein patterns, particularly with the presence of 36–38 kDa proteins. However, the precise relationship between protein pattern, serovar, genotype, and virulence potential is complex. Heterogeneity of *H. parasuis* LPS has been demonstrated by SDS-PAGE patterns and immunoblotting with monoclonal antibodies, but LPS patterns have not been associated with virulence (Zucker et al. 1994, 1996; Hueller et al. 1999). Filamentous structures presumed to be fimbriae have been demonstrated on some *H. parasuis* strains, but their role in adhesion or pathogenicity remains to be defined (Münch et al. 1992).

A cell-associated neuraminidase that may function as a virulence factor has been characterized for *H. parasuis* (Lichtensteiger and Vimr 1997, 2003). The future understanding of virulence factors and differences among *H. parasuis* strains lies in newer molecular techniques, such as differential display reverse transcription-polymerase chain reaction (DDRT-PCR), which has recently been used in a search for virulence-associated genes (Hill et al. 2003). The development of new molecular techniques has made significant contributions to an understanding of the epidemiology within a herd and between related herds (reviewed by Oliveira and Pijoan 2004b). Although there is a high genetic diversity among strains affecting unrelated herds, only 2–3 prevalent strains are normally involved in mortality within a herd or related herds (Rafiee et al. 2000; Ruiz et al. 2001; Oliveira et al. 2003a, 2004c). These prevalent strains may persist in affected herds for periods of up to 1 year (Oliveira et al. 2003a, 2004c).

PATHOGENESIS

To overcome the influence of natural infection and maternal antibodies, experimental challenge models using CDCD or naturally farrowed, colostrum-deprived pigs have been developed (Rapp-Gabrielson et al. 1995; Oliveira et al. 2003b). Vahle et al. (1995) examined sequential events in infection by inoculating CDCD pigs intranasally with a virulent strain of *H. parasuis*. Within 12 hours postinoculation, *H. parasuis* was isolated from the nasal cavity and trachea; within 36 hours, from blood cultures; and at 36–108 hours, from systemic tissues. Early colonization of the middle and caudal nasal cavity and trachea was also demonstrated by immunohistochemistry and transmission electron microscopy (Vahle et al. 1997). Colonization was associated with purulent rhinitis, focal loss of cilia, and acute cell swelling within the nasal and tracheal mucosa. In vitro infection of nasal turbinate explants also resulted in marked reduction in ciliary activity and damage to ciliated epithelial cells (Vahle 1996). Bacterial cells were not closely associated with cilia or epithelium, and the mechanism of colonization or cellular destruction was not defined. The observation by these investigators that *H. parasuis* preferentially colonizes the nasal cavity and trachea, and not the tonsil, is in concordance with the ability to isolate *H. parasuis* from the nasal cavity, but not tonsil or lung specimens, from slaughterhouse pigs (Møller et al. 1993). Other studies, however, have demonstrated that *H. parasuis* may not only be isolated from the tonsil of healthy pigs (Oliveira et al. 2001a; Raßbach 1992), but it can also be detected in tonsillar tissue by immunoperoxidase stain and electron microscopic examination (Amano et al. 1994). A recent study suggests that prior infection of the nasal cavity with *Bordetella bronchiseptica* may increase nasal colonization by *H. parasuis* (Brockmeier 2004). However, the role of increased colonization by *H. parasuis* on pathogenesis of infection still remains to be defined.

Mucosal injury may enhance invasion. Microbial and host factors involved with systemic infection are not known; however, the virulence of some strains is remarkable. Intratracheal inoculation of less than 100 colony-forming units of strains representing several serovars caused systemic disease and death in CDCD pigs within a few days (Rapp-Gabrielson et al. 1995). Bacteremia is apparent in pigs in the early stages of infection (Vahle et al. 1995). Septicemic lesions consist of petechiae or ecchymoses in the liver, kidney, and meninges; high levels of endotoxin are detected in plasma, and fibrinous thrombi are present in many organs (Amano et al. 1994). Subsequent replication at multiple serosal surfaces produces the typical fibrinosuppurative polyserositis, polyarthritis, and meningitis observed in field cases (Amano et al. 1994; Vahle et al. 1995). Endotoxin shock and disseminated intravascular coagulation (DIC) may be involved in acute deaths (Amano et al. 1997). Pneumonia was not prominent in one challenge model, even though *H. parasuis* was isolated from the lung (Vahle et al. 1997). Pneumonia was also not evident following inoculation of the reference strains of serovars 1, 4, or 5 (Amano et al. 1994). Differing observations on the ability of *H. parasuis* to produce pneumonia may be due to differences per se in the challenge models, the doses administered, or pathogenic potential of the strains examined.

CLINICAL SIGNS AND LESIONS

Clinical presentation is dependent on the location of inflammatory lesions. In naive herds or pigs, onset is rapid, occurring a few days after exposure. Clinical signs include pyrexia and apathy followed by inappetence and anorexia. Dyspnea, pain (evidenced by squealing), swollen joints, lameness (Figure 40.2A), tremor, incoordination, cyanosis, recumbency, and death may follow. Abortion in gilts and chronic lameness in boars may be sequelae to acute infection. Even if infection of gilts is controlled by antibiotic treatment, pigs in subsequent farrowings may experience severe disease (Menard and Moore 1990). In conventional herds, chronic infections in nursery pigs may result in poorly performing pigs. Cough, dyspnea, weight loss, lameness, and rough hair coat are the primary clinical signs.

Primary macroscopic lesions are a serofibrinous to fibrinopurulent exudate at single or multiple serosal surfaces, including the peritoneum, pericardium, and pleura (Figure 40.2B); articular surfaces, particularly the carpal and tarsal joints, and the meninges may also be involved (Hjärre 1958; Amano et al. 1994). Microscopically, the exudate consists of fibrin, neutrophils, and lesser numbers of macrophages (Figure 40.3) (Vahle et al. 1995). Less commonly, *H. parasuis* infection may result in acute septicemic disease in which cyanosis, sub-

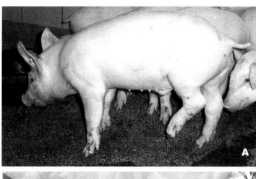

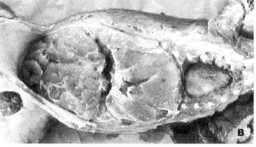

40.2. *Clinical signs and macroscopic lesions characteristic of* Haemophilus parasuis *systemic infection. (A) Lameness. (B) Polyserositis characterized by fibrinous exudate on serosal surfaces (peritoneum and pericardium).*

cutaneous and pulmonary edema, and death can occur without the typical serosal inflammation (Riley et al. 1977; Peet et al. 1983; Desrosiers et al. 1986). Fasciitis and myositis (Hoefling 1991) and purulent rhinitis (Gois et al. 1983; Vahle et al. 1995) have also been reported.

DIAGNOSIS

Diagnosis is usually based on herd history, clinical signs, and necropsy. Bacterial isolation, necessary for confir-

mation, is not always successful. This is due in part to the fragility and fastidious growth requirements of *H. parasuis* relative to other bacteria that may also be present in the specimen. Retrospective analysis of submissions to diagnostic laboratories in Ontario indicate that the true incidence of disease may be tenfold higher than reported, due in part to the inability to confirm the presence of *H. parasuis* from submitted specimens (Miniats et al. 1986). Detection of *H. parasuis* in clinical specimens by PCR or in-situ hybridization is useful for diagnosis when isolation is negative (Segalés et al. 1997; Calsamiglia et al. 1999; Oliveira et al. 2001b; Jung and Chae 2004; Jung et al. 2004). Although these newer molecular techniques may help define the role of *H. parasuis* in the disease process, they are not widely available as diagnostic tools. PCR must be interpreted with caution since the technique does not differentiate between virulent and avirulent organisms. Isolation is still necessary for further characterization of field isolates by serotyping and genotyping (Oliveira and Pijoan 2004b). Necropsies should be performed not only on pigs with severe clinical signs and lesions but also on pigs in the acute phase of disease, prior to administration of antibiotics. Isolation rates are considerably higher when samples are collected from euthanized pigs rather than from pigs found dead (Oliveira et al. 2002). The best chance for isolation is by culturing several serosal surfaces or exudates, cerebrospinal fluid, and heart blood, even if lesions are mild or not apparent. *H. parasuis* can be recovered from these fluids when inoculated into a transport medium prior to shipment to the diagnostic laboratory (Mendez-Trigo and Trigo 1996; del Rio et al. 2003a). Although somewhat laborious for routine diagnosis, special dilution techniques followed by plating on selective media containing antibiotics have been used successfully for culturing *H. parasuis* in high numbers from

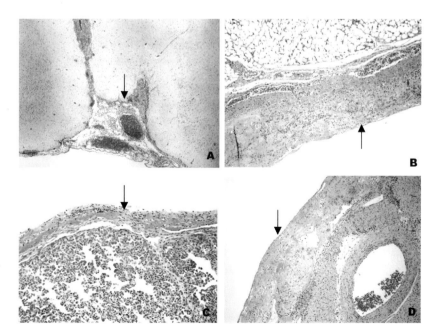

40.3. *Microscopic lesions characteristic of* Haemophilus parasuis *systemic infection. (A) Brain, meningitis. (B) Synovial membrane, arthritis. (C) Lung, pleuritis. (D) Heart, pericarditis. Arrows indicate fibrinous exudate containing inflammatory cells on the surface of affected organs.*

Table 40.3. Differential biochemical reactions of swine NAD-dependent *Pasteurellaceae*

Biochemical Characteristic	*Haemophilos parasuis*	Other NAD-dependent Pasteurellaceae				
		Actinobacillus pleuropneumoniae	*Actinobacillus minor*	*Haemophilus* Taxon C	*Actinobacillus porcinus*	*Actinobacillus indolicus*
Urease	−	+	+	−	−	−
Hemolysis	−	+	−	−	−	−
Indole	−	−	−	−	−	+
Fermentation of						
Glucose	+	+	+	+	±	+
Lactose	−	−	+	−	±	±
Sucrose	+	+	+	+	±	+
Mannitol	−	+	−	−	±	±
Xylose	−	+	±	−	±	±
L-Arabinose	−	−	−	+	±	−
Raffinose	−	−	+	+	±	+

Sources: Møller and Kilian 1990; Rapp-Gabrielson and Gabrielson 1992; Møller et al. 1996; Kielstein et al. 2001.

Note: *A. minor* was formerly known as *Haemophilus* taxon "Minor Group"; *A. porcinus* was formerly known as *Haemophilus* sp. taxons D or E; *A. indolicus* was formerly known as *Haemophilus* sp. taxon F. Taxon C has infrequently been isolated from swine.

Key: + indicates greater than 90% of isolates are positive; −, less than 10% of isolates positive; ±, variable reactions among isolates.

respiratory specimens (Møller and Kilian 1990; Møller et al. 1993; Kirkwood et al. 2001). The use of defibrinated horse blood and tryptose blood agar base, rather than bovine or sheep blood and trypticase soy agar, also appears to enhance growth.

Biochemical tests are required to distinguish *H. parasuis* from other NAD or V factor–dependent organisms belonging to the family *Pasteurellaceae* that have been isolated from swine (Table 40.3). Occasionally misidentified as *H. parasuis*, these other NAD-dependent organisms are present in high numbers in the nasal cavity, tonsils, or lungs and are generally believed to be of low pathogenic potential (Møller and Kilian 1990; Møller et al. 1993; Chiers et al. 2001). However, recent analysis of *A. minor, A. porcinus*, and *A. indolicus* strains indicate that it is not uncommon for these organisms to be isolated in pure culture from lungs with inflammatory changes and that their possible role in respiratory disease should be reevaluated (Kielstein and Wuthe 1998; Kielstein et al. 2001).

Several different strains, distinguishable by genotype or serovar may be present in a herd, or even in different specimens from a single pig (Smart et al. 1989; Rapp-Gabrielson and Gabrielson 1992; Rapp-Gabrielson 1993; Kirkwood et al. 2001; Oliveira et al. 2003a). Thus, recovery from systemic sites or gross lesions is the only assurance that the isolate obtained is involved in the disease process. Serotyping and genotyping, critical to an understanding of the epidemiology of the disease outbreak and immune response to infection or vaccination, are available only at a few diagnostic laboratories.

Differential diagnosis should include septicemic bacterial infections caused by *Streptococcus suis, Erysipelothrix rhusiopathiae, Actinobacillus suis, Salmonella choleraesuis* var. kunzendorf, and *Escherichia coli. Mycoplasma hyorhinis* polyserositis and arthritis in 3–10-week-old pigs produces lesions similar to *H. parasuis*. The signifi-

cance of *H. parasuis* in bronchopneumonia can be ascertained only after identification of other viral and bacterial pathogens that may be involved in the multifactoral disease process.

TREATMENT

Prophylactic use of antibiotics or therapeutic oral medication may be of little value in severe *H. parasuis* outbreaks (Madsen 1984; Wiseman et al. 1989; Menard and Moore 1990). High antibiotic doses should be administered parenterally as soon as clinical signs have manifested, and all pigs in the affected group, not just those showing signs, should be treated (Desrosiers et al. 1986). Penicillin has been considered the drug of choice, but one study reported an increasing resistance to penicillin has been reported (Kielstein and Leirer 1990). Most *H. parasuis* strains are also sensitive in vitro to ampicillin, ceftiofur, ciprofloxacin, enrofloxicin, erythromycin, florphenicol, gentamicin, spectinomycin, tiamulin, tilmicosin, and potentiated sulfas (Kielstein 1985; Trigo et al. 1996; Vonaltrock 1998; Wissing et al. 2001; Aarestrup et al. 2004). In some regions, a number of strains show higher resistance to tetracycline, erythromycin, streptomycin, kanamycin, gentamicin, sulfonamide, and lincosamide (Trigo et al. 1996; Wissing et al. 2001). Oral amoxicillin, either administered through the water or as a feed additive, may be the drug of choice, but is effective mostly when given before clinical signs become apparent.

PREVENTION AND IMMUNITY

Because nasal mucosa of baby pigs may be colonized before 1 week of age, elimination of *H. parasuis* by early weaning alone is unlikely to be successful. Clark et al. (1994) evaluated several medicated early-weaning strategies and found that *H. parasuis* could be eliminated only when parenteral and oral administration of high doses of antibiotics to baby pigs was a part of the treatment. Elimination of *H. parasuis* from a herd may not be desirable, inasmuch as subsequent mixing of naive pigs with pigs harboring *H. parasuis* during later stages in production may result in a disease course with devastating economic losses. Introduction of new breeding stock from a herd with a different health background should include isolation and acclimation periods long enough to allow for development of protective immunity from either vaccination or natural exposure.

Maternal and natural immunity are critical factors for controlling the disease process (Nielsen and Danielsen 1975; Blanco et al. 2004). Swine previously exposed to nonpathogenic *H. parasuis* strains develop resistance to subsequent challenge with virulent strains (Nielsen 1993). Vaccination of gilts resulted in protective maternal immunity for up to 4 weeks when weaned piglets were challenged with the same serovar contained in the bacterin (Solano et al. 1998; Solano-Aguilar et al. 1999; Baumann and Bilkei 2002; Hoffmann and Bilkei 2002). Because of the septicemic nature of the disease, antibodies are probably a major protective immune mechanism. Tadijine et al. (2004b) characterized two mononoclonal antibodies that recognized an OM protein epitope or an LPS-associated polysaccharide epitope, both of which were common to all *H. parasuis* isolates. They demonstrated that both antibodies were involved in protecting mice against lethal infection and that antibodies to these same epitopes occurred in sera from naturally infected swine.

Controlled exposure has been proposed as an alternative technique to control disease in the field (Pijoan et al. 1997; Oliveira et al. 2001a, 2004c). The main objective of this technique is to expose young piglets to a low dose of the prevalent *H. parasuis* strains involved in herd mortality while pigs are still protected by maternal immunity, thus allowing the piglet to develop natural immunity. Although this technique has been shown to effectively reduce nursery mortality, there are legitimate concerns regarding the safety of exposing young pigs to live, virulent *H. parasuis*. Sow vaccination may reduce the risks of systemic infection in exposed piglets. Concurrent PRRS virus infection may predispose pigs to systemic infection by the *H. parasuis* strain used for colonization (Oliveira et al. 2004d).

There are numerous reports of successful disease control by vaccination with commercial or herd-specific (autogenous) bacterins (Nielsen and Danielsen 1975; Riising 1981; Wiseman et al. 1989; Menard and Moore 1990; Schimmel et al. 1992; Kirkwood et al. 2001; Takahashi et al. 2001). There are also instances where bacterins are not efficacious, and these may be due to lack of cross-protection for the strain or serovar involved in the disease process or when the timing of vaccination is inappropriate. Cross-protection against other virulent

strains is not always evident in experimental challenge models (Miniats et al. 1991; Kielstein and Raßbach 1991; Rapp-Gabrielson et al. 1997). Although cross-protection is primarily a concern for commercial bacterins, autogenous bacterins may also lack efficacy because of the presence of more than one strain or serovar or the subsequent introduction of a new strain into the herd. Several factors should be taken into account when selecting isolates to be included in autogenous bacterins. Isolates recovered from systemic sites are preferred and genotyping can be used to define the clusters of genetically related strains affecting the herd. A representative isolate from each prevalent cluster should be included in the autogenous bacterin. Isolates recovered from new clinical cases should be genotyped and compared with those included in the vaccine (Oliveira et al. 2002, 2004c).

Efficacy of vaccination against challenge with different strains of the same serovar, as well as cross-protection against some heterologous serovars, has been demonstrated. A commercial bacterin containing *H. parasuis* serovars 4 and 5 has been shown to protect against experimental challenge with strains representing serovars 12, 13, or 14, but not against serovar 2 (Rapp-Gabrielson et al. 1996, 1997). Lack of cross-protection between serovar 2 and 5 bacterins was also reported by Takahashi et al. (2001). A bacterin containing *H. parasuis* serovar 5 that is commercially available in Europe showed some cross-protection against serovars 1, 12, 13, and 14 (Bak and Riising 2002).

Strains representing nine serovars, as well as nontypeable strains, have been demonstrated to be virulent. Demonstration that virulent strains may not protect against challenge with different strains of the same serovar, or even against challenge with the homologous strain, indicates that the protective antigens may not be identical to the virulence factors or the type-specific antigens (Kielstein and Raßbach 1991; Rapp-Gabrielson et al. 1997). Because of the heterogeneity of strains with pathogenic potential and the current lack of understanding of protective antigens and virulence factors, it is unlikely that any bacterin will provide cross-immunity against all strains of etiologic significance in the swine population. Control programs may include vaccination and antibiotic treatments but also should address management practices to reduce or eliminate other respiratory pathogens, tighten weaning age and pig flow, and eliminate mixing of pigs at all stages of production.

REFERENCES

Aarestrup FM, Seyfarth AM, Angen Ø. 2004. Antimicrobial susceptibility of *Haemophilus parasuis* and *Histophilus somni* from pigs and cattle in Denmark. Vet Microbiol 101:143–146.

Amano H, Shibata M, Kajio N, Morozumi T. 1994. Pathologic observations of pigs intranasally inoculated with serovar 1, 4, and 5 of *Haemophilus parasuis* using immunoperoxidase method. J Vet Med Sci 56:639–644.

———. 1996. Pathogenicity of *Haemophilus parasuis* serovars 4 and 5 in contact-exposed pigs. J Vet Med Sci 58:559–561.

Amano H, Shibata M, Takahashi K, Sasaki Y. 1997. Effects of endotoxin pathogenicity in pigs with acute septicemia of *Haemophilus parasuis* infection. J Vet Med Sci 59:451–455.

Angen Ø, Svensmark B, Mittal KR. 2004. Serological characterization of Danish *Haemophilus parasuis* isolates. Vet Microbiol 103:255–258.

Baehler JF, Burgisser H, de Meuron P A, Nicolet J. 1974. Infection à *Haemophilus parasuis* chez le porc. Schweiz Arch Tierheilkd 116:183–188.

Bak H, Riising H-J. 2002. Protection of vaccinated pigs against experimental infections with homologous and heterologous *Haemophilus parasuis*. Vet Record 151:502–505.

Bakos K, Nilsson A, Thal E. 1952. Untersuchungen über Haemophilus suis. Nord Vet-Med 4:241–255.

Barigazzi G, Valenza F, Bollo E, Guarda F, Candotti P, A Raffo, Foni E. 1994. Anatomohistopathological features related to *Haemophilus parasuis* infection in pigs. Proc Int Congr Pig Vet Soc 13:235.

Baumann G, Bilkei G. 2002. Effect of vaccinating sows and their piglets on the development of Glässer's disease induced by a virulent strain of *Haemophilus parasuis* serovar 5. Vet Record 151:18–21.

Bertschinger HU, Nicod B. 1970. Untersuchungen über die Nasenflora bei Schweinen Vergleich zwischen SPF-Herden und schwedisch sanierten Herden. Schweiz Arch Tierheilkd 112:493–499.

Biberstein EL, White, DC. 1969. A proposal for the establishment of two new Haemophilus species. J Med Microbiol 2:75–78.

Blackall PJ, Rapp-Gabrielson VJ, Hampson DJ. 1996. Serological characterization of *Haemophilus parasuis* isolates from Australian pigs. Aust Vet J 73:93–95.

Blackall PJ, Trott DJ, Rapp-Gabrielson V, Hampson DJ. 1997. Analysis of *Haemophilus parasuis* by multilocus enzyme electrophoresis. Vet Microbiol 56:125–134.

Blanco I, Galina-Pantoja L, Oliveira S, Pijoan C, Sanchez C, Canals A. 2004. Comparison between *Haemophilus parasuis* infection in colostrums-deprived and sow-reared piglets. Vet Microbiol. 103:21–27.

Bloch IJM. 1985. Beitrag zur Epidemiologie, Serologie und Polyacrylamid-Gelelektrophorese von *Haemophilus parasuis*. Diss. Univ Bern.

Brockmeier SL. 2004. Prior infection with *Bordetella bronchiseptica* increases nasal colonization by *Haemophilus parasuis* in swine. Vet Microbiol 99:75–78.

Calsamiglia M, Pijoan C, Solano G, Rapp-Gabrielson V. 1999. Development of an oligonucleotide-specific capture plate hybridization assay for detection of *Haemophilus parasuis*. J Vet Diagn Invest 11:140–145.

Chiers K, Haesebrouck F, Mateusen B, Van Overbeke I, Ducatelle R. 2001. Pathogenicity of *Actinobacillus minor*, *Actinobacillus indolicus* and *Actinobacillus porcinus* strains for gnotobiotic pigs. J Vet Med B 48:127–131.

Clark LK, Hill MA, Kniffen TS, Van Alstine W, Stevenson G, Meyer KB, Wu CC, Scheidt AB, Knox K, Albregts S. 1994. An evaluation of the components of medicated early weaning. Swine Health and Production 2:5–11.

Cooper VL, Doster AR, Hesse RA, Harris NB. 1995. Porcine reproductive and respiratory syndrome: NEB-1 PRRSV infection did not potentiate bacterial pathogens. J Vet Diagn Invest 7:313–320.

Cu HP, Nguyen NN, Do NT. 1998. Prevalence of *Haemophilus* sp infection in the upper respiratory tract of pigs and some characteristics of the isolates. Khoa Hoc Ky Thuat Thu Y 5:88–93.

de la Puente Redondo VA, Méndez JN, García del Blanco N, Boronat NL, Gutiérrez Martín CB, Rodríguez Ferri EF. 2003. Typing of *Haemophilus parasuis* strains by PCF-RFLP analysis of the *tbpA* gene. Vet Microbiol 92:253–262.

De Ley J, Mannheim W, Mutters R, Piechulla K, Tytgat R, Segers P, Bisgaard M, Frederiksen W, Hinz KH, Vanhoucke M. 1990. Inter- and intrafamilial similarities of rRNS cistrons of the Pasteurellaceae. Int J Sys Bacteriol 40:126–137.

del Rio ML, Gutiérrez B, Gutiérrez CB, Monter JL, Rodriguez Ferri EF. 2003a. Evaluation of survival of *Actinobacillus pleuropneumoniae* and *Haemophilus parasuis* in four liquid media and two swab specimen transport systems. Am J Vet Res 64: 1176–1180.

del Rio ML, Gutiérrez CB, Rodríguez Ferri EF. 2003b. Value of indirect hemagglutination and coagglutination tests for serotyping *Haemophilus parasuis*. J Clin Microbiol 41:880–882.

Desrosiers R, Phaneuf JB, Broes A. 1986. An outbreak of atypical Glässer's disease in Quebec. Proc Int Congr Pig Vet Soc 9:277.

Dewhirst FE, Paster BJ, Olsen I, Fraser GJ. 1992. Phylogeny of 54 representative strains of species in the family Pasteurellaceae as determined by comparison of 16S rRNA sequences. J Bacteriol 174:2002–2013.

Docic M, Bilkei G. 2004. Prevalence of *Haemophilus parasuis* serotypes in large outdoor and indoor pig units in Hungary/ Romania/Serbia. Berl Münch Tierärztl Wschr 117:271–273.

Glässer K. 1910. Untersuchungen über die Schweineseuche mit besonderer Berücksichtigung ihrer Ätiologie and Pathologie. Dtsch Tierärztl Wschr 18:729–733.

Gois M, Barnes HJ, Ross RF. 1983. Potentiation of turbinate atrophy in pigs by long-term nasal colonization with Pasteurella multocida. Am J Vet Res 44:372–378.

Harris DL, Ross RF, Switzer WP. 1969. Incidence of certain microorganisms in nasal cavities of swine in Iowa. Am J Vet Res 30:1621–1624.

Hill CE, Metcalf DS, MacInnes JI. 2003. A search for virulence genes of *Haemophilus parasuis* using differential display RT-PCR. Vet Microbiol 96:189–202.

Hjärre A. 1958. Enzootic virus pneumonia and Glässer's disease of swine. Adv Vet Sci 4:235–263.

Hjärre A, Wramby G. 1943. Über die fibrinöse Serosa-Gelenkentzündung (Glässer) beim Schwein. Z Infektionskr Parasitenkd Krankheit Hyg Haustiere 60:37–64.

Hoefling DC. 1991. Acute myositis associated with *Haemophilus parasuis* in primary SPF sows. J Vet Diagn Invest 3:354–355.

Hoffmann CR, Bilkei G. 2002. The effect of a homologous bacterin given to sows prefarrowing on the development of Glässer's disease in postweaning pigs after i.v. challenge with *Haemophilus parasuis* serotype 5. Dtsch Tierarztl Wochenschr 109:271–276.

Hueller E, Gottschaldt J, Drexler S. 1999. Immunoblot assays for differentiation of *Haemophilus parasuis*. Tierarztl Umschau 54:331–335.

Jung K, Chae C. 2004. In-situ hybridization for the detection of *Haemophilus parasuis* in naturally infected pigs. J Comp Path 130:294–298.

Jung K, Ha Y, Kim S-H, Chae C. 2004. Development of polymerase chain reaction and comparison with in situ hybridization for the detection of *Haemophilus parasuis* in formalin-fixed paraffin-embedded tissues. J Vet Med Sci 66:841–845.

Kielstein P. 1985. Zur Glässerschen Krankheit und Chemotherapeutika-Empfindichkeit ihres Erregers. Mh Vet-Med 40:801–809.

———. 1991. Zur Glässerschen Krankheit des Schweines Untersuchungen über Zusammenhänge zwischen serologischen Eigenschaften, Kapselausbildung und Virulenz von Haemophilus-parasuis-Stämmen. Mh Vet-Med 46:137–142.

Kielstein P, Leirer R. 1990. Zur Glässerschen Krankheit des Schweines—Ätiologisch-epizootiologische Untersuchungen zum Erregerspektrum. Mh Vet-Med 45:577–582.

Kielstein P, Rapp-Gabrielson VJ. 1992. Designation of 15 serovars of *Haemophilus parasuis* based on immunodiffusion using heat-stable antigen extracts. J Clin Microbiol 30:862–865.

Kielstein P, Raßbach A. 1991. Serologische Typisierung und Nachweis immunogener Kreuzreaktionen von *Haemophilus parasuis* (Glässersche Krankheit). Mh Vet-Med 46:586–589.

Kielstein P, Wuthe H-H. 1998. Isolation of *Actinobacillus pleuropneumoniae, Haemophilus parasuis* and related bacteria from the organs of pigs in Schleswig-Holstein. Tierärztl Umschau 53:250–258.

Kielstein P, Wuthe H-H, Angen Ø, Mutters R, Ahrens P. 2001. Phenotypic and genetic characterization of NAD-dependent Pasteurellaceae from the respiratory tract of pigs and their possible pathogenetic importance. Vet Microbiol 81:243–255.

Kilian M. 1976. A taxonomic study of the genus Haemophilus, with the proposal of a new species. J Gen Microbiol 93:9–62.

Kirkwood RN, Rawluk SA, Cegielski AC, Otto AJ. 2001. Effect of pig age and autogenous sow vaccination on nasal mucosal colonization of pigs by *Haemophilus parasuis*. J. Swine Health Prod 9:77–79.

Kobayashi H, Morozumi T, Miyamoto C, Shimizu M, Yamada S, Ohashi S, Kubo M, Kimura K, Mitani K, Ito N, Yamamota K. 1996. Mycoplasma hyorhinis infection levels in lungs of piglets with porcine reproductive and respiratory syndrome (PRRS). J Vet Med Sci 58:109–113.

Kobisch M, Desmettre P. 1980. Hemophilose du porc: Pouvoir pathogène expérimental de deux souches d'*Haemophilus parasuis*. Rec Méd Vét 156:219–224.

Kott BE. 1983. Chronological Studies of Respiratory Disease in Baby Pigs. M.S. thesis, Iowa State Univ, Ames.

Lecce JG. 1960. Porcine polyserositis with arthritis: Isolation of a fastidious pleuropneumonialike organism and Haemophilus influenzae suis. Ann NY Acad Sci 79:670–676.

Lichtensteiger CA, Vimr ER. 1997. Neuraminidase (sialidase) activity of *Haemophilus parasuis*. FEMS Microbiol Lett 152:269–274.

——. 2003. Purification and renaturation of membrane neuraminidase from *Haemophilus parasuis*. Vet Microbiol 93:79–87.

Little TWA. 1970. Haemophilus infection in pigs. Vet Rec 87:399–402.

Madsen P. 1984. Atypical outbreaks of Glässer's disease in Danish pig herds. Proc Int Congr Pig Vet Soc 8:107.

Menard J, Moore C. 1990. Epidemiology and management of Glässer's disease in SPF herds. In Proc 21st Annu Meet Am Assoc Swine Pract, Denver, pp. 187–200.

Mendez-Trigo AV, Trigo E. 1996. Viability of *Haemophilus parasuis* in tissues, exudates and pure culture swabs. Proc Int Congr Pig Vet Soc 14:314.

Miniats OP, Smart NL, Metzger K. 1986. Glässer's disease in southwestern Ontario. I. A retrospective study. Proc Int Congr Pig Vet Soc 9:279.

Miniats OP, Smart NL, Rosendal S. 1991. Cross protection among *Haemophilus parasuis* strains in immunized gnotobiotic pigs. Can J Vet Res 55:37–41.

Møller K, Andersen LV, Christensen G, Kilian M. 1993. Optimization of the detection of NAD dependent Pasteurellaceae from the respiratory tract of slaughterhouse pigs. Vet Microbiol 36:261–271.

Møller K, Fussing V, Grimont PAD, Paster BJ, Dewhirst FE, Kilian M. 1996. *Actinobacillus minor* sp. nov., *Actinobacillus porcinus* sp. nov., and *Actinobacillus indolicus* sp. nov., three new V factor–dependent species from the respiratory tract of pigs. Int J Syst Bacteriol 46:951–956.

Møller K, Kilian M. 1990. V factor–dependent members of the family Pasteurellaceae in the porcine upper respiratory tract. J Clin Microbiol 28:2711–2716.

Morikoshi T, Kobayashi K, Kamino T, Owaki S, Hayashi S, Hirano S. 1990. Characterization of *Haemophilus parasuis* isolated in Japan. Jpn J Vet Sci 52:667–669.

Morozumi T, Nicolet J. 1986a. Morphological variations of *Haemophilus parasuis* strains. J Clin Microbiol 23:138–142.

——. 1986b. Some antigenic properties of *Haemophilus parasuis* and a proposal for serological classification. J Clin Microbiol 23:1022–1025.

Morozumi T, Pauli U, Braun R, Nicolet J. 1986. Deoxyribonucleic acid relatedness among strains of *Haemophilus parasuis* and other Haemophilus spp. of swine origin. Int J System Bacteriol 36:17–19.

Müller G, Köhler H, Diller R, Raßbach A, Berndt A, Schimmel D. 2003. Influences of naturally occurring and experimentally induced porcine pneumonia on blood parameters. Res Vet Sci 74:23–30.

Münch S, Grund S, Krüger M. 1992. Fimbriae and membranes on *Haemophilus parasuis*. Zentralbl Veterinarmed (B) 39:59–64.

Narita M, Kawashima K, Matsuura S, Uchimura A, Miura Y. 1994. Pneumonia in pigs infected with pseudorabies virus and *Haemophilus parasuis* serovar 4. J Comp Path 110:329–339.

Nicolet J, Morozumi T, Bloch I. 1986. Proposal for a serological classification of *H. parasuis*. Proc Int Congr Pig Vet Soc 9:260.

Nielsen R. 1993. Pathogenicity and immunity studies of *Haemophilus parasuis* serotypes. Acta Vet Scand 34:193–198.

Nielsen R, Danielsen V. 1975. An outbreak of Glässer's disease: Studies on etiology, serology and the effect of vaccination. Nord Vet-Med 27:20–25.

Oliveira S, Batista L, Torremorell M, Pijoan C. 2001a. Experimental colonization of piglets and gilts with systemic strains of *Haemophilus parasuis* and *Streptococcus suis* to prevent disease. Can J Vet Res 65:161–167.

Oliveira S, Galina L, Pijoan C. 2001b. Development of a PCR test to diagnose *Haemophilus parasuis* infections. J Vet Diagn Invest 13:495–501.

Oliveira S, Pijoan C, Morrison R. 2002. Role of *Haemophilus parasuis* in nursery mortality. Proc Allen D. Leman Swine Conf, p. 111.

Oliveira S, Blackall PJ, Pijoan C. 2003a. Characterization of the diversity of *Haemophilus parasuis* field isolates by the use of serotyping and genotyping. Am J vet Res 64:435–442.

Oliveira S, Galina L, Blanco I, Canals A, Pijoan C. 2003b. Naturally farrowed, artificially-reared pigs as an alternative model for experimental infection by *Haemophilus parasuis*. Can Vet J 67:146–150.

Oliveira S, Pijoan C. 2004a. Computer-based analysis of *Haemophilus parasuis* protein fingerprints. Can J. Vet Res 68:71–75.

——. 2004b. *Haemophilus parasuis*: New trends on diagnosis, epidemiology and control. Vet Microbiol 99:1–12.

Oliveira S, Pijoan C, Morrison R. 2004c. Evaluation of *Haemophilus parasuis* control in the nursery using vaccination and controlled exposure. J Swine Health and Production 12(3):123–128.

Oliveira S, Mahlberg J, Simonson R. 2004d. Safety of controlled exposure to *Haemophilus parasuis*: The role of sow vaccination and PRRSV infection. Proc Int Congr Pig Vet Soc 18:89.

Peet RL, Fry J, Lloyd J, Henderson J, Curran J, Moir D. 1983. *Haemophilus parasuis* septicaemia in pigs. Aust Vet J 60:187.

Pijoan C, Torremorell M, Solano G. 1997. Colonization patterns by the bacterial flora of young pigs. Proc Am Assoc Swine Pract, pp. 463–464.

Pöhle D, Johannsen U, Kielstein P, Raßbach A, Wiegand M. 1992. Investigations on pathology and pathogenesis of *Haemophilus parasuis* infection of swine. Proc Int Congr Pig Vet Soc 12:335.

Rafiee M, Bara M, Stephens CP, Blackall PJ. 2000. Application of ERIC-PCR for the comparison of isolates of *Haemophilus parasuis*. Aust Vet J 78:846–849.

Rafiee M, Blackall PJ. 2000. Establishment, validation and use of the Kielstein-Rapp-Gabrielson serotyping scheme for *Haemophilus parasuis*. Aust Vet J 78(3):172–174.

Rapp VJ, Ross RF, Nicolet J. 1986. Characterization of the outer membrane proteins of *Haemophilus parasuis*. Proc Int Congr Pig Vet Soc 9:262.

Rapp-Gabrielson VJ. 1993. *Haemophilus parasuis*: The association of serovar with prevalence, pathogenicity, and immunogenicity. Proc Allen D Leman Swine Conf, St. Paul 20:31–33.

Rapp-Gabrielson VJ, Gabrielson DA. 1992. Prevalence of *Haemophilus parasuis* serovars among isolates from swine. Am J Vet Res 53:659–664.

Rapp-Gabrielson VJ, Gabrielson DA, Musser JM. 1992a. Phenotypic and genotypic diversity of *Haemophilus parasuis*. Proc Int Congr Pig Vet Soc 12:334.

Rapp-Gabrielson VJ, Gabrielson DA, Schamber GJ. 1992b. Comparative virulence *of Haemophilus parasu*is serovars 1 to 7 pguinea pigs. Am J Vet Res 53:987–994.

Rapp-Gabrielson VJ, Kocur GJ, Clark JT, Muir SK. 1995. Virulence of different serovars of *Haemophilus parasuis* for cesarean-derived, colostrum-deprived pigs. In Haemophilus, Actinobacillus, and Pasteurella. W Donachie, FA Lainson, JC Hodgson, eds. New York: Plenum Press, p. 204.

——. 1997. *Haemophilus parasuis*: Immunity in swine following vaccination. Vet Med 92:83–90.

Rapp-Gabrielson VJ, Kocur G, Clark J, Muir S, White R. 1996. Efficacy and duration of immunity of the *Haemophilus parasuis* fractions of Suvaxyn RespiFend MH/HPS. Proc Int Congr Pig Vet Soc 14:300.

Raßbach A. 1992. Biochemical and serological typing of *Haemophilus parasuis*. Monatsh Veterinaermed 47:637–641.

Riising HJ. 1981. Prevention of Glässer's Disease through Immunity to *Haemophilus parasuis*. Zentralbl Veterinarmed (B) 28:630–638.

Riley MGI, Russell EG, Callinan RB. 1977. *Haemophilus parasuis* infection in swine. J Am Vet Med Assoc 171:649–651.

Rosner H, Kielstein P, Müller W, Rohrmann B. 1991. Beziehung zwischen Serotyp, Virulenz und SDS-PAGE Proteinmustern von *Haemophilus parasuis*. Dtsch Tierärztl Wschr 98:327–330.

Rúbies X, Kielstein P, Costa Ll, Riera P, Artigas C, Espuña E. 1999. Prevalence of *Haemophilus parasuis* serovars isolated in Spain from 1993 to 1997. Vet Microbiol 66:245–248.

Ruiz A, Oliveira S, Torremorell M, Pijoan C. 2001. Outer membrane proteins and DNA profiles in strains of *Haemophilus parasuis* recovered from systemic and respiratory sites. J Clin Microbiol 39:1757–1762.

Schimmel D, Hogg A, Uhlemann J. 1992. Prevention of *Haemophilus parasuis* infection with an inactivated vaccine. Proc Int Congr Pig Vet Soc 12:336.

Schimmel D, Kielstein P, Hass R. 1985. Zur serologische Typisierung von *Haemophilus parasuis*. Arch Exp Vet Med, Leipzig 39:944–947.

Segalés J, Domingo M, Balasch M, Solano GI, Pijoan, C. 1998. Ultrastructural study of porcine alveolar macrophages infected in vitro with porcine reproductive and respiratory syndrome (PRRS) virus, with and without *Haemophilus parasuis*. J Comp Path 118:231–243.

Segalés J, Domingo M, Solano GI, Pijoan C. 1997. Immunohistochemical detection of *Haemophilus parasuis* serovar 5 in formalin-fixed, paraffin-embedded tissues of experimentally infected swine. J Vet Diagn Invest 9:237–243.

——. 1999. Porcine reproductive and respiratory syndrome virus and *Haemophilus parasuis* antigen distribution in dually infected pigs. Vet Microbiol 64:287–297.

Smart NL, Miniats OP, MacInnes JI. 1988. Analysis of *Haemophilus parasuis* isolates from southern Ontario swine by restriction endonuclease fingerprinting. Can J Vet Res 52:319–324.

Smart NL, Miniats OP, Rosendal S, Friendship R. 1989. Glässer's disease and prevalence of subclinical infection with *Haemophilus parasuis* in swine in southern Ontario. Can Vet J 30:339–343.

Solano G, Bautista E, Molitor T, Segalés J, Pijoan, C. 1998. Effect of procine reproductive and respiratory syndrome virus infection on the clearance of *Haemophilus parasuis* by porcine alveolar macrophages. Can J Vet Res 62:251–256.

Solano G, Ségales J, Collins J, Molitor T, Pijoan, C. 1997. Porcine reproductive and respiratory syndrome virus (PRRSv) interaction with *Haemophilus parasuis*. Vet Microbiol 55:247–257.

Solano-Aguilar GI, Pijoan C, Rapp-Gabrielson V, Collins J, Carvalho LF, Winkelman N. 1999. Protective role of maternal antibodies against *Haemophilus parasuis* infection. Am J Vet Res 60:81–87.

Tadjine M, Mittal KR, Bourdon S, Gottschalk M. 2004a. Development of a new serological test for serotyping *Haemophilus parasuis* isolates and determination of their prevalence in North America. J Clin Microbiol 24:839–840.

——. 2004b. Production and characterization of murine monoclonal antibodies against *Haemophilus parasuis* and study of their protective role in mice. Microbiol 150:3935–3945.

Takahashi K, Nagai S, Yagihashi T, Ikehata T, Nakano Y, Senna K, Maruyama T, Murofushi J. 2001. A cross-protection experiment in pigs vaccinated with *Haemophilus parasuis* serovars 2 and 5 bacterins, and evaluation of a bivalent vaccine under laboratory and field conditions. J Vet Med Sci 63:487–491.

Trigo E, Mendez-Trigo AV, Simonson R. 1996. Antimicrobial susceptibility profiles of *Haemophilus parasuis*: A retrospective study from clinical cases submitted during 1994 and 1995 to a veterinary diagnostic laboratory. Proc Int Congr Pig Vet Soc 14:313.

Turni C, Blackall PJ. 2005. Comparison of the indirect haemagglutination and gel diffusion test for serotyping *Haemophilus parasuis*. Vet Microbiol 106:145–151.

Vahle JL. 1996. Pathogenesis of *Haemophilus parasuis* infection in swine. Ph.D. diss., Iowa State Univ, Ames.

Vahle JL, Harness JS, Andrews JJ. 1995. Experimental reproduction of *Haemophilus parasuis* infection in swine: Clinical, bacteriological, and morphologic findings. J Vet Diagn Invest 7:476–480.

Vahle JL, Haynes JS, Andrews JJ. 1997. Interaction of *Haemophilus parasuis* with nasal and tracheal mucosa following intranasal inoculation of cesarean derived colostrum deprived (CDCD) swine. Can J Vet Res 61:200–206.

Vonaltrock A. 1998. Occurrence of bacterial agents in lungs of pigs and evaluation of their resistance to antibiotics. Berl Münch Tierärztl Wschr 111:164–172.

Wiseman B, Harris DL, Glock RD, Wilkins L. 1989. Management of seedstock that is negative for *Haemophilus parasuis*. In Proc 20th Annu Meet Am Assoc Swine Pract, Des Moines, pp. 23–25.

Wissing A, Nicolet J, Boerlin P. 2001. Die aktuelle antimikrobielle resistenzsituation in der schweizerischen veterinärmedizen. Schweiz Arch Tierheilk 143:503–510.

Zucker B, Krüger M, Rehak E, Horsch F. 1994. Untersuchungen zur Lipopolysaccharidestruktur von *Haemophilus parasuis*-Stämmen in der SDS-PAGE. Berl Münch Tierärztl Wschr 107:78–81.

Zucker BA, Baghian A, Truax R, O'Reilly KL, Storz J. 1996. Detection of strain-specific antigenic epitopes of the lipo-oligosaccharide of *Haemophilus parasuis* by use of monoclonal and polyclonal antibodies. Am J Vet Res 57:63–67.

41 Leptospirosis

W. A. Ellis

Leptospirosis is a cause of reproductive loss in breeding herds and has been reported in swine from all parts of the world; however, knowledge of the incidence and economic impact of the disease is largely confined to the intensive pig industries of the Northern Hemisphere, Australia, New Zealand, Argentina, and Brazil.

Endemic infection in a herd of swine may produce little evidence of clinical disease, but when it is first introduced into a susceptible breeding herd, or during periods of waning herd immunity, it can cause very appreciable losses through abortion, the full-term birth of dead pigs or of weak pigs of reduced viability, or infertility.

Leptospires persist in the kidneys and genital tracts of carrier swine and are excreted in urine and genital fluids. Survival outside the host is favored by warm, moist conditions. Transmission is by direct or indirect contact with a carrier animal.

Interruption of transmission from an infected pig or other host to the pig is the critical factor in control.

Leptospirosis is an occupational zoonosis of those who work with pigs.

ETIOLOGY

Leptospirosis of swine is a disease caused by a variety of morphologically similar, but antigenically and genetically distinct, small, motile, aerobic spirochetes belonging to the genus *Leptospira*. They are thin, helical, motile, gram-negative organisms that are often hooked at one or both ends. They spin constantly on their long axis. They range in length from about 6 to 20 µm, with an amplitude of approximately 0.1–0.15 µm and a wavelength of about 0.5 µm. Under adverse nutritional conditions, leptospires may be greatly elongated, whereas under conditions such as high salt concentrations or in aging culture or tissues, leptospires may form coccoid forms of about 1.5–2 µm in diameter (Faine 1994). They divide by binary fission. They stain poorly with aniline dyes. Unstained cells are visible only by dark-field microscopy. In a suitable liquid environment, motility is

accomplished by rotating along the long axis, but this changes to an undulating action in semisolid media. They require special media containing mammalian serum or albumin for cultivation.

The major structural components are an outer envelope, which surrounds a cell wall or peptidoglycan complex, and two polar endoflagella (originating subterminally at each end).

The taxonomy of the leptospires has been through a period of change which continues to cause considerable confusion to those not intimately acquainted with the subject. Until recently a single genus *Leptospira* was recognized in the family *Leptospiraceae*. Two groupings were recognized within the genus: those found in animal species (the parasitic strains) and those found in water (the saprophytic strains). These two groupings, which were referred to as the *interrogans* and *biflexa* complexes, can be differentiated by their growth requirements and biochemical reactions. Only the parasitic strains are of medical and veterinary interest.

For taxonomic purposes and as an aid to epidemiological studies, the parasitic leptospires were divided into serogroups on the basis of antigenic relationships as determined by cross-agglutination reactions and were further subdivided into serovars by agglutination-absorption patterns. About 23 serogroups are recognized, containing approximately 212 serovars.

The advent of genetic typing methods has provided rapid, reproducible typing protocols. The current recommendations on the taxonomy of leptospires (Ellis 1995) recognized eight species of pathogenic leptospires within the family *Leptospiraceae*. They are *Leptospira interrogans, L. borgpetersenii, L. inadai, L. kirschneri, L. noguchii, L. meyer, L. weilii,* and *L. santarosai*.

The species definition is based on a level of DNA-DNA homology of at least 70% and 5% or less divergence in DNA relatedness. Taxonomy at the subspecific level continues to be based on serovars as defined by Dikken and Kmety (1978), but other valid methods which give results comparable to conventional serotyping can be used for their identification. Such methods include monoclonal antibody agglutination profiles, factor analysis, and analyses in which restriction-fragment length polymorphisms or rRNA gene restriction patterns are used in pulsed-field gel electrophoresis analyses. The term "type" is used to indicate strain differences at the subserovar level (Ellis 1995).

Molecular Biology

The genus *Leptospira* is characterized by a guanine plus cytosine (G+C) ratio of 35–41 mol% in its chromosomal DNA, depending on species. The published genome size has varied between 3100 and 5000 kb depending on the techniques used to measure it and reflecting differences between strains. The *Leptospira interrogans* serovars *icterohaemorrhagiae* and *pomona* have two circular chromosomes: the large (4400–4600 kb) and the small (350 kb) replicons are regarded as chromosomal because the essential asd gene is located on the smaller unit. *Leptospira interrogans* strains contain two 23S and 16S rRNA genes but only one 5S rRNA gene. The 5S rRNA gene is highly conserved among the pathogenic leptospires.

There are differences in the global distribution of some of the *Leptospira* species: *L. interrogans*, *L. borgpetersenii*, and *L. kirschneri* have a worldwide distribution, whereas *L. noguchii* and *L. santarosai* are found mainly in North and South America, and *L. weilii* is found mainly in China and eastern Asia. Strains that cause disease in pigs are found mainly in the *L. interrogans* and *L. borgpetersenii* species.

EPIDEMIOLOGY

The epidemiology of swine leptospirosis is potentially very complicated, since swine can be infected by any of the pathogenic serovars. Fortunately, only a small number of serovars will be endemic in any particular region or country. Furthermore, leptospirosis is a disease that shows a natural nidality, and each serovar tends to be maintained in specific-maintenance hosts. Therefore, in any region, pigs will be infected by serovars maintained by pigs or by serovars maintained by other animal species present in the area. The relative importance of these incidental infections is determined by the opportunity that prevailing social, management, and environmental factors provide for contact and transmission of leptospires from other species to pigs.

Pigs act as maintenance hosts for serovars belonging to the *Pomona*, Australis, and *Tarassovi* serogroups, while strains belonging to the *Canicola*, *Icterohaemorrhagiae*, and *Grippotyphosa* serogroups are among the more commonly identified incidental infections in swine.

Pomona Infection

Serovar *pomona* has been the most common serovar isolated from pigs worldwide. Infection with this serovar has been extensively studied and it provides a suitable model with which to illustrate general concepts of swine leptospirosis. Many strains of serovar *pomona*, especially those of type kennewicki found in the United States and Canada, are adapted to swine. Serovar *pomona* has been the cause of widespread clinical disease in swine in North and South America, Australia, New Zealand, parts of Asia, and Eastern and Central Europe and is endemic in many of these regions. Such strains are apparently absent from the more westerly parts of Europe. Furthermore, not all strains of serovar *pomona* are adapted to pigs nor are the other serovars of the *Pomona* serogroup, but they have rodent hosts (Sebek et al. 1983).

In parts of North America, the prevalence of *pomona* infection in pigs has fallen from the high levels observed in the 1950s and early 1960s: no carriers were detected in a 1989 meat-plant survey carried out in Iowa (Bolin and Cassells 1992). In contrast, Baker et al. (1989) recovered serovar *pomona* (type kennewicki) from almost 10% of pigs in a small survey in Canada.

Leptospires have a particular affinity for the kidneys of infected pigs, where they persist, multiply, and are voided in urine. This characteristic is very important in the transmission of infection.

Infection is introduced into a susceptible herd by three possible routes: the introduction of infected stock, exposure to a contaminated environment, or contact with an alternative infected animal vector (Hathaway 1983). Carrier pigs are probably the most common route of introduction. Replacement gilts (Edwards and Daines 1979) or infected boars (Kemenes and Suveges 1976) have been identified as important means of introducing infection.

The importance of free-living species as possible sources of *pomona* infection of pigs depends on geographical location. In North America, the skunk has been incriminated as a source of *pomona* outbreaks in pigs (Mitchell et al. 1966).

Once *pomona* has been introduced into a pig population, a high prevalence of infection is established. Only low infective doses are required to transmit infection (Chaudhary et al. 1966a, b). If direct contact is prevented, indirect contact through contaminated effluent, water, or soil ensures transmission (Michna 1970; Buddle and Hodges 1977; Kingscote 1986). The presence of moisture is critical for indirect transmission; the organisms cannot withstand dessication, but when infected urine is deposited in damp soil or water with a pH around or slightly on the alkaline side, the organisms may survive for extended periods (Mitscherlich and Marth 1984).

During the initial herd infection, clinical disease may occur in all ages of sows.

Following the initial establishment of infection, an endemic cycle typical of that in a maintenance host population is set up (Hathaway 1981). Piglets are passively protected in the first weeks of life by colostrum-derived immunoglobulins from infected dams (Fish et al. 1963; Bolt and Marshall 1995a). The duration of this passive protection depends primarily on the quantity of immunoglobulins received in colostrum (Chaudhary et al. 1966b). A study of grower pigs in New Zealand has shown that leptospiral infection becomes apparent in piglets from 12 weeks of age, and by slaughter up to 90% may be infected. The intensity of leptospiruria is greatest in the first 3–4 weeks of infection, after which it declines and becomes intermittent (Bolt and Marshall 1995a, b). Infection between groups of fattening pigs is often by urine-contaminated effluent from a common drainage system (Buddle and Hodges 1977).

In herds with endemic infection, clinical disease is usually restricted to gilts that either have been reared in isolation since weaning and reintroduced into the herd or, more commonly, have been brought in from an uninfected herd.

Tarassovi Infection

There is much less information available on the epidemiology of *tarassovi* infection in pigs. The pig acts as a maintenance host for some strains of *tarassovi* found in Eastern Europe and Australia. In these regions, it does not spread as rapidly in a pig population as does *pomona* (Kemenes and Suveges 1976), but endemic infection is readily maintained (Ryley and Simmons 1954b; Kemenes and Suveges 1976).

Many strains of *tarassovi* have been recovered from free-living animals (Anon. 1966, 1975) and these may give rise to incidental pig infections. For example, *tarassovi* has not been recovered from swine in the United States, but there is serologic evidence of infection in pigs (Cole et al. 1983) in the southeastern states, where it has been isolated from racoons, skunks, and opossums (McKeever et al. 1958; Roth 1964).

Australis Infection

Serovar *bratislava* and to a lesser extent the closely related serovar *muenchen* have emerged as major swine-maintained leptospiral infections in the last few years. Serologic data have indicated widespread *bratislava* infection in Germany (Weber and Fenske 1978), the United Kingdom (Hathaway and Little 1981; Hathaway et al. 1981), Czechoslovakia (Propopcakova et al. 1981), the Netherlands (Bercovich et al. 1983), Sweden (Sandstedt and Engvall 1985), Denmark (Jensen and Binder 1989; Nissen 1989), the United States (Hanson 1985, 1987), Canada (Kingscote 1988), Austria (Loimayr 1990), Australia (Chappel et al. 1992), Brazil (Oliveira et al. 1994), and South Africa (Potts et al. 1995). There is, as yet, no information from Russia but it would be reasonable to assume that infection is now present in all major pig-rearing countries.

Serovar *bratislava* was first recovered from a pig in the Netherlands by Hartmann et al. (1975) (Ellis 1992) and has now been recovered from pigs in the United

Kingdom (Ellis et al. 1986a, b, c), the United States (Ellis and Thiermann 1986; Bolin and Cassells 1990, 1992), and Germany (Schonberg et al. 1992).

The epidemiology of these strains is poorly understood. There are specific pig-adapted strains, strains that are maintained by pigs, dogs, horses, and hedgehogs, and strains that are found only in wildlife.

Two very distinct serologic profiles may be seen in endemically infected herds. In indoor sow units infected with pig-adapted strains of *bratislava*, the prevalence of sows with antibody titers of greater than 1:100 in the microscopic agglutination test (MAT) is usually very low, although many sows will have titers of less than 1:100. This is thought to result from infection being primarily due to venereal transmission. In contrast, in units where the sows are kept outside, the seroprevalences (≥1:100) may be greater than 50%. This is thought to be due to the sows being infected systemically as a result of exposure to infected rodent urine.

Although the renal-carrier state does become established, urinary excretion is poor compared with *pomona* excretion, and transmission within the fattening house is inefficient. Important additional carrier sites have been identified, namely, the upper genital tracts of sows and boars (Ellis et al. 1986b, c; Power 1991; Bolin and Cassells 1992). Venereal transmission is thought to play an important role in the spread of *bratislava* infection.

Canicola Infection

Although organisms belonging to the *Canicola* serogroup have been recovered from swine in at least 11 countries (Hanson and Tripathy 1986), little is known of the epidemiology of *canicola* infection in pigs. The dog is the recognized maintenance host for this serovar and is the probable vector whereby this serovar enters a piggery, although a report from Peru (Paz-Soldan et al. 1991) incriminates wildlife as the source of an outbreak in sows. The long period of leptospiruria observed in infected pigs (at least 90 days) (Michna 1962) and the ability of *canicola* to survive for up to 6 days in undiluted pig urine (Michna 1962) suggest that there would be an opportunity for intraspecies transmission, but no studies have been done on this subject (Hathaway 1983).

Icterohaemorrhagiae Infection

Serologic evidence of *Icterohaemorrhagiae* serogroup infection has been reported in many countries but few isolations have been made from pigs (Hathaway 1985). It appears that both serovars *copenhageni* and *icterohaemorrhagiae* may be involved. The maintenance host for these serovars is the brown rat (*Rattus norvegicus*), and it is probable that *copenhageni* and *icterohaemorrhagiae* are introduced to susceptible stock via an environment contaminated with infected rat urine. Field investigation suggests that transmission between swine is inefficient (Hathaway 1985). Schnurrenberger et al. (1970) found that urinary excretion lasted less than 35 days in naturally infected pigs, while Fennestad and Borg-Petersen (1966) failed to demonstrate leptospiruria in experimentally infected pigs. Low prevalences of renal infection have been found in those microbiological surveys in which Icterohaemorrhagiae strains have been recovered; Hathaway et al. (1981) reported a 0.7% prevalence in England, and McErlean (1973) found a 0.4% prevalence in Ireland. It is believed, in the absence of supporting isolation data, that vaccine-induced antibodies are responsible for the seroprevalences of *icterohaemorrhagiae* observed in the United States.

Grippotyphosa Infection

Serovar *grippotyphosa* infection is maintained by wildlife hosts, and incidental infection of pigs gives rise to low prevalences of antibodies in swine in various regions, particularly Eastern and Central Europe and the United States. It has been recovered from pigs in the former USSR (Gorshanova 1964) and the United States (Hanson et al. 1965, 1971).

Hardjo Infection

Serovar *hardjo* infection is maintained by cattle worldwide, and where cattle and pigs come in close contact, the opportunity arises for infection in pigs to occur. There are now reports of the isolation of *hardjo* from pigs in the United Kingdom (Hathaway et al. 1983; Ellis et al. 1986a) and the United States (Bolin and Cassells 1992). Persistence in renal tissue was not a feature of experimental infection (Hathaway et al. 1983); therefore, intraspecies transmission is unlikely.

Sejroe Infections

Serovar *sejroe,* which is maintained by small rodents, has also been isolated from swine in Europe (Brandis 1956; Fuzi et al. 1957; Combiesco et al. 1958), and another serovar in this group (serovar *balcanica*) has been recovered from swine in the former USSR (Matveeva et al. 1977).

PATHOGENESIS

The most important route of natural infection has not been determined; however, it is thought to be via the mucous membranes of the eye, mouth, or nose (Alston and Broom 1958; Alexander et al. 1964; Michna and Campbell 1969). Infection via the vaginal route is also possible (Ferguson and Powers 1956; Chaudhary et al. 1966a). Transmission of leptospires through milk from an infected dam has been demonstrated experimentally (Tripathy et al. 1981). A period of bacteremia, which may last for a week, begins 1 or 2 days after infection. During this period leptospires can be isolated from most organs of the body and also from cerebrospinal fluid. This primary bacteremic phase ends with the appearance of circulating antibodies, which are detectable usually after 5–10 days (Hanson and Tripathy 1986). A secondary bacteremic period (after 15–26 days) has been reported in experimental *hardjo* infection (Hathaway et al. 1983).

Antileptospiral agglutinins appear at detectable levels in the blood at approximately 5–10 days after infection and reach maximum levels at around 3 weeks (Ryley and Simmons 1954b; Ferguson and Powers 1956; Morse et al. 1958). Peak titers vary considerably (1:1000 to 1:100,000 in the MAT), and these may be maintained for up to 3 weeks, after which a gradual decline occurs. Low titers may be detectable for several years in many animals.

Following the period of leptospiremia, the leptospires localize in the proximal renal tubules, where they multiply and are voided in the urine. The duration and intensity of urinary shedding vary from pig to pig and with the infecting serovar. In the case of *pomona* infection, the intensity of excretion is highest during the first month of shedding, when more than a million leptospires may be present in each milliliter of urine (Morse et al. 1958); leptospiruria is very constant during this period (Hodges et al. 1979). A variable period of intermittent, low-intensity leptospiruria then ensues, and this may last for up to 2 years in some cases (Ryley and Simmons 1954a; Morse et al. 1958; Mitchell et al. 1966). Low levels of antibody may be detected in the urine of pigs (Morse et al. 1958), but the immunologic mechanism whereby infection is ultimately eliminated from the kidneys is not known.

Leptospires also localize in the uterus of pregnant sows, and abortion, production of stillborn pigs, and neonatal disease frequently result from intrauterine infections occurring in the last half of the gestation period. Abortions and stillbirths usually occur 1–4 weeks following infection of the gilt or sow (Hanson and Tripathy 1986), by which time most sows have developed detectable antibody titers. Since pig fetuses are capable of producing antibodies during the latter stages of gestation, some stillborn piglets will have detectable titers.

The pathogenesis of reproductive disease is poorly understood, but some authors believe that transplacental infection, occurring during the very limited period of maternal leptospiremia, is the sole cause (Fennestad and Borg-Petersen 1966). While this may be true for systemic infections such as *pomona*, the low antibody titers detected in sows aborting *bratislava*-infected fetuses has led to the hypothesis that infection occurs as a result of waning uterine immunity being unable to prevent transplacental infection by leptospires present in the genital tract. The possibility of transplacental infection during leptospiremia appears to increase with the stage of pregnancy (Wrathall 1975). From midpregnancy onward, it is likely that the majority of fetuses in a litter at risk will become infected. Fennestad and Borg-Petersen (1966) have suggested that horizontal transmission to littermates not infected during the period of maternal leptospiremia may also occur. Once the placental barrier is breached, septicemia results in large numbers of leptospires in all fetal tissues (Preston and Morter 1960). It is unlikely that placental insufficiency plays a role in fetal death (Wrathall 1975); abortion is probably initiated by toxic products released from dead and autolyzing fetuses.

An additional feature seen in *bratislava* infection but not reported for the other swine leptospiral infections is the persistence of leptospires in the oviduct and uterus of nonpregnant sows (Ellis et al. 1986c; Ellis and Thiermann 1986; Bolin and Cassells 1992) and in the genital tracts of boars (Ellis et al. 1986b).

CLINICAL SIGNS

The vast majority of swine leptospiral infections are subclinical. Two groups of pigs are most likely to experience clinical infections: the young piglet and the pregnant sow.

Acute Leptospirosis

This phase usually coincides with the period of bacteremia (Morse et al. 1958; Sleight and Lundberg 1961; Chaudhary et al. 1966a, b). In experimental infections, many pigs exhibit transient anorexia, pyrexia, and listlessness at this time (Hanson and Tripathy 1986). However, the mild nature of these signs means that in natural infections, especially in endemically infected herds where perhaps only one or two animals may be affected, this phase of infection usually goes unrecognized.

There have been a few reports of jaundice and hemoglobinuria in naturally occurring outbreaks (Ferguson et al. 1956), particularly in cases of infection in piglets under 3 months of age by strains belonging to the Icterohaemorrhagiae serogroup (Klarenbeek and Winsser 1937; Field and Sellers 1951; Urban and Androsov 1976). A high proportion of these undergo spontaneous recovery within a week of when symptoms develop. The small number of such reports suggests that this more severe form of disease is rare.

Chronic Leptospirosis

Abortions, stillbirths, and the birth of weak piglets of reduced viability are primary signs of chronic leptospirosis, particularly *pomona* infection, in pigs (Bohl et al. 1954; Fennestad and Borg-Petersen 1966) and it is this aspect of leptospirosis that can cause considerable economic loss. Weak litters have been reported as a feature of Icterohaemorrhagiae infection (Neto et al. 1997).

Information as to the importance of leptospirosis as a cause of abortion in national swine herds is not available, and if it were, it must vary from country to country depending on prevalence, epidemiological, and management factors, including the implementation of control measures. From the limited information available, it would appear that even in countries where vaccination has been widely practiced, leptospirosis is a common cause of swine abortion. In Ontario, for example, 6% of swine abortions were attributed to *pomona* infection (Anon. 1986). Endemic *tarassovi* infection was considered to be the cause of a 3% abortion rate in herds in Poland investigated by Wandurski (1982). Acute outbreaks can still give rise to severe losses; Saravi et al. (1989) described an outbreak in a herd in which 19% of pregnant sows aborted, while the number of dead piglets/sow rose from 8% prior to the outbreak to 28% during the outbreak. Differences in strain pathogenicity also contribute to different prevalences of clinical abortion in infected herds (Nagy 1993).

A very high prevalence of serovars belonging to the Australis serogroup has been observed in aborted pig litters in part of the United Kingdom. Ellis et al. (1986a) isolated either serovar *bratislava* or *muenchen* from 71% of the litters they examined. Similar strains have also been recovered from aborted piglets in the United States (Bolin and Cassells 1990), where a high prevalence in aborted fetuses has also been noted (Bolin et al. 1991). Rehmtulla et al. (1992) reported fetal *bratislava* infection following abortions in 16% of sows in a herd in Ontario. Egan (1995) reported fluorescent antibody test (FAT) positive prevalences ranging from 5% to 23% in diagnostic submissions in Ireland. Published experimental evaluations of the significance of such microbiological findings are not available. There has, however, been an absence of significant isolations of other abortifacient agents from these cases, and the farrowing rate and the number of live piglets born/sow improve significantly following either *bratislava* vaccination (Frantz et al. 1989) or the use of an antibiotic medication program (Ellis 1989). Van Til and Dohoo (1991) failed to demonstrate a relationship between positive serology and stillbirths.

Following abortions due to *pomona*, there does not appear to be any subsequent limitation on reproductive performance, even in pigs that remain infected for long periods (Ferguson and Powers 1956; Mitchell et al. 1966; Kemenes and Suveges 1976).

Infertility is a feature of *bratislava* infection. An analysis of serologic and clinical data by Hathaway and Little (1981) has shown a statistically significant relationship between Australis serogroup titers and infertility in sows. Similar associations have been observed by Jensen and Binder (1989) and Van Til and Dohoo (1991). Split-herd trials, carried out using a *bratislava* bacterin, have demonstrated significant improvements in sow fertility (Frantz et al. 1989).

LESIONS

The main pathological changes are essentially the same for all infections, with the primary lesion being damage to the membranes of the endothelial cells of small blood vessels.

In acute leptospirosis there are no pathognomonic gross changes. Pathological changes in acute *pomona* infection are very limited, reflecting the mild nature of acute clinical disease. Hanson and Tripathy (1986) reported little gross or histopathological change in swine killed during the acute phase of leptospirosis. Burnstein and Baker (1954) reported that petechial and ecchymotic hemorrhages could be seen in the lungs of some pigs, and histological examinations have revealed minor renal tubular damage, focal liver necrosis, lymphocytic infiltration of the adrenal glands, and meningoencephalitis with perivascular lymphocytic infiltration (Burnstein and Baker 1954; Sleight et al. 1960; Chaudhary et al. 1966a).

In chronic leptospirosis, lesions are confined to the kidneys and consist of scattered small gray foci, often surrounded by a ring of hyperemia. Microscopic examination shows these lesions to be a progressive focal interstitial nephritis (Burnstein and Baker 1954; Langham et al. 1958; Cheville et al. 1980). The interstitial leukocytic infiltrations, which consist mainly of lymphocytes, macrophages, and plasma cells, may be extensive in some areas. Focal damage may also involve glomeruli and renal tubules. Some affected glomeruli are swollen, some atrophic, and others are replaced by fibrosis. The Bowman's capsule may be thickened, containing eosinophilic granular material (Langham et al. 1958). Tubular changes involve atrophy, hyperplasia, and the presence of necrotic debris in the lumen in some areas. Occasionally, petechial hemorrhages may be present in interstitial spaces.

Older lesions mainly consist of fibrosis and interstitial infiltration. Chronic lesions with accompanying acute inflammatory changes are still noticeable as long as 14 months postinfection (Morter et al. 1960).

Experimental studies indicate leptospires can invade the mammary gland of pigs and produce a mild, focal nonsuppurative mastitis (Tripathy et al. 1981).

The gross pathology of fetuses aborted as a sequela of *pomona* infection is nonspecific and includes edema of various tissues, serous or bloodstained fluid in body cavities, and sometimes petechial hemorrhages in the renal cortex (Ryley and Simmons 1954b; Fennestad and Borg-Petersen 1966; Wrathall 1975). These changes are probably the result of intrauterine autolysis. Jaundice may be seen in some aborted piglets (Hathaway et al. 1983). Focal necrosis, presenting as small grayish-white spots, is a frequent finding in the liver (Ryley and Simmons 1954b; Fish et al. 1963; Fennestad and Borg-Petersen 1966). Histological examination may reveal small foci of interstitial nephritis.

Placentas from aborted fetuses are grossly normal (Fish et al. 1963; Fennestad and Borg-Petersen 1966).

DIAGNOSIS

A diagnosis of leptospirosis in swine may be required not only for the clinician to confirm leptospirosis as a cause of clinical disease but also for other reasons, such as (1) the assessment of the infection and/or the immune status of a herd for the purposes of a control or eradication program on either a herd or a national basis; (2) epidemiological studies; or (3) a determination of the infectivity status of an individual animal to assess its suitability for international trade or for introduction into an uninfected herd.

The mild, often inapparent, clinical signs of acute leptospirosis make clinical diagnosis difficult; therefore, diagnosis is usually based on the results of laboratory procedures.

Laboratory diagnostic procedures for leptospirosis fall into two groups. The first group consists of tests for antibody detection; the second contains the tests for the demonstration of leptospires in pig tissues. The selection of tests to be carried out depends on the purpose for which a diagnosis is to be made and the resources available.

Serologic Tests

Serologic testing is the most widely used method for diagnosing leptospirosis, and the MAT (Cole et al. 1980; Faine 1982) is the standard serologic test. The minimum antigen requirements are that the test should employ representative strains of all the serogroups known to exist in the particular country, plus those known to be maintained by pigs elsewhere.

The MAT is used primarily as a herd test. To obtain useful information, at least 10 animals or 10% of the herd, whichever is the greater (Cole et al. 1980), should be tested. A retrospective diagnosis of both acute leptospirosis and *pomona* abortion may be made when the majority of affected animals have titers of 1:1000 or greater. Increasing the sample size and sampling a number of different cohorts markedly improve epidemiological information, investigations of clinical disease, assessments of vaccination needs, and public health tracebacks.

As an individual-animal test, the MAT is very useful in diagnosing acute infection; rising antibody titers in paired acute and convalescent serum samples are diagnostic. The presence of antibody in fetal serum is diagnostic of leptospiral abortion.

The MAT has severe limitations in the diagnosis of chronic infection in individual pigs, both in the diagnosis of abortion and in the identification of renal or genital carriers. Infected animals may have MAT titers below the widely accepted minimum significant titer of 1:100 (Ellis et al. 1986b, c).

Other serologic tests have been described for use in pigs, especially ELISA-based tests, but none of these have gained widespread acceptance for use as diagnostic tests.

Demonstration of Leptospires in Pig Tissues

The isolation of leptospires from, or their demonstration in, the internal organs (such as liver, lung, brain) and body fluids (blood, cerebrospinal, thoracic, and peritoneal) of clinically affected animals gives a definitive diagnosis of acute clinical disease or, in the case of a fetus, a diagnosis of leptospiral abortion and probable chronic infection of its mother.

Their presence in the male or female genital tract, the kidney, or urine, in the absence of evidence of generalized infection, is diagnostic of chronic infection. Failure to demonstrate leptospires in the urine of a pig does not rule out the possibility of the animal being a chronic renal carrier; it merely indicates that the pig was not excreting detectable numbers of leptospires at the time of testing.

Isolation. Isolation, especially from clinical material, is difficult and time-consuming and is a job for laboratories specializing in the identification of isolates. Isolation from renal carriers is very useful in epidemiological studies to determine which serovars are present in an animal species or in a particular group of animals or geographic location.

The isolation of leptospires is the most sensitive method of demonstrating their presence, provided that antibiotic residues are absent, that tissue autolysis is not advanced, and that tissues for culture have been stored at a suitable temperature (4°C) and, in the case of urine, at a suitable pH since collection.

Culture should be carried out in a semisolid (0.1–0.2% agar) bovine serum-albumin medium containing either Tween 80 (Johnson and Harris 1967) or a combination of Tween 80 and Tween 40 (Ellis 1986), and preferably a small amount of fresh rabbit serum (0.4–2%) if the more fastidious leptospires such as *bratislava* are to be isolated. A dilution culture method should be used (Ellis 1986). Contamination may be controlled by a variety of selective agents (e.g., 5-fluorouracil, nalidixic acid, fosfomycin, and a cocktail of rifamycin, polymyxin, neomycin, 5-fluorouracil, bacitracin, and actidione). The use of selective agents will reduce the chance of isolation where there are only small numbers of viable leptospires. Culture media containing 5-fluorouracil at levels between 200 and 500 µg/mL should be used as transport media for the submission of samples (Ellis 1990).

Cultures should be incubated at 29–30°C for at least 12 weeks, preferably for 26 weeks (Ellis 1986). They should be examined by dark-ground microscopy every 1–2 weeks.

Other Methods of Demonstrating Leptospires. Leptospires do not stain satisfactorily with the aniline dyes, and silver-staining techniques lack sensitivity and specificity (Baskerville 1986). Dark-ground microscopy of fetal fluids or urine has been widely used in the diagnosis of leptospirosis and can be a useful tool in the hands of an experienced diagnostician, but many tissue artifacts can be mistakenly identified as leptospires.

The demonstration of leptospires by immunochemical tests (immunofluorescence, immunoperoxidase, and immunogold) is more suited to most laboratory sit-

uations; however, these tests are "number-of-organisms" dependent and lack the sensitivity of culture. They provide no information as to the infecting serovar (Ellis 1990) and require high-IgG-titer antileptospire sera, which are not available commercially. Immunofluorescence is the method of choice for the diagnosis of fetal leptospirosis. There have been a number of polymerase chain reaction methods published, but so far these have failed to deliver the promised increase in sensitivity which the underlying technology should theoretically deliver (Taylor et al. 1997).

PREVENTION AND CONTROL

Interruption of transmission from an infected pig or other host to a pig is the critical factor in control. Control of leptospirosis depends on the combined use of three strategies: antibiotic therapy, vaccination, and management. Unfortunately, not all these options are available in every country; for example, vaccines are not available in many Western European countries, including the United Kingdom, and problems of antibiotic residues may make the use of antibiotic therapy difficult in other situations. In the United States, the most useful antibiotic for leptospiral control/treatment programs, streptomycin, is no longer available for veterinary use. Control programs must therefore be modified to meet local conditions.

Vaccination induces immunity of relatively short duration. Immunity to infection is probably never 100% and, at best, lasts little more than 3 months (Kemenes and Suveges 1976; Ellis et al. 1989); immunity to clinical disease is believed to last somewhat longer, although the exact duration is not known. Vaccination will markedly reduce the prevalence of infection in a herd (Wrathall 1975; Kemenes and Suveges 1976) but will not eliminate infection (Hodges et al. 1976; Edwards and Daines 1979; Cargill and Davos 1981). Given the widespread use of tetracycline medication of feed in parts of Europe to control *bratislava* infection and all the attendant residue problems, there is an urgent need for the marketing of an effective *bratislava* vaccine in Europe.

Antibiotics alone will not eliminate pig-maintained leptospiral infections from the individual carrier animal or control infection in herds. Despite claims by some authors that either systemic streptomycin at 25 mg/kg body weight (Dobson 1974; Alt and Bolin 1996) or oral tetracyclines at levels of 800 g/ton of feed (Stalheim 1967) will eliminate carriers, others have reported that these regimes do not work (Doherty and Baynes 1967; Hodges et al. 1979). Recent work into the use of alternative antibiotic therapy regimes indicates that oxytetracycline (40 mg/kg for 3 or 5 days), tylosin (44 mg/kg for 5 days), or erythromycin (25 mg/kg for 5 days) may be effective in eliminating *pomona* from the kidneys of experimentally infected pigs (Alt and Bolin 1996).

The main management factor in the control of leptospirosis is the prevention of direct or indirect contact with free-living vectors or other domestic stock. Strict biosecurity should be implemented and rodent control programs instigated in and around the production complex. When faced with an outbreak of clinical disease, the best option is to treat both affected and at-risk stock with streptomycin at 25 mg/kg body weight, to immediately vaccinate the at-risk stock, and then to introduce a regular vaccination program. If vaccination is not an available option, then a feed medication program, using either chlor- or oxytetracycline at 600–800 g/ton of feed, should be introduced. This ration is fed either continuously or on a 1-month-on/1-month-off basis. Alternatively, it may be fed for two periods of 4 weeks in the year, preferably one in the spring and the other in the autumn.

The use of artificial insemination is an important tool in the control of *bratislava* infection.

ZOONOSIS

Leptospirosis is an important occupational zoonosis of those who work with pigs, especially farmers and those involved in slaughtering pigs. Pigs are now being produced for intended xeno grafting. It is important to remember the potential risk to recipients posed by pig-associated leptospirosis (Bjoersdorff et al. 1995).

REFERENCES

Alexander AD, Yager RH, Keefe TJ. 1964. Leptospirosis in swine. Bull Off Epizoot 61:273–304.

Alston JM, Broom JC. 1958. Leptospirosis in Man and Animals. Edinburgh: E. and S. Livingstone, pp. 65–75.

Alt DP, Bolin CA. 1996. Preliminary evaluation of antimicrobial agents for treatment of *Leptospira interrogans* serovar *pomona* infection in hamsters and swine. Am J Vet Res 57:59–62.

Anon. 1966. Zoonoses Surveillance: Leptospiral Serotype Distribution Lists. USDHEW, Atlanta, Ga.

——. 1975. Zoonoses Surveillance: Leptospiral Serotype Distribution Lists according to Host and Geographic Area. July 1966–July 1973. USDHEW, Atlanta, Ga.

——. 1986. Diagnosis of abortions, V.L.S., Guelph. Can Vet J 27:A20.

Baker IF, McEwan SA, Prescott JF, Meek AH. 1989. The prevalence of leptospirosis and its association with multifocal interstitial nephritis in swine at slaughter. Can J Vet Res 53:290–294.

Baskerville A. 1986. Histological aspects of diagnosis of leptospirosis. In The Present State of Leptospirosis Diagnosis and Control. Dordrecht, Netherlands: Martinus Nijhoff, pp. 33–43.

Bercovich Z, Spek CW, Comvalius-Adriaan I. 1983. Occurrence of antibodies to various serotypes of *Leptospira interrogans* among swine in the Netherlands between 1975 and 1980. Tidjschr Diergeneeskd 108:133–138.

Bjoersdorff A, Korsgren O, Feinstein R, Andersson A, Tollemar J, Malmborg A-S, Ehrnst A, Groth CG. 1995. Microbiological characterization of porcine fetal islet-like cell clusters for intended clinical xenografting. Xenotransplantation 2:26–31.

Bohl EH, Powers TE, Ferguson LC. 1954. Abortions in swine associated with leptospirosis. J Am Vet Med Assoc 124:262.

Bolin CA, Cassells JA. 1990. Isolation of *Leptospira interrogans* serovar *bratislava* from stillborn and weak pigs in Iowa. J Am Vet Med Assoc 196:1601–1604.

——. 1992. Isolation of *Leptospira interrogans* serovars *bratislava* and *hardjo* from swine at slaughter. J Vet Diag Invest 4:87–89.

Bolin CA, Cassells JA, Hill HT, Frantz JC, Nielsen JN. 1991. Reproductive failure associated with *Leptospira interrogans* serovar *bratislava* infection of swine. J Vet Diag Invest 3:152–154.

Bolt I, Marshall RB. 1995a. The epidemiology of *Leptospira interrogans* serovar *pomona* in grower pig herds. NZ Vet J 43:10–15.

——. 1995b. The epidemiology of *Leptospira interrogans* serovar *pomona* in grower pig herds. NZ Vet J 43:204.

Brandis H. 1956. Über Leptospirosen durch den type *L. saxkoebing*. Klin Wochenschr 34:521.

Buddle JR, Hodges RT. 1977. Observations on some aspects of the epidemiology of leptospirosis in a herd of pigs. NZ Vet J 25:56, 65–66.

Burnstein T, Baker JA. 1954. Leptospirosis in swine caused by *Leptospira pomona*. J Infect Dis 94:53–54.

Cargill CF, Davos DE. 1981. Renal leptospirosis in vaccinated pigs. Aust Vet J 57:236–238.

Chappel RJ, Ellis WA, Adler B, Amon L, Millar BD, Zhu SS, Prime RW. 1992. Serological evidence for the presence of *Leptospira interrogans* serovar *bratislava* in Australian pigs. Aust Vet J 69:119–120.

Chaudhary RK, Fish NA, Barnum DA. 1966a. Experimental infection with *Leptospira pomona* in normal and immune piglets. Can Vet J 7:106–112.

——. 1966b. Protection of piglets from immunised sows via colostrum against experimental *Leptospira pomona* infection. Can Vet J 7:121–127.

Cheville NF, Huhn R, Cutlip RC. 1980. Ultrastructure of renal lesions in pigs with acute leptospirosis caused by *Leptospira pomona*. Vet Pathol 17:338–351.

Cole JR, Ellinghausen HC, Rubin HL. 1980. Laboratory diagnosis of leptospirosis of domestic animals. Proc US Anim Health Assoc 83:189–199.

Cole JR, Hall RF, Ellinghausen HC, Pursell AR. 1983. Prevalence of leptospiral antibodies in Georgia cattle and swine, with emphasis on *Leptospira interrogans* serovar *tarassovi*. Proc US Anim Health Assoc 87:199–210.

Combiesco D, Sturdza N, Sefer M, Radu I. 1958. Recherches sur les leptospirosis. Arch Roum Pathol Exp Microbiol 17:245.

Dikken H, Kmety E. 1978. Serological typing methods of leptospires. Methods in Microbiology 11:259–307.

Dobson KJ. 1974. Eradication of leptospirosis in commercial pig herds. Aust Vet J 50:471.

Doherty PC, Baynes ID. 1967. The effects of feeding oxytetracycline on leptospira in pigs infected with *L. pomona*. Aust Vet J 43:135–137.

Edwards JD, Daines D. 1979. A leptospirosis outbreak in a piggery. NZ Vet J 27:247–248.

Egan J. 1995. Porcine leptospirosis. Irish Vet J 48:399, 401–402.

Ellis WA. 1986. The diagnosis of leptospirosis in farm animals. In The Present State of Leptospirosis Diagnosis and Control. Dordrecht, Netherlands: Martinus Nijhoff, pp. 13–31.

——. 1989. *Leptospira* Australis infection in pigs. Pig Vet J 22:83–92.

——. 1990. Leptospirosis. In OIE Manual of Recommended Diagnostic Techniques and Requirements for Biological Products for List A and B Diseases, vol. 2, sec. 7, pp. 1–11. Paris.

——. 1992. Leptospirosis. In Diseases of Swine, 7th ed. AD Leman, BE Straw, WL Mengeling, S D'Allaire, DJ Taylor. eds. Ames: Iowa State Univ Press, pp. 529–535.

——. 1995. International Committee on Systematic Bacteriology Subcommittee on the Taxonomy of *Leptospira*. Int J Systematic Bacteriol 45:872–874.

Ellis WA, Thiermann AB. 1986. Isolation of *Leptospira interrogans* serovar *bratislava* from sows in Iowa. Am J Vet Res 47:1458–1460.

Ellis WA, McParland PJ, Bryson DG, Cassells JA. 1986a. Prevalence of *leptospira* infection in aborted pigs in Northern Ireland. Vet Rec 118:63–65.

——. 1986b. Boars as carriers of leptospires of the Australis serogroup on farms with an abortion problem. Vet Rec 118:563.

Ellis WA, McParland PJ, Bryson DG, Thiermann AB, Montgomery J. 1986c. Isolation of leptospires from genital tract and kidneys of aborted sows. Vet Rec 118:294–295.

Ellis WA, Montgomery JM, McParland PJ. 1989. An experimental study with a *Leptospira interrogans* serovar *bratislava* vaccine. Vet Rec 125:319–321.

Faine S. 1982. Guidelines for the control of leptospirosis. Offset Pub no. 67. Geneva: WHO.

——. 1994. *Leptospira* and Leptospirosis. Boca Raton: CRC Press.

Fennestad KL, Borg-Petersen C. 1966. Experimental leptospirosis in pregnant sows. J Infect Dis 116:57–66.

Ferguson LC, Powers TE. 1956. Experimental leptospirosis in pregnant swine. Am J Vet Res 17:471–477.

Ferguson LC, Lococo S, Smith HR, Handy AH. 1956. The control and treatment of swine leptospirosis during a naturally occurring outbreak. J Am Vet Med Assoc 129:263–265.

Field HI, Sellers KC. 1951. *Leptospira icterohaemorrhagiae* infection in piglets. Vet Rec 63:78–81.

Fish NA, Ryu E, Hulland TJ. 1963. Bacteriological and pathological studies of natural and experimental swine abortion due to *Leptospira pomona*. Can Vet J 4:317–327.

Frantz JC, Hanson LE, Brown AL. 1989. Effect of vaccination with a bacterin containing *Leptospira interrogans* serovar *bratislava* on the breeding performance of swine herds. Am J Vet Res 50:1044–1047.

Fuzi M, Alfoldy Z, Kiszel J, Raditz I. 1957. Die Leptospiren-Infection der Feldnagetiere in einem Gebiet von Westungarn. Acta Microbiol Acad Sci Hung 4:155–156.

Gorshanova EN. 1964. Domestic animals as a source of leptospirosis in Dagestan. J Microbiol (Moscow) 41:120.

Hanson LE. 1985. Report of the committee on leptospirosis. Proc US Anim Health Assoc 90:217.

——. 1987. *Bratislava*—A newly recognised leptospiral serovar in swine. Swine Consultant (Spring):1–8.

Hanson LE, Reynolds HA, Evans LB. 1971. Leptospirosis in swine caused by serovar *grippotyphosa*. Am J Vet Res 32:855.

Hanson LE, Schnurrenberger PR, Marshall RB, Scherrick GW. 1965. Leptospiral serotypes in Illinois cattle and swine. Proc US Livest Sanit Assoc 69:164.

Hanson LE, Tripathy DN. 1986. Leptospirosis. In Diseases of Swine, 6th ed. AD Leman, B Straw, RD Glock, WL Mengeling, RHC Penny, E Scholl, eds. Ames: Iowa State Univ Press, pp. 591–599.

Hartmann EG, Brummelman B, Dikken H. 1975. *Leptospirae* of serotype lora of the serogroup Australis isolated for the first time from swine in the Netherlands. Tidjschr Diergeneeskd 100:421–425.

Hathaway SC. 1981. Leptospirosis in New Zealand: An ecological view. NZ Vet J 29:109–112.

——. 1983. Leptospirosis in Pigs in England. FRCVS thesis. Royal College Vet Surgeons, London.

——. 1985. Porcine leptospirosis. Pig News Inf 6:31–34.

Hathaway SC, Little TWA. 1981. Prevalence and clinical significance of leptospiral antibodies in pigs in England. Vet Rec 108:224–228.

Hathaway SC, Little TWA, Stevens AE. 1981. Serological and bacteriological survey of leptospiral infection in pigs in southern England. Res Vet Sci 31:169–173.

Hathaway SC, Ellis WA, Little TWA, Stevens AE, Ferguson HW. 1983. *Leptospira interrogans* serovar *hardjo* in pigs: A new host parasite relationship in the United Kingdom. Vet Rec 113:153–154.

Hodges RT, Stocker RP, Buddle JR. 1976. *Leptospira interrogans* serotype *pomona* infection and leptospiruria in vaccinated pigs. NZ Vet J 24:37–39.

Hodges RT, Thompson J, Townsend KG. 1979. Leptospirosis in pigs: The effectiveness of streptomycin in stopping leptospiruria. NZ Vet J 27:124–126.

Jensen AM, Binder M. 1989. Serological reactions for leptospires in reproductive failure in Danish pigs. Is there a connection? A preliminary investigation. Dansk Vet 72:1181–1187.

Johnson RC, Harris VG. 1967. Differentiation of pathogenic and saprophytic leptospires. 1. Growth at low temperatures. J Bacteriol 94:27–31.

Kemenes F, Suveges T. 1976. *Leptospira*-induced repeated abortion in sows. Acta Vet Hung 26:395–403.

Kingscote BF. 1986. Leptospirosis outbreak in a piggery in southern Alberta. Can Vet J 27:188–190.

——. 1988. Leptospiral serovars in Canada. Can Vet J 29:70–71.

Klarenbeek A, Winsser J. 1937. Ein Fall von spontaner Weilscher Krankheit bei Ferkeln. Dtsch Tierärztl Wochenschr 45:434–435.

Langham RF, Morse EV, Morter RL. 1958. Experimental leptospirosis. V. Pathology of *Leptospira pomona* infection in swine. Am J Vet Res 19:395–400.

Loimayr V. 1990. Survey for antibodies to *Leptospira* in Austrian pigs. Wiener Tierarztl Monatsschr 77:60.

Matveeva AA, Sakharova PV, Sharban EK, Dragomir AV. 1977. [Etiology of leptospires in animals in the Moldavian Republic, USSR]. Veterinariya (Moscow) 1:61–63.

McErlean BA. 1973. The isolation of *leptospirae* from the kidneys of bacon pigs. Irish Vet J 27:185–186.

McKeever S, Gorman GW, Chapman JF, Galton MM, Powers DK. 1958. Incidence of leptospirosis in wild mammals from southwestern Georgia with a report of new hosts of six serotypes of leptospires. Am J Trop Med Hyg 7:646.

Michna SW. 1962. Abortion in the sow due to infection by *Leptospira canicola*: A preliminary report. Vet Rec 74:917–919.

——. 1970. Leptospirosis. Vet Rec 86:484–496.

Michna SW, Campbell RSF. 1969. Leptospirosis in pigs: Epidemiology, microbiology and pathology. Vet Rec 84:135–138.

Mitchell D, Robertson A, Corner AH, Boulanger P. 1966. Some observations on the diagnosis and epidemiology of leptospirosis in swine. Can J Comp Med 30:211–217.

Mitscherlich E, Marth EH. 1984. Microbial Survival in the Environment. Berlin: Springer-Verlag, pp. 202–218.

Morse EV, Bauer DC, Langham RF, Lang RW, Ullrey DE. 1958. Experimental leptospirosis. IV. Pathogenesis of porcine *Leptospira pomona* infections. Am J Vet Res 19:388–394.

Morter EV, Morse EV, Langham RF. 1960. Experimental leptospirosis. VII. Re-exposure of pregnant sows with *Leptospira pomona*. Am J Vet Res 21:95.

Nagy G. 1993. Comparative pathogenicity study of *Leptospira interrogans* serovar *pomona* strains. Acta Vet Hung 41:315–324.

Neto JSF, Vasconelles SV, Ito FH, Moretti ASA, Camargo CA, Sakamoto SM, Marangon Turilli C, Martini M. 1997. *Leptospira interrogans* serovar icterohaemorrhagiae seropositivity and the reproductive performance of sows. Prev Vet Med 31:87–93.

Nissen OD. 1989. Leptospirosis in pigs: A review of the literature and a study of the development of titres against *L. bratislava* in two herds. Dansk Vet 72:619–635.

de Oliveira SJ, Borowski SM, Barcellos DESN. 1994. Serological evidence of infection by *Leptospira bratislava* as the cause of reproductive disorders in pigs. Ciencia-Rural 24:345–348.

Paz-Soldan SV, Dianderas MT, Windsor RS. 1991. *Leptospira interrogans* serovar *canicola*: A causal agent of sow abortions in Arequipa, Peru. Trop Anim Hlth Prodn 23:233–240.

Potts AD, Lotter C, Robinson JTR. 1995. Serological prevalence of leptospiral antibodies in pigs in South Africa. Onderstepoort J Vet Res 62:281–284.

Power SB. 1991. Diagnosing *leptospira* in pigs. Vet Rec 128:43.

Preston KS, Morter RL. 1960. Rapid laboratory confirmation of clinical diagnosis of *Leptospira pomona* infection in pregnant sows. Allied Vet 31:104–107.

Propopcakova H, Pospisil R, Cislakova L, Kozak M. 1981. Determination of antibodies to leptospirosis in animals and man in eastern Slovakia in the past ten years. Veterinarstvi 31:275–277.

Rehmtulla AJ, Prescott JF, Nicholson VM, Bolin CA. 1992. *Leptospira bratislava* infection in aborted pigs in Ontario. Can Vet J 33:344–345.

Roth EE. 1964. Leptospirosis in wildlife in the United States. Proc Am Vet Med Assoc 101:211.

Ryley JW, Simmons GC. 1954a. *Leptospira pomona* as a cause of abortion and neonatal mortality in swine. Queens J Agric Sci 11:61–74.

——. 1954b. Leptospirosis of pigs with special reference to birth of dead pigs and neonatal mortality. Aust Vet J 30:203–208.

Sandstedt K, Engvall A. 1985. Serum antibodies to *Leptospira bratislava* in Swedish pigs and horses. Nord Vet Med 37:312–313.

Saravi MA, Molinar R, Soria EH, Barriola JL. 1989. Serological and bacteriological diagnosis, and reproductive consequences of an outbreak of porcine leptospirosis caused by a member of the *Pomona* serogroup. Res Sci Tech Off Int Epix 8:709–718.

Schnurrenberger PR, Hanson LE, Martin RJ. 1970. Long term surveillance of leptospirosis on an Illinois farm. Am J Epidemiol 92:223–239.

Schonberg A, Hahnhey B, Kampe U, Schmidt K, Ellis WA. 1992. The isolation and identification of *Leptospira interrogans* serovar *bratislava* from a pig in Germany. J Vet Med Series B 39:362–368.

Sebek Z, Treml F, Valova M. 1983. Experimental infection with the virulent central European murine *Leptospira pomona* strain in the pig. Folia Parasitol 30:269–275.

Sleight SD, Lundberg AM. 1961. Persistence of *Leptospira pomona* in porcine tissues. J Am Vet Med Assoc 139:455–456.

Sleight SD, Langham RF, Morter RL. 1960. Experimental leptospirosis: The early pathogenesis of *Leptospira pomona* infection in young swine. J Infect Dis 106:262–269.

Stalheim OHV. 1967. Chemotherapy of renal leptospirosis in swine. Am J Vet Res 28:161–166.

Taylor MJ, Ellis WA, Montgomery JM, Yan K-T, McDowell SWJ, Mackie DP. 1997. Magnetic immuno-capture PCR assay (MIPA): Detection of *Leptospira borgpetersenii* serovar *hardjo*. Vet Micro 56:135–145.

Tripathy DN, Hanson LE, Mansfield ME, Thilsted JP. 1981. Pathogenesis of *Leptospira pomona* in lactating sows and transmission to piglets. Proc US Anim Health Assoc 85:188.

Urban VP, Androsov VA. 1976. [Titer of leptospiral antibodies as a function of time and course of infectious process.] Dokl Vses Acad Sci-Khoz Nauk 2:39–42.

Van Til LD, Dohoo IR. 1991. A serological survey of leptospirosis in Prince Edward Island swine herds and its association with infertility. Can J Vet Res 55:352–355.

Wandurski A. 1982. Effect of infections with various serotypes of *Leptospira interrogans* on the fertility of swine. Med Weter 38:218–220.

Weber B, Fenske G. 1978. Unterschungen zur *Leptospira bratislava* Infection beim Schwein. Monatsh Vet Med 33:652–656.

Wrathall AE. 1975. Reproductive Disorders in Pigs. Anim Health Rev Ser no. 11. Commonwealth Agricultural Bureaux.

42 Mycoplasmal Diseases

Eileen L. Thacker

Mycoplasma hyopneumoniae and the pneumonia associated with it remain a concern to the swine industry throughout the world. *M. hyopneumoniae*, associated with enzootic pneumonia, is also considered to play a primary role in the porcine respiratory disease complex (PRDC), a continuing problem to swine producers. Other important pathogenic mycoplasmas include *M. hyorhinis,* which induces polyserositis and arthritis, and *M. hyosynoviae,* also a cause of arthritis in grow-finish pigs. Although the majority of other swine mycoplasmas, including *M. flocculare, M. sualvi, M. hopharyngis,* and several species of *Acholeplasma* can be isolated from swine, they appear to be nonpathogenic.

MYCOPLASMAL PNEUMONIA OF SWINE

Both Mare and Switzer in the U.S. (1965) and Goodwin et al. in the U.K. (1985) isolated *M. hyopneumoniae* in 1965. Since that time the role of *M. hyopneumoniae* in the induction of chronic pneumonia in pigs throughout the world continues to be problematic to the swine industry. Pneumonia caused by *M. hyopneumoniae* alone is mycoplasmal pneumonia. However, enzootic pneumonia is the most common term used because it describes the epidemiology pattern of the disease in combination with the various other etiological agents or lesions involved. Enzootic pneumonia is characterized by infection with *M. hyopneumoniae* and other pathogenic bacteria, such as *Pasteurella multocida, Streptococcus suis, Haemophilus parasuis,* or *Actinobacillus pleuropneumoniae* (APP). When combined with porcine respiratory and reproductive syndrome virus (PRRSV), porcine circovirus type 2 (PCV2) and/or swine influenza virus (SIV), a syndrome known as the porcine respiratory disease complex (PRDC) has emerged as a serious health problem to the swine industry. Infection with *M. hyopneumoniae,* independent of terminology, is associated with respiratory disease and reduced productivity in pigs.

Etiology

Culture and isolation of *M. hypneumoniae* is slow and complex. It can be grown in medium (Friis 1975); however, culture and identification is tedious, time consuming, and often unsuccessful. Contamination by other bacteria or other mycoplasmas, especially *M. hyorhinis,* will often preclude successful culture and isolation of the organism. Media and methods for isolation of *M. hyopneumoniae* were reviewed by Ross and Whittlestone (1983).

In culture, *M. hyopneumoniae* grows slowly compared to other porcine mycoplasmas, producing turbidity and an acid color shift to the media 3–30 days after inoculation of the media. Inoculation of solid agar medium and incubation in a 5–10% carbon dioxide atmosphere results in barely visible colonies after 2–3 days incubation. The organism must be differentiated from other swine mycoplasmas, and the nonpathogenic *M. flocculare* has many morphological, growth, and antigenic similarities to *M. hyopneumoniae.*

Antigenic diversity between *M. hyopneumoniae* isolates was first identified by Frey (1992) and further supported by Artiushin and Minion (1996) and Kokotovic (1999). Recent studies have further demonstrated differences in virulence between field isolates of *M. hyopneumoniae* (Strait et al. 2003; Vicca et al. 2002, 2003).

Epidemiology

Transmission of *M. hyopneumoniae* by carrier swine is the most common source of infection in field conditions. Isolation of the organism in nasal samples from infected pigs was demonstrated by Goodwin (1972). More recently, the use of polymerase chain reaction assays (PCR) have confirmed the presence of the organism in the nasal cavity of infected pigs (Calsamiglia et al. 1999, 2000; Kurth et al. 2002; Mattsson et al. 1995)). In addition, it was demonstrated that transmission of the organism can occur between penmates, independent of age (Etheridge et al. 1979; Piffer and Ross 1984). The slow growth characteristics and fastidious nature of *M. hyopneumoniae* would suggest that transmission between herds would be difficult. However, numerous researchers have documented the infection or reinfection of herds. As early as 1985, Goodwin found that herds that were less than 3.2 km apart could infect each other (Goodwin 1985). A number of studies of the Danish specific pathogen free (SPF) systems found that most reinfections occurred in the autumn and winter and when SPF herds were close to non-SPF herds (Jorsal and Thomsen 1988). More recently, risk factors identified with reinfection of *M. hyopneumoniae*-free herds in Switzerland include the presence of finishing farms, large mixed breeding-finishing farms, infected neighbors, and the close proximity of pig transport parking sites to the farm (Hege et al. 2002). Airborne transmission of *M. hyopneumoniae* has also been documented (Stark et al. 1998; Thomsen 1992).

The transmission of *M. hyopneumoniae* in many herds occurs by sow-to-pig exposure (Calsamiglia and Pijoan 2000; Rautiainen and Wallgren 2001). After infection is established, transmission between penmates occurs. Differences in exposure times as well as production systems have been investigated and identified (Sibila et al. 2004; Vicca et al. 2002). These studies demonstrated that numerous factors including housing styles and ventilation, management practices including stocking density, climatic conditions, and 1- or 2-site production systems versus 3-site systems can influence the transmission and dynamics of disease within a herd. In the majority of herds, transmission among penmates occurs at weaning. In continuous-flow systems, *M. hyopneumoniae* and other respiratory pathogens may be transmitted in large numbers at that time. However, overt signs of mycoplasmal pneumonia are typically not observed in pigs under 6 weeks of age, although all ages of pigs are susceptible (Piffer and Ross 1984). Exceptions to the typical age of pneumonia has been shown to occur experimentally in the presence of PRRSV, where an increase in the percentage of mycoplasmal pneumonia occurred within 10 days of experimental infection with *M. hyopneumoniae* (Thacker et al. 1999). Use of early weaning strategies, where pigs are weaned at 7–10 days of age and removed to an isolated site significantly reduced, but does not always completely eliminate, the vertical transmission from sows (Dritz et al. 1996).

The incidence of mycoplasmal pneumonia varies between countries. A recent survey of U.S. swine populations in the National Animal Health Monitoring Survey (NAHMS) (USDA 2001) found that swine producers in the U.S. felt *M. hyopneumoniae* was a concern in 19.6% in nursery pigs on 29% of the farms surveyed. In large swine operations with more than 10,000 pigs, mycoplasma associated disease was important in 52.7% of the sites with nursery pigs and 68% sites with finisher pigs. A diagnosis of *M. hyopneumoniae* was made in over 50% of the sites. Other countries have indicated the prevalence of herds with pneumonia consistent with mycoplasma ranging between 38% and 100% (Guerrero 1990). The exact prevalence of pneumonia due to *M. hyopneumoniae* is often difficult to ascertain due to the complication of co-infections with other respiratory pathogens including *P. multocida,* PRRSV, SIV and PCV2.

Eradication strategies for *M. hyopneumoniae* have been implemented in various countries with differing success. An eradication program using partial depopulation, consisting of a 2-week period during which no animals younger than 10 months were allowed on the farm, has been used successfully in a number of European countries including Switzerland, Denmark, Sweden, and Finland (Baekbo et al. 1996; Heinonen et al. 1999; Rautiainen et al. 2001; Zimmerman et al. 1989). In a follow-up to the Swiss eradication program, it was determined that 2.6% of the farms became reinfected, which is a considerable reduction over the time prior to the implementation of the eradication program (Hege et al. 2002). However, the reinfection rate in Switzerland that attempted eradication on a national level is indicative of the difficulty in successful eradicating the organism on a wide scale basis.

Economic losses due to mycoplasmal pneumonia have been associated with reduced daily weight gain (DWG), increased mortality, reduced feed efficiency and increased costs due to medication. A review article found that the DWG was reduced from 2.8% to 44.1% in 24 different studies (Straw et al. 1989). Pointon et al. (1985) found the growth rate of pigs in contact with *M. hyopneumoniae*-infected pigs was reduced by 12.7%. Information related to the exact amount of economic loss and percentage of pneumonia can often be difficult to interpret. Scheidt et al. (1990) found no correlation between average daily gain and severity of pneumonia at slaughter. Paisley et al. (1993) reported that mycoplasma-like pneumonia, as well as other respiratory lesions, was related to reduced mean daily gain. However, they concluded that lesions present at slaughter were responsible for only 9–27% of the variation and suggested that the remaining variation was due to factors such as environment, feed, genetics, and management systems.

Pathogenesis

The pathogenesis of *M. hyopneumoniae* is complex and consists of two separate methods of causing disease and affecting the overall health of the host. Colonization of the airways by *M. hyopneumoniae* begins with the binding of the organism to the cilia of epithelial cells in the airways of the pig (Zielinski and Ross 1992). Although the exact method of adherence of the organism to the cilia has not been fully identified, a number of proteins involved with adhesion have been identified. A protein, P97, has been recognized by Zhang, et al. (1994, 1995) to be involved in adherence of *M. hyopneumoniae* to the cilia, because monoclonal antibodies to this protein can block adherence to the organism in vitro. While P97 has been recognized as important in adherence to the cilia, vaccination against this protein alone has not produced protection against clinical disease or colonization in vivo (King et al. 1997). The P97 gene has been cloned and the binding region has been identified (Hsu et al. 1997; Hsu and Minion 1998). However, it has been determined that variation in this gene due to the addition or subtraction of repeated amino acids may result in alteration of the protein, making recognition by the immune system and thus immunization difficult (Wilton et al. 1998). Other glycoproteins (Chen et al. 1998) and cell surface features are probably also involved in the binding of the organism to the cilia (Zielinski and Ross 1992). Colonization of the cilia by *M. hyopneumoniae* results in ciliostasis, clumping and loss of cilia (DeBey and Ross 1994), and loss of epithelial cells and bronchial goblet cells (DeBey et al. 1992). Colonization of the airways by *M. hyopneumoniae* results in a significant reduction in the ability of mucociliary apparatus to function and clear the airways of debris and invading pathogens, especially bacteria. This is thought to be an important mechanism for the increased colonization of the airways by respiratory bacteria, including *P. multocida, B. bronchiseptica, A. pleuropneumoniae, A. pyogenes,* and other bacteria. This co-infection of *M. hyopneumoniae* with bacteria results in enzootic pneumonia.

The virulence factors associated with *M. hyopneumoniae* are largely unknown and appear to be extremely complex. The genome of one isolate has recently been sequenced (Dr. F. C. Minion, Iowa State University, personal communication), which should facilitate the identification of the genes and proteins that are important in the induction of disease and immunity. Virulence factors that contribute to attachment/colonization, cytotoxicity, competition for substrates, and evasion and modulation of the respiratory immune system remain unknown. The various mechanisms of pathogenesis involved with *M. hyopneumoniae* infection are probably not due to a single gene, but rather to a multitude of gene products that will need to be identified.

The complex, chronic pathogenesis of *M. hyopneumoniae*-mediated respiratory disease appears dependent on the alteration or modulation of the respiratory immune response. Immunopathologic changes are a major component of mycoplasmal pneumonia, although little is known about the mechanisms of how the organism induces the immune and inflammatory responses associated with disease. The microscopic lesions associated with mycoplasmal pneumonia are characterized by an infiltration of the peribronchiolar and perivascular areas with mononuclear cells consisting of both macrophages and lymphocytes. This infiltration of both B and T lymphocytes over time can result in the formation of lymphoid nodules with germinal-like centers. The infiltration of mononuclear cells in association with *M. hyopneumoniae* infection impacts all of the components of the immune system, including macrophages from the innate immune system and B and T lymphocytes of the adaptive immune response. Pulmonary alveolar macrophages infected with both *M. hyopneumoniae* and APP were shown to have reduced phagocytic capability (Caruso and Ross 1990). *M. hyopneumoniae*-infection also induces macrophages to produce proinflammatory cytokines, including interleukin (IL)-1, IL-6, IL-8, and tumor necrosis factor (TNF) alpha, both in vivo (Asai et al. 1993, 1994; Thacker et al. 2000) and in vitro (Thanawongnuwech et al. 2001). Recent research has demonstrated that IL-10 and IL-12 levels are also increased in the bronchoalveolar lavage fluid 28 days after experimental infection with *M. hyopneumoniae* (Thanawongnuwech and Thacker 2003). Production of proinflammatory cytokines increases the inflammation in the lung, which further reduces the respiratory immune system's ability to control other pathogens in the respiratory tract. Although an inflammatory response is important in the control of pathogens, the tissue injury and disease subsequent to *M. hyopneumoniae* infections appears to be caused more by the response from the host than the organism itself.

In addition to affecting macrophages, *M. hyopneumoniae* has an impact on both B and T lymphocytes. Evidence of the immunosuppressive effect of *M. hyopneumoniae* to nonspecific mitogens has been reported (Kishima and Ross 1985). A subsequent study found nonspecific stimulation (mitogenic) of lymphocytes by the organism (Messier and Ross 1991). Tajima et al. (1984) further confirmed the role of the immune system in the pathogenesis of mycoplasmal pneumonia by demonstrating that the pneumonia was less severe in thymectomized pigs treated with antithymocyte serum and inoculated with *M. hyopneumoniae*. These results suggest that a cell-mediated immune mechanism may be important in the development of pneumonia. However, in the same study *M. hyopneumoniae* was isolated from the spleen of one of the thymectomized pigs, indicating that containing and controlling invasion and systemic spread of the organism by T lymphocytes is crucial in preventing systemic spread of the organism. The alterations of the various effector cells in the respiratory immune system by *M. hyopneumoniae* in infected pigs is probably important in the ability of the organism to persist and cause disease in pigs.

Onset of mycoplasmal pneumonia may be dependent on the intensity of infection and the number of organisms that colonize the respiratory tract and the presence of other pathogens in the respiratory tract that contribute to disease. Recent research has determined that different isolates have different virulence capabilities that influence their ability to induce disease (Strait et al. 2003; Vicca et al. 2003). The incubation period for experimental infection as well as acute infections in the field is 10–14 days. Under natural field conditions it is more difficult to pinpoint the exact time of infection and thus the incubation period. Disease has been reported to occur as early as 2 weeks of age (Holmgren 1974), but more commonly it spreads slowly within the herd, and pigs begin showing clinical disease associated with mycoplasmal pneumonia at 3–6 months of age.

An important role of *M. hyopneumoniae* in swine respiratory disease is its interaction with other pathogens. Infections with *M. hyopneumoniae* alone induce a mild chronic pneumonia; however, in conjunction with other pathogens; the respiratory disease becomes a severe problem consistent with PRDC in the field. Numerous studies have investigated the impact of co-infections of other pathogens and *M. hyopneumoniae*. In most cases, it is the co-infecting organism that has an increased severity and potentially duration of disease associated with *M. hyopneumoniae*. Ciprian et al. (1994) did a nice review of the interaction of *M. hyopneumoniae* with the various bacteria of the respiratory tract. Enzootic pneumonia, attributed to *M. hyopneumoniae*, is centered on the interaction with other bacteria, including *P. multocida* and APP. With secondary bacterial infections, the pneumonia consistent with *M. hyopneumoniae* infection appears more severe resulting in enzootic pneumonia. In contrast, combination with viral respiratory pathogens, including PRRSV and PCV2, has changed the character of respiratory disease and has resulted in the term porcine respiratory disease complex (PRDC). In a first study investigating the interaction of *M. hyopneumoniae* and PRRSV, Van Alstine (1996) did not see a strong interaction between the two. However, since that time, Thacker et al. (1999) demonstrated that the viral pneumonia induced by PRRSV was significantly increased in both severity and duration when both pathogens were present. In this study, it was found that the presence of PRRSV resulted in increased acute mycoplasmal pneumonia. Similar findings were observed in the presence of pseudorabies virus (PRV) (Shibata et al. 1998). Recently it has been demonstrated that *M. hyopneumoniae* increases the pneumonia associated with concurrent infection with PCV2 (Opriessnig et al. 2003). In contrast, the interaction of *M. hyopneumoniae* with SIV lacks the interaction observed with the other viruses, and although the severity of pneumonia at the peak of infection is increased, the potentiation observed with PRRSV and PCV2 did not occur (Thacker et al. 2001). This interaction with other pathogens is probably the most important role that *M. hyopneumoniae* plays in swine respiratory disease.

Clinical Signs

Mycoplasmal pneumonia is chronic in nature with a high morbidity and a low mortality. Clinically it is characterized by a dry, nonproductive cough, although the presence or absence of cough is variable with individual animals. Experimentally, onset of clinical signs characterized by coughing, occurs within 7–14 days post infection; however, with natural infection clinical disease onset is less predictable (Robert 1974; Sorensen et al. 1997; Vicca et al. 2002). Onset of clinical signs in a herd tends to be gradual, with coughing within the herd lasting weeks to months. The presence of other clinical symptoms, such as fever, decreased appetite, labored breathing or prostration, is due to secondary pathogens. Many pigs with mycoplasmal pneumonia may appear unthrifty and feed intake is reduced, but overall the pigs remain normal in appearance.

Lesions

The macroscopic lesions of mycoplasmal pneumonia consist of purple to gray areas of consolidation of the cranial-ventral portions of the lung. The lesions tend to be in the ventral portions of the cranial and middle lobes, the accessory lobe, and the cranial ventral portions of the caudal lobes of the lungs; however, they can be spread throughout the lungs in severe cases. In the absence of secondary infections, the lesions tend to be focal and fairly well demarcated. In the presence of other organisms, the lesions become more diffuse and depending on the agent, difficult to differentiate from the other pathogens. When the lung tissue is cut, the consistency of the lung is thick and heavy although not excessively firm. A catarrhal exudate is often present in the airways. The regional lymph nodes are usually firm and enlarged.

Microscopic lesions are characteristic of a chronic pneumonia. Early in the disease process, accumulations of neutrophils in the airways are present microscopically. As the disease progresses, lymphocytes and monocytes infiltrate the peribronchiolar, peribronchial, and perivascular regions. Interstitial pneumonia may also be observed, with airways filled with cellular debris. Alveoli may contain eosinophilic fluid consistent with edema and increased numbers of mononuclear and polymorphonuclear cells. More advanced lesions can consist of lymphoid nodules associated with the airways. In recovering lesions, alveoli are collapsed and emphysematous and lymphoid nodules are common. The severity of the microscopic lesions increases with increased numbers of secondary pathogens as well as in pigs housed in poor environments with inadequate management strategies. Neither macroscopic nor the microscopic lesions are specific for *M. hyopneumoinae*, and other respiratory pathogens, including bacterial invaders and swine influenza virus (SIV) must be ruled out.

Diagnosis

Macroscopic lesions associated with mycoplasmal pneumonia combined with the onset of clinical disease and coughing lead to the suspicion of *M. hyopneumoniae* infection. It is important to remember however that the clinical signs, macroscopic and microscopic lesions, are not specific for mycoplasmal pneumonia, so other differential assays must be done to confirm the role of the organism in respiratory disease in a herd.

The pathogenesis of disease due to *M. hyopneumoniae* makes accurate diagnosis of the organism challenging. The organism's location on the mucosal surface of the respiratory tract, gene expression variation and ability to modulate the respiratory immune response can make the diagnosis of mycoplasma pneumonia difficult. Although culture and isolation are considered the "gold standards" for detecting *M. hyopneumoniae,* isolation of the organism is difficult due to its requirement for specialized media and its slow growth properties, often requiring 4–8 weeks to grow to measurable levels (Friis 1975). Difficulty in culturing the organism is increased by the additional requirement for swine serum negative for *M. hyopneumoniae* antibodies. Due to the slow growth in culture, contamination by other swine mycoplasmas or bacteria may preclude the growth and isolation of *M. hyopneumoniae.* Combined, these factors make isolation and growth of the organism expensive, difficult and impractical. Culture is not recommended as a diagnostic technique and failure to isolate the organism under field conditions should not be used to deny the presence of the organism within a herd.

Serology is the most common tool used to determine the presence or absence of an organism within a herd situation and *M. hyopneumoniae* is no exception. However, as with most diagnostics associated with *M. hyopneumoniae*, interpretation of serological results can be challenging. Numerous studies have compared the various assays as well as their association with lung lesions and protection against disease. Originally complement fixation (CF) assays were used to detect antibodies to *M. hyopneumoniae.* However in several comparison studies, it was determined that an indirect ELISA assay was more efficacious at detecting antibody than the CF assay (Bereiter et al. 1990; Piffer et al. 1984). Currently, ELISA assays are the most commonly used assay to detect antibodies to the organism. Serology is best suited to screening for infected herd status or evaluating vaccine responses. Care must be taken in their use on an individual animal basis, as well as in evaluating for vaccine compliance. Three ELISA assays are currently used in the United States to detect mycoplasmal serum antibodies. Indirect ELISA assays include the Tween-20 assay (Bereiter et al. 1990; Nicolet et al. 1980) and the HerdCheck *Mycoplasma hyopneumoniae* ELISA assay (Idexx Laboratories, Westbrook, Maine). The DAKO *Mycoplasma hyopneumoniae* ELISA (DAKO corporation, Carpenteria, California) is a blocking ELISA based on an antigenic internal protein. A recent study using serum from experimentally infected pigs found that all three assays had excellent specificity in recognizing antibody negative samples and thus few false positive results are observed (Erlandson et al. 2002). In contrast, the sensitivity of the assays was low and ranged from 37–49%. This low sensitivity results in a low negative predictive value and a high percentage of false negative results. Of the assays assessed, the DAKO ELISA was the most con-

sistent in identifying infected pigs; however, a combination of assays appeared to improve the predictive ability of the tests. Sorensen et al. (1997) found similar results of high specificity and low sensitivity in *M. hyopneumoniae* ELISA assays. In addition, recent research has found that the assays varied in their ability to detect antibodies induced in pigs experimentally infected with different field isolates of the organism (Strait et al. 2003; Vicca et al. 2002). To further complicate the serological diagnosis of *M. hyopneumoniae*, *M. flocculare* antibodies can cross-react with a number of the serological assays and must be considered in the diagnostic workup within a farm. A study of nine naturally infected Danish swine herds found that most pigs seroconverted in the growing-to-finishing units and the association of lung lesions at slaughter and seroconversion was complex (Andreasen et al. 2000, 2001). It was demonstrated that pigs seroconverting to *M. hyopneumoniae* close to slaughter had the highest percentage of pneumonia and early seroconversions appeared to be related to pleuritic lesions in the cranio-ventral regions of the lung (Andreasen et al. 2001). In addition, concurrent infection with PRRSV (Thacker et al. 1999), SIV (Thacker et al. 2001), or PCV2 (Opriessnig et al. 2003) appear to increase *M. hyopneumoniae* antibody levels. Antibody levels following vaccination with *M. hyopneumoniae* bacterins may vary depending on the vaccine, the infection status of the pig, and the serological assay used (Erlandson et al. 2002; Thacker 2001). No correlation between vaccine-induced antibody levels and protection from colonization and disease has been observed (Djordjevic et al. 1997; Thacker et al. 1998).

In addition to assessing serum samples for the presence of antibodies to *M. hyopneumoniae*, colostrum has been used to document freedom of a herd from infection (Rautiainen et al. 2000). Detection of antibodies in colostrum occurred weeks prior to clinical outbreak of mycoplasmal pneumonia in one case (Sorensen et al. 1993). However, sampling colostrum within the first 2 hours after farrowing is required for the most accurate detection of antibodies, which decreases the practicality under typical field situations. In addition, it has been demonstrated that parity is important in the accurate detection of antibodies in colostrums, with high-parity sows being a better source for the detection of antibodies to assess the herd status (Rautiainen et al. 2000).

Accurate diagnosis of *M. hyonpneumoniae* has increased with the development of polymerase chain reaction (PCR) assays (Artiushin et al. 1993; Calsamiglia et al. 1999; Harasawa et al. 1991; Mattson et al. 1995; Stark et al. 1998; Stemke 1997; Stemke et al. 1994; Verdin et al. 2000). The various collection sites and potential uses of PCR to detect infection accurately have been investigated (Calsamiglia and Pijoan 2000; Calsamiglia et al. 2000, Kurth et al. 2002; Sorensen et al. 1997). On the basis of these studies, lung tissue and bronchial washings appear to be among the most reliable collection sites, and detection of the organism from the nasal cavity appears more variable. To increase the sensitivity of the assay, nested PCR assays using two sets of primers are typically used. This results in an assay capable of picking up as few as four to five organisms. Although the ability to detect these low numbers of organisms may assist in the detection of *M. hyopneumoniae* on a herd basis, the potential for contamination may be problematic. It has been documented that PCR assays are capable of detecting the organism in the air of production units housing pigs infected with *M. hyopneumoniae* (Stark et al. 1998). In addition, recent research investigating the variability of the genetics of different field isolates of *M. hyopneumoniae* has documented potential differences in our ability to detect the organism through the use of PCR (Strait et al. 2003). These results suggest that additional research is required to determine the accuracy of detection of *M. hyopneumoniae* by PCR under field conditions.

Detection of *M. hyopneumoniae* by either fluorescent antibody (FA) or immunohistochemistry (IHC) assays is typically performed in diagnostic laboratories (Amanfu et al. 1983; Opriessnig et al. 2003). Frozen tissues are required to detect *M. hyopneumoniae* by FA assay, making sample collection problematic in the field. In situ hybridization of fixed tissues has also been described, although used less commonly (Kwon and Chae 1999). Because in situ hybridization and IHC assays can be performed on fixed tissues, these assays are more practical for samples collected on the farm. It is critical that the samples collected for all of these assays include airways with ciliated epithelial cells so the organism can be detected.

Ultimately the assay used to diagnose *M. hyopneumoniae* is dependent on whether it is to determine infection status as an aid in determining intervention strategy timing or to assess whether a herd is free of the organism in eradication protocols. Serology alone would be a poor choice to confirm that a herd is negative for *M. hyopneumoniae*, and PCR assays are not usually required to determine timing of vaccination or therapy, which can be based primarily on the occurrence of clinical disease. Sorensen et al. (1997) compared duration of disease and evaluation of four diagnostic assays, including serology and PCR following experimental challenge. He reported similar predictive values between all of the assays. Thus, for the greatest degree of accuracy on detecting the organism, multiple diagnostic procedures are probably required. The sensitivity and specificity of each of the assays should be considered both for accurate interpretation of clinical signs and serological and PCR test results, and according to the information required by the veterinarian and producer.

Treatment

Antibiotics against *M. hyopneumoniae* can help control the disease, but do not eliminate the organism from the respiratory tract nor heal existing lesions. A number of studies have assessed the efficacy of a number of antibiotics, including various quinolones (Hannan et al. 1989), tylosin, oxytetracycline (Cooper et al. 1993), and tilmicosin (Thacker et al. 2001), among others using a number of different testing systems (Tanner et al. 1993; Ter Laak et al. 1991; Williams 1978; Wu et al. 1997) to evaluate the susceptibility of each antimicrobial agent in vitro. In these studies, the quinolones tended to be highly effective; tiamulin, danfloxacin, chlortetracycline, lincomycin, tilmicosin, and other antibiotics were active against the organism, but many of these appeared to mycoplasmastatic rather than 'cidal. However, care must be taken when comparing in vitro antibiotic studies on *M. hyopneumoniae* to their performance in the pig, due to the location of the organism on the cilia within the airways. In order for an antibiotic to be effective against the organism, it must be able to achieve significant levels within the mucous and fluids of the respiratory tract.

Studies assessing antibiotic efficacy in vivo have also been performed, occasionally with conflicting results. *M. hyopneumoniae* lacks a cell wall, which precludes the effectiveness of antibiotics that would interfere with cell wall synthesis, such as penicillin, ampicillin, amoxicillin, and cephalosporin. Other antibiotics that would have little efficacy against *M. hyopneumoniae* include polymyxin, erythromycin, streptomycin, trimethoprim, and sulphonamides. The ability of *M. hyopneumoniae* to develop resistance to antibiotics is unknown; however, it has been reported in the field that resistance to the tetracyclines can occur (Maes et al. 1996). Tiamulin has been reported to reduce the severity of experimentally induced and naturally acquired mycoplasmal pneumonia (Hannan et al. 1982). In a separate study, Ross and Cox (1988) failed to observe beneficial effects of tiamulin on macroscopic or microscopic lesions or *M. hyopneumoniae* antigens detected by FA. Research has demonstrated that use of chlortetracycline in the feed administered prior to challenge reduces both the severity of pneumonia as well as the number of organisms (Thacker et al. 2001). Other studies have demonstrated the beneficial effects of tiamulin (Hsu et al. 1983), tilmicosin and tylosin (Mateusen et al. 2001), and doxycycline (Bousquet et al. 1998) on weight gain and clinical disease. However, these were field trials, and pigs were infected with multiple pathogens making assessment of antibiotic impact on *M. hyopneumoniae* more difficult to interpret. However, results of antibiotic use in the treatment of *M. hyopneumoniae* are often disappointing because the organisms tend to reappear after the medication is discontinued. In addition, infection with secondary pathogens makes therapy more challenging and often results in the need to use multiple antibiotics to control all of the various pathogens associated with respiratory disease. The successful use of combination therapies with antibiotics has also been reported (Burch et al. 1986; Stipkovits et al. 2001).

Antibiotics as a therapy for mycoplasmal pneumonia are best used during periods of stress in the life of the pig, including weaning or mixing. Knowing the other pathogens present in the respiratory tract is critical for the success of therapy as well as determining the optimal timing for the best results. Administration of medication prior to or early following exposure to the organism is also important for success in using medication as an aid in controlling mycoplasmal pneumonia. Overall, prevention of the development of mycoplasmal pneumonia is the only effective method for decreasing the economic impact of *M. hyopneumoniae* within a swine herd.

Prevention

Effective prevention and control of mycoplasmal pneumonia, enzootic pneumonia, or PRDC is based on providing an optimal environment for the pigs, which includes adequate quality of air, ventilation, ambient temperature, and the appropriate number of animals housed in the available space. Management practices such as all in/all out pig flow, medicated and segregated early weaning, and multisite operations further facilitate control of respiratory disease associated with *M. hyopneumoniae* infection. In addition, Maes et al. (1996) recommended other management strategies that help limit the impact of *M. hyopneumoniae* on pig production. These include a balanced and stable sow herd with fewer than 30% replacement gilts; closing the herd or minimizing the number of sources used to procure pigs; multisite production; biosecurity to prevent the spread and introduction of disease; reduction of stress on pigs; optimal stocking density; and adequate ventilation, air quality and room temperature.

Eradication has become a goal for many production systems. The Swiss have used a program referred to earlier to eradicate the organism from the country (Zimmerman et al. 1989). Other protocols for eradication of the organism within a herd include medicated early weaning protocols where the sow is treated with antibiotics and the pigs weaned at 6 days of age (Alexander et al. 1980), and segregated early weaning with the use of multisite operations to decrease significantly the number of organisms transmitted from the sow to the pigs (Harris 1990). Using pigs that have been produced by cesarean section–derived, colostrum-deprived (CDCD) pigs to repopulate a herd is the only method guaranteed to produce *M. hyopneumoniae*-free pigs consistently. In all cases, reexposure and reinfection have been problems in maintaining *M. hyopneumoniae*-free pigs.

Vaccines against *M. hyopneumoniae*, produced from adjuvanted whole-cell or membrane preparations are commonly used to control the clinical disease associated with mycoplasmal pneumonia. Numerous commercial vaccines are now used throughout the United States and the world. More than 85% of the herds in the U.S. vaccinate with mycoplasma vaccine (USDA 2001). Numerous studies have been performed demonstrating the efficacy of these vaccines under both field and experimental settings. Currently in the U.S. both single- and dual-dose vaccination protocols are used successfully to control disease. The appropriate use of either of these strategies is based on a number of factors, including overall health of the farm, time of clinical disease associated with *M. hyopneumoniae*, level of maternal antibodies, and circulation of PRRSV virus in the herd.

The economic benefit of mycoplasma vaccination has been demonstrated in a number of studies (Dohoo and Montgomery 1996; Jensen et al. 2002; Maes et al. 1999). Analysis of the immune response induced by *M. hyopneumoniae* bacterins has demonstrated reduction in percentage of lung lesions, production of serum antibodies, production of local IgG and IgA in the respiratory tract, and reduction of proinflammatory cytokines (Djordjevic et al. 1997; Kobisch et al. 1987; Kristensen et al. 1981; Messier et al. 1990; Ross et al. 1984; Sheldrake et al. 1993; Thacker et al. 1998, 2000). In addition, the effectiveness of antibiotic use in conjunction with vaccination has been demonstrated as an efficacious method to reduce the clinical disease associated with *M. hyopneumoniae* infection (Mateusen et al. 2001, 2002). Vaccine failure has been reported in the field and the impact of maternal antibodies has been investigated. It appears that maternal antibody levels against *M. hyopneumoniae* inhibit vaccine efficacy only if levels of antibodies are very high (Jayappa et al. 2001; Thacker et al. 1998, 2000; Thacker and Thacker 2001). However, a major cause of decreased mycoplasma vaccine efficacy is the presence of PRRSV during or shortly after vaccination (Thacker et al. 2000). Vaccination against *M. hyopneumoniae* reduced the increased severity of PRRSV pneumonia in conjunction with mycoplasmal pneumonia; however, the presence of PRRSV, either through infection or use of a modified live vaccine, significantly decreased the efficacy of the vaccine against *M. hyopneumoniae*-induced disease. The current vaccines are effective in reducing the clinical disease associated with mycoplasmal pneumonia including percentage of lung lesions and coughing; however, they do not prevent colonization of the organism in the host (Thacker et al. 2000). Investigation of new vaccines is actively occurring, including the use of aerosol and feed-based vaccines as well as subunit vaccines (Fagan et al. 1996, 2001; Frey et al. 1994; Lin et al. 1991; Murphy et al. 1993).

M. HYORHINIS

Polyserositis, arthritis, and otitis are clinical disorders associated with *M. hyorhinis* infection. The organism is ubiquitous within the swine population and also a common cell contaminant in cultured cell lines from humans and all species of animals.

Etiology

If present, *M. hyorhinis* is typically the first mycoplasma that grows in culture when investigating mycoplasmal diseases in pigs. The protocol and media for isolation and growth of *M. hyorhinis* is well summarized by Ross and Whittlestone (1983). The presence of the organism in pigs frequently prevents the isolation of other mycoplasmas.

Epidemiology

M. hyorhinis is a common pathogen in swine production units, with pigs becoming infected from either the sows or older pigs in system. Ross and Spear (1993) demonstrated that the organism could be isolated from the nasal secretions of 10% of sows and 30–40% of weanling pigs. It is considered a normal member of the upper airways of young pigs (Ross and Young 1993). Following exposure, the organism spreads quickly through the upper respiratory tract and can frequently be isolated from the lungs and eustachian tube. The majority of infected pigs have no apparent clinical disease, although many clinical diseases, including pneumonia, arthritis, polyserositis, eustachitis, and otitis, have been described in conjunction with *M. hyorhinis* infection.

Pathogenesis

Little is known about the pathogenesis of *M. hyorhinis*. Like *M. hyopneumoniae*, *M. hyorhinis* adheres to ciliated epithelial cells within the upper and lower respiratory tract of pigs. Little is known about the virulence factors of *M. hyorhinis*. Within the respiratory tract, pneumonia has been reported to be associated with some strains of *M. hyorhinis* (Ross 1992). In addition, infection with *M. hyorhinis* can result in otitis media (Kazama et al. 1989; Morita et al. 1999). The presence of the organism in the auditory tube may impair the mucociliary apparatus as the organism adheres to the cilia of the epithelial cells. This enables ascending infection with other bacteria such as *P. multocida* and *A. pyogenes*. Co-infection of the respiratory tract with other pathogens, including PRRSV (Kawashima et al. 1996) or *B. bronchiseptica* (Gois et al. 1977) has been suggested as being important for the increased respiratory disease that occasionally occurs with *M. hyorhinis* infection.

Although *M. hyorhinis* is a common inhabitant of the respiratory tract of pigs, much of the disease is associated with invasion of the organism systemically resulting in polyserositis and arthritis. The mechanism that enables the *M. hyorhinis* to leave the respiratory tract and induce systemic disease is currently unknown, although the presence of other pathogens or stress may facilitate the spread of the organism systemically. Once systemic, the organism produces polyserositis and polyarthritis in pigs less than 8 weeks of age, and infection in 3–6-month-old pigs typically results in only arthritis (Potgieter et al. 1972; Potgieter and Ross 1972).

Isolation of the organism from areas of polyserositis or arthritis is most successful during the acute stages of disease. It may be possible to isolate the organism later in infection and the organism has been shown to persist as long as 6 months in some joints. In a study of arthritis in Canada, 56 of 153 joints with arthritis were positive for bacteria and 5 of those were a *Mycoplasma* sp, with 3 confirmed as *M. hyorhinis* (Hariharan et al. 1992). This suggests that, although infection with the organism is potentially capable of inducing arthritis in pigs, it is not a frequent cause. Genetic differences in the susceptibility of pigs to experimental inoculation with *M. hyorhins* has been suggested and appears to be related to the production of proinflammatory cytokines (Magnusson et al. 1998; Reddy et al. 2000).

Clinical Signs

The polyserositis associated with *M. hyorhinis* infection generally occurs in 3–10-week-old pigs, although occasionally it can occur in older animals. Typically evidence of disease occurs 3–10 days after exposure or the precipitating cause of the systemic spread of the organism. Pigs become unthrifty in appearance with roughened hair coat, slight fever, depression, reduced appetite, reluctance to move, difficulty breathing, abdominal tenderness, lameness, and swollen joints. The acute clinical signs begin to resolve after 10–14 days depending on the severity of the clinical disease. Some pigs continue to do poorly or die acutely. If arthritis is involved, lameness and swollen joints will persist for 2–3 months, although many pigs will remain lame up to 6 months later. In addition, conjunctivitis has been associated with *M. hyorhinis* infection (Friis 1976).

Lesions

The polyserositis of the acute phase of the disease consists of fibrinopurulent pericarditis, pleuritis, and occasionally peritonitis. Over time, the membrane lesions consist of fibrous adhesions and thickened, cloudy, rough serosal membranes. Acute arthritis is associated with painful and swollen joints with increased amounts of serosanguineous synovial fluid. The synovial membranes are swollen and hyperemic. Over time, the synovial fluid increases in amount and fibrous adhesions occur. The lesions appear less active, although erosion of cartilaginous surfaces and pannus formation may occur.

Otitis due to *M. hyorhinis* is characterized by the appearance of mycoplasmas among the cilia in the auditory canal.

Diagnosis

The diagnosis of clinical disease in association with *M. hyorhinis* is commonly made by the appearance of the serofibrinous to fibinopurulent lesions, although other pathogens such as *H. parasuis* and *S. suis* can cause similar lesions. The organism can be isolated during the acute and subacute stages of disease. Freshly necropsied animals will increase the success in isolating the organism as autolysis reduces the chances of culturing *M. hyorhinis*.

PCR assays capable of detecting *M. hyorhinis* have been used to assist in differentiating the various mycoplasma species isolated from field cases; however, they are not routinely performed as a diagnostic procedure (Taylor et al. 1984, 1985).

Treatment

In vitro antibiotic susceptibility for *M. hyorhinis* has been shown to many antibiotics. However, treatment of clinically affected animals is usually unsuccessful because the majority of the lesions are chronic in nature and elimination of the organism does little to reduce the adhesions and inflammation. Treatment with tylosin or lincomycin may be beneficial (Ross 1992).

Prevention

Control programs should stress preventing the other medical conditions that may predispose the animals to the systemic spread of *M. hyorhinis*. No published information is available on the ability of antibiotics to reduce clinical disease and no vaccine is currently available on a commercial basis.

M. HYOSYNOVIAE ARTHRITIS

M. hyosynoviae-induced arthritis has been recognized throughout the world with reports from the United States (Ross and Duncan 1970), England (Blowey 1993; Roberts et al. 1972), Germany (Ross et al. 1977) and Denmark (Nielsen et al. 2001). It was demonstrated in 1995 that 8–9% of synovial fluid samples from Danish slaughter pigs with nonpurulent arthritis were positive for the organism (Buttenshon 1995), and Friis et al. (1992) isolated the organism from 20% of arthritic lesions of pigs in a Danish abattoir.

Etiology

A review of isolation techniques and the media required for isolating *M. hyosynoviae* are reported in Ross and Karmon (1970). Isolation of the organism is often complicated because of overgrowth by *M. hyorhinis* and bacteria. A selective media has been described that facilitates the ability to isolate *M. hyosynoviae* in the presence of *M. hyorhinis* (Friis 1979). Recent research has identified genetic variation between isolates of the organism with several genotypically distinct variants occurring in a single herd (Kokotovic et al. 1999, 2002).

Epidemiology

M. hyosynoviae colonizes the respiratory tract of pigs (Friis et al. 1991) and is primarily located in the upper portions (Ross and Spear 1973). The organism can persist in carrier swine indefinitely in the tonsils (Friis et al. 1991; Ross and Spear 1973). Although present in infected sows, the organism is not transmitted to the pigs until 4–8 weeks of age (Ross and Spear 1973). Large numbers of the organism are shed only during the acute phase of infection and only intermittently from persistently infected sows (Ross and Spear 1973). It is unknown why the organism can't be isolated from pigs younger than 4 weeks of age; however, it does allow pigs to be obtained that are free of the organism.

Following infection of a few pigs at 4–8 weeks of age, it is thought the organism is spread throughout the pens from either acute or chronically infected animals (Hagedorn-Olsen et al. 1999). The rate of spread may be related to environmental factors as well as stocking density.

Pathogenesis

The acute phase of infection with *M. hyosynoviae* lasts 1–2 weeks, during which time the organism spreads systemically to the joints and various tissues throughout the body. Arthritis can occur after an incubation period of 4–9 days and the mycoplasma can be isolated from the joints during the acute phase, which is 1–2 weeks after the occurrence of lameness and typically 2–3 weeks post exposure. The subacute and chronic phases occur 3–16 weeks after clinical arthritis, during which time the tonsils remain infected and viable organisms can persist in joint and lymph nodes. Infection of pigs from chronically infected animals through pen contact may not result in the systemic spread of the organism, but infect the tonsils only. This suggests that animals are initially infected through the tonsils, which may then result in systemic spread (Hagedorn-Olsen et al. 1999). In a study by Hagedorn-Olsen et al. (1999), septicemia was found in 90% of experimentally infected pigs, 12 of 23 pigs developed clinical arthritis, and 20% of the joints from which the organism was isolated appeared normal, demonstrating that infection does not always result in clinical disease. Differences in genetics, body structure, management practices, and environment appear to play a role in determining whether clinical arthritis will result following infection with *M. hyosynoviae* (Ross 1973). Osteochondrosis or trauma-induced bursal lesions (Nielsen et al. 2001) may predispose pigs to arthritis induced by *M. hyosynoviae*.

Clinical Signs

Clinical lameness associated with *M. hyosynoviae* typically occurs in 3–5-month-old pigs. The lameness appears acutely and may occur in more than one leg. One study found only hindlegs were involved in clinical lameness associated with the organism (Nielsen et al. 2001). Rectal temperatures remain normal, and pigs may exhibit a slight reduction in appetite with an accompanying weight loss. Often soft fluctuating to no joint swelling is observed, with no evidence of suppurative arthritis.

Acute signs persist for 3–10 days after which the

lameness gradually decreases in severity. Many animals recover with no further lameness or may exhibit stiffness of motion. Continued clinical signs are often due to osteochondrosis as well as *M. hyosynoviae*-induced arthritis. Mortality is low and morbidity ranges form 1–50% in affected herds (Ross 1992).

Lesions

Proliferation, swelling, edema, and hyperemia of synovial membranes are common in *M. hyosynoviae*-infected joints. Increased volumes of synovial fluid that is serofibrinous to serosanguineous in nature are frequently observed. Lame pigs may have cloudy to brownish-colored synovial fluid. The periarticular tissues surrounding the affected joint are often edematous. In chronic phases the joint membranes may be thickened with fibrosis with pannus formation occurring. Cartilaginous changes may be associated with either *M. hyosynoviae* infection or due to osteochondrosis. Pseudocysts or calluses on the cranial surface of the carpal joint or the plantar and lateral surface of the tarsal joint may occur (Nielsen et al. 2001). Microscopically, acute lesions are characterized by edema, hyperemia, hyperplasia of synovial cells, and perivascular infiltration with mononuclear cells, including lymphocytes, monocytes, and macrophages. As the infection progresses, increased numbers of plasma cells and lymphocytes are present, followed by fibrosis as the joint heals (Hagedorn-Olsen et al. 1999).

Diagnosis

Acute lameness in 10–20-week-old pigs that is not responsive to penicillin is suggestive of *M. hyosynoviae* (Ross 1992). Isolation of the organism from the joint that exhibits lesions consistent with *M. hyosynoviae* infection is required for a definitive diagnosis. Animals with a disease profile consistent with *M. hyosynoviae* infection and in the acute phase of the disease should be selected for diagnostic procedures. Joint fluids from several animals should be collected from live animals or at slaughter or necropsy.

Serology can be used to detect antibodies to the organism. Both complement fixation and ELISA assays have been described, although these assays are not generally available in the U.S. (Hagedorn-Olsen et al. 1999; Zimmermann and Ross 1982). Pigs with subclinical infections may develop antibodies in the absence of disease, so the use of paired serum samples collected during the acute and subacute or chronic phase of disease should be used to ascertain that the antibody levels are increasing with the clinical disease.

Treatment

An in vitro study demonstrated that enrofloxacin, lincomycin, tetracycline, and tiamulin are all active against the *M. hyosynoviae* (Aarestrup and Friis 1998). In the same study, isolates collected between 1968–1971 appeared to be highly susceptible to tylosin activity, and isolates collected in 1995–1996 were divided between highly susceptible and relatively resistant, suggesting the development of resistance to tylosin by some isolates (Aarestrup and Friis 1998). Earlier studies had documented that *M. hyosynoviae* was sensitive to tylosin, lincomycin (Zimmermann and Ross 1975), and valnemulin (Hannan et al. 1997). In addition, Burch et al. (1984) demonstrated that the use of tiamulin and lincomycin was effective in improving production parameters and reducing lameness in a herd that was experiencing clinical disease associated with *M. hyosynoviae*. However, in a study of 9 Danish herds, treatment had no apparent impact on the outcome of clinical disease, with the majority of lameness resolving independent of the antibiotic therapy used (Nielsen et al. 2001).

MYCOPLASMA HAEMOSUIS (SUIS) (EPERYTHROZOON SUIS)

With the advent of molecular biology, *Eperythrozoon suis* has recently been reclassified as a member of the Mollicutes family based on the physical characteristic of the organism and the 16s ribosomal RNA gene sequences. Initially renamed *Mycoplasma suis,* it has been proposed to be called *M. haemosuis* and will be used in this chapter (Neimark et al. 2002). Independent of name, the organism remains the cause of anemia in pigs.

Etiology

M. haemosuis was originally observed as "a rickettsia-like or anaplasmosis-like disease in swine" characterized by icteroanemia, respiratory distress, weakness and fever occurring in 2–8-month-old pigs (Doyle 1932). In 1950, Splitter and Williamson described the organism responsible for the clinical disease observed earlier by Doyle and named the organism *Eperythrozoon suis* because of its similarity to similar organisms in cattle and sheep. Originally described as two species, *E. suis* and *E. parvum* due to differences in appearance, it was later determined that they were the same organism at different stages of maturity (Liebich and Heinritzi 1992; Zachary and Basgall 1985).

M. haemosuis were originally classified in the family Anaplasmataceae due to biologic and phenotypic characteristics that were not consistent with regular bacteria (Moulder 1974). However, there was always a suspicion that they were a member of the class Mollicutes based on their lack of intracellular parasitism, small size, lack of cell wall, resistance, and susceptibility to tetracyclines (Tanaka et al. 1965). This was confirmed in 1997 when Rikihisa, et al. (1997) sequenced the 16s rRNA gene sequences of the organsims. The gene sequences were found to have little in common with other Rickettsial organisms, instead being closer to other mycoplasmal species (Johansson et al. 1999). As a result, it was proposed that *E. suis* be named *Mycoplasma suis* (Neimark et al. 2002). However, rather than naming the organism after the species it was suggested that the name *M. haemosuis* be used (Neimark et al. 2001).

M. haemosuis is round to oval with an average diameter of 0.2–2 μm that adheres to the surface of erythrocyte membranes (Liebich and Heinritzi 1992; Zachary and Basgall 1985). It has not been cultured in media in the absence of cells to date.

Epidemiology

The disease has been reported to be widespread in the Midwestern U.S. (Splitter 1950a). Smith et al. (1977) tested 10,000 swine sera and found approximately 20% of the animals were seropositive at a titer of 40 or more using an indirect hemagglutination assay (IHA) (Smith and Rahn 1975). Morbidity ranges from 10–60% and mortality may reach up to 90% in association with acute disease (Anthony et al. 1962). Morbidity due to subclinical infection is much lower as is mortality and difficult to measure. Recently a PCR assay has been developed and a small study found that 29% of the serum of 60 pigs tested were positive for the organism (Messick 2004). Clinical disease is often closely associated with outbreaks of other infectious diseases present in the herd.

Transmission of the organism can be through direct exposure by oral uptake of blood and blood components by such practices such as licking wounds, cannibalism, or uptake of blood-contaminated urine. Indirect transmission also occurs by means of vectors, including ectoparasites and blood-sucking insects, and by nonliving vectors such as contaminated needles, surgical instruments, or snares. Transmission by semen occurs only in the case of blood contamination and thus is rare (Heinritzi 1999).

The incubation period in experimentally infected and splenectomized pigs is between 3 and 30 days. This results in an acute phase of the disease. However, a carrier state that can recrudesce is also possible (Splitter 1950b).

Pathogenesis

The initial decrease in PCV, total RBC count, and hemoglobin concentration observed with *M. haemosuis* infection is due to massive parasitism of RBC. The resulting reduction in RBC numbers may contribute to the development of anemia and bilirubinemia. Infected RBCs are more fragile, have altered membranes, and are recognized as abnormal and removed from the circulation by the spleen. In addition to the direct damage to RBC membranes, the host immune response appears to play a role in both acute and chronic forms of the anemia associated with *M. haemosuis*. This is due to the presence of autoantibodies present to the RBCs (Smith 1992). The production of cold-reacting agglutinins is directed at sialoglycoconjugates on the RBC membranes (Feizi and Loveless 1996). It has been suggested that the host's immune response may exacerbate the hemolytic episodes.

A prerequisite for RBC agglutination is some type of membrane injury and blood from pigs with both spontaneous and experimentally produced infection agglutinated in the cold (Hoffman et al. 1981). The mechanism used by *M. haemosuis* to adhere to RBCs is unknown.

In the acute phase, an increased bleeding potential is observed occasionally resulting in a consumptive coagulopathy. The greater the number of RBCs affected by the organism, the more striking the changes. Similar effects on blood coagulation are not observed with latent infection with *M. haemosuis* (Plank and Heinritzi 1990). During acute infection, hypoglycemia and blood acidosis can occur due to the metabolic activity of the organism (Heinritzi 1999).

In addition to the changes in the RBCs, research has demonstrated that *M. haemosuis* infection results in a transient hyperglobulinemia that increases the IHA titers. Lymphocyte responses to the nonspecific mitogens, phytohemagglutinin, pokeweed, and *E. coli* lipopolysaccharide was reduced after massive parasitemia. This may be one of the mechanisms for the increased occurrence of diseases of the respiratory and enteric tracts observed following infection (Zachary and Smith 1985). Further support of the impact that the organism has on the immune response is demonstrated by the increased difficulty in controlling other diseases in *M. haemosuis*-infected herds (Henry 1979).

Clinical outbreaks may increase in frequency in infected herds, but eventually a certain equilibrium is reached between the organism and the pigs that results in minimal disease that can be attributed directly to *M. haemosuis*. This equilibrium can be disrupted by other pathogens, stress, or inadequate management practices resulting in a clinical outbreak, which makes management critical in controlling the disease in an infected herd. The primary importance of a *M. haemosuis* infection within a herd is the impact the infection has on production parameters.

Clinical Signs

M. haemosuis infection can cause acute hemolytic disease and death in young pigs, prepartum sows, and stressed weaned and feeder pigs (Henry 1979; Smith 1992). Pigs of any age can exhibit disease in association with *M. haemosuis*. Pallor, fever, occasional icterus, and cyanosis of the extremities, especially the ears, are observed clinically during the acute phases of the disease. More commonly, mild anemia and poor growth rates are observed in weaned and feeder pigs. Infection of sows may result in fever, anorexia, lethargy, decreased mild production, and poor maternal behavior. Clinical disease in sows typically occurs within 3–4 days of introduction to the farrowing room or immediately after farrowing.

Chronic infections in animals with low or undetectable numbers of parasites results in uthriftiness, pallor, and occasionally skin hypersensitivities characterized by urticaria. Chronic *M. haemosuis* infections have been associated with decreased reproduction, resulting in sows with anestrus, delayed estrus, early embryonic death, and abortions. However, Zinn et al. (1983) found no appreciable impact on sow reproductive performance, but did see a reduced rate of gain in pigs farrowed from sows with high IHA titers.

In all cases, secondary bacterial or viral infections, poor management strategies, including overcrowding, poor environmental conditions, and the presence of parasites contribute to the severity of disease associated with *M. haemosuis* infection. Frequent injections and vaccinations can also be an important factor in spread of the organisms as well as subsequent reinfection. The use of oral treatment with tetracycline in treatment of other diseases can mask the clinical signs.

Diagnosis

Diagnosis is based on clinical signs, hematology results, demonstration of the organism, IHA assays for antibodies, and PCR. Prior to the development of PCR assays, the best diagnostic test to detect or confirm latent infection in carrier animals was by splenectomizing a potentially infected pig or by inoculation of a splenectomized pig with blood from suspected pigs.

Serological assays include the IHA assay (Smith and Rahn 1975). The production of antibodies occurs in waves, with each reinfection or recrudescent episode resulting in the production of new antibodies. However, the antibody titers persist only 2–3 months resulting in frequent false negative results (Heinritzi 1999).

More recently a PCR assay has been developed that is more sensitive and allows increased detection of pigs that are either carriers or subclinically infected (Messick et al. 1999).

Treatment

The treatment of choice is oxytetracycline at a dose of 20–30 mg/kg administered parenterally (Heinritzi 1999). Acutely ill pigs require parenteral treatment due to lack of adequate feed consumption. Administration of oxytetracycline at times of stress or treatment in infected herds may help prevent acute disease. However, treatment does eliminate the organism from the pig. Oral chlortetracycline therapy can reduce the incidence of anemia, although will not prevent outbreaks. Supportive therapy and iron injections (200 mg iron dextran/pig) will help recovery and minimize mortality.

Prevention

Supportive and prophylactic measures should be included with therapy (Claxton and Klunish 1975). Stopping the spread of the organism and preventing reinfection are critical to controlling disease in the herd. Parasitic control and hygiene are critical for disease control. Transmission by needles and surgical instruments must be minimized by changing needles between sows and litters.

No vaccines are available and if a herd is *M. haemosuis*-free, new additions should also be from herds negative for the organism. Negative status can be assumed if serologic or PCR tests from serum of pigs in the farrowing unit are negative or if transfusion from at least 10 blood samples into splenectomized pigs has no effect.

OTHER MYCOPLASMAS FROM SWINE

A number of mycoplasmas are present in swine that are of less importance to the industry than those discussed earlier in this chapter. These include mycoplasmas that are typically in other species, strains that are not normally associated with disease in swine, and acholepasmas, which are common in a wide variety of animals and plants.

A species of mycoplasma that is frequently isolated from swine, but considered nonpathogenic is *M. flocculare*. It was first isolated from the respiratory tract of pigs in Denmark (Friis 1972). Since that time, the organism has been isolated by researchers in the U.K., Sweden, and the U.S. (Armstrong and Friis 1981). It was demonstrated that *M. flocculare* is capable of inducing lymphocytic infiltrations in the nasal tissues and peribronchial areas (Friis 1973). These findings were later confirmed by Armstrong et al. (1987). However the role of *M. flocculare* in respiratory disease in the field remains poorly defined. *M. flocculare* is of primary importance to the swine industry due to its antigenic similarities to *M. hyopneumoniae*, which can complicate their differentiation both antigenically following culture and isolation and more importantly, serologically (Bereiter et al. 1990). However, it has been confirmed using molecular techniques that the two organisms differ genetically (Blank and Stemke 2001).

Infection of the genitourinary tract with mycoplasmas in many animal species is common; however, little evidence has been presented reporting similar findings in swine. Shin et al. (2003) demonstrated a cytopathic species of *M. hyorhinis* that was thought to be a cause of abortions in sows.

Other species of mycoplasmas that have been isolated from swine include *M. sualvi, M. hyopharyngis, M. arginini, M. bovigenitalium, M. buccale, M. gallinarum, M. iners, M. mycoides,* and *M. salivarium.* In addition to mycoplasmas, Acholeplasmas have occasionally been isolated from the respiratory tract of swine (Gois et al. 1969). Acholeplasmas differ from Mycoplasmas by having a larger genome and being capable of growing in media that lacks sterols (Ross 1992). No importance in their presence of pigs has been demonstrated.

REFERENCES

Aarestrup FM, Friis NF. 1998. Antimicrobial susceptibility testing of Mycoplasma hyosynoviae isolated from pigs during 1968 to 1971 and during 1995 and 1996. Vet Microbiol 61:33–39.

Alexander TJ, Thornton K, Boon G, Lysons RJ, Gush AF. 1980. Medicated early weaning to obtain pigs free from pathogens endemic in the herd of origin. Vet Rec 106:114–119.

Amanfu W, Weng CN, Ross RF, Barnes HJ. 1984. Diagnosis of *Mycoplasmal pneumoniae* of swine: Sequential study by direct immunofluorescence. Am J Vet Res 45:1349–1352.

Andreasen M, Mousing J, Krogsgaard Thomsen L. 2001. No simple association between time elapsed from seroconversion until slaughter and the extent of lung lesions in Danish swine. Prev Vet Med 52:147–161.

Andreasen M, Nielsen, Baekbo P, Willeberg P, Botner A. 2000. A longitudinal study of serological patterns of respiratory infections in nine infected Danish swine herds. Prev Vet Med 45:221–235.

Anthony H, Kelley D, Nelson D, et al. 1962. Suppressing *eperythrozoon* infection in swine. Vet Med Small Anim Clin 57:702–703.

Armstrong CH, Friis NF. 1981. Isolation of *Mycoplasma flocculare* from swine in the United States. Am J Vet Res 42:1030–1032.

Armstrong CH, Sands-Freeman L, Freeman MJ. 1987. Serological, pathological and cultural evaluations of swine infected experimentally with *Mycoplasma flocculare*. Can J Vet Res 51:185–188.

Artiushin S, Minion FC. 1996. Arbitrarily primed PCR analysis of *Mycoplasma hyopneumoniae* field isolates demonstrates genetic heterogeneity. Int J Syst Bacteriol 46:324–328.

Artiushin S, Stipkovits L, Minion FC. 1993. Development of polymerase chain reaction primers to detect *Mycoplasma hyopneumoniae*. Mol Cell Probes 7:381–385.

Asai T, Okada M, Ono M, Irisawa T, Mori Y, Yokomizo Y, Sato S. 1993. Increased levels of tumor necrosis factor and interleukin 1 in bronchoalveolar lavage fluids from pigs infected with *Mycoplasma hyopneumoniae*. Vet Immunol Immunopathol 38:253–260.

Asai T, Okada M, Ono M, Mori Y, Yokomizo Y, Sato S. 1994. Detection of interleukin-6 and prostaglandin E2 in bronchoalveolar lavage fluids of pigs experimentally infected with *Mycoplasma hyponeumoniae*. Vet Immunol Immunopathol 44:97–102.

Baekbo P, Kooij D, Mortensen S, Barfod K, Mousing J. 1996. Economic evaluation of national eradication and control strategies for *Mycoplasma hyopneumoniae* in Denmark. Acta Vet Scand Suppl 90:63–65.

Bereiter M, Young TF, Joo HS, Ross RF. 1990. Evaluation of the ELISA and comparison to the complement fixation test and radial immunodiffusion enzyme assay for detection of antibodies against *Mycoplasma hyopneumoniae* in swine serum. Vet Microbiol 25:177–192.

Blank WA, Stemke GW. 2001. A physical and genetic map of the *Mycoplasma flocculare* ATCC 277\ chromosome reveals large genomic inversions when compared with that of *Mycoplasma hyopneumoniae* strain J(T). Int J Syst Evol Microbiol 51:1395–1399.

Blowey RW. 1993. *Mycoplasma hyosynoviae* arthritis. Pig Veterinary Journal 30:72–76.

Bousquet E, Pommier P, Wessel-Robert S, Morvan H, Benoit-Valiergue H, Laval A. 1998. Efficacy of doxycycline in feed for the control of pneumonia caused by *Pasteurella multocida* and *Mycoplasma hyopneumoniae* in fattening pigs. Vet Rec 143:269–272.

Burch DG, Jones GT, Heard TW, Tuck RE. 1986. The synergistic activity of tiamulin and chlortetracycline: In-feed treatment of bacterially complicated enzootic pneumonia in fattening pigs. Vet Rec 119:108–112.

Buttenshon J, Svensmark B, Kyrval J. 1995. Non-purulent arthritis in Danish slaughter pigs. I. A study of field cases. J Vet Med A 42:633–641.

Calsamiglia M, Collins JE, Pijoan C. 2000. Correlation between the presence of enzootic pneumonia lesions and detection of *Mycoplasma hyopneumoniae* in bronchial swabs by PCR. Vet Microbiol 76:299–303.

Calsamiglia M, Pijoan C. 2000. Colonisation state and colostral immunity to *Mycoplasma hyopneumoniae* of different parity sows. Vet Rec 146:530–532.

Calsamiglia M, Pijoan C, Trigo A. 1999. Application of a nested polymerase chain reaction assay to detect *Mycoplasma hyopneumoniae* from nasal swabs. J Vet Diagn Invest 11:246–251.

Caruso JP, Ross RF. 1990. Effects of *Mycoplasma hyopneumoniae* and *Actinobacillus (Haemophilus) pleuropneumoniae* infections on alveolar macrophage functions in swine. Am J Vet Res 51:227–231.

Chen JR, Lin JH, Weng CN, Lai SS. 1998. Identification of a novel adhesin-like glycoprotein from *Mycoplasma hyopneumoniae*. Vet Microbiol 62:97–110.

Ciprian A, Cruz TA, de la Garza M. 1994. *Mycoplasma hyopneumoniae*: Interaction with other agents in pigs, and evaluation of immunogens. Arch Med Res 25:235–9.

Claxton M, Kunish J. 1975. Eperythrozoonosis in swine. Iowa State Vet 37:82–83.

Cooper AC, Fuller JR, Fuller MK, Whittlestone P, Wise DR. 1993. In vitro activity of danofloxacin, tylosin and oxytetracycline against mycoplasmas of veterinary importance. Res Vet Sci 54:329–334.

DeBey MC, Jacobson CD, Ross RF. 1992. Histochemical and morphologic changes of porcine airway epithelial cells in response to infection with *Mycoplasma hyopneumoniae*. Am J Vet Res 53:1705–1710.

DeBey MC, Ross RF. 1994. Ciliostasis and loss of cilia induced by *Mycoplasma hyopneumoniae* in porcine tracheal organ cultures. Infect Immun 62:5312–5318.

Djordjevic SP, Eamens GJ, Romalis LF, Nicholls PJ, Taylor V, Chin J. 1997. Serum and mucosal antibody responses and protection in pigs vaccinated against *Mycoplasma hyopneumoniae* with vaccines containing a denatured membrane antigen pool and adjuvant. Aust Vet J 75:504–511.

Dohoo IR, Montgomery ME. 1996. A field trial to evaluate a *Mycoplasma hyopneumoniae* vaccine: Effects on lung lesions and growth rates in swine. Can Vet J 37:299–302.

Doyle L. 1932. A rickettsia-like or anaplasmos-like disease in swine. J Am Vet Med Assoc 8:668–671.

Dritz SS, Chengappa MM, Nelssen JL, Tokach MD, Goodband RD, Nietfeld JC, Staats JJ. 1996. Growth and microbial flora of non-medicated, segregated, early weaned pigs from a commercial swine operation. J Am Vet Med Assoc 208:711–715.

Erlandson K, Thacker B, Wegner M, Evans R, Thacker E. 2002. Evaluation of three serum antibody ELISA tests for *Mycoplasma hyopneumoniae*. Proc 17th Congr Int Pig Vet Soc, Ames, Iowa, p. 249.

Etheridge JR, Cottew GS, Lloyd LC. 1979. Isolation of *Mycoplasma hyopneumoniae* from lesions in experimentally infected pigs. Aust Vet J 55:356–359.

Fagan PK, Djordjevic SP, Eamens GJ, Chin J, Walker MJ. 1996. Molecular characterization of a ribonucleotide reductase (nrdF) gene fragment of *Mycoplasma hyopneumoniae* and assessment of the recombinant product as an experimental vaccine for enzootic pneumonia. Infect Immun 64:1060–1064.

Fagan PK, Walker MJ, Chin J, Eamens GJ, Djordjevic SP. 2001. Oral immunization of swine with attenuated *Salmonella typhimurium* aroA SL3261 expressing a recombinant antigen of *Mycoplasma hyopneumoniae* (NrdF) primes the immune system for a NrdF specific secretory IgA response in the lungs. Microb Pathog 30:101–110.

Feizi T, Loveless RW. 1996. Carbohydrate recognition by *Mycoplasma pneumoniae* and pathologic consequences. Am J Resp Crit Care Med 154:S133–S136.

Frey J, Haldimann A, Kobisch M, Nicolet J. 1994. Immune response against the L-lactate dehydrogenase of *Mycoplasma hyopneumoniae* in enzootic pneumonia of swine. Microb Pathog 17:313–322.

Frey J, Haldimann A, Nicolet J. 1992. Chromosomal heterogeneity of various *Mycoplasma hyopneumoniae* field strains. Int J Syst Bacteriol 42:275–280.

Friis NF. 1972. Isolation and characterization of a new porcine mycoplasma. Acta Vet Scand 13:284–286.

Friis NF. 1973. The pathogenicity of *Mycoplasma flocculare*. Acta Vet Scand 14:344–346.

Friis NF. 1975. Some recommendations concerning primary isolations of *Mycoplasma suipneumoniae* and *Mycoplasma flocculare*. Nord Vet Med 27:337–339.

Friis NF. 1976. A serologic variant of *Mycoplasma hyorhinis* recovered from the conjunctiva of swine. Acta Vet Scand 17:343–353.

Friis NF. 1979. Selective isolation of slowly growing acidifying mycoplasmas from swine and cattle. Acta Vet Scand 20:607–609.

Friis NF, Ahrens P, Larsen H. 1991. *Mycoplasma hyosynoviae* isolation from the upper respiratory tract and tonsils of pigs. Acta Vet Scand 32:425–429.

Friis NF, Hansen KK, Schirmer AL, Aabo S. 1992. *Mycoplasma hyosynoviae* in joints with arthritis in abattoir baconers. Acta Vet Scand 33:205–210.

Gois M, Cerny M, Rozkosny V, Sovadina J. 1969. Studies on the epizootiological significance of some species of mycoplasma isolated from nasal swabs and lungs of pigs. Zentralbl Veterinarmed B 16:253–265.

Gois M, Kuksa F, Sisak F. 1977. Experimental infection of gnotobiotic piglets with *Mycoplasma hyorhinis* and *Bordetella bronchiseptica*. Zentralbl Veterinarmed B 24:89–96.

Goodwin RF. 1972. Isolation of *Mycoplasma suipneumoniae* from the nasal cavities and lungs of pigs affected with enzootic pneumonia or exposed to this infection. Res Vet Sci 13:262–267.

Goodwin RF. 1985. Apparent reinfection of enzootic-pneumonia-free pig herds: Search for possible causes. Vet Rec 116:690–694.

Guerrero RJ. 1990. Respiratory disease: An important global problem in the swine industry. Proc Congr Int Pig Vet Soc, Lausanne, Switzerland, p. 98.

Hagedorn-Olsen T, Basse A, Jensen TK, Nielsen NC. 1999. Gross and histopathological findings in synovial membranes of pigs with experimentally induced *Mycoplasma hyosynoviae* arthritis. Apmis 107:201–210.

Hagedorn-Olsen T, Nielsen NC, Friis NF. 1999. Induction of arthritis with *Mycoplasma hyosynoviae* in pigs: Clinical response and re-isolation of the organism from body fluids and organs. Zentralbl Veterinarmed A 46:317–325.

Hagedorn-Olsen T, Nielsen NC, Friis NF, Nielsen J. 1999. Progression of *Mycoplasma hyosynoviae* infection in three pig herds. Development of tonsillar carrier state, arthritis and antibodies in serum and synovial fluid in pigs from birth to slaughter. Zentralbl Veterinarmed A 46:555–564.

Hannan PC, Bhogal BS, Fish JP. 1982. Tylosin tartrate and tiamutilin effects on experimental piglet pneumonia induced with pneumonic pig lung homogenate containing mycoplasmas, bacteria and viruses. Res Vet Sci 33:76–88.

Hannan PC, O'Hanlon PJ, Rogers NH. 1989. In vitro evaluation of various quinolone antibacterial agents against veterinary mycoplasmas and porcine respiratory bacterial pathogens. Res Vet Sci 46:202–211.

Hannan PC, Windsor HM, Ripley PH. 1997. In vitro susceptibilities of recent field isolates of *Mycoplasma hyopneumoniae* and *Mycoplasma hyosynoviae* to valnemulin (Econor), tiamulin and enrofloxacin and the in vitro development of resistance to certain antimicrobial agents in *Mycoplasma hyopneumoniae*. Res Vet Sci 63:157–160.

Harasawa R, Koshimizu K, Takeda O, Uemori T, Asada K, Kato I. 1991. Detection of *Mycoplasma hyopneumoniae* DNA by the polymerase chain reaction. Mol Cell Probes 5:103–109.

Hariharan H, MacDonald J, Carnat B, Bryenton J, Heaney S. 1992. An investigation of bacterial causes of arthritis in slaughter hogs. J Vet Diagn Invest 4:28–30.

Harris D. 1990. Isolated weaning. Large Animal Veterinarian 45:10–13.

Hege R, Zimmermann W, Scheidegger R, Stark KD. 2002. Incidence of reinfections with *Mycoplasma hyopneumoniae* and *Actinobacillus pleuropneumoniae* in pig farms located in respiratory-disease-free regions of Switzerland—Identification and quantification of risk factors. Acta Vet Scand 43:145–156.

Heinonen M, Autio T, Saloniemi H, Tuovinen V. 1999. Eradication of *Mycoplasma hyopneumoniae* from infected swine herds joining the LSO 2000 health class. Acta Vet Scand 40:241–252.

Heinritzi K. 1999. Eperythrozoonosis. In *Diseases of Swine,* 8th ed. B Straw, S D'Allaire, WL Mengeling, DJ Taylor, eds.. Ames: Iowa State University Press, pp. 413–418.

Henry SC. 1979. Clinical observations on eperythrozoonosis. J Am Vet Med Assoc 174:601–603.

Hoffman R, Schimd DO, Hoffmann-Fezer G. 1981. Erythrocyte antibodies in porcine eperythrozoonosis. Vet Immunol Immunopathol 2:111–119.

Holmgren N. 1974. An indirect haemagglutination test for detection of antibodies against *Mycoplasma hyopneumoniae* using formalinized tanned swine erythrocytes. Res Vet Sci 16:341–346.

Hsu FS, Yeh TP, Lee CT. 1983. Tiamulin feed medication for the maintenance of weight gains in the presence of mycoplasmal pneumonia in swine. J Anim Sci 57:1474–1478.

Hsu T, Artiushin S, Minion FC. 1997. Cloning and functional analysis of the P97 swine cilium adhesin gene of *Mycoplasma hyopneumoniae*. J Bacteriol 179:1317–1323.

Hsu T, Minion FC. 1998. Identification of the cilium binding epitope of the *Mycoplasma hyopneumoniae* P97 adhesin. Infect Immun 66:4762–4766.

Jayappa H, Davis R, Rapp-Gabrielson V, Wasmoen T, Thacker E, Thacker B. 2001. Evaluation of the efficacy of *Mycoplasma hyopneumoniae* bacterin following immunization of young pigs in the presence of varying levels of maternal antibodies. Proc Amer Assoc of Swine Veterinarians, Nashville, Tennessee, pp. 237–241.

Jensen CS, Ersboll AK, Nielsen JP. 2002. A meta-analysis comparing the effect of vaccines against *Mycoplasma hyopneumoniae* on daily weight gain in pigs. Prev Vet Med 54:265–278.

Johansson KE, Tully JG, Bolske G, Pettersson B. 1999. *Mycoplasma cavipharyngis* and *Mycoplasma fastidiosum*, the closest relatives to *Eperythrozoon* spp. and *Haemobartonella* spp. FEMS Microbiol Lett 174:321–326.

Jorsal SE, Thomsen BL. 1988. A Cox regression analysis of risk factors related to *Mycoplasma suipneumoniae* reinfection in Danish SPF herds. Acta Vet Scand 29:436–438.

Kawashima K, Yamada S, Kobayashi H, Narita M. 1996. Detection of porcine reproductive and respiratory syndrome virus and *Mycoplasma hyorhinis* antigens in pulmonary lesions of pigs suffering from respiratory distress. J Comp Pathol 114:315–323.

Kazama S, Yagihashi T, Seto K. 1989. Preparation of *Mycoplasma hyopneumoniae* antigen for the enzyme-linked immunosorbent assay. Can J Vet Res 53:176–181.

King KW, Faulds DH, Rosey EL, Yancey, Jr RJ. 1997. Characterization of the gene encoding Mhp1 from *Mycoplasma hyopneumoniae* and examination of Mhp1's vaccine potential. Vaccine 15:25–35.

Kishima M, Ross RF. 1985. Suppressive effect of nonviable *Mycoplasma hyopneumoniae* on phytohemagglutinin-induced transformation of swine lymphocytes. Am J Vet Res 46:2366–2368.

Kobisch M, Quillien L, Tillon JP, Wroblewski H. 1987. The *Mycoplasma hyopneumoniae* plasma membrane as a vaccine against porcine enzootic pneumonia. Ann Inst Pasteur Immunol 138:693–705.

Kokotovic B, Friis NF, Ahrens P. 2002. Characterization of *Mycoplasma hyosynoviae* strains by amplified fragment length polymorphism analysis, pulsed-field gel electrophoresis and 16S ribosomal DNA sequencing. J Vet Med B Infect Dis Vet Public Health 49:245–252.

Kokotovic B, Friis NF, Jensen JS, Ahrens P. 1999. Amplified-fragment length polymorphism fingerprinting of Mycoplasma species. J Clin Microbiol 37:3300–3307.

Kristensen B, Paroz P, Nicolet J, Wanner M, de Weck AL. 1981. Cell-mediated and humoral immune response in swine after vaccination and natural infection with Mycoplasma hyopneumoniae. Am J Vet Res 42:784–788.

Kurth KT, Hsu T, Snook ER, Thacker EL, Thacker BJ, Minion FC. 2002. Use of a Mycoplasma hyopneumoniae nested polymerase chain reaction test to determine the optimal sampling sites in swine. J Vet Diagn Invest 14:463–469.

Kwon D, Chae C. 1999. Detection and localization of Mycoplasma hyopneumoniae DNA in lungs from naturally infected pigs by in situ hybridization using a digoxigenin-labeled probe. Vet Pathol 36:308–313.

Liebich HG, Heinritzi K. 1992. [Light and electron microscopic studies of Eperythrozoon suis]. Tierarztl Prax 20:270–274.

Lin SY, Tzan YL, Weng CN, Lee CJ. 1991. Preparation of enteric-coated microspheres of Mycoplasma hyopneumoniae vaccine with cellulose acetate phthalate: (II). Effect of temperature and pH on the stability and release behaviour of microspheres. J Microencapsul 8:537–545.

Maes D, Deluyker H, Verdonck M, Castryck F, Miry C, Vrijens B, Verbeke W, Viaene J, de Kruif A. 1999. Effect of vaccination against Mycoplasma hyopneumoniae in pig herds with an all-in/all-out production system. Vaccine 17:1024–1034.

Maes D, Verdonck M, Deluyker H, de Kruif A. 1996. Enzootic pneumonia in pigs. Vet Quart 18:104–109.

Magnusson U, Wilkie B, Mallard B, Rosendal S, Kennedy B. 1998. Mycoplasma hyorhinis infection of pigs selectively bred for high and low immune response. Vet Immunol Immunopathol 61:83–96.

Mare CJ, Switzer WP. 1965. New Species: Mycoplasma Hyopneumoniae; a Causative Agent of Virus Pig Pneumonia. Vet Med Small Anim Clin 60:841–846.

Mateusen B, Maes D, Hoflack G, Verdonck M, de Kruif A. 2001. A comparative study of the preventive use of tilmicosin phosphate (Pulmotil premix) and Mycoplasma hyopneumoniae vaccination in a pig herd with chronic respiratory disease. J Vet Med B Infect Dis Vet Public Health 48:733–741.

Mateusen B, Maes D, Van Goubergen M, Verdonck M, de Kruif A. 2002. Effectiveness of treatment with lincomycin hydrochloride and/or vaccination against Mycoplasma hyopneumoniae for controlling chronic respiratory disease in a herd of pigs. Vet Rec 151:135–140.

Mattsson JG, Bergstrom K, Wallgren P, Johansson KE. 1995. Detection of Mycoplasma hyopneumoniae in nose swabs from pigs by in vitro amplification of the 16S rRNA gene. J Clin Microbiol 33:893–897.

Messick JB. 2004. Hemotrophic mycoplasmas (hemoplasmas): A review and new insights into pathogenic potential. Vet Clin Pathol 33:2–13.

Messick JB, Cooper S, Huntley M. 1999. Development and evaluation of a polymerase chain reaction assay using the 16S rRNA gene for detection of Erperythrozoon suis infection. J Vet Diagn Invest 11:229–236.

Messier S, Ross RF. 1991. Interactions of Mycoplasma hyopneumoniae membranes with porcine lymphocytes. Am J Vet Res 52:1497–1502.

Messier S, Ross RF, Paul PS. 1990. Humoral and cellular immune responses of pigs inoculated with Mycoplasma hyopneumoniae. Am J Vet Res 51:52–58.

Morita T, Ohiwa S, Shimada A, Kazama S, Yagihashi T, Umemura T. 1999. Intranasally inoculated Mycoplasma hyorhinis causes eustachitis in pigs. Vet Pathol 36:174–178.

Moulder J. 1974. Order I. Rickettsiales. In Bergey's Manual of Determinative Bacteriology, 8th ed. R Buchannan, N Gibbons, eds. Baltimore: The Williams & Wilkins Co, pp. 882–890.

Murphy D, Van Alstine WG, Clark LK, Albregts S, Knox K. 1993. Aerosol vaccination of pigs against Mycoplasma hyopneumoniae infection. Am J Vet Res 54:1874–1880.

Neimark H, Johansson KE, Rikihisa Y, Tully JG. 2001. Proposal to transfer some members of the genera Haemobartonella and Eperythrozoon to the genus Mycoplasma with descriptions of 'Candidatus Mycoplasma haemofelis,' 'Candidatus Mycoplasma haemomuris,' 'Candidatus Mycoplasma haemosuis,' and 'Candidatus Mycoplasma wenyonii.' Int J Syst Evol Microbiol 51:891–899.

——. 2002. Revision of haemotrophic Mycoplasma species names. Int J Syst Evol Microbiol 52:683.

Nicolet J, Paroz P, Bruggmann S. 1980. Tween 20 soluble proteins of Mycoplasma hyopneumoniae as antigen for an enzyme linked immunosorbent assay. Res Vet Sci 29:305–309.

Nielsen EO, Nielsen NC, Friis NF. 2001. Mycoplasma hyosynoviae arthritis in grower-finisher pigs. J Vet Med A Physiol Pathol Clin Med 48:475–486.

Opriessnig T, Thacker E, Yu S, Evans R, Strait E, Vincent A, Halbur P. 2003. Presented at the 84th Annual Meeting of Conference of Research Workers in Animal Diseases, Chicago, IL, November 9–11, 2003.

Paisley LG, Vraa-Andersen L, Dybkjaer L, Moller K, Christensen G, Mousing J, Agger JF. 1993. An epidemiologic and economic study of respiratory diseases in two conventional Danish swine herds. Acta Vet Scand 34:319–344.

Piffer IA, Ross RF. 1984. Effect of age on susceptibility of pigs to Mycoplasma hyopneumoniae pneumonia. Am J Vet Res 45:478–481.

Piffer IA, Young TF, Petenate A, Ross RF. 1984. Comparison of complement fixation test and enzyme-linked immunosorbent assay for detection of early infection with Mycoplasma hyopneumoniae. Am J Vet Res 45:1122–1126.

Plank G, Heinritzi K. 1990. Disseminierte intravasale Gerinnung bei der Eperythrozoonose des Schweines. Berl Munch Tierarztl Wochenschr 103:13–18.

Pointon A, Byrt D, Heap P. 1985. Effect of enzootic pneumonia of pigs on growth performance. Aust Vet J 62:13–18.

Potgieter LND, Frey ML, Ross RF. 1972. Chronological Development of Mycoplasma hyorhinis and Mycoplasma hyosynoviae Infections in cultures of a swine synovial cell strain. Can J Comp Med 36:145–149.

Potgieter LND, Ross RF. 1972. Demonstration of Mycoplasma hyorhinis and Myocoplasma hyosynoviae in lesions of experimentally infected swine by immunofluorescence. Am J Vet Res 33:99–105.

Rautiainen E, Oravainen J, Virolainen JV, Tuovinen V. 2001. Regional eradication of Mycoplasma hyopneumoniae from pig herds and documentation of freedom of the disease. Acta Vet Scand 42:355–364.

Rautiainen E, Tuovinen V, Levonen K. 2000. Monitoring antibodies to Mycoplasma hyopneumoniae in sow colostrum—A tool to document freedom of infection. Acta Vet Scand 41:213–225.

Rautiainen E, Wallgren P. 2001. Aspects of the transmission of protection against Mycoplasma hyopneumoniae from sow to offspring. J Vet Med B Infect Dis Vet Public Health 48:55–65.

Reddy NRJ, Wilke BN, Borgs P, Mallard B. 2000. Cytokines in Mycoplasma hyorhinis-induced arthritis in pigs bred selectively for high and low immune responses. Infect Immun 68:1150–1155.

Rikihisa Y, Kawahara M, Wen B, Kociba G, Fuerst P, Kawamori F, Suto C, Shibata S, Futohashi M. 1997. Western Immunoblot Analysis of Haemobartonell amuris and Comparison of 16S rRNA Gene Sequences of H. muris, H. felis, and Eperuthrozoon suis. J Clin Microbiol 35:823–829.

Roberts DH. 1974. Experimental infection of pigs with Mycoplasma hyopneumoniae (suipneumoniae). Br Vet J 130:68–74.

Roberts DH, Johnson CT, Tew NC. 1972. The isolation of Mycoplasma hyosynoviae from an outbreak of porcine arthritis. Vet Rec 90:307–309.

Ross R. 1992. Mycoplasmal diseases. In Diseases of Swine, 7th ed. AD Leman, B Straw, WL Mengeling eds. Ames: Iowa State University Press, pp. 537–551.

Ross RF. 1973. Predisposing factors in *Mycoplasma hyosynoviae* arthritis in swine. J Infect Dis 127:Suppl:S84–s86.

Ross RF, Cox DF. 1988. Evaluation of tiamulin for treatment of mycoplasmal pneumonia in swine. J Am Vet Med Assoc 193:441–446.

Ross RF, Duncan JR. 1970. *Mycoplasma hyosynoviae* arthritis of swine. J Am Vet Med Assoc 157:1515–1518.

Ross RF, Karmon JA. 1970. Heterogeneity among strains of *Mycoplasma granularum* and identification of Mycoplasma hyosynoviae, sp. n. J Bacteriol 103:707–713.

Ross RF, Spear ML. 1973. Role of the sow as a reservoir of infection for *Mycoplasma hyosynoviae*. Am J Vet Res 34:373–378.

Ross RF, Weiss R, KirchhoffH. 1977. Demonstration of *M. hyorhinis* and *M. hyosynoviae* in arthritis joints of swine. Zentralbl Veterinarmed B 24:741–745.

Ross RF, Whittlestone P. 1983. Recovery of, identification of, and serological response to porcine mycoplasmas. Methods in Mycoplasmology 2:115–127.

Ross RF, Young TF. 1993. The nature and detection of mycoplasmal immunogens. Vet Microbiol 37:369–380.

Ross RF, Zimmermann-Erickson BJ, Young TF. 1984. Characteristics of protective activity of *Mycoplasma hyopneumoniae* vaccine. Am J Vet Res 45:1899–1905.

Scheidt AB, Mayrose VB, Hill MA, Clark LK, Cline TR, Knox K, Runnels LJ, Frantz S, Einstein ME. 1990. Relationship of growth performance to pneumonia and atrophic rhinitis detected in pigs at slaughter. J Am Vet Med Assoc 196:881–884.

Sheldrake RF, Romalis LF, Saunders MM. 1993. Serum and mucosal antibody responses against *Mycoplasma hyopneumoniae* following intraperitoneal vaccination and challenge of pigs with *M hyopneumoniae*. Res Vet Sci 55:371–376.

Shibata I, Okada M, Urono K, Samegai Y, Ono M, Sakano T, Sato S. 1998. Experimental dual infection of cesarean-derived, colostrum-deprived pigs with *Mycoplasma hyopneumoniae* and pseudorabies virus. J Vet Med Sci 60:295–300.

Shin JH, Joo HS, Lee WH, Seok HB, Calsamig M, Pijoan C, Molitor TW. 2003. Identification and characterization of cytopathogenic *Mycoplasma hyorhinis* from swine farms with a history of abortions. J Vet Med Sci 65:501–509.

Sibila M, Calsamiglia M, Vidal D, Badiella L, Aldaz A, Jensen JC. 2004. Dynamics of *Mycoplasma hyopneumoniae* infection in 12 farms with different production systems. Can J Vet Res 68:12–18.

Smith A. 1992. Eperythrozoonosis. In Diseases of Swine, 7th ed. B Straw, WL Mengeling, S D'Allaire, DJ Taylor, eds. Ames: Iowa State University Press, pp. 470–474.

Smith AR, Rahn T. 1975. An indirect hemagglutination test for the diagnosis of *Eperythrozoon suis* infection in swine. Am J Vet Res 36:1319–1321.

Sorensen KJ, Botner A, Madsen ES, Strandbygaard B, Nielsen J. 1997. Evaluation of a blocking Elisa for screening of antibodies against porcine reproductive and respiratory syndrome (PRRS) virus. Vet Microbiol 56:1–8.

Sorensen V, Ahrens P, Barfod K, Feenstra AA, Feld NC, Friis NF, Bille-Hansen V, Jensen NE, Pedersen MW. 1997. *Mycoplasma hyopneumoniae* infection in pigs: Duration of the disease and evaluation of four diagnostic assays. Vet Microbiol 54:23–34.

Sorensen V, Barfod K, Feld NC, Vraa-Andersen L. 1993. Application of enzyme-linked immunosorbent assay for the surveillance of *Mycoplasma hyopneumoniae* infection in pigs. Rev Sci Tech 12:593–604.

Splitter EJ. 1950a. *Eperythrozoon Suis* n. sp. and *Eperythrozoon Parvum* n. sp., two new blood parasites of swine. Science 111:513–514.

——. 1950b. *Eperythrozoon suis*, the etiologic agent of icteroanemia or an anaplasmosis-like disease in swine. Am J Vet Res 11.

Splitter EJ, Williamson RL.1950c. Eperythrozoonosis in swine; A preliminary report. J Am Vet Med Assoc 116(878):360–364.

Stark KD, Nicolet J, Frey J. 1998. Detection of *Mycoplasma hyopneumoniae* by air sampling with a nested PCR assay. Appl Environ Microbiol 64:543–548.

Stemke GW. 1997. Gene amplification (PCR) to detect and differentiate mycoplasmas in porcine mycoplasmal pneumonia. Lett Appl Microbiol 25:327–330.

Stemke GW, Phan R, Young TF, Ross RF. 1994. Differentiation of *Mycoplasma hyopneumoniae, M flocculare*, and *M hyorhinis* on the basis of amplification of a 16S rRNA gene sequence. Am J Vet Res 55:81–84.

Stipkovits L, Miller D, Glavits R, Fodor L, Burch D. 2001. Treatment of pigs experimentally infected with *Mycoplasma hyopneumoniae, Pasteurella multocida*, and *Actinobacillus pleuropneumoniae* with various antibiotics. Can J Vet Res 65:213–222.

Strait E, Madsen ML, Minion FC, Thacker EL. 2003. Presented at the In Conf Res Worker in Anim Dis Abstract, Chicago, IL, November 9–11.

Straw B, Tuovinen V, Bigras-Poulin M. 1989. Estimation of the cost of pneumonia in swine herds. J Am Vet Med Assoc 195:1702–1706.

Tajima M, Yagihashi T, Nunoya T, Takeuchi A, Ohashi F. 1984. *Mycoplasma hyopneumoniae* infection in pigs immunosuppressed by thymectomy and treatment with antithymocyte serum. Am J Vet Res 45:1928–1932.

Tanaka H, Hall WT, Sheffield JB, Moore DH. 1965. Fine structure of *Haemobartonella muris* as compared with *Eperythrozoon coccoides* and *Mycoplasma pulmonis*. J Bacteriol 90:1735–1749.

Tanner AC, Erickson BZ, Ross RF. 1993. Adaptation of the Sensititre broth microdilution technique to antimicrobial susceptibility testing of *Mycoplasma hyopneumoniae*. Vet Microbiol 36:301–306.

Taylor MA, Wise KS, McIntosh MA. 1984. Species-specific detection of *Mycoplasma hyorhinis* using DNA probes. Isr J Med Sci 20:778–780.

——. 1985. Selective detection of *Mycoplasma hyorhinis* using cloned genomic DNA fragments. Infect Immun 47:827–8

Ter Laak EA, Pijpers A, Noordergraaf JH, Schoevers EC, Verheijden JH. 1991. Comparison of methods for in vitro testing of susceptibility of porcine Mycoplasma species to antimicrobial agents. Antimicrob Agents Chemother 35:228–233.

Thacker B, Boettcher T, Anderson T, Thacker E, Young T. 1998. The influence of passive immunity on serological responses to *Mycoplasma hyopneumoniae* vaccination. Proc.15th Int Pig Vet Soc Congress, Birmingham, England, July 5–9, 1998, p. 154.

Thacker B, Thacker E, Halbur P, Minion F, Young T, Erickson B, Thanawongnuwech R. 2000. The influence of maternally-derived antibodies on *Mycoplasma hyopneumoniae* infection. Proc 16th Int Pig Vet Soc Cong, Melbourne, Australia, p. 454.

Thacker BJ, Thacker EL. 2001. Influence of maternally-derived antibodies on the efficacy of a *Mycoplasma hyopneumoniae* bacterin. Proc Amer Assoc of Swine Vets An Mtg, Nashville, Tennessee, pp. 513–515.

Thacker EL. 2001. Immunology of the porcine respiratory disease complex. Vet Clin North Am Food Anim Pract 17:551–565.

Thacker EL, Halbur PG, Ross RF, Thanawongnuwech R, Thacker BJ. 1999. *Mycoplasma hyopneumoniae* potentiation of porcine reproductive and respiratory syndrome virus-induced pneumonia. J Clin Microbiol 37:620–627.

Thacker EL, Thacker BJ, Boettcher TB, Jayappa H. 1998. Comparison of antibody production, lymphocyte stimulation, and protection induced by four commercial *Mycoplasma hyopneumoniae* bacterins. J Swine Health Prod 6:107–112.

Thacker EL, Thacker BJ, Janke BH. 2001. Interaction between *Mycoplasma hyopneumoniae* and swine influenza virus. J Clin Microbiol 39:2525–2530.

Thacker EL, Thacker BJ, Kuhn M, Hawkins PA, Waters WR. 2000. Evaluation of local and systemic immune responses induced by intramuscular injection of a *Mycoplasma hyopneumoniae* bacterin to pigs. Am J Vet Res 61:1384–1389.

Thacker EL, Thacker BJ, Wolff T. 2001. Efficacy of Aureomycin (chlortetracycline) granular premix against experimental *Mycoplasma hyopneumoniae* challenge. Proc Amer Assoc of Swine Vets, Nashville, Tennessee, pp. 83–85.

Thacker EL, Thacker BJ, Young TF, Halbur BG. 2000. Effect of vaccination on the potentiation of porcine reproductive and respiratory syndrome virus (PRRSV)-induced pneumonia by *Mycoplasma hyopneumoniae*. Vaccine 18:1244–1252.

Thacker EL, Young TF, Erickson BZ, DeBey MC. 2001. Evaluation of tilmicosin's ability to prevent adherence of *Mycoplasma hyopneumoniae* to cilia using a differentiated swine epithelial culture system. Veterinary Therapeutics 2:293–300.

Thanawongnuwech R, Thacker EL. 2003. Interleukin-10, interleukin-12, and interferon-gamma levels in the respiratory tract following *Mycoplasma hyopneumoniae* and PRRSV infection in pigs. Viral Immunol 16:357–367.

Thanawongnuwech R, Young TF, Thacker BJ, Thacker EL. 2001. Differential production of proinflammatory cytokines: In vitro PRRSV and *Mycoplasma hyopneumoniae* co-infection model. Vet Immunol Immunopathol 79:115–127.

Thomsen BL, Jorsal SE, Andersen S, Willeberg P. 1992. The Cox regression model applied to risk factor analysis of infections in the breeding and multiplying herds in the Danish SPF system. Prev Vet Med 12:287–297.

USDA. 2001. Part I: Reference of Swine Health and Management in the United States, 2000, National Animal Health Monitoring System. Fort Collins, CO. #N338.0801

Van Alstine WG, Stevenson GW, Kanitz CL. 1996. Porcine reproductive and respiratory syndrome virus does not exacerbate *Mycoplasma hyopneumoniae* infection in young pigs. Vet Microbiol 49:297–303.

Verdin E, Saillard C, Labbe A, Bove JM, Kobisch M. 2000. A nested PCR assay for the detection of *Mycoplasma hyopneumoniae* in tracheobronchiolar washings from pigs. Vet Microbiol 76:31–40.

Vicca J, Maes D, Thermote L, Peeters J, Haesebrouck F, de Kruif A. 2002. Patterns of *Mycoplasma hyopneumoniae* infections in Belgian farrow-to-finish pig herds with diverging disease-course. J Vet Med B Infect Dis Vet Public Health 49:349–353.

Vicca J, Stakenborg T, Maes D, Butaye P, Peeters J, de Kruif A, Haesebrouck F. 2003. Evaluation of virulence of *Mycoplasma hyopneumoniae* field isolates. Vet Microbiol 97:177–190.

Williams PP. 1978. In vitro susceptibility of *Mycoplasma hyopneumoniae* and *Mycoplasma hyorhinis* to fifty-one antimicrobial agents. Antimicrob Agents Chemother 14:210–213.

Wilton JL, Scarman AL, Walker MJ, Djordjevic SP. 1998. Reiterated repeat region variability in the ciliary adhesin gene of *Mycoplasma hyopneumoniae*. Microbiology 144 (Pt 7):1931–1943.

Wu CC, Shryrock TR, Lin TL, Fleck M. 1997. Testing antimicrobial susceptibility against *Mycoplasma hyopneumoniae* in vitro. J Swine Health Prod 5:227–230.

Zachary JF, Basgall EJ. 1985. Erythrocyte membrane alterations associated with the attachment and replication of *Eperythrozoon suis*: A light and electron microscopic study. Vet Pathol 22:164–170.

Zachary JF, Smith AR. 1985. Experimental porcine eperythrozoonosis: T-lymphocyte suppression and misdirected immune responses. Am J Vet Res 46:821–830.

Zhang Q, Young TF, Ross RF. 1994. Microtiter plate adherence assay and receptor analogs for *Mycoplasma hyopneumoniae*. Infect Immun 62:1616–1622.

———. 1995. Identification and characterization of a *Mycoplasma hyopneumoniae* adhesin. Infect Immun 63:1013–1019.

Zielinski GC, Ross RF. 1992. Morphologic features and hydrophobicity of the cell surface of *Mycoplasma hyopneumoniae*. Am J Vet Res 53:1119–1124.

———. 1993. Adherence of *Mycoplasma hyopneumoniae* to porcine ciliated respiratory tract cells. Am J Vet Res 54:1262–1269.

Zimmerman W, Odermatt W, Tschudi P. 1989. Enzootic Pneumonia (EP): The partial depopulation of sow farms reinfected with EP as an alternative to the complete depopulation. Schweiz Arch Tierheilkd 1989:179–191.

Zimmermann BJ, Ross RF. 1975. Determination of sensitivity of *Mycoplasma hyosynoviae* to tylosin and selected antibacterial drugs by a microtiter technique. Can J Comp Med 39:17–21.

———. 1982. Antibody response of swine experimentally infected with *Mycoplasma hyosynoviae*. Vet Microbiol 7:135–146.

Zinn GM, Jesse GW, Dobson AW. 1983. Effect of eperythrozoonosis on sow productivity. J Am Vet Med Assoc 182:369–371.

43 Pneumonic Pasteurellosis

Carlos Pijoan

Pneumonic pasteurellosis, the result of *Pasteurella multocida* infection of the lung, is the common final stage of enzootic pneumonia or porcine respiratory disease complex (PRDC). This syndrome is one of the most common and costly diseases of pigs, especially when they are raised under confinement. Published data suggest that pneumonic lesions at slaughter are very common, even in well-managed herds. Reports on the prevalence of pigs with pneumonic lesions at slaughter has varied from as low as 30% to as high as 80% in various studies through the years. Recent data from the United States found a prevalence of 75% of pigs with pneumonia and 13% with pleuritis in a sample of 6634 pigs inspected, with all herds studied showing some animals with lesions (Bahnson 1994), which highlights pneumonia as the most frequent lesion seen at slaughter.

Pneumonia in pigs also appears to be a very costly disease, although the actual cost has been difficult to calculate and has varied widely in published results. Noyes et al. (1990) performed a radiographic study of pigs' lungs in a commercial herd in order to evaluate lifetime pneumonia and found a significant correlation between the extent of lifetime pneumonic lesions and the weight of the animals at 180 days. Bahnson (1994) compared batches of finishing pigs sent to slaughter. The batch with the highest pneumonia scores had a 7.8% lower rate of gain than the batch with the lowest score, a difference that has considerable economic impact.

Pneumonic pasteurellosis occurs worldwide and in all climates and husbandry conditions. Specific-pathogen-free (SPF) schemes, especially at the national level, do achieve a degree of control, presumably through the eradication of *Mycoplasma hyopneumoniae*. However, *P. multocida,* which is a common inhabitant of the pig's nasal flora, is extremely difficult to eradicate and can be found in most high-health-status herds, such as SPF or minimal-disease herds. Since pasteurellae can interact directly with other agents, elimination of mycoplasmas does not give an absolute guarantee of controlling pneumonia.

A more recent strategy for raising high-health-status pigs has been to use a combination of segregation of the offspring together with early weaning. This program of segregated early weaning (SEW) has been extremely successful in controlling and minimizing most of the common diseases that affect the pig. However, its impact on pneumonic pasteurellosis has been variable. In most farms and groups of pigs, pneumonia at slaughter has decreased to negligible levels. However, some farms have presented with severe pneumonia during the late finishing stages, around 16–18 weeks of age. This late pneumonia has been attributed mostly to infection by *M. hyopneumoniae,* but *P. multocida* is also commonly isolated. SEW, at least when used with weaning at 15 days, does not eliminate *P. multocida* from the offspring. Elimination of *M. hyopneumoniae* is more variable and unpredictable, probably dependent on sow immunity, and is most probably the predisposing trigger for pneumonia in these systems.

ETIOLOGY

P. multocida is a gram-negative coccobacillus, 0.5–1 4× 1–2 μm in size. The organism is a facultative anaerobe, growing well in most enriched media. It is oxidase positive, nonmotile, indole positive, and urease negative. It does not grow well in MacConkey and is nonhemolytic and does not require X and V factors. These reactions are helpful in differentiating *P. multocida* from a group of closely related bacteria that are also involved in pulmonary diseases of pigs, namely, *P. haemolytica, Actinobacillus suis,* and *A. pleuropneumoniae.*

P. multocida has five capsular serotypes, A, B, D, E, and F of which A, B, and D have been reported in swine. Serotype B however, is atypical in that it produces a much more severe disease. It is also rare, confined to regions of Southeast Asia, China, and India (Verma 1988). It has not been reported from natural outbreaks in pigs in North America or Europe. The most common serotype isolated from pneumonic lungs is A, although a variable proportion of serotype D strains is also found

(Pijoan et al. 1983a, 1984; Kielstein 1986; Hoie et al. 1991; Rubies et al. 1996). *P. multocida* also has 16 somatic serotypes; strains of serotypes 3 and 5 are commonly detected in pigs, with strains A:3, A:5, D:5, and D:3 being the most prevalent, in that order.

Virulence Factors

The virulence factors of *P. multocida* are not well defined. In particular, the importance of the dermonecrotic toxin (DNT) is unresolved. This toxin is central to the production of atrophic rhinitis (see Chapter 34) when only toxigenic strains of *P. multocida* are involved in the disease. Toxigenic strains of *P. multocida* from lungs were first reported by Pijoan et al. (1984). Since then, a number of authors have found increasing numbers of toxigenic strains (both type A and type D) in pneumonic lungs. Some reports (Kielstein 1986; Iwamatsu and Sawada 1988) show that between 25% and 45% of strains isolated from lungs are toxigenic. Kielstein (1986) found that toxigenic strains were frequently isolated from acute cases but not from slaughterhouse lungs, suggesting enhanced virulence. However, Baekbo (1988) postulated that toxigenicity was not important in determining the virulence of *P. multocida* in experimentally infected animals.

The role, if any, of toxigenicity in pneumonic pasteurellosis is still under debate. For example, Hoie et al. (1991) found that 94% of serotype A and 90% of serotype D isolates from pneumonic lungs were toxigenic. In contrast, Rubies et al. (1996) found no toxigenic strains (either A or D) in 218 isolates from pneumonic lungs in Spain.

The capsule appears to be an important virulence factor, especially in serotype A, for it may help the organism avoid phagocytosis by alveolar macrophages, at least in vitro. Maheswaran and Thies (1979) reported that *P. multocida* uptake by swine alveolar macrophages was very low, even in the presence of opsonins. Similar results were found by Fuentes and Pijoan (1986). More recent work, however, suggests that little capsule is expressed when the organisms are grown under iron-restricted conditions (Jacques et al. 1994). These growth conditions mimic the scenario found in vivo. Thus, the relevance of the capsule to virulence may have been overestimated in the past.

Some strains of *P. multocida* are able to produce pleuritis and abscessation in experimentally infected pigs (Pijoan and Fuentes 1987). The virulence factors that distinguish these strains from less virulent pneumonic strains are not defined. However, Iwamatso and Sawada (1988) found that strains of serotype D or toxigenic strains (of both serotypes) were associated with abscesses but not with pleuritis.

Mucosal Colonization

The colonization of mucous surfaces by *P. multocida* has received some attention lately, as it is of paramount im-

portance in understanding the pathogenesis of this organism. Jacques (1987) found that both serotypes A and D adhered poorly to isolated tracheal epithelial cells, although serotype A strains were more adherent. He later showed that serotype A strains adhered mostly to ciliated epithelial cells. Pijoan and Trigo (1989) also found sparse colonization by serotype A and D strains but found that serotype D strains adhered mostly to nonciliated cells. Trigo and Pijoan (1988) and later Issacson and Trigo (1995) found that some strains, in particular toxigenic ones, had detectable pili on their surface, although the role of these structures in adhesion is still under debate. In contrast to their poor attachment to epithelial surfaces, *P. multocida* strains have been shown to attach readily to nasal mucus, raising questions as to where normal attachment and colonization take place.

The presence of capsule has been shown to decrease the attachment of *P. multocida* to respiratory tract mucus, as well as to cultured tracheal rings (Jacques et al. 1993). On the other hand, the same group has reported that preinfection of tracheal rings with *Bordetella bronchiseptica* enhanced subsequent attachment by *P. multocida* (Dugal et al. 1992). Some other authors, however, have had difficulties in confirming that *P. multocida* attached to immobilized mucus (Issacson and Trigo 1995).

Mucosal colonization of suckling pigs is becoming a very important issue in SEW systems. It has been postulated (Pijoan 1995) that pigs weaned early (at 15 days of age or less) are not homogeneously colonized with organisms such as *P. multocida* and *M. hyopneumoniae*. As a result, pigs are weaned into isolated nurseries in populations that have a variable prevalence of colonized animals. Populations with low prevalence of colonization are at risk of developing severe clinical disease, because some pigs in the population will become infected very late, at a time when no maternal immunity is available. This could explain why SEW systems sometimes present with delayed PRDC (the "18-week wall") (Dee 1997).

EPIDEMIOLOGY

The epidemiology of *P. multocida* is not well understood. The organism is present in practically all herds and can be readily isolated from the nose and tonsils of normal, healthy individuals. Transmission of the disease by aerosols has been postulated but is unlikely to be of importance. Baekbo and Nielsen (1988) measured airborne *P. multocida* in herds suffering from atrophic rhinitis. They were able to isolate the organism in 29 of 44 herds studied. However, the low number of organisms isolated (144 CFU/mL) led them to conclude that there was no relationship between the number of organisms recovered and the severity of the clinical problem.

Although aerosol transmission may occasionally occur within the herd, it is probable that nose-to-nose contact is the common route of infection. Both vertical and horizontal transmission occur, although within farms most transmission appears to be horizontal, with one strain predominating in pneumonic lungs (Zhao et al. 1993). This suggests the existence of *P. multocida* strains of variable virulence, with one of the more virulent strains producing most of the disease within a population. External sources of the organism include mice and other rodents, although chickens and chicken manure have also been postulated as sources. These are probably not common sources of the organism in modern swine farms, however.

PATHOGENESIS

Experimental infections with *P. multocida* are very difficult to produce. Healthy pigs will readily tolerate large doses of organisms instilled intranasally or even intratracheally. Pulmonary clearance is very effective, and the bacteria cannot be reisolated 30 minutes after challenge. Recent work demonstrating that little capsule is present in vivo has clarified the apparent disparity between the poor phagocytosis observed in vitro and the ready clearance of bacteria found in healthy animals. Experimental models of the disease have used serotype B organisms (Farrington 1986), previous infections with immunosuppressive virus or mycoplasmas (Fuentes and Pijoan 1986; Ciprian et al. 1988), or massive instillation of infected fluids into the lung (Hall et al. 1988). This has led to the conclusion that *P. multocida* is not a primary agent of pneumonia but rather follows infections with other agents. Vaccination against hog cholera virus (Pijoan and Ochoa 1978) and infection with Aujezsky's virus (Fuentes and Pijoan 1987) or *M. hyopneumoniae* (Ciprian et al. 1988) have all been shown to predispose the pig to superinfections with *P. multocida*. In contrast, porcine reproductive and respiratory syndrome (PRRS) virus could not be shown to interact with *P. multocida* in the production of pneumonia (Carvalho et al. 1997).

Once established, the organism stimulates a rapid suppurative reaction, characterized by neutrophil infiltration. This is probably a host reaction to bacterial lipopolysaccharide, which stimulates the release of inflammatory cytokines. Death is uncommon, probably the result of endotoxic shock and respiratory failure.

CLINICAL SIGNS

The clinical signs vary in severity depending on the strain of *P. multocida* involved, together with the immune status of the animals.

Acute Form

This form is most commonly associated with serotype B strains. It is rare and is never seen in Europe or North America. The animals show dyspnea, labored breathing with abdominal "thumps" (sudden contractions of the abdomen), prostration, and high fever (up to 42.2°C, 108°F). Mortality may be high (5–40%) in these cases;

dead and moribund animals may show purplish discoloration of the abdominal region, suggesting endotoxic shock.

Subacute Form

This is associated with *P. multocida* strains that produce pleuritis. In these cases, cough and abdominal breathing can be detected in grower or finishing pigs up to market weight. Cough in this age pig is usually the hallmark of severe disease. Clinically, this form of the disease is very similar to pleuropneumonia due to *A. pleuropneumoniae* (see Chapter 33). The main distinguishing feature is that pleuritic pasteurellosis rarely results in sudden death. Rather, pigs become extremely emaciated but may survive for a long time. Recently, outbreaks of PRDC in finishing pigs (about 16–18 weeks of age) on farms using SEW methods has resulted in cough and abdominal breathing in pigs but usually not pleuritis (Dee 1997).

Chronic Form

This is the most common form of the disease, characterized by occasional cough, thumping, and low or nonexistent fever. Animals affected are usually in the later stages of the nursery or are growers (10–16 weeks of age). The signs are indistinguishable from those following *M. hyopneumoniae* infections, for *P. multocida* causes the continuation and exacerbation of primary mycoplasmosis.

LESIONS

Lesions of *P. multocida* are confined to the thoracic cavity and are superimposed on those of *M. hyopneumoniae*. Typically, anteroventral consolidation of the lung is seen, together with froth in the trachea. There is a clear line of demarcation between affected and healthy lung tissue. The affected portion of the lung will have discoloration ranging from red to grayish-green, depending on the course of the infection (Figure 43.1).

Severe cases may present varying degrees of pleuritis and abscessation. Pleural adhesions to the thoracic wall are common in these cases, and the pleura has a translucent, dry appearance (Figures 43.2, 43.3). This is useful in differentiating pneumonic pasteurellosis from actinobacillus pleuropneumonia, in which moist, yellowish pleural adhesions with massive fibrin infiltration are more common (Pijoan 1989).

Histologically, a lobular, exudative bronchopneumonia is found. Severe bronchopneumonia, alveolar epithelial hyperplasia, and the presence of abundant neutrophils are seen with mucopurulent exudate in the bronchial lumen and in alveolar spaces. These lesions are not specific to *P. multocida* infections and are similar for most bacterial pneumonias.

Evidence has also been presented for a relationship between pasteurella-induced bronchopneumonia and the presence of disseminated focal nephritis (Butten-

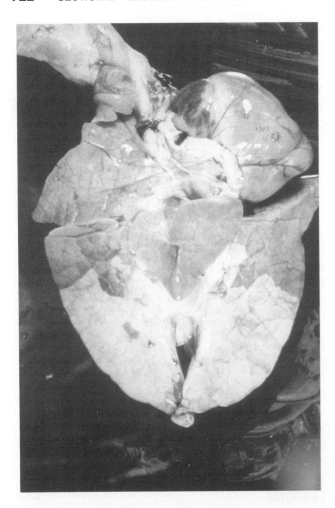

43.1.   *Pneumonic pasteurellosis. Lung consolidation is anteroventral with a clear demarcation line between affected and healthy tissue.*

schon 1991). The author concluded that the two diseases are connected by a process of dissemination from the pulmonary lesions.

DIAGNOSIS

Since the lesions of *P. multocida* infection are not pathognomonic, they cannot be used as the only criteria to establish a definite diagnosis. The history of the outbreak, histopathology, and isolation of the organism should be used to confirm the original presumptive diagnosis. Serology has not proven effective for diagnosis, and no serologic test is routinely available for *P. multocida* infections.

P. multocida is a relatively easy organism to culture, provided proper specimens are submitted to the laboratory. Specimens yielding the best isolations include swabs of tracheobronchial exudate and affected lung tissue obtained from the border area between affected and normal tissue. Nasal swabs have also been shown to be good samples for isolation of *P. multocida* (Schoss and Alt 1995). Swabs should be immersed in an appropriate transport medium, such as Stuart's. Lung samples should be obtained as aseptically as possible. All samples should be refrigerated (but not frozen) until cultured.

Culture of *P. multocida* can be successfully achieved in laboratories with minimal facilities. Good-quality specimens will yield the organism on direct culture onto blood agar or glucose agar plates. If the samples are more contaminated, they can be serially diluted tenfold in brain-heart infusion (BHI) broth, grown overnight, and then plated (Pijoan et al. 1983b). Alternatively, selective media can be used: Ackermann et al. (1994) successfully isolated *P. multocida* from tonsils and turbinates of adult pigs using blood agar with 3.75 U/mL of bacitracin, 5 µg/mL clindamycin, 0.75 µg/mL gentamicin, and 2.25

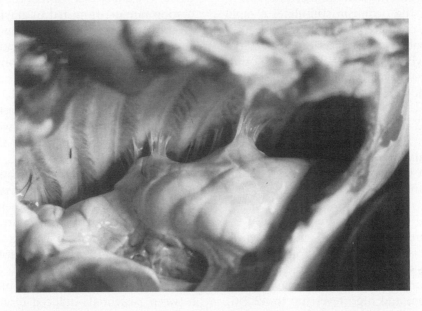

43.2.   *Pleural adhesions of lung to the thoracic wall in a case of pleuritic pasteurellosis. Note that the pleura has a translucent, dry aspect.*

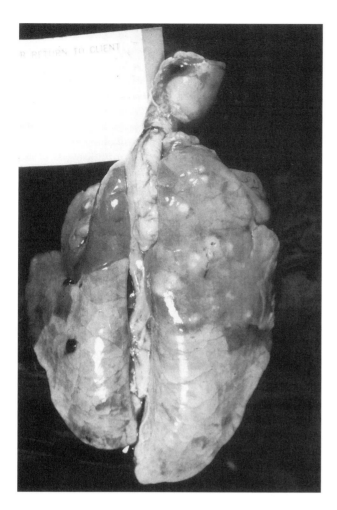

43.3. *Lung from a case of pleuritic pasteurellosis. Note anteroventral, well-demarcated lesions, together with the presence of multiple abscesses. There is extensive interlobar adhesion.*

μg/mL of amphotericin B. Isolation can also be enhanced by injecting the specimen intraperitoneally into mice and then recovering the pasteurellae 24 hours later from liver and ascitic fluid.

Differential diagnosis must include influenza virus, *A. pleuropneumoniae, B. bronchiseptica, Salmonella choleraesuis,* and pure *M. hyopneumoniae* infections. Accurate clinical differentiation based on the epidemiology and lesions can be readily achieved for some of these conditions but may be difficult in cases of influenza, *B. bronchiseptica,* or *M. hyopneumoniae.* In these cases, histology and bacterial culture will be needed. Ramirez and Pijoan (1982) and Straw (1986a) have published tables for the differential diagnosis of these conditions.

TREATMENT

Treatment of *P. multocida* field infections with antibiotics is usually difficult or unsuccessful. This is partly due to widespread antibiotic resistance in *P. multocida* isolates in the United States and also to difficulties in

achieving adequate antibiotic concentrations in consolidated, pneumonic lung.

A variety of antibiotics and antibiotic combinations have been commonly used (Farrington 1986). These include parenteral antibiotics such as oxytetracycline, 11 mg/kg; long-acting oxytetracycline, 20 mg/kg; procaine penicillin, 66,000 units/kg; benzathine penicillin, 32,000 units/kg; tiamulin, 10–12.5 mg/kg; and ampicillin, 6.6 mg/kg. Many of these drugs, however, are becoming increasingly less efficient due to widespread antibiotic resistance. Treatment via feed antibiotics has also been suggested, although, as in the case of other pneumonias, it is probably not very effective.

Cote et al. (1991) found some plasmid-mediated resistance to streptomycin and sulfonamides among 29 field isolates investigated. Gutierrez Martin and Rodriguez Ferri (1993) studied 59 Spanish isolates, finding good activity with penicillins, aminoglycosides, tetracyclines, erythromycin, colistin, and rifampicin, with some resistance to tylosin, vancomycin, and tiamulin. They reported that third-generation cephalosporins and fluorinated quinolones were the most effective drugs. Raemdonck et al. (1994) found good minimum inhibitory concentrations (MIC) for danofloxacin, ceftiofur, and trimethoprim-sulfonamide; they found variable to high resistance to erythromycin, gentamicin, lincomycin, oxytetracyclines, and spectinomycin. Finally, Salmon et al. (1995) tested isolates from several countries and found the best activity with cephalosporins and enrofloxacin, with poor activity shown in vitro by erythromycin, sulfamethazine, spectinomycin, and lincomycin.

The effectiveness of all these antimicrobials will vary considerably depending on strain susceptibility. Since *P. multocida* readily exhibits resistance to various antimicrobials, antibiograms should be performed before instituting treatment.

As in other respiratory infections, antibiotics are more effective when used as prophylactic, rather than therapeutic, agents. Tetracyclines alone, tetracyclines combined with sulfamethazine or sulfathiazole or penicillin, and tylosin combined with sulfamethazine have been recommended for this purpose. It is probable that the most effective compound in these mixtures is sulfamethazine. This antimicrobial has been the focus of controversy over residues. Because of this, its use has been severely limited and monitored. Tiamulin (40 ppm in feed) has been shown, in a number of trials, to improve average daily gain. However, since pneumonic lesions are not significantly reduced by this antibiotic (Pott and Edwards 1990), the mode of action by which these improvements are obtained is unclear. Tiamulin has been found to be of variable effectiveness against *P. multocida.* It is therefore probable that its main effect in pneumonia lies in the control of *M. hyopneumoniae.*

Some new antibiotics with claims for *P. multocida* treatment are not available in the United States but are used extensively in other countries. These include injectable lincomycin-spectinomycin, some cephalosporins, and various quinolones including enrofloxacin and danofloxacin. Injectable ceftiofur is available in the United States, however, and it has been shown by a number of authors to have good activity against *P. multocida*.

PREVENTION

Management Approaches

Since antibiotic therapy is often unsuccessful and even when successful may not prove cost-effective, prevention of pneumonia has received much attention. Prevention is usually obtained through changes in management. The management techniques that result in decreased pneumonia have been reviewed by several authors (Pijoan 1986; Straw 1986b). Caution must be taken when implementing these recommendations, since they derive mostly from retrospective epidemiological studies and not from experimental data. Also, they are intended to reduce pneumonia as a whole (and other respiratory problems) and do not differentiate between conditions of different etiology.

Management changes can be directed either at modifying the pigs' environment or at reducing the possibilities of spreading the organism.

Environmental changes such as increasing ventilation flow rate, decreasing ammonia, and minimizing temperature fluctuations and dust are usually recommended. Some of these recommendations are antagonistic; increasing airflow, especially in winter, results in a decrease of both temperature and humidity, with an increase in dust. Most of these changes have not proven valuable in controlled, experimental conditions. Noyes et al. (1986) found that decreasing ventilation below minimal recommended levels (0.5 CFM/pig) had no effect on weaned pigs inoculated with both *B. bronchiseptica* and *P. multocida*. Similarly, Rafai et al. (1987) found that cold stress, even though it reduced immune function in suckling pigs, had no effect on the course of an experimental *P. multocida* infection. Environmental changes frequently entail extensive remodeling. They are, therefore, expensive to institute and maintain. It is not clear that these changes are cost-effective in terms of reducing respiratory disease.

On the other hand, considerable improvement may be obtained by instituting management changes that reduce the spread of the organism. These include the following:

1. Segregated early weaning: SEW has a major impact on pneumonia and, when properly done, will reduce or eliminate pneumonia from most groups of pigs. This is probably based on the control of *M. hyopneumoniae*, which in many herds is virtually eliminated. Early weaning probably has less effect on *P. multocida*, since it has been shown that pigs are colonized as early as 10 days of age. Occasional farms or groups of pigs will experience acute outbreaks of pneumonia.

2. All-in/all-out production: In farms where SEW is not possible, efforts should be made to institute an all-in/all-out production program. Several workers have shown that this type of production system markedly decreases the incidence of pneumonia.

3. Closed herds: Minimizing the purchase of outside pigs, especially fatteners, will result in a decrease of pneumonia and other respiratory conditions. However, the pressure to improve genetics in modern farms has forced most producers to purchase their breeding animals. It has become increasingly important to evaluate the health status of the farm from which these animals are purchased, in order to minimize the probability of introducing disease.

4. Minimal mixing and sorting: This is a source of stress to the pigs, while also intensifying the probabilities of disease transmission. Pigs should be mixed as few times as possible during their productive life.

5. Reduction in building and pen size: Smaller rooms and smaller pens both have been shown to reduce levels of pneumonia. Rooms should have a maximum of 250 pigs, and pens a maximum of 20–25 pigs each. This again is difficult to achieve in modern farms. However, the recent trend of building wean-to-finish barns, where pigs are only mixed once, at weaning, will probably have a positive effect in decreasing pneumonia.

6. Reduction in animal density: Decreasing animal density has been shown by many authors to reduce levels of pneumonia. It is important therefore to find a reasonable compromise between densities that are appropriate for the animals' health and those that maximize returns on the building's cost.

Vaccination

Although several killed vaccines for the prevention of pneumonic pasteurellosis are available, their effectiveness is questionable. Since no reliable model of experimental disease exists, potency testing is usually performed in mice. It is doubtful, therefore, that this model truly replicates the disease in the pig. Under field conditions, clinicians frequently have disappointing results with these vaccines, and they do not appear to be cost-effective.

Some modern approaches to vaccination against *P. multocida* have been reported recently. The use of purified lipopolysaccharide (LPS) antigen and the use of *aro* A gene deletion mutants both resulted in protection against homologous, but not heterologous, challenge (Adler et al. 1996). The use of a cloned, 87 kDa outer-membrane protein had similar limitations (Ruttolo and Adler 1996). Cross-protection has been reported in chickens with the use of a protein preparation from cells grown under iron-deprived conditions, which mimic the in vivo environment (Wang and Glisson 1994). However, none of these fraction vaccines are commercially available or have been tested in pigs, where the disease is not septicemic as it is in chickens and mice. Therefore, there is at present no successful commercial vaccine against *P. multocida* in the pig.

OTHER PASTEURELLA INFECTIONS IN PIGS

Several authors have sporadically isolated *P. haemolytica*–like organisms from cases of severe necrotizing pleuropneumonia. The lesions seen are similar to those found in *A. pleuropneumoniae* infections but tend to be less severe. In this regard, they are also similar to lesions reported from *A. suis*. A new nicotinamide adenine dinucleotide (NAD)-independent biotype of *A. pleuropneumoniae* has now been recognized, and it is very probable that many of these severe pneumonias are related to these two organisms rather than to *P. hemolytica*.

All these organisms are very similar and differ in minor biochemical reactions such as indole formation or V-factor requirement. Bisgaard (1984) did a comprehensive study of these strains and concluded that they differed from *P. haemolytica* sensu stricto. Since the lesions produced (and the serologic reactions) are indistinguishable from *A. pleuropneumoniae,* it is possible that some field outbreaks have been misdiagnosed. At present, it is very difficult to assess the true prevalence and economic impact of these strains.

REFERENCES

Ackermann MR, Debey MC, Register KC, Larson JL, Kinyon JM. 1994. Tonsil and turbinate colonization by toxigenic and nontoxigenic strains of *Pasteurella multocida* in conventionally raised swine. J Vet Diag Invest 6:375–377.

Adler B, Chancellor R, Hamchampa P, Hunt M, Ruffolo C, Strugnell R, Wapling D. 1996. Immunity and vaccine development in *Pasteurella multocida* infections. J Biotechnol 44(1–3):139–144.

Baekbo P. 1988. Pathogenic properties of *Pasteurella multocida* in the lungs of pigs. Proc Int Congr Pig Vet Soc 10:58.

Baekbo P, Nielsen JP. 1988. Airborne *Pasteurella multocida* in pig fattening units. Proc Int Congr Pig Vet Soc 10:51.

Bahnson BB. 1994. Enzootic Pneumonia of Swine: Epidemiology and Effect on the Rate of Gain. Ph.D. diss. Univ Minnesota.

Bisgaard M. 1984. Comparative investigations of *Pasteurella haemolytica* sensu stricto and so-called *P. haemolytica* isolated from different pathological lesions in pigs. Acta Pathol Microbiol Immunol Scand (B) 92:203–207.

Buttenschon J. 1991. Statistical evidence for a link between pleuropneumonia and disseminated focal nephritis in pigs. Zentralblatt für Vet Reihe A 38(4):287–299.

Carvalho L, Segales J, Pijoan C. 1997. Effect of PRRS virus on subsequent *Pasteurella multocida* challenge in pigs. Vet Microbiol (in press).

Ciprian A, Pijoan C, Cruz T, Camacho J, Tortora J, Colmenares G, Lopez-Revilla R, Garza M De la. 1988. *Mycoplasma hyopneumoniae* increases the susceptibility of pigs to experimental *Pasteurella multocida* pneumonia. Can J Vet Res 52:434–438.

Cote S, Harel J, Higgins R, Jacques M. 1991. Resistance to antimicrobial agents and prevalence of R plasmids in *Pasteurella multocida* from swine. Am J Vet Res 52(10):1653–1657.

Dee SA. 1997. Porcine respiratory disease complex: The "18 week wall." In Proc Am Assoc Swine Pract (Quebec), pp. 465–466.

Dugal F, Belanger M, Jacques M. 1992. Enhanced adherence of *Pasteurella multocida* to porcine tracheal rings preinfected with *Bordetella bronchiseptica*. Can J Vet Res 56(3):260–264.

Farrington DO. 1986. Pneumonic pasteurellosis. In Diseases of Swine, 6th ed. AD Leman, B Straw, RD Glock WL Mengeling, RHC Penny, E Scholl, eds. Ames: Iowa State Univ Press, p. 436.

Fuentes M, Pijoan C. 1986. Phagocytosis and killing of *Pasteurella multocida* by pig alveolar macrophages after infection with pseudorabies virus. Vet Immunol Immunopathol 13:165–172.

——. 1987. Pneumonia in pigs induced by intranasal challenge exposure with pseudorabies virus and *Pasteurella multocida*. Am J Vet Res 48:1446–1448.

Gutierrez Martin CB, Rodriguez Ferri EF. 1993. In vitro susceptibility of *Pasteurella multocida* strains isolated from swine to 42 antimicrobial agents. Int J Med Microbiol Virol Parasitol Dis 279(3):387–393.

Hall W, Bane D, Kilroy C, Essex-Sorlie D. 1988. A model for the induction of pneumonia caused by *Pasteurella multocida* type A. Proc Int Congr Pig Vet Soc 10:59.

Hoie S, Falk K, Lium BM. 1991. An abbatoir survey of pneumonia and pleuritis in slaughter weight swine from 9 selected herds. IV. Bacteriological findings in chronic pneumonic lesions. Acta Vet Scand 32(3):395–402.

Issacson RE, Trigo E. 1995. Pili of *Pasteurella multocida* of porcine origin. FEMS Microbiol Letters 132(3):247–251.

Iwamatsu S, Sawada T. 1988. Relationship between serotypes, dermonecrotic toxin production of *Pasteurella multocida* isolates and pneumonic lesions of porcine lungs. Jpn J Vet Sci 50:1200–1206.

Jacques M. 1987. Adherence of *Pasteurella multocida* to porcine upper respiratory tract cells. Current Microbiol 15:115–119.

Jacques M, Belanger M, Diarra MS, Dargis M, Malouin F. 1994. Modulation of *Pasteurella multocida* capsular polysaccharide during growth under iron-restricted conditions and in vivo. Microbiol 140 (Pt 2):263–270.

Jacques M, Kobisch M, Belanger M, Dugal F. 1993. Virulence of capsulated and noncapsulated *Pasteurella multocida* and their adherence to porcine respiratory tract cells and mucus. Infect Immun 61(11):4785–4792.

Kielstein P. 1986. On the occurrence of toxin-producing *Pasteurella multocida* strains in atrophic rhinitis and in pneumonias of swine and cattle. J Vet Med (B) 33:418–424.

Maheswaran S, Thies E. 1979. Influence of encapsulation on phagocytosis of *Pasteurella multocida* by bovine neutrophils. Infect Immun 26:76–81.

Noyes E, Feeney D, Pijoan C. 1990. Comparison of the effect of pneumonia detected during a lifetime with pneumonia detected at slaughter on growth in swine. J Am Vet Med Assoc 197:1025–1029.

Noyes E, Pijoan C, Jacobson L. 1986. Ventilating environment for the weaned pig. Proc Int Congr Pig Vet Soc 9:401.

Pijoan C. 1986. Respiratory system. In Diseases of Swine, 6th ed. AD Leman, B Straw, RD Glock, WL Mengeling, RHC Penny, E Scholl, eds. Ames: Iowa State Univ Press, pp. 152–162.

——. 1989. Pleuritis effect on growth underestimated. Int Pig Lett 9:17–19.

——. 1995. Diseases of high-health pigs: Some ideas on pathogenesis. In Proc A Leman Conf (Minnesota), pp. 16–17.

Pijoan C, Fuentes M. 1987. Severe pleuritis associated with certain strains of *Pasteurella multocida* in swine. J Am Vet Med Assoc 191:823–826.

Pijoan C, Lastra A, Ramirez C, Leman A. 1984. Isolation of toxigenic strains of *Pasteurella multocida* from lungs of pneumonic swine. J Am Vet Med Assoc 185:522–523.

Pijoan C, Morrison RB, Hilley HD. 1983a. Serotyping of *Pasteurella multocida* isolated from swine lungs collected at slaughter. J Clin Microbiol 17:1074–1076.

——. 1983b. Dilution technique for isolation of *Haemophilus* from swine lungs collected at slaughter. J Clin Microbiol 18:143–145.

Pijoan C, Ochoa G. 1978. Interaction between a hog cholera vaccine strain and *Pasteurella multocida* in production of porcine pneumonia. J Comp Pathol 88:167–170.

Pijoan C, Trigo E. 1989. Bacterial adhesion to mucosal surfaces with special reference to *Pasteurella multocida* isolates from atrophic rhinitis. Can J Vet Sci 54:516–521.

Pott J, Edwards J. 1990. Beneficial effects of tiamutin administered in feed at 40 ppm to pigs with enzootic pneumonia. Proc Int Congr Pig Vet Soc 11:86.

Raemdonck DL, Tanner AC, Tolling ST, Michener SL. 1994. Antimicrobial susceptibility of *Actinobacillus pleuropneumoniae*, *Pasteurella multocida* and *Salmonella choleraesuis* isolates from pigs. Vet Rec 134:5–7.

Rafai P, Neumann R, Leonhardt W, Frenyo L, Rudas P, Fodor L, Boros G. 1987. Effect of environmental temperature on pigs infected with *Pasteurella multocida* type A. Acta Vet Hung 35:211–223.

Ramirez N, Pijoan C. 1982. Diagnostico de las Enfermedades del Cerdo. RR Necoechea, C Pijoan, eds. Mexico City: Necoechea and Pijoan, p. 227.

Rubies X, Casal J, Fernandez J, Pijoan C. 1996. Transmission of *Pasteurella multocida* clones in a swine pyramid structure. Proc Int Congr Pig Vet Soc 14:243.

Ruttolo CG, Adler B. 1996. Cloning, sequencing, expression and protective capacity of the oma 87 gene encoding the *Pasteurella* multocida 87-kilodalton outer membrane antigen. Infect Immun 64(8):316–317.

Salmon SA, Watts JL, Case CA, Hoffman LJ, Wegener HC, Yancey RJ, Jr. 1995. Comparison of MICs of Ceftiofur and other antimicrobial agents against bacterial pathogens of swine from the United States, Canada and Denmark. J Clin Microbiol 33(9):2435–2444.

Schoss P, Alt M. 1995. Are nasal swabs appropriate for the diagnosis of bacterial pneumonia agents? Dtsch Tierarztl Wochen 102(11):427–430.

Straw BE. 1986a. Differential diagnosis of swine diseases. In Diseases of Swine, 6th ed. AD Leman, B Straw, RD Glock, WL Mengeling, RHC Penny, E Scholl, eds. Ames: Iowa State Univ Press, p. 214.

——. 1986b. A look at factors that contribute to the development of swine pneumonia. Vet Med (Aug):747–755.

Trigo E, Pijoan C. 1988. Presence of pili in *Pasteurella multocida* strains associated with atrophic rhinitis. Vet Rec 122:19.

Verma ND. 1988. *Pasteurella multocida* B:2 in haemorrhagic septicaemia outbreak in pigs in India. Vet Rec 123:63.

Wang C, Glisson JR. 1994. Passive cross-protection provided by antisera directed against in vivo expressed antigens of *Pasteurella multocida*. Avian Dis 38(3):506–514.

Zhao G, Pijoan C, Murtaugh MP. 1993. Epidemiology of *Pasteurella multocida* in a farrow-to-finish swine herd. Can J Vet Res 57(2):136–138.

44 Proliferative Enteropathies

Steven McOrist and Connie J. Gebhart

Proliferative enteropathies (PE; also known as *ileitis*) are a group of acute and chronic conditions of widely differing clinical signs but with a common underlying pathological change visible at necropsy: a thickening of the mucosa of the small intestine and colon. Histologically, the affected tissues show marked proliferation of immature epithelial cells of the intestinal crypts, forming a hyperplastic to adenoma-like mucosa. These proliferating cells invariably contain numerous intracytoplasmic *Lawsonia intracellularis*, an obligate intracellular bacterium.

In growing pigs with uncomplicated proliferation of the mucosa, the condition is chronic proliferative enteropathy, also known as *porcine intestinal adenomatosis (PIA)* or *ileitis*. In some pigs, these changes can be mild and subclinical or, alternatively, can have additional changes superimposed on this basic lesion, including a necrotic enteritis, a granulomatous regional ileitis, or an acute proliferative hemorrhagic enteropathy (PHE, Rowland and Lawson 1975). The chronic, subclinical and acute hemorrhagic forms of PE are now important enteric diseases in the modern pig industry.

The lesions of PE were first described in pigs in Ames, Iowa, by Biester and others in the 1930s (Biester and Schwarte 1931; Biester et al. 1939) and were subsequently found to occur in other major pig-raising areas throughout the world, but it was not until 1973 that Alan Rowland and Gordon Lawson, investigating major outbreaks occurring in Scotland, developed a productive research program (Rowland and Rowntree 1972; Rowland and Lawson 1974). They found that whenever these proliferative changes in pigs were studied either ultrastructurally or using silver stains, intracellular bacteria were consistently present within the abnormal proliferating cells (Rowland and Lawson 1974). These bacteria lie free in the apical cytoplasm of infected epithelial cells and are not membrane-bound during the important stages of infection. The identity of these bacteria and their etiologic role in PE in pigs were finally resolved in 1993 with successful culture of the intracellular organism and the reproduction of the disease in pigs using a pure culture of this agent (Lawson et al. 1993; McOrist et al. 1993). Also in 1993, its taxonomic position was clarified (Gebhart et al. 1993); its definitive name is *Lawsonia intracellularis* (McOrist et al. 1995a).

Pathological changes closely resembling porcine PE and caused by intracellular Lawsonia species have been described in a wide range of host species as single case reports, including in macaques (Klein et al. 1999; Cooper and Gebhart 1998). However despite obvious infection opportunities, no case of PE or Lawsonia infection has been detected in humans. Natural disease outbreaks are reported in the laboratory hamster (Frisk and Wagner 1977; Williams et al. 1996; Lavoie et al. 2000), in the laboratory rabbit (Schoeb and Fox 1990; Duhamel et al. 1998), in deer (Drolet et al. 1996), and in ratite birds (Cooper et al. 1997; Lemarchand et al. 1997), but importantly, other farm birds and wild-type mice appear resistant (Collins et al. 1999; McOrist et al. 2003a). Experimental transmission studies, in situ immunostaining and DNA analysis across species have demonstrated that the one bacterial species can infect the intestinal cells of a wide variety of host species (Lawson and Gebhart 2000). The common infection among laboratory rabbits hampers simple production of specific polyclonal antibody. However, there is currently no evidence to link these other hosts directly with the onset of disease in farmed pigs. The disease has been detected in wild pigs (Sus scrofa) living in central Europe (Tomanova et al. 2002).

ETIOLOGY

The cause of PE is the obligately intracellular bacterium, *L. intracellularis*, which preferentially grows within the cytoplasm of intestinal epithelial cells. This bacterial growth is invariably accompanied by localized proliferation of infected immature crypt epithelial cells. It has not as yet been cultivated in cell-free media, due to a metabolic requirement for preformed mitochondrial triphosphates or a similar energy source. Some earlier literature refers to the intracellular bacterium as a Campylobacter-like organism; however, that designation was based only on its morphologic similarity to that genus.

L. intracellularis forms curved to straight vibrioid-shaped rods with either tapered or rounded ends and measure 1.25–1.75 μm in length by 0.25–0.43 μm in width. It has a typical gram-negative trilaminar outer envelope. No fimbriae or spores have been detected. A long, single, polar flagellum and darting motility has been observed in some isolates co-cultured on cell lines, but only when the bacteria are located extracellularly. It has a small, single circular genome and 3 plasmids, totalling 1.72 million bp and 1,324 orf. It possesses the small genome, cell-dependent respiration, low G+C%, and significant expression of the gro EL heat shock proteins commonly seen in other symbiont intracellular bacteria (Dale et al. 1998; McOrist and Gebhart 2004). Despite being placed in the Desulfovibrionaceae family on DNA sequence analysis, it does not appear to have sulfate reduction capacity. In vitro culture of *L. intracellularis* requires co-culture on a transformed cell line such as intestinal epithelial cells, in a microaerobic atmosphere of 82.2% nitrogen, 8.8% carbon dioxide, and 8% oxygen at 37°C (Stills 1991; Lawson et al. 1993). Isolates of *L. intracellularis* from pigs and those from a variety of origins and other host species (hamster, horse, deer) show a very high degree (>98%) of similarity among DNA sequences in key taxonomic sites and in their outer membrane proteins, indicating that a single "strain" of *L. intracellularis* may occur (Cooper et al. 1997; Al-Ghamdi 2003).

Experimental transmission studies using pure cultures of *L. intracellularis* as oral-challenge inocula for conventional pigs and using gnotobiotic pigs predosed with a minimal bacterial flora of nonpathogenic enteric species have resulted in reproduction of the specific lesions of PE (McOrist et al. 1993, 1994). Exposure of pigs to crude, or partially filtered, homogenized diseased mucosa resulted in reproduction of specific intestinal lesions and clinical disease in early challenge trials (Roberts et al. 1977; Mapother et al. 1987; McOrist and Lawson 1989a). This strategy was later revived into a well-chararacterized mucosal homogenate challenge exposure model for reproduction of PE in conventional pigs (Winkelman et al. 2002; Guedes and Gebhart 2003a, b). Intestinal lesions that develop as a result of artificial exposure to various isolates have had all the characteristics of the field disease, including the presence of mucosal proliferation and intracellular bacteria (McOrist et al. 1993; Guedes and Gebhart 2003a, b). *L. intracellularis* isolates derived from American or European origins and from acute or chronic lesions have proved capable of producing typical chronic or acute PE lesions (Mapother et al. 1987; Knittel et al. 1996), indicating that the differing clinical expression of PE cases

(PIA, subclinical, PHE) are due to dosage and host response differences, not to separate bacterial strains.

EPIDEMIOLOGY

The disease is worldwide in distribution and occurs commonly in all pig-raising regions and in all pig farm management systems, including outdoor ones (McOrist et al. 2003b). The incidence of lesions in pigs at normal slaughter age is generally low, at 0.7–2.0%, and therefore unreliable for farm monitoring (Rowland and Hutchings 1978; Christensen and Cullinane 1990; Jensen et al. 1999).

The development and widespread use of Lawsonia-specific PCR suitable for fecal samples and serology methods has enabled a clearer understanding of the widespread prevalence and epidemiology of PE on pig farms. Recent surveys in Europe, Asia, and the Americas have indicated that practically all pig farms have at least a low level of infection and that some 20–40% of pig farms have a notable level of clinical and/or subclinical cases (Moller et al. 1998; Kim et al. 1998; Stege et al. 2000; Bane et al. 2001; Jacobsen et al. 2003; Marsteller et al. 2003).

Comparison of management systems with the onset of infection indicates that on pig farms with age-separation of groups (so-called multisite farm systems) *L. intracellularis* infection occurs rarely in breeding stock and is usually delayed in grower-finishers until they are 12–20 weeks old (Just et al. 2001; Bronsvoort et al. 2001; Chouet et al. 2003). This delayed infection may be associated with the onset of PIA or PHE cases, but antibiotic usage may complicate this simplistic pattern.

In contrast, on single-site farms with a continuous pig flow between different groups (so-called farrow-to-finish systems) there is early postweaning infection at approximately 5 to 7 weeks old, with frequent occurrence of related subclinical and clinical problems (PIA). Infection of piglets probably occurs soon after maternally derived passive immunity wanes, via positive feces exposure. The infection can then amplify over the next few weeks in groups of postweaned "nursery" pigs. In these farms, levels of recent exposure of at least 10% are also evident among healthy breeding females of all parities, with some (<5%) of these exposed sows shedding detectable *L. intracellularis* in their feces. Where group housing of breeding females occurs, this rate of recent exposure consistently rises above 30%, presumably due to higher contamination of the bedding (Stege et al. 2000; Chouet et al. 2003).

It is likely that the environment of many pig farms, particulary the grower-finisher areas, contains a sustained level of *L. intracellularis* infection "embedded" in the fecal material, fomites, pens, insects, and walkways in the buildings. This acts to reintroduce the infection to many new groups of pigs at various ages. However, even with use of the best diagnostic tests, it can be difficult to establish exactly when a group infection and/or its related clinical outbreak of ileitis starts on any given farm (Hammer 2004). In other words, the infection can build up slowly or quickly, with variations in the time of disease onset on different farms and, importantly, on the same farm between different groups in the same building or pens (Philips et al. 1998; Hammer 2004). The highest levels of exposure in all farms are usually seen in older finisher pigs (Moller et al. 1998; Marsteller et al. 2003). Transmission of positive feces from this contaminated area to other areas of a farm, such as those containing breeding animals, would occur more commonly on single-site farms. Modes of this transmission probably include passive transfer of feces on boots or fomites, such as within rodent feet. Although cross-species transmission of *L. intracellularis* infection has been demonstrated experimentally, an active role of infected vectors has not yet been clearly demonstrated on any *L. intracellularis*–infected farm.

Clinically important outbreaks of acute PHE are now very apparent and frequent, probably due to the persistence of this obvious and often fatal disease in the face of "high health" strategies, such as multisite farms and medicated early weaning (Guedes et al. 2002a). Particular management situations are thought to lend themselves to outbreaks of acute PHE. Young adults (4–12 months old) within boar and gilt performance testing stations, gilts within breeding programs that involve transportation to new units, and the movement and mixing of boars and gilts into breeding groups are commonly associated with PE outbreaks. Although this often partly reflects changes in exposure and use of antibiotics at these times, the occurrence of major stressors, such as extreme weather conditions, is a common feature prior to many outbreaks.

Overall epidemiologic features of PE include: *L. intracellularis* can remain viable in feces at 5 to 15°C for 2 weeks (Collins et al. 2000), the infectious dose is relatively low (McOrist et al. 1993; Guedes et al. 2003) and fecal excretion may be high in some infected "spreader" pigs (Smith and McOrist 1997; Guedes et al. 2002a). Sanitation methods are incompletely understood. Of 6 disinfectants tested in one study (Collins et al. 2000), only quaternary ammonium (3% cetrimide QA) and iodine-based (1% povidone-iodine) compounds showed full bactericidal activity. Isolates appeared somewhat resistant to a 0.33% phenolic mixture. In herds with endemic chronic PE, feces from infected pigs or on the boots of workers can clearly provide the likely source of new infections. Rigorous removal of feces from boots and between batches of pigs in buildings capable of complete "all-in/all-out" is likely to be more effective at control of PE than reliance on slatted floors and sunken pits for feces removal (Smith et al. 1998; Bane et al. 2001). It is possible but not considered likely that feces from infected gilts or sows are responsible for regular transmission to their progeny.

PATHOGENESIS

PE can be reproduced by exposing susceptible pigs to *L. intracellularis* or to diseased mucosa containing these intracellular bacteria (Roberts et al. 1977; McOrist and Lawson 1989; McOrist et al. 1993, 1994; Guedes and Gebhart 2003a). In typical oral challenge exposure studies of postweaned pigs (4 weeks old) with a standard inoculum of 10^8 *L. intracellularis* bacteria, numerous intracellular bacteria can be visualized in the developing proliferative intestines and feces 1–3 weeks following inoculation with a peak of infection and lesions 3 weeks after challenge. In most of these pigs, intestinal infection, proliferative lesions and excretion persists for approximately 4 weeks, but in some exposed pigs, excretion may persist for at least 10 weeks (Smith and McOrist 1997; Guedes et al. 2002a). At the peak of infection 3 weeks after challenge, moderate diarrhea and histologic lesions of PE are usually observed in 50% and 100%, respectively, of animals challenged with this inoculum. Infection and lesions in the large intestine generally occur a week or two after small intestinal infection following oral challenge (Guedes and Gebhart 2003b). Naive pigs of a wide age range (neonates to grower-finishers) are susceptible to oral challenge.

PE develops initially as a progressive proliferation of immature epithelial cells populated by numerous intracellular bacteria. In most cases, no significant inflammatory reaction occurs and the organisms remain in the epithelium at this stage. In severe cases of PE, *L. intracellularis* can also be observed in the mesenteric lymph node and tonsils (Roberts et al. 1980; Jensen et al. 2001), but these appear to be secondary sites. In vivo and in vitro studies have elucidated some of the early events in bacteria-cell interaction (McOrist et al. 1989b, 1995b; Lawson et al. 1995). Bacteria associate with the cell membrane and then quickly enter the enterocyte via an entry vacuole. Specific adhesins or receptors have not been identified, but *L. intracellularis* may possess a type III secretion system. The entry vacuole rapidly breaks down (within 3 hours), and the bacteria flourish and multiply free (not membrane-bound) within the cytoplasm. The entry of bacteria into cells is dependent on cell, but not necessarily bacterial, viability—that is, a type of induced phagocytosis (Lawson et al. 1995). The mechanism whereby the bacteria cause infected cells to fail to mature, but continue to undergo mitosis and form hyperplastic crypts, is not yet understood fully. It may reflect an inhibition of the normal crypt cell differentiation process, as regulated locally at the crypt neck. *L. intracellularis*–infected intestinal crypts can become enormously elongated and often branched. Loss of body protein and amino acids into the intestinal lumen and the reduced nutrient absorption by the intestinal mucosa lacking mature enterocytes are the likely causes of the reduction in weight gain and feed conversion efficiency seen in pigs affected with chronic uncomplicated

PE lesions (Rowan and Lawrence 1982; Gogolewski et al. 1991).

Early lesions contain very few infiltrating inflammatory cells, probably not above the normal for pig intestines (McOrist et al. 1992). Affected epithelial cells contain a large accumulation of intracellular IgA (Lawson et al. 1979; McOrist et al. 1992), and intestinal lavages contain a high level of Lawsonia-specific IgA (Guedes et al. 2002c). Macrophage ingestion of *L. intracellularis* in developing lesions probably leads to a typical Th1 type immune cell response in the lamina propria (McOrist et al. 1992; MacIntyre et al. 2003). Both cell-mediated and humoral responses occur in the blood of affected pigs (McOrist and Lawson 1993; Knittel et al. 1998; Guedes and Gebhart 2003b). These are first detectable 2 weeks after exposure and can persist for up to 3 months in acutely infected pigs (Guedes et al. 2002c). It is therefore likely that animals exposed to *L. intracellularis* show a specific immune response.

Degenerative and reparative changes may be superimposed on the basic enterocyte proliferation, probably due to local secondary bacterial infections. Inflammatory changes range from a superficial fibrinous reaction to extensive, deep, coagulative necrosis, which is the lesion of necrotic enteritis. In some pigs a substantial granulation tissue reaction may occur, leading to fibrous tissue infiltration and muscular hypertrophy, which is the lesion of regional ileitis.

Acute hemorrhagic PE (PHE) is marked by severe bleeding into the lumen of the intestine, but with underlying lesions of chronic PE. The hemorrhage occurs concurrently with the widespread degeneration and desquamation of many epithelial cells and leakage from the capillary bed. PHE has been reproduced in older naive pigs, challenged once with a high dose of *L. intracellularis*, indicating a host rather than bacterial effect. The pathogenesis of this lesion has not yet been determined fully.

CLINICAL SIGNS

Clinical cases of chronic PE are observed most commonly in the postweaned pig between 6 and 20 weeks of age. In many cases of chronic PE in growing pigs, the clinical signs are slight to subclinical, and little more is seen than variation in pig performance with a failure to sustain growth despite normal feed intake. Ileal lesions are a consistent feature of these pigs. In some pigs there may be a degree of anorexia, characterized by curiosity about food but refusal to eat. Thus, affected animals vary from the clinically unremarkable to those showing marked dullness and apathy. Diarrhea, when present, is generally moderate, with loose, sloppy to watery stools of normal grey-green color; this is probably a feature of only a proportion of pigs affected with chronic PE. Blood or mucus are not features of chronic PE diarrhea. When chronic or subclinical PE is suspected in a herd,

milder cases can be relatively common but difficult to detect. Therefore, such farms should be inspected for apparent wasting of well-grown animals with anorexia and irregular diarrhea, with variable sizes of growing pigs in a group. Records should be carefully examined to detect changes in average weight gains and feed conversion efficiency in the postweaned group (Roberts et al. 1979; Gogolewski et al. 1991). More severely affected cases are often associated with varying degrees of inflammatory or necrotic change in the affected mucosa, and those that develop necrotic enteritis show severe loss of condition and often scour persistently.

Unlike chronic PE, cases of acute hemorrhagic PE occur more commonly in young adults 4–12 months old, such as breeding gilts, and present a clinical picture of acute hemorrhagic anemia. Black tarry feces are often the first visible clinical sign and these may become loose. However, some animals die without fecal abnormality and show only marked pallor. Probably around half of the animals clinically affected will die, the remainder recovering over some weeks. Pregnant animals that are clinically affected may abort, the majority within 6 days of the onset of clinical signs, with some residual reproductive losses possible (McOrist et al. 1999). Progeny from acutely affected breeding females are not protected from acquiring PE (Guedes et al. 2002a).

In most cases of uncomplicated chronic PE, recovery occurs 4–10 weeks after the onset of clinical signs with a return of appetite and growth rate to normal levels. However, although progress to slaughter weight can take place despite extensive lesions (Rowland and Hutchings 1978; Jensen et al. 1999), there will be a reduction in average weight gain, causing a significant extension of the time pigs take to reach market weight, with a consequent cost burden. The increase in feed required per unit weight gain in affected pigs is also a major cost in extra feed requirements. Careful feed and weight measurements during challenge studies have established that average weight gains are reduced 6–20% in affected pigs, and the increase in feed required per unit gain is 6–25%, compared to normal pigs (Gogolewski et al. 1991; McOrist et al. 1996b, 1997). The costs in increased "variation" in a group of pigs destined for breeding programs or a specific market target can be significant. The economic losses due to PE have been estimated from its negative impacts on slaughter weight, feed conversion efficiency, space utilization, breeding problems, and morbidity-mortality effects, totaling at from U.S. $0.50 to over U.S. $1 per affected growing pig, depending on the variable prices for pigs, building spaces and feed (McOrist et al. 1997; Veenhuizen et al. 2002).

LESIONS

Chronic PE

Chronic PE in growing pigs occurs most commonly in the terminal 50 cm of the small intestine and the upper

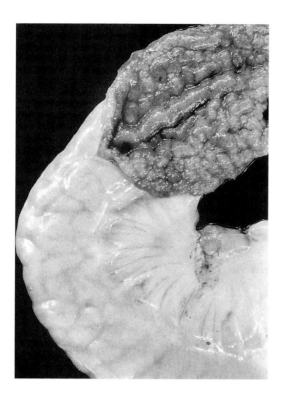

44.1. *Chronic PE. Ileum showing thickened, ridged mucosa.*

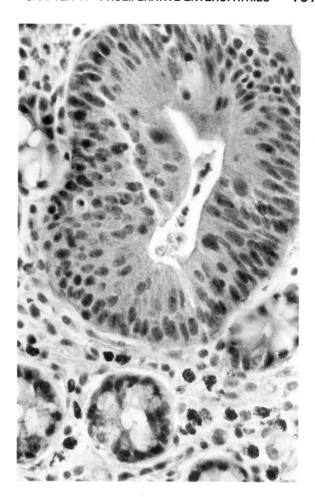

44.2. *Chronic PE, ileum. High-power micrograph showing marked enlargement of affected intestinal crypts, 5–10 epithelial cells thick, compared with adjacent normal crypt (H&E; ×400).*

third of the proximal colon. In severe cases, the lesions will extend to the jejunum, cecum, and lower large intestine. The magnitude of the proliferation varies widely, but in the developed lesions the wall is visibly thickened and the overall diameter increased. In minor lesions, the area of the terminal ileum that is 10 cm proximal from the ileocecal valve should be carefully examined as the most likely site of infection. Care is needed to distinguish minor lesions from contracted mucosa over the Peyer's patches. Some subserosal and mesenteric edema is common, and the normal corrugated pattern of the serosal surface is emphasized. The mucosal surface is moist but not mucoid, sometimes with flecks of inflammatory exudate loosely adherent. The affected mucosa itself is thrown into deep folds, longitudinal or transverse (Figure 44.1); similar changes in the large intestine may result in apparent plaque or polyp formation.

Histologically, the mucosa is composed of enlarged, branching crypts lined with immature epithelial cells. Compared to normal crypts, which are 1 cell layer thick, affected crypts are often 5, 10, or more cells thick (Figure 44.2). Numerous mitotic figures occurring throughout the crypt are evident. Other nuclei of affected cells may appear as enlarged vesicular structures or densely staining elongated spindles. Goblet cells are absent, and their reappearance in deep glands is an indication of impending resolution. In uncomplicated disease, the lamina propria is normal.

Silver staining, specific immunostaining or electron

microscopy of affected intestinal sections reveals intracellular *L. intracellularis*, often in considerable numbers, lying in the apical cytoplasm of the affected epithelial cells (Figure 44.3). In recovering lesions, the organisms become aggregated and may be extruded in degenerate cells into the lumen or be consumed by activated macrophages in the lamina propria. Many cases show little evidence of inflammatory reaction. The recovering lesions are notable for the resumption of development of a population of mature epithelium, with goblet cells in the deep crypts, and a rapid disappearance of the adenomatous cells from the surface (McOrist et al. 1996a).

Necrotic Enteritis

This is evident as coagulative necrosis with marked inflammatory exudation superimposed on an established lesion of PE. Yellow-gray cheesy masses that adhere tightly to the jejunal-ileal mucosa are present and may closely follow the original thickened mucosal architecture for some distance. Histologically, the coagulative necrosis is clearly defined, with fibrin deposits and degenerative inflammatory cells. Diagnosis is confirmed

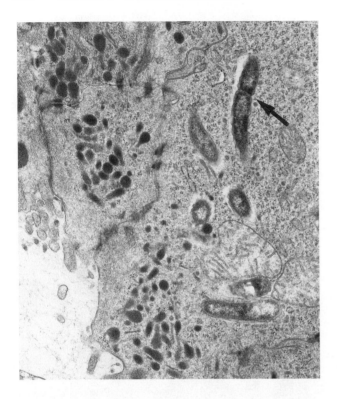

44.3. *Chronic PE. Intestinal epithelial cell of ileum. Apical cytoplasm containing several* L. intracellularis *organisms lying free in the cytoplasm and undergoing division (arrow) (uranyl acetate and lead citrate; original magnification ×10,000).*

by the presence of remnants of the proliferative epithelium observed in the deep layers.

Regional Ileitis

This is recognized as a smoothly contracted, almost rigid length of lower small intestine; hence the traditional name "hose pipe gut" (Figure 44.4). The mucosa may contain ulceration, with granulation tissue and islands of surviving mucosa adjacent. The most striking feature is hypertrophy of the outer muscle coats. Regional ileitis lesions are now considered relatively rare.

Acute Hemorrhagic PE

Hemorrhagic PE generally affects the terminal ileum and colon. The affected intestine is thickened, dilated, and somewhat turgid with serosal edema. The lumen of the ileum and colon usually contains one or more formed blood clots, often with no other bloody fluids or feed contents evident. The rectum may contain black, tarry feces of mixed blood and digesta (Figure 44.5). The mucosal surface of the affected portion of intestine shows little gross damage except for the marked hyperplastic thickening. Bleeding points, ulcers, or erosions are not observed. Histological examination demonstrates extensive degeneration, congestion, and hemorrhage within the proliferative epithelium. There is marked accumulation of bloody cellular debris containing numerous *L. intracellularis* organisms above the af-

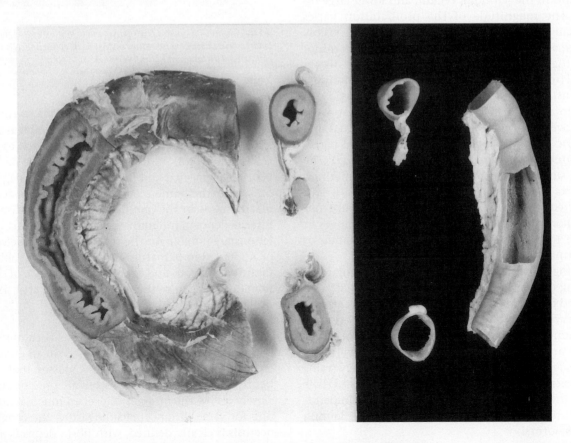

44.4. *Regional ileitis. Small intestine showing marked muscular hypertrophy. Normal intestine adjacent.*

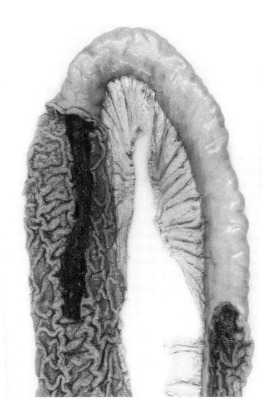

44.5. *Acute hemorrhagic PE. Small intestine showing thickened mucosa and blood clot in lumen.*

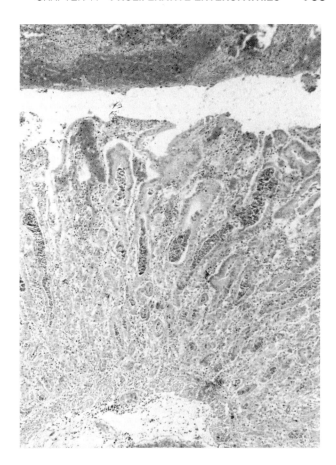

44.6. *Acute hemorrhagic PE, ileum. Micrograph of mucosa showing widespread degeneration of mucosal crypts with hemorrhage on the surface.*

fected mucosa and in the lumina of affected intestinal crypts (Figure 44.6).

DIAGNOSIS

Because of the difficulty of culturing *L. intracellularis*, it has been necessary to develop alternative methods for its detection. Confirmation of a clinical diagnosis of PE may be obtained by demonstration of *L. intracellularis* in feces, either by a PCR assay using *L. intracellularis*-specific primers (Jones et al. 1993) or by using specific hyperimmune rabbit polyclonal antibody or, preferably, a specific anti–*L. intracellularis* monoclonal antibody (McOrist et al. 1987; Guedes and Gebhart 2003c) incorporated into immunoassay techniques. Pigs with active lesions are usually found to be excreting the agent over several weeks (Knittel et al. 1998; Kim et al. 1998; Guedes et al. 2002c). However, fecal analysis is unlikely to prove sufficiently sensitive for the diagnosis of all infections. The PCR assay can detect 10^2–10^5 organisms per gram of feces, depending on the DNA extraction method and type of assay used (nested or direct). Animals 6–10 weeks old usually have the highest prevalence rates for screening of single-site farms. Older animals are usually sampled only during outbreaks of acute PE. Feces should be stored at 4°C or below for either test.

Methods described for the serologic diagnosis of PE have employed whole bacterial antigen incorporated into an indirect immunofluorescence assay (Lawson et al. 1988; Knittel et al. 1998) or an immunoperoxidase assay (Guedes et al. 2002b). Those assays used bacteria extracted from affected intestines or cultured *L. intracellularis*. Results from serologic assays suggest that the serum antibody response in pigs to *L. intracellularis* is specific and involves IgM and IgG. Although detectable antibody responses relate well to the presence of lesions, exposure to infection may not induce significant seroconversion in all cases. Although blood collection is considerably more time-consuming than feces collection, the serotests are probably cheaper to perform and more amenable to high throughputs.

At necropsy, the use of modified Ziehl-Neelsen stain or the Giminez stain on mucosal smears to demonstrate the intracellular organisms is a simple presumptive technique, requiring minimal time and equipment (Love et al. 1977). Histopathological examination of affected tissues will reveal the distinctive morphology of the proliferative lesions. Specific identification of *L. intracellularis* in these lesions can be achieved by immunohistochemical staining of fixed embedded tissues (Lawson et al. 1985; McOrist et al. 1987; Guedes et al. 2002c). In the absence of specific immunological reagents, silver-staining techniques will clearly show the presence of intracellular bacteria (Figure 44.7). Modifications of the Warthin-

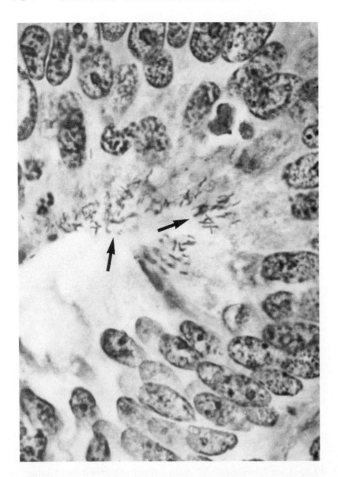

44.7. *Chronic PE, ileum. Micrograph of enlarged mucosal crypt showing numerous intracellular bacteria (arrows) in the apical cytoplasm of epithelial cells (Warthin-Starry silver stain; original magnification ×2000).*

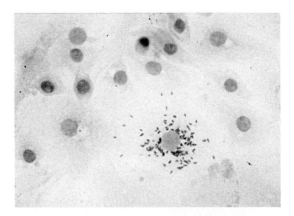

44.8. Culture of L. intracellularis. *Micrograph of IPEC-J2 pig intestinal epithelial cells, one of which contains numerous intracellular bacteria in the cytoplasm. Immunoperoxidase stain incorporating Lawsonia-specific monoclonal antibody.*

Starry silver impregnation technique (Young 1969) are satisfactory for routine use. The affected crypts need to be examined carefully at high magnifications due to the small size of *L. intracellularis*. Where electron microscopic facilities are available, the presence of the intracellular organism can be confirmed.

Cultivation of the obligate intracellular *L. intracellularis* in the laboratory requires establishment of a suitable cell line, such as IEC-18 rat enterocytes or IPEC-J2 pig enterocytes and the addition of purified *L. intracellularis* from pig intestines in the presence of antibiotics to retard the growth of other bacteria (Lawson et al. 1993; McOrist et al. 1995b). Maintenance and passage of the organism in co-culture require suitable microaerobic atmospheres and cell lysis conditions, respectively (Lawson et al. 1993). Most cells in a monolayer are typically infected with around 50 cytoplasmic bacteria (Figure 44.8), causing no apparent cytopathic effect.

TREATMENT AND PREVENTION

In vitro evaluations via a cell culture approach of the minimum inhibitory concentration of 20 antimicrobial agents and the minimum bactericidal concentration of 10 of these suggested a rather broad range of antibiotic groups with potential activity against *L. intracellularis* (McOrist et al. 1995c; McOrist and Gebhart 1995). However, challenge exposure and controlled field evaluations of treatment and prevention measures in commercial pigs have indicated that macrolides, lincosamides, and pleuromutilins are the most effective antibiotics, when given at an adequate dosage rate per kg of bodyweight (McOrist et al. 1996b, 1997; Walter et al. 2001; Schwartz et al. 1999; Winkelman et al. 2002). In the U.S., some quinoxalines are also available and effective. Acquired resistance to these active drug groups has not been proven in *L. intracellularis* (McOrist 2000). Apparent medication failures with these drugs are most likely to occur in pigs with ileitis that are underdosed on a bodyweight basis, such as breeding pigs with a low feed intake, or when pigs are medicated before or after actual peaks of infection. Antimicrobial drugs now known to be inherently ineffective against *L. intracellularis* in clinical cases of PE include the penicillins, bacitracin, aminoglycosides such as neomycin, virginiamycin, and the ionophores. Nonantibiotic therapies such as copper or zinc compounds or feed acidifiers have also shown no evidence of efficacy.

Various approaches to medication are possible, depending on the age and type of pigs involved. Treatment of acute PE in breeding herds requires a vigorous approach. Treatment needs to include both the clinically affected and the in-contact animals (which may be the whole herd). The preferred treatment would be tiamulin (120 ppm) or tylosin (100 ppm) for 14 days, delivered orally via a water-soluble formulation or an in-feed premix or by intramuscular injection of an equivalent dose to affected and in-contact pigs.

Severe chronic clinical disease manifested as wasting pigs with or without necrotic enteritis will often appear to be moderated by the use of tylosin, lincomycin, or tiamulin (or carbadox where available). If sufficient numbers of clinical cases are occurring in growing pigs, the removal of affected animals to separate accommodation, with supportive therapy, may limit losses. Controlled field trials now suggest that incorporation of in-feed or water-soluble antibiotics for control achieves best results if given just prior to the peak period of *L. intracellularis* infection; on many single-site farms this is around 8–11 weeks of age (McOrist et al. 1999, 2000). Medication of older pigs, such as breeding stock, is not likely to eliminate the infection from their progeny or from other groups. Because infection and PE disease can vary in the time of onset on different farms and between batches on the same farm, in-feed antibiotics for treatment might be added too late to stop damaging clinical signs and poor performance (Hammer 2004). Alternatively, if they are added too early, groups of "clean" pigs are not getting the chance to develop active immunity to the disease and may remain naive and susceptible to later severe acute PE cases.

Despite the short time since the elucidation of the cause of PE, its endemic nature, major economic impact, and variable time of onset persuasively indicate that a vaccine approach is the most logical for long lasting control. Oral administration of a single low titer dose ($10^{4.9}$ TCID^{50}/dose) of an attenuated live vaccine (Enterisol Ileitis, Boehringer Ingelheim) to young pigs provided significant levels of protective immunity against subsequent challenge with virulent heterologous *L. intracellularis* (Kroll et al. 2004). This was confirmed by a significant reduction ($p < 0.05$) in the primary parameter of gross and microscopic lesions in the ileum of vaccinates. This protection was independent of the route of oral administration chosen (individual oral drench or drinking water delivery to a group). Significantly improved weight gains and reduced fecal shedding of *L. intracellularis* were also noted after vaccine administration, particularly if given via drinking water. This vaccine has rapidly grown to widespread usage where available, with no safety concerns identified. Killed or subunit vaccine types are not available.

Where vaccine is unavailable, animals such as replacement breeding stock that are to be introduced into infected transport situations or into infected premises could be allowed a period of exposure followed by therapeutic levels of antimicrobial agents to impede the occurrence of clinical disease. The preferred treatment would be tiamulin (120 ppm), tylosin (100 ppm) or lincomycin (110 ppm), delivered orally via a stabilized in-feed premix for 14 days. Following the transport or on-farm period of exposure, no more than 2–3 weeks should elapse before the introduction of antibiotics (Love and Love 1977). Such an approach is most suited to the management of acute PE in young adult animals. However, even with this type of program, PE may occur in medicated animals following the end of therapy.

It remains a matter of concern that acute and chronic PE continue to be serious problems in high-health-status, minimal-disease herds, often with early weaning and high-quality commercial breeding lines in place. It cannot be overemphasized that in most conventional herds, the absence of clinical PE, even over a period of years, is no guarantee of freedom from the infection and disease. Apparently clean animals from such herds may be responsible for the introduction of PE into a hitherto uncontaminated environment, often followed by an explosive outbreak of acute hemorrhagic PE and later by a low level of endemic chronic PE.

REFERENCES

Al-Ghamdi M. 2003. Repetitive element based polymerase chain reaction analysis of *Lawsonia intracellularis* isolates obtained from various animal species. PhD thesis, University of Minnesota.

Bane D, Neumann E, Gebhart CJ, Gardner I. 2001. Porcine proliferative enteropathy: A case control study in swine herds in the United States. J Swine Health Prod 9:155–158.

Biester HE, Schwarte LH. 1931. Intestinal adenoma in swine. Am J Pathol 7:175–185.

Biester HE, Schwarte LH, Eveleth DF. 1939. Studies on a rapidly developing intestinal adenoma in a pig. Am J Pathol 15:385–389.

Bronsvoort M, Norby B, Bane DP, Gardner IA. 2001. Management factors associated with seropositivity to *Lawsonia intracellularis* in U.S. swine herds. J Swine Health Prod 9:285–290.

Chouet S, Prieto C, Mieli L, Veenhuizen MF, McOrist S. 2003. Patterns of exposure to *Lawsonia intracellularis* infection on European pig farms. Vet Rec 152:14–17.

Christensen NH, Cullinane LC. 1990. Monitoring the health of pigs in New Zealand abattoirs. NZ Vet J 38:136–141.

Collins AM, Love RJ, Jasni S, McOrist S. 1999. Attempted infection of mice, rats and chickens by porcine strains of *Lawsonia intracellularis*. Aust Vet J 77:120–122.

Collins AM, Love RJ, Pozo J, Smith SH, McOrist S. 2000. Studies on the ex vivo survival of *Lawsonia intracellularis*. J Swine Health Prod 8:211–215.

Cooper DM, Gebhart CJ. 1998. Comparative aspects of proliferative enteritis. J Am Vet Med Assoc 212:1446–1451.

Cooper DM, Swanson DL, Barns SM, Gebhart CJ. 1997b. Comparison of the 16S ribosomal DNA sequences from the intracellular agents of proliferative enteritis in a hamster, deer, and ostrich with the sequence of a porcine isolate of *Lawsonia intracellularis*. Int J Syst Bacteriol 47: 635–639.

Cooper DM, Swanson DL, Gebhart CJ. 1997a. Diagnosis of proliferative enteritis in frozen and formalin-fixed, paraffin-embedded tissues from a hamster, horse, deer and ostrich using a *Lawsonia intracellularis*–specific multiplex PCR assay. Vet Microbiol 54:47–62.

Dale CJH, Moses EJ, Ong C, Morrow CJ, Reed MB, Hasse D, Strugnell RA. 1998. Identification and sequencing of the groE operon and flanking genes of *Lawsonia intracellularis*: Use in phylogeny. Microbiology 144:2073–2084.

Drolet R, Larochelle D, Gebhart CJ. 1996. Proliferative enteritis associated with *Lawsonia intracellularis* (ileal symbiont intracellularis) in white-tailed deer. J Vet Diagn Invest 8:250–253.

Duhamel GE, Klein EC, Elder RO, Gebhart CJ. 1998. Subclinical proliferative enteropathy in sentinel rabbits associated with *Lawsonia intracellularis*. Vet Pathol 35:300–303.

Frisk CS, Wagner JE. 1977. Experimental hamster enteritis: An electron microscopic study. Am J Vet Res 38:1861–1868.

Gebhart CJ, Barns SM, McOrist S, Lin G-F, Lawson GHK. 1993. Ileal symbiont intracellularis, an obligate intracellular bacterium of porcine intestines showing a relationship to Desulfovibrio species. Int J Syst Bacteriol 43:533–538.

Gogolewski RP, Cook RW, Batterham ES. 1991. Suboptimal growth associated with porcine intestinal adenomatosis in pigs in nutritional studies. Aust Vet J 68:406–408.

Guedes RMC, Gebhart CJ. 2003a. Comparison of intestinal mucosa homogenate and pure culture of the homologous *Lawsonia intracellularis* isolate in reproducing proliferative enteropathy in swine. Vet Microbiol 93:159–166.

——. 2003b. Onset and duration of fecal shedding, cell-mediated and humoral immune responses in pigs after challenge with a pathogenic isolate or attenuated vaccine strain of *Lawsonia intracellularis*. Vet Microbiol 91:135–145.

——. 2003c. Preparation and characterization of polyclonal and monoclonal antibodies against Lawsonia intracelluilaris. J Vet Diagn Invest 15:438–446.

Guedes RMC, Gebhart CJ, Armbruster G, Roggow BD. 2002a. Serologic follow-up of a repopulated swine herd after an outbreak of proliferative hemorrhagic enteropathy. Can J Vet Res 66:258–263.

Guedes RMC, Gebhart CJ, Winkelman NL, Mackie-Nuss RA. 2002b. A comparative study of an indirect fluorescent antibody test and an immunoperoxidase monolayer assay for the diagnosis of porcine proliferative enteropathy. J Vet Diagn Invest 14:420–423.

Guedes RMC, Gebhart CJ, Winkelman NL, Mackie-Nuss RA, Marsteller TA, Deen J. 2002c. Comparison of different methods for diagnosis of porcine proliferative enteropathy. Can J Vet Res 66:99–107.

Guedes RMC, Winkelman NL, Gebhart CJ. 2003. Relationship between the severity of porcine proliferative enteropathy and the infectious dose of *Lawsonia intracellularis*. Vet Rec 153:432–433.

Hammer JM. 2004. The temporal relationship of fecal shedding of *Lawsonia intracellularis* and seroconversion in field cases. J Swine Health Prod 12:29–33.

Jacobsen M, Segerstad CH, Gunnarsson A, Fellstrom C, Klingenberg KV, Wallgren P, Jensen-Waern M. 2003. Diarrhoea in the growing pig—A comparison of clinical, morphological and microbial findings between animals from good and poor performance herds. Res Vet Sci 74:163–169.

Jensen TK, Moller K, Christensen G, Leser TD, Jorsal SE. 1999. Monitoring ileitis and *Lawsonia intracellularis* in abattoir pigs. Vet Rec 145:613–615.

Jensen TK, Moller K, Lindecrona R, Jorsal SE. 2000. Detection of *Lawsonia intracellularis* in the tonsils of pigs with proliferative enteropathy. Res Vet Sci 68:23–26.

Jones GF, Ward GE, Murtaugh MP, Lin G, Gebhart CJ. 1993. Enhanced detection of intracellular organism of swine proliferative enteritis, ileal symbiont intracellularis, in feces by polymerase chain reaction. J Clin Microbiol 31:2611–2615.

Just S, Thoen CO, Thacker BJ, Thompson JU. 2001. Monitoring of *Lawsonia intracellularis* by indirect serum immunofluorescence assay in a commercial swine production system. J Swine Health Prod 9:57–61.

Kim O, Kim B, Chae C. 1998. Prevalence of *Lawsonia intracellularis* in selected pig herds in Korea as determined by PCR. Vet Rec 143:587–589.

Klein EC, Gebhart CJ, Duhamel GE. 1999. Fatal outbreaks of proliferative enteritis caused by *Lawsonia intracellularis* in young colony-raised rhesus macaques. J Med Primatol 28:11–18.

Knittel JP, Jordan DM, Schwartz KJ, Janke BH, Roof MB, McOrist S, Harris DL. 1998. Evaluation of antemortem polymerase chain reaction and serologic methods for detection of *Lawsonia intracellularis*–infected pigs. Am J Vet Res 59:722–726.

Knittel JP, Larson DI, Harris DL, Roof MB, McOrist S. 1996. United States isolates of *Lawsonia intracellularis* from porcine proliferative enteropathy resemble European isolates. J Swine Health Prod 4:119–122.

Kroll J, Roof MB, McOrist S. 2004. Evaluation of protective immunity in pigs following oral administration of an avirulent live vaccine of *Lawsonia intracellularis*. Am J Vet Res 65:559–565.

Lavoie JP, Drolet R, Parsons D, Leguilette R, Sauvageau R, Shapiro J, Houle L, Halle G, Gebhart CJ. 2000. Equine proliferative enteropathy: A cause of weight loss, colic, diarrhoea and hypoproteinaemia in foals on three breeding farms in Canada. Equine Vet J 32:418–425.

Lawson GHK, Gebhart CJ. 2000. Proliferative enteropathy. J Comp Pathol 122:77–100.

Lawson GHK, Mackie RA, Smith DGE, McOrist S. 1995. Intracellular multiplication of ileal symbiont intracellularis depends on host cell function and actin polymerisation. Vet Microbiol 45:339–350.

Lawson GHK, McOrist S, Rowland AC, Roberts L, McCartney E. 1988. Serological diagnosis of the porcine proliferative enteropathies: Implications for aetiology and epidemiology. Vet Rec 122:554–557.

Lawson GHK, McOrist S, Sabri J, Mackie RA. 1993. Intracellular bacteria of porcine proliferative enteropathy: Cultivation and maintenance in vitro. J Clin Microbiol 31:1136–1142.

Lawson GHK, Rowland AC. 1974. Intestinal adenomatosis in the pig: A bacteriological study. Res Vet Sci 17:331–336.

Lawson GHK, Rowland AC, MacIntyre N. 1985. Demonstration of a new intracellular antigen in porcine intestinal adenomatosis and hamster proliferative ileitis. Vet Microbiol 10(4):303–313.

Lawson GHK, Rowland AC, Roberts L, Fraser G, McCartney E. 1979. Proliferative haemorrhagic enteropathy. Res Vet Sci 27:46–51.

Lemarchand TN, Tully TN, Shane SM, Duncan DE. 1997. Intracellular Campylobacter-like organisms associated with rectal prolapse and proliferative enteroproctitis in emus (Dromaius novaehollandiae). Vet Pathol 34:152–156.

Love RJ, Love DN. 1977. Control of proliferative haemorrhagic enteropathy in pigs. Vet Rec 100:473.

Love RJ, Love DN, Edwards MJ. 1977. Proliferative haemorrhagic enteropathy in pigs. Vet Rec 100:65–68.

MacIntyre N, Smith DGE, Shaw DJ, Thomson JR, Rhind SM. 2003. Immunopathogenesis of experimentally induced proliferative enteropathy in pigs. Vet Pathol 40:421–432.

Mapother ME, Joens LA, Glock RD. 1987. Experimental reproduction of porcine proliferative enteritis. Vet Rec 121:533–536.

Marsteller TA, Armbruster G, Bane DP, Gebhart CJ, Muller R, Weatherford J, Thacker B. 2003. Monitoring the prevalence of *Lawsonia intracellularis* IgG antibodies using serial sampling in growing and breeding swine herds. J Swine Health Prod 11:127–130.

McOrist S. 2000. Antimicrobial activity against obligate intracellular bacteria: A comparison of clinical and in vitro efficacy. Trends Microbiol 8:483–487.

McOrist S, Barcellos DE, Wilson RJ. 2003b. Global patterns of porcine proliferative enteropathy. Pig J 51:26–35.

McOrist S, Boid R, Lawson GHK. 1989a. Antigenic analysis of Campylobacter species and an intracellular Campylobacter-like organism associated with the porcine proliferative enteropathies. Infect Immun 57:957–962.

McOrist S, Boid R, Lawson GHK, McConnell I. 1987. Monoclonal antibodies to intracellular Campylobacter-like organisms of the porcine proliferative enteropathies. Vet Rec 121:421–422.

McOrist S, Gebhart CJ. 1995. In vitro testing of antimicrobial agents for proliferative enteropathy (ileitis). J Swine Health Prod 3:146–149.

——. 2004. *Genus Lawsonia* McOrist, Gebhart, Boid and Barns 1995a[VP]. In Bergey's Manual of Systematic Bacteriology, 2nd edition. GM Garrity, ed. Baltimore: Williams and Wilkins.

McOrist S, Gebhart CJ, Boid R, Barns SM. 1995a. Characterization of *Lawsonia intracellularis* gen. nov., sp. nov., the obligately intracellular bacterium of porcine proliferative enteropathy. Int J Syst Bacteriol 45:820–825.

McOrist S, Jasni S, Mackie RA, Berschneider HM, Rowland AC, Lawson GHK. 1995b. Entry and release of the bacterium ileal symbiont intracellularis in cultured enterocytes. Res Vet Sci 59:255–260.

McOrist S, Jasni S, Mackie RA, MacIntyre N, Neef N, Lawson GHK. 1993. Reproduction of porcine proliferative enteropathy with pure cultures of ileal symbiont intracellularis. Infect Immun 61:4286–4292.

McOrist S, Keller L, McOrist AL. 2003a. Search for *Lawsonia intracellularis* and Bilophila wadsworthia in malabsorption-diseased chickens. Can J Vet Res 67:232–234.

McOrist S, Lawson GHK. 1989. Reproduction of proliferative enteritis in gnotobiotic piglets. Res Vet Sci 46:27–33.

——. 1993. Interactions of porcine lymphocytes with Campylobacter-like organism membranes purified from proliferative enteropathy. Vet Microbiol 34:381–388.

McOrist S, Lawson GHK, Rowland AC, MacIntyre N. 1989b. Early lesions of proliferative enteritis of pigs and hamsters. Vet Pathol 26:260–264.

McOrist S, MacIntyre N, Stokes CR, Lawson GHK. 1992. Immunocytological responses in the porcine proliferative enteropathies. Infect Immun 60:4184–4191.

McOrist S, Mackie RA, Lawson GHK. 1995c. Antimicrobial susceptibility of ileal symbiont intracellularis isolated from pigs with porcine proliferative enteropathy. J Clin Microbiol 33:1314–1317.

McOrist S, Mackie RA, Neef N, Aitken I, Lawson GHK. 1994. Synergism of ileal symbiont intracellularis and gut flora in the reproduction of porcine proliferative enteropathy. Vet Rec 134:331–332.

McOrist S, Morgan J, Veenhuizen MF, Lawrence K, Kroger HW. 1997. Oral administration of tylosin phosphate for treatment and prevention of proliferative enteropathy in pigs. Am J Vet Res 58:136–139.

McOrist S, Muller Wager A, Kratzer D, Sjosten CG. 2000. Therapeutic efficacy of water-soluble lincomycin-spectinomycin powder against porcine proliferative enteropathy in a European field study. Vet Rec 146:61–65.

McOrist S, Roberts L, Jasni S, Rowland AC, Lawson GHK, Gebhart CJ, Bosworth B. 1996a. Developed and resolving lesions in porcine proliferative enteropathy: Possible pathogenetic mechanisms. J Comp Pathol 115:35–45.

McOrist S, Smith SH, Green LE. 1997. Estimate of direct financial losses due to porcine proliferative enteropathy. Vet Rec 140:579–581.

McOrist S, Smith SH, Klein T. 1999. Monitored control programme for proliferative enteropathy on British pig farms. Vet Rec 144:202–204.

McOrist S, Smith SH, Shearn MFH, Carr MM, Miller DJS. 1996b. Treatment and prevention of porcine proliferative enteropathy with oral tiamulin. Vet Rec 139:615–618.

Moller K, Jensen TK, Jorsal SE, Leser TD, Carstensen B. 1998. Detection of *Lawsonia intracellularis*, Serpulina hyodysenteriae, weakly beta-haemolytic intestinal spirochaetes, Salmonella enterica, and haemolytic Esherichia coli from swine herds with and without diarrhoea among growing pigs. Vet Microbiol 62:59–72.

Philips RC, Geiger JO, Karhoff K. 1998. Evaluation of the use of *Lawsonia intracellularis* indirect fluorescent antibody test (IFA) in a large production system. Proc Allen D Leman Conf 25:5–6.

Roberts L, Lawson GHK, Rowland AC, Laing AH. 1979. Porcine intestinal adenomatosis and its detection in a closed pig herd. Vet Rec 104:366–368.

Roberts L, Rowland AC, Lawson GHK. 1977. Experimental reproduction of porcine intestinal adenomatosis and necrotic enteritis. Vet Rec 100:12–13.

——. 1980. Porcine intestinal adenomatosis: Epithelial dysplasia and infiltration. Gut 21:1035–1040.

Rowan TG, Lawrence TLJ. 1982. Amino-acid digestibility in pigs with signs of porcine intestinal adenomatosis. Vet Rec 110:306–307.

Rowland AC, Hutchings DA. 1978. Necrotic enteritis and regional ileitis in pigs at slaughter. Vet Rec 103:338–339.

Rowland AC, Lawson GHK. 1974. Intestinal adenomatosis in the pig: Immunofluorescent and electron microscopic studies. Res Vet Sci 17:323–330.

——. 1975. Porcine intestinal adenomatosis: A possible relationship with necrotic enteritis, regional ileitis and proliferative haemorrhagic enteropathy. Vet Rec 97:178–180.

Rowland AC, Rowntree PGM. 1972. A haemorrhagic bowel syndrome associated with intestinal adenomatosis in the pig. Vet Rec 91:235–241.

Schoeb TR, Fox JG. 1990. Enterocolitis associated with intraepithelial Campylobacter-like bacteria in rabbits. Vet Pathol 27:73–80.

Schwartz K, Knittel J, Walter D, Roof M, Anderson M. 1999. Effect of oral tiamulin on the development of porcine proliferative enteropathy in a pure-culture challenge model. J Swine Health Prod 7:5–11.

Smith SH, McOrist S. 1997. Development of persistent intestinal infection and excretion of *Lawsonia intracellularis* by piglets. Res Vet Sci 62:6–10.

Smith SH, McOrist S, Green LE. 1998. Questionnaire survey of proliferative enteropathy on British pig farms. Vet Rec 142:690–693.

Stege H, Jensen TK, Moller K, Baekbo P, Jorsal SE. 2000. Prevalence of intestinal pathogens in Danish finishing pig herds. Prev Vet Med 46:279–292.

Stills HR. 1991. Isolation of an intracellular bacterium from hamsters (Mesocricetus auratus) with proliferative ileitis and reproduction of the disease with a pure culture. Infect Immun 59:3227–3236.

Tomanova K, Bartak P, Smola J. 2002. Detection of *Lawsonia intracellularis* in wild pigs in the Czech Republic. Vet Rec 151:765–767.

Veenhuizen MF, Elam TE, Soenksen N. 2002. Porcine proliferative enteropathy: Diagnosis and impact. Comp Contin Educ Pract Vet 24:S10–S15.

Walter D, Knittel J, Schwartz K, Kroll J, Roof M. 2001. Treatment and control of porcine proliferative enteropathy using different tiamulin delivery methods. J Swine Health Prod 9:109–115.

Williams NM, Harrison LR, Gebhart CJ. 1996. Proliferative enteropathy in a foal caused by *Lawsonia intracellularis*-like bacterium. J Vet Diagn Invest 8:254–256.

Winkelman NL, Crane JP, Elfring GD, Kratzer D, Meeuwse DM, Dame KJ, Buckham SL, Gebhart CJ. 2002. Lincomycin-medicated feed for the control of porcine proliferative enteropathy (ileitis) in swine. J Swine Health Prod 10:106–110.

Young BJ. 1969. A reliable method for demonstrating spirochaetes in tissue sections. J Med Lab Technol 26:248–252.

45 Salmonella

R. W. Griffith, K. J. Schwartz, and D. K. Meyerholz

Members of the genus *Salmonella* are notorious for their ability to infect a broad range of hosts, which is a major factor in their success as pathogens. Taylor and McCoy (1969) observed that salmonellae have been isolated from virtually all vertebrate hosts from which they have been sought, with the possible exception of fish in unpolluted waters. Although many of the more than 2400 salmonella serotypes have a broad host range and are widely distributed, several serotypes are quite adapted to a single host species, most notably *S. typhi* (humans), *S. dublin* (bovine), and *S. choleraesuis* (swine). Many serotypes are not associated with overt disease and appear to have limited host and geographical range.

Salmonella infections of swine are of concern for two major reasons. The first is the clinical disease (salmonellosis) in swine that may result, and the second is that swine can be infected with a broad range of salmonella serotypes that can be a source of infection of pork products.

Salmon and Smith (1886) first associated salmonellae with disease when they described *S. choleraesuis* as the putative cause of classical swine fever (hog cholera). The identification and, in many swine-producing areas, eradication of the viral etiology of classical swine fever, relegated *S. choleraesuis* to an opportunistic pathogen in swine. The dramatic increase in salmonellosis during the 1980s in North America underscored the pathogenic potential of *S. choleraesuis* for swine.

Disease associated with host-adapted *S. choleraesuis* is referable to septicemia, enterocolitis, or bacteremic localization as pneumonia and hepatitis (Baskerville and Dow 1973) or occasionally as meningitis (Reynolds et al. 1967; McErlean 1968), encephalitis (Wilcock and Olander 1977c), and abortion (Schwartz and Daniels 1987). Only a handful of other serotypes are associated with disease in swine, usually as a cause of enterocolitis, the most notable being *S. typhimurium*. Reported rarely, *S. typhisuis* is associated with caseous lymphadenitis (Barnes and Bergeland 1968).

ETIOLOGY

The genus *Salmonella* is a morphologically and biochemically homogeneous group of gram-negative, motile, non–spore-forming, facultatively anaerobic bacilli with peritrichous flagella. The reservoir for salmonellae is, typical of the family *Enterobacteriaceae*, the intestinal tract of warm-blooded and cold-blooded animals.

Salmonellae are hardy and ubiquitous bacteria. They multiply at 7–45°C; survive freezing and desiccation well; and persist for weeks, months, or even years in suitable organic substrates. Salmonellae were reported to survive in meat-meal fertilizer for 8 months (Mittermeyer and Foltz 1969) and in manure oxidation ditches for 47 days (Will et al. 1973). Survival is greatly shortened below pH 5.0 (Henry et al. 1983). Numerous reports of prolonged survival in water have been cited (Williams 1975; Wray and Sojka 1977; Pokorny 1988). The bacteria are readily inactivated by heat and sunlight as well as by common phenolic, chlorine, and iodine-based disinfectants (Rubin and Weinstein 1977). Ability to survive in the environment, as well as prolonged carrier states in innumerable hosts, ensures the widespread distribution of this genus worldwide.

Techniques for isolation of salmonellae vary widely, depending on the nature of the suspect material and sometimes with the specific serotypes sought. In sewage, feed, and polluted water, where salmonella numbers are likely to be low compared to other organisms, well-documented and sometimes elaborate techniques of pre-enrichment, selective enrichment, and selective plating are commonly used (Groves et al. 1971; Edwards and Ewing 1972; Skovgaard et al. 1985; Vassiliadis et al. 1987). It is important to note that some of the enrichment media are detrimental to the growth of certain serotypes of salmonellae. For example, Rappaport-Vassiliadis is commonly used for enrichment of food and environmental samples but is known to restrict the growth of those serotypes that are host-adapted. Occasionally enrichment techniques may be necessary for the isolation of salmonellae from tissues or feces of carrier animals in which numbers are low, but in clinically affected animals the populations are such that direct plating of internal organs on routine selective and differential enteric media such as brilliant green agar and MacConkey agar are usually adequate (Committee on Salmonella 1969). The isolation of salmonellae is not sufficient for definitive diagnosis of salmonellosis, particularly if elaborate isolation techniques are required, since subclinical infections and environmental contamination are common. Isolation techniques for various types of specimens are detailed in most standard texts on clinical microbiology. Epidemiological investigations of zoonotic outbreaks occasionally demand more sophisticated techniques of phage typing, plasmid characterization, mapping of outer-membrane proteins (OMP), or DNA analysis to trace a specific isolant.

S. choleraesuis is the type species for the genus *Salmonella* as described by Salmon, although it is now more commonly isolated as the hydrogen sulfide–producing variant *kunzendorf*. There is considerable disagreement over the nomenclature of the genus *Salmonella* and several proposals for altering it have been made. Convention is to refer to each of the over 2400 distinct serotypes as though it is a species. Serotype identification uses the Kauffmann-White schema, based on antigenic differences in somatic (O), surface or capsular (Vi), phase 1 flagellar, and phase 2 flagellar antigens determined by agglutination serology. Complete serotyping is laborious and is available at only a few reference laboratories. Most laboratories use commercially available antisera to determine the O antigen groups of isolates for rapid and preliminary identification. The serogroup designation will help predict the serotype present or, at least, can be used to rule out those serotypes found in other serogroups (Table 45.1).

In contrast to the large number of serotypes isolated from carcasses and pork products, disease in swine is almost always caused by either the hydrogen sulfide–producing variant of *S. choleraesuis* variety *kunzendorf* or by *S. typhimurium*. The former has been and continues to be the most frequent serotype causing disease in swine (Levine et al. 1945; Lawson and Dow 1966; Morehouse 1972; Wilcock et al. 1976; Mills and Kelly 1986; Schwartz and Daniels 1987; Schwartz 1997a), generally manifested as septicemia.

S. typhimurium is the second most frequently isolated serotype from diseased swine, usually associated with enterocolitis. Disease caused by *S. typhimurium* occurs with greater than expected frequency in what could be considered unusually clean herds: university research herds, testing stations, closed specific pathogen free (SPF) herds, or purebred breeding herds (Heard et al. 1965; Gooch and Haddock 1969; Lynn et al. 1972).

Table 45.1. Serogroups of selected salmonella serotypes and ranking of frequency of isolation from diseased pigs, swine sources, and humans

Serogroup	Serotype	Isolations from Diseased Pigs (Schwartz 1997a)	Isolations from Swine Sources (Ferris and Frerichs 1996)	Isolations from Humans (CDC 1996)
A	*S. paratyphi A*			
B	*S. typhimurium*	3	5	3
	S. typhimurium var. copenhagen	2	3	2
	S. derby		1	
	S. agona		4	6
	S. schwarzengrund		10	
	S. hadar			7
	S. saint paul			
	S. heidelberg	4	6	4
C$_1$	*S. choleraesuis*		7	
	S. choleraesuis var. kunzendorf	1	2	
	S. mbandaka		9	
	S. typhisuis			
	S. montevideo			8
	S. oranienburg			9
	S. infantis			
	S. thompson			10
C$_2$	*S. newport*			5
	S. muenchen			
D$_1$	*S. dublin*			
	S. typhi			
	S. enteritidis			1
	S. pullorum			
E$_1$	*S. anatum*		8	
E$_2$	*S. newington*			
E$_4$	*S. senftenberg*			
G$_2$	*S. worthington*			

Presumably, this is because of introduction to a previously immunologically naive population, a situation occurring with increasing frequency in modern production units using age-segregated rearing. This organism is also frequently isolated as a sequel to other enteric or debilitating diseases.

Localized epizootics of disease caused by the biochemically atypical *S. typhisuis* have been reported in the American Midwest (Barnes and Bergeland 1968; Andrews 1976) and at least historically in Europe (Barnes and Sorensen 1975). This organism grows poorly in standard selective media for salmonella isolation, but the disease produced by *S. typhisuis* is so characteristic that outbreaks are not likely to remain unnoticed (Barnes and Bergeland 1968).

Other serotypes are occasional causes of disease in swine but are usually transient and associated with predisposing factors, including other intestinal disturbances or disease, circumstances that allow immunologically naive pigs to be exposed to very large doses, or debilitated and immunologically compromised pigs. A variety of serotypes may be isolated from diarrheic piglets in the immediate postweaning period, but most are usually associated with concurrent enteric pathogens, inappropriate diets, poor hygiene and environment, or debilitation. The isolation of uncommon serotypes of salmonellae from diarrheic pigs generally warrants further diagnostic investigation. *Salmonella heidelberg* has been associated with postweaning diarrhea, with lesions more typical of enterotoxigenic diarrheal disease than typical salmonellosis (Reed et al. 1985). Reports of naturally occurring disease, such as those for *S. dublin* (Lawson and Dow 1966; McErlean 1968) and *S. enteritidis* (Reynolds et al. 1967), should support the isolation of the offending serotype with clinical and pathologic evidence of salmonellosis. In the case of both *S. dublin* and *S. enteritidis*, the reports were of meningitis in suckling pigs.

EPIDEMIOLOGY

The reservoir for salmonellae is the intestinal tract of warm- and cold-blooded animals. Salmonellae have mastered virtually all of the attributes necessary to ensure wide distribution, including abundant reservoir hosts, efficient fecal shedding from carrier animals, persistence within the environment, and the effective use of transmission vectors (feed, fomites, vehicles, etc.). Inapparent, long-term carriers that can shed salmonellae in feces continuously or intermittently, often in high numbers, are common in most host species. Shedding of the organism can be exacerbated by a long list of stressors, including commingling of pigs, transportation, concurrent diseases, and food deprivation.

The epidemiology of salmonella infections in swine is two relatively separate problems: salmonella infection of pork carcasses and retail products and infections that cause salmonellosis in swine. Infection of swine by one or more serotypes is common, but primary clinical disease caused by serotypes other than *S. choleraesuis* or *S. typhimurium* is uncommon. It is important to understand that swine can be infected with a variety of serotypes that do not cause disease in swine but do represent a source of infection for pork products.

Extrapolation of epidemiological data from experimental studies where a single serotype with predetermined dose is administered to naive healthy pigs is not likely to represent field situations, where there are multiple serotypes, varying doses, intermittent exposures, variable host resistance, many management variables, and various intercurrent infections and diseases. Similarly, disease prevalence surveys must be carefully scrutinized to be sure that infection is not equated with disease, that multiple isolations are recorded from a single source, and that a source of infection is not inaccurately implicated.

Salmonellae in Pork

Data collected from various countries indicate salmonellae to be present in 0–48% of carcasses (Riley 1970; Nottingham et al. 1972; McCaughey et al. 1973; Gustafson et al. 1976; Tacal and Lawrence 1980; Morse and Hird 1984; Jayarao et al. 1989; Carr et al. 1996) and 0–30% of retail pork products (Gooch and Goo 1971; Surkiewicz et al. 1972; Roberts et al. 1975; Banks and Board 1983; Silas et al. 1984; Fukushima et al. 1987; Anon. 1994). The marked variation is probably due, in part, to real variation in contamination and, in part, to differences in methods of survey and methods of meat processing. The high level of infection demonstrated in some of the studies is apparently the result of abattoir cross-contamination in holding pens prior to slaughter. There also may be some mechanical transfer of contamination among carcasses by dehairing machines, scalding tanks, and polishers (Galton et al. 1954; Hansen et al. 1964; Kampelmacher et al. 1965; Williams and Newell 1970; Michaud 1978; Morgan et al. 1987). Although much of the salmonella contamination of pork products occurs within abattoirs, infected pigs leaving the farm are considered the original source of abattoir infections. The stress of transport and feed deprivation increases shedding from inapparent carriers, which then contaminate the environment of the truck and abattoir (Williams and Newell 1970). The prevalence of infection within the group continues to increase with increasing length of stay in the pens prior to slaughter, rising by about 50% for each 24-hour period (Craven and Hurst 1982; Morgan et al. 1987). It should be noted that *S. choleraesuis* is rarely associated with contamination of carcasses and pork products, although this may be an artifact of the isolation methods used. Although unusual as a cause of human disease, *S. choleraesuis* is particularly severe when it does occur (Cherubin 1980).

There is currently an explosion of investigational

activity related to issues of food safety, including salmonella contamination of a variety of foods. Salmonellosis is considered to be one of the most common food-borne illnesses in humans. There has been an increased public awareness of microbiological hazards of food and improved monitoring. Although salmonella contamination of poultry and beef products exceeds that of pork, salmonella control programs in swine will continue to be a primary focus of food safety initiatives. Salmonella reduction programs are becoming commonplace, with long-range goals to include the production and marketing of salmonellae-free pork products. Numerous, dynamic programs are in place utilizing hazard analysis and critical control point (HACCP) principles. Those programs that have been in place for a sufficient period of time, such as the Danish program, have significantly reduced the rate of salmonella infection in pork products (Nielsen et al. 1995). Fortunately, most of the methods useful for preharvest salmonella reduction in swine populations are related to sound management practices that also improve the overall health of a swine operation. The Danish program using serology to identify salmonella-infected herds and thereby control the introduction of shedding swine into the abbatoir has not been as successful as originally hoped.

Salmonellosis in Swine

Most salmonellosis outbreaks occur in intensively reared weaned pigs, and although disease in adults and suckling pigs is infrequent, infection is not (Gooch and Haddock 1969; Wilcock et al. 1976). The low frequency of salmonellosis in suckling pigs presumably results from lactogenic immunity, since neonatal swine are susceptible to oral challenge with salmonellae and develop a disease comparable to that in weaned pigs (Wilcock 1978). Disease occurs worldwide but varies markedly in estimated prevalence, morbidity, and mortality. This may be from incautious extrapolation of data gathered from microbiological surveys applied to actual disease incidence. In one correlative study in Indiana in 1974–1975, salmonellosis accounted for 19% of 327 consecutive porcine necropsies (Wilcock et al. 1976). In contrast, Hooper and Troutt (1971) reported that salmonella infection was considered the major disease process in only 2% of samples submitted in Missouri between 1967 and 1969. During a 4-year period in Ireland, salmonellosis was the diagnosis in 4.4% of 2180 swine necropsies (Lawson and Dow 1966). In Taiwan, salmonellae were isolated from about 10% of scouring pigs and 48% of fatal diarrheas or septicemias in weaned pigs (Hsu et al. 1983). A survey of diagnostic submissions to the Iowa State University Veterinary Diagnostic Laboratory from 1994 through 1996 revealed salmonellae to be present in 11% of 9109 porcine pneumonia cases, 9% of 3320 enteric cases, and 58% of 1612 cases of porcine bacterial septicemia (Schwartz 1997a).

Host-adapted *S. choleraesuis,* isolated almost exclusively from diseased swine, is the most common cause of salmonellosis in swine, and is usually manifested as septicemia. Midwestern U.S. diagnostic laboratories and veterinarians reported an increasing frequency of salmonellosis due to *S. choleraesuis* from 1981 to 1990 and a decreasing frequency from 1991 to 1997 (Schwartz 1997b). The recent decrease in the Midwest is likely due to improvements in swine management and husbandry and the advent of efficacious attenuated live vaccines. Regional variation in salmonellosis incidence is loosely correlated to pig density, husbandry practices, and, in particular, commingling of pigs of different ages and/or origins.

S. typhimurium accounts for most of the remaining cases of salmonellosis in swine. This serotype has worldwide distribution and is not host-specific. Enterocolitis is the primary disease referable to this serotype, most commonly seen in pigs with concurrent debilitating illnesses, in conditions of poor hygiene that allow exposure to high doses of the organism, or where immunologically naive pigs are exposed to sufficiently large doses. The latter situation appears to be more frequently encountered with modern production systems utilizing age-segregated production.

The attribution of primary pathogenic status to other serotypes should be made with caution. Most other serotypes are transient, sporadic causes of disease and often cannot be associated with disease experimentally without unique, qualifying criteria. *S. heidelberg* has been associated with catarrhal enterocolitis in young pigs, with enterotoxigenic properties leading to accumulations of large amounts of fluid in the small intestine and colon as a rather unusual presentation of salmonellosis (Reed et al. 1985).

Sources of Infection

The number of potential sources of salmonella infection for a population of swine is seemingly endless. A task force study in the United States did not reach a consensus as to the most important source of salmonellae for pigs (Bixler 1978), in large part due to the diversity and the biology of the genus *Salmonella*. In general, the source of salmonellae virulent for swine is most likely to be other swine or environments contaminated by swine. *S. choleraesuis* is the most frequent porcine isolate from clinically ill pigs, but it is a very infrequent isolate from pig feeds or nonporcine salmonella reservoirs. The conclusion seems clear that infected, shedding pigs and contaminated environments are the major sources of new infections of *S. choleraesuis*. Vertical (dam to offspring) and horizontal transmission both occur. Feed contamination and nonporcine species have not been implicated as a source of *S. choleraesuis* infection of swine.

The source of infection for other serotypes is less clear, since the host and vector range for salmonellae is broad and they have amazing capability to persist in environments outside the host. For serotypes other than *S. choleraesuis*, pigs should be thought of as biological filters for the low numbers of various salmonella serotypes present in feed, water, or litter contaminated by birds, rodents, or other animals. There may be exceptions to this; for example, *S. derby* seems to be very common in some abattoir surveys of swine. Evidence linking sources of contamination to primary clinical outbreaks, without other concurrent diseases or predisposing conditions, is generally lacking. Feed containing ingredients of animal origin is widely accepted as a source of salmonella infection to herds, but it should be emphasized that ingredients of vegetable origin can also be a source of salmonellae-contaminated feed. Water is not as likely a source of infection unless surface water is used for consumption or pigs have access to recycled lagoon water. Birds, insects, rodents, and pets can all act as carriers, as can bedding and litter (Allred et al. 1967; Williams et al. 1969; Nape and Murphy 1971). In a survey in the United States, salmonellae were isolated from feed or feed ingredients from 14 of 30 farms and 36 of 1228 samples (Harris et al. 1997). The isolation of salmonellae from feed was significantly associated with the lack of bird-proofing, with on-farm feed preparation, and with the housing of pigs in facilities other than total confinement, for all stages of production. Interestingly, salmonella isolation from complete feeds was more frequent from pelleted feeds than from ground feed. No *S. typhimurium* was isolated from feed samples in this study.

Transmission, Shedding, and Carrier State

Because of the dynamic relationship between salmonellae, host, and environment, and because infection does not equate with disease, definitive statements regarding transmission, shedding, and carrier states are apt to be misinterpreted, if not erroneous. Salmonella transmission and shedding within differing populations of animals in an endless variety of environmental, feeding, and management situations result in countless unique situations that cannot be experimentally reproduced. In general, fecal-oral transmission is the most likely mode of transmission of virulent salmonellae. Salmonella can be recovered from the intestinal tract of pigs within several minutes of oral exposure. Transmission can occur from pig to pig, contaminated environment to pig, or dam to offspring. Oral-pharyngeal secretions may contain salmonellae, largely due to the fact that tonsils become rapidly contaminated with salmonellae following oral transmission. This may allow nose-nose transmission. Aerosolized secretions, feces, or contaminated dust particles make the potential for aerosol transmission for short distances quite real.

Salmonella infection of swine herds is much more common than disease. Longitudinal Dutch studies suggest that about 25% of herds are never infected, 24% are constantly infected, and 50% are infected most of the time. There appear to be infection cycles, with the endemic salmonellae having an ecological advantage over newly introduced salmonella serotypes. Infection occurs in the first weeks after arrival or commingling and reaches a maximum of 80–100% prevalence within another 2–3 weeks. About 5–30% of the pigs are still excreting salmonellae at the end of the finishing period. In 1995, the National Animal Health Monitoring Service (NAHMS) reported 30–60% of U.S. herds infected with at least one serotype of *Salmonella*, with the greatest percentage of postive herds found in the southeastern United States and in herds marketing greater than 10,000 head annually.

During acute disease, pigs will shed up to 10^6 *S. choleraesuis*/g feces (Smith and Jones 1967) or 10^7 *S. typhimurium* (Gutzmann et al. 1976). The minimum disease-producing dose of either serotype has not been established in field situations, but disease is difficult to reproduce experimentally at low doses. There is one report of moderate disease following oral inoculation of 10^6 cells (Dawe and Troutt 1976), but most authors report successful experimental disease production with doses of 10^8–10^{11} cells unless pigs are artificially stressed by injection of dexamethasone or in some other manner. Pigs infected with 10^3 organisms remained clinically normal but uninoculated pigs in the same pen did become clinically ill (Gray et al. 1996). It is likely that dose (and perhaps virulence) is magnified when pigs are infected and sequential (pig-to-pig) transmission occurs in field situations, so that the initial infective dose in the field is considerably less than that required in experimental situations. High animal density, stress of transport, and intercurrent nutritional or infectious disease are assumed to increase the shedding by carriers as well as the susceptibility of exposed pigs (Committee on Salmonella 1969). Pigs with nondetectable shedding of salmonellae can begin shedding within hours of an applied stress. The transmission demonstrated between feeder pigs also occurs between pigs during market transport and lairage at abattoirs, with infection rates proportional to time spent in transport and lairage (Hurd et al. 2001a; Hurd et al. 2001b). It is likely that catecholamines are released in association with stress, resulting in decreased gastric acid production and increased intestinal motility. Increases in stomach pH increase the likelihood that salmonellae will survive passage through the stomach and will access and replicate in the intestine and colon.

Outbreaks of salmonellosis are usually characterized by spread from pen to pen. Situations of spread from pen to distant pen are likely because of vectors or caretaker transmission. When all animals sicken simultaneously, a common source such as feed, bedding, water, or a contaminated environment should be suspected. Salmonella infections tend to be more prevalent in continuous-flow systems than in barns managed by principles of all-in/all-out. Prevalence is also higher in barns with open flush-gutters than in those with slotted floors, with the highest rates of infection observed in outdoor finishing systems (Davies et al. 1997).

Numerous studies in a variety of host species with a potpourri of serotypes have demonstrated prolonged carrier states following infection. The pattern of shedding and the duration of the carrier state after clinically apparent disease have been studied only in group-housed pigs with no barrier to repeated reinfection (Wilcock and Olander 1978; Wood et al. 1989). After experimental infection, *S. typhimurium* was isolated from feces daily during the first 10 days post infection and frequently during the next 4–5 months. When slaughtered 4–7 months after initial infection, over 90% of pigs were positive for *S. typhimurium* in the mesenteric lymph node, tonsil, cecum, or feces (Wilcock and Olander 1978; Wood et al. 1989; Wood and Rose 1992; Fedorka-Cray et al. 1994). *S. newport* has been shown to persist in mesenteric lymph nodes for 28 weeks. Infection of individual animals may be relatively short-lived (less than 8 weeks), but organisms may circulate within a population and between pigs and the environment for extended periods of time.

S. choleraesuis given by either the intranasal or the intragastric route has been demonstrated to persist within ileocolic junction, lymph nodes, tonsils, lungs, and colon for at least 12 weeks (Gray et al. 1995). Infection with low doses of *S. choleraesuis* produced a shorter period of infection than infection with moderate or high doses. *S. choleraesuis* has been shown to persist for at least 3 months in wet feces and 6 months in desiccated feces.

The influence of antibiotics on the frequency and duration of shedding of salmonellae in pigs has received little attention. In human enteric salmonellosis, the use of antibiotics has long been recognized to prolong the carrier state (Dixon 1965; Aserkoff and Bennett 1969). In pigs with enterocolitis, antibiotics do not reduce the duration or the magnitude of fecal shedding, but neither are they reported to prolong or intensify shedding (Finlayson and Barnum 1973; DeGeeter et al. 1976; Gutzmann et al. 1976; Wilcock and Olander 1978; Jones et al. 1983; Jacks et al. 1988). In contrast, vigorous antibacterial therapy early in the course of septicemia caused by *S. choleraesuis* may significantly reduce the magnitude and duration of fecal shedding (Jacks et al. 1981).

PATHOGENESIS

The clinical and pathological features of salmonella infections are extremely variable. Severity is influenced by serotype, virulence, natural and acquired host resistance, and route and quantity of the infective dose. Over 200 virulence factors have been associated with salmonellae but few have been completely characterized. Generally, those that promote virulence in pathogenic salmonellae are involved in adhesion, invasion, cytotoxicity, and resistance to intracellular killing, often working in combination to promote disease. Despite distinct differences in clinical signs, many parallels can be drawn between *S. choleraesuis* and *S. typhimurium* when discussing pathogenesis.

Although large doses (greater than 10^7) are required to induce disease experimentally, intraluminal replication may be important with small inocula. Disease is facilitated by factors such as peristaltic impairment, interference with intestinal flora, and elevation of gastric pH (Clarke and Gyles 1993). Replication to about 10^7 organisms/g of intestinal content is required for lesion production in pigs infected with *S. typhimurium*, a finding that probably also applies to other serotypes causing enterocolitis. Alterations in normal intestinal defenses by antibiotic-induced changes in normal flora or cold-induced alteration in intestinal motility may reduce the amount of replication required for disease or increase the ease of salmonella replication (Bohnhoff et al. 1954). Infection with *S. choleraesuis* may not require such massive luminal proliferation as prerequisite for disease, because it is inherently more invasive than other serotypes, can infect via the pharyngeal tonsil, and regularly causes signs of septicemia 24–72 hours before the onset of diarrhea (Smith and Jones 1967; Cherubin et al. 1974; Wilcock 1979; Reed et al. 1986).

The ability to invade is a requirement for pathogenesis and is encoded by a serotype-specific plasmid (Helmuth et al. 1985). Removal of this plasmid results in a lack of ability to invade but has no effect on ingestion or killing by murine macrophages, LPS production, or serum resistance (Gulig and Curtiss 1987). During the invasion process there is induction of synthesis of new proteins that probably enhance intracellular survival (Finlay et al. 1989). Peroxidase-antiperoxidase immunoenzymatic labeling and immunogold labeling techniques have demonstrated that *S. typhimurium* has a low tendency to invade the enteric mucosa and does not have a predilection for any specific intestinal location. While many epithelial cell types (enterocytes, M-cells, goblet cells) in the jejunum and ileum may be invaded, the predominant portal of entry into the submucosa may occur at Peyer's patches (Meyerholz et al. 2002; Meyerholz et al. 2003; Schauser et al. 2004). *S. choleraesuis* locates preferentially in the colon on the luminal surface of ileal M cells of Peyer's patches (Pospischil et al. 1990). Invasion is by endocytosis by M cells of gut-associated lymphoid tissue as well as enterocytes. Attachment of the bacteria to epithelial receptors triggers microfilament-controlled uptake, vacuole formation, vacuole transport through the cell cytoplasm, and entry into the lamina propria via exocytosis through the basement membrane (Takeuchi 1967; Takeuchi and Sprinz 1967). Passage through the epithelium causes mild and transient enterocyte damage. Salmonellae can synthesize over 30 proteins that are selectively induced during infection of macrophages, making them facultative intracellular bacteria (similar to *Brucella, Mycobacterium,* and *Listeria*) that can survive within macrophages and neutrophils in the lamina propria (Roof et al. 1992a, b). Spread to mesenteric lymph nodes is rapid, occurring within 2 hours of inoculation of ligated intestinal loops or 24 hours after oral challenge (Reed et al. 1985, 1986). Knockout mice (CD18⁻) have been used to show that CD18⁺ phagocytes are important in the dissemination of the organism to the spleen and liver (Vazquez-Torres et al. 1999). Two leading cell candidates for this systemic transport are the macrophages and dendritic cells (Vazquez-Torres et al. 2000). Recent in vitro work has suggested that dendritic cells are capable of producing tight junction proteins to penetrate the epithelium and sample luminal bacteria including *Salmonella* (Rescigno et al. 2001). Concurrent with bacillary spread is the appearance of an acute, predominantly macrophagic, inflammatory reaction and prominent microvascular damage with thrombosis within the lamina propria and submucosa. Other routes of systemic invasion may be important. When administered intranasally to esophagotomized pigs, *S. choleraesuis* demonstrated primary colonization of the lung within 4 hours (Fedorka-Cray et al. 1995; Gray et al. 1995).

Early intestinal inflammation is considered a key feature of pathogenesis for enteric forms of salmonellosis. Neutrophil recruitment and transmigration across the epithelium is considered the most significant component (McCormick et al. 1995). Caspase-1 can act as a proinflammatory agent by cleaving interleukin-1 beta and interleukin-18 into active molecules (Fantuzzi and Dinarello 1999). SipA has also been shown to contribute to the inflammatory response by activation of phosphokinase C (Lee et al. 2000). Salmonella-induced activation of inflammatory mediators such as nuclear factor kappa B and phosphokinase C results in basolateral secretion of interleukin-8 and apical secretion of pathogen-elicited epithelial chemoattractant (Eaves-Pyles et al. 1999; Lee et al. 2000). These molecules act as chemokines promoting the transepithelial migration of neutrophils into the intestinal lumen (Gewirtz et al. 1999). In contrast, several studies using rabbits, monkeys, calves, or pigs have demonstrated fluid secretion independent of mucosal necrosis or inflammation (Giannella et al. 1973; Rout et al. 1974; Kinsey et al. 1976; Clarke and Gyles 1987). These studies present evidence that, at least early in the disease, the diarrhea is the result of decreased sodium resorption and increased chloride secretion due to cholera-like and shiga-like enterotoxins. Secretion stimulated by prostaglandins elaborated by endotoxin-stimulated neutrophils may also be important (Stephen et al. 1985). Toxic effects of certain OMPs, as well as lipid A associated with the LPS, are also important mediators of cell damage. Survival within phagocytes is an important attribute of virulent salmonellae, the mechanism of which is not clear. Salmonellae which possess smooth LPS, O side chains, and a complete LPS core are more resistant to phagocyte killing.

Mucosal inflammation and necrosis, as well as septicemia, occur in concert with the diarrhea but perhaps independently of it. Microvascular thrombosis and endothelial necrosis in the submucosa and lamina propria are consistent early lesions in porcine salmonellosis (Lawson and Dow 1966; Wilcock et al. 1976; Jubb et al. 1993; Reed et al. 1986), probably in response to locally produced endotoxin. Salmonellae are not directly associated with the damaged vessels but direct the events from the protected intracellular niche of macrophages in the surrounding submucosa or lamina propria (Takeuchi and Sprinz 1967). Mucosal ischemia as a result of the microvascular thrombosis is probably a major contributor to the mucosal necrosis so typical of salmonellosis in all species. The second major contribution to mucosal necrosis is probably from the chemical products of mucosal inflammation. The systemic signs and lesions of septicemic salmonellosis, in swine almost exclusively *S. choleraesuis* infection, are most commonly attributed to endotoxemia from bacterial dissemination. The complex biology of endotoxin is beyond the scope of this chapter, and readers should consult Wolff (1973), Elin and Wolff (1976), or Cybulsky et al. (1988). Briefly, endotoxin interacts with plasma and with leukocytes to initiate inflammation and fever. Most of the effects are mediated by interleukin-1, a lymphokine produced by macrophages stimulated by the endotoxin (Rubin and Weinstein 1977). Endotoxins have either direct effects on tissue or effects via an array of cytokine mediators.

CLINICAL SIGNS, PATHOLOGICAL FINDINGS, AND DIAGNOSIS

The clinical signs of porcine salmonellosis are referable to septicemia or to enterocolitis, and this section describes each syndrome separately. Pigs surviving acute septicemia may develop clinical signs due to bacteremic localization: pneumonia, hepatitis, enterocolitis, and, occasionally, meningoencephalitis. Pigs initially suffering from enterocolitis may later develop chronic wasting disease or, occasionally, rectal stricture.

The most available salmonella diagnostic method is bacterial isolation and identification, which, along with compatible lesions, remains the basis for diagnosis. Other tests using more sophisticated technology, including polymerase chain reaction (PCR), are not required for routine diagnosis. PCR currently has value as a screening tool but has a relatively high cost and currently lacks sensitivity without preenrichment. Detection of salmonellae does not constitute diagnosis of salmonellosis.

Serology is becoming increasingly available, usually in the form of an ELISA test. Most tests use surface antigens such as OMP or LPS. These tests, some of which use mixed antigens containing both OMP and LPS or antigens from several serotypes, thus far appear to lack specificity and sensitivity for individual-animal diagnosis but are useful for herd screening (Baum et al. 1996). A mixed-ELISA test using meat juice at slaughter to detect antibody to a broad range of serotypes has been useful in categorizing the level of salmonella infection in herds in Denmark (Nielsen et al. 1995; Mousing et al. 1997).

Septicemic Salmonellosis

This form of disease, usually caused by *S. choleraesuis*, occurs mainly in weaned pigs less than 5 months of age but may be seen occasionally in market swine, suckling piglets, or adult breeding stock either as a septicemia or as a cause of abortion.

Clinical Signs.   Pigs ill with *S. choleraesuis* are inappetent, lethargic, febrile with temperatures of 105–107°F (40.5–41.6°C) and may have a shallow, moist cough with slight expiratory dyspnea. Icterus may be apparent. The first evidence of disease may be finding pigs reluctant to move, huddled in the corner of a pen, or even dead, with cyanosis of extremities and abdomens. Diarrhea is not usually a feature of septicemic salmonellosis until the third or fourth day of disease, when watery yellow feces may be seen. In most outbreaks, the case fatality rate is high; morbidity is variable but is usually less than 10%. Outbreaks are frequently associated with stressful situations. The duration of the disease in individual pigs, as well as the duration and severity of each epizootic, is unpredictable but will be prolonged without successful intervention. Evaluation of therapeutic regimens in naturally occurring outbreaks is dif-ficult, making response to therapy a poor diagnostic criterion. Disease spread is by ingestion of contaminated feces or nasopharyngeal secretions, with an incubation period ranging from 2 days to at least several weeks. Surviving pigs may remain carriers and fecal shedders for at least 12 weeks.

Gross Lesions.   Lesions at necropsy include cyanosis of ears, feet, tail, and ventral abdominal skin; congestion progressing to infarction of gastric fundic mucosa; splenomegaly with less severe hepatomegaly; and moist, swollen gastrohepatic and mesenteric lymph nodes. Lungs are firm and resilient, diffusely congested, often with interlobular edema and perhaps hemorrhage; cranioventral bronchopneumonia is not uncommon. Icterus can be severe, although not consistently present (Fig. 45.1). An inconsistent, subtle lesion is miliary, random white foci of necrosis in the liver. In pigs surviving the first few days of disease there may be serous to necrotic enterocolitis. The features of the intestinal lesion are described more fully in the section on salmonella enterocolitis. Petechial hemorrhages, when present, are usually best seen in the renal cortex or on the epicardium.

Microscopic Lesions.   The most diagnostic lesion of systemic salmonellosis is the presence of paratyphoid nodules in the liver. These are clusters of histiocytes amid foci of acute coagulative hepatocellular necrosis, corresponding to the white foci seen grossly. These lesions are often present (Lawson and Dow 1966) and unique for this disease, although other agents can produce suppurative or necrotic foci in liver. Other lesions typical of salmonellosis include fibrinoid thrombi in

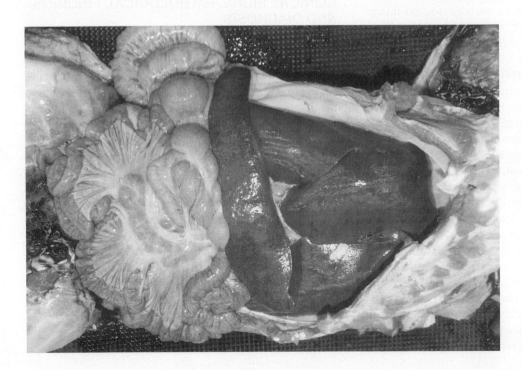

45.1. *Splenomegaly, hepatomegaly, and swollen mesenteric lymph nodes from* S. choleraesuis *infection.*

venules of gastric mucosa, in cyanotic skin, in glomerular capillaries, and less regularly in pulmonary vessels. There is hyperplasia of reticular cells of spleen and lymph nodes as well as generalized swelling of endothelial cells and histiocytes typical of gram-negative sepsis. A similar diffuse histiocytic interstitial pneumonia is present in lung. A complete discussion of the pathology of septicemic salmonellosis can be found in Lawson and Dow (1966) and Jubb et al. (1993).

Diagnosis. The diagnosis of septicemic salmonellosis cannot be made on the basis of clinical signs alone, which are similar to those of other causes of septicemia in pigs, particularly *Erysipelothrix rhusiopathiae, Streptococcus suis, Actinobacillus suis,* or death due to classical swine fever or *Actinobacillus pleuropneumoniae.* Gross lesions of splenomegaly, hepatomegaly, lymphadenopathy, interstitial pneumonia, or focal hepatic necrosis are very suggestive of septicemic salmonellosis, but are not seen in every case. In most situations, definitive diagnosis requires the isolation of large numbers of salmonellae from tissues of affected pigs, almost invariably *S. choleraesuis* var. *kunzendorf.* Samples of lung, liver, or spleen often yield pure cultures of the organism on brilliant green, bismuth sulfite, blood agar, or MacConkey agar. Enrichment techniques are seldom required unless the organs have been contaminated by feces or careless handling or have autolysis, in which case tetrathionate broth at 42–43°C is the enrichment medium of choice. Selenite broth is inhibitory for *S. choleraesuis* and should be avoided (Edwards and Ewing 1972). Attempts to isolate salmonellae from animals that have received antimicrobial therapy are often unrewarding. Intestine or feces are not reliable specimens for isolation of the organism in pigs with acute septicemia. Differential diagnosis must include agents associated with the particular systems affected, including those that may cause septicemia, pneumonia, hepatitis, encephalitis, or enterocolitis (Schwartz 1991).

Salmonella Enterocolitis

Salmonellosis manifested as enterocolitis is most frequent in pigs from weaning to about 4 months of age. Disease may be acute or chronic and can usually be ascribed to *S. typhimurium* (including variety copenhagen) or, less frequently, to *S. choleraesuis.* Although isolation of other serotypes of salmonellae from pigs with diarrhea occurs with some frequency, implication of serotypes other than *S. choleraesuis, S. typhimurium,* and perhaps *S. heidelberg* as primary pathogens should be done with caution.

Clinical Signs. The initial clinical sign is watery yellow diarrhea, initially without blood or mucus. The disease may spread rapidly to involve most pigs in a pen within a few days. The initial diarrhea in an individual pig usually lasts 3–7 days, but it typically may recur for second and third bouts, giving the impression of a waxing and waning diarrheal disease of several weeks' duration. Blood may appear sporadically in the feces but rarely with the profuseness typical of swine dysentery or hemorrhagic porcine proliferative enteropathy (PPE). Affected pigs are febrile, have decreased feed intake, and are dehydrated, paralleling the severity and duration of the diarrhea. Mortality usually is low and occurs only after several days of diarrhea, presumably as the result of hypokalemia and dehydration. Most pigs make complete clinical recovery but a portion may remain as carriers and intermittent shedders for at least 5 months. A few pigs may remain unthrifty and, occasionally, may develop rectal strictures.

Gross Lesions. In pigs that have died of diarrhea, the major lesion is focal or diffuse necrotic enteritis, colitis, or typhlitis. The lesion is seen as adherent gray-yellow debris on the red, roughened mucosal surface of an edematous spiral colon, cecum, or ileum (Fig. 45.2). Colon and cecal contents are bile stained and scant, often with

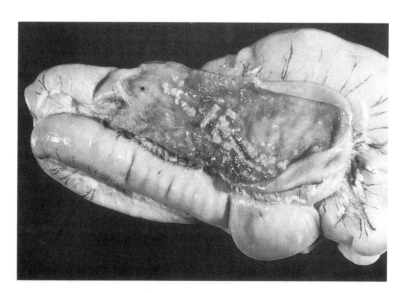

45.2. *Coalescing colonic ulcers from* S. typhimurium *infection.*

black or sandlike gritty material. Mesenteric lymph nodes, especially ileocecal nodes, are greatly enlarged and moist. The gross lesion may extend to involve the descending colon and rectum. The necrosis may be seen as sharply delineated button ulcers, particularly in resolving lesions. Necrotic ileitis has historically been attributed to several agents, including *Salmonella,* but in confirmed cases of salmonellosis, ileal involvement usually is seen as reddening and slight roughening of the mucosa, suggesting mild superficial necrosis. Salmonellae associated with necrotic enteritis may be a sequel to PPE. Lesions of septicemia may be present in those cases involving *S. choleraesuis.* In cases of *S. typhimurium* enterocolitis, the liver and spleen are not enlarged except by terminal congestion.

Microscopic Lesions. The typical enteric lesion is necrosis of cryptal and surface enterocytes that varies from focal to diffuse. The lamina propria and submucosa contain numerous macrophages and moderate numbers of lymphocytes; neutrophils are numerous only in the very early lesions. Thrombi containing fibrin, platelets, and leukocytes are numerous (Fig. 45.3). The necrosis frequently extends to involve muscularis mucosa, submucosa, and lymphoid follicles. *Balantidium coli* is commonly present in necrotic debris of chronic cases. In the ileum, necrosis is usually quite superficial and is often seen as villous atrophy. The Peyer's patches may be necrotic in acute disease, but in pigs dying of the naturally occurring disease, lymphoid hypertrophy or even regenerative hyperplasia is more common. The liver may contain paratyphoid nodules but not with the consistency or the necrosis usually seen in the septicemic disease. A more complete discussion of the pathology can be found in Wilcock et al. (1976), Reed et al. (1986), and Jubb et al. (1993).

Diagnosis. The differential diagnosis of diarrhea in weaned pigs must include salmonellosis, swine dysentery, and PPE due to *Lawsonia intracellularis*. Other viral, bacterial, or parasitic diseases capable of causing diarrhea include rotaviral and coronaviral enteritis, postweaning colibacillosis, trichuriasis, and coccidiosis. Salmonellosis concurrently present with other diseases is not uncommon.

Typical acute swine dysentery is distinguished from salmonellosis on the basis of the mucoid and bloody diarrhea in otherwise alert swine with dysentery, contrasted with depression and profuse yellow diarrhea of salmonellosis. PPE may be seen as acute intestinal hemorrhage or acute to chronic diarrhea with mucosal proliferation or necrosis. Differentiation among the three diseases at necropsy is primarily by recognition of differences in lesion distribution rather than by differences in character. Salmonellosis is usually in colon and occasionally small intestine, may be focal, and always involves marked mesenteric lymphadenopathy. The lesion of swine dysentery is diffuse, shallow, and restricted to large intestine; lymph node enlargement is absent or mild. In PPE ileal involvement usually overshadows the milder colonic lesions, and the mucosa underlying the necrotic membrane is markedly hyperplastic (Table 45.2). Whipworms (*Trichuris suis*) may also cause diffuse mucohemorrhagic colitis.

The diagnosis of salmonellosis is confirmed by microbiological and histological examination. The wide distribution of environmental salmonellae makes isolation alone unreliable for disease diagnosis, and a positive isolation should always be supported by appropriate lesions before a diagnosis of salmonellosis is made. A pool of ileum and ileocecal lymph node should enable detection of virtually all active or recently recovered cases, although tissues such as tonsil or cecal wall will usually yield positive cultures as well (Wilcock et al. 1976; Wood et al. 1989). From live animals, large (10 g) aliquots of feces or pharyngeal tonsil scrapings are preferable to rectal swabs for isolation, with tetrathionate enrichment the method of choice.

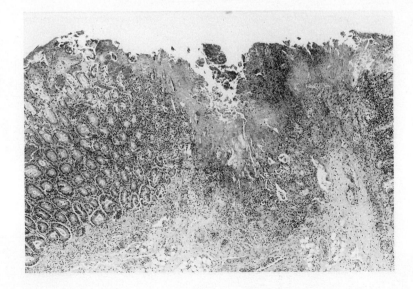

45.3. *Histological section showing deep colonic ulceration and inflammation from* S. typhimurium *infection.*

Table 45.2. Differential diagnosis of enterocolitis in swine at necropsy

Condition	Ileal Lesion	Colonic Lesion	Ileocecal Nodes	Extraintestinal Lesions
Salmonellosis	Mild, usually no pseudo-membrane	Focal to diffuse, deep necrotic lesions	Always enlarged two to five times normal	Variable, gastric infarction, interstitial pneumonitis, miliary hepatic necrosis
Swine dysentery	Absent	Superficial and usually diffuse necrosis, blood and/or mucus	Often normal, slight enlargement	None except gastric fundic infarction in natural deaths
Porcine proliferative enteritis	Varies from hemorrhagic to necrotic or proliferative	Milder than in the ileum, usually only the proximal spiral colon	Variable with stage of disease	None

Other Syndromes

Salmonellae are occasionally involved in disease outbreaks in which the clinical signs may not suggest salmonellae as the etiologic diagnosis. Outbreaks of neurologic disease resembling classical swine fever or pseudorabies have been reported (Wilcock and Olander 1978), and brain lesions sometimes occur with septicemic salmonellosis. The lesion in the brain is necrotic vasculitis and perivascular granulomatous lesions resembling typical paratyphoid nodules (Fig. 45.4). Rectal strictures in growing pigs have been ascribed to defective healing of ulcerative proctitis caused by *S. typhimurium* (Wilcock and Olander 1977a, b). The stricture reportedly represents fibrosis in an area of persistent ischemia, with the rectum predisposed because of a normally precarious blood supply (Fig. 45.5).

Infection with the fastidious, swine-adapted serovar *S. typhisuis* causes a relatively specific chronic syndrome of diarrhea and wasting in which caseous lymphadenitis, histiocytic interstitial pneumonia, or suppurative bronchopneumonia is added to the typical necrotic colitis (Barnes and Bergeland 1968; Andrews 1976; Fenwick and Olander 1987). In some pigs the intestinal lesions may have healed, leaving the lymphoid and pulmonary lesions to be distinguished from tuberculosis and infection with *Arcanobacterium pyogenes* (Barnes and Sorensen 1975).

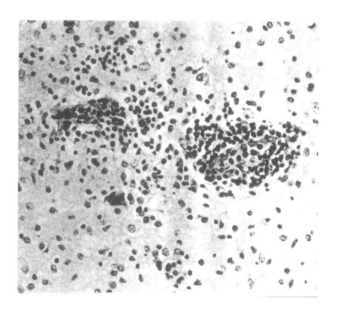

45.4. *Histological section showing vasculitis and perivascular granulomatous inflammation in the brain stem from* S. choleraesuis *encephalitis.*

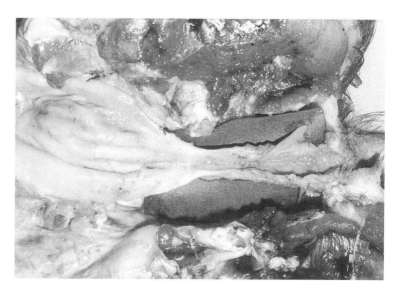

45.5. *Rectal stricture at necropsy.*

TREATMENT

With either septicemic or enteric salmonellosis, the goals of treatment in an outbreak of salmonellosis are to minimize the severity of clinical disease, prevent spread of infection and disease, and prevent recurrence of the disease in the herd. With salmonellosis the attainment of these goals is particularly difficult. Both *S. choleraesuis* and *S. typhimurium* are often resistant in vitro to many antibacterial agents used in swine (Barnes and Sorensen 1975; Wilcock et al. 1976; Blackburn et al. 1984; Schultz 1989; Fales et al. 1990; Schwartz 1997a). During clinical disease, the organism inhabits a protected intracellular niche inaccessible to many common antibacterials. The use of various antibiotics to treat enteric salmonellosis is widely advocated (Morehouse 1972; Barnes and Sorensen 1975; Blood et al. 1979), but much of the information to support this recommendation has been taken from trials designed to test the prophylactic efficacy of drugs, not their therapeutic efficacy. Thus, pigs on medicated feed, when inoculated orally with salmonellae, have the antibiotic already present in the gastrointestinal tract to interact with the salmonellae, resulting in milder disease because of what amounts to a decreased inoculum. In the few trials designed specifically to test antibacterial drug efficacy against clinical enteric salmonellosis, such therapy was considered to have little merit (Heard et al. 1968; Gutzmann et al. 1976; Olson et al. 1977; Wilcock and Olander 1978). Although not therapeutic, oral medications may decrease efficiency of transmission and have a prophylactic effect on pigs not yet affected. Antimicrobials are ordinarily administered at maximum permissible levels in feed or, preferably, water. Ideally, the choice of antibacterial agent should be based on in vitro susceptibility testing of isolates from each outbreak. Since medication often must be initiated before such results are available, choices must be based on previous experience and results of controlled trials.

In contrast, vigorous therapy early in the course of septicemia caused by *S. choleraesuis* has been reported to significantly reduce the duration and severity of disease (Jacks et al. 1981). In that report, therapy was initiated after inoculation but prior to the onset of clinical signs. Evaluation of efficacy under field conditions is difficult because of the unpredictability of the disease and because husbandry changes often accompany the use of antibacterials in an outbreak. Reports and practitioner communications from the American Midwest, however, suggest that visibly affected animals respond to aggressive therapy with parenteral antimicrobials (Schwartz 1991). Mass medication of the population at risk to decrease severity of disease and transmission of salmonellae is also widely practiced. The choice of an appropriate antimicrobial is aided by antibiograms and previous herd experience. In the absence of either, amikacin, gentamicin, neomycin, apramycin, ceftiofur, and trimethoprim-sulfonamide are effective in vitro against most isolates (Barnes and Sorensen 1975; Wilcock et al. 1976; Mills and Kelly 1986; Schultz 1989; Evelsizer 1990; Fales et al. 1990, Schwartz 1997b). Antiinflammatory agents are sometimes administered to critically ill animals to combat the effects of endotoxin (Schwartz and Daniels 1987; Schultz 1989; Evelsizer 1990).

Most salmonella antimicrobial resistance is plasmid-mediated. Of concern is the recent emergence of an *S. typhimurium* definitive type 104 (DT 104), isolated primarily from bovine and human populations, that has chromosomally integrated multiple antimicrobial resistance (Low et al. 1997). This isolate has a higher morbidity and mortality in humans than other *S. typhimurium* organisms and is increasing in prevalence in human and bovine populations. Carrier swine are generally asymptomatic. Although evidence linking emergence of such isolates to veterinary medical practices is generally lacking, the impact will affect public health initiatives as well as the availability of therapeutic agents for food-producing animals. It should be emphasized that salmonella control programs that rely strictly on antimicrobials are doomed to failure.

In addition to antimicrobial therapy, the successful treatment of salmonellosis relies heavily on routine husbandry procedures recommended for control of infectious diseases. The diarrheic pig contaminates its environment and is the single most important source of infection for other pigs. Removal and isolation of sick animals, minimizing exposure to infective material by scrupulous pen sanitation, frequent cleaning of water bowls, and restriction of animal or staff movement from potentially contaminated to clean areas are necessary. Efforts to modify management and environment to decrease crowding and stress and increase pig comfort are essential adjuncts to specific therapy.

PREVENTION

Prevention of infection of swine with salmonellae is not currently possible. Infection does not necessarily result in disease, and pigs may not sicken with disease until severely stressed long after initial exposure. The control of disease expression rests on efforts to minimize the exposure dose and to maximize pig resistance. The carrier pig and contaminated feed or environment are the most significant sources of infection to pigs, and pigs are most likely to develop disease during periods of stress or when exposed to massive numbers of salmonellae. The commingling and transport of weanling pigs from different sources to finishing farms enhance activation of latent carriers and ensure exposure of stressed pigs to salmonellae (Allred 1972). The source of host-adapted *S. choleraesuis*, which is rarely, if ever, isolated from feed or feed ingredients, would seem to be limited to carrier pigs and facilities previously contaminated with this serotype. The fact that many outbreaks occur in facilities with good sanitation suggests that other stresses probably contribute to occurrence of the disease. Management practices that allow filling of grower and finishing rooms with single-source and single-age pigs are beneficial. Minimizing the variety of stresses often involved in acute outbreaks requires constant attention to details of management and husbandry, including proper animal density; dry, comfortable pens and temperatures; and adequate ventilation. On farms with enzootic disease, modifications to the facility and environment and implementation of management practices that emphasize all-in/all-out production should precede a prophylactic drug program. Antibiotics are probably useful as aids in preventing occurrence of disease when used prophylactically, but their use will not prevent infection and when relied upon for prevention of disease will eventually fail.

Nutritional approaches to prevent or alleviate swine salmonellosis include feeding of propionic or other volatile fatty acids, mannose, lactose, probiotics, and heavy metals. Although all of these practices are based on a sound theoretical basis and are reported to be successful experimentally or in other species, evidence for their efficacy in swine is lacking. Anecdotal reports suggest acidification of rations or water to be of some benefit.

As with other facultative intracellular bacteria, live vaccines that stimulate cell-mediated immunity are the most likely to be protective for salmonellae in swine. Historically, an attenuated live *S. choleraesuis* vaccine was used widely in the United Kingdom for many years but was withdrawn when *S. choleraesuis* infection decreased in that country to negligible proportions. Recently, the introduction of effective and safe modified live attenuated vaccines for *S. choleraesuis* has had a major impact on the occurrence of systemic salmonellosis in North America. The isolates used in these vaccines are either naturally occurring avirulent *S. choleraesuis* or are derived from repeated passage through porcine neutrophils, the product of which was demonstrated to have been cured of a 50 kb virulence plasmid necessary for intracellular survival (Roof et al. 1992b; Kramer et al. 1987, 1992). When given at weaning, vaccine protected pigs for at least 20 weeks (Roof and Doitchinoff 1995) against homologous serotypes, with some cross-protection suggested with heterologous serotypes.

Partial protection can be obtained with bacterins, primarily because of the nonspecific mitogenic and immunostimulant effect of LPS (Fenwick et al. 1986). Killed vaccines for *S. typhimurium* are safe, but the bulk of the evidence suggests that they have little efficacy in preventing disease following strong challenge because resistance to disease rests primarily on cell-mediated immunity (Collins 1974; Davies and Kotlarski 1976). Extrapolation of information from experience in humans (Hornick et al. 1970; Welliver and Ogra 1978) and calves (Bairey 1978) suggests, however, that use of a po-

tent killed vaccine may increase the dose necessary to cause disease and may offer some protection from septicemic salmonellosis, in which humoral immunity may play a role.

Monitoring herds for salmonellae has not been commonly practiced. The detection of carrier animals is difficult because of the unpredictability of fecal shedding. The detection of salmonellae by bacterial culture of feces and tonsils of diarrheic pigs in the nursery would likely be the most rewarding for identification of infected herds. However, even repeated negative fecal or tonsilar cultures do not guarantee that a herd or individual is not a salmonella carrier and thus a potential shedder. The use of salmonella serology can determine if an animal has had previous exposure to salmonellae, but this has little relevance to the carrier status or to the probability of shedding. Food safety concerns have stimulated renewed interest in serology as a method to determine the salmonella infection status of groups of market swine. This technology offers the possibility of sensitive and specific methods to identify infected herds, but it is not yet useful for determining the infection status of individual pigs.

REFERENCES

Allred JN. 1972. Comments on salmonellosis in swine. J Am Vet Med Assoc 160:601–602.
Allred JN, Walker JW, Beal VC, Germaine FW. 1967. A survey to determine the salmonella contamination rate in livestock and poultry feeds. J Am Vet Med Assoc 151:1857–1860.
Andrews JJ. 1976. *Salmonella typhisuis* infection in swine. In Proc North Cent Conf Vet Lab Diagn, p. 7.
Anon. 1994. Annual Report on Zoonoses in Denmark. Copenhagen: Ministry of Agriculture and Fisheries, Danish Veterinary Service, Danish Zoonosis Centre.
Aserkoff B, Bennett JV. 1969. Effect of antibiotic therapy in acute salmonellosis on the fecal excretion of salmonellae. N Engl 281:636–640.
Bairey MH. 1978. Immunization of calves against salmonellosis. J Am Vet Med Assoc 173:610–613.
Banks JG, Board RG. 1983. The incidence and level of contamination of British fresh sausages and ingredients with salmonellas. J Hyg (Lond) 90:213–223.
Barnes DM, Bergeland ME. 1968. *Salmonella typhisuis* infection in Minnesota swine. J Am Vet Med Assoc 152:1766–1769.
Barnes DM, Sorensen DK. 1975. Salmonellosis. In Diseases of Swine, 4th ed. HW Dunne, AD Leman, eds. Ames: Iowa State Univ Press, pp. 554–564.
Baskerville A, Dow C. 1973. Pathology of experimental pneumonia in pigs produced by *Salmonella choleraesuis*. J Comp Pathol 83:207–215.
Baum DH, Harris DL, Nielsen B, Fedorka-Cray PJ, Homan WH, Rankin RA. 1996. Comparison of the Danish MIX-ELISA to culture for the detection of Salmonella in finishing pigs at or near slaughter. In ISU Swine Res Rep, p. 177.
Bixler WB. 1978. FDA salmonella control activities for animal feeds and feed ingredients. In Proc Nat Salmonellosis Sem, Washington, D.C.
Blackburn BO, Schlater LK, Swanson MR. 1984. Antibiotic resistance of members of the genus *Salmonella* isolated from chickens, turkeys, cattle, and swine in the United States during October 1981 through September 1982. Am J Vet Res 45:1245–1249.

Blood DC, Henderson JA, Radostits OM. 1979. Veterinary Medicine, 4th ed. London: Baillière Tindall, pp. 476–486.

Bohnhoff M, Drake BL, Miller C. P. 1954. Effect of streptomycin on susceptibility of intestinal tract to salmonella infection. Proc Soc Exp Biol Med 86:133–137.

Carr MA, Bawcom DW, Miller MF, Ramsey CB, Thompson LD. 1996. Microbiology of Pig Carcasses. 1st Int Symp Ecology of Salmonella in Pork Products, NADC, Ames, Iowa.

Centers for Disease Control and Prevention (CDC). 1996. Annual Summary, Salmonella Surveillance.

Cherubin CE. 1980. Epidemiologic assessment of antibiotic resistance in salmonella. In CRC Handbook Series in Zoonosis, I Sect D. JH Steele, ed. pp. 173–200.

Cherubin CE, Neu HC, Imperato PJ, Harvey RP, Bellen N. 1974. Septicemia with nontyphoid salmonella. Medicine 53:365–376.

Clarke RC, Gyles CL. 1987. Virulence of wild and mutant strains of *Salmonella typhimurium* in ligated intestinal segments of calves, pigs, and rabbits. Am J Vet Res 48:504–510.

——. 1993. Salmonella. In Pathogenesis of Bacterial Infections in Animals, 2d ed. Ames: Iowa State Univ Press, pp. 133–153.

Collins FM. 1974. Vaccines and cell-mediated immunity. Bacteriol Rev 38:371–402.

Committee on Salmonella. 1969. An evaluation of the salmonella problem. Washington, D.C.: Nat Acad Sci.

Craven JA, Hurst DB. 1982. The effect of time in lairage on the frequency of salmonella infection in slaughtered pigs. J Hyg (Camb) 88:107–111.

Cybulsky MI, Chan MKW, Movat HZ. 1988. Biology of disease: Acute inflammation and microthrombosis induced by endotoxin, interleukin-1, and tumor necrosis factor and their implication in gram-negative infection. Lab Invest 58:365–378.

Davies PR, Morrow WEM, Jones FT, Deen J, Fedorka-Cray PJ, Gray JT. 1997. Risk of shedding Salmonella organisms by market-age hogs in a barn with open-flush gutters. J Am Vet Med Assoc 210:386–389.

Davies R, Kotlarski I. 1976. The role for antibody in the expression of cellular immunity to *Salmonella typhimurium* C5. Aust J Exp Biol Med Sci 54:207–219.

Dawe DL, Troutt HF. 1976. Treatment of experimentally induced salmonellosis in weanling pigs with trimethoprim and sulfadiazine. Proc Int Congr Pig Vet Soc 4:M4.

Degeeter MH, Stahl GL, Geng S. 1976. Effect of lincomycin on prevalence, duration and quantity of *Salmonella typhimurium* excreted by swine. Am J Vet Res 37:525–529.

Dixon JMS. 1965. Effect of antibiotic treatment on duration of excretion of *Salmonella typhimurium* by children. Br Med J 2:1343–1345.

Eaves-Pyles T, Szabo C, Salzman AL. 1999. Bacterial invasion is not required for activation of NF-kappa beta in enterocytes. Infect Immun 67:800–804.

Edwards PR, Ewing WH. 1972. Identification of Enterobacteriaceae, 3d ed. Minneapolis: Burgess, pp. 146–207.

Elin RJ, Wolff SM. 1976. Biology of endotoxin. Ann Rev Med 27:127–141.

Evelsizer R. 1990. Salmonellosis in Grow-Finish pigs. Minnesota Swine Conf Vet, St. Paul.

Fales WH, Maddox CW, Oakman JK. 1990. Antimicrobial susceptibility of *Salmonella choleraesuis* from Missouri swine. In 33d Annu Meet AAVLD, Denver, Colo.

Fantuzzi G, Dinarello CA. 1999. Interleukin-18 and interleukin-1 beta: Two cytokine substrates for ICE (capsase-1). J Clin Immunol 19:1–11.

Fedorka-Cray PJ, Kelley LC, Stabel TJ, Gray JT, Laufer JA. 1995. Alternate routes of invasion may affect pathogenesis of *Salmonella typhimurium*. Infect Immun 63:2658–2664.

Fedorka-Cray PJ, Whipp SC, Isaacson RE, Nord N, Lager K. 1994. Transmission of *Salmonella typhimurium* to swine. Vet Micro 41:333–344.

Fenwick BS, Cullor JS, Osburn BI, Olander HJ. 1986. Mechanisms involved in protection provided by immunization against core lipopolysaccharides of *E. coli*. J strain from lethal Haemophilus pleuropneumonia in swine. Infect Immun 53:296–302.

Fenwick BW, Olander HJ. 1987. Experimental infection of weanling pigs with *Salmonella typhisuis*: Effect of feeding low concentrations of chlortetracycline, penicillin, and sulfamethazine. Am J Vet Res 48:1568–1573.

Ferris K, Frerichs W. 1996. Summary of Salmonella Isolated from Swine. Ames, Iowa: Nat Vet Services Laboratories.

Finlay BB, Heffron F, Falkow, S. 1989. Epithelial cell surfaces induce Salmonella proteins required for bacterial adherence and invasion. Science 243:940–943.

Finlayson M, Barnum DA. 1973. The effect of chlortetracycline feed additive on experimental salmonella infection of swine and antibiotic resistance transfer. Can J Comp Med 37:139–146.

Fukushima H, Hoshina K, Nakamura R, Ito Y. 1987. Raw beef, pork and chicken in Japan contaminated with *Salmonella* sp., *Campylobacter* sp., *Yersinia enterocolitica* and *Clostridium perfringens*: A comparative study. Zentralbl Bakteriol Mikrobiol Hyg 184:60–70.

Galton MM, Smith WV, McElrath HB, Hardy AB. 1954. Salmonella in swine, cattle, and the environment of abattoirs. J Infect Dis 95:236–245.

Gewirtz AT, Siber AM, Madara JL, McCormick BA. 1999. Orchestration of neutrophil movement by intestinal epithelial cells in response to *Salmonella typhimurium* can be uncoupled from bacterial internalization. Infect Immun 67:608–617.

Giannella RA, Formal SB, Dammin GJ Collins H. 1973. Pathogenesis of salmonellosis: Studies of fluid secretion, mucosal invasion, and morphologic reaction of the rabbit ileum. J Clin Invest 52:441–453.

Gooch JM, Goo V. 1971. Frequency of Salmonella isolation in selected foods of animal origin, Hawaii: The red meat processor's role in salmonella prevention. In Proc Nat Salmonellosis Sem, Washington, D.C.

Gooch JM, Haddock RL. 1969. Swine salmonellosis in a Hawaiian piggery. J Am Vet Med Assoc 154:1051–1054.

Gray JT, Fedorka-Cray PJ, Stabel TJ, Ackermann MR. 1995. Influence of inoculation route on the carrier state of *Salmonella choleraesuis* in swine. Vet Micro 47:43–59.

Gray JT, Stabel TJ, Fedorka-Cray PJ. 1996. Effect of dose on the immune response and persistence of *Salmonella choleraesuis* in swine. Am J Vet Res 57:313–319.

Groves BI, Fish NA, Mitchell WR. 1971. The occurrence of salmonella infection in market swine in Ontario. Can Vet J 12:11–15.

Gulig PA, Curtiss R. 1987. Plasmid associated virulence of *Salmonella typhimurium*. Infect Immun 55:2891–2901.

Gustafson RH, Kobland JD, Langner PH. 1976. Incidence and antibiotic resistance of salmonella in market swine. Proc Int Congr Pig Vet Soc 4:M2.

Gutzmann F, Layton H, Simiins K, Jarolmen H. 1976. Influence of antibiotic-supplemented feed on the occurrence and persistence of *Salmonella typhimurium* in experimentally infected swine. Am J Vet Res 37:649–655.

Hansen R, Rogers R, Emge S, Jacobs NJ. 1964. Incidence of Salmonella in the hog colon as affected by handling practices prior to slaughter. J Am Vet Med Assoc 145:139–140.

Harris IT, Fedorka-Cray PJ, Gray JT, Thomas LA, Ferris K. 1997. Prevalence of Salmonella organism in swine feed. J Am Vet Med Assoc 210:382–385.

Heard TW, Jennett NE, Linton AH. 1968. The control and eradication of salmonellosis in a closed pig herd. Vet Rec 82:92–99.

Heard TW, Linton AH, Penny RHC, Wilson MR. 1965. *Salmonella typhimurium* infection in a hysterectomy-produced herd of pigs. Vet Rec 77:1276–1279.

Helmuth R, Bunge C, et al. 1985. Epidemiology of virulence-associated plasmids and outer membrane protein patterns within several common Salmonella serotypes. Infect Immun 48:175–182.

Henry DP, Frost AJ, Samuel JL, O'Boyle DA, Thomson RH. 1983. Factors affecting the survival of Salmonella and *Escherichia coli* in anaerobically fermented pig waste. J Appl Bacteriol 55:89–95.

Hooper BE, Troutt HF. 1971. Swine salmonellosis. In Proc Carbadox: Synthetic Antibacterial Agent, Kansas City, pp. 83–101.

Hornick RB, Griesman SE, Woodward TE. 1970. Typhoid fever: Pathogenesis and immunologic control. N Engl J Med 283:735–746.

Hsu FS, Chueck LL, Shen YM. 1983. Isolation, serotyping and drug resistance of salmonellae in scouring pigs in Taiwan. Chung Hua Min Kuo Wei Sheng Wu Chi Mien I Hsueh Tsa Chih 16:283–290.

Isaacson RE. 1996. Persistent colonization of pigs by *Salmonella typhimurium* and effects of transportation related stress on the shedding of *Salmonella typhimurium*. In 1st Int Symp Ecology of Salmonella in Pork Products, NADC, Ames, Iowa.

Jacks TM, Frazier E, Judith FR, Olson G. 1988. Effect of efrotomycin in feed on the quantity, duration, and prevalence of shedding and antibacterial susceptibility of *Salmonella typhimurium* in experimentally infected swine. Am J Vet Res 49:1832–1835.

Jacks TM, Welter CJ, Fitzgerald GR, Miller BM. 1981. Cephamycin C treatment of induced swine salmonellosis. Antimicrob Agents Chemother 19:562–566.

Jayarao BM, Biro G, Kovacs S, Domjan H, Fabian A. 1989. Prevalence of Salmonella serotypes in pigs and evaluation of a rapid, presumptive test for detection of Salmonella in pig faeces. Acta Vet Hung 37:39–44.

Jones FT, Langlois BE, Cromwell GL, Hays VW. 1983. Effect of feeding chlortetracycline or virginiamycin on shedding of salmonellae from experimentally infected swine. J Anim Sci 57:279–285.

Jubb KVF, Kennedy PC, Palmer NC. 1993. Pathology of Domestic Animals. San Diego: Academic Press.

Kampelmacher EH, Guinee PAM, Van Keulen A. 1965. Prevalence of salmonellosis in pigs fed decontaminated and normal feeds. Zentralbl Veterinärmed (B) 12:258–267.

Kinsey MD, Dammin GJ, Formal SB, Giannella RA. 1976. The role of altered intestinal permeability in the pathogenesis of salmonella-diarrhea in the rhesus monkey. Gastroenterology 71:429–434.

Kramer TT, Pardon P, Marly J, Bernard S. 1987. Conjunctival and intramuscular vaccination of pigs with a live avirulent strain of *Salmonella choleraesuis*. Am J Vet Res 48:1072–1076.

Kramer TT, Roof MB, Matheson RR. 1992. Safety and efficacy of an attenuated strain of *Salmonella choleraesuis* for vaccination of swine. Am J Vet Res 53:444–448.

Lawson GHK, Dow C. 1966. Porcine salmonellosis. J Comp Pathol 76:363–371.

Levine ND, Peterson EH, Graham R. 1945. Studies on swine enteritis. II. Salmonella and other enteric organisms isolated from diseased and normal swine. Am J Vet Res 6:241–246.

Lee CA, Silva M, Siber AM, Kelly AJ, Galyov E, McCormick BA. 2000. A secreted salmonella protein induces a proinflammatory response in epithelial cells, which promotes neutrophil migration. Proc. Natl. Acad. Sci. USA 97:12283–12288.

Low JC, Angus M, Hopkins G, Munro D, Rankin SC. 1997. Antimicrobial resistance of *Salmonella enterica* typhimurium DT104 isolates and investigation of strains with transferable apramycin resistance. Epid Infect 118:97–103.

Lynn M, Dobson AW, McClune EL, Dorn CR. 1972. A study of *Salmonella typhimurium* infection in a swine-testing station. Vet Med Small Anim Clin 67:1022–1027.

McCaughey WG, McClelland TG, Roddy RM. 1973. Salmonella isolations in pigs. Vet Rec 92:191–194.

McCormick BA, Miller SI, Carnes D, Madara JL. 1995. Transepithelial signaling to neutrophils by salmonellae: A novel virulence mechanism for gastroenteritis. Infect Immun 63:2302–2309.

McErlean BA.1968. *Salmonella dublin* meningitis in piglets. Vet Rec 82:257–258.

Meyerholz DK, Stabel TJ. 2003. Comparison of early ileal invasion by *Salmonella enterica* serovars Choleraesuis and Typhimurium. Vet Pathol 40(4):371–375.

Meyerholz DK, Stabel TJ, Ackermann MR, Carlson SA, Jones BD, Pohlenz J. 2002. Early epithelial invasion by *Salmonella enterica* serovar Typhimurium DT104 in the swine ileum. Vet Pathol 39(6):712–720.

Michaud RP. 1978. Contributory Sources of Salmonella in the Environment of Swine Slaughterhouses. M.S. thesis, Univ Guelph.

Mills KW, Kelly BL. 1986. Antibiotic susceptibilities of swine *Salmonella* isolants from 1979 to 1983. Am J Vet Res 47:2349–2350.

Mittermeyer FC, Foltz VD. 1969. Salmonella survey of plant foods used in and around the home. Appl Microbiol 18:682–683.

Morehouse LG. 1972. Salmonellosis in swine and its control. J Am Vet Med Assoc 160:594–601.

Morgan IR, Krautil FL, Craven JA. 1987. Effect of time in lairage on caecal and carcass salmonella contamination of slaughter pigs. Epidemiol Infect 98:323–330.

Morse JW, Hird DW. 1984. Bacteria isolated from lymph nodes of California slaughter swine. Am J Vet Res 45:1648–1649.

Mousing J. Thode Jensen P, Bager F, Feld N, Nielsen B, Nielsen JP, Bech-Nielsen S. 1997. Nation-wide *Salmonella enterica* surveillance and control in Danish slaughter swine herds. Prev Vet Med 29:247–261.

Nape WF, Murphy C. 1971. Recovery of salmonellae in feed mills, using terminally heated and regularly processed animal protein. J Am Vet Med Assoc 159:1569–1572.

Nielsen B, Baggesen D, Bager F, Haugegaard J, Lind P. 1995. The serological response to *Salmonella* serovars *typhimurium* and *infantis* in experimentally infected pigs: The time course followed with an indirect anti-LPS ELISA and bacteriological examinations. Vet Microbiol 47:205–218.

Nottingham PM, Penney N, Wyborn R. 1972. Salmonella infection in calves and other animals. III. Further studies with pigs and calves. NZ J Agric Res 15:279–283.

Olson LD, Rodebaugh DE, Morehouse LG. 1977. Comparison of furazolidone and carbadox in the feed for treatment of *Salmonella choleraesuis* in swine. Am J Vet Res 38:1471–1477.

Pokorny J. 1988. Survival and virulence of salmonellae in water. J Hyg Epidemiol Microbiol Immunol 32:361–366.

Pospischil A, Wood RL, Anderson TD. 1990. Peroxidase-antiperoxidase and immunogold labeling of *Salmonella typhimurium* and *Salmonella choleraesuis* var kunzendorf in tissues of experimentally infected swine. Am J Vet Res 51:619–624.

Reed WM, Olander HJ, Thacker HL. 1985. Studies on the pathogenesis of *Salmonella heidelberg* infection in weanling pigs. Am J Vet Res 46:2300–2310.

——. 1986. Studies on the pathogenesis of *Salmonella typhimurium* and *Salmonella choleraesuis* var. kunzendorf infection in weanling pigs. Am J Vet Res 47:75–83.

Rescigno M, Urbano M, Valzasina B, Francolini M, Rotta G, Bonasio R, Granucci F, Kraehenbuhl JP, Ricciardi-Castagnoli P. 2001. Dendritic cells express tight junction proteins and penetrate gut epithelial monolayers to sample bacteria. Nat Immunol 2:361–367.

Reynolds IM, Miner PW, Smith RE. 1967. *Salmonella enteritidis* from porcine meningitis: A case report. Cornell Vet 58:180–185.

Riley MGI. 1970. The incidence of salmonellosis in normal slaughtered pigs in Australia. Aust Vet J 46:40–43.

Roberts D, Boag K, Hall MLM, Shipp CR. 1975. The isolation of salmonella from British pork sausage and sausage meat. J Hyg (Camb) 75:173–184.

Roof MB, Doitchinoff DD. 1995. Safety, efficacy, and duration of immunity induced in swine by use of an avirulent live *Salmonella choleraesuis*-containing vaccine. Am J Vet Res 56:39–44.

Roof MB, Kramer TT, Kunesh JP, Roth JA. 1992b. In vivo isolation of *Salmonella choleraesuis* from porcine neutrophils. Am J Vet Res 53:1333–1346.

Roof MB, Kramer TT, Roth JA, Minion CF. 1992a. Characterization of a *Salmonella choleraesuis* isolate after repeated neutrophil exposure. Am J Vet Res 53:1328–1332.

Rout WR, Formal SB, Giannella RA, Dammin GJ. 1974. Pathophysiology of Salmonella diarrhea in the rhesus monkey: Intestinal transport, morphologic and bacteriological studies. Gastroenterology 67:59–70.

Rubin RH, Weinstein L. 1977. Salmonellosis. New York: Stratton Intercontinental Medical Book Corp., p. 25.

Salmon DE, Smith T. 1886. The bacterium of swine plague. Am Mon Microbiol J 7:204.

Schauser K, Olsen JE, Larsson LI. 2004. Immunocytochemical studies of *Salmonella typhimurium* invasion of procine jejunal epithelial cells. J Med Microbiol 53(7):691–695.

Schultz RA. 1989. Salmonellosis—The Problem—How Do We Handle It? Proc Am Assoc Swine Prod, Des Moines, Iowa.

Schwartz KJ. 1991. Salmonellosis in swine. Compend Contin Educ 13(1):139–148.

——. 1997a. A summary of 1994–1996 Annual Reports of the Iowa State University Veterinary Diagnostic Laboratory, Ames, Iowa.

——. 1997b. Salmonellosis. Proc AASP, Quebec City, Quebec.

Schwartz KJ, Daniels G. 1987. Salmonellosis. Proc Minnesota Swine Herd Health Prog Conf, Univ Minnesota.

Silas JC, Carpenter JA, Reagan JO. 1984. Update: Prevalence of Salmonella in pork sausage. J Anim Sci 59:122–124.

Skovgaard N, Christensen SG, Culistani AW. 1985. Salmonellas in Danish pigs: A comparison of three isolation methods. J Hyg (Lond) 95:69–75.

Smith HW, Jones JET. 1967. Observations on experimental oral infection with *Salmonella dublin* in calves and *Salmonella choleraesuis* in pigs. J Pathol 93:141–156.

Stephen J, Wallis TS, Starkey WG, Candy DCA, Osborne MP, Huddon S. 1985. Salmonellosis: In retrospect and prospect. In Microbial Toxins and Diarrhoeal Diseases. Ciba Foundation Symposium. London: Pitman.

Surkiewicz BF, Johnston RW, Elliott EP, Simmons ER. 1972. Bacteriologic survey of fresh pork sausage produced at establishments under federal inspection. Appl Microbiol 23:515–520.

Tacal JV, Lawrence W. 1980. A survey for salmonella among market swine in southern California, 1980. Calif Vet 11:15–18.

Takeuchi A. 1967. Electron-microscopic studies of experimental salmonella infection. I. Penetration into the intestinal epithelium by *Salmonella typhimurium*. Am J Pathol 50:109–136.

Takeuchi A, Sprinz H. 1967. Electron microscopic studies of experimental salmonella infection in the preconditioned guinea pig. II. Response of the intestinal mucosa to the invasion by *Salmonella typhimurium*. Am J Pathol 51:137–161.

Taylor J, McCoy JH. 1969. Salmonella and Arizona infections and intoxications. In Foodborne Infections and Intoxications. New York: Academic Press, pp. 3–71.

Vassiliadis P, Mavromati C, Trichopoulus D, Kalapothaki V, Papadakis J. 1987. Comparison of procedures based upon Rappaport-Vassiliadis medium with those using Muller-Kauffmann medium containing Teepol for the isolation of *Salmonella* sp. Epidemiol Infect 99:143–147.

Vazquez-Torres A, Jones-Carlson J, Baumler AJ, Falkow S, Valdivia R, Brown W, Le M, Berggren R, Parks WT, Fang FC. 1999. Extraintestinal dissemination of Salmonella by CD18-expressing phagocytes. Nature 401:804–808.

——. 2000. Salmonella pathogenesis: The Trojan horse or the New York shuttle? Gastroenterol 118:803–805.

Welliver RC, Ogra PL. 1978. Importance of local immunity in enteric infection. J Am Vet Med Assoc 173:560–564.

Wilcock BP. 1978. Experimental *Klebsiella* and *Salmonella* infection in neonatal swine. Can J Comp Med 43:100–106.

——. 1979. Serotype-associated virulence factors in porcine salmonellosis. Conf Res Workers, Anim Dis Res Inst, Ottawa.

Wilcock BP, Armstrong CH, Olander HJ. 1976. The significance of the serotype in the clinical and pathologic features of naturally occurring porcine salmonellosis. Can J Comp Med 40:80–88.

Wilcock BP, Olander HJ. 1977a. The pathogenesis of porcine rectal stricture. I. Observations on the naturally occurring disease and its association with salmonellosis. Vet Pathol 14:36–42.

——. 1977b. The pathogenesis of porcine rectal stricture. II. Experimental salmonellosis and rectal stricture. Vet Pathol 14:43–55.

——. 1977c. Neurologic disease in naturally occurring *Salmonella choleraesuis* infection in pigs. Vet Pathol 14:113–120.

——. 1978. Influence of oral antibiotic feeding on the duration and severity of clinical disease, growth performance and pattern of shedding in swine inoculated with *Salmonella typhimurium*. J Am Vet Med Assoc 172:472–477.

Will LA, Diesch SL, Pomeroy BX. 1973. Survival of *Salmonella typhimurium* in animal manure disposed in a model oxidation ditch. Am J Public Health 63:322–336.

Williams CB. 1975. Environmental considerations in salmonellosis. Vet Rec 93:317–321.

Williams LP, Newell KW. 1970. Salmonella excretion in joy-riding pigs. Am J Public Health 50:926–929.

Williams LP, Vaughn JP, Scott A, Blanton V. 1969. A ten-month study on salmonella contamination in animal protein meals. J Am Vet Med Assoc 155:167–174.

Wolff SM. 1973. Biologic effects of bacterial endotoxins in man. J Infect Dis 128(Suppl):159–164.

Wood RL, Pospischil A, Rose R. 1989. Distribution of persistent *Salmonella typhimurium* infection in internal organs of swine. Am J Vet Res 50:1015–1021.

Wood RL, Rose R. 1992. Populations of *Salmonella typhimurium* in internal organs of experimentally infected carrier swine. Am J Vet Res 53:653–658.

Wray C, Sojka WJ. 1977. Reviews of progress in dairy science: Bovine salmonellosis. J Dairy Res 44:383–425.

46 Porcine Colonic Spirochetosis / Intestinal Spirochetosis

David J. Hampson and G. E. Duhamel

Porcine colonic spirochetosis (PCS), also known as porcine intestinal spirochetosis, is a spirochete-associated colitis that occurs mainly in weaner and grower pigs. The disease results from infection with a weakly hemolytic anaerobic intestinal spirochete that is distinct from *Brachyspira hyodysenteriae*, the agent of swine dysentery (Taylor et al. 1980; Zuerner et al. 2004). The spirochete causing PCS is now named *Brachyspira pilosicoli* (Ochiai et al. 1997), although it has also been referred to as "*Anguillina coli*" (Lee et al. 1993), "*Serpulina coli*" (Duhamel et al. 1993), a group IV weakly hemolytic intestinal spirochete (Fellström and Gunnarsson 1995) and, most recently, *Serpulina pilosicoli* (Trott et al. 1996a).

Infection with *B. pilosicoli* usually causes a mild to moderate typhlocolitis accompanied with either watery diarrhea or stools with the consistency of "wet cement," sometimes containing mucus. Based on the severity and extent of the colonic damage, affected pigs display variable loss of condition and reduced growth rate. Individual infected pigs may show increased time to reach market weight, thus disrupting efficient production flow through commercial units (Duhamel 1998).

A common histologic feature in the early phase of PCS is the presence of focal areas of inflammation in the cecum, colon, and/or rectum, where large numbers of spirochetes may be found attached by one cell end to the apical surface of the epithelium, forming a "false brush border" (Taylor et al. 1980; Girard et al. 1995) (Figure 46.1). This characteristic attachment of *B. pilosicoli* also is found in natural disease in other hosts, including humans (Trivett-Moore et al. 1998), nonhuman primates (Duhamel et al. 1997; Duhamel et al. 2003), dogs (Duhamel et al. 1996), domestic chickens (Trampel et al. 1994; McLaren et al. 1997; Stephens and Hampson 2001), and various species of wild birds (Webb et al. 1997; Jansson et al. 2001). Because isolation of *B. pilosicoli* from feces does not always correlate with the presence of diarrhea or end-on epithelial attachment of the spirochetes, the significance of identifying the spirochete needs to be interpreted in the context of a complete diagnostic investigation (Thomson et al. 1998). Experimental challenge studies in susceptible pigs have clearly shown that *B. pilosicoli* is associated with all of the clinical and pathological changes seen in spontaneous PCS (reviewed by Duhamel 2001).

PCS was first described by Taylor and colleagues (1980), who challenged 7- to 8-week-old susceptible weaned pigs with a weakly beta-hemolytic intestinal spirochete (strain P43/6/78^T). The pigs developed a mucoid diarrhea containing flecks of blood, and lesions of colitis. This spirochete initially was thought to be a strain of the nonpathogenic weakly beta-hemolytic intestinal spirochete *Brachyspira innocens*, but it is now recognized as the type strain of the species *B. pilosicoli*. PCS with or without end-on attachment of spirochetes to the colonic mucosa has since been experimentally reproduced in pigs in several independent investigations, using other strains of *B. pilosicoli* besides P43/6/78^T (e.g., Trott et al. 1996b; Thomson et al. 1997; Duhamel 1998; Jensen et al. 2000; Jensen et al. 2004a). PCS is increasingly recognized as an important cause of colitis worldwide. Reasons for this include the increased availability of improved diagnostic methods for differentiation of *B. pilosicoli* from other intestinal spirochetes, the withdrawal of routine antimicrobial growth promoters that might otherwise have been supressing the growth of *B. pilosicoli*, and the fact that other major intestinal diseases such as salmonellosis and swine dysentery are now better controlled in many countries (Duhamel 1996). It is likely that at least some of the cases of "nonspecific colitis" reported in the United Kingdom may have been caused by *B. pilosicoli*, although a noninfectious, diet-responsive colitis also appears to exist (Wood 1991). PCS has been reported in most major pig-producing countries, including Australia (Hampson 1990; Lee et al. 1993), Belgium (Castryck et al. 1997; Hommez et al 1998a), Brazil (Barcellos et al. 2000a), Canada (Jacques et al. 1989; Girard et al. 1995), Denmark (Møller et al. 1998), Finland (Heinonen et al. 2000), France (Pronost et al. 1999), Germany (Verspohl et al. 2001), Korea (Choi

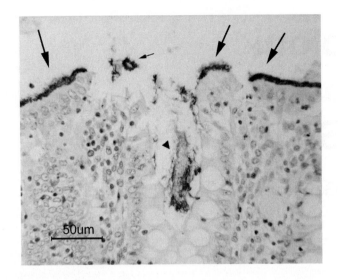

46.1. *Light photomicrograph of the colonic epithelium obtained from a pig with spontaneous porcine colonic spirochetosis and stained by immunohistochemistry. A dark fringe of spirochetes attached by one cell end along the brush border of epithelial cells (big arrows) and free in the mucin in the lumen of the crypt opening (arrowhead). Note a raft of spirochetes attached to necrotic epithelial cells sloughing into the lumen (small arrow). Brachyspira-specific monoclonal antibody to FlaB periplasmic flagellar core proteins followed by the avidinbiotin-alkaline phosphatase complex method.*

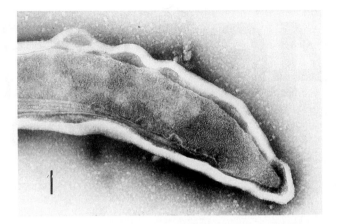

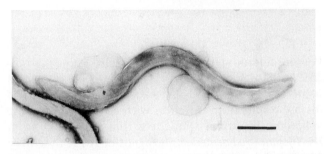

46.2. *(A) Electron photomicrograph of magnified cell end of Brachy-spira pilosicoli strain P43/6/78^T showing pointed tip, five periplasmic flagella, and insertion discs (marker bar = 0.1 μm). (B) Photomicrograph of a whole cell of P43/6/78^T showing the spiral morphology of the spirochete (marker bar = 0.5 μm).*

et al. 2002), Spain (de Arriba et al. 2002), Sweden (Fell-ström et al. 1996), the United Kingdom (Taylor et al. 1980; Thomson et al. 1998; Thomson et al. 2001), and the United States (Ramanathan et al. 1993; Duhamel et al. 1995a). Much of the research concerning PCS has been undertaken in the last decade, and many important aspects of the disease are still poorly understood, including detailed epidemiology, virulence determinants of the spirochete, and pathogenesis of infection—including the role of host immune and inflammatory responses. The overall economic impact of PCS also has not been critically evaluated.

ETIOLOGY

Brachyspira pilosicoli is the etiologic agent of PCS (by definition), but, in the field, mixed infections with other enteric pathogens frequently occur. *B. pilosicoli* has a characteristic spirochete morphology and a general appearance similar to other species in the genus *Brachyspira* (formerly *Serpulina*). It is 6–10 μm long, 0.25–0.30 μm wide, and characteristically has 4–7 periplasmic flagella attached at each cell end, and pointed ends (Figure 46.2). The spirochete has a pronounced corkscrew like motility that helps it penetrate and move through mucus overlying the colonic epithelium. The outer envelope of the spirochete contains a semirough type lipooligosaccharide, and this is serologically heterogeneous among different strains (Lee and Hampson 1999). A number of outer membrane proteins and lipoproteins of *B. pilosicoli*

have been described, but more work is needed to define their potential role in disease, including whether they may be involved in attachment and/or in generating protective immunity (reviewed by Trott et al. 2001).

Brachyspira pilosicoli is cultured under the same anaerobic conditions as those described for *B. hyodysenteriae* (see Chapter 48). After 3–5 days incubation on trypticase soy blood agar, *B. pilosicoli* forms a thin spreading surface haze surrounded by a zone of weak beta-hemolysis. For isolation, plates containing colistin (25 μg/ml), vancomycin (25 μg/ml), and spectinomycim (400 μg/ml) are widely used (CVS; Jenkinson and Wingar 1981). The inclusion of rifampicin and spiramycin, sometimes recommended for the isolation of *B. hyodysenteriae*, inhibits the growth of *B. pilosicoli* and thus is not recommended (Duhamel and Joens 1994; Duhamel et al. 1995b; Trott et al. 1996c). Slicing the agar prior to primary inoculation, as reported for *B. hyodysenteriae* (Olson 1996), can improve the recovery of *B. pilosicoli*. However, by contrast with *B. hyodysenteriae*, a zone of enhanced hemolysis, or ring phenomenon, is not usually seen with *B. pilosicoli*. Once isolated, the spirochete grows readily in various liquid media, such as in a prereduced anaerobically sterilized (PRAS) medium based on trypticase soy broth (Kunkle et al. 1986) and in Brain Heart Infusion broth.

In the last decade, the taxonomy of the porcine intestinal spirochetes has undergone considerable revision (Hampson and Trott 1995; Hampson and Stanton 1997). Currently there are four species of weakly beta-hemolytic anaerobic spirochetes recognized as colonizing pigs, of which only *B. pilosicoli* is confirmed to be a pathogen. Other porcine intestinal spirochetes of unusual phenotypes and uncertain taxa also have been reported (Thomson et al. 2001). Although *B. pilosicoli* contains a copy of the *hlyA* gene that encodes a hemolysin in *B. hyodysenteriae* (Hsu et al. 2001), it is believed that this is either not expressed in *B. pilosicoli* or expressed in a form that results in reduced hemolytic activity (Zuerner et al. 2004).

Until recently the four named weakly hemolytic *Brachyspira* species colonizing pigs belonged to the genus *Serpulina,* but in 1997 the strongly hemolytic *Serpulina hyodysenteriae* and weakly hemolytic *S. innocens* and *S. pilosicoli* were transferred to the genus *Brachyspira* (Ochiai et al. 1997; Validation list 1998). Unfortunately, two weakly beta-hemolytic spirochete species of pigs, *Serpulina intermedia* and *Serpulina murdochii* (Stanton et al. 1997), were not officially transferred. Nevertheless, by general agreement among spirochete scientists, they are now "unofficially" referred to as *Brachyspira intermedia* and *Brachyspira murdochii* (Hampson 2000). These four species of weakly hemolytic intestinal spirochete have a similar appearance on blood agar and can be differentiated only by biochemical and genetic typing techniques. *B. innocens*, *B. intermedia*, and *B. murdochii* have not been shown to cause disease in experimentally infected conventional pigs and are generally considered to be nonpathogenic commensals in pigs (Lee et al. 1993; Jensen et al. 2000). On the other hand, certain strains of avian *B. intermedia* are pathogenic in commercial chickens (Hampson and McLaren 1999), and a porcine strain caused cecal damage in experimentally infected 1-day-old chicks (Trott and Hampson 1998). Additionally, *B. intermedia* can cause lesions when inoculated into isolated porcine colonic loops (Binek and Szynkiewicz 1984) and on occasions has been associated with diarrhea in pigs in the field (Fellström and Gunnarsson 1995). Overall, however, it remains doubtful whether *B. intermedia* is a cause of enteric disease in pigs. Some strains of *B. innocens* isolated from pigs with diarrhea have been shown to cause diarrhea and lesions when inoculated into gnotobiotic pigs (Neef et al. 1994), but again whether or not they are capable of causing significant disease under field conditions (for example, under certain specialized circumstances) remains uncertain. The identification of virulence determinants among *Brachyspira* species should help resolve some of these questions. Currently, the main significance of the commensal weakly hemolytic intestinal spirochetes is that their presence may complicate attempts to diagnose PCS and/or swine dysentery. Recently, a *Brachyspira*-like spirochete was found associated with lesions of colitis in experimentally infected pigs in Finland. Surprisingly, this spirochete hybridized with a nucleic acid probe against *Leptospira* but not with a *Brachyspira* probe (Jensen et al. 2004b). The significance of this finding is not clear, but if such organisms exist and are widespread they also could complicate attempts to diagnose spirochete-associated colitis.

EPIDEMIOLOGY

The detailed epidemiology of PCS has not been fully determined. Infection is believed to occur by the fecal/oral route, and, as previously shown with swine dysentery, PCS in naive herds may be introduced by carrier pigs. *B. pilosicoli* can persist in the environment; therefore, the disease can recur between batches of pigs if the premises are not adequately cleaned and disinfected. In fact, *B. pilosicoli* can survive in spiked feces kept at different temperatures for longer than *B. hyodysenteriae* (Barcellos et al. 2000b). Oxberry et al. (1998) showed that *B. pilosicoli* can survive in lake water at 4°C for 66 days, again surviving longer than *B. hyodysenteriae*. Other studies have shown that *B. pilosicoli* remains viable for 119 days in soil and 210 days both in soil with 10% pig feces and in pig feces kept at 10°C (Boye et al. 2001). The spirochete is susceptible to many commonly used disinfectants, but the efficacy of some of these products is reduced in the presence of organic matter, such as feces (Corona-Barrera et al. 2004a).

Various studies have demonstrated that *B. pilosicoli* may be isolated from pigs during any period of the growing stage, but infection is most common and significant in weaner and grower pigs. Lack of availability of serologic assays has hampered progress in determining antibody titers indicative of exposure in live animals. Instead, detection of *B. pilosicoli* in live animals is usually accomplished by bacteriological culture of feces as described above, followed by identification of suspected bacterial growth using amplification of *Brachyspira* species-specific nucleotide sequences by the polymerase chain reaction (PCR), as described below.

Using these detection techniques, the prevalence of *B. pilosicoli* among herds in different geographic regions has been estimated. In a study in Sweden, *B. pilosicoli* was isolated from 6 of 7 (85.6%) herds with diarrhea, and from only 1 of 8 herds without diarrhea (Fellström et al. 1996). In a survey conducted in the U.K. between 1992 and 1996 that involved 85 pig farms with colitis and diarrhea, *B. pilosicoli* was identified as the primary etiological agent on 21 (25%) units, and formed part of a mixed infection on another 23 (27%) units (Thomson et al. 1998). In a follow-up investigation conducted between 1997 and 1999 on 98 farms with problems of diarrhea and enterocolitis, *B. pilosicoli* was the primary etiologic agent in 18 (18.4%) units, and was involved as part of a mixed infection in 24 (24.5%) units—indicating that PCS continues to be a significant problem in the U.K. (Thomson et al. 2001). In Denmark, *B. pilosicoli* was isolated from 10 of 72 (13.9%) herds with diarrhea and from none of 26 herds where diarrhea was not a problem (Møller et al. 1998). In a subsequent study of 79 randomly selected herds, 15 (19.0%) were found to contain grower pigs colonized by *B. pilosicoli*, with these having a within-herd prevalence rate of 5–10% (Stege et al. 2000). In a survey conducted in Finland in 1997, *B. pilosicoli* was isolated from 14 of 50 (28%) high health status farms (Heinonen et al. 2000), whereas a survey conducted in 1998 in Brazil revealed *B. pilosicoli* in the feces of growers in 7 of 17 (41.2%) farms where diarrhea was a problem (Barcellos et al. 2000a). A recent study from Sweden revealed that the presence of *B. pilosicoli* and *L. intracellularis* was significantly associated with herds having poor performance in growing pigs (Jacobson et al. 2003). Collectively, these studies indicate that a variable, but often very high, proportion of farms that have persistent diarrhea are also infected with *B. pilosicoli*, whereas farms without diarrhea have very low or no infection. The specific prevalence values obtained in individual surveys must be interpreted with caution, because they can be influenced by several factors, including the concurrent administration of antibiotics, the age of the pigs examined, the methods of collection and handling of specimens, the limitations of culture and identification methods used, and the degree of contamination with other fecal organisms, all of which can affect the ability to detect *B. pilosicoli*.

Relatively few detailed epidemiologic studies have examined the within–herd pattern of *B. pilosicoli* infection. Recently, Oxberry and Hampson (2003) conducted cross-sectional and cohort studies on two Australian farms with PCS. Their study demonstrated that the on-farm epidemiology of *B. pilosicoli* can be highly variable. The prevalence on farm A (>2,000 sows) was 2.4%, with infection largely confined to grower/finisher pigs. All isolates obtained were identical—a situation that resembles swine dysentery, where all infections on a farm usually can be attributed to a single strain of *B. hyodysenteriae*.

On farm B, an 80-sow research farm that received replacement pigs from farm A, the prevalence among growers and finishers was 12.2%, and weaners also were infected. Here, not only was the prevalence higher, but the 10 isolates obtained were genetically heterogeneous, comprising seven different genetic types. The results were consistent with those from a small farm investigated in an earlier study, where nine genotypes of *B. pilosicoli* were identified among 14 isolates obtained from different pigs (Trott et al. 1998). The presence of multiple *B. pilosicoli* genotypes within certain farms might explain why PCS commonly recurs in convalescent animals or in those that have been treated with antimicrobials. In such cases, reinfection may be with a different strain, possibly having different antigenic determinants, antimicrobial susceptibilities, or potential to colonize and cause disease. Porcine strains of *B. pilosicoli* with different pathogenic potentials probably do exist (Thomson et al. 1997; Jensen et al. 2004a).

The extensive genetic diversity of strains from within the species *B. pilosicoli* is well established (Lee and Hampson 1994). Members of the species apparently are capable of undergoing genetic recombination and rearrangements (Trott et al. 1998; Zuerner et al. 2004), perhaps in part associated with the activity of a generalized transducing bacteriophage (Stanton et al. 2003). A recent study of strain diversity among isolates from pig herds in Finland revealed that most farms had their own distinct genotypes of *B. pilosicoli*, whilst it was rare to find the same genotype on different farms (Fossi et al. 2003). Interestingly, the within-farm genotypes appeared fairly stable, because three farms that were re–examined after 3 years still had the same genotypes of *B. pilosicoli* present.

In the study of Oxberry and Hampson (2003), on farm B, *B. pilosicoli* also was detected in chickens, effluent pond water, and wild ducks on the effluent pond. An isolate from the pond belonged to the same genetic type as one from a pig, a finding consistent with a previous observation suggesting that feral waterbirds may contaminate water supplies and so represent a potential source of *B. pilosicoli* infection for pigs (Oxberry et al. 1998). Although it is well established that rodents can be persistent carriers of *B. hyodysenteriae*, they appear less likely to serve as a biologic reservoir of *B. pilosicoli*. To date there appears to be only one report of a natural infection of a feral mouse with *B. pilosicoli* (Fellström et al. 2004). The apparent rarity of this occurrence may relate to the fact that it is difficult to obtain colonization of laboratory mice with *B. pilosicoli* unless they receive specialized diets that increase fermentation in the large intestine (Sacco et al. 1997; Jamshidian et al. 2004).

In addition to pigs, a wide range of animal species may be naturally infected with *B. pilosicoli* (reviewed by Duhamel 2001), and typical clinical signs and lesions associated with PCS have been recorded in all host species, including humans. Although isolates from pigs, dogs, birds, and humans are genetically closely related (Lee and Hampson 1994; Trott et al. 1998), clear evidence for zoonotic transmission has not been obtained. Nevertheless, human strains of *B. pilosicoli* can cause disease when inoculated into conventional pigs (Trott et al. 1996b) and can colonize 1-day-old chicks (Duhamel et al. 1995a; Trott et al. 1995; Muniappa et al. 1997; Muniappa et al. 1998; Trott and Hampson 1998) and adult chickens (Jamshidi and Hampson 2003). Therefore, the potential for cross-transmission of *B. pilosicoli* between humans and animals cannot be discounted. Colonization of humans with *B. pilosicoli* is usually associated with either an immunocompromised state or poor hygiene, such as occurs in developing communities where fecal contamination of water supplies is often found (Margawani et al. 2004; Munshi et al. 2004). Consequently, industry workers who are healthy are unlikely to be at risk of developing disease from contact with pigs with PCS.

PATHOGENESIS

The pathogenesis of PCS is not well understood but is thought to differ from swine dysentery in several aspects (Johnston et al. 1999). Infection is often associated with the presence of large numbers of spirochetes attached by one cell end to the luminal surface of colonic and cecal epithelial cells. Additionally, the colitis associated with PCS is usually much less severe than swine dysentery and resembles the early stages of that disease.

As with swine dysentery, *B. pilosicoli* colonization and/or expression of disease can be influenced by the pig's diet. An analysis of risk factors on farms revealed that reduced prevalences can result from using home-mixed and/or nonpelleted diets (Stege et al. 2001). Reducing the energy and protein content of the diet also has alleviated clinical problems (Spearman et al. 1988; Wilkinson and Wood 1987). Addition of carboxymethylcellulose to a weaner pig diet, to experimentally increase the viscosity of the intestinal contents, enhanced colonization with *B. pilosicoli* (Hopwood et al. 2002). The authors speculated that high levels of soluble nonstarch polysaccharide ("soluble fiber"), such as are present in grains like barley and rye, may similarly increase viscosity and enhance *B. pilosicoli* colonization. Consistent with this, pigs fed diets based on cooked white rice (highly digestible and low in soluble fiber) have shown reduced colonization with *B. pilosicoli* compared to pigs fed conventional diets (Hampson et al. 2000; Lindecrona et al. 2004). In the study of Lindecrona and co-workers (2004), feeding pigs a pelleted diet rather than meal increased the risk of colonization, but feeding fermented liquid feed or lactic acid did not influence colonization.

In order to be able to colonize, *B. pilosicoli* cells need to be able to penetrate and move through the mucus overlying the colonic mucosa. Cells of *B. pilosicoli* are motile, but are not attracted to colonic mucin in the same way as are virulent strains of *B. hyodysenteriae* (Milner and Sellwood 1994), and their chemotactic response appears to be modulated by the presence of certain substrates in the growth medium (Witters and Duhamel 1999). Pigs convalescent from PCS have serum IgG antibodies to a membrane lipoprotein of *B. pilosicoli* that is homologous to MglB, the glucose and galactose transport and chemoreceptor lipoprotein present in the pathogenic spirochetes *Borrelia burgdorferi*, the cause of Lyme disease, and *Treponema pallidum*, the syphilis spirochete (Zhang et al. 2000). As this protein is involved in motility-regulated signal transduction of the spirochete and is recognized by pigs recovered from PCS, it must be expressed during infection, perhaps during scavenging of glycoconjugate present in colonic mucin. Hence it likely plays a role in mucosal association.

Following experimental inoculation, *B. pilosicoli* may be shed in the feces within 2–7 days, although the incubation period may range up to 20 days. In the initial stage of infection, *B. pilosicoli* cells can adhere in large numbers to the surface of cecal and colonic epithelial cells, resulting in effacement of the microvilli and disruption of the terminal web microfilaments. Attachment occurs to only mature apical enterocytes between crypt units, and spirochetes do not attach to immature cells deeper within intestinal crypts (Trott et al. 1996b). Epithelial cell damage results in an increase in the crypt cell mitotic rate, crypt elongation, and the replacement of the mature columnar epithelium by squamous or cuboidal cells. Erosion of the epithelium is evident grossly as small adherent nodules on the surface of the mucosa (Figure 46.3).

B. pilosicoli cells have been observed inside dilated colonic crypts (Trott et al. 1996b), invading through tight junctions between colonic enterocytes, within

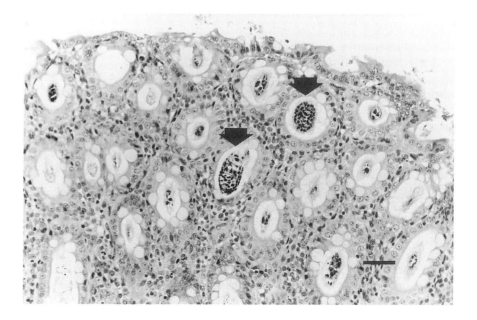

46.3. *Colonic mucosa of a chronic case of porcine colonic spirochetosis. Note the coalescing erosions accompanied by mucosal hyperemia and hemorrhage.*

goblet cells (Thomson et al. 1997), and within the lamina propria (Duhamel 2001). The presence of *B. pilosicoli* within crypts and the lamina propria is associated with neutrophilic exocytosis (crypt abscesses) and colitis characterized by edema, with a mixed infiltrate of neutrophils and lymphocytes within the lamina propria and occasionally extending further into the gut wall. In chronic infections, the lamina propria is infiltrated with large numbers of monocytes, lymphocytes, and plasma cells (Duhamel 2001). Invasion has been observed both concurrent with and independent of attachment of spirochete cells to the epithelium. In humans, *B. pilosicoli* has been isolated from the bloodstream of individuals with severe clinical disease or impaired immunity, in association with colitis (Trott et al. 1997; Kanavaki et al. 2002). Although a systemic spread or spirochetemia with *B. pilosicoli* has not been directly observed in pigs, its occurrence cannot be excluded.

The epithelial damage followed by local invasion and subsequent colitis combine to cause an increase in the water content of the cecal and colonic contents, together with excess mucus production and occasionally flecks of blood. Erosion of the epithelium leading to replacement by immature cells may reduce available surface area of the colon for absorption of water, electrolytes, and volatile fatty acids, and consequently affect feed conversion efficiency and weight gain (Duhamel 1998; Thomson et al. 1997).

Besides the "virulence life-style" genes of *B. pilosicoli* involved in motility and chemotaxis, other virulence determinants that might contribute to the disease have yet to be identified. A search for the attachment and invasion determinants encoded by the *inv, ail,* and *yadA* genes of *Yersinia enterocolitica*, the *eae* gene from enteropathogenic *Escherichia coli*, and a virulence plasmid of *Shigella flexneri* failed to identify similar genes in *B. pilosicoli* (Hartland et al. 1998). Although the attachment of *B. pilosicoli* to epithelial cells has been confirmed using intestinal epithelial cell lines in vitro, to date putative adhesins or host cell receptors have not been identified (Muniappa et al. 1998). At least three different protease activities, including a subtilisin-like serine protease similar to that of other gram-negative bacteria have been found in the membrane of *B. pilosicoli* (Muniappa and Duhamel 1997; Dassanayake et al. 2004). However, the role of these enzymes in disease, if any, has not been determined. Identification of virulence determinants in *B. pilosicoli* has been hampered by a lack of genomic information for this spirochete. Furthermore, unlike the case with *B. hyodysenteriae*, no successful gene inactivation experiments have been described for *B. pilosicoli*.

The host immune mechanisms that may be directed against *B. pilosicoli* have not been determined. In early studies, agglutinating serum antibodies were demonstrated in pigs recovered from experimental infection (Taylor et al. 1980). The development of serum IgG antibodies against whole cell extracts and membrane preparations of *B. pilosicoli* has been recorded 2–7 weeks after challenge inoculation of conventional weaned pigs (Zhang et al. 1999; Zhang et al. 2000; Zhang and Duhamel 2002). However, in another study, significant titers against whole cell preparations of *B. pilosicoli* were not found within 18 days following experimental infection of pigs, even though colonization and mild colitis were present (Hampson et al. 2000).

Gnotobiotic pigs (Neef et al. 1994), 1-day-old chicks (Duhamel et al. 1995a; Trott et al. 1995; Muniappa et al. 1998; Trott and Hampson 1998), adult chickens (Jamshidi and Hampson 2003), and mice (Sacco et al. 1998; Jamshidian et al. 2004) have been used as experimental models of *B. pilosicoli* infection. In various experimental infections of conventional pigs, between 17% and 100% of pigs have become infected, with 17–67% developing diarrhea and 8–100% exhibiting lesions of colitis (reviewed by Duhamel 2001). Not all colonized or diseased pigs have shown end-on attachment of spirochetes to the colonic epithelium (Thomson et al. 1997).

CLINICAL SIGNS

PCS has a clinical presentation similar to other forms of colitis and to the early stages of swine dysentery. It is commonly seen in the immediate postweaning period and in recently mixed growers placed on a new diet, but can be observed in finishers and occasionally pregnant sows and recently introduced breeding stock. PCS may affect groups of pigs of the same age in a unit or be present in pigs of mixed age on the same farm. It is not uncommon to observe various manifestations of PCS in weaners, growers, and finishers on the same farm. As a result of the large functional capacity of the cecum and colon, not all infected animals develop diarrhea; however, subclinical infections still may result in depressed growth rates.

The first clinical signs are hollowing of the flanks and the passage of loose, sometimes sticky feces that adhere to the pen floor. The consistency of the feces then changes to that of wet cement or porridge and may take on a glistening appearance. These may be the only clinical signs observed in finishers. Weaner and grower pigs usually develop a watery to mucoid diarrhea which is green or brown in color and occasionally characterized by thick tags of mucus and, rarely, flecks of blood. Diarrhea is usually self-limiting and lasts between 2 and 14 days, although some animals may relapse and again develop clinical signs after convalescence or treatment.

Affected pigs appear unthrifty, have fecal staining of the perineum, have a tucked-up appearance, and are sometimes febrile, but usually continue to eat. Pigs with PCS may have concurrent illness, particularly intestinal diseases such as swine dysentery, salmonellosis, or proliferative enteropathy. Mixed infections occur commonly in the field (Duhamel et al. 1995a; Girard et al. 1995; Møller et al. 1998; Thomson et al. 1998; Stege et al. 2000; Stege et al. 2001; Thomson et al. 2001). Pigs with uncomplicated PCS that develop loose feces may show significant loss of condition, decreased feed conversion, and delays in reaching market weight (Thomson et al. 1997; Thomson et al. 1998). Mortality is generally not a feature of PCS.

LESIONS

Gross Lesions

Gross lesions associated with PCS are limited to the cecum and colon and may be very subtle, particularly in the early stages of the disease. Postmortem examination soon after the onset of clinical signs often reveals a flaccid, fluid-filled cecum and colon with an edematous serosal surface and enlarged mesenteric and colonic lymph nodes. The large intestinal contents are abundant and watery green or occasionally yellow and frothy. Mild congestion and hyperemia of the mucosal surface might be apparent, with occasional erosions and necrotic foci. Inflammation in the later stages may result in multifocal erosive, ulcerative, or mucohemorrhagic colitis, but it is not as severe as that observed in swine dysentery. The mucosa becomes thickened, and local ecchymotic or petechial hemorrhages may be apparent on the surface. In chronic cases and in resolving lesions, the hemorrhages are covered by small tags of adherent fibrin, necrotic material, and digesta, which appear as conical scales adherent on the surface of the mucosa (see Figure 46.3). This material may be dislodged by rinsing, and can be found as a deposit after decanting the washings (Johnston et al. 1999).

Microscopic Lesions

PCS has been described as a catarrhal, multifocal, erosive or ulcerative colitis. Lesions are generally confined to the mucosa and submucosa, but may extend into the muscularis. The mucosa is thickened, edematous, and occasionally hyperemic and is characterized by the presence of dilated, elongated intestinal crypts filled with mucus, cellular debris, and degenerate inflammatory cells (Figure 46.4). The crypt cell mitotic rate is increased, and immature, cuboidal, or squamous epithelium may be present on the surface of the mucosa between crypt units. Where columnar epithelium is still present on the surface of the colon, it may be covered by a dark fringe of spirochetes attached by one cell end (see Figure 46.1). Silver stains (Muniappa et al. 1997), and more specifically either immunohistochemical staining with specific antibodies (Webb et al. 1997) or fluorescent in situ hybridization with specific oligonucleotide probes (Boye et al. 1998; Jensen et al. 2000), can be used to confirm the presence of spirochetes attached to the surface of colonic enterocytes, within dilated intestinal crypts, and occasionally within the lamina propria. The protozoan *Balantidium coli* is often seen in large numbers on the surface of the colon in pigs with PCS (Taylor et al. 1980; Trott et al. 1996b).

Electron Microscopy

Using transmission electron microscopy, polar-attached spirochetes with 4–7 periplasmic flagella may be observed invaginated into the terminal web cytoplasm, effacing microvilli and disrupting microfilaments without penetrating the host cell plasmalemma (Figure 46.5). Scanning electron microscopy reveals the adherent spirochetes as a patchy fringe on the surface of

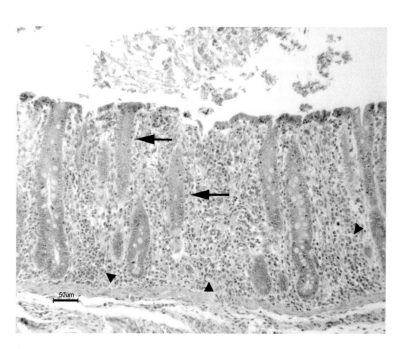

46.4. *Light photomicrograph of a colon obtained from a pig 21 days after intragastric inoculation with B. pilosicoli. Note the overall loss of crypt columns accompanied with hyperplasia of the remaining crypt epithelium (arrows) and diffuse infiltration of the lamina propria between crypt units by large numbers of mixed mononuclear inflammatory cells, mostly macrophages and lymphocytes (arrowheads). Hematoxylin and eosin.*

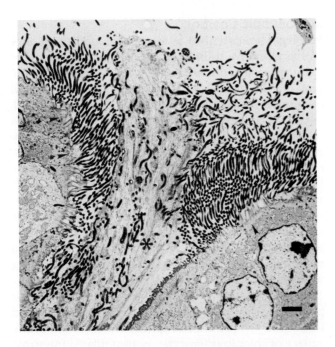

46.5. *Transmission electron photomicrograph of colon obtained from a pig with spontaneous porcine colonic spirochetosis. Note attachment of large numbers of spirochetes by one of their ends to the apical membrane of enterocytes causing effacement of the microvilli and rarefaction of terminal web microfilaments (arrowheads). Many spirochetes are associated with the mucin at the opening and extending inside the lumen of the crypt (asterisk). Uranyl acetate and lead citrate; Bar = 2.5 μm (Reproduced from Johnston et al. 1999, with permission).*

colonic epithelial cells. Spirochetes also may be observed invading between epithelial cells in the extrusion zone between adjacent crypt units (Duhamel 1996).

DIAGNOSIS

PCS should be suspected when typical clinical signs of mucoid or porridge-like diarrhea without blood and no mortality are found in weaned pigs. The clinical signs of PCS are difficult to differentiate from those associated with the proliferative enteropathies caused by *Lawsonia*

intracellularis. In addition to proliferative enteropathy, PCS may occur concurrently with a number of other intestinal infections, including salmonellosis, postweaning colibacillosis, swine dysentery, yersiniosis, and trichuriasis. All of these should be considered in the differential diagnosis of PCS, as well as nonspecific colitis, an apparently diet-related condition possibly associated with a form of hypersensitivity to pelleted feed (Smith and Nelson 1987).

To obtain a diagnosis, postmortem examination of several affected pigs, including routine histologic and bacteriologic examination, should be undertaken (Johnston et al. 1999). Fecal samples for culture and/or PCR for *Brachyspira* spp. and other pathogens also should be obtained from a cross-section of affected pigs. Swabs taken directly from the colonic wall can be used to prepare wet smears for viewing by phase contrast microscopy, or they can be fixed and Gram-stained, in both cases to look for the presence of large numbers of spirochetes that might suggest a spirochetal etiology. In histologic sections from the cecum and particularly the colon, the presence of spirochetes attached to the colonic mucosa is diagnostic for PCS, but this change is not observed in every case of the disease. Other histologic lesions associated with PCS are often nonspecific, and a definitive diagnosis of PCS requires demonstration of *B. pilosicoli* by bacteriologic culture and/or PCR. While waiting for confirmation of results, medication should be initiated, because sometimes it can take 1–2 weeks to obtain a definitive diagnosis.

The four species of weakly beta-hemolytic spirochetes colonizing pigs can be differentiated from one another and from *B. hyodysenteriae* using a number of simple biochemical tests outlined in Table 46.1. Unfortunately, these tests generally require the growth of pure cultures, a process which can take several weeks to achieve, particularly if the initial plates are heavily contaminated with other fecal flora. In addition, the existence of isolates with unusual phenotypes, such as hippurate negative strains of *B. pilosicoli* (Fossi et al. 2004), can make interpretation difficult. Generally, laboratory

Table 46.1. Differentiation of the five recognized groups of porcine intestinal spirochetes by their hemolyis pattern on Trypticase Soy blood agar, biochemical reactions and utilization of sugars.

Test	B. hyodysenteriae	B. intermedia	B. innocens	B. murdochii	B. pilosicoli
Hemolysis	strong	weak	weak	weak	weak
Indole	+[a]	+	−	−	−[a]
Hippurate	−	−	−	−	+[b]
API-ZYM	1	1	2	3	4
D-ribose	−	−	−	−	+

+positive reaction; − negative reaction
[a]Indole negative strains of *B. hyodysenteriae* and indole positive strains of *B. pilosicoli* have been recorded.
[b]Hippurate negative strains of *B. pilosicoli* have been recorded.
1 = alpha-glucosidase positive, alpha-galactosidase negative.
2 = alpha-glucosidase positive or negative, alpha-galactosidase positive.
3 = alpha-glucosidase negative, alpha-galactosidase negative.
4 = variable reactions, including positive reactions for both enzymes, beta-glucosidase negative.

confirmation of *B. pilosicoli* can be accomplished using strength of beta-hemolysis, hippurate hydrolysis, metabolism of ribose, and lack of beta-glucosidase activity in the API-ZYM profile (Fellström and Gunnarsson 1995; Trott et al. 1996c). Nowadays, diagnosis is more usually supported by the use of specific polymerase chain reaction (PCR) tests.

Several PCR assays that are based on either a unique 16S rRNA gene sequence (Park et al. 1995; Fellström et al. 1997; Muniappa et al. 1997), a 23S rDNA sequence (Leser et al. 1997), or the NADH oxidase gene (Atyeo et al. 1999) specific for *B. pilosicoli* have been described. When applied to growth harvested from the primary isolation plate, the combined culture/PCR technique is more sensitive than culture alone and can significantly reduce the time taken for a diagnosis, even if there is a large amount of contamination with other fecal microbiota (Atyeo et al. 1998). A recent improvement in diagnosis involves the use of a duplex PCR for the simultaneous detection of both *B. pilosicoli* and *B. hyodysenteriae,* which is applied directly to DNA extracted from the feces (La et al. 2003). Potentially this can be used to give a diagnosis on the day of sample submission. The duplex PCR has been further modified to introduce a *Lawsonia intracellularis* component in the reaction, increasing the range of potential pathogens that it can detect in a single fecal sample (La et al. 2004). When using these fecal PCRs, it is usual also to culture the samples to obtain isolates, so that these can be used for strain-typing and/or determining their antimicrobial susceptibilities.

As previously mentioned, another recent adjunct to diagnosis has been the development of a fluorescent in situ hybridization (FISH) technique, which uses fluorescent oligonucleotide probes specific for sequences present in the 16S or 23S rRNA of *B. pilosicoli* (Boye et al. 1998; Jensen et al. 2000). The advantage of this technique is that identification and localization of the spirochetes associated with the intestinal mucosa can be done simultaneously. Localization of intestinal spirochetes in formalin-fixed and de-paraffinized tissue sections also has been accomplished using immunohistochemical staining with a *Brachyspira*-specific mouse monoclonal antibody (MAB) to FlaB periplasmic flagellar core proteins and the avidin-biotin-alkaline phosphatase complex method (Fisher et al. 1997; Webb et al. 1997; Johnston et al. 1999). These techniques are particularly useful in a research setting when investigating aspects of the pathogenesis of PCS.

A number of other schemes have been developed to detect and/or identify species of weakly hemolytic intestinal spirochetes of swine, as well as *B. hyodysenteriae,* without the need for culture and biochemical analysis. These involve PCR amplification of specific gene sequences, followed by restriction enzyme digestion of the products to give species-specific banding patterns after gel electrophoresis. Genes that have been used in this way include the 16S rRNA gene (Stanton et al. 1997), the 23S rRNA gene (Barcellos et al. 2000c; Thomson et al. 2001), and the NADH-oxidase gene (Rohde et al. 2002). Indirect fluorescent antibody tests using MABs that have been raised against specific outer-membrane proteins of *B. pilosicoli* also have potential for diagnostic use on feces (Lee and Hampson 1995; Tenaya et al. 1998). Unfortunately, a MAB-based immunomagnetic separation of *B. pilosicoli* from feces did not improve sensitivity of detection above those achieved with standard culture followed by PCR (Corona-Barrara et al. 2004b).

Typing of individual strains of *B. pilosicoli* can provide important epidemiologic information to help devise control measures. Early studies used multilocus enzyme electrophoresis (MLEE) to differentiate intestinal spirochete isolates into species and strains (Lee et al. 1993; Stanton et al. 1996), but this time-consuming technique is no longer commonly used. Pulsed field gel electrophoresis now is the most commonly used strain typing technique for *B. pilosicoli* and gives better strain discrimination than MLEE (Atyeo et al. 1996; Trott et al. 1998; Fossi et al. 2003).

As a result of significant serologic cross-reactivity among the weakly beta-hemolytic intestinal spirochetes, to date no reliable tests are available to measure species-specific serum antibody titers.

TREATMENT AND CONTROL

Although treatment and control of PCS are largely modeled on procedures developed for swine dysentery, some modifications are necessary because of the lesser economic impact of PCS on pig production. No effective vaccines have been developed to date. An autogenous bacterin vaccine induced good systemic antibody titers, but vaccinated pigs still became colonized and developed diarrhea after experimental challenge (Hampson et al. 2000).

Implementation of rational antimicrobial therapy can reduce *B. pilosicoli* infection and maximize productivity while improving the welfare of pigs raised under intensive management. Affected pigs should be treated by water or feed medication at similar levels and lengths of time as recommended for the treatment of swine dysentery (Chapter 48). Parenteral treatment may sometimes be warranted for severely ill pigs.

Although information on the in vitro antimicrobial susceptibility of *B. pilosicoli* is relatively limited, a number of antimicrobials that are effective against *B. hyodysenteriae,* including tiamulin, valnemulin, carbadox, dimetridazole, and to a lesser extent lincomycin, have been shown to have low minimum inhibitory concentration (MIC) values when tested against collections of porcine *B. pilosicoli* isolates (Trott et al. 1996c; Cizek et al. 1998; Duhamel et al. 1998; Hommez et al. 1998b; Fossi et al. 1999; Kinyon et al. 2002; Brooke et al. 2003). Fewer isolates have been found to be susceptible to tylosin (Cizek et al. 1998; Hommez et al. 1998b; Kinyon et al. 2002). Olaquindox has been shown to have MIC values of less than 1.0 μg/mL against *B. pilosicoli*, and the organism could not be isolated from herds previously receiving olaquindox in the feed at 100 ppm (Fellström et al. 1996). However, despite its preventive attributes, the use of this agent is now very limited. Resistance to single antimicrobials, particularly tylosin, or to combinations of antimicrobials commonly used for treatment of PCS have been recorded (Kinyon et al. 2002). Of great concern is the recent emergence of *B. pilosicoli* strains resistant to tiamulin among field isolates obtained from pigs in Finland (Fossi et al. 1999) and North America (Kinyon et al. 2002).

Management strategies, particularly those aimed at limiting access of pigs to environments contaminated with manure, can be used to reduce the impact of PCS. Implementation of an all-in/all-out system ("batch production") rather than a continuous flow system of production reduces the risk of infection (Stege et al. 2001). Improved pen hygiene can reduce transmission. Where practical, modification to the diet composition and/or physical form may help control the impact of the infection. The addition of zinc oxide in the feed at 3 kg/tonne can help control PCS (Love 1996). This method also has been effective in controlling uncomplicated cases of nonspecific colitis (Kavanagh 1992). Interestingly, in laying hens, the addition of 50 ppm zinc bacitracin to the diet actually enhanced colonization with *B. pilosicoli* (Jamshidi and Hampson 2002), but whether the same occurs in pigs is not known.

The methods described in Chapter 48 for the elimination of swine dysentery also may be effective for PCS, but because PCS is less severe and has less economic impact than swine dysentery, it generally does not warrant such drastic procedures. Fossi et al. (2001) reported eradicating *B. pilosicoli* from a 60-sow herd by tiamulin treatment, followed by relocation of the breeding herd, thorough cleaning and disinfection of the premises, and then returning the adult animals to the original location. This protocol would be more difficult to follow in larger herds, and the existence of reservoir hosts for *B. pilosicoli*, such as feral waterbirds, presents an ongoing threat of reintroduction of PCS.

Where PCS becomes endemic in a herd, regular periods of treatment with antimicrobials in the feed or water may be required to prevent sudden increases in morbidity due to recent introduction of naive pigs, change of diet, or other periods associated with stress.

As a result of the current global nature of the pig industry and the limited number of available antimicrobial agents with demonstrated efficacy against *B. pilosicoli*, the potential for emergence of resistant strains has become an international concern. To assist future control of PCS, a high priority should be given to monitoring the antimicrobial resistance patterns of *B. pilosicoli*, to improving understanding of the basic mechanisms of resistance, and to investigating the feasibility of producing vaccines or other methods to help control the disease.

REFERENCES

Atyeo RF, Oxberry SL, Combs BG, Hampson DJ. 1998. Development and evaluation of polymerase chain reaction tests as an aid to diagnosis of swine dysentery and intestinal spirochaetosis. Lett Appl Microbiol 26:126–130.

Atyeo RF, Oxberry SL, Hampson DJ. 1996. Pulsed-field gel electrophoresis for sub-specific differentiation of *Serpulina pilosicoli* (formerly "*Anguillina coli*"). FEMS Microbiol Lett 141:77–81.

Atyeo RF, Stanton TB, Jensen NS, Suriyaarachichi DS, Hampson DJ. 1999. Differentiation of *Serpulina* species by NADH oxidase (*nox*) gene comparisons and *nox*-based polymerase chain reaction tests. Vet Microbiol 67:49–62.

Barcellos DE, de Uzeda M, Ikuta N, Lunge VR, Fonseca AS, Kader II, Duhamel GE. 2000c. Identification of porcine intestinal spirochetes by PCR-restriction fragment length polymorphism analysis of ribosomal DNA encoding 23S rRNA. Vet Microbiol 75:189–198.

Barcellos DE, Mathiesen MR, de Uzeda M, Kader II, Duhamel GE. 2000a. Prevalence of *Brachyspira* species isolated from diarrhoeic pigs in Brazil. Vet Rec 146:398–403.

Barcellos DE, Mathiesen MR, Duhamel GE. 2000b. Effect of temperature on survival of pathogenic intestinal spirochetes in spiked pig feces. Proc 16th Congr Int Pig Vet Soc, p. 44.

Binek M, Szynkiewicz Z. 1984. Physiological properties and classification of strains of *Treponema* sp. isolated from pigs in Poland. Comp Immunol Microbiol Infect Dis 7:141–148.

Boye M, Baloda, SB, Leser TD, Møller K. 2001. Survival of *Brachyspira hyodysenteriae* and *B. pilosicoli* in terrestrial microcosms. Vet Microbiol 81:33–40.

Boye M, Jensen TK, Møller K, Leser TD, Jorsal SE. 1998. Specific detection of the genus *Serpulina*, *S. hyodysenteriae* and *S. pilosicoli* in porcine intestines by fluorescent rRNA *in situ* hybridization. Mol Cell Probes 12:323–330.

Brooke CJ, Hampson DJ, Riley TV. 2003. In vitro antimicrobial susceptibility of human isolates of *Brachyspira pilosicoli*. Antimicrob Agents Chemother 47:2354–2357.

Castryck A, Hommez J, Miry C, Lein A. 1997. Porcine intestinal spirochaetosis caused by *Serpulina pilosicoli* in Belgium. Vlaams Diergen Tijdschrift 66:125–128.

Choi C, Han DU, Kim J, Cho WS, Chung HK, Jung T, Yoon BS, Chae C. 2002. Prevalence of *Brachyspira pilosicoli* in Korean pigs, determined using a nested PCR. Vet Rec 150:217–218.

Cizek A, Smola J, Mádr P. 1998. In vitro activity of six antidysenteric drugs on *Serpulina hyodysenteriae* and *S. pilosicoli* strains isolated in the Czech Republic. Proc 15th Congr Int Pig Vet Soc, p. 135.

Corona-Barrera E, Smith DG, Murray B, Thomson JR. 2004a. Efficacy of seven disinfectant sanitisers on field isolates of *Brachyspira pilosicoli*. Vet Rec 154:473–474.

Corona-Barrera E, Smith DGE, La T, Hampson DJ, Thomson JR. 2004b. Immunomagnetic separation of the intestinal spirochaetes *Brachyspira pilosicoli* and *Brachyspira hyodysenteriae* from porcine faeces. J Med Microbiol 53:301–307.

Dassanayake RP, Caceres NE, Sarath G, Duhamel GE. 2004. Biochemical properties of membrane-associated proteases of *Brachyspira pilosicoli* isolated from humans with intestinal disorders. J Med Microbiol 53:319–323.

de Arriba ML, Vidal AB, Carvajal A, Pozo J, Martinez A, Duhamel GE, Rubio P. 2002. First confirmation of porcine colonic spirochaetosis caused by *Brachyspira pilosicoli* in Iberian pigs in Spain. Vet Rec 150:250–251.

Duhamel GE. 1996. Porcine colonic spirochaetosis caused by *Serpulina pilosicoli*. Misset Pigs, May (Enteric Diseases Suppl):10–13.

——. 1998. Colonic spirochaetosis caused by *Serpulina pilosicoli*. Large Anim Prac 19:14–22.

——. 2001. Comparative pathology and pathogenesis of naturally acquired and experimentally induced colonic spirochetosis. Anim Health Res Rev 2:3–17.

Duhamel GE, Elder RO, Muniappa N, Mathiesen MR, Wong VJ, Tarara RP. 1997. Colonic spirochetal infections in nonhuman primates that were associated with *Brachyspira aalborgi*, *Serpulina pilosicoli*, and unclassified flagellated bacteria. Clin Infect Dis 25 Suppl 2:S186–S188.

Duhamel GE, Hunsaker BD, Mathiesen MR, Moxley RA. 1996. Intestinal spirochetosis and giardiasis in a Beagle pup with diarrhea. Vet Pathol 33:360–362.

Duhamel GE, Joens LA. 1994. Laboratory procedures for diagnosis of swine dysentery. American Association of Veterinary Laboratory Diagnosticians Inc., USA.

Duhamel GE, Kinyon JM, Mathiesen MR, Murphy DP, Walter D. 1998. In vitro activity of four antimicrobial agents against North American isolates of porcine *Serpulina pilosicoli*. J Vet Diag Invest 10:350–356.

Duhamel GE, Mathiesen MR, Schafer RW, Ramanathan M, Johnston JL. 1993. Description of a new species of spirochete, *Serpulina coli* sp. nov. associated with intestinal spirochetosis of swine and human beings. In Conf Res Worker Anim Dis Abstract, p. 14.

Duhamel GE, Muniappa N, Gardner I, Anderson MA, Blanchard PC, DeBey BM, Mathiesen MR, Walker RL. 1995a. Porcine colonic spirochaetosis: A diarrhoeal disease associated with a newly recognized species of intestinal spirochaete. Pig J 35:101–110.

Duhamel GE, Muniappa N, Mathiesen MR, Johnson JL, Toth J, Elder RO, Doster AR. 1995b. Certain canine weakly beta-hemolytic spirochetes are phenotypically and genotypically related to spirochetes associated with human and porcine intestinal spirochetosis. J Clin Microbiol 33:2212–2215.

Duhamel GE, Stryker CJ, Lu G, Wong VJ, Tarara RP. 2003. Colonic spirochetosis of colony-raised rhesus macaques associated with *Brachyspira* and Helicobacter. Anaerobe 9:45–55.

Fellström C, Gunnarsson A. 1995. Phenotypic characterisation of intestinal spirochaetes isolated from pigs. Res Vet Sci 59:1–4.

Fellström C, Landen A, Karlsson M, Gunnarsson A, Holmgren N. 2004. Mice as a reservoir of *Brachyspira hyodysenteriae* in repeated outbreaks of swine dysentery in a Swedish fattening herd. Proc 18th Congr Int Pig Vet Soc, p. 280.

Fellström C, Pettersson B, Johansson K, Lundenheim N, Gunnarsson A. 1996. Prevalence of *Serpulina* species in relation to diarrhea and feed medication in pig-rearing herds in Sweden. Am J Vet Res 57:807–811.

Fellström C, Pettersson B, Thompson J, Gunnarsson A, Persson M, Johansson K. 1997. Identification of *Serpulina* species associated with porcine colitis by biochemical analysis and PCR. J Clin Microbiol 35:462–467.

Fisher, L. N.; Duhamel, G. E.; Westerman, R. B.; and Mathiesen, M. R. 1997. Immunoblot reactivity of polyclonal and monoclonal antibodies with periplasmic flagellar proteins FlaA1 and FlaB of porcine *Serpulina* species. Clin Diagn Lab Immunol 4:400–404.

Fossi M, Heinonen M, Pohjanvirta T, Pelkonen S, Peltoniemi AT. 2001. Eradication of endemic *Brachyspira pilosicoli* infection from a farrowing herd: A case report. Anim Health Res Rev 2:53–57.

Fossi M, Pohjanvirta T, Pelkonen S. 2003. Molecular epidemiological study of *Brachyspira pilosicoli* in Finnish sow herds. Epidemiol Infect 131:967–973.

Fossi M, Pohjanvirta T, Sukura A, Heinikainen S, Lindecrona R, Pelkonen S. 2004. Molecular and ultrastructural characterization of porcine hippurate-negative *Brachyspira pilosicoli*. J Clin Microbiol 42:3153–3158.

Fossi M, Saranpaa T, Rautiainen E. 1999. In vitro sensitivity of the swine *Brachyspira* species to tiamulin 1995–1997. Acta Vet Scand 40:355–358.

Girard C, Lemarchand T, Higgins R. 1995. Porcine colonic spirochetosis: A retrospective study of eleven cases. Can Vet J 36:291–294.

Hampson DJ. 1990. New developments in research on swine dysentery and spirochaetal colitis. Pig News Info 12:233–235.

——. 2000. The Serpulina story. Proc 16th Congr Int Pig Vet Soc, pp. 1–5.

Hampson DJ, McLaren AJ. 1999. Experimental infection of layer hens with *Serpulina intermedia* causes reduced egg production and increased faecal water content. Avian Pathol 28:113–117.

Hampson DJ, Robertson ID, La T, Oxberry SL, Pethick DW. 2000. Influences of diet and vaccination on colonisation of pigs by the intestinal spirochaete *Brachyspira* (*Serpulina*) *pilosicoli*. Vet Microbiol 73:75–84.

Hampson DJ, Stanton TB. 1997. Intestinal Spirochaetes in Domestic Animals and Humans. England: CAB International.

Hampson DJ, Trott DJ. 1995. Intestinal spirochaetal infections of pigs: An overview and an Australian perspective. In Manipulating Pig Production V. DP Hennessy, PD Cranwell, eds. Canberra: Australasian Pig Science Association, pp. 139–169.

Hartland EL, Mikosza ASJ, Robins-Browne R, Hampson DJ. 1998. Examination of *Serpulina pilosicoli* for attachment and invasion determinants of Enterobacteria. FEMS Microbiol Lett 165:59–63.

Heinonen M, Fossi M, Jalli J-P, Saloniemi H, Tuovinen V. 2000. Detectability and prevalence of *Brachyspira* species in herds rearing health class feeder pigs in Finland. Vet Rec 146:343–347.

Hommez J, Castryck F, Haesebrouck F, Devriese LA. 1998a. Identification of porcine *Serpulina* strains in routine diagnostic bacteriology. Vet Microbiol 62:163–169.

Hommez J, Devriese LA, Castryck F, Miry C, Lein A, Haesebrouck F. 1998b. Susceptibility of different *Serpulina* species in pigs to antimicrobials agents. Vlaams Diergen Tijdschrift 67:32–35.

Hopwood DE, Pethick DW, Hampson DJ. 2002. Increasing the viscosity of the intestinal contents stimulates proliferation of enterotoxigenic *Escherichia coli* and *Brachyspira pilosicoli* in weaner pigs. Br J Nutr 88:523–532.

Hsu T, Hutto DL, Minion FC, Zuerner RL, Wannemuehler MJ. 2001. Cloning of a beta-hemolysin gene of *Brachyspira* (*Serpulina*) *hyodysenteriae* and its expression in *Escherichia coli*. Infect Immun 69:706–711.

Jacques M, Girard C, Higgins R, Goyette G. 1989. Extensive colonization of the porcine colonic epithelium by a spirochete similar to *Treponema innocens*. J Clin Microbiol 27:1139–1141.

Jacobson M, Hard af Segerstad C, Gunnarsson A, Fellström C, de verdier Klingenberg K, Wallgren P, Jensen-Waern, M. 2003. Diarrhoea in the growing pig—A comparison of clinical, morphological and microbial findings between animals from good and poor performance herds. Res Vet Sci 74:163–169.

Jamshidi A, Hampson DJ. 2002. Zinc bacitracin enhances colonisation by the intestinal spirochaete *Brachyspira pilosicoli* in experimentally infected layer hens. Avian Pathol 31:293–298.

——. 2003. Experimental infection of layer hens with a human isolate of *Brachyspira pilosicoli*. J Med Microbiol 52:361–364.

Jamshidian M, La T, Phillips ND, Hampson DJ. 2004. *Brachyspira pilosicoli* colonisation in experimentally infected mice can be facilitated by dietary means. J Med Microbiol 53:313–318.

Jansson, DS, Bröjer C, Gavier-Widén D, Gunnarsson A, Fellström C. 2001. *Brachyspira* spp. (*Serpulina* spp.) in birds: A review and results from a study of Swedish game birds. Anim Health Res Rev 2:93–100.

Jenkinson SR, Wingar CR. 1981. Selective medium for the isolation of *Treponema hyodysenteriae*. Vet Rec 109:384–385.

Jensen TK, Boye M, Møller K. 2004a. Extensive intestinal spirochaetosis in pigs challenged with *Brachyspira pilosicoli*. J Med Microbiol 53:309–312.

Jensen TK, Fossi M, Boye M. 2004b. Demonstration of a *Leptospira*-like spirochaete associated with colitis in weaned pigs. Preliminary results. 18th Proc Congr Int Pig Vet Soc, p. 325.

Jensen TK, Møller K, Boye M, Leser TD, Jorsal SE. 2000. Scanning electron microscopy and fluorescent in situ hybridization of experimental *Brachyspira (Serpulina) pilosicoli* infection in growing pigs. Vet Pathol 37:22–32.

Johnston T, Duhamel GE, Mathiesen MR, Walter D, Smart N, Dewey C. 1999. Recent advances in diagnosing and controlling porcine colonic spirochetosis. Compend Food Anim Med Manag 21:S198–S207.

Kanavaki S, Mantadakis E, Thomakos N, Pefanis A, Matsiota-Bernard P, Karabela S, Samonis G. 2002. *Brachyspira (Serpulina) pilosicoli* spirochetemia in an immunocompromised patient. Infection 30:175–177.

Kavanagh, N. T. 1992. Non-specific colitis: Observations on methods of control and prevention at farm level. Proc 12th Congr Int Pig Vet Soc, p. 522.

Kinyon JM, Murphy D, Stryker C, Turner V, Holck JT, Duhamel G. 2002. Minimum inhibitory concentration for US swine isolates of *Brachyspira pilosicoli* to valnemulin and four other antimicrobials. Proc 17th Congr Int Pig Vet Soc, p. 50.

Kunkle RA, Harris DL, Kinyon JM. 1986. Autoclaved liquid medium for propagation of *Treponema hyodysenteriae*. J. Clin Microbiol 24:669–671.

La T, Collins AM, Phillips ND, Oksa A, Hampson DJ. 2004. Evaluation of a multiplex-PCR for the detection of *Brachyspira hyodysenteriae*, *Brachyspira pilosicoli* and *Lawsonia intracellularis* in pig faeces. Proc 18th Congr Int Pig Vet Soc, p. 283.

La T, Phillips ND, Hampson DJ. 2003. Development of a duplex PCR assay for detection of *Brachyspira hyodysenteriae* and *Brachyspira pilosicoli* in pig feces. J Clin Microbiol 41:3372–3375.

Lee BJ, Hampson DJ. 1995. A monoclonal antibody reacting with the cell envelope of spirochaetes isolated from cases of intestinal spirochaetosis in pigs and humans. FEMS Microbiol Lett 131:179–184.

——. 1999. Lipooligosaccharide profiles of *Serpulina pilosicoli* strains, and their serological cross-reactivities. J Med Microbiol 48:411–415.

Lee JI, Hampson DJ, Lymbery AJ, Harders SJ. 1993. The porcine intestinal spirochaetes: Identification of new genetic groups. Vet Microbiol 34:273–285.

Lee JI, Hampson DJ. 1994. Genetic characterisation of intestinal spirochaetes and their association with disease. J Med Microbiol 40:365–371.

Leser TD, Møller K, Jensen TK, Jorsal SE. 1997. Specific detection of *Serpulina hyodysenteriae* and potentially pathogenic weakly haemolytic porcine intestinal spirochaetes by polymerase chain reaction targeting 23S rDNA. Mol Cell Probes 11:363–372.

Lindecrona RH, Jensen TK, Møller K. 2004. Influence of diet on the experimental infection of pigs with *Brachyspira pilosicoli*. Vet Rec 154:264–267.

Love R. 1996. *Serpulina pilosicoli* colitis in grower pigs. Aust Assoc Pig Vet News 20:6.

Margawani KR, Robertson ID, Brooke JC, Hampson DJ. 2004. Prevalence, risk factors and molecular epidemiology of *Brachyspira pilosicoli* in humans on the island of Bali, Indonesia. J Med Microbiol 53:325–332.

McLaren AJ, Trott DJ, Swayne DE, Oxberry SL, Hampson DJ. 1997. Genetic and phenotypic characterization of intestinal spirochetes colonizing chickens and allocation of known pathogenic isolates to three distinct genetic groups. J Clin Microbiol 35:412–417.

Milner JA, Sellwood R. 1994. Chemotactic response to mucin by *Serpulina hyodysenteriae* and other porcine spirochetes: Potential role in intestinal colonization. Infect Immun 62:4095–4099.

Møller K, Jensen TK, Jorsal SE, Leser TD, Carstensen B. 1998. Detection of *Lawsonia intracellularis, Serpulina hyodysenteriae,* weakly beta-haemolytic intestinal spirochaetes, *Salmonella enterica,* and haemolytic *Escherichia coli* from swine herds with and without diarrhoea among growing pigs. Vet Microbiol 62:59–72.

Muniappa N, Duhamel GE. 1997. Outer membrane-associated serine protease of intestinal spirochaetes. FEMS Microbiol Lett 154:159–164.

Muniappa N, Mathiesen MR, Duhamel GE. 1997. Laboratory identification and enteropathogenicity testing of *Serpulina pilosicoli* associated with porcine colonic spirochetosis. J Vet Diag Invest 9:165–171.

Muniappa N, Ramanathan MR, Tarara MP, Westerman RB, Mathiesen MR, Duhamel GE. 1998. Attachment of human and rhesus *Serpulina pilosicoli* to cultured cells and comparison with a chick infection model. J Spiro Tick-borne Dis 5:44–53.

Munshi MA, Traub RJ, Robertson ID, Mikosza ASJ, Hampson DJ. 2004. Colonization and risk factors for *Brachyspira aalborgi* and *Brachyspira pilosicoli* in humans and dogs on tea-estates in Assam, India. Epidemiol Infect 132:137–144.

Neef NA, Lysons RJ, Trott DJ, Hampson DJ, Jones PW, Morgan JM. 1994. Pathogenicity of porcine intestinal spirochetes in gnotobiotic pigs. Infect Immun 62:2395–2403.

Ochiai S, Adachi Y, Mori K. 1997. Unification of the genera *Serpulina* and *Brachyspira*, and proposals of *Brachyspira hyodysenteriae* comb. nov., *Brachyspira innocens* comb. nov. and *Brachyspira pilosicoli* comb. nov.. Microbiol Immunol 41:445–452.

Olson LD. 1996. Enhanced isolation of *Serpulina hyodysenteriae* by using sliced agar media. J Clin Microbiol 34:2937–2941.

Oxberry SL, Hampson DJ. 2003. Epidemiological studies of *Brachyspira pilosicoli* in two Australian piggeries. Vet Microbiol 93:109–120.

Oxberry SL, Trott DJ, Hampson DJ. 1998. *Serpulina pilosicoli*, water birds and water: Potential sources of infection for humans and other animals. Epidemiol Infect 121:219–225.

Park NY, Chung CY, McLaren AJ, Atyeo AJ, Hampson DJ. 1995. Polymerase chain reaction for identification of human and porcine spirochaetes recovered from cases of intestinal spirochaetosis. FEMS Microbiol Lett 125:225–230.

Pronost S, Baluti-Osako M, Dumontier S, Leguennec J, Fortier G, Moalic PY. 1999. Apports de la PCR pour l'identification des souches de *Brachyspira* pathogenes chez le porc. Rev Méd Vét 150:803–808.

Ramanathan M, Duhamel GE, Mathiesen MR, Messier S. 1993. Identification and partial characterization of a group of weakly ß-hemolytic spirochetes of swine distinct from *Serpulina innocens*. Vet Microbiol 37:53–64.

Rohde J, Rothkamp A, Gerlach GF. 2002. Differentiation of porcine *Brachyspira* species by a novel nox PCR-based restriction fragment length polymorphism analysis. J Clin Microbiol 40:2598–2600.

Sacco RE, Trampel DW, Wannemuehler MJ. 1997. Experimental infection of C3H mice with avian, porcine and human isolates of *Serpulina pilosicoli*. Infect Immun 65:5349–5353.

Smith WJ, Nelson EP. 1987. Grower scour/non-specific colitis. Vet Rec 121:334.

Spearman JG, Nayar G, Sheridan M. 1988. Colitis associated with *Treponema innocens* in pigs. Can Vet J 29:747.

Stanton TB, Fournie-Amazouz E, Postic D, Trott DJ, Grimont PAD, Baranton G, Hampson DJ, Saint Girons I. 1997. Recognition of two new species of intestinal spirochetes: *Serpulina intermedia* sp. nov. and *Serpulina murdochii* sp. nov. Int J System Bacteriol 47:1007–1012.

Stanton TB, Thompson MG, Humphrey SB, Zuerner RL. 2003. Detection of bacteriophage VSH-1 svp38 gene in *Brachyspira* spirochetes. FEMS Microbiol Lett 224:225–229.

Stanton TB, Trott DJ, Lee JI, McLaren AJ, Hampson DJ, Paster BJ, Jensen NS. 1996. Differentiation of intestinal spirochaetes by multilocus enzyme electrophoresis and 16S rRNA sequence comparisons. FEMS Microbiol Lett 136:181–186.

Stege H, Jensen TK, Møller K, Bækbo P, Jorsal SE. 2000. Prevalence of intestinal pathogens in Danish finishing pig herds. Prev Vet Med 46:279–292.

——. 2001. Risk factors for intestinal pathogens in Danish finishing pig herds. Prev Vet Med 50:153–164.

Stephens CP, Hampson DJ. 2001. Intestinal spirochaete infections in chickens: A review of disease associations, epidemiology and control. Anim Health Res Rev 2:101–110.

Taylor DJ, Simmons JR, Laird HM. 1980. Production of diarrhoea and dysentery in pigs by feeding pure cultures of a spirochaete differing from *Treponema hyodysenteriae*. Vet Rec 106:326–332.

Tenaya IWM, Penhale JP, Hampson DJ. 1998. Preparation of diagnostic polyclonal and monoclonal antibodies against outer envelope proteins of *Serpulina pilosicoli*. J Med Microbiol 47:317–324.

Thomson JR, Smith WJ, Murray BP. 1998. Investigations into field cases of porcine colitis with particular reference to infection with *Serpulina pilosicoli*. Vet Rec 142:235–239.

Thomson JR, Smith WJ, Murray BP, McOrist S. 1997. Pathogenicity of three strains of *Serpulina pilosicoli* in pigs with a naturally acquired intestinal flora. Infect Immun 65:3693–700.

Thomson JR, Smith WJ, Murray BP, Murray D, Dick JE, Sumption KJ. 2001. Porcine enteric spirochete infections in the UK: Surveillance data and preliminary investigation of atypical isolates. Anim Health Res Rev 2:31–36.

Trampel DW, Jensen NS, Hoffman LJ. 1994. Cecal spirochaetosis in commercial laying hens. Avian Dis 38:895–898.

Trivett-Moore NL, Gilbert GL, Law CLH, Trott DJ, Hampson DJ. 1998. Isolation of *Serpulina pilosicoli* from rectal biopsy specimens showing evidence of intestinal spirochetosis. J Clin Microbiol 36:261–265.

Trott DJ, Alt DP, Zuerner RL, Wannemuehler MJ, Stanton TB. 2001. The search for *Brachyspira* outer membrane proteins that interact with the host. Anim Health Res Rev 2:19–30.

Trott DJ, Hampson DJ. 1998. Evaluation of day-old specific pathogen-free chicks as an experimental model for pathogenicity testing of intestinal spirochaete species. J Comp Path 118:365–381.

Trott DJ, Huxtable CR, Hampson DJ. 1996b. Infection of newly weaned pigs with human and porcine strains of *Serpulina pilosicoli*. Infect Immun 64:4648–4654.

Trott DJ, Jensen NS, Saint Girons I, Oxberry SL, Stanton TB, Lindquist D, Hampson DJ. 1997. Identification and characterisation of *Serpulina pilosicoli* isolates recovered from the blood of critically-ill patients. J Clin Microbiol 35:482–485.

Trott DJ, McLaren AJ, Hampson DJ. 1995. Pathogenicity of human and porcine intestinal spirochaetes in day-old specific pathogen free chicks: An animal model of intestinal spirochaetosis. Infect Immun 63:3705–3710.

Trott DJ, Mikosza ASJ, Combs BG, Oxberry SL, Hampson DJ. 1998. Population genetic analysis of *Serpulina pilosicoli* and its molecular epidemiology in villages in the Eastern Highlands of Papua New Guinea. Int J System Bacteriol 48:659–668.

Trott DJ, Stanton TB, Jensen NS, Duhamel GE, Johnson JL, Hampson DJ. 1996a. *Serpulina pilosicoli* sp. nov.: The agent of porcine intestinal spirochetosis. Int J System Bacteriol 46:206–215.

Trott DJ, Stanton TB, Jensen NS, Hampson DJ. 1996c. Phenotypic characteristics of *Serpulina pilosicoli*, the agent of intestinal spirochaetosis. FEMS Microbiol Lett 142:209–214.

Validation list no. 64. 1998. Int J Syst Bacteriol 48:327–328.

Verspohl J, Feltrup C, Thiede S, Amtsberg G. 2001. Diagnosis of swine dysentery and spirochaetal diarrhea: Part III: Results of cultural and biochemical differentiation of intestinal *Brachyspira* spec. by routine culture from 1997 to 1999. Dtsch tierärztl Wschr 108:67–69.

Webb DM, Duhamel GE, Mathiesen MR, Muniappa N, White A. 1997. Cecal spirochetosis associated with *Serpulina pilosicoli* in captive juvenile ring-necked pheasants. Avian Dis 41:997–1002.

Wilkinson JD, Wood EN. 1987. Grower scour/non-specific colitis. Vet Rec 121:406.

Witters NA, Duhamel GE. 1999. Motility-regulated mucin association of *Serpulina pilosicoli*, the agent of colonic spirochetosis of humans and animals. Adv Exp Med Biol 473:199–205.

Wood EN. 1991. Fashionable and future diseases. Pig Vet J 27:193–197.

Zhang P, Cheng X, Duhamel GE. 2000. Cloning and DNA sequence analysis of an immunogenic glucose/galactose MglB lipoprotein homologue from *Brachyspira pilosicoli*, the agent of colonic spirochetosis. Infect Immun 68:4559–4565.

Zhang P, Duhamel GE. 2002. Serum antibody responses of pigs following challenge with *Brachyspira pilosicoli*. Proc 17th Congr Int Pig Vet Soc, p. 188.

Zhang P, Witters NA, Duhamel GE. 1999. Recovery from infection elicits serum IgG antibodies to specific *Serpulina pilosicoli* outer membrane antigens (SPOMA). Adv Exp Med Biol 473:191–197.

Zuerner RL, Stanton TB, Minion FC, Li C, Charon NW, Trott DJ, Hampson DJ. 2004. Genetic variation in *Brachyspira*: chromosomal rearrangements and sequence drift distinguish *B. pilosicoli* from *B. hyodysenteriae*. Anaerobe 10:229–237.

47 Streptococcal Diseases

Robert Higgins and Marcelo Gottschalk

Several streptococcal species can be found in tonsils, intestines, and genital tracts of clinically healthy pigs, and some of them are potential pathogens. Among species considered as part of the intestinal microflora in swine, are *S. hyointestinalis* (Devriese et al. 1988), *S. suis, S. alactolyticus* (*S. intestinalis*), and *S. bovis* (Devriese et al. 1994b). *S. suis, S. porcinus*, and *S. dysgalactiae* subsp. *equisimilis* (Vieira et al. 1998) are generally found in tonsils (Devriese et al. 1994b). Vaginal microflora may comprise some of the above mentioned species, as well as *S. hyovaginalis* and *S. thoraltensis* (Devriese et al. 1997). Members of the genus *Enterococcus* such as *E. faecalis, E. faecium, E. durans, E. hirae*, and *E. villorum* are also important members of the intestinal microflora.

In this chapter, the different pathological conditions associated with streptococci and enterococci are presented. A particular emphasis was put on the infections caused by *S. suis* because of their importance in the swine industry during the last 15 years. Efforts were made to synthesize the more recent knowledge about the different aspects of these infections, particularly pathogenesis, clinical signs, diagnosis, and prevention. Importance was also given to the fact that *S. suis* is a zoonotic agent with severe consequences, and that its presence in a wide range of animal species and birds may influence the epidemiology and the control of the infection in swine. Comments about infections caused by other streptococci, such as *S. porcinus* (Lancefield groups E, P, U, and V), *S. dysgalactiae* subsp. *equisimilis* (Lancefield groups C, G, and L), have been included, as well as a discussion of diarrhea associated with enterococci.

INFECTIONS CAUSED BY *STREPTOCOCCUS SUIS*

Etiology and Prevalence

New alpha-hemolytic streptococci from septicemic infections in pigs were first biochemically and serologically characterized by de Moor between 1956 and 1963 as new Lancefield groups R, S, RS, and T (de Moor 1963). In England, Elliott (1966) suggested that de Moor's group S was similar to his PM *Streptococcus* and that both belonged to Lancefield's group D; he proposed the name *Streptococcus suis* serotype 1. In 1975, Windsor and Elliott isolated other porcine streptococci which corresponded to de Moor's group R and named them *S. suis* serotype 2. Isolates reacting with both antisera against serotypes 1 and 2 were designated serotype ½ (originally RS group). Isolations of streptococci belonging to group T from tonsillar, vaginal, and preputial swabs were reported by Clifton-Hadley in 1984. The Lancefield group T reference strain was designated *S. suis* serotype 15 in 1989 (Gottschalk et al. 1989).

Between 1983 and 1995, a total of 32 new serotypes were described, out of a total number of 35 serotypes (Perch et al. 1983; Gottschalk et al. 1989; Gottschalk et al. 1991b; Higgins et al. 1995). Reference strains originated from diseased pigs except for capsular type 14, a human isolate, capsular types 17, 18, 19, and 21 isolated from clinically healthy pigs, capsular types 20 and 31 from diseased calves, and type 33 from a diseased lamb (Gottschalk et al. 1989; Higgins et al. 1995). The designation of *S. suis* as a new bacterial species was made official in 1987 by Kilpper-Balz and Schleifer. This species appeared genetically distinct and displayed no specific relationship with other streptococcal species examined (Chatellier et al. 1998). Genetic diversity among members of the *S. suis* species is important (Chatellier et al. 1999; Hampson et al. 1993), and this should be taken into account in diagnosis, surveillance, and control of the disease.

Initial reports of *S. suis* infections were published by Jansen and Van Dorssen in the Netherlands (1951) and by Field et al. (1954) in England. Since then, *S. suis* has been reported in all countries where the swine industry is important, and for more than 15 years, infections associated with this microorganism have been observed in both traditional and modern intensive swine operations. Most *S. suis* organisms isolated from diseased pigs belong to a limited number of serotypes, often those between 1 and 8 (Galina et al. 1992; Higgins and Gottschalk 2001; Hogg et al. 1996; Kataoka et al. 1993; Reams et al. 1996). Although serotype 2 isolates predominate in most countries, the situation may be different depending on the geographical location. For example, the prevalence of this serotype recovered from diseased animals in Canada remained relatively low (below 25%) during the last 10 years (Higgins and Gottschalk 2001). This situation is very different from that observed in some European countries, where serotype 2 was frequently isolated in France, Italy, and Spain (Berthelot-Hérault et al. 2000; Wisselink et al. 2000). In this regard, it may be hypothesised that European and North American serotype 2 strains of *S. suis* possess a different virulence potential (Gottschalk and Segura 2000). In Japan, serotype 2 was also the most prevalent serotype (28%) (Kataoka et al. 1993).

Some strains belonging to less common serotypes have also been associated with severe cases of infection. Serotype 9 was reported to be most frequently isolated in Belgium, The Netherlands and Germany (Wisselink et al. 2000) and associated with outbreaks of septicemia, meningitis, and pneumonia in weaned pigs (Orr et al. 1989; Gogolewski et al. 1990). In the United Kingdom, serotype 14 is frequently isolated from piglets presenting clinicopathological findings similar to those associated with serotype 2 (Heath and Hunt 2001). The number of untypeable isolates is in general relatively low (Higgins and Gottschalk 2001). Most of the time, these isolates are recovered from sporadic cases of disease. It seems that there is no justification at the present time for the characterization of new serotypes.

Serotype 2 can also be isolated from clinically healthy pigs, but its prevalence has been reported to be low. British authors showed that in four herds without any history or clinical signs of the disease, two were negative for the presence of type 2, one had a prevalence of 1.5%, and another a prevalence of 20% (Clifton-Hadley et al. 1984). This is in accordance with Canadian studies that reported the presence of this serotype in relatively low number of herds without clinical signs of infection and in a low number of piglets within these herds (Brisebois et al. 1990; Monter Flores et al. 1993). However, the prevalence of a specific serotype may also be underestimated due to the lack of sensitivity of the isolation method used in these studies.

Hogg et al. (1996) noted a higher prevalence of serotypes 9–34 from nasal and vaginal swabs than from tissues taken from diseased pigs. It is noteworthy that several serotypes may be present in the same animal. In one study, 31% of pigs had only one serotype of *S. suis* in their nasal cavities, 38% had two or three serotypes, and 6% had more than four serotypes (Monter Flores et al. 1993). Isolation of multiple serotypes also has to be taken into consideration in diseased animals (see the section on diagnosis).

Epidemiology

Natural Habitat. The natural habitat of *S. suis* is the upper respiratory tract (particularly the tonsils and nasal cavities) and the genital and alimentary tracts of pigs (Devriese et al. 1994b; Hogg et al. 1996; Baele et al. 2001; Cloutier et al. 2003). *S. suis* is also increasingly isolated from a wide range of animal species and birds (Higgins et al. 1990b, 1995; Kataoka et al. 1993; Devriese et al. 1994a), and this may affect some epidemiological aspects of this infection. Finally, its presence in the environment is transitory (see the next section).

Transmission. Transmission of the infection between herds usually occurs by the movement of healthy carrier animals. The introduction of carrier pigs harboring virulent strains (breeding gilts, boars, weaners) into a non-infected herd may result in the subsequent onset of disease in weaners and/or growing pigs in recipient herds. Sows infect their own piglets during the birth process and probably through the respiratory route (Clifton-Hadley et al. 1986b; Robertson et al. 1991; Amass et al. 1997; Cloutier et al. 2003). It appears that although most weaned piglets carry *S. suis* strains, only a few of them carry strains capable of inducing the disease after weaning (Torremorell et al. 1998; Cloutier et al. 2003). It has been reported for serotype 2 and 5 that, even though different strains within the same serotype are present in the herd, only one of them is usually responsible for the clinical cases (Torremorell et al. 1998; Cloutier et al. 2003). For other serotypes, such as serotype 1/2, strains isolated from diseased animals seem to be similar to those recovered from carrier animals in herds without clinical disease (Martinez et al. 2002). Horizontal transmission seems to be significant especially in the presence of clinical signs, with a considerably higher number of bacteria in the environment that would increase transmission either by aerosol or direct contact. Aerosol transmission without nose-to-nose contact has been demonstrated for *S. suis* serotype 2 (Berthelot-Hérault et al. 2001).

S. suis also appears to be also transmitted via fomites (Robertson et al. 1991; Dee and Corey 1993). *S. suis* types 1 and 2 were isolated from the feed troughs of piglets and sows (Robertson et al. 1991). Enright et al. (1987) demonstrated that flies can carry *S. suis* type 2 for at least 5 days and can contaminate materials on which they feed for at least 4 days. Thus, flies could spread infection within farms and between farms. The importance of other animal species or birds as reservoirs or vectors of the infection has still to be determined. Carriage by humans also seems possible (Sala et al. 1989).

Survival in the Environment. Studies on the survival of *S. suis* in the environment have only been carried out with serotype 2. This organism survived in water at 4°C for 1–2 weeks. In experimentally inoculated feces, it survived at 0°C, 9°C, and 22–25°C for 104, 10, and 8 days, respectively, and in dust for 54, 25, and 0 days, respectively. Thus, at a summertime or weaner-accommodation temperature of 22–25°C, the organism could survive about 8 days in feces but less than 24 hours in dust (Clifton-Hadley and Enright 1984). *S. suis* serotype 2 was shown to survive in pig carcasses left rotting on farms. Survival time was 6 weeks at 4°C and 12 days at 22–25°C, potentially providing a source of infection for indirect spread by, for example, birds, rats, mice, or dogs (Clifton-Hadley et al. 1986c).

With regard to the cleaning of infected pens, disinfectants and cleaners commonly used in piggeries can kill *S. suis* type 2 in less than 1 minute, even at concentrations in distilled water less than those recommended by the manufacturers (Clifton-Hadley and Enright 1984; Robertson et al. 1991). The presence of dirt and organic material protects some organisms from the action of chemical disinfectants, and hence, removal of surface dirt from pens is an important part of the disinfection procedure. *S. suis* type 2 has survived for up to 2 hours at 50°C, but only 10 minutes at 60°C. Hot water may be used, but water from heated pressure washers cools rapidly on pen surfaces and is usually below 50°C. Thus, its value is in diluting contaminating microorganisms and washing away surface dirt rather than in killing by heat (Clifton-Hadley and Enright 1984).

Clinical Signs and Lesions

Even when the pig carrier rate is near 100%, the incidence of the disease varies from period to period and is usually less than 5% (Clifton-Hadley et al. 1986a). However, in the absence of treatment, mortality rates can reach 20% (Cloutier et al. 2003). In most cases, affected animals are generally between 5 and 10 weeks of age, but cases in pigs up to 32 weeks of age and a few hours old have also been described (Nielsen et al. 1975; Reams et al. 1996; MacInnes and Desrosiers 1999; Lapointe et al. 2002; Cloutier et al. 2003). Reams et al. (1996) indicated that in 75% of *S. suis* cases reported in United States, pigs were aged of 16 weeks or less. The earliest sign is usually a rise in rectal temperature to as high as 42.5°C. This may occur initially without any other obvious signs. It is accompanied by a detectable bacteremia or pronounced septicemia, which, if untreated, may persist for up to 3 weeks. During this period, there is usually a fluctuating fever and variable degrees of inappetence, depression, and shifting lameness (Clifton-Hadley et al. 1984).

In peracute cases, pigs may be found dead with no premonitory signs. Meningitis is the most striking feature and the one on which a presumptive diagnosis is usually based. Early nervous signs include incoordination and adoption of unusual stances, which soon progress to inability to stand, paddling, opisthotonus, convulsions, and nystagmus (Staats et al. 1997). The eyes are often staring, with reddening of mucous mem-

branes. Septicemia, arthritis, and pneumonia are less remarkable manifestations of the disease, and a tentative diagnosis may be difficult to make. Among other manifestations of *S. suis* infections, there are endocarditis, rhinitis, abortions, and vaginitis (Sanford and Tilker 1982; Sihvonen et al. 1988). In North America, *S. suis* is, by far, the infectious agent most frequently isolated from cases of endocarditis in pigs. Affected pigs may die suddenly or show various levels of dyspnea, cyanosis, and wasting.

In the United Kingdom, infections due to *S. suis* serotype 2 were primarily associated with septicemia and meningitis in weaned pigs (Windsor and Elliott 1975). In North America, early reports indicated that *S. suis* was predominantly isolated from cases of pneumonia (Koehne et al. 1979; Sanford and Tilker 1982; Erickson et al. 1984). Years later, reports from the United Kingdom mentioned septicemia, meningitis, and polyarthritis, but rarely pneumonia (MacLennan et al. 1996; Heath et al. 1996), whereas pulmonary lesions still predominated in North America (Reams et al. 1994, 1996; Hogg et al. 1996). In the Netherlands, *S. suis* type 2 was associated with pneumonia in 42% of the cases, followed by meningitis, endocarditis, and polyserositis in 18%, 18%, and 10%, respectively (Vecht et al. 1985). *S. suis* isolates belonging to serotypes other than 2 have been recovered from cases of bronchopneumonia in Argentina (Vena et al. 1991), Denmark (Perch et al. 1983), the Netherlands (Vecht et al. 1985), Belgium (Hommez et al. 1986), Finland (Sihvonen et al. 1988), Australia (Gogolewski et al. 1990), Canada (Higgins et al. 1990a; Gottschalk et al. 1991a, b), and the United States (Reams et al. 1994). The role of *S. suis* as a primary agent of pulmonary lesions, in the absence of other pathogens, is still controversial (Staats et al. 1997); so far, only one report indicated the presence of fibrinous pleurisy and bronchopneumonia in specific-pathogen–free piglets experimentally infected with *S. suis* serotype 2 (Berthelot-Hérault et al. 2001). In general, it is considered that neither clinical signs nor gross lesions are associated with specific serotypes (Reams et al. 1996).

Significant microscopic lesions are usually limited to the lung, brain, heart, and joints (Reams et al. 1994). The predominant lesions are neutrophilic meningitis and choroiditis, with hyperemic meningeal blood vessels, fibrinopurulent or suppurative epicarditis and suppurative bronchopneumonia (Sanford and Tilker 1982; Erickson et al. 1984; Reams et al. 1994, 1996). Evidence of encephalitis, edema, and congestion of the brain may be present (Staats et al. 1997). The choroid plexus may have disruption of the plexus brush border and fibrin and inflammatory cell exudates may be present in the ventricles (Staats et al. 1997). Interstitial pneumonia is also seen and is considered a lesion secondary to septicemia (Reams et al. 1994). Microscopic lesions do not seem to be associated with serotype (Reams et al. 1994). Rare cases of fibrinohemorrhagic pneumonia and septal necrosis have been seen, and it is suggested that certain strains of *S. suis* may cause vascular lesions (Reams et al. 1995). In this regard, it has been reported that hemolysin-positive strains are toxic for endothelial cells (Charland et al. 2000; Vanier et al. 2004). Unusual lesions of hemorrhagic and necrotizing myocarditis and subacute meningoencephalitis and meningoencephalomyelitis have also been reported by Sanford (1987a, b). In cases of arthritis, the carpal and tarsal joints are most commonly affected (Windsor and Elliot 1975).

Virulence Factors and Pathogenesis of the Infection

Most studies on *S. suis* virulence factors have been carried out with serotype 2 strains. Although there is confusion in the description of virulence, researchers agree on the existence of virulent and avirulent strains of this serotype (Gottschalk and Segura 2000). Different opinions or versions about the definition of the virulence of *S. suis* have contributed to hampering the studies on virulence factors of this bacterial species, because the concept of "virulence" may differ depending on the experimental infection model that is used. In fact, there is no universally accepted model, and different research groups use different animal species, pigs with different health status and different ages, different routes of infection, or variable bacterial doses. (Gottschalk et al. 1999a). As a consequence, important discrepancies exist in the literature regarding even the virulence of the same strain (Gottschalk et al. 1999a). One of the most important practical applications of the identification of virulence factors is their use as "virulence markers" to differentiate virulent from avirulent strains. So far, there is no such universal virulence marker for *S. suis*.

Despite the fact that knowledge on virulence factors is limited, the most important candidates in *S. suis* serotype 2 are the capsular polysaccharide (CPS), virulence-related proteins, such as the muramidase-released protein (MRP) and the extracellular factor (EF), the hemolysin or suilysin, and some adhesins (Gottschalk and Segura 2000). The CPS is an important antiphagocytic factor, and these findings significantly changed the studies on the pathogenesis of the meningitis (see below). Despite the fact that the CPS was shown to be a major virulence factor, most avirulent strains are encapsulated indicating that other virulence factors are essential (Charland et al. 1998).

The MRP and EF proteins were originally associated with virulence (Vecht et al. 1991). Variants of these proteins were later described with a series of phenotypes that can be found in several serotypes (Smith et al. 1997). A certain association of these proteins with virulence in European strains seems to exist, and most isolates harboring these factors are virulent. However, the absence of one or both of these proteins cannot necessarily be associated with a lack of virulence. In fact, some European and most virulent North American iso-

lates do not produce these factors (Quessy et al. 1994; Galina et al. 1996; Gottschalk et al. 1998; Berthelot-Hérault et al. 2000). Similar observations have been made with the suilysin, a thiol-activated hemolysin produced by some strains of *S. suis* (Jacobs et al. 1994; Gottschalk et al. 1995). Although some authors reported a high association between virulence and the presence of this toxin (Staats et al. 1999; Tarradas et al. 2001), others showed that this hemolysin is absent in most North American virulent isolates (Gottschalk et al. 1998). Segers et al. (1998) also reported that the suilysin was present in 95% of the strains isolated in Eurasia, but only in 7% of the strains from North America. As is the case for the MRP and EF proteins, a certain association between the presence of the suilysin and virulence may be established, since avirulent suilysin-positive strains have never been reported so far (Gottschalk and Segura 2000). Isogenic mutants lacking either the MRP and EF proteins or the suilysin have been obtained and shown to be as virulent for pigs as the respective parent strain (Smith et al. 1997; Allen et al. 2001).

Adhesins, such as hemagglutinins (Haataja et al. 1993; Tikkanen et al. 1996), an albumin-binding protein (Quessy et al. 1997), an IgG-binding protein (Serhir et al. 1993) and a fibronectin-binding protein (de Greeff et al. 2002), have also been suggested as potential virulence factors. These binding proteins may participate in the establishment of the infection, but their role in the pathogenesis of *S. suis* infections remains to be confirmed.

The mechanisms that enable *S. suis* to disseminate throughout the animal are not well understood. The bacterium could spread systemically from the nasopharynx, occasionally resulting in septicemia and death (Gottschalk and Segura 2000). Both palatine and pharyngeal tonsils are considered as possible portals of entry for *S. suis* with subsequent hematogenous or lymphogenous spread (Madsen et al. 2002). An early theory suggested uptake of bacteria by monocytes, intracellular survival, and invasion of the central nervous system (CNS) by the Trojan horse theory (Williams and Blakemore 1990). Studies carried out by flow cytometry are controversial, with high (Busque et al. 1998) or low (Lun and Willson 2004) levels of phagocytosis. However, most studies carried out during the last decade suggest that bacteria may also use (an)other mechanism(s) to disseminate. It seems that most bacteria remain extracellular and the number of monocytes containing bacteria in septicemic pigs is low (≤2%) (Williams and Blakemore 1990). In addition, the CPS would confer antiphagocytic properties to *S. suis* (Charland et al. 1998; Smith et al. 1999). It is possible that bacteria travel either free in circulation or even externally attached to monocytes (modified Trojan horse theory) (Gottschalk and Segura 2000; Segura and Gottschalk 2002). Bacteria can then reach the CNS via the endothelial cells that form the brain blood barrier

(BBB). It has been recently reported that *S. suis* is able to invade porcine brain microvascular endothelial cells (Vanier et al. 2004). On the other hand, interactions of bacteria with polarized epithelial cells of the choroid plexus (another important cell component of the BBB) may be the consequence of pressure of high-grade constant bacteremia. In fact, disruption of the plexus brush border, with fibrin and inflammatory cell exudates present in the ventricules has been described during natural and experimentally induced *S. suis* meninigitis (Williams and Blakemore 1990). Further studies of interactions between *S. suis* and epithelial cells from the choroid plexus might bring new and relevant information. Finally, studies have pointed out that the inflammatory exudate itself may be detrimental in some cases and have recommended treatment with antiinflammatory medications (Tunkel et al. 1990). In this regard, *S. suis* has been described as being able to induce an important release of proinflammatory cytokines (Gottschalk and Segura 2000; Segura et al. 2002).

Diagnosis

From Diseased Pigs. Presumptive diagnosis of *S. suis* infections is generally based on clinical signs, age of animals, and macroscopic lesions. Confirmation is achieved by the isolation of the infectious agent and microscopic lesions in tissues. When feasible, collection of more than one alpha-hemolytic colony from different tissues of the same animal or from different animals in the same herd is recommended, because multiple serotypes and strains of *S. suis* can be involved (Reams et al. 1996). Amass et al. (1997) suggested periodic culture of CSF from pigs with meningitis to ensure that the strain(s) of *S. suis* causing meningitis in the herd have not changed. This could be very helpful when vaccination is considered. Since *S. suis* may be recovered even from healthy lung tissues (Mwaniki et al. 1994), isolates from tissues other than lungs should be preferred in septicemic cases. In respiratory case accessions, isolation of other infectious agents such as *Pasteurella multocida*, *Actinobacillus pleuropneumoniae*, or *Arcanobacterium pyogenes* is frequent, but pure cultures of *S. suis* are also isolated (Higgins et al. 1990a; Galina et al. 1992). Direct detection of *S. suis* from infected tissues has also been studied. *In situ* hybridization with a probe detecting (without differentiating) serotypes 1–31 was used for detection of *S. suis* in formalin-fixed, paraffin-embedded tissue sections of brain, endocardium, and lung from *S. suis* infected pigs. In addition, immunohistochemical methods for the detection (without differentiation) of serotypes 2 and 1/2 were also reported (Boye et al. 2000). Detection of some serotypes of *S. suis* by PCR has also been reported (Wisselink et al. 2002a). However, these methods are not used in routine diagnosis.

After isolation, biochemical identification of *S. suis* isolates is possible with a minimum of tests when serotyping is available (Higgins and Gottschalk 1990).

Devriese et al. (1991) suggested the use of only two tests on pig isolates: amylase positive and Voges-Proskauer (acetoin) negative. However, this simplified identification scheme can be used only for isolates recovered from diseased or dead pigs and from sites other than the upper respiratory tract.

Serotyping is still an important part of the routine diagnostic procedure. It can be carried out by different techniques, but many laboratories have adopted the coagglutination technique. Since the majority of typeable isolates belong to serotypes 1–8 and 1/2, it is advisable for diagnostic laboratories to only use antisera corresponding to those serotypes and to send untypeable isolates to a reference laboratory (Higgins and Gottschalk 1990; Hogg et al. 1996). Some isolates cross-react with more than one antiserum using the coagglutination, as well as the capsular reaction, tests. The most important cross reactions are serotype 1/2 isolates with antisera against serotypes 1 and 2, and serotype 1 isolates with antiserum against serotype 14 (Gottschalk et al. 1989; Gottschalk and Segura 2000).

Genetic tools could be of valuable help in distinguishing individual isolates of *S. suis*, in establishing the origin of the infection in a given herd, in monitoring the kinetics of an outbreak, or in ensuring that the right strain is included in a vaccine. It was demonstrated that an important diversity existed among *S. suis* isolates even for those belonging to the same serotype (Mogollon et al. 1990). Genomic fingerprinting has allowed the identification of outbreak isolates of *S. suis* serotypes 2 and 5 (Mogollon et al. 1991; Cloutier et al. 2003). One study carried out with isolates from diseased pigs from different regions of Brazil showed the presence of a clonal atypical isolate (Martinez et al. 2003). Conversely, for herds affected with serotype 1/2 strains, clinical manifestations of the disease were more likely to be the result of inherent herd factors than the virulence of a specific isolate (Martinez et al. 2002). Overall, the great genetic heterogeneity of the clinical strains of *S. suis*, the isolation of different strains within the same herd, and the predominance of particular strains in some herds are evidence that infection by *S. suis* is a dynamic process and reinforce the idea that the epidemiology of *S. suis* infection is very complex (Vela et al. 2003). Isolates from different geographical origins seem to be genotypically different. In fact, strains of *S. suis* serotype 2 from Europe (presenting a MRP', EF', suilysin' phenotype) seem to be different from North American strains, which are negative for these markers (Chatellier et al. 1999).

From Clinically Healthy Pigs. As mentioned before, *S. suis* is considered a normal inhabitant of the upper respiratory tract (Baele et al. 2001). Detection of *S. suis* from tonsils has no practical utility. These sites are highly contaminated and traditional bacterial isolation presents a low sensitivity (Gottschalk et al. 1999b). The presence of *S. suis* in high numbers in nasal cavities may reflect an active transmission of the infection rather than a carrier state (Cloutier et al. 2003). In this regard, it has been reported that the use of selective isolation using immunomagnetic beads coated with serotype 2 specific antibodies significantly increased the isolation rate of this serotype from tonsils when compared to the standard isolation technique (Gottschalk et al. 1999b). This technique has also been used with serotype 5 infected herds (Cloutier et al. 2003). Wisselink et al. (1999) described a PCR for the detection of virulent strains of serotype 1 and 2 from tonsils, but based on the phenotypes EF and MRP, which are not present in North America. Untypeable isolates recovered from tonsils or nasal cavities must be confirmed as being *S. suis* by genetic methods (Okwumabua et al. 2003), since biochemical identification may be misleading.

Different serologic tests for the detection of antibodies against *S. suis* have been evaluated (del Campo Sepulveda et al. 1996; Kataoka et al. 1996). However, these tests are not useful to differentiate infected from noninfected herds and cannot be used routinely. It has been reported that the use of an ELISA test using a protein extract of *S. suis* (homologous strain present in the herd) as coating antigen presented high interest. The development of a strain-specific ELISA allowed the evaluation of the serologic profiles of the maternal antibody levels in piglets to decide the time of vaccination as well as the induction of antibodies after either natural infection or vaccination (Lapointe et al. 2002; Cloutier et al. 2003).

Treatment

The choice of the best antibacterial agent against *S. suis* infections must be based on several criteria such as the susceptibility of the organism, the type of infection, and the mode of administration. Using the Kirby-Bauer method, susceptibility of *S. suis* isolates to penicillin appeared to be high (Kataoka et al. 2000; Han et al. 2001; Marie et al. 2002). The determination of minimal inhibitory concentrations allowed the demonstration of a large number of isolates moderately susceptible to penicillin, but the sensitivity rate to amoxicillin and ampicillin was around 90% (Shryock et al. 1992; Dee et al. 1993; Turgeon et al. 1994). It is now recommended that penicillin be used only in cases where sensitivity tests have shown that *S. suis* is sensitive. Different authors have reported a high degree of resistance of *S. suis* isolates to some antibacterial agents such as tetracycline, clindamycin, erythromycin, kanamycin, neomycin, and streptomycin (Estoepangestie and Lämmler 1993; Dee et al. 1993; Reams et al. 1993; Turgeon et al. 1994). Susceptibility to trimethoprim-sulfamethoxazole appeared to be variable (Sanford and Tilker 1989; Shryock et al. 1992; Turgeon et al. 1994; Kataoka et al. 2000). A Danish study showed a significant serotype-associated difference in the susceptibility to macrolides and tetracycline and demonstrated an increase in resistance

among *S. suis* isolates recovered during the last years to the two most commonly used antimicrobial agents (tylosin and tetracycline) in pig production in Denmark (Aarestrup et al. 1998). Marie et al. (2002) also described a higher proportion of resistance among non-serotype 2 isolates of *S. suis*. On the other hand, Han et al. (2001) did not find any correlation between antimicrobial susceptibility and serotype. MacInnes and Desrosiers (1999) suggested that ampicillin, ceftiofur, gentamicin, tiamulin and a combination of trimethoprim and a sulfonamide would seem to be the most useful antibacterial products for parenteral treatment.

Prompt recognition of the early clinical signs of streptococcal meningitis followed by immediate parenteral treatment of affected pigs with an appropriate antibiotic is currently the best method to maximize pig survival (Amass et al. 1997). Pigs in the early stages of meningitis may be difficult to detect, and groups of pigs should be checked 2–3 times daily. Affected pigs hold their ears back, squint their eyes, or exhibit dog-sitting (Amass et al. 1997). Adjunctive therapy with an antiinflammatory agent is recommended for treatment of *S. suis* meningitis in pigs (Amass et al. 1997). In a segregated early-weaning (SEW) program where postweaning meningitis associated with *S. suis* was observed, excellent results were obtained when piglets, in the very early stages of the disease, were injected with both penicillin and dexamethasone (Clark 1995). In peracute forms of the disease, the response to antibiotic treatment can be poor and it is sometimes advisable to treat all the pigs in a pen when one is affected or found dead (MacInnes and Desrosiers 1999).

Treatment can also be administered via the drinking water or in medicated feed. However, due to the method of spread of the disease, treatment needs to be started very quickly. Whichever method of medication is to be used, it is important that treatment is continued for at least 5 days (Denicourt and Le Coz 2000).

Prevention

Control of Predisposing Factors. *S. suis* is an example of an emerging infection associated with the intensification of the swine industry. Multiple factors are involved, and among them are the health status of the herd (such as concomitant infections and immunosuppression), the degree of virulence of the *S. suis* strains involved, and the quality of the environment and of the management. It was also reported that minimizing variation in weaning age, with concurrent use of an autogeneous vaccine and antibiotic at processing and weaning, appeared to contribute to a decrease in nursery mortality (Villani 2003).

Overcrowding, poor ventilation, excessive temperature fluctuations, and mixing of pigs with an age spread of more than 2 weeks seem to be the most important stress factors involved in the development of *S. suis* infection in susceptible pigs (Dee et al. 1993). Management practices such as all-in/all-out pig flow can help reduce the incidence of the disease. Dividing large buildings into smaller rooms can help minimize temperature fluctuations and the age spread between pigs. Cleaning each room between groups of pigs reduces buildup of microorganisms and improves health status, average daily gain, and feed conversion (Dee et al. 1993).

It is likely that concomitant viral infections could potentiate the development of lesions in infections due to *S. suis*. Iglesias et al. (1992) concluded that clinical disease associated with *S. suis* type 2 was enhanced by concomitant infection with pseudorabies virus. In North America, swine practitioners generally agree with the concept that the infection with the porcine reproductive and respiratory syndrome virus (PRRSV) significantly increases the susceptibility of animals to secondary infections, such as those caused by *S. suis*. This was confirmed by experimental infections (Galina et al. 1994; Thanawongnuwech et al. 2000). In addition, Feng et al. (2001) clearly demonstrated that in utero infection by PRRSV makes piglets more susceptible to infection and disease following challenge by *S. suis* type 2.

Production Technologies. Medicated early weaning and SEW have been used to improve the health status of pigs and to eliminate some infectious organisms (Alexander et al. 1980). It is now accepted that although early weaning can succeed in controlling diseases such as pleuropneumonia and swine dysentery, its capacity to reduce or eliminate early colonizers, such as *S. suis, Haemophilus parasuis,* and *Actinobacillus suis*, is questionable (Pijoan 1996). Control of these problems requires aggressive use of new diagnostic techniques, such as serum profiling, together with some manipulation of sow immunity and disease transmission in the nursery (Pijoan 1996). Other procedures, such as nursery depopulation, are under evaluation (Dee and Joo 1997).

Antimicrobial Preventive Medication. Antimicrobial preventive medication of groups of pigs via feed or water against *S. suis* infections must be based on several considerations. Bioavailability, route of administration (feed or water), competition (overcrowded pens), and serum concentration needed to kill *S. suis* have to be considered prior to prophylactic antimicrobial treatment (del Castillo et al. 1995; Amass et al. 1997).

Procaine penicillin incorporated into the feed was reported to significantly reduce the prevalence of streptococcal meningitis within a herd (McKellar et al. 1987). Oral administration of procaine penicillin G resulted in measurable systemic concentrations, although it is known that in humans, only about one-third of an orally administered dose is absorbed from the intestinal tract. Higher plasma concentrations are obtained with an equivalent dose of phenoxymethyl penicillin (McKellar et al. 1987). Del Castillo et al. (1995) indicated that of all types of oral treatments with penicillin, only

penicillin V in water given to fasted piglets could reach serum concentrations greater than the target concentrations selected for *S. suis* isolates. In the same conditions, penicillin G concentrations were much lower and hardly stayed above the target serum level. In the presence of food, only penicillin V reached the target level, but only in a few piglets. Thus, penicillin should exclusively be orally administered through drinking water to reduce the interference in absorption due to feed (del Castillo et al. 1995).

Amoxicillin is also an antibiotic of choice, since it rapidly achieves high plasma levels, diffuses well into the extracellular space, and most *S. suis* strains present low MIC (Denicourt and Le Coz 2000). In addition, persistence of amoxicillin in lymph nodes and tonsils may be relevant to control pathogens such as *S. suis*. Other authors have reported less conclusive results using experimentally infected animals (Halbur et al. 2000; Schmitt et al. 2001). In these studies, the use of ampicillin and penicillin G did not significantly reduce disease in animals exposed to a co-infection with *S. suis* and SRRPV. Ceftiofur treatment was the only regimen that significantly reduced mortality, recovery of *S. suis* from tissues at necropsy and severity of gross lung lesions.

Immunization. Until now, most vaccines used in the field to protect against *S. suis* infections have been commercial autogenous bacterins and results have been inconsistent (Reams et al. 1996; Torremorell et al. 1997; Halbur et al. 2000). The exact reasons for vaccine failure are still unknown, but possible explanations are degradation of protective antigens or loss of antigenicity of the bacteria caused by heat or formalin processing (Holt et al. 1990a), production of antibodies to antigens not associated with virulence factors (Holt et al. 1988), and weak immunogenicity of the capsulated bacteria (del Campo Sepulveda et al. 1996). Since affected animals are in general between 6 and 10 weeks old, interference with maternal antibodies should be taken into consideration. This was demonstrated by Lapointe et al. (2002) with a serotype 1/2 *S. suis* strain in an autogenous vaccine using sonicated bacteria. The serologic profile revealed that antibody levels against the *S. suis* serotype 1/2 strain varied considerably among 2- and 4-week-old pigs. Differences in antibody levels among piglets in these age groups could be attributed to differences in maternal antibody levels and/or in the rate of absorption of maternal antibodies by the piglets. In that study, it was clear that animals with the lowest levels of antibodies against the strain of *S. suis* serotype 1/2 responded more effectively to vaccination (Lapointe et al. 2002). In addition, the adjuvant used seems to play an important role. Wisselink et al. (2001) showed that a bacterin with a water-in-oil emulsion as an adjuvant presented better results than the same bacterin but with aluminium hydroxide-based adjuvant.

Live avirulent strains have also been tested. Protection was obtained in pigs following the inoculation of live avirulent *S. suis* serotype 2 strains (Holt et al. 1988; Busque et al. 1997). On the other hand, a live acapsular mutant was shown to fail to provide protection (Wisselink et al. 2002b). Since in some cases, live *S. suis* strains appear to induce a protection similar to that produced by live virulent strains, it is suggested that the important immunogens may be different from *S. suis* virulence factors (Gottschalk and Segura 2000). The use of a reduced dose of virulent *S. suis* also showed good protective results although some residual virulence was observed (Schmitt et al. 2001).

The importance of humoral immunity was well established by succeeding in passively transferring protection against *S. suis* type 2 (Holt et al. 1988, Andresen and Tegtmeier 2001). The role of antibodies against the capsule is still controversial. It was demonstrated that pigs experimentally or naturally infected with *S. suis* type 2 produced only low levels of antibodies against the capsular polysaccharide (del Campo Sepulveda et al. 1996). Andresen and Tegtmeier (2001) obtained high titers of antibodies against the CPS in one of two horses immunized for more than 40 weeks with whole cells of *S. suis* serotype 2. On the other hand, Wisselink et al. (2002b) showed that antibodies against the CPS and other bacterial components are essential for full protection against homologous challenge.

Studies have shown that different *S. suis* type 2 proteins could induce a good protection (Holt et al. 1990b; Quessy et al. 1994). A vaccine using MRP and EF proteins completely protected pigs against a challenge with virulent *S. suis* serotype 2 strains (Wisselink et al. 2001). These results disagree with those presented by Jacobs et al. (1996), who also reported that the suilysin was the only protein giving complete protection against *S. suis* infection. However, as mentioned, these three proteins are not present in all virulent strains (Quessy et al. 1994; Galina et al. 1996; Gottschalk et al. 1998; Berthelot-Hérault et al. 2000).

Most studies have been carried out with piglets. However, vaccination of sows and gilts has also been proposed and shown to be effective to a certain extent (Torremorell et al. 1997; Amass et al. 2000).

Finally, and based on the fact that systemic strains of *S. suis* are rarely found colonizing the upper respiratory tract of sows and gilts, and that a small number of piglets reach the nursery colonized with the herd's systemic strains, it has been suggested that early colonization of young pigs with the systemic strain can be used as a method for disease prevention (Torremorell et al. 1999; Oliveira et al. 2001). These authors showed that although both colonization protocols were successful in getting the piglets colonized, direct inoculation of 5-day-old piglets with the herd's systemic strain of *S. suis* tended to be more effective in reducing the morbidity and mortality than the colonization of piglets by nose-to-nose contact with inoculated sows (Oliveira et al. 2001).

Eradication

Attempts to eradicate the infection have focused only on serotype 2. Medicated early weaning (Alexander et al. 1980) is in general poorly effective, since *S. suis* is a very early colonizer (Torremorell et al. 1998). According to Clifton-Hadley et al. (1986b), only depopulation and restocking with clean pigs will ensure eradication of the infection, and in most herds this is not economic. Mills (1996) described the procedures that were used to establish a purebred minimal-disease herd from gilts found to be carriers of a virulent strain of *S. suis* type 2. Amass et al. (1996), on the other hand, did not recommend such an approach. They emphasized optimization of management and environment of pigs coupled with strategic medication of clinically ill animals for control and prevention of mortality caused by streptococcosis.

Cesarean section can be used to derive pigs free of *S. suis* from infected dams. Strict biosecurity measures are needed and they must include eliminating rodents and flies (Amass et al. 1997).

Considering that the infection is transmitted during farrowing, disease is often associated with respiratory problems and with multiple *S. suis* serotypes, that some less common serotypes are more and more involved in severe outbreaks, that reliable diagnostic or monitoring tools such as serology will not be available in the short term, and, finally, that *S. suis* is now isolated from a wide range of animal species and birds, it would appear reasonable to direct research efforts toward control measures rather than eradication.

Infection in Humans

S. suis is a zoonotic agent which deserves attention. Since the first description in Denmark in 1968 (Perch et al. 1968), nearly 200 human cases of *S. suis* infection have been reported. Several reports indicate "Lancefield group R streptococci"; these cases must be considered as *S. suis* since the latter terminology has been abandoned (Gottschalk and Segura 2000). In general, the *S. suis* disease is considered a rare event in man; however, it has been reported to be "one of the major causes of meningitis in adults in Hong Kong" (Chau et al. 1983). Most cases are caused by serotype 2 strains; but cases due to serotype 4 (one case) and serotype 14 (two cases) strains have also been observed (Gottschalk and Segura 2000; Watkins et al. 2001). Two recently found *S. suis* serotype 1 cases in humans remain to be confirmed because the serotype of these strains was only established using biochemical criteria and was not confirmed with a serologic reaction using specific sera (Kopic et al. 2003). Unfortunately, these isolates are no longer viable to confirm the serotype (J. Kopic, personal communication 2004).

Cases have been reported in The Netherlands, Denmark, Italy, Germany, Belgium, United Kingdom, France, Spain, Sweden, Ireland, Austria, Hungary, Hong Kong, Croatia, Japan, Singapore, Taiwan, New Zealand,

and Argentina (Gottschalk 2004). In the United Kingdom and France, this infection has been listed as an Industrial Disease in 1983 and 1995, respectively (Walsh et al. 1992; Pedroli et al. 2003). Mysteriously, although human cases have been observed in Canada (Michaud et al. 1996), none has been reported in the United States. It seems that the lack of reports on this disease in humans in the U.S. is most probably due to the misidentification of the microorganism (Gottschalk 2004). Even though *S. suis* field isolates readily grow on media employed for culturing meningitis causing bacteria, many laboratories working in human diseases are not aware of this microorganism and it is usually misidentified as enterococci, *Streptococcus pneumoniae, Streptococcus bovis,* viridans group streptococci, or even *Listeria* spp. (Lütticken et al. 1986; Michaud et al. 1996). In many cases, the initial gram stain diagnosis of the cerebrospinal fluid (CSF) specimen is pneumococcal meninigitis.

In man, *S. suis* usually produces a purulent or nonpurulent meningitis (Lütticken et al. 1986). In addition, endocarditis, cellulitis, rhabdomyolysis, arthritis, pneumonia, and endopthalmitis have also been reported (Gottschalk 2004). Severe cases of sepsis with shock, multiple organ failure, disseminated intravascular coagulation, and associated purpura fulminans, which lead to death within hours, have also been described (François et al. 1998). One of the most striking features of the infection is the consequence of deafness following *S. suis* meningitis (Lütticken et al. 1986). *S. suis* meningitis may have been missed in the past because of such confusion. *S. suis* infection in humans is observed more frequently in intensive pig farming areas or where people live in close contact with pigs (Strangmann et al. 2002). In fact, in nearly all reported cases, patients had close contact with pigs—as farmers, butchers, abattoir workers—or handled pork products (Arends and Zanen 1988). One documented case of a veterinary surgeon has been reported (Walsh et al. 1992). The most frequent transmission route is through skin abrasions or cuts, although in many cases, no skin laceration could be shown (Michaud et al. 1996). The finding that liquid soap inactivates *S. suis* type 2 in less than 1 minute at a dilution in water of 1 in 500 suggests that washing with soap and water would be a satisfactory way of removing skin contamination (Clifton-Hadley and Enright 1984). Since *S. suis* type 2 can survive in carcasses at 4°C for 6 weeks, chilled or frozen meat could be a hazard long after being butchered.

Information about the occurrence and frequency of human colonization by *S. suis* is scarce, with most data coming from abattoir workers (Strangmann et al. 2002; Sala et al. 1989). In New Zealand, relatively high antibody titer against *S. suis* serotype 2 were reported in people with occupational contact with the pig industry (Robertson and Blackmore 1989). However, these data should be taken with caution since no standardized serological test to detect *S. suis* antibodies exists.

In general, *S. suis* isolates from humans are phenotypically and genotypically similar to those recovered from pigs (Berthelot-Hérault et al. 2002) and they are also susceptible to beta-lactams. Gentamicin appeared also very active against *S. suis*, and a combination with penicillin is recommended in human cases of endocarditis due to this agent (Trottier et al. 1991).

INFECTIONS CAUSED BY BETA-HEMOLYTIC STREPTOCOCCI

Streptococcus porcinus

The name *Streptococcus porcinus* was proposed in 1984 by Collins et al. (1984) to represent streptococci of serological groups E, P, U, and V, which formed a single DNA-DNA homology group. *S. porcinus* has a unique phenotypic profile in addition to serologic differences that can be used to help identify the species. By rRNA sequencing, *S. porcinus* is closely related to the other beta-hemolytic streptococci, such as groups A, B, and C (Facklam et al. 1995).

S. porcinus group E has been associated, particularly in the United States, with a contagious clinical entity in growing pigs known as streptococcal lymphadenitis, jowl abscesses, or cervical abscesses. Transmission is possible by contact, drinking water, or ingestion of food contaminated by abscess discharge or infected feces. The organisms enter the swine host through the mucosa of the pharyngeal or tonsillar surfaces and are carried to the lymph nodes, primarily of the head and neck region, where abscesses are formed (Wessman 1986). Losses due to this disease in the United States were important in the 1960s, but its incidence has since declined. The disease is not recognized as an important economic entity in other countries, where the bacterium represents only a few percent of the microorganisms isolated from abscesses in swine (Wessman 1986). A report of an outbreak from Spain mentioned that 80% of 50 feeder pigs had mandibular and retropharyngeal purulent lymphadenitis (Real et al. 1992). Antibiotic treatment is not usually successful in abscessed swine or in elimination of carriers. Resistance to tetracycline has been recently reported (Facklam et al. 1995; Lämmler and Bahr 1996). Vaccination is possible but has not been widely used since the condition is not widespread.

S. porcinus group E can be isolated from tonsils, pharynx, and nasal cavities of clinically healthy pigs. It is also occasionally found in the vaginal mucus of sows and in the semen and prepuce of boars. It is considered to be more of a secondary invader than a primary pathogen in conditions such as pneumonia, enteritis, encephalitis, and arthritis (Wessman 1986). It was isolated in Canada from the lungs of a 2-year-old pig affected with an abscessative pneumonia, along with other bacterial agents (A. Désilets, personal communication 1995).

S. porcinus groups P, U, and V were isolated by

Hommez et al. (1991) from pig lungs, genital organs, and brains. However, no histological lesions could be associated with their presence. *S. porcinus* groups P and V were associated with abortions in pigs (Plagemann 1988; Lämmler and Bahr 1996). Hommez et al. (1991) cited a report of Hinterdorfer et al. (1990), in which *S. porcinus* group P was associated with hemorrhagic tracheitis in pigs.

Katsumi et al. (1997) found *S. porcinus* in 1.6% of slaughtered pigs with lesions of endocarditis. In 1998, the same authors reported that on a total of 170 beta-hemolytic streptococci isolated from lesions in slaughtered pigs, 22.4% were identified as *S. porcinus*. Of those, 3.0% belonged to group E, 3.0% to group P, 8.2% to group U, and 8.2% were ungroupable (Katsumi et al. 1998).

Streptococcus dysgalactiae subsp. *equisimilis*

In 1984, Farrow and Collins, using DNA-DNA hybridization, DNA base composition, and biochemical tests, indicated that *Streptococcus dysgalactiae*, *S. equisimilis*, and streptococci of Lancefield serologic groups C, G, and L were a single species. In 1996, Vandamme et al. proposed that the name *S. dysgalactiae* subsp. *dysgalactiae* be used for strains of animal origin, and the name *S. dysgalactiae* subsp. *equisimilis* be used for human isolates. However, in 1998, Vieira et al., based on multilocus enzyme electrophoresis typing and genomic DNA relatedness, proposed a new classification for these organisms: alpha- and non-hemolytic streptococci of Lancefield group C are defined as *S. dysgalactiae* subsp. *dysgalactiae*, and beta-hemolytic streptococci belonging to groups C, G, or L are named *S. dysgalactiae* subsp. *equisimilis*.

In swine, members of the *S. dysgalactiae* subsp. *equisimilis* species are all beta-hemolytic streptococci. Although members of the normal flora, they are considered the most important beta-hemolytic streptococci involved in lesions in pigs, and these agents were judged to be of etiological significance in autopsy reports (Hommez et al. 1991). *S. dysgalactiae* group C streptococci are common in nasal and throat secretions, tonsils, and vaginal and preputial secretions (Jones 1976). Vaginal secretions and milk from postparturient sows are the most likely sources of infection for the piglets (Woods and Ross 1977). Streptococci enter the bloodstream via skin wounds, the navel, and tonsils. A bacteremia or septicemia occurs, and the organisms then settle in one or more tissues, giving rise to arthritis, endocarditis, or meningitis. Insufficient consumption of colostrum or milk or inadequate levels of antibodies, especially in gilts, may predispose to disease (Windsor 1978).

Infection is usually first seen in pigs between 1 and 3 weeks of age. Joint swelling and lameness are the most obvious and persistent clinical signs. Elevated temperatures, lassitude, roughened hair coat, and inappetence may also be noted. Early lesions consist of periarticular edema; swollen, hyperemic synovial membranes; and turbid synovial fluid. Necrosis of articular cartilage may be seen 15–30 days after onset and may become more severe. Fibrosis and multiple focal abscessation of periarticular tissues and hypertrophy of synovial villi also occur. In lame pigs, up to 12 weeks of age, the causative agents of arthritis were, in decreasing order, *S. dysgalactiae* subsp. *equisimilis* (26.3%), *Staphylococcus hyicus* (24.6%), *Arcanobacterium pyogenes* (13.2%), *S. aureus* (7.9%), and *Haemophilus parasuis* (7.9%), and most of the pigs culled for arthritis were under 6 weeks of age (Hill et al. 1996). Hommez et al. (1991) mentioned that *S. dysgalactiae* is frequently isolated from pigs, in which the organisms cause septicemia, arthritis, or valvular endocarditis. In 1997, Katsumi et al. reported the isolation of *S. dysgalactiae* from lesions of endocarditis in 15.2% of slaughtered pigs, and *S. suis* was present in 25.7% of the animals. In 1998, Katsumi et al. mentioned that during a 7-year period, 77.6% of beta-hemolytic streptococci isolated from slaughtered pigs belonged to the *S. dysgalactiae* species. Of those, 45.8% belonged to Lancefield group C, 25.3% to group L, and 6.5% to group G.

Since baby pigs are virtually assured of being exposed to *S. dysgalactiae*, effective preventive measures should be followed. Adequate intake of colostrum may ensure that the piglets receive protective antibodies. Traumatic injuries to the feet and legs should be minimized by reducing the abrasiveness of the floor surface in the nursing area. Beta-hemolytic streptococci are sensitive to beta-lactam antibiotics. Long-acting antibacterial agents may be beneficial, and treatment should be given before the inflammatory process is well advanced (Sanford and Higgins 1992). There are no recent reports about vaccination against groups C or L streptococci. Autogenous bacterins have been used, and a reduction in incidence of arthritis has been reported when sows were vaccinated before farrowing (Woods and Ross 1977).

Enteritis Associated with Enterococci in Piglets

Some enterococcal species that show typical adhesion to the apical surface of the enterocytes of the small intestine of young animals have been described as associated with diarrhea in different animal species (Vancanneyt et al. 2001). Cases have been reported in piglets between 2 and 20 days of age. Most cases were sporadic (Johnson et al. 1983; Drolet et al. 1990), but an outbreak included 90% of the piglets in 16 of 20 litters (Cheon and Chae 1996). Taxonomic studies have shown that most of these enterococci are members of the *E. faecium* species group, mainly *E. durans* and *E. hirae*. In 2001, Vancanneyt et al. reported that some of the *E. hirae* or *E. hirae*-like isolates retrieved from piglets were genetically different from the reference strains and should be represented by a new species, *E. villorum*.

Enterococci are known as part of the intestinal flora, but some strains have the capacity to colonize the mucosal surface of the small intestine extensively. The pathogenesis of enteric disease associated with adherent enterococci is unclear. Adherence occurs with the help of fibrillar projections (Tzipori et al. 1984), and diarrhea is not associated with enterotoxin production or substantial mucosal injury (Cheon and Chae 1996). A decreased activity of brush border digestive enzymes such as lactase and alkaline phosphatase would interfere with digestion and absorption of the brush border (Drolet et al. 1990; Cheon and Chae 1996). Because of the natural resistance of enterococci to some antibacterial agents, antimicrobial susceptibility testing is advised before the institution of a treatment. Due to the lack of knowledge about the clinical and epidemiological aspects of this infection, preventive measures are difficult to establish.

REFERENCES

Aarestrup FM, Rasmusse n SR, Artursson K, Jensen NE. 1998. Trends in the resistance to antimicrobial agents of *Streptococcus suis* isolates from Denmark and Sweden. Vet Microbiol 63:71–80.

Alexander TJL, Thornton K, Boon G, Lysons RJ, Gush AF. 1980. Medicated early weaning to obtain pigs free from pathogens endemic in the herd of origin. Vet Rec 106:114–119.

Allen AG, Bolitho S, Lindsay H, Khan S, Bryant C, Norton P, Ward P, Leigh J, Morgan J, Riches H, Eastty S, Maskell D. 2001. Generation and characterization of a defined mutant of *Streptococcus suis* lacking suilysin. Infect Immun 69:2732–2735.

Amass SF, San Miguel P, Clark LK. 1997. Demonstration of vertical transmission of *Streptococcus suis* in swine by genomic fingerprinting. J Clin Microbiol 35:1595–1596.

Amass SF, Stevenson G, Vyverberg B, Huxford T, Knox K, Grote LA. 2000. Administration of a homologous bacterin to sows prefarrowing provided partial protection against streptococcosis in their weaned pigs. Swine Health Prod 8:217–219.

Amass SF, Wu CC, Clark LK. 1996. Evaluation of antibiotics for the elimination of the tonsillar carrier state of *Streptococcus suis* in pigs. J Vet Diagn Invest 8:64–67.

Andresen L, Tegtmeier C. 2001. Passive immunization of pigs against experimental infection with *Streptococcus suis* serotype 2. Vet Microbiol 81:331–344.

Arends JP, Zanen HC. 1988. Meningitis caused by *Streptococcus suis* in humans. Rev Infect Dis 10:131–137.

Baele M, Chiers K, Devriese LA, Smith HE, Wisselink HJ, Vaneechoutte M, Haesebrouck F. 2001. The gram-positive tonsillar and nasal flora of piglets before and after weaning. J App Microbiol 91:997–1003.

Berthelot-Hérault F, Gottschalk M, Labbe A, Cariolet R, Kobisch M. 2001. Experimental airborne transmission of *Streptococcus suis* capsular type 2 in pigs. Vet Microbiol 82:69–80.

Berthelot-Hérault F, Marois C, Gottschalk M, Kobisch M. 2002. Genetic diversity of *Streptococcus suis* strains isolated from pigs and humans as revealed by pulsed-field gel electrophoresis. J Clin Microbiol 40:615–619.

Berthelot-Hérault F, Morvan H, Kéribin AM, Gottschalk M, Kobisch M. 2000. Production of muraminidase-released protein (MRP), extracellular factor (EF) and haemolysin by field isolates of *Streptococcus suis* capsular types 2, ½, 9, 7 and 3 isolated from swine in France. Vet Res 31:473–479.

Boye M, Feenstra AA, Tegtmeier C, Andresen LO, Rasmussen SR, Bille-Hansen V. 2000. Detection of *Streptococcus suis* by *in situ*

hybridization, indirect immunofluorescence, and peroxidase-antiperoxidase assays in formalin-fixed, paraffin-embedded tissue sections from pigs. J Vet Diagn Invest 12:224–232.

Brisebois LM, Charlebois R, Higgins R, Nadeau M. 1990. Prevalence of *Streptococcus suis* in four to eight week old clinically healthy piglets. Can J Vet Res 54:174–177.

Busque P, Higgins R, Caya F, Quessy S. 1997. Immunization of pigs against *Streptococcus suis* serotype 2 infection using a live avirulent strain. Can J Vet Res 61:275–279.

Busque P, Higgins R, Senechal S, Marchand R, Quessy S. 1998. Simultaneous flow cytometric measurement of *Streptococcus suis* phagocytosis by polymorphonuclear and mononuclear blood leukocytes. Vet Microbiol 63:229–238.

Charland N, Harel J, Kobisch M, Lacasse S, Gottschalk M. 1998. *Streptococcus suis* serotype 2 mutants deficient in capsular expression. Microbiology 144:325–32.

Charland N, Nizet V, Rubens CE, Kim KS, Lacouture S, Gottschalk M. 2000. *Streptococcus suis* serotype 2 interactions with human brain microvascular endothelial cells. Infect Immun 68:637–43.

Chatellier S, Gottschalk M, Higgins R, Brousseau R, Harel J. 1999. Relatedness of *Streptococcus suis* serotype 2 isolates from different geographical origins as evaluated by molecular fingerprinting and phenotyping. J Clin Microbiol 37:362–366.

Chatellier S, Harel J, Zhang Y, Gottschalk M, Higgins R, Devriese L, Brousseau R. 1998. Phylogenetic diversity of *Streptococcus suis* strains of various serotypes as revealed by 16S rRNA gene sequence comparison. Int J Syst Bacteriol 48:581–589.

Chau PY, Huang CY, Kay R. 1983. *Streptococcus suis* meningitis. An important underdiagnosed disease in Hong Kong. Med J Aust 1:414–417.

Cheon D-S, Chae C. 1996. Outbreak of diarrhea associated with *Enterococcus durans* in piglets. J Vet Diagn Invest 8:123–124.

Clark LK. 1995. SEW:Program, problems, performances, potential profits and methods of implementation for various herd sizes. In Proc 36th George A. Young Swine Conf, pp. 1–14.

Clifton-Hadley FA. 1984. Studies of *Streptococcus suis* type 2 infection in pigs. Vet Res Comm 8:217–227.

Clifton-Hadley FA, Alexander TJL, Enright MR. 1986a. Diagnosis of *Streptococcus suis* infection in pigs. Proc Pig Vet Soc 14:27–34.

——. 1986b. The epidemiology, diagnosis, treatment and control of *Streptococcus suis* type 2 infection. In Proc Am Assoc Swine Pract, pp. 473–491.

Clifton-Hadley FA, Alexander TJL, Enright MR, Guise J. 1984. Monitoring herds for *Streptococcus suis* type 2 by sampling tonsils of slaughter pigs. Vet Rec 115:562–564.

Clifton-Hadley FA, Enright MR. 1984. Factors affecting the survival of *Streptococcus suis* type 2. Vet Rec 114:585–587.

Clifton-Hadley FA, Enright MR, Alexander TJL. 1986c. Survival of *Streptococcus suis* type 2 in pig carcasses. Vet Rec 118:275.

Cloutier G, D'Allaire S, Martinez G, Surprenant C, Lacouture S, Gottschalk M. 2003. Epidemiology of *Streptococcus suis* serotype 5 infection in a pig herd with and without clinical disease. Vet Microbiol 97:135–51.

Collins MD, Farrow JAE, Katic V, Kandler O. 1984. Taxonomic studies on streptococci of serological groups E, P, U and V: Description of *Streptococcus porcinus* sp. nov. Syst Appl Microbiol 5:402–413.

Dee SA, Corey MM. 1993. The survival of *Streptococcus suis* on farm and veterinary equipment. Swine Hlth Prod 1:17–20.

Dee SA, Joo HS. 1997. Elimination of PRRS virus: Is it possible? In Proc 28th Annu Meet Am Assoc Swine Pract, pp. 393–397.

de Greeff A, Buys H, Verhaar R, Dijkstra J, van Alphen L, Smith HE. 2002. Contribution of fibronectin-binding protein to pathogenesis of *Streptococcus suis* serotype 2. Infect Immun 70:1319–25.

del Campo Sepulveda EM, Altman E, Kobisch M, D'Allaire S, Gottschalk M. 1996. Detection of antibodies against *Streptococcus suis* capsular type 2 using a purified capsular polysaccharide antigen-based indirect ELISA. Vet Microbiol 52:113–125.

del Castillo J, Martineau GP, Messier S, Higgins R. 1995. The use of pharmacokinetics to implement penicillin prophylaxis for streptococcal diseases. In Proc Allen D. Leman Swine Conf, Minnesota, pp. 93–96.

de Moor CE. 1963. Septicaemic infections in pigs caused by haemolytic streptococci of new Lancefield groups designated R, S and T. Antonie van Leeuwenhoek 29:272–280.

Denicourt M, Le Coz P. 2000. *Streptococcus suis* 2000 update: Nine strategic and practical steps to quickly understand *Streptococcus suis* infection and disease. GP Martineau (Editor). Virbac.

Devriese LA, Ceyssens K, Hommez J, Kilpper-Balz R, Schleifer KH. 1991. Characteristics of different *Streptococcus suis* ecovars and description of a simplified identification method. Vet Microbiol 26:141–150.

Devriese LA, Haesebrouck F, De Herdt P, Dom P, Ducatelle R, Desmidt M, Messier S, Higgins R. 1994a. *Streptococcus suis* infections in birds. Avian Pathol 23:721–724.

Devriese LA, Hommez J, Pot B, Haesebrouck F. 1994b. Identification and composition of the streptococcal and enterococcal flora of tonsils, intestines and faeces of pigs. J Appl Bacteriol 77:31–36.

Devriese LA, Kilpper-Balz AR, Schleifer KH. 1988. *Streptococcus hyovaginalis* sp. nov. From the gut of swine. Int J Syst Bacteriol 38:440–441.

Devriese LA, Pot B, Vandamme P, Kersters K, Collins MD, Alvarez N, Haesebrouck F, Hommez J. 1997. *Streptococcus hyovaginalis* sp. nov. And *Streptococcus thoraltensis* sp. nov., from the genital tract of sows. Int J Syst Bacteriol 47:1073–1077.

Drolet R, Higgins R, Jacques M. 1990. L'entéropathie associée à *Enterococcus (Streptococcus) durans* chez le porcelet. Méd Vét Québec 20:114–115.

Elliott SD. 1966. Streptococcal infection in young pigs. I. An immunological study of the causative agent (PM streptococcus). J Hyg Camb 64:205–212.

Enright MR, Alexander TJL, Clifton-Hadley FA. 1987. Role of houseflies (*Musca domestica*) in the epidemiology of *Streptococcus suis* type 2. Vet Rec 121:132–133.

Erickson ED, Doster AR, Pokorny TS. 1984. Isolation of *Streptococcus suis* from swine in Nebraska. J Am Med Vet Assoc 185:666–668.

Estoepangestie S, Lämmler C. 1993. Distribution of capsular types 1 to 28 and further characteristics of *Streptococcus suis* isolates from various European countries. Zentrbl Bakteriol 279:394–403.

Facklam R, Elliott J, Pigott N, Franklin AR. 1995. Identification of *Streptococcus porcinus* from human sources. J Clin Microbiol 33:385–388.

Farrow JAE, Collins MD. 1984. Taxonomic studies on streptococci of serological groups C, G and L and possibly other taxa. System Appl Microbiol 5:483–493.

Feng W, Laster SM, Tompkins M, Brown T, Xu JS, Altier C, Gomez W, Benfield D, McCaw MB. 2001. *In utero* infection by porcine reproductive and respiratory syndrome virus is sufficient to increase susceptibility of piglets to challenge by *Streptococcus suis* type II. J Virol 75:4889–4895.

Field HI, Buntain D, Done JT. 1954. Studies on piglet mortality. I. Streptococcal meningitis and arthritis. Vet Rec 66:453–455.

François B, Gissot V, Ploy MC, Vignon P. 1998. Recurrent septic shock due to *Streptococcus suis*. J Clin Microbiol 36:2395.

Galina L, Collins JE, Pijoan C. 1992. Porcine *Streptococcus suis* in Minnesota. J Vet Diagn Invest 4:195–196.

Galina L, Pijoan C, Sitjar M, Christianson WT, Rossow K, Collins JE. 1994. Interaction between *Streptococcus suis* serotype 2 and porcine reproductive and respiratory syndrome virus in specific pathogen-free piglets. Vet Rec 134:60–64.

Galina L, Vecht U, Wisselink HJ, Pijoan C. 1996. Prevalence of various phenotypes of *Streptococcus suis* isolated from swine in the U.S.A. based on the presence of muraminidase-released protein and extracellular factor. Can J Vet Res 60:72–74.

Gogolewski RP, Cook RW, O'Connell CJ. 1990. *Streptococcus suis* serotypes associated with disease in weaned pigs. Austr Vet J 67:202–204.

Gottschalk M. 2004. Porcine *Streptococcus suis* strains as a potential source of infections in humans: An underdiagnosed problem in North America? Swine Health Prod. In press.

Gottschalk M, Higgins R, Jacques M, Beaudoin M, Henrichsen J. 1991a. Isolation and characterization of *Streptococcus suis* capsular types 9–22. J Vet Diagn Invest 3:60–65.

——. 1991b. Characterization of six new capsular types (23 through 28) of *Streptococcus suis*. J Clin Microbiol 29:2590–2594.

Gottschalk M, Higgins R, Jacques M, Mittal, KR, Henrichsen J. 1989. Description of 14 new capsular types of *Streptococcus suis*. J Clin Microbiol 27:2633–2635.

Gottschalk M, Higgins R, Quessy S. 1999a. Dilemma of the virulence of *Streptococcus suis*. J Clin Microbiol 37:4202–4203.

Gottschalk M, Lacouture S, Dubreuil JD. 1995. Characterization of *Streptococcus suis* capsular type 2 haemolysin. Microbiology 141:189–195.

Gottschalk M, Lacouture S, Odierno L. 1999b. Immunomagnetic isolation of *Streptococcus suis* serotypes 2 and $\frac{1}{2}$ from swine tonsils. J Clin Microbiol 37:2877–81.

Gottschalk M, Lebrun A, Wisselink H, Dubreuil JD, Smith H, Vecht U. 1998. Production of virulence-related proteins by Canadian strains of *Streptococcus suis* capsular type 2. Can J Vet Res 62:75–79.

Gottschalk M, Segura M. 2000. The pathogenesis of the meningitis caused by *Streptococcus suis*: The unresolved questions. Vet Microbiol 76:259–272.

Haataja S, Tikkanen K, Liukkonen J, François-Gerard C, Finne J. 1993. Characterization of a novel bacterial adhesion specificity of *Streptococcus suis* recognizing blood group P receptor oligosaccharides. J Biol Chem 268:4311–431.

Halbur P, Thanawongnuwech R, Brown G, Kinyon J, Roth J, Thacker E, Thacker B. 2000. Efficacy of antimicrobial treatments and vaccination regimens for control of porcine reproductive and respiratory syndrome virus and *Streptococcus suis* coinfection of nursery pigs. J Clin Microbiol 38:1156–1160.

Hampson DJ, Trott DJ, Clarke IT, Mwaniki CG, Robertson ID. 1993. Population structure of Australian isolates of *Streptococcus suis*. J Clin Microbiol 31:2895–2900.

Han DU, Choi C, Ham HJ, Jung JH, Cho WS, Kim J, Higgins R, Chae C. 2001. Prevalence, capsular type and antimicrobial susceptibility of *Streptococcus suis* isolated from slaughter pigs in Korea. Can J Vet Res 65:151–155.

Heath PJ, Hunt BW. 2001. *Streptococcus suis* serotypes 3 to 28 associated with disease in pigs. Vet Rec 148:207–208.

Heath PJ, Hunt BW, Duff JP, Wilkinson JD. 1996. *Streptococcus suis* serotype 14 as a cause of pig disease in the UK. Vet Rec 139:450–451.

Higgins R, Gottschalk M. 1990. An update on *Streptococcus suis* identification. J Vet Diagn Invest 2:249–252.

——. 2001. Distribution of *Streptococcus suis* capsular types in 2000. Can Vet J 42:223.

Higgins R, Gottschalk M, Beaudoin M. 1990a. *Streptococcus suis* infection in swine: A sixteen-month study. Can J Vet Res 54:170–173.

Higgins R, Gottschalk M, Boudreau M, Lebrun A, Henrichsen J. 1995. Description of six new *Streptococcus suis* capsular types. J Vet Diagn Invest 7:405–406.

Higgins R, Gottschalk M, Fecteau G, Sauvageau R, De Guise S, Du Tremblay D. 1990b. Isolation of *Streptococcus suis* from cattle. Can Vet J 31:529.

Hill BD, Corney BG, Wagner TM. 1996. Importance of *Staphylococcus hyicus* subsp. *hyicus* as a cause of arthritis in pigs up to 12 weeks of age. Aust Vet J 73:179–181.

Hinterdorfer F, Köfer J, Hahn G. 1990. Streptokokkenisolate aus Untersuchungsmaterial von Schweinen in der Steiermark. Wiener Tierartzl Monatsschr 77:153–157.

Hogg A, Amass SF, Hoffman LJ, Wu CC, Clark LK. 1996. A survey of *Streptococcus suis* isolations by serotype and tissue of origin. In Proc Am Assoc Swine Pract, pp. 79–81.

Holt ME, Enright MR, Alexander TJL. 1988. Immunization of pigs with live cultures of *Streptococcus suis* type 2. Res Vet Sci 45:345–352.

———. 1990a. Immunization of pigs with killed cultures of *Streptococcus suis* type 2. Res Vet Sci 48:23–27.

———. 1990b. Protective effects of sera raised against different fractions of *Streptococcus suis* type 2. J Comp Path 103:85–94.

Hommez J, Devriese LA, Castryck F, Miry C. 1991. Beta-hemolytic streptococci from pigs: Bacteriological diagnosis. J Vet Med (B) 38:441–444.

Hommez J, Devriese LE, Henrichsen J, Castryck F. 1986. Identification and characterization of Streptococcus suis. Vet Microbiol 11:349–355.

Iglesias JG, Trujano M, Xu J. 1992. Inoculation of pigs with *Streptococcus suis* type 2 alone or in combination with pseudorabies virus. Am J Vet Res 53:364–367.

Jacobs AAC, Loeffen PLW, van den Berg AJG, Storm P. 1994. Identification, purification, and characterization of a thiol-activated hemolysin (suilysin) of *Streptococcus suis*. Infect Immun 62:1742–1748.

Jacobs AAC, van den Berg AJG, Loeffen PLW. 1996. Protection of experimentally infected pigs by suilysin, the thiol-activated haemolysin of *Streptococcus suis*. Vet Rec 139:225–228.

Jansen EJ, Van Dorssen CA. 1951. Meningoencephalitis bij varkens door streptococcen. Tijdschr Diergeneeskd 76:815–832.

Johnson DD, Duimstra JR, Gates CA, McAdaragh JP. 1983. Streptococcal colonization of pig intestine. In Proc Vet Infect Dis Org, Saskatoon, Canada, pp. 292–298.

Jones JET. 1976. The carriage of beta-hemolytic streptococci by healthy pigs. Br Vet J 132:276–283.

Kataoka Y, Sugimoto C, Nakazawa M, Morozumi T, Kashiwazaki M. 1993. The epidemiological studies of *Streptococcus suis* infections in Japan from 1987 to 1991. J Vet Med Sci 55:623–626.

Kataoka Y, Yamashita T, Sunaga S, Imada Y, Ishikawa H, Kishima M, Nakazawa M. 1996. An enzyme-linked immunosorbent assay (ELISA) for the detection of antibody against *Streptococcus suis* type 2 in infected pigs. J Vet Med Sci 58:369–372.

Kataoka Y, Yoshida T, Sawada T. 2000. A 10-year survey of antimicrobial susceptibility of *Streptococcus suis* isolates from swine in Japan. J Vet Med Sci 62:1053–1057.

Katsumi M, Kataoka Y, Takahashi T, Kikuchi N, Hiramune T. 1997. Bacterial isolation from slaughtered pigs associated with endocarditis, especially the isolation of *Streptococcus suis*. J Vet Med 59:75–78.

———. 1998. Biochemical and serological examination of beta-hemolytic streptococci isolated from slaughtered pigs. J Vet Med 60:129–131.

Kilpper-Balz R, Schleifer KH. 1987. *Streptococcus suis* sp. nov.; nom. rev. Int J Syst Bacteriol 37:160–162.

Koehne G, Maddux RL, Cornell WD. 1979. Lancefield group R streptococci associated with pneumonia in swine. Am J Vet Res 40:1640–1641.

Kopic J, Paradzik MT, Pandak, N. 2003. *Streptococcus suis* infection as a cause of severe illness: 2 cases from Croatia. Scand J Infect Dis 34:683–709.

Lämmler C, Bahr K-H. 1996. Characterization of *Streptococcus porcinus* serogroup P isolated from an aborted fetus of a pig. Med Sci Res 24:177–178.

Lapointe L, D'Allaire S, Lebrun A, Lacouture S, Gottschalk M. 2002. Antibody response to an autogenous vaccine and serologic profile for *Streptococcus suis* capsular type 1/2. Can J Vet Res 66:8–14.

Lun S, Willson PJ. 2004. Expression of green fluorescent protein and its application in pathogenesis studies of serotype 2 *Streptococcus suis*. J Microbiol Methods 56:401–412.

Lütticken R, Temme N, Hahn G, Bartelheimer EW. 1986. Meningitis caused by *Streptococcus suis*: Case report and review of the literature. Infection 14:181–185.

MacInnes JI, Desrosiers R. 1999. Agents of the "suis-ide diseases" of swine: *Actinobacillus suis*, *Haemophilus parasuis*, and *Streptococcus suis*. Can J Vet Res 63:83–89.

MacLennan M, Foster G, Dick K, Smith WJ, Nielsen B. 1996. *Streptococcus suis* serotypes 7, 8 and 14 from diseased pigs in Scotland. Vet Rec 139:423–424.

Madsen LW, Svensmark B, Elvestad K, Aalbaek B, Jensen H.E. 2002. *Streptococcus suis* serotype 2 infection in pigs: New diagnostic and pathogenetic aspects. J Comp Path 126:57:65.

Marie J, Morvan H, Berthelot-Herault F, Sanders P, Kempf I, Gautier-Bouchardon AV, Jouy E, Kobisch M. 2002. Antimicrobial susceptibility of *Streptococcus suis* isolated from swine in France and from humans in different countries between 1996 and 2000. J Antimicrob Chemother 50:201–209.

Martinez G, Harel J, Lacouture S, Gottschalk M. 2002. Genetic diversity of *Streptococcus suis* serotypes 2 and ½ isolates recovered from carrier pigs in closed herds. Can J Vet Res 66:240–248.

Martinez G, Pestana de Castro AF, Ribeiro Pagnani KJ, Nakazato G, Dias da Silveira W, Gottschalk M. 2003. Clonal distribution of an atypical MRP', EF*, and suilysin' phenotype of virulent *Streptococcus suis* serotype 2 strains in Brazil. Can J Vet Res 67:52–55.

McKellar QA, Baxter P, Taylor D, Bogan JA. 1987. Penicillin therapy of spontaneous streptococcal meningitis in pigs. Vet Rec 121:347–350.

Michaud S, Duperval R, Higgins R. 1996. *Streptococcus suis* meningitis: First case reported in Quebec. Can J Infect Dis 7:329–331.

Mills G. 1996. Establishing a *Streptococcus suis* type II-free herd by a combination of medication and removal of piglets at birth. Irish Vet J 49:674–677.

Mogollon JD, Pijoan C, Murtaugh MP, Collins JE, Cleary. 1991. Identification of epidemic strains of *Streptococcus suis* by genomic fingerprinting. J Clin Microbiol 29:782–787.

Mogollon JD, Pijoan C, Murtaugh MP, Kaplan EL, Collins JE, Cleary PP. 1990. Characterization of prototype and clinically defined strains of *Streptococcus suis* by genomic fingerprinting. J Clin Microbiol 28:2462–2466.

Monter Flores JL, Higgins R, D'Allaire S, Charette R, Boudreau M, Gottschalk M. 1993. Distribution of the different capsular types of *Streptococcus suis* in nineteen swine nurseries. Can Vet J 34:170–171.

Mwaniki CG, Robertson ID, Hampson DJ. 1994. The prevalence of *Streptococcus suis* type 2 in Western Australian piggeries. Austr Vet J 71:385–386.

Nielsen NC, Bille N, Larsen JL, Svendsen J. 1975. Preweaning mortality in pigs. 7. Polyarthritis. Nord Vet Med 27:529–543.

Okwumabua O, O'Connor M, Shull E. 2003. A polymerase chain reaction (PCR) assay specific for *Streptococcus suis* based on the gene encoding the glutamate dehydrogenase. FEMS Microbiol Lett 218:79–84.

Oliveira S, Batista L, Torremorell M, Pijoan C. 2001. Experimental colonization of piglets and gilts with systemic strains of *Haemophilus parasuis* and *Streptococcus suis* to prevent disease. Can J Vet Res 65:161–167.

Orr J, Copeland S, Chirino-Trejo M. 1989. *Streptococcus suis* type 9 outbreak in swine. Can Vet J 30:680.

Pedroli S, Kobisch M, Beauchet O, Chaussinand JP, Lucht F. 2003. Bactériémie à *Streptococcus suis*. Presse Med 32:599–601.

Perch B, Kristjansen P, Skadhange KN. 1968. Streptococci pathogenic for man. Acta Pathol Microbiol Scand B 74:69–76.

Perch B, Pedersen KB, Henrichsen J. 1983. Serology of capsulated streptococci pathogenic for pigs: Six new serotypes of *Streptococcus suis*. J Clin Microbiol 17:993–996.

Pijoan C. 1996. Bacterial respiratory pathogens: What is their impact? In Proc 4th Annu Swine Dis Conf Swine Pract, pp. 45–47.

Plagemann O. 1988. *Streptococcus porcinus* as a cause of abortion in swine. Zentrbl Vet B 35:770–772.

Quessy S, Dubreuil D, Caya M, Létourneau R, Higgins R. 1994. Comparison of pig, rabbit and mouse IgG response to *Streptococcus suis* serotype 2 proteins and active immunization of mice against the infection. Can J Vet Res 58:220–223.

Quessy S, Busque P, Higgins R, Jacques M, Dubreuil JD. 1997. Description of an albumin binding activity for *Streptococcus suis* serotype 2. FEMS Microbiol Lett 147:245–250.

Real F, Ferrer O, Rodriguez JL. 1992. Purulent streptococcal lymphadenitis in swine. Vet Rec 131:151–152.

Reams RY, Glickman LT, Harrington DD, Bowersock TL, Thacker HL. 1993. *Streptococcus suis* infection in swine: A retrospective study of 256 cases. Part I. Epidemiologic factors and antibiotic susceptibility patterns. J Vet Diagn Invest 5:363–367.

Reams RY, Glickman LT, Harrington DD, Thacker HL, Bowersock TL. 1994. *Streptococcus suis* infection in swine: A retrospective study of 256 cases. Part II. Clinical signs, gross and microscopic lesions, and coexisting microorganisms. J Vet Diagn Invest 6:326–334.

Reams RY, Harrington DD, Glickman LT, Thacker HL, Bowersock TL. 1995. Fibrinohemorrhagic pneumonia in pigs naturally infected with *Streptococcus suis*. J Vet Diagn Invest 7:406–408.

——. 1996. Multiple serotypes and strains of *Streptococcus suis* in naturally infected swine herds. J Vet Diagn Invest 8:119–121.

Robertson ID, Blackmore DK. 1989. Occupational exposure to *Streptococcus suis* type 2. Epidemiol Inf 103:157–164.

Robertson ID, Blackmore DK, Hampson DJ, Fu ZF. 1991. A longitudinal study of natural infection of piglets with *Streptococcus suis* types 1 and 2. Epidemiol Infect 107:119–126.

Sala V, Colombo A, Gerola L. 1989. Infection risks of *Streptococcus suis* type 2 localizations in slaughtered swine. Arch Vet Italiano 40:180–184.

Sanford SE. 1987a. Gross and histopathological findings in unusual lesions caused by *Streptococcus suis* in pigs. I. Cardiac lesions. Can J Vet Res 51:481–485.

——. 1987b. Gross and histopathological findings in unusual lesions caused by *Streptococcus suis* in pigs. II. Central nervous system lesions. Can J Vet Res 51:486–489.

——. 1989. *Streptococcus suis*: A strategic update. In Proc Am Assoc Swine Pract, pp. 193–195.

Sanford SE, Higgins R. 1992. Streptococcal diseases. In Diseases of Swine 7th ed. AD Leman, BE Straw, WL Mengeling, S D'Allaire, DJ Taylor, eds. Ames: Iowa State Univ Press, pp. 588–598.

Sanford SE, Tilker AME. 1982. *Streptococcus suis* type II–associated diseases in swine: Observations of a one-year study. J Am Med Vet Assoc 181:673–676.

——. 1989. *Streptococcus suis* antimicrobial susceptibility. Can Vet J 30:679.

Schmitt CS, Halbur PG, Roth JA, Kinyon JM, Kasorndorkbua C, Thacker B. 2001. Influence of ampicillin, ceftiofur, attenuated live PRRSV vaccine, and reduced dose *Streptococcus suis* exposure on disease associated with PRRSV and *S. suis* coinfection. Vet Microbiol 78:29–37.

Segers RP, Kenter T, de Haan LA, Jacobs AA. 1998. Characterisation of the gene encoding suilysin from *Streptococcus suis* and expression in field strains. FEMS Microbiol Lett 167:255–261.

Segura M, Gottschalk M. 2002. *Streptococcus suis* interactions with the murine macrophage cell line J774: Adhesion and cytotoxicity. Infect Immun 70:4312–4322.

Segura M, Vadeboncoeur N, Gottschalk M. 2002. CD14-dependent and -independent cytokine and chemokine production by human THP-1 monocytes stimulated by *Streptococcus suis* capsular type 2. Clin Exp Immunol 127:243–54.

Serhir B, Higgins R, Foiry B, Jacques M. 1993. Detection of immunoglobulin-G-binding proteins in *Streptococcus suis*. J Gen Microbiol 139:2953–2958.

Shryock TR, Mortensen JE, Rhoads SL. 1992. Antibiotic susceptibility in *Streptococcus suis*. Curr Therap Res 52:419–424.

Sihvonen L, Kurl DN, Henrichsen J. 1988. *Streptococcus suis* isolated from pigs in Finland. Acta Vet Scand 29:9–13.

Smith HE, Damman M, van der Velde J, Wagenaar F, Wisselink HJ, Stockhofe-Zurwieden N, Smits MA. 1999. Identification and characterization of the cps locus of *Streptococcus suis* serotype 2: The capsule protects against phagocytosis and is an important virulence factor. Infect Immun 67:1750–1756.

Smith HE, Wisselink HJ, Stockhofe-Zurwieden N, Vecht U, Smits MM. 1997. Virulence markers of *Streptococcus suis* type 1 and 2. Adv Exp Med Biol 418:651–5.

Staats JJ, Feder I, Okwumabua O, Chengappa MM. 1997. *Streptococcus suis*: Past and present. Vet Res Comm 21:381–407.

Staats JJ, Plattner BL, Stewart GC, Changappa MM. 1999. Presence of the *Streptococcus suis* suilysin gene and expression of MRP and EF correlates with high virulence in *Streptococcus suis* type 2 isolates. Vet Microbiol 70:201–211.

Strangmann E, Fröleke H, Kohse KP. 2002. Septic shock caused by *Streptococcus suis*: Case report and investigation of a risk group. Int J Hyg Environ Health 205:385–392.

Tarradas C, Borge C, Arenas A, Maldonado A, Astorga R, Miranda A, Luque I. 2001. Suilysin production by *Streptococcus suis* strains isolated from diseased and healthy carrier pigs in Spain. Vet Rec 148:183–184.

Thanawongnuwech R, Brown GB, Halbur PG, Roth JA, Royer RL, Thacker BJ. 2000. Pathogenesis of porcine reproductive and respiratory syndrome virus-induced increase in susceptibility to *Streptococcus suis* infection. Vet Pathol 37:143–152.

Tikkanen K, Haataja S, Finne J. 1996. The galactosyl-(alpha-1-4)-galactose-binding adhesin of *Streptococcus suis*: Occurrence in strains of different hemagglutination activities and induction of opsonic antibodies. Infect Immun 64:3659–3665.

Torremorell M, Calsamiglia M, Pijoan C. 1998. Colonization of suckling pigs by *Streptococcus suis* with particular reference to pathogenic serotype 2 strains. Can J Vet Res 62:21–26.

Torremorell M, Pijoan C, Dee S. 1999. Experimental exposure of young pigs using a pathogenic strain of *Streptococcus suis* serotype 2 and evaluation of this method for disease protection. Can J Vet Res 1999. 63:269–275.

Torremorell M, Pijoan C, Trigo E. 1997. Vaccination against *Streptococcus suis*: Effect on nursery mortality. Swine Health Prod 5:139–143.

Trottier S, Higgins R, Brochu G, Gottschalk M. 1991. A case of human endocarditis due to *Streptococcus suis* in North America. Rev Infect Dis 13:1251–1252.

Tunkel AR, Wispelwey B, Scheld M. 1990. Bacterial meningitis: Recent advances in pathophysiology and treatment. Ann Intern Med 112:610–614.

Turgeon PL, Higgins R, Gottschalk M, Beaudoin M. 1994. Antimicrobial susceptibility of *Streptococcus suis* isolates. Br Vet J 150:263–269.

Tzipori S, Hayes J, Sims L, Withers M. 1984. *Streptococcus durans*: An unexpected enteropathogen of foals. J Infect Dis 150:589–593.

Vancanneyt M, Snauwaert C, Cleenwenk I, Baele M, Descheemaeker P, Goossens H, Pot B, Vandamme P, Swings J, Haesebrouck F, Devriese LA. 2001. *Enterococcus villorum* sp. nov., an enteroadherent bacterium associated with diarrhea in piglets. Int J Syst Evol Microbiol 51:393–400.

Vandamme P, Pot B, Falsen E, Kersters K, Devriese LA. 1996. Taxonomic study of Lancefield streptococcal groups C, G and L (*Streptococcus dysgalactiae*) and proposal of S. *dysgalactiae* subsp. *equisimilis* subsp. nov. Int J Syst Bacteriol 46:774–781.

Vanier G, Segura M, Friedl P, Lacouture S, Gottschalk M. 2004. Invasion of porcine brain microvascular endothelial cells by *Streptococcus suis* serotype 2. Infect Immun 72:1441–9.

Vecht U, van Leengoed LAMG, Verheijen ERM. 1985. *Streptococcus suis* infections in pigs in the Netherlands (Part I). Vet Quart 7:315–321.

Vecht U, Wisselink HJ, Jellema ML, Smith HE. 1991. Identification of two proteins associated with virulence of *Streptococcus suis* type 2. Infect Immun 59:3156–3162.

Vela AI, Goyache J, Tarradas C, Luque I, Mateos A, Moreno M.A, Borge C, Perea JA, Dominguez L, Fernandez-Garayzabal JF. 2003. Analysis of genetic diversity of *Streptococcus suis* clinical isolates from pigs in Spain by pulsed-field gel electrophoresis. J Clin Microbiol 41:2498–2502.

Vena MM, Miquet JM, Isern S. 1991. *Streptococcus suis* isolated from an outbreak of pig pneumonia. Vet Arg 8:316–319.

Vieira VV, Teixeira LM, Zahner V, Momen H, Facklam RR, Steigerwalt AG, Brenner DJ, Castro ACD. 1998. Genetic relationships among the different phenotypes of *Streptococcus dysgalactiae* strains. Int J Syst Bacteriol 48:1231–1243.

Villani D. 2003. A retrospective evaluation of actions taken to control *Streptococcus suis* infection. J Swine Healh Prod 11:27–30.

Walsh B, Williams AE, Satsangi J. *Streptococcus suis* type 2: Pathogenesis and clinical disease. Rev Med Microbiol 1992. 3:65–71

Watkins EJ, Brooksby P, Schweiger MS, Enright SM. 2001. Septicaemia in a pig-farm worker. The Lancet 357:38.

Wessman GE. 1986. Biology of the group E streptococci: A review. Vet Microbiol 12:297–328.

Williams A, Blakemore WF. 1990. Pathogenesis of meningitis caused by *Streptococcus suis* type 2. J Infect Dis 162:474–481.

Windsor RS. 1978. Streptococcal infections in young pigs. Vet Annu 18:134–143.

Windsor RS, Elliott SD. 1975. Streptococcal infection in young pigs. IV. An outbreak of streptococcal meningitis in weaned pigs. J Hyg Camb 75:69–78.

Wisselink HJ, Joosten JJ, Smith HE. 2002a. Multiplex PCR assays for simultaneous detection of six major serotypes and two virulence-associated phenotypes of *Streptococcus suis* in tonsillar specimens from pigs. J Clin Microbiol 40:2922–2929.

Wisselink HJ, Reek FH, Vecht U, Stockhofe-Zurwieden N, Smits MA, Smith HE. 1999. Detection of virulent strains of *Streptococcus suis* type 2 and highly virulent strains of *Streptococcus suis* type 1 in tonsillar specimens of pigs by PCR. Vet Microbiol 67:143–157.

Wisselink HJ, Smith HE, Stockhofe-Zurwieden N, Peperkamp K, Vecht U. 2000. Distribution of capsular types and production of muramidase-released protein (MRP) and extracellular factor (EF) of *Streptococcus suis* strains isolated from diseased pigs in seven European countries. Vet Microbiol 74:237–48.

Wisselink HJ, Stockhofe-Zurwieden N, Hilgers L, Smith HE. 2002b. Assessment of protective efficacy of live and killed vaccines based on non-encapsulated mutant of *Streptococcus suis* serotype 2. Vet Microbiol 84:155–168.

Wisselink HJ, Vecht U, Stockhofe-Zurwieden N, and Smith HE. 2001. Protection of pigs against challenge with virulent *Streptococcus suis* serotype 2 strains by a muramidase-released protein and extracellular factor vaccine. Vet Rec 148:473–477.

Woods RD, Ross RF. 1977. Immunogenicity of experimental *Streptococcus equisimilis* vaccines in swine. Am J Vet Res 38:33–36.

48 Swine Dysentery

David J. Hampson, C. Fellström, and Jill R. Thomson

Swine dysentery (SD) is a mucohemorrhagic colitis affecting pigs primarily during the grow-finish period. The disease can be severe and may cause significant economic loss. SD has been reported worldwide and remains problematic in many major swine-rearing countries. The primary etiologic agent of SD is the strongly beta-hemolytic anaerobic intestinal spirochete *Brachyspira hyodysenteriae*. An emerging issue of concern to veterinarians is the existence of *B. hyodysenteriae* isolates with reduced susceptibility to a number of antimicrobial agents that were formerly effective for the control of SD. The presence of such isolates on certain piggeries, and their possible spread, reduces the options available for controlling SD.

ETIOLOGY

Intestinal Spirochetes and Swine Dysentery

The spirochetal etiology of SD was conclusively demonstrated in the early 1970s (Taylor and Alexander 1971; Glock and Harris 1972), when the causal strongly beta-hemolytic anaerobic spirochete was identified and named *Treponema hyodysenteriae* (Harris et al. 1972). Subsequently, the spirochete was transferred to a new genus *Serpula* (Stanton et al. 1991), then to *Serpulina* (Stanton 1992), and is now classified in the genus *Brachyspira* as *Brachyspira hyodysenteriae* (Ochiai et al. 1997; Validation list 1998). This genus includes four other named species of intestinal spirochete (all weakly beta-hemolytic) that colonize swine, as well as at least four other named or suggested *Brachyspira* species that are known to colonize other animal species or humans (Hampson 2000). Of the porcine intestinal spirochetes, besides *B. hyodysenteriae* only *Brachyspira pilosicoli* is confirmed to be pathogenic in swine, causing an often-mild colitis called "porcine colonic spirochetosis" or "porcine intestinal spirochetosis" (see Chapter 46). The other three species, *Brachyspira innocens, Brachyspira intermedia* and *Brachyspira murdochii* are generally considered to be nonpathogenic commensals in swine. *B. inter-media* occasionally has been suspected of causing diarrhea in pigs (Fellström et al. 1996), and it is known to cause wet litter and reduced egg production in adult chickens (Stephens and Hampson 2001).

B. hyodysenteriae produces typical signs and lesions of SD when orally inoculated into conventional or specific pathogen free pigs (Taylor and Alexander 1971; Glock and Harris 1972; Harris et al. 1972). Lesions also can be produced with pure cultures of *B. hyodysenteriae* in porcine colonic segments prepared by surgical anastomosis (Hughes et al. 1975), and in isolated ligated porcine colonic loops (Whipp et al. 1978). Mice are frequently used as an experimental model of SD (Joens and Glock 1979). The spirochete has been recovered from naturally infected rheas (a large flightless South American bird) in the United States, in which it causes a necrotizing typhlocolitis (Jensen et al. 1996). Strongly hemolytic spirochetes identified as *B. hyodysenteriae* recently have been isolated from Mallard ducks in Sweden, but whether they cause disease in this species is unclear (Jansson et al. 2004).

Characteristics of *B. hyodysenteriae*

Brachyspira hyodysenteriae is a gram-negative, oxygen-tolerant, anaerobic spirochete. It is 6–8.5 µm long, 320–380 nm in diameter, loosely coiled (Figure 48.1), motile, and

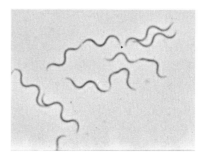

48.1. *Cells of* Brachyspira hyodysenteriae *as viewed under a phase contrast microscope.*

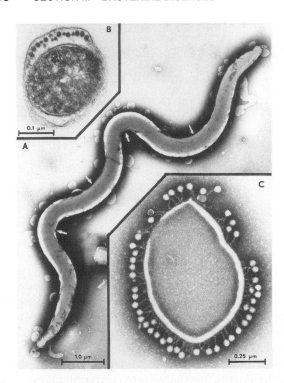

48.2. *Electron micrographs of* B. hyodysenteriae. *(A)* B. hyodysenteriae *from the intestinal mucosa of a pig acutely affected with SD. The spirochete is negatively stained with potassium phosphotungstate. Arrows indicate areas of cross-over of periplasmic flagella (A. E. Ritchie and L. N. Brown, unpublished data, 1974). (B)* B. hyodysenteriae *in thin section. Transverse aspect illustrating diameters of periplasmic flagella and apposition to the outer envelope. The differences in periplasmic flagella diameter are presumably due to different stages of morphogenic assembly (A. E. Ritchie and L. A. Joens, unpublished data, 1978). (C) Bacteriophages ubiquitously associated with* B. hyodysenteriae, *in potassium phosphotungstate negative stain illustrating uniform morphology and close proximity of the receptor sites on a fragment of the outer envelope (Ritchie et al. 1978).*

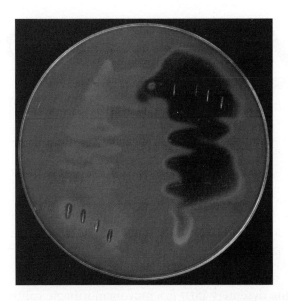

48.3. *Blood agar plate showing zones of clear beta-hemolysis around* B. hyodysenteriae *(right) and weak beta-hemolysis around* B. innocens *(left).*

strongly beta-hemolytic on blood agar. It has 7–14 periplasmic flagella inserted at each cell end, and these overlap at the middle of the protoplasmic cylinder. The whole cell, including the periplasmic flagella, is covered by a loose outer membrane (Figure 48.2).

B. hyodysenteriae grows slowly in an anaerobic environment at 37–42°C on trypticase soy agar and on similar agar plates that are fortified with 5–10% defibrinated blood (usually ovine or bovine). After 3–5 days, the spirochetes can be seen as a low flat haze of growth surrounded by a zone of strong beta-hemolysis (Figure 48.3.). The hemolysis can be enhanced by cutting slices into the agar at the time of inoculation (Olson 1996). Different combinations of antibiotics may be incorporated into the agar to make selective plates for isolation of the spirochete from feces (see diagnosis section).

B. hyodysenteriae can be propagated in various anaerobic broth media. Broths are incubated at 37–42°C, and are usually gently agitated on a reciprocal shaker. Growth of 10^8–10^9 cells per mL can be achieved within 2–3 days in the prereduced anaerobic trypticase soy

broth medium of Kunkle et al. (1986), and also in brain heart infusion broth containing 10% (v/v) fetal bovine serum (Stanton and Lebo 1988). The latter authors showed that the addition of 1% O_2 to the anaerobic culture atmosphere enhances growth. *B. hyodysenteriae* can utilize oxygen with the aid of enzymes such as nicotinamide adenine dinucleotide, reduced [NADH] oxidase (Stanton 1997).

Stanton (1997) published a comprehensive description of the metabolic activities of *B. hyodysenteriae* and related intestinal spirochetes. Useful features that can help distinquish *B. hyodysenteriae* from other intestinal spirochete species include their ability to produce indole, their enzymic profile in the commercial API-ZYM kit, and the presence of strong beta-hemolysis (Fellström et al. 1997). Some comparative features of *B. hyodysenteriae* and other porcine spirochetes are tabulated in Chapter 46. It must be emphasized that none of these phenotypic properties can be completely relied upon to provide identification, because strains of intestinal spirochetes with unusual phenotypes are occasionally encountered (Thomson et al. 2001). For example, indole negative strains of *B. hyodysenteriae* recently have been described (Fellström et al. 1999), whilst *B. intermedia* is also indole positive.

The outer envelope of *Brachyspira hyodysenteriae* contains lipooligosaccharide (LOS: a semirough form of the more usual lipopolysaccharide [LPS] of gram-negative bacteria) (Halter and Joens 1988). Baum and Joens (1979) extracted LOS from *B. hyodysenteriae* using hot phenol/water, and used agar gel diffusion to react it with serum from rabbits that had been hyperimmunized with *B. hyodysenteriae*. Doing this, they were able to classify a set of 13 isolates into four LOS serotypes.

Subsequent work uncovered the existence of considerably more antigenic diversity among LOS extracted from other isolates, and the typing system was extended to include new serotypes. The system was then modified to include a number of serogroups, some of which also contained individual serovars (Hampson et al. 1989). The serogroup is identified using unabsorbed sera, and the serovar is then identified using cross-absorbed sera. Currently 11 serogroups are recognized (Hampson et al. 1997). There is no indication that the virulence of an isolate correlates with its serotype, although LOS antigens appear important in stimulating protective immunity (see later section).

A number of attempts have been made to identify outer envelope proteins from *B. hyodysenteriae* (e.g., Chatfield et al. 1988; Joens et al. 1993), mainly in the course of attempts to identify potentially immunogenic molecules for use in vaccine production. Extraction of the outer membrane with Triton X-114 is considered the preferred method to reduce cellular contamination (Sellwood and Bland 1997), although osmotic lysis followed by isopycnic centrifugation also may result in spirochetal extracts that are free of cytoplasmic and flagellar contaminants (Trott et al. 2001). Well-characterized outer membrane lipoproteins include the 16 kDa "SmpA" (Thomas and Sellwood 1993), which has been renamed BmpA (Lee et al. 2000), and the 29.7 kDa BmpB (Lee et al. 2000). BmpB has also been referred to as BlpA, with the encoding gene sequence *blpA* being identified as a component of a locus designated *blpGFEA,* encoding four tandem paralogous *B. hyodysenteriae* genes encoding lipoproteins all of approximately 30 kDa (Cullen et al. 2003). A 39 kDa variable surface protein, encoded by eight linked gene copies, and possibly involved in immune avoidance, also has been described (Gabe et al. 1998; McCaman et al. 2003). A periplasmic ATP-binding cassette involved in iron importation has been characterized, which includes at least three lipoproteins (Dugourd et al. 1999).

Genomic Organization and Population Genetics

A physical and genetic map of the chromosome of the type strain of *B. hyodysenteriae* (B78[T]) has been prepared (Zuerner and Stanton 1994). The chromosome is circular and is estimated to be about 3.2 Mbp in size, compared to about 2.45 Mbp for *B. pilosicoli* (Zuerner et al. 2004). Ritchie et al. (1978) demonstrated several different types of bacteriophages on the surfaces of cultures of *B. hyodysenteriae* and *B. innocens* (see Figure 48.2). A generalized transducing bacteriophage (VSH-1) from *B. hyodysenteriae* has been purified and characterized (Humphrey et al. 1997) and is believed to be important in transferring host genes between cells.

Analysis of the population structure of *B. hyodysenteriae* using multilocus enzyme electrophoresis (MLEE) has shown that the species is quite diverse, that it contains numerous genetically distinct strains, and that it includes at least four subgroups with similar phenotypes (including virulence) (Lee et al. 1993). Subsequent analysis of new MLEE data was used to deduce that the species is recombinant, and that it has an epidemic population structure (i.e., epidemic clones exist, which may be widespread) (Trott et al. 1997). In a study using pulsed-field gel electrophoresis (PFGE) to analyze strains from individual farms, it was shown that over the course of several years new strains of *B. hyodysenteriae* may emerge as variants of the original parent strain (Atyeo et al. 1999a). Other than the occurrence of random mutational and recombination events, bacteriophages such as VSH-1 may contribute to this on-farm "micro-evolution" of strains through transduction of new sequences from other *Brachyspira* species or strains. New strains that emerge could have altered phenotypic properties, potentially including altered antimicrobial susceptibility, colonization potential, or virulence. Drifts in antigenicity of surface LOS among isolates on the same farm over a number of years have been recorded (Combs et al. 1992). Interestingly, chromosomal rearrangements and sequence drift also contribute to differences observed between the genomes of *B. hyodysenteriae* and *B. pilosicoli* (Zuerner et al. 2004).

Virulence Attributes

Virulence attributes of *B. hyodysenteriae* are likely to consist of a set of virulence "lifestyle" factors involved in initial colonization and fitness for survival in the microenvironment adjacent to the mucosa of the large intestine, as well as "essential" virulence factors that are required for lesion production. Avirulent isolates of *B. hyodysenteriae* that colonize pigs but do not induce disease have been described in the U.K. and Australia (Lysons et al. 1982; Lee et al. 1993; Thomson et al. 2001), and a study of these may help to define *B. hyodysenteriae* virulence factors. Some of these avirulent isolates have been reported to have a reduced motility in porcine mucus (Milner and Sellwood 1994), suggesting that motility is important in efficient colonization. Recent analysis of other avirulent isolates suggests that some lack a homologue of the *mglB* gene, encoding the glucose-galactose lipoprotein, which is believed to be a chemoreceptor in glucose and galactose chemotaxis (Walker et al. 2002). Both chemotaxis and motility are likely to be important mechanisms in allowing *B. hyodysenteriae* to associate with the gut mucosa (Kennedy et al. 1988). The role of motility in colonization has been confirmed in experiments where *B. hyodysenteriae* strains with disruptions introduced to their flagella genes (*flaA* and *flaB*) had both reduced motility and a reduced ability to colonize (Rosey et al. 1996; Kennedy et al. 1996).

Another likely "lifestyle" virulence factor is the NADH oxidase activity of *B. hyodysenteriae,* which is believed to enhance the spirochete's ability to colonize the colonic mucosa by protecting it from oxygen toxicity. Consistent with this, *B. hyodysenteriae* strains with an inactivated *nox* gene show a reduced ability both to colonize swine and to cause disease (Stanton et al. 1999).

The hemolytic activity of *B. hyodysenteriae* is considered to be associated with its virulence, and the hemolysin is probably an "essential" virulence factor. Unfortunately, there has been considerable confusion about the nature of the hemolysin(s) involved. Various early studies suggested that *B. hyodysenteriae* hemolysins had molecular weights of 19 kDa, 68 kDa or 74 kDa (reviewed by ter Huurne and Gaastra 1995). The hemolysin or hemolysins were oxygen-stable and resemble another carrier-dependent toxin, streptolysin S. Purified hemolysin is cytotoxic for a number of tissue culture cell lines and to primary pig cells (Kent and Lemcke 1984). It has been shown to damage epithelial cells in porcine ligated intestinal loops (Lysons et al. 1991) and in the murine cecum (Hutto and Wannemuehler 1999). Three different genes (*tlyA*, *tlyB*, and *tlyC*) encoding putative hemolysins of *B. hyodysenteriae* were originally described, based on their ability to induce a hemolytic phenotype in *Escherichia coli* (ter Huurne et al. 1994). More recently, a distinct gene (*hlyA*) has been characterized that encodes an 8.93 kDa polypeptide of *B. hyodysenteriae*, which has hemolytic activity (Hsu et al. 2001). It now appears that the *tly* genes may be regulatory elements, rather than encoding hemolysins themselves. Nevertheless, inactivation of *tlyA* has been shown to reduce both the hemolytic activity and the virulence of *B. hyodysenteriae* (Hyatt et al. 1994). These results emphasize the likely role of hemolysin(s) in the virulence of *B. hyodysenteriae*.

LOS from *B. hyodysenteriae* has some of the same biological properties as LPS from other gram-negative bacteria and is likely to contribute to the pathology observed in SD. Nuessen et al. (1982) showed that *B. hyodysenteriae* LOS extracted by phenol/water was toxic for mouse peritoneal macrophages, increased uptake of red blood cells by murine peritoneal cells via Fc and C3 receptors, acted as a mitogen for murine splenocytes, and generated chemotactic factors in fresh swine serum. Greer and Wannemuehler (1989b) found that endotoxin extracted from *B. hyodysenteriae* by butanol/water had more biological activity than the LOS extracted by phenol/water. It induced interleukin-1 and tumor necrosis factor from murine peritoneal cells and augmenting natural killer activity. Nevertheless, these authors also found that the biological activities of LOS and endoxin from *B. hyodysenteriae* and *B. innocens* were similar, and therefore may not account for the different pathogenic potential of the two species (Greer and Wannemuehler 1989a). Subsequent in vivo studies in mice and pigs demonstrated that *B. hyodysenteriae* endotoxin also can induce production of proinflammatory cytokines such as interleukin-6 (Nibbelink et al. 1997). Other evidence that *B. hyodysenteriae* LOS has a poten-

tial role in virulence came from studies where the outcome of infection in C3H/HeJ mice (hyporesponsive to LPS) was compared to the response in C3H/HeB mice (normal responders) (Nuessen et al. 1983). Lesions were produced in the colons of endotoxin-sensitive mice but not in endotoxin-resistant mice. Nibbelink and Wannemuehler (1991) subsequently obtained similar results and again concluded that the host's response to LOS influences their susceptibility to *B. hyodysenteriae*.

EPIDEMIOLOGY

Distribution of SD

SD is known to have a worldwide distribution, although the incidence of disease varies in different countries and regions, and alters with time. For example, in 1993 Mapother reported that 11% of U.S. herds showed serological evidence of infection with *B. hyodysenteriae*, with there being a 33% prevalence in the major pig producing state of Iowa. Now, even though there have been no recent surveys conducted, there is a general consensus that SD is much less common in the U.S. In part, this reduction in incidence may have resulted from rapid alterations in production systems, with the establishment of new high-health-status herds in nontraditional swine-rearing states, and with larger units, multisite production, and early-weaning systems now predominating.

In contrast to the U.S., SD still seems to be a relatively common and important problem in Europe. In the U.K., a postal survey of 105 pig units conducted in 1996 indicated that 50.5% had had scour problems in grower-finisher pigs in the last 3 years, and overall 10.5% had had a diagnosis of SD made (Pearce 1999). In a separate survey of 85 U.K. pig units where colitis was a problem, conducted in the period 1992–1996, *B. hyodysenteriae* was the primary etiological agent in 6 units (7%), and was isolated with other etiological agents of colitis in 3 other units (3.5%) (Thomson et al. 1988). Subsequently, in the period 1997–1999, Thomson et al. (2001) surveyed another 98 units with colitis problems, and found *B. hyodysenteriae* alone in 13% of these, and forming part of a mixed infection in another 16% of the units. In Denmark, among 72 units with diarrhea problems, 10 (14%) had *B. hyodysenteriae* infection, while the spirochete was not isolated from pigs on another 26 units where diarrhea was not a problem (Møller et al. 1998). In a subsequent study, examining samples from growing pigs in 79 randomly selected herds, only 2 herds (2.5%) were infected with *B. hyodysenteriae*, with a within-herd prevalence of 25–30% (Stege et al. 2000). In Sweden, a survey of diagnostic submissions over the period 1996–2003 indicated that SD remains a substantial ongoing clinical problem (Råsbäck et al. 2004). In parts of Europe, particularly where there are large numbers of pig units in close proximity to each other, the disease may be more widespread. In Poland, fecal samples from 8 of 23 (34.8%) herds with diarrhea were positive for *B.*

hyodysenteriae (Plawinska et al. 2004). In Spain, fecal samples from 86 of 225 (38.3%) herds with diarrhea contained *B. hyodysenteriae*, with a within–herd prevalence of 45.4% (Carvajal et al. 2003). Among 17 herds with diarrhea in Brazil, 6 (35.3%) were infected with *B. hyodysenteriae* (Barcellos et al. 2000a). In Australia, the disease occurs less commonly than it did 10 years ago, but it is still entrenched in certain large units.

There is little published information about the prevalence of SD in other parts of the world, although the disease is certainly present and is highly likely to be causing problems. For example, SD is reported to have been increasing in incidence in Thailand in recent years, possibly as a result of increased governmental regulations on antimicrobial use (Prapasarakul et al. 2004). Concerns have been expressed elsewhere that the incidence of clinical cases of SD will increase in association with restrictions on growth promoter use and the reduced availability and efficacy of other antimicrobials. It is likely that these agents currently may be masking disease in some infected piggeries.

Patterns of Disease in Infected Herds

SD is most commonly observed in grower and finisher pigs, with the disease especially becoming evident a few weeks after pigs are moved from the nursery. This coincides with removal of antimicrobial agents that are frequently administered to weaner pigs to control respiratory and enteric diseases. The disease also is seen in weaners, and may occur in adults, particularly in sows reared outdoors, and occasionally in suckling piglets.

On endemically infected piggeries, clinical signs of SD often recur in a cyclic manner. In large groups of affected pigs, symptoms in individual pigs and in the group as a whole may reappear at 3–4-week intervals. This reappearance often occurs after removal of therapeutic levels of drugs from the water or feed. Asymptomatic pigs also may develop diarrhea following management procedures, such as moving them to new pens, mixing with different animals, weighing, or a change in feed. Stresses such as overcrowding, and exposure to extreme changes in environmental temperatures also may precipitate disease. Where antibiotic medication is routine, any cause of loss of appetite, such as pneumonia, stops the intake of drug and the animal can then succumb to SD. Many pigs that survive the acute phase of the disease do recover from SD, and are capable of resisting subsequent challenge. However, chemotherapy during the acute phase may not allow the pig to initiate an immune response.

In outbreaks of SD, morbidity in weaner pigs may approach 90% and mortality may be 30%, depending on the effectiveness of treatment. The severity in chronically affected herds may be mild, and disease may not be clinically evident, particularly if the herd is being medicated. Under experimental conditions in which pigs are not treated, mortality may reach 50%. The occurrence

and severity of experimentally induced SD is related to a number of things, including the amount of stress on the pig, the quantity of infectious inoculum administered, the growth-phase of the culture (with active log-phase inoculum being most infectious), the diet, the group size, and the weight of the pig (Jacobson et al. 2004).

Sources of Infection

On an endemically infected piggery, transmission of infection to susceptible pigs occurs primarily by ingestion of fecal material that originates either from clinically affected pigs or from asymptomatic pigs that are colonized by the spirochete. This sort of transmission is especially likely to occur in single-site, farrow-to-finish herds with continuous flow and poor on-farm biosecurity. Experimentally, transmission has been accomplished by exposure of susceptible pigs to previously infected animals that have had no clinical signs for 70 days (Songer and Harris 1978). *B. hyodysenteriae* in feces may be transmitted by animal caretakers who did not change clothing or footwear between isolation units containing diseased and healthy pigs. Transmission between pens is also likely to occur in older housing systems where open channels draining excreta run between pens. The infectious nature of this material is emphasized by the fact that lagoon water containing effluent of a herd affected with SD produced the disease when administered to susceptible pigs (Glock et al. 1975).

B. hyodysenteriae is relatively resistant in the environment of a pig house, particularly in feces in moist conditions. For example, Chia and Taylor (1978) demonstrated that *B. hyodysenteriae* will survive in dysenteric feces diluted in water for 48 days at between 0°C and 10°C, although it survived for only 7 days at 25°C, and less than 24 hours at 37°C. In a more recent study, *B. hyodysenteriae* survived for 10 days in soil held at 10°C, but this increased to 78 days in soil in the presence of 10% pig feces, and was 112 days in pure pig feces (Boye et al. 2001). Under laboratory conditions, *B. hyodysenteriae* survives at minus 80°C for more than 10 years.

Other potential reservoirs of infection on a piggery include feral and other animals. For example, *B. hyodysenteriae* was isolated from the feces of a dog that frequented pens containing pigs affected with SD (Songer et al. 1978). The organism also has been isolated from field mice captured on farms on which there were pigs affected with the disease (Joens and Kinyon 1982; Fellström et al. 2004). Hampson et al. (1991) isolated *B. hyodysenteriae* from the cecum of a wild rat living on an Australian piggery where SD was present. Mice probably represent a greater risk for recycling of infection than rats, since experimentally inoculated mice shed *B. hyodysenteriae* in their feces for over 180 days (Joens 1980), and rats apparently shed it for only 2 days (Chia 1977). Under experimental conditions, pigs exposed to the feces of infected mice developed clinical symptoms of SD within 11 days after the first contact with mouse feces (Joens 1980). *B. hyodysenteriae* has also been isolated from the feet and feces of seagulls frequenting outdoor pig herds in the U.K. (J. R. Thomson, unpublished data). This suggests that transmission of infection between neighboring units by birds is a risk, particularly in outdoor farming systems.

Most new outbreaks of SD are associated with the introduction of asymptomatic carrier pigs into a herd, particularly where these new animals are not quarantined and/or treated prophylactically. However, outbreaks of the disease also occur in herds with no history of introduction of new animals. In these cases infection may be introduced through contaminated feed or animal trucks, or by visitors or others who have had contact with pigs on infected farms. When investigating risk factors for SD, Robertson et al. (1992) found a high odds ratio for infection for both allowing visitors onto farms, and there being rodents present. On the other hand, provision of boots and protective clothing for visitors, and the presence of security fencing around piggeries were protective. Interestingly, the use of home-mixed feed and acquisition of replacement breeders from the same source each year also both were protective.

Molecular Epidemiology

In recent years there has been an increased interest in understanding the molecular epidemiology of *B. hyodysenteriae* infections, particularly in the context of the need to understand and control the dissemination of problematic strains with reduced susceptibility to antimicrobials. The earliest strain-typing method used was serotyping, based on the LOS antigens (Baum and Joens 1979). It soon became apparent that a large number of serologically distinct strains of *B. hyodysenteriae* existed, with, for example, 91 Australian isolates being divided into eight serogroups (Combs et al. 1992). Interest in serotyping was stimulated by the finding that immunity against *B. hyodysenteriae* infection in a porcine colonic-loop model was largely LOS-serotype specific (Joens et al. 1983). In turn, this meant that bacterin vaccines would have to contain strains of the appropriate serotypes for use in a particular area, so these serotypes had to be determined. Subsequently, the use of bacterin vaccines for control of SD has not had great commercial success, so interest in serotyping has waned. Studies using MLEE showed that strains with the same serotype were not necessarily closely related genetically, and closely related strains were not necessarily of the same serotype (Lee et al. 1993). Other DNA-based typing techniques that have been applied to study the molecular epidemiology of *B. hyodysenteriae* include DNA restriction endonuclease analysis (Combs et al. 1992; Harel et al. 1994), DNA restriction fragment polymorphism analysis (Fisher et al. 1997), random amplification of polymorphic DNA (Dugourd et al. 1996), and pulsed-field gel electrophoresis (PFGE) (Atyeo et al. 1999a). The latter technique now is most frequently applied, and, although DNA banding

patterns for *B. hyodysenteriae* are usually not as clear as those for *B. pilosicoli*, PFGE has proved very useful for epidemiological studies—such as tracing strains with reduced susceptibility to tiamulin (Karlsson et al. 2004). All techniques have shown the species to be made up of large numbers of genetically distinct strains. In contrast to the situation with *B. pilosicoli*, generally only one strain of *B. hyodysenteriae* is found on a given infected piggery (Combs et al. 1992). Where two strains are found, one may have emerged as a variant of the original strain (Atyeo et al. 1999a, b). In two separate studies, strain-typing techniques have been used to demonstrate the presence of the same strain of *B. hyodysenteriae* in pigs and rats (Hampson et al. 1991) and pigs and mice (Fellström et al. 2004) on infected piggeries.

FINANCIAL IMPACT

SD causes considerable financial loss due to mortality, decreased growth rate, poor feed conversion, and expenses for treatment. Less tangible costs arise from the necessity to implement preventative measures in herds that do not have the disease, and particularly from the disruption to the supply and movement of pigs when the disease becomes introduced into stock in large breeding company herds. In the latter situation, the company's losses potentially can be enormous. There have been no recent evaluations of these costs, but older figures illustrate how expensive this disease can be. For example, Cutler and Gardiner (1988) considered it to be the most costly endemic pig disease in Australia. Lysons (1983) calculated that in-feed medication for SD cost £1.50–£5.00 ($2.60–8.60) per pig. Wood and Lysons (1988) demonstrated that the feed-conversion efficiency ratio in an infected herd deteriorated by 0.58, a cost increase of £7.31 ($12.60) per pig sold, and the cost of medication was £1.38 ($2.40) per pig. Walter and Kinyon (1990) found that the cost of medicating an infected herd was $8.30 per pig marketed, and that medication costs were reduced to US$0.08 per pig after eradication. Polson et al. (1992) projected the financial impact of SD via four simulation scenarios: SD-free, endemic SD, eradication by medication and disinfection, and total depopulation/repopulation. Net present value, internal rate of return, and benefit/cost ratio were calculated for each simulation scenario over a 10-year period. The profit margin per 100 kg liveweight produced was as follows: SD-free, $7.44; endemic SD, $1.67; eradication, $4.93; and depopulation/repopulation, $0.07. Ten years ago, total national losses to the U.S. swine industry were estimated to be $115.2 million (Duhamel and Joens 1994).

PATHOGENESIS

The pathogenesis of SD is complex and not completely understood. An important feature of the infection is the fact that various species of anaerobic bacteria that normally form part of the microbiota of the swine colon and cecum act synergistically with *B. hyodysenteriae*, facilitating spirochete colonization and augmenting inflammation and lesion production (Whipp et al. 1979; Joens et al. 1981). The diet consumed by pigs has a strong influence on the density and composition of the colonic microbiota (Durmic et al. 1998; Leser et al. 2000). Consistent with this, and consistent with there being a role for some other members of the normal microbiota in full expression of SD, it has been reported that colonization of *B. hyodysenteriae* can be inhibited by feeding pigs highly digestible diets that result in reduced fermentative activity in the large intestine (Pluske et al. 1996, 1998; Siba et al. 1996). Colonization of the ceca of mice with *B. hyodysenteriae* also can be influenced by diet and by the composition of the microbiota (Suenaga and Yamazaki 1984; Nibblink and Wanneumuehler 1992). Nevertheless, emphasizing the complexity of this situation, similar changes in the colonic microenvironment and/or inhibition of spirochetal colonization in pigs have not always been obtained using experimental diets designed to inhibit *B. hyodysenteriae* colonization (Durmic et al. 2000; Lindecrona et al. 2003).

Pigs become affected with SD following ingestion of dysenteric feces containing *B. hyodysenteriae*. Under experimental conditions an inoculum of 10^5 colony-forming units (cfu) is usually sufficient to produce SD (Kinyon et al. 1977), although much higher dose rates (e.g., 10^{10} cfu) often are used for experimental challenge (e.g., Hampson et al. 1993). Optimal colonization is achieved using actively motile bacterial cells in mid-log phase and repeating the oral challenge daily over 2 or 3 days. Presumably the bacteria normally survive the acidic environment of the stomach protected in feces, and eventually they arrive at the large intestine.

As previously discussed under "Virulence Attributes," spirochetal proliferation and colonization of the mucosa in the large intestine require a number of specialized bacterial features. These include the ability of *B. hyodysenteriae* to survive in the anaerobic environment of the large intestine, to utilize available substrate, to penetrate and move through viscous mucus down a chemotactic gradient into the crypts, and to avoid potential oxygen toxicity at the surface of the colonic mucosa. In infected pigs, the spirochetes may be seen close to epithelial cells in the lumen and crypts of the cecum and colon (Wilcock and Olander 1979a, b). At these sites they stimulate an outpouring of mucus into the lumen. Clinical signs and lesions of SD start to develop as numbers of spirochetes reach $10^6/\text{cm}^2$ of mucosa (Hughes et al. 1977; Whipp et al. 1979). Spirochetes first appear in the feces 1–4 days before diarrhea commences (Kinyon et al. 1977). At this time, there is a shift in the composition of the rest of the colonic microflora, from predominantly gram-positive bacteria in healthy animals, to mainly gram-negative organisms in pigs with dysentery (Pohlenz et al. 1984).

It is not known whether spirochetal attachment to epithelial cells is an important feature of the disease. Both Knoop et al. (1979) and Bowden et al. (1989) demonstrated in vitro attachment of *B. hyodysenteriae* to animal cell cultures. Bowden et al. (1989) concluded that the *B. hyodysenteriae* binding adhesins for cultured Henlé intestinal epithelial (HIE 407) cells contain sialic acid residues. In these studies, cellular damage and invasion of the cultured cells did not occur. Although *B. hyodysenteriae* can be seen within epithelial cells, particularly goblet cells, and in the lamina propria of tissues with typical lesions, this invasion does not seem to be essential for lesion production (Glock et al. 1974).

Although the mechanism of tissue destruction in SD has not been fully elucidated, the hemolysin(s) and LOS of *B. hyodysenteriae* may play a role (see section on virulence). These toxic substances presumably act locally to disrupt the adjacent epithelial barrier in the colon, resulting in epithelial sloughing and subsequent submucosal invasion by spirochetes as well as other secondary bacteria and the protozoan *Balantidium coli*. *B. hyodysenteriae* does not invade beyond the lamina propria of the large intestine, and the lack of *B. hyodysenteriae* and significant lesions in other organs implies that the entire pathogenesis of the disease can be directly attributed to the enteric lesions (Kinyon et al. 1980). The primary systemic effects of typical SD are the result of fluid and electrolyte imbalance induced by enteritis. The pathogenesis of peracute deaths is not known, but may be attributable to endotoxin release.

A series of studies have been conducted on the pathophysiology of SD (Argenzio et al. 1980; Argenzio 1981; Schmall et al. 1983). These have shown that, in contrast to what might be expected from histologic interpretations, the diarrhea observed in pigs with SD is not the result of increased mucosal permeability and leakage of protein and extracellular fluid from blood to lumen because of increased tissue hydrostatic pressures. Instead, the fluid loss appears to be the result of colonic malabsorption as a consequence of the failure of the epithelial transport mechanisms to actively transport sodium and chloride ions from lumen to blood. Furthermore, cyclic adenosine monophosphate (cAMP) and cyclic guanosine monophosphate (cGMP) levels in colonic mucosa of infected pigs were normal, but their response to a stimulus (theophylline) was markedly attenuated. Thus, these studies strongly suggest that an enterotoxin and/or prostaglandins released from the inflamed mucosa are not involved in the production of diarrhea. Therefore, the pathogenesis of dysentery is unlike the diarrhea induced by enterotoxigenic *E. coli* or *Salmonella* spp. Consistent with this, Whipp et al. (1978) reported that sterile filtrates of broth cultures of *B. hyodysenteriae* failed to cause fluid accumulation in ligated colonic loops of pigs or in sucking mice. Furthermore, sterile filtrates did not produce changes in Y-1 adrenal cells. Inactivated whole cells and sonically disrupted suspensions of *B. hy-*

odysenteriae also do not cause lesions or fluid accumulation in ligated colonic segments of pigs.

Studies of small-intestinal function in infected pigs indicated that the glucose-stimulated fluid-absorptive mechanism was intact and that no additional small-intestinal secretory component was present. Therefore, the fluid losses are exclusively the result of failure of the colon to reabsorb the animals' own endogenous secretions. Because as much as 30–50% of the extracellular fluid volume of these animals, in the form of endogenous secretions, is presented daily to the colon for absorption, colonic absorptive failure alone is sufficient to explain the progressive dehydration and death associated with the disease. These studies also imply that oral glucose-electrolyte solutions would be useful as a therapeutic measure in restoring these extracellular fluid losses.

CLINICAL SIGNS

The incubation period of SD is variable. Specific reports range from 2 days to 3 months, but the disease usually occurs within 10–14 days in naturally exposed pigs. Diarrhea is the most consistent sign, but the severity may be quite variable. The disease usually spreads gradually through an infected herd, with new animals being affected daily. The course varies not only between individual animals within a herd but also between herds.

Occasional animals are peracutely affected and die after a period of a few hours with little or no evidence of diarrhea. The first evidence of the disease in most animals is soft, yellow to gray feces. Partial anorexia and increased rectal temperature of 104–105°F (40–40.5°C) may be evident in some animals. A few hours to a few days following infection, large amounts of mucus and often flecks of blood are found in the feces. As the diarrhea progresses, watery stools containing blood, mucus, and shreds of white mucofibrinous exudate are seen with concurrent staining of the perineum. The majority of animals recover over a period of several weeks, but their growth rate remains depressed. Where prolonged diarrhea occurs it leads to dehydration with increased thirst, and affected animals become weak, incoordinated, and emaciated. Where death occurs it is associated with dehydration, acidosis, and hyperkalemia. The cause of occasional peracute deaths is not known.

Suckling pigs are not commonly affected, except in older piglets in gilt litters where the gilt has not been exposed to *B. hyodysenteriae*, and in piglets in newly infected herds. Infected piglets may have catarrhal enteritis without hemorrhage.

LESIONS

Gross Lesions

Pigs that have died from SD are often emaciated and may have a rough hair coat with fecal staining. Dehydration is usually evident. A consistent characteristic is the presence of lesions in the large intestine but not in the small intestine, often with a sharp line of demarcation at the ileocecal junction.

Typical changes in the acute stages of SD include hyperemia and edema of the walls and mesentery of the large intestine. Mesenteric lymph nodes may be swollen and small amounts of clear ascitic fluid may be present. White, slightly raised foci on the serosa, particularly in subacute or chronic infections are caused by aggregates of mononuclear cells, mainly lymphocytes in the submucosa that form part of the inflammatory reaction. There is obvious swelling of the mucosa, with loss of the typical rugose appearance. The mucosa is usually covered by mucus and fibrin with flecks of blood, and the colonic contents are soft to watery and contain exudate.

As the condition progresses, the amount of edema within the wall of the large intestine may decrease. Mucosal lesions may become more severe with increased fibrin exudation and may form thick, mucofibrinous pseudomembranes containing blood. As lesions become more chronic, the mucosal surface is usually covered by a thin, dense, fibrinous exudate, often giving the appearance of marked necrosis, which is quite superficial. Lesions can be found in clinically healthy pigs and appear as discrete areas of reddening of the mucosa, usually covered with some mucus, but with colon contents of normal consistency.

The distribution of lesions within the large intestine varies. In some instances the entire organ may be involved, while at other times only certain segments may be affected. Lesions tend to become more diffuse in the later stages of the disease.

Other lesions may include hepatic congestion and hyperemia or congestion of the gastric fundus. However, these lesions are also associated with other diseases and are not specific for SD. The stomach may be full.

Microscopic Lesions

The only significant microscopic lesions are found in the cecum, colon, and rectum. Typical acute lesions include obvious thickening of the mucosa and submucosa due to vascular congestion and extravasation of fluids and leukocytes. There is also hyperplasia of goblet cells, and the epithelial cells at the base of the crypts may be elongated and hyperchromic in appearance. The spirochetes may enter goblet cells in the colonic crypts, and penetrate intercellular gaps in the epithelium (Sueyoshi and Adachi 1990). There is an associated loss of cohesion between colonic enterocytes, with subsequent necrosis and shedding of the epithelium. The organisms may attach to the lumenal surface and enter these disrupted epithelial cells. Increased numbers of various types of leukocytes may be present in the lamina propria, with excessive accumulation of neutrophils in and around capillaries near the lumen. Some spirochetes also may be observed in the lamina propria, particularly around blood vessels. Bleeding occurs from small vessels

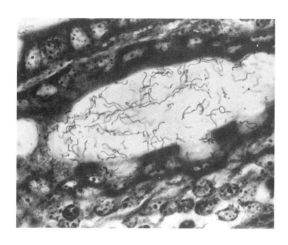

48.4. B. hyodysenteriae *in colonic crypt and epithelium (Warthin-Starry; ×750).*

located under areas of eroded epithelium, which also may be invaded by other members of the colonic microbiota. Blood becomes trapped in the overlying mucus, producing the typical blood-flecked appearance of the colonic contents in the acute stages of the disease.

Later changes include accumulation of large amounts of fibrin, mucus, and cellular debris in mucosal crypts and on the lumenal surface of the large intestine. Superficial necrosis of the mucosa may be extensive, but deep ulceration is not typical. Increased numbers of neutrophils may be seen throughout the lamina propria. Large spirochetes with the appearance of *B. hyodysenteriae* are found in the lumen and within crypts at all stages of the disease but are most numerous in the acute phase (Figure 48.4).

Chronic changes are not particularly specific, with less hyperemia and edema being present. There is often more advanced superficial necrosis of the mucosa, which usually has a thick, fibrinous pseudomembrane.

Ultrastructural changes during the early stages of SD

have been characterized. Large numbers of spirochetes with the appearance of *B. hyodysenteriae* are found at the lumenal surface and within crypts (Figure 48.4). Adjacent epithelial cells have lesions, including destruction of microvilli, swelling of the mitochondria and endoplasmic reticulum, loss of other organelles, and decreased density. As damage becomes more pronounced, the epithelial cells often shrink and become dark. *B. hyodysenteriae* invade epithelial cells, goblet cells, and the lamina propria, and may be found in large clusters within some epithelial cells (Figure 48.5), suggesting that intracellular multiplication may occur (Taylor and Blakemore 1971; Glock et al. 1974).

Hematology

Hematologic changes in SD include marked alterations in many measurable factors. Total leukocyte counts may increase, but not consistently. A marked left shift usually occurs, with high numbers of immature neutrophils in circulation. Other changes include early transient increases in erythrocyte sedimentation rates and fibrinogen levels. Packed-cell volumes vary but do not indicate significant blood loss, and total plasma protein may be elevated as a result of dehydration. Serum glutamic-oxaloacetic transaminase levels remain normal.

The most significant changes occur in blood electrolytes. Serum sodium, chloride, and bicarbonate levels decrease, and a marked metabolic acidosis develops, which may be fatal. Terminal hyperkalemia may be noted, and together with acidemia may be a significant cause of death (Glock 1971).

IMMUNITY

Pigs that have recovered from SD may be protected against subsequent experimental challenge with *B. hyodysenteriae* for up to 17 weeks (Olson 1974; Joens et al. 1979). Nevertheless, a proportion of recovered pigs (7–43%) remain susceptible (Jenkins 1978; Joens et al.

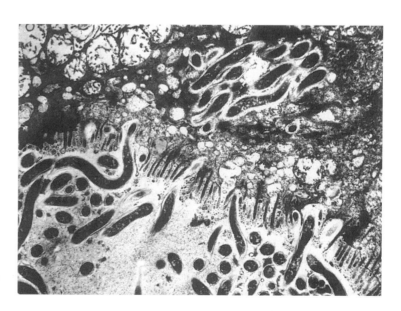

48.5. *Electron photomicrograph of* B. hyodysenteriae *invading a colonic epithelial cell (Glock and Harris 1972).*

1979; Rees et al. 1989a), and about 10% may become fully protected only after two previous bouts of disease (Rees et al. 1989a).

As previously stated, immunity to *B. hyodysenteriae* appears to be quite strongly serotype-specific, directed against LOS antigens present in the cell envelope (Joens et al. 1983). Following experimental infection or vaccination with a bacterin vaccine, there is some limited protection against serotypes of *B. hyodysenteriae* other than those to which the animals have been exposed (Kennedy et al. 1992; Nuessen and Joens 1982; Parizek et al. 1985). This suggests that besides being targeted at LOS antigens, protective immune responses also are directed against other spirochetal components that are common to isolates of different serotypes.

Changes occur in both antibody titers and in cell-mediated immunity in pigs with SD, but their importance is unclear. Titers of serum IgG against *B. hyodysenteriae* correlate with the duration of clinical signs, and IgA titers in colonic washes are indicative of recent exposure (Rees et al. 1989b). Neither of these titers is strongly correlated with protection from developing SD (Joens et al. 1982; Fernie et al. 1983; Rees et al. 1989b). Other studies suggest that complement components, in conjunction with immune serum, may be involved in the clearance of *B. hyodysenteriae* from the colon (Joens et al. 1985). Cell-mediated immunity also may be involved in protection, since there is evidence of inhibition of peripheral blood leukocyte migration, a delayed hypersensitivity response, and a T cell proliferative response to *B. hyodysenteriae* antigens in pigs convalescent from SD (Jenkins et al. 1982; Kennedy et al. 1992). In contrast, in mouse models of the disease, no significant changes in T cell subsets in the lamina propria were observed (Nibbelink and Wannemuehler 1990). It seems unlikely that there are immune-mediated components to the lesions of SD, because in mouse models the changes observed in numbers of mast cells in the lamina propria are not correlated with lesion development (Nibbelink and Wannemuehler 1990). Recent studies have identified CD8αα cell proliferation in pigs recovered from SD (Waters et al. 2000a). Most recently, Jonasson et al. (2004) investigated levels of circulating leukocytes and lymphocyte subpopulations in pigs before and after experimentally induced SD. By comparing results from pigs that did or did not succumb to disease, the authors deduced that γδ T cells and CD8+ cells may be associated with susceptibility to infection, and monocytes and CD4+ CD8+ T cells appear to be the major responding lymphocytes. Further work is required to understand the mechanisms involved in host immunity to *B. hyodysenteriae*.

DIAGNOSIS

Clinical Features

The diagnosis of SD depends primarily on differentiating the condition from other potential causes of diarrhea. Factors that should be considered include history, clinical signs, gross lesions, microscopic lesions, as well as isolation or detection of *B. hyodysenteriae*.

SD may occur as a persistent problem within a herd, with phases of increased or decreased severity. Diagnostic problems are most likely to occur in a herd in which the disease has not been previously diagnosed. History may be helpful because it is not unusual to have an outbreak following the introduction of new (carrier) animals into the herd. Other situations that disrupt the normal environment may also precipitate outbreaks in herds that have been exposed to *B. hyodysenteriae* but in which the overt disease has not been detected.

Clinical signs such as depression, dehydration, and diarrhea with mucus and/or blood in the feces are quite suggestive but offer only presumptive evidence. Temperature increases are too moderate and inconsistent to be of any diagnostic benefit. Hematologic changes as previously described are characteristic, but not sufficiently unique to be of any great differential value.

Necropsy and Histopathological Findings

In acutely infected animals the essential finding at necropsy is diffuse enteritis limited to the large intestine. Mucofibrinous exudate and free blood in the lumen are characteristic of SD, but not pathognomonic. Typical microscopic lesions of mucosal edema and microfibrinous enteritis with superficial erosion, particularly if associated with the presence of numerous spirochetal bacteria, are very suggestive of SD. The organisms can best be demonstrated by staining with Warthin-Starry, Victoria blue 4-R, or Goodpasture stains.

Laboratory Diagnosis

Sample Selection. Diagnostic samples are best taken from several acutely affected animals that have not been medicated. Colonic contents from recently necropsied animals are optimal, but fecal samples obtained from several animals with mucohemorrhagic diarrhea are also satisfactory. Where disease is mild or subclinical, it may be necessary to examine very large numbers of fecal samples before a positive specimen is identified. Fellström et al. (2001) have recommended pooling batches of five rectal swabs to increase the sensitivity of detection in such herds. Samples should be transported to the laboratory with care taken not to let them dry out. Serum samples from convalescent or slaughter-age animals can also be taken where there is access to a laboratory that can evaluate them for specific antibody titers.

Visual Examination of Samples. It is usual to conduct direct examination of smears prepared on slides from colonic mucosa or feces of pigs suspected of being affected with SD looking for the presence of characteristic spirochetal bacteria. Clearly, this cannot distinguish between *B. hyodysenteriae*, the pathogenic *B. pilosicoli*, or other commensal spirochetes. Workers in the United

Kingdom have traditionally utilized an absorbed antiserum in an indirect fluorescent antibody test to detect *B. hyodysenteriae* in such smears (Hunter and Saunders 1977). Unfortunately, even with extensive cross-absorption, it is technically difficult to prepare standard high titer polyclonal sera that are specific for *B. hyodysenteriae,* so false positive reactions can occur using this method. The use of specific monoclonal antibodies, as described by Lee and Hampson (1996), should improve this situation. Unfortunately, attempts to use this monoclonal antibody bound to magnetic beads to extract *B. hyodysenteriae* from feces has not increased the sensitivity of detection over that obtained with other currently used diagnostic techniques (Corona-Barrera et al. 2004).

Culture and Identification. A definitive diagnosis of SD requires specific demonstration of *B. hyodysenteriae* in the colonic mucosa or feces. This has traditionally been done by anaerobic culture, followed by examination of phenotypic properties of the organism. Optimal culture media and conditions are as described earlier under "Characteristics of *B. hyodysenteriae,*" but with the addition of 400 µg/mL spectinomycin and 25 µg/mL each of colistin and vancomycin to the agar to make the medium selective (Jenkinson and Wingar 1981). Alternatively, a more selective medium with lower concentrations of the previous three antimicrobials, but with 25 µg/mL spiramycin and 12.5 µg/mL rifampin also added, is frequently used (Kunkle and Kinyon 1988). Recently it has been suggested that isolation can be improved by briefly preincubating the sample in a selective broth medium prior to plating out (Calderado et al. 2001).

Pigs acutely affected with SD possess large numbers (10^8–10^9/g) of *B. hyodysenteriae* in their colonic mucosa and feces, and these are readily isolated. By contrast, pigs that are asymptomatic may only shed the organism periodically at detectable levels in their feces. Furthermore, medications commonly used to treat or prevent SD may reduce the number of organisms below culturally detectable levels. Therefore, caution must be used in interpreting the results of negative culture results, particularly from fecal samples.

On primary isolation, *B. hyodysenteriae* produces zones of strong beta hemolysis in which colonies are hard to distinguish, but a film of growth in the hemolytic zone is grossly visible. As a routine, plates without evidence of beta hemolysis should be further incubated anaerobically and observed at 48-hour intervals for up to 10 days. False negative culture results can occur for a number of reasons, including inappropriate sample handling or storage between collection and culture—for example, high temperature or freezing, drying out, or delay during transport.

Phenotypic Tests for *B. hyodysenteriae.* After a strongly hemolytic spirochete is isolated, it is usual to examine selected biochemical properties, as described

earlier under "Characteristics of *B. hyodysenteriae.*" It is important to obtain a pure culture of the isolate before phenotypic characterization, which can prove difficult unless microbiology technicians are highly experienced in this field. Mixed spirochete species can be present within the confluent culture growth, and exacting procedures are required to clone individual isolates to purity. Antigen detection–based methods have been described that also may help to confirm an isolate's identity, although these largely have been superceded by PCR testing. Methods include using a fluorescent antibody test with absorbed antiserum (as described for fecal smears), a growth-inhibition test (Lemcke and Burrows 1979), and a rapid slide agglutination test (Burrows and Lemcke 1981).

Nucleic Acid-Based Techniques. In an attempt to increase the sensitivity of detection from clinical material, and to improve the identification process of spirochetal isolates, nucleic acid probes and polymerase chain reaction (PCR) amplification of specific sequences have been developed for *B. hyodysenteriae* and other intestinal spirochetes. Probes have been used to detect 10^5 cells of *B. hyodysenteriae* per gram of pig feces (Jensen et al. 1990), but the technique is quite technically difficult and time-consuming. The use of probes in fluorescent in situ hybridization (FISH) on fixed colonic tissue is, however, a potentially useful tool for examining aspects of the pathogenesis of SD (Boye et al. 1998). The PCR is a simpler technique and generally can detect many fewer organisms. The most usual targets for DNA amplification are the 23S rRNA gene (Leser et al. 1997) and the NADH oxidase gene (Atyeo et al. 1999b). The PCR is usually conducted on growth harvested from the primary isolation plate. Even under these circumstances, where results are obtained in 3–5 days, PCR offers a more rapid, sensitive, and specific approach to diagnosis than does the more routine method of isolation followed by biochemical identification of the spirochetes (Atyeo et al. 1998). Use of PCR on growth from the primary isolation plates also is compatible with obtaining spirochetal isolates for subsequent antimicrobial sensitivity testing and/or strain typing, where required.

Another PCR-based methodology that can be used to detect and identify intestinal spirochetes to species level involves amplification of portions of specific genes, followed by restriction enzyme digestion of the products to give species-specific banding patterns after gel electrophoresis. Genes that have been used in this way include the 16S rRNA gene (Stanton et al. 1997a), the 23S rRNA gene (Barcellos et al. 2000b; Thomson et al. 2001), and the NADH-oxidase gene (Rohde et al. 2002). Unfortunately, in the U.K. "atypical" isolates of *B. hyodysenteriae* have been obtained that fail to amplify in this 23S rDNA PCR (Thomson et al. 2001).

Recently, the basic PCR test has been streamlined, such that it can be conducted as a duplex reaction identifying both *B. hyodysenteriae* and *B. pilosicoli* in DNA extracted directly from fecal samples (La et al. 2003). Potentially this test gives the opportunity to obtain same-day results, and it is also specific and highly sensitive for detection when applied to spiked fecal samples. It is anticipated that these tests will be improved further by the impending introduction of real-time PCR for *Brachyspira* species.

Molecular-based methods can be used to detect *B. hyodysenteriae* DNA in samples where spirochetes are dead on arrival at the laboratory (spirochetes are present in the sample but show lack of motility). In this case direct extraction of DNA from feces for PCR testing can be done in addition to attempted bacterial culture.

Serologic Assays. Several serologic tests have been reported that detect antibodies to *B. hyodysenteriae* in serum of experimentally affected pigs (reviewed by La and Hampson 2001). Generally these tests have not been based on species-specific antigens and consequently have had low specificity and/or sensitivity. Tests have included microtiter agglutination (Joens et al. 1978), indirect fluorescent antibody, passive hemolysis (Jenkins et al. 1976), and enzyme-linked immunosorbent assays (ELISAs) using various plate-coating antigens (Burrows et al. 1984). The most useful ELISA has used LOS as plate-coating antigen (Joens et al. 1982; Egan et al. 1983). This type of ELISA has proved helpful for use in identifying infected herds, but not for detection of individual pigs with SD. LOS-based ELISA systems also have the disadvantage that they require a knowledge of the serotypes of organisms present in the herds to be tested (Mhoma et al. 1992) so that the appropriate LOS can be used as plate-coating antigen, and consequently they are now rarely used. Recently, an ELISA using recombinant BmpB (the 29.7 Kda outer membrane lipoprotein of *B. hyodysenteriae*) as the plate-coating antigen has been described (La and Hampson 2001). Further work is required to evaluate this ELISA under field conditions before it can be made available for more general use.

Differential Diagnosis

A number of enteric diseases may be confused with SD. Also it is important to realize that SD often occurs concurrently with infections with other enteric pathogens (Møller et al. 1998; Thomson et al. 1998). Proliferative enteropathy caused by *Lawsonia intracellularis* may clinically resemble the signs of SD. However, unlike proliferative enteropathy, SD does not affect the small intestine. A definitive diagnosis of proliferative enteropathy depends on a positive PCR test from feces, herd serology, and/or demonstration of typical pathology including the presence of *L. intracellularis* in crypt enterocytes.

Salmonellosis, in particular infection with *Salmonella enterica* serovar Choleraesuis, easily can be confused with SD because clinical signs and lesions may be quite similar. Hemorrhage or necrosis in parenchymatous organs and lymph nodes may be expected with salmonellosis but not with SD. Mucosal lesions may be found in the small intestine with salmonellosis but not with uncomplicated SD. Deep ulcerative enteric lesions are also much more typical of salmonellosis. The definitive diagnosis depends on lack of *B. hyodysenteriae* in the mucosa of the large intestine and the isolation of *Salmonella* serovars from the intestine or other organs such as lymph nodes or spleen. The mere isolation of *Salmonella* does not constitute a positive diagnosis, since both normal animals and animals with SD may harbor these bacteria.

Trichuriasis may be differentiated on the basis of the presence of numerous *Trichuris suis* in the large intestine and the lack of *B. hyodysenteriae*. Concurrent infections can occur, and possible potentiation of SD by *T. suis* has been postulated.

Gastric ulcers and other hemorrhagic conditions may cause the presence of blood in the feces and confusion with SD. These conditions are easily differentiated at necropsy since they generally involve the anterior digestive tract. Feces also tend to be "tarry" due to digestion of the blood.

"Colitis" is a diet-related disease syndrome of growing pigs that can resemble SD both in clinical signs and in postmortem appearance (Lysons et al. 1988). There has been some confusion over this condition, and some reported cases actually might have been colonic spirochetosis/intestinal spirochetosis, caused by infection with *Brachyspira pilosicoli* (see Chapter 46). Typically, weaner or grower/finisher pigs aged 7 weeks or more are affected. They may develop a watery scour, or sometimes just soft feces, and lose body condition. Lesions are confined to the colon. In the early stages of the disease, the large intestine is filled with liquid contents and there is a mild reddening of the colon. Pigs in which the disease persists can become thin, excrete mucus in the feces, and have a mucofibrinous exudate on the mucosal surface of the colon. To eliminate SD from the diagnosis, it is necessary to autopsy pigs in the early stages of the disease and to carry out extensive screening for the presence of *B. hyodysenteriae*. Clearly, colonic spirochetosis represents the most difficult differential diagnosis, since it so closely resembles mild cases of SD. Although it responds to similar treatment, an accurate diagnosis is important because, in general, it has much less economic impact in individual herds than SD. Furthermore, it appears that aspects of the epidemiology of colonic spirochetosis differ from those described for SD (see Chapter 46).

TREATMENT AND CONTROL

Principles of Antimicrobial Treatment

Prior to implementing medication, the diagnosis of SD should be confirmed. At the same time it is important to have a clear idea of the overall goal of the treatment and to have a long-term strategy for dealing with the disease on the farm. Eradication should be the preferred option, and this is discussed in a later section.

At present there are only a few effective drugs available for treatment of SD, and in recent years it has become increasingly evident that the development of resistance of *B. hyodysenteriae* strains to antimicrobials such as pleuromutilins presents a potential long-term threat to the pig industry. Therefore, the use of such drugs must be restricted to specific therapy and, specifically, they should be reserved for attempts to eradicate the disease or for use in cases where other drugs or control measures are not effective.

The route of administration of antimicrobials is also an important consideration. Severely affected animals may require parental (intramuscular) treatment for, e.g., 3 days; however, in most cases medication via the drinking water for 5–7 days is the preferable way of treating acute SD. If medication via the water is not possible, in-feed medication for 7–10 days may be considered, although this has the disadvantage that affected animals may have a low feed intake. Medication of acute SD should always be accomplished by free access to drinking water, with or without supplementation with electrolytes. Treatment of acute SD may be followed by in-feed medication at subtherapeutic levels for 2–4 weeks to prevent reinfection.

Medication should be used in conjunction with management practices that reduce the risk of reinfection of medicated pigs and spread of infection to other groups or batches. All-in/all-out management of pig buildings with thorough cleaning and disinfection between batches is an important part of the control process. Ideally, affected batches should be moved to clean buildings at the end of the course of SD medication, thereby breaking the cycle of infection. Careful disposal of infected bedding materials, the use of boot scrubbers and disinfectant footbaths, cleaning and disinfection of equipment used in infected areas and changing of protective clothing are all vital parts of successful control procedures. Furthermore, because outbreaks of SD are often associated with conditions that produce stress, such as pig handling, crowding, transportation, severe weather conditions or dietary changes, it is important to minimize these stresses where possible. Attention also should be paid to the form and composition of the diet, to determine whether this might be predisposing to disease expression (see section on pathogenesis).

A list of the four drugs most commonly used for the treatment of SD—tiamulin, valnemulin, tylosin, and lincomycin—together with their dose rates and potential side effects, is presented in Table 48.1. Based on consideration of pharmacokinetic properties and in vitro susceptibility data, it appears that the pleuromutilins

Table 48.1. Dosage level, duration of administration and side effects for the four drugs most commonly used for the treatment of SD

Drug	Dosage and duration	Side effects
Tiamulin	10mg/kg bw; im for 1–3 days.	Rare: erythema. Local reactions at the injection site. Lethal side effects may occur in combination with ionophors.
	8mg/kg bw; po for 5–7days in drinking water.	
	Or: in-feed medication with 100 ppm for 7–10 days, followed by 30–40 ppm for 2–4 weeks.	
Valnemulin	In-feed medication 3–4 mg/kg bw for 1–4 weeks.	Adverse effects, including lethargy, depression, erythema, edema, pyrexia, ataxia, anorexia, and deaths have been reported. Lethal side effects may occur in combination with ionophors.
Tylosin	10mg/kg bw; im twice daily for 3–5 days.	Diarrhea, pruritus, erythema rectal edema, and prolapse have been reported.
	Or: 5–10 mg/kg bw; po in drinking water for 5–7 days.	
	Followed by: in-feed medication with 100 grams per ton feed for 3 weeks, followed by in-feed medication 40 grams per ton feed.	
Lincomycin	8mg/kg bw; po in drinking water. Not to be used for more than 10 days and not for use in swine weighing more than 250 pounds (115 kg).	Rare
	In-feed medication 100 grams per ton feed for 3 weeks or until signs of disease disappear, followed by 40 grams per ton. Not for use in swine weighing more than 250 pounds (115 kg).	

Note: The information in this table is an abbreviated summary of product labeling. For information regarding withdrawal times (which vary extensively between countries), review national regulations and product labels. bw = body weight, im = intramuscular, po = per os (oral).

(tiamulin, valnemulin) are the most suitable antimicrobials available for the treatment of SD (Kitai et al. 1979; Messier et al. 1990; Rønne and Szancer 1990; Walter and Kinyon 1990; Weber and Earley 1991; Binek et al. 1994; Molnar 1996; Cizek et al. 1998; Karlsson et al. 2003). Unfortunately, in several countries such as the U.K. (Gresham et al. 1998), the Czech Republic (Lobova et al. 2004) and Sweden (SVARM 2004), a decreased susceptibility to tiamulin among *B. hyodysenteriae* isolates has been reported. Strains with high MICs to pleuromutilins also have been reported from Germany (Rohde et al. 2004). The mechanism(s) of tiamulin resistance by *B. hyodysenteriae* are not known; however, one study indicates that resistance emerges slowly in vitro (Karlsson et al. 2001). Another recent study showed that tiamulin usage was sufficient to select several clones of *B. hyodysenteriae* with decreased tiamulin susceptibility on different farms in Germany (Karlsson et al. 2004). Therefore, to reduce the risk of emerging resistance to pleuromutilins, and if herd records or MIC determinations indicate that other drugs are effective for treatment of SD in a specific herd, such drugs should be preferred over pleuromutilins. The other two commonly used drugs, tylosin and lincomycin, have the disadvantage that high levels of resistance to them have been reported in *Brachyspira* spp., for example by Smith et al. (1991), Binek et al. (1994), Rønne and Szancer (1994), Hommez et al. (1998) and Karlsson et al. (2002, 2003). Macrolide and lincosamide resistance is caused by a single point mutation in the 23S rRNA gene, and tylosin resistance develops within 2 weeks in vitro (Karlsson et al. 1999).

Many other antibacterials, such as bacitracin, spiramycin, gentamicin, dimetridazole, ronidazole, virginiamycin, olaquindox, and carbadox have been used more or less successfully over the years in the treatment and prevention of SD. Unfortunately, the development of resistance by *B. hyodysenteriae* to several of those substances has been reported, and the availability of others is now much reduced internationally. For example, carbadox and olaquindox have been withdrawn from use in the European Union (EU) and in several other countries, while dimetridazole and ronidazole are no longer available either in the EU or the U.S.A. Olaquindox and carbadox usually have low MICs against *B. hyodysenteriae*. Nevertheless, their pharmacokinetic properties result in low concentrations of the drugs in relevant parts of the gastrointestinal tract, and this makes them unsuitable for the treatment of SD—although they work well as an effective prophylaxis (de Graaf et al. 1988).

Hopefully, new drugs, or old substances that have been modified to improve their efficiency, will become available to replace these antimicrobials. For example, acetylisovaleryltylosin (aivlosin), a new macrolide antibiotic, recently was shown to prevent clinical SD, as well as to treat the disease when it was used for in-feed medication (Tasker et al. 2004).

Serious losses also may be prevented, even in exposed herds, by the use of growth promoters with antibacterial potential such as salinomycin and monensin (ionophores). It should be noted, though, that toxicity occurs when ionophores are used with pleuromutilins or with other drugs that potentially interfere with hepatic metabolism. For example, severe side effects have been reported when salinomycin was mixed in the feed with pleuromutilins (Kavanagh 1992). Growth promoters with potential antibacterial effects have the disadvantage that they may mask disease in apparently SD-free herds. They should not be used as a substitute for good management.

Control of Vectors

Studies using strain detection techniques have strongly indicated that mice and rats can act as a reservoir for *B. hyodysenteriae* in pig herds (Hampson et al. 1991; Fellström et al. 2004). Consequently, lack of efficient rodent control may be an important explanation for failures in SD eradication programs. The role of birds as possible vectors for *B. hyodysenteriae* is unclear, but should not be ignored. *B. hyodysenteriae* or isolates similar to *B. hyodysenteriae* are commonly found in the feces of Swedish mallards (Jansson et al. 2004). Whether these avian isolates are capable of causing disease in pigs is not known, although it was not possible to induce SD in pigs challenged with rhea isolates of *B. hyodysenteriae* (Stanton et al. 1997b). Mechanical transmission of infectious material by birds and other possible wildlife vectors is an important risk factor in outdoor pig units where effective control is impossible.

Vaccination for SD

To date vaccination has not played a large role in the control of SD, mainly because of the limited efficacy and availability of such vaccines. Even if available, it is unlikely that they would be used prophylactically in herds free of SD unless there was a perception that the herds were at a high risk of introducing the disease. Generally, if appropriate vaccines were available, they could be used to help manage SD. For example, in herds that were intended to be eradicated, vaccines could be used prior to this to help reduce shedding and environmental contamination. In other infected herds, vaccines could be used to replace or supplement current antimicrobial usage. This would reduce overall herd antimicrobial consumption, and remove selective pressures that might lead to the development of resistance in spirochete strains.

Bacterin vaccines are available commercially in some countries, and may provide a degree of protection against SD (Fernie et al. 1983; Parizek et al. 1985; Hampson et al. 1993; Diego et al. 1995; Waters et al. 2000b). Unfortunately, they tend to be LOS serogroup-specific, which then requires the use of autogenous or multivalent bacterins. Furthermore, they are relatively difficult and costly to produce on a large scale because of the fastidious growth requirements of the spirochete. One publication reported that immunization with a *B. hyodysenteriae* bacterin actually exacerbated dysentery (Olson et al. 1994). A commercial proteinase-digested bacterin may offer a better level of protection than conventional bacterins, although the cellular immune responses generated by it in pigs were not different from those in bacterin-vaccinated pigs (Waters et al. 2000b).

Several attempts have been made to develop either attenuated or genetically modified live avirulent strains of *B. hyodysenteriae* as vaccines for SD. Naturally avirulent or low-virulence strains have been used experimentally (Hudson et al. 1976), sometimes in combination with bacterins (Lysons et al. 1986), while modified strains have been produced by inducing mutations in genes affecting motility (Rosey et al. 1996; Kennedy et al. 1997), hemolysis (Hyatt et al. 1994), and protection from oxygen toxicity (Stanton et al. 1999). These strains may have a reduced ability to colonize the large intestine, and, probably for this reason, have produced limited protective immunity. To date, none have become commercially available as live vaccines.

The use of recombinant subunit vaccines for the control of SD is an attractive alternative, since the products would be well defined (essential for registration purposes) and relatively easy to produce on a large scale. A recombinant 38-kDa flagellar protein from *B. hyodysenteriae* used as a trial vaccine failed to prevent *B. hyodysenteriae* colonization in pigs (Gabe et al. 1995), but recently the immunogenic 29.7 kDa outer-membrane lipoprotein of *B. hyodysenteriae*, designated BmpB, provided a 50% reduction in incidence of disease in pigs that were vaccinated and then experimentally infected (La et al. 2004). Although protection was not complete, it appears that recombinant vaccines have potential for use in this context. Apart from identifying appropriate recombinant vaccine candidates, a major issue is how to deliver them to pigs in a way to optimize protective immunity in the large intestine. Many different strategies are being considered, but as yet there is no consensus on how best to do this. The large intestine is a difficult site to protect, and ideally a vaccine would prevent colonization rather than just limit the extent of lesion formation. This requires the production of a persistent and effective local immune response.

Elimination of SD

Eradication Programs without Depopulation. In herds with SD, elimination of the disease should always be the aim, both because of the devastating effect of SD on feed-conversion efficiency and for animal welfare reasons. Furthermore, herds with SD represent a potential risk of disease for other pig herds, and a high consumption of antibacterials in infected herds increases the risk of development of antibacterial resistance and spread of resistant strains. Elimination programs have not always proved successful (Muirhead 1984; Wood and Lysons 1988), so, to improve the chances of success, considerable effort must be put into planning, organizing, and achieving the full understanding and cooperation of all personnel involved. Generally, eradication becomes more difficult as herd size increases and as the company operation becomes larger and more complex. Wood and Lysons (1988) suggested that provided that there was a careful selection of herds the chances of an eradication program succeeding were around 80–90%. The cost for elimination of SD has been estimated to be recovered in 6–12 months through improved production and reduced drug usage (Windsor and Simmons 1981; Christensen et al. 1987; Wood and Lysons 1988). Hence successful eradication is of considerable long-term financial benefit to the producer.

Attempts to eliminate SD without total depopulation of pigs from the unit is not recommended unless an effective antimicrobial agent against *B. hyodysenteriae* isolates from the unit is available. It is also important to establish a source of replacement breeding stock that is guaranteed to be free from SD (e.g., herds officially certified as free from the disease). Alternatively, a system of isolation and medication of all replacement stock is necessary before permitting entry to the unit. The introduction of *B. hyodysenteriae* into pig herds primarily occurs with carrier pigs and, unfortunately, at present there are no reliable methods of detecting carrier pigs from infected herds.

Depending on the herd structure, the production model (e.g., batch or continuous production), economical considerations, etc., eradication can be performed in several different manners. These vary from intensive medication of all pigs for a short period, to introduction of medicated-early-weaning and multisite production, through to an ongoing program performed by emptying and disinfecting each herd unit in a cycle, and thereafter introducing medicated animals to cleaned and disinfected units. The eradication period for the latter method may last for several months. General guidelines, partly adopted from Harris and Glock (1981), Baekbo (1998), and Løvens Kemiske Fabrik (1998) follow:

1. The diagnosis should be verified by culture, biochemical tests, and/or PCR.
2. Since the herd may be infected by more than one clone of *B. hyodysenteriae*, several isolates should be tested for their susceptibility to antibacterials available for use in an eradication program. Susceptibility testing should use agar dilution or broth dilution to establish minimum inhibitory concentration (MIC) values. In most cases pleuromutilins will be the agents of choice.
3. Herds practicing a continuous production system should be encouraged to change their production to a planned system based on batch production before the eradication program is performed.
4. The eradication program should be performed during a warm season since the survival time of *B. hyo-*

dysenteriae in the environment is reduced and the efficiency of disinfectants is improved at higher temperatures.

5. The number of animals in the herd should be reduced to as few as possible. Ideally, all weaners, growers, and finishers should be removed from the herd before the start of the program.

6. An efficient rodent and insect control program should be introduced and protective measures taken to stop wild birds from entering buildings where pigs are housed.

7. Dogs and cats should not be allowed within the herd area. Alternatively they should not be allowed to leave the house where they are kept and should be included in the medication program.

8. All possible sanitary measures to reduce environmental contamination with potentially infectious spirochetes should be taken, including thorough cleaning and disinfecting of all areas where pigs are housed or with which they have contact, the watering and feeding systems, all equipment, etc. Cleaning should be performed by high pressure washing with hot water to remove organic matter, followed by disinfection. *B. hyodysenteriae* is sensitive to most of the commonly used disinfectants. Where slatted floors are present, the slats have to be lifted before cleaning/disinfection. Slurry tanks must be emptied and subjected to the same cleaning and disinfection procedures. Effective cleaning and disinfection may be particularly problematic in outdoor production units or units where grower pigs are housed in shelters and bedded on straw or rice hulls over an earth floor. Relocation of cleaned and disinfected outdoor huts to fresh fields and burning any remaining organic material at the old location followed by ploughing and reseeding the ground should be effective in eliminating infection.

9. All sows, gilts, and boars should be medicated through the drinking water or feed for a minimum of 14 days and introduced into cleaned and disinfected buildings. Piglets born during the medication period should be weaned and finished offsite, receiving parenteral treatment with the antimicrobial agent of choice at weaning. All sow and boar accommodation, including the farrowing accommodation must be thoroughly cleaned and disinfected during the medication period. Ideally the program of cleaning should be started in advance of medication so that the buildings are empty for at least 2 weeks after completion of disinfection. Piglets born after the sows have completed the 14-day medication period can be weaned and finished onsite.

10. All replacement of stock should be stopped during the eradication program.

11. Outdoor lots that have held pigs affected with SD should remain free of pigs for a substantial time period (see Sources of Infection). Any liquid feces, such as in pits and lagoons, should be considered to contain infectious *B. hyodysenteriae* for several months, and lagoon water should not be used for recycling until an appropriate time period of 2–3 months has elapsed after an elimination program has been completed.

Depopulation/Repopulation with SD-Free Stock. Total depopulation, cleanup, disinfection, and repopulation with SD-free stock to reestablish an ongoing pig operation should not be made without accurate financial calculations (Wood and Lysons 1988). However, in some situations this alternative is the only method available to eliminate *B. hyodysenteriae* from the herd. The general guidelines described for elimination without depopulation should be carefully followed. Financial evaluations comparing medication/disinfection methods with depopulation/repopulation methods were made by Polson et al. (1992). Elimination without depopulation was financially more attractive than the depopulation/repopulation method. However, the probability of successful eradication would certainly influence the choice of eradication method.

Prevention of SD

Herds that have been established as free of SD and are either closed or maintained in a closed pyramid will remain free of SD if situated in an isolated location and precautions are taken to prevent contamination by feces from carrier pigs or by vectors, especially rodents and birds. Infectious materials may also be carried into a herd by fomites such as workers' boots, farm implements, and feed or animal trucks. However, introduction of new stock represents by far the greatest hazard. A reliable history of the source herd is the only assurance of safety, since no reliable methods of detecting carrier pigs from infected herds exist. Research efforts are being directed at various methods of identification of carrier animals, and it is hoped that sensitive and specific serologic tests or other detection methods will be available in the future. To avoid introduction of SD and other diseases into herds, purchased animals should always be kept in quarantine for at least 3 weeks. Quarantine is a highly recommended procedure, since clinical signs often appear in subclinically affected animals as a result of transportation. During quarantine, the newly purchased animals can be treated to eliminate *B. hyodysenteriae* from the intestinal tract.

ACKNOWLEDGMENTS

The authors wish to acknowledge Professors D. L. Harris and R. D. Glock for their input into earlier versions of this chapter, on which the current chapter was based.

REFERENCES

Argenzio RA. 1981. Glucose-stimulated fluid absorption in the pig small intestine: An approach to oral fluid therapy in swine dysentery. Am J Vet Res 41:2000–2006.

Argenzio RA, Whipp SC, Glock RD. 1980. Pathophysiology of swine dysentery: Colonic transport and permeability studies. J Infect Dis 142:676–684.

Atyeo RF, Oxberry SL, Combs BG, Hampson DJ. 1998. Development and evaluation of polymerase chain reaction tests as an aid to diagnosis of swine dysentery and intestinal spirochaetosis. Lett Appl Microbiol 26:126–130.

Atyeo RF, Oxberry SL, Hampson DJ. 1999a. Analysis of *Serpulina hyodysenteriae* strain variation and its molecular epidemiology using pulsed field gel electrophoresis. Epidemiol Infect 123:133–138.

Atyeo RF, Stanton TB, Jensen NS, Suriyaarachichi DS, Hampson DJ. 1999b. Differentiation of *Serpulina* species by NADH oxidase (*nox*) gene comparisons and *nox*-based polymerase chain reaction tests. Vet Microbiol 67:49–62.

Baekbo P. 1998. Sanering for sygdomme-danske erfaringer. VeterinärInformation 4:16–19.

Barcellos DE, de Uzeda M, Ikuta N, Lunge VR, Fonseca AS, Kader II, Duhamel GE. 2000b. Identification of porcine intestinal spirochetes by PCR-restriction fragment length polymorphism analysis of ribosomal DNA encoding 23S rRNA. Vet Microbiol 75:189–198.

Barcellos DE, Mathiesen MR, de Uzeda M, Kader II, Duhamel GE. 2000a. Prevalence of *Brachyspira* species isolated from diarrhoeic pigs in Brazil. Vet Rec 146:398–403.

Baum DH, Joens LA. 1979. Serotypes of beta-hemolytic *Treponema hyodysenteriae*. Infect Immun 25:792–796.

Binek M, Wojcik U, Szyncikwicz Z, Jakubowski T. 1994. Dynamics of susceptibility of *Serpulina hyodysenteriae* to different chemotherapeutics in vitro. In Proc 13th Congr Int Pig Vet Soc, p. 203.

Bowden CA, Joens LA, Kelley LM. 1989. Characterization of the attachment of *Treponema hyodysenteriae* to Henlé intestinal cells in vitro. Am J Vet Res 50:1481–1485.

Boye M, Baloda SB, Leser TD, Moller K. 2001. Survival of *Brachyspira hyodysenteriae* and *B. pilosicoli* in terrestrial microcosms. Vet Microbiol 81:33–40.

Boye M, Jensen TK, Moller K, Leser TD, Jorsal SE. 1998. Specific detection of the genus *Serpulina*, *S. hyodysenteriae* and *S. pilosicoli* in porcine intestines by fluorescent rRNA *in situ* hybridization. Mol Cell Probes 12:323–330.

Burrows MR, Lemcke RM. 1981. Identification of *Treponema hyodysenteriae* by a rapid slide agglutination test. Vet Rec 108:187–189.

Burrows MR, Lysons RJ, Rowlands GJ, Lemcke RM. 1984. An enzyme-linked immunosorbent assay for detecting serum antibody to *Treponema hyodysenteriae*. In Proc 8th Congr Pig Vet Soc, p. 186.

Calderaro A, Merialdi G, Perini S, Ragni P, Guegan R, Dettori G, Chezzi C. 2001. A novel method for isolation of *Brachyspira (Serpulina) hyodysenteriae* from pigs with swine dysentery in Italy. Vet Microbiol 80:47–52.

Carvajal A, De Arriba ML, Rodriguez H, Vidal AB, Rubio P. 2003. Prevalence of *B. hyodysenteriae* and *B. pilosicoli* infections amongst Spanish swine herds with diarrhoea. In Proc 2nd Int Conf Colonic Spirochaetal Infections in Animals and Humans, Eddleston, Scotland, p. 43.

Chatfield SN, Fernie DS, Penn C, Dougan G. 1988. Identification of the major antigens of *Treponema hyodysenteriae* and comparison with those of *Treponema innocens*. Infect Immun 56:1070–1075.

Chia SP. 1977. Studies of the survival of *Treponema hyodysenteriae* and the epidemiology of swine dysentery. M.V.S. thesis, Univ Glasgow, Scotland.

Chia SP, Taylor DJ. 1978. Factors affecting the survival of *Treponema hyodysenteriae* in dysenteric pig feces. Vet Rec 103:68–70.

Christensen F, Lind O, Schou J, Sørensen L, Szancer J. 1987. III. Sanering Medicinsk behandling med Tiamutin 2% premix kombineret med tømning af staldene—Produktionsøkonomisk vurdering. Dansk Veterinærtidskrift 70:890–897.

Cizek A, Smola J, Mádr P. 1998. *In vitro* activity of six anti-dysenteric drugs on *Serpulina hyodysenteriae* and *S. pilosicoli* strains isolated in the Czech Republic. In Proc 15th Congr Int Pig Vet Soc, p. 135.

Combs BG, Hampson DJ, Harders SJ. 1992. Typing of Australian isolates of *Treponema hyodysenteriae* by serology and by DNA restriction endonuclease analysis. Vet Microbiol 31:273–285.

Corona-Barrera E, Smith DGE, La T, Hampson DJ, Thomson JR. 2004. Immunomagnetic separation of the intestinal spirochaetes *Brachyspira pilosicoli* and *Brachyspira hyodysenteriae* from porcine faeces. J Med Microbiol 53:301–307.

Cullen PA, Coutts SA, Cordwell SJ, Bulach DM, Adler B. 2003. Characterization of a locus encoding four paralogous outer membrane lipoproteins of *Brachyspira hyodysenteriae*. Microbes Infect 5:275–283.

Cutler R, Gardiner I. 1988. A blue print for pig health research. Australian Pig Research Council, Canberra.

de Graaf GJ, Jager LP, Baars AJ, Spierenburg TJ. 1988. Some pharmacokinetic observations of carbadox medication in pigs. Vet Q 10:34–41.

Diego R, Lanza I, Carvajal A, Rubio P, Carmenes P. 1995. *Serpulina hyodysenteriae* challenge of fattening pigs vaccinated with an adjuvanted bivalent bacterin against swine dysentery. Vaccine 13:663–667.

Dugourd D, Jacques M, Bigras-Poulin M, Harel J. 1996. Characterization of *Serpulina hyodysenteriae* isolates of serotype 8 and 9 by random amplification of polymorphic DNA analysis. Vet Microbiol 48:305–314.

Dugourd D, Martin C, Rioux CR, Jacques M, Harel J. 1999. Characterization of a periplasmic ATP-binding cassette iron import system of *Brachyspira (Serpulina) hyodysenteriae*. J Bacteriol 181:6948–6957.

Duhamel GE, Joens, LA. 1994. Laboratory Procedures for Diagnosis of Swine Dysentery. American Association of Veterinary Laboratory Diagnosticians, Inc., USA.

Durmic Z, Pethick DW, Mullan BP, Schulze H, Accioly JM, Hampson DJ. 2000. Extrusion of wheat or sorghum and/or addition of exogenous enzymes to pig diets influences the large intestinal microbiota but does not prevent development of swine dysentery following experimental challenge. J Appl Microbiol 89:678–86.

Durmic Z, Pethick DW, Pluske JR, Hampson DJ. 1998. Changes in bacterial populations in the colon of pigs fed different sources of dietary fibre, and the development of swine dysentery after experimental challenge. J Appl Microbiol 85:574–582.

Egan IT, Harris DL, Joens LA. 1983. Comparison of the microtitration agglutination test and the enzyme-linked immunosorbent assay for the detection of herds affected with swine dysentery. Am J Vet Res 44:1323–1328.

Fellström C, Karlsson M, Pettersson B, Zimmerman U, Gunnarsson A, Aspan A. 1999. Emended descriptions of indole negative and indole positive isolates of *Brachyspira (Serpulina) hyodysenteriae*. Vet Microbiol 70:225–238.

Fellström C, Landen A, Karlsson M, Gunnarsson A, Holmgren N. 2004. Mice as a reservoir of *Brachyspira hyodysenteriae* in repeated outbreaks of swine dysentery in a Swedish fattening herd. In Proc 18th Congr Int Pig Vet Soc, p. 280.

Fellström C, Pettersson B, Johansson K, Lundenheim N, Gunnarsson A. 1996. Prevalence of *Serpulina* species in relation to diarrhea and feed medication in pig-rearing herds in Sweden. Am J Vet Res 57:807–811.

Fellström C, Pettersson B, Thompson J, Gunnarsson A, Persson M, Johansson K. 1997. Identification of *Serpulina* species associated with porcine colitis by biochemical analysis and PCR. J Clin Microbiol 35:462–467.

Fellström C, Zimmerman U, Aspan A, Gunnarsson A. 2001. The use of culture, pooled samples and PCR for identification of herds infected with *Brachyspira hyodysenteriae*. Anim Health Res Rev 2:37–43.

Fernie DS, Ripley PH, Walker PD. 1983. Swine dysentery: Protection against experimental challenge following single dose parenteral immunisation with inactivated *Treponema hyodysenteriae*. Res Vet Sci 35:217–221.

Fisher LN, Mathiesen MR, Duhamel GE. 1997. Restriction fragment length polymorphism of the periplasmic flagellar *flaA1* gene of *Serpulina* species. Clin Diagn Lab Immunol 4:681–686.

Gabe JD, Chang R-J, Sloiany R, Andrews WH, McCaman MT. 1995. Isolation of extracytoplasmic proteins from *Serpulina hyodysenteriae* B204 and molecular cloning of the *flaB1* gene encoding a 38-kilodalton flagellar protein. Infect Immun 63:142–148.

Gabe JD, Dragon E, Chang R, McCaman MT. 1998. Identification of a linked set of genes in *Serpulina hyodysenteriae* (B204) predicted to encode closely related 39-kilodalton extracytoplasmic proteins. J Bacteriol 180:444–448.

Glock RD. 1971. Studies on the etiology, hematology and pathology of swine dysentery. Ph.D. diss., Iowa State Univ.

Glock RD, Harris DL. 1972. Swine dysentery. II. Characterization of lesions in pigs inoculated with *Treponema hyodysenteriae* in pure and mixed culture. Vet Med Small Anim Clin 67:65–68.

Glock RD, Harris DL, Kluge JP. 1974. Localization of spirochetes with the structural characteristics of *Treponema hyodysenteriae* in the lesions of swine dysentery. Infect Immun 9:167–178.

Glock RD, Vanderloo KJ, Kinyon JM. 1975. Survival of certain pathogenic organisms in swine lagoon effluent. J Am Vet Med Assoc 166:277–278.

Greer JM, Wannemuehler MJ. 1989a. Comparison of the biological responses produced by lipopolysaccharide and endotoxin of *Treponema hyodysenteriae* and *Treponema innocens*. Infect Immun 57:717–723.

———. 1989b. Pathogenesis of *Treponema hyodysenteriae*: Induction of interleukin-1 and tumour necrosis factor by a treponema butanol/water extract (endotoxin). Microbiol Pathol 7:279–288.

Gresham AC, Hunt BW, Dalziel RW. 1998. Treatment of swine dysentery—Problems of antibiotic resistance and concurrent salmonellosis. Vet Rec 619.

Halter MR, Joens LA. 1988. Lipooligosaccharides from *Treponema hyodysenteriae* and *Treponema innocens*. Infect Immun 56:3152–3156.

Hampson DJ. 2000. The Serpulina story. In Proc 16th Congr Int Pig Vet Soc, pp. 1–5.

Hampson DJ, Atyeo RF, Combs BG. 1997. Swine dysentery. In Intestinal Spirochaetes in Domestic Animals and Humans. DJ Hampson, TB Stanton, eds. CAB International, England, pp. 175–209.

Hampson DJ, Combs BG, Harders SJ, Connaughton ID, Fahy VA. 1991. Isolation of *Treponema hyodysenteriae* from a wild rat living on a piggery. Aust Vet J 68:308.

Hampson DJ, Mhoma JRL, Combs BG, Buddle JR. 1989. Proposed revisions to the serological typing systems for *Treponema hyodysenteriae*. Epidemiol Infect 102:75–84.

Hampson DJ, Robertson ID, Mhoma JRL. 1993. Experiences with a vaccine being developed for the control of swine dysentery. Aust Vet J 70:18–20.

Harel J, Belanger M, Forget C, Jacques M. 1994. Characterisation of *Serpulina hyodysenteriae* isolates of serotypes 8 and 9 from Quebec by restriction endonuclease fingerprinting and ribotyping. Can J Vet Res 58:302–305.

Harris DL, Glock RD. 1981. Swine dysentery. In Diseases of Swine (5th edition). AD Leman, RD Glock, WL Mengeling, RHC Penny, E. Scholl, B Straw, eds. Ames: Iowa State Univ Press.

Harris DL, Glock RD, Christensen CR, Kinyon JM. 1972. Swine dysentery. I. Inoculation of pigs with *Treponema hyodysenteriae*

(new species) and reproduction of the disease. Vet Med Small Anim Clin 67:61–64.

Hommez J, Devriese LA, Castryck F, Miry C, Lein A, Haesebrouck F. 1998. Susceptibility of different *Serpulina* species in pigs to antimicrobial agents. Vlaams Diergen Tijds 67:32–35.

Hsu T, Hutto DL, Minion FC, Zuerner RL, Wannemuehler MJ. 2001. Cloning of a beta-hemolysin gene of *Brachyspira (Serpulina) hyodysenteriae* and its expression in *Escherichia coli*. Infect Immun 69:706–711.

Hudson MJ, Alexander TJ, Lysons RJ, Prescott JF. 1976. Swine dysentery: Protection of pigs by oral and parenteral immunisation with attenuated *Treponema hyodysenteriae*. Res Vet Sci 21:366–367.

Hughes R, Olander HJ, Kanitz DL, Qureshi S. 1977. A study of swine dysentery by immunofluorescence and histology. Vet Pathol 14:490–507.

Hughes R, Olander HJ, Williams CB. 1975. Swine dysentery: Pathogenicity of *Treponema hyodysenteriae*. Am J Vet Res 36:971–977.

Humphrey SB, Stanton TB, Jensen NS, Zuerner RL. 1997. Purification and characterization of VSH-1, a generalized transducing bacteriophage of *Serpulina hyodysenteriae*. J Bacteriol 179:323–329.

Hunter D, Saunders CN. 1977. Diagnosis of swine dysentery using an absorbed fluorescent antiserum. Vet Rec 101:303–304.

Hutto DL, Wannemuehler MJ. 1999. A comparison of the morphologic effects of *Serpulina hyodysenteriae* or its beta-hemolysin on the murine mucosa. Vet Pathol 36:412–422.

Hyatt DR, ter Huurne AAHM, Van Der Zeist BAM, Joens L.A. 1994. Reduced virulence of *Serpulina hyodysenteriae* hemolysin-negative mutants in pigs and their potential to protect pigs against challenge with a virulent strain. Infect Immun 62:2244–2248.

Jacobson M, Fellström C, Lindberg R, Wallgren P, Jensen-Waern M. 2004. Experimental swine dysentery: Comparison between infection models. J Clin Microbiol 53:273–280.

Jansson DS, Johansson KE, Olofsson T, Råsbäck T, Vagsholm I, Pettersson B, Gunnarsson A, Fellström C. 2004. *Brachyspira hyodysenteriae* and other strongly beta-haemolytic and indole-positive spirochaetes isolated from mallards (*Anas platyrhynchos*). J Med Microbiol 53:293–300.

Jenkins EM. 1978. Development of resistance to swine dysentery. Vet Med Small Animal Clin 73:931–936.

Jenkins EM, Mohammad A, Klesius PH. 1982. Evaluation of cell-mediated immune response to *Treponema hyodysenteriae*. In Proc 6th Congr Pig Vet Soc, p. 41.

Jenkins EM, Sinhi PP, Vance RT, Reese GL. 1976. Passive hemolysis test for antibody to *Treponema hyodysenteriae*. Infect Immun 14:1106–1107.

Jenkinson SR, Wingar CR. 1981. Selective medium for the isolation of *Treponema hyodysenteriae*. Vet Rec 109:384–385.

Jensen NS, Casey TA, Stanton TB. 1990. Detection and identification of *Treponema hyodysenteriae* by using oligonucleotide probes complementary to 16S rRNA. J Clin Microbiol 28:2717–2721.

Jensen NS, Stanton TB, Swayne DE. 1996. Identification of the swine pathogen *Serpulina hyodysenteriae* in rheas (*Rhea americana*). Vet Microbiol 52:259–269.

Joens LA. 1980. Experimental transmission of *Treponema hyodysenteriae* from mice to pigs. Am J Vet Res 41:1225–1226.

Joens LA, Deyoung DW, Glock RD, Mapother ME, Cramer JD, Wilcox iii HE. 1985. Passive protection of segmented swine colonic loops against swine dysentery. Am J Vet Res 46:2369–2371.

Joens LA, Glock RD. 1979. Experimental infection in mice with *Treponema hyodysenteriae*. Infect Immun 25:757–760.

Joens LA, Glock RD, Whipp SC, Robinson IM, Harris, D. L. 1981. Location of *Treponema hyodysenteriae* and synergistic anaerobic bacteria in colonic lesions on gnotobiotic pigs. Vet Microbiol 6:69–77.

Joens LA, Harris DL, Baum DH. 1979. Immunity to swine dysentery in recovered pigs. Am J Vet Res 40:1352–1354.

Joens LA, Harris DL, Kinyon JM, Kaeberle ML. 1978. Microtitration agglutination for detection of *Treponema hyodysenteriae* antibody. J Clin Microbiol 8:293–298.

Joens LA, Marquez MR, Halter M. 1993. Comparison of outer-membrane fractions of *Serpulina (Treponema) hyodysenteriae*. Vet Microbiol 35:119–132.

Joens LA, Nord NA, Kinyon JM, Egan IT. 1982. Enzyme-linked immunosorbent assay for detection of antibody to *Treponema hyodysenteriae* antigens. J Clin Microbiol 15:249–252.

Joens LA, Whipp SC, Glock RD, Nuessen ME. 1983. Serotype-specific protection against *Treponema hyodysenteriae* infection in ligated colonic loops of pigs recovered from swine dysentery. Infect Immun 39:460–462.

Jonasson R, Johannisson A, Jacobson M, Fellström C, Jensen-Waern M. 2004. Differences in lymphocyte subpopulations and cell counts before and after experimentally induced swine dysentery. J Med Microbiol 53:267–272.

Karlsson M, Aspan A, Landen A, Franklin A. 2004. Further characterization of porcine *Brachyspira hyodysenteriae* isolates with decreased susceptibility to tiamulin. J Med Microbiol 53:281–285.

Karlsson M, Fellström C, Gunnarsson A, Landen A, Franklin A. 2003. Antimicrobial susceptibility testing of porcine *Brachyspira (Serpulina)* species isolates. J Clin Microbiol 41:2596–604.

Karlsson M, Fellström C, Heldtander MU, Johansson KE, Franklin A. 1999. Genetic basis of macrolide and lincosamide resistance in *Brachyspira (Serpulina) hyodysenteriae*. FEMS Microbiol Lett 172:255–260.

Karlsson M, Gunnarsson A, Franklin A. 2001. Susceptibility to pleuromutilins in *Brachyspira (Serpulina) hyodysenteriae*. Anim Health Res Rev 2:59–65.

Karlsson M, Oxberry SL, Hampson DJ. 2002. Antimicrobial susceptibility testing of Australian isolates of *Brachyspira hyodysenteriae* using a new broth dilution method. Vet Microbiol 84:123–133.

Kavanagh NT. 1992. Salinomycin toxicity in pigs. Pig Vet J 28:116–118.

Kennedy MJ, Rosey EL, Frank RK, Jensen NS, Stanton TB. 1996. Generation, characterization and virulence testing of NADH oxidase defective mutants of *Serpulina hyodysenteriae*. Abstr B105. New Orleans: American Society for Microbiology.

Kennedy MJ, Rosey EL, Yancey Jr RJ. 1997. Characterization of *flaA*- and *flaB*-mutants of *Serpulina hyodysenteriae*: Both flagellin subunits, FlaA and FlaB, are necessary for full motility and intestinal colonization. FEMS Microbiol Lett 153:119–128.

Kennedy MJ, Rosnick DK, Ulrich RG, Yancey RJ. 1988. Association of *Treponema hyodysenteriae* with porcine intestinal mucosa. J Gen Microbiol 134:1565–1567.

Kennedy MJ, Rosnick DK, Ulrich RG, Yancey Jr RJ. 1992. Identification and immunological characterisation of the major immunogenic antigens of serotypes 1 and 2 of *Serpulina hyodysenteriae*. In Proc 12th Congr Int Pig Vet Soc, p. 273.

Kent KA, Lemcke RM. 1984. Purification and cytotoxic activity of a haemolysin produced by *Treponema hyodysenteriae*. In Proc 8th Congr Int Pig Vet Soc, p. 185.

Kinyon, JM, Harris DL, Glock RD. 1977. Enteropathogenicity of various isolates of *Treponema hyodysenteriae*. Infect Immun 15:638–646.

———. 1980. Isolation of *Treponema hyodysenteriae* from experimentally infected pigs at various intervals post-inoculation. In Proc 6th Congr Int Pig Vet Soc, p. 232.

Kitai K, Kashiwazaki M, Adachi Y, Kume T, Arakawa A. 1979. In vitro activity of 39 antimicrobial agents against *Treponema hyodysenteriae*. Antimicrob Agents Chemother 15:392–395.

Knoop FC, Schrank GD, Ferraro FM. 1979. In vitro attachment of *Treponema hyodysenteriae* to mammalian epithelial cells. Can J Microbiol 25:399–405.

Kunkle RA, Harris DL, Kinyon JM. 1986. Autoclaved liquid medium for propagation of *Treponema hyodysenteriae*. J Clin Microbiol 24:669–671.

Kunkle RA, Kinyon JM. 1988. Improved selective medium for the isolation of *Treponema hyodysenteriae*. J Clin Microbiol 26:2357–2360.

La T, Hampson DJ. 2001. Serologic detection of *Brachyspira (Serpulina) hyodysenteriae* infections. Anim Health Res Rev 2:45–52.

La T, Phillips ND, Hampson DJ. 2003. Development of a duplex PCR assay for detection of *Brachyspira hyodysenteriae* and *Brachyspira pilosicoli* in pig feces. J Clin Microbiol 41:3372–3375.

La T, Phillips ND, Reichel MP, Hampson DJ. 2004. Protection of pigs from swine dysentery by vaccination with recombinant BmpB, a 29.7 kDa outer-membrane lipoprotein of *Brachyspira hyodysenteriae*. Vet Microbiol 102:97–109.

Lee BJ, Hampson DJ. 1996. Production and characterisation of a monoclonal antibody to *Serpulina hyodysenteriae*. FEMS Microbiol Lett 136:193–197.

Lee JI, Hampson DJ, Combs BG, Lymbery AJ. 1993. Genetic relationships between isolates of *Serpulina (Treponema) hyodysenteriae*, and comparison of methods for their subspecific differentiation. Vet Microbiol 34:35–46.

Lee BJ, La T, Mikosza ASJ, Hampson DJ. 2000. Identification of the gene encoding BmpB, a 30 kDa outer envelope lipoprotein of *Brachyspira (Serpulina) hyodysenteriae*, and immunogenicity of recombinant BmpB in mice and pigs. Vet Microbiol 76:245–257.

Lemcke RM, Burrows MR. 1979. A disc growth-inhibition test for differentiating *Treponema hyodysenteriae* from other intestinal spirochetes. Vet Rec 104:548–551.

Leser TD, Lindecrona RH, Jensen TK, Jensen BB, Møller K. 2000. Changes in bacterial community structure in the colon of pigs fed different experimental diets and after infection with *Brachyspira hyodysenteriae*. Appl Environ Microbiol 66:3290–3296.

Leser TD, Møller K, Jensen TK, Jorsal SE. 1997. Specific detection of *Serpulina hyodysenteriae* and potentially pathogenic weakly haemolytic porcine intestinal spirochaetes by polymerase chain reaction targeting 23S rDNA. Mol Cell Probes 11:363–372.

Lindecrona RH, Jensen TK, Jensen BB, Leser TD, Jiufeng W, Møller K. 2003. The influence of diet on the development of swine dysentery upon experimental infection. Anim Sci 76:81–87.

Lobova D, Smola J, Cizek A. 2004. Decreased susceptibility to tiamulin and valnemulin among Czech isolates of *Brachyspira hyodysenteriae*. J Med Microbiol 53:287–291.

Løvens Kemiske Fabrik. 1998. In Plan för sanering av svinedysenteri. Løvens kemiske Fabrik, Industriparken 55, 2750 Ballerup.

Lysons RJ. 1983. European perspectives on the control of swine dysentery. Proc Annu Meet Am Assoc Swine Pract, p. 179.

Lysons RJ, Burrows MR, Debney TG, Bew J. 1986. Vaccination against swine dysentery—An effective novel method. In Proc 9th Congr Int Pig Vet Soc, p. 180.

Lysons RJ, Kent KA, Bland AP, Sellwood R, Robinson WP, Frost AJ. 1991. A cytotoxic haemolysin from *Treponema hyodysenteriae*: A probable virulence determinant in swine dysentery. J Med Microbiol 34:97–102.

Lysons RJ, Lemcke RM, Bew J, Burrows MR, Alexander TJL. 1982. An avirulent strain of *Treponema hyodysenteriae* isolated from herds free of swine dysentery. In Proc 7th Congr Int Pig Vet Soc, p. 40.

Lysons RJ, Lemcke RM, Duncan AL. 1988. "Colitis" of pigs—An emerging disease. In Proc 10th Congr Int Pig Vet Soc, p. 141.

Mapother ME. 1993. An Estimate of the Prevalence of Swine Dysentery in U.S. Swine Herds during 1989–1991. Survey, National Animal Health Monitoring System, National Veterinary Services Laboratory, U.S. Dept Agric, Washington, D.C.

McCaman MT, Auer K, Foley W, Gabe JD. 2003. *Brachyspira hyodysenteriae* contains eight linked gene copies related to an expressed 39-kDa surface protein. Microbes Infect 5:1–6.

Messier S, Higgins R, Moore C. 1990. Minimal inhibitory concentrations of five antimicrobials against *Treponema hyodysenteriae* and *Treponema innocens*. J Vet Diagn Invest 2:330–333.

Mhoma JRL, Hampson DJ, Robertson ID. 1992. A serological survey to determine the prevalence of *Treponema hyodysenteriae* in Western Australia. Aust Vet J 69:81–84.

Milner JA, Sellwood R. 1994. Chemotactic response to mucin by *Serpulina hyodysenteriae* and other porcine spirochetes: Potential role in intestinal colonization. Infect Immun 62:4095–4099.

Møller K, Jensen TK, Jorsal SE, Leser TD, Carstensen B. 1998. Detection of *Lawsonia intracellularis, Serpulina hyodysenteriae,* weakly beta-haemolytic intestinal spirochaetes, *Salmonella enterica,* and haemolytic *Escherichia coli* from swine herds with and without diarrhoea among growing pigs. Vet Microbiol 62:59–72.

Molnar L. 1996. Sensitivity of strains of *Serpulina hyodysenteriae* isolated in Hungary to chemotherapeutic drugs. Vet Rec 138:158–160.

Muirhead MR. 1984. With precise planning and implementation, swine dysentery can be eliminated from a herd. Int Pig Lett 4:1–3.

Nibbelink SK, Sacco RE, Wannemuehler MJ. 1997. Pathogenicity of *Serpulina hyodysenteriae*: In vivo induction of tumor necrosis factor and interleukin-6 by a serpulinal butanol/water extract (endotoxin). Microb Pathog 23:181–187.

Nibbelink SK, Wannamuehler MJ. 1990. Effect of *Treponema hyodysenteriae* infection on mucosal mast cells and T cells in the murine caecum. Infect Immun 58:88–92.

———. 1991. Susceptibility of inbred mouse strains to infection with *Serpula (Treponema) hyodysenteriae*. Infect Immun 59:3111–3118.

———. 1992. An enhanced murine model for studies of *Serpulina (Treponema) hyodysenteriae* pathogenesis. Infect Immun 60:3433–3436.

Nuessen ME, Birmingham JR, Joens LA. 1982. Biological activity of a lipopolysaccharide extracted from *Treponema hyodysenteriae*. Infect Immun 37:138–142.

Nuessen ME, Joens LA. 1982. Serotype-specific opsonisation of *Treponema hyodysenteriae*. Infect Immun 38:1029–1032.

Nuessen ME, Joens LA, Glock RD. 1983. Involvement of lipopolysaccharide in the pathogenicity of *Treponema hyodysenteriae*. J Immun 131:997–999.

Ochiai S, Adachi Y, Mori K. 1997. Unification of the genera *Serpulina* and *Brachyspira*, and proposals of *Brachyspira hyodysenteriae* comb. nov., *Brachyspira innocens* comb. nov. and *Brachyspira pilosicoli* comb. nov. Microbiol Immunol 41:445–452.

Olson LD. 1974. Clinical and pathological observations on the experimental passage of swine dysentery. Can J Comp Med 28:7–13.

———. 1996. Enhanced isolation of *Serpulina hyodysenteriae* by using sliced agar medium. J Clin Microbiol 34:2937–2941.

Olson LD, Dayalu KI, Schlink GT. 1994. Exacerbated onset of dysentery in swine vaccinated with inactivated adjuvanted *Serpulina hyodysenteriae*. Am J Vet Res 55:67–71.

Parizek R, Stewart R, Brown K, Blevins D. 1985. Protection against swine dysentery with an inactivated *Treponema hyodysenteriae* bacterin. Vet Med 80:80–86.

Pearce GP. 1999. Epidemiology of enteric disease in grower-finisher pigs: A postal survey of pig-producers in England. Vet Rec 144:338–342.

Plawinska J, Jakubowski T, Rzewuska M, Binek M. 2004. Occurrence of *Lawsonia intracellularis* and *Brachyspira* spp. infection in swine suffering from diarrhea. In Proc 18th Congr Int Pig Vet Soc, p. 287.

Pluske JR, Durmic Z, Pethick DW, Mullan BP, Hampson DJ. 1998. Confirmation of the role of non-starch polysaccharides and resistant starch in the expression of swine dysentery in pigs following experimental infection. J Nutr 128:1737–1744.

Pluske JR, Siba PM, Pethick DW, Durmic Z, Mullan BP, Hampson DJ. 1996. The incidence of swine dysentery in pigs can be reduced by feeding diets that limit the amount of fermentable substrate entering the large intestine. J Nutr 126:2920–2933.

Pohlenz JF, Whipp SC, Robinson IM, Fagerland JA. 1984. A hypothesis on the pathogenesis of *Treponema hyodysenteriae* induced diarrhoea in pigs. In Proc 8th Cong Int Pig Vet Soc, p. 178.

Polson DD, Marsh WE, Harris DL. 1992. Financial considerations for individual herd eradication of swine dysentery. In Proc 12th Congr Int Pig Vet Soc, p. 510.

Prapasarakul N, Niyomthom W, Tripipat T, Tummarak P, Sukchai S, Thanawongnuwech R. 2004. In vitro activity of antimicrobial agents against *B. hyodysenteriae* isolates from pigs with recurrent dysentery in Thailand. In Proc 18th Congr Int Pig Vet Soc, p. 553.

Råsbäck T, Melin L, Lundeheim N, Gunnarson A, Fellström C. 2004. Isolation of *Brachyspira* species in Swedish pig herds with diarrhoea 1996–2003. In Proc 18th Congr Int Pig Vet Soc, p. 286.

Rees AS, Lysons RJ, Stokes CR, Bourne FJ. 1989a. Antibody production in the colon during infection with *Treponema hyodysenteriae*. Res Vet Sci 47:263–269.

———. 1989b. The effect of parental immunization on antibody production in the pig colon. Vet Immunol Immunopathol 47:263–269.

Ritchie AE, Robinson IM, Joens LA, Kinyon JM. 1978. A bacteriophage for *Treponema hyodysenteriae*. Vet Rec 102:34–35.

Robertson ID, Mhoma JRL, Hampson DJ. 1992. Risk factors associated with the occurrence of swine dysentery in Western Australia: Results of a postal survey. Aust Vet J 69:92–93.

Rohde J, Kessler M, Baums CG, Amtsberg G. 2004. Comparison of methods for antimicrobial susceptibility testing and MIC values for pleuromutilin drugs for *Brachyspira hyodysenteriae* isolated in Germany. Vet Microbiol 102:25–32.

Rohde J, Rothkamp A, Gerlach GF. 2002. Differentiation of porcine *Brachyspira* species by a novel nox PCR-based restriction fragment length polymorphism analysis. J Clin Microbiol 40:2598–2600.

Rønne H, Szancer J. 1990. In vitro susceptibility of Danish field isolates of *Treponema hyodysenteriae* to chemotherapeutics in swine dysentery (SD) therapy. In Proc 11th Congr Int Pig Vet Soc, p. 126.

Rosey EL, Kennedy MJ, Yancey RJ. 1996. Dual *flaA1 flaB1* mutant of *Serpulina hyodysenteriae* expressing periplasmic flagella is severely attenuated in a murine model of swine dysentery. Infect Immun 64:4154–4162.

Schmall MS, Argenzio RA, Whipp SC. 1983. Pathophysiologic features of swine dysentery: Cyclic nucleotide-independent production of diarrhea. Am J Vet Res 44:1309–1316.

Sellwood R, Bland AP. 1997. Ultrastructure of intestinal spirochaetes. In Hampson DJ and Stanton TB (editors). Intestinal Spirochaetes in Domestic Animals and Humans. CAB International, England, pp. 109–149.

Siba PM, Pethick DW, Hampson DJ. 1996. Pigs experimentally infected with *Serpulina hyodysenteriae* can be protected from developing swine dysentery by feeding them a highly digestible diet. Epidem Infect 116:207–216.

Smith SC, Muir T, Holmes M, Coloe PJ. 1991. In-vitro antimicrobial susceptibility of Australian isolates of *Treponema hyodysenteriae*. Aust Vet J 68:408–409.

Songer JG, Glock RD, Schwartz KJ, Harris DL. 1978. Isolation of *Treponema hyodysenteriae* from sources other than swine. J Am Vet Med Assoc 172:464–466.

Songer JG, Harris DL. 1978. Transmission of swine dysentery by carrier pigs. Am J Vet Res 39:913–916.

Stanton TB. 1992. Proposal to change the genus designation *Serpula* to *Serpulina* gen. nov. containing the species *Serpulina hyodysenteriae* comb. nov. and *Serpulina innocens* comb. nov. Int J Syst Bacteriol 42:189–190.

———. 1997. Physiology of ruminal and intestinal spirochaetes. In Hampson DJ and Stanton TB (editors). Intestinal Spirochaetes in Domestic Animals and Humans. CAB International, England, pp. 7–45.

Stanton TB, Fournie-Amazouz E, Postic D, Trott, DJ. Grimont PAD, Baranton G, Hampson DJ, Saint Girons I. 1997a. Recognition of two new species of intestinal spirochetes: *Serpulina intermedia* sp. nov. and *Serpulina murdochii* sp. nov.. Int J System Bacteriol 47:1007–1012.

Stanton TB, Jensen NS, Bosworth BT, Kunkle RA. 1997b. Evaluation of the virulence of rhea *S. hyodysenteriae* strains for swine. First International Virtual Conference on Infectious Diseases of Animals, USA. http://www.nadc.usda.gov/virtconf/subpost/posters/I00006.htm.

Stanton TB, Jensen NS, Casey TA, Dewhirst FE, Paster BJ. 1991. Reclassification of *Treponema hyodysenteriae* and *Treponema innocens* in a new genus, *Serpula*, gen. nov., as *Serpula hyodysenteriae* comb. nov. and *Serpula innocens* comb. nov. Int J Syst Bacteriol 41:50–58.

Stanton TB, Lebo DF. 1988. *Treponema hyodysenteriae* growth under various culture conditions. Vet Microbiol 18:177–190.

Stanton TB, Rosey EL, Kennedy MJ, Jensen NS, Bosworth BT. 1999. Isolation, oxygen sensitivity, and virulence of NADH oxidase mutants of the anaerobic spirochete *Brachyspira* (*Serpulina*) *hyodysenteriae*, etiologic agent of swine dysentery. Appl Environ Microbiol 65:5028–5034.

Stege H, Jensen TK, Møller K, Baekbo P, Jorsal SE. 2000. Prevalence of intestinal pathogens in Danish finishing pig herds. Prev Vet Med. 46:279–292.

Stephens CP, Hampson DJ. 2001. Intestinal spirochaete infections in chickens: A review of disease associations, epidemiology and control. Anim Health Res Rev 2:101–110.

Suenaga I, Yamazaki T. 1984. Experimental *Treponema hyodysenteriae* infection in mice. Zent Bakt Microbiol Hyg A 257:348–356.

Sueyoshi M, Adachi Y. 1990. Diarrhea induced by *Treponema hyodysenteriae*: A young chick cecal model for swine dysentery. Infect Immun 58:3348–3362.

SVARM. 2004. Swedish Veterinary Antimicrobial Resistance Monitoring. The National Veterinary Institute (SVA), Sweden. ISSN 1650–6332.

Tasker JB, Burrows MR, Kavanagh JB. 2004. Use of aivlosin in feed for treatment and prevention of swine dysentery. In Proc 18th Congr Int Pig Vet Soc, p. 18.

Taylor DJ, Alexander TJL. 1971. The production of dysentery in swine by feeding cultures containing a spirochaete. Br Vet J 127:58–61.

Taylor DJ, Blakemore WF. 1971. Spirochaetal invasion of the colonic epithelium in swine dysentery. Res Vet Sci 12:177–179.

ter Huurne AAHM, Gaastra W. 1995. Swine dysentery: More unknown than known. Vet Microbiol 46:347–360.

ter Huurne AAHM, Muir S, Van Houten M, Van der Zeijst BAM, Gaastra W, Kusters JG. 1994. Characterization of three putative *Serpulina hyodysenteriae* hemolysins. Microbiol Pathogen 16:269–282.

Thomas W, Sellwood R. 1993. Molecular cloning, expression, and DNA sequence analysis of the gene that encodes the 16-kilodalton outer membrane lipoprotein of *Serpulina hyodysenteriae*. Infect Immun 61:1136–1140.

Thomson JR, Smith WJ, Murray BP. 1998. Investigations into field cases of porcine colitis with particular reference to infection with *Serpulina pilosicoli*. Vet Rec 142:235–239.

Thomson JR, Smith WJ, Murray BP, Murray D, Dick JE, Sumption KJ. 2001. Porcine enteric spirochete infections in the UK: Surveillance data and preliminary investigation of atypical isolates. Anim Health Res Rev 2:31–36.

Trott DJ, Alt DP, Zuerner RL, Wannemuehler MJ, Stanton TB. 2001. The search for *Brachyspira* outer membrane proteins that interact with the host. Anim Health Res Rev 2:19–30.

Trott DJ, Oxberry SL, Hampson DJ. 1997. Evidence for *Serpulina hyodysenteriae* being recombinant, with an epidemic population structure. Microbiol 143:3357–3365.

Validation list no. 64. 1998. Int J Syst Bacteriol 48:327–328.

Walker CA, Sumption KJ, Murray BP, Thomson JR. 2002. The *MglB* gene, a possible virulence determinant of porcine *Brachyspira* species. In Proc 17th Congr Int Pig Vet Soc, p. 68.

Walter DH, Kinyon JM. 1990. Recent MIC determination of six antimicrobials for *Treponema hyodysenteriae* in the United States; use of tiamulin to eliminate swine dysentery from two farrow to finish herds. In Proc 11th Congr Int Pig Vet Soc, p. 129.

Waters WR, Hontecillas R, Sacco RE, Zuckermann FA, Harkins KR, Bassaganya-Riera J, Wannemuehler MJ. 2000a. Antigen-specific proliferation of porcine CD8alphaalpha cells to an extracellular bacterial pathogen. Immunology 101:333–341.

Waters WR, Pesch BA, Hontecillas R, Sacco RE, Zuckermann FA, Wannemuehler MJ. 2000b. Cellular immune responses of pigs induced by vaccination with either a whole cell sonicate or pepsin-digested *Brachyspira* (*Serpulina*) *hyodysenteriae* bacterin. Vaccine 18:711–719.

Weber FH, Earley DL. 1991. Novel method for measuring growth of *Treponema hyodysenteriae* and its application for monitoring susceptibility of clinical isolates to antimicrobial agents. Antimicrob Agents Chemother 35:2012–2015.

Whipp SC, Harris DL, Kinyon JM, Songer JG, Glock RD. 1978. Enteropathogenicity testing of *Treponema hyodysenteriae* in ligated colonic loops of swine. Am J Vet Res 39:1293–1296.

Whipp SC, Robinson IM, Harris DL, Glock RD, Mathews PJ, Alexander TJL. 1979. Pathogenic synergism between *Treponema hyodysenteriae* and other selected anaerobes in gnotobiotic pigs. Infect Immun 26:1042–1047.

Wilcock BD, Olander HJ. 1979a. Studies on the pathogenesis of swine dysentery. I. Characterization of the lesions in colons and colonic segments inoculated with pure cultures or colonic content containing *Treponema hyodysenteriae*. Vet Pathol 16:450–465.

———. 1979b. Studies on the pathogenesis of swine dysentery. II. Search for a cytotoxin in spirochetal broth cultures and colon content. Vet Pathol 16:567–573.

Windsor EN, Simmons JR. 1981. Investigation into the spread of swine dysentery in 25 herds of East Anglia and assessment of its significance in five herds. Vet Rec 122:482–484.

Wood EN, Lysons RJ. 1988. The financial benefit from the eradication of swine dysentery. Vet Rec 121:277–279.

Zuerner RL, Stanton TB. 1994. Physical and genetic map of the *Serpulina hyodysenteriae* B78 chromosome. J Bacteriol 176:1087–1092.

Zuerner RL, Stanton TB, Minion FC, Li C, Charon NW, Trott DJ, Hampson DJ. 2004. Genetic variation in *Brachyspira*: Chromosomal rearrangements and sequence drift distinguish *B. pilosicoli* from *B. hyodysenteriae*. Anaerobe 10:229–237.

49 Tuberculosis

Charles O. Thoen

Tuberculosis continues to cause significant economic losses to swine producers throughout the world. Although tuberculosis due to *Mycobacterium bovis* has been nearly eradicated in many developed countries, lesions continue to be reported in the cervical and mesenteric lymph nodes of swine during meat inspection. Available information indicates that 30–50% of the carcasses of slaughter swine from some large confined herds have granulomatous lesions from which *M. avium* complex serovars were isolated (Pritchard et al. 1977). The processing of tuberculous swine carcasses is costly and results in significant economic losses. Regulations of the Meat and Poultry Inspection Program of the USDA require that unaffected portions of swine carcasses with tuberculous lesions in more than one primary site, such as cervical and mesenteric lymph nodes, be cooked at 170°F (76.7°C) for 30 minutes before being approved for human food (National Archives and Records Services 1973). The value of a cooked carcass is only about 20–25% of the value of a carcass not cooked. In processing plants where facilities are not available for cooking, the carcass is condemned and there is no salvage value. The public health significance of *Mycobacterium avium* complex infections has been recognized. Of special interest are reports on the isolation of some of the same serovars of *M. avium* complex from patients with acquired immune deficiency syndrome and from swine (Chin et al. 1994; Komijn et al. 1999).

There has been no direct campaign to eradicate tuberculosis in swine. It was once believed that the campaign to eradicate bovine tuberculosis, which was started in 1917, would result in a reduction of the disease in swine in the United States. However, the percentage of swine with tuberculous lesions continued to increase for a number of years (Table 49.1).

ETIOLOGY

Swine are susceptible to infection with *M. avium* complex, *Mycobacterium tuberculosisc* complex, and *M. bovis*.

M. avium complex serovars 1, 2, 4, and 8 are the most common isolates from tuberculous lesions in swine in the United States (Mitchell et al. 1975; Thoen et al. 1975). At least 15 other *M. avium* complex serovars have been isolated from swine in the United States (Thoen et al. 1975) as well as in other countries: Australia (Tammemagi and Simmons 1971), Brazil (Pestana de Castro et al. 1978), Denmark (Jorgensen 1978), France, Germany (Meissner et al. 1978), Hungary (Szabo et al. 1975), Japan (Nishimori et al. 1995; Yugi et al. 1972), South Africa (Kleeberg and Nel 1973), and the Czech Republic (Matlova et al. 2004). These reports indicate the worldwide distribution of tuberculosis in swine due to *M. avium* complex. The similarity of *M. avium* and so-called *M. intracellulare* has led to the proposal that the latter be considered serovars of *M. avium* complex (*M. avium ss aviium–M. avium ss intracellulare*) (Wolinsky and Schaefer 1973; Thoen et al. 1984); this has been done in this chapter.

Molecular techniques including restriction fragment length polymorphism (RFLP) and serotyping have been shown to be reliable for identifying *M. avium* complex isolated from swine (Thorensen and Saxegaard 1993; Ritacco et al. 1998; Komijn et al. 1999; Pavlik et al. 2000). *Mycobacterium avium* complex (serovars 1, 2, and 3) occur mainly in birds but also in swine and humans, whereas serovars 4–6 and 8–11 are found in swine and humans. Molecular evidence supports a proposal to refer to human/porcine type of *M. avium* as *M. avium ss hominus-suis* (Mijs et al. 2002).

The decrease in prevalence of tuberculosis in swine in the United States is largely attributable to a lowering of the incidence of tuberculosis in poultry, which in turn is the result of the increasing practice of maintaining all-pullet flocks of chickens (Table 49.1). The control of tuberculosis in swine is thus incidental to and a beneficial but secondary effect of a changing practice of poultry husbandry. However, tuberculosis has been observed in large confined swine herds, in which the infection is caused by *M. avium* complex serovars 4, 6, and 8.

Table 49.1. Prevalence of tuberculosis in swine in the United States as determined by inspection in abattoirs under federal supervision

Year	Number Slaughtered	Percent Tuberculosis[a]	Percent Condemned[b]
1912	34,966,378	4.69	0.12
1917	40,210,847	9.89	0.19
1922	34,416,439	16.38	0.20
1927	42,650,443	13.54	0.14
1932	45,852,422	11.38	0.08
1937	36,226,309	9.48	0.08
1942	50,133,871	7.96	0.026
1947	47,073,370	8.50	0.023
1952	63,823,263	4.40	0.015
1956	66,781,940	4.76	0.010
1962	67,109,539	2.25	0.008
1968	72,325,507	1.35	0.005
1972	83,126,396	0.85	0.007
1978	71,805,911	0.75	0.006
1983	79,992,743	0.41	0.003
1989	82,110,688	0.67	0.002
1995	94,490,329	0.21	0.003

Sources: Data compiled from USDA 1922, 1973, 1979, 1984, 1990, 1996; Feldman 1963.

[a]Includes all carcasses with evidence of tuberculosis, varying in extent from only small foci in cervical lymph nodes to generalized involvement.

[b]Includes carcasses with evidence of generalized tuberculosis.

The problem has been associated with the use of sawdust and peat for litter contaminated with *M. avium* complex (Dalchow and Nassal 1979; Songer et al. 1980; Pavlick 2000).

EPIDEMIOLOGY

Because swine are not routinely tested with tuberculin, the only sources of information on the prevalence and geographic distribution of tuberculosis in this species are the data obtained from meat inspection records. On this basis an increase in the rate of infection occurred in the United States until 1922 (Table 49.1). During 1922, 16.38% of all swine slaughtered under federal supervision had tuberculous lesions; in 0.2%, the disease was so extensive that the entire carcass was condemned. Since 1922, there has been a gradual decline; by 1995, the prevalence had decreased to 0.21%, with only 0.003% having evidence of generalized tuberculous disease.

Data on the prevalence of tuberculosis in swine from meat inspection records may be misleading because the diagnoses are made on the basis of the macroscopic appearance of lesions (Figure 49.1). A certain number of tuberculous infections will escape detection because the lesions are not grossly visible. Avian tubercle bacilli have been isolated from tonsils (Feldman and Karlson 1940) and lymph nodes of apparently normal swine (Langenegger and Langenegger 1981).

In studies in the United States and Canada, where presumably tuberculous lymph nodes of swine were col-

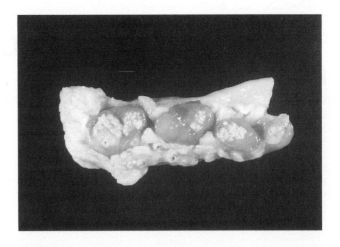

49.1. *Tuberculous lesions in a mesenteric lymph node of a pig at slaughter (Thoen 1994).*

lected at abattoirs and examined bacteriologically, a varying percentage failed to yield tubercle bacilli (Table 49.2). Similar observations have been made by workers in Australia (Clapp 1956), Denmark (Plum 1946; Jorgensen et al. 1972), England (Cochin 1943), Finland (Vasenius 1965), France (LaFont and LaFont 1968), and Germany (Retzlaff 1966; Dalchow and Nassal 1979). The failure to demonstrate tubercle bacilli in lesions that appear grossly to be tuberculous may be due to inadequacy in present-day methods for isolating tubercle bacilli, occurrence of healed processes that contain no viable tubercle bacilli, or cause of the lesions by some microorganism other than tubercle bacilli, such as *Rhodococcus equi* or *R. sputi* (to be discussed later).

Sources of Infection and Their Control

Swine are susceptible to infection with serovars of *M. avium* complex, *M. tuberculosis*, and *M. bovis*. The occurrence of tuberculosis in swine, therefore, is in part related to the opportunity for direct or indirect contact with tuberculous cattle, humans, and fowl or the organism in the environment.

Mycobacterium bovis is not a frequent cause of tuberculosis in swine in localities where the disease in cattle is controlled by a campaign of eradication. In the United States and Canada, for example, *M. bovis* is rarely found in lesions of swine (Table 49.2). In Great Britain during 1952–1955, the bovine type of tuberculosis in swine gradually declined concurrently with the eradication of the disease in cattle. The percentage of avian-type infection increased from 44% during the first 5 years of the study to 92% for the last 5 years (Lesslie et al. 1968). However, the occasional finding of *M. bovis* in swine is a reminder that the disease in cattle is a constant threat. Efforts to eradicate bovine tuberculosis should not be diminished.

Where tuberculosis does occur in cattle, the infection may be transmitted to swine by the feeding of un-

Table 49.2. Summary of data compiled from reports in North America on the occurrence of tubercle bacilli in tuberculous lymph nodes of swine

Reference	Date[a]	Origin of Swine	Specimens	Avian Only	Mammalian Only	Mixed	None[b]
Van Es	1925b	Nebraska	248	74.6	4.4	5.6	15.4
Van Es and Martin	1925b	Michigan	14	92.9	None	7.1	None
Mitchell et al.	1934b	Canada	96	38.5	None	None	61.5
Feldman	1938b	Southeastern Minnesota	30[c]	80.0	6.6 (bovine)	None	13.3
Feldman	1939b	Minnesota	75[d]	46.6	16.0 (human)	None	37.3
Feldman and Karlson	1940b	Minnesota	89	61.8	None	None	38.2
Pullin	1946b	Eastern Canada	232	44.8	0.9 (bovine)	None	54.3
Bankier	1946b	Alberta, Canada	102	88.0	1.0 (bovine)	None	11.0
Karlson and Thoen	1971b	Minnesota	36	72.0	None	None	28.0
Thoen et al.	1975b	United States	2036	76.0	<1.0	<1.0	22.0
Pritchard et al.	1977b	Idaho	31	80.0	None	None	None
Cole et al.	1978b	Georgia	112	53.6	None	None	46.4
Margolis et al.	1994b	Pennsylvania	125	70	None	None	26

Note: Specimens obtained from abattoirs under federal supervision.
[a]Several papers indicated that the work was done from 1 to 2 years before publication.
[b]Tubercle bacilli not demonstrated by cultural or animal inoculation tests.
[c]Selected cases of generalized tuberculosis; some of the specimens were portions of lung, liver, or spleen.
[d]Garbage-fed swine.

pasteurized milk and dairy by-products. Feces of tuberculous cattle may contain viable tubercle bacilli; this provides an obvious hazard where swine and cattle are maintained in a common feedlot.

The practice of feeding swine the offal from abattoirs or uncooked garbage is obviously unwise, because such material may contain tuberculous material from beef carcasses. Fichandler and Osborne (1966) described an epizootic of tuberculosis in a herd of swine in Connecticut that was fed improperly cooked offal from tuberculous cattle. A serious outbreak of avian tuberculosis in a swine-feeding establishment in Denmark was traced to the improper cooking of offal from poultry plants (Biering-Sorensen 1959). *Mycobacterium tuberculosis* is occasionally isolated from tuberculous lesions in swine. No person known to have active tuberculosis should be permitted to have contact with swine or other animals.

Uncooked garbage is a potential means of transmitting tuberculosis to swine. Feldman (1939) recorded that 75 (28.4%) of 264 garbage-fed swine were found to have tuberculous lesions at the time of slaughter. Of these, 47 contained tubercle bacilli, of which 35 were avian type and 12 were human type. It was concluded that garbage may contain the offal of tuberculous chickens and that material from tuberculous human patients is not properly disposed of. The frequent occurrence of *M. avium* complex in lesions limited to the cervical and mesenteric lymph nodes in naturally infected swine indicates that infection usually occurs by ingestion. Janetschke (1963) found that the primary complex involved the alimentary tract in 97.3% of 1000 carcasses with tuberculous lesions; a pulmonary route of infection was noted in only 2.7%, as indicated by involvement of the bronchial lymph nodes.

Schalk et al. (1935) found that swine contracted tuberculosis when placed on ground that had not been occupied by tuberculous chickens for the previous 2 years. Viable and pathogenic avian tubercle bacilli were found in the soil and litter of a chicken cage after 4 years. Schalk and coworkers concluded that soil contaminated by feces of tuberculous fowl is the most important source of infection for swine. No success was obtained in controlling the disease merely by use of the tuberculin test and elimination of reactors, because the soil remained contaminated. They recommended that an ideal program to control avian tuberculosis is to rear young birds on clean ground and to dispose regularly of all fowl more than 1 year old.

Schliesser and Weber (1973) studied the survival of *M. avium* complex in sawdust. At 18–22°C, the survival time of two virulent strains was 153–160 days, and the survival time of two avirulent strains was 169–214 days. The survival times were greatly reduced when the contaminated sawdust was maintained at 37°C.

Wild birds may be incriminated as a source of *M. avium* infections in swine. Tuberculosis was found in starlings on a farm with a high incidence of tuberculosis in the swine but where no poultry had been kept for 8 years (Bickford et al. 1966). Tuberculosis due to *M. avium* has been found in various wild birds, some of which frequent feedlots (Thoen 1997).

The close contact of sows and slaughter pigs in yards and feeding pens provides opportunity for transmission of tuberculosis from animal to animal (Alfredsen and Skjerve 1993). The occurrence of intestinal lesions (Figure 49.2) allows spread of tubercle bacilli in feces. Feldman and Karlson (1940) and Pullar and Rushford (1954) demonstrated avian tubercle bacilli in the tonsils

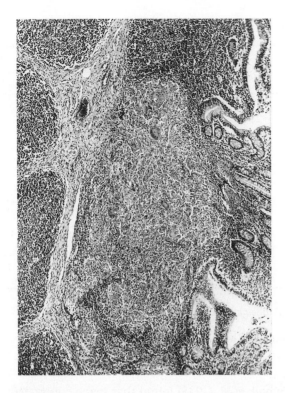

49.2. *Submucosal tuberculous lesion due to avian tubercle bacilli in the intestinal tract of the pig. The lesion appears to be extending toward the surface, where it may ulcerate and discharge bacilli into the lumen. Diffuse cellular proliferation with little necrosis is typical of avian tubercle bacillus infection in swine (H&E; ×50).*

of pigs. The latter workers suggested that this may be a source of infection for other animals. Smith (1958) found *M. aviam* in apparently normal lymph nodes of 7% of swine, 5% of sheep, and 5% of cattle but was unable to find them in adult normal chickens; he suggested, therefore, that domestic mammals may contract *M. avium* from each other as well as from tuberculous fowl.

Pulmonary, uterine, and mammary tuberculous lesions in swine constitute sources of infection for other animals. Jorgensen et al. (1972) described an enzootic of pulmonary tuberculosis resulting from *M. avium* in pigs. Lesslie and Birn (1967) found *M. avium* in the udder or milk of 18 cows and concluded that such animals may be a source of *M. avium* in pigs. Bille and Larsen (1973) reported congenital infection in swine caused by *M. avium*, suggesting that infected pregnant sows may have a role in the transmission of this infection. Sigurdardottir et al. (1994) reported granulomatous enteritis due to *M. avium* in a pig.

Where sawdust is used for bedding, serovars 4 and 8 of *M. avium* complex have been isolated from lesions in swine as well as from the sawdust. Reactions to avian and bovine tuberculin have been reported in boars exposed to sawdust from which *M. avium* or other nonphotochromogenic mycobacteria were isolated (Fodstad 1977). Schliesser and Weber (1973) found that *M. avium* would

survive as long as 214 days in sawdust. In Hungary, Szabo et al. (1975) found that the incidence of tuberculous adenitis in swine was greater when sawdust was used as litter; when the use of sawdust was discontinued, the occurrence of such lesions decreased significantly. Dalchow and Nassal (1979) recorded that the same serovars of *M. avium* complex as found in swine could be isolated from sawdust. These workers also reported that sawdust could contain infectious mycobacteria even after 4 years of storage. Songer et al. (1980) investigated herds of swine in Arizona and found in at least one herd that the source was sawdust and wood shavings.

Investigations conducted in the Czech Republic and Slovakia indicate that *M. avium* complex serotype 8 may be spread by adult flies (Fischer et al. 2001).

PATHOGENESIS

The development of disease in swine depends on the ability of the tubercle bacillus to multiply within tissues of the host and to induce a host response. Although acid-fast bacilli initially encounter granulocytes and humoral components, activated mononuclear macrophages are considered to be more important in protection of the host against mycobacteria.

The capacity of *M. avium* to produce progressive disease may be related to certain complex lipids present in the cell wall, such as the glycopeptidolipids (previously referred to as C-mycosides) localized in the exterior portion of the cell envelope (Rastogi and Barrow 1994). However, it appears that the effect of these components alone or together on phagolysosome fusion cannot account for virulence. Available information suggests that a combination of toxic lipids and factors released by virulent tubercle bacilli may cause disruption of the phagosome, interfere with phagolysosome formation, alter the release of hydrolytic enzymes from the attached lysosomes, and/or inactivate the lysosomal enzymes released into the cytoplasmic vacuole (Thoen and Bloom 1995). Certain serovars of *M. avium* are susceptible to bactericidal mechanisms of macrophages; however, the importance of reactive nitrogen intermediates and oxygen radicals in macrophages of swine exposed to virulent tubercle bacilli remains to be elucidated (Thoen and Barletta 2004). Although the mechanisms by which mycobacteria produce disease in swine have not been clearly defined, experimental studies in piglets revealed that nonspecific esterase activity was elevated in mononuclear macrophages of lymph nodes 7 days following inoculation of *M. avium* complex serovar 8 (Momotani et al. 1980). Granulomas of varying stages were observed in mesenteric and mandibular lymph nodes and intestinal mucosa at 14 days postinoculation. In other investigations, sensitized lymphocytes and detectable mycobacterial antibodies have been reported to occur at 14–28 days post exposure to *M. avium* or *M. bovis* (Muscoplat et al. 1975; Thoen et al. 1979a).

LESIONS

Tubercle Bacilli

Detailed discussions of the pathological anatomy of tuberculosis in swine may be found in Pallaske (1931), Feldman (1938a), Francis (1958), and Kramer (1962). As seen in the abattoirs, tuberculous lesions in swine are usually limited to lymph nodes of the cervical and the mesenteric regions. The lesions vary in appearance from small, yellowish white, caseous foci a few millimeters in diameter to diffuse enlargement of the entire node (Figure 49.1). The disease may be localized in one group of nodes or may involve a number of lymph nodes along the digestive tract.

Gross differentiation between tuberculous adenitis caused by avian tubercle bacilli and that caused by mammalian tubercle bacilli is difficult, but in general, some features are characteristic of each. In an infection of avian origin the lymph nodes may be enlarged and firm with no discrete purulent foci, or there may be one or more soft caseous areas with indistinct borders. Calcification is seldom demonstrable. The cut surface of the lesion has a neoplastic appearance with a few caseous foci. Although there may be diffuse fibrosis, there is little tendency to encapsulation. Relatively large areas of caseation may be present and occasionally will involve the entire lymph node. The lesions due to tubercle bacilli of the avian type are generally not easily enucleated. In contrast, when the infection is due to *M. bovis* or *M. tuberculosis* the lesions tend to be well encapsulated and are relatively easy to separate from the surrounding tissue. In addition, calcification is usually prominent in lesions. The individual foci appear to be discrete and caseous. These distinctions are by no means absolute, and there are many variations in the gross appearance of tuberculous lesions in lymph nodes of swine.

Clapp (1956) examined, by bacteriological procedures, 420 lymph nodes (mostly submaxillary) designated as tuberculous upon meat inspection. There was some association between the gross appearance and the cause. Localized lesions that were not easily enucleated and large, dry calcareous processes involving an entire lymph node were usually due to *M. avium*. Indistinctly mottled and streaked lesions, large encapsulated purulent abscesses, and lesions that could be easily enucleated were usually not caused by tubercle bacilli. Some of these yielded *Corynebacterium equi*, now reclassified as *Rhodococcus equi* (Goodfellow et al. 1982), which Clapp considered important in producing tuberculosis-like lymphadenitis in swine. In the series of 420 specimens, only 5 were from swine with generalized tuberculosis, and all of these were associated with *M. bovis and M. avium*. Microscopically, the changes induced in swine tissues are characterized by diffuse proliferation of epithelioid cells and giant cells. There may be some necrosis and calcification, especially in older lesions, but cal-

cification is not usually prominent. Similar changes are observed in sows and slaughter pigs (Thoen et al. 1976b). Proliferation of connective-tissue elements accompanies the process. Lesions caused by mammalian tubercle bacilli have a tendency to become encapsulated by a well-developed zone of connective tissue (Figure 49.3). In addition, there is often early caseation and marked calcification (Karlson and Thoen 1971). However, consistent histopathological differentiation between lesions caused by mammalian and avian tubercle bacilli is not possible (Himes et al. 1983).

Generalized tuberculosis in swine is not commonly seen. In most instances it is from infection with *M. bovis,* but it may also result from the *M. avium* (Feldman 1938b; Jorgensen et al. 1972). The extent and character of generalized involvement vary from the occurrence of a few small foci in several organs to extensive nodular processes involving the liver, spleen, lungs, kidneys, and many lymph nodes. Generalized lesions from infection with *M. avium* tend to be diffuse. The cut surface is usually smooth, and there is no great tendency toward encapsulation by fibrosis. There may be foci of caseation, but calcification is not pronounced. Lesions resulting from infection with mammalian tubercle bacilli, however, are likely to be discrete, caseous, and well circumscribed by fibrosis. Calcification is prominent.

Bacteria Other than Tubercle Bacilli

Various species of mycobacteria other than tubercle bacilli have been isolated from swine and other animals in different countries, but reports of such are few and usually concern only sporadic cases (Schliesser 1976). The significance of finding *M. kansasii, M. xenopi,* or *M. fortuitum* is not clear. It may be important, however, to learn if animals and humans become infected from the same sources (Thoen and Williams 1994). Of potential importance is the recovery of *M. chelonei* from swine because this bacterium has been isolated from prosthetic heart valves that were prepared from swine (Thoen and Himes 1977).

In Norway, *M. avium paratuberculosis* was isolated by culture from lesions in the mesenteric lymph nodes of swine as well as from normal swine that were closely associated with a herd of cattle in which Johne's disease was present (Ringdal 1963). This microorganism was isolated in the United States from a slaughter pig (Thoen et al. 1975b). Jorgensen (1969) and Larsen et al. (1971) found that swine may be infected with *M. avium ss paratuberculosis* after oral administration of the organism. *M. xenopi* was isolated from tissues of slaughtered swine that originated in the southeastern region of the United States (Jarnagin et al. 1971). Another rare finding was the isolation of *M. microti,* from lymph nodes of three swine (Huitema and Jaartsveld 1967).

Mention must be made of the occurrence of *R. equi* in localized lesions that cannot be easily differentiated from tuberculous processes either macroscopically or

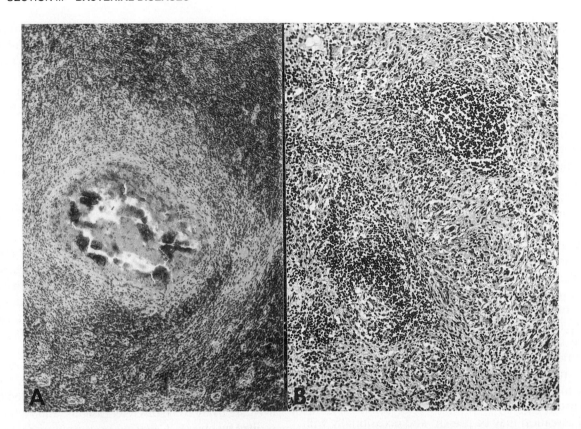

49.3. *Tuberculous changes in cervical lymph nodes of swine. (A) Mammalian tubercle bacillus infection. Peripheral fibrosis, necrosis, and calcification are typical of lesions due to bovine or human types of tubercle bacilli (H&E; ×40). (B) M. avium infection. Diffuse cellular proliferation with little necrosis (H&E; ×95).*

histologically (Feldman et al. 1940). Holth and Amundsen (1936) in Norway reported that of 162 tuberculous lymph nodes from swine, only 103 yielded tubercle bacilli (97 were typed, with 80 avian and 16 human strains and 1 bovine strain). Of the other 59, 38 contained a variably acid-fast "coccobacillus." The acid-fastness, however, was not constant and was lost on subculture. The presence of this microorganism in localized tuberculosis-like lesions in swine was soon confirmed by other Scandinavian workers. Ottosen (1945) has shown that *R. equi* occurs more frequently in the soil of hog pens than elsewhere. In Denmark, Plum (1946) studied a large number of tuberculous lymph nodes from swine and concluded that it is difficult for inspectors in abattoirs to differentiate between tuberculosis and *R. equi* infection. Barton and Hughes (1980) recorded 32 reports of *R. equi* infection in swine. *R. equi* expressing a 20 kDa antigen has been observed in all pig isolates, and 2 of 5 plasmids from pig isolates were the same as those from human isolates, suggesting that the source of infection for humans may be pigs or the pig environment (Takai et al. 1996).

Rhodococcus sputi has been isolated from tuberculosis lesions in the mesenteric lymph nodes of swine (Tsukamura et al. 1988).

DIAGNOSIS

A clinical diagnosis of tuberculosis in swine is presumptive at best. Generally, the tuberculous lesions are limited to small foci in a few lymph nodes of the digestive tract. It is difficult to conceive that such nonprogressive morbid changes may elicit signs detectable by physical examination. In extensive tuberculous infection, signs may be suggestive of an infectious disease, but the symptoms and changes are not sufficiently characteristic to establish a diagnosis of tuberculosis.

The necropsy and histopathological appearance of tuberculosis in swine has been described. Although the morbid changes are sufficiently characteristic to permit a tentative diagnosis of tuberculosis, they are not specific. The great similarity between localized tuberculous lesions and those associated with *R. equi* and other bacteria has already been discussed. Also, chronic granulomatous lesions may be difficult to differentiate grossly because of parasitic nodules and neoplasms.

Enzyme-linked immunosorbent assay (ELISA) has been described for detecting antibodies in swine infected with *M. avium* complex (Thoen et al. 1979a, b). Positive ELISA reactions were observed in pigs experimentally infected and in those naturally infected. The

ELISA is a rapid test that can be automated and may be of value in testing replacement breeding animals.

The mere demonstration of acid-fast bacilli in exudates or in lesions may be misleading. Some workers have recorded that *R. equi* is acid-fast in smears of necrotic material from lymph nodes of swine (Ottosen 1945). Acid-fast microorganisms other than tubercle bacilli have been isolated from swine (Karlson and Feldman 1940; Brandes 1961).

The characteristic pathological features of tuberculosis in swine and the presence of acid-fast microorganisms in such lesions provide important indications on which to base a diagnosis of tuberculosis. However, an unequivocal diagnosis can be made on the basis of bacteriological procedures designed for the isolation, identification by biochemical and seroagglutination tests, and/or by molecular techniques (Kaneene and Thoen 2004).

Tuberculin Test

The tuberculin test for the diagnosis of tuberculosis in swine appears to be a useful procedure on a herd basis. Of the various techniques described for this test in swine, the operator should select the method that proves by experience to be most suitable. Separate simultaneous tests with *M. avium* and *M. bovis* tuberculin must be made (Thoen and Karlson 1970). A number of investigators have found that some tuberculous swine may fail to react to the intradermal tuberculin test. Therefore, tests should be repeated in a herd in which animals with positive reactions have been found and excluded.

The intradermal test, usually on the ear or vulva, may be employed. Because swine are susceptible to infection with *M. tuberculosis* complex and *M. avium* complex, avian and mammalian tuberculin should be used. Fichandler and Osborne (1966) described an extensive outbreak of *M. bovis* in swine in which animals reacted to mammalian tuberculin by developing erythema and swelling of the ear, compared with slight reactions to the *M. aviam* tuberculin.

Feldman (1938a) recommended the use of 0.2 mL 25% Old Tuberculin applied into the dermis on the dorsal surface of the ear, slightly anterior to the base. A positive reaction is indicated in 24 hours by a flat, reddish swelling up to 3 cm in diameter, which in 48 hours reaches its maximal intensity. At this time the erythema and swelling are more pronounced; the central area becomes hemorrhagic, and ulceration may occur. McDiarmid (1956) described a means of testing swine in which restraint is not necessary. While the animals are feeding from a trough, 0.1 mL tuberculin is injected at a right angle into the skin at the junction of the ear and neck using a needle only 3.5 mm long. With this short needle, most of the tuberculin is deposited in the skin. Reactions are recorded in 48 hours. A positive reaction varies from "puffy" edema to inflammation, with purple discoloration and necrosis. McDiarmid used

Weybridge purified protein derivative (PPD), which, according to Paterson (1949), has 3 mg protein/mL for mammalian tuberculin and 0.8 mg protein/mL for *M. aviam*.

Lanz (1955) recommended injecting the tuberculin in the skin of the back about 10–20 cm caudal to the shoulders and slightly to the right of the midline. This was easier and less time-consuming than trying to use the ear. A dose of 0.1 mL PPD (as used for cattle in Switzerland) is injected intradermally. A positive reaction reaches its peak in 72 hours and consists of a painful erythematous swelling 22–35 mm in diameter. As determined by necropsy, no false-negative or atypical reactions were found among 316 animals.

Lesslie et al. (1968), using Weybridge PPD, tested 84 White pigs from a herd known to have tuberculosis. The avian tuberculin was given in injections of 0.1 mL, each containing 2500 tuberculin units (TU); and the mammalian tuberculin was given in injections of 0.1 mL, each containing 10,000 TU. The injections were made simultaneously, each at the base on an ear; in 48–72 hours a positive reaction was recorded when the reaction consisted of edema and erythema. Guinea pigs experimentally sensitized with *M. avium* serovars 3, 4, 5, 6, 8, and 9 each reacted similarly to tuberculin prepared from serovars 2 and 7 (Anz et al. 1970). Swine experimentally infected with *M. avium* serovars 4 and 8 reacted well to the USDA avian Old Tuberculin and to PPD prepared from *M. avium* serovar 1 (Thoen et al. 1976a; Thoen et al. 1979b).

At present, intradermal injection of PPD tuberculin in the dorsal surface of the ear is the recommended procedure for applying the tuberculin test in swine. The injection site should be observed at 48 hours.

PREVENTION

The eradication of tuberculosis in swine, as well as in other species, is dependent on the availability of an economical and specific means of detecting infected animals. Additional information is needed to determine adequate measures for cleaning and disinfecting the premises where *M. avium* complex persists in the soil, in buildings, or on equipment. Also, we need to know how long these organisms will remain viable in the environment. Investigations also should be made to determine the sources and modes of transmission of the different serovars of *M. avium* complex.

REFERENCES

Alfredsen S, Skjerve E. 1993. An abattoir-based case-control study of risk factors for mycobacteriosis in Norwegian swine. Prev Vet Med 15:253–259.

Anz W, Lauterback D, Meissner G, Willers I. 1970. Vergleich von Sensitin-Testen an Meerschweinchen mit Serotyp und Huhnervirulenz bei *M. avium-* and *M. intracellulare-Stammen.* Zentralbl Bakteriol (Orig A) 215:536–549.

Bankier JC. 1946. Tuberculous lesions of swine. II. Survey of lesions found in the prairie provinces, especially in Alberta. Can J Comp Med 10:250–253.

Barton MD, Hughes KL. 1980. *Corynebacterium equi*: A review. Vet Bull 50:65–80.

Bickford AA, Ellis GH, Moses HE. 1966. Epizootiology of tuberculosis in starlings. J Am Vet Med Assoc 149:312–318.

Biering-Sorensen, U. 1959. Ophobning af tilfaelde af aviaer tuberkulose I en svinebesaetning. Medd Dan Dyrlaegeforen 42:550–552.

Bille, N, Larsen JL. 1973. Porcine congenital infection due to *Mycobacterium tuberculosis typus avium*: Report of a case. Nord Vet Med 25:139–143.

Brandes T. 1961. Zur makroskopischen Unterscheidung zwischen tuberkulosen und tuberkuloseahnlichen Veranderungen in den Mesenterial-lymphoknoten des Schweines. Arch Lebensmittelhyg 12:53–56.

Chin DP, Hopwell PC, Yajko DM, Vittinghoff E, Horsburgh CR, Hadley WK, Stone EN, Nassos PS, Ostroff SM, Jacobson MA, Matkin CC, Reingold AL. 1994. *Mycobacterium avium* complex in the respiratory or gastrointestinal tract and the risk of *M. avium* complex bacterium in patients with human immunodeficiency virus infection. J Infect Dis 169:289–295.

Clapp KH. 1956. Tuberculosis-like lesions in swine in South Australia. Aust Vet J 32:110–113.

Cochin E. 1943. Tubercle bacilli in lesions of the submaxillary lymph nodes of swine. J Comp Pathol 53:310–314.

Cole JR, Sangster LT, Thoen CO, Pursell AR, Williams DJ, DuBois PR, McDaniel HT. 1978. Mycobacteriosis in a Georgia swine herd. In Proc 21st Meet Am Assoc Vet Lab Diagn, pp. 195–208.

Dalchow W, Nassal J. 1979. Mykobakteriose beim Schwein durch Sagemehleinstreu. Tierärztl Umsch 34:253–261.

Dvorska L, Bartos M, Ostadal O, Kaustova J, Matlova L, Pavlik I. 2002. IS1311 and IS1245 Restriction fragment length polymorphism analyses, serotypes, and drug susceptibilities of *Mycobacterium avium* complex isolates obtained from a human immunodeficiency virus-negative patient. Jour Clin Microbiol 40(10):3712–3719.

Feldman WH. 1938a. Avian Tuberculosis Infections. Baltimore: Williams & Wilkins.

——. 1938b. Generalized tuberculosis of swine due to avian tubercle bacilli. J Am Vet Med Assoc 92:681–685.

——. 1939. Types of tubercle bacilli in lesions of garbage-fed swine. Am J Public Health 29:1231–1238.

——. 1963. Tuberculosis. In Diseases Transmitted from Animals to Man, 5th ed. TG Hull, ed. Springfield, Ill.: Charles C. Thomas, p. 5.

Feldman WH, Karlson AG. 1940. Avian tubercle bacilli in tonsils of swine. J Am Vet Med Assoc 96:146–149.

Feldman WH, Moses HE, Karlson AG. 1940. *Corynebacterium equi* as a possible cause of tuberculosis-like lesions of swine. Cornell Vet 30:465–481.

Fichandler PD, Osborne AD. 1966. Bovine tuberculosis in swine. J Am Vet Med Assoc 148:167–169.

Fischer O, Matlova L, Dvorska L, Svastova P, Bartl J, Melicharek I, Weston RT, Pavlik I. 2001. Diptera as vectors of mycobacterial infections in cattle and pigs. Med Vet Entomol 15(2):208.

Fodstad FH. 1977. Tuberculin reactions in bulls and boars sensitized with atypical mycobacteria from sawdust. Acta Vet Scand 18:374–383.

Francis J. 1958. Tuberculosis in Animals and Man: A Study in Comparative Pathology. London: Cassell, p. 177.

Goodfellow M, Beckham AR, Feldman WH, Barton MD. 1982. Numerical classification of *Rhodococcus equi*. J Appl Bacteriol 53:199–207.

Himes EM, Miller LD, Thoen CO. 1983. Swine tuberculosis: Histologic similarities of lesions from which *Mycobacterium tuberculosis*, *M. avium* complex or *M. bovis* was identified. In Proc 26th Meet Am Assoc Vet Lab Diagn, pp. 63–76.

Holth H, Amundsen H. 1936. Fortsattle undersokelser over baciltypene ved tuberkulose hos svinet pa Ostlandet. Nor Vet Tidsskr 48:2–17.

Huitema H, Jaartsveld FHJ. 1967. *Mycobacterium microti* infection in a cat and some pigs. Antonie van Leeuwenhoek 33:209–212.

Janetschke P. 1963. Über die tuberkulose beim Schwein. Monatsschr Veterinärmed 18:860–864.

Jarnagin JL, Richards WD, Muhm RL, Ellis EM. 1971. The isolation of *Mycobacterium xenopi* from granulomatous lesions in swine. Am Rev Respir Dis 104:763–765.

Jorgensen JB. 1969. Paratuberculosis in pigs: Experimental infection by oral administration of *Mycobacterium paratuberculosis*. Acta Vet Scand 10:275–287.

——. 1978. Serological investigation of strains of *Mycobacterium avium* and *Mycobacterium intracellulare* isolated in animal and non-animal sources. Nord Vet Med 30:155–162.

Jorgensen JB, Haarbo K, Dam A, Engbaek HC. 1972. An enzootic of pulmonary tuberculosis in pigs caused by *M. avium*. I. Epidemiological and pathological studies. Acta Vet Scand 13:56–57.

Kaneene JB, Thoen CO. 2004. Tuberculosis. Jour Amer Vet Med Assoc 224(5):685–691.

Karlson AG, Feldman WH. 1940. Studies on an acid-fast bacterium frequently present in tonsillar tissue of swine. J Bacteriol 39:461–472.

Karlson AG, Thoen CO. 1971. *Mycobacterium avium* in tuberculous adenitis of swine. Am J Vet Res 32:1257–1261.

Kleeberg HH, Nel EE. 1973. Occurrence of environmental atypical mycobacteria in South Africa. Ann Soc Belg Med Trop 53:405–417.

Komijn RE, de Haas PEW, Schneider MME, Eger T, Nieuwenhuijs JHM, van den Hoek RJ, Bakker D, van Zijd Erveld FG, van Soolingen D. 1999. Prevalence of *Mycobacterium avium* in slaughter pigs in The Netherlands and comparison of IS1245 restriction fragment length polymorphism patterns of porcine and human isolates. Jour Clin Microbiol 37(5):1254–1259.

Kramer H. 1962. Zur Beurteilung tuberkuloseahnalicher Veranderungen in den Gekroslymphknoten des Schweines unter besonderer Beruchsichigung der bakterioskopisher Prufung. Arch Lebensmittelhyg 13:264–271.

LaFont P, LaFont J. 1968. Étude microbiologique des adenites cervicales du porc. II. Adenites a mycobacteries atypiques. Rec Méd Vét 144:611–630.

Langenegger CH, Langenegger J. 1981. Prevalence and distribution of serotypes of mycobacteria of the MAIS-complex isolated from pigs in Brazil. Pesqui Vet Bras 1:75–80.

Lanz E. 1955. Über die Tuberkulose und die intrakutane Tuberkulinisierung beim Schwein. Schweiz Arch Tierheilkd 97:229–245.

Larsen AB, Moon HW, Merkal RS. 1971. Susceptibility of swine to *Mycobacterium paratuberculosis*. Am J Vet Res 32:589–595.

Lesslie IW, Birn KJ. 1967. Tuberculosis in cattle caused by the avian type tubercle bacillus. Vet Rec 80:559–564.

Lesslie IW, Birn KJ, Stuart P, O'Neill PAF, Smith J. 1968. Tuberculosis in the pig and the tuberculin test. Vet Rec 83:647–651.

Margolis MJ, Hutchinson LJ, Kephart KB, Hattel AL, Whitlock RH, Payeur JB. 1994. Results of using histologic examination and acid-fast staining to confirm a diagnosis of swine mycobacteriosis made on the basis of gross examination. JAVMA 204:1571–1572.

Matlova L, Dvorska L, Palecek K, Maurenc L, Bartos M, Pavlik I. 2004. Impact of sawdust and wood shavings in bedding on pig tuberculous lesions in lymph nodes, and IS1245 RFLP analysis of *Mycobacterium avium* subsp. *hominissuis* of serotypes 6 and 8 isolated from pigs and environment. Vet Microbiol 102:227–236.

McDiarmid A. 1956. Tuberculin testing of pigs. Vet Rec 68:298–299.

Meissner G, Viallier J, Coullioud D. 1978. Identification serologique de 1590 souches de *Mycobacterium avium* isolées en

France et en Allemagne Federale. Ann Microbiol (Paris) 129A:131–137.

Mijs W, de Haas P, Rossau R, van Der Laan T, Rigouts L, Portaels F, van Soolingen D. 2002. Molecular evidence to support a proposal to reserve the designation *Mycobacterium avium* subsp. Avium for bird-type isolates and '*M. avium* subsp. *Hominissuis*' for the human/porcine type of *M. avium*. Int J System Evolutionary Microbiol 52:1505–1518.

Mitchell CA, Walker RVL, Humphrey FA. 1934. Types of tubercle bacilli found in swine of two accredited areas. In Rep Vet Dir Gen Dep Agric Can, pp. 43–44.

Mitchell MD, Huff IH, Thoen CO, Himes EM, Howder JW. 1975. Swine tuberculosis in South Dakota. J Am Vet Med Assoc 167:152–153.

Momotani E, Yokomizo Y, Shoya S, Nakamura K, Yugi H. 1980. Experimental granuloma formation with *Mycobacterium intracellulare* in HPCD piglets. J Tokyo Vet Zootec Sci 29:25–32.

Muscoplat CC, Thoen CO, Chen AW, Rakich PM, Johnson DW. 1975. Development of specific lymphocyte immunostimulation and tuberculin skin reactivity in swine infected with *Mycobacterium bovis* and *Mycobacterium avium*. Am J Vet Res 36:1167–1171.

National Archives and Records Services. 1973. Code of Federal Regulations: Animal and Animal Byproducts. Title 9, chap. 3, subchap. A, pt. 311. Washington, D.C.: Gen Serv Adm.

Nishimori K, Eguchi M, Nakaoka Y, Onodera Y, Ito T, Tanaka K. 1995. Distribution of IS901 in strains of *Mycobacterium avium* complex from swine using IS901 detecting primers that discriminate between *M. avium* and *Mycobacterium intracellulare*. Clin Microbiol 33:2102–2106.

Ottosen HE. 1945. Undersogelser over Corynebacterium Magnusson-Holth, specielt med Henblik paa dens serologiske Forhold. A/S Carl. Fr Mortensen, Copenhagen.

Pallaske G. 1931. Studien zum Ablauf, zur Pathogenese und pathologischen Anatomie der Tuberkulose des Schweines. Beitrag zum Vergleichenden Studium der Tiertuberkulose. Z Infektioskr Parasitenkd Krankheit Haustiere 39:211–260.

Paterson AB. 1949. Tuberculosis in animals other than cattle. III. Vet Rec 61:880–881.

Pavlik I, Svastova P, Bartl J, Dvorska L, Rychlik I. 2000. Relationship between IS901 in the *Mycobacterium avium* complex strains isolated from birds, animals, humans, and the environment and virulence for poultry. Clin Diag Lab Immunol 7(2):212–217.

Pestana de Castro AF, Campedelli Filho O, Waisbich E. 1978. Opportunistic mycobacteria isolated from the mesenteric lymph nodes of apparently healthy pigs in São Paulo, Brazil. Rev Microbiol (Brazil) 9:74–83.

Plum N. 1946. Om Vaerdien af den Makroskopiske Diagnose af de Holthske Processer. Maandsskr Dyrlaegeforen 58:27–37.

Pritchard WD, Thoen CO, Himes EM, Muscoplat CC, Johnson DW. 1977. Epidemiology of mycobacterial lymphadenitis in an Idaho swine herd. Am J Epidemiol 106:222–227.

Pullar EM, Rushford BH. 1954. The accuracy of the avian intradermal tuberculin test in pigs. Aust Vet J 30:221–231.

Pullin JW. 1946. Tuberculous lesions of swine. I. Survey of lesions found in eastern Canada. Can J Comp Med 10:159–163.

Rastogi N, Barrow WW. 1994. Cell envelope constituents and the multifaceted nature of *Mycobacterium avium* pathogenicity and drug resistance. Res Microbiol 145:243–252.

Retzlaff N. 1966. Histologische Untersuchungen an Lymphknoten von mit Mykobakterien infizierten Schlachtschwein. Arch Lebensmittelhyg 17:56–62.

Ringdal G. 1963. Johne's disease in pigs. Nord Vet Med 15:217–238.

Ritacco V, Kremer K, van der Laan T, Pijnenburg JEM, de Haas PEW, van Soolingen D. 1998. Use of IS901 and IS1245 in RFLP typing of *Mycobacterium avium* complex: relatedness among serovar reference strains, human and animal isolates. Int J Tuberc Lung Dis 2(3):242–251.

Schalk AF, Roderick LM, Foust HL, Harshfield GS. 1935. Avian Tuberculosis: Collected Studies. ND Agric Exp Stn Tech Bull 279.

Schliesser T. 1976. Vorkommen und Bedeutung von Mycobakterien bei Tieren. Zentralbl Bakteriol (Orig A) 235:184–194.

Schliesser T, Weber A. 1973. Untersuchungen über die Tenazitzt von Mykobakterien der Gruppe III nach Runyon in Sagemehleinstreu. Zentralbl Veterinärmed (B) 20:710–714.

Sigurdardottir OG, Nordstoga K, Baustad B, Saxegaard F. 1994. Granulomatous enteritis in a pig caused by *Mycobacterium avium*. Vet Pathol 31:274–276.

Smith HW. 1958. The source of avian tuberculosis in the pig (letter to the editor). Vet Rec 70:586.

Songer JG, Bicknell EJ, Thoen CO. 1980. Epidemiological investigations of swine tuberculosis in Arizona. Can J Comp Med 44:115–120.

Szabo I, Tuboly S, Szecky A, Kerekes J, Udvardy N. 1975. Swine lymphadenitis due to *Mycobacterium avium* and atypical mycobacteria. II. Studies on the role of littering in mycobacterial lymphadenitis incidence in large-scale pig units. Acta Vet Acad Sci Hung 25:77–83.

Takai S, Fukunaga N, Ochiai S, Imai Y, Sasaki Y, Tsubaki S, Sekizaki T. 1996. Identification of intermediately virulent *Rhodococcus equi* isolate from pigs. Clin Microbiol 34:1034–1037.

Tammemagi L, Simmons GC. 1971. Pathogenicity of *Mycobacterium intracellulare* to pigs. Aust Vet J 47:337–339.

Thoen CO. 1994. *Mycobacterium avium* infections in animals. Res Microbiol 145(3):173–177.

——. 1997. Avian tuberculosis. In Diseases of Poultry, 10th ed. BW Calnek, WM Reid, HW Yoder, Jr, eds. Ames: Iowa State Univ Press.

Thoen CO, Armbrust AL, Hopkins MP. 1979a. Enzyme-linked immunosorbent assay for detecting antibodies in swine infected with *Mycobacterium avium*. Am J Vet Res 40:1096–1099.

Thoen CO, Barletta RG. 2004. *Mycobacterium*. In Pathogenesis of Bacterial Infections in Animals. Third Edition. Chapter 6. CL Gyles, JF Prescott, JG Songer, CO Thoen, eds. Ames: Blackwell Publishing, pp. 69–76.

Thoen CO, Bloom BR. 1995. Pathogenesis of *Mycobacterium bovis*. In *Mycobacterium bovis* Infection in Animals and Humans. CO. Thoen, JH Steele, eds. Ames: Iowa State Univ Press, pp. 3–14.

Thoen CO, Himes EM. 1977. Isolation of *Mycobacterium chelonei* from a granulomatous lesion in pig. J Clin Microbiol 6:81–83.

Thoen CO, Himes EM, Karlson AG. 1984. *Mycobacterium avium* complex. In The Mycobacteria: A Sourcebook. GP Kubica, LG Wayne, eds. New York: Marcel Dekker.

Thoen CO, Himes EM, Weaver DE, Spangler GW. 1976b. Tuberculosis in brood sows and pigs slaughtered in Iowa. Am J Vet Res 37:775–778.

Thoen CO, Jarnagin JL, Richards WD. 1975. Isolation and identification of mycobacteria from porcine tissues: A three-year summary. Am J Vet Res 36:1383–1386.

Thoen CO, Johnson DW, Himes EM, Menke SB, Muscoplat CC. 1976a. Experimentally induced *Mycobacterium avium* serotype 8 infection in swine. Am J Vet Res 37:177–181.

Thoen CO, Karlson AG. 1970. Epidemiologic studies on swine tuberculosis. In Proc US Anim Health Assoc, pp. 459–464.

Thoen CO, Owen WJ, Himes EM. 1979b. *Mycobacterium avium* serotype 4 infection in swine. In Proc 83d Annu Meet US Anim Health Assoc, pp. 468–479.

Thoen CO, Williams DE. 1994. Tuberculosis, tuberculoidoses and other mycobacterial infections. In Handbook of Zoonoses, 2d ed. G W Beran, ed. Boca Raton, Fla.: CRC Press, pp. 41–60.

Thorensen OF, Saxegaard F. 1993. Comparative use of DNA probes for *Mycobacterium avium* and *Mycobacterium intracellulare* and serotyping for identification and characterization of animal isolates of the *M. avium* complex. Vet Microbiol 34:83–88.

Tsukamura M, Komatsuzaki C, Sakai R, Kaneda K, Kudo K, Seino A. 1988. Mesenteric lymphadenitis of swine caused by *Rhodococcus sputi*. J Clin Microbiol 26:155–157.

USDA. 1922. Yearbook of Agriculture. Washington, D.C.

——. 1973. Statistical Summary. Federal Meat and Poultry Inspection for Calendar Year 1972. MPI-1.

——. 1979. Statistical Summary. Federal Meat and Poultry Inspection for Calendar Year 1978. MPI-1.

——. 1984. Statistical Summary. Federal Meat and Poultry Inspection for Calendar Year 1983. MPI-1.

——. 1990. Statistical Summary. Federal Meat and Poultry Inspection for Calendar Year 1989. MPI-1.

——. 1996. Statistical Summary. Federal Meat and Poultry Inspection for Calendar Year 1995.

Van Es L. 1925. Tuberculosis of Swine. Univ Nebr Agric Exp Stn Circ 25.

Vasenius H. 1965. Tuberculosis-like lesions in slaughter swine in Finland. Nord Vet Med 17:17–21.

Wolinsky E, Schaefer WB. 1973. Proposed numbering scheme for mycobacterial serotypes of agglutination. Int F Syst Bacteriol 23:182–183.

Yugi H, Nemoto H, Watanabe K. 1972. Serotypes of *Mycobacterium intracellulare* of porcine origin. Nat Inst Anim Health Q (Tokyo) 12:168–169.

50 Miscellaneous Bacterial Infections

David J. Taylor

Anthrax

Anthrax is relatively rare in swine compared to sheep and cattle, which are highly susceptible. Swine may become infected, however, along with other species of farm animals and may become important as a reservoir of infection.

Since anthrax is a zoonosis, infections in swine are a threat to human health. Infected swine represent a hazard to the farmworker and veterinarian, to the abattoir worker, and to those preparing and eating contaminated pig products. The importance of this relatively rare disease in swine is increased by the public health requirement for abattoir disinfection and the disposal of carcasses after the discovery of an infected animal at meat inspection. Meat processors are becoming unwilling to slaughter pigs from infected farms, retailers are increasingly concerned about their duty to consumers, and the safe disposal of manures can be a major problem. These factors add a wider importance to the disease.

Anthrax is present throughout the world, and the FAO-WHO report (1973) indicates that the disease occurred in swine in every continent during 1972. The incidence remains low and sporadic, but the disease presents a local problem in some areas.

ETIOLOGY

Anthrax is caused by *Bacillus anthracis,* a large grampositive, aerobic, spore-forming, nonmotile rod. The individual bacilli are 1–5 µm in diameter and 3–8 µm long. When observed in tissue from an infected animal, the organisms are commonly in short chains surrounded by a well-developed capsule. Under suitable aerobic conditions, spores highly resistant to disinfectants, heat, and desiccation may be produced.

B. anthracis grows very luxuriantly on most common laboratory media. On blood agar plates, colonies can usually be detected within 12 hours. After 24 hours at 37°C, the colonies have a "ground glass" appearance, with irregular, wavy borders that give them the "medusa head" characteristic. No hemolysis is produced on blood agar; this is useful in distinguishing the colonies from those of certain nonpathogenic species of the genus (Norberg 1953). The colony of *B. anthracis* growing on blood agar on primary isolation possesses a stickiness that can be readily detected by touching with the bacteriological loop. The colonial growth tends to adhere to the loop and forms tenacious threads.

Bacteria in these colonies do not produce capsules unless grown on special media or in 5% carbon dioxide but do produce spores. *B. anthracis* may be distinguished from other members of the genus by biochemical tests. Those of use in differentiating the organism from related bacilli are listed in the section on diagnosis below. *B. anthracis* is pathogenic to laboratory animals and humans. Culture should not be attempted unless appropriate safety precautions such as safety cabinets and adequate disposal facilities are available. Personnel handling the organism should be vaccinated.

EPIDEMIOLOGY

Anthrax is generally considered a soilborne infection in cattle, sheep, and horses. Animal-to-animal spread does not commonly occur, but rather, *B. anthracis* is deposited in the soil or the environment by the infected animal at the time of or following death. Spores are formed by some of the organisms, and these highly resistant bodies may remain viable for years, even under adverse conditions. Subsequently, the spores may be ingested by susceptible animals and anthrax may develop.

Swine can presumably become infected in this manner; however, because of the small number of spores likely to be picked up and the higher degree of resistance in swine, infection probably occurs only rarely. Rather, anthrax in swine generally occurs following ingestion of feed that contains a large number of *B. anthracis* or viable spores. Swine that are permitted to eat the carcass of an animal dead of anthrax may consume large numbers of organisms and may therefore become infected. The use of bonemeal or other animal products containing spores of *B. anthracis* in feed is the most common source of infection in swine. Davies and Harvey (1955) isolated *B. anthracis* from 5 of 41 cargoes of bonemeal shipped to England from the Near and Middle East. Direct cultural methods were unsuccessful, but the authors isolated the organism from guinea pigs that were first protected from the various anaerobic species common in bonemeal by means of clostridial antisera and antitoxins and that were then injected with a concentrated infusion from the bonemeal specimen.

The role of feed contaminated with spores of *B. anthracis* in the transmission of anthrax can be illustrated by a brief account of the 1952 outbreak that occurred in the midwestern United States (Ferguson 1986). Anthrax was confirmed on a farm in southern Ohio in February 1952, and further outbreaks occurred in rapid succession in widely separated areas. Within a week of the recognition of the first case, feed was incriminated as the source of infection. A number of feed companies were involved, but all had incorporated bonemeal obtained from a company in Columbus, Ohio, which had processed part of a shipment of 100 tons of raw bonemeal obtained from Belgium into a meat scrap concentrate. The companies purchased the concentrate and included it in many hundreds of tons of swine feed sold throughout Ohio and adjoining states. The organism was isolated from the raw bonemeal and from the meat scrap concentrate but not from any of the finished feeds.

The organism appears to be spread in wet-feed systems but rarely affects more than 1–2 animals in an infected herd. This was the classic picture, but accounts of continuing outbreaks exist (Jackson 1967; Jackson and Taylor 1989; Edgington 1990). The outbreak referred to by Jackson and Taylor (1989) and Edgington (1990) occurred in a 500-sow unit and persisted for 14 weeks, resulting in at least 18 cases in sows, suckling pigs, and weaned pigs. The development of disease in weaners may have been delayed by maternal immunity in this continuing outbreak. The origin of the outbreak was considered to be feed, but the disease persisted within the herd in spite of antimicrobial treatment. Persistence may have been in carrier pigs or as spores in slurry and housing. The role of flies in persistence and transmission was not clear, although recent studies in the United States indicate that biting flies (*Stomoxys calcitrans*) and mosquitoes (*Aedes aegyptii* and *A. taeniorhynchus*) transmit the disease experimentally 4 hours after feeding (Turell and Knudson 1987). Ticks (*Dermacentor marginatus*) were shown to harbor the organism for 76 days at 4°C and for 35 days at 22–25°C in the former Soviet Union (Akhmerov et al. 1982).

PATHOGENESIS

B. anthracis has two major sets of pathogenic determinants: a protective capsule composed of a polymer of d-glutamic acid and the complex exotoxin. Molecular biology studies have shown that toxin production results from the possession of a 110 MDa plasmid and that capsulation is related to the possession of a smaller 60 MDa plasmid (Uchido et al. 1985; Mikesell et al. 1983). The exotoxin (Smith et al. 1955; Harris-Smith et al. 1958; Davis et al. 1973) is composed of three fractions and is produced when bacteria reach $5–10 \times 10^6$ organisms per milliliter of blood. The toxins share the same binding unit—the protective antigen (PA)—and are binary toxins. PA binds to cell surfaces and is activated by a host protease, allowing edema factor (EF) and lethal factor (LF) to enter cells. EF is a calmodulin-dependent adenylate cyclase and affects neutrophils, preventing the respiratory burst and thus protecting the organisms. It is also responsible for the progressive hyperglycemia and the severe terminal hypoglycemia seen in animals with the septicemic form. LF appears to be a zinc-dependent protease affecting macrophages. All three toxins are needed to produce typical anthrax.

The organism appears to enter the pig through the gut or tonsil. Septicemic disease is rare, and the organism multiplies locally, resisting phagocytosis by means of the polyglutamic acid capsule. Edema is commonly produced locally. Neutrophils and other phagocytes are killed by EF, and organisms multiply until LF is produced, resulting in the death of the animal as a result of its effect on the mitochondria. Immunity against anthrax is associated with antibodies against the exotoxin (PA) (Sargeant et al. 1960; Thorne et al. 1960). Antibody to the cell wall may be produced but is not protective.

CLINICAL SIGNS

The first indications of an outbreak of the disease may be an increase in mortality. Investigation of these extra deaths may indicate the presence of anthrax and the clinical signs described below may be identified. Three forms of anthrax have been observed in swine: pharyngeal, intestinal, and septicemic. The usual portal of entry is the oral cavity, and invasion occurs in the tonsils or mucosa of the pharynx. In some cases the infection may remain localized in the lymph nodes of this region, and the disease is classified as pharyngeal. In other cases the organisms may pass into the intestinal tract, where primary invasion may also occur. When *B. anthracis* is not localized but gains access to the general circulation, the septicemic form of the disease develops.

The clinical signs commonly observed in pharyngeal anthrax are cervical edema and dyspnea. General depression, inappetence, and vomiting are commonly seen. Fever with temperatures to 41.7°C may occur, but it is not consistent, and in some affected swine the temperature may be subnormal. Death follows in many of the swine within 24 hours after the cervical edema is noticed. It is not uncommon for swine to recover even in the absence of treatment. The swelling may disappear gradually, and complete recovery appears to occur; however, such animals may continue to remain carriers of *B. anthracis*.

Clinical signs of intestinal anthrax are not as obvious as those in the pharyngeal form. In severe cases an acute digestive disturbance may be evident, with vomiting, complete loss of appetite, and diarrhea with bloody feces. Death may follow in the most severely affected swine; however, recovery occurs in many affected with the milder forms (Brennan 1953). When 50 pigs were infected in an experimental study (Redmond et al. 1997), 33 developed anorexia, lethargy, dullness, shivering, constipation, loose feces, blood in the feces, and ataxia at some point between 1 and 8 days after infection. Only 2 died. Fever did not exceed 41.9°C, peaking 48 hours after infection.

Intestinal anthrax has been reported only rarely in the United States. Many cases may be unrecognized because of the usual practice of avoiding a complete necropsy of animals suspected of anthrax. It is possible that some of the animals dying of pharyngeal anthrax may also have had lesions in the intestinal tract. Brennan (1953) reported that intestinal anthrax was the most common form of the disease seen in the 1952 outbreak of anthrax in England.

Septicemic anthrax is the highly acute form that results from the entrance of *B. anthracis* into the bloodstream, followed by rapid reproduction of the organisms throughout the body. Death frequently occurs in animals so affected, without any period of illness being noticed by the owner. In swine it is the uncommon form of the disease. Walker et al. (1967) reported the presence of viable spores of *B. anthracis* in the lungs of dwarf swine for as long as 7 days following respiratory exposure. These authors suggested that resistance of swine may be related to some mechanism that inhibits germination of the spores. Of 30 swine examined at necropsy during the anthrax outbreak of 1952 in Ohio, only 3 had the enlarged, dark spleen so characteristically seen in cattle. It is possible that young pigs develop septicemia more frequently than older swine (Ferguson 1986).

LESIONS

In the interests of controlling anthrax, complete necropsy of animals is strongly discouraged. Pigs with anthrax may not be identified before necropsy because the disease is relatively rare. Large pigs which have died from the disease may have a bloody discharge from the nose (Edgington 1990), and small ones may appear very pale and dehydrated. The cervical region is edematous, but otherwise no superficial lesions are evident. Incision of the region reveals an extensive infiltration of the tissues with fluid, which is usually straw colored but may

appear pink or hemorrhagic. The tissue, containing large amounts of fluid, may appear to possess a gelatinous consistency. The tonsils are usually covered with a fibrinous exudate, or extensive necrotic changes may be evident. The pharyngeal mucosa is frequently inflamed and swollen.

The mandibular and suprapharyngeal lymph nodes are enlarged to several times their normal size. The cut surface of the affected node may vary in color from deep brick red to strawberry red. In more chronic cases the color may be grayish yellow, indicative of necrotic changes in the node. In cases of the septicemic and intestinal forms the carcass may be opened before anthrax is suspected. The intestinal form is more common and there is usually copious pinkish peritoneal fluid, which may clot on exposure to air. The small intestine is usually inflamed, with fibrinous adhesions on the serous surface. The mesenteric lymph nodes may be swollen, hemorrhagic, or necrotic, and edema of the mesentery is common. The intestinal mucosa is covered with a diphtheritic membrane and may be hemorrhagic. The intestinal wall may be grossly thickened. In the septicemic form little may be seen other than the presence of bloodstained fluid in the peritoneal cavity and local petechiation. In some cases the spleen is enlarged and there may be marked petechiation of the kidney. Small abscesses may be present in the lymph nodes of recovered pigs (Redmond et al. 1997).

Microscopic lesions in the lymph nodes usually consist of hemorrhage and necrosis with encapsulated bacilli. These may also be seen in the necrotic diphtheritic lesions of the intestinal mucosa and in the capillaries of any organ in septicemia.

DIAGNOSIS

Anthrax should be suspected when swine show cervical edema and dyspnea. However, erysipelas or malignant edema from *Clostridium septicum* may also provoke similar clinical signs. In malignant edema, the edema will often be more prominent in the shoulders or axillary spaces. The edematous fluid and enlarged cervical or mesenteric lymph nodes, as seen on necropsy, are very suggestive of anthrax. When the carcass has been opened, the presence of bloodstained fluid in the peritoneum, petechiation of the kidney or serosal surfaces, enlargement of the spleen, and thickening and inflammation of the small intestine should lead to suspicion of anthrax. A history of the type of feed products eaten by the affected swine is always of value.

The accurate diagnosis of anthrax is very important and in most cases is dependent upon the isolation and identification of *B. anthracis*.

Microscopic Examination
Impression smears and cultures should be made from the cut surfaces of the cervical lymph nodes, spleen,

mesenteric lymph nodes, intestinal mucosa, or kidney as appropriate, and peritoneal fluid should also be sampled when present. Smears should be fixed in Zenker's fluid, which kills spores, or by low heat, which does not, and then stained by polychrome methylene blue for 2 minutes and washed with water. The bacilli of anthrax appear as square-ended blue rods in a pinkish capsule. In smears made from decayed carcasses, other bacilli may be present, and where antimicrobial treatment has been given, the bacilli may be present only as capsules or in aberrant forms. The failure to find anthrax bacilli immediately should not rule out the disease, as up to 30 minutes' examination may be required. Peritoneal fluid is more often positive than splenic smears in septicemia. Slides and reagents used for diagnosis should be disposed of by incineration or formaldehyde fixation.

Spores are not observed in slides prepared from fresh tissue or from freshly cut surfaces. Spore-forming anaerobes are frequently encountered in tissues of animals that have been dead several hours prior to necropsy. Differentiation is important in such cases, and the following points are helpful. Spores are rarely seen in *B. anthracis* in fresh-tissue preparations, whereas spores are regularly seen in clostridia. In the latter organism the rod is usually slightly enlarged by the spore. Capsules are very rarely observed in the clostridia, and any capsules seen do not stain purple with polychrome methylene blue.

Cultural Studies

B. anthracis grows readily on many common media and is characterized by very rapid colonial development. Typical colonies can be observed after 12–18 hours of incubation. This rapid growth is useful in differentiating *B. anthracis* from other pathogens.

B. anthracis is readily cultured from the enlarged lymph nodes, and it may also be demonstrated from the surrounding connective tissue in some cases. In the occasional septicemic case the organisms can be isolated from the blood, spleen, or liver—in fact, from essentially any tissue of the body. Since *B. anthracis* grows more rapidly than most of the saprophytic bacteria likely to be encountered, except other species of *Bacillus*, one should always examine the cultures after incubation for 12–18 hours.

Suspect colonies can be identified as *B. anthracis* by their biochemical characters using API systems or by the absence of hemolysis, lack of motility, growth on chloral hydrate agar, and susceptibility to anthrax phage. Final confirmation of pathogenic *B. anthracis* depends on the inoculation of culture into scratches on the footpad of a guinea pig or mouse under strict containment. All cultures and any experimental animals should be fixed in formaldehyde and incinerated.

Serology

A competitive enzyme immunosorbent assay (EIA) has been described (Turnbull et al. 1986, 1992) to identify the presence of IgG antibody to PA, and PA may be assayed in serum in pigs which have died using the capture EIA (Turnbull 1990).

CONTROL

Control of the spread of anthrax differs significantly from control of most of the other important animal diseases. The highly resistant spore formed by *B. anthracis* accounts for this difference. Some swine may become inapparent carriers, but there is little evidence to indicate that this forms an important source of infection to susceptible animals. Otherwise, animals that become infected do show clinical signs and generally develop an acute disease that terminates in death within a few days. Transmission from animal to animal rarely occurs, but soil contaminated by the organisms serves as a source from which susceptible animals subsequently ingest the spores. Because of this common form of transmission, anthrax can be controlled by preventing susceptible animals from contacting viable spores of *B. anthracis*.

Van Ness and Stein (1956) pointed out the importance of soil types in the survival of anthrax spores. The principal areas of enzootic anthrax are regions characterized by soils high in nitrogen and with adequate calcium. Where such soil types are lacking (e.g., central and eastern United States), anthrax does not appear to persist.

The spores can survive for years under a variety of environmental conditions. In the unopened carcasses of animals dead of anthrax, few spores are formed except at the body openings. When the animal is opened for a complete necropsy or when carnivorous animals are permitted to eat the carcass, there is usually extensive spore formation as the heavily infected blood and viscera are exposed to the oxygen of the air. For this reason, the orifices and any cuts in a carcass should be covered with disinfectant-soaked cotton wool to prevent sporulation and spread of infection. The most productive control measures include the complete destruction of the carcasses of animals dead of anthrax by incineration or deep burial.

When an animal dies in the open, it is generally recommended that it be burned on the spot. If the animal must be moved, the carcass must be placed on a sled or some other vehicle that can be thoroughly disinfected and then hauled, not dragged, to an area for disposal. If burning is not an option, deep burial can be used. The carcass should be covered with lime and at least 4 feet (1.25 m) of soil. When carefully completed, these methods will minimize the chances of transmission of the infection.

Disinfection can be achieved with 5% freshly prepared sodium hydroxide or, more controllably, with 10% formaldehyde and the use of appropriate respirators. Only disinfectants capable of inactivating anthrax spores, such as those containing glutaraldehyde and formaldehyde, should be used. Disinfectants should be used prior to clearing up infected premises, and contaminated articles should be burned. Exposed surfaces should be scrubbed or pressure washed with the disinfectant.

Edgington (1990) gives an account of the procedure adopted in depopulating and disinfecting a chronically infected 500-sow unit from which purchasers would no longer take pigs. All 5000 pigs were slaughtered and burned, all 300,000 gallons (1,364,000 L) of slurry were disinfected with 10% formaldehyde and disposed of in an approved toxic-waste site, and the buildings were formaldehyde-fumigated and cleaned—at a cost of £1,000,000 (US $1,700,000). Similar precautions may have to be adopted in contaminated meat plants to safeguard public health.

Following the outbreaks of anthrax in the midwestern United States in 1952, which were conclusively traced to imported bonemeal, regulations were established that prohibit the importation of raw bonemeal into the United States (Stein 1953). Comparable preventive legislation was adopted in Canada (Moynihan 1963). Bonemeal processed by an acceptable steam treatment may be imported under these regulations. In addition to this federal regulation, some states have laws pertaining to the operation of rendering plants and the use of animal products in feed. These regulations have proved effective. Similar regulations apply in most developed countries.

TREATMENT

Treatment of animals infected with *B. anthracis* is possible. Since swine may develop a chronic form of the disease, treatment can be successfully administered in some cases. In the outbreak in Ohio in 1952, penicillin in oil was used at a dosage level of 10,000 units/lb (22,000 units/kg) body weight. According to Ferguson (1986), pigs that were showing clinical signs of anthrax recovered completely after this treatment, and the losses were reduced considerably when the disease was recognized early in its course. Anthrax antiserum in doses of 20–75 mL was also used in treatment of a limited number of animals. The results were comparable to those following treatment with penicillin in that the pigs in the early stages of anthrax recovered promptly. Oxytetracycline is effective against *B. anthracis* and may be used parenterally in daily doses of 4.4–11.0 mg/kg body weight. Edgington (1990) reported the successful use of penicillin, oxytetracycline, and chlortetracycline:sulfonamide:penicillin combinations to treat or suppress infection but had to withdraw treatment from animals intended for slaughter. Following the study of Redmond et al. (1997), it is clear that infection may persist for up to 21 days after infection in a population, and this factor must be considered before carcasses are submitted for human consumption.

PREVENTION

Kaufmann et al. (1973) evaluated the Sterne strain anthrax vaccine, an avirulent spore vaccine, in an outbreak of the disease in Louisiana. The results supported the efficacy of the vaccine in swine, but the number involved was too small to provide significant data for this species. Similar findings were obtained by Jackson (1967) in a continuing outbreak in the United Kingdom. Immunization of swine would probably reduce incidence of infection when they are exposed to massive doses of *B. anthracis*. Immunization on a large scale has not been recommended, however, since swine possess a level of natural resistance adequate to prevent the disease except following heavy exposure to *B. anthracis*.

Human infection can be prevented by the safe disposal of all contaminated carcasses, articles, and fluids on the farm by the methods outlined above. Persons exposed to the infection can be given prophylactic antimicrobials such as penicillin and tetracyclines, and any cases can be treated with them. Where longer-term exposure is likely, vaccination should be carried out.

REFERENCES

Akhmerov DS, Kusov VN, Chernova AA. 1982. Survival of *Bacillus anthracis* in the tick *Dermacentor marginatus*. Rep Kaganskii Vet Inst, pp. 101–103.

Brennan ADJ. 1953. Anthrax, with special reference to the recent outbreak in pigs. Vet Rec 65:255.

Davies DG, Harvey RW. S. 1955. The isolation of *Bacillus anthracis* from bones. Lancet 2:86.

Davis BD, Dulbecco R, Eisen NH, Ginsberg HS, Wood WB, McCarty M. 1973. Microbiology, 2d ed. New York: Harper & Row.

Edgington AB. 1990. An outbreak of anthrax in pigs: A practitioner's account. Vet Rec 127:321–324.

FAO/WHO. 1973. Animal Health Yearbook for 1972. Rome: FAO.

Ferguson LC. 1986. Anthrax. In Diseases of Swine, 6th ed. AD Leman, B Straw, RD Glock, WL Mengeling, RHC Penny, E Scholl, eds Ames: Iowa State Univ Press, pp. 622–627.

Harris-Smith PW, Smith H, Keppie J. 1958. Production in vitro of the toxin of *Bacillus anthracis* previously recognised in vivo. J Gen Microbiol 19:91.

Jackson WT. 1967. Anthrax in pigs—A series of deaths. State Vet J 22:67–71.

Jackson WT, Taylor KC. 1989. Anthrax in pigs—A series of deaths. State Vet J 43:119–125.

Kaufmann AF, Fox MD, Kolb RC. 1973. Anthrax in Louisiana, 1971: An evaluation of the Sterne strain anthrax vaccine. J Am Vet Med Assoc 163:442.

Mikesell P, Ivins BE, Ristroph JD, Dreier TM. 1983. Evidence for plasmid mediated toxin production in *Bacillus anthracis*. Infect Immun 39:371–376.

Moynihan WA. 1963. Anthrax in Canada. Can Vet J 4:283.

Norberg BK. 1953. Continued investigations of some important characteristics in anthrax-like microorganisms as viewed from a point of view of differential diagnosis. Nord Vet Med 5:915.

Redmond C, Hall GA, Turnbull PCB, Gillgan JS. 1997. Experimentally assessed public health risks associated with pigs from farms experiencing anthrax. Vet Rec 141:244–247.

Sargeant K, Stanley JL, Smith H. 1960. The serological relationship between purified preparations of factors I and II of the anthrax toxin produced in vivo and in vitro. J Gen Microbiol 22:219.

Smith H, Keppie J, Stanley JL. 1955. The chemical basis of the virulence of *Bacillus anthracis*. V. The specific toxin produced by *B. anthracis* in vivo. Br J Exp Pathol 36:460.

Stein CD. 1953. A review of anthrax in livestock during 1952 with reference to outbreaks in the first eight months of 1953. In Proc US Livest Sanit Assoc, p. 101.

Thorne CB, Molnar DM, Strange RE. 1960. Production of toxin in vitro by *Bacillus anthracis* and its separation into two components. J Bacteriol 79:450.

Turell MJ, Knudson GB. 1987. Mechanical transmission of *Bacillus anthracis* by stable flies (*Stomoxys calcitrans*) and mosquitoes (*Aedes aegyptii* and *Aedes taeniorhynchus*). Infect Immun 55:1859–1861.

Turnbull PCB. 1990. Salisbury Medical Bulletin. In Proc Int Workshop on Anthrax, Apr 11–13, 1989, Winchester. 68. Special Suppl, p. 53.

Turnbull PCB, Broster MG, Carman JA, Manchee RJ, Melling J. 1986. Development of antibodies to protective antigen and lethal factor components of anthrax toxin in humans and guinea pigs and their relevance to protective immunity. Infect Immun 52:356–363.

Turnbull PCB, Doganay M, Lindeque PM, Aygen B, McLaughlin J. 1992. Serology and anthrax in humans, livestock, and Etosha National Park wildlife. Epidemiol Infect 108:299–313.

Uchido I, Sekizaki T, Hashimoto K, Terakado N. 1985. Association of the encapsulation of *Bacillus anthracis* with a 60 Megadalton plasmid. J Gen Microbiol 131:363–367.

Van Ness G, Stein CD. 1956. Soils of the United States favorable for anthrax. J Am Vet Med Assoc 128:7.

Walker JS, Klein F, Lincoln RE, Fernelius AL. 1967. A unique defense mechanism against anthrax demonstrated in dwarf swine. J Bacteriol 93:2031.

Melioidosis (*Burkoldaria pseudomallei* Infection)

Melioidosis is a chronic bacterial infection of pigs in tropical and subtropical regions such as those of Asia and northern Australia. Pigs may become infected by *Burkoldaria* (formerly *Pseudomonas*) *pseudomallei,* which is a short, gram-negative rod, 0.8 by 1.5 µm, that produces rough or mucoid colonies on a wide variety of laboratory media. It is present in water and soil in tropical and subtropical areas and may infect pigs when water supplies are contaminated. Infection is often clinically inapparent but has been associated with clinical signs (Olds and Lewis 1955; Omar et al. 1962; Laws and Hall 1964; Rogers and Andersen 1970; Veljanov et al. 1994). Clinical signs include a raised rectal temperature (40–42°C, 104–108°F) for up to 4 days, unsteady gait, lameness or weakness, slight nasal discharge, and subcutaneous swellings of the limbs. Deaths may occur but are rare in adults, in which abortions and uterine discharges have been recorded.

Lesions are found in slaughter pigs in which clinical signs have not been seen and in those that have died from the disease. They consist of large abscesses in the lungs, liver, spleen, kidney, and mesenteric and subcutaneous lymph nodes. The organism can be isolated from them. Melioidosis may be suspected on clinical grounds especially when prolonged raised rectal temperatures and unsteady gait are associated with subcutaneous swellings of the limbs. More frequently, diagnosis is based on the creamy abscesses found at slaughter or on the bacteriological results needed to confirm the presence of *B. pseudomallei* (Ketterer et al. 1986; Veljanov et al. 1994). A hypersensitivity test resembling a tuberculin test (the melioidin test) and serum-agglutination and complement-fixation tests have all been described and can be used to confirm a diagnosis in the live pig.

Treatment with tetracyclines has been described, and the disease can be prevented by use of clean or chlorinated water supplies and preventing access to contaminated soil. As the disease is of public health importance, infected carcasses should be disposed of safely.

REFERENCES

Ketterer PJ, Webster WR, Shield J, Arthur RJ, Blackall PJ, Thomas AD. 1986. Melioidosis in intensive piggeries in South Eastern Queensland. Aust Vet J 63:146–149.

Laws L, Hall WTK. 1964. Melioidosis in animals in North Queensland. IV. Epidemiology. Aust Vet J 40:309–314.

Olds, R. J., and Lewis, F. A. 1955. Melioidosis in a pig. Aust Vet J 31:273–274.

Omar AR, Cheah KK, Mahendranathan T. 1962. Observations on porcine melioidosis in Malaya. Br Vet J 118:421–429.

Rogers RJ, Andersen DJ. 1970. Intrauterine infection of a pig by *Pseudomonas pseudomallei*. Aust Vet J 46:292.

Veljanov D, Vesselinova A, Nicolova S, Kussovski V, Najdenski H. 1994. Experimental *Pseudomonas pseudomallei* infection of pigs. Proc Int Congr Pig Vet Soc 13:236.

Chlamydiae

Chlamydiae are small intracellular bacteria that cause disease in many mammalian species and are widespread in birds. They have been demonstrated in cases of conjunctivitis, enteritis, pneumonia, pleurisy, pericarditis, arthritis, orchitis, uterine infections, and abortion in pigs. Recent work on chlamydiae in pigs has shown that at least three species are involved (*Chlamydophila psittaci, C. pecorum, Chlamydia trachomatis*); the development of reliable tissue culture methods and the use of immunoperoxidase staining of tissue sections, DNA probes, and, more recently, polymerase chain reaction (PCR) methods have demonstrated that the organisms are relatively common in pig populations. The literature prior to 1983 was reviewed comprehensively by Stellmacher et al. (1983), and the account in the present chapter draws on earlier work only where it is relevant to current knowledge.

ETIOLOGY

Chlamydiae are gram-negative bacteria that can multiply only inside living cells. They are unusual among bacteria in that they exist outside the cell only as an inactive, trypsin-resistant, infectious particle 0.2–0.3 μm (200–300 nm) in diameter known as an elementary body (Figure 50.1). This body has an electron-dense core packed with DNA and surrounded by a trilaminar cytoplasmic membrane, outside which lies a further trilaminar envelope and then a cell wall with projections that may be associated with attachment to cells. The outer-membrane proteins of the chlamydiae have been studied in considerable detail, and sequences of the genes coding for outer-membrane protein A (*ompA*) have been obtained (Kaltenbroeck and Storz 1992; Kaltenbroeck et al. 1993; Anderson et al. 1996). These sequences have contributed to the current species classification and are now widely used in diagnosis. *C. psittaci* contains a plasmid, and DNA sequences of it have also been identified in *C. pecorum*.

Within 6–9 hours after an elementary body has entered a cell, it forms a reticulate body 1 μm (1000 nm) in diameter. This body divides by binary fission to form further reticulate bodies in an inclusion within the host cell. At this stage the infected host cell may divide to give infected daughter cells, which may account for latent infections seen in animal hosts. Within 20 hours of the first division of the reticulate body, some begin to mature into elementary bodies. The chlamydial inclusions may occupy up to three-quarters of the cell volume and contain up to 10,000 elementary bodies. *C. trachomatis* produces glycogen inclusions in cells at this stage; *C. psittaci* and *C. pecorum* do not. Infected cells may lyse to release the elementary bodies or these may be budded from persistently infected cells.

Chlamydiae can be grown in the laboratory by inoculation of the yolk sac of 6- to 8-day-old embryonated hen eggs and in neonatal mice. Most laboratories now use cell cultures, usually McCoy or L929 cells, in which the chlamydiae grow readily. Some strains and species can be maintained in Vero cells. In some cases, isolation can be improved by treatment of the cells, using irradiation or cycloheximide (1 μm/mL), and by centrifugation of the chlamydiae onto the cells.

The different species of chlamydiae and biotypes within them can be distinguished by their differential growth in cell cultures in the presence of tissue culture medium supplemented with amino acids such as arginine, isoleucine, and methionine (Johnson 1984) and by the presence of inclusions or the time taken to develop in a particular cell line. The main methods of dif-

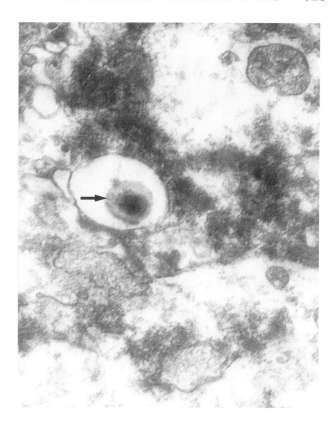

50.1. *Electron micrograph of elementary body (arrow) of* Chlamydophila *sp. in an aborted placenta (original magnification ×52,500).*

ferentiation are now (1) antigenic, based on differences between the outer-membrane proteins detected using monoclonal antibodies in immunoperoxidase, immunofluorescence, or ELISA methods, and (2) nucleic acid based, using genomic and *ompA* sequences for PCR (Anderson et al. 1996; Kaltenbroek and Storz 1992; Kaltenbroeck et al. 1993).

EPIDEMIOLOGY

The recent development of methods to differentiate the three species of chlamydiae present in pigs has raised a number of questions about the epidemiology of infections with these species in the pig. All three species are found in other animals or birds, and experimental infections show that *C. psittaci* from species such as sheep can be transmitted to pigs and sometimes produces lesions (Harris et al. 1984; Vasquez-Cisneros et al. 1994). *C. psittaci* occurs in many avian species and is particularly common in pigeons and doves but may occur in almost any bird. Some mammals such as sheep, cattle, and rodents may be infected. All these species may form a reservoir of *C. psittaci* infection for the pig. The relationship between *C. pecorum* and *C. trachomatis* infections of other mammalian species and the pig has not yet been explored in detail. All chlamydiae can survive for considerable lengths of time as elementary bodies in the environment, where they are resistant to drying. The major routes of transmission of *C. psittaci* to pigs are by inhalation of aerosols of elementary bodies, either fresh or in dust, from respiratory, genital tract, or enteric infections; by ingestion of contaminated feed; and by contact, particularly venereal in the case of genital tract infections. The exact methods by which *C. pecorum* and *C. trachomatis* are transferred are not yet clear but are probably similar, with the fecal-oral route being of importance for enteric infections and transmission by flies or dust being involved in *C. trachomatis* conjunctivitis (Rogers et al. 1993).

Chlamydial infection in the pig has been reported from the United States (Willigan and Beamer 1955; Pospischil and Wood 1987), Britain (Wilson and Plummer 1966; Harris 1976), Rumania (Sorodoc et al. 1961), Germany (Stellmacher et al. 1983), and more recently from other countries. The early serologic surveys suggested that complement-fixing and microagglutinating antibodies were present in up to 23% of slaughter pigs (Wilson and Plummer 1966). Most antibody titers were low (1:8–1:128), but titers as high as 1:1024 were recorded (Wilson and Plummer 1966). More recent surveys using immunoperoxidase staining of histological sections of gut suggest that chlamydial inclusions can be found in up to 67% of piglets (Zahn et al. 1995) and 99% of finishing pigs (Szeredi et al. 1996). Serum antibody surveys of the same finishing animals using an ELISA method confirmed antibody in 82.6%, but the complement-fixation test (CFT) detected antibody in only 28.6%, a figure similar to that of Wilson and Plummer (1966). It is clear, therefore, that infection with chlamydiae is widespread among pigs.

Studies of the distribution of infection within infected herds suggest that infection can occur in animals of every age group. Samples from which chlamydiae have been isolated include semen samples from boars; fetuses, both live and aborted; sows; lungs, joints, and organs such as liver and spleen from piglets; store pigs; and pigs at slaughter. Enteric infection is uncommon in piglets of less than 4 weeks of age (6.9%) and more common (41.8%) in piglets aged more than 4 weeks (Zahn et al. 1995), and conjunctival infection was recorded by Rogers et al. (1993) as associated with clinical signs between 2 and 8 weeks of age. The presence of low levels of antibody in piglets may suggest maternal antibody transfer. The possibility of transmission of intestinal chlamydiae to humans from slaughter pigs was raised by Szeredi et al.(1996).

PATHOGENESIS

Experimental infections were carried out with "*C. psittaci*" or "chlamydiae" prior to the identification of the presence of three species of chlamydiae in pigs. The account which follows uses the term "*C. psittaci*" unless there is evidence that the organisms were of the other species.

Elementary bodies of *C. psittaci* enter by the respiratory, oral, or genital routes and enter epithelial cells, in which they multiply or are taken up by macrophages and distributed to lymph nodes. Infection may be local at the portal of infection and remain inapparent or latent; may cause local disease such as pneumonia, enteritis, or disturbances of reproduction; or may become generalized. *C. psittaci* isolates of avian, bovine, ovine, and porcine origin have been used in experimental infections; but strains of porcine origin appear to be most virulent for the pig, provided they have not become yolk sac or tissue culture adapted.

There appears to be some adaptation of strains to the method of transmission, in that strains of genital origin (Kielstein et al. 1983) do not appear to cause severe pneumonia, and parenteral inoculation was found necessary to reproduce arthritis with an arthritis isolate. Pneumonia has been consistently produced by intranasal or intratracheal inoculation with porcine strains (Kielstein et al. 1983; Martin et al. 1983; Stellmacher et al. 1983; Rogers et al. 1996), but infection was found to spread consistently to other organs. An acute exudative or interstitial pneumonia with peribronchiolar cellular cuffing and a lobular distribution occurs within 4–8 days of infection. Lesions are fully developed by 8–12 days postinfection and are largely resolved by 4 weeks after infection, although infection may still be present in the lungs. Similar lesions were produced in germfree pigs by Rogers et al. (1996) using a *C. trachomatis*–like isolate from a case of pneumonia. They identified mild multifocal rhinitis and diarrhea in addition to the pneumonic changes. Rogers and Anderson (1996) infected gnotobiotic piglets with isolates from diarrheic pigs to produce diarrhea after 4–5 days which lasted for 8 days. The apical part of the villus appeared to be colonized in the distal jejunum and ileum, with little or no infection in the colon. Villous atrophy developed and this was later followed (7–10 days postinfection) by mild focal serositis.

Contact infections suggest that natural infection is normally less severe and that reinfection after 3–4 weeks results in little or no further disease. This development of immunity is accompanied by development of complement-fixing antibodies to *C. psittaci*, which appear within 2 weeks and remain detectable for a variable period. Information on the time course of antibody detectable by ELISA and indirect immunofluorescence is lacking.

In genital infections, infected semen given to sows has resulted in the birth of weak piglets and continued shedding of chlamydiae for up to 20 months.

CLINICAL SIGNS

Many chlamydial infections are inapparent, but consistent features of respiratory tract and generalized infections include an incubation period of 3–11 days followed by inappetence and a rise in rectal temperature to 39–41°C. Dyspnea, pneumonia and conjunctivitis may occur and may persist for 4–8 days. Evidence of pleurisy or pericarditis may be detected by auscultation, and articular involvement by lameness in one or more joints. In slaughter pigs, polyarthritis associated with synovitis has been reported. Other disturbances of gait include weakness in piglets and nervous signs in pigs of all age groups. Fatal infections are most commonly reported in younger animals.

Diarrhea has been reported to be associated with chlamydial infection (Pospischil and Wood 1987) and can be produced experimentally in gnotobiotic pigs with isolates from diarrheic animals (Rogers and Anderson 1996), but retrospective analysis of cases by Nietfeld et al. (1997) failed to confirm that infection (demonstrated by immunoperoxidase staining of the intestinal epithelium) was statistically associated with diarrhea. Many reports deal with genital tract infection and disturbances in reproduction. In the boar, infection is associated with orchitis, epididymitis, and urethritis; while infections in gilts and sows have resulted in late abortions and the birth of dead or weak piglets. Serologic and isolation studies suggest that many genital tract infections are clinically inapparent.

LESIONS

Lesions in which *C. psittaci* has been demonstrated often contain other agents, and many descriptions of the lesions found in field cases may not take into account the presence of agents such as mycoplasmas or viruses. The large body of work on respiratory disease suggests that lung lesions are distributed posteriorly in most cases, although occasional patches of pneumonia may occur in the anterior lobes (Harris et al. 1984).

Lesions are irregular and raised, are of firm consistency, extend deep into the lung tissue, are limited by lobular boundaries, and are clearly demarcated from adjacent grossly normal tissue. Early lesions are pale red, becoming grayish as they age. Enlarged bronchial lymph nodes may be present. The microscopic findings include thickening of the alveolar septae by capillaries, septal edema, and neutrophils in peribronchial and subepithelial sites. Neutrophils and macrophages are common in the alveolar lumina, and in some areas this exudate occludes terminal bronchioles. Edema and massive epithelial cell shedding have been reported in severely affected lung lobules (Martin et al. 1983). Foci of type II pneumocyte hypertrophy and hyperplasia and vacuolated pneumocytes and bronchial epithelium have been reported in *C. trachomatis*–like experimental infection (Rogers et al. 1996). Peribronchiolar accumulations of plasma cells, lymphocytes, and macrophages are also common. There appears to be no pleurisy in experimental infections, and no gross changes in other organs were reported beyond enlargement of the bron-

chial lymph nodes. Antigen can be demonstrated in bronchial and bronchiolar epithelial cells and in pneumocytes in experimental studies (Rogers et al. 1996) and in field cases (Done et al. 1992).

The other lesions reported to occur in field cases include pericarditis, pleurisy, hemorrhages of kidney and bladder, and enlargement of the spleen. There is little doubt that synovitis accompanies the arthritic changes and that orchitis in boars is accompanied by interstitial edema and tubular degeneration. Aborted piglets may be mummified; stillborn or weak piglets may have lung, liver, or enteric lesions. The organism has been isolated from pseudomembranous colitis in experimental *S. typhimurium* infections (Pospischil and Wood 1987), and extensive studies of pig intestines by immunoperoxidase (Zahn et al. 1995; Pospischil et al. 1996; Szeredi et al. 1996; Nietfeld et al. 1997) confirm the distribution of the inclusions in the small-intestinal villi in piglets and in the large-intestinal intercrypt epithelium in finisher pigs. Lesions in experimentally infected gnotobiotic piglets included watery colon contents with flakes of undigested curd, villous atrophy, lymphangitis, and multifocal necrosis of the apical portion of the villi (Rogers and Anderson 1996).

DIAGNOSIS

The clinical signs of chlamydial infection are not distinctive, but it must be considered as a possible cause of pneumonia, polyarthritis, enteritis, late abortion, stillbirths, mummified piglets, and orchitis. The gross lesions in the lung may be suggestive of chlamydial infection, but any firm diagnosis involves laboratory tests. These are serologic: complement fixation using heat-stable *C. psittaci* antigen, and ELISA using tissue culture antigen (Szeredi et al. 1996); microscopic agglutination (Wilson and Plummer 1966); and indirect immunofluorescence. Complement-fixing antibodies should ideally be found to rise in paired serum samples, but the presence of high levels of antibody (1:256) may be sufficient. As only low levels of complement-fixing antibodies may arise from infections in sites such as the respiratory, enteric, and genital tracts, the absence of high levels of complement-fixing antibody does not rule out chlamydiae as a cause of disease.

Chlamydiae may be detected in smears of discharges or postmortem specimens and in histological specimens after staining by Giemsa's method. The organisms are tiny (0.2–1.0 μm) and are present in large numbers in cells. A more satisfactory method is to use Koster's stain in which a fixed smear is stained for 5 minutes with carbol fuchsin, decolorized for 30 seconds with 0.25% acetic acid, and counterstained for 1 minute with 1% aqueous Loeffler's methylene blue. The chlamydiae appear as clusters of intracellular red dots against a blue background (Figure 50.2). Most specific of all is the

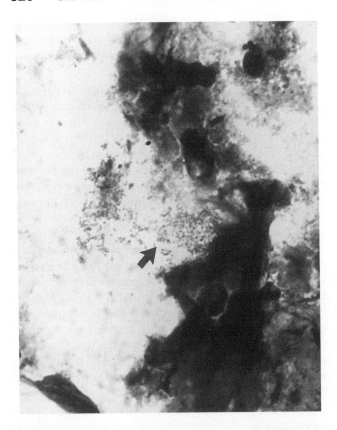

50.2. *Photomicrograph of elementary bodies of* Chlamydia *sp. (arrow) in aborted placenta (original magnification ×1200).*

immunofluorescence test using specific fluorescein-conjugated antibody to *C. psittaci* to demonstrate infected cells. Immunoperoxidase tests have been described (Chasey et al. 1981), and the immunoperoxidase staining of fixed tissue sections is now standard and appears to be the most sensitive method of detection (Szeredi et al. 1996) in tissue. Many laboratories are using PCR tests to confirm the presence of the three species in feces and tissue specimens. Primers include genomic DNA sequences, 16S rRNA gene sequences, *ompA* gene sequences, and plasmid sequences.

Isolation can also be carried out by the inoculation of young mice and of 6- to 8-day fertile hen eggs. More than one subculture may be necessary before infection can be detected. Cell cultures using L929 or McCoy cell lines treated with cycloheximide (1 µg/mL) may be inoculated by centrifugation (Farmer et al. 1982) in tissue culture medium at pH 7.0. Inclusions are at a maximum after 48 hours of incubation at 35–37°C.

Transport media for chlamydiae should contain streptomycin (50–100 mg/L) or gentamicin (10–20 mg/L) with vancomycin (100 µg/mL) and nystatin (25 mg/L). Samples can be stored at 4°C or at −70°C. Handling *C. psittaci* is dangerous, and severe human infections and death can result. Appropriate safety precautions should be observed.

TREATMENT

A number of antimicrobials have some effect on *C. psittaci* in vitro, but the most satisfactory compounds for treatment are the tetracyclines. Treatment for inadequate times may result in relapse; for complete elimination or suppression of infection to the latent state, 21-day treatment should be given at the therapeutic level. Tetracycline, oxytetracycline, and chlortetracycline can all be used in drinking water or feed. Long-acting oxytetracycline injections are useful for treating individual infected animals.

PREVENTION

Pigs should be prevented from coming into contact with infected pigs, other mammalian species, and bird droppings. Infected pigs should be maintained in separate air and drainage spaces from susceptible animals. Any infected breeding stock should be used only after tetracycline treatment or kept with other infected stock in isolation until sufficient uninfected animals are available to replace them. Disinfection with phenols and formalin fumigation will eliminate elementary bodies from buildings.

REFERENCES

Anderson IE, Baxter SIF, Dunbar S, Rae AG, Philips HL, Clarkson MJ, Herring AJ. 1996. Analyses of the genomes of chlamydial isolates from ruminants and pigs support the adoption of the new species *Chlamydia pecorum*. Int J Syst Bacteriol 46:245–251.

Chasey D, Davis P, Dawson M. 1981. Immunoperoxidase detection of *Chlamydia ovis* in experimentally infected cell culture. Br Vet J 137:634–638.

Done SH, McGill I, Spencer Y, Simmons J. 1992. *Chlamydia psittaci* and necrotizing interstitial pneumonia. Proc Int Congr Pig Vet Soc 12:341.

Farmer H, Chalmers WSK, Woolcock PR. 1982. *Chlamydia psittaci* isolated from the eyes of domestic ducks (*Anas platyrhynchos*) with conjunctivitis and rhinitis. Vet Rec 110:59.

Harris JW. 1976. Chlamydial antibodies in pigs in Scotland. Vet Rec 98:505–506.

Harris JW, Hunter AR, Martin DA. 1984. Experimental chlamydial pneumonia in pigs. Comp Immun Microbiol Infect Dis 7:19–26.

Johnson FWA. 1984. Isolation of *C. psittaci* from nasal and conjunctival exudate of a cat. Vet Rec 114:342–344.

Kaltenbroeck B, Kousoulas KG, Storz J. 1993. Structures of and allelic diversity and relationships among the major outer membrane protein (*ompA*) genes of the four chlamydial species. J Bacteriol 175:487–502.

Kaltenbroeck B, Storz J. 1992. Biological properties and genetic analysis of the *ompA* locus in chlamydia isolated from swine. Am J Vet Res 53:1482–1487.

Kielstein P, Stellmacher H, Horsch F, Martin J. 1983. Zur ChlamydienInfektion des Schweines. I. Mitteilung zur experimentellen Chlamydien-Pneumonie des Schweines. Arch Exp Veterinärmed 37:569–586.

Martin J, Kielstein P, Stellmacher P, Horsch F. 1983. Zur Chlamydien Infektion des Schweines. II. Mitteilung: Pathologische-histologische Besonderhect der experimentellen Chlamydien Pneumonie des Schweines. Arch Exp Veterinärmed 37:939–949.

Nietfeld JC, Leslie-Steen P, Zeman DH, Nelson D. 1997. Prevalence of intestinal chlamydial infection in pigs in the Midwest as determined by immunoperoxidase staining. Am J Vet Res 58:260–264.

Pospischil A, Thoma R, Schiller I, Sydler T, and Guscetti, F. 1996. Chlamydia in pigs. Pig J 37:9–13.

Pospischil A, Wood RL. 1987. Intestinal Chlamydia in pigs. Vet Pathol 24:568–570.

Rogers DG, Anderson AA. 1996. Intestinal lesions caused by two swine chlamydia isolates in gnotobiotic pigs. J Vet Diagn Invest 8:433–440.

Rogers DG, Anderson AA, Hogg A, Nielson DL, Huebert MA. 1993. Conjunctivitis and keratoconjunctivitis associated with chlamydias in swine. J Am Vet Med Assoc 203:1321–1323.

Rogers DG, Anderson AA, Hunsaker BD. 1996. Lung and nasal lesions caused by a swine chlamydial isolate in gnotobiotic pigs. J Vet Diagn Invest 8:45–55.

Sorodoc G, Surdan C, Sarateanu D. 1961. Cercetari asupra identificarii virusului pneumoniei enzootice a porcilor. Stud Cerc Inframicrobiol 12 (Suppl):355–364.

Stellmacher H, Kielstein P, Horsch F, Martin J. 1983. Zur Bedeutung der Chlamydien-Infektion des Schweines unter besonder Berucksichtigung der Pneumonien. Monatsh Veterinärmed 38:601–606.

Szeredi L, Schiller I, Sydler T, Guscetti F, Heinen E, Corboz L, Eggenberger E, Jones GE, Pospischil A. 1996. Intestinal chlamydia in finishing pigs. Vet Pathol 33:369–374.

Vasquez-Cisneros C, Wilsmore AJ, Bolle E. 1994. Experimental infections of pregnant sows with ovine chlamydia strains. Vet Microbiol 42:383–387.

Willigan DA, Beamer PD. 1955. Isolation of transmissible agent from pericarditis of swine. J Am Vet Med Assoc 126:118–122.

Wilson MR, Plummer PA. 1966. A survey of pig sera for the presence of antibodies to the P.L.V. group of organisms. J Comp Pathol 76:427–433.

Zahn I, Szeredi L, Schiller I, Straumann Kunz U, Buergi E, Guscetti F, Heinen E, Corboz L, Sydler T, Pospischil A. 1995. Immunologischer nachweis von *Chlamydia psittaci/pecorum* und *Chlamydia trachomatis* im Ferkel Darm. J Vet Med Series B 42:266–276.

Actinobacillus suis

Septicemia and death caused by *Actinobacillus suis* and occasionally by *A. equuli* in suckling and recently weaned pigs have been reported sporadically from several pig-rearing countries (Van Dorssen and Jaartsveld 1962; Cutlip et al. 1972; Windsor 1973; Mair et al. 1974; MacDonald et al. 1976). *A. suis* outbreaks resembling erysipelas have been reported in older pigs and sows in Canada (Miniats et al. 1989), and the organism has also been the cause of disease resembling pleuropneumonia in older pigs in the United States (Yaeger 1996) and the United Kingdom. Most outbreaks occur as sudden death of one or several piglets in one, two, or, rarely, multiple litters in individual herds. Infection with *A. suis* is probably widespread but disease is seldom reported.

ETIOLOGY

A. suis is a gram-negative, nonmotile, nonencapsulated, aerobic, and facultative anaerobic coccobacillus, 0.5–3 μm long and about 0.8 μm in diameter. Filamentous forms occur. Grayish, adherent, circular, translucent colonies measuring 1–2 mm form on blood agar within 24 hours. On horse blood agar, colonies are surrounded by a narrow but distinct zone of alpha hemolysis, and on calf and sheep blood agars, by a wide zone of beta (complete) hemolysis. The organism grows on MacConkey agar. Biochemically, *A. suis* can be differentiated from other related bacteria isolated from pigs by its ability to produce catalase, oxidase, and urease; hydrolysis of esculin; and acid production without gas from arabinose, lactose, salicin, and trehalose, but not from mannitol or sorbitol. Its biochemistry and antigenicity have recently been studied by Bada et al. (1996). Distinction from isolates of *A. pleuropneumoniae* biotype II is difficult but can be achieved biochemically and using DNA analysis. *A.*

equuli differs from *A. suis* by being nonhemolytic; producing acid from mannitol but not from arabinose, cellulose, and salicin; and not splitting esculin. *A. suis* is pathogenic for mice; *A. equuli* is not. *A. suis* and *A. equuli* are killed within 15 minutes at 60°C and are sensitive to most disinfectants. They die out within a few days in culture and pathologic material.

EPIDEMIOLOGY

A. suis can be carried in the tonsils and nostrils of healthy pigs of any age and in the vaginas of apparently healthy sows (Ross et al. 1972). Clinical disease occurs in neonates and suckling pigs up to and just after weaning age, and less commonly in sows and mature swine (Miniats et al. 1989; Sanford et al. 1990). With the separation of pigs and horses in modern farming systems, infection in pigs by *A. equuli* seems to have diminished.

Outbreaks of clinical disease associated with *A. suis* infection occur more frequently in minimal-disease and other high-health-status herds (Miniats et al. 1989; Sanford et al. 1990), possibly because the lack of immunity in these pigs allows virulent *A. suis* organisms to express their pathogenic potential, but the organism can be recovered from herds in which disease is not apparent.

PATHOGENESIS

The pathogenesis of *A. suis* infection has not been defined. Infection probably occurs via the upper respiratory tract, and the disease has been reproduced by intranasal inoculation (Fenwick et al. 1996), although invasion through abrasions in the skin and mucous membranes is also likely. In susceptible animals, septic emboli then spread rapidly to multiple organs and tissues throughout the body and either are trapped in vessels or adhere to vessel walls, forming microcolonies surrounded by areas of hemorrhage and necrosis. Virulence factors of *A. suis* have not been specifically determined, but lipopolysaccharide, polysaccharides in the cell wall, outer-membrane proteins, and, in some strains, a 104 kDa hemolysin (ApxI) are all potential virulence factors likely to be involved in pathogenesis. Antibodies to ApxI have been demonstrated in the sera of pigs which have recovered from experimental infection (Fenwick et al. 1996). Pigs may die within 15 hours of infection.

CLINICAL SIGNS

Sudden death of suckling piglets, 2 days to 4 weeks old, in one or more litters is often the first indication of an outbreak of actinobacillosis. Deaths in piglets are sometimes mistakenly attributed to crushing. Cyanosis, petechial hemorrhages, fever (up to 40°C, 104°F), and panting, sometimes accompanied by shaking and/or paddling, may be seen prior to death in suckling pigs. Congestion of extremities (leading to necrosis of feet, tail, and ears) and swollen joints may occur. In weaned pigs, anorexia, fever, a persistent cough, respiratory distress (Yaeger 1996) and pneumonia are reported; recovered animals may remain unthrifty. In outbreaks in mature animals, fever, round and rhomboid erythematous skin lesions, inappetence, and sudden deaths are characteristic, but mortality is usually low. Metritis, meningitis, and abortion have been reported in sows. The disease may be confused with erysipelas, especially when skin lesions develop, and with pleuropneumonia when respiratory signs are present.

LESIONS

The most striking gross lesions are petechial to ecchymotic hemorrhages in any of the following organs: lung, kidney, heart, liver, spleen, skin, and intestines. The lesions are especially prominent and most frequently seen in the lung, where lobular necrosis and serofibrinous exudates also occur (Figure 50.3). Increased serous or serofibrinous exudates may occur in the thorax and the pericardium. Pleurisy, pericarditis, and miliary abscesses in the lung, liver, skin, mesenteric lymph nodes, and kidney may be seen in older suckling or weaned pigs. The pneumonic lesions may resemble those of pleuropneumonia. Arthritis (Van Dorssen and Jaartsveld 1962; Odin 1994) and valvular endocarditis (Jones and Simmons 1971) have been reported. In mature animals, numerous round, rhomboid, or irregular skin lesions are common.

Histologically, bacterial thromboemboli with accompanying fibrinohemorrhagic necrosis in randomly scattered vessels in the lung, liver, kidney, skin, spleen, heart, pericardium, meninges, and brain are characteristic (Figure 50.4). Bacterial emboli may be surrounded by radiating eosinophilic clublike colonies. These are most obvious in the lung, where there may be large coalescing areas of necrosis.

DIAGNOSIS

Sudden mortality in suckling pigs in individual litters in herds with previous *A. suis* outbreaks usually indicates a new outbreak. The gross lesions of hemorrhages and necrosis in the lung and/or skin and kidney and splenic enlargement are suggestive of *A. suis* infection. In mature pigs, fever, inappetence, and skin lesions resembling erysipelas, especially in herds already vaccinated against erysipelas, should raise a suspicion of *A. suis*. Microscopic lesions consisting of bacterial emboli, necrosis, and inflammatory cells in the lung and other organs are also suggestive. Diagnosis, however, depends on isolation of *A. suis* or *A. equuli* from the lesions. *A. suis* infection should be considered when pleuropneumonia is suspected in herds thought to be free from that disease. In these herds it may cause mild or atypical lung lesions and give rise to antibody to ApxI but not to the cytotoxin of *A. pleuropneumoniae* or to its somatic antigens (Fenwick et al. 1996). *A suis* can usually be isolated from the tonsils of piglets aged 2–10 days in such herds.

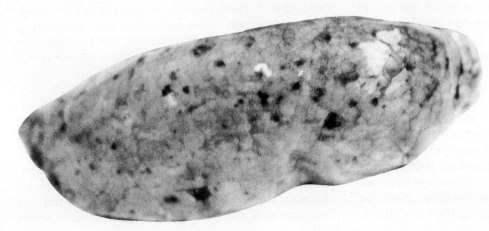

50.3. *Lung of 3-day-old piglet with actinobacillosis. Note the hemorrhages.*

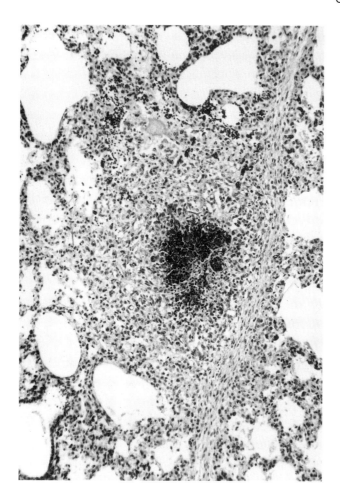

50.4. *Photomicrograph of a microabscess in the lung as shown in Fig. 50.3. Note the microcolonies of bacteria (H&E; original magnification ×110).*

TREATMENT

A. suis is sensitive to most commonly used antibiotics. Since outbreaks in suckling pigs are so acute and unpredictable, however, treatment is usually too late. In older pigs, responses to treatment with ampicillin (5 mg/kg) orally or parenterally, injectable benzathine-procaine penicillin G ($2.25–3.0 \times 10^6$ IU/kg) intramuscularly (IM), injectable procaine penicillin ($1.8–2.4 \times 10^6$ IU/kg) IM, or in-feed medication with oxytetracycline hydrochloride (550 g/ton) and/or streptomycin for periods up to 1 week have all been excellent.

PREVENTION

Autogenous bacterins have not been critically evaluated but have been used in herds with repeated *A. suis* outbreaks with apparent success.

REFERENCES

Bada R, Mittal KR, Higgins R. 1996. Biochemical and antigenic relationships between porcine and equine strains of *Actinobacillus suis*. Vet Microbiol 51:393–396.

Cutlip RC, Amtower WC, Zinober MR. 1972. Septic embolic actinobacillosis of swine: A case report and laboratory reproduction of the disease. Am J Vet Res 33:1621–1626.

Fenwick B, Rider M, Chengappa M, Montarz J. 1996. Cross protective immunity between *Actinobacillus suis* and *A. pleuropneumoniae*. Proc Int Congr Pig Vet Soc 14:373.

Jones JET, Simmons JR. 1971. Endocarditis in the pig caused by *Actinobacillus equuli*: A field and an experimental case. Br Vet J 127:25–29.

MacDonald DW, Hewitt MP, Wilton GS, Rawluk S, Childs L. 1976. *Actinobacillus suis* infections in Alberta swine, 1973–1975: Pathology and bacteriology. Can Vet J 17:251–254.

Mair NS, Randall CJ, Thomas GW, Harbourne JF, McCrea CT, Cowl KP. 1974. *Actinobacillus suis* infection in pigs: A report of four outbreaks and two sporadic cases. J Comp Pathol 84:113–119.

Miniats OP, Spinato MT, Sanford SE. 1989. *Actinobacillus suis* septicemia in mature swine: Two outbreaks resembling erysipelas. Can Vet J 30:943–947.

Odin M. 1994. Les infections a *Actinobacillus suis* au Quebec: une étude retrospective de 22 cas. Méd Vét du Quebec 24:61–65.

Ross RF, Hall JE, Orning AP, Dale SE. 1972. Characterization of an Actinobacillus isolated from the sow vagina. Int J Syst Bacteriol 22:39–46.

Sanford SE, Josephson GKA, Rehmtulla AJ, Tilker AME. 1990. *Actinobacillus suis* infection in pigs in southwestern Ontario. Can Vet J 31:443–447.

Van Dorssen CA, Jaartsveld FHJ. 1962. *Actinobacillus suis* (novo species), a bacterium occurring in swine. Tijdschr Diergeneeskd 87:450–458.

Windsor RS. 1973. *Actinobacillus equuli* infection in a litter of pigs and a review of previous reports on similar infections. Vet Rec 92:178–180.

Yaeger MJ. 1996. An outbreak of *Actinobacillus suis* septicemia in grow/finish pigs. J Vet Diagnost Invest 8:381–383.

Yeasts

Yeasts are fungi that are normally single celled but can form filaments (or pseudohyphae). Some can sporulate to produce resistant spores. They occur in the food of the pig and in dusts. Some species are commonly found on the skin and mucous membranes. In certain situations, yeasts of a number of species (but principally *Candida albicans*) may be isolated from inflammatory lesions of the oral cavity, gastrointestinal tract, urogenital tract, and skin. Their isolation from such lesions is often associated with use of therapeutic antimicrobials, especially in piglets. Yeasts belonging to the genus *Malassezia,* possibly *M. pachydermatis,* are present in the ears and on the skin of pigs, but their role in disease at these sites is not known. They can reach high numbers when skin or ear lesions develop, but so little is currently known about them and their role in disease that they will not be considered further.

Yeasts may also form a major part of the diet of the

pig, as either yeast wastes from brewing or distilling or yeast grown and treated specifically as a component of rations. These yeasts can provide high protein and, in particular, high lysine. Traces of paraffin waxes have been found in the fat of pigs fed on yeasts grown on that substrate, and there are some reports of diarrhea and increased kidney weights in yeast-fed pigs. Most reports indicate that inclusion of yeasts in the ration does not adversely affect the health of pigs.

ETIOLOGY

Yeasts identified in infections in pigs belong to a number of genera. Those of the genus *Candida* are most commonly isolated, although species of *Torulopsis, Trichosporon, Rhodotorula, Pichia, Pityrosporum,* and *Cryptococcus* have been recorded. *Cryptococcus neoformans* has been isolated from cryptococcosis in pigs, but the disease is rare in this species and occurs only where the organism is commonly found in other livestock.

Candida albicans is the species of *Candida* most frequently reported; but *C. tropicalis, C. pseudotropicalis, C. brumptii, C. sloofii, C. rugosa, C. lipolytica, C. krusei,* and *C. scottii* have been isolated from lesions or feces of apparently healthy pigs. Since *C. albicans* is associated most frequently with specific lesions, both it and its relationship to these lesions will be described here.

Candida spp. are spherical cells, 2.5–6 μm in diameter. They reproduce by budding (blastospores) and chlamydospores, which bud from filaments (or pseudohyphae) on chlamydospore agar, particularly under reduced oxygen tension at 25°C (Carter 1979). Pseudohyphae and oval yeast forms are found in lesions. *Candida* spp. grow readily on Sabouraud agar, malt agar, and often on blood agar incubated aerobically. They form 1–2 mm, creamy white, opaque, circular colonies within 24–48 hours at 37°C and within 2–4 days at 25°C. *C. albicans* produces chlamydospores and germ tubes but no pellicle when grown in broth and ferments glucose, maltose, and galactose but not sucrose or lactose. It is not known to produce toxins, although there have been suggestions that it can produce keratolytic enzymes in the presence of glucose.

EPIDEMIOLOGY

C. albicans has been identified in the bedding, feed, and water supplies of pigs. It occurs on the skin and in the oral cavity, stomach, and intestines of normal pigs in small numbers. It can be shed in the feces and exhaled in droplets by animals with oral infections. It may be isolated from the feces of birds, rodents, and other animal species and may cause disease in those species, which may become sources of the organism for pigs. Organisms in the environment may multiply in moist conditions in the presence of suitable substrates such as spilled meal or garbage.

PATHOGENESIS

C. albicans appears to colonize debilitated skin surfaces and lesions on other mucous surfaces. The predisposing factors appear to include the effects of artificial rearing of piglets (Osborne et al. 1960) and chronic enteritis often associated with treatment with broad-spectrum antimicrobials. Gastric ulcers appear to be colonized by yeasts rather than initiated by them, and cutaneous candidiasis often results from exposure to continually warm moist conditions that are accompanied by poor hygiene and food residues (Reynolds et al. 1968).

Invasion of mucous surfaces appears to follow accumulation of yeast forms on the debilitated surface and develops with pseudohyphal invasion of the superficial layers of the epithelium. Systemic invasion is rare and the inflammatory response to infection is slight.

CLINICAL SIGNS

Yeasts have been implicated in chronic gastroenteritis in piglets, gastric ulceration, and cutaneous and oropharyngeal infections. Piglets are often 3–5 days old (more commonly, 7–14 days) before yeast infection complicates the underlying problem. The clinical signs of gastroenteritis complicated by yeasts are not specific, but there is often a history of dullness, inappetence, vomiting, and chronic diarrhea that may be grayish or blackish depending on the diet and has failed to respond to the use of broad-spectrum antibiotics such as tetracyclines. Piglets may die after 10–14 days of illness. In many cases there are characteristic yellowish white, circular, 2–5 mm lesions on the tongue and hard palate, which resemble colonies of *C. albicans* on artificial media. When scraped off, no macroscopic changes are seen beneath them. Cutaneous candidiasis often presents as a moist gray exudate on the surface of the skin of the abdomen with little or no effect on the hair in early lesions, but later resulting in hair loss and thickening of the skin. Affected animals are often kept in moist conditions and exposed to food residues.

LESIONS

Piglets with candidiasis are often in poor condition with chronic diarrhea. There may be lesions in the oral cavity and throughout the gastrointestinal tract. These consist of white specks and circular patches 2–5 mm in diameter on the dorsum of the tongue, less frequently on the pharynx, and sometimes on the soft or hard palate. These patches may coalesce to form larger areas of pseudomembranous material that may occlude the lumen of the esophagus. The lesions may extend down the esophagus and may be seen on the gastric mucosa. There may be small hemorrhages in the cardiac area and white pseudomembranous lesions in the esophageal area. Descriptions of the lesions distal to the stomach are rarely published, but in heavily infected animals they resemble those of chronic enteritis, with villous atrophy and thickening of the mucosa. When the white pseudomembranous material is removed, congestion of the mucosal surface may be seen, but ulceration is rare. In older pigs, *C. albicans* may be isolated from gastric ulcers, but these do not differ grossly from uninfected ones. Gross lesions may be seen in cutaneous candidiasis and include a grayish surface deposit, thickening of the skin, and hair loss.

Microscopic lesions include the presence of numerous yeasts on the epithelial surface, with pseudohyphal filaments visible as 1.5–2.0 µm deeply staining threads in the epithelium. In lesions on the tongue, yeast cells and pseudohyphae may be seen in cavities beneath the papillae. They may also be present in large numbers in the periphery of infected gastric ulcers. Degenerative changes are frequently present in the infected epithelium. They include desquamation of epithelial cells, capillary dilation, edema of the submucosa or dermis (depending on the epithelial surface attached), and presence of inflammatory cells. These are neutrophils in the early lesions, later (in 4- to 5-day-old lesions) accompanied by eosinophils, macrophages, plasma cells, and lymphocytes.

DIAGNOSIS

In piglets the appearance of the white 2–5 mm lesions in the oral cavity may suggest that candidiasis is present, but diarrhea and association of infection with gastric ulceration may not be identified on clinical grounds. Skin changes may also suggest a diagnosis of candidiasis. A history of chronic enteritis and broad-spectrum antibiotic use or housing in moist conditions is often suggestive of candidiasis.

Confirmation of diagnosis is based on demonstration of the organism concerned in the lesions or, in life, isolation of large numbers from the feces. The presence of yeasts in lesions of the intestine may be established by their demonstration in Gram-stained smears in which oval or round, gram-positive, often budding, 2.5–6 µm cells may be seen (Figure 50.5). Similar bodies may be seen in histological sections stained by hematoxylin and eosin or, more easily, stained by periodic acid-Schiff or silver stains such as Grocott's (Figure 50.6). None of these allow the complete identification of the organism.

Yeasts may be isolated using Sabouraud's agar with or without chloramphenicol (Carter 1979). Some, such as *C. albicans*, will grow readily on horse blood agar. Incubation at 25°C yields colonies 1–2 mm in diameter after 3–4 days, but incubation at 37°C can allow colonies to be identified within 24–48 hours. The genera can be separated using characters such as shape of the cells, presence or absence of pseudomycelium, presence or absence of capsule, production of chlamydospores, ability to split urea, and other characters (Carter 1979). Many yeast species may be identified in culture using commercial biochemical strips such as the API Yeast series.

Isolation of large numbers of yeasts from lesions may confirm a diagnosis of candidiasis, but their isolation in small numbers from the skin, vagina, or feces and intestines of clinically normal pigs may not be significant.

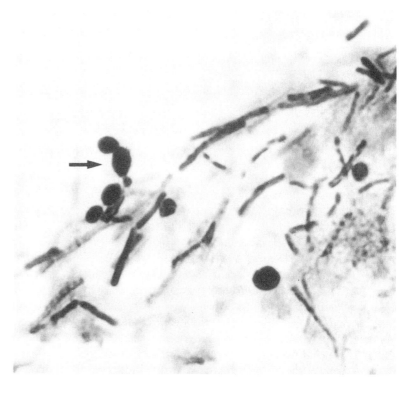

50.5. Photomicrograph of yeast cells (arrow) from the ileal mucosa in a 10-day-old piglet (Gram; original magnification ×1200).

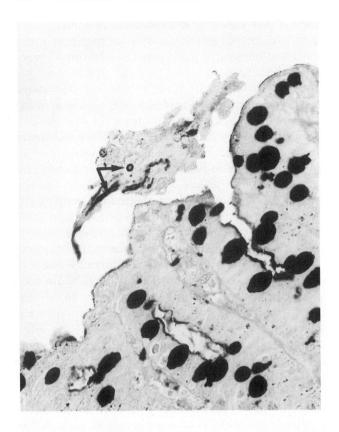

50.6. *Photomicrograph of yeast cells and pseudohyphae adjacent to the ileal mucosa in a 10-day-old piglet (Grocott; original magnification ×400).*

TREATMENT

C. albicans and other yeasts are sensitive in vitro to a number of compounds such as nystatin, miconazole, and amphotericin B, but only nystatin and ampho-tericin B have been used in treatment (Osborne et al. 1960). Nystatin suppressed the clinical signs but did not eliminate infection. Amphotericin B may be effective in young piglets given at a rate of 0.5 mg/kg twice daily. In many instances, correction of underlying disease or husbandry factors is sufficient. Cleaning up waste food and providing a dry environment caused resolution of cutaneous candidiasis (Reynolds et al. 1968). Treatment should also include discontinuation of the use of broad-spectrum antibiotics and their replacement with narrow-spectrum ones if they are a factor in yeast colonization. Animals with cutaneous candidiasis may also be scrubbed with suitable detergent or with hexetidine-based shampoos.

PREVENTION

Pigs should be maintained in warm, dry, clean conditions, and accumulations of moist fermenting food should be prevented. Enteric diseases in piglets should be treated with appropriate antimicrobials, and lengthy treatment with broad-spectrum antibiotics should be avoided. Disinfection of pens and pen fittings can be carried out using formaldehyde vapor or 2% formaldehyde; cleaning and drying of the pens will reduce levels of yeasts to normal background levels.

REFERENCES

Carter GR. 1979. Diagnostic Procedures in Veterinary Bacteriology and Mycology, 3d ed. Springfield: Charles C. Thomas, chap. 30.

Osborne AD, McCrae MR, Manners MJ. 1960. Moniliasis in artificially reared pigs and its treatment with nystatin. Vet Rec 72:237–241.

Reynolds IM, Miner P, Smith RE. 1968. Cutaneous candidiasis on swine. J Am Vet Med Assoc 152:182–186.

Yersinias

A number of species of *Yersinia* have been isolated from pigs, and reports of association between infection and clinical disease are increasing. *Y. enterocolitica* has increasingly become recognized as a cause of human food poisoning and enteritis since the late 1960s, and the pig is an important source. There are reports in the literature of many surveys of pig carcasses, offal, and feces for the presence of *Y. enterocolitica* (Doyle et al. 1981; Schiemann and Fleming 1981; Hunter et al. 1983). Results of these surveys show that infection is distributed worldwide in pigs, and serotypes considered pathogenic to humans are commonly present. This relationship to human disease has stimulated a number of reports of pathogenic determinants (Mosimbale and Gyles 1982) that have been demonstrated in *Y. enterocolitica* in both porcine and human isolates, and it seems clear from the work of Kwaga and Iversen (1993) that the pig and human strains are identical. Further reports deal with the antigenic relationships between *Yersinia* spp. and *Brucella* spp., since infections with certain strains of the former can cause interference with serologic tests for both *B. abortus* and *B. suis*. This interference is described in Chapter 35.

Infection in pigs is usually inapparent, but *Y. pseudotuberculosis* and *Y. enterocolitica* have been isolated from pigs with fever, enteritis, and diarrhea.

ETIOLOGY

Yersinias are aerobic or facultatively anaerobic, gramnegative coccobacilli (or short rods), 1.2 μm in length and 0.5–1.0 μm in diameter. They are nonmotile at 37°C, but some are motile at lower temperatures. Species isolated from pigs include *Y. pseudotuberculosis*, *Y. pseudotuberculosis* subsp. *pestis* (the plague bacillus), *Y. enterocolitica*, *Y. intermedia*, *Y. fredrikensii*, and *Y. kristensenii*. Only two species (*Y. pseudotuberculosis* and *Y. enterocolitica*) have yet been associated with clinical disease in pigs.

Yersinias may be isolated in routine media, upon which they appear as grayish 1–2 mm colonies within 24–48 hours and as similar-sized non-lactose-fermenting colonies on MacConkey agar. The species are distinguished by biochemical tests. *Y. pseudotuberculosis* is motile at 22°C, grows on citrate media at 22°C, splits urea, and does not ferment sucrose or raffinose but does ferment mannose. *Y. pseudotuberculosis* subsp. *pestis* is negative for all these characters. *Y. enterocolitica* is also motile and splits urea but ferments sucrose and does not grow on citrate or ferment mannose. Individual species can be divided into biotypes and serotypes. Capsules, attachment antigens, and enterotoxins have been described in organisms of this genus.

Y. enterocolitica has been subdivided into at least 46 O groups and at least 5 biotypes. Of these, most human infections are associated with biotype 2, O9 and biotype 4, O3. Biotype 1, O8 is also associated with some human infections. *Y. enterocolitica* organisms of a number of O groups have been recorded from pigs. The actual O groups isolated may vary from one part of a country to another (Schiemann and Fleming 1981) but include O3, O5, O6, O7, O8, O9, O13, O18, and O46.

EPIDEMIOLOGY

Y. enterocolitica is found throughout the world and has been recorded from pigs in many countries (Bockemuhl et al. 1979; Cantoni et al. 1979; Barcellos and Castro 1981; Doyle et al. 1981; Schiemann and Fleming 1981; Hunter et al. 1983). Infection may not be general, since not all herds are infected (Christensen 1980). It persists on the tonsils of infected pigs for long periods and is shed in the feces of infected pigs for up to 30 weeks. It has been shown to be transmitted to human food and elsewhere on farms by flies (Fukushima et al. 1979). Feed has been found to be infected, and studies of the dissemination of infection in pig facilities (Fukushima et al. 1983) indicate that infection is transmitted from contaminated pens, in which infection can persist for 3 weeks. Other studies suggest that feces can remain infected for up to 12 weeks and that, in suitable substrates, the organism may multiply at 20–22°C. It appears that transmission from pig to pig is via fecal contamination of accommodation, water, and feed.

Y. pseudotuberculosis is less commonly demonstrated in America than in Europe or Japan and is less commonly identified in pigs than *Y. enterocolitica*. It is commonly found in rodents, which probably represent the main source of infection for pigs.

Y. pseudotuberculosis subsp. *pestis* may infect wild pigs in California, presumably from infection present in rodents (Clark et al. 1983).

PATHOGENESIS

Y. enterocolitica has been shown to infect pigs orally, to multiply and be found in the feces within 2–3 weeks of infection, and to disappear from the feces within 30 weeks (Fukushima et al. 1984). No clinical signs or lesions were described and none were found following infection of 6 pigs with the isolate obtained from the clinical outbreak described above. Experimental studies by Nielsen et al. (1996) have confirmed that infection of the feces may be found between 5 and 21 days after infection and that tonsillar carriage persists longer. A serum antibody response develops by 19 days after infection and has disappeared by 70 days postinfection. Studies in suckling mice have indicated that 10 of the 12 pig isolates tested produced enterotoxin and that one isolate could produce fluid in piglet gut loops. The Sereny test for invasiveness was negative in typical pig strains (Mosimbale and Gyles 1982). Pig isolates harbor the virulence plasmid (Kwaga and Iversen 1993) and possess the capsular material considered essential for pathogenicity and detected using the Congo red magnesium oxalate test. Studies by Erwerth and Natterman (1987) suggest that oral infection is followed by establishment of infection in the tonsils and the development of enteritis in the ileum and large intestine. Similar colonization was reported by Schiemann (1988) and has also been reproduced by Shu et al. (1995a, b) and Shu et al. (1997), who demonstrated that small-intestinal infection in piglets led to microabscesses at the base of the villi and to reductions in the levels of intestinal lactases (Shu et al. 1997) and depressed growth (Shu et al. 1995b).

CLINICAL SIGNS

Clinical disease has been associated only with *Y. enterocolitica* and *Y. pseudotuberculosis*. *Y. pseudotuberculosis* subsp. *pestis* is clearly capable of producing serologic reactions (Clark et al. 1983), but no clinical disease has been described.

Y. enterocolitica was isolated in profuse culture from outbreaks of diarrhea in weaned pigs from which no other infectious agents could be recovered. Mild fever (to 39.4°C, 103°F) was present, and the diarrhea contained no blood or mucus and was blackish in color. Clinical signs resembling those described above have been seen in animals receiving tylosin or lincomycin. Bloodstained mucus may also be found in some diarrheic feces and on solid feces passed by penmates. The organism has been isolated from the rectal mucosa in cases of rectal stricture. Experimental infections in suckling piglets result in anorexia, vomiting, diarrhea, and reduction in weight gain (Shu et al. 1995a).

Y. pseudotuberculosis has been associated with clinical signs by Morita et al. (1968), who described an outbreak in Japan. Affected pigs were dull and showed inappetence; bloodstained diarrhea; and edema of eyelids, lower face, and dependent parts of the abdomen. Diarrhea was also observed by Barcellos and Castro (1981). Neef and Lysons (1994) were able to reproduce diarrhea in 4 of 9 pigs infected with a colitis isolate of *Y. pseudotuberculosis*. The organism has been isolated from pigs with the rectal stricture syndrome.

LESIONS

The lesions caused by *Y. enterocolitica* infection have been described in detail by Erwerth and Natterman (1987) and consist of catarrhal enteritis in the small and large intestines. Microcolonies of the organism can be seen in the disrupted intestinal epithelium, and in pigs with rectal lesions, bacterial penetration and inflammation reach the muscularis mucosae. Shu et al. (1995a) confirmed this finding for the small intestine and describe the presence of microabscesses at the bases of the villi.

Lesions of *Y. pseudotuberculosis* have been described (Morita et al. 1968). They resembled those of pseudotuberculosis in other species, with miliary gray-white spots on the liver and spleen and swollen gray-white mesenteric lymph nodes. A catarrhal and diphtheritic change was described in the colon and rectum, as edema and ascites also occurred. Microscopic lesions included necrotic foci containing masses of bacteria surrounded by a thin layer of granulation tissue in the lung, liver, spleen, mesenteric lymph nodes, and lymphoid follicles of the large intestine. Similar findings were made by Neef and Lysons (1994), who noted the penetration of the microabscesses into the lamina propria. *Y. pseudotuberculosis* was isolated from the liver, spleen, lungs, duodenum, rectum, and mesenteric lymph nodes by Morita et al. (1968). *Y. pseudotuberculosis* can also be isolated from inflammatory lesions of the rectal mucosa similar to those described above.

DIAGNOSIS

The clinical signs are not distinctive, but the occurrence of mild fever and blood and mucus on solid feces can indicate yersinia infection in the absence of swine dysentery. Where rectal stricture is common, the organism may be responsible for diarrhea in younger age groups, and the organism may be involved in the "colitis" syndrome of mild diarrhea in growing pigs. Diagnosis of infection with most *Yersinia* spp. in pigs depends upon isolation of the organism and its identification. Serology has been used to identify *Y. pseudotuberculosis* subsp. *pestis* (Clark et al. 1983), but most accounts of yersinia infections suggest that although agglutinating antibody may result from infection, isolation methods are adequate for diagnosis. The indirect ELISA developed by Nielsen et al. (1996) for *Y. enterocolitica* O3 may be of value in the field but may not detect infections by other serotypes. *Y. pseudotuberculosis* can readily be isolated at 37°C on blood and MacConkey agar from lesions of the type described by Morita et al. (1968) and so may *Y. enterocolitica*. Most isolation methods for all yersinias involve use of a cold enrichment technique in which tissues or samples under investigation are placed in phosphate-buffered saline M/15 at pH 7.6 at 4°C for 6 weeks, with subculture at 3 and 6 weeks onto a selective medium (Hunter et al. 1983). The selective medium may be MacConkey agar incubated at 30°C or a specific medium for *Y. enterocolitica*. These methods may be used for direct isolation. Media are described by Hunter et al. (1983) and six are reviewed by Catteau et al. (1983). Recent studies by food microbiologists have resulted in a range of tests, such as the immunomagnetic separation and polymerase chain reaction technique of Rasmussen et al. (1995), which can detect as few as 200 cells per gram of feces.

TREATMENT

There is at present no general indication for the treatment of yersinia infections, since clinical signs are so rare. In vitro studies suggest that isolates are often sensitive to oxytetracycline, furazolidone, neomycin, sulfonamides, and spectinomycin. Tetracyclines have been used in feed to eliminate infection and clinical signs.

PREVENTION

Since spread of *Y. enterocolitica* from pig to pig appears to occur from contact with feces, hygiene coupled with housing groups of pigs in separate drainage areas will reduce infection. Control of flies and rodents and disinfection of pens before restocking will reduce transmission. Morita et al. (1968) found that pseudotuberculosis could be prevented by excluding birds and rodents. Current requirements for the control of *Y. enterocolitica* in pig meat concentrate on the removal of the tonsil at slaughter, so control programs have not been developed for the live animal. Control may be required when serologic cross-reaction in the brucellosis test is identified in herds selling breeding stock. The findings of Nielsen et al. (1996) suggest that serologic reactions peak at 33 days postinfection and have disappeared by 70 days postinfection, so pigs may be treated or managed at the time of infection to prevent the development of antibody or held and retested after antibody levels have declined.

REFERENCES

Barcellos DESN de, Castro AFP de. 1981. Isolation of *Yersinia pseudotuberculosis* from diarrheas in pigs. Br Vet J 137:95–96.

Bockemuhl J, Schmitt H, Roth J, Saupe E. 1979. Die jahreszeitliche Haufigkeit der Ausscheidung von *Yersinia enterocolitica* im Kot gesunder Schlachtschweine. Zentralbl Bakteriol (Orig A) 224:494–505.

Cantoni C, D'Aubert S, Buogo A, Guizzardi F. 1979. *Yersinia enterocolitica* nelli feci di suino. Arch Vet Ital 30:134–136.

Catteau M, Krembel C, Wauters G. 1983. Isolement de *Yersinia enterocolitica* de langues de porc. Rec Méd Vét 159:89–94.

Christensen SG. 1980. *Yersinia enterocolitica* in Danish pigs. J Appl Bacteriol 48:377–382.

Clark RK, Jessup DA, Hird DW, Rupanner R, Meyer ME. 1983. Serologic survey of California wild hogs for antibody against selected zoonotic disease agents. J Am Vet Med Assoc 183:1248–1259.

Doyle MP, Hugdahl MB, Taylor SL. 1981. Isolation of *Yersinia enterocolitica* from porcine tongues. Appl Environ Microbiol 41:661–666.

Erwerth W, Natterman H. 1987. Histopathologische Untersuchengen bei der experimentellen oralen *Yersinia enterocolitica* Infektion des Jung-schweines. Monatsh Vet 42:319–324.

Fukushima H, Ito Y, Saito K, Tsubokura M, Otsuki K. 1979. Role of the fly in the transport of *Yersinia enterocolitica*. Appl Environ Microbiol 38:1009–1010.

Fukushima H, Nakamura R, Ito Y, Saito K. 1984. Ecological studies of *Yersinia enterocolitica*. II. Experimental infection with *Y. enterocolitica* in pigs. Vet Microbiol 9:375–389.

Fukushima H, Nakamura R, Ito Y, Saito K, Tsubokura M, Otsuki K. 1983. Ecological studies of *Y. enterocolitica* in pigs. I. Dissemination of *Y. enterocolitica* in pigs. Vet Microbiol 8:469–483.

Hunter D, Hughes S, Fox E. 1983. Isolation of *Yersinia enterocolitica* from pigs in the United Kingdom. Vet Rec 112:322–323.

Kwaga J, Iversen JO. 1993. Plasmids and outer membrane proteins of *Yersinia enterocolitica* and related species of swine origin. Vet Microbiol 36:205–214.

Morita M, Nakamatsu M, Goto M. 1968. Pathological studies on pseudotuberculosis rodentium. III. Spontaneous swine cases. Jpn J Vet Sci 30:233–239.

Mosimbale F, Gyles CL. 1982. The pathogenicity of *Yersinia enterocolitica* strains isolated from various sources for four test systems. Can J Comp Med 46:70–75.

Neef NA, Lysons RJ. 1994. Pathogenicity of a strain of *Yersinia pseudotuberculosis* isolated from a pig with porcine colitis syndrome. Vet Rec 135:58–63.

Nielsen B, Heisel C, Wingstrand A. 1996. Time course of the serological response to *Yersinia enterocolitica* O:3 in experimentally infected pigs. Vet Microbiol 48:293–303.

Rasmussen HN, Rasmussen OF, Christensen H, Olsen JE. 1995. Detection of *Yersinia enterocolitica* O:3 in fecal samples and tonsil swabs from pigs using immunomagnetic separation and polymerase chain reaction. J Appl Bacteriol 78:563–568.

Schiemann DA. 1988. The pathogenicity of *Yersinia enterocolitica* for piglets. Can J Vet Res 52:325–330.

Schiemann DA, Fleming CA. 1981. *Yersinia enterocolitica* isolated from throats of swine in eastern and western Canada. Can J Microbiol 27:1326–1333.

Shu D, Simpson HV, Xu RJ, Mellor DJ, Reynolds GW, Alley MR, Fenwick SG, Marshall R B. 1995a. Impact of *Yersinia enterocolitica* enteritis on disaccharidase activity and small intestinal morphology in colostrum-deprived newborn piglets. New Zealand Vet J 45:27–36.

Shu D, Simpson HV, Xu RJ, Mellor DJ, Reynolds G. W, Marshall RB. 1995b. Effects of *Yersinia enterocolitica* infection on growth of the body and internal organs in newborn colostrum-deprived piglets. Biology of the Neonate 67:360–369.

———. 1997. Experimental infection of newborn piglets with *Yersinia enterocolitica*: An animal model of enteritis. New Zealand Vet J 43:50–56.

Staphylococci

Staphylococci are ubiquitous. They are present on every pig farm and involved in a wide range of lesions in pigs of all ages. The most easily recognized are those of exudative epidermitis caused by *Staphylococcus hyicus* and described in Chapter 39. Few, if any, of the other lesions can be unequivocally identified as being staphylococcal on clinical grounds; in the majority, staphylococcal involvement must be confirmed by laboratory means. In addition to their association with pig disease, some of the staphylococci that infect the pig, notably *S. aureus*, may be involved in human food poisoning if carcasses are contaminated or abscesses are present.

ETIOLOGY

Staphylococci are gram-positive, 0.5–1.5 μm in diameter, forming grapelike clusters when grown in serum broth or seen in pus. They grow primarily in aerobic conditions but can also grow anaerobically, are oxidase-negative but produce catalase, and metabolize a wide variety of sugars. They produce a wide range of enzymes and some toxins. The species are distinguished by the presence of enzymes such as coagulase, DNAase, he-

molysins, and phosphatase and by the ability to utilize a variety of sugars. Major species reported from the pig are *S. aureus*, *S. hyicus*, and *S. epidermidis*, although *S. saprophyticus* has also been described.

S. aureus is the only species apart from *S. hyicus* to be consistently isolated from lesions in pigs. It forms yellowish-white, opaque, circular, domed colonies, 1–2 mm in diameter, on blood agar after 24 hours of incubation. These colonies may be surrounded by a zone of complete hemolysis, caused by alpha hemolysins, on horse blood agar. On sheep blood agar, the ring of complete hemolysis is surrounded by a wider area of incomplete hemolysis caused by beta hemolysins; this becomes complete on cooling of the plate. In addition to these hemolysins, the organism produces coagulase, DNAase, proteinases, hyaluronidase, and toxins that include the alpha toxin and the enterotoxins. Both have been demonstrated in strains of porcine origin (Engvall and Schwan 1983); protein A (Takeuchi et al. 1995) and polysaccharide capsules are also present. Isolates of *S. aureus* can be identified by phage typing and plasmid profiling, and those of public health significance may readily be traced. *S. aureus* is fairly resistant to drying but is readily inactivated by heat. It is sensitive to a wide range of disinfectants, such as phenols, hypochlorites, iodine, and iodophors.

EPIDEMIOLOGY

S. aureus is widely distributed in the environment and has been recovered from pig feces, food, water following contamination of drinkers, pen floors and walls, and the air in pig facilities. The organism can be isolated from a wide range of hosts, including birds, rodents, dogs, cats, and humans. The extent to which isolates from lesions in pigs are of nonporcine origin is not yet known. Porcine strains capable of enterotoxin production have been identified on carcasses and represent a source of infection or possible food poisoning to humans (Engvall and Schwan 1983).

The pig is probably the major source of infection for other pigs; *S. aureus* can be isolated from the skin, oral cavity, upper respiratory tract, prepuce, vagina, and gut of healthy pigs on a very wide scale. Transmission of the organism may be by aerosol to the upper respiratory tract, directly by skin contact, or indirectly by contact with contaminated walls or fittings. Ingestion of *S. aureus* from food, contaminated water, or litter is common. Venereal contact may be responsible for some genital infections; local invasion of the mammary gland, navel, and skin lesions is common.

PATHOGENESIS

S. aureus appears to multiply on damaged mucosal surfaces or skin and can invade to cause bacteremia. In some cases, such as neonatal septicemia, animals may become fevered and die, but bacteremia usually leads to formation of multiple abscesses. These may occur in bones to give osteomyelitis; in joints; on the heart valves to give vegetative endocarditis; and in the liver, kidney, or lymph nodes. Vegetative endocarditis may give rise to septic emboli that cause abscess formation and infarction in the kidney. Most of these systemic infections occur in neonates or piglets and take 7–10 days to develop. They are also present in apparently normal pigs at slaughter. Abscesses contain neutrophils and microcolonies of bacteria in all stages of multiplication and heal by fibrosis.

Mastitis, vaginitis, and metritis appear to result from ascending infection. Abortion has been associated with the demonstration of serum antibody to alpha hemolysin in the sow (Kohler and Wille 1980), but the importance of this and other toxins in abortion is not known.

In enteric infection, experimental studies have shown that staphylococcal enterotoxin A will cause emesis within 90–180 minutes when given orally in doses of 40–50 μg (Taylor et al. 1982). Larger doses can cause behavioral changes, including inappetence, restlessness, and staggering. The piglet is clearly susceptible, but the ability of enteric staphylococcal infections to produce enterotoxin in vivo is not known.

CLINICAL SIGNS

The presence of *S. aureus* infection cannot readily be suspected on clinical grounds. *S. aureus* has been isolated from a wide variety of syndromes. Most of these occur in individual animals, and disease rarely spreads from animal to animal. It can cause neonatal septicemia and is often identified in small, hairy, stunted piglets of 7–10 days of age with umbilical abscesses, polyarthritis, and signs of cardiac enlargement due to vegetative endocarditis. It is a cause of subcutaneous abscesses associated with abrasions and foot lesions, especially in piglets. These often result in arthritis of the distal phalangeal joints, enlargement of the hoof, and sinus formation at the coronary band. Creamy pus is often seen to exude from the abscesses.

S. aureus has been isolated from enteritis in piglets and in older animals and from the rectal mucosa of animals with lesions of rectal stricture. No particular features of diarrhea are associated with staphylococci except that the enteritis is often chronic and antibiotic treatment may have been given. The organism is also present in a small percentage of cases of mastitis and has been isolated from pigs with metritis and agalactia. The only reason to suspect staphylococcal involvement may be the presence of a creamy white or bloodstained pus, but this often contains other organisms. It has also been isolated from aborted fetuses and placentas (Kohler and Wille 1980).

LESIONS

No gross lesions may be seen in piglet septicemia. In chronic infections, an inflamed mucosa may be associated with staphylococcal infection, but there is no specific feature that allows their identification with staphylococcal infection. Abscesses may occur in the umbilicus, liver, lungs, lymph nodes, spleen, kidneys, joints, and bones in osteomyelitis; bone abscesses may give rise to pathologic fractures, especially when in the vertebrae. Body cavities (peritoneal cavity, pericardial cavity, uterine lumen) may contain pus, especially in young animals, following umbilical infection. *S. aureus* is only one cause of such lesions. Both gross and microscopic lesions of mastitis may be found in the mammary glands, and in some cases fibrosis may be considerable. Occasionally, a granulomatous mass with fibrosis may be found in the abdominal cavity of piglets that have died after castration. In all cases, confirmation that the lesions are staphylococcal depends on demonstration of the organisms.

DIAGNOSIS

The clinical signs resulting from multiple abscess formation in individual pigs may be suggestive, and similar suspicions may arise from the postmortem findings.

Confirmation of involvement of staphylococci rather than *Arcanobacterium pyogenes* or streptococci in abscesses and arthritis is obtained from Gram-stained smears of the pus in which gram-positive cocci may be seen singly or in clusters. Only the isolation of staphylococci in culture confirms that they are involved. *S. aureus* can be isolated readily on blood and MacConkey agar, and its identity can be confirmed by coagulase and DNAase tests and by its ability to ferment mannitol. Isolates may be phage typed if this is considered relevant, and any toxins produced may be identified.

In most abscesses the absence of other bacteria must be confirmed before *S. aureus* is considered to be the sole cause; exclusion of other agents is even more important in diseases at mucous surfaces.

TREATMENT

Individual abscesses may be opened surgically after skin cleaning and disinfection, but most treatments rely on antimicrobial treatment. Since *S. aureus* infection is an individual-animal problem, there is usually no need to treat the whole group. Parenteral treatment with an appropriate formulation and prompt treatment at any age can prevent the development of large and potentially extensive and fatal abscesses. The use of feed medication as a prophylactic cannot be justified unless a severe problem has been identified, since the development of antimicrobial resistance in staphylococci is likely to favor them over other organisms after a brief period during which they are suppressed. The use of bacterins has been described, but they are not widely available or extensively used.

REFERENCES

Engvall A, Schwan O. 1983. Isolation and partial characterization of bacteria recovered from abscesses of normally slaughtered pigs. Acta Vet Scand 24:74–83.

Kohler B, Wille H. 1980. Bakteriologische Untersuchungen bei abortierten Schweinfeten unter Berucksichtigung der ätiologischen Bedeutung von *Staphylococcus aureus*. Monatsch Veterinärmed 35:506–510.

Takeuchi S, Matuda K, Sasano K. 1995. Protein A in *Staphylococcus aureus* isolates from pigs. J Vet Med Sci 57:581–582.

Taylor SL, Schlunz LR, Beerey JT, Cliver DO, Bergdoll MS. 1982. Emetic action of staphylococcal enterotoxin A on weanling pigs. Infect Immunol 36:1263–1266.

Actinobaculum (Actinomyces-Eubacterium-Corynebacterium) suis

Soltys and Spratling (1957) isolated, anaerobically, a diphtheroid bacterium from the urine and diseased tissue of adult pigs in the United Kingdom affected with cystitis and pyelonephritis and named it *Corynebacterium suis*. Soltys (1961) described the characteristics of *C. suis* in more detail. *C. suis* was subsequently assigned to the genus *Eubacterium* (Wegienek and Reddy 1982), Actinomyces (Ludwig et al. 1992), and finally *Actinobaculum* Lawson et al. 1997).

A. suis infection associated with urinary tract disease in sows has been reported from Canada (Percy et al. 1966), Norway (Aalvik 1968), Holland (Dijkstra 1969; Frijlink et al. 1969; Narucka and Westendorp 1972), Denmark (Larsen 1970, 1973), Hong Kong (Munro and Wong 1972), Australia (Glazebrook et al. 1973), Switzerland (Schallibaum et al. 1976), Finland (Kauko et al. 1977), Malaysia (Too et al. 1985), Germany (Muller et al. 1986; Waldmann 1987), Brazil (De Oliveira et al. 1988), and the United States (Walker and MacLachlan 1989). Disease caused by *A. suis* occurs in small outbreaks or individual sows, but carriage is much more widespread. The main features of the organism and the disease are described below.

ETIOLOGY

A. suis is a gram-positive pleomorphic rod, 2–3 μm long and 0.3–0.5 μm wide; the organism tends to be larger in tissues than in cultures. In tissues and cultures it occurs in the form of so-called Chinese letters and in a palisade fashion. It is nonmotile and does not form spores.

A. suis grows well on blood agar under anaerobic conditions. Colonies are evident at 2 days, having a diameter of 2–3 mm; they then begin to flatten and develop a characteristic dry, gray, opaque surface with a crenated edge; some colonies attain a size of 4–5 mm in 5–6 days. There is no hemolysis. Growth on nutrient agar, even after subculture, is poor. In liquid media such as cooked meat broth and brain-heart infusion, slight turbidity is produced in 2–4 days; growth is more luxuriant in trypticase soy broth and is further enhanced by the addition of urea to a final concentration of 1.2% (w/v). The addition of maltose to either solid or liquid media improves growth. Although *A. suis* has always been described as an anaerobic organism, prolonged aerobic incubation on blood agar results in the development of colonies within 5–10 days; on subculture, aerobically, colonies are evident in 1–3 days.

The organism is relatively inactive when subjected to conventional biochemical tests. Most strains ferment maltose and xylose and hydrolyze starch but do not attack other commonly used "sugars"; all produce urease. Catalase, methyl red, Voges-Proskauer, indole, and nitrate-reduction tests are negative. Coagulated serum and egg medium are not liquefied. A slight alkalinity is produced in litmus milk.

EPIDEMIOLOGY AND PATHOGENESIS

Most male pigs aged 6 months or more harbor *A. suis* in the preputial diverticulum, which may become colonized when pigs are only a few weeks old. Uninfected males are readily infected when they are housed with carrier males (Jones and Dagnall 1984). The organism may be found on the floors of pens occupied by male pigs. Carr and Walton (1990) have isolated *A. suis* from the footwear of handlers working with boars but not from those working in the farrowing area. Only rarely is it found in the vagina of healthy females, but it may be that existing cultural techniques are insufficiently sensitive to demonstrate its presence there. There are no reports of *A. suis* being isolated from any sites in the pig other than the urogenital tract.

Cystitis and pyelonephritis caused by *A. suis* mainly affect adult females. Infection of the bladder and kidneys is by the ascending route. Most cases occur within 1–3 weeks of mating, suggesting that predisposing factors are operating at this time. Wendt et al. (1994) suggest that these may include infection with other organisms, because of a requirement for erosion of mature vesical epithelial cells to allow attachment by *A. suis*. Water restriction and the presence of crystalluria may also predispose to infection (Wendt and Sobestiansky 1995). The disease may become clinically evident at any time in the breeding cycle of the sow (e.g., after parturition), and in such cases it is not always clear whether infection of the urinary tract is recent or whether there has been a recrudescence of previously existing disease.

Studies on the adhesive properties of *A. suis* have been reported by Larsen et al. (1986). They have demonstrated that some strains are heavily fimbriated and are able to adhere to the epithelial cells of the porcine bladder; their findings support the hypothesis that glycoconjugates are specific receptor sites for the attachment of *A. suis*. Infection of the ureters and kidneys follows infection of the bladder.

CLINICAL SIGNS AND LESIONS

Hematuria is the main sign in the acute phase. As the disease progresses, there is loss of weight. Some sows may die suddenly, apparently from acute renal failure.

Inflammatory reactions in the mucosa of the urethra, bladder, and ureters may be catarrhal, fibrinopurulent, hemorrhagic, or necrotic. Affected kidneys often have irregular yellow areas of degeneration in the parenchyma that are visible on the surface. The renal pelvis may be dilated and contain mucoid fluid in which flakes of necrotic debris and altered blood are present. The medullary pyramids often show yellow or dark green to black foci of necrosis. The ureters are often dilated and filled with reddish purulent urine. There are no related lesions elsewhere in the body.

DIAGNOSIS

Diagnosis is based on clinical signs and bacteriological examination of urine. *A. suis* is easily seen in Gram-stained films, often with other bacteria, notably streptococci. For cultural examination it is essential to incubate the medium (e.g., blood agar), which has been inoculated with urine or other appropriate material, anaerobically for 4 days. Results of cultural procedures should not be reported as negative before that time. Rapid diagnosis can be achieved by the use of immunofluorescent techniques (Schallibaum et al. 1976; Kauko et al. 1977). A selective medium for the isolation of *A. suis* has been described by Dagnall and Jones (1982). Wendt and Amstberg (1995) evaluated the possibility of using serology to detect infection and tested indirect immunofluorescence in diagnosis. They found that antibody did not appear until 3 weeks after hemorrhagic cystitis had occurred and that when a titer of ++ at 1/16 was used as an endpoint to give 100% specificity, the sensitivity was only 79%. There was no relationship between antibody level and the degree of renal damage.

TREATMENT AND PREVENTION

A. suis is sensitive in vitro to several antibiotics, including penicillin and tetracyclines. Administration of antibiotics is frequently effective, at least in the short term. However, relapses commonly occur, and often it is best to advise early slaughter of affected animals. Prolonged treatment for 20 days with ampicillin given at 20 mg/kg may be used (Wendt and Sobestiansky 1995), and enrofloxacin given for 10 days at 10 mg/kg may also be effective. In Wendt and Sobestiansky's studies (1995), pigs with lesions confined to the bladder recovered with antimicrobial treatment alone, but those with renal damage required infusion therapy for recovery.

There are no proven methods of prevention. *A. suis* may be transmitted from boars to sows at the time of mating. Culling of carrier boars has been suggested as a method of preventing infection of sows; this does not seem worthwhile, because replacement boars will almost certainly be infected. Culling might be of value if there are "pathogenic" and "nonpathogenic" strains of *A. suis*, but there is no evidence that such different strains exist. Currently, the only means of attempting prevention of the disease is to administer antibiotics to sows immediately after service or, if outbreaks of the disease are economically serious, to use artificial insemination.

REFERENCES

Aalvik B. 1968. *Corynebacterium suis* isolert fra et tilfelle av pyelonefritt hos purke. Nord Vet Med 20:319–320.

Carr J, Walton JR. 1990. Investigation of the pathogenic properties of *Eubacterium (Corynebacterium) suis*. Proc Int Congr Pig Vet Soc 11.

Dagnall GJR, Jones JET. 1982. A selective medium for the isolation of *Corynebacterium suis*. Res Vet Sci 32:389–390.

De Oliveira SJ, Barcellos DESN, Borowski SM. 1988. Urinary tract infections in two pig breeding herds, with emphasis on the presence of *Corynebacterium suis*. Proc Int Congr Pig Vet Soc 10.

Dijkstra RG. 1969. Cysto-pyelonefritis bij varkens verzoorzaakt door *Corynebacterium suis*. Tijdschr Diergeneeskd 94:393–394.

Frijlink GPA, Van Dijk JE, Goudswaard J. 1969. Een hemorragische-necrotiserende cystopyelonefritis bij een drachtige zeug, veroorzaakt door *Corynebacterium suis*. Tijdschr Diergeneeskd 94:389–393.

Glazebrook JS, Donaldson-Wood C, Ladds PW. 1973. Pyelonephritis and cystitis in sows associated with *Corynebacterium suis*. Aust Vet J 49:546.

Jones JET, Dagnall GJR. 1984. The carriage of *Corynebacterium suis* in male pigs. J Hyg (Camb) 93:381–388.

Kauko L, Schildt R, Sandholm M. 1977. *Corynebacterium suis* emakoiden pyelonefritin aiheuttajana suomessa. Suom Elainl 83:489–492.

Larsen JL. 1970. *Corynebacterium suis* infektioner hos svin. Nord Vet Med 22:422–431.

———. 1973. Et enzootisk udbrud af cystitis og pyelonephritis forarsaget af *Corynebacterium suis*. Medlemsbl Dan Dyrlaege-foren 56:509–515.

Larsen JL, Hogh P, Hovind-Hougen K. 1986. Haemagglutinating and hydrophobic properties of *Corynebacterium (Eubacterium) suis*. Acta Vet Scand 27:520–530.

Lawson PA, Falsen E, Akervall E, Vandamme P, and Collins MD. 1997. Characterization of some *Actinomyces*-like isolates from human clinical specimens: reclassification of *Actinomyces suis* (Soltys and Spratling) as *Actinomyces suis* comb nov and description of *Actinobaculum schaalii*. Int J Syst Bacteriol 47:899–903.

Ludwig W, Kirchof G, Weizenegger M, Weiss N. 1992. Phylogenetic evidence for the transfer of *Eubacterium suis* to the genus *Actinomyces* as *Actinomyces suis* comb nov. Int J Syst Bacteriol 42:161–165.

Muller E, Pozvari M, Merkt M. 1986. Zum Vorkommen von blutig-eitrigen Harnblasen und Nierenentzundungen bei Zuchtsauen in Verbindung mit *Corynebacterium suis*. Prakt Tierärztl 67:1081–1083.

Munro R, Wong F. 1972. First isolation of *Corynebacterium suis* in Hong Kong. Br Vet J 128:29–32.

Narucka U, Westendorp JF. 1972. *Corynebacterium suis* in pigs. Neth J Vet Sci 4:86–92.

Percy DH, Ruhnke HL, Soltys MA. 1966. A case of infectious cystitis and pyelonephritis of swine caused by *Corynebacterium suis*. Can Vet J 7:291–292.

Schallibaum M von, Hani H, Nicolet J. 1976. Infektion des Harn-traktes beim Schwein mit *Corynebacterium suis*: Diagnosis met Immunofluoreszenz. Schweiz Arch Tierheilkd 118:329–334.

Soltys MA. 1961. *Corynebacterium suis* associated with specific cystitis and pyelonephritis in pigs. J Pathol 81:441–446.

Soltys MA, Spratling FR. 1957. Infectious cystitis and pyelonephritis of pigs: A preliminary communication. Vet Rec 69:500–504.

Too HL, Chooi KF, Bahaman AR. 1985. Cystitis in a sow due to *Corynebacterium suis*. Kajian Veterinar 17:155–156.

Waldmann KH. 1987. Die Pyelozystitis der Zuchtsau. Tierärztl Prax 15:263–267.

Walker RL, MacLachlan JJ. 1989. Isolation of *Eubacterium suis* from sows with cystitis. J Am Vet Med Assoc 195:1104–1107.

Wegienek J, Reddy CA. 1982. Taxonomic study of *Eubacterium suis* (nom. rev.) Comb. nov. Int J Syst Bacteriol 32:218–228.

Wendt M, Amstberg G. 1995. Untersuchungen zum Nachweis von Antikorpen gegen *Eubacterium suis* beim Schwein. Schweiz Arch für Tierheilkd 137:129–136.

Wendt M, Liebhold M, Drommer W. 1994. Rasterelektronenmikr-oskopische Untersuchungen an der Harnblase von Sauen unter besonderer Berucksichtigung einer *Eubacterium suis*–Infektion. J Vet Med Ser B 41:126–138.

Wendt M, Sobestiansky J. 1995. Untersuchungen zur Therapie von Harnwegs-infektionen bei Sauen. Dtsch Tierärztl Wochenschr 102:21–22.

Rhodococcus equi

Rhodococcus equi is associated with granulomatous lymphadenitis affecting the lymph nodes of the head and neck of the pig. The lesions can be confused at slaughter with those of tuberculosis, and the organism is important for this reason rather than as a cause of clinical disease.

ETIOLOGY

The organism was first isolated from the pneumonic lungs of a foal by Magnusson (1923) and was given the name *Corynebacterium equi*; it is now called *Rhodococcus equi*. This gram-positive coccobacillus is a member of the nocardioform actinomycete group (Goodfellow et al. 1982). In common with other members of *Rhodococcus*, *R. equi* produces pinkish colonies on solid media. The mycolic acids of *R. equi* have a chain length of 34–48 C, and the DNA base composition is 66–72 mol% guanine plus cytosine. Chemical properties used in defining the species were summarized by Goodfellow (1987).

Isolation of *R. equi* from clinical samples is easily achieved by aerobic culture on routine media at 37°C, although the optimum temperature is 28–30°C. Selective media, such as that developed by Woolcock et al. (1979), are required for fecal isolation. Colonies are slow growing, requiring 48 hours to reach a size of 2–4 mm. The typical colony is irregularly round, buff-pink, smooth, and mucoid, although colonial variation is common within and between strains (Mutimer and Woolcock 1981). *R. equi* is biochemically unreactive. It is not proteolytic and does not ferment carbohydrates. *R. equi* is catalase positive, usually urease positive, and oxidase negative. The API ZYM system has been found helpful in bacterial identification (Mutimer and Woolcock 1982). *R. equi* is not hemolytic but, in conjunction with the phospholipase D of *Corynebacterium pseudotuberculosis* or the beta toxin of *Staphylococcus aureus,* produces complete hemolysis of sheep and cattle erythrocytes (Prescott et al. 1982). Semipurification of this factor, known as "equi factor," has indicated that cholesterol oxidase is the major constituent (Linder and Bernheimer 1982).

R. equi possess an abundant acidic polysaccharide capsule, which is the basis for several serotyping schemes. Prescott (1981) has identified 7 serotypes, of which serotype 1 is the most frequently isolated in Canada, Australia, and India. Japanese workers have identified 27 serotypes, with the most common being equivalent to Prescott serotype 1 (Nakazawa et al. 1983). There is no relationship between capsular serotype and origin of the isolates. The capsular polysaccharides of 4 Prescott serotypes have been purified.

Recent studies of this species have confirmed that isolates from pigs possess a virulence-associated protein (vapA) that is encoded by a virulence plasmid. Takai et al. (1996) confirmed the presence of 79–95 kb plasmids coding for a 20 kDa virulence protein.

EPIDEMIOLOGY AND PATHOGENESIS

R. equi is primarily a soil resident. Environmental distribution favors soils enriched with herbivore manure, since fecal matter potentiates bacterial multiplication (Barton and Hughes 1984). *R. equi* is also a transient in the intestinal tract of many species, including pigs, cattle, deer, horses, sheep, goats, and wild birds (Woolcock et al. 1979; Carman and Hodges 1987). Being an obligate aerobe, *R. equi* is not likely to be a member of the normal flora. The bacterium is found in soil samples collected from arable land that has not pastured animals for many years, emphasizing its durability. *R. equi* is present in dust and even in cobwebs of farm buildings in areas where it occurs. *R. equi* is relatively resistant to chemical disinfectants, such as treatment with 2.5% oxalic acid and 0.5% sodium hydroxide over periods of 15–60 minutes (Karlson et al. 1940).

Little is known of the epidemiology or pathogenesis of the naturally occurring disease in swine. As in horses, *R. equi* infection is likely to be acquired from the environment (Woolcock et al. 1980). Ingestion is the normal mode of exposure in foals (Takai et al. 1986a), leading to the development of solid protective immunity in the majority of animals (Prescott et al. 1980; Chirino-Trejo et al. 1987). A similar situation probably occurs in swine housed on pasture or in yards contaminated with *R. equi*, as the bacterium is readily isolated from the feces of such pigs (Barton and Hughes 1984). Several slaughterhouse studies have also demonstrated recovery of *R. equi* from normal cervical and submaxillary lymph nodes at rates varying from 7% to 35% (Mutimer and Woolcock 1980; Takai et al. 1986b), although the organism may now be less common, as Takai et al. (1996) recovered it from only 3.1% of 1832 swine in Japan. However, no epidemiological studies have been carried out to correlate infection rates, disease prevalence, and environmental contamination of *R. equi* on pig farms, as has been done for horses. There have been suggestions that isolates from pigs differ somewhat from those from horses and that some pig isolates resemble those from humans.

Takai et al. (1996) speculated that some human cases may be of porcine origin.

The way in which *R. equi* causes granulomatous lymphadenitis of the head and neck in the pig is not clear. *R. equi* can be recovered from normal nodes, and there are accounts of failure to reproduce the nodal lesions experimentally (Karlson et al. 1940; Cotchin 1943). *Mycobacterium* spp. may also be recovered in some cases. It is possible that the severity of the lesions reflects the possession of the virulence-associated protein, which may vary from strain to strain, the degree of immunity present when infection took place, or the duration of the infection at sampling. However, *R. equi* typically produces a granulomatous tissue reaction in lymph nodes of other species, consistent with its action as a facultative intracellular pathogen (Yager 1987).

R. equi has been associated with serious clinical disease, including one outbreak of oral abscesses and one of pneumonia (Thal and Rutqvist 1959; Rao et al. 1982), but pigs are extremely resistant to experimental infection. Following aerosolization, *R. equi* is cleared from the lungs very slowly, but clinical signs and pathological lesions of pneumonia are minimal despite exposure to 107 organisms on 7 consecutive days (Zink and Yager 1987). Pneumonia has, however, been induced by intratracheal inoculation of fluid inocula (Thal and Rutqvist 1959).

LESIONS

Lymphadenitis causes no significant clinical signs; lesions are detected only at slaughter. Affected submandibular and cervical nodes are enlarged, containing multiple yellow-tan foci, often in a subcapsular location. Caseation and calcification of these foci sometimes occur. Histologically, the lesion is a granulomatous lymphadenitis. Similar lesions reported in the mesenteric lymph nodes have yielded *Rhodococcus sputi* on culture (Tsukamura et al. 1988).

DIAGNOSIS

Diagnosis is at postmortem. Microbiological identification of *R. equi* is necessary for it is not possible to differentiate the gross lesions of *R. equi*–induced lymphadenitis from those caused by *Mycobacterium* spp.

TREATMENT AND PREVENTION

R. equi–induced disease is not sufficiently important to necessitate antemortem diagnosis and treatment in swine. Therapy, which in foals requires long-term administration of rifampicin and erythromycin, is not feasible on economic grounds. While some economic loss may accrue from condemnation at slaughter, there are no studies that indicate the extent of this loss and there appears to be no incentive to institute control measures.

These would in any case be difficult; an effective vaccine is presently unavailable.

REFERENCES

Barton MD, Hughes KL. 1984. Ecology of *Rhodococcus equi.* Vet Microbiol 9:65–76.

Carman MG Hodges, RT. 1987. Distribution of *Rhodococcus equi* in animals, birds and from the environment. NZ Vet 35:114–115.

Chirino-Trejo JM, Prescott JF, Yager JA. 1987. Protection of foals against experimental *Rhodococcus equi* pneumonia by oral immunization. Can J Vet Res 51:444–447.

Cotchin E. 1943. *Corynebacterium equi* in the submaxillary lymph nodes of swine. J Comp Pathol 53:298–309.

Goodfellow M. 1987. The taxonomic status of *Rhodococcus equi.* Vet Microbiol 14:205–209.

Goodfellow M, Beckham AR, Barton MD. 1982. Numerical classification of *Rhodococcus equi* and related actinomycetes. J Appl Bacteriol 53:199–207.

Karlson AG, Moses HR, Feldman WH. 1940. *Corynebacterium equi* (Magnusson, 1923) in the submaxillary lymph nodes of swine. J Infect Dis 67:243–251.

Linder R, Bernheimer AW. 1982. Enzymatic oxidation of membrane cholesterol oxidase in relation to lysis of sheep erythrocytes by corynebacterial enzymes. Arch Biochem Biophys 213:395–404.

Magnusson H. 1923. Spezifische Infektiose Pneumonie beim Fohlen: Ein neurer Eitererreger beim Pferde. Arch Wiss Prakt Tierheilk 50:22–38.

Mutimer MD, Woolcock JB. 1980. *Corynebacterium equi* in cattle and pigs. Vet Q 2:25–27.

——. 1981. Some problems associated with the identification of *Corynebacterium equi.* Vet Microbiol 6:331–338.

——. 1982. API ZYM for identification of *Corynebacterium equi.* Zentralbl Bakteriol Hyg Abt (Orig C3):410–415.

Nakazawa M, Kubo M, Sugimoto C, Isayama Y. 1983. Serogrouping of *Rhodococcus equi.* Microbiol Immunol 27:837–846.

Prescott JF. 1981. Capsular serotypes of *Corynebacterium equi.* Can J Comp Med 45:130–134.

Prescott JF, Lastra M, Barksdale L. 1982. *Equi* factors in the identification of *Corynebacterium equi* Magnusson. J Clin Microbiol 16:988–990.

Prescott JF, Ogilvie TJH, Markham RJF. 1980. Lymphocyte immunostimulation in the diagnosis of *Corynebacterium equi* pneumonia of foals. Am J Vet Res 41:2073–2075.

Rao MS, Zaki S, Keshavamurthy BS, Singh KC. 1982. An outbreak of an acute *Corynebacterium equi* infection in piglets. Indian Vet J 59:487–488.

Takai S, Fukunaga N, Ochiai S, Imal Y, Sasaki Y, Tsubaki S, Sekizaki T. 1996. Identification of intermediately virulent *Rhodococcus equi* isolates from pigs. J Clin Microbiol 34:1034–1037.

Takai S, Ohkura H, Watanabe Y, Tsubaki S. 1986a. Quantitative aspects of fecal *Rhodococcus (Corynebacterium) equi* in foals. J Clin Microbiol 23:794–796.

Takai S, Takeuchi T, Tsubaki S. 1986b. Isolation of *Rhodococcus (Corynebacterium) equi* and atypical mycobacteria from the lymph nodes of healthy pigs. Jpn J Vet Sci 48:445–448.

Thal E, Rutqvist L. 1959. The pathogenicity of Corynebacterium equi for pigs and small laboratory animals. Nord Vet Med 11:298–304.

Tsukamura M, Komatsuzaki C, Sakai R, Kane-da K, Kudo T, Seino A. 1988. Mesenteric lymphadenitis of swine caused by *Rhodococcus sputi.* J Clin Microbiol 26:155–157.

Woolcock JB, Farmer AMT, Mutimer MD. 1979. Selective medium for *Corynebacterium equi* isolation. J Clin Microbiol 9:640–642.

Woolcock JB, Mutimer MD, Farmer AMT. 1980. Epidemiology of *Corynebacterium equi* in horses. Res Vet Sci 28:87–90.

Yager JA. 1987. The pathogenesis of *Rhodococcus equi* pneumonia in foals. Vet Microbiol 14:225–232.

Zink MC, Yager JA. 1987. Experimental infection of piglets by aerosols of *Rhodococcus equi.* Can J Vet Res 51:290–296.

Arcanobacterium pyogenes

Arcanobacterium pyogenes, previously known as *Actinomyces pyogenes,* and even earlier as *Corynebacterium pyogenes,* is a common cause of suppurative lesions in pigs throughout the world. Infection is opportunistic, resulting from the invasion of skin or mucous membranes by resident *A. pyogenes.* Clinical disease can result from vertebral osteomyelitis, arthritis, pneumonia, endocarditis, mastitis, and subcutaneous and deep-tissue abscesses.

ETIOLOGY

A. pyogenes is a small gram-positive pleomorphic rod. There is marked morphologic variation between and within strains. Growth is enhanced by the addition of serum or blood to media and occurs under both aerobic and anaerobic conditions. The optimal temperature for growth is 37°C. Colonies are translucent and small, taking 48 hours to reach a diameter of 1 mm. *A. pyogenes* colonies are surrounded by a narrow zone of complete hemolysis after 24 hours on blood agar. Strains isolated from pigs are more hemolytic than those isolated from cattle. *A. pyogenes* produces a hemolysin and an exotoxin that is dermonecrotic in rabbits and guinea pigs and lethal following intravenous injection in rabbits and mice (Lovell 1944). Glucose is fermented by all strains, but other carbohydrate reactions are variable. In general, porcine strains are more biochemically active than bovine strains (Roberts 1968; Tainaka et al. 1983). *A. pyogenes* is proteolytic, a series of serine proteases with molecular masses of 69, 59, and 55 kDa being produced along with one of 108 kDa that is only produced by pig strains (Takeuchi et al. 1995).

A. pyogenes had been classified into the genus *Actinomyces* by Collins and Jones (1982), chiefly on the basis of cell wall composition. The guanine-cytosine content of DNA is 58 mol%. Identification of *Arcanobacterium pyogenes* is rapid and reliable with the API 20 Strep system (Morrison and Tillotson 1988). Recent studies of vaginal isolates have allowed the differentiation of *Arcanobacterium hyovaginalis* (Collins et al. 1993).

EPIDEMIOLOGY AND PATHOGENESIS

Arcanobacterium pyogenes is common on the mucous membranes of the upper respiratory tract and genital tract of several animal species, including the pig. Disease is therefore the result of endogenous infection and is sporadic, requiring some predisposing event, such as trauma, to initiate the process. For *A. pyogenes* to cause subcutaneous lesions, devitalized or inflamed tissue is an apparent prerequisite, since the inoculation of *A. pyogenes* subcutaneously does not, per se, lead to abscesses. Infection is often secondary. Tail biting may lead to abscessation and suppurative osteomyelitis, retention of the fetal membranes may lead to endometritis and infertility, lacerations of the mammary gland may lead to mastitis and arthritis, umbilical cord contamination may lead to omphalophlebitis, and iatrogenic abscesses may result from faulty injection or castration techniques. Local extension may produce pelvic lymphadenitis and peritonitis. *A. pyogenes* may act as a secondary invader in preexisting pneumonia.

Bacteremic spread from infective foci results in a variety of lesions, including embolic pneumonia, endocarditis, arthritis, and vertebral osteomyelitis. Experimental intravenous inoculation of *A. pyogenes* shows bacterial localization within the marrow of vertebral body epiphyses, initiating osteolysis, abscessation, and the formation of osteophytes (Vladutiu et al. 1982). Valvular endocarditis may result from bacteremia following tail-biting lesions (Van den Berg et al. 1981). *A. pyogenes* is occasionally recovered from fetuses and fetal membranes, but its role in abortion has not been established. Some of these isolates may be *A. hyovaginalis*.

A. pyogenes, as denoted by its name, causes suppurative lesions. Surprisingly little, however, is known of the virulence factors important in disease causation. Both the hemolytic protein exotoxin and protease have been proposed as toxic factors (Kume et al. 1983). *A. pyogenes* also binds alpha-2 macroglobulin (Lammler et al. 1985), a property that could interfere with local regulation of inflammation.

CLINICAL SIGNS AND LESIONS

The clinical signs are very variable, since *A. pyogenes* is responsible for a range of pathological lesions. Some, such as endocarditis and adhesive peritonitis, may be fatal. Others, such as vertebral osteomyelitis leading to posterior paralysis, may necessitate euthanasia. Suppurative osteomyelitis generally affects the vertebral bodies, leading to transverse pathological fractures, vertebral collapse, and compression of the spinal cord. Lameness results from polyarthritis or from cellulitis and periarthritis. However, many lesions, including subcutaneous and intramuscular abscesses, are clinically inapparent and are discovered only at postmortem or slaughter. Such abscesses vary from a few millimeters to

several centimeters in size, usually have a thick fibrous capsule, and contain a yellow-green pus of variable consistency. Mastitis may be confined to one gland or may involve several.

DIAGNOSIS

Diagnosis in individual cases requires the demonstration of the organism in lesional material and confirmation by laboratory culture and identification. Carcass abscesses typically yield mixed cultures, including clostridia, *Bacteroides* spp., *Propionibacterium granulosum*, *Pasteurella multocida*, and unidentified anaerobes (Hara 1980; Jones 1980). Diagnosis of infection within a herd has been attempted serologically using an immunodiffusion test for antibody to *A. pyogenes* protease (Takeuchi et al. 1979). However, in a slaughterhouse survey, only 34.4% of pigs with abscesses had an antiprotease titer (Hara 1980).

TREATMENT

A. pyogenes is sensitive to a wide range of antimicrobial agents, including penicillin, tetracycline, and erythromycin. Some strains have been shown to be resistant to sulfonamides and trimethoprim. In vivo sensitivity does not necessarily reflect in vitro sensitivity, for the physicochemical properties of chronic abscesses tend to protect the bacteria from the action of antimicrobial drugs. Abscesses may be removed surgically.

PREVENTION

Surveys of serum antibodies to *A. pyogenes* protease show that approximately one-third of pigs are positive (Hara 1980). Antitoxin antibodies are also demonstrable and may increase with age. However, mice vaccinated with preparations of whole cells with or without toxoid or even given live organisms are not adequately protected against subsequent challenge (Derbyshire and Matthews 1963; Durner and Werner 1983). There is no effective vaccine available for swine. Prevention requires management of the environment to reduce or abolish the various conditions that predispose the development of *A. pyogenes* lesions. The treatment of sows with antimicrobials such as tetracyclines in the food prior to farrowing and throughout weaning can eliminate infection and reduce vulval discharges (Taylor 1984).

REFERENCES

Collins MD, Jones D. 1982. Reclassification of *Corynebacterium pyogenes* (Glage) in the genus *Actinomyces*, as *Actinomyces pyogenes* comb. nov. J Gen Microbiol 128:901–902.
Collins MD, Stubbs S, Hommez J, Devriese LA. 1993. Molecular taxonomic studies of *Actinomyces*-like bacteria isolated from purulent lesions in pigs and description of *Actinomyces hyovaginalis* sp. nov. Int J Syst Bacteriol 43:471–473.

Derbyshire JB, Matthews PRJ. 1963. Immunological studies with *Corynebacterium pyogenes* in mice. Res Vet Sci 4:537–542.

Durner K, nd Werner B. 1983. Untersuchungen zur Immunogenitat und zu den Pathogenitatsfaktoren von *Corynebacterium pyogenes*. Arch Exp Vet Med Leipzig 37:541–547.

Hara F. 1980. A study on pig pyogenic infections: Results of clinical, pathological, bacteriological and serological examinations of slaughtered pigs. Bull Azabu Uni Vet Med 1:187–202.

Jones, J. E. T. 1980. Observations on the bacterial flora of abscesses in pigs. Br Vet J 136:343–348.

Kume, T, Tainaka, M, Saito, M, Hiruma, M, Nishio, S, Kashiwazaki, M, Mitani, K, and Nakajima, Y. 1983. Research on experimental *Corynebacterium pyogenes* infections in pigs. Kitasato Arch Exp Med 56:119–135.

Lammler C, Chhatwal GS, Blobel H. 1985. Binding of a_2-macroglobulin and haptoglobin to *Actinomyces pyogenes*. Can J Microbiol 31:657–659.

Lovell R. 1944. Further studies on the toxin of *Corynebacterium pyogenes*. J Pathol Bacteriol 56:525–529.

Morrison JRA, Tillotson GS. 1988. Identification of *Actinomyces (Corynebacterium) pyogenes* with the API 20 Strep system. J Clin Microbiol 26:1865–1866.

Roberts RJ. 1968. Biochemical reactions of *Corynebacterium pyogenes*. J Pathol Bacteriol 95:127–130.

Tainaka M, Kume T, Takeuchi S, Nishio S, Saito M. 1983. Studies on the biological and serological properties of *Corynebacterium pyogenes* infection in pigs by immunodiffusion test with protease antigen. Nat Inst Anim Health Q (Tokyo) 19:77–82.

Takeuchi S, Azuma R, Nakajima Y, Suto T. 1979. Diagnosis of *Corynebacterium pyogenes* infection in pigs by immunodiffusion test with protease antigen. Nat Inst Anim Health Q (Tokyo) 19:77–82.

Takeuchi S, Kaidoh T, Azuma R. 1995. Assay of proteases from *Actinomyces pyogenes* isolated from pigs and cows by zymography. J Vet Med Sci 57:977–979.

Taylor DJ. 1984. Clinical and bacteriological effects of antimicrobial therapy on naturally-occurring post-partum vulval discharge in sows. Proc Int Congr Pig Vet Soc 8:151.

Van den Berg J, Narucka U, Nouws JFM, Okma BD, Peelen JPJ, Soethout AEE. 1981. Lesions in slaughtered animals. II. Inflammation of the tail and embolic pneumonia in pigs. Tijdschr Diergeneeskd 106:407–410.

Vladutiu O, Florescu S, Murgu I. 1982. Research in the pathogenetic mechanisms of osteophytosis in pyobacillary polyarthritis. Arch Vet 16:75–95.

IV Miscellaneous Conditions

51 Behavioral Problems

P. H. Hemsworth and Greg M. Cronin

Most behavioral differences between wild and domestic animals, including farm animals, are quantitative rather than qualitative in character and best explained in differences in response thresholds (Price 2003). Once a species has become adapted to its captive environment, reproduction and growth efficiency are generally improved through better nutrition and health, reduced energy expenditure, and, in some cases, reduced stress in this captive or domestic environment. Behavioral problems by definition involve behavioral changes as a consequence of either environmental or genetic change that compromise the fitness of the animals, and thus in the case of farm animals, we can consider that behavioral problems compromise the animals' production efficiency, health, and welfare.

The term "abnormal behavior" in domestic animals often refers to behavior that either is not in the animal's natural repertoire of behavior or differs in its pattern, frequency, or context from what is considered normal. This issue of "what is natural or normal?" in domestic species is a contentious one, and it is simpler and perhaps less ambiguous to use the term *behavioral problem* and define it as a behavior that compromises the animals' production efficiency, health, and welfare. Such a definition incorporates implications for the animal, other animals, and the animal owner or caretaker. This review will focus on the major behavioral problems in commercial pigs, with the objective of recommending possible solutions to improve the productivity, health, and welfare of these pigs.

AGGRESSION

Agonistic behaviors are behaviors that occur in response to a conflict; may include offense, defense, submissive, or escape components (including dispersal, although this behavior is not possible in pig housing systems in which pigs are contained in pens or relatively small paddocks); and consist of contact (e.g., biting or pushing) or noncontact (e.g., body postures, gestures or vocaliza-

tions) behaviors. Aggressive behaviors strictly refer to attack and actual fighting and thus include parallel pressing, head-to-head knocks, levering, and bites in pigs (Fraser and Broom 1996).

An important behavioral trait that influenced the domestication of ungulate and galliform species was their social organization: these species had the ability to live in relatively large groups without marked year-round territoriality (Stricklin and Mench 1987). This trait has been further affected through artificial selection during domestication; the formation of social hierarchies and the tendency for subordinates to avoid dominant animals is considered an important mechanism that functions to control aggression in situations of limited resources (e.g., space and feed). Nevertheless social instability is an important social stressor for livestock. For instance, entire male pigs are reported to grow much less efficiently during the finisher phase of production than their genetic capability (De Haer and Merks 1992). The high level of aggression and social instability characteristic of entire boars in groups, was eliminated by application of an immuno-castration vaccine (Improvac), with concomitant improvement in feed intake and growth during the last few weeks of the finisher phase (Cronin et al. 2003).

In addition to aggression caused by competition over resources, such as feed, and meetings between unacquainted animals, some aggression in farm animals may function to maintain distance between individual animals (Fraser and Rushen 1987). Research on farm animals generally indicates that both increases in group size and decreases in space are associated with increased aggression, and high levels of aggression in pigs has been shown to lead to physical injury, including lameness, and acute stress and, if unresolved, chronic stress with consequences on immunity, disease, and productivity.

The results of growth studies on growing pigs generally indicate depressions in growth performance, either decreases in growth rate or increases in feed-to-gain ratio, with decreasing space allowance and increasing group

847

size (Kornegay and Notter 1984; Chapple 1993), with space allowance perhaps having the greater impact.

Reducing space in terms of either floor space or pigs per feeder will eventually reduce the growth performance of growing pigs (see Gonyou 2001), presumably through stress and/or access to feed. Reductions in space allowance may not be accompanied by changes in aggression since restrictions in space may restrict specific behavioral patterns, such as the species-specific motor patterns utilized in aggressive encounters. Indeed, Barnett et al. (1993) suggested that the reduced aggression observed in gestating gilts housed in narrow pens was due to insufficient space to fight using aggressive motor patterns such as parallel pressing. These adverse effects of space are generally a consequence of either stress or aggression and, in turn, injury and stress limiting growth in suboptimal social environments. Such effects also have obvious welfare implications. Since space requirements change with an animal's size, the following allometric expression has proven to be useful in estimating space allowance to maximize growth over a wide range of liveweights (Gonyou 2001): space allowance is calculated when the constant 0.035 is multiplied by body weight$^{0.667}$, with space allowance expressed as square meters and liveweight in kilograms.

Several studies have also examined the effects of space allowance on breeding female pigs (see Barnett et al. 2001). There is evidence of a chronic stress response and reduced reproductive performance if space allowance is insufficient. For example, elevated basal cortisol concentrations have been reported in breeding gilts in groups of six with a floor space allowance of 1 m^2/pig or less (Hemsworth et al. 1986a; Barnett et al. 1992). While the former study indicated that there may be reproductive performance advantages of housing at 3 m^2/pig rather than 2 m^2/pig, the physiological criteria indicated no differences between these space allocations. Weng et al. (1998) reported increased aggression and injuries in sows with decreasing space allowance and recommended a space allowance between 2.4 and 3.6 m^2/sow for groups of six pregnant sows.

While some research has indicated that increasing group sizes up to 80 will increase aggression and reduce growth in growing pigs (e.g., Petherick and Blackshaw 1987; Spoolder et al. 1999), other research has suggested no effect at least on growth if pigs are given ample space and the opportunity for ad libitum feed (e.g., Kornegay and Notter 1984; McConnell et al. 1987). Morrison et al. (2003) observed that growing pigs in groups of 200 on deep litter had a higher incidence of agonistic interactions per pig than pigs in groups of 20 on partially slatted concrete floors.

Mixing small groups of pigs results in vigorous fighting within the first 24 h, and by 48 h the dominance hierarchy can generally be identified (Meese and Ewbank 1973). Although olfactory, auditory, and visual cues have been suggested as important cues in individual pig

recognition, it is still uncertain how the mechanism of individual animal recognition operates in pigs (Fraser and Broom 1997). Conventional thinking has been that small groups form stable social hierarchies and that as group size increases and individual animal recognition declines, aggression will increase. This has led to the widespread view in the literature that if animals regularly encounter unfamiliar animals in large groups in confined areas, aggression will increase with adverse effects on production and welfare. For instance, it is commonly believed that the total number of group members that can be recognized or remembered by each individual is 20 to 30 in pigs (Fraser and Broom 1997).

In contrast, there is recent evidence in laying hens and broiler chickens (Pagel and Dawkins 1997; Estevez 1998; Nicol et al. 1999) that aggression may actually decline as group size substantially increases with either total pen space or space per animal remaining constant. It is possible that the greater resources in very large groups, such as total and free space and availability of preferred lying areas, may reduce the need to form dominance hierarchies that function to control aggression in situations of limited resources. Pagel and Dawkins (1997) have also argued that if animals are able to adjust their behavior according to the size of the group, they may abandon all attempts to establish dominance hierarchies. Hughes et al. (1997) also suggested that animals might be more socially tolerant in large groups. While the effects of varying the size of small groups have been studied, neither maximal nor optimal group sizes have been identified for most livestock (Stricklin and Mench 1987).

There is some evidence that group size affects sow reproduction and welfare. Barnett et al. (1984, 1986) found that housing sexually mature gilts in pairs resulted in elevated basal cortisol concentrations compared to housing in groups of 4–8 with a similar space allowance. Both large group size (24 vs. 8 gilts) and small group size (3 vs. 9, 17, or 27 gilts) may reduce the expression of estrus (Christenson and Ford 1979; Christenson and Hruska 1984), while increasing group size and concomitantly decreasing space allowance may also reduce the expression of estrus in gilts (Cronin et al. 1983). Broom et al. (1995) compared sows in groups of 5 fed in stalls and a group of 38 sows with an electronic feeding station and while there was increased aggression in the larger group, particularly after initial mixing, any differences in aggression and stereotypies had disappeared by the fourth parity. Olsson et al. (1994) reported increased injuries as group size increased. Some limited research by Taylor et al. (1997) has shown varying group sizes, of 5, 10, 20, and 40 sows with a space allowance of 2.0 m^2/sow, had no effects on reproductive performance (farrowing rate and litter size). Although aggression immediately after mixing increased as group size increased, the number of lesions during gestation were similar across treatments. In the same study, reducing space allowance for groups of 10 sows from 2.0 to 1.2 m²/sow increased aggression. Further research is required to determine the optimum space allowance and group size for pregnant pigs. There are no data on space allowance and group size interactions for adult female pigs.

The design of the group pen will affect gilt and sow aggression. Petherick et al. (1987) have shown some advantages of partial stalls in reducing aggression around feeding in pens of group-housed pigs. However, whether the reduced aggression was due to individual feeding or the provision of escape areas was not determined. Barnett et al. (1992) subsequently demonstrated welfare advantages of partial stalls within group pens based on a reduction in aggression immediately after grouping unfamiliar pigs and in the longer term by feeding in the partial stalls. Feeding in the partial stalls also resulted in long-term benefits, based on lower free cortisol concentrations and a higher cell-mediated immunity. However, a subsequent study examining effects of pen design in reducing aggression in groups showed no benefits of partial stalls within pens either in the short term or subsequently (Barnett et al. 1993), although in that study the pigs were not fed in the stalls. Thus, it would appear that partial stalls may confer advantages in reducing aggression if the pigs are routinely fed in the partial stalls. Similar design modifications—that is, incorporating stalls into group pens—have also been reported (Edwards 1985). Pen shape has some effects on aggression (Barnett et al. 1993). Aggression was less in rectangular pens than square pens as a result of grouping unfamiliar pigs, provided the space allowance was 1.4.m²/pig; the benefits were lost in larger pens providing 3.4 m²/pig. However, Olsson et al. (1994) recommended against using long narrow pens with liquid feeding on the basis of competition and variable intakes.

Aggression among recently grouped unfamiliar gilts and sows has obvious welfare and reproductive disadvantages. In spite of the research to date on minimizing aggression when grouping unfamiliar pigs, there are few rigorous recommendations. In reviewing the literature, Barnett et al. (2001) suggested that aggression can be reduced in gilts by

1. Modifying pen size and shape on the basis that pigs require a minimum space in which to fight
2. Modifying pen design on the basis that the provision of escape areas reduces aggression
3. Preexposing pigs to their new pen
4. Grouping after dark, on the basis that it is the "normal" sleeping time, or providing feed ad libitum on the basis that restrictively fed pigs may prefer to feed than fight
5. Using masking odors on the basis that anosmic pigs show reduced aggression
6. Using "mood-altering" drugs on the basis of their positive effects in animal models

However, all or some of these methods may be effective in only postponing aggression rather than reducing it. There are few rigorous recommendations and this subject needs further research to allow industry to manage group housing of sows successfully, and thus minimize risks to welfare and reproduction. In particular, the effects of and interactions between factors such as space allowance, group size, pen shape, and features on pig welfare require thorough investigation.

As recognized by Barnett et al. (2001), both stall and group housing during gestation have advantages and disadvantages for the sow. A combination of these housing systems may optimize sow reproduction and welfare. For example, group housing of sows at mating and during mid-late pregnancy when social contact (Barnett and Hemsworth 1991) and space and exercise (Barnett et al. 2001), respectively, may be important, and individual housing of sows early in pregnancy when the control of nutrition may affect embryo mortality and aggression may affect conception (Barnett et al. 2001). There may also be opportunities to improve the design of these systems, such as "turning around" stalls for periods of individual housing (Barnett and Taylor 1995) and providing feeding stalls during the period of group housing (Barnett et al. 1992).

FEAR OF HUMANS

Stockperson interactions with livestock have been shown in a number of livestock industries to influence the welfare and productivity of farm animals (see Hemsworth and Coleman 1998). While many of these human interactions may appear mild and harmless, research in many livestock industries has shown that the frequent use of some routine behaviors by stockpeople can surprisingly result in farm animals becoming highly fearful of humans. Labor savings that have occurred through facility design and automation have generally reduced the human contact that pigs receive in modern production units. Consequently, opportunities for positive human contact are probably reduced and this, together with the fact that many routine husbandry tasks undertaken by stockpeople often contain aversive elements, may lead to the stockperson's interactions being biased toward negative ones.

Studies in the swine industry have shown, first, substantial variation between farms in the animals' fear of humans and, second, significant sequential relationships between the stockperson's attitudes and behavior toward their animals and the fear of humans and productivity of pigs farm animals (Coleman et al. 1998; Hemsworth et al. 1981; Hemsworth et al. 1989b). For example, negative attitudes to handling, such as beliefs that considerable verbal and physical effort is required to move pigs and that pigs do not require petting and stroking, were correlated or associated with a high percentage of negative behaviors used by stockpeople in handling pigs. Negative tactile behaviors by stockpeople that were recorded included forceful hits and slaps as well as audible slaps and pushes while positive tactile behaviors included pats, strokes, and the hand of the stockperson resting on the back of the animal. Furthermore, a high percentage of negative behaviors used by stockpeople correlated with high fear levels in pigs. Surprisingly, high levels of fear of humans were best predicted at the farm when the classification of negative behaviors included not only forceful hits and slaps, but also negative behaviors used with less force, such as moderate slaps and pushes. This highlights the sensitivity of pigs to moderate negative interactions by humans, something that is not intuitively obvious to most of us.

Laboratory studies indicate that the likely mechanism responsible for the adverse effects of high fear on the productivity of pigs is a chronic stress response. Handling treatments that result in high fear levels, similar to those often seen in the swine industry, have been consistently shown to stress pigs as evidenced by a sustained elevation in the stress hormone cortisol (see Hemsworth and Coleman 1998). These stress effects of negative handling also accompany depressions in growth and reproductive performance (see Hemsworth and Coleman 1998).

Studies in the swine industry have shown that it is possible to improve the attitudinal and behavioral profiles of stockpeople and, in turn, reduce the level of fear and improve the productivity and welfare of commercial pigs (Hemsworth et al. 1994, Coleman et al. 2000). This approach in which cognitive-behavioral training is used to improve the attitudes and behavior of stockpeople has been described in detail by Hemsworth and Coleman (1998), but basically this type of training involves retraining people in terms of their behavior by, first, targeting both the attitudes that underlie the behavior and the behavior in question and, second, maintaining these changed attitudes and behavior. This process of inducing behavioral change is really a comprehensive procedure in which all the personal and external factors that are relevant to the behavioral situation are explicitly targeted. Clearly there is a strong case for introducing this training in the swine industry. A commercial multimedia training program called "ProHand," which targets the attitudes and behavior of the swine stockperson, is available and is currently used in Australia, New Zealand, and the U.S. (see website www.animal-welfare.org.au for details). A similar training program is also available for swine stockpeople at abattoirs.

Recent research has also shown the potential value of selecting stockpeople using screening aids to predict the performance of stockpeople. The results of research by Coleman et al. (2000) and Coleman (2001) have shown that a number of job-related characteristics, such as empathy and attitudes toward animals and toward aspects of work, may be useful in identifying inexperienced people who are likely to be good stockpeople. Therefore such tests could be assembled into a kit for use in selection in the swine industry. In addition to assisting in selecting stockpeople, assessing the key job-related characteristics of stockpeople may also provide the swine industry with a good opportunity to monitor the potential impact of individual stockpeople on animal welfare. Screening aids such as attitude and job motivation questionnaires may identify both weakness in individual stockpeople and specific training needs for these individuals.

There is a clear need to reduce the limitations that human-animal interactions impose on the productivity and welfare of commercial pigs. Appropriate strategies to recruit and train stockpeople in the swine industry will be integral in safeguarding the productivity and welfare of commercial pigs.

A crude assessment of differences in the level of fear of humans by pigs between units or farms can be made by observing in a standard manner the behavior of pigs in the presence of humans. For example, for units that house sows in gestation stalls, observation of the avoidance responses of sows to a human approaching in a standard manner and placing his or her hand in the front of the stall may provide consultants or managers with a useful technique to assess the relative fear levels across a number of units.

TAIL BITING

Although the incidence of tail biting appears to be highly variable, the problem is widespread with its incidence probably increasing with intensification of pig production (Smith and Penny 1986). The incidence of tail biting is generally lower in outdoor and straw-based housing systems (Schroder-Petersen and Simonsen 2001). The pathology of tail biting has been described by Smith and Penny (1986), and van Putten (1969) lists the possible consequences of tail biting as restlessness, poor growth, possible paralysis and mortality due to infections, and condemnation of the carcass. There have been few experimental studies conducted on tail biting because it is difficult to reliably induce, and consequently its cause(s) is poorly understood.

Outbreaks of tail biting have been attributed to numerous factors, including crowding, poor ventilation, interruption in feed or water supply, poor quality diets, absence of straw and breed type (Smith and Penny 1986; van Putten 1969, Fraser 1987a). The underlying causation of tail biting is poorly understood, but van Putten (1969) argues that an outbreak of tail biting originates from the chewing and rooting of penmates that generally occur with groups of pigs. These low-intensity behaviors are probably a result of the pig's natural tendency to root and chew on objects in its environment, but the behaviors are directed toward other pigs at least partly because of a lack of more suitable objects in a commercial pig pen (van Putten 1969). Tail biting and aggression may occur when pen space is restricted (Jensen 1971; Bryant and Ewbank 1972; Randolph et al. 1981) and Beattie et al. (1996, 2000) showed that enriching the environment with the provision of straw reduced tail biting and persistent nosing of penmates, while increasing exploratory behaviors.

Since the tail is easy to chew and the chewing may not initially provoke an attack by the recipient because the distal half of the tail is relatively insensitive, it is the tail that is most likely to receive a wound. According to van Putten (1969), it is the vigorous tail waving, due to the irritation of a wound, that attracts further biting by other penmates as well as by the original biter. Fraser (1987b) has proposed that an attraction to blood from the wound may also lead to an escalation of tail biting. The large idiosyncratic differences between pigs in the degree of attraction to blood (Fraser 1987a, b) could explain the variable incidence of tail biting.

Removal of the distal half of the tail is a common industry practice: the remaining section of the tail is sufficiently sensitive to chewing to cause the recipient pig to respond (Fraser and Broom 1997). While clipping of the tail may reduce the incidence of tail biting, it may only mask the underlying problem. Attention to ventilation, temperature control, space allowances, feed trough space and drinking facilities may reduce the frequency of low-intensity chewing of penmates (Fraser 1987b; Fraser and Broom 1997), and the provision of distractions such as straw or other chewable objects may be beneficial (van Putten 1969). Injured animals obviously should be removed from the pen and the biter(s) should be identified if possible and housed separately from the group to avoid further occurrences of biting.

EAR AND FLANK BITING

As with tail biting, the cause(s) of outbreaks of these behaviors is poorly understood. However, the origins of outbreaks of ear and flank biting may be similar to those of outbreaks of tail biting: chewing and rooting penmates in an impoverished environment and reduced space may lead to a wound on the ear or a lesion on the flank, which in turn stimulates an outbreak of more biting by penmates. The pathology of ear and flank biting has been described by Smith and Penny (1986).

Treatment and control should be similar to that suggested for tail biting.

BELLY-NOSING

The nosing of the belly or the region between the hind legs of other pigs by weaned piglets, often in flat-deck cages, has been reported by a number of authors (see Fraser and Broom 1997). Belly-nosing for long periods may lead to inflammation of the nipples, umbilicus, penis or scrotum of the recipient.

Since access to straw has been shown to reduce its incidence (Beattie et al. (1996, 2000), the provision of straw or other chewable materials may reduce the incidence of belly-nosing in piglets. Early weaning is implicated in the incidence of belly-nosing (Fraser 1978; Gonyou et al. 1998).

PEN FOULING

The excretory behavior of penned pigs indicates that they have highly localized excretory habits (Baxter 1984), and although many pens are designed with specific excreting areas such as partly slatted areas or dung passages, this does not guarantee the use of these areas by pigs for excretion (Baxter 1989). Only limited research has been conducted on the excretory behavior of pigs; however, Petherick (1983) and Baxter (1984, 1989) have suggested that the main factors affecting the excretory behavior of pigs are security and the thermal environment.

Although objective data are limited, Baxter (1989) proposed a set of rules that can be utilized when designing a pig pen; those rules relating to excretory behavior can be considered when addressing a problem of pen fouling:

1. Pigs will choose a dry, warm, draft-free area in which to rest.
2. Pigs will not choose to rest in areas subject to commotion and disturbance such as around *ad libitum* feeders, drinkers, and grooming points.
3. Pigs will rarely excrete in the area chosen for resting, but they will excrete in any space that is left after the resting area has been established.
4. Pigs may choose to lie in wet, excretory areas if environmental temperatures are high enough to raise their body temperatures to their upper critical level.
5. Pigs will tend to defecate next to walls or corners of the excretory space where they have some protection when they adopt the somewhat unstable posture during excretion. Subordinates may be displaced from an overcrowded excretory area and may then excrete anywhere; this may give rise to a new focus for excretion.
6. A minimum of two drinkers should be provided in every pen, since competition for the drinker (as with feeders) may cause commotion, which in turn may encourage pigs to excrete away from the disturbance.

STEREOTYPIES

Stereotypic behavior can be defined as those behaviors that consist of morphological invariant movements that are regularly repeated, have no obvious function, or are unusual in the context of their performance (Cronin et al. 1986). Examples of these behaviors are bar biting, sham chewing, head weaving, chain chewing or rooting, and excessive drinking (Cronin and Wiepkema 1984).

Numerous authors have proposed explanations for stereotypies in pigs, and these proposed causes range from frustration of feeding to lack of environmental stimulation (Barnett and Hemsworth 1990). Stereotypies shown by pregnant sows in a range of housing systems have been studied by Vieuille-Thomas et al. (1995). The proportion of sows developing stereotypies did not differ between stall-housed and tethered sows (90 vs. 94%) but was lower in group-housed than stall-housed sows (66 vs. 93%). Stereotypies shown by tethered sows mainly involved actions directed against the physical environment, such as licking and rubbing, whereas group-housed and stall-housed sows mainly displayed biting and vacuum oral (self-directed) activities (e.g., vacuum chewing, sucking, and yawning/mouth stretching).

While the cause(s) of the stereotypies is unclear, the function is even less clear and indeed controversial. Some authors have proposed that the occurrence of stereotypies is indicative of poor welfare: it has been suggested that the welfare of the animal is at risk if the stereotypies occur for 10% of the animal's waking life (Broom 1983) and if they occur in more than 5% of all animals (Wiepkema 1983). In contrast, there is limited evidence that some stereotypies may be adaptive for the animal. For example, evidence of either associations between changes in stress physiology, indicative of reduced stress, and stereotypic behavior or that the prevention of stereotypies leads to changes in stress physiology, indicative of increased stress, suggests the adaptive value of these behaviors (Cooper and Nicole 1991). Furthermore, Loijens et al. (1999) reported a negative association between the intensity of stereotypy performance and the density of naloxone binding sites (evidence of opiate receptors) in the hippocampus of tether housed sows. This finding, together with the subsequent finding that individual differences in the density of opioid receptors in the hypothalamus and the hippocampus in sows were related to behavioral and heart rate responses of the pigs in stressful situations (Loijens et al. 2002), adds to the speculation that different individuals may have different coping strategies, and stereotypic behavior may be thus adaptive for some animals in stressful situations. While the latter findings support an association between stereotypies and endogenous opioid activity (e.g., Cronin et al. 1986; Kennes et al. 1988; Zanella et al. 1996), other authors do not support this coping hypothesis (see Dantzer 1991; Rushen 1993). Furthermore, not all stereotypies are a response to stress since Mason (1991) has shown that different forms of stereotypies may have different causes. As concluded by Rushen (1993), the adaptive value of many oral stereotypies may relate to their effects on digestive processes rather than in response to stress.

Therefore, with our present knowledge of the cause and function of stereotypies, there are substantial difficulties in interpreting the implications of stereotypies for the welfare and productivity of pigs, except for those stereotypies that result in physical damage—e.g., the development of lesions in stall-housed sows that persistently rub their tail roots from side to side against stall fittings (Ewbank 1978).

MATERNAL BEHAVIOR

A significant proportion of live-born piglets do not survive the lactation period and a number of factors, such as the physical and climatic environments, health, and nutrition appear to be responsible (see Chapter 62). While savaging and overlying of piglets by sows may account for up to a third of preweaning losses (Cutler et al. 1989), the contribution of changes in maternal behavior of sows to preweaning mortality has received surprisingly little research attention.

Savaging of piglets is more common in primiparous sows (Harris and Gonyou 2003) and the savaging attempt is often directed to only the first-born piglet (English et al. 1984; Spicer et al. 1985). Anecdotal observations suggest that the presence of multiparous (experienced) sows in the farrowing room in the vicinity of nulliparous sows helps calm the inexperienced sows and may contribute to a lower likelihood of savaging. Sows that savage their litters, however, are more likely to be those mated at low body weights (Spicer et al. 1985). Although the cause(s) of savaging is unknown, Pomeroy (1960) suggested that pain and fear predisposed gilts to savage their piglets, while Luescher et al. (1989) suggested that additional factors may be involved, such as the inability of sows to isolate themselves and perform nest-building activities, climatic stress, and human interference during parturition. Some nulliparous sows savage the entire litter. While savaging was responsible for increased mortality in piglets born outside the working hours of the piggery staff (Spicer et al. 1986), this could be reduced if farrowing rooms were continuously lit (Harris and Gonyou 2003). In cases in which the stockperson is on hand when savaging occurs, massage of the sow's udder by the stockperson, an injection of a suitable tranquillizer (e.g., Azaperone) (English et al. 1984) followed by separation of piglets from the sow until farrowing is complete is usually all that is needed to settle the sow.

While malnutrition or illness of piglets may be implicated in many cases of overlying (English et al. 1984), many overlain piglets show no evidence of preexisting illness (Spicer et al. 1985). If a high incidence of overlying is suspected, consideration should be given to the recommendations made by Cutler et al. (Chapter 62) for the provision of a suitable thermal environment for the sow and litter.

The possibility that piglet mortality may be affected by disturbances to the maternal behavior of sows has been demonstrated in an increasing number of studies. Cronin and van Amerongen (1991) found that the provision of straw to and a hessian cover over the farrowing crates of primiparous sows, in order to simulate a completed farrowing nest, reduced preweaning mortality. It is also of interest that the sows in this treatment were more responsive to distress vocalizations of their piglets. Similarly, Cronin et al. (1993) found the addition of small amounts of sawdust to the farrowing crates of young sows (parity 1–3) reduced both the incidence of intrapartum deaths (litter size alive of 10.5 vs. 10.0) and overlying during and 6 hours after parturition (2% vs. 21% of sows). The authors proposed that the provision of sawdust stimulated prepartum activity in younger sows which may have promoted the process of parturition and the development of maternal behavior. While Thodberg et al. (2002) reported that sows appeared calmer before parturition in farrowing pens in which prepartum "nesting" behavior was stimulated, Cronin et al. (1998) found that small, narrow farrowing pens appeared to interfere with the sows' prefarrowing nesting behavior, with consequent increases in sow restlessness during and after farrowing and piglet mortality. These limited results indicate that it may be possible to improve maternal behavior in order to reduce preweaning mortality by modifying the physical environment at parturition, and clearly further research is warranted on maternal behavior.

LOW LEVELS OF SEXUAL BEHAVIOR IN THE BOAR

While there is little documented evidence on poor sexual behavior in commercial boars, experience from artificial insemination centers and commercial piggeries indicate that up to 49% of culled boars are unable to copulate or copulate at sufficient frequency (Melrose 1966). This situation may not have changed much today. Low levels of sexual behavior result from either low sexual motivation or poor mating competency. The latter, if not too serious, may be overcome in some situations where matings are supervised and assisted by stockpeople. Poor mating competency leading to reduced mating success may lead in turn to poor sexual motivation.

Poor Mating Competency

Locomotor and penile injuries may not physically allow the achievement of copulation or may inhibit copulation because of pain (Christensen 1953), while injury sustained during copulation may produce a psychological effect for some time after physical recovery has occurred, again inhibiting copulation. Prevention of locomotor and penile injuries should include attention to the design and maintenance of the accommodation and mating areas, appropriate supervision and assistance at mating or semen collection, and selection for heritable conformational traits of the feet and legs. (See Physical Environment at Mating for a discussion on a suitable

arena for mating.) Poor orientation of the mounting response, such as head mounting, is often seen in the young boar. However, proper orientation is probably a learned response, and if the boar is of satisfactory sexual motivation, mating competency should improve with the positive reinforcement of copulation.

Social Environment

Research has shown that the social environment around the time of puberty can have long-term effects on the sexual behavior of the boar. Isolation of young postpubertal boars from 6–9 months of age from female pigs has been shown to depress their subsequent sexual behavior in a series of mating tests (Hemsworth et al. 1983). This has clear implications for boars used in natural mating but may also have implications for boars used for semen collection, although sexual motivation above a low level may be less critical because of the moderate collection frequency generally required. Housing young postpubertal boars within several meters of females should provide them with sufficient female contact to promote their subsequent sexual behavior. The effects on the sexual behavior of boars of housing near mature boars or near a semen collection area in which olfactory, visual, and auditory stimulation are provided are unknown. However, the interest in using exogenous hormones such as PGF2α to expedite the training of young sexually inexperienced boars for semen collection suggests the need to improve our understanding in this area (Kozink et al. 2002).

Isolation of mature boars from female pigs will also depress their sexual behavior (Hemsworth et al. 1977); however, this effect is not permanent, and housing these isolated boars near females will restore their sexual behavior within 4 weeks. The estrous status of the females does not influence the effectiveness of females in stimulating the sexual behavior of mature boars (Hemsworth 1982). It appears that olfactory and perhaps auditory stimuli from the female are most likely involved in stimulating the sexual behavior of mature boars in natural mating situations (Hemsworth 1982).

As with the social environment around puberty, the social environment during rearing also appears to exert a long-term and perhaps even permanent effect on the sexual behavior of boars. Young boars up to 30 weeks of age require social contact, particularly tactile contact with other pigs, in order to develop high levels of sexual behavior (Hemsworth 1982). Failure to provide young boars with this contact will depress their subsequent sexual behavior. It is recommended that prepubertal boars that may eventually be selected for breeding should be kept in groups for as long as practical, so that sexual behavior develops normally. Young boars kept in groups also display a fully coordinated mating response at an earlier age than boars reared individually (Thomas et al. 1979). If it is necessary to measure individual feed intake, separate feeding stalls could be provided in the group pens. Alternatively, since limited tactile contact with neighboring pigs through wire-mesh walls is sufficient for boars to develop normal levels of sexual behavior (Hemsworth 1982), young boars can be reared in individual pens with wire-mesh or barred divisions.

Physical Environment at Mating

The implications of the physical environment at mating for the reproductive performance of the pig are often neglected. A common practice in intensive units is to mate pigs in the boar's accommodation pen, even though the physical conditions for mating may be far from ideal. For example, the pens are often small and the floors may be slippery, yet research has demonstrated the importance of physical conditions at mating on the sexual behavior of the boar. Hemsworth et al. (1989a) found that the percentage of mating tests that resulted in copulations was lower for pigs mating in the boar's accommodation pen than for those mating in a specific mating pen that had a large, dry, nonslip floor. The sexual behavior of the gilts in the two treatments was similar, but there was a consistent trend between treatments to differ in average time taken by the boars to mount suggesting that the low mating rate of pigs in the boar pen may have been mediated through an effect on the sexual behavior of the boar rather than that of the gilt. The authors concluded that the sexual motivation of the boars may have been adversely affected by the poor physical conditions at the time of mating when matings occurred in the boars' accommodation pens. This study highlights the importance of mating conditions for boars used for both natural matings and semen collection. It is recommended that natural matings should be conducted in separate, specially designed pens with a large floor area (minimum dimension of 2.5 m) to provide the boar with good access to the female's rear quarters; a nonslip floor surface, not abrasive to the animal's feet, that should be kept dry; and an area free of obstructions or other features, such as damaged or wire-mesh walls, that may trap the leg of an unbalanced boar. Similar principles should apply to the area for semen collection.

To minimize moving the pigs, it is useful to have an area adjacent to the boar pens that can be used for both estrus detection and mating. A group of females can be briefly held in this area while the back-pressure test (or riding test, see later) is conducted, and those in estrus can be separated and mated in this pen. Research indicates that gilts detected and mated in such an area have larger litters than those mated in the boar's accommodation pen (Hemsworth et al. 1991). If there is insufficient space available to build a mating pen, a number of these features of a mating pen can be incorporated into the boar pens. For example, pen floors should be properly maintained and a light application of sawdust or straw prior to mating may overcome a slippery floor.

In "hand-mating" systems, the stockperson has a critical role in providing supervision and assistance at mating and in fact may be able to overcome the limitations of some mating systems. Stockpeople have an important role at the time of estrus detection and mating, particularly in terms of avoiding stress and injury to the sexually unreceptive female from a vigorously courting boar, providing the boar with good access to the rear quarters of the receptive female, assisting intromission to maximize the chances of mating, steadying the partners when there is a problem with their footing (e.g., slippery floor, slatted floor, etc.), and identifying those matings with a short duration of ejaculation (i.e., those where a repeat copulation should be attempted if the female is still sexually receptive).

An example of poor supervision that may compromise reproductive performance is found in observations on supervised matings in a large intensive piggery in Australia (Hemsworth, unpublished data). These observations found that one-third of the copulations by gilts and sows had mean durations of ejaculation of 2.5 and 3.2 minutes, respectively, and repeat copulations immediately following these copulations were not attempted. The number of sperm ejaculated during short copulations such as these may be insufficient to consistently achieve high fertility (Thiengtham 1991) and thus proper supervision in these cases may have enabled identification of most of these short copulations to allow a repeat copulation if the female was still receptive. Grigoriadis et al. (2000) has shown the importance of the quality of matings on the fertility of gilts in a dynamic group mating system.

Genetic and Climatic Factors

Evidence from other species (e.g., domestic fowl, McCollom et al. 1971), together with breed comparisons of boars (Einarsson 1968), suggests that the sexual behavior of the boar may have a heritable basis. Elevated environmental temperatures may reduce the sexual behavior of the boar, but this effect is generally only temporary (Winfield et al. 1981), and conducting matings during the cooler times of the day (e.g., early morning) should avoid this problem. Insulation, adequate ventilation, and sprinkler cooling in the mating shed should minimize the adverse effects of high external temperatures.

LOW LEVELS OF SEXUAL BEHAVIOR IN THE FEMALE PIG

Low levels of sexual behavior in female pigs will result in problems with estrus detection and sexual receptivity. It is generally recognized by pig producers that there is more difficulty in mating gilts than in mating sows (English et al. 1982), and thus this section concentrates on gilts; however, most of the principles considered apply to the sow. The literature indicates that in addition to delayed puberty, poor detection of estrus contributes to mating difficulties in commercial gilts (Hemsworth 1982). The incidence and consequences of poor sexual receptivity in those gilts detected in estrus are unknown, although this condition does occur (Cronin et al. 1982). Nevertheless, problems with sexual receptivity and detection of estrus should be considered together, since receptivity or the standing response is generally the criterion used in the main procedures for detecting estrus (e.g., use of boars or the back-pressure test).

Boar Contact

The most common procedure for detecting estrus other than the use of boars is the back-pressure test (BPT) or riding test (Signoret 1970). Females reacting to pressure on their back by displaying the "standing" or lordosis response for at least 10 seconds are generally classified as being sexually receptive (Hemsworth et al. 1988). The efficiency of this procedure depends on the female receiving intense boar contact at the time of testing. Signoret (1970) reported that the maximum percentage of gilts displaying the standing response to the BPT in the absence of boars was 59% between 24 and 36 hours after the start of estrus. This percentage increased to 90% by providing the gilts with auditory and olfactory contact with boars and further increased to 100% with the addition of visual and tactile contact with boars. Similarly, Hemsworth et al. (1984) demonstrated the importance of intense contact with the boar at the time of conducting the BPT. Testing gilts at a distance of 1 m or more from the boar, which presumably reduced the amount of boar contact, reduced the efficiency of the test (52% of postpubertal gilts detected in estrus compared to 90% when gilts were tested adjacent to boars). Therefore, intense boar contact at the time of testing is vital in achieving a high efficiency with the BPT. Reducing boar contact at the time of detection will reduce sexual receptivity in estrous females. Langendijk et al. (2003) have shown the importance of boars in eliciting sexual receptivity, oxytocin release, and, in turn, uterine activity in estrous sows, and thus the stimulation from boars may be critical in situations that are suboptimal for fertilization, such as during seasonal infertility (Pena et al. 1998).

While it appears that boar contact has an important role in stimulating the female's sexual behavior, there are situations where continuous stimulation from the boar may adversely affect sexual behavior. Research (Hemsworth et al. 1984, 1986a, 1988) has shown that housing postpubertal gilts adjacent to boars, with a wire-mesh wall separating them, generally results in a low estrus detection rate with the BPT (e.g., 53% vs. 93% for gilts housed near but not adjacent to boars, Hemsworth et al. 1988). It has been proposed that habituation by gilts to the important boar stimuli (e.g., auditory and olfactory stimuli), which facilitate the standing response of the estrous female to pressure on her back (Signoret 1970), is responsible for this detection problem (Hemsworth et al. 1988). Housing gilts adjacent to boars, which is not uncommon in the industry, may also produce problems in detecting estrus when boars are used for detection (Hemsworth et al. 1987). The results of these studies indicate that housing postpubertal gilts adjacent to boars, with a wire-mesh or barred wall separating them, may adversely affect the sexual behavior of the gilts to the extent that there are difficulties in detecting estrus. Housing weaned sows adjacent to boars does not adversely affect the detection of estrus, possibly because there is insufficient time for habituation to the boar stimuli to occur before the onset of estrus (Hemsworth and Hansen 1990).

Another behavioral problem that may arise through excessive boar stimulation is prolonged boar stimulation at the time of detection. Observations on the sexual receptivity of estrous gilts exposed for an extended period to boars during estrus detection with the BPT indicate that many estrous females may become temporarily refractory to this stimulation, resulting in failure to display the standing response. Levis and Hemsworth, (unpublished data), in studying the behavioral responses of estrous gilts to repeated testing about every 5 minutes, found that the percentage of females standing for the BPT declined from 100% when initially tested to 65% when tested 21 minutes later. This reduction in the sexual receptivity of estrous gilts with frequent stimulation may be due to sexual refractiveness, similar to the sexual refractiveness that occurs in both males and females after copulation. This observation has implication for those situations where females may be tested with the BPT or a boar for estrus over an extended period, but mating or insemination is delayed. There is the possibility that repeated stimulation over an extended period at estrus detection may result in estrous females temporarily experiencing a decline in their sexual receptivity before they can be either detected in estrus or mated.

There is substantial variability in the industry in procedures that use a boar to detect estrous females and yet these procedures have received little research attention. Hughes et al. (1985) reported that 6- to 7-month-old boars provide female pigs with less sexual stimulation than older boars. They found that while only 38% of estrous gilts displayed an immediate standing response to the mounting attempts of young boars, the artificial provision of olfactory and auditory stimulation from older boars increased this percentage to 59%. When stockpeople rely on boars for estrus detection, it is therefore essential that the stockpeople adequately supervise the detection and promptly address any detection problems. Stockpeople need to be particularly vigilant when young boars are used, or when there is variation in the motivation of boars, distractions to the boar's courtship when testing occurs in an unfamiliar location for the boar, and insufficient time and opportunity for the boar to test each female when females are tested in groups. A useful addition to procedures which directly rely on boars for estrus detection is for the stockperson to concurrently use the BPT.

Space Allowance and Group Size

As discussed earlier, there is limited evidence that space allowance and, to a lesser extent, group size of group-housed gilts may influence the efficiency of detecting estrus. Hemsworth et al. (1986b) examined the effects of housing groups of adult postpubertal gilts (6 pigs/group) with a space allowance of 1, 2, or 3 m²/gilt on sexual behavior. A lower percentage of gilts was detected in estrus when housed with a space allowance of 1 m²/gilt than with a space allowance of 2 or 3 m²/gilt (88% vs. 100% and 100%). A significant sustained increase in plasma-free-corticosteroid concentrations in gilts housed with a space allowance of 1 m²/gilt suggests that a chronic stress response may have reduced sexual receptivity. Clearly more comprehensive research is required, but in the meantime it is suggested that postpubertal gilts and weaned sows around the time of mating should be provided with at least 2 m²/animal.

Several studies have examined the effects of group size, however the effects of group size on the sexual behavior of female pigs appear equivocal, perhaps because of suboptimal space allowances in these studies (Hemsworth and Barnett 1990). There are the suggestions from these results that there may be problems in detecting estrus in small groups (groups of 3, Christenson 1984), large groups (groups of 24, Christenson and Ford 1979), and groups of 50 or more (Cronin et al. 1983). The interaction between group size and space allowance must be examined to clarify the optimal social and spatial conditions for group-housed gilts.

Subordinate pair-housed sows show lower levels of sexual receptivity to boars than dominant pair-housed sows or individually housed sows (Pedersen et al. 2003). Although the number of animals studied was low, there were no adverse effects reported on the reproductive performance of these subordinate animals housed in groups. Nevertheless these results further highlight the need for vigilance by stockpeople in detecting estrus in situations in which social effects may impact on the sexual behavior of gilts and sows.

Climatic Environment

Several studies have reported seasonal variation in the rate of detecting estrus in gilts. Christenson (1981) observed that a higher proportion of ovulating gilts were undetected in late summer than in the remainder of the year (16.7 and 8.4%, respectively). Cronin et al. (1983) reported that in the spring there was a lower percentage of unmated postpubertal gilts at 35 weeks of age that had not been detected in estrus than at other times of the year (3.2 and 6.5%, respectively). The effects of photoperiod and temperature are confounded in these two studies.

There is some limited evidence that indicates that increased environmental temperatures may affect sexual behavior of gilts. In two of three trials, Warnick et al. (1965) reported that a total of 3 out of 13 gilts (23.1%) were not detected in estrus at an ambient temperature of 32°C although all had ovulated. In only one of a series of experiments reported by Godfrey et al. (1983), increased temperatures (38°C for 10 hours and 32° for 14 hours) reduced the percentage of gilts detected in estrus (21 vs. 4% for control); however, it was not determined whether ovulatory activity or detection of estrus was affected. Several studies reported that the duration of detected estrus was reduced by high temperatures (see review by Paterson and Pett 1987).

REFERENCES

Barnett JL, Cronin GM, McCallum TH, Newman EA. 1993. Effects of pen size/shape and design on aggression when grouping unfamiliar adult pigs. Appl Anim Behav Sci 36:111–122.

——. 1994. Effects of food and time of day on aggression when grouping unfamiliar adult pigs. Appl Anim Behav Sci 39:339–347.

Barnett JL, Cronin GM, Winfield CG, Dewar AM. 1984. The welfare of adult pigs: The effects of five housing treatments on behaviour, plasma corticosteroids and injuries. Appl Anim Behav Sci 12:209–232.

Barnett JL, Hemsworth PH. 1990. The validity of physiological and behavioural measures of animal welfare. Appl Anim Behav Sci 25:177–187.

——. 1991. The effects of individual and group housing on sexual behaviour and pregnancy in pigs. Anim Reprod Sci 25:265–273.

Barnett JL, Hemsworth PH, Cronin GM, Jongman EC, and Hutson GD. 2001. A review of the welfare issues for sows and piglets in relation to housing. Aust J Agric Res 52:1–28.

Barnett JL, Hemsworth PH, Cronin GM, Newman EA, McCallum TH, Chilton D. 1992. Effects of pen size, partial stalls and method of feeding on welfare-related behavioural and physiological responses of group-housed pigs. Appl Anim Behav Sci 34:207–220.

Barnett JL, Hemsworth PH, Winfield CG, Hansen C. 1986. Effects of social environment on welfare status and sexual behaviour of female pigs. I. Effects of group size. Appl Anim Behav Sci 16:249–257.

Barnett JL, Taylor IA. 1997. Sequential versus concurrent feeding on acute and chronic stress responses in pigs. In Livestock Environment V, volume II. ERW Bottcher, SJ Hoff, eds. American Society of Agricultural Engineers, Michigan, pp. 607–612.

Baxter SH. 1984. Intensive Pig Production: Environmental Management and Design. London: Granada, pp. 210–254.

——. 1989. Designing the pig pen. In Manipulating Pig Production II. Australasian Pig Science Association, Werribee, Australia, pp. 191–206.

Beattie VE, O'Connell NE, Kilpatrick DJ, Moss BW. 2000. Influence of environmental enrichment on welfare–related behavioural and physiological parameters in growing pigs. Anim Sci 70:443–450.

Beattie VE, Walker N, Sneddon IA. 1996. An investigation of the effect of environmental enrichment and space allowance on the behaviour and production of growing pigs. Appl Anim Behav Sci 48:151–158.

Broom DM. 1983. Stereotypies as animal welfare indicators. In Indicators Relevant to Farm Animal Welfare. D Smith, ed. The Hague: Martinus Nijhoff, pp. 81–87.

Broom DM, Mendl MT, Zanella AJ. 1995. A comparison of the welfare of sows in different housing conditions. Animal Science 61:369–385.

Bryant MJ, Ewbank R. 1972. Some effects of stocking rate and group size upon agonistic behaviour in groups of growing pigs. Brit Vet J 128:64–70.

Chapple RP. 1993. Effect of stocking arrangement on pig performance. In Manipulating Pig Production. ES Batterham, ed. Australasian Pig Science Association, Vol. 4, pp. 87–104.

Christensen NO. 1953. Impotentia coeundi in boars due to arthrosis deformans. 15th Int Vet Congr, Part I, Vol. 2, pp. 742–745; Part II, pp. 332–333.

Christenson RK. 1981. Influence of confinement and season of the year on puberty and estrus activity of gilts. J. Anim Sci 52:313–320.

Christenson RK, Ford JJ. 1979. Puberty and estrus in confinement-reared gilts. J Anim Sci 49:743–751.

Christenson RK, Hruska RL. 1984. Influence of number of gilts per pen on estrous traits in confinement reared gilts. Theriogenology 22:313–320.

Coleman GJ, Hemsworth PH, Hay M, Cox M. 1998. Predicting stockperson behaviour towards pigs from attitudinal and job-related variables and empathy. Appl Anim Behav Sci 58:63–75.

——. 2000. Modifying stockperson attitudes and behaviour towards pigs at a large commercial farm. Appl Appl Anim Behav Sci 66:11–20.

Cooper JJ, Nicole CJ. 1991. Stereotypic behaviour affects environmental preference in bank voles, Clethrionomys glareolus. Anim Behav 41:971–977.

Cronin GM, Dunshea FR, Butler KL, McCauley I, Barnett JL, Hemsworth PH. 2003. The effects of immuno- and surgical-castration on the behaviour and consequently growth of group-housed, male finisher pigs. Appl Anim Behav Sci 81:111–126.

Cronin GM, Dunsmore B, Lesbon E. 1998. The effects of farrowing nest size and width on sow and piglet behaviour and piglet survival. Appl Anim Behav Sci 60:331–345.

Cronin GM, Hemsworth PH, Winfield CG. 1982. Oestrous behaviour in relation to fertility and fecundity of gilts. Anim Reprod Sci 5:117–125.

Cronin GM, Hemsworth PH, Winfield CG, Muller B, Chamley WA. 1983. The incidence of, and factors associated with, failure to mate by 245 days of age in the gilt. Anim Reprod Sci 5:199–205.

Cronin GM, Schirmer BN, McCallum TH, Smith JA, Butler KL. 1993. The effects of providing sawdust to pre-parturient sows in farrowing crates on sow behaviour, the duration of parturition and the occurrence of intra-partum stillborn piglets. Appl Anim Behav Sci 36:301–315.

Cronin GM, van Amerongen G. 1991. The effect of modifying the farrowing environment on sow behaviour and growth of piglets. Appl Anim Behav Sci 30:287–298.

Cronin GM, Wiepkema PR. 1984. An analysis of stereotyped behaviour in tethered sows. Ann Rech Vet 15:263–270.

Cronin GM, Wiepkema PR, van Ree JM. 1986. Endorphins implicated in stereotypies of tethered sows. Experientia 42:198–199.

Cutler RS, Spicer EM, Prime RW. 1989. Neonatal mortality: The influence of management. In Manipulating Pig Production. II. Werribee, Australia: Australasian Pig Science Association, pp. 122–126.

de Haer LCM, Merks JWM. 1992. Patterns of daily food intake in growing pigs. Anim Prod 54:95–104.

Dantzer R. 1991. Stress, stereotypies and welfare. Behav Process 25:95–102.

Edwards SA. 1985. Group housing systems for dry sows. Farm Building Progress 80:19–22.

Einarsson S. 1968. Fertility and serving ability of Swedish Landrace and Swedish Yorkshire boars. Nord Vet Med 20:616–621.

Estevez I. 1998. Broiler chickens: A tolerant social system? Etologia 5:19–29.

English PR, Smith WJ, MacLean A. 1984. The Sow—Improving Her Efficiency, 2nd ed. Suffolk: Farming Press Limited, pp. 186–218.

Ewbank R. 1978. Stereotypies in clinical veterinary practice. 1st World Congr Ethol Appl Zootech, Madrid, pp. 499–502.

Fraser AF, Broom DM. 1996. Farm Animal Behaviour and Welfare. Third Edition. UK: CAB International.

Fraser D. 1978. Observations on the behavioural development of suckling and early-weaned piglets during the first six weeks after birth. Anim Behav 26:22–30.

——. 1987a. Mineral-deficient diets and the pig's attraction to blood: Implications for tail biting. Can J Anim Sci 76:909–918.

——. 1987b. Attraction to blood as a factor in tail biting by pigs. Appl Anim Behav Sci 17:61–68.

Fraser D, Rushen J. 1987. Aggressive behaviour. Vet Clin North Am: Food Animal Practice 3:285–305.

Godfrey NW, Mercy AR, Emmus Y. 1983. The effect of high ambient temperature on reproductive performance in gilts. Proc Aust Pig Ind Res Comm Workshop Reprod, Tasmania, Australia.

Gonyou HW. 2001. The social behaviour of pigs. In Social Behaviour in Farm Animals. LJ Keeling, HW Gonyou, eds. Oxon UK: CAB International, pp. 147–176.

Gonyou HW, Beltranena E, Whittington DL, Patience JF. 1998. The behaviour of pigs weaned at 12 and 21 days of age from weaning to market. Can J Anim Sci. 78:517–523.

Grigoriadis DF, Edwards SA, English PR, Davidson FM. 2000. The reproductive behaviour of pigs in a dynamic service system for gilts. Appl Anim Behav Sci 66:203–216

Harris MJ, Gonyou HW. 2003. Savaging behaviour in domestic gilts: A study of seven commercial farms. Can J Anim Sci 83:435–444.

Hemsworth PH. 1982. Social environment and reproduction. In Control of Pig Reproduction. DJA Coles, GR Foxcroft, eds. London: Butterworth, pp 585–601.

Hemsworth PH, Barnett JL. 1990. Behavioural responses affecting gilt and sow reproduction. J Reprod Fert Suppl 40:343–354.

Hemsworth PH, Barnett JL, Coleman GJ. 1993. The human-animal relationship in agriculture and its consequences for the animal. Anim Welf 2:33–51.

Hemsworth PH, Barnett JL, Coleman CJ, Hansen C. 1989b. A study of the relationships between the attitudinal and behavioural profiles of stockpersons and the level of fear of humans and reproductive performance of commercial pigs. Appl Anim Behav 23:301–314.

Hemsworth PH, Barnett JL, Hansen C, Winfield CG. 1986b. Effects of social environment on welfare status and sexual behaviour of female pigs. II. Effects of space allowance. Appl Anim Behav Sci 16:259–267.

Hemsworth PH, Brand A, Willems PJ. 1981. The behavioural response of sows to the presence of human beings and their productivity. Livestock Prod. Sci. 8:67–74.

Hemsworth PH, Coleman GJ. 1998. Human-Livestock Interactions: The Stockperson and the Productivity and Welfare of Intensively-farmed Animals. Oxon UK: CAB International.

Hemsworth PH, Coleman GJ, Barnett JL. 1994. Improving the attitude and behaviour of stockpeople towards pigs and the consequences on the behaviour and reproductive performance of commercial pigs. Appl Anim Behav Sci 39:349–362.

Hemsworth PH, Cronin GM, Hansen, G, Winfield CG. 1984. The effects of two oestrus detection procedures and intense boar stimulation near the time of oestrus on mating efficiency of the female pig. Appl Anim Behav Sci 12:339–347.

Hemsworth PH, Hansen C. 1990. The effects of continuous boar contact on oestrus detection rate of weaned sows. Appl Anim Behav Sci 28:281–285.

Hemsworth PH, Hansen C, Coleman GJ, Jongman EC. 1991. The influence of conditions at the time of mating on reproduction of commercial pigs. Appl Anim Behav Sci 30:273–285.

Hemsworth PH, Hansen C, Winfield CG. 1989a. The influence of mating conditions on the sexual behaviour of male and female pigs. Appl Anim Behav Sci 23:207–214.

Hemsworth PH, Winfield CG, Barnett JL, Hansen C, Schirmer B, Foote M. 1987. The efficiency of boars to detect oestrous females housed adjacent to boars. Appl Anim Behav Sci 19:81–87.

Hemsworth PH, Winfield CG, Barnett JL, Schirmer B, Hansen C. 1986a. A comparison of the effects of two oestrus detection procedures and two housing systems on the oestrus detection rate of female pigs. Appl Anim Behav Sci 16:345–351.

Hemsworth PH, Winfield CH, Beilharz RG, Galloway DB. 1977. Influence of social conditions post-puberty on the sexual behaviour of the domestic male pig. Anim Prod 25:305–309.

Hemsworth PH, Winfield CH, Hansen C, Makin AW. 1983. The influence of isolation from females and mating frequency on the sexual behaviour and semen quality of young post-pubertal boars. Anim Prod 37:49–52.

Hemsworth PH, Winfield CG, Tilbrook AJ, Hansen C, Barnett JL. 1988. Habituation to boar stimuli: Possible mechanism responsible for the reduced detection rate of oestrous gilts housed adjacent to boars. Appl Anim Behav Sci 19:255–264.

Hughes BO, Carmichael NL, Walker AW, Grigor PN. 1997. Low incidence of aggression in large flocks of laying hens. Appl Anim Behav Sci 154:215–234.

Hughes PE, Hemsworth PH, Hansen C. 1985. The effects of supplementary olfactory and auditory stimuli on the stimulus value and mating success of the young boar. Appl Anim Behav Sci 14:245–252.

Jensen AH. 1971. Biological implications of intensive swine rearing systems. J Anim Sci 32:560–565.

Kennes D, Ödberg FO, Bouquet Y, de Rycke PH. 1988. Changes in naloxone and haloperidol effects during the development of captivity-induced jumping stereotypy in bank voles. European J of Pharmacol 153:19–24.

Kornegay ET, Notter DR. 1984. Effects of floor space and number of pigs per pen on performance. Pig News Information 5:23–33.

Kozink DM, Estienne MJ, Harper AF, Knight JW. 2002. The effect of lutalyse on the training of sexually inexperienced boars for semen collection. Theriogenology 58:1039–1045.

Langendijk P, Bouwman EG, Schams D, Soede NM, Kemp B. 2003. Effects of different sexual stimuli on oxytocin release, uterine activity and receptive behaviour in estrous sows. Theriogenology 59:849–861.

Loijens LWS, Schouten WGP, Wiepkema PR, Wiegant VM. 1999. Brain opioid receptor density relates to stereotypies in chronically stressed pigs. Stress 3:17–26.

———. 2002. Brain opioid receptor density reflects behavioural and heart rate responses in pigs. Physiol & Behavior 76:579–587.

Luescher UA, Friendship RM, Lissemore KD, McKeown DB. 1989. Clinical ethology in food animal practice. Appl Anim Behav Sci 22:191–214.

Mason GJ. 1991. Stereotypies: A critical review. Anim. Behav. 41:1015–1037.

McCollom RE, Siegel PB, van Krey HP. 1971. Responses to androgen in lines of chickens selected for mating behaviour. Horm Behav 2:31–42.

McConnell JC, Eargle JC, Waldorf RC. 1987. Effects of weaning weight, co-mingling, group size and room temperature on pig performance. J Anim Sci 65:1201–1206.

Meese GB, Ewbank R. 1973. The establishment and nature of the dominance hierarchy in the domesticated pig. Anim Behav 21:326–334.

Melrose DR. 1966. A review of progress and of possible developments in artificial insemination of pigs. Vet Rec 78:159–168.

Morrison RS, Hemsworth PH, Cronin GM, Campbell RG. 2003. The social and feeding behaviour of growing pigs in deep-litter, group housing systems. Appl Anim Behav Sci 82:173–188.

Nicol CJ, Knowles NG, Parkman TG, Wilkins LJ. 1999. Differential effects of increased stocking density, mediated by increased flock size, on feather pecking and aggression in laying hens. Appl Anim Behav Sci 65:137–152.

Olsson AC, Svendsen J, Reese D. 1994. Housing of gestating sows in long narrow pens with liquid feeding: Function studies and grouping routines in five sow pools. Swedish J Agricultural Research 24:131–141.

Paterson AM, Pett DH. 1987. The role of high ambient temperature in seasonal infertility in the sow. In Manipulating Pig Production. Werribee, Australia: Australasian Pig Science Association, pp. 48–52.

Pagel M, Dawkins MS. 1997. Peck orders and group sizes in laying hens: "Future contracts" for nonaggression. Behavioural Processes 40:13–25.

Pedersen LJ, Heiskanen T, Damm BI. 2003. Sexual motivation in relation to social rank in pair-housed sows. Anim Reprod Sci 75:39–53.

Pena FJ, Dominguez JC, Carbajo M, Anel L, Alegre B. 1998. Treatment of swine summer infertility syndrome by means of oxytocin under field conditions. Theriogenology 49:829–836.

Petherick CJ, Blackshaw JK. 1987. A review of the factors influencing the aggressive and agonistic behaviour of the domestic pig. Aust J Agric Res 27:605–611.

Petherick JC. 1983. A biological basis for the design of space in livestock housing. In Farm Animal Housing and Welfare. ESH Baxter, MR Baxter, JAC MacCormack, eds. The Hague: Martinus Niijhoff, pp. 103–120.

Petherick JC, Bodero DAV, Blackshaw JK. 1987. The use of partial barriers along the feed trough in a group housing system for non-lactating sows. Farm Buildings and Engineering 4:32–36.

Pomeroy RW. 1960. Infertility and neonatal mortality in the sow: Neonatal mortality and foetal development. J Agric Sci (U.K.) 54:31–56.

Price EO. 2003. Animal Domestication and Behavior. Wallingford, Oxon, UK: CAB International, pp. 180.

Randolph JH, Cromwell GL, Stahly TS, Kratzer DD. 1981. Effects of group size and space allowance on performance and behaviour of swine. J Anim Sci 53:922–927.

Rushen J. 1993. The coping hypothesis of stereotypic behaviour. Anim Behav 45:613–615.

Schroder-Petersen DL, Simonsen HB. 2001. Tail biting in pigs. Vet J 162:196–210.

Signoret JP. 1970. Swine behaviour in reproduction. In Effect of Disease and Stress on Reproductive Efficiency in Swine. Extension Service, Univ of Nebraska, pp. 28–45.

Smith WJ, Penny RHC. 1986. Behavioural problems, including vices and cannibalism. In Diseases of Swine, 6th ed. AD Leman, B Straw, RD Glace, WL Mengeling, RHC Penny, E Scholl, eds. Ames: Iowa State Univ Press, pp. 761–722.

Spicer EM, Driesen SJ, Fahy VA. 1986. Causes of preweaning mortality on a large intensive piggery. Aust Vet J 63:71–75.

Spicer EM, Driesen SJ, Fahy VA, Horton BJ. 1985. Trauma, overlay and savaging. Aust Adv Vet Sci, p. 122.

Spoolder HAM, Edwards SA, Corning S. 1999. Effects of group size and feeder space allowance on welfare in finishing pigs. Anim Sci 69:481–489.

Stricklin WR, Mench JA. 1987. Social Organisation. In Farm Animal Behaviour. EO Price, ed. York, PA: Maple-Vail Book Manufacturing Group, pp. 307–322.

Taylor IA, Barnett JL, Cronin GM. 1997. Optimum group size for pigs. In Livestock Environment V, Volume II. RW Bottcher, SJ Hoff, eds. Michigan, USA: American Society of Agricultural Engineers, pp. 965–971.

Thiegtham J. 1991. The distribution of spermatozoa over time in the ejaculate of boars, semen output and sexual behaviour and the effects of sexual stimulation. Master of Agricultural Science Thesis, The University of Melbourne, Australia.

Thodberg K, Jensen KH, Herskin MS. 2002. Nest building and farrowing in sows: Relation to the reaction pattern during stress, farrowing environment and experience. Appl Anim Behav Sci 77:21–42.

Thomas HR, Kattesh HG, Knight JW, Gwazdauskas FC, Meacham TN, Kornegay ET. 1979. Effects of housing and rearing on age of puberty and libido in boars. Anim Prod 28:231–243.

van Putten G. 1969. An investigation of tail-biting among fattening pigs. Br. Vet J 125:511–517.

Vieuielle-Thomas C. 1995. Stereotypies in pregnant sows: Indications of influence of the housing system on the patterns expressed by the animals. Appl Anim Behav Sci 44:19–27.

Warnick AE, Wallace HD, Palmer AZ, Sosa E, Duerre DJ, Caldwell VE. 1965. Effect of temperature on early embryo survival in gilts. J Anim Sci 24:89–92.

Weng RC, Edwards SA, English PR. 1998. Behaviour, social interactions and lesion score of group-housed sows in relation to floor space allowance. Appl Anim Behav Sci 59 307–316.

Wiepkema PR. 1983. On the significance of ethological criteria for the assessment of animal welfare. In Indicators Relevant to Farm Animal Welfare. D Smith, ed. The Hague: Martinus Nijhoff, pp.71–79.

Winfield CG, Hemsworth PH, Galloway DB, Makin AW. 1981. Sexual behaviour and semen characteristics of boars: Effects of high temperature. Agric Anim Husb 21:39–45.

Zanella AJ, Broom DM, Hunter JC Mendl MT. 1996. Brain opioid receptors in relation to stereotypies, inactivity, and housing in sows. Physiol & Behav 59:769–775.

52 Coccidia and Other Protozoa

David S. Lindsay and J. P. Dubey

Coccidia (*Isospora suis* and *Eimeria* spp.)

Coccidia are obligatory intracellular protozoan parasites. *Eimeria, Isospora, Cryptosporidium, Toxoplasma*, and *Sarcocystis* are important genera of protozoal parasites of mammals and birds. Domestic animals may be infected with several species of coccidia but usually only a few species are pathogenic for a given host.

ETIOLOGY

The number of valid species of intestinal coccidia that infect swine is unknown because most are known only from the sporulated oocyst stage. Levine and Ivens (1986) list 13 named species of *Eimeria* and 3 species of *Isospora* from swine. *Isospora suis, I. almataensis*, and *I. neyrai* are the species of *Isospora* described from swine. *Isospora almataensis* and *I. neyrai* are known only from oocysts in the feces and have not been observed in the United States; they probably are not valid species. Neonatal coccidiosis caused by *I. suis* is the most important protozoal disease of swine. Although the causative agent, *I. suis*, was described from pigs in 1934 (Biester and Murray 1934), it was not until the middle 1970s that clinical coccidiosis was recognized as a disease problem in nursing pigs (Sangster et al. 1976). In 1978, it was demonstrated that *I. suis* was the cause of piglet coccidiosis in natural cases, and coccidiosis was experimentally reproduced in nursing pigs (Stuart et al. 1978). Neonatal piglet coccidiosis has a cosmopolitan distribution and is found anywhere pigs are raised in confinement.

Life cycle of *I. suis*

Coccidial life cycles are divided into three phases: sporogony, excystation, and endogenous development (Figure 52.1). Each coccidial phase is unique for each species and knowledge of life cycle phases is important in diagnosis, treatment, prevention, and control of coccidiosis.

Sporogony is the process by which the oocyst (environmentally resistant stage) develops from the unsporulated noninfectious stage passed in the feces to the infective stage (Figure 52.2). Proper temperature and moisture must be present for sporulation to take place. The oocysts of *I. suis* sporulate rapidly at temperatures between 20°C and 37°C (Lindsay et al. 1982). The supplemental heat of between 32°C and 35°C provided by producers for newborn piglets favors rapid development (within 12 hours) of *I. suis* oocysts in the farrowing crate. Oocysts are most sensitive to killing when in the unsporulated state and during sporulation. Once the oocysts are sporulated, they are resistant to most disinfectants. When fully sporulated, the oocysts of *I. suis* and all other *Isospora* species contain two sporocysts, each with four sporozoites.

Excystation is the phase of the life cycle that occurs immediately after the infectious oocysts are ingested. Passage through the stomach alters the oocyst wall and allows bile salts and digestive enzymes to activate the sporozoites. The activated sporozoites leave the sporocyst and oocyst and are freed into the intestinal lumen. The sporozoites then penetrate enterocytes and begin the endogenous phase of parasite multiplication.

The endogenous stages of the life cycle of *I. suis* occur in cytoplasm of enterocytes throughout the small intestine, with most stages being present in the jejunum and ileum. Occasionally, in heavy infections, parasites can be found in the cecum and colon as well. Coccidial stages are usually located on the distal portions of the villi and are in a parasitophorous vacuole below the host-cell nucleus (Lindsay et al. 1980). In severe clinical or experimental cases, stages may also be located in crypt enterocytes.

There are two distinct types of asexual stages in the endogenous life cycle of *I. suis*. Sporozoites enter enterocytes and become binucleated type 1 meronts, which

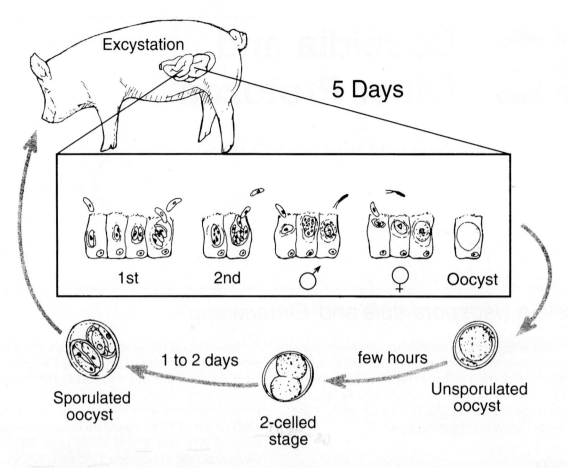

52.1. *Life cycle of* Isospora suis.

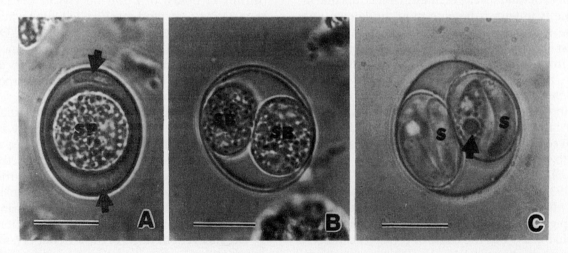

52.2. *Oocysts of* Isospora suis *in fecal flotations. Bar = 10 μm. (A) Freshly excreted Unsporulated oocyst. Note the hazy bodies (arrows) and the sporont (SP). (B) Oocyst several hours after excretion. Note that 2 sporoblasts (SB) are present. (C) Sporulated oocyst approximately 1 day after excretion. Note the sporozoites (S) and residual body (arrow) in the sporocysts (Modified from Lindsay et al. 1982).*

divide by endodyogeny in about 24 hours; each meront produces two type 1 merozoites. The characteristic side-by-side appearance of these type 1 merozoites is useful in diagnosis because none of the swine *Eimeria* species divide by endodyogeny. Several divisional cycles by endodyogeny can occur and produce cells with many

type 1 merozoites. Type 2 meronts are multinucleated and form type 2 merozoites, which may be seen as early as 1 day postinoculation (PI). Type 2 merozoites are smaller than type 1 merozoites. Sexual stages consist of microgamonts, which produce biflagellated microgametes, and uninucleate macrogamonts. The microgametes fertilize the macrogamonts, and an oocyst is formed. These sexual stages also may be seen 4 days PI, whereas oocysts are first seen in the feces 5 days PI (rarely 4 days).

Immunity to *Isospora suis*

Pigs that have been infected with *I. suis* and recover are resistant to challenge infection (Stuart et al. 1982b). These challenged pigs excrete no or very few oocysts (in contrast to initial infection) and do not develop clinical signs. Administration of corticosteroids (methylprednisolone acetate) does not cause these previously exposed pigs to reexcrete oocysts, suggesting good immunity has developed. Colostral antibodies against *I. suis* do not protect piglets from developing clinical coccidiosis (Taylor 1984). Serum antibodies peak about 1 week after primary infection, and a secondary antibody response occurs following challenge infection. Serum antibodies against *I. suis* do not recognize sporozoites of *E. debliecki, E. neodebliecki, E. scabra,* or *E. porci* from pigs in an indirect fluorescent antibody test.

Pigs have age-related differences in susceptibility to experimental infection and disease (Stuart et al. 1982a; Koudela and Kucerova 1999). Pigs that are 1–2 days old develop much more severe disease than do pigs inoculated with an identical number of oocysts at 2 or 4 weeks of age.

Clinical Signs

Signs of disease occur in formerly healthy nursing pigs between 7 and 11 days of age (Stuart et al. 1978). Yellowish to grayish diarrhea is the major clinical sign. The feces are initially loose or pasty and become more fluid as the infection progresses. Piglets become covered with the liquid feces, causing them to stay damp and have a rancid odor of sour milk. The piglets usually continue to nurse, develop a rough hair coat, become dehydrated, and have depressed weight gains (Lindsay et al. 1985). Litters within the farrowing house vary in the degree to which they demonstrate clinical signs, and not all piglets within a litter are equally affected. Morbidity is usually high but mortalities are usually moderate. Concurrent bacterial, viral, or other parasitic infections may lead to extreme mortalities and complicate diagnosis.

Occasionally *I. suis* oocysts are present in the feces of recently weaned pigs, some of which may have diarrhea. Although this indicates a patent infection, whether or not *I. suis* is the etiologic agent of the diarrhea is unknown because of complicating factors such as diet and other management changes that occur at weaning. There is a report that *I. suis* caused postweaning diarrhea in 5- to 6-week-old piglets (Nilsson 1988). Diarrhea began 4–7 days after the piglets were weaned. Morbidity was high (80–90%) but mortalities were rare. *I. suis* infections do not cause disease in finishing pigs or in breeding stock.

Pathologic Changes

Experimental studies have shown that the degree of disease is dependent on the number of sporulated *I. suis* oocysts that a piglet ingests (Stuart et al. 1980). Inoculation of 200,000 or more oocysts usually produces severe disease and moderate to extreme mortalities (Stuart et al. 1980; Lindsay et al. 1985). Inoculation of fewer oocysts generally produces clinical disease characterized principally by diarrhea but few or no mortalities.

Necropsy examination may demonstrate gross lesions of neonatal coccidiosis characterized by a fibrinonecrotic membrane in the jejunum and ileum, but this is seen only in severely infected piglets. Hemorrhage is not seen even in extreme cases of natural infections or in experimental infections where large numbers of oocysts are given.

Microscopic lesions consist of villous atrophy, villous fusion, crypt hyperplasia, and necrotic enteritis (Stuart et al. 1980). The usual tall columnar enterocytes at the tips of the villi may be destroyed, exposing the underlying lamina propria, or they may be replaced by flattened immature enterocytes. The functional ability for absorption is diminished in this altered epithelium, resulting in fluid loss and diarrhea. Immunohistochemical studies indicate that infection alters carbohydrate residues on the enterocystes (Choi et al. 2003). Lesions develop about 4 days PI and are associated with the presence of the asexual stages. In most natural cases few parasites are present in the sections and most of these parasites are asexual stages. In severe cases piglets may succumb to coccidiosis before the sexual stages are produced. The extent of microscopic lesions produced is dependent on the number of *I. suis* oocysts a pig ingests.

The role of viral and bacterial copathogens with *I. suis* has been examined experimentally (Baba and Gaffer 1985; Vitovec et al. 1991). The responses of gnotobiotic and conventional pigs to *I. suis* and rotavirus infection are similar (Vitovec et al. 1991). The degree of observed clinical disease is more severe when the two pathogens are administered concurrently than when either is given singly. Both the virus and the parasite prefer to develop in the enterocytes on the central and distal portion of the villi in the small intestine, and competition for a suitable host cell is believed to be the cause for the observed increase in clinical disease and microscopic lesions. An established *I. suis* infection will interfere with the establishment of a *Salmonella typhimurium* infection (Baba and Gaffer 1985). The increased gut motility and destruction of host cells probably interfere with the bacterium's ability to colonize the intestinal mucosa.

DIAGNOSIS

Diarrhea in nursing pigs 7–14 days of age that does not respond to antibiotic treatment is suggestive of neonatal *I. suis* infection. Other agents such as enteropathogenic *Escherichia coli,* transmissible gastroenteritis virus, rotavirus, *Clostridium perfringens* type C, and *Strongyloides ransomi* should be considered in the differential diagnosis.

Diagnosis of *I. suis* is best achieved by finding *I. suis* oocysts in the feces of clinically affected piglets (Figure 52.2A, B). This is the quickest method available for diagnosis. Fecal smears or fecal flotations should be made from several litters within the farrowing house that have been showing clinical signs for 2–3 days, because diarrhea starts about a day before oocysts are passed and peak oocyst production occurs about 2–3 days after clinical signs develop. Piglets excrete oocysts in several phases and may be negative during these phases. Pasty fecal samples are likely to contain more oocysts than are liquid samples. The oocysts of *I. suis* have characteristic structures called "hazy bodies" between the oocyst wall and the sporont (Figure 52.2A). These are diagnostic for *I. suis* because none of the oocysts of the swine *Eimeria* species have this structure (Lindsay et al. 1982). Additionally, some of the oocysts may be in the two-celled sporoblast stage (Figure 52.2B), which is also diagnostic for *I. suis.* Fecal fat may make identification of oocysts in Sheather's sugar flotation preparations difficult. A solution of saturated sodium chloride and glucose (500 g of glucose in 1000 ml saturated sodium chloride solution) has been recommended as an alternative flotation medium (Henriksen and Christensen 1992).

Demonstration of developmental stages (Figure 52.3A–D) in mucosal smears can be used in the diagnosis of *I. suis* infection (Lindsay et al. 1983). The intestinal mucosa should be scraped with a scalpel or coverslip using just enough pressure to dislodge villi, and the scrapings should be prepared as a smear on a glass microscope slide. The smears are then stained with any of a number of routine blood stains.

The presence of paired type 1 merozoites (Figure 52.3D) is diagnostic. Other asexual stages (such as binucleated type 1 meronts or type 2 meronts and merozoites) and sexual stages (microgamonts and macrogamonts) will probably be present also, but their identification is more difficult and not needed for diagnosis.

Histologic diagnosis of *I. suis* in tissue sections is possible (Lindsay et al. 1983). As with mucosal smears, demonstration of paired type 1 merozoites is diagnostic (Figure 52.3E–H). The multinucleated type 2 meronts of *I. suis* are elongated and are often found in the same host cell. Finally, the macrogamonts of *I. suis* lack the characteristic eosinophilic wall-forming bodies seen in *Eimeria species.*

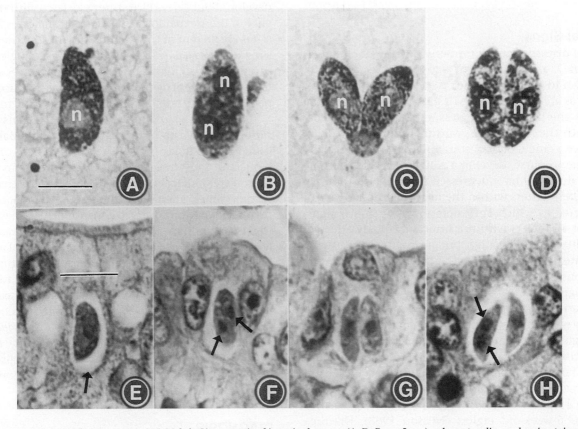

52.3. *Diagnostic stages of* Isospora suis *in Wright's Giemsa-stained intestinal smears (A–D: Bar = 5 μm) or hematoxylin- and eosin-stained histological sections (E–H: Bar = 10 μm). (A) Zoite with a single nucleus (n). (B) Type 1 meront, which has two nuclei (n). (C) Dividing type 1 meront. Note the nuclei (n). (D) Paired type 1 merozoites. Note that each has a single nucleus (n). (E) Zoite in a parasitophorous vacuole (arrow). (F) Type 1 meront. Note that two nuclei (arrows) are present. (G) Paired type I merozoites. (H) Host cell with a type 1 meront (arrows label nuclei) and a type 1 merozoite. (Modified from Lindsay et al. 1980.)*

PCR (Ruttkowski et al. 2001) and autofluorescence (Daugschies et al. 2001) of oocysts are other methods that can be used to diagnose *I. suis* infection. These methods are limited to use by diagnostic laboratories using specialized equipment.

EPIDEMIOLOGY

Eimeria Species

Eight species of *Eimeria* occur in swine in the United States (Vetterling 1965). Reports of coccidiosis in swine caused by *Eimeria* species are rare (Hill et al. 1985). Experimental studies have demonstrated that inoculation of 3-day-old nursing pigs with up to 5 million oocysts of *Eimeria debliecki* does not cause clinical disease and that inoculation of up to 10 million oocysts does not cause disease in 4-week-old weaned pigs (Lindsay et al. 1987). Similar results were obtained in 2- to 3-month-old pigs given 4 million oocysts of *E. debliecki* (Vitovec and Koudela 1990).

Eimeria spinosa is not pathogenic for pigs under experimental conditions (Koudela and Vitovec 1992). Reports of natural cases of *E. spinosa* associated disease in weaned pigs suggest that this species can cause disease under appropriate conditions in the field (Lindsay et al. 2002, Yaeger et al. 2003). Coccidia vary in their inherent abilities to cause disease, and it appears that the *Eimeria* species infecting swine are generally nonpathogenic.

Isospora suis

Once *I. suis* coccidiosis was recognized as a problem in nursing pigs, most veterinarians and researchers assumed that piglets were infected by ingesting *I. suis* oocysts from the sow's feces. However, studies have failed to confirm this assumption. Surveys of the swine population in the United States indicate that *Eimeria* infections are common (60–95%) in animals raised in lots or in the wild, but less than 3% of the animals sampled excrete oocysts of *I. suis* (Vetterling 1966; Lindsay et al. 1984). One study examined the species of oocysts excreted by sows on farms with and without a history of *I. suis* infections in nursing pigs; sows on all the farms underwent gestation on dirt lots (Lindsay et al. 1984). The study reported that 82% of the sows on farms with a history of coccidiosis had *Eimeria* infections but no detectable *I. suis* infections. The sows from farms with no history of neonatal coccidiosis had an infection rate of 95% with *Eimeria* species and less than 1% with *I. suis*.

In the United States, Stuart and Lindsay (1986) examined the transmission of *I. suis* on two farms in Georgia. Daily fecal samples were collected rectally from sows typically 1 week prior to farrowing, the day of farrowing, and for about 1 week after farrowing. Colostrum and placentas from several sows were examined microscopically for parasites. A coccidiostat (amprolium HC1, Amprol 25% feed grade) was given to half of the sows on each farm. *Eimeria* species were the only coccidia seen in the feces of sows. None of the sows given amprolium HC1 had oocysts in fecal samples at farrowing. No parasitic stages were seen in the colostrum or placentas examined. On Farm 1, 7 of 12 litters from nontreated sows and 9 of 12 litters from treated sows developed clinical coccidiosis. On Farm 2, all litters from nontreated sows and 11 of 12 litters from treated sows developed clinical coccidiosis. *I. suis* was the only species of coccidia seen in these piglets.

The results of these studies indicate that sows are not the primary source of *I. suis* infection for nursing pigs. It is still not known how *I. suis* becomes established on a farm; once it is established, it is probably transmitted through contaminated farrowing crates. The temperature (32–35°C) and moisture in the farrowing crate favor rapid sporulation of *I. suis*. High temperatures (32–35°C) may inhibit sporulation of the *Eimeria* species and could explain the absence of these species in nursing pigs.

TREATMENT AND CONTROL

Anticoccidials

Sows do not appear to be a major source of infection for nursing pigs; therefore, using anticoccidial drugs in the sow's ration is of little value in controlling neonatal coccidiosis. Early studies that reported success with treating sows probably are due to improved sanitation once the producers were made aware that their pigs had coccidiosis. Studies that demonstrate anticoccidial activity of drugs in weaned or finishing pigs are of no value in predicting the ability of these drugs to control disease in nursing pigs. Addition of anticoccidial drugs to the drinking water of piglets or mixing drugs in oral iron may be beneficial in treating coccidiosis, but there is no way to ensure that every piglet gets a therapeutic/preventive dose. There are no controlled studies that have documented the effectiveness of this type of treatment. Individual dosing is still the best way to ensure that each piglet gets a proper dose of anticoccidial drug.

Toltrazuril, a triazinon antiprotozoal not available in the United States, appears promising as an effective means of preventing coccidiosis in nursing piglets (Driesen et al. 1995). Toltrazuril (Baycox 5% suspension) was given orally at 20–30 mg/kg as a single dose to 3- to 6-day-old piglets on five farms with coccidiosis problems. Coccidiosis was reduced from 71% to 22% in treated litters. The severity of diarrhea and oocyst excretion was reduced in toltrazuril-treated piglets. Experimentally, toltrazuril was effective in reducing clinical signs and oocyst production at a single 20 mg/kg dose given to 5-day-old pigs that had been inoculated at 3 days of age (Mundt et al. 2003). Toltrazuril's excellent activity is probably based on its ability to kill asexual and sexual stages of coccidia and because it is slowly released from tissues of treated animals.

Controlled studies conducted to date in nursing pigs

have not identified other effective coccidiostats. Amprolium, furazolidone and monensin are not effective against neonatal procine coccidiosis.

Sanitation

Improved attention to sanitation has been the most successful method for reducing losses due to neonatal coccidiosis in pigs (Ernst et al. 1985; Stuart and Lindsay 1986). A good sanitation program entails thorough cleaning of the crates to remove organic debris, disinfection with bleach (at least 50%) or ammonia compounds for several hours or overnight, and steam-cleaning. Buildings should be empty of animals when disinfecting is being done. Ventilation should be adequate to prevent excessive exposure of workers to fumes of bleach or ammonia, or a chemical mask must be worn by workers. Producers should limit access to farrowing crates by workers to avoid crate-to-crate contamination with oocysts carried on boots or clothing. Likewise, pets should be prevented from entering the farrowing house and spreading oocysts from crate to crate on their paws. Rodent populations should be controlled to prevent these animals from mechanically transmitting oocysts.

Facilities need to be sanitized after every farrowing. Producers should be made aware that even though clinical disease is under control, the potential for future outbreaks is still present. In some cases, outbreaks of moderate clinical disease have developed in the first farrowing after sanitation was not done (Ernst et al. 1985).

Toxoplasmosis (*Toxoplasma gondii*)

Toxoplasmosis is caused by infection with *Toxoplasma gondii,* a protozoan parasite related to the coccidia. Infections are common in humans and animals. Postnatally, animals or humans become infected by ingesting food and water contaminated with sporulated *T. gondii* oocysts or by consuming meat containing tissue cysts. Cats (and other felines) are the only animals that can excrete resistant oocysts in their feces and are important in the transmission of *T. gondii* to pigs and other animals (Figure 52.4). Tissue cysts are found mainly in many edible tissues of infected animals, and they contain bradyzoites in various slowly multiplying stages (Figure 52.5B). Tissue cysts remain viable in the tissues for many years and probably the life of the animal. After ingestion, oocysts or bradyzoites can survive passage through the stomach. Once in the intestine of the host, sporozoites or bradyzoites change into a fast-multiplying stage called tachyzoites (Figure 52.5A). Tachyzoites multiply in the lamina propria of the intestine and eventually spread throughout the body. Prenatal infection may occur if the mother is infected during pregnancy. Tachyzoites from the mother's blood may cross to the fetus via the placenta. Tachyzoites cause tissue damage and eventually develop into the bradyzoite stage and form tissue cysts. Toxoplasmosis is a zoonosis, and pork is considered a major meat source of human infection in the United States (Dubey 1990).

Clinical Signs

Most infections in swine are subclinical (Dubey 1986). Abortions due to *T. gondii,* although uncommon, may occur in sows infected during pregnancy. Transplacentally infected pigs may be born premature, dead, or weak, or they may die soon after birth. Pigs that live may develop diarrhea, incoordination, tremors, or cough. Few reports exist on clinical disease in pigs that acquire infection postnatally, but epizootics of clinical toxoplasmosis have been observed in both young and adult pigs (Dubey et al. 1979; Dubey and Beattie 1988). Experimental studies indicate that ingestion of *T. gondii* oocysts by pigs is more likely to produce clinical disease than ingestion of tissue cysts (Dubey 1986). Severity of disease is dependent upon the number of oocysts ingested. Older animals are less likely to develop clinical disease.

Pathologic Changes

Pathologic changes are associated with necrosis of host tissue caused by the rapidly multiplying tachyzoites (Figure 52.6). Ingestion of oocysts is more likely to give rise to intestinal lesions than is ingestion of tissue cysts. Enteritis, lymphadenitis, splenitis, hepatitis, pneumonitis, and less frequently myositis and encephalitis are seen in naturally infected pigs (Dubey 1986).

DIAGNOSIS

Methods of diagnosis include bioassays of tissues in cats or mice, serology, and histology. Bioassays are the most sensitive but are costly and time-consuming, and few laboratories perform these tests. Several serologic tests are available for determining antibodies to *T. gondii* in pigs. These include the Sabin-Feldman dye test (DT), indirect hemagglutination test, direct agglutination (DAG) test, latex agglutination test, indirect fluorescent antibody test, and ELISA. The DAG test is the most sensitive and specific for the detection of latent *T. gondii* infection in swine (Dubey et al. 1995a). Although finding *T. gondii* antibody in adult pigs only means exposure to *T. gondii,* finding antibody in a fetus indicates congenital infection because maternal antibodies are not transferred to the fetus in pigs. Histologic examination of tissues may be utilized for a presumptive diagnosis based

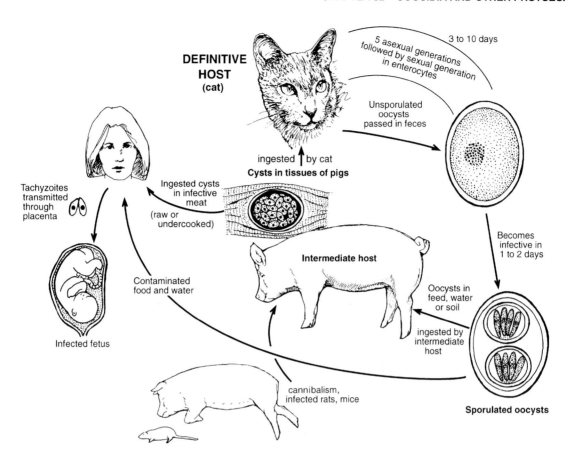

52.4. *Life cycle of* Toxoplasma gondii.

on lesion characteristics and parasite structure following routine histologic staining of tissue sections or identification of organisms in impression smears stained with Giemsa or other blood stains (Figure 52.5A). *Toxoplasma gondii* tachyzoites are lunate and about the size of a red blood cell. Tissue cysts are oval to round, up to 70 μm in diameter, and contain many bradyzoites (Figure 52.5B). For a definitive diagnosis if parasites are found in tissue sections, specific immunohistochemical tests (peroxidase-antiperoxidase test, avidin-biotin complex test) can be used.

EPIDEMIOLOGY

The prevalence of congenital *T. gondii* infection in pigs is less than 0.01%. Prevalence of *T. gondii* antibodies in feeder pigs (younger than 6 months) is much lower (3–5%) than in sows (15–20%) based on large-scale surveys in Illinois (Weigel et al. 1995; Dubey et al. 1995b). The presence of *T. gondii*-infected cats and infected rodents were identified as the main sources of *T. gondii* infection for pigs (Weigel et al. 1995). Cats become infected with *T. gondii* by ingesting infected animals (rodents, birds) soon after weaning. Therefore, infected juvenile cats are considered to be the main source of *T. gondii* for farm pigs. Cats generally acquire good immu-

nity to *T. gondii*, and cats that have excreted oocysts once are less likely to excrete oocysts again (Dubey et al. 1986).

TREATMENT AND CONTROL

Because porcine toxoplasmosis is usually subclinical, little is known about the treatment of the disease (Dubey 1986). In general, drugs used to treat toxoplasmosis in humans have been effective. These include pyrimethamine or trimethoprim in combination with a systemically active sulfonamide.

Control of *T. gondii* infection in pigs is important because of public-health concerns over human infections. Toxoplasmosis causes mental retardation and loss of vision in congenitally infected children. Following experimental infection, viable tissue cysts of *T. gondii* can be found in most commercial cuts of pork, and studies have shown that the tissue cysts will be viable for at least 2.5 years (Dubey 1988). Freezing (−12°C) for 3 days or cooking pork until internal temperature reaches 60°C will kill tissue cysts in pork (Dubey et al. 1990). Low-dose gamma irradiation (0.5 kGy cessium 137) kills tissue cysts in pork.

Prevention of *T. gondii* infection in pigs can be achieved by practicing good husbandry. There is no vac-

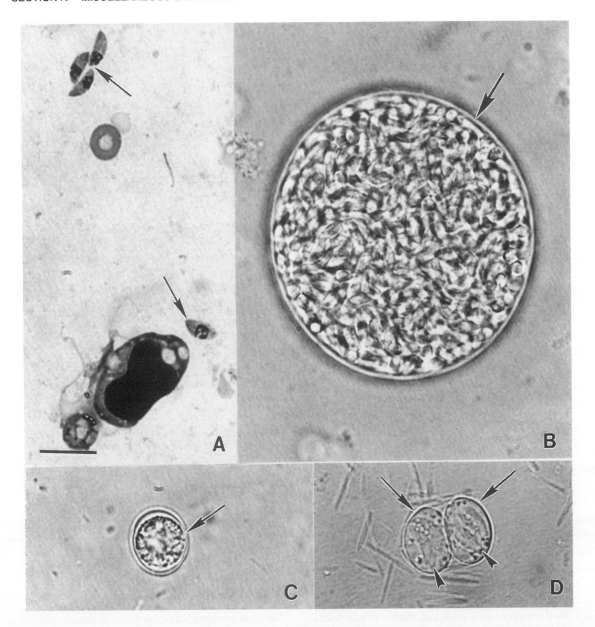

52.5. Toxoplasma gondii *stages in smears of tissues of animals. Bar = 10 μm. (A) Tachyzoites from lung (arrows), Giemsa stain. (B) Tissue cyst from brain, unstained. Note hundreds of bradyzoites enclosed in a thin cyst wall (arrow). (C) Unsporulated oocyst (arrow) from cat feces, unstained. (D) Sporulated oocyst from cat feces, unstained. Note two sporocysts (arrows). The sporozoites are barely visible (arrowheads).*

cine. To prevent oocyst-induced infections, cats should never be allowed in buildings where pigs are housed or where feed is stored. Rodenticides should be used to control rodents and eliminate this possible source of tissue cysts. Any pigs that die should be removed promptly to prevent cannibalism. Wild-animal carcasses or uncooked garbage should never be fed to pigs. Feed should be kept covered to prevent cats from defecating in it.

Sarcocystosis

Sarcocystis spp. are coccidia parasites that have a two-host life cycle (Figure 52.7). Three species use pigs as the intermediate host and form tissue cysts (sarcocysts) in the pig muscles. *Sarcocystis miescheriana* has a pig-dog life cycle and is the only species found in the United States. Dogs excrete infective stages (sporocysts) in their feces. The other species are *S. suihominis*, which uses the human as the definitive host, and *S. porcifelis*, which uses the cat as the definitive host (Dubey et al. 1989). Surveys indicate that from 3–18% of commercial breed-

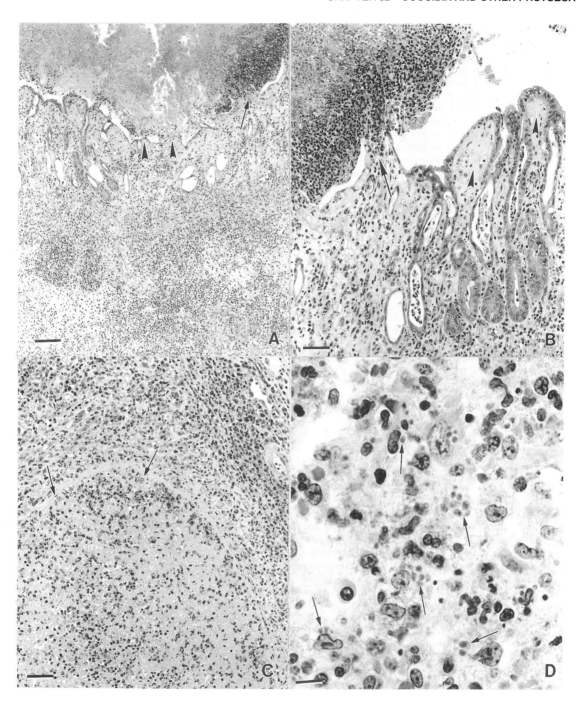

52.6. *Lesions in the small intestine (A,B) and mesenteric lymph node (C, D) in a pig 9 days after ingesting 100,000* Toxoplasma gondii *oocysts (Hematoxylin and eosin stain). (A) Pseudomembranous necrotic enteritis. Note severe inflammation involving the entire width of the intestine, shortening of the villi (arrowheads), and attachment of desquamated intestinal contents to the epithelium (arrow). Bar = 10 μm. (B) Higher power of an area marked by an arrow in A. Note attachment of pseudomembrane to intestinal lamina propria (arrow) and necrosis of the lamina propria at tips of the villi (arrowhead). Bar = 25 μm. (C) Necrosis and depletion of lymphocytes. Numerous tachyzoites are present but only a few (arrows) are visible at this magnification. Bar = 25 μm. (D) High power of C. Note numerous tachyzoites (arrows). Bar = 10 μm.*

ing sows and 32% of wild swine examined in the United States have *Sarcocysitis* infection (Dubey and Powell 1994). There are no reports of naturally occurring clinical disease due to *Sarcocystis* infection in swine (Dubey et al. 1989). Experimental infections indicate that *S. mi-*

escheriana can cause abortion, death, dyspnea, weight loss, muscle tremors, and purpura of the skin. *Sarcocystis* infection in swine can be prevented by eliminating their exposure to canine feces. To prevent exposure in dogs, they should not be allowed to consume pig carcasses.

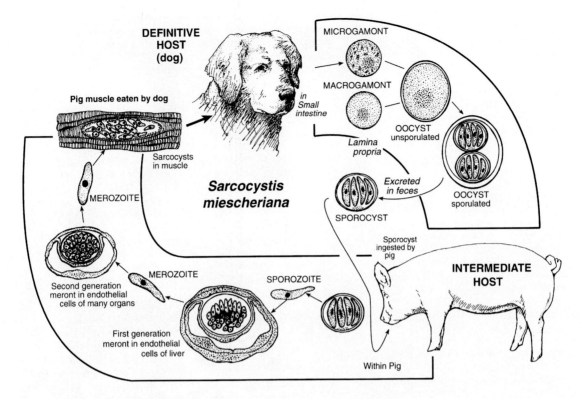

52.7. *Life cycle of* Sarcocystis miescheriana.

Cryptosporidiosis

Members of the genus *Cryptosporidium* differ from conventional coccidia that infect animals in that they develop in the microvillous border of enterocytes rather than deep down in the host-cell cytoplasm (Figure 52.8). Additionally, oocysts of *Cryptosporidium* are completely sporulated when excreted in the feces and contain four sporozoites and no sporocysts (Upton and Current 1985).

Cryptosporidiosis is caused by infection with *Cryptosporidium parvum,* which is a recognized zoonosis. Recent molecular and animal infectivity studies indicate that pigs are host for other species of *Cryptosporidium* referred to as "pig genotypes" (Enemark et al. 2003; Ryan et al. 2003) that are different from *C. parvum*. The prevalence of *C. parvum* compared to pig genotype infections in pigs is not known. Human infections with pig genotypes are rare (Xiao et al. 2002), and pigs do not appear to be a major source of infection for humans.

CLINICAL SIGNS AND PATHOLOGIC CHANGES

Porcine cryptosporidiosis is usually subclinical and not a major production problem (Sanford 1987). If clinical signs are present, they consist of nonhemorrhagic diarrhea, usually in pigs younger than 12 weeks (Sanford 1987).

Microscopic lesions associated with cryptosporidial infection in pigs are minimal or absent. The parasites are found in the jejunum, ileum, cecum, and colon, with most parasites being in the ileum. When lesions are present, they consist of mild villous atrophy and invasion of the lamina propria by large numbers of mononuclear inflammatory cells and fewer eosinophils (Sanford 1987). Microvilli in the area of the parasites may be displaced or hypertrophic.

EPIDEMIOLOGY AND DIAGNOSIS

Pigs are infected by ingesting oocysts in contaminated feed, from the environment, or in water. There is no seasonal pattern to the prevalence of infection (Sanford 1987).

Diagnosis can be achieved by finding the developmental stages of the parasite in histologic sections. The parasites are 2–6 μm and basophilic and appear to be embedded in the microvillous border of the enterocytes. Diagnosis can also be made by finding the characteristic oocysts in fecal flotations, but molecular methods are needed for speciation. The oocysts are small, 5.0 by 4.5 μm, and have a pinkish color and residual body when observed with light microscopy. Sheather's sugar solution is the flotation medium of choice; a microscope

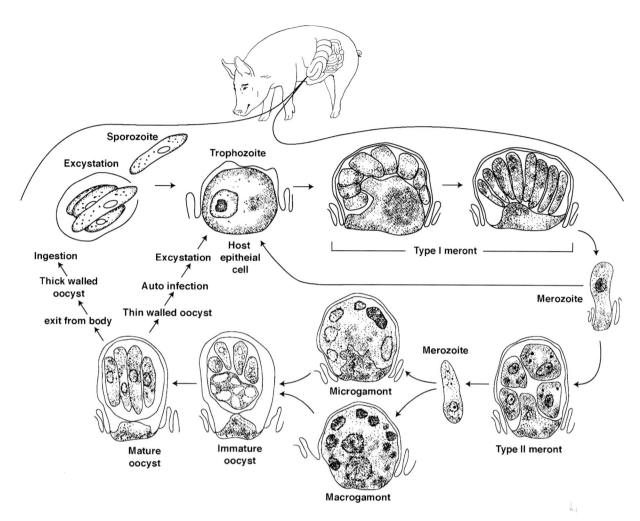

52.8. *Life cycle of* Cryptosporidium.

equipped with good objectives is needed to identify the oocysts in flotations. It is important to remember that in fecal flotations, the cryptosporidial oocysts will be in a slightly higher plane of focus than other coccidial oocysts. Several methods of staining fecal samples and examining for oocysts have been developed but these are not practical for use in pigs. Several serologic methods such as enzyme-linked immunosorbent assay (ELISA) and indirect fluorescent antibody test (IFAT) have been developed for estimating the prevalence of cryptosporidial exposure, but these tests are not currently in widespread use.

TREATMENT AND CONTROL

There is no treatment for cryptosporidial infection. Sanitation methods used to control *I. suis* coccidiosis should also prove effective against cryptosporidial infections.

Other Protozoa of Minor Importance or Potentially Transmissible to Humans

GIARDIA

Giardia species are flagellated protozoan that cause fatty diarrhea in humans and companion animals. *Giardia* cysts contain four nuclei, median bodies, and are about 12 micrometers in length. These cysts can be found in the feces of many mammalian species, including pigs.

The trophozoites of *Giardia* live in the lumen of the small intestine, usually the upper small intestine. They have two nuclei and an adhesive disk by which they attach to enterocytes. They are not considered pathogenic for pigs (Koudela et al. 1991). Molecular analysis of *Giardia* isolates obtained from pigs indicates that human infective *Giardia* may be found in pigs and that "Livestock" infective genotypes can be found in pigs (Ey et al. 1997). The role of pigs in the transmission of *Giardia* to humans is not presently known.

MICROSPORIDIA

Microsporidia are in the phylum Microspora. These organisms infect both vertebrates and invertebrates. They are intracellular pathogens and can be found in a variety of locations in the host's body. Human and animal infections with the well-known *Encephalitozoon cuniculi* were recognized prior to the AIDS pandemic. However, overall awareness of this phylum as important parasites of warm-blooded animals came about only after the advent of AIDS. Hosts are infected by ingestion of spores passed in the urine or feces. The polar tube penetrates a cell, and the sporoplasm, containing the nucleus, is passed through the tube into the host cell. Inside the host cell the parasite replicates asexually until the host cell bursts, releasing newly formed spores. Most microsporidia are small (1 to 4 micrometers) and resemble bacteria when examined unstained with light microscopy.

Clinical microsporidiosis has not been reported in pigs. Pigs are naturally infected with *Enterocytozoon bieneusi* (Breitenmoser et al. 1999), an important cause of chronic diarrhea in AIDS patients. Self-limiting diarrhea occurs in immuonocompetent patients. Several different genotypes of *Ent. bieneusi* occur in pigs and humans. An 18-month long survey of pigs from a slaughterhouse in Massachusetts revealed that 32% of the pigs were positive for *Ent. bieneusi* using a PCR test (Buckholt et al. 2002). Human infective genotypes were also isolated from the feces of these pigs.

Experimental infections of gnotobiotic pigs with *Ent. bieneusi* did not result in clinical signs (Kondova et al. 1998). Pigs excreted spores for at least 50 days. *Enterocytozoon bieneusi* was detected in enterocytes and feces of experimentally infected gnotobiotic pigs.

BALANTIDIUM COLI

Balantidium coli is the only important ciliate found in pigs and in humans. It is transmitted by cysts that are excreted in the host's feces. The cysts are 50 to 70 µm in diameter and contain a macronucleus and a micronucleus. No division occurs in the cyst. Trophozoites are covered in short cilia, are up to 100 µm in length, and also contain a macronucleus and a micronucleus. Trophozoites are usually found in the lumen of the large intestine. Most infections in swine and humans are subclinical. Individual infection rates approaching 100% can be found in weaned pigs and breeding stock on farms where *B. coli* is present (Hindsbo et al. 2000).

REFERENCES

Baba E, Gaffer SM. 1985. Interfering effect of *Isospora suis* infections on *Salmonella typhimurium* infection in swine. Vet Parasitol 17:271–278.

Biester HE, Murray C. 1934. Studies in infectious enteritis of swine. VIII. *Isospora suis*, new species in swine. J Am Vet Med Assoc 85:207–219.

Breitenmoser AC, Mathis A, Burgi E, Weber R, Deplazes P. 1999. High prevalence of *Enterocytozoon bieneusi* in swine with four genotypes that differ from those identified in humans. Parasitology 118:447–453.

Buckholt MA, Lee JH, Tzipori S. 2002. Prevalence of *Enterocytozoon bieneusi* in swine: An 18-month survey at a slaughterhouse in Massachusetts. Appl Environ Microbiol 68:2595–2599.

Choi BY, Sohn YS, Choi C, Chae, C. 2003. Lectin histochemistry for glycoconjugates in the small intestines of piglets naturally infected with *Isospora suis*. J Vet Med Sci 65:389–392.

Daugschies A, Bialek R, Joachim A, Mundt HC. 2001. Autofluorescence microscopy for the detection of nematode eggs and protozoa, in particular *Isospora suis*, in swine faeces. Parasitol Res 87:409–412.

Driesen SJ, Fahy VA, Carland PG. 1995. The use of toltrazuril for the prevention of coccidiosis in piglets before weaning. Aust Vet J 72:139–141.

Dubey JP. 1986. A review of toxoplasmosis in pigs. Vet Parasitol 19:181–223.

——. 1988. Long-term persistence of *Toxoplasma gondii* in tissues of pigs inoculated with *T gondii* oocysts and effect of freezing on viability of tissue cysts in pork. Am J Vet Res 49:910–913.

——. 1990. Status of toxoplasmosis in pigs in the United States. J Am Vet Med Assoc 196:270–274.

Dubey JP, Beattie CP. 1988. Toxoplasmosis of Animals and Man. Boca Raton: CRC Press.

Dubey JP, Kotula AW, Sharar A, Andrews CD, Lindsay DS. 1990. Effect of high temperature on infectivity of *Toxoplasma gondii* tissue cysts in pork. J Parasitol 76:201–204.

Dubey JP, Murrell KD, Hanbury RD, Anderson WR, Doby PB, Miller H0. 1986. Epidemiologic findings on a swine farm with enzootic toxoplasmosis. J Am Vet Med Assoc 189:55–56.

Dubey JP, Powell EC. 1994. Prevalence of *Sarcocystis* in sows from Iowa. Vet Parasitol 52:151–155.

Dubey JP, Speer CA, Fayer R. 1989. Sarcocystis of Animals and Man. Boca Raton: CRC Press.

Dubey JP, Thulliez P, Weigel RM, Andrews CD, Lind P, Powell EC. 1995a. Sensitivity and specificity of various serologic tests for detection of *Toxoplasma gondii* infection in naturally infected sows. Am J Vet Res 56:1030–1036.

Dubey JP, Weigel RM, Siegel AM, Thulliez P, Kitron UD, Mitchell MA, Mannelli A, Mateus-Pinilla NE, Shen SK, Kwok 0CH, Todd KS. 1995b. Sources and reservoirs of *Toxoplasma gondii* infection on 47 swine farms in Illinois. J Parasitol 81:723–729.

Dubey JP, Weisbrode SE, Sharma SP, Al-Khalidi NW, Zimmerman JL, Gaafar SM. 1979. Porcine toxoplasmosis in Indiana. J Am Vet Med Assoc 174:604–609.

Enemark HL, Ahrens P, Bille-Hansen V, Heegaard PM, Vigre H, Thamsborg SM, Lind P. 2003. *Cryptosporidium parvum*: Infectivity and pathogenicity of the 'porcine' genotype. Parasitology 126:407–416.

Ernst JV, Lindsay DS, Current WL. 1985. Control of *Isospora suis*-induced coccidiosis on swine farms. Am J Vet Res 46:643–645.

Ey PL, Mansouri M, Kulda J, Nohynkova E, Monis PT, Andrews RH, Mayrhofer G. 1997. Genetic analysis of *Giardia* from hoofed farm animals reveals artiodactyl-specific and potentially zoonotic genotypes. J Eukaryot Microbiol 44:626–635.

Henriksen SA, Christensen JPB. 1992. Demonstration of *Isospora suis* oocysts in faecal samples. Vet Rec 131:443–444.

Hill JE, Lomax LG, Lindsay DS, Lynn BS. 1985. Coccidiosis caused by *Eimeria scabra* in a finishing hog. J Am Vet Med Assoc 186:981–982.

Hindsbo O, Nielsen CV, Andreassen J, Willingham AL, Bendixen M, Nielsen MA, Nielsen NO. 2000. Age-dependent occurrence of the intestinal ciliate *Balantidium coli* in pigs at a Danish research farm. Acta Vet Scand 41:79–83.

Kondova I, Mansfield K, Buckholt MA, Stein B, Widmer G, Carville A, Lackner A, Tzipori S. 1998. Transmission and serial propagation of *Enterocytozoon bieneusi* from humans and Rhesus macaques in gnotobiotic piglets. Infect Immun 66:5515–5519.

Koudela B, Kucerova S. 1999. Role of acquired immunity and natural age resistance on course of *Isospora suis* coccidiosis in nursing piglets. Vet Parasitol 82:93–99.

Koudela B, Nohynkova E, Vitovec J, Pakandl M, Kulda J. 1991. *Giardia* infection in pigs: Detection and in vitro isolation of trophozoites of the *Giardia intestinalis* group. Parasitology 102:163–166.

Koudela B, Vitovec J. 1992. Biology and pathogenicity of *Eimeria spinosa* in experimentally infected pigs. Int. J Parasitol 22:651–656.

Levine ND, Ivens V. 1986. The Coccidian Parasites (Protozoa, Apicomplexa) of Artiodactyla. Illinois Biological Monographs 55. Champaign: Univ Illinois Press.

Lindsay DS, Blagburn BL, Boosinger TR. 1987. Experimental *Eimeria debliecki* infections in nursing and weaned pigs. Vet Parasitol 25:39–45.

Lindsay DS, Current WL, Ernst JV. 1982. Sporogony of *Isospora suis* of swine. J Parasitol 68:861–865.

Lindsay DS, Current WL, Ernst JV, Stuart BP. 1983. Diagnosis of neonatal porcine coccidiosis caused by Isospora suis. Vet Med Small Anim Clin 78:89–95.

Lindsay DS, Current WL, Taylor JR. 1985. Effects of experimental *Isospora suis* infection on morbidity, mortality and weight gains of nursing pigs. Am J Vet Res 46:1511–1512.

Lindsay DS, Ernst JV, Current WL, Stuart BP, Stewart TB. 1984. Prevalence of oocysts of *Isospora suis* and *Eimeria* spp. from sows on farms with and without a history of neonatal coccidiosis. J Am Vet Med Assoc 185:419–421.

Lindsay DS, Neiger R, Hildreth M. 2002. Porcine enteritis associated with *Eimeria spinosa* Henry, 1931 infection. J Parasitol 88:1262–1263.

Lindsay DS, Stuart BP, Wheat BF, Ernst JV. 1980. Endogenous development of the swine coccidium *Isospora suis*. J Parasitol 66:771–779.

Mundt HC, Daugschies A, Wustenberg S, Zimmermann M. 2003. Studies on the efficacy of toltrazuril, diclazuril and sulphadimidine against artificial infections with *Isospora suis* in piglets. Parasitol Res 90:S160–S162.

Nilsson O. 1988. *Isospora suis* in pigs with postweaning diarrhoea. Vet Rec 122:310–311.

Ruttkowski B, Joachim A, Daugschies A. 2001. PCR-based differentiation of three porcine *Eimeria* species and *Isospora suis*. Vet Parasitol 95:17–23.

Ryan UM, Samarasinghe B, Read C, Buddle JR, Robertson ID, Thompson RC. 2003. Identification of a novel *Cryptosporidium* genotype in pigs. Appl Environ Microbiol 69:3970–3974.

Sanford SE. 1987. Enteric cryptosporidial infection in pigs: 184 cases (1981–1985). J Am Vet Med Assoc 190:695–698.

Sangster LT, Seibold HR, Mitchell FE. 1976. Coccidial infections in suckling pigs. Proc Am Assoc Vet Lab Diagn 19:51–55.

Stuart BP, Gosser HS, Allen CB, Bedell DM. 1982a. Coccidiosis in swine: Dose and age response to *Isospora suis*. Can J Comp Med 46:317–320.

Stuart BP, Lindsay DS. 1986. Coccidiosis in swine. Vet Clin North Am Food Anim Pract 2:455–468.

Stuart BP, Lindsay DS, Ernst JV. 1978. Coccidiosis as a cause of scours in baby pigs. Proc Int Symp Neonatal Diarrhea 2:371–382.

Stuart BP, Lindsay DS, Ernst JV, Gosser HS. 1980. *Isospora suis* enteritis in piglets. Vet Pathol 17:84–93.

Stuart BP, Sisk DB, Bedell DM, Gosser HS. 1982b. Demonstration of immunity against *Isospora suis* in swine. Vet Parasitol 9:185–191.

Taylor JR. 1984. Immune response of pigs to *Isospora suis* (Apicomplexa, Eimeriidae). Ph.D. thesis. Auburn Univ, Auburn, Ala.

Upton SJ, Current WL. 1985. The species of *Cryptosporidium* infecting mammals. J Parasitol 71:625–629.

Vetterling JM. 1965. Coccidia (Protozoa: Eimeriidae) of swine. J Parasitol 51:887–912.

———. 1966. Prevalence of coccidia in swine from six localities in the United States. Cornell Vet 56:155–166.

Vitovec J, Koudela B. 1990. Pathologenicity and ultrastructural pathology of *Eimeria debliecki* in experimentally infected pigs. Folia Parasitol 37:193–199.

Vitovec J, Koudela B, Kudweis M, Stephanek J, Smid B, Dvorak R. 1991. Pathogenesis of experimental combined infections with *Isospora suis* and rotavirus in conventional and gnotobiotic pigs. J Vet Med B 38:215–226.

Weigel RM, Dubey JP, Siegel AM, Kitron UD, Mannelli A, Mitchell MA, Mateus-Pinifia NE, Thuffiez P, Shen SK, Kwok CH, Todd K. 1995. Risk factors for transmission of *Toxoplasma gondii* on swine farms in Illinois. J Parasitol 81:736–741.

Xiao L, Bern C, Arrowood M, Sulaiman I, Zhou L, Kawai V, Vivar A, Lal AA, Gilman RH. 2002. Identification of the *Cryptosporidium* pig genotype in a human patient. J Infect Dis 185:1846–1848.

Yaeger MJ, Holtcamp A, Jarvinen JA. 2003. Clinical coccidiosis in a boar stud. J Vet Diagn Invest 15:387–389.

53 External Parasites

C. Cargill and Peter R. Davies

The importance of external parasites in swine production varies greatly among regions because of differences in climate and systems used to raise pigs. Unquestionably, the mite *Sarcoptes scabiei* var. *suis* is the most important external parasite of swine worldwide. Other external parasites include demodectic mites, lice, fleas, mosquitoes, flies, and ticks. Mites and ticks belong to the class Arachnida and are characterized by having four pairs of legs. Lice, fleas, flies, and mosquitoes belong to the class Insecta.

External parasites produce a range of clinical signs in pigs. Rubbing, scratching, and skin lesions, which are secondary to irritation, are the most common. Some parasites also cause significant economic effects due to reduced growth rate, reduced feed efficiency, and loss of carcass value at slaughter. The risk of chemical residues in meat is also increased because many products used to treat external parasites have a long withholding period and treatment of animals can complicate routine market and culling decisions. Furthermore, some external parasites are implicated in the transmission of pathogenic organisms.

SARCOPTIC MANGE

The mite *Sarcoptes scabiei* var. *suis*, the cause of sarcoptic mange, is the most important ectoparasite of swine throughout the world. Mange is considered the most detrimental skin disease affecting pigs, because of the economic losses from reduced growth rates and feed efficiency in growing pigs and decreased fertility in breeding sows (Zimmermann and Kircher 1998; Kessler et al. 2003). Its economic importance tends to be underestimated, especially by pig producers who fail to check for encrustations in the ears of sows and to recognize the importance of clinical signs in growing pigs.

Two clinical forms of the disease are recognized: a hyperkeratotic form (sometimes referred to as *chronic mange*) that most commonly affects multiparous sows and a pruritic or hypersensitive form that affects grow-

ing pigs. Earlier descriptions of sarcoptic mange referred to hyperkeratotic mange and described encrusted skin lesions from which mites were readily isolated (McPherson 1960; Sheahan 1970). More recent studies have shown that the hypersensitive form is the more common in growing pigs and is characterized by the development of delayed and immediate hypersensitive reactions to the mites. (Davis and Moon 1990a,b,c; Alonso de Vega et al. 1998; Cargill 2001, 2002).

Distribution

Sarcoptic mange mites are ubiquitous in swine herds, unless eliminated by specific eradication procedures (Yeoman 1984). Herd prevalence estimates of between 43% and 95% have been reported in numerous countries, including Australia, Belgium, Canada, the former Republic of Czechoslovakia, Denmark, France, Great Britain, Italy, Japan, Mexico, the Netherlands, Scotland, Spain, Sweden, and the United States (Wooten-Saadi et al. 1987b; Smeets et al. 1989; Horie 1990; McMullin et al. 1990; Davies et al. 1991a; Hasslinger and Resch 1992; Klopfenstein et al. 1992; McMullin et al. 1992; Mendez de Vigo et al. 1992; Garcia et al. 1994; Gualandi et al. 1994; Davies et al. 1996b). In many studies herd prevalences of 70–90% were recorded, with animal prevalences within herds ranging from 20% to 95%. As recently as 2003, herd prevalence in the U.S.A. and Canada was quoted at 29% and 38%, respectively (Melancon 2003).

Etiology and Life Cycle

Sarcoptes scabiei is a small, grayish-white, eight-legged arthropod, from the class *Arachnidia*, order *Acariana*, belonging to the family *Sarcoptidae* (Hill 1997). The mite is circular, approximately 0.5 mm in length, and just visible to the naked eye when placed on a dark background. When viewed under a dissecting microscope, the mite readily moves away from bright light. It has four pairs of short stumpy legs, some of which are provided with long unjointed pedicles that terminate in sucker like or-

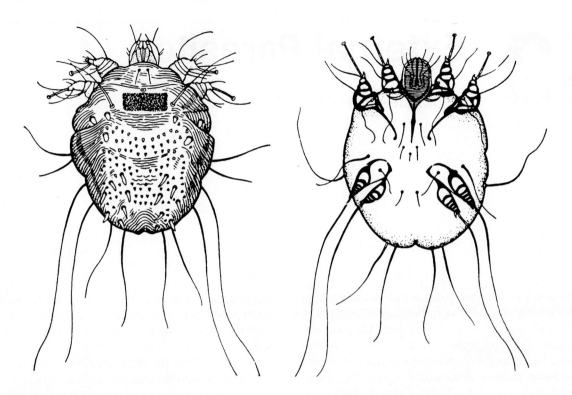

53.1. Sarcoptes scabiei, *the sarcoptic mange mite. Female, dorsal view (left) and ventral view (right). (From Belding 1952. Courtesy Appleton-Century-Crofts.)*

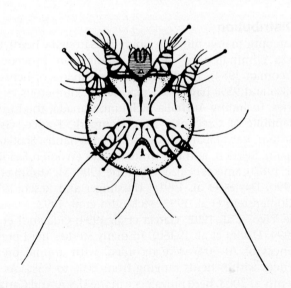

53.2. Sarcoptes scabiei, *the sarcoptic mange mite. Male, ventral view. (From Belding 1952. Courtesy Appleton-Century-Crofts.)*

gans. These pedicles occur on the first two pairs of legs in the female and on the first, second, and fourth pairs in the male (Figures 53.1, 53.2).

Mites are permanent parasites in the epidermis, where eggs, larvae, nymphs, and adults all develop. The mites burrow by extra-oral digestion of the stratum corneum, and then consume cells of the stratum granulosum and stratum spinosum (Davis and Moon 1990a). After females mate, they lay 40–50 eggs in tunnels carved into the upper two-thirds of the epidermis and die approximately 30 days after maturity (Hill 1997). The eggs hatch in 3–5 days, larvae molt to nymphs, and then nymphs molt to adults, all within the tunnels. Mating occurs in the molting pockets or near the skin surface, after which the ovigerous females initiate new burrows. Reproduction can occur only on the host, and the entire cycle from egg to ovigerous female requires 10–25 days. Most studies in the pig suggest that most of the mite activity is confined to the inner surface of the ear (Walton 1967; Sheahan 1975; Davis and Moon 1990a, d). Although material from ear scrapings taken from an animal with an established infestation may contain very large numbers of mites, mites may be difficult to find on other parts of the body (Bogatko 1974; Cargill and Dobson 1979a). Using tissues dissected from mite-infested pigs, Magee (1974) demonstrated that mites burrow no deeper than the epidermis and make burrows parallel to the skin surface.

Epidemiology

Hyperkeratotic encrustations in the ears of multiparous sows are the main reservoir of mites within a herd. Boars, although less important with the increasing use of AI, can also be a source of infestation in breeding herds because they tend to be treated less often than sows. Although extensive hyperkeratotic lesions may occur on the body and hindlegs of adult animals (Martineau et al. 1984), only a small percentage of animals are affected in this manner. Hyperkeratotic lesions are occasionally visible in the ears and on the body of growing pigs, especially where control measures for mange are poor. In most herds, mite populations are maintained within the ears of sows, and piglets become infested during suckling. Spread between sows and boars and between litters is mainly by direct contact between pigs, but according to Stegeman et al. (2000) the transmission of mites is slow. They estimated that the transmission of mange in housed pigs to be in the order of 0.06 new infestations for each infested pig per day. The newly fertilized adult female mite is thought to be the main means of spread and maximum opportunity for spread exists when groups of pigs huddle. Pig management practices such as group housing of sows, continuous-flow management systems for growing pigs, and current trends towards larger group sizes of growing pigs will facilitate the spread of mites.

Although environmental spread is much less important than direct contact between animals, pigs have become infested when placed in pens for as little as 24 hours immediately after infested pigs were removed from the pens (Smith 1986). Although mites have been kept alive for 3 weeks under optimum laboratory conditions (Soulsby 1968), survival of mites and eggs away from the host is limited. Their viability is reduced by desiccation and can be improved artificially by placing them in media such as mineral oil (Davis and Moon 1987). In our experience mites die within a few minutes in direct sunlight and after several hours in temperatures above 28°C. Even in colder climates mites do not appear to survive for more than 12 days in a piggery at temperatures of 7–18°C and relative humidity of 65–75% (Mikhalochkina 1975). In warmer climates, clinical evidence of sarcoptic mite hypersensitivity could not be demonstrated when noninfested pigs were exposed on repeated occasions to contaminated bedding vacated 3 days previously in either autumn or spring (Cargill and Dobson 1977). This was supported by laboratory experiments which demonstrated that mites did not survive longer than 96 hours at temperatures of less than 25°C, longer than 24 hours from 25–30°C, and less than 1 hour at temperatures above 30°C (Cargill and Dobson 1977). The prevalence and severity of sarcoptic mange have also been reported to increase in cooler months and decrease in warmer months (Davies et al. 1991b; Elbers et al. 1992; Davies et al. 1996b). Other species do not appear to play a role in porcine scabies (Magee 1974), and transmission from one herd to another usually occurs when pigs with subclinical infestations are moved.

The results of several studies indicate that only a small percentage of growing pigs will harbor significant numbers of mites on the internal surface of the pinna. In a study of 187 clinically healthy pigs (Bogatko 1974), mites could not be observed in skin scrapings from the head and neck region although 18% of skin scrapings from the luminal surface of the ears were positive. In other studies, the prevalence of mites in the ears was five times higher in groups of pigs with hypersensitive skin lesions compared to pigs without lesions (Hollanders and Vercruysse 1990). Davies et al. (1996b) found that the number of pigs in a group with positive skin scrapings was positively correlated with the level of papular dermatitis in the group at slaughter. The prevalence of positive skin scrapings ranged from 3–63%. In a group of pigs where 47% had signs of hypersensitive mange and 5% had hyperkeratotic mange, mites were found in 33% of hypersensitive pigs but in 81% of pigs with hyperkeratotic mange (Kambarage 1993). Although the level of pruritus in groups of pigs appears to be positively correlated with the number of pigs that are positive for mites, the presence of mites on individual pigs appears to be negatively correlated with the degree of pruritus and hypersensitivity (Cargill et al. 1996a). The level of immune hypersensitivity in individual pigs appears to affect both the host behavior and the development of encrusted lesions (Davis and Moon 1990b). It would appear that within a group of pigs there are two populations. A smaller population of pigs harbors significant numbers of mites, but do not develop a severe form of hypersensitive mange, and a larger population of pigs harbors few mites, but develops a marked hypersensitivity reaction (Davies et al. 1996a). In this latter population the number of mites declines over time as the level of hypersensitivity increases (Cargill and Dobson 1979a; Cargill and Wegiel 2000; Davis and Moon 1990a). Regular exposure to mites from penmates maintains the allergic reaction and clinical signs in the hypersensitive animals (Cargill and Wegiel 2000).

Economic Importance

The production effects of sarcoptic mange have been previously reviewed by Davies (1995). Based on our current understanding of the pathogenesis of mange, deaths are unlikely in the absence of concurrent disease (Davies 1995), although mortalities may occur in cases with severe hyperkeratotic lesions (Pullar 1941). Field studies indicate that improved mange control will improve milk production, reduce piglet mortalities due to overlying, and increase weaning weights (Hewett and Heard 1982; Schultz 1986; Martelli and Beghian 1990). However, other studies have failed to confirm these findings (Dalton and Ryan 1988; Arends et al. 1990) but have demonstrated that feed utilization efficiency improved following prefarrowing treatment of sows. The variations in results could have been due to differences in the degree of infestation in the herds (Davies 1995). Other economic effects include downgrading and trimming of carcasses at slaughter and damage to pens and fixtures caused by rubbing pigs.

The most significant economic effect of sarcoptic mange is reduced growth rate and feed efficiency in growing pigs (Cargill et al. 1997); the level of economic loss may be underestimated by producers who fail to appreciate the severity of clinical signs. The effect of sarcoptic mange on growth rate has been investigated in a number of studies, by comparing experimentally infested pigs with noninfested controls (Sheahan 1974; Cargill and Dobson 1979b; Wooten et al. 1986; Davies 1995) or by comparing treated with untreated pigs (Sheahan and Kelly 1974; Hewett 1985; Alva-Valdes et al. 1986; Wooten-Saadi et al. 1987a; Arends et al. 1990; Martelli and Beghian 1990). Although some results are conflicting, where growth rate was measured over a period of 12 weeks or greater, or from less than 20 to more than 60 kg liveweight, the majority of studies demonstrate growth rate suppression of between 4.5% and 12%. In one study, the growth rate in infested pigs was decreased by 8% (Wooten-Saadi et al. 1987a), and in another study (Davies 1995) reductions in growth rate in infested pigs ranged from zero up to 5.7% and were associated with the severity of papular dermatitis among groups. In a recent report by Elbers et al. (2000), infested pigs grew significantly slower, with a reduced feed efficiency of 2%, when compared with the control. Smets et al. (1999) also showed that breeding sows needed 5% less feed after eradication of mange. In the same herd, returns to estrus were reduced by 4.5%, pigs born alive increased by 0.33 piglets per litter, and pigs weaned increased by 1.34 piglets per sow per year. In addition to effects on production performance, financial loss is also incurred in treatment costs (acaricides and labor), carcass downgrading, and due to the risk of chemical treatment residues in meat products.

Interaction between sarcoptic mange and other diseases has also been suggested (Yeoman 1984; Gaafer et al. 1986) but no objective reports are available.

Clinical Signs, Pathogenesis, and Lesions

Pruritus is the most consistent clinical sign of sarcoptic mange. Following infestation, intermittent body scratching may be observed in piglets born to an infested sow or in older pigs coming into contact with mites for the first time. True generalized pruritus occurs from 2–11 weeks after infestation (Sheahan 1974; Cargill and Dobson 1979a). This variation is similar to that reported in human scabies, where the period between exposure and the development of pruritus ranges from 9–10 days to 4–6 weeks (Sheahan and Kelly 1974). Following exposure, pigs go through several phases, which include a nonresponse phase, a delayed-type hypersensitivity phase, a delayed- and immediate-type hypersensitivity phase, and finally an immediate-type hypersensitivity phase (Davis and Moon 1990a). The development of pruritus and the intensity of rubbing will depend on the number of mites in the initial exposure and the level of ongoing exposure. When pigs were exposed to either low (100) or high doses (1000) of mites, the development of delayed-type hypersensitivity, but not the development of immediate-type hypersensitivity, was found to be dose dependent (Davis and Moon

1990a). Desensitization has not been documented but field evidence suggests that it occurs.

The pattern and chronological order of clinical events are similar in both natural and experimental infestations (Sheahan 1974, 1975; Cargill and Dobson 1979a; Cargill and Wegiel 2000). Pigs develop encrusted lesions that are rich in mites, especially on the luminal surface of the pinnae (Figure 53.3). These plaquelike lesions may coalesce to cover up to 70% of the surface of the pinnae but will regress with time as hypersensitivity develops. The epidermal changes and sequence of events have been well documented by Morsy et al. (1989), using electron microscopy. It has been suggested that papular lesions of human scabies may result from unsuccessful burrowing of immature mites that fail to survive to adulthood (Green 1989).

Focal erythematous skin papules associated with hypersensitivity occur in most animals as encrustations regress. The papules occur primarily on the rump, flank, and abdomen (Cargill and Dobson 1979a). Histologically, they contain large numbers of eosinophils, mast cells, and lymphocytes but no evidence of mites. Immunoglobulin-secreting cells increase to a peak in the 2–5 weeks after infestation and then subside substantially after a few weeks (Morsy and Gaafar 1989). Repeated or multiple infestations result in only a small increase in immunoglobulin-secreting cells. The development of pruritus is signified by rubbing, which in severe cases results in the proliferation of connective tissue and keratinization, leading to hair loss, abrasions, and thickening of the skin, especially over the flanks of animals that rub frequently.

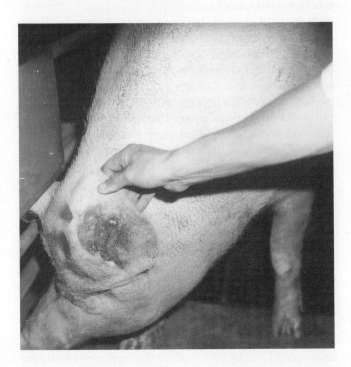

53.3. *Photograph of the ear of a sow with encrustation caused by sarcoptic mange mites.*

Lesions of hyperkeratotic mange are most common in mature animals. In growing animals they occur mainly in pigs that fail to develop the typical hypersensitivity response after infestation. The lesions, seen as thick asbestos-like scabs that are loosely attached to the skin, are very rich in mites and occur most frequently in the ears. The scabs may progressively cover the head, neck, and other parts of the body, although this is uncommon.

An interrelationship among immunity, inadequate nutrition, poor management, and hyperkeratotic sarcoptic mange has been noted. Hyperkeratotic mange has been described as a disease of poor management, and it is considered to be more common in poorly fed pigs. Studies have shown that low-protein diets and iron deficiency are associated with reduced hypersensitivity and a greater proportion of animals with hyperkeratotic mange (Sheahan 1974; Cargill and Dobson 1979a). The overall clinical picture is substantially influenced by the effectiveness of treatment and herd management. The influence of concurrent disease in the development of sarcoptic mange has not been elaborated.

Diagnosis

Sarcoptic mange is present in most herds unless they have been derived from specific pathogen free (SPF) sources or special measures have been taken to eradicate the parasite. Rubbing in growing pigs with small red papules on the body is the most obvious indication of sarcoptic mange. The small size of the parasite and its intracutaneous location, in combination with nonspecific signs (including pruritus), can make the diagnosis of scabies difficult to confirm (Smets and Vercruysse 2000). The majority of pigs in an infested herd may be subclinically infested and may not manifest obvious clinical signs of the disease (Kessler et al. 2003).

Diagnosis is confirmed by demonstrating the presence of mites within a herd, but the sensitivity of the methods available is low and the results depend on the location of the scrapings and the number of samples (Smets et al. 1999, Deckert et al. 2000). The best method is to use a flashlight to examine the luminal surface of the ears of breeding animals for encrusted lesions. About 1–2 cm² of the lesion can be removed and examined for mites. Mites can be observed by breaking the material onto a sheet of black paper and gently removing it after a few minutes, leaving mites adhering to the paper by the suckers on their feet. Mites can be observed directly or with a magnifying glass (Brakenridge 1958). A more sensitive technique is to break down scabs with 10% potassium hydroxide and observe them under a low-power microscope. Large numbers of mites can be collected from encrusted ear lesions by vibrating material in a petri dish over low heat for 6–24 hours. This will cause mites to emerge in great numbers and adhere to the bottom of the dish (Sheahan and Hatch 1975).

The severity of sarcoptic mange in a herd can be assessed by quantifying the level of pruritus in various groups of pigs. This is achieved by calculating a rubbing index (RI) (Pointon et al. 1995; Cargill et al. 1997; Cargill 2001). A group of 25–30 pigs is observed for 15 minutes and the number of rubbing and scratching episodes is divided by the number of pigs in the group to give the RI. An RI of greater than 0.1 indicates the need to review mange control programs. Increased stocking density will reduce the RI, whereas wetting pigs will increase the RI. Although other, confounding factors need to be identified before using an RI with confidence to compare pigs on different farms, it does provide a simple means of assessing mange control programs on individual farms (Cargill et al. 1997).

Examination of carcasses at slaughter for papular lesions also provides a simple and objective method for assessing the prevalence and severity of sarcoptic mange in growing pigs. The causal association between sarcoptic mites and papular dermatitis was first suggested by Flesja and Ulvesaeter (1979) and was confirmed by Davies et al. (1991a). The original method for scoring lesions was described by Pointon et al. (1987, 1992), and categories were defined according to the severity of dermatitis (Pointon et al. 1999). Although the specificity of score 2 and 3 lesions is greater than 0.98, the specificity of score 1 lesions ranges from 0.7 to 0.9 (Davies et al. 1996b). In order to improve specificity, a modified scoring system has been recently introduced in Australia where minor spotting, which may be caused by insect bites and bedding, is ignored. Score 1 lesions include mild dermatitis about the shoulders, underline, and rump up to a more generalized distribution of mild lesions over the back and moderately dense lesions about the shoulders, underline, and rump. Score 2 lesions include a generalized distribution of moderately dense lesions over the back and dense lesions over shoulders, underline, and rump, and worse. Hollanders et al. (1995) have also suggested modifying the scoring system in a similar way to improve specificity. However, it is also important to validate and quantify the association between skin lesions and sarcoptic mange on a regional and geographic basis and to ensure repeatability among the observers recording lesions (Cargill et al. 1997). This will allow interpretation of the lesions in a herd regardless of the system used to record lesions.

Recently, several enzyme-linked immunosorbent assays (ELISAs), which detect antibodies to *S. scabiei* in serum, have been used as diagnostic tools (Bornstein and Wallgren 1997; Bornstein et al. 2000; Deckert et al. 2000; Vercruysse and Smets 2000; Zalunardo et al. 2000). Although individual sensitivity varies from 29–64%, as a herd test, sensitivity approaches 95% (Deckert et al. 2000). Specificity of the antibodies in individual pigs ranges from 78–97% (Smets and Vercruysse 2000). Results of serological tests are affected by the stage of the disease process. Specific antibodies are not detectable until 5–7 weeks post-infestation or approximately 3–4 weeks following the onset of clinical signs of mange (Bornstein and Zakrisson 1993). Furthermore, following treatment and elimination of mites from heavily infested animals, detectable antibodies may persist for up to 9–12 months (Smets and Vercruysse 2000). Serological responses are also affected by the infective dose (Bornstein et al. 1994) and age of the pigs. Although antibodies can persist for at least 10 months in naturally infested sows following treatment (Bornstein et al. 1994), the half-life of specific antibody appears to be significantly shorter (less than 2 months) in younger pigs (Bornstein and Wallgren 1997). The ELISA has also been used to validate the efficacy of eradication programs (Jacobson et al. 1999; Cargill et al. 2004).

Differential diagnosis from other skin conditions is important. Conditions that can be confused with mange include parakeratosis, exudative epidermitis, niacin and biotin deficiencies, dermatomycosis, swinepox, sunburn, and photosensitization. The role of mosquitoes and other insects in the differential diagnosis of papular dermatitis must also be considered. Occasionally in mange-free herds, ear scrapings may reveal the presence of mites and mite eggs but not clinical disease. That may occur when old straw is used for bedding.

Treatment, Control, and Eradication

Failure to control sarcoptic mange is due in part to the covert nature of the disease and to a failure to understand the epidemiology of mange. Commonly farmers regard rubbing, the main clinical sign of hypersensitive mange, as normal. Several strategies are open to producers to reduce the economic effects of mange.

Establishment and Maintenance of Mange-Free Pig Populations. The establishment and maintenance of mange-free herds and populations is facilitated by three important facts. First, piglets are born free of mites and become infested through contact with infested sows or older growing pigs. Second, the mites are highly host-specific and survive poorly away from the pig. Third, modern acaricides are very effective. Mange-free herds can be established with cesarean-derived pigs, by depopulation and repopulation from mange-free stock, by segregated rearing of treated pigs, and by eradication using avermectins and other products. Biosecurity measures, which focus on careful scrutiny of, and minimization of, sources of incoming stock are usually adequate to prevent introduction of the parasite. In a number of countries, major breeding-stock suppliers maintain mange-free herds, and large populations of pigs in integrated production systems have been kept free of the parasite for many years. This should be the goal of most farms.

The Dutch mange-free certification scheme is an excellent example of how to eradicate sarcoptic mange from a large number of farms (Rambags et al. 1998, 2000). The scheme relies on treatment programs de-

signed for individual farms, and freedom is validated using slaughter checks and serology.

Treatment. The key to the successful eradication and control of mange is correct use of acaricides. In our experience, the majority of registered acaricides will keep mange under control, and even eradicate it, provided the correct dosage and treatment schedules are used. The acaricides available for treating sarcoptic mange have received considerable attention. Older remedies include crankcase oil, diesel oil, and lime sulfur (Dobson and Davies 1992). Oil mixtures are more effective than water-soluble products because oil assists in softening the hard scab; oil mixtures are still useful either as an alternative treatment or in conjunction with insecticides. The first insecticides used were mainly sprays of either organochlorinated hydrocarbons (lindane and toxaphene) or organophosphate compounds (malathion, trichlorfon, and diazinon) (Table 53.1). Because of their toxicity, chlorinated hydrocarbons have been deregistered in many countries and should no longer be used. Although the organophosphates are not as effective, they have shorter withholding periods than the chlorinated hydrocarbons and are safer. More recently developed acaricides include phosmet, used as a pour-on, amitraz used as a spray, and the avermectins (ivermectin, doramectin, and moxidectin), which are given as injections or, in the case of ivermectin, can also be given orally in the feed. The precise products available depend on the legislation of the country in question. Instructions on dilutions, withholding periods, dangers, and any precautions given by the manufacturer must be followed carefully.

Amitraz, used as a 0.1% spray (Johansson et al. 1980) and phosmet formulated as a 20% oily pour-on and applied at the rate of 1 mL/10 kg body weight (Hewett and Heard 1982) have been shown to be effective. In the case of phosmet, it is recommended that a small amount of the product be placed in the inner aspect of each ear.

The avermectins are broad-spectrum antiparasiticides effective against most internal parasites, as well as lice and sarcoptic mange mites, with varying levels of persistence (Arends et al. 1999; Cargill et al. 2000). Ivermectin can be given orally at 300–500 µg/kg (Lee et al. 1980; Alva-Valdes et al. 1984), and all the avermectins can be given by either subcutaneous (SC) or intramuscular (IM) injection at 300 µg/kg body weight (Courtney et al. 1983; Martineau et al. 1984; Dalton and Ryan 1988; Ohba et al. 1989; Satyavir and Chhabra 1992; Seaman et al. 1993; Hollanders et al. 1995; Cargill et al. 1996a; Logan et al. 1996; Yazwinski et al. 1997). They are more efficient because of their systemic action and ease of administration.

Eradication. Eradication of sarcoptic mange is possible if a sound program is developed. Keller et al. (1972) eradicated sarcoptic mange from six SPF herds, which be-

Table 53.1. Guidelines for chemical treatment of external parasites of swine

Chemical	Concentration	Parasites Affected	Directions for use
Amitraz	0.1% solution	Mites	Spray pigs and surroundings, repeat in 7 days.
Ciodrin	0.25%	Lice	Spray, repeat in 14 days.
Coumphos (Co-Ral)	0.06% solution	Lice, horn flies	Spray.
	0.12% solution	Ticks (*Amblyomma, Dermacentor, Ixodes*)	Treat wounds.
	0.24% solution	Mites	Apply to pigs; simultaneously apply 20g/m^2 to fresh bedding.
	1% dust	Screwworm, blowflies	Apply to ears and adjacent areas of head.
	5% dust	Lice	
		Ear ticks	
Diazanon	0.05% emulsion	Lice, mites	Spray 3 times at 10–day intervals
Dioxathion (Delnav)	0.15% solution	Lice, Ticks (*Amblyomma, Dermacentor, Ixodes*)	Spray or dip. Do not treat sows within 2 weeks of farrowing or while lactating. Do not repeat treatment within a 2-week period.
Doramectin	IM injection	Lice, mites, fleas	300 μg/kg body weight
Ivermectin	SC injection	Lice, mites, fleas	300 μg/kg body weight
	Orally in feed		300–500 (g/kg body weight
Lindane	0.06% emulsion	Lice, sarcoptic mites	Dip or spray. Do not use benzene hexachloride.
	1% dust	Fleas	
	3% formulated in smear, paste, or pressurized aerosol	Fleas, screwworm, blowflies	Dust head, neck, and back. Treat all wounds.
Malathion	0.05% emulsion	Lice, ticks, mites	Spray.
	6% dust	Fleas, lice	Dust thoroughly.
	2.5% emulsion	Houseflies, stable flies, fleas,	Spray environment.
Moxidectin	SC injection, pour-on	Lice, mites, fleas	300 μg/kg body weight
Phosmet	20% oily solution	Mites	Pour 1ml/10kg body weight along back. Place some in each ear.
Polysulfide	2% solution	Sarcoptic mites	Spray.
Primiphos (Actelic 50 EC)	Powder	Control of fleas	Sprinkle through straw bedding (check withholding period).
Rabon	2% solution	Houseflies, stable flies, lice	Spray 4.5L/12–14g/m^2.
Ronnel (Korlan)	0.25% emulsion	Lice	Spray.
	5% granules	Lice	Apply to bedding 25g/m^2.
	5% pressurized aerosol	Screwworm, blowflies	Treat wounds.
Roteneone	1% powder	Fleas	Dust head, neck, and back.
Toxaphene	0.5% emulsion	Lice, ticks, mites	Spray.
Trichlorfon (Neguvon)	0.125% emulsion	Houseflies, stable flies, mites	Spray environs (avoid feed and water).

Source: Based on compilation by Bennet (1975) and Dobson and Davies (1992).
Note: It is important to follow the manufacturer's recommendations and observe the withholding period specified for each chemical.

came infested accidentally. All pigs were treated three to four times with diazinon and lindane at 9- to 15-day intervals, and the environment was sprayed. Dobson and Cargill (1979) achieved eradication by washing sows in oil and using two treatments of trichlorfon at 7-day intervals prior to farrowing and isolating progeny from untreated pigs. Courtney et al. (1983), Henriksen et al. (1987), White and Ryan (1987), Dalton and Ryan (1988), and Reddin (1997) eradicated sarcoptic mange from herds with a single SC injection of ivermectin, but Alva-Valdes et al. (1984) and Thomas et al. (1986) were unsuccessful with either a single oral treatment of ivermectin at 300 or 500 μg/kg or with three SC injections of 300 μg/kg within a month. Subsequently Ebbesen (1998) eradicated mange in three farrow to finish herds by medicating the breeding herd and all weaned pigs on the farm orally for 16 days with ivermectin and injecting

piglets twice 14 days apart. Prefarrowing treatment of sows will prevent the transmission of mites to their progeny (Firkins et al. 2001) and mites have been eliminated from pigs using single or double administrations of an avermectin (Jacobson et al. 2000), as well as a single injection of doramectin (Jensen et al. 2002). More recently Cargill et al. (2004) described three eradication programs based on treatment of the breeding herd only, using either oral or injectable formulations of ivermectin. Sows were treated twice prefarrowing and progeny were reared in isolation. Boars were treated whenever sows were medicated. Eradication was validated using slaughter checks and serology, as described in the Dutch eradication program (Rambags et al. 1998, 2000).

Eradication programs involve several key points. If the whole herd is to be treated, all marketable pigs must be sold before each treatment to reduce the cost, and the withholding period for the chemical must be observed. All pigs are treated twice at the recommended interval for the acaricide used. If only the sow herd is to be treated, two options are available. All sows and boars can be treated at the recommended interval, or individual sows can be treated prefarrowing and moved to clean pens or crates. If the latter approach is taken, boars should be treated every 3 months, and the progeny of treated sows must be isolated from the progeny of untreated sows. Eradication is made easier in growing pigs by changing from a continuous-flow management system to an all-in/all-out system, such as age-segregated-rearing or multiple-site production. However, changing the management system must be combined with effective prefarrowing treatment of sows. All of these approaches can be effective and are justified economically.

Control. Mange control involves identification of animals with chronic mange so that they can receive systematic and regular treatment to protect the younger animals in the herd. All control programs must target the breeding herd. Mercier et al. (2002) demonstrated that a single dose of ivermectin (300 μg ivermectin/kg live weight) administered to the sows 8 days before farrowing was very effective in preventing the transmission of mites to piglets. Any animals with extensive hyperkeratotic lesions in the ears and over the body should be culled, and the remainder of the sows treated either simultaneously or alternatively in segregated groups prior to farrowing. The boars should be treated every 3–6 months to prevent the spread of mites at mating. Piglets born to sows that are free of mites and housed in clean pens will remain free of mites unless they are exposed to infested pigs after weaning (Cargill et al. 2004). If mange is present in both breeding and growing pigs, the whole herd must be treated along with all introductions into the herd. Contaminated bedding should be removed and the environment sprayed with insecticide. Humans who handle infested pigs can also transfer mites to uninfested animals on their clothing (Mock 1997). Therefore, it is important that workers work with only one herd (infested or uninfested) or change clothes and shower before moving onto work with another herd.

DEMODECTIC MANGE

In contrast to sarcoptic mange, demodectic mange is relatively unimportant in pigs. It is a condition identified occasionally at meat inspection and is seldom reported as a clinical entity in the field.

Distribution throughout the world and in pig populations is not well documented. It has been reported in many countries, including Australia, the United States, Kenya, New Zealand, and several European and Pacific island countries.

The agent of swine demodectic mange is the mite *Demodex phylloides* (Figure 53.4). This spindle-shaped

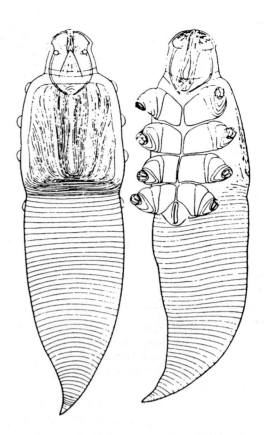

53.4. Demodex phylloides, *the demodectic mange mite. Female, dorsal view (left) and ventral view (right). (From Hirst 1922. British Museum. Economic series 13.)*

mite measures about 0.25 mm in length and has four pairs of short, stumpy legs. It lives in the hair follicles, and for this reason the condition is often referred to as follicular mange. The life cycle of the mite is not well understood. The female lives in the hair follicle and lays spindle-shaped eggs, from which larvae with three pairs of legs hatch. The larval stage progresses through three nymphal instars to the adult (Soulsby 1968). Approximately 2 weeks are required to complete the life cycle, and the life span of the adult is 1–2 months.

Transmission of the mites is probably by direct contact of pigs, but it is difficult to produce artificial infestations. The parasites are able to survive for several days off the host in moist surroundings and up to 21 days under experimental conditions in pieces of skin kept moist and cool (Nutting 1976). However, the mites will live for only 1 or 2 days if removed from the host tissue and can be killed by desiccation in as little as 1 hour at 20°C on the skin surface.

Lesions observed are red pinpoint foci around the snout and eyelids, along the underside of the neck and abdomen, and inside the thighs (Walton 1967). Later, the lesions may take on a more scaly nodular appearance, particularly in the area of the mammary gland and flanks. These nodules resemble old pox lesions and when incised contain a thick, white, cheeselike material with innumerable mites (Harland et al. 1971). Mites have been recovered in scrapings from the eyelids of swine that have shown no gross signs of infestation (Nutting et al. 1975) and most infestations are probably asymptomatic.

Diagnosis of the condition is confirmed by demonstration of *D. phylloides* in the lesions. Although there are no reports of successful treatment of pigs with any form of medication, either topical or systemic, both ivermectin and amitraz have been used successfully in dogs (Murthy et al. 1993). Severely affected animals should be culled from the herd.

LICE

Lice in pigs are readily observed and often blamed for damage due to mange because both conditions cause irritation and rubbing. Herds treated routinely to effectively control mange seldom carry significant lice populations, and many are probably free of lice. The sole species of lice that affects pigs (*Haematopinus suis*) belongs to the suborder Anoplura and has piercing and sucking mouthparts. It is grayish brown in color and has black markings. The females are about 6 mm long and the males slightly smaller (Figure 53.5). The pig louse is distributed almost worldwide. A survey of market pigs in Indiana in 1980–81 demonstrated lice in 22.5% of 821 herds surveyed (Wooten-Saadi et al. 1987b), but the parasite is likely to be much less prevalent in contemporary production systems.

The life cycle of *H. suis* was described by Florence (1921). The adult female lays 3–4 eggs (nits) each day, to a total of up to 90 over a period of about 25 days. Each egg is about 1–2 mm long and is attached by clear cement to the hair. Eggs hatch in 12–20 days. The nymphs develop through three instars, all of which feed on blood that is generally from a tender part of the body such as the inner surface of the ear. The third instar nymphs develop into adults. The whole cycle takes 23–30 days (Walton 1967) and epidemiology is uncomplicated. The pig louse is host-specific and cannot live for more than 2–3 days away from the host.

Lice are found on all parts of the body but particularly in the folds of the skin around the neck, jowl, and flanks, and on the inner surfaces of the legs. They often shelter inside the ears, where they are sometimes seen in "nests." The method of spread is by direct contact among pigs during huddling, although clean pigs placed in a yard just vacated by lousy pigs can become infested.

The economic importance of lice has not been critically evaluated to the same extent as sarcoptic mange has. However, it is known that heavy infestations result in anemia in young pigs and may affect growth rate and efficiency of food conversion. One estimate of reduced growth was 50 g/day (Hiepe and Ribbeck 1975), though Davis and Williams (1986) failed to demonstrate any such effect. Lice have always been considered vectors of

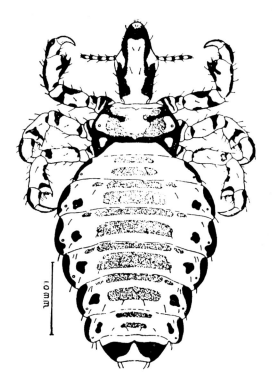

53.5. Haematopinus suis, *the pig louse. (From Whitehead 1942. Macdonald College Farm Bull 7.)*

swinepox. It has also been reported that hides from pigs with lice are rendered unsuitable for manufacture into high-grade leather (Hiepe and Ribbeck 1975).

Diagnosis

Lice should always be considered in the differential diagnosis of pruritus in pigs. Infestation can be confirmed by identifying adult lice on the body and nits attached to the lower parts of hairs. Examination inside the ears of a number of breeding animals will assist in finding lice if they are present and will enable differential diagnosis from sarcoptic mange.

Treatment and Control

Treatment and control of lice are readily achieved because the parasites live on the skin surface and can survive for only a few days away from their host.

Therapeutic agents may be applied to the pig in the form of sprays, pour-ons, and dusting powders. Control can also be assisted by placing granules containing insecticides in the bedding. Pour-ons and powders have the advantage that pigs do not have to be sprayed in cold weather.

The older treatments of diesel oil and crankcase oil applied to the pig either directly or from rubbing posts are of limited value and have been largely superseded by insecticides of the organochloride and organophosphorus compounds, which are effective and easier to apply. Several of the organophosphorus compounds, such as rabon, ciodrin, ronnel, coumaphos, and methoxychlor, are suitable for lice control but are less commonly registered for treatment of sarcoptic mange (refer to Table 53.1). In addition, avermectins have been shown to be effective in controlling lice (Barth and Brokken 1980).

Control and eradication strategies listed for sarcoptic mange apply equally to the treatment of lice. These include special attention to the ears, treatment of the boars, multiple treatment of sows prior to farrowing, segregation of clean and untreated animals if all the herd is not treated at one time, and treatment of all introduced animals. Eradication of lice by thorough treatment of the whole herd is an achievable goal.

FLEAS

Fleas are not host-specific and will parasitize any convenient mammal or bird to obtain a blood meal. The two fleas most commonly associated with swine are *Pulex irritans*, the human flea, and the stickfast flea *Echidnophaga gallinacea. Ctenocephalides canis*, the dog flea and *C. felis*, the cat flea, also occasionally infest young swine. *Tunga penetrans*, the chigger flea, has been associated with pigs in Africa.

The distribution of fleas in nature is wide, but they are seldom a serious problem in the well-managed piggery. These wingless insects are 2–4 mm in length, have a thick, brown chitinous exoskeleton, and have powerful legs.

Life cycles are similar for all flea species. The female lays eggs about 0.5 mm long, which drop off the host into the animal bedding. Larvae hatch in 2–16 days and feed on dry blood, feces, and other organic material. With moderate temperature and high humidity, the larvae mature in 1–2 weeks and pass through a pupal stage. The whole life cycle takes as little as 18 days but may take in excess of 1 year depending on environmental conditions (Soulsby 1968).

Only the adult flea is parasitic in that it requires periodic blood meals. The stickfast flea differs from the others, spending most of its adult life on a host animal.

Fleas can survive for many months in the absence of a host. Survival is dependent on whether they are fed and the degree of moisture in the environment. Under optimal conditions the human flea can live for over 2 years.

Although fleas appear to be relatively unimportant in pig production, severe infestations have been reported recently in outdoor pig herds in New Zealand (Dobinson 2000). Clinical signs recorded were bright red discoloration of the skin, fleabite marks over the mammary glands, edema of the prepuce in boars, and sows spending more time in wallows. Because infestations occurred primarily over summer, it was difficult to determine whether production losses were flea- or weather-related. An allergic dermatitis similar to that described in dogs has also been described in pigs, and its signs resemble those seen in the allergic form of sarcoptic mange (Nesbitt and Schmitz 1978).

T. penetrans infestation has been reported as being associated with agalactia in sows in the Republic of Zaire (Verhulst 1976). Clinical examination showed that the ovigerous females (chiggers) were localized in the teats and obstructed the ducts. This produced agalactia and death of piglets. An outbreak of *T. penetrans* was also reported in Tanzania in which adult pigs were affected around the feet, snout, and scrotum (Cooper 1967).

Diagnosis and Treatment

Diagnosis of flea infestation is not easy, because adult fleas may leave the host, and larvae and eggs are difficult to find. The bites are not readily differentiated from those of mosquitoes, lice, and mites, so the presence of those other parasites should be carefully checked before a diagnosis is made. Infestation of humans during contact with pigs is also a good diagnostic aid (Dobinson 2000).

The range of chemicals used to treat and control fleas include many of the products listed for other external parasites. According to Dobinson (2000), amitraz, coumpaphos, maldison, doramectin, and ivermectin have all been used successfully to treat pigs and their bedding. However, although pigs are easily treated, ridding the environment of fleas is more difficult. Control is based on the location and treatment of the flea-breeding area, but it is important to use chemicals with published withholding periods so that pigs can be held in a chemical-free environment for the appropriate period before slaughter. Although litter, bedding, dirt, and manure should be removed and burned, this is not always practical until the pigs are moved. Environmental control has been achieved with primiphos and chlorpyrifos (Dobinson 2000) or 2.5% malathion.

MOSQUITOES

Mosquitoes, although considered primarily pests of humans, also attack livestock, causing discomfort and irritation. In some cases the affected carcasses of pigs must be skinned at slaughter.

Aedes spp. have been observed attacking swine in large numbers in Florida (Bennett 1975; Becker and Gross 1987). In South Australia the same species has bred in brackish pools of seawater left by high tides and has caused troubles in nearby piggeries (Dobson 1973). Lesions appeared on several or all the pigs within a pen in the form of raised edematous weals on the legs and abdomen. These tended to disappear spontaneously within 1–2 days but made pigs unacceptable for marketing at the time. Control was achieved by regular spraying with diazinon in the late evening. Mosquito screening and insect repellents are also helpful in minimizing the problem. Where possible, the breeding ground of the mosquitoes should be identified. The larvae can be destroyed by either draining water reservoirs or covering the surface with oil. A wide range of insecticides has been used successfully in breeding grounds.

Mosquitoes have a seasonal distribution, with populations disappearing in most temperate regions during winter. Mosquitoes are important vectors in the transmission of Japanese encephalitis virus, especially in rice-growing areas (Wada and Smith 1988). Vaccination has proved unsuccessful, and pigs must be separated from rice fields to prevent them from acting as amplifier hosts. Mosquitoes can also mechanically transmit porcine reproductive and reproductive syndrome virus (PRRSV), but do not serve as a biological vector of the virus (Otake et al. 2003a, 2002). The virus can also reside in the intestinal tract of the mosquito for up to 6 hours, but does not survive on the exterior surface of the insect. Mosquitoes also transmit *Mycoplasma haemosuis* between pigs (Prullage et al. 1993).

FLIES

Flies are important in pig production for several reasons, and they tend to be used as a measure of hygiene by local health authorities. Some flies annoy animals by their vicious bite, and others act only as a vehicle for transmission of infectious disease. Some species are associated with myiasis, that is, invasion of the tissues of animals by fly larvae.

The common housefly (*Musca domestica*) is ubiquitous and most active in summer. It prefers to breed either in the feces of animals or in decaying organic matter. The housefly is well known for its ability to transfer pathogenic bacteria mechanically via its hairy feet and legs or by regurgitation of fluid from its crop. It can also act as the intermediate host of several worm parasites of domestic animals, and it may act as a disseminator of the eggs of many others (Soulsby 1968). It has been demonstrated experimentally that it is capable of spreading hog cholera (HC) virus (Morgan and Miller 1976) and *Streptococcus suis* (Enright et al. 1987) from infected to susceptible pigs.

The stable fly (*Stomoxys calcitrans*) is about the size of the housefly, but it prefers to breed in moist, decaying vegetable matter such as straw and hay. Flies are most abundant in summer and prefer fairly strong light rather than dark stables or houses. Both male and female are bloodsuckers of humans and animals. When present in large numbers, the stable fly may become a source of annoyance, resulting in weight loss. However, Campbell et al. (1984) were not able to demonstrate reduced gain or feed conversion experimentally. The stable fly can also act as a vector of infectious organisms, including HC and *Mycoplasma haemosuis* (Prullage et al. 1993).

Horseflies of the Tabanidae family are large, robust flies with clear, powerful wings. The common breeding place is on the leaves of plants in the vicinity of water. Horseflies are active in summer, particularly on hot, sultry days. They attack animals, including pigs, by biting and feeding on blood (Tidwell et al. 1972). They are capable of transmitting infectious diseases, including HC (Tidwell et al. 1972).

Blackflies of the family Simuliidae, also known as buffalo gnats, occur in all parts of the world and can be troublesome in warm countries. They breed in streams below the surface of running water. They may cause inappetence and attack the legs, abdomen, head, and ears, resulting in vesicles and papules. Considerable numbers of stock have been killed in European countries. Grafner et al. (1976) reported the death of 3 sows and severe illness in another 27, together with reduced growth rate, in pigs in Germany.

Screwworm flies of the family Calliphoridae cause myiasis in humans and animals. *Cochliomyia hominovora* is present in Latin America, and *Chrysomya bezziana*, the Old World screwworm fly, occurs in Africa and southern Asia. The adult fly is 10–15 mm long and has a metallic green sheen to its thorax and abdomen. It has three longitudinal stripes on the thorax. It breeds in wounds on live animals, and each female lays 150–500 eggs at the edge of a wound. Larvae hatch in 10–12 hours and mature in 3–6 days, after which they leave the host to pupate in the ground. The pupal period lasts from 3 days to several weeks, depending on prevailing temperatures. Hibernation occurs most commonly in the pupal stage (Soulsby 1968).

Most cases of myiasis occur in rainy weather. Maggots penetrate the wound tissue, which they liquefy and thus extend the lesion. There is a foul-smelling exudate and deaths can occur. Loss can be prevented if surgical wounds are avoided during the fly season and prompt attention is given to lacerations and injuries. Wounds can be protected from myiasis by the application of a prophylactic wound dressing. Smear 62 (containing diphenylamine, benzol, turkey red oil, and lampblack) or, alternatively, EQ335 (containing 3% lindane and 35% pine oil) will protect wounds for at least 3 days (Bennett 1975). After wounds are invaded by larvae, they may be effectively treated with pressurized aerosols containing coumaphos, lindane, or ronnel (refer to Table 53.1). The larvae in wounds can be killed if penetration is not too deep.

Blowflies of the subfamily Calliphorinae differ from screwworm flies in that they deposit their eggs in necrotic wounds. Secondary blowflies deposit their eggs only on necrotic wounds that have been previously struck by either primary blowflies or screwworm flies. The damage caused by blowflies is similar to but less severe than that caused by screwworms. Treatment and prevention are similar.

Houseflies can also mechanically transmit PRRSV, but as with mosquitoes, do not serve as biological vectors of the virus. According to Otake et al. (2004, 2003b), the virus also resides in the intestinal tract of the housefly for up to 12 hours, but not on the exterior surface of the fly.

Control

Fly control in all piggeries must be a continuing exercise in summer months. The aim is to prevent flies from breeding and to destroy adult flies. Breeding of flies can be prevented by regular removal of dung. At temperatures of 25°C or more, the life cycle of the housefly takes only 15 days; hence frequent cleaning is important. Manure should be removed at least weekly and spread thinly on soil to kill eggs and larvae by desiccation. Dung should be disposed of in the center of effluent ponds rather than at the edge, where flies can breed. A number of methods can be used to destroy flies within pig sheds. Insecticides are effective in the form of sprays, baits, or vapors strips (refer to Table 53.1). Some insecticides such as trichlorfon, given to pigs as a medication for internal parasites, are effective in destroying both the larvae and adult flies that settle on dung from treated pigs.

Sprays are applied to walls, ceilings, and pen partitions within sheds. With some insecticides, stock and feed may need to be removed first. Space or aerosol sprays (foggers) used twice daily with knockdown insecticides are also effective. Baits applied to clean concrete surfaces and pen divisions are effective and usually contain insecticides such as ronnel, diazinon, malathion, trichlorfon, and dichlorvos.

Fly electrocutors offer an automatic nonchemical method of controlling flies. Screens on openings help limit the number of flies entering buildings but can be impractical. Electric-light traps can be used as an auxiliary in fly control but are considered more efficient for midges rather than flies (Schmidt 1987).

TICKS

Ticks infest many species of mammals and birds and are generally not host-specific. Compared with grazing species, in which ticks and tick-borne diseases are of major economic importance, pigs are not commonly parasitized by ticks, and ticks essentially do not occur on pigs raised in confinement. The ticks of potential importance to pigs are of the suborder Ixodoidia, which includes two large families, the Ixodidae (or hard tick) and the Argasidae (or soft tick).

In the United States the following ticks have been reported as occurring on swine:

Ixodidae
- *Dermacentor andersoni* (Rocky Mountain spotted fever tick)
- *D. variabilis* (American dog tick or wood tick)
- *D. nitens* (tropical horse tick)
- *Amblyomma maculatum* (Gulf Coast tick)
- *Ixodes scapularis* (black-legged tick or shoulder tick)

Argasidae
- *Ornithodoros turicata* (relapsing fever tick)
- *Otobius megnini* (spinose ear tick)

In Australia, *I. holocyclus,* the dog paralysis tick, has been known to cause death in suckling pigs (Seddon 1968). In general, species of ticks are adapted to specific ranges of temperature and humidity, and the reader should seek local information to assist in identifying specific species.

Life cycles of ticks are characterized by the stages of egg, larva (seed tick), nymph, and adult. The six-legged seed tick, on hatching from the egg, climbs onto grass or shrubs, and waits until a suitable host passes. It attaches itself to the host and engorges with lymph and blood. It then molts and an eight-legged nymph emerges. This feeds on the host and molts to become an adult tick. After mating, the female drops off the host, lays her eggs, and dies.

The main economic importance of ticks for all species is their ability to act as vectors in disease transmission. Pathogens transmitted by ticks include protozoa, rickettsias, and viruses. African swine fever virus, when introduced experimentally to the tick *Ornithodoros moubata,* could be recovered 50 weeks after infection (Greig 1972). Therefore, ticks could be of significance in the spread of viral diseases from wild pigs to domestic animals.

Diagnosis

The diagnosis of tick infestation is based on the known location of ticks and the access of pigs to these areas. Ticks are readily seen by gross visual examination. Although found on any part of the body, they are more often seen around the ears, neck, and flanks. The tick differs from other arthropod parasites in that it is attached to its host. The size and appearance vary according to the degree of blood engorgement. A careful check should be made in the ear for the *Otobius* ear tick.

Treatment and Control

The treatment and control of ticks in pigs are seldom problems. If only a few ticks are present, these can be removed manually and the pigs confined away from infested pasture. Many insecticides are effective as a spray or dip. Toxaphene as a 0.5% spray is recommended because it will protect against reinfestation for 2 weeks or longer (McIntosh and McDuffie 1956). Other effective acaricides include coumaphos, dioxathion, and malathion (refer to Table 53.1). A 5% coumaphos dust has been used effectively in the ears to control the spinose ear tick.

REFERENCES

Aiello SE. 1998. The Merck Veterinary Manual, 8th ed. Whitehouse Station, NJ: Merck & Co., Inc.

Alonso de Vega F, Mendez de Vigo J, Ortiz Zanches J, Martinez-Carrasco Pleite C, Albaladejo Serrano A, Ruiz de Ybanes Carnero MR. 1998. Vet Parasitol 76:203–209.

Alva-Valdes R, Wallace DH, Benz GW, Foster AG, Holste JE. 1984. Efficiency of ivermectin against the mange mite *Sarcoptes scabiei* var. *suis* in pigs. Am J Vet Res 45:2113–2114.

Alva-Valdes R, Wallace DH, Foster AG, Ericsson GF, Wooden JW. 1986. The effects of sarcoptic mange on the productivity of confined pigs. Vet Med 81:258–260.

Arends JJ. 1991. Managing mange, losses to the swine industry may reach $230 million annually. Lg Anim Vet 46:6–10.

Arends JJ, Skogerboe TL, Ritzhaupt LK. 1999. Persistent efficacy of doramectin and ivermectin against experimental infestations of *Sarcoptes scabiei* var. *suis* in swine. Vet Parasitol 82(1):71–79.

Arends JJ, Stanislaw CM, Gerdon D. 1990. Effects of sarcoptic mange on lactating swine and growing pigs. J Anim Sci 68:1495–1499.

Barth D, Brokken ES. 1980. The activity of 22, 23-dihydroavermectin B1 against the pig louse, Haematopinus *suis*. Vet Rec 106:388.

Becker HN, Gross TL. 1987. Porcine allergic dermatitis caused by insect bites. Agri-Pract 8:8–10.

Belding DL. 1952. Textbook of Clinical Parasitology. New York: Appleton-Century-Crofts.

Bennett DG. 1975. External parasites. In Diseases of Swine, 4th ed. HW Dunne, AD Leman, eds. Ames: Iowa State Univ Press.

Bogatko W. 1974. Studies in the occurrence of *Sarcoptes scabiei* in clinically healthy pigs. Med Weter 30:38.

Bornstein S, Eliasson-Selling L, Naslund K, Wallgren P. 2000. Evaluation of a serodiagnostic ELISA for swine sarcoptic mange. Proc Int Pig Vet Soc Cong 2000, p 269.

Bornstein S, Fellstrom C, Thebo P, Wallgren P. 1994. Eradication of sarcoptic mange in a herd of pigs monitored by skin scrapings and ELISA. Proc Int Pig Vet Soc Cong 1994, p 251.

Bornstein S, Wallgren P. 1996. Serum antibody responses to *Sarcoptes scabiei* infections in young pigs following acaricidal treatment. Proc Int Pig Vet Soc Cong 14:355.

———. 1997. Serodiagnosis of sarcoptic mange in pigs. Vet Rec 141:8–12.

Bornstein S, Zakrisson G. 1993. Clinical picture and antibody response in pigs infected by *Sarcoptes scabiei* var *suis*. Veterinary Dermatology 4:123–131.

Brakenridge DT. 1958. Mange in pigs. A survey. NZ Vet J 6:166–167.

Campbell JB, Boxler DJ, Danielson DM, Cvenshaw MA. 1984. Effects of house and stable flies on weight gain and feed efficiency by feeder pigs. S West Entomol 9:273–274.

Cargill C. 2001. La gale sarcoptique chez le porc—Conséquences économiques, aspects cliniques, outils diagnostiques, contrôle et éradication. In Actualités en Production Porcine—Association Francaise de Medicine Veterinaire Porcine, pp. 13–20.

———. 2002. Sarcoptic mange in pigs—Economic effects, clinical patterns, diagnostic tools, control and eradication. 69th Philippine Veterinary Medical Association Annual Conference, Pampanga, The Philippines, pp. 75–78.

Cargill C, Sandeman M, Garcia R, Homer D. 2002. The efficacy of top-dressing sow rations pre-farrowing with Ivomec powder. Proc Int Pig Vet Soc Cong, Ames, Iowa, p. 271.

———. 2004. Three mange eradication programs based on breeding herd treatment only—Validated by slaughter check and ELISA assay. Proc Int Pig Vet Soc Cong, Hamburg, Germany (in press).

Cargill C, Wegiel J. 2000. The progression and epidemiology of a natural infestation of sarcoptic mange in growing pigs. Proc Int Pig Vet Soc Cong, Melbourne Australia, p. 264.

Cargill CF, Davies P, Carmichael I, Hooke F, Moore M. 1996a. Treatment of sarcoptic mite infestation and mite hypersensitivity in pigs with injectable doramectin. Vet Rec 138:468–471.

Cargill CF, Dobson KJ. 1977. Field and experimental studies of sarcoptic mange in pigs in South Australia. Proc 54th Annu Conf Aust Vet Assoc, p. 129.

———. 1979a. Experimental *Sarcoptes scabiei* infestation in pigs. I. Pathogenesis. Vet Rec 104:11–14.

———. 1979b. Experimental *Sarcoptes scabiei* infestation in pigs. II. Effects on production. Vet Rec 104:33–36.

Cargill CF, Pointon AM, Davies P, Garcia R. 1997. Using slaughter inspections to evaluate sarcoptic mange infestation of finishing swine. J Parasitol 70:191–200.

Cargill CF, Pointon AM, Moore M, Garcia R. 1996b. A retrospective evaluation based on slaughter monitoring of using ivermectin to control and eradicate sarcoptic mange. Proc Int Pig Vet Soc Cong 14:356.

Cooper JE. 1967. An outbreak of Tunga penetrans in a pig herd. Vet Rec 80:365–366.

Courtney CH, Ingalls WL, Stitzlein SL. 1983. Ivermectin for the control of swine scabies: Relative values of prefarrowing treatment of sows and weaning treatment of pigs. Am J Vet Res 44:1220–1223.

Dalton PM, Ryan WG. 1988. Productivity effects of pig mange and control with ivermectin. Vet Rec 122:307–308.

Davies PR. 1995. Sarcoptic mange and production performance of swine: A review of the literature and studies of associations between mite infestation, growth rate and measures of mange severity in growing pigs. Vet Parasitol 60:249–264.

Davies PR, Garcia R, Gross S. 1996a. Preliminary evidence of parasite aggregation in swine sarcoptic mange. Proc Int Pig Vet Soc Cong 14:354.

Davies PR, Moore MJ, Pointon AM. 1991a. Sarcoptic mite hypersensitivity and skin lesions in slaughtered pigs. Vet Rec 128:516–518.

———. 1991b. Seasonality of sarcoptic mange in South Australia. Aust Vet J 68:390–392.

Davies PR, Sahnson PB, Grass JJ, Marsh WE, Garcia R, Melancon J, Dial GD. 1996b. Evaluation of the monitoring of papular dermatitis lesions in slaughtered swine to assess sarcoptic mite infestation. Vet Parasitol 62:143–153.

Davis DP, Moon RD. 1987. Survival of *Sarcoptes scabiei* in three media and at three temperatures. J Parasitol 73:661–662.

———. 1990a. Density of itch mite, *Sarcoptes scabiei* (Acari: Sarcoptidae), and temporal development of cutaneous hypersensitivity in swine mange. Vet Parasitol 36:285–293.

———. 1990b. The dynamics of swine mange infestation. J Med Entomol 27:727–737.

———. 1990c. Pruritis and behaviour of pigs infested with itch mites *Sarcoptes scabiei* (Acari: Sarcoptidae). J Econ Entomol 83:1439–1445.

———. 1990d. Density and location of *Sarcoptes scabiei* on experimentally infected pigs. J Med Entomol 27:391–398.

Davis DP, Williams RE. 1986. Influence of hog lice, *Haematopinus suis*, on blood components, behaviour, weight gain and feed efficiency of pigs. Vet Parasitol 22:307–314.

Deckert A, Nixon R, Diagenault J, Pentney P, Dewey C. 2000. The evaluation of Bommeli ELISA SARCOPTEST for *Sarcoptes scabiei* var.*suis* and the prevalence of mange in Ontario, Canada.Proc Int Pig Vet Soc Cong, Melbourne, Australia 17–20 September, 2000, p. 268.

Dobinson S. 2000. Approaches to the control of fleas in outdoor piggeries. Proc Australian Association of Pig Veterinarians. Perth, p. 71–74.

Dobson KJ. 1973. External parasites of pigs: Mosquitoes. Univ Sydney Post Grad Comm Vet Sci Proc 19:349.

Dobson KJ, Cargill CF. 1979. Epidemiology and economic consequence of sarcoptic mange in pigs. Proc 2d Int Symp Vet Epidemiol Econ. Canberra: Aust Gov Pub Serv, p. 401.

Dobson KJ, Davies PR. 1992. External parasites. In Diseases of Swine, 7th ed. AD Leman, BE Straw, WL Mengeling, S D'Allaire, DJ Taylor, eds. Ames: Iowa State Univ Press, pp. 668–679.

Ebbesen T. 1998. Eradication of Sarcoptic Mange in farrow to finish herds with Ivomec vet premix and Ivomec vet. inj. Proc Int Pig Vet Soc Cong, Birmingham England, p. 120.

Elbers ARW, Rambags PGM, van der Heijden HMJF, Hunneman WA. 2000. Production performance and pruritic behaviour of pigs naturally infected by *Sarcoptes scabiei* var. *suis* in a contact transmission experiment. Vet Quart 22:145–149.

Elbers ARW, Teilen MJM, Snidjers JMA. 1992. Epidemiological studies on lesions in finishing pigs in the Netherlands. 1. Prevalence, seasonality and interrelationship. Prev Vet Med 14:217–231.

Enright MR, Alexander TJL, Clifton-Hadley FA. 1987. Role of houseflies (*Musca domestica*) in the epidemiology of *Streptococcus suis* type 2. Vet Rec 121:132–133.

Firkins LD, Jones CJ, Keen DP, Arends JJ, Thompson L, King VL, Skogerboe TL. 2001. Preventing transmission of *Sarcoptes scabiei* var. *suis* from infested sows to nursing piglets by a prefarrowing treatment with doramectin injectable solution. Vet Parasitol 99(4):323–330.

Flesja KI, Ulvesaeter HO. 1979. Pathological lesions in swine at slaughter. 1. Baconers. ACTA Vet Scand 20:498–514.

Florence I. 1921. The Hog Louse *Haematopinus suis linne*, Its Biology, Anatomy and Histology. Cornell Univ Agric Exp Stn Mem 51.

Frick W, Kraus H, Danneberg HD. 1974. Results of ectoparasite control on pigs at district level. Monatsh Veterinaermed 29:612.

Gaafer SM, Arends JJ, Hogg A, Holscher KH, Williams RE. 1986. An integrated program using Taktic to control mange in swine. J Agric Entomol 3:374–381.

Garcia R, Piche C, Davies PR, Gross S. 1994. Prevalence of sarcoptic mange mites and dermatitis in slaughter pigs in North America and Western Europe. Proc Int Pig Vet Soc Cong 13:250.

Grafner G, Zimmermann H, Karge E, Munch J, Ribbeck R, Hiepe T. 1976. Occurrence and harmful effects of the black flies in the Schwerin district of East Germany. Angew Parasitol 17:2.

Green MS. 1989. Epidemiology of scabies. Epidemiol Rev 11:126–150.

Greig A. 1972. The localisation of African swine fever virus in the tick *Ornithodoros moubata porcinus*. Arch Gesamte Virusforsch 39:24C.

Gualandi GL, Boni P, Varisco E, Paiaro R, Garcia R, Gross S. 1994. Study of the prevalence of sarcoptic mange in pigs at slaughterhouses in major swine production areas in northern Italy. Proc Int Pig Vet Soc Cong 13:246.

Harland EC, Simpson CF, Neal FC. 1971. Demodectic mange of swine. J Am Vet Med Assoc 159:1752–1754.

Hasslinger MA, Resch J. 1992. Studies on endoparasite and ectoparasite infestation in slaughter pigs. Proc Int Pig Vet Soc Cong 12:375.

Henriksen SA, Ebbesen TJ, Nielsen KV. 1987. Eradication of mange from a large sow and slaughter pig herd. Dansk Vet Tidsskr 70:575–579.

Hewett GR. 1985. Phosmet for the systemic control of pig mange in growing pigs. Vet Parasitol 18:265–268.

Hewett GR, Heard TW. 1982. Phosmet for the systemic control of pig mange. Vet Rec 111:558.

Hiepe T, Ribbeck R. 1975. The pig louse (*Haematopinus suis*). Angew Parasitol 16(Suppl).

Hill SD. 1997. The Economic Importance of Insects. London: Chapman and Hall.

Hollanders W, Harbers AHM, Huige JCM, Monster P, Rambags PGM, Hendrickx WML. 1995. Control of *Sarcoptes scabiei* var. *suis* with ivermectin: Influence on scratching behaviour of fattening pigs and occurrence of dermatitis at slaughter. Vet Parsitol 58:117–127.

Hollanders W, Vercruysse J. 1990. Sarcoptic mite hypersensitivity: A cause of dermatitis in fattening pigs at slaughter. Vet Rec 126:308–310.

Horie PF, De La. 1990. Prevalence of sarcoptic mange in fattening pigs: Results of a French survey. Proc Int Pig Vet Soc Cong 11:320.

Jacobson M, Bornstein S, Wallgren P. 1999. The efficacy of simplified eradication strategies against sarcoptic mange mite infections in swine herds monitored by an ELISA. Vet Parasitol 81(3):249–258.

Jensen JC, Nielsen LH, Arnason T, Cracknell V. 2002. Elimination of mange mites *Sarcoptes scabiei* var. *suis* from two naturally infested Danish sow herds using a single injection regime with doramectin. Acta Vet Scand 43(2):75–84.

Johansson LE, Nilsson O, Olevall O. 1980. Amitraz (Taktik) for the control of pig mange. Nord Vet Med 32:161–164.

Kambarage DM. 1993. Diagnosis of sarcoptic mange in pigs: Clinical examination and mite recovery as diagnostic methods in determination of disease status. Zimbabwe Vet J 24:31–36.

Keller H, Eckert J, Trepp HC. 1972. Eradication of sarcoptic mange in pigs. Schweiz Arch Tierheilkd 114:573–582.

Kessler E, Matthes H-F, Schein E, Wendt M. 2003. Detection of antibodies in sera of weaned pigs after contact infection with *Sarcoptes scabiei* var. *suis* and after treatment with an antiparasitic agent by three different indirect ELISAs. Vet. Parasitol 114:63–73.

Klopfenstein C, Piche C, D'Allaire S, Villeneuve A, Bahnson PB, Gross S. 1992. Survey of the prevalence of sarcoptic mange and dermatitis in slaughter pigs in Quebec, Canada. Proc Int Pig Vet Soc Cong 11:323.

Lee RP, Dooge DJD, Preston JM. 1980. Efficiency of ivermectin against *Sarcoptes scabiei* in pigs. Vet Rec 107:503–505.

Logan NB, Weatherly AJ, Jones RM. 1996. Activity of doramectin against nematode and arthropod parasites of swine. Vet Parasitol 66:87–94.

Magee JC. 1974. Studies on *Sarcoptes scabiei* on swine in Iowa. Proc North Cent Branch Entomol Soc Am 29:125.

Martelli P, Beghian MA. 1990. Pig mange: Economical impact of pour-on treatment. Proc Int Pig Vet Soc Cong 11:323.

Martineau GP, Vaillancourt J, Frechette JL. 1984. Control of *Sarcoptes scabiei* infestation with ivermectin in a large intensive breeding piggery. Can Vet J 25:235–238.

McIntosh A, McDuffie WC. 1956. Ticks that affect domestic animals and poultry. In Animal Diseases. Yearbook of Agriculture. Washington, D.C.: USDA, p. 157.

McMullin PF, Guise J, Cuthbertson C, Jones MA. 1992. A survey of *Sarcoptes scabiei* var. *suis* in finishing pigs in Great Britain. Proc Int Pig Vet Soc Cong 12:373.

McMullin PF, Jones PGH, Hale CJ, Jones MA, Ryan WG. 1990. A survey of sarcoptic mange in cull sows in Great Britain. Proc Int Pig Vet Soc Cong 11:318.

McPherson EA. 1960. Sarcoptic mange in pigs. Vet Rec 72:869–870.

Melancon J. 2003. Prevalence of mange (*Sarcoptes scabiei*) in the Northern USA and Canadian Swine Belt. Merial Veterinary Bulletin MVB-03-020.

Mendez de Vigo J, Garcia R, Gutierrez JF, Diez-Banos P, Gomez-Butista M, Alonsa de Vego F. 1992. Study of the prevalence of sarcoptic mange in pigs at slaughterhouses in major swine-production areas in Spain. Proc Int Pig Vet Soc Cong 12:374.

Mercier P, Cargill CF, White CR. 2002. Preventing transmission of sarcoptic mange from sows to their offspring by injection of ivermectin effects on swine production. Vet Parasitol 110:25–33.

Mikhalochkina EI. 1975. Resistance of Sarcoptes *suis* to environmental factors. Uch Zap Vitebsk Vet Inst 28:179.

Mock DE. 1997. Lice, Mange and Another Swine Insect Problems. Kansas State University.

Morgan NO, Miller LD. 1976. Muscidae (Diptera): Experimental vectors of hog cholera virus. J Med Entomol 12:657.

Morsy GH, Gaafar SM. 1989. Responses of immunoglobulin-secreting cells in the skin of pigs during *Sarcoptes scabiei* infestation. Vet Parasitol 33:165–175.

Morsy GH, Turek JJ, Gaafar SM. 1989. Scanning electron microscopy of sarcoptic mange lesions in swine. Vet Parasitol 31:281–288.

Murthy TVR, Rao R, Gaafar AA. 1993. Therapeutic trial of demodectic mange in dogs with amitraz and ivermectin. Indian Vet J 17:28–29.

Nesbitt GH, Schmitz JA. 1978. Fleabite allergic dermatitis: A review and survey of 330 cases. J Am Vet Med Assoc 173:282–288.

Nutting WB. 1976. Hair follicle mites (*Demodex* spp.) of medical and veterinary concern. Cornell Vet 66:214–231.

Nutting WB, Kettle PR, Tenquist JD, Whitten L. 1975. Hair follicle mites (*Demodex* spp.) in New Zealand. NZ J Zool 2:219–222.

Ohba S, Toriumi H, Takeishi M, Noda R. 1989. Efficacy of ivermectin against live mites and eggs of *Sarcoptes scabiei* in pigs. Jap J Vet Sc 51:981–985.

Otake S, Dee SA, Moon RD, Rossow KD, Trincado C, Farnham M, Pijoan C. 2003b. Survival of porcine reproductive and respiratory syndrome virus in houseflies. Can J Vet Res 67(3):198–203.

Otake S, Dee SA, Moon RD, Rossow KD, Trincado C, Pijoan C. 2003a. Evaluation of mosquitoes, *Aedes vexans,* as biological vectors of porcine reproductive and respiratory syndrome virus. Can J Vet Res 67(4):265–270.

Otake S, Dee SA, Moon RD, Rossow KD, Trincado C, Pijoan C. 2004. Studies on the carriage and transmission of porcine reproductive and respiratory syndrome virus by individual houseflies (*Musca domestica*). Vet Rec 17:154(3):80–85.

Otake S, Dee SA, Rossow KD, Moon RD, Pijoan C. 2002. Mechanical transmission of porcine reproductive and respiratory syndrome virus by mosquitoes, *Aedes vexans* (Meigen). Can J Vet Res. 66(3):191–5. Erratum in Can J Vet Res 66(4):294.

Pointon AM, Cargill CF, Slade J. 1995. Skin disease. In The Good Health Manual for Pigs. J. Ferguson, ed. Canberra, Australia: Pig Research and Development Corp, pp. 113–115.

Pointon AM, Davies PR, Bahnson PB. 1999. Disease surveillance at slaughter. In Diseases of Swine 8th ed. BE Straw, S D'Allaire, WL Mengeling, DJ Taylor, eds. Ames: Iowa State Univ Press, pp. 1111–1132.

Pointon AM, Farrell M, Cargill CF, Heap P. 1987. A pilot health scheme for Australian conditions. Univ Sydney Post Grad Comm Vet Sci Proc 95:743–777.

Pointon AM, Mercy AR, Backstrom L, Dial GD. 1992. Disease surveillance at slaughter. In Diseases of Swine, 7th ed. AD Leman, BE Straw, WL Mengeling, S D'Allaire, DJ Taylor, eds. Ames: Iowa State Univ Press, pp. 968–987.

Prullage JB, Williams RE, Gaafar SM. 1993. On the transmissibility of *Eperythrozoon suis* by *Stomoxys calcitrans* and *Aedes aegypti*. Vet Parsitol 50:125–135.

Pullar EM. 1941. Mange or scabies in pigs. J Agric Victoria Aust 39:99–104.

Rambags PGM, Elbers ARW, van der Heijden HMJF, Hunneman WA. 2000. The Dutch mange free (*Sarcoptes scabiei* var *suis*) certification programme: Evaluation and update after a transmission experiment. Proc Int Pig Vet Soc Cong, Melbourne Australia, p. 267.

Rambags PGM, Vesseur PC, van der Heijden HMJF. 1998. Mange (*Sarcoptes scabiei* var *suis*) eradication programme and possibilities for certification in Dutch farms. Proc Int Pig Vet Soc Cong, Birmingham England, p. 123.

Reddin J. 1997. Eradication of mange from pig herds. In Pig Production. Univ Sydney Post Grad Comm Vet Sci Proc (in press).

Satyavir S, Chhabra MB. 1992. Comparative efficacy of ivermectin and fenvalerate against sarcoptic mange in pigs. Indian Vet J 69:1037–1040.

Schmidt U. 1987. Use of electric light traps to control insects in a piggery. Fleischwirtschaft 68:1421–1425. Cited in Pig News Inf 9:1660 (abstr).

Schultz R. 1986. Mange costs millions. Hog Farm Management, Apr, p. 17.

Seaman JT, Thompson DR, Barrick RA. 1993. Treatment with ivermectin of sarcoptic mange in pigs. Aust Vet J 70:307–308.

Seddon HR. 1968. Sarcoptic mites: Sarcoptic mange. In Diseases of Domestic Animals in Australia. II. Arthropod Infestations, 2d ed. HE Albiston, reviewer. Commonw Dep Health Serv Publ 7, p. 98.

Sheahan BJ. 1970. Sarcoptic mange in Irish pigs: A survey. Ir Vet J 24:201–203.

——. 1974. Experimental *Sarcoptes scabiei* infection in pigs: Clinical signs and significance of infection. Vet Rec 94:202–209.

——. 1975. Pathology of *Sarcoptes scabiei* infection in pigs. I.

Naturally occurring and experimentally induced lesions. II. Histological, histochemical and ultrastructural changes at skin test sites. J Comp Pathol 85:87–110.

Sheahan BJ, Hatch C. 1975. A method for isolating large numbers of *Sarcoptes scabiei* from lesions in the ears of pigs. J Parasitol 61:350.

Sheahan BJ, Kelly EP. 1974. Improved weight gains in pigs following treatment for sarcoptic mange. Vet Rec 95:169–170.

Smeets JFM, Snijders JMA, Gruys E. 1989. Dermatitis in slaughter pigs: Occurrence, pathology and economic significance. Tijdschr Diergeneeskd,114:603–610.

Smets K, Neirynck W, Vercruysse J. 1999. Eradication of sarcoptic mange from a Belgian pig breeding farm with a combination of injectable and in-feed ivermectin. Vet Rec 145:721–724.

Smets K, Vercruysse J. 2000. Evaluation of different methods for the diagnosis of scabies in swine. Vet Parasitol 90:137–145.

Smith HJ. 1986. Transmission of *Sarcoptes scabiei* in swine by fomites. Can Vet J 27:252–254.

Soulsby EJL. 1968. Helminths, arthropods and protozoa of domesticated animals. In Monnig's Veterinary Helminthology and Entomology, 6th ed. London: Bailliere, Tindall and Cassell.

Stegeman JA, Rambags PG, van der Heijden HM. 2000. Experimental quantification of the transmission of *Sarcoptes scabiei* var.*suis* among finishing pigs. Vet Parasitol 93:57–67.

Taylor DJ. 1999. Pig Diseases, 7th ed. Great Britain: St. Edmundsbury Press Ltd.

Thomas P, Bicknell SR, Hamlet EJ, Janowicz J, Griffiths P, Wherton C, Ross DB. 1986. Porcine sarcoptic mange, an eradication project: A preliminary report. Proc Pig Vet Soc 15:496.

Tidwell MA, Dean WD, Combs GA, Anderson DW, Cowart WD, Axtell RC. 1972. Transmission of hog cholera virus by horseflies (*Tabanidae: Diptera*). Am J Vet Res 33:615–622.

Vercruysse J, Smets K. 2000. The diagnosis of swine mange: A European perspective. Proc Int Pig Vet Soc Cong, Melbourne Australia, p. 266.

Verhulst A. 1976. *Tunga penetrans* (*Sarcopsylla penetrans*) as a cause of agalactia in sows in the Republic of Zaire. Vet Rec 98:384.

Wada Y, Smith WH. 1988. Strategies for the control of Japanese encephalitis in rice production systems in developing countries. Proc Workshop on Res and Training Needs in the Field of Integrated Vector-borne Disease Control. Manilla, Philippines: Int Rice Inst, pp. 153–160.

Walton GS. 1967. The young pig ectoparasitic infestations. Vet Rec 80(Clin Suppl)9:11–13.

White MEC, Ryan WG. 1987. Control of an outbreak of pig mange with ivermectin. Vet Rec 121:496.

Wooten EL, Blecha F, Broce AB, Pollman DS. 1986. The effect of sarcoptic mange on growth performance, leukocytes and lymphocyte proliferative responses in pigs. Vet Parsitol 22:315–325.

Wooten-Saadi EL, Broce AB, Stevenson JS, Nelson JL. 1987a. Growth performance and behavioral patterns of pigs infested with sarcoptic mites. J Econ Entomol 80:625–628.

Wooten-Saadi EL, Towell-Vail CA, Williams RE, Gaafar SM. 1987b. Incidence of *Sarcoptes scabiei* and *Haematopinus suis* on swine in Indiana. J Econ Entomol 80:1031–1034.

Yazwinski TA, Tucker C, Featherston H, Johnson Z, Wood-Huels N. 1997. Endectocidal efficacies of doramectin in naturally parasitized pigs. Vet Parasitol 70(1–3):123–128.

Yeoman GH. 1984. Pig mange: New concepts in control. In The Vet Ann, 14th ed. FWG Hill, ed. Bristol: Wright-Scientechnia, pp. 132–137.

Zalunardo M, Cargill C, Sandeman. 2000. Serological confirmation of mange eradication in pigs. Proc Int Pig Vet Soc Cong, Melbourne Australia, p. 270.

Zimmerman W, Kircher P. 1998. Serologische Bestandesuntersuchung und Sanierungsüberwachung der *Sarcoptes scabiei* var.*suis* Infektion: Erste vorläufige Resultate. Schwiez Arch Tierhielk 140:513–517.

54 Gastric Ulcers

Robert M. Friendship

This chapter focuses on ulceration of the pars oesophagea, the non-glandular region of the pig's stomach surrounding the esophageal entrance. This syndrome is distinct from ulceration of the fundic and pyloric regions. Often erosions in the glandular area of the stomach are associated with systemic diseases such as salmonellosis, erysipelas, or hog cholera infection. On the whole, ulceration of the pars oesophagea is the far more common and important of the two conditions and can lead to sudden death from acute intragastric hemorrhage or to chronic ill thrift. In addition to "gastric ulceration," various terms have been used to describe this condition, including "esophagogastric ulceration" (Driesen et al. 1987), "gastroesophageal ulceration" (Deen 1993), "proventricular ulcer" (Ito et al. 1974), and "ulcerative gastric hemorrhage" (Hannan and Nyhan 1962).

The first description of pars oesophageal ulceration was made in 1897 (McIntosh 1897), but little attention was paid to this condition until modern husbandry practices were adopted. Epizootic outbreaks of pars oesophageal ulceration began to occur in North America and Europe in the late 1950s (Thoonen and Hoorens 1961; Curtin et al. 1963; Griffing 1963; Muggenburg et al. 1964) concurrent with new developments in housing and feeding. Wherever in the world the introduction of confinement rearing and the use of grain-based processed rations have occurred, the problem of gastric ulcers has arisen. This syndrome is of economic significance, and its relative importance is increasing despite a growing knowledge of the risk factors and therapeutic procedures.

ETIOLOGY

The exact cause or causes of gastric ulceration is not completely understood, but many of the risk factors are well known. A list of some of the factors that have been reported to be associated with gastric ulceration in pigs are presented in Table 54.1.

There is considerable interaction between many of these factors, particularly in their effect on the fluidity of the stomach content, the speed of passage of ingesta through the stomach, and whether or not the stomach contains feed. Generally, factors that increase the firmness of the stomach content help prevent gastric lesions and factors that cause increased fluidity of the contents increases the risk of ulcers (Nielsen and Ingvartsen 2000).

Fine particle size of feed has been shown to increase the prevalence of gastric lesions (Mahan et al. 1966; Reimann et al. 1968; Maxwell et al. 1970, 1972; Hedde et al. 1985; Potkins and Lawrence 1989a; Wondra et al. 1995a; Ayles et al. 1996a). In addition, pelleting of feed may also increase the likelihood of ulcers developing (Griffing 1963; Chamberlain et al. 1967; Potkins and Lawrence 1989b). The prevalence and severity of ulcers vary with the cereal component of the diet. Generally, oats and barley appear to have a sparing effect (Reese et al. 1966) and corn and wheat tend to be more ulcerogenic (Smith and Edwards 1996).

The method by which the grain is processed affects the prevalence of ulcers. Grain that is ground using a hammer mill tends to be more ulcerogenic than if a roller mill is used (Wondra et al. 1995b; Nielsen and Ingvartsen 2000). Feed particle size is affected by grain component, milling procedure, and processing. Grains such as wheat are more likely to shatter during grinding and result in finer particle size compared to oats or barley. If grain is processed using a roller mill, there is less chance of the grain kernel shattering and creating "fines."

In addition, the pelleting process causes a further decrease in particle size. Neilsen and Ingvartsen (2000) showed that, in general, barley and rolling prevented stomach lesions while wheat grinding and pelleting increased the prevalence and severity of ulcers. The overall effect of a feed with very fine particle size is that the stomach content is very fluid and the emptying time is relatively rapid (Regina et al. 1999), and as a result, the pH gradient between the neutral proximal part of the stomach and the acidic distal region is lost.

Table 54.1. Risk factors associated with ulceration of the *pars oesophagea* in swine

Nutrition	Housing/Management	Other
Feed particle size	Confinement rearing	Season
Type of grain	Herd size	Concurrent disease
Milling	Mixing pigs	Parturition
Pelleting	Overcrowding	Heredity
Grinding vs. rolling	Holding and transport	Somatotropin
Heat processing	Feeding regimen	Histamine
Lack of fiber		*Helicobacter* infection
Vitamin E/Se deficiency		Porcine circovirus type II
Rancid fat		
Withdrawal of feed		

The method of feeding may be as important as feed processing and composition. A major risk factor of ulcer development is an interruption of feed intake (Henry 1996). Fasting of pigs has been a consistent method of experimentally producing gastric lesions (Pocock et al. 1968; Lawrence et al. 1998). Various workers have noted dramatic increases in ulcer severity and prevalence at slaughter in pigs examined after a 24-hour holdover period compared to pigs from the same herds slaughtered on the day of arrival at the abattoir (Chamberlain et al. 1967; Straw et al. 1992; Davies et al. 1994; Lawrence et al. 1998). There is at least one study that documented no association between a 24-hour feed withdrawal and an increased prevalence or severity of ulcers (Eisemann et al. 2002). Presumably, there is an interaction between factors affecting stomach emptying such as feed particle size and the effect of feed withdrawal that can explain the differences in findings between these studies.

Feeding regimen can influence ulcer development, although much of the work in this area is contradictory. For instance, Blackshaw et al. (1980) found fewer ulcer lesions in pigs fed twice daily than in pigs fed ad libitum, whereas Robert et al. (1991) found a similar prevalence of ulcers in pigs fed ad libitum and pigs fed twice daily but noted that ulcers were less severe in ad libitum–fed pigs. One can speculate that stability in the feeding regimen is critical and ultimately more important than whether pigs are routinely fed once a day, twice a day, or ad libitum.

Interruption of normal feed intake commonly occurs on almost all farms because of mechanical problems or human error. Periods of transition in feeding patterns such as when gilts are transferred to the breeding herd from a finishing barn or when sows approach the time of parturition, should be viewed as high risk for ulcerogenic events (Henry 1996). Hot weather resulting in dramatic reduction in feed intake is associated with gastric ulcer outbreaks (Deen 1993).

It is likely that factors such as acute infectious disease and season influence ulcer development in a similar manner to management practices that interrupt feed intake. Acute respiratory disease is associated with an increased likelihood of gastric ulceration (Dionissopoulos

et al. 2001). In addition to respiratory disease causing inappetence, it is possible that increased levels of histamine as a result of infection could play a role, in that histamine is a powerful stimulant of gastric acid secretion. Injection of histamine has been shown to experimentally produce ulceration of the pars oesophagea (Muggenburg et al. 1966; Huber and Wallin 1965; Hedde et al. 1985). Experimental infection of gnotobiotic pigs with various viral pathogens, including porcine reproductive and respiratory syndrome virus, does not result in gastric ulceration; however, experimental infection of porcine circovirus type II has caused gastric lesions (Harms et al. 2001).

There has been considerable interest in finding an infectious cause of porcine gastric ulcers similar to the situation in humans. *Helicobacter*-like organisms have been identified in the glandular region of the stomach (Mendes et al. 1990) and appear to be widespread in the pig population (Grasso et al. 1996; Magras et al. 1999; Melnichouk et al. 1999). Whereas some workers have observed a correlation between the presence of these bacteria and the prevalence and severity of gastric ulcers (Barbosa et al. 1995; Queiroz et al. 1996), other researchers have not (Magras et al. 1999; Melnichouk et al. 1999).

Inoculations of *Helicobacter*-like organisms from pigs and *Helicobacter pylori* from humans have both been used to infect gnotobiotic pigs (Krakowka et al. 1995). These organisms colonize and cause irritation and lesions in the glandular region, but have not been shown to cause ulceration of the pars oesophagea. More work is necessary to clearly understand what significance these organisms have in the pig, but it is unlikely *Helicobacter* play such a significant role in ulceration of the para oesophagea of the pig compared to their importance in human peptic ulcer disease. It should be noted that the stomach ulcer problem in pigs is more like the human condition "oesophageal-gastric reflux disease" than peptic ulcer disease.

Before *H. pylori* became recognized as the main cause of gastric ulceration in humans, the accepted theory was that ulcers were caused by excessive acid secretion stimulated by stress. This theory has been examined extensively in pigs. The onset of the first cases of porcine gastric ulcers occurred at the time of confinement rearing and increased intensification were first adopted. Certain studies have shown that the prevalence increases as herd size increases (Christensen and Cullinane 1990) and as stocking density increases (Pickett et al. 1969). However, there are other studies contradicting the belief that overcrowding is a risk factor (Driesen et al. 1987; Eisemann and Argenzio 1999a). It is likely that factors such as available feeder space and environmental temperature interact with stocking density to cause these contradictory results. Research clearly demonstrates that ulceration of the pars oesophagea is not mediated by glucocorticoids (Zamora et al. 1980). Chronic elevation of corticosteroids in response to stressful conditions has been shown under controlled trials to not result in an increase in ulcer prevalence or severity (Jensen et al. 1996).

Genetic susceptibility may play a role in ulcer development. Researchers have reported a link between fast growth rate and/or low backfat and a high prevalence of gastric ulcers (Berruecos and Robinson 1972; Grondalen and Vangren 1974). It has also been reported that injection of swine with porcine somatotropin causes an increase in prevalence and severity of ulcers (Smith and Kasson 1991).

In summary, many of the factors associated with an increased risk of ulcer development are closely tied to economic competitiveness such as the use of finely ground feed and fast-growing, lean genetics. Therefore, steps to reduce the prevalence of gastric ulcers need to be carefully balanced between economic considerations and welfare concerns.

EPIDEMIOLOGY

Gastric ulceration is common and widespread. Table 54.2 presents findings of various studies worldwide. Abattoir surveys demonstrate that the prevalence of stomach lesions, including parakeratosis, erosions, and ulcers, often approaches 90% when pigs are managed using modern confinement husbandry practices (Driesen et al. 1987). There is great herd-to-herd variation in prevalence and severity. Ulceration of the pars oesophagea can affect any age of pig but the highest rate of ulceration occurs in pigs 3–6 months of age. Mortality due to gastric ulceration among grower-finisher pigs has been reported to be about 1–2% on some farms, with much higher levels occurring sporadically (Deen 1993; Melnichouk 2002). Sows at the time of parturition are also a relatively high risk group. Examination of culled sows revealed 60% with stomach lesions and 10–15% with ulcerations (Hessing et al. 1992; O'Sullivan et al. 1996). Frequently, sow stomachs have extensive scar tissue, indicating previous severe ulcerative episodes. Gastric ulceration has been reported as a common cause of sow mortality (Sanford et al. 1994; Chagnon et al. 1991).

PATHOGENESIS

The pars oesophagea has a cornified stratified squamous epithelium and does not secrete protective mucus. It is generally assumed that chronic insult of this sensitive tissue results in hyperplasia of epithelial cells and thickening from layers of 10–20 cells to layers of 60–80 cells or more and keratinization (Driesen et al. 1987; Roels et al. 1997). Rapid cell development results in the production of immature cells, and the thickened layers of cells tend to outgrow their nutrient supply. As a consequence, the tight junctions between epithelial cells break down, allowing digestive juices access to underlying tissues. Initially, superficial layers of epithelium are lost, but if the insult continues, deeper erosions develop and affect the lamina propria and, eventually, the muscularis mucosa and submucosa. Erosion and damage can spread rapidly, destroying the entire pars oesophageal region. Ulceration ends abruptly at the junction of the glandular portion and the pars oesophagea,

Table 54.2.   Abattoir surveys of the worldwide prevalence of lesions of the *pars oesophagea*

Reference	Country	Pigs Examined	% with Lesions
Jensen and Frederick 1939	USA	20,000	5
Curtin et al. 1963	USA	443	86
Griffing 1963	USA	610	91
Pocock 1966	Canada	198	69
Bivin et al. 1974	Brazil	3,113	78
Ito et al. 1974	Japan	73	100
Kowács 1974	Hungary	13,400	13
Szemerédi and Solá 1979	Cuba	2,457	20
Driesen et al. 1987	Australia	5,000	99
Christensen and Cullinane 1990	New Zealand	2,661	32
Straw et al. 1992	USA	600	65
Elbers et al. 1995a	Netherlands	274	75
Elbers et al. 1995a	Netherlands	184	89
Guise et al. 1997	UK	1,242	80
Robertson et al. 2002	Australia	15,741	80

resulting in a thick inflammatory ridge of edematous tissue separating normal and damaged areas.

There is still uncertainty as to the exact mechanism of insult that causes injury to the relatively unprotected pars oesophagea. In all likelihood there are several mechanisms that can cause tissue damage and various factors that might weaken the defensive barrier protecting the stratified squamous mucosa.

Because gastric ulceration is commonly associated with conditions that cause greater fluidity of the contents of the stomach and therefore a breakdown of the pH gradient between the distal and proximal portions, it is reasonable to assume that the increased acidity of the proximal stomach is a key factor in causing tissue damage. However, the stratified squamous mucosa of the pars oesophagea is relatively resistant to injury from HCl alone (Argenzio and Eisemann 1996). Studies have shown that pigs fed finely ground diets and/or are fasted tended to have high concentrations of bile acids in the proximal stomach (Lang et al. 1998). In vitro studies of pig tissue have shown that a combination of low pH and a conjugated bile salt concentration of ≥ 1 mmol/l can induce extensive tissue damage (Lang et al. 1998). Similarly, short chain fatty acids produced at relatively high concentrations by bacteria in the proximal portion of the stomach may be implicated in causing gastric ulceration, in that these acids can diffuse rapidly across tissue barriers as the luminal pH is reduced (Argenzio and Eisemann 1996).

It has been hypothesized that as HCl concentrations are increased, more of the short chain fatty acids would become undissociated, augmenting their rate of absorption. Lesions in the pars oesophagea were produced experimentally by feeding a carbohydrate-enriched diet to gnotobiotic pigs and inoculating the pigs with two different fermentative commensal bacteria, *Lactobacillus sp* and *Bacillus sp* (Krakowka et al. 1998). The importance of short chain fatty acids in causing gastric ulcers under farm conditions is uncertain. Generally, diets associated with producing the highest level of short chain fatty acids are the coarse-ground rations and nonulcerogenic finely ground diets (Argenzio 1999).

It is possible that in addition to the production of short chain fatty acids and the breakdown of the pH gradient caused by increased fluidity of the stomach contents and thus the combination of bile and HCl contacting the pars oesophagea, there may be other factors that interact with these agents. One obvious possibility is the hypersecretion of HCl which might occur with histamine release (Muggenburg et al. 1966) or by other mechanisms. It has been suggested that *Helicobacter sp* may play a role in ulcer development by somehow inducing excess acid secretion (Yeomans and Kolt 1996). However, hyperacid secretion has not been observed in trials using experimental *Helicobacter sp* infection (Krakowka et al. 1995 1998).

Diet may influence the defensive mechanisms of the pars oesophagea. Gastric ulcers have been observed in association with deficiencies of vitamin E or selenium (Van Vleet et al. 1970) presumably due to increased generation of reactive oxygen metabolites. In a recent study, focusing on the antioxidant defense system in stratified squamous mucosa, pigs fed a finely ground diet were found to produce higher levels of peroxides than pigs fed a coarse ration (Eisemann and Argenzio 1999a, b). These authors speculate that the generation of prooxidants and the antioxidant defense system may play a role in the predilection of gastric ulcers.

CLINICAL SIGNS

Ulceration occurs rapidly and the progression from normal pars oesophagea to complete ulceration may take less than 24 hours. Clinical signs tend to reflect the degree of blood loss associated with the gastric lesion. Frequently, a pig that had appeared to be healthy only a few hours earlier is found dead and the carcass is extremely pale. If blood loss occurs more slowly, signs associated with anemia will be apparent, such as paleness, lethargy, weakness, increased respiratory rate, and anorexia. In addition, black tarry feces may be noted, and some pigs show signs of abdominal pain by grinding their teeth and arching their backs. Vomiting may occur. Rectal temperatures of affected pigs are often below normal.

Sporadic outbreaks of gastric ulceration tend to occur among grower-finisher pigs, and frequently when one pig has suddenly died, careful observation will reveal others in the group that are showing signs of anemia. When ulceration occurs without significant blood loss, animals will generally appear to be in normal health. Evidence that subclinical ulceration reduces growth rate is inconsistent. Various researchers have attempted to correlate severity of stomach lesions at slaughter with growth performance during the grower-finisher phase. Certain studies have found no relationship (Pocock et al. 1969; Backstrom et al. 1981), whereas Elbers et al. (1995a) observed a 50–75 g per day decrease in growth rate for pigs with ulcers versus pigs with normal stomachs. This last result is in agreement with findings of a trial that followed pigs using endoscopic examination to measure gastric lesions (Ayles et al. 1996b).

Ulcers can occur rapidly and heal quickly, making it difficult to relate lesions at slaughter with performance during the grower-finisher stage. Evidence of past ulceration can sometimes be seen as cicatrization and a reduction in size of the pars oesophagea. In extreme cases, the pars oesophagea is entirely destroyed, and stenosis of the esophagus at its entry to the stomach occurs. Pigs afflicted with stenosis are observed to vomit shortly after eating but are hungry and therefore will immediately resume eating. These pigs tend to grow more slowly than penmates despite maintaining good appetites.

LESIONS

Lesions associated with ulceration of the pars oesophagea rarely extend into the contiguous esophagus or the glandular region of the stomach. Ulcerations and erosions of the pars oesophagea may involve only a small portion or all of the gastric squamous mucosa. The most common site for ulceration is at the junction of the pars oesophagea and the cardiac mucosa (Penny and Hill 1973). The normal epithelium of the pars oesophagea is smooth, white, and glistening and is easily distinguished from the surrounding glandular mucosa. It is believed that lesions usually progress from parakeratosis that causes a thickened, rough appearance to fissuring and peeling that result in erosion and eventually ulceration.

Frequently, the pars oesophagea is yellowish as a result of bile staining, particularly when the surface is rough and thickened due to parakeratosis. This type of corrugated surface may flake and peel off readily. When ulceration involves the entire pars oesophagea, the lesion has a punched-out or crater-like appearance with elevated ridges. The floor of the ulcer may be so smooth that it is misinterpreted as normal (Barker et al. 1993). The relationship between gross and microscopic lesions has been investigated by Embaye et al. (1990), who concluded that, generally, gross appearance was directly related to microscopic findings. However, these researchers found that in 155 apparently normal stomachs, 32% showed histologic evidence of parakeratosis, 30% had minor erosive lesions, and microscopically 23% had severe ulceration.

Gross evaluation of stomach lesions is commonly incorporated into an abattoir surveillance program to monitor disease status. To examine the pars oesophagea, the stomach should be incised along the greater curvature and inverted. Emptying the contents and rinsing the stomach before examination will improve the accuracy of the inspection. Various classification schemes have been used to grade stomach lesions at slaughter (Christensen and Cullinane 1990; Ayles et al. 1996a), and an example of such a system is presented in Table 54.3.

Histologically, the lesion is the result of thickening and parakeratosis, with nucleated cells present on the mucosal surface. Rete pegs and proprial papillae are elongated, and neutrophils and eosinophils are often present at the tips of the proprial papillae. Epithelial

Table 54.3. Classification of stomach lesions at slaughter

Severity	Description
Grade 0	Normal, shiny, white, glistening surface over entire *pars oesophagea*
Grade 1	Evidence of parakeratosis such as thickening, roughened surface, corrugation, yellow color
Grade 2	Erosions of the epithelium, particularly at the border of the cardiac region
Grade 3	Active ulcers and cicatrization

separation and erosion usually occur beneath a band of cells with cytoplasmic pallor and nuclear degeneration (Embaye et al. 1990). Ulcers of the pars oesophagea usually involve only the submucosa, but they may advance to the muscularis externa and occasionally to the serosa (Barker et al. 1993).

In the case of a pig that has died acutely of gastric ulceration, postmortem diagnosis is usually straightforward. The carcass is typically pale but in good body condition. The stomach may contain clotted and unclotted blood and fibrinous exudate enclosing a variable amount of food. Blood may be found in the intestine as well. A blood clot may be adhered to the surface of the ulcer, which is generally deep and extensive in the case of a fatal hemorrhagic episode.

Gastric ulcers can heal by granulation and reepithelialization. Scarring can occur and, if extensive, may lead to occlusion of the esophageal opening into the stomach.

DIAGNOSIS

Often diagnosis is accomplished on the basis of gross postmortem findings and clinical history. Typically, only one or two animals in a large group of grower-finisher pigs are noticed to be ill or are found dead. Lesions in the stomach are readily observed and generally diagnostic. Determining the prevalence and severity of ulcer lesions in the remaining animals in a herd or group poses more of a diagnostic challenge. Mild to moderate blood loss occurring over a period of several days or weeks will result in anemia and poor performance. Various conditions causing anemia need to be considered, including blood loss from tail biting, abdominal bleeding from other organs, swine dysentery, proliferative ileitis, hemorrhagic bowel syndrome, and possibly dietary deficiencies.

Anemia associated with porcine reproductive and respiratory syndrome (PRRS) has been reported (Rathje et al. 1996). Slaughter checks (Elbers et al. 1995a) and necropsy information from pigs that die of various causes can help determine the extent to which ulceration of the pars oesophagea is a clinical problem in a herd. Care must be taken in interpreting necropsy data to determine disease prevalence in that an association exists between acute respiratory disease and gastric ulceration (Dionissopoulos et al. 2001).

Occasionally, swine practitioners are asked to make a diagnosis on an individual animal when sacrificing the animal in order to perform a postmortem examination is not an option, such as in the case of a valuable breeding boar or sow. Clinical signs of anemia and the presence of digested blood in the stool are suggestive of a gastric ulcer, but definitive diagnosis requires endoscopy (Kowalczyk et al. 1968; Mackin et al. 1997). Modern portable endoscopes are practical tools in the diagnosis of gastric ulcers in swine. They can be used to determine the specific phase in production when ulceration is occurring without sacrificing pigs. Early erosive lesions are easily distinguished as red lesions against the white background of the pars oesophageal surface. At postmortem, these lesions are commonly overlooked because of the lack of contrast (Mackin et al. 1997).

TREATMENT

Early intervention is important for successfully treating pigs with gastric ulceration. This is usually hampered by the rapid onset of the problem and the difficulty in diagnosing subclinical disease in the live animal. Pigs that are observed to be pale and weak should be segregated from penmates to avoid injury from bullying. If severe blood loss has occurred, euthanasia should be a consideration.

If a specific risk factor can be identified as a probable contributing cause, then steps should be taken to change the factor. For instance, replacing finely ground pelleted feed with a moderately coarse mash feed has been shown to result in healing (Ayles et al. 1996a). Similarly, nutritional deficiencies such as vitamin E deficiency should be immediately corrected, and concurrent respiratory disease must be treated with appropriate medication.

In the case of expensive breeding stock, one might initiate more extensive treatment than mere pen separation and symptomatic care. Parenteral administration of glucose with electrolytes and vitamin K or 8% gelatin has been recommended as an initial response (Kowalczyk 1975). A blood transfusion (of 1–2 liters of blood in an hour for animals weighing 150–200 kg) should be performed as soon as possible. Parenteral preparations of iron and B-complex vitamins to stimulate hemopoiesis and appetite are generally administered to pigs recovering from severe blood loss.

Numerous pharmaceutical agents have been used in an attempt to neutralize acid, reduce gastric secretions, and/or promote ulcer healing. Various antacid preparations have been studied for their ability to neutralize gastric acid. Sodium bicarbonate is the most commonly used, but with conflicting results. Gamble et al. (1967) found no effect on ulcer severity by feeding 3% $NaHCO_3$, whereas Wondra et al. (1995c) demonstrated a slight improvement with inclusion of 1% $NaHCO_3$ in the ration. Southern et al. (1993) found an increase in stomach lesions when 1% $NaHCO_3$ was fed. The ingestion of sodium bicarbonate in small amounts over time can result in an increase in acid secretion, and this may nullify the advantages of its buffering capability. Nonabsorbable antacids such as aluminum hydroxide and magnesium silicate may be preferable to sodium bicarbonate because they act more slowly and with a more prolonged effect. If buffering agents are to be used, there is good rationale to add them to the water rather than the feed (Ange et al. 2000).

Reduction of acid production should be a goal in treating the individual pig with ulceration of the pars oesophagea. Histamine H_2-receptor antagonists, including cimetidine, ranitidine, famotidine, and nizatidine, have been considered potentially useful drugs. In addition to inhibiting histamine-evoked gastric acid secretion, cimetidine and ranitidine also appear to effectively control upper gastrointestinal bleeding in humans. Unfortunately, researchers (Hedde et al. 1985) have shown that histamine H_2-receptor antagonists do not reduce the incidence or severity of ulcers associated with finely ground feed. Likewise, ranitidine (150 mg per day) administered by injection, three times per day, does not alleviate ulcers in porcine somatotropin-treated swine (Baile et al. 1994). Intramuscular administration of cimetidine (4.3 mg/kg) or ranitidine (0.75 mg/kg) causes gastric pH to rise above 3.5 for only about 2 hours in swine, compared to a much longer time in humans (Sangiah et al. 1990), possibly explaining the poor response in pigs.

The inhibitors of H^+/K^+ ATPase (the proton pump in parietal cells) such as omeprazole (Friendship et al. 2000) and trioprazole (Adelstein et al. 1988) may be more useful agents in treating swine gastric ulcers. These benzinidazole compounds have been shown to successfully reduce severity and prevalence of ulcers in swine treated with porcine somatotropin (Baile et al. 1994). The E-type prostaglandins are widely used in human treatment. These drugs reduce acid secretion and promote mucus secretion. They have not been found to be effective in alleviating ulcer development in swine (Baile et al. 1994). However, other cytoprotectants may be more useful. Various inert and insoluble protectives such as bismuth subcarbonate, kaolin, and pectin have been used in an attempt to coat the ulcerated area and promote healing. Sucralfate, an aluminum salt of sulfated sucrose which adheres to ulcers and erosions and promotes healing while preventing further attacks, has been shown to prevent ulceration in bile duct–ligated pigs (Stapleton et al. 1989). However, the addition of 1 or 4 mg sucralfate per 3 kg of a finely ground pelleted diet fed to somatotropin-treated swine failed to alleviate ulcers of the pars oesophagea (Baile et al. 1994).

The role of *Helicobacter* spp. in swine gastric ulceration is unclear and may not be important. In humans, the recurrence rate of patients with *H. pylori* is 40–80% per year but is reduced to 0–4% when *H. pylori* is eradicated. The treatment for human *Helicobacter* infection is complex, involving the use of three or four pharmaceutical agents. For example, a patient may be prescribed a 1-week course of omeprazole (20 mg bid), bismuth subsalicylate (2 tabs qid), metronidazole (250 mg qid), and tetracycline (500 mg qid) (Chiba 1996). It is not likely appropriate to consider this regimen in swine practice. Even if it can be proven that infection with *Helicobacter* spp. is a factor in swine disease, reinfection from environmental sources may make eradication an impractical approach in preventing the recurrence of gastric ulcers under farm conditions.

PREVENTION

Treatment for the most part is prohibitively expensive, laborious, and often unsuccessful. In addition, early diagnosis of gastric ulcer disease is difficult. Therefore, prevention of stomach lesions is generally considered the most appropriate approach to handling this problem. A cost-benefit analysis of the prevention program is important in determining what action should be taken to reduce losses from gastric ulcers on a particular farm. The risk factors and the losses from disease will vary from herd to herd, and each case needs to be considered separately. In general, it is very easy to overreact to the loss of one or two animals and institute changes that reduce overall herd performance and result in economic losses that far outweigh the benefits of reduced ulcer prevalence. For example, changing feed particle size from fine to coarse, decreasing the stocking density, and removing growth promotants from the ration are all common recommendations (Kowalczyk 1975), but each will have a significant effect on growth rate and/or feed efficiency.

On the other hand, the swine industry needs to be concerned about the welfare implications of a high level of stomach lesions and must take steps to decrease the prevalence if possible. Many causative factors and complex interactions of nutrition, environment, and management contribute to the expression of this disease, but a coordinated effort—although difficult by feed providers, owners, production personnel, and herd veterinarians—can result in feed preparation standards and management that limit gastric ulceration as a swine production problem without reducing animal performance (Henry 1996). The use of roller mills instead of grinding feed appears to be one of the best methods of reducing ulcers (Nielsen and Ingvartsen 2000).

The feed industry must endeavor to produce a pellet that contains grain particles of a uniform and appropriate size, prepared at a proper temperature. Feed production practices that incorporate flour or "fines" in pellets increase the risk of ulcers. Likewise, high temperatures during pelleting might result in gelatinization of starches and therefore be more ulcerogenic. The addition of fat to the diet, if allowed to become rancid, can also contribute to an ulcer problem. Addressing these concerns can lead to better feed efficiency and reduce the incidence of gastric ulcers.

Feeding practices must be carefully monitored. An interruption of feed intake appears to be a major contributing factor to ulcer formation. Blocked feeders or waterers, heat stress, unpalatable feed, or the presence of vomitoxin in the feed can lead to ulcer problems. Good management practices can minimize the occurrence and influence of these factors.

Various attempts have been made to incorporate protective substances in swine feeds to prevent ulcer development. Increasing levels of antioxidants such as vitamin E and selenium beyond physiological requirements does not appear to be useful (Davies 1993). There is some evidence to suggest that the inclusion of vitamin U (methylmethionine sulphonium) reduces the prevalence and severity of ulcers (Hegedus et al. 1983; Elbers et al. 1995c). Alfalfa has been used at levels of up to 9%, because it is high in vitamins E and K, as well as a source of increased fiber. Alfalfa was not effective in reducing the level of severity of ulcers in pigs treated with porcine somatotropin (Baile et al. 1994). The production of sunflower hulls to diets was shown to be effective in reducing lesions (Dirkzwager et al. 1998).

Products that reduce gastric emptying have been examined and found somewhat effective, at least in an experimental setting. Melatonin has been reported to slow gut motility and when included at levels as low as 2.5 g/ton results in less ulcer development (Ayles et al. 1996b). Similarly, diets containing sodium polyacrylate are retained for longer periods of time in the stomach of swine, and gastric ulceration is reduced (Yamaguchi et al. 1981). There may be circumstances in which various therapeutic agents are useful for treatment or prevention, but because of the many contributing factors and the interactions of these factors, it is unlikely that a single pharmaceutical product or management technique will be found that completely prevents gastric ulceration caused by various combinations of factors in different herds.

REFERENCES

Adelstein GW, Yen CH, Haack RA, Yu S, Gullikson G, Price DV, Anglin C, Decktor DL, Tsai H, Keith RH. 1988. Substituted 2-[(2-Benzimidazolylsulfinyl) methyl] anilines as potential inhibitors of H⁺/K⁺ ATPase. J Med Chem 31:1215–1220.

Ange KD, Eisemann JH, Argenzio RA, Almond GW, Blikslager AT. 2000. Effects of feed physical form and buffering solutes on water disappearance and proximal stomach pH in swine. J Anim Sci 78:2344–2352.

Argenzio RA. 1999. Comparative pathophysiology of nonglandular ulcer disease: A review of experimental studies. Equine Vet J (Suppl) 29:19–23.

Argenzio RA, Eisemann S. 1996. Mechanisms of acid injury in porcine gastroesophageal mucosa. Am J Vet Res 57:564–573.

Ayles HL, Ball RO, Friendship RM, Bubenik GA. 1996b. The effect of graded levels of melatonin on performance and gastric ulcers in pigs. Can J Anim Sci 76:607–611.

Ayles HL, Friendship RM, Ball RO. 1996a. Effect of dietary particle size on gastric ulcers, assessed by endoscopic examination, and relationship between ulcer severity and growth performance of individually fed pigs. Swine Health and Production 4:211–216.

Backstrom L, Crenshaw T, Shenkman D. 1981. Gastric ulcers in swine. Effects of dietary fiber, corn particle size, and preslaughter stress. Am J Vet Res 42:538–543.

Baile CA, Buonomo FC, McLaughlin CL, Vineyard BD. 1994. Benzimidazoles for alleviating stomach ulcers in swine. Patent Application No. PCT/US93/05692. Publication No. WO94/01107.

Barbosa AJA, Silva JCP, Nogueira AMMF, Pasilino E, Jr, Miranda CR. 1995. Higher incidence of gastric ulcer of the pars oesophagea. Vet Pathol 32:134–139.

Barker IK, VanDreumel AL, Palmer N. 1993. The alimentary system. In Pathology of Domestic Animals (4th edition) Volume 2. KVF Jubb, PC Kennedy, RN Palmer , eds. San Diego: Academic Press, pp. 65–72.

Berruecos JM, Robinson OW. 1972. Inheritance of gastric ulcers in swine. J Anim Sci 35:20–23.

Bivin WS, Lombardo De Barros LS, Salles De Barros C, Nogueira Dos Santos M. 1974. Gastric ulcers in Brazilian swine. J Am Vet Med Assoc 164:405–407.

Blackshaw JK, Cameron RDA, Kelly WR. 1980. Effect of feeding regimen on gastric ulceration of the pars oesophagea of intensively raised pigs. Aust Vet J 56:384–386.

Chagnon M, D'Allaire S, Drolet R. 1991. A prospective study of sow mortality in breeding herds. Can J Vet Res 55:180–185.

Chamberlain CC, Merrimann GM, Lidvall ER, Gamble CT. 1967. Effects of feed processing method and diet form on the incidence of esophagogastric ulcers in swine. J Anim Sci 26:72–75.

Chiba N. 1996. *H. pylori*—An evidence-based approach. Medicines of N Am (Nov/Dec), pp. 57–65.

Christensen NH, Cullinane LC. 1990. Monitoring the health of pigs in New Zealand abattoirs. NZ Vet J 38:136–141.

Curtin TM, Goetsch GD, Hollandbeck R. 1963. Clinical and pathological characterization of esophagogastric ulcers in swine. J Am Vet Med Assoc 143:854–860.

Davies PR. 1993. Gastric ulcers in pigs and humans: Comparative aspects of etiology and risk factors. In Proc A. D. Leman Swine Conf, Univ Minnesota, pp. 129–135.

Davies PR, Grass JJ, Marsh WE, Bahnson PB, Dial GD. 1994. Time of slaughter affects prevalence of lesions of the pars esophagea of pigs. Proc Int Congr Pig Vet Soc 13:471.

Deen J. 1993. The problem of gastroesophageal ulcers: A field problem. In Proc A. D. Leman Swine Conf, pp. 137–138.

Dionissopoulos L, deLange CFM, Dewey CE, MacInnes JI, Friendship RM. 2001. Effect of health management strategy during rearing on grower-finisher pig performance and selected indicators of immune system stimulation. Can J Anim Sci 81:563–566.

Dirkzwager A, Elbers ARW, Vanderaar P, Vos JH. 1998. Effect of particle size and addition of sunflower hulls diets on the occurrence of oesophagogastric lesions and performance in growing-finishing pigs. Livestock Prod Sci 56:53–60.

Driesen SJ, Fahy VA, Spicer EM. 1987. Oesophagogastric ulcers. In Proc Pig Production (Sydney Univ) 95:1007–1017.

Eisemann JH, Argenzio RA. 1999a. Effects of diet and housing density on growth and stomach morphology in pigs. J Anim Sci 77:2709–2714.

——. 1999b. Effect of diets differing in propensity to promote gastric lesions on defense systems in gastric mucosae. J Anim Sci 77:2715–2720.

Eisemann JH, Morrow WEM, See MT, Davies PR, Zering K. 2002. Effect of feed withdrawal prior to slaughter on prevalence of gastric ulcers in pigs. J Amer Vet Med Assoc 220:503–506.

Elbers ARW, Hessing MJC, Tielen MJM, Vos JH. 1995a. Growth and oesophagogastric lesions in finishing pigs offered pelleted feed ad libitum. Vet Rec 136:588–590.

Elbers ARW, Vos JH, Hunneman WA. 1995b. Effect of hammer mill screen size and addition of fibre or *S*-methylmethionine-sulphonium chloride to the diet on the occurrence of oesophagogastric lesions in fattening pigs. Vet Rec 137:290–293.

Embaye H, Thomlinson SR, Lawrence TLJ. 1990. Histopathology of oesophagogastric lesions in pigs. J Comp Pathol 103:253–264.

Friendship RM, Melnichouk SI, Dewey CE. 2000. The use of omeprazole to alleviate stomach ulcers in swine during periods of feed withdrawal. Can Vet J 41:925–928.

Gamble CT, Chamberlain CC, Merriman GM, Lidvall ER. 1967. Effect of pelleting, pasture, and selected diet ingredients on incidence of esophagogastric ulcers in swine. J Anim Sci 26:1054–1058.

Grasso GM, Ripabelli G, Sammarco MI, Ruberto A, Iannetto G. 1996. Prevalence of Helicobacter-like organisms in porcine gastric mucosa: A study of swine slaughtered in Italy. Comp Immun Microbiol Infect Dis 19:213–217.

Griffing WJ. 1963. A study of etiology and pathology of gastric ulcers in swine. Diss Abstr 24:1581–1582.

Grondalen T, Vangen O. 1974. Gastric ulcers in pigs selected for leanness or fatness. Norw Vet Med 25:50–53.

Guise HJ, Carlyle WWH, Penny RHC, Abbott TA, Riches HL, Hunter EJ. 1997. Gastric ulcers in finishing pigs: Their prevalence and failure to influence growth rate. Vet Rec 141:563–566.

Hannan J, Nyhan JF. 1962. The use of some vitamins in the control of ulcerative gastric haemorrhage in pigs. Vet J 16:196–197.

Harms PA, Sorden SD, Halbur PG, Bolin S, Lager K, Morozov I, Paul PS. 2001. Experimental reproduction of severe disease in CD/CD pigs concurrently infected with type 2 porcine circovirus and PRRSV. Vet Pathol 38:428–539.

Hedde RD, Lindsey TO, Parrish RC, Daniels HD, Morgenthien EA, Lewis HB. 1985. Effect of diet particle size and feeding of H2-receptor antagonists on gastric ulcers in swine. J Anim Sci 61:179–186.

Hegedus M, Bokori J, Tamás J. 1983. Oesophagogastric ulcer in swine and vitamin U. II. Nature of vitamin U. Acta Vet Hungarica 31:155–163.

Henry SC. 1996. Gastric ulcers: Feed management is top priority for prevention. Large Anim Vet, pp. 8–11.

Hessing JJC, Geudeke MJ, Scheepens CJM, Tielen MJM, Schouten WGP, Wiepkema PR. 1992. Slijmvliesveranderingen in de pars oesophagea bij varkens: Prevalentie en de invloed van stress. Tijdschr voor Diergeneeskd 117:445–450.

Huber WG, Wallin RF. 1965. Experimental production of porcine gastric ulcers. Vet Med 60:551–558.

Ito T, Miura S, Tanimura J. 1974. Pathological studies on proventricular ulcer in swine. Jpn J Vet Sci 36:263–272.

Jensen KH, Pedersen LJ, Nielsen EK, Heller KE, Ladewig J, Jørgensen E. 1996. Intermittent stress in pigs: Effects on behaviour, pituitary-adrenocortical axis, growth, and gastric ulceration. Physiol and Behaviour 59(4/5):741–748.

Jensen LB, Frederick LD. 1939. Spontaneous ulcer of the stomach in several domestic animals. J Am Vet Med Assoc 95:167–169.

Kowács F. 1974. Occurrence of stomach ulcers in pigs in Hungary. Magyar Állatorvosok Lapja 29:226–229.

Kowalczyk T. 1975. Gastric ulcers. In Diseases of Swine (4th edition). HW Dunne, AD Leman, eds. Ames: Iowa State Univ Press, pp. 978–1010.

Kowalczyk T, Tanaka Y, Muggenburg BA, Olson WG, Morrissey JE. 1968. Endoscopic examination of the swine's stomach. Am J Vet Res 29:729–736.

Krakowka S, Eaton KA, Rings DM. 1995. Occurrence of gastric ulcers in gnotobiotic piglets colonized by *Helicobacter pylori*. Infect Immunol 63:2352–2355.

Krakowka S, Easton KA, Rings DM, Argenzio RA. 1998. Production of gastroesophageal erosions and ulcers (GEU) in gnotobiotic swine monoinfected with fermentative commensal bacteria and fed high carbohydrate diet. Vet Pathol 35:274–282.

Lang J, Blikslager A, Regina D, Eisemann J, Argenzio RA. 1998. Synergistic effect of hydrochloric acid and bile acids on the pars esophageal mucosa of the porcine stomach. Amer J Vet Res 59:1170–1176.

Lawrence BV, Anderson DB, Adeola O, Cline TR. 1998. Changes in pars esophageal tissue appearance of the porcine stomach in response to transportation, feed deprivation, and diet composition. J Anim Sci 76:788–795.

Mackin AJ, Ayles HL, Friendship RM, Ball RO, Wilcock BP. 1997. Development and evaluation of endoscopic technique permitting rapid visualization of the cardiac region of the porcine stomach. Can J Vet Res 61:121–127.

Magras C, Cantet F, Koffi G, Ilet F, Mégraud F, Federighi M. 1999. *Helicobacter sp* dans l'estomac des porco charcutiers: Un problème de santé publique? J Rech Porcine en France 31:395–399.

Mahan DC, Pickett RA, Perry TW, Curtis TM, Featherston WR, Beeson WM. 1966. Influence of various nutritional factors and physical form of feed on esophagogastric ulcers in swine. J Anim Sci 25:1019–1023.

Maxwell CV, Reimann EM, Hoekstra WG, Kowalczyk T, Benevenga NJ, Grummer RH. 1970. The effect of dietary particle size on lesion development and on the contents of various regions of the stomach. J Anim Sci 30:911–922.

———. 1972. Use of tritiated water to assess *in vivo* the effect of dietary particle size on the mixing of stomach contents in swine. J Anim Sci 34:213–216.

McIntosh D. 1897. Diseases of Swine. Donahue, Chicago, p. 40.

Melnichouk SI. 2002. Mortality associated with gastric ulceration in swine. Can Vet J 43:23–225.

Melnichouk SI, Friendship RM, Dewey CE, Bildfell RJ, Smart N. 1999. Helicobacter-like organisms in the stomach of pigs with and without gastric ulceration. Swine Health Prod 7:201–205.

Mendes EN, Queiroz DM, Rocha GA, Nogueira AM, Carvalho AC, Lage AP, Barbosa AJ. 1990. Ultrastructure of a spiral micro-organism from pig gastric mucosa (*Gastrospirillum suis*). J Med Microbiol 33:61–66.

Moran ET. 1982. Comparative Nutrition of Fowl and Swine: The Gastrointestinal Systems. Office of Educ Pract, Univ Guelph, pp. 48–67.

Muggenburg BA, Kowalczyk T, Reese NA, Hoekstra WG, Grummer RH. 1966. Experimental production of gastric ulcers in swine by histamine in mineral oil-bees wax. Am J Vet Res 27:292–299.

Muggenburg BA, McNutt SH, Kowalczyk T. 1964. Pathology of gastric ulcers in swine. Am J Vet Res 25:1354–1365.

Nielsen EK, Ingvartsen KL. 2000. Effects of cereal disintegration method, feeding method, and straw as bedding on stomach characteristics including ulcers and performance in growing pigs. Acta Agric Scand A 50:30–38.

O'Sullivan T, Friendship RM, Ball RO, Ayles H. 1996. Prevalence of lesions of the pars oesophageal region of the stomach of sows at slaughter. In Proc Am Assoc Swine Practitioners, pp. 151–153.

Penny RHC, Hill FWG. 1973. Abattoir observations of ulceration of the stomach of the pig. Vet Annu 14:55–60.

Pickett RA, Fugate WH, Harrington RB, Perry TW, Curtain TM. 1969. Influence of feed preparation and number of pigs per pen on performance and occurrence of esophagogastric ulcers in swine. J Anim Sci 28:837–841.

Pocock EF. 1966. Gastric Ulcers in Swine. M.Sc. thesis, Univ Guelph.

Pocock EF, Bayley HS, Roe CK. 1968. Relationship of pelleted, autoclaved, and heat expanded corn or starvation to gastric ulcers in swine. J Anim Sci 27:1296–1302.

Pocock EF, Bayley HS, Slinger SJ. 1969. Dietary factors affecting the development of esophagogastric ulcers in swine. J Anim Sci 29:591–597.

Potkins ZV, Lawrence TLJ. 1989a. Oesophagogastric parakeratosis in the growing pig: Effects of the physical form of barley-based diets and added fibre. Res in Vet Sci 47:60–67.

———. 1989b. Rate of development of oesophagogastric parakeratosis in the growing pig: Some effects of finely ground barley diets, genotype, and the previous husbandry. Res Vet Sci 47:68–74.

Queiroz DMM, Rocha GA, Mendes EN, Moura SB, Oliveira AMR, Mirandoa D. 1996. Association between *Helicobacter* and gastric ulcer disease of the pars esophagea in swine. Gastroenterol 111:19–27.

Rathje J, Halbur PG, Hagemoser WA, Paul PS. 1996. Effect of porcine reproductive and respiratory syndrome virus (PRRSV) on blood and bone marrow. In Proc Am Assoc Swine Practitioners, pp. 171–177.

Reese NA, Muggenburg BA, Kowalczyk T, Grummer RH, Hoekstra WG. 1966. Nutritional and environmental factors influencing gastric ulcers in swine. J Anim Sci 25:14–20.

Regina DC, Eisemann JH, Lang JA, Argenzio RA. 1999. Changes in gastric contents in pigs fed a finely ground and pelleted or coarsely ground meal diet. J Anim Sci 77:2721–2729.

Reimann EM, Maxwell CV, Kowalczyk T, Benevenga NJ, Grummer RH, Hoekstra WG. 1968. Effects of fineness of grind of corn on gastric lesions and contents of swine. J Anim Sci 27:992–999.

Robert S, Matte JJ, Girard CL. 1991. Effect of feeding regimen on behaviour of growing-finishing pigs supplemented or not supplemented with folic acid. J Anim Sci 69:4428–4436.

Robertson ID, Accioly JM, Moore KM, Driesen SJ, Pethick DW, Hampson DJ. 2002. Risk factors for gastric ulcers in Australian pigs at slaughter. Pre Vet Med 53:292–303.

Roels S, Ducatelle R, Broekaert D. 1997. Keratin pattern in hyperkeratotic and ulcerated gastric pars oesophagea in pigs. Res Vet Sci 62:165–169.

Rokkjaer M, Sogaard H, Kruse A, Amdrup E. 1977. Bile induced chronic gastric ulcer in swine. World J Surgery 1:371–379.

Sanford SE, Josephson GKA, Rehmtulla AS. 1994. Causes of sudden death in sows submitted to a diagnostic laboratory over a 1-year period: A prospective study. Proc Int Congr Pig Vet Soc 13:476.

Sangiah S, Amouzadeh HR, Barron S, Maxwell C, Mauromoustakos A. 1990. Effects of cimetidine and ranitidine on basal gastric pH, free and total acid content in pigs. Res Vet Sci 49:279–282.

Smith VG, Kasson CW. 1991. The interrelationship between crude protein and exogenous porcine somatotropin on growth, feed, and carcass measurements of pigs. J Anim Sci 69:571–577.

Smith WJ, Edwards SA. 1996. Ulceration of the pars oesophagea—The role of a factor in wheat. Proc Int Congr Pig Vet Soc 14:693.

Southern LL, Watkins KL, French DD. 1993. Effect of dietary sodium bicarbonate on growth, liver, copper concentration and incidence of gastric ulceration in pigs fed excess dietary copper. Int J Vet Nutrition Res 63:45–47.

Stapleton GN, Marks IN, Fourie AJ, McLeod H, Hickman R, Mall A, Terblanche J. 1989. Sucralfate in the prevention of porcine experimental peptic ulceration. Am J Med 86:21–22.

Straw B, Henry S, Nelssen J, Doster A, Moxley R, Rogers D, Webb D, Hogg A. 1992. Prevalence of lesions in the pars esophagea of normal and sick pigs. Proc Int Congr Pig Vet Soc 12:386.

Szemerédi G, Solá A. 1979. Role of meteorological factors in the development of oesophageal gastric ulcers in pigs under tropical conditions. Magyar Állatorvosok Lapja 34:176–178.

Thoonen J, Hoorens J. 1961. Meagulcera in de pars oesophea big varkens. Vlaams Diergeneeskd Tijdschr 30:79–92.

Van Vleet JF, Carlton W, Olander HJ. 1970. Hepatosis dietetica and mulberry heart disease associated with selenium deficiency in Indiana swine. J Am Vet Med Assoc 157:1208–1219.

Wondra KJ, Hancock JD, Kennedy GA, Hines RH, Behnke KC. 1995a. Reducing particle size of corn in lactation diets from 1,200 to 400 micrometers improves sow and litter performance. J Anim Sci 73:421–426.

Wondra KJ, Hancock JD, Behnke KC, Hines RH. 1995c. Effects of dietary buffers on growth performance, nutrient digestibility, and stomach morphology in finishing pigs. J Anim Sci 73:414–420.

Wondra KJ, Hancock JD, Behnke KC, Stark CR. 1995b. Effects of mill type and particle size uniformity on growth performance, nutrient digestibility, and stomach morphology in finishing pigs. J Anim Sci 73:2564–2573.

Yamaguchi M, Takemoto T, Sakamoto K, Asano T, Uchimura M, Masuda I. 1981. Prevention of gastric ulcers in swine by feeding of sodium polyacrylate. Am J Vet Res 42:960–962.

Yeomans ND, Kolt SD. 1996. *Helicobacter heilmannii* (formerly *Gastrospirillium*): Association with pig and human gastric pathology. Gastroenterol 111:244–259.

Zamora CS, Reddy VK, Frandle KA, Samson MD. 1980. Effect of prednisone on gastric blood flow in swine. Am J Vet Res 41:885–888.

55 Internal Parasites

T. Bonner Stewart and Phillip G. Hoyt

Internal parasites are ever present and must be considered in the economic production of pork. Infectious diseases are spread quickly through a herd and are often easily recognized by the presence of moribund or dead pigs. The internal nematodes, more specifically the worms, can also kill, but loss of appetite, reduction in rate of gain, poor feed utilization, and the potentiation of other pathogens that may be present are the more common results of parasitism. The less-than dramatic performance problems cannot be easily related directly to parasite infection or measured in terms of economic losses. Condemnation of parts of and even entire carcasses due to parasites can be dramatic and is easily documented; however, the more important losses come from insidious depressant effects of parasites on feed intake, daily gain, and feed conversion.

Controlled trials with single-species infections with the more common parasites of swine have shown that all of the nematode infections resulted in a reduction in average daily gain (ADG) of infected pigs compared to their controls. Similarly, the feed to gain ratio (F/G) for the infected pigs increased compared to control pigs. Differences at low levels of infection ranged from 2% to 21% reduction in ADG and from 3% to 6% increase in F/G for the infected pigs compared to their controls. At higher levels of infection, deaths occurred (Stewart 1996) Losses vary greatly in relation to geographic region, type of housing, management, nutrition, pig breed and strain, and species of parasite. The impact of swine parasites and the need for research have been reviewed (Stewart et al. 1985a), as well as the economic losses in production (Stewart and Hale 1988; Kennedy et al. 1988)

In a survey in the United States, based on examination of fecal samples from 84 hog farms judged to have good management in 15 states, the prevalence of *A. suum* was 70% (Kennedy et al. 1988). Utilizing available statistical data (U.S. Department of Agriculture) and calculating performance data on the basis of experimental low ascarid infections, the estimated loss in 1994 from ascarid infections was $174 million (Stewart 1996).

Most schemes for parasite control have been aimed at reducing condemnation of livers caused by *A. suum* or *Stephanurus dentatus*: for example, the "McLean County" system developed in the midwestern United States (Raffensperger and Connely 1927), the "Profit" program in North Carolina (Behlow and Batte 1974), and the "Gilt-Only" system developed in Georgia (Stewart et al. 1964). These systems incorporated sanitation, anthelmintics, and management, singly or in combination, to reduce condemnation and production losses. All anthelmintics introduced for swine since the 1950s have been highly efficacious against *A. suum,* yet it is still the most prevalent swine worm parasite in the world. Incidently, this is also true of *A. lumbricoides* of humans.

More recently, biological systems of control have been researched. For example, daily doses of 5×10^4 units of chlamydospores of the microfungus *Duddingtonia flagrans* fed in feed over a 2-month period to pastured pigs infected with known number of *Oesophagostomum dentatum* and *Hyostrongylus rubidus* resulted in lower herbage numbers of infective larvae of both species compared to the control pigs not receiving the microfungus (Nansen et al. 1996).

The organization of this chapter is by anatomic system infected by the important cosmopolitan parasites, beginning with the stomach. Other parasites are discussed in the section on miscellaneous parasites. The distribution, morphology, life cycle, pathology, and diagnosis of each parasite and, where appropriate, other special effects such as immune response, public health significance, and economic importance are discussed. Separate sections are included on prevention and on anthelmintic compounds currently being used and those under development.

STOMACH

Hyostrongylus rubidus

The trichostrongyloid nematode *Hyostrongylus rubidus*, the red stomach worm of pigs, becomes concentrated in the lesser curvature in the fundic area of the stomach of pigs. The adult worms are less than 10 mm in length and are bright red when first removed from the host. They are essentially parasites of pastured animals.

Morphology. These slender red worms have cuticular striation (Figure 55.2). Males are 4–7 mm and females 5–9 mm in length. Males have a pair of short spicules and a bursa. The female vulva is located on the midposterior half of the body. Cervical papillae are present. The eggs are typical strongyle type and are in the 16- to 32-cell stage when passed in the feces. They are thin-shelled and measure 60–76 by 30–38 μm (Figure 55.1F).

Life Cycle. Eggs develop on the ground into infective larvae (L_3) in about 7 days. After ingestion, the infection becomes patent in about 21 days. The L_3 enter pits of the gastric glands, where they remain for about 2 weeks as they go through two molts, returning to the lumen as L_5, young adults. Larvae can remain in the mucosa for several months in a histotrophic stage similar to that of *Ostertagia* of cattle and sheep and cause formation of small nodules.

Pathology. Infections usually are not pathogenic, but if enough worms are present, hyperemia, catarrhal gastritis, submucosal edema, hyperplasia of the gastric gland area, erosion of the mucosa, and ulcer formation may result (Porter 1940; Kendall et al. 1960; Stockdale et al. 1973). *H. rubidus* is a bloodsucker; and in herds with clinical hyostrongylosis, emaciation and pallor of the skin and mucous membranes may be apparent in adult animals (Davidson et al. 1968; Appert and Taranchon 1969). Clinically inapparent infections can lead to reduced weight gains, feed conversion, and N balance (Dey-Hazra et al. 1972; Stewart et al. 1985b).

Diagnosis. The eggs are almost indistinguishable from those of *Oesophagostomum* spp. in both size and morphology, although *H. rubidus* eggs are more advanced in development. Larval culture is a better method of differentiation (Homer 1967).

SMALL INTESTINE

Strongyloides ransomi

Strongyloides ransomi, the small-intestinal threadworm, is a rhabditoid nematode of cosmopolitan distribution. Its prevalence and importance are greater in the warmer climatic regions, where it is an important parasite of suckling pigs.

Morphology. Only parthogenetic females are present in the parasitic generation. Adults are practically microscopic, measuring 3.3–4.5 mm in length. The filariform esophagus occupies about a third of the total body length. The vulva is located near the middle of the body.

The thin-shelled eggs passed in the feces contain larvae and measure 45–55 by 26–35 μm (Figure 55.1A).

Life Cycle. Larvated eggs that pass in the feces hatch in a few hours into L_1 rhabditiform larvae. These may develop either directly into infective larvae (homogonic cycle) or into males and females (heterogonic cycle), which in turn will produce infective larvae. In the homogonic cycle, infective larvae can appear in a little more than a day. In the heterogonic cycle, infective larvae can appear in 2.5 days. Different routes of infection have been proven for *S. ransomi*: percutaneous, oral, transcolostral, and prenatal.

Percutaneous penetration by larvae produces patency in 6–10 days after infection. Larvae enter the bloodstream, proceed to the lungs, undergo tracheal migration, and are swallowed. Oral infections are possible when the ingested larvae penetrate the mucous membranes and migrate to the lungs, L_3 being killed by gastric juices.

Transcolostral infection may also occur, by 4 days after birth. This is considered the primary means of infection of neonates in the southeastern United States. Larvae in the sow colostrum differ physiologically from L_3 and pass through the stomach and develop into adults in the small intestine without migration. Larvae responsible for infection of the neonates are sequestered in the mammary fat of the sow and apparently are mobilized and included in the colostrum (Moncol 1975; Stewart et al. 1976).

Prenatal infection producing patency in suckling pigs as early as 2–3 days after birth can occur. Larvae from the sow accumulate in various tissues of the fetus during the latter part of pregnancy, and complete migration to the small intestine of the newborn rapidly after birth.

Pathology. Diarrhea followed by progressive dehydration is the usual sign. In heavy infections, death generally occurs before pigs are 10–14 days old, but stunting and unthriftiness are the more usual sequelae of *S. ransomi* infection. No pathognomonic lesions are associated with field cases of strongyloidosis (Stewart et al. 1968). Larvae apparently can be distributed widely in most tissues of the body and lesions are dependent on the number of larvae and host response (Stone and Simpson 1967).

Immune Response. Breed differences in susceptibility to *S. ransomi*, which appear to be genetic (Johnson et al. 1975), have been reported. Duroc pigs were less susceptible to effects of infection than Hampshire pigs, and the F_1 cross of the two breeds was intermediate in response. Murrel and Urban (1983) showed that enteral exposure of pigs infected with milk larvae produced protective immunity to subsequent subcutaneous inoculation with *S. ransomi* L_3.

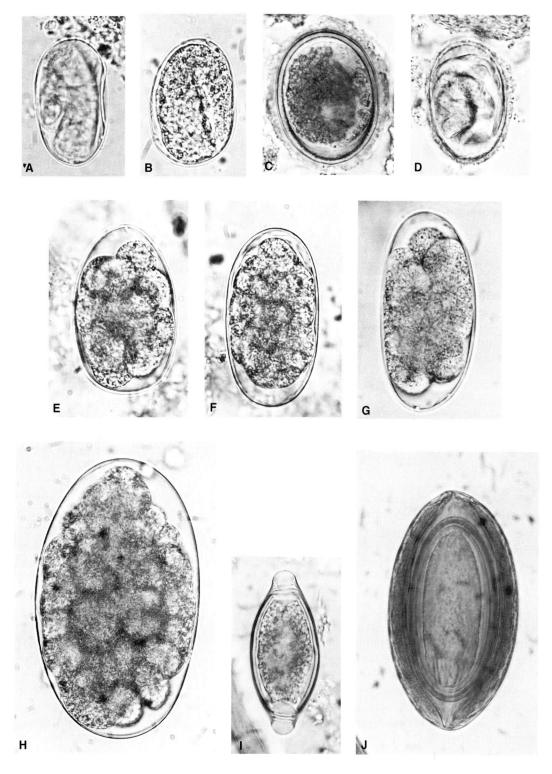

55.1. *(A)* Strongyloides *egg, thin-shelled, lacking one of three layers, and larvated; (B)* Ascarops *egg, larvated and similar morphologically to those of* Physocephalus *and* Gongylonema; *(C) the* Ascaris *egg has an outer proteinaceous layer, often missing; (D)* Metastrongylus *egg;* *(E)* Oesophagostomum *egg; (F)* Hyostrongylus *egg; (G)* Globocephalus *egg; (H)* Stephanurus dentatus *egg passed in the urine; (I)* Trichuris *egg;* *(J)* Macracanthorhynchus *egg. (All eggs photographed and printed at the same magnification.)*

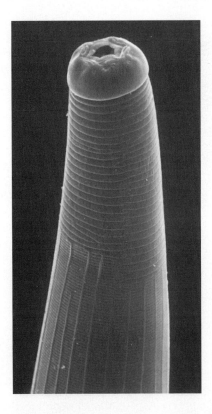

55.2. *Scanning electron micrograph of anterior of* Hyostrongylus rubidus *showing cuticular striations.*

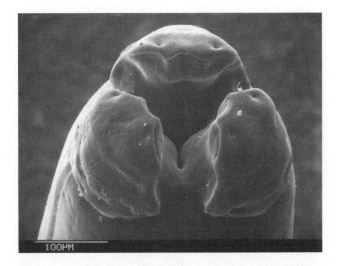

55.3. *The three lips of* Ascaris suum. *Note sensory papillae and denticles on edges of lips.*

Diagnosis. Identification of eggs in feces or finding the adults in the small intestine at necropsy, with a history of diarrhea and unthriftiness, confirms a diagnosis of strongyloidosis; however, care must be taken because clinical disease can be confused with colibacillosis and coccidiosis.

Ascaris suum

Ascaris suum, the large roundworm of swine, is an ascaridoid (ascarid) nematode of cosmopolitan distribution. It is the most common gastrointestinal worm parasite in pigs, with a prevalence of 50–75%. It is more common in growing pigs than in mature pigs. Although now recognized as a separate species, the large roundworm of humans, *A. lumbricoides*, was thought to be the same as that in pigs.

Morphology. Ascarids are large, stout-bodied, pinkish-yellow nematodes with three prominent lips surrounding the mouth (Figure 55.3. Females are 20–40 cm long, and the males 15–25 cm. The male tail is conical and bent ventrally. Males have two stout spicules. The female vulva is anterior to the middle of the body. Eggs are thick-shelled and brownish yellow with a mammillated proteinaceous coating on the exterior, and they measure 50–80 by 40–60 μm. The eggs are unsegmented when passed in feces (Figure 55.1C)

Life Cycle. The life cycle is direct and involves a hepatotracheal migration route. Eggs are laid in the intestine of the pigs and pass out in the feces. At room temperature the L_1 appeared in the egg at 17–22 days; the L_2 appeared at 22–27 days; and the L_3 first appeared on day 27 (Geenen et al. 1999). Additional time is needed for eggs to become infective, and they may remain infective for 7 years or longer in protected areas of lots and pastures.

When ingested, infective eggs hatch in the digestive tract. The liberated L_3 penetrate the intestinal wall and generally pass via the hepatic portal system to the liver. A few, however, may pass via the lacteals to the mesenteric lymph nodes; others may even be found in the peritoneal cavity and other locations. Most larvae are in the liver by the first or second day after ingestion and in the lungs by days 4–7. From day 8 to day 10 after infection, larvae leave the lungs by penetrating the bronchioles, are coughed up into the trachea, and are swallowed. By 10–15 days after infection the L_3 have returned to the small intestine and molted to L_4. At this time, some L_4 are spontaneously eliminated from the small intestine into the cecum and colon. L_4 molt to young adults (L_5) 21–30 days after ingestion of eggs. The prepatent period is 40–53 days. Female ascarids are phenomenal egg producers capable of laying hundreds of thousand to nearly 2 million eggs per day. The eggs are sticky and are easily transported by cockroaches and other arthropods, birds, boots, etc. Most disinfectants have no effect on the eggs, but heat (steam) and direct sunlight are effective in destroying their viability.

Most adults live in pigs only about 6 months, at which time they begin to be expelled, but pigs may continue to carry a light infection for a year or longer. In foreign hosts as in humans or domesticated and laboratory animals, larvae may migrate but are generally unable to develop to adults in the intestine and are expelled in the feces if they reach the digestive system.

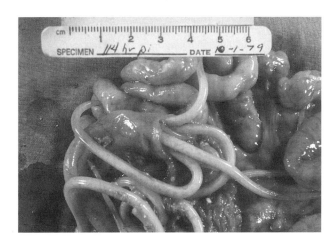

55.4. Ascaris *emerging from a tear in the gut wall. (Photo by Mark Martinez.)*

Pathology. The larvae migrate through the liver and cause hemorrhagic foci which microscopically show mild eosinophilic infiltration and a few, small lymphoid nodules in portal areas. On repeated exposure to larvae, there is an increase in connective tissue, infiltrating eosinophils, and dilation of lymphatics, which grossly appear as whitish spots, commonly referred to as "milk spots." Such lesions disappear within 25 days. In the lungs, migrating larvae cause verminous pneumonia, which may result in death if large numbers of larvae are involved. Clinical signs are those of pneumonia. Pigs have an asthmatic cough ("thumps") and may breathe with difficulty. Hemorrhagic foci of various sizes are present. There may be an exudate, edema and emphysema with secondary bacterial pneumonia. Migration of *A. suum* larvae markedly enhances the pathogenicity of swine influenza as well as viral pneumonia.

Adult worms compete with the host for nutrients and interfere with absorption of nutrients by the host. They may occlude and rupture the small intestine (Figure 55.4). In addition, adults may migrate into the common bile duct and occlude it, causing icterus.

Immune Response. Acquired resistance can be induced in pigs by oral inoculation with infective eggs or L_3 pulmonary larvae (Eriksen 1982: Stewart et al. 1985c). The presence of adults or late larval ascarids can prevent development of additional larval stages (Stewart and Rowell 1986). High levels of protective immunity based on the number of lung larvae recovered after challenge with 10,000 larvae following repeated experimental or natural exposure was shown by Urban et al. (1989). Protective immunity was not altered by strategic anthelmintic treatment that prevented growth retardation of pigs constantly exposed to natural infection. Sterilizing immunity is transitory, and periodic boosting or anthelmintic treatment is necessary to eliminate both intestinal worms and lesions during the growing-finishing period (Urban et al. 1988, 1989). The intestine

is considered important as a defense mechanism in preventing larval penetration of the gut mucosa (Bindseil 1970), and it has been shown that the intestinal phase of ascarids can induce circulating antibodies without prior somatic migration (Leigh-Brown and Harpur 1974). Protective immunity is characterized by antibody in serum and in intestinal washings (Urban et al. 1984).

Economic Importance. Ascariasis is undoubtedly the most important parasitism of pigs worldwide. The effects of ascarids on the performance of pigs were detailed by Spindler in 1947 and by many others since then. Controlled experimental single infections at different levels with the ubiquitous *A. suum* showed that low levels of infection depress feed intake and daily gain with a concomitant increase in maintenance cost; at higher levels of infection, depression in feed conversion also occurs. Periodic analyses of metabolic functions during the prepatent period showed a significant effect on nitrogen (N) metabolism on days 33–37, coincident with rapid growth of the immature worms in the small intestine. The average number of worms recovered at slaughter ranged from 13–18, although the infecting doses in the studies ranged from 600–60,000 (Hale et al. 1985). Such lack in correlation between infecting numbers and establishment of adults has been observed many times (Schwartz 1959; Andersen et al. 1973). Losses from condemnation of parts and lowered performance of pigs in the United Sates were calculated at more than $385 million annually (Levine 1980). More recently, losses due solely to lowered feed conversion from low-level *A suum* infections were estimated at $155 million for 1987 in the United States (Stewart and Hale 1988). There are no estimates of the value of losses incurred from the potentiation or exacerbation of other diseases by migrating ascarid larvae, or the effect of different management practices or nutritional levels (Underdahl 1958; Zimmerman et al. 1973).

Diagnosis. Typical eggs in fecal flotation or "milk spot" liver lesions at necropsy are diagnostic. In heavy infections the adult worms can be seen and felt in the intact intestine. In areas where the kidney worm is endemic, liver lesions must be differentiated because early *S. dentatus* lesions can be confused with those produced by *A. suum*.

Trichinella spiralis

Probably all mammalian species are susceptible to *Trichinella spiralis* infection, although natural cycles seem climatically based. In the Temperance Zone the usual cycle has swine and bears as natural hosts (Schad et al. 1984), and in the Arctic Zone polar bears and grizzly bears (Kim 1983) and walrus (MacLean et al. 1989) are natural hosts. Other species, including humans, are involved incidently. Trichinellosis is found less frequently in the Tropics. Regulation of garbage feeding to swine, public health programs, and recently improved trichinoscopic and serodiagnostic techniques have reduced the incidence of this infection.

Morphology. The life stage most frequently observed is the encysted (L_1) in muscle fibers. These cysts are 400–600 µm long and 250 µm in diameter. Prior to skeletal muscle fiber penetration, (L_1) may be found in the circulatory system. Adult females occur in the lamina propria of the small intestine, have a stichosome type esophagus, produce larvated eggs in utero and are 3–4 mm long and 60 µm in diameter. Adult males are rarely seen but are about one-half the size of females.

Life Cycle. Muscle cysts are ingested and digested in the stomach and small intestine, and L_1 are liberated into the small intestine. Molting from L_1 to L_5 then occurs in 2–6 days. Intracellular infection of enterocytes with adults was demonstrated in mice by electron microscopy (Wright 1979). Males die soon after mating and females burrow into lymph spaces, depositing larvae. Larvae are numerous in the blood from 8–25 days post infection; these L_1 penetrate the sarcolemma of skeletal muscle fibers throughout the body and become encysted by 3 months. Although calcification of cysts begins at 6–9 months, L_1 remain viable for up to 11 years, demonstrating the symbiotic relationship between L_1 and host muscle fiber, the "nurse cell" (Despommier 1990). Modes of transmission in swine herds include cannibalism, tail biting, scavenging on carcasses of dead farm cats (Hanbury et al. 1986), feeding on raw garbage, the presence of hog lots on covered garbage dumps (Zimmerman et al. 1962), and eating wild animal carcasses such as raccoon and fox (Kazacos 1986; Campbell 1988).

Pathology. *Trichinella* is much less pathogenic for swine than for rats and humans. Experimental infections in pigs caused decreased weight gains and intense muscle pain, but most of these infected pigs recovered with rapid weight gain (Scholtens et al. 1966); in experimentally infected miniature pigs, eosinophilia and hypergammaglobulinemia were observed (Beck and Anfinson (1965). Clinical illness has not been described for natural infection with the muscle fiber cyst and infiltration of eosinophils is often the lesion observed.

Immune Response. Experimental inoculation of pigs with *T. spiralis* excretory-secretory products induced moderate but variable degrees of immunity to subsequent challenge per os with doses of 2500–2700 L_1. These pigs harbored fewer adult worms, and the fecundity of female worms recovered (measured by shedding of newborn larvae) was significantly lower than that of females recovered from control pigs (Gamble et al. 1986). Prospects for potential use of targeted vaccine in an integrated control program for swine trichinosis are being investigated (Murrel 1985).

Diagnosis. Federal, until recently state, meat inspection regulations have not included examination for *Trichinella*, but procedures for diagnosis would be by digestion of muscle at slaughter or by enzyme-linked immunosorbent assay (ELISA) for serologic detection of *Trichinella*-specific antibodies (Gamble et al. 1983). A pooled-sample digestion method using 5–6 g diaphragm samples from lots of 20 pig carcasses has been adopted by several European countries but not by the U.S. Department of Agriculture (Zimmerman 1967). These pooled samples are digested and homogenized using 1% pepsin/1% HCL and a mixing action which simulates peristaltic motion of the stomach (using a stomacher device). Analysis of pooled samples can be accomplished in 1.5 hours (Oliver et al. 1985).

An ELISA test using an excretory antigen for diagnosis of trichinosis was evaluated in the field with sera from herds with ongoing transmission of *T. spiralis* (Murrell et al. 1986). Results showed a high sensitivity of 93–96% with sera from infected pigs. Of those that were false-negative, five-sixths had fewer than 5.0 larvae per gram (LPG). This should prove to be a major technique for antemortem diagnosis in herd screening.

Public Health. In Europe, trichinoscopic examination of pork appears to have practically eliminated *T. spiralis* from domestic swine. Incidence of swine trichiniasis in the United States was 0.125% in 1966–1970 (Zimmerman and Zinter 1971). Pork, mainly prepared sausage, apparently is the major source of human trichinellosis, accounting for 73.2% of 254 cases for which source was identified (USDHHS 1976). There are close to 40 million potential exposures each year based on the estimated number of infected pigs, the estimated number of human cases is 300,000, the majority of which cases cause no symptoms of infection (Leighty 1974). Non-pork products included meat from walrus, black bear, and horses and ground beef (James 1989), with beef likely adulterated with pork. Small custom slaughterhouses are important epidemiologically, for these often prepare fresh, whole dressed pork for social occasions where one animal is consumed by many persons (Schad et al. 1985). There have been several recent small epidemics among Indo-Chinese immigrants in the United States (USDHHS 1982); an update on trichinosis surveillance in the United States appeared in 1988 (USDHHS 1988).

In the United States, educating the public to recognize the hazard and to cook pork adequately to kill the organisms, and requiring freezing of manufactured pork products that need cooking have been the two principal patterns used by federal and state meat inspection programs (Leighty 1974). A more concerted effort to identify herds with active infections in order to provide a "safe" product was initiated by the state of Illinois with the introduction of a Trichinosis Control Act in 1986. The pooled-sample digestion and ELISA technique are employed to identify and subsequently to quarantine, depopulate, and indemnify those herds found infected. Other states, such as North Carolina, are following suit with use of a semiautomatic ELISA to screen hogs in a packing plant at the rate of 400/hour; all recorded positives then are screened by the diaphragm technique.

For chemotherapy, ivermectin was confirmed as having no antiparasitic activity, whereas excellent efficacy was reported for albendazole. Calf thymus extract, cyclosporin A, and the experimental compound luxabendazole have also been proven efficacious (James 1989).

CECUM AND COLON

Trichuris suis

Pigs and wild boars are considered the natural hosts of *Trichuris suis*, although primates, including humans, may be infected with *T. suis*. Whipworms are distributed widely and are a fairly common problem in swine.

Morphology. Adult females measure 6–8 cm long and males half that length. This trichuroid has a unique morphology, with the anterior or esophageal portion 0.5 mm in diameter and extending two-thirds of the body length. The esophagus is a stichosome-type consisting of a column of spiraling stichocytes, one cell layer in thickness. A microscopic lancet protrudes from the stoma in all stages. Glandular and muscular components are interspersed along the esophagus. The posterior third of the body is thicker, 0.65 mm, protrudes into the lumen and contains the midgut of the worm and its reproductive tract. Bipolar thick-shelled eggs may be seen in the uterus of the female, and a single copulatory spicule in the male. Eggs are 60 by 25 μm, yellow to brown, and in the one-cell stage (Figure 55.1I).

Life Cycle. The eggs passed in the feces require 3–4 weeks to reach infectivity, still in the L_1 stage, and can remain infective for as long as 6 years. Infective eggs hatch in the small intestine and cecum, with the released L_1 penetrating cells lining the crypts. A histotrophic phase persists for 2 weeks with gradual larval migration from the deeper lamina propria to the submucosa. Luminal development begins the third week post infection with the posterior body coming into view and the anterior end remaining buried in the mucosa (Figure 55.5). Meanwhile, four molts have occurred, prepatency is 6–7 weeks, and life span 4–5 months (Beer 1973).

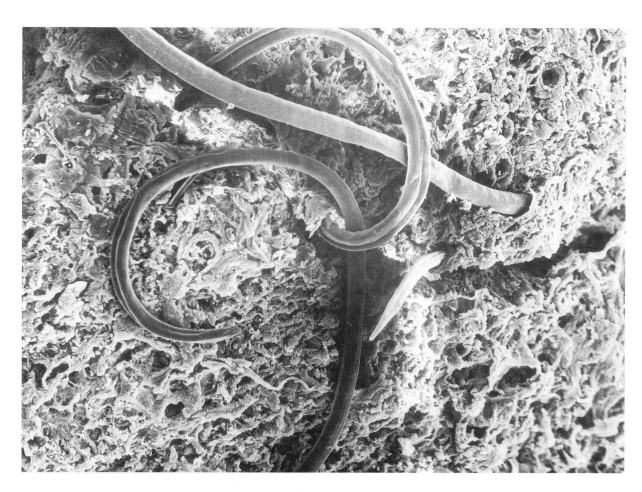

55.5. Trichuris *worm. Note intracellular penetration (Batte et al. 1977.)*

Pathology. *Trichuris* infections cause enterocyte destruction, ulceration of the mucosal lining, loss of capillary blood, and probably secondary bacterial infection. Thus, trichuriosis must be considered in the differential diagnosis of swine dysentery complex that does not respond to antibiotic therapy. The spectrum of gross lesions may be edema with formation of nodules containing exudates surrounding portions of worms to formation of a fibrinonecrotic membrane. Erosion of capillary beds and vasodilation results in hemorrhage, anemia, and hypoalbuminemia. Clinical signs include anorexia, mucoid to bloody diarrhea, dehydration, and death.

Immune Response. Susceptibility with accompanying clinical signs is up to 6 months of age, although mature hogs may show clinical infection when stressed. Light infections persist, allowing intermittent shedding of eggs. Infection of pigs with *Trichuris suis* was shown to induce suppression of mucosal immunity to resident bacteria and is linked to the pathogenesis of necrotic proliferative colitis (Mansfield and Urban 1996).

Diagnosis. Clinical signs, including bloody scouring, are presumptive. Eggs in stools and whipworms at necropsy are confirmative. Trichurids are sporadic egg layers therefore, little significance can be given to number of eggs per gram (EPG).

Oesophagostomum spp.

Oesophagostomum spp. are strongyloid nematodes, of which *O. dentatum* and *O. quadrispinulatum* are the most common in occurrence. *O. brevicaudum* occurs in the southeastern United States and other areas with similar climates. Two other species, *O. granatensis* in Europe and *O. georgianum* in the southeastern United States, are probably morphovariants of *O. dentatum* (Raynaud et al. 1974; Stewart and Gasbarre 1989).

Morphology. Adult *Oesophagostomum* have stout, slightly curved bodies; females are 1–2 cm long and males are slightly shorter. Species differentiation is by shape of esophagus, shape of buccal capsule, and length of tail and spicules (Figure 55.6). Eggs are 70 by 40 µm, morulated when passed, thin-shelled, and typically strongyloid (Figure 55.1E).

Life Cycle. The preparasitic cycle is of the strongylid type, with L$_1$ emerging from eggs and ensheathed L$_3$ appearing by 1 week. Larvae can survive on pastures for up to 12 months. Swine are infected by ingesting L$_3$ from contaminated pastures, by mechanical transmission by psychodid flies (midges), or from rats with encysted larvae (Jacobs and Dunn 1968). The L$_3$ enter the mucosa of the cecum and colon and molt to L$_4$, remain for 2 weeks, causing small nodules, and emerge into the lumen, molt to L$_5$, and reach patency in 3 weeks after ingestion.

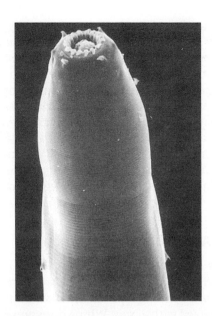

55.6. *Scanning electron micrograph of anterior of* Oesophagostomum brevicaudum.

Pathology. Formation of nodules from the cecum to the rectum is the major change (Taffs 1966). The sequelae are petechiation at the point of entry of the L$_3$ (Jacobs 1969); focal thickening of the mucosa consisting of lymphocytes, macrophages, and esosinophils; and then presence of luminal nodules by day 4. Encysted larvae may be found in the muscularis mucosa (McCracken and Ross 1970). By 1 week, nodules are up to 8 mm in diameter and plugged with yellow to black necrotic debris. Walls of the cecum and colon become edematous from extensive thrombosis of lymphatics; there is possibly a localized fibrinonecrotic membrane. Resolution begins the second week with some remnants of nodules and scarring. Secondary infection may occur and enhance clinical signs of depression, anorexia, and scouring.

Immunity. There is no apparent age immunity (Taffs 1956), but pigs over 3 months seem more susceptible (Haas et al. 1972). A periparturient rise of EPG is maintained through lactation with a subsequent expulsion of worms (Connan 1967; Haas et al. 1972).

RESPIRATORY TRACT

Metastrongylus spp.

Species include *M. apri (elongatus)*, *M. pudendotectus* and *M. salmi*, which occur in the bronchi and bronchioles, especially in the diaphragmatic lobes, and exclusively in swine. Although *M. apri* is the most common, all occur worldwide and natural infections occur more often with two species present.

Morphology. Adults are slender and white, with females 50 mm in length and males 25 mm; males have paired spicules, Mucoid deposits around these adults makes it

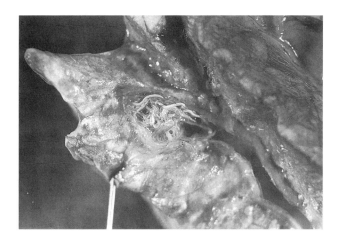

55.7. *Cluster of* Metastrongylus *worms in a terminal bronchiole of the diaphragmatic lobe of the lung. (Photo by Blaise Brazos.)*

difficult to separate individuals. Eggs are larvated, thick-shelled, and measure 40–50 µm (Figure 55.1D).

Life Cycle. Larvated eggs are coughed up, swallowed, and passed in feces. Earthworms ingest these eggs, which then hatch, and L_1 migrate to the heart. Infective larvae appear in 10 days and hogs rooting in the soil eat the infected worms. These L_3 penetrate the wall of the intestine and are transported to the mesentery lymph nodes, where they molt to L_4. These L_4 are then swept through the right heart to the lungs (Figure 55.7) and molt to L_5, with patency in 4 weeks.

Pathology. Dissecting the bronchioles reveals mucoid plugs in the diaphragmatic lobes of the lungs; these are adults and eggs. Parasites, mucus, and cellular exudate cause occlusion and induce atelectasis, observed as coughing or "thumps." Apparently *Mycoplasma hyopneumoniae* is not transmitted with *Metastrongylus* via earthworms (Preston and Switzer 1976). Fewer parasites seem to occur in breeding stock.

Diagnosis. It is difficult to find *Metastrongylus* eggs in a fecal exam, but it is important to look for "fuzzy" areas in which eggs are held in mucus. At necropsy, lungworms can be extruded by clipping the posteroventral margins or the tip of the diaphragmatic lobes of the lungs.

URINARY TRACT

Stephanurus dentatus

The kidney worm is a strongyloid nematode of swine. Domestic and feral pigs raised on soil in warm climates are most often infected. In the United States, endemicity is from the Carolinas to southern Missouri, with interstate transport accounting for the worm's appearance as far north as Canada (Smith and Hawkes 1978).

Morphology. Adults are thick-bodied with black and white mottling from contents of the reproductive and intestinal tracts showing through the cuticle; they are 1–3 cm long by 2 mm in diameter. The strongylid eggs are ellipsoidal, thin-walled, morulated, and measure 120 by 70 µm (Figure 55.1H).

Life Cycle. Kidney worms are found in cysts in perirenal fat with fistulous openings into the ureters, in the kidney, and in ectopic sites such as the pancreas, lumbar muscles, spinal cord, and lungs. Eggs are voided, with the greatest numbers found at first urination from overnight accumulation in the bladder. Eggs may hatch in 1–2 days; molt to infective L_3 in 3–5 days; and survive for several months in warm, moist, shaded conditions. They are invasive by ingestion, skin penetration, and infected earthworms (Tromba 1955; Batte et al. 1960). Prenatal infection also has been reported (Batte et al. 1966).

Infective L_3 migrate from the small intestine to the mesenteric lymph nodes and molt to L_4, which move through portal veins to the liver (Lichtenfels and Tromba 1972). Bronchiole lymph nodes, lungs, pancreas, and spleen also may be infected by L_3 (Waddell 1969). In the liver, L_4 increase from 0.4 to 6.0 mm, molt to L_5 in 2–4 months, and then leave the liver (Lichtenfels and Tromba 1972). They migrate through the body cavity to perirenal and mesenteric fat. Patency is uncommon before 9–12 months, and eggs are shed for 3 years after initial infection (Batte et al. 1966).

Pathology. Gross pathological changes may be found where there is migration. Mesentery lymph nodes are edematous and swollen; liver changes include inflammation, eosinophilia, abscessation, and extensive fibrosis, making this infection easily differentiated from ascarid migration. Similar lesions can be seen in other organs. Nodules are formed in perirenal fat, and fistulous tracts are present along the ureters. Posterior paralysis has been associated with migration around the spinal cord.

Diagnosis. Worms, abscessation, and liver scarring can be seen at necropsy. Eggs in urine are confirmatory antemortem.

Economic Consideration. At least 95% of liver condemnations are due to kidney worms and ascarids in hogs in the southeastern United States (Batte et al. 1975). Marked reduction in growth rate and feed efficiency was shown in pigs infected experimentally (Hale and Marti 1983).

MISCELLANEOUS PARASITES

Three spiruroid nematodes that require dung beetles as intermediate hosts infect pigs: *Ascarops strongylina* and

Physocephalus in the stomach and *Gongylonema pulchrum* under the epithelial layer of the esophagus and tongue. The two thick stomach worms cause a gastritis if present in large numbers. For aesthetic reasons, tongues for human consumption should be scalded and the skin peeled off to remove *G. pulchrum*. The eggs of these spiruroids are thick-shelled. Eggs of *Ascarops* measure 34–40 by 18–22 µm (Figure 55.1B); eggs of *Physocephalus* measure 31–39 by 12–17µm; and eggs of *Gongylonema* measure 57–59 by 30–34 µm.

The hookworm of swine, *Globocephalus urusubulatus*, of cosmopolitan distribution, is more common in the southern part of the United States in feral and pastured swine. It apparently is not as common or pathogenic as hookworms of carnivores and has received little attention. The eggs are typically strongyloid and measure 52–56 by 26–35 µm (Figure 55.1G). *Macracanthorhynchus hirudinaceus,* the thorny-headed worm of swine, is an acanthocephalan. It attaches to the ileal portion of the small intestine and causes nodular lesions, which are sometimes invaded by secondary organisms. Occasionally the gut wall is perforated by the proboscis, and peritonitis results. Eggs measure 110 by 65 µm, are brown, and have a three-layered shell (Figure 55.1J). A beetle is the required intermediate host.

Two trichostrongylid nematodes, commonly parasites of ruminants, can be found in pigs: *Trichostrongylus axei* in the stomach and *T. colubriformis* in the small intestine.

Of public importance, *Taenia solium* (*Cysticercus cellulosae*) has humans as the host for the adult tapeworm as well as the potential host for the cysticercus. Swine are the natural intermediate host. Humans are usually infected with a single worm; the adult measuring 3–5 m long, and with an armed rostellum. Gravid proglottids are 12 by 6 mm, have a single, lateral genital pore, and contain taeniid eggs 42 µm in diameter. Following ingestion of proglottids by swine, cysticerci develop in skeletal and cardiac muscles, measuring up to 18 mm in diameter. These are infective by 2–3 months and remain so for 2 years; prepatency in humans is 2 months. Cysticercosis in swine and taeniasis in humans are usually of no clinical significance, but cysticercosis in humans is life threatening, because cysticerci become space-occupying lesions in the central nervous system and have unrestricted growth with no outer limiting membrane (racemose).

Swine may also be infected with *Fasciola hepatica* and *Echinococcus granulosus* in the liver but with no apparent clinical problems. These infected swine are found in endemic areas where there is common pasture use with sheep.

The ciliated protozoan *Balantidium coli* is found primarily in the cecum and anterior colon of swine as a commensal. The motile form is pleomorphic, 30–150 µm by 25–120 µm, and 45–65 µm in diameter. Reproduction is by binary fission, resistant cysts are formed. *B. coli* feeds on starch, bacteria, and ingesta, including nematode eggs. It is a secondary invader into mucosal lesions by other invaders and produces hyaluronidase, which enlarges lesions. Humans, other primates, and dogs have been found clinically affected in zoos and in areas near hog farms. *B. coli* may cause an explosive bloody diarrhea in these species.

PREVENTION

Parasite control methods may be broadly categorized as either preventive or therapeutic. Those parasites requiring an intermediate host can be successfully prevented by removing pigs from contact with the intermediate hosts—for example, dung beetles and earthworms. Therefore, maintaining pigs on concrete will prevent infection with the spiruroids, acanthocephalans, and metastrongyloids. An added benefit would also be the reduction or prevention of infection by other parasites, such as *Hyostrongylus*, *Globocephalus*, and *Trichostrongylus*, that require pasture conditions for transmission.

Good sanitation is a critical element in controlling parasitic infections. The major mode of transmission of internal parasites is through contamination of food, soil, or bedding with feces or urine. Since parasite eggs need moisture and warmth to develop and survive, direct sunlight or dry conditions shorten egg and larval survival. Thorough cleaning of buildings, pens, and equipment with detergent and steam is the best way to control parasite eggs and larvae Steam penetrates cracks and crevices and kills the tiny eggs and larvae. The common disinfectants used on the farm do not kill eggs of parasites such as ascarids.

Since parasites compete with the host for available nutrients, adequate nutrition aids in reducing the adverse effects on feed efficiency and average daily gain. It has been shown that increasing the protein and vitamins in the feed affects the performance of parasitized pigs by increasing the average daily gain and feed efficiency (Stewart et al. 1969).

A management system in which only gilts are used as breeders has been shown to be effective in eradicating kidney worms. This is possible because of the lengthy prepatent period of 6 months or longer and the fact that only animals 2 years old or older pass kidney worm eggs in significant numbers. Selling breeders as soon as first litters are weaned and maintaining boars separately or replacing them with young stock will prevent contamination of the premises. Eradication can be achieved in 2 years or less by using the "gilt-only" system (Stewart et al. 1964).

TREATMENT

Therapeutic treatment of pigs with anthelmintics may present only a temporary solution, unless the conditions under which the parasites were acquired are altered. No drug is effective against all parasites, and the tissue damage prior to patency results in slower growth rates and increased nutrient requirements. A good management system will incorporate practices, such as sanitation, genetic selection, and nutrition, to prevent infections and will not use treatment as the sole method of controlling parasites. The choice of anthelmintic is dependent on the parasite species present and the relative cost of the products. Routine surveillance and strategic treatment for parasites is advisable on farms with a previous history of clinical disease. Treatment reduces the number of egg-producing parasites and keeps further premise contamination to a minimum.

The use of chemical agents such as pyrantel tartrate fed for several weeks can be helpful under lot or pasture conditions to control infections and reduce lesions from ascarids and nodular worms. Prophylactic use of pyrantel or repetitive treatments with fenbendazole reduces worm populations and also appears to stimulate immunity against *Ascaris suum* (Southern et al. 1989; Stankiewicz and Jeska 1990).

Treatment of sows 10–14 days before farrowing with ivermectin has been shown to be effective in preventing transmission of *Strongyloides ransomi* from sows to their piglets. Such treatment of sows is also beneficial in preventing transmission of *Sarcoptes scabiei*.

Anthelmintics

From 1960–1996 several new classes of anthelmintic compounds were developed, approved by the Food and Drug Administration for use in swine, and marketed in formulations for administration in water or feed and by injection. The spectrum of activity varies by compound, with some effective against a few target species and others broader in effect.

Macrocyclic Lactones. Avermectins are derived from fermentation products of *Streptomyces avermitilis*. The mode of action is to stimulate the release of the inhibitory neurotransmitter gamma-aminobutyric acid (GABA) in target organisms. This inhibits neuromuscular transmission, leading to paralysis and death. The spectrum of activity includes internal and external parasites, including *Ascaris*, *Oesophagotomum*, and *Metastrongylus*, with less effect on *Trichuris* and excellent effect on *Haematopinus* (sucking lice) and *Sarcoptes*.

Ivermectin is available as an injectable formulation and as a feed additive. The injectable formulation is approved for the control of *A. suum*, *Hyostrongylus rubidus*, *Oesophagostomum* spp., *S. ransomi* (adults and somatic larvae), *Metastrongylus* spp., *Haematopinus suis*, and *Sarcoptes scabiei* var. *suis*. It has an 18-day slaughter withdrawal. The feed formulation is approved for the control of *A. suum*, *Ascarops strongylina*, *H. rubidus*, *Oesophagostomum* spp., *S. ransomi* (adults and somatic larvae), *Metastrongylus* spp., *Stephanurus dentatus*, *Haematopinus suis*, and *Sarcoptes scabiei* var. *suis*. It has a 5-day slaughter withdrawal.

In a series of controlled trials doramectin, which is available in an injectable form, was shown to have an efficacy of 98% or greater against *H. rubidus*, *A. suum*, *S. ransomi*, *Oesophagostomum dentatum*, *Oesophagostomum quadrispinulatum*, *Stephanurus dentatus*, and *Metastrongylus* spp., but its efficacy against *Trichuris suis* varied (Logan et al. 1996). In two controlled studies the efficacy of doramectin against *T. suis* was 54% in mixed-species infections and 95% in single-species infections. In both types of population, efficacy was greater for female than for male worms (Stewart et al. 1996a). The efficacy of doramectin against *S. dentatus* was 100% against worms in all locations (Stewart et al. 1996b). It is approved for the control of *A. suum*, *O. dentatum*, *O. quadrispinulatum*, *S. ransomi*, *H. rubidus*, *Metastrongyulus* spp., *S. dentatus*, *S. scabiei* var. *suis*, and *H. suis*. It has a 24-day slaughter withdrawal.

Moxidectin, a milbemycin related to the avermectins, has experimentally been shown to have efficacy as a pour-on against *A. suum*, *Oesophagostomum* spp., and *Metastrongylus* spp. with a variable efficacy against *Trichuris* (Stewart et al. 1999). Currently there is no approved formulation for swine in the United States.

Benzimidazole Carbamates. There are several efficacious compounds among the benzimidazole carbamates, but only fenbendazole (FBZ) is approved for use in swine in the United States. The progenitor of this class of anthelmintics is thiabendazole (TBZ), which has been available since the early 1960s. At 50 mg/kg body weight, TBZ had a greater than 95% efficacy against *Hyostrongylus*, *Strongyloides*, and *Oesophagostomum* but much less activity against ascarids and whipworms. Commercially, it was used in a paste form given therapeutically in a single oral dose for *Strongyloides* infections in baby pigs. Its pharmacologic action is to block nematode fumarate reductase activity. Absorption is a passive diffusion through the cuticle of the worm. TBZ has little solubility in water; therefore, only a small amount is rapidly absorbed from the intestinal tract. Its metabolites are excreted completely in feces and urine within 3 days. There is negligible mammalian toxicity, with 20 times the therapeutic dose producing no adverse effects.

FBZ was approved for use in swine in the United States in 1984. It is known to be effective against ascarids, whipworms, nodular worms, lungworms, and larval and adult kidney worms (Batte 1977). It is more potent than TBZ, especially against ascarids. Pharmacologic activity is inhibition of glucose uptake from luminal fluid of the nematode gut, which results in an inability of the parasite to produce adenosine triphosphate (ATP). Parasites are expelled over a 2- to 3-day period following treatment. FBZ may also affect fumarate reductase. It is administered in feed over a 3-day period (Corwin et al. 1984). It is approved for the control of *A. suum*, *O. dentatum*, *O. quadrispinulatum*, *H. rubidus*,

Metastrongylus apri, Metastrongylus pudendotectus, T. suis, and *S. dentatus*. No slaughter withdrawal is required. Although approved for *T. suis*, its efficacy is variable (Marti et al. 1978).

Imidazothiazoles. Levamisole was introduced in the late 1960s and demonstrated a broad range of activity in the removal of gastrointestinal, respiratory, and urinary tract nematodes. It has good efficacy against *Ascaris*, *Strongyloides, Hyostrongylus,* and *Oesophagostomum* and low efficacy against *Trichuris* (Marti et al. 1978). It has also demonstrated efficacy against *Stephanurus* (Stewart et al. 1977).

Levamisole has a paralyzing effect by blocking ganglionic transmission, with a rapid expulsion of living worms. It also blocks the metabolic pathway responsible for formation of ATP at the site of fumarate reduction and succinate oxidation. Parasites expelled from the proximal gut are decomposed and may not be apparent in the feces.

Only the hydrochloride form is approved for use in swine and is administered in the feed or water at 8 mg/kg body weight. Levamisole hydrochloride is marketed in a pelleted ready-to-use form with a dehydrated alfalfa carrier or as a powder for use in drinking water. It is intended to be consumed within a 24-hour period. It is highly soluble in water and is rapidly absorbed from the gastrointestinal tract, with 40% excreted in the urine in 12 hours and 41% in the feces over 8 days. It is approved for the control of *A. suum, Oesophagostomum* spp., *Metastrongylus* spp., and *S. ransomi*. It has a 72-hour slaughter withdrawal.

Resistance to levamisole and cross-resistance to pyrantel in swine *Oesophagostomum* spp. has been reported in Denmark (Bjorn et al. 1990).

Organophosphate Compounds. Dichlorvos is the only organophosphate compound approved for use as a swine anthelmintic. It was the first broad-spectrum compound for use in swine, with good efficacy against *Ascaris, Oesophagostomum, Trichuris,* and *Hyostrongylus* with slightly lower efficacy against *Strongyloides* (Marti et al. 1978).

Dichlorvos inhibits nematode cholinesterase, leading to interference with neuromuscular transmission (Knowles and Cassida 1966). Nematode cholinesterase is removed by complexing with the organophosphate, whereas host cholinesterase may fail to complex, thus providing a margin of safety for the treated host. Dichlorvos is rapidly absorbed from the gastrointestinal tract and detoxified by the liver. Metabolites do not persist as tissue residues. Dichlorvos should not be given within a few days of other organophosphates, other anthelmintics, or modified live virus vaccines. There apparently are no adverse effects upon conception or gestation. The compound causes increased intestinal peristalsis.

Dichlorvos is a unique organophosphate in that it can be incorporated into polyvinyl chloride pellets which allow for slow release of the volatile active ingredient from these undigestible units during passage along the intestinal tract. Slow release allows for continued effect in the cecum, thereby producing the desired removal of whipworms. This also provides greater safety for an otherwise toxic compound, since the host can then detoxify dichlorvos as it is absorbed over a 2- to 3-day period. Dichlorvos is administered in the feed, mixed with one-third the regular ration. The recommended dose is 11.2–21.6 mg/kg body weight. It is approved for the control of *A. suum, Oesophagostomum* spp., *T. suis,* and *Ascarops strongylina*. There is no slaughter withdrawal when used at the recommended dosages.

Tetrahydropyrimidines. Pyrantel tartrate is the only tetrahydropyrimidine approved for swine and was introduced as a broad-spectrum anthelmintic compound in 1966. It is efficacious in the removal of adult and infective larval stages of *Ascaris, Oesophagostomum,* and *Hyostrongylus*.

Pyrantel acts as a neuromuscular blocking agent by depolarization of synapses. The musculature contracts irreversibly. The powdered premix is given at a single therapeutic dose level of 22 mg/kg body weight with an overnight fast or as a prophylactic measure at 96 g/ton of feed. For maximum effect against luminal forms, it is administered dry in the feed to minimize absorption. It is most commonly used as a continuous dewormer in feed for starter and growing pigs and is given in combination with carbadox, which promotes growth. It has a great margin of safety and can be used concurrently with organophosphate insecticides. It is not recommended for use in severely debilitated animals because of more pronounced nicotinic activity. It is approved for the control of *A. suum* and *Oesophagostomum* spp., an aid in the prevention of larval migration and establishment of *A. suum*, and an aid in the prevention of establishment of *Oesophagostomum*. There is a 24-hour slaughter withdrawal. Resistance of swine *Oesophagostomum* spp. has been reported in Denmark (Roepstorff et al. 1987).

Piperazine Salts. An older generation of antiparasitic drugs includes piperazine salts. Piperazine compounds are still widely used, being efficacious in removal of ascarids and nodular worms. Up to 100% of the lumen-dwelling stages may be eliminated with a single treatment, but mature worms are more susceptible than earlier stages. A second treatment is recommended 2 months later to remove emerging larval stages.

Piperazine is a diethylenediamine, with the hexahydrate formed in water. It is readily absorbed from the proximal region of the gastrointestinal tract. Some of the base is metabolized in tissues, with 30–40% excreted in the urine. The pharmacologic effect is an anticholinergic action at the myoneural junction, producing a neuromuscular block. In addition, succinic acid production is inhibited. These combined activities produce an overall narcotic effect. Affected parasites are passively removed by intestinal peristalsis and voided live in the host feces. There are no known contraindications, and the compound can be given to animals with gastrointestinal distress.

Piperazine salts are administered in the feed or water. For example, piperazine citrate is given as a 1-day medication in feed, and the hexahydrate form is used in drinking water because of its suitability for storage in solution. Medicated feed or water should be consumed in an 8- to 12-hour period; therefore, withholding feed or water the previous night is beneficial. The recommended dosage is 275–440 mg/kg body weight. It is approved for the control of *A. suum* and *Oesophagostomum* spp. There is a 21-day slaughter withdrawal.

REFERENCES

References to publications prior to 1975 cited in the text are not included but can be found in the 8th edition of this book.

Batte EG. 1977. Evaluation of fenbendazole as a swine anthelmintic. Vet Med Small Anim Clin 73:1183–1186.

Batte EG, McLamb RD, Vestal TJ. 1975. Swine parasites: Causes of liver condemnation. Vet Med Small Anim Clin 70:809–812.

Bjorn H, Roepstorff A, Waller PJ, Nansen P. 1990. Resistance to levamisole and cross-resistance between pyrantel and levamisole in *Oesophagostomum quadrispinulatum* and *Oesophagostomum dentatum* of pigs. Vet Parasitol 37:21–30.

Campbell WC. 1988. Trichinosis revisited—Another look at modes of transmission. Parasitol Today 4:83–86.

Corwin RM, Pratt SE, Muser RK. 1984. Evaluation of fenbendazole as as extended anthelmintic treatment regimen for swine. J Am Vet Med Assoc 185:58–59.

Despommier DD. 1990. *Trichinella spiralis*: The worm that would be a virus. Parasitol Today 6:193–196.

Eriksen L. 1982. Experimentally induced resistance to *Ascaris suum* in pigs. Nord Vet Med 34:177–1887.

Gamble HR, Anderson WR, Graham CE, Murrell KD. 1983. Diagnosis of swine trichinosis by enzyme-linked immunosorbent assay (ELISA) using an excretory-secretory antigen. Vet Parasitol 13:349–361.

Gamble HR, Murrell KD, Marti HP. 1986. Inoculation of pigs against *Trichinella spiralis*, using larval excretory-secretory antigens. Am J Vet Res 47:2396–2399.

Geenen PL, Bresciani J, Boes J, Pedersen A, Eriksen L, Fagerholm H-P, Nansen P. 1999. The morphogenesis of *Ascaris suum* to the infective third stage larvae within the egg. J Parasitol 85:616–622.

Hale OM, Marti OG. 1983. Infuence of an experimental infection of swine kidney worm (*Stephanurus dentatus*) on performance of pigs. J Anim Sci 56:616–620.

Hale OM, Stewart TB, Marti OG. 1985. Influence of an experimental infection of *Ascaris suum* on performance of pigs. J Anim Sci 60:220–225.

Hanbury RD, Doby BP, Miller HO, Murrell KD. 1986. Trichinosis in a herd of swine: Cannibalism as a major mode of transmission. J Am Vet Med Assoc 188:1155–1159.

James ER. 1989. ICT7: The 1988 *Trichinella* Olympics. Parasitol Today 5:66–67.

Johnson JC Jr, Stewart TB, Hale OM. 1975. Differential response of Duroc, Hampshire, and crossbred pigs to a superimposed infection with the intestinal threadworm, *Strongyloides ransomi*. J Parasitol 61:517–524.

Kazacos KR. 1986. Trichinosis. J Am Vet Med Assoc 188:1272–1275.

Kazacos KR, Gamble HR, Brown J. 1986. Field evaluation of the enzyme-linked immunosorbent assay for swine trichinosis: Efficacy of the excretory-secretory antigen. Am J Vet Res 47:1046–1049.

Kennedy TJ, Bruce DJ, Marchiondo AA, et al. 1988. Prevalence of swine parasites in major hog producing areas of the United States. Agri-Pract 9:25–32.

Kim WC. 1983. Geographic distribution and prevalence. pp.445–500. In Trichinella and Trichinosis. WC Campbell, ed. New York: Plenum Press.

Levine ND. 1980. Nematode Parasites of Domestic Animals and of Man. 2d. Ed. Minneapolis: Burgess Publishing Co., p. 477.

Logan NB, Weatherley AJ, Jones RM. 1996. Activity of doramectin against nematodes and arthropod parasites of swine. Vet Parasitol 66:87–94.

Mansfield LS, Urban JF. The pathogenesis of necrotic proliferative colitis in swine is linked to whipworm induced suppression of mucosal immunity to resident bacteria. Vet Imm Immunopath 50:1–17.

Marti OG, Stewart TB, Hale OM. 1978. Comparative efficacy of fenbendazole, dichlorvos, and levamisole HCL against Gastrointestinal nematodes of pigs. J Parasitol 64(6):1028–1031.

McLean JP, Vialett J, Law C, Staudt M. 1989. Trichinosis in the Canadian Arctic: Report of five outbreaks and a new clinical syndrome. J Inf Dis 160:513–520.

Moncol DJ. 1975. Supplement to the life history of *Strongyloides ransomi* Schwartz and Alicata ,1930 (Nematoda: Strongyloididae) of pigs. Proc Helminthol Soc Wash 42:86–92.

Murrell KD. 1985. Strategies for the control of human trichinosis transmitted by pork. Food Technol 39:65–68.

Murrell KD, Anderson WR, Schad GA, Hanbury RD, Nansen P, Larsen M, Roepstorff A, Gronvold J, Wolstrup J, Henriksen SA. 1996. Control of *Oesophagostomum dentatum* and *Hyostrongylus rubidus* in outdoor-reared pigs by daily feeding with microfungus *Duddingtonia flagrans*. Parasitol Res 82:580–584.

Murrell KD, Urban JF Jr. 1983. Induction of immunity by transcolostrally-passed *Strongyloides ransomi* larvae in neonatal pigs. J Parasitol 69:74–77.

Oliver DG, Hanbury RD, Van Houwellin CD. 1985. Proc 89th Annu Meet US Anim Health Assoc, Milwaukee.

Preston KS, Switzer WP. 1976. Failure of lungworm-larvae-infected earthworms to transmit mycoplasmal pneumonia in swine. Vet Microbiol 1:15–18.

Roepstorff A, Bjorn H, Nansen P. 1987. Resistance of *Oesophagostomum* spp. in pigs to pyrantel citrate. Vet Parasitol 24:229–239.

Schad GA, Leiby DA, Duffy DH, Murrell KD. 1985. Swine trichinosis in New England slaughterhouses. Am J Vet Res 46:2008–2010.

Schad GA, Leiby DA, Murrell KD. 1984. Distribution, prevalence and intensity of *Trichinella spiralis* infection in furbearing mammals of Pennsylvania. J Parasitol 70:372–377.

Smith HJ, Hawkes AR. 1978. Kidney worm infection in feral pigs in Canada with transmission to domestic swine. Can Vet J 19:30–43.

Southern LL, Stewart TB, Bodak-Koszalka E, Leon DL, Hoyt PG, Bessette ME. 1989. Effect of fenbendazole and pyrantel tartrate on the induction of protective immunity in pigs naturally or experimentally infected with *Ascaris suum*. J Anim Sci 67:628–634.

Stankiewicz M, Jeska EL. 1990. Evaluation of pyrantel-tartrate abbreviated *Ascaris suum* infections for development of resistance in young pigs against migrating larvae. Int J Parasitol 20:77–81.

Stewart TB. 1996. Losing millions to the insidious parasites. Pigs, June, pp.6–7.

Stewart TB, Batte EG, Connell HE, Corwin RM, Ferguson DL, Gamble HR, Murrell KD, Prestwood AK, Stuart BP, Wheat BE. 1985a. Research needs and priorities for swine internal parasites in the United States. Am J Vet Res 46:1029–1033.

Stewart TB, Fincher GT, Marti OG, McCormick WC. 1977. Efficacy of levamisole against the swine kidney worm, Stephanurus dentatus. J Am Vet Med Assoc 38(12):2081–2083.

Stewart TB, Fox MC, Wiles SE. 1996a. Doremectin efficacy against gastrointestinal nematodes of pigs. Vet Parasitol 66:101–108.

——. 1996b. Doramectin efficacy against the kidney worm, *Stephanurus dentatus in sows*. Vet Parasitol 66:95–99.

Stewart TB, Gasbarre LC. 1989. The veterinary importance of nodular worms (*Oesophagostomum* spp.). Parasitol Today 5:209–213.

Stewart TB, Hale OM. 1988. Losses to internal parasites in swine production. J Anim Sci 66:1548–1554.

Stewart TB, Hale OM, Johnson JC. 1969. Failure of parasitized gilt and barrow pigs on different planes of nutrition to respond alike to a superimposed infection with *Strongyloides ransomi*. J Parasitol 55:1055–1062.

Stewart TB, Hale OM, Marti OG. 1985b. Experimental infections with *Hyostrongylus rubidus* and the effects on performance of growing pigs. Vet Parasitol 17:219–227.

Stewart TB, Rowell TJ. 1986. Susceptibility of fourth-stage *Ascaris suum* larvae to fenbendazole and to host response in the pig. Am J Vet Res 47:1671–1673.

Stewart TB, Southern LL, Gibson RB, Simmons LA. 1985c. Immunization of pigs against *Ascaris suum* by sequential experimental infections terminated with fenbendazole during larval migration. Vet Parasitol 17:319–326.

Stewart TB, Wiles SE, Miller JE, Rulli RD. 1999. Efficacy of moxidectin 0.5% pour-on against swine nematodes. Vet Parasitol 87:39–44.

Urban JF Jr, Alizadeh HA, Romanowski RD. 1984. Acquired gut immunity to the large roundworm (*Ascaris suum*) of swine. Proc Int Congr Pig Vet S 8:2001.

——. 1988. *Ascaris suum*: Development of intestinal immunity to infective second-stage larvae in swine. Exp Parasitol 66:66.

Urban JF Jr, Romanowski RD, Steele NC. 1989. Influence of helminth parasite exposure and strategic application of anthelmintics on the development of immunity and growth of swine. J Anim Sci 67:1668–1677.

U.S. Dept Health and Human Services (USDHHS). 1976. Public Health Services, Centers for Disease Control, Atlanta, Georgia. Morb Mortal Wkly Rep 25:393.

——. 1982.Public Health Services, Centers for Disease Control, Atlanta, Georgia, Morb Mortal Wkly Rep 31:61.

——. 1988. Public Health Services, Centers for Disease Control, Atlanta, Georgia, Morb Mortal Wkly Rep 37:1–8. Control, Atlanta, Georgia. Morb Mortal Wkly Rep 37:1–8.

Wright KA. 1979. *Trichinella spiralis*: An intracellular parasite in the intestinal phase. J Parasitol 65:441–445.

56 Occurrence of Mycotoxins in Grains and Feeds

G. D. Osweiler

Mycotoxins are secondary metabolites of mold growth in grains or forages. They result from stress or altered conditions of fungal growth related to a variety of plant and environmental factors. Most mycotoxin problems in veterinary medicine involve the feed grains (e.g., corn, wheat, milo, cottonseed). Fungal growth requires a readily available carbohydrate (supplied by grains), adequate moisture, oxygen, and appropriate temperatures (often 12–25°C; Wilson and Abramson 1992). Plant or fungal stressors (e.g., drought, high ambient temperatures, insect damage, mechanical harvest damage, and reduced plant vigor) predispose crop plants to infestation by toxigenic fungi with subsequent mycotoxin production (Richard and Cole 1989; Ominski et al. 1994). Environmental and plant stress factors are sometimes used by plant pathologists to predict mold infestations and probable mycotoxin production.

Although specific fungi are associated with mycotoxin formation, simple visual or cultural examination of grain or feed cannot be used to determine safety for animals. Many toxigenic strains of molds can occur in grains without the production of mycotoxins, and there is little correlation between spore counts or degree of fungal growth and presence of mycotoxins. Conversely, absence of molds does not mean that a feed is safe from mycotoxins, since high temperature and pressure during milling may reduce fungal populations so that mold growth is not apparent. However, the common mycotoxins are resistant to the temperatures that kill molds and may persist in feeds when there is no evidence of fungal contamination (Osweiler et al. 1985).

Two general categories of fungi recognized are field fungi and storage fungi (Christensen and Kaufmann 1965; Wilson and Abramson 1992). Field fungi grow in crops prior to harvest. Fusarium spp. are recognized as a source of common mycotoxins. They require high relative humidity (>70%) and grain moisture (>23%) for growth. Field fungi often cause death of ovules, shriveling of seeds or kernels, and weakening or death of embryos. The grading term for this effect is "weathering."

The field fungi grow poorly after harvest because storage to prevent spoilage precludes these conditions, and growth and toxin production appear not to occur readily if dry grain is remoistened (Christensen and Kaufmann 1965).

Storage fungi include the genera Aspergillus and Penicillium, which account for several mycotoxins important in swine production. These fungi may grow and produce mycotoxins even when moisture content ranges from 14–18% and at temperatures that vary from 10–50°C. Aspergillus flavus, normally considered a storage fungus, often produces significant concentrations of aflatoxin in crops prior to harvest.

Mycotoxins occur sporadically both seasonally and geographically (Pier 1981). Certain geographic regions are considered at high risk for specific mycotoxins. This regional predilection may be strongly influenced, however, by local conditions such as early frost, drought, and insect damage. In addition, long-distance transport of grains and finished feeds, as well as blending of grains, damage in transit, and improper storage, can obscure regional differences.

Environmental and management conditions may influence mycotoxin production and animal exposure to mycotoxins. Mycotoxin concentrations are higher in grain that is damaged, light, or broken, which occurs, for example, in screenings. When screenings are fed on the farm or sold locally at harvest time, there may be increased exposure to high concentrations of mycotoxins; grain producers who also have a farrowing operation may give lower-quality grain to sows for short periods of time during harvest. Grain that is slightly above optimum moisture for storage may continue to respire and produce water; eventually a portion of the storage bin will achieve free-moisture levels supportive of mold growth and toxin production. Alternating warm and cool temperatures during fall and spring may favor moisture migration and condensation within a storage bin. Each time a fungal-contaminated grain is cracked or ground, the protective seed coat is broken and the

Table 56.1.   Conditions for Fungal Growth and Synthesis of Common Mycotoxins

Fungal Source	Grains Most Affected	Optimal Temperature	Moisture Requirements	Mycotoxin Produced	Agronomic Influences
Aspergillus flavus *A. parasiticus*	Corn, peanuts, cottonseed, milo	24–35°C	ERH 80–85% EMC 17%	Aflatoxin	Drought, insect damage increase risk
Fusarium roseum	Corn, wheat, barley	7–21°C	EMC 24%	Deoxynivalenol	Alternating warm and cool growing season
Claviceps purpurea	Rye, wheat, triticale, oats, barley	Likely moderate to cool during seed formation	Moist, humid conditions favor production	Ergot	Warm humid conditions, wind and insects favor spread of ergot infection
Fusarium moniliforme *F. proliferatum*	Corn	Likely moderate temperatures <25°C	Probable EMC> 20%	Fumonisin	Dry and hot growing conditions followed by moist autumn
Aspergillus ochraceus *Penicillium viridicatum*	Corn, wheat, barley, rye	12–25°C Can produce toxin at 4°C	ERH 85% EMC 19–22%	Ochratoxin	Lower temperatures favor increase toxin yield
Fusarium sporotrichiodes	Corn, barley, milo, wheat,	8–15°C	EMC 22–26%	T-2 Toxin	Alternating cool and warm conditions; overwintered crops.
Fusarium roseum	Corn, wheat	7–21°C	EMC 24%	Zearalenone	Alternating high and low temperatures during maturation

ERH = Equilibrium Relative Humidity; EMC = Equilibrium Moisture Content.

grain is susceptible to molding. Feed stored in warm, humid conditions such as a nursery may mold and produce mycotoxins within only a few days. Table 56.1 shows the fungi and their growth conditions that favor production of specific mycotoxins.

INTOXICATION BY MYCOTOXINS

The most important factor in toxicosis is access to contaminated grain by a susceptible animal. Dietary deficiencies of protein, selenium, and vitamins have been suggested as predisposing factors in mycotoxicosis, but well-documented examples are rare. Drugs that reduce or enhance foreign-compound metabolism could influence response to mycotoxins, since most common mycotoxins are metabolized to intermediate or final products that differ in toxicity from the parent mycotoxin (Osweiler et al. 1985; Beasley et al. 1986). This type of drug interaction is more likely with aflatoxins and ochratoxin than with the trichothecenes.

Combinations of some mycotoxins may potentiate the action of one another, or at least exert an additive effect. One example of this is the combination of aflatoxin and ochratoxin (Huff et al. 1988; Harvey et al. 1989a). Currently there is little evidence that common mycotoxins act synergistically. Fortunately, conditions for production of several mycotoxins concurrently in the same grain appear to be relatively uncommon.

Some mycotoxins are reported to alter immune function under certain conditions. Aflatoxins, some trichothecenes, and ochratoxin A have been demonstrated to be immunosuppressive in domestic or laboratory animals. Common diseases influenced by aflatoxin under experimental conditions include swine erysipelas,

swine dysentery, and salmonellosis. Generally, immunosuppressive effects of aflatoxins and trichothecenes are seen only at concentrations that cause subtle or chronic changes typical of the mycotoxin. Marin et al. 2002, reported that 4 weeks feeding of 280 ppb aflatoxin reduced weight gain in swine while also increasing leukocyte count and raising serum gamma globulin. This same study demonstrated that immune response to *Mycoplasma agalactiae* was reduced and that cytokine mRNA expression in phytohemagglutinin-stimulated blood cells was associated with decreased proinflammatory factors, IL-1 beta and TNF-alpha, but increased antiinflammatory IL-10 cytokine expression. Because the mycotoxin interaction is usually expressed as the infectious disease, mycotoxin-facilitated disease is difficult to detect or confirm. Normal immune function is expected to return after exposure to the toxin ends (Pier 1981; Panangala et al. 1986; Richard and Cole 1989).

CLINICAL MYCOTOXICOSES

Clinical response of swine to mycotoxins may be acute, subacute, or chronic and is both dose and time dependent, similar to other chemical toxins. For known mycotoxins of clinical importance, response is usually subacute or chronic and the presenting signs are often subtle and vague. Many times problems are expressed only as alterations of the reproductive cycle, reduced feed intake, slow growth, or impaired feed efficiency. Nevertheless, an understanding of the range of effects for specific mycotoxins is important in differential diagnosis and evaluation of clinical prognosis for mycotoxin diseases. Common mycotoxins affecting swine are summarized in Table 56.2.

Table 56.2. Major Features of Mycotoxins That Commonly Affect Swine

Mycotoxin	Most Susceptible	Clinical Effects	Lesions	Diagnostic Specimens and Tests	Therapy and/or Prevention	Residue Concerns
Aflatoxin	Piglets, feeder pigs	Reduced growth, hepatotoxicosis Immune dysfunction	Hepatic necrosis, bile duct hyperplasia	Aflatoxin in feed; AF M1 in liver or urine	Vitamin E and selenium supplements Aluminosilicate in diet	Residues occur in liver and milk for <3 weeks
DON	Feeder pig, Finishers Sows	Feed refusal, reduced growth	Weight loss	DON >1 ppm in diet	Change feed	Not likely to cause residues
Fumonisin	All	Pulmonary edema, dyspnea, cyanosis, 2–4 hrs to death. Abortion in sows. Hepatic damage	Pulmonary edema, hepatosis	Histological lesions of pulmonary edema or hepatosis; FB1 in feed	Change feed; treat for liver damage; avoid grain screenings in diet	Residues brief, most likely in liver and kidney
Diacetoxy-Scirpenol or T-2 Toxin	Feeder pig, Finishers Sows	Feed refusal Diarrhea Leucopenia Oral ulceration Immune suppression	Oral ulcers, gastric ulcers, lymphoid and thymic depletion	Histological lesions of ulceration, lymphopenia, leucopenia, feed analysis	Change feed and treat for diarrhea/ulcers	Not likely to cause residues
Ergot	Sows Nursing pigs	Agalactia with piglet starvation Peripheral gangrene	Piglet starvation Peripheral gangrene	Ergot bodies or alkaloids in urine or diet; peripheral vascular lesions	Avoid ergot in grain	Residues brief, not likely to be significant
Ochratoxin	All	Reduced growth Polydipsia, polyuria, renal failure	Gastric ulcers Pale swollen kidneys	Histological evidence of gastric ulcers and renal tubular damage or fibrosis	Change feed; low protein diet for kidney damage recovery	High probability of persistent residues
Zearalenone	Prepuberal gilts Cycling sows Young boars	Hyperestrogenism in young gilts Pseudopregnancy, delayed cycling, early embryonic death Reduced libido	Vulvovaginitis, Vaginal keratinization Retained Corpora lutea Reduced testicular size	Histological lesion of vaginal keratinization; Elevated serum progesterone; Zearalenone in feed	Change feed; treat gilts for prolapse Administer 10 mg PGF2α to pseudopregnant sows	Rapidly excreted in urine; low residue probability

917

Aflatoxins

Aspergillus flavus and *A. parasiticus* produce aflatoxins in grains and oilseeds both in storage and before harvest. Although many areas of North America have conditions supportive of aflatoxin production, conditions leading to aflatoxin production often occur in the southeastern United States (Richard and Cole 1989).

Aflatoxins B_1, B_2, G_1, and G_2 occur in grains. When Aflatoxin B_1 (AFB$_1$) is metabolized by mammals, it occurs in milk or urine as aflatoxin M_1. Aflatoxin B_1 is the most abundant and most toxic fraction under natural contamination (Jelinik et al. 1989; Richard and Cole 1989).

Aflatoxin B_1 is metabolized by liver microsomal mixed-function oxidases to form at least seven metabolites. The major metabolite of aflatoxin is an epoxide, which binds covalently to nucleic acids and proteins and is believed to be responsible for causing hepatic cancer as well as toxic signs and lesions. Impairment of protein synthesis and subsequent inability to mobilize fats result in characteristic early lesions of hepatic fatty change and necrosis, as well as reduced growth rate. Animals on protein-deficient diets are more susceptible to aflatoxin, and increased dietary protein will protect against aflatoxin effects on weight gain (Coffey et al. 1989).

Toxicity of aflatoxin is affected by dosage, length of exposure, animal species, and age of animal. Acute toxicosis is uncommon. The single oral dose LD50 for swine is 0.62 mg/kg body weight; dietary levels of 2–4 parts per million (ppm) are associated with acute fatal toxicosis, while rations containing 260 ppb for several weeks were associated only with reduced growth rate (Allcroft 1969). Exposure to low or moderate concentrations in feed for several weeks is a common circumstance of exposure. Combined evidence from experimental reports, field cases, and my personal experience suggests that concentrations of naturally occurring aflatoxins above 300 ppb fed for a period of several weeks will likely cause reduced growth and feed efficiency (Allcroft 1969; Cook et al. 1989; Harvey et al. 1988, 1989c; Richard and Cole 1989; Dilkin et al. 2003).

The experimental threshold dietary concentration for clinical effects varies widely. Young swine are more susceptible to aflatoxins than finishing hogs or adults, and mitigating factors may include dietary protein level, vitamin A deficiency, and inadequate selenium intake. Effects of aflatoxins may be both time and dosage dependent. Liver lesions have been reported caused by concentrations as low as 140 ppb fed for 12 weeks in 18–64 kg swine, and 690 ppb was associated with mild liver lesions in 64–91 kg finishing hogs (Allcroft 1969). In my experience, prolonged feeding of aflatoxin at concentrations above 400 ppb can cause microscopic liver lesions. Dilkin et al. 2003, fed 50 (ppb) of Aflatoxin B_1 to weaned piglets for 28 days. Body weight gain and feed consumption were not affected, and there were no gross or microscopic lesions found. In addition, no evidence of changes in complete blood count or clinical chemistry were detected. Marin et al. (2002) fed Aflatoxin B_1 (AFB$_1$) to weanling pigs at 140 and 280 ppb for 28 days. AFB$_1$ at 280 ppb caused significant decrease in weight gain, but caused no effect on total red blood cell count, differential leukocyte count, total globulin, albumins, or total protein concentration in serum. However, gamma globulin was significantly increased at both 140 ppb and 280 ppb. The lower concentration of AFB$_1$ (140 ppb) resulted in reduced average daily gain that was not statistically significant (P <.05). Aflatoxin at 50 ppb when fed concurrently with 30 ppm Fumonisin B_1 (FB$_1$) caused decreased feed consumption and reduced feed conversion (Dilkin et al. 2003), but effects were attributed mainly to FB$_1$. Much higher dietary concentrations of FB$_1$ have resulted in significant clinical and pathological effects. Harvey et al. (1995a, b) fed 2.5 ppm AFB$_1$ to 17.5 kg barrows for 35 days. Body weight, gain, and feed consumption were significantly (P <0.05) decreased by AF. Aflatoxin increased serum gamma glutamyl transferase (GGT) activity and total iron concentration and decreased urea nitrogen concentration and unsaturated iron-binding capacity. Aflatoxin increased relative liver weight and resulted in liver that was pale, rubbery, and resistant to cutting. Characteristic hepatic necrosis and degeneration, accompanied by bile duct proliferation resulted from aflatoxin feeding. When 100 ppm of Fumonisin B_1 (FB$_1$) was fed with 2.5 ppm AFB$_1$, mitogen-induced lymphoblastogenic stimulation index was decreased by aflatoxin and FB$_1$ diets, and the combination diet significantly decreased cell-mediated immunity compared to single toxin diets. Thus AFB$_1$ and FB$_1$ in culture material, singly or in combination, can adversely affect clinical performance, serum biochemical, hematologic, and immunologic values and induce lesions in growing barrows. One should remember that the dosages of this study were very high and do not commonly occur under natural conditions.

Clinical signs of acute to subacute toxicosis are depression and anorexia. Anemia, ascites, icterus, and hemorrhagic diarrhea may develop. Coagulopathy characterized by hypoprothrombinemia may occur. Enzymes associated with hepatocellular damage are elevated, including aspartate aminotransferase, alanine aminotransferase, alkaline phosphatase, and gamma glutamyl transferase. Other serum clinical chemistry changes observed have been decreases in serum total iron-binding capacity, total protein, albumin, cholesterol, blood urea nitrogen, and glucose (Harvey et al. 1989c). Total bilirubin, icterus index, sulfobromophthalein clearance, prothrombin time, and partial thromboplastin time are also elevated in clinical aflatoxicosis (Panangala et al. 1986).

Gross lesions associated with porcine aflatoxicosis include pale tan or clay-colored liver with centrilobular hemorrhages, subserosal petechial to ecchymotic hemorrhages, and intestinal and colonic hemorrhages. As the course of aflatoxicosis progresses, the liver becomes yellow and fibrosis develops, characterized by a firm, hard liver with accentuated lobular pattern. The yellow discoloration of icterus occurs at serosal and mucosal surfaces (Cook et al. 1989; Harvey et al. 1989b).

Microscopic alterations are useful for diagnostic purposes and generally include hepatocyte vacuolization, necrosis, and fatty change, which is more predominant around central veins. As disease progresses to subacute or chronic, hepatomegalocytosis, including multiple nuclei is seen. Interlobular fibrosis and characteristic biliary hyperplasia develop in chronic cases (Cook et al. 1989; Harvey et al. 1988). Full evaluation and diagnosis of aflatoxicosis should include a search for the characteristic lesions.

Significant reproductive effects of aflatoxin in swine have not been documented. Sows fed aflatoxin have maintained normal reproduction through four successive gestations at dietary concentrations of 500 and 700 ppb. Although gestation and farrowing were normal, piglets nursing these sows had reduced growth rate due to aflatoxin excretion in the milk (Armbrecht et al. 1972; McKnight et al. 1983).

Aflatoxins are recognized as immunosuppressive agents in many species. Aflatoxin is an immunomodulating agent that acts primarily on cell-mediated immunity and phagocytic cell function (Bondy and Pestka 2000). Piglets nursing on sows exposed to AFB_1 may be immunocompromised. Sows fed diets containing either 800 or 400 ppb purified AFB_1 throughout gestation and lactation had B_1 and M_1 residues in milk 5 and 25 days after parturition, at approximately 1000-fold lower than that in the feed and with increases during the 25 days after parturition. Lymphoproliferative response to mitogens was reduced and monocyte-derived macrophages failed to efficiently produce superoxide anions after oxidative burst stimulation in vitro. Ability of macrophages to phagocytose red blood cells was not compromised, but granulocytic cells showed a reduction of chemotactic response in vitro to chemoattractant bacteria factor and casein (Silvotti et al. 1997).

Residues of aflatoxin M_1 occur in tissues, milk, and urine of swine but are not persistent. Dietary concentrations of 400 ng/g resulted in tissue residues of 0.05 ppb or less, and these rapidly disappeared when aflatoxin feeding stopped (Trucksess et al. 1982).

Diagnosis of aflatoxicosis should be considered when acute icterus, hemorrhages, or coagulopathy are not explained by other causes. Chronic signs of slow growth, malnutrition, and persistent low-grade infectious diseases should also suggest investigation for aflatoxicosis. Characteristic liver lesions and clinical chemistry changes would strongly suggest aflatoxicosis. Chemical analysis of the ration and grain supply may identify aflatoxin, but sometimes the grain that initiated a chronic problem is no longer available or representative. Any grain sampling should be representative (see the section Prevention and Management of Mold

and Mycotoxin Problems for sampling procedure). Examination of suspect grain sample under ultraviolet light has long been a screening approach. This simple procedure identifies kojic acid, a metabolite produced by aflatoxin-producing fungi. However, it may falsely implicate some samples and should never be relied upon without a confirmatory chemical analysis for AFB_1.

Aflatoxicosis is generally a herd problem and not amenable to individual animal treatment. Specific practical antidotes for affected animals are not available. Work in poultry has shown some benefit from increased dietary selenium. Increased dietary levels of high-quality protein and supplementation with vitamins (A, D, E, K, and B complex) are recommended (Coppock and Swanson 1986; Coffey et al. 1989). Hydrated sodium calcium aluminosilicate (HSCAS) at 0.5% in the diet provided substantial protection against loss of gain and occurrence of lesions induced by dietary aflatoxin in swine (Harvey et al. 1989c). Treatment of grain with anhydrous ammonia for 10–14 days has reduced aflatoxin concentration in grain. Swine accept ammoniated grain and their growth is comparable to controls. Presently, this method of treatment has not been cleared by the U.S. Food and Drug Administration.

Since aflatoxin may compromise the immune system, animals with concurrent infectious diseases should be aggressively treated with appropriate antimicrobial therapy and passive immunization if appropriate. However, specific studies with the antibiotics lincomycin and tylosin added to aflatoxin-contaminated diets neither decreased or enhanced the detrimental effects of aflatoxicosis in growing swine (Harvey et al. 1995b).

Ochratoxin and Citrinin

Ochratoxin is a fungal nephrotoxin produced by *Aspergillus ochraceus* and *Penicillium viridicatum*. Citrinin, also a nephrotoxin, is produced by *P. citrinum*. Based on clinical and pathologic effects in swine, both toxins can be considered together. Toxins are associated with corn, barley, rye, and wheat, most commonly from eastern and northern Europe, Canada, and the northern United States (Jelinik et al. 1989; Juszkiewicz et al. 1992). Significant concentrations of ochratoxin can occur at temperatures as low as 4°C. Ochratoxin A has been prevalent in Denmark and is associated with the feeding of barley and oats (Carlton and Krogh 1979). In the United States, at least one case has been documented in swine fed contaminated corn (Cook et al. 1986). A survey of Romanian slaughter pigs revealed that 98% of serum samples were positive for ochratoxin A (OTA) at concentrations as high as 13.4 ng/g, although 85% of samples contained less than 5 ng OTA per ml. Measurable levels of OTA occurred in 75–80% of swine liver and kidney. (Curturi et al. 2001).

Toxicity appears related to binding of OTA in specific receptors for organic ion transporters of the renal tubule (Huessner et al. 2002). The mechanism of action appears

Table 56.3. Clinical guide to mycotoxins in swine

Toxin	Category of Swine	Dietary Level	Clinical Effect
Aflatoxins	Growing-finishing	<100 ppb	No clinical effect
		200–400 ppb	Reduced growth and feed efficiency; possible immunosuppression
		400–800 ppb	Microscopic liver lesions, cholangiohepatitis; increased serum liver enzymes; immunosuppression
		800–1200 ppb	Reduced growth; decreased feed consumption, rough hair coat; icterus, hypoproteinemia
	Brood sows and gilts	>2000 ppb	Acute hepatosis and coagulopathy; deaths in 3–10 days
		500–750 ppb	No effect on conception; deliver normal piglets that grow slowly due to aflatoxin in milk
Ochratoxin and Citrinin	Finishing	200 ppb	Mild renal lesions seen at slaughter; reduced weight gain
		1000 ppb	Polydipsia; reduced growth; azotemia and glycosuria
		4000 ppb	Polydipsia and polyuria
	Sows and gilts	3–9 ppm	Normal pregnancy when fed first month
Trichothecenes T-2 and DAS	Growing-finishing	1 ppm	No effect
		3 ppm	Decreased feed consumption
		10 ppm	Decreased feed consumption; oral/dermal irritation; immunosuppression
		20 ppm	Complete feed refusal, vomiting
Deoxynivalenol (DON, vomitoxin)	Growing-finishing	1 ppm	No clinical effect; minimal (10%) reduction in feed consumption
		5–10 ppm	25–50% reduction in feed consumption; taste aversion to same diet
		20 ppm	Complete feed refusal
Zearalenone	Prepuberal gilts	1–3 ppm	Estrogenic; vulvovaginitis, prolapse in prepuberal gilts
	Cycling sows and gilts	3–10 ppm	Retained corpora lutea; anestrous; pseudopregnancy
	Pregnant sows	>30 ppm	Early embryonic death when fed 1–3 weeks post mating
Ergot	All swine	0.1%	Reduced weight gain
	Sows last trimester	0.3%	Gangrene of ears, tail, feed
		3.0%	Decreased feed consumption
		0.3%	Agalactia, reduced piglet birth weight; piglet starvation
Fumonisins	All swine	25 ppm	Minimal changes in clinical chemistry – increased AST, AP
		50–75 ppm	Minimal reduction in feed intake; possible mild hepatosis
		75–100 ppm	Reduced feed intake, reduced weight gain; hepatosis with icterus and increased bilirubin and GGT
		>100 ppm	Acute pulmonary edema after 3–5 days consumption; survivors develop hepatosis

to result from a combination of inhibition of phenylalanine metabolizing enzymes, inhibition of adenosine triphosphate (ATP) production, and accumulation of lipid peroxidation (Marquardt and Frohlich 1992). Resulting effects on protein synthesis may be related to inhibition of phenylalanine metabolism. Immunosuppressive effects are associated with a combination of suppressed lymphocyte proliferation and interference with the complement system (Bondy and Pestka 2000).

In swine, principal effects are manifest on proximal renal tubules. Ochratoxin A at 1 mg/kg body weight is lethal in 5–6 days. Concentrations of 1 ppm in the diet for 3 months cause polydipsia, polyuria, reduced growth, and lowered feed efficiency. Levels as low as 200 ppb for several weeks cause detectable renal lesions. Additional clinical signs are diarrhea, anorexia, and dehydration. Sometimes no clinical signs are noted and the only effect observed is the appearance of pale, firm kidneys at slaughter, commonly associated with ochratoxin in endemic areas such as Denmark and Sweden.

Clinical pathology changes include increases in blood urea nitrogen, plasma protein, packed-cell volume, aspartate aminotransferase, and isocitric dehydrogenase, as well as increased urinary glucose and protein.

Citrinin, ochratoxin, and penicillic acid are synergistic and primarily produce nephrosis characterized by necrosis of the proximal convoluted tubules, followed by interstitial fibrosis. Liver damage, characterized by fatty change and necrosis, may be present but is less severe than for other primary hepatoses. Gastric ulceration is a characteristic and consistent lesion in prolonged clinical cases (Szczech et al. 1973; Carlton and Krogh 1979). Boars given 20 μg OTA per os for 6 weeks had reduced ejaculation volume, initial viability, and progressive motility. Viability, initial forward motility, and motility after 24 hours were significantly reduced during a 24-hour storage period (Biro et al. 2003).

Diagnosis should include demonstration of the toxin and/or its metabolite, ochratoxin alpha, in feed or fresh kidney. A simple HPLC method recently reported can detect from 0.3–3 ng ochratoxin A or B (Curturi and Gareis 2001). The approximate half-life for ochratoxin A in swine tissue is 3–5 days, and little or no ochratoxin can be found in kidneys 30 days after ochratoxin exposure ceases (Carlton and Krogh 1979). Mildly affected animals may recover if removed promptly from the contaminated feed. However, if the clinical course is prolonged, recovery is slow.

Trichothecenes

The trichothecenes include at least 148 structurally related compounds. Those of known veterinary importance are produced by Fusaria, especially *F. graminearum* and *F. sporotrichioides*. This group of sesquiterpene toxins has an epoxide group that is responsible for most toxic effects. The three receiving most attention world wide are T-2 toxin, diacetoxyscirpenol (DAS), and deoxynivalenol (DON, vomitoxin). Even though much work has been done with the macrocyclic trichothecenes, T-2 and DAS, in swine, they rarely occur at toxic concentrations in North American grains.

Trichothecenes are metabolized in two phases. Initially (phase 1) oxidation and hydrolysis create transformation products that are then conjugated with glucuronic acid. In phase 2 the epoxide ring of trichothecenes is cleaved by gastrointestinal microflora (Bauer 1995; Beasley et al. 1986). Deoxynivalenol undergoes no extensive metabolism; only deoxynivalenol glucuronide and the de-epoxide product are produced. Serum, bile, and urine may contain DON after experimental feeding of as little as 4.3 ppm dietary DON. However, de-epoxy DON is found only in urine (Doll et al. 2003). The glucuronide is rapidly excreted, mainly in urine, and does not accumulate in plasma (Eriksen et al. 2003).

Trichothecenes can cause direct skin irritation and necrosis, profound lymphoid depletion, gastroenteritis, diarrhea, shock, cardiovascular failure, and death from experimental direct dosing. Chronic administration causes hematopoietic suppression and eventual pancytopenia. In addition, they are immunosuppressants (Coppock et al. 1985; Beasley 1993; Lundeen et al. 1986). Although T-2 and DAS are potent toxins, their strong tendency to induce feed refusal and/or vomiting in swine makes them somewhat self-limiting as toxins, except as potential causes of reduced feed consumption.

DON has great economic importance in world wide feed grain use because it is established as a common mycotoxin of corn, barley and wheat and is well documented as a cause of feed refusal or reduced feed intake in swine (Trenholm et al. 1984; Russell et al. 1990; Bohm 1992; Bergsjo et al. 1993; Rotter et al. 1996). In corn, DON occurs at low levels during some harvest seasons, with an incidence as high as 50%. Grain contamination in other grains and in other parts of the world also occurs (Hietaniemi and Kumpulainen 1991). Swine begin to reduce voluntary feed consumption at DON concentrations of 1 ppm or more, and feed refusal may be complete at concentrations in excess of 10 ppm (Young et al. 1983; Pollman et al. 1985; Bohm 1992; Bergsjo et al. 1992; Rotter et al. 1996).

Many studies have demonstrated only feed refusal with concurrent health effects in swine that are consistent with effects of reduced nutrient intake (Lun et al. 1985). Among a variety of blood chemistry parameters in pigs fed DON, only alpha-globulin and possibly cortisol were altered in animals fed diets containing DON. Other sporadic differences appeared to be due to differences in feed intake; hematologic and blood chemistry tests are of limited value in diagnosing low-level dietary DON in swine (Prelusky et al. 1994a). At low dosages of DON, hematological, clinical, and immunological changes are transitory and decrease as compensatory/adaptation mechanisms are established (Rotter et al. 1994). Effects of a 3.5 mg DON/kg diet included increased liver weights, decreased serum proteins and albumin, and a temporary fall in packed-blood-cell volume, serum calcium, and serum phosphorus. No other effects on hematological, biochemical, or immunological parameters occurred (Bergsjo et al. 1993). Diets containing 3.0 mg DON/kg fed for 28 days appeared associated with increased skin temperature, depressed feed intake, reduction in thyroid size, and apparent hyperplasia and increased mucosal folding of the esophageal portion of the stomach. Serum T4 (thyroxine) levels were increased at 7 and 28 days of exposure. Other changes reported were elevated serum albumin levels, decreased alpha-globulin levels, increased albumin/globulin ratio, and delayed titer response to immunization with sheep red blood cells. An increase in the segmented neutrophil count was observed (Rotter et al. 1994).

Recent work has shown that DON in swine causes conditioned taste aversion, and flavoring agents will be ineffective in inducing swine to consume contaminated grain (Osweiler et al. 1990). Others have shown that T-2 toxin, closely related to DON, may affect brain neurotransmitters, such as serotonin or dopamine, contributing to feed refusal and lethargy (MacDonald et al. 1988). A number of studies have implicated changes in brain neurochemistry as a factor in feed refusal and/or vomiting induced by DON or T-2 toxin. Central serotoninergic (5-hydroxytryptamine [5HT]) pathways are believed to be involved in the mechanisms of anorexia and/or emesis evoked by DON (Prelusky et al. 1992). Low-level DON exposure (30 μg/kg intragastric [IG]) caused a rapid and sustained increase in cerebrospinal fluid 5-hydroxyindoleacetic acid (5HIAA) for up to 20 hours post dosing, indicating that elevated brain serotonin turnover related to DON exposure is important in the decreased feed intake of animals fed DON (Prelusky 1993, 1996). DON causes elevated norepinephrine and depressed dopamine concentrations, while levels of 5HT increase initially and then drop significantly at 8 hours. However, DON has only weak affinity for 5HT receptors, suggesting that relatively high concentrations of the toxin are needed for this effect, and there may be other mechanisms of interaction with serotoninergic receptors at the central level. Feeding grain contaminated with 5.5 ppm DON and 0.5 ppm 15-acetyl DON, 26.8 ppm Fusaric Acid, and 0.4 ppm zearalenone caused an expected reduction in feed intake and weight gain (Swamy et al. 2002). In addition, there were significantly reduced concentrations of dopamine in the hypothalamus and pons as well as concentration of dihydroxyindoleacetic acid and norepinephrine in the pons. Prelusky (1997) found that infusion of DON by intraperitoneal osmotic pump caused a more prolonged and sustained decrease in weight gain than an equivalent dietary exposure. Pigs fed DON tend to recover weight gain significantly after the initial 3 days of exposure to dietary DON. This was interpreted as evidence that the effect of DON on weight gain is due to more than just reduced feed intake. Although several neurochemical changes caused by DON are compatible with known neurochemical changes for chemical-induced anorexia, the feed refusal effects of acute DON exposure need further clarification.

Diagnosis of mycotoxin-related feed refusal presents a difficult problem to the clinician. Other toxins, drugs, concurrent disease, inclement weather, and reduced water intake may contribute to feed refusal. There is no apparent detectable effect of DON on plasma levels of brain neurotransmitters at DON doses that cause vomiting in swine. Thus, sampling of peripheral blood would not predict the central serotoninergic effects associated with DON toxicosis (Prelusky 1994). Since trichothecenes are rapidly metabolized, diagnosis by analysis of tissue or blood samples is rarely possible or practical. Fortunately, due to rapid metabolism and excretion, significant residues of trichothecene mycotoxins in edible swine tissues are unlikely (Bauer 1995). Often the DON concentration detected chemically in feed is insufficient to fully explain feed refusal. One should remember that feed concentrations are approximations, that sampling is never completely representative, and that many factors in the herd and environment may not be apparent to either the clinician or the producer.

Treatment of DON toxicosis with drugs has been studied very little. Antiemetics that are specific serotonin (5HT)-receptor antagonists (ICS 205-930, BRL 43694 A) have been shown to prevent DON-induced vomiting in swine. Anticholinergic compounds were moderately effective at high dosages by acting directly at the emetic center. However, antihistaminic and antidopaminergic antiemetics without anticholinergic activity were not effective anti-emetics against DON (Prelusky and Trenholm 1993).

Attempts to prevent DON effects have centered on feeding adsorbents or on chemical or physical means of detoxification. These have included calcium aluminosilicate, bentonite, and sodium bisulfite. None of these have been successful in an economic and practical way. Recently, Avantaggiato et al. (2004) have shown in an in vitro gastrointestinal model significant reduction in intestinal absorption of DON and Nivalenol. With 2% activated carbon (charcoal) there was a reduction of absorption from 51% to 28% for DON and from 21% to 12% for Nivalenol. If the in vitro model is confirmed effective in feeding trials, this could offer another alternative to adsorption prophylaxis against DON. Feeding of yeast cell wall polymer (a glucomannan polymer, GM polymer) prevented some of the known effects of trichothecenes on brain neurochemistry and serum Ig concentrations (Swamy et al. 2002). Another novel detoxification method was described in which contents of the large intestine of chickens (CLIC) incorporated into swine diets reduced the feed refusal effects of 2.1 ppm dietary DON (He et al. 1993). Anaerobic incubation of swine colonic contents with DON demonstrated degradation of the epoxide ring of DON (Kollarczik et al. 1994). Additional data (Eriksen et al. 2002) has shown that different gastrointestinal microfloras of swine have different capacities to metabolize trichothecenes. They found that intestinal de-epoxidation ability is common on some Swedish swine farms, and that this characteristic may be transferred between pigs in a herd. These studies may suggest future means for management or prevention of the feed refusal effects from DON. Physical decontamination of deoxynivalenol from barley was recently demonstrated by use of an abrasive pearling procedure, which removed 66% of DON with loss of only 15% of the grain mass (House et al. 2003). This method could provide a practical means for reducing DON contamination to a manageable level in years of widespread crop contamination.

Zearalenone (F-2 Toxin)

Fusarium graminearum (F. roseum) produces zearalenone, an estrogenic mycotoxin in corn, milo, and wheat. *Fusarium roseum* can produce either zearalenone or deoxynivalenol (Diekman and Green 1992). High moisture (23–25%) is required for growth. Under laboratory conditions, optimum production of zearalenone occurs when *F. graminearum* is incubated at a water activity $(a[w]) = 0.97$ for 2 weeks at 28°C followed by 4 weeks at 12°C (Jimenez et al. 1996). Poorly dried ear corn and alternating high and low ambient temperatures favor zearalenone production (Christensen and Kaufmann 1965). Often it is produced in the field prior to harvest.

Zearalenone is a substituted resorcyclic acid lactone similar in structure to the anabolic agent zearanol used in cattle. As an estrogen, zearalenone binds competitively to estrogen receptors of the uterus, mammary gland, liver, and hypothalamus. It will cause hypertrophy of the uterus and cornification of vaginal epithelium. Zearalenone is rapidly absorbed from the intestine and is metabolized to alpha- and beta-zearalenol and alpha- and beta-zearalanol and then conjugated with glucuronic acid for excretion in bile and urine (Gajecki 2002; Meyer et al. 2000).

Clinical signs vary with dosage and age of swine exposed. In prepuberal gilts, concentrations as low as 1–5 ppm in the ration cause vulvovaginitis, which is characterized by tumescence and edema of the vulva and vagina and precocious mammary development. Tenesmus is common, occasionally with resultant rectal prolapses (Osweiler 2000). Zearalenone at clinically effective dosage in sexually immature gilts is reported to have caused ovarian follicle atresia and apoptotic-like changes in granule cells. Intensified cell proliferation was observed in both uterus and oviduct (Obremski et al. 2003). Prepuberal gilts fed 2 ppm for up to 90 days attained normal sexual maturity with no adverse effects on subsequent reproductive function (Green et al. 1990; Rainey et al. 1990).

Reproductive effects of zearalenone on mature cycling sows are quite different from the effects seen in prepuberal gilts. As with other estrogens, zearalenone is luteotropic in swine, and dietary concentrations of 3–10 ppm can induce anestrus in sows if consumed during the middle portion of the estrous cycle. Since estrogens are luteotropic in swine, the probability of abortion in the last two trimesters of gestation appears very unlikely. Anestrus and elevated serum progesterone persist for several months; long after exposure to zearalenone has stopped (Edwards et al. 1987).

Fewer pigs per litter are seen in sows given high dietary concentrations of zearalenone. The susceptible period for reduced litter size appears to be in the preimplantation stage at 7–10 days post-mating (Long et al. 1983; Diekman and Long 1989). Zearalenone fed at 1 mg zearalenone/kg body weight (equivalent to approximately 60 ppm dietary zearalenone) on days 7 through 10 after mating resulted in mild blastocyst degeneration by day 11 and advanced degeneration by day 13. Viability of individual embryos is apparently not maintained beyond 21 days. During this time period zearalenone did not cause morphologic changes in the endometrium that could be associated with hyperestrogenism (height of the endometrial luminal epithelium and morphology of secretory vesicles in the endometrial glandular epithelium) (Long et al. 1992). Zearalenone at 22.1 ppm in the ration of breeding gilts caused a decrease in the number of corpora lutea, a decrease in ovarian weight, a decrease in the number of live embryos, and an increase in the number of deadborn piglets and abortions (Kordic et al. 1992).

Piglets born to sows receiving zearalenone may have enlarged external genitalia and uteri. Zearalenone and its metabolites, alpha and beta zearalenol, are present in milk of exposed sows and may contribute to estrogenic effects in piglets (Palyusik et al. 1980; Dacasto et al. 1995). A perinatal hyperestrogenic syndrome reported in swine herds and by experimental verification included lower conception rate, increased numbers of repeat breeders, decreased litter size, and increased numbers of stillbirths. Clinical signs in neonatal gilts were swelling of the vulva and teats and edematous infiltration of the perineal region, ventral abdomen, and umbilicus, usually accompanied by exudative, crusted inflammation and necrosis of the teats. An increase in splayleg and trembling piglets has been reported. Lesions of hyperestrogenism included enlargement of

the ovary and uterus, ovarian follicle maturation, glandular proliferation of the endometrium, and epithelial proliferation in the vagina (Vanyi et al. 1994). Swine diets containing 2 ppm zearalenone from day 30 of gestation through weaning did not adversely affect reproduction in sows. Estrogenic effects on testes and on uterine and ovarian weights were observed in the piglets at 21 days of age, but subsequent breeding performance was not affected (Yang et al. 1995).

Preputial enlargement may occur in boars exposed to zearalenone. Young boars may have reduced libido and decreased testicular size, but mature boars are unaffected by concentrations of zearalenone as high as 200 ppm (Ruhr et al. 1983; Young and King 1983).

Differential diagnosis of zearalenone toxicosis should include estrogenic feed additives and natural estrogens such as coumestrol in mature alfalfa. Suspect rations of corn should first be analyzed for the presence of zearalenone, then for other estrogens. Feed samples available at the time of anestrus or return to service may not represent the contaminated feed that initiated the problem.

Treatment of zearalenone toxicosis depends on the nature of the effect and the age and reproductive status of swine. Removal of the feed from prepuberal gilts will allow regression of signs within 3–7 days. Medical and surgical treatment of vaginal and rectal prolapse may be necessary. For mature, nongravid sows with anestrus, administration of one 10 mg dose of prostaglandin $F_{2\alpha}$ or two 5 mg doses on successive days is useful in eliminating retained corpora lutea (B. N. Day, personal communication, 1982; Green et al. 1991). Dehydrated alfalfa has experimentally shown some protection from zearalenone-induced enlargement of the uterus of gilts (James and Smith 1982; Smith 1992), although the high concentrations needed (>20%) are not considered practical in swine diets. Activated charcoal or cholestyramine has been used at 2% in an in vitro gastrointestinal model system to evaluate its binding effect on zearalenone. Both activated charcoal and cholestyramine reduced absorption of zearalenone from 32% to 5% and 16%, respectively (Avantaggiato et al. 2003). The dramatic reduction caused by activated charcoal could be useful for contaminated grain if feeding trials are also effective.

Ergot

Ergot, *Claviceps purpurea,* is a parasitic fungus that affects cereal grains, especially rye, oats, and wheat. The fungus invades the grass ovary, forming a dark elongated body (sclerotium), which produces alkaloids that cause gangrene and reproductive interference. Major toxic alkaloids include ergotamine, ergotoxine, and ergometrine; total ergot alkaloid content commonly ranges from 0.2–0.6% of sclerotia weight. The U.S. Department of Agriculture has set a tolerance of 0.3% ergot in grain (Christensen and Kaufmann 1965).

Gangrenous ergotism is the result of a combination of vasoconstriction and endothelial damage, leading to prolonged ischemia of appendages and eventually gangrene. Because venous and lymphatic drainage remains intact, the gangrene is "dry" in nature. Signs occur over a period of days or weeks and include depression, reduced feed intake, rapid pulse and respiration, and general ill thrift. Lameness may occur, most commonly in rear limbs, and in advanced cases necrosis and sloughing of the tail, ears, and hooves can occur. Signs may be exacerbated by cold weather.

Ergot alkaloids affect reproduction indirectly by causing agalactia. Pregnant gilts fed either 0.3% or 1% sclerotia during gestation had low piglet birth weights, low piglet survival, and poor piglet weight gains. Agalactia occurred in 50% of gilts fed 0.3% sclerotia in the gestation and lactation rations (Nordskog and Clark 1945; Wiernusz and Schneider 1984). The agalactia induced is noninflammatory and results from the well-known ability of ergot to inhibit prolactin release in late gestation (Whitacre and Threlfall 1981). Both experimental and clinical evidence indicates that ergot in rations of pregnant sows is not generally a cause of abortion, and swine exposed to ergot during late gestation routinely suffer agalactia but rarely abortion (Osweiler et al. 1985).

Reduced weight gain may be caused by as little as 0.1% ergots in the ration. Higher levels (3.0%) have been implicated in feed wastage and slow growth (Roers et al. 1974).

Differential diagnosis should include zearalenone or other estrogenic factors, bacterial infections, and mastitis-metritis-agalactia syndrome. If the clinical signs suggest ergotism, grains should be examined for the presence of significant amounts of ergot sclerotia. In the case of ground or processed feeds, feed microscopy or chemical analysis for ergot alkaloids may be necessary to confirm the diagnosis.

Treatment of ergotism is general and supportive. Gangrenous areas should be cleaned and treated locally and secondary infections controlled with broad-spectrum antibiotics. Removal of the feed is followed by improvement within 2 weeks for gangrenous effects. When agalactia has occurred, milk production returns 3–7 days after feed is changed. In the interim, supplemental nutrition and milk replacers may be used to save the piglets.

Fumonisins

Fusarium moniliforme and *F. proliferatum* fungi are ubiquitous in white and yellow corn worldwide (Bezuidenhoudt et al. 1988; Steyn 1995; Shephard et al. 1996; Gelderblom et al. 1988). Recently, these fungi have been identified as the source of the fumonisin mycotoxins. Swine consuming fumonisins have been affected by the disease generally known as porcine pulmonary edema (PPE). Corn screenings contaminated with the fumonisin mycotoxins are the most likely source of fumonisin toxicosis (Harrison et al. 1990; Ross et al. 1991; Osweiler et al. 1992; Ross et al. 1992).

Fumonisins appear to be produced when corn is stressed by moderate drought followed by persistent rainfall or high humidity late in development, but full knowledge of the inciting conditions remain to be determined. Since corn screenings contain the highest concentrations of fumonisins, producers should be advised to clean poor-quality corn to remove damaged kernels before feeding.

Fumonisins commonly present in corn are fumonisin B_1 (FB$_1$), fumonisin B_2 (FB$_2$), and fumonisin B_3 (FB$_3$). They are water-soluble, heat-stable, and alkaline-resistant aliphatic hydrocarbons with a terminal amine group and two tricarboxylic acid side chains (Steyn 1995). The number and position of hydroxyl groups on the aliphatic hydrocarbon determine the structure as FB$_1$, FB$_2$, or FB$_3$; the first two are of approximately equal toxicity, while FB$_3$ is much less toxic.

In South Africa, fumonisin-contaminated corn is associated with esophageal cancer in a well-defined geographic area (Bezuidenhoudt et al. 1988). The fumonisins are known tumor promoters leading to precancerous liver nodules after appropriate initiation. Chronic fumonisin consumption by swine has experimentally caused esophageal hyperplasia and hepatic neoplasia (Casteel et al. 1993, 1994).

Acute PPE has been associated with increases in pulmonary intravascular macrophages and increased pulmonary arterial pressure (Smith et al. 1996). These responses have been hypothesized to lead to pulmonary edema either by increased pulmonary hydrostatic pressure or by pulmonary capillary endothelial cell damage.

Fumonisins are poorly absorbed orally (3–6% of ingested dose), and most ingested fumonisins remain in the gastrointestinal tract. Once absorbed, they are excreted readily and rapidly in both bile and urine (Prelusky et al. 1994b). Persistent tissue residues after toxicological or accidental exposure appear unlikely, but more work is needed to clarify the toxicokinetics of fumonisins.

Mechanism of Action and Toxicity. Fumonisins inhibit the enzyme-mediated conversion of sphinganine to sphingosine, thus raising the sphinganine/sphingosine (SA/SO) ratio and potentially interfering with cell cycle control and cell function (Norred et al. 1992; Riley et al. 1993; Ramasamy et al. 1995). FB1 affects several cell signaling proteins including protein kinase C (PKC), a serine/threonine kinase involved in a number of signal transduction pathways that include cytokine induction, carcinogenesis, and apoptosis (Gopee and Sharma 2004). Fumonisin B1 appears also to inhibit ceramide synthase in the sphingolipid signaling pathway on the ascending aortic impedance spectrum of pigs. This is associated with inhibition of myocardial L-type calcium channels with a decrease in cardiac contractility, left heart failure, and pulmonary edema (Constable et al. 2003). The result clinically in pigs is massive pulmonary edema and hydrothorax. Smith et al. (2000) concluded that fumonisin-induced pulmonary edema is caused by left-sided heart failure and not by altered endothelial permeability. Interestingly, Zomborszky-Kovacs et al. (2002) reported that very low concentrations of FB_1 fed for 8 weeks resulted in chronic pulmonary changes of connective tissue proliferation, in the subpleural and interlobular connective tissue of lungs and in peribronchial and peribronchiolar areas. Whether there is a relationship ranging from more acute to chronic low dose studies relative to porcine pulmonary edema is not clear from current literature.

More than 120 ppm dietary fumonisins for 4–10 days produces acute PPE (Haschek et al. 1992; Osweiler et al. 1992; Colvin et al. 1993). Surviving swine develop subacute hepatic toxicosis in 7–10 days. Dietary levels of more than 50 ppm cause hepatosis within 7–10 days. Although 25 ppm or less causes no apparent clinical effects, mild microscopic hepatic lesions are documented for dietary levels as low as 23 ppm (Moetlin et al. 1994). The serum SA/SO ratio has been altered experimentally by diets with as low as 5 ppm fumonisins, although the clinical relevance of this change is not known (Riley et al. 1993; Moetlin et al. 1994). FB_1 and FB_2 are similarly toxic to swine, and they appear to occur at a relatively constant ratio in field-contaminated corn (P. F. Ross, personal communication, 1996). FB_3 appears to be nearly nontoxic to swine (G. D. Osweiler, unpublished data).

Fumonisins have been evaluated for their potential interactions with aflatoxins and deoxynivalenol (DON). Effects of aflatoxins and fumonisins were found to be additive when fed together, except for the variables cholinesterase and alkaline phosphatase, which showed a synergistic response to aflatoxins and FB_1 (Harvey et al. 1995). For a combination of FB_1 and DON, the effect on most variables was additive. However, for body weight, weight gain, hepatic weight, and mean corpuscular hemoglobin concentration, the responses were interactive in a greater-than-additive manner (Harvey et al. 1996).

Clinical Signs and Lesions. Dietary concentrations of fumonisins greater than 120 ppm are likely to cause acute interstitial pulmonary edema and hydrothorax, with attack rates up to 50% and case fatality rates of 50–90%. Initially there is lethargy, restlessness, depression, and dermal hyperemia. Mild salivation, dyspnea, open-mouth breathing, posterior weakness, recumbence, and moist rales develop rapidly, followed by cyanosis, weakness, and death. Initial signs begin after 4–7 days of continuous fumonisin consumption (Colvin and Harrison 1992; Osweiler et al. 1992). Once signs appear, death usually occurs in 2–4 hours. Sur-

vivors may develop hepatic disease. Feeding fumonisins at concentrations from 75–100 ppm for 1–3 weeks, without development of pulmonary edema, causes hepatic disease characterized by icterus, anorexia, ill thrift, and weight loss (Osweiler et al. 1993).

Serum chemistry analyses show elevated concentrations of gamma glutamyl transferase (GGT), aspartate amino transferase (AST), alkaline phosphatase (ALP), lactate dehydrogenase (LDH), cholesterol, and bilirubin. Early increases in the serum enzymes and cholesterol are followed by increased GGT and serum bilirubin accompanied by clinical icterus (Osweiler et al. 1992; Colvin et al. 1993; Moetlin et al. 1994).

Based on current evidence, fumonisins are not considered potent immunosuppressants in swine. One study has shown transient reduction in lymphocyte blastogenesis and delayed titer response to pseudorabies vaccine (Osweiler et al. 1993). Others have also reported decreased lymphoblastogenesis (Harvey et al. 1995, 1996). Tornyos et al. (2003) determined humoral and cell-mediated immune response to FB_1. Pigs were fed a high dose (100 mg/animal/day for 8 days) or in a low concentration for a longer period (1, 5, and 10 ppm for 3–4 months), and then vaccinated against Aujeszky's disease with inactivated vaccine. Specific and nonspecific in vitro cellular immune response was measured by the lymphocyte stimulation test (LST) induced by PHA-P, Con A, LPS, and inactivated suspension of the Aujeszky's disease virus. Humoral immune response—e.g., specific antibody titer—was measured by virus neutralization (VN). None of the immunological parameters examined showed significant differences between groups. They concluded that fumonisin B_1 had no significant effect on the humoral and cellular specific and nonspecific immune response.

The characteristic lesion of PPE is pulmonary edema and hydrothorax with 200–350 mL of clear, cell-free, straw-colored thoracic transudate. Lungs are heavy and wet with wide seams (3–10 mm) of interlobular edema. Bronchioles, bronchi, and trachea are relatively clear with little alveolar edema (Haschek et al. 1992; Osweiler et al. 1992; Colvin et al. 1993; Moetlin et al. 1994; Palyusik and Moran 1994). Acidophilic, fibrillar material is found in alveoli and interlobular lymphatics, and hyalinized alveolar capillary thrombi may be present. Increased numbers of pulmonary intravascular macrophages (PIM) filled with osmiophilic material have been reported by electron microscopy. This response is hypothesized to result from phagocytosis of damaged cellular components. Pancreatic necrosis and hepatosis with disrupted hepatic architecture, increased mitotic figures in hepatocytes, apoptosis and single-cell hepatic necrosis are typical lesions of subacute fumonisin toxicosis (Haschek et al. 1992). Chronic exposure can include fibrosis, hepatic hyperplastic nodules and medial hypertrophy of small pulmonary arteries.

Abortions are common 1–4 days after onset of acute

signs (Osweiler et al. 1992; Becker et al. 1995), presumably due to fetal anoxia caused by severe pulmonary edema in the dam. Concentrations of 100 ppm FB_1 fed in the last 30 days of gestation did not cause abortion, fetal abnormalities, or infertility in sows (G. D. Osweiler, unpublished data). Persistent clinical signs or continuing reproductive problems after exposure is stopped have not been reported.

Diagnosis. Clinical signs of acute respiratory distress with high mortality and lesions of interstitial edema and hydrothorax suggest fumonisin toxicosis. A history of consumption of corn screenings or poor-quality corn is typical. Serum chemistry changes and elevated serum SA/SO ratios are expected, and the acute liver enzymes usually peak at from 4–7 days after initial exposure, while bilirubin and GGT continue to increase for 1–2 weeks if sublethal exposure continues. Serum SA/SO ratio is the most sensitive indicator of fumonisin exposure and appears unique to the fumonisins (Riley et al. 1993; Moetlin et al. 1994). However, this assay is currently not widely available as a diagnostic test. Many diagnostic and commercial laboratories can detect and quantitate fumonisins in corn and feeds, but routine chemical analysis to detect fumonisins in tissues is not available, and the metabolism and excretion rate of fumonisins from oral exposures are unknown but likely very rapid (Prelusky et al. 1994a).

Treatment and Management. There is no antidote to the toxin itself. The very acute and massive changes of PPE do not allow for effective symptomatic and supportive therapy. Because clinical signs appear after days to weeks of exposure, oral detoxification is usually not useful. Liver damage from fumonisin toxicosis may be lessened by appropriate supportive care.

Analysis of corn or feeds for fumonisins can identify a source and help in estimating the risk from a specific feedstuff (Ross et al. 1991). Contaminated corn should be cleaned and the good-quality grain analyzed to demonstrate that a safe level of fumonisins has been reached.

Fumonisins are potential human and animal carcinogens, and their eventual regulation in foodstuffs seems likely.

PREVENTION AND MANAGEMENT OF MOLD AND MYCOTOXIN PROBLEMS

When mycotoxicosis occurs or is suspected, the first action should be to change the source of feed. This may be beneficial, even when a specific mycotoxin cannot be identified. A thorough inspection of the grain storage bins, mixing equipment, and feeders may reveal caking, molding, or musty odors. All contaminated feed should be removed and the equipment cleaned. Additionally, walls and containers should be washed with a dilute so-

lution of hypochlorite (laundry bleach) to reduce contaminating fungi. All equipment should be completely dry before fresh feed is added.

Any suspect feed should be analyzed to determine if known mycotoxins were present. Although spore counts or fungal cultures alone do not confirm a diagnosis, they may give some indication of the potential for mycotoxin production. With this information, the swine producer can better formulate a preventive program.

If storage conditions are adverse or if grain moisture is too high, use of a mold inhibitor may be advisable. Most commercial mold inhibitors are based on an organic acid such as propionic acid and are effective in reducing or delaying mold growth. Mold inhibitors do not destroy preformed toxins, which commonly may have formed in the field prior to harvest. Except for ammoniation (not yet approved by the Food and Drug Administration) to destroy aflatoxin, there are no practical commercial treatments that effectively destroy preformed mycotoxins.

Dilution of contaminated grain with clean grain is commonly used to reduce mycotoxin effects; this is not an approved procedure for aflatoxin. For any mycotoxin problem, dilution may reduce exposure initially, but care must be taken that wet or contaminated grain does not introduce new fungi and conditions that eventually lead to the entire mixture being contaminated.

Mycotoxin contamination may not be suspected until most or all of a contaminated feed is consumed. A prudent practice is to save a representative sample of all grains and feeds purchased and hold them in stable condition until swine are marketed or at least a month past when the feed was consumed. When questions about feed quality arise later, these samples may be valuable in documenting whether specific feeds were involved in a problem.

Samples of feeds or grain should be representative of the entire supply. Representative sampling can best be done after feed is ground and mixed by passing a cup through the moving auger stream at frequent intervals, mixing these samples thoroughly, and saving a 4.5 kg (10-pound) sample for analysis (Davis et al. 1980). Alternatively, probe sampling of large bins may give some idea of contamination levels. Bins should be probed in at least 6–10 perimeter locations and 2–4 central locations for each 1.8 m (6 feet) of bin height. High-moisture samples should be either dried to 12% moisture or stored frozen. Long-term storage is recommended in paper bags permanently marked with the date and source of the feed or grain, and samples should be held in a dry, clean location.

Mycotoxins present formidable challenges to the swine producer and veterinarian. Diagnosis is sometimes difficult and effective therapy is virtually lacking. A sound and practical preventive program should be a part of every swine management system.

REFERENCES

Allcroft R. 1969. Aflatoxicosis in farm animals. In Aflatoxin. LA Goldblatt, ed. New York: Academic Press.

Armbrecht BH, Wiseman HG, Shalkopf T. 1972. Swine aflatoxicosis II. The chronic response in brood sows fed sublethal amounts of aflatoxin and the reaction in their piglets. Environ Physiol Biochem 2:77–85.

Avantaggiato G, Havenaar R, Visconti A. 2003. Assessing the zearalenone-binding activity of adsorbent materials during passage through a dynamic in vitro gastrointestinal model. Food Chem Toxicol 41(10):1283-1290.

——. 2004. Evaluation of the intestinal absorption of deoxynivalenol and nivalenol by an in vitro gastrointestinal model, and the binding efficacy of activated carbon and other adsorbent materials. Food Chem Toxicol 42:817–824.

Bauer J. 1995. The metabolism of trichothecenes in swine. Dtsch Tierärztl Wochenschr 102:50–52.

Beasley VR. 1993. Trichothecenes. In Current Veterinary Therapy 3: Food Animal Practice, 3d ed. Philadelphia: WB Saunders, pp. 332–333.

Beasley VR, Swanson SP, Corley RA, Buck WB, Koritz GD, Burmeister HR. 1986. Pharmacokinetics of the trichothecene mycotoxin, T2 toxin in swine and cattle. Toxicon 24:13–23.

Becker BA, Pace L, Rottinghaus GE, Shelby R, Misfeldt M, Ross PF. 1995. Effects of feeding fumonisin B_1 in lactating sows and their suckling pigs. Am J Vet Res 56:1253–1258.

Bergsjo B, Langseth W, Nafstad I, Jansen JH, Larsen HJ. 1993. The effects of naturally deoxynivalenol-contaminated oats on the clinical condition, blood parameters, performance and carcass composition of growing pigs. Vet Res Commun 17(4):283–294.

Bergsjo B, Matre T, Nafstad I. 1992. Effects of diets with graded levels of deoxynivalenol on performance in growing pigs. Zentralbl Veterinärmed A 39:752–758.

Bezuidenhoudt SC, Wentzel A, Gelderblom WCA. 1988. Structure elucidation of the fumonisins, mycotoxins from Fusarium moniliforme. J Chem Soc Chem Commun, pp. 743–745.

Biro K, Barna-Vetro I, Pecsi T, Szabo E, Winkler G, Fink-Gremmels J, Solti L. 2003. Evaluation of spermatological parameters in ochratoxin A-challenged boars. Theriogenology 60:199–207.

Bohm J. 1992. The significance of the mycotoxins deoxynivalenol, zearalenone and ochratoxin A for agricultural domestic animals. Arch Tierernähr 42(2):95–111.

Bondy GS, Pestka JJ. 2000. Immunomodulation by fungal toxins. J Toxicol Environ Health B Crit Rev 3:109–143.

Carlton WW, Krogh P. 1979. Ochratoxins: A review. In Conference on Mycotoxins in Animal Feeds and Grains Related to Animal Health. National Technical Information Service, Springfield, VA, pp. 165–287.

Carson TC. 1999. Toxic minerals, chemicals, plants, and gases. In Diseases of Swine, 8th edition. B Straw, S D'Allaire, WL Mengeling, DJ Taylor, eds. Ames: Iowa State Univ Press, pp. 783–796.

Casteel SW, Turk JR, Cowart RP, Rottinghaus GE. 1993. Chronic toxicity of fumonisin in weanling pigs. J Vet Diagn Invest 5:413–417.

Casteel SW, Turk JR, Rottinghaus GE. 1994. Chronic effects of dietary fumonisin on the heart and pulmonary vasculature of swine. Fund Appl Toxicol 23:518–24.

Christensen CM, Kaufmann HH. 1965. Deterioration of stored grains by fungi. Annu Rev Phytopathol 3:69–84.

Coffey MT, Hagler WM, Cullen JM. 1989. Influence of dietary protein, fat and amino acids on the response of weanling swine to aflatoxin B_1. J Anim Sci 67:465–472.

Colvin BM, Cooley AJ, Beaver RW. 1993. Fumonisin toxicosis in swine: Clinical and pathologic findings. J Vet Diagn Invest 5:232–241.

Colvin BM, Harrison LR. 1992. Fumonisin-induced pulmonary edema and hydrothorax in swine. Mycopathologia 117:79–82.

Constable PD, Smith GW, Rottinghaus GE, Tumbleson ME, Haschek WM. 2003. Fumonisin-induced blockade of ceramide synthase in sphingolipid biosynthetic pathway alters aortic input impedance spectrum of pigs. Am J Physiol Heart Circ Physiol 284:H2034-2044.

Cook WO, Osweiler GD, Anderson TD, Richard JL. 1986. Ochratoxicosis in Iowa swine. J Am Vet Med Assoc 188:1399–1402.

Cook WO, Van Alstine WG, Osweiler GD. 1989. Aflatoxicosis in Iowa swine: Eight cases (1983–1985). J Am Vet Med Assoc 194:554–558.

Coppock RW, Gelberg HB, Hoffman WE, Buck WB. 1985. The acute toxicopathy of intravenous diacetoxyscirpenol (Anguidine) administration in swine. Fund Am Appl Toxicol 5:1034–1049.

Coppock RW, Swanson SP. 1986. Aflatoxins. In Current Veterinary Therapy 2: Food Animal Practice, 2d ed. Philadelphia: W. B. Saunders, pp. 363–366.

Dacasto M, Rolando P, Nachtmann C, Ceppa L, Nebbia C. 1995. Zearalenone mycotoxicosis in piglets suckling sows fed contaminated grain. Vet Hum Toxicol 37(4):359–361.

Davis ND, Dickens JW, Freie JW, Hamilton PB, Shotwell OL, Wiley TD, Fulkerson JF. 1980. Protocols for surveys, sampling, postcollection handling and analysis of grain samples involved in mycotoxin problems. J Assoc Off Anal Chem 63:95–102.

Diekman MA, Green ML. 1992. Mycotoxins and reproduction in domestic livestock. J Anim Sci 70:1615–1627.

Diekman MA, Long GG. 1989. Blastocyst development on days 10 or 14 after consumption of zearalenone by sows on days 7 to 10 after breeding. Am J Vet Res 50:1224–1227.

Dilkin P, Zorzete P, Mallmann CA, Gomes JD, Utiyama CE, Oetting LL, Correa B. 2003. Toxicological effects of chronic low doses of aflatoxin B(1) and fumonisin B(1)-containing Fusarium moniliforme culture material in weaned piglets. Food Chem Toxicol 41:1345–1353.

Doll S, Danicke S, Ueberschar KH, Valenta H, Schnurrbusch U, Ganter M, Klobasa F, Flachowsky G. 2003. Effects of graded levels of Fusarium toxin contaminated maize in diets for female weaned piglets. Arch Tierernahr 57:311–334.

Edwards S, Cantley TC, Rottinghaus GE, Osweiler GD, Day BN. 1987. The effects of zearalenone on reproduction in swine. 1. The relationship between ingested zearalenone dose and anestrus in non-pregnant, sexually mature gilts. Theriogenology 28:43–57.

Eriksen GS, Pettersson H, Johnsen K, Lindberg JE. 2002. Transformation of trichothecenes in ileal digesta and faeces from pigs. Arch Tierernahr 57:263–274.

Eriksen GS, Pettersson H, Lindberg JE. 2003. Absorption, metabolism and excretion of 3-acetyl DON in pigs. Arch Tierernahr 57:335–345.

Gajecki M. 2002. Zearalenone—Undesirable substances in feed. Pol J Vet Sci 5:117–122.

Gelderblom WCA, Jaskiewicz K, Marasas WFO, Thiel PG, Horak RM, Vleggaar R, Kriek NRJ. 1988. Fumonisins—Novel mycotoxins with cancer-promoting activity produced by Fusarium moniliforme. Appl Environ Microbiol 54:1806–1811.

Gopee NV, Sharma RP. 2004. Selective and transient activation of protein kinase C alpha by fumonisin B1, a ceramide synthase inhibitor mycotoxin, in cultured porcine renal cells. Life Sci 74:1541–1559.

Green ML, Diekman MA, Malayer JR, Scheidt AB, Long GG. 1990. Effect of prepubertal consumption of zearalenone on puberty and subsequent reproduction of gilts. J Anim Sci 68:171–178.

Green ML, Stouffer DK, Scheidt AB, Long GG, Diekman MA. 1991. Evaluation of use of progesterone to counteract zearalenone toxicosis during early pregnancy in gilts. Am J Vet Res 52(11):1871–1874.

Harrison LR, Colvin BM, Green JT, Newman LE, Cole JR Jr. 1990. Pulmonary edema and hydrothorax in swine produced by fumonisin B$_1$, a toxic metabolite of Fusarium moniliforme. J Vet Diagn Invest 2:217–221.

Harvey RB, Edrington TS, Kubena LF, Corrier DE, Elissalde MH. 1995b. Influence of the antibiotics lincomycin and tylosin on aflatoxicosis when added to aflatoxin-contaminated diets of growing swine. J Vet Diagn Invest 7:374–379.

Harvey RB, Edrington TS, Kubena LF, Elissalde MH, Casper HH, Rottinghaus GE, Turk JR. 1996. Effects of dietary fumonisin B1–containing culture material, deoxynivalenol-contaminated wheat, or their combination on growing barrows. Am J Vet Res 57:1790–1794.

Harvey RB, Edrington TS, Kubena LF, Elissalde MH, Rottinghaus GE. 1995a. Influence of aflatoxin and fumonisin B$_1$–containing culture material on growing barrows. Am J Vet Res 56:1668–1672.

Harvey RB, Huff WE, Kubena LF, Corrier DE, Phillips TD. 1988. Progression of aflatoxicosis in growing barrows. Am J Vet Res 49:482–487.

Harvey RB, Huff WE, Kubena LF, Phillips TD. 1989a. Evaluation of diets contaminated with aflatoxin and ochratoxin fed to growing pigs. Am J Vet Res 50:1400–1404.

Harvey RB, Kubena LF, Huff WE, Corrier DE, Clark DE, Phillips TD. 1989b. Effects of aflatoxin, deoxynivalenol, and their combinations in the diets of growing pigs. Am J Vet Res 50:602–607.

Harvey RB, Kubena LF, Phillips TD, Huff WE, Corrier DE. 1989c. Prevention of aflatoxicosis by addition of hydrated sodium calcium aluminosilicate to the diets of growing barrows. Am J Vet Res 50:416–420.

Haschek WM, Moetlin G, Ness DK, Harlin KS, Hall WF, Vesonder RF, Peterson RE, Beasley VR. 1992. Characterization of fumonisin toxicity in orally and intravenously dosed swine. Mycopathologia 117:83–96.

He P, Young LG, Forsberg C. 1993. Microbially detoxified vomitoxin-contaminated corn for young pigs. J Anim Sci 71(4):963–967.

Hietaniemi V, Kumpulainen J. 1991. Contents of Fusarium toxins in Finnish and imported grains and feeds. Food Addit Contam 8(2):171–181.

Huff WE, Kubena LF, Harvey RB, Doerr JA. 1988. Mycotoxin interactions in poultry and swine. J Anim Sci 66:2351–2355.

James LJ, Smith TK. 1982. Effect of dietary alfalfa on zearalenone toxicity and metabolism in rats and swine. J Anim Sci 55:110–117.

Jelinik CF, Pohland AE, Wood GE. 1989. Worldwide occurrence of mycotoxins in foods and feeds—An update. J Assoc Off Anal Chem 71:1176–1179.

Jimenez M, Manez M, Hernandez E. 1996. Influence of water activity and temperature on the production of zearalenone in corn by three Fusarium species. Int J Food Microbiol 29:417–421.

Juszkiewicz T, Piskorska M, Pliszczynska J. 1992. Occurrence of mycotoxins in animal feeds. J Environ Pathol Toxicol, Oncol 11:211–215.

Kollarczik B, Gareis M, Hanelt M. 1994. In vitro transformation of the Fusarium mycotoxins deoxynivalenol and zearalenone by the normal gut microflora of pigs. Nat Toxins 2:105–110.

Kordic B, Pribicevic S, Muntanola-Cvetkovic M, Mikolic P, Nikolic B. 1992. Experimental study of the effects of known quantities of zearalenone on swine reproduction. J Environ Pathol Toxicol Oncol 11:53–55.

Long GG, Diekman MA, Tuite JF, Shannan GM, Vesonder RF. 1983. Effect of Fusarium roseum (Giberella zea) on pregnancy and the estrous cycle in gilts fed molded corn on days 7–17 postestrus. Vet Res Commun 6:199–204.

Long GG, Turek J, Diekman MA, Scheidt AB. 1992. Effect of zearalenone on days 7 to 10 post-mating on blastocyst development and endometrial morphology in sows. Vet Pathol 29:60–67.

Lun AK, Young LG, Lumsden JH. 1985. The effects of vomitoxin and feed intake on the performance and blood characteristics of young pigs. J Anim Sci 61:1178–1185.

Lundeen GR, Poppenga RH, Beasley VR, Buck WB, Tranquilli WJ, Lambert RJ. 1986. Systemic distribution of blood flow during T-2 toxin induced shock in swine. Fund Appl Toxicol 7:309–323.

MacDonald EJ, Cavan DR, Smith TK. 1988. Effect of acute oral doses of T-2 toxin on tissue concentrations of biogenic amines in the rat. J Anim Sci 66:434–441.

Marin DE, Taranui, Bunaciu RP, PascaleF, Tudor DS, Avram N, Sarca M, Cureu I, Criste RD, Suta V, Oswald IP. 2002. Changes in performance, blood parameters, humoral and cellular immune responses in weanling piglets exposed to low doses of aflatoxin. J Anim Sci 80(5):1250–1257.

Marquardt RR, Frohlich AA. 1992. A review of recent advances in understanding ochratoxicosis. J Anim Sci 70:3968–3976.

McKnight CR, Armstrong WD, Hagler WM, Jones EE. 1983. The effects of aflatoxin on brood sows and the newborn pigs. J Anim Sci 55(Suppl 1):104.

Meyer K, Usleber E, Martlbauer E, Bauer J. 2000. Occurrence of zearalenone, alpha- and beta-zearalenol in bile of breeding sows in relation to reproductive performance. Berl Munch Tierarztl Wochenschr 113:374–379.

Moetlin GK, Haschek WM, Ness DK, Hall WF, Harlin KS, Schaeffer DJ, Beasley VR. 1994. Temporal and dose-response features in swine fed corn screenings contaminated with fumonisin mycotoxins. Mycopathologia 126:27–40.

Nordskog AW, Clark RT. 1945. Ergotism in pregnant sows, female rats, and guinea pigs. Am J Vet Res 6:107–116.

Norred WP, Wang E, Yoo H, Riley RT, Merrill AH Jr. 1992. In vitro toxicology of fumonisins and the mechanistic implications. Mycopathologia 117:73–78.

Obremski K, Gajecki M, Zwierzchowski W, Zielonka L, Otrocka-Domagala I, Rotkiewicz T, Mikolajczyk A, Gajecka M, Polak M. 2003. Influence of zearalenone on reproductive system cell proliferation in gilts. Pol J Vet Sci 6:239–245.

Ominski KH, Marquardt RR, Sinha RN, Abramson KH. 1994. Ecological aspects of growth and mycotoxin production in storage fungi. In Mycotoxins in Grain: Compounds Other Than aflatoxin. JD Miller, HL Trenholm, eds. St. Paul: Eagan Press, pp. 287–312.

Osweiler GD. 2000. Mycotoxins: Contemporary Issues of Food Animal Health and Productivity. Vet Clin North Am Food Anim Pract 15:33–46.

Osweiler GD, Carson TL, Buck WB, Van Gelder GA. 1985. Mycotoxicoses. In Clinical and Diagnostic Veterinary Toxicology, 3d ed. Dubuque, Iowa: Kendall Hunt, pp. 409–442.

Osweiler GD, Hopper DL, Debey BM. 1990. Taste aversion in swine induced by deoxynivalenol. J Anim Sci 68(Suppl 1):403.

Osweiler GD, Ross PF, Wilson TM, Nelson PE, Witte ST, Carson TL, Rice LG, Nelson HA. 1992. Characterization of an epizootic of pulmonary edema in swine associated with fumonisin in corn screenings. J Vet Diagn Invest 4:53–59.

Osweiler GD, Schwartz KJ, Roth JR. 1993. Effect of fumonisin contaminated corn on growth and immune function in swine. (Abstr.) Midwestern Sec, Am Soc Anim Sci. Mar 30, Des Moines, Iowa.

Palyusik M, Harrach B, Mirocha CJ, Pathre SV. 1980. Transmission of zearalenone into porcine milk. Acta Vet Acad Sci Hung 28:217–222.

Palyusik M, Moran EM. 1994. Porcine pulmonary edema with hydrothorax: A review. J Environ Pathol Toxicol Oncol 13:63–66.

Panangala VS, Giambrone JJ, Diener UL, Davis ND, Hoerr FJ, Mitra A, Schultz RD, Wilt GR. 1986. Effects of aflatoxin on the growth, performance and immune responses of weanling swine. Am J Vet Res 47:2062–2067.

Pier AC. 1981. Mycotoxins and animal health. Adv Vet Sci Comp Med 25:185–243.

Pollman DS, Koch BA, Seitz LM. 1985. Deoxynivalenol-contaminated wheat in swine diets. J Anim Sci 60:239–247.

Prelusky DB. 1993. The effect of low-level deoxynivalenol on neurotransmitter levels measured in pig cerebral spinal fluid. J Environ Sci Health B 28:731–761.

——. 1994. The effect of deoxynivalenol on serotoninergic neurotransmitter levels in pig blood. J Environ Sci Health B 29:1203–1218.

——. 1996. A study on the effect of deoxynivalenol on serotonin receptor binding in pig brain membranes. J Environ Sci Health B 31:1103–1117.

——. 1997. Effect of intraperitoneal infusion of deoxynivalenol on feed consumption and weight gain in the pig. Nat Toxins 5:121–125.

Prelusky DB, Gerdes RG, Underhill KL, Rotter BA, Jui PY, Trenholm HL. 1994a. Effects of low-level dietary deoxynivalenol on haematological and clinical parameters of the pig. Nat Toxins 2:97–104.

Prelusky DB, Trenholm HL. 1993. The efficacy of various classes of anti-emetics in preventing deoxynivalenol-induced vomiting in swine. Nat Toxins 1:296–302.

Prelusky DB, Trenholm HL, Savard ME. 1994b. Pharmacokinetic fate of 14C-labelled fumonisin B_1 in swine. Nat Toxins 2:73–80.

Prelusky DB, Yeung JM, Thompson BK, Trenholm HL. 1992. Effect of deoxynivalenol on neurotransmitters in discrete regions of swine brain. Arch Environ Contam Toxicol 22:36–40.

Rainey MR, Tubbs RC, Bennett LW, Cox NM. 1990. Prepubertal exposure to dietary zearalenone alters hypothalamohypophyseal function but does not impair postpubertal reproductive function of gilts. J Anim Sci 68:2015–2022.

Ramasamy S, Wang E, Hennig B, Merrill AH Jr. 1995. Fumonisin B_1 alters sphingolipid metabolism and disrupts the barrier function of endothelial cells in culture. Toxicol Appl Pharmacol 133:343–348.

Richard JL, Cole RJ, eds. 1989. Mycotoxins: Economic and health risks. Council for Agricultural Science and Technology, Task Force Report No. 116. Ames, Iowa, pp. 1–99.

Riley RT, An NH, Showker JL, Yoo HS, Norred WP, Chamberlain WJ, Wang E, Merrill AH Jr, Moetlin G, Beasley VR. 1993. Alteration of tissue and serum sphinganine to sphingosine ratio: An early biomarker of exposure to fumonisin-containing feeds in pigs. Toxicol Appl Pharmacol 118:105–112.

Roers JE, Harrold RL, Haugse CN, Vinusson WE. 1974. Barley rations for baby pigs. Farm Research Nov–Dec, North Dakota Agriculture Experiment Station.

Ross PF, Rice LG, Osweiler GD, Nelson PE, Richard JL, Wilson TM. 1992. A review and update of animal toxicoses associated with fumonisin-contaminated feeds and production of fumonisins by Fusarium isolates. Mycopathologia 117:109–114.

Ross PF, Rice LG, Plattner RD, Osweiler GD, Wilson TM, Owens DL, Nelson HA, Richard JL. 1991. Concentrations of fumonisin B_1 in feeds associated with animal health problems. Mycopathologia 114:129–35.

Rotter BA, Prelusky DB, Pestka JJ. 1996. Toxicology of deoxynivalenol (vomitoxin). J Toxicol Environ Health 48:1–34.

Rotter BA, Thompson BK, Lessard M, Trenholm HL, Tryphonas H. 1994. Influence of low-level exposure to Fusarium mycotoxins on selected immunological and hematological parameters in young swine. Fund Appl Toxicol 23(1):117–124.

Ruhr LP, Osweiler GD, Foley CW. 1983. Effect of the estrogenic mycotoxin zearalenone on reproductive potential in the boar. Am J Vet Res 44:483–485.

Russell L, Cox DF, Larsen G, Bodwell K, Nelson CE. 1990. Incidence of molds and mycotoxins in commercial animal feed mills in seven Midwestern states, 1988–1989. J Anim Sci 69:5–12.

Shephard GS, Thiel PG, Stockenstrom S, Sydenham EW. 1996. Worldwide survey of fumonisin contamination of corn and corn-based products. J AOAC Int 79:671–687.

Silvotti L, Petterino C, Bonomi A, Cabassi E. 1997. Immunotoxicological effects on piglets of feeding sows diets containing aflatoxins. Vet Rec 141:469–472.

Smith GW, Constable PD, Eppley RM, Tumbleson ME, Gumprecht LA, Haschek-Hock WM. 2000. Purified fumonisin B(1) decreases cardiovascular function but does not alter pulmonary capillary permeability in swine. Toxicol Sci 56(1):240–249.

Smith GW, Constable PD, Haschek WM. 1996. Cardiovascular responses to short-term fumonisin exposure in swine. Fund and Appl Toxicol 33(1):140–148.

Smith GW, Constable PD, Tumbleson ME, Rottinghaus GE, Haschek WM. 1999. Sequence of cardiovascular changes leading to pulmonary edema in swine fed culture material containing fumonisin. Am J Vet Res 60:1292–300.

Smith GW, Constable PD, Smith TK. 1992. Recent advances in the understanding of Fusarium trichothecene mycotoxicoses. J Anim Sci 70:3989–3993.

Steyn PS. 1995. Mycotoxins, general view, chemistry and structure. Toxicol Lett 82–83:843–851.

Swamy HV, Smith TK, MacDonald EJ, Boermans HJ, Squires EJ. 2002. Effects of feeding a blend of grains naturally contaminated with Fusarium mycotoxins on swine performance, brain regional neurochemistry, and serum chemistry and the efficacy of a polymeric glucomannan mycotoxin adsorbent. J Anim Sci 80:3257–3267.

Szczech GM, Carlton WW, Tuite J, Caldwell R. 1973. Ochratoxin A toxicosis in swine. Vet Pathol 10:347–364.

Tornyos G, Kovacs M, Rusvai M, Horn P, Fodor J, Kovacs F. 2003. Effect of dietary fumonisin B1 on certain immune parameters of weaned pigs. Acta Vet Hung 51:171–9.

Trenholm HL, Hamilton RMG, Friend DW, Thompson BK, Hartin KE. 1984. Feeding trials with vomitoxin (deoxynivalenol)-contaminated wheat: Effects on swine, poultry, and dairy cattle. J Am Vet Med Assoc 185:527–531.

Trucksess MW, Stoloff L, Brumley WC, Wilson DM, Hale OM, Sangster T, Miller DM. 1982. Aflatoxicol and aflatoxins B_1 and M_1 in the tissues of pigs receiving aflatoxin. J Assoc Off Anal Chem 65:884–887.

Vanyi A, Bata A, Glavits R, Kovacs F. 1994. Perinatal oestrogen syndrome in swine. Acta Vet Hung 42:433–446.

Whitacre MD, Threlfall WR. 1981. Effects of ergocryptine on plasma prolactin, luteinizing hormone, and progesterone in the periparturient sow. Am J Vet Res 42:1538–1541.

Wiernusz ML, Schneider N. 1984. Effects of feeding ergot-contaminated rye diets on swine gestation and lactation. In Proc 1984 George A. Young Conf, Lincoln, Nebr.

Wilson DM, Abramson D. 1992. Mycotoxins. In Storage of Cereal Grains and Their Products. DB Sauered. American Association of Cereal Chemists, St. Paul, pp. 341–389.

Yang HH, Aulerich RJ, Helferich W, Yamini B, Chou KC, Miller ER, Bursian SJ. 1995. Effects of zearalenone and/or tamoxifen on swine and mink reproduction. J Appl Toxicol 15:223–232.

Young LG, King GJ. 1983. Prolonged feeding of low levels of zearalenone to young boars. J Anim Sci 57(Suppl 1):313–314.

Young LG, McGirr L, Valli VE, Lumsden JH, Lun A. 1983. Vomitoxin in corn fed to young pigs. J Anim Sci 57:655–664.

Zomborszky-Kovacs M, Vetesi F, Horn P, Repa I, Kovacs F. 2002. Effects of prolonged exposure to low-dose fumonisin B_1 in pigs. J Vet Med B Infect Dis Vet Public Health 49:197–201.

57 Nutrient Deficiencies and Excesses

D. E. Reese and P. S. Miller

Proper nutrition is the foundation for sustained economic and environmental viability of any pork producing operation. Pigs perform best and excrete less manure nutrients when they consume diets that contain the correct amount and balance of essential nutrients. Occasionally pigs consume diets that contain insufficient or excessive amounts of one or more nutrients. The effects range from mild (slight, unnoticed reductions in weight gain and feed efficiency) to marked (obvious clinical and subclinical symptoms, including death).

The relationship between a nutrient deficiency and excess varies among nutrients (Figure 57.1). The absolute difference (the range of tolerance) between the nutrient intake associated with overcoming a deficiency (i.e., requirement) and the intake associated with a toxicity may be large (e.g., water-soluble vitamins) or small (e.g., selenium). This observation is critical in as much as it represents the window of safety for a particular nutrient.

This chapter presents clinical symptoms (outwardly apparent) and subclinical symptoms (evident only by necropsy or clinical methodology) of nutrient deficiencies and excesses that have occurred in pigs. Although it is rare today to observe symptoms of a single nutrient deficiency or excess, the recognition of faulty nutrition should be part of an overall approach to solving problems in swine operations.

The information presented herein was derived from research results with pigs and, in most instances, obtained by varying the intake of one nutrient at a time. However, nutrient interactions occur and it is unclear if the information would apply when multiple deficiencies or excesses of nutrients exist (e.g., when a vitamin and trace mineral mix is not added to the diet properly).

On farms today, vitamin and mineral deficiencies are less likely to occur than excesses. This is because diets are routinely fortified with vitamins and minerals. Also, it is important to consider that many of the nutrient deficiency symptoms reported here were observed in pigs fed purified or semipurified diets. This was necessary in order to provide a diet that contained a very low level of the nutrient of interest so deficiency symptoms could be observed. Ingredients used in practical swine diets contain a variety of essential nutrients (NRC 1998) which, even without recommended nutrient fortifications, would prevent the appearance of some symptoms.

CAUSES OF NUTRIENT DEFICIENCIES

Reduced Feed Intake

Pigs should consume a certain quantity of essential nutrients daily for optimum performance. Because diets are often formulated on a concentration basis, lower-than-expected feed intake by pigs could result in a nutrient deficiency. This situation is most commonly observed in gestating sows and breeding boars when feed intake is restricted to control weight gain, and in lactating sows, because they may consume less feed than needed for optimum performance. Furthermore, growing pigs with a high genetic capacity for lean-tissue accretion sometimes have reduced feed intake.

Low Nutrient Bioavailability in Ingredients

Nutrients present in ingredients are not fully available to the pig for maintenance, growth, and(or) lactation. The portion of the nutrient in the ingredient that is absorbed in a form utilizable by the pig is said to be bioavailable. The amount of that nutrient that is bioavailable depends primarily on the nutrient source. For example, the phosphorus in dicalcium phosphate is much more bioavailable than the phosphorus in grain and plant protein supplements. In these ingredients, the phosphorus is bound in a phytate complex and is not fully released during digestion. Thus, a phosphorus deficiency could occur if bioavailability is not considered in diet formulation. On the other hand, some feed ingredients contain nutrients that have a low bioavailability but that still release sufficient amounts of nutrients to meet the animal's requirement. It should be

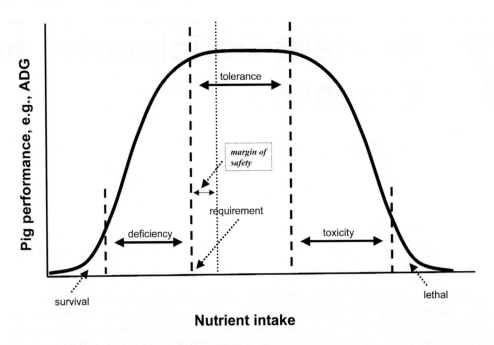

57.1. *Idealized relationship between pig performance (e.g., average daily gain) and nutrient intake.*

noted that estimates of bioavailability are relative to a reference ingredient or ingredients; therefore, one should closely examine the nature of the reference ingredients.

Variability in Nutrient Content of Ingredients
Deviations in the nutrient content of ingredients from expected or "book" values can result in nutrient deficiencies if not taken into account in diet formulations. For example, samples of corn from 15 states in the USA contained between 0.24% and 0.31% lysine; for soybean meal the range was from 2.7%–3.0% (NCR-42 1992). More variability has been reported for vitamins, and this has been attributed to agronomic, harvest, storage, and processing conditions (Hoffman-La Roche 1991).

Diet Formulation and Preparation Errors
There are a number of possible mistakes in diet formulation and preparation that can result in nutrient deficiencies. These include using the incorrect quantity or the wrong ingredients in the diet and not cleaning the mixer properly between batches. In addition, nutrient deficiencies can occur when commercial feed products that are not designed to complement each other are used to prepare the diet. Haphazard additions of an extra package of minerals to a diet already adequately fortified may cause certain minerals to interfere with the utilization of others, resulting in deficiencies. Furthermore, according to Traylor et al. (1994), cutting short the time the feed mixer runs can cause significant variation in the nutrient content of the final diet and reduce pig performance.

Variation in Nutrient Requirements of Pigs
Pigs have varying potentials for lean growth and reproduction and therefore have different nutrient requirements. For example, a given level of dietary lysine may be seemingly adequate for diseased, low-lean-gain pigs but deficient for high-health, high-lean-gain pigs (Williams et al. 1997). Stahly et al. (1991) also demonstrated that increasing the dietary lysine density improved performance to a greater extent as the lean-growth capacity of different genotypes increased, indicating a genotype by lysine density interaction. Moreover, within a contemporary group of pigs, some may show deficiency symptoms while others do not (Cunha 1977), indicating the need to carefully observe individual pigs for symptoms of nutrient deficiencies.

Nutrient Excesses
All essential nutrients must be digested and utilized by the pig to avoid deficiencies. To facilitate this process, it is important to maintain a proper balance of nutrients in the diet. There are common absorption sites for many nutrients in the small intestine. Thus, a high dietary concentration of one nutrient can impair the passage of another nutrient through the absorption sites and cause a deficiency. In addition, an excess of one nutrient can cause the formation of certain chemical complexes which are poorly absorbed. The more frequent nutrient interactions that can cause problems in practical situations are between calcium and phosphorus, calcium and zinc, and copper, iron, and zinc. In some cases, a nutrient excess can be associated with the deficiency symptom of the interacting nutrient it is .

SYMPTOMS OF NUTRIENT DEFICIENCIES

Clinical and subclinical deficiency symptoms for several nutrients are presented in Tables 57.1, 57.2, and 57.3. There is wide variation in the amount of time that elapses before symptoms of nutrient deficiency begin to appear. For example, it takes 4–6 months for pigs fed a vitamin D–deficient diet to develop symptoms of a deficiency (NRC 1998), whereas a salt deficiency will be evident in a few days (Patience and Zijlstra 2001).

Nutrient requirements for swine were published by the NRC (1998). These can serve as a guide in formulating swine diets to minimize the occurrence of nutrient deficiencies. Because several factors are known to influence nutrient requirements (NRC 1998), it is prudent to add a margin of safety to these requirements to ensure optimum animal performance (Reese et al. 2000).

CAUSES OF NUTRIENT EXCESSES

Excessive Feed Intake

Sometimes gestating females and breeding boars are given more feed than they need for optimum performance. Consequently, they consume too much energy and get excessively heavy and fat, which reduces reproductive performance and longevity.

Diet Preparation Errors

The same mistakes in diet preparation that can cause nutrient deficiencies can also cause nutrient excesses.

Poor Water Quality

Water may contain large amounts of several minerals, some of which may be contributed to the water by industrial wastes and other sources of pollution (NRC 1980) and by natural mineral deposits. Few studies have been conducted to investigate nutrient excesses caused by consuming poor-quality water. However, it appears pigs can tolerate water containing high levels of total dissolved solids (5000 ppm) after a period of adaptation (Reese et al. 2000).

Contaminated Mineral Supplements

Mineral supplements, such as dicalcium phosphate and defluorinated rock phosphate, are added to swine diets to correct the deficiencies in diets formulated with grains and protein supplements. Often these mineral supplements contain elements other than those of primary interest. For example, defluorinated rock phosphate contains 3.27% and .84% sodium and iron, respectively (NRC 1998). In addition, some phosphorus sources may contain high levels of aluminum and fluorine, and some sources of calcium contain large amounts of magnesium and iron. Also, some zinc and copper sources may be contaminated with lead and cadmium (D. A. Hill, personal commmunication, 1997). These "extra" elements will not normally pose a prob-lem to the pig if their contribution to the diet is accounted for during formulation. The type and amount of the "other" elements the mineral supplement contains depend on the raw material from which the supplement was made and the type of processing (NRC 1980).

SYMPTOMS OF NUTRIENT EXCESSES AND TOLERANCE LEVELS

Symptoms of excessive nutrient intake and estimated tolerance levels for several nutrients are presented in Tables 57.4, 57.5, and 57.6. Because many minerals interact with each other during the digestive and utilization processes, a high intake of one mineral (e.g., calcium) can result in a deficiency of another mineral (e.g., phosphorus or zinc). To solve this kind of problem, either reduce the dietary level of calcium, for example, or increase the level of phosphorus and(or) zinc in the diet.

Copper (at 250 ppm as copper sulfate) and zinc (at 3000 ppm as zinc oxide) are unique in that they promote additional growth in young growing pigs at dietary concentrations which far exceed the nutritional requirement for these nutrients (Hill and Spears 2001). However, like other minerals, too much copper or zinc in the diet will produce deleterious effects (see Table 57.5).

According to Lewis (2001) the deleterious effects of consuming incorrect amounts of amino acids have been classified into at least two main types: toxicity and imbalance. Toxicities result from the consumption of a large excess of an individual amino acid. Imbalances are also caused by excessive intake(s) of (an) amino(s), but in this case the excess exacerbates a deficiency of the most limiting amino acid in the diet. An imbalance is corrected by the appropriate addition of that amino acid. Under practical conditions, toxicities and imbalances would be caused only by mistakes in formulation or manufacturing of a diet with crystalline amino acids. The only amino acids currently available in feed-grade form are lysine, tryptophan, threonine and methionine.

With the exception of the study by Wahlstrom and Libal (1974) where supplemental lysine and methionine were evaluated, the effects of excess levels of amino acids reported in Table 57.6 were observed when the amino acid of interest was added to a basal diet considered to be adequate in all essential amino acids. In other words, a constant level of soybean meal was maintained in the basal and amino acid–supplemented diets.

Wahlstrom and Libal (1974) added DL-methionine (0.2%) to a diet that contained less soybean meal than the basal diet. They observed a reduction in pig performance at a lower level of added methionine than other researchers have reported because they exacerbated a lysine deficiency (i.e., caused an amino acid imbalance). Nevertheless, according to Baker (1977), pigs appear to be particularly sensitive to excess methionine in the diet. It is important to recognize that there is probably a

Table 57.1. Signs of vitamin deficiencies in swine

Nutrient	Clinical Signs	Subclinical Signs	Reference
Vitamin A	Incoordination; lordosis; paralysis of rear limbs; night blindness; congenital defects; reduced weight gain; respiratory disfunction; roughness of skin; tilting of head; eye discharge; stillborn pigs; aborted fetuses with cleft palate, harelip, and deformed hind legs; impaired spermatogenesis; increased embryonic mortality	Retarded bone growth; increased cerebrospinal fluid pressure; degeneration of sciatic and femoral nerves; minimal visual purple; atrophy of epithelial layers of genital tract; decreased plasma vitamin A	NRC 1979, 1998; Ullrey 1991; Darroch 2001
Vitamin D	Rickets; osteomalacia; tetany; reduced weight gain; stiffness and lameness; posterior paralysis	Lack of bone calcification and proliferation of epiphyseal cartilage; rib and vertebra fracture; low plasma calcium, magnesium, and inorganic phosphorus; elevated serum alkaline phosphatase	NRC 1979; Cunha 1977; Crenshaw 2001
Vitamin E	Lactation failure; reduced litter size; extended parturition time; weak pigs at birth; sudden death (fast-growing pigs); postweaning diarrhea	Liver necrosis (hepatosis dietetica); cardiac muscle degeneration (mulberry heart); increased fluid in pericardial sac; gastric ulcers; anemia; yellow discoloration of fat tissue; skeletal degeneration; increased serum glutamic oxalo-acetic transaminase and glutamic pyruvic transaminase; reduced prothrombin time, serum vitamin E, and immune response; testicular degeneration	NRC 1998; Mahan 1991, 2001
Vitamin K (menadione)	Pale newborn pigs with loss of blood from umbilical cord; massive subcutaneous hemorrhage; hematomas in ears; enlarged, blood-filled joints; sudden death following dicoumarin intake; blood in urine	Increased prothrombin and blood-clotting time; internal hemorrhage; anemia due to blood loss	NRC 1979, 1998; Fritschen et al. 1971; Crenshaw 2001
Biotin	Excessive hair loss, skin ulcerations, and dermatitis; exudate around eyes; inflammation of the mucous membranes of the mouth; transverse cracking of the hooves; cracking and bleeding of footpads; spasticity of hind legs; diarrhea; reduced litter size	Reduced serum biotin	NRC 1998; Dove and Cook 2001
Choline	Reduced weight gain, litter size, and farrowing rate; rough hair coat; unbalanced and staggering gait	Fatty infiltration of liver and kidney; reduced red blood cell count, hematocrit, and hemoglobin; increased plasma alkaline phosphatase	NRC 1998
Folic acid	Reduced weight gain and litter size; fading hair color	Normocytic and macrocytic anemia; leukopenial thrombopenia; reduced hematocrit; bone marrow hyperplasia	NRC 1998; Dove and Cook 2001
Niacin	Anorexia; reduced weight gain; rough hair coat; hair loss; severe diarrhea; dermatitis; vomiting	Buccal mucosa ulcerations, ulcerative gastritis; inflammation and necrosis of cecum and colon; normocytic anemia	NRC 1998
Pantothenic acid	Anorexia; reduced weight gain; dry skin; rough hair coat; hair loss; unusual gait (goose-stepping); impaired sow reproductivity	Edema and necrosis of intestinal mucosa; increased connective tissue invasion of the submucosa; loss of nerve myelin; degeneration of dorsal root ganglion, fatty liver; enlarged adrenal glands; atrophic ovaries; infantile uteri; reduced immune response; intramuscular hemorrhage	NRC 1998; Dove and Cook 2001
Riboflavin	Reduced weight gain; cataracts; seborrhea; stiffness of gait; vomiting; hair loss; reduced farrowing rate; anestrus; higher piglet mortality	Increased blood neutrophil granulocytes; discolored liver and kidney tissue; fatty liver; collapsed follicles; degenerating ova; degenerating myelin of the sciatic and brachial nerves; elevated blood erythrocyte glutathione reductase activity coefficient; reduced immune response	NRC 1998; Dove and Cook 2001
Vitamin B_1 (thiamin)	Anorexia; reduced weight gain; occasional vomiting; sudden death	Cardiac hypertrophy; bradycardia; increased plasma pyruvate; reduced body temperature; myocardial degeneration; flabby heart	NRC 1998; Dove and Cook 2001

Table 57.1. (*continued*)

Nutrient	Clinical Signs	Subclinical Signs	Reference
Vitamin B$_6$ (pyridoxine)	Anorexia; reduced weight gain; convulsions; exudate development around eyes; ataxia; vomiting; coma; death	Microcytic hypochromic anemia; elevated serum iron and gamma globulin; fatty infiltration of liver; reduced albumin, hemoglobin, red blood cells, lymphocytes	NRC 1998; Dove and Cook 2001
Vitamin B$_{12}$	Anorexia; reduced weight gain, litter size, and pig birth weight; hypersensitivity; rough hair coat; dermatitis; hind leg incoordination	Normocytic anemia; increased neutrophil and reduced lymphocyte count; enlarged liver	NRC 1998; Dove and Cook 2001
Vitamin C (ascorbic acid)[a]	None documented	None documented	Dove and Cook 2001

[a]Synthesized from d-glucose and related compounds in pigs. No deficiency signs have been observed; however, reports of improved pig performance from vitamin C additions to practical diets exist.

greater tolerance level of feed-grade forms of amino acids when they are added to a diet which contains an adequate quantity of the 10 essential amino acids than when they are added individually to a low-protein diet.

For some nutrients, no documentation was found to indicate a tolerance level, because no adverse effects from an excessive intake have been reported in swine. Thus, when "none documented" appears in the tables, one should not assume that the nutrient is completely safe for swine. There are reports of magnesium and potassium toxicity in other species (NRC 1980), as well as for niacin, vitamin K, vitamin E, and pyridoxine (NRC 1987). In general the vitamins that have not been observed to cause adverse reactions in swine are relatively safe at dietary concentrations much greater than the requirement. This is especially true for the "B vitamins" (e.g., riboflavin, folic acid), which are not extensively stored in the body and excesses are readily excreted in the urine.

Estimated tolerance for a nutrient is defined as the dietary concentration, when fed for a limited time, that is not likely to impair pig performance and should not produce unsafe residues in pork (NRC 1980). Although the tolerance level will vary with the age and physiological condition of the animal (NRC 1980), only one tolerance level is given in the tables for each nutrient, except where information was deemed sufficient to give more. The tolerance values listed may not represent the actual tolerance levels for production situations. Many of the research trials on which the tolerance levels were based were conducted for a limited time period using nutrient sources that may have different bioavailabilities from those used in practical swine diets. "Not determined" in the tables means insufficient data were available to suggest a tolerance level.

INVESTIGATING A POSSIBLE FEED-RELATED DISORDER

Good production records combined with close, daily observation of animals are important in identifying problems caused by faulty nutrition. Monitor gain, feed intake and feed efficiency, because they are typically impacted by many feed-related disorders. After it is apparent that growth performance is impaired or several animals appear abnormal, it is important to consider what aspects of feeding and nutrition could be a problem. Generally, feed-related disorders are caused by inadequate feed intake or impaired feed quality.

Feed Intake
Many feed-related problems on farms occur because pigs do not consume enough feed. For example, access to feed by lactating sows and growing pigs is too often restricted. Feed access is often restricted because of human error, feed bridging in the bins or feeders, or equipment failure. Other reasons for inadequate feed intake are water quantity or quality problems, overcrowding, and poor feeder space and design. Eliminate the possibility that inadequate feed intake may be causing suspected feed-related disorders before investigating feed quality.

Feed Quality
If a feed-related disorder can not be explained by inadequate feed intake, look for possible feed quality problems. Observe for evidence of foreign contamination such as dirt, stones, rodent droppings, and other indicators such as color and odor. A significant change in color may indicate a change in ingredients (which is not necessarily a problem) or it may suggest improper processing such as overheating. Beware of moldy or mycotoxin-contaminated feed. Also, feed quality may be impaired because it contains too little or too much of one or more nutrients.

Nutrient deficiencies and excesses are seldom severe enough on farms to cause clinical or subclinical signs in pigs; however, some have occurred under practical conditions. Selenium/vitamin E, amino acid, biotin (in sows), zinc, phosphorus, and salt deficiencies have been observed. Problems with excess amounts of selenium, vitamin A and D, copper, and zinc have been seen.

Table 57.2. Signs of mineral deficiencies in swine

Nutrient	Clinical Signs	Subclinical Signs	Reference
Calcium	Rickets; osteomalacia; low calcium tetany; humped back or camelback syndrome; reduced weight gain; stiffness of gait; lameness; enlarged and painful joints; spontaneous fractures; posterior paralysis (downer sow syndrome)	Reduced bone breaking strength; low plasma calcium level; elevated serum phosphorus and alkaline phosphatase; reduced bone mineralization	NRC 1979; Peo 1991; Crenshaw 2001
Chromium[a]	None documented	None documented	Hill and Spears 2001
Copper	Anorexia; reduced weight gain; bowing of legs; spontaneous fractures; ataxia	Microcytic, hypochromic anemia; leucopenia; reduced serum ceruloplasmin; reduced erythrocyte life span; aortic rupture; cardiac hypertrophy	Miller 1991; NRC 1998; Hill and Spears 2001
Iodine	Goiter; sows farrow weak, hairless pigs	Enlarged, hemorrhagic thyroid; hyperplasia of follicular epithelium of thyroid; reduced plasma protein-bound iodine	Hill and Spears 2001
Iron	Reduced feed intake, weight gain, and feed efficiency; rough hair coat; pallor; wrinkled skin; labored breathing; death	Hypochromic, microcytic anemia; enlarged heart and spleen; enlarged fatty liver; ascites; reduced serum iron, percent transferrin saturation and hemoglobin (≤ 7 g/100 mL); thin, watery blood; reduced disease resistance	NRC 1979, 1998; Miller 1991; Hill and Spears 2001
Magnesium	Hyperirritability; muscular twitching; reluctance to stand; weak pasterns; loss of equilibrium; tetany; death	Low serum magnesium and calcium; reduced bone magnesium	NRC 1979, 1998
Manganese	Lameness; enlarged hock joints with crocked and shorten legs; increased fat deposition; resorbed fetuses; small, weak pigs born; reduced milk production; irregular or absent estrous cycles; delayed postweaning estrus	Replacement of cancellous bone with fibrous tissue; early closure of distal epiphyseal plate; low serum manganese and alkaline phosphatase	NRC 1979, 1998; Hill and Spears 2001
Phosphorus	Reduced weight gain and feed efficiency; rickets; osteomalacia; spontaneous fractures; posterior paralysis (downer sow syndrome)	Reduced bone breaking strength and mineralization; elevated serum calcium and alkaline phosphatase; enlarged costochondral junction (beading); reduced serum inorganic phosphorus	NRC 1979; Koch and Mahan 1986; Hall et al. 1991; Crenshaw 2001
Potassium	Anorexia; reduced weight gain; rough hair coat; emaciation; ataxia; inactivity	Reduced heart rate; increased PR, QRS, and QT intervals on electrocardiogram; multifocal myocardial necrosis	Van Vleet and Ferrans 1986; NRC 1998; Patience and Zijlstra 2001
Selenium	Sudden death; reduced milk production; prolonged farrowing time; weak progeny; postweaning diarrhea; lower sperm production and motility; sperm tail abnormalities	Liver necrosis (hepatosis dietetica); cardiac muscle degeneration (mulberry heart); increased fluid in pericardial sac; gastric ulcers; skeletal degeneration; increased serum glutamic oxalo-acetic transaminase and glutamic pyruvic transaminase; reduced prothrombin time and immune response; reduced serum and skeletal muscle selenium; reduced glutathione peroxidase activity	Ullrey 1987; NRC 1998; Mahan 2001
Sodium and chloride	Reduced feed intake, weight gain, and feed efficiency; low water intake; unthriftiness; reduced pig birth weight and litter size; extended weaning-to-estrus interval; increased attraction to blood and possibly tail-biting	Reduced plasma sodium and chloride (sodium deficiency); elevated plasma potassium (sodium deficiency); elevated plasma urea nitrogen (sodium and chloride deficiency); elevated plasma total protein and albumin (sodium deficiency)	Honeyfield et al. 1985; Fraser 1987; Cromwell et al. 1989; Seynaeve et al. 1996; Patience and Zijlstra 2001
Zinc	Anorexia; reduced weight gain and feed efficiency; parakeratosis; extended parturition time; increased stillbirth rate; reduced litter size and pig birth weight; alopecia; poor wound healing	Reduced serum, tissue, and milk zinc; reduced serum albumin and alkaline phosphatase; reduced thymus weight; retarded testicle development; deleted fat depots; serous atrophy of fat; depletion of thymocytes; keratinization of tongue and esophagus; cardia of stomach; reduced immune response	Kalinowski and Chavez 1986; Miller 1991; NRC 1998; Hill and Spears 2001

[a]Supplemental chromium (from chromium tripicolinate, chromium propionate, or chromium-L-methionine) has improved growth performance, muscling, and litter size (Southern and Payne 2003).

Table 57.3.   Deficiency signs for other nutrients and dietary components in swine

Item	Clinical Signs	Subclinical Signs	Reference
Energy	Weakness; low body temperature; reduced weight gain and loss of body weight; impaired sow reproductivity; coma; death	Hypoglycemia; loss of subcutaneous fat; elevated hematocrit and serum cholesterol; reduced blood glucose, calcium, and sodium	NRC 1979; Pettigrew and Tokach 1991
Fat (linoleic acid)	Dermatitis; hair loss; necrosis of skin	Small gallbladder; elevated triene/tetraene in tissue lipids	NRC 1979; ARC 1981
Protein/amino acids	Reduced feed intake, weight gain, and feed efficiency; unthriftiness; impaired sow and boar reproductivity; increased carcass backfat, feed wastage, and attraction to blood (possibly tail-biting)	Kwashiorkor-like symptoms in baby pigs, including reduced serum protein and albumin, anemia, gross edema, and increased liver lipids; increased plasma urea; reduced resistance to bacterial infection	NRC 1979, 1998; Baker and Speer 1983; Pettigrew and Tokach 1991; Fraser et al. 1991; Lewis 1992
Water	Reduced feed intake and weight gain; dehydration; possible salt poisoning; increased respiration; diarrhea in piglets; death	Elevated hematocrit and plasma electrolytes; loss of temperature regulation; tissue dehydration; crystalluria; proteinuria; bacteriuria; cystitis	NRC 1979; Madec et al. 1986; Thacker 2001

To facilitate identification of the nutrient(s) to focus on when troubleshooting suspected feed-related problems, use Table 57.7 as an initial screen. In this table the clinical symptoms presented in Tables 52.1–52.6 are arranged in alphabetical order. Locate the clinical symptom observed and determine the nutrient(s) that may be involved. For example, if pig feed intake is impaired, find "anorexia/reduced feed intake" in Table 57.7 for a list of nutrients that may be involved in decreased feed intake. If additional clinical symptoms are observed, use them to help narrow the list to fewer nutrients. Subsequently refer to the subclinical symptoms in Tables 57.1–57.6 to help make a more definite diagnosis. It is important to remember that some of the clinical symptoms in Table 57.7 may be caused by factors other than faulty nutrition (i.e., environment, infectious disease, etc.). Finally, collect a sample of the feed and analyze it for the nutrient(s) suspected to be involved.

Sampling Procedures

When sampling feeds for laboratory analysis, it is essential to get a representative sample; otherwise, the results may be misleading. The sampling technique will be most accurate by using a grain probe; it allows deep penetration into feeders, bags, and other containers while sampling. If a probe is not available, use your hand or a cup on a pole.

Obtain samples from feeders to maximize the chance of identifying a feed quality problem. Take a sample from at least one out of every two feeders, inserting the probe at two different locations. If you use your hand for sampling, be sure to insert your arm to elbow depth to obtain a sample. When sampling directly from the mixer or unloader, grab 10 single handfuls of feed per ton at various intervals as the feed is unloaded, except for the initial and final outputs. Collect the samples in a large, clean container and mix thoroughly. Obtain two

.5 kg samples and seal each in individual, clearly marked and dated containers. Heavy plastic bags, plastic containers with lids and clean, widemouthed jars are excellent for storing samples. Submit one sample to the laboratory and keep the other in the freezer until the analysis is complete.

Interpreting Laboratory Results

Even if the feed sampled was made to perfection, there are errors in sampling and laboratory analyses that at best can only be minimized. These errors can cause differences in nutrient levels between what the laboratory reports and producer expects. Generally there is no need for concern as long as analyzed nutrient values are not significantly different from the calculated nutrient content of the diet. Comparing analyzed values to the calculated nutrient content of the diet is an essential step in interpreting laboratory results.

Calculate the nutrient content of the finished feed from the diet formula, appropriate feed labels, and nutrient contents of ingredients. Compare those values to the "as-fed," "as-is," or "as-received" values from the laboratory report.

How much difference can there be between the calculated and analyzed values before it is appropriate to conclude there is a feed quality problem? The expected amount of variation associated with sampling and laboratory analyses for some nutrients is shown in Table 57.8 (for phosphorus, 13%). From these values and the calculated nutrient content of the diet, an expected range for the amount of that nutrient in the diet can be estimated. For example, assume the calculated phosphorus content of a diet is .65%. To allow for normal sampling and laboratory variation, the acceptable range of phosphorus levels in the diet will be from .57 to .73%:

.65% × .13 = .08; .65% − .08% = .57%; .65% + .08% = .73%

Table 57.4. Signs of vitamin excess and estimated tolerance level in swine

Nutrient	Clinical Signs	Subclinical Signs	Estimated Dietary Tolerance Level[a]	Reference
Vitamin A[b]	Reduced feed intake and weight gain; skeletal malformation; rough hair coat; hyperirritability; incoordination; blood in urine and feces; joint pain and swelling; skin thickening; death	Bone lesions; internal hemorrhage; bone fractures; reduced spinal fluid pressure, liver and serum tocopherol and uronic acid in joint cartilage; increased blood clotting time	20,000 IU/kg (growing pig) 40,000 IU/kg (breeding herd)	NRC 1987; Blair et al. 1992, 1996; Darroch 2001
Vitamin D[c]	Reduced feed intake, feed efficiency and weight gain; rough hair coat; lameness; stiffness; arching of the back; paralysis; vomiting; death	Reduced liver, radius, and ulna weight; calcification in aorta, heart, kidney, and lung; hypercalcemia; hyperphosphatemia; osteoporosis; hemorrhagic gastritis	22,000 IU/kg (<60 days)[d] 2,200 IU/kg (>60 days)[d]	Long 1984; Hancock et al. 1986; NRC 1987, 1998; Crenshaw 2001
Vitamin E	None documented	None documented	Not determined[e]	Mahan 2001
Vitamin K (menadione)	None documented	None documented	500 mg/kg	NRC 1998; Crenshaw 2001
Biotin	None documented	None documented	0.2–0.5 mg/kg	NRC 1998; Dove and Cook 2001
Choline	Reduced feed intake and weight gain[f]	None documented	Not determined	Dove and Cook 2001
Folic acid	None documented	None documented	Not determined	Dove and Cook 2001
Niacin	None documented	None documented	Not determined	Dove and Cook 2001
Pantothenic acid	None documented	None documented	Not determined	Dove and Cook 2001
Riboflavin	None documented	None documented	Not determined[g]	Campbell and Combs 1990a; Dove and Cook 2001
Vitamin B_1 (thiamin)	None documented	None documented	Not determined[h]	Dove and Cook 2001
Vitamin B_6 (pyridoxine)	None documented	None documented	Not determined[i]	Dove and Cook 2001
Vitamin B_{12}	None documented	None documented	Not determined	Dove and Cook 2001
Vitamin C (ascorbic acid)	None documented	None documented	Not determined[j]	Dove and Cook 2001

[a]When higher dietary levels were provided certain clinical and subclinical signs were either observed or could appear under experimental conditions. These levels may not represent actual tolerance levels in production situations and they generally apply to growing pigs allowed ad libitum access to feed.

[b]Increased dietary levels of vitamins D, E, and K may reduce vitamin A toxicity.

[c] Toxicity is reduced when the diet is low in calcium or high in vitamin A.

[d]Applies to vitamin D_3. Vitamin D_2 is significantly more toxic.

[e]Feeding ≤1000 IU/kg of feed has not caused any ill effects in growing swine.

[f]Observed when 2000 mg/kg choline was fed throughout the nursery, growing, and finishing phases (Southern et al. 1986)

[g]No ill effects were observed when 37 kg pigs were fed diets supplemented with 0.1, 0.3, 0.5, and 0.7% riboflavin for 70 days.

[h]100 mg/kg has been fed to young pigs with no ill effects.

[i]No detrimental effects were observed when a diet containing 9.2 mg/kg was fed to early weaned pigs.

[j]No adverse effects were observed when a diet containing 10 g/kg was fed to young pigs.

If the analyzed value falls within the acceptable range (e.g., between .57% and .73%), a feed quality problem associated with that nutrient probably does not exist. However, if the level of all or any one of the nutrients falls outside the acceptable range and proper sampling procedures were used, submit a portion of the retained sample to the same or another laboratory for a repeat analysis. If the results from the second analysis also fall outside the normal range, a feed quality problem may exist. Review the causes of nutrient deficiencies and excesses presented earlier in this chapter to help determine an explanation for the quality problem. Again it is important to remember that a nutrient deficiency may be manifested by the antagonism or excess of another nutrient. Therefore, deficiency symptoms may be observed in the presence of seemingly adequate dietary nutrient concentrations. This situation is most likely to occur between zinc and copper and calcium and zinc.

PREVENTING NUTRIENT DEFICIENCIES AND EXCESSES

Emphasis should be placed on reducing the opportunity for pigs to consume diets with inadequate or excessive

Table 57.5. Signs of mineral excess and estimated tolerance level in swine

Nutrient	Clinical Signs	Subclinical Signs	Estimated Dietary Tolerance Level[a]	Reference
Calcium	Reduced feed intake, weight gain and feed efficiency; parakeratosis[b]	Elevated plasma calcium; increased prothrombin clotting time[c]	1.0%	NRC 1980; Foley et al. 1990; Hall et al. 1991; Crenshaw 2001
Chromium	Anorexia; diarrhea; depression; inactivity; labored breathing; tremors[d]	None documented	3,000 ppm (oxide) 1,000 ppm (chloride)	Vishnyakov et al. 1985; Hill and Spears 2001
Cobalt[e]	Anorexia; reduced weight gain; stiff-legged; humped back; incoordination; muscle tremors	Anemia	10 ppm	NRC 1980, 1998; Hill and Spears 2001
Copper	Anorexia; reduced weight gain; bloody feces; jaundice; death	Anemia; yellow appearance to liver; internal hemorrhage; ulceration of esophageal zone of stomach; pulmonary edema; elevated liver and kidney copper; reduced hemoglobin	250 ppm[f]	NRC 1980, 1998; Cromwell et al. 1983; Miller 1991; Hill and Spears 2001
Iodine	Reduced feed intake and weight gain	Decreased blood hemoglobin and liver iron	400 ppm	NRC 1980; Miller 1991; Hill and Spears 2001
Iron	Reduced feed intake, weight gain, and feed efficiency; profuse diarrhea; incoordination; shivering; tetanic convulsions; labored breathing; coma; dyspnea; drowsiness; death; rickets[g]	Edema of stomach wall; hyperemia; extensive mucosal necrosis; pallor of skeletal muscles; swollen kidneys; epicardial hemorrhage; hypopericardium; hydrothorax; severe degeneration of muscle and nephrosis; necrosis of liver; reduced disease resistance	3,000 ppm <100 mg[h]	NRC 1980, 1998; Miller 1991
Magnesium	None documented	None documented	0.3%	NRC 1998
Manganese	Reduced feed intake and weight gain; stiffness	Reduced hemoglobin	400 ppm	NRC 1980, 1998
Phosphorus	Reduced weight gain and feed efficiency	Urinary calculi; osteodystropia fibrosa; metastic calcification in soft tissue	0.9%[i]	Hall et al. 1991; Crenshaw 2001
Potassium	None documented	Abnormal electrocardiogram	3%	Patience and Zijlstra 2001
Selenium[j]	Anorexia; reduced feed intake and weight gain; hair loss; separation of hoof and skin at coronary band; reduced conception rate and litter size; pigs small, weak, or dead at birth; labored breathing; vomiting; prostration; frothing at month; abnormal staggering movement; muscle twitching; squeal when approached; spinal paralysis; death	Degenerative changes in liver and kidney; pulmonary edema; elevated serum selenium and glutamic oxaloacetic transaminase; high liver selenium; fatty infiltration of liver	0.5 ppm[k]	Mahan 1991, 2001; NRC 1998; Kim and Mahan 2001
Sodium and chloride	Anorexia; weight loss; edema; nervousness; weakness; staggering; diarrhea; epileptic seizures; paralysis; death		8%[l]	NRC 1998; Pretzer 2000; Patience and Zijlstra 2001
Zinc	Reduced weight gain, feed intake, feed efficiency, litter size, and pig weight at weaning; arthritis; lameness; depression	Hemorrhage in axillary spaces; gastritis; osteochondrosis in sows; increased liver zinc; decreased liver iron and copper	3,000 ppm (weanling pigs)[m] 1,000 ppm (carbonate)	Poulsen 1995; NRC 1998; Hill and Spears 2001

[a]When higher dietary levels were provided certain clinical and subclinical signs were observed under experimental conditions. These levels may not represent actual tolerance levels in production situations and they generally apply to growing pigs allowed ad libitum access to feed.
[b]With limited dietary zinc.
[c]In the absence of supplemental vitamin K in the diet.
[d]Trivalent chromium given via stomach tube (3g/kg body weight) to 60-day-old pigs.
[e]Selenium, vitamin E, and cysteine have provided some protection against excessive levels of cobalt.
[f]250 ppm has resulted in symptoms of excess when fed throughout the starter, growing, and finishing phases and when dietary iron, zinc, and sulfur intake was limited. Nursery pigs can tolerate diets with 500 ppm as copper sulfate for 28 days.
[g]Increasing dietary phosphorus has alleviated the rickets.
[h]As iron dextran administrated IM to pigs born from vitamin E-deficient dams.
[i]The amount of calcium in the diet is important. A deficiency of calcium may lower the tolerance level.
[j]Chronic selenosis can be treated by supplementing the diet with 40 ppm arsenic or 50–100 ppm arsenilic acid (Osweiler et al. 1985).
[k]Tolerance may be higher, but less than 5 ppm.
[l]Assumes ample water supplies are available. Water restriction will lower the tolerance level.
[m]As zinc oxide for a maximum of 35 days.

Table 57.6. Symptoms of excess and estimated tolerance level for other nutrients and dietary components in swine

Nutrient	Clinical Signs	Subclinical Signs	Estimated Dietary Tolerance Level[a]	Reference
Energy	Reduced sow feed intake in lactation[b]; increased carcass backfat; reduced embryo survival[c]	Impaired development of mammary secretory tissue; elevated plasma nonesterified fatty acid level; reduced plasma insulin	Variable	Kirkwood and Thacker 1988; Weldon et al. 1991, 1994a, 1994b; Australian Agricultural Council 1987
Fat	Increased carcass backfat	Soft carcass fat[d]	Variable	Wood et al. 1994; Azain 2001
Protein	Reduced weight gain, feed efficiency, and carcass backfat; mild diarrhea	Increased plasma urea	Not determined	Hansen and Lewis 1993; Dewey 1993; Chen et al. 1995; NRC 1998
Lysine	Reduced weight gain and feed efficiency[e]	None documented	Not determined[f]	Wahlstrom and Libal 1974; Edmonds et al. 1987; Goodband et al. 1989; Campbell and Combs 1990b.
Methionine	Reduced weight gain, feed intake and feed efficiency	None documented	Variable[g]	Wahlstrom and Libal 1974; Edmonds et al. 1987; Edmonds and Baker 1987; Campbell and Combs 1990c; Van Heugten et al. 1994
Threonine	Reduced feed intake and weight gain	None documented	1%	Edmonds et al. 1987; Edmonds and Baker 1987
Tryptophan	Reduced feed intake, weight gain, and feed efficiency; diarrhea	None documented	1% (100 kg pigs) 2% (10 kg pigs)	Edmonds et al. 1987; Edmonds and Baker 1987; Chung et al. 1991

[a]When higher dietary levels were provided, certain clinical and subclinical signs were observed under experimental conditions. These levels may not represent actual tolerance levels in production situations and they generally apply to growing pigs allowed ad libitum access to feed. Variable indicates tolerance levels are generally known, but they are too situation-dependent to describe here.

[b]Result of excessive energy intake during gestation.

[c]Result of excessive energy intake during rearing, the estrus cycle, and early pregnancy.

[d]Occurs when high iodine number (highly unsaturated) fat(s) is present in the diet.

[e]When provided as L-lysine acetate (4% of the diet) to 28-day-old pigs for 16 days.

[f]L-lysine≈HCL (0.7% of the diet) provided to 31 kg pigs for 85 days did not affect performance. In addition, L-lysine≈HCL (1.03% of the diet) provided to 61 kg pigs for 50 days did not affect performance.

[g]Tolerance level appears to be impacted by pig age and dietary amino acid concentration and ingredient composition. The tolerance level is less than 0.2% added DL-methionine in finishing pigs fed a lysine-deficient diet. However, no ill effects were observed in nursery pigs fed diets containing 1 or 1.08% DL-methionine.

levels of nutrients. Proper nutrition ensures that the goals of economy, performance, health, and environmental stewardship are realized.

Meet The Pigs' Nutrient Requirements

Several factors, including gender, age, season, and genotype affect nutrient requirements of pigs. Therefore, it is important to monitor pig performance (e.g., rate of lean gain, feed intake, etc.) on individual farms and formulate diets based on observed production rather than using a general set of nutrient recommendations. In addition, as pigs grow their nutrient requirements decrease when expressed as a percentage of the diet. Thus, as pigs approach market weight they should be fed diets that contain a lower density of nutrients. This is commonly called "phase feeding." In typical phase-feeding programs, pigs growing from 25–120 kg would be fed four or more different diets. Also, because barrows consume more feed than gilts during the growing-finishing

period, amino acid requirements (percent of the diet) for barrows are lower. Thus, it is recommended that barrows be separated from gilts and fed diets containing different amino acids densities (Reese et al. 2000). Nutrient recommendations for various classes of swine were provided by NRC (1998) and Reese et al. (2000). Typically, separate requirements for barrows and gilts relative to other nutrients are not provided.

Implement a Quality Control Program

Monitor the nutrient content of ingredients and finished feeds on a periodic basis to help prevent problems associated with faulty nutrition. Collect samples carefully to ensure they are representative and submit them to a reputable laboratory for analysis. It is not practical to analyze ingredients and diets for all the nutrients pigs require. Instead, analyze for the major nutrients provided by an ingredient or contained in the diet. In general, these include crude protein, calcium, and phos-

Table 57.7. A summary of clinical signs associated with nutrient deficiencies and excesses in swine

Clinical Signs	Caused by a Deficiency of:	Caused by an Excess of:
Aborted fetuses	Vitamin A	...
Anestrus	Riboflavin, manganese, energy, protein/amino acids	...
Anorexia/reduced feed intake	Niacin, pantothenic acid, vitamin B$_1$, vitamin B$_6$, vitamin B$_{12}$, copper, iron, potassium, sodium and chloride, zinc, protein/amino acids, water	Vitamin A, vitamin D, chromium, cobalt, copper, iodine, iron, manganese, selenium, zinc, calcium, sodium and chloride, energy (in gestation sows), methionine, threonine, tryptophan
Ataxia	Vitamin B$_6$, copper, potassium	...
Blood-filled joints	Vitamin K	...
Blood, increased attraction to	Sodium and chloride, protein/amino acids	...
Bloody feces	...	Copper
Bloody urine and feces	...	Vitamin A
Breathing, labored	Iron	Chromium, iron, selenium
Coma	Vitamin B$_6$, energy	Iron
Congenital defects	Vitamin A	...
Death	Vitamin B$_6$, magnesium, energy, water, iron	Vitamin A, vitamin D, iron, selenium, sodium and chloride, copper
Death, sudden	Vitamin E, selenium, vitamin B$_1$	
Dehydration	Water	...
Depression	...	Chromium, zinc
Dermatitis	Biotin, niacin, linoleic acid, vitamin B$_{12}$, pantothenic acid	...
Diarrhea	Niacin, biotin, selenium, vitamin E, water	Chromium, iron, protein, tryptophan, sodium and chloride
Embryo survival, reduced	Vitamin A	Energy
Epileptic seizures	...	Sodium and chloride
Eye discharge	Vitamin A, biotin, vitamin B$_6$	...
Farrowing rate, reduced	Choline, pantothenic acid, riboflavin, energy, protein/amino acids	Selenium
Feed efficiency, reduced	Iron, phosphorus, sodium and chloride, zinc, protein/amino acids	Calcium, phosphorus, iron, zinc, vitamin D, protein, lysine, methionine, tryptophan
Fractures, spontaneous	Calcium, copper, phosphorus	...
Frothing at mouth	...	Selenium
Gait, goose-stepping	Pantothenic acid	...
Gait, stiff and stilted	Riboflavin, calcium	Cobalt, manganese
Goiter	Iodine	...
Hair coat, rough	Choline, niacin, pantothenic acid, vitamin B$_{12}$, iron, potassium	Vitamin A, vitamin D
Hair loss (alopecia)	Biotin, niacin, pantothenic acid, riboflavin, linoleic acid, zinc	Selenium
Hemorrhage, subcutaneous	Vitamin K	...
Hoof cracks	Biotin	...
Hoof, skin separate at coronary band	...	Selenium
Humped back	Calcium	Cobalt, vitamin D
Hypersensitivity/irritability	Vitamin B$_{12}$, magnesium	Vitamin A, sodium and chloride
Inactivity	...	Potassium, chromium
Incoordination/staggering movement	Vitamin A, vitamin B$_{12}$, choline	Vitamin A, cobalt, iron selenium, sodium and chloride
Joints, enlarged	Calcium, manganese	Vitamin A
Lactation failure	Vitamin E, selenium	...
Lameness	Vitamin D, manganese, calcium	Vitamin D, zinc
Legs, bowed	Copper, manganese	...
Litter size, reduced	Vitamin A, vitamin E, biotin, choline, folic acid, pantothenic acid, vitamin B$_{12}$, sodium and chloride, selenium, zinc, manganese, energy, protein/amino acids	Selenium, zinc
Milk production, reduced	Manganese, selenium	...
Night blindness	Vitamin A	...
Osteomalacia	Vitamin D, calcium, phosphorus	...
Pallor	Iron	...
Parakeratosis	Zinc	Calcium
Paralysis	Vitamin A, vitamin D, calcium, phosphorus	Vitamin D, selenium, sodium and chloride
Parturition time, extended	Vitamin E, selenium, zinc	...

(continued)

941

Table 57.7. (*continued*)

Clinical Signs	Caused by a Deficiency of:	Caused by an Excess of:
Piglets, born weak and small	Vitamin E, riboflavin, vitamin B_{12}, manganese, zinc, selenium, protein/amino acids	Selenium
Piglets, born hairless and weak	Iodine	. . .
Piglets, born pale and bleeding	Vitamin K	. . .
Prostration	. . .	Selenium
Rickets	Vitamin D, calcium, phosphorus	Iron
Skeletal malformation	. . .	Vitamin A
Sperm motility, reduced	Selenium	. . .
Sperm tail abnormalities	Selenium	. . .
Sperm production, reduced	Selenium, protein/amino acids, vitamin A	. . .
Stillbirths, increased	Vitamin A, zinc	. . .
Tail-biting	Sodium and chloride, protein/amino acids	. . .
Tetany	Vitamin D, calcium, magnesium	Iron
Tremors, muscle	. . .	Chromium, cobalt, selenium
Ulcers, gastric	Vitamin E, selenium	. . .
Vomiting	Riboflavin, niacin, vitamin B_6, vitamin B_1	Vitamin D, selenium
Water intake, reduced	Sodium and chloride	. . .
Weaning to estrus interval, extended	Sodium and chloride, manganese, energy, protein/amino acids	. . .
Weight gain, reduced	Vitamin A, vitamin D, choline, folic acid, niacin, pantothenic acid, riboflavin, vitamin B_1, vitamin B_6, vitamin B_{12}, calcium, copper, iron, phosphorus, sodium and chloride, zinc, potassium, energy, protein/amino acids, water	Vitamin A, vitamin D, choline, calcium, cobalt, copper, iodine, iron, manganese, phosphorus, selenium, zinc, protein, lysine, methionine, threonine, tryptophan

Table 57.8. Analytical variations[a]

Item	Variation, %	Example	
		Calculated level	Normal range
Crude protein	±3	16%	15.5–16.5%
Lysine	±20	.7%	.56–.84%
Calcium	±26	.70%	.52–.88%
Phosphorus	±13	.65%	.57±.73%
Copper	±25	250 ppm	188–313 ppm
Zinc	±20	100 ppm	80–120 ppm
Selenium	±25	.3 ppm	.23–.38 ppm
Vitamin A	±30	5,500 IU/kg	3,850–7,150 IU/kg

[a]Adapted from AAFCO 2004.

phorus for complete diets. Analyze protein supplements for crude protein and refer to NRC (1998) for coefficients to estimate amino acids from crude protein content. Analyze for calcium, phosphorus, at least one trace mineral (e.g., zinc), and vitamin A or E in base mixes and premixes. Compare the analyzed values to the expected nutrient content of the ingredient or diet when interpreting the results.

In situations where animals are not performing as expected, it is sometimes appropriate to collect a water sample for chemical analysis. Some commercial laboratories offer a "livestock suitability" test which includes an analysis for various minerals. Minerals from water should not substitute for quantities recommended in the feed. Furthermore, when water contains a higher-than-normal mineral content, always compare the pig's daily requirement for that mineral to that which would

be consumed through the water. Then decide whether the mineral content of the diet should be adjusted to prevent a problem with mineral excess. Often the mineral contribution from water is minute compared to the pig's requirement, and thus no adjustment in the mineral concentration of the diet is warranted.

Adopt Good Feed-Manufacturing Practices

These include using products according to the manufacturer's directions, operating the mixer properly, and using a reliable set of scales to weigh feed ingredients. The bulk density or test weight of ingredients is variable; thus, adding ingredients to the diet on a volume basis is not recommended (Reese and Brumm 1992). In addition, be sure all feed ingredients are clearly labeled and that the mill area is kept clean. Monitor ingredient purchases and usage to ensure feed is being prepared according to specifications. Also, use feed within 30 days of manufacture.

Maximize Nutrient Intake and Minimize Nutrient Excretion

Only a portion of the nutrient content of a feed ingredient and(or) diet is available to the pig. The inefficiencies of digestion and metabolism are associated with nutrients excreted in the feces and urine, respectively. Therefore, to account for the variability of nutrient availability among feedstuffs (especially by-product feedstuffs), diets should be formulated based on digestible nutrient content (i.e., apparent digestibility or true ileal digestibility). In addition, nutrient concentration for amino acids, minerals, and vitamins can be corrected according to estimates for relative bioavailability (see Ammerman et al. 1995). Relative bioavailabilities of nutrients from several ingredient sources have been reported by NRC (1998).

Blend Adulterated Feed

Feed that contains higher-than-intended levels of a nutrient(s) is sometimes identified before it is offered to pigs. Often the adulterated feed can be handled as a new ingredient and used to manufacture other diets.

CONCLUSION

Pigs will exhibit certain symptoms when they are not provided optimum nutrition. The challenges for producers and their advisors are to ensure that pigs continually receive the correct balance and amount of all essential nutrients and effectively monitor for and recognize symptoms of faulty nutrition.

REFERENCES

AAFCO. 2004. Official Publication Association of American Feed Control Officials Incorporated. Association of American Feed Control Officials.

Ammerman CB, Baker DH, Lewis AJ. 1995. Bioavailability of Nutrients for Animals. Amino Acids, Minerals and Vitamins. Academic Press, NY.

ARC. 1981. The Nutrient Requirements of Pigs. 2d ed. Slough, England: Commonwealth Agricultural Bureaux.

Australian Agricultural Council Pig Subcommittee. 1987. Feeding Standards for Australian Livestock-Pigs. Editorial and Publishing Unit, CSIRO Australia.

Azain MJ. 2001. Fat in swine nutrition. In Swine Nutrition. AJ Lewis, LL Southern, eds. Boca Raton: CRC Press, pp. 95–105.

Baker DH. 1977. Sulfur in Nonruminant Nutrition. West Des Moines, Iowa: National Feed Ingredients Assoc.

Baker DH, Speer VC. 1983. Protein-amino nutrition of nonruminant animals with emphasis on the pig: Past, present and future. J Anim Sci 57(Suppl 2):284–299.

Blair R, Aherne FX, Doige CE. 1992. Tolerance of growing pigs for dietary vitamin A, with special reference to bone integrity. Int J Vitamin and Nutrition Res 62:130–133.

Blair R, Facon M, Bildfell RJ, Owen BD, Jacob JP. 1996. Tolerance of young pigs for dietary vitamin A and ß-carotene, with special reference to the immune response. Can J Anim Sci 76:121–126.

Campbell DR, Combs GE. 1990a. The influence of excess riboflavin supplementation on performance of growing-finishing pigs. Univ Florida 35th Annu Swine Field Day Res Report AL-1990-4:14–17.

——. 1990b. The influence of excess lysine supplementation on performance of growing-finishing pigs. Univ Florida 35th Annu Swine Field Day Res Report AL-1990-1:1–4.

——. 1990c. The influence of excess methionine supplementation on performance of starting pigs. Univ Florida 35th Annu Swine Field Day Res Report AL-1990-3:9–13.

Chen HY, Miller PS, Lewis AJ, Wolverton CK, Stroup WW. 1995. Changes in plasma urea concentration can be used to determine protein requirements of two populations of pigs with different protein accretion rates. J Anim Sci 73:2631–2639.

Chung TK, Gelberg HB, Dorner JL, Baker DH. 1991. Safety of L-tryptophan for pigs. J Anim Sci 69:2955–2960.

Crenshaw TD. 2001. Calcium, phosphorus, vitamin D, and vitamin K in swine nutrition. In Swine Nutrition. AJ Lewis, LL Southern, eds. Boca Raton: CRC Press, pp. 187–212.

Cromwell G, Hall LDD, Combs GE, Hale OM, Handlin DL, Hitchcock JP, Knabe DA, Kornegay ET, Lindemann MD, Maxwell CV, Prince TJ. 1989. Effects of dietary salt level during gestation and lactation on reproductive performance of sows: A cooperative study. J Anim Sci 67:374–385.

Cromwell GL, Stahly TS, Monegue HJ. 1983. High levels of copper as a growth stimulant in starter diets for weaning pigs. Univ Kentucky Swine Res Report Progress Report, 274:14.

Cunha TJ. 1977. Swine Feeding and Nutrition. New York: Academic Press.

Darroch CS. 2001. Vitamin A in swine nutrition. In Swine Nutrition. AJ Lewis, LL Southern, eds. Boca Raton: CRC Press, pp. 263–280.

Dewey CE. 1993. Ration-induced diarrhea in grower pigs. Swine Health and Prod 1(2):16–21.

Dove CR, Cook DA. 2001. Water-soluble vitamins in swine nutrition. In Swine Nutrition. AJ Lewis, LL Southern, eds. Boca Raton: CRC Press, pp. 315–355.

Edmonds MS, Baker DH. 1987. Amino acid excesses for young pigs: Effects of excess methionine, tryptophan, threonine or leucine. J Anim Sci 64:1664–1671.

Edmonds MS, Gonyou HW, Baker DH. 1987. Effects of excess levels of methionine, tryptophan, arginine, lysine or threonine on growth and dietary choice in the pig. J Anim Sci 65:179–185.

Foley MK, Galloway ST, Luhman CM, Faidley TD, Beitz DC. 1990. Influence of dietary calcium and cholecalciferol on composition of plasma lipids in young pigs. J Nutrition 120(1):45–51.

Fraser D. 1987. Mineral-deficient diets and the pig's attraction to blood: Implications for tail-biting. Can J Anim Sci 67(4):909–918.

Fraser D, Bernon DE, Ball RO. 1991. Enhanced attraction to blood by pigs with inadequate dietary protein supplementation. Can J Anim Sci 71:611–619.

Fritschen RD, Grace OD, Peo ER Jr. 1971. Bleeding pig disease. Nebraska Swine Report EC 71-219:22–23.

Goodband RD, Hines RH, Nelssen JL, Kropf DH, Stoner GR. 1989. The effects of excess dietary lysine additions on growth performance and carcass characteristics of finishing pigs. Kansas State Univ Swine Day Proc Report of Progress 581:125–127.

Hall DD, Cromwell GL, Stahly TS. 1991. Effects of dietary calcium, phosphorus, calcium:phosphorus ratio and vitamin K on performance, bone strength and blood clotting status of pigs. J Anim Sci 69:646–655.

Hancock JD, Peo ER Jr, Lewis AJ, Crenshaw JD, Moser BD. 1986. Vitamin D toxicity in young pigs. J Anim Sci 63(Suppl 1):268.

Hansen BC, Lewis AJ. 1993. Effects of dietary protein concentration (corn:soybean meal ratio) on the performance and carcass characteristics of growing boars, barrows, and gilts: Mathematical descriptions. J Anim Sci 71:2122–2132.

Hill GM, Spears JW. 2001. Trace and ultratrace elements in swine nutrition. In Swine Nutrition. AJ Lewis, LL Southern, eds. Boca Raton: CRC Press, pp. 229–261.

Hoffman-La Roche. 1991. Vitamin Nutrition for Swine. Animal Health and Nutrition Department. Nutley, NJ: Hoffmann-La Roche.

Honeyfield DC, Froseth JA, Barke RJ. 1985. Dietary sodium and chloride levels for growing-finishing pigs. J Anim Sci 60:691–698.

Kalinowski J, Chavez ER. 1986. Low dietary zinc intake during pregnancy and lactation of gilts. 1. Effects on the dam. Can J Anim Sci 66(1):201–216.

Kim YY, Mahan DC. 2001. Comparative effects of high dietary levels of organic and inorganic selenium on selenium toxicity of growing-finishing pigs. J Anim Sci 79:942–948.

Kirkwood RN, Thacker PA. 1988. Nutritional factors affecting embryo survival in pigs (results and speculations). Pig News and Infor 9(1):15–21.

Koch ME, Mahan DC. 1986. Biological characteristics for assessing low phosphorus intake in finishing swine. J Anim Sci 62:163–172.

Lewis AJ. 1992. Determination of the amino acid requirements of animals. In Modern Methods in Protein Nutrition and Metabolism. S Nissen, ed. San Diego: Academic Press, pp. 67–85.

———. 2001. Amino acids in swine nutrition. In Swine Nutrition. AJ Lewis, LL Southern. Boca Raton: CRC Press, pp. 131–150.

Long GG. 1984. Acute toxicosis in swine associated with excessive dietary intake of vitamin D. J Amer Vet Med Assoc 184(2):164–170.

Madec F, Cariolet R, Dantzer R. 1986. Relevance of some behavioral criteria concerning the sow (motor activity and water intake) in intensive pig farming and veterinary practice. Ann Rech Vet 17:177–184.

Mahan DC. 1991. Vitamin E and selenium in swine nutrition. In Swine Nutrition. ER Miller, DE Ullrey, AJ Lewis, eds. Stoneham: Butterworth-Heinemann, pp. 193–214.

———. 2001. Selenium and vitamin E in swine nutrition. In Swine Nutrition. AJ Lewis, LL Southern, eds. Boca Raton: CRC Press, pp. 281–314.

Miller ER. 1991. Iron, copper, zinc, manganese, and iodine in swine nutrition. In Swine Nutrition. ER Miller, DE Ullrey, AJ Lewis, eds. Stoneham: Butterworth-Heinemann, pp. 267–284.

NCR-42 Committee on Swine Nutrition. 1992. Variability among sources and laboratories in chemical analysis of corn and soybean meal. J Anim Sci 70(Suppl 1):70.

NRC. 1979. Nutrient Requirements of Swine. 8th rev. ed. Washington, D.C.: National Academy Press.

———. 1980. Mineral Tolerance of Domestic Animals. Washington, D.C.: National Academy Press.

———. 1987. Vitamin Tolerance of Animals. Washington DC: National Academy Press.

———. 1998. Nutrient Requirements of Swine. 10th rev. ed. Washington, D.C.: National Academy Press.

Osweiler GD, Carson TL, Buck WB. 1985. Clinical and Diagnostic Veterinary Toxicology, 3d ed. Dubuque, Iowa: Kendall/Hunt, pp. 132–142.

Patience JF, Zijlstra RT. 2001. Sodium, potassium, chloride, magnesium, and sulfur in swine nutrition. In Swine Nutrition. AJ Lewis, LL Southern, eds. Boca Raton: CRC Press, pp. 213–2227.

Peo ER Jr. 1991. Calcium, phosphorus, and vitamin D in swine nutrition. In Swine Nutrition. ER Miller, DE Ullrey, AJ Lewis, eds. Stoneham: Butterworth-Heinemann, pp. 165–182.

Pettigrew JE, Tokach MD. 1991. Nutrition and female reproduction. Pig News and Infor 12(4):559–562.

Poulsen HD. 1995. Zinc oxide for weanling piglets. Acta Agric Scand 45(1):159–167.

Pretzer SD. 2000. Diarrhea in gilts caused by excessive dietary sodium chloride. Swine Health Prod 8(4):181–183.

Reese DE, Brumm MC. 1992. Mixing Quality Pig Feed. Univ Nebraska NebGuide G88-892-A.

Reese DE, Thaler RC, Brumm MC, Lewis AJ, Miller PS, Libal GW. 2000. Nebraska and South Dakota Swine Nutrition Guide. Univ Nebraska EC-95-273-C.

Seynaeve MR, De Wilde R, Janssens G, De Smet B. 1996. The influence of dietary salt level on water consumption, farrowing, and reproductive performance on lactating sows. J Anim Sci 74:1047–1055.

Southern LL, Brown DR, Werner DD, Fox MC. 1986. Excess supplemental choline for swine. J Anim Sci 62:992–996.

Southern LL, Payne RL. 2003. Role of chromium in swine nutrition explored. Feedstuffs 75(34):11–24.

Stahly TS, Cromwell GL, Terhune D. 1991. Responses of high, medium and low lean growth genotypes to dietary amino acid regimen. J Anim Sci 69(Suppl 1):364.

Thacker PA. 2001. Water in swine nutrition. In Swine Nutrition. AJ Lewis, LL Southern, eds. Boca Raton: CRC Press, pp. 381–398.

Traylor SL, Hancock JD, Behnke KC, Stark CR, Hines RH. 1994. Uniformity of mixed diets affects growth performance in nursery and finishing pigs. J Anim Sci 72(Suppl 1):59.

Ullrey DE. 1987. Biochemical and physiological indicators of selenium status in animals. J Anim Sci 65:1712–1726.

———. 1991. Vitamins A and K in swine nutrition. In Swine Nutrition. ER Miller, DE Ullrey, AJ Lewis, eds. Stoneham: Butterworth-Heinemann, pp. 215–233.

Van Heugten E, Spears JW, Coffey MT, Kegley EB, Qureshi MA. 1994. The effect of methionine and aflatoxin on immune function in weanling pigs. J Anim Sci 72:658–664.

Van Vleet JF, Ferrans VJ. 1986. Myocardial diseases of animals. Am J Pathol 124(1):98–178.

Vishnyakov SI, Levantovskii SA, Morozov VV, Ryzhkova GF. 1985. Toxicity for Swine of Trivalent Chromium Compounds. Veterinariya, Moscow, USSR No 5, 69–70. Abstract no 2657 in Pig News and Infor 6(4):496.

Wahlstrom RC, Libal GW. 1974. Gain, feed efficiency and carcass characteristics of swine fed supplemental lysine and methionine in corn-soybean meal diets during the growing and finishing periods. J Anim Sci 38:1261–1266.

Weldon WC, Lewis AJ, Louis GF, Kovar JL, Geisemann MA, Miller PS. 1994a. Postpartum hypophagia in primiparous sows. I. Effects of gestation feeding level on feed intake, feeding behavior, and plasma metabolite concentrations during lactation. J Anim Sci 72:387–394.

Weldon WC, Lewis AJ, Louis GF, Kovar JL, Miller PS. 1994b. Postpartum hypophagia in primiparous Sows. II. Effects of feeding level during gestation and exogenous insulin on lactation feed intake, glucose tolerance, and epinephrine-stimulated release of nonesterified fatty acids and glucose. J Anim Sci 72:395–403.

Weldon WC, Thulin AJ, MacDougald OA, Johnston LJ, Miller ER, Tucker HA. 1991. Effects of increased dietary energy and protein during late gestation on mammary development in gilts. J Anim Sci 69:194–200.

Williams NH, Stahly TS, Zimmerman DR. 1997. Effect of level of chronic immune system activation on the growth and dietary lysine needs of pigs fed from 6 to 112 kg. J Anim Sci 75:2481–2496.

Wood JD, Wiseman J, Cole DJA. 1994. Control and manipulation of meat quality. In Principles of Pig Science. DJA Cole, J Wiseman, M Varley, eds. Nottingham: Nottingham Univ Press, pp. 433–456.

58 Porcine Stress Syndrome

P. J. O'Brien and Ron O. Ball

Porcine stress syndrome (PSS) is a well-known concern in the swine industry. The genetic mutation responsible for PSS is widespread and commercially important and produces dramatic features. In swine homozygous for the gene causing PSS, effects are conspicuous: heavy muscling and leanness (decreased fat deposition), predisposition to postmortem muscle deterioration, and a susceptibility to stress and anesthetic agents that may produce death and severe loss of pork quality. The PSS mutation was first captured in Pietrain swine in Belgium by selection and development for extreme muscularity, formerly referred to as "double-muscling" or *culard*. In the early 1950s, the PSS gene began to spread rapidly throughout the intensive swine industry worldwide until it reached near-epidemic proportions. Its spread was fueled by the demand for increased lean-meat production and decreased fat deposition but disregard for poor meat quality.

The heavy muscling is associated with other economically beneficial traits (leanness and increased growth efficiency) but also with economically deleterious traits: stress susceptibility and predisposition to development of inferior pork quality. The expression of the deleterious susceptibilities, however, is highly variable since it can be modified by environmental and managemental factors.

There is reasonably good understanding of the pathophysiological basis of the abnormalities associated with the PSS gene (O'Brien 1987, 1995; O'Brien et al. 1990a). They reflect inappropriate and excessive metabolic and contractile responses to all forms of stimulation of skeletal muscle. This includes stimulation associated with exertional, thermal, and social stressors—especially during transport and mixing of swine—and the electrical, mechanical, and anoxic stimulation occurring with stunning and exsanguination at slaughter. PSS is the first genetic disease for which the molecular basis is known and the mutation identified and for which a DNA-based diagnostic test is used on a wide, international, and commercial scale. The PSS mutation occurs in the *ryr-1* gene (first known as the *Hal* gene) coding for the calcium-release channel (ryanodine receptor) of sarcoplasmic reticulum of skeletal muscle.

CLINICAL SIGNS

Ludvigsen (1953, 1954) first reported an often fatal syndrome, occurring in Danish swine, characterized by increased temperature, dyspnea, muscle twitches, and light cyanosis. It was also associated with the exertional, thermal, and social stress of transporting and processing swine for slaughter. The syndrome resulted in pale, "juicy," sour-smelling pork, which he called *muskeldegeneration*. In the late 1950s this condition was recognized in other countries and described as *la myopathie exudative dépigmentaire du porc* in France (Henry et al. 1955), pale, soft, and exudative (PSE) pork in the United States (Judge et al. 1959; Briskey et al. 1959a; Briskey 1964), "back muscle necrosis" in Belgium (Thoonen and Hoorens 1960), and "white muscle condition" in England (Lawrie 1960).

The condition was found to be associated with pigs that were "stress-susceptible" (Judge et al. 1967, 1968; Forrest et al. 1968). When excited in a warm environment, they developed marked metabolic and respiratory acidosis, oxygen desaturation of venous blood, and tachycardia and tachypnea which progressed to cardiac and respiratory failure. Postmortem, their muscle was extremely PSE. The clinical syndrome was further described and named "porcine stress syndrome" (PSS) (Topel et al. 1968). In Europe, it was referred to as "acute stress syndrome" (Allen et al. 1970a), "malignant hyperthermia syndrome" (Eikelenboom and Minkema 1974), or "acute back muscle necrosis" (Thoonen and Hoorens 1960; Bickhardt et al. 1975; Bradley et al. 1979). PSS was also noted to occur on-farm and to be associated with other social stressors, including mixing, fighting, and mating. Topel et al. (1968) noted that rapid tail tremors were often the first sign, followed by dyspnea progressing to open-mouthed breathing, hyperthermia, irregular skin blanching and erythema, reluctance to move, collapse, and death within as little as a few minutes of the stress, and rigor mortis occurring almost immediately postmortem.

Pharmacologic induction in pigs of a fatal syndrome with a genetic basis was first recognized during anesthesia of Landrace pigs for experimental surgery using depolarizing muscle relaxants such as succinylcholine (Hall et al. 1966; Harrison 1994) and volatile anesthetics such as halothane (Harrison et al. 1968). Malignant hyperthermia rapidly developed, characterized by muscle rigidity, "blotchy blueness" of the skin, and circulatory failure with gross metabolic and respiratory acidosis. The similarity of this malignant hyperthermia syndrome to PSS was soon recognized (Eikelenboom and Sybesma 1969; Sybesma and Eikelenboom 1969; Allen et al. 1970a), and a halothane challenge test was developed as a field test for identification of swine with susceptibility to PSS (Christian 1974) and formation of PSE pork (Eikelenboom and Minkema 1974) and gained widespread, international use (Webb 1980). Induction of malignant hyperthermia has also been reported using α-adrenergic agents $5HT_{2A}$ serotonin receptor agonists (Hall et al. 1977b; Löscher et al. 1990; Fiege et al. 2003) and high doses of ryanodine receptor agonists such as 4-chloro-m-cresol (Wappler et al. 1999).

EPIDEMIOLOGY

Origin

Occurrence of PSE pork was reported in the German literature in the early twentieth century (Wismer-Pedersen 1969). It was associated with inbreeding, the stress of management and transport, and acute heart failure (Hupka 1939). The mutation was first recognized and concentrated in swine near the small village of Pietrain in the province of Brabant in Belgium about 1920 (Ollivier 1980; Porter 1993). It was used to create the Pietrain breed, which was based on crossings of swine of the local (Normand) and Berkshire breeds (Porter 1993). With the development of demand for high-quality fresh meat, the leanness (decreased fat deposition) and muscularity of the Pietrain gained greater importance, and it was recognized as a breed, with a Belgium herd book being established in 1953 (Porter 1993). Recent haplotype DNA sequence analyses (Fujii et al. 1991) and extensive DNA testing throughout the world (O'Brien et al. 1993; Vögeli et al. 1993, 1994; McPhee et al. 1994; Lackovic et al. 1997; Yun et al. 1998; Bastos et al. 2000; Morioka 2002; EuiKyung and YeonSoo 2002; Sabre et al. 2003) confirm that PSS arose from a single founder pig.

Spread

The PSS mutation apparently spread from Belgium to adjacent Germany, France, and the Netherlands, and to other European countries. It may have spread to the United States via Danish Landrace, which were imported into the United States in 1934, released to the public in 1950, and became important in establishing the American Landrace herd (Porter 1993). In the United States, the PSS gene first became well known in Ohio's Poland China breed, where the mutation might also have been introduced from its Berkshire ancestry (Lynch 1914), which it has in common with the Pietrain breed. During the Second World War, due to the development of vegetable fats and consequent decrease in demand for lard, the Poland China began to be bred for a leaner carcass (Porter 1993). By the late 1950s this breed was recognized for its high incidence of PSE pork (Judge et al. 1959; Briskey 1964), by the mid-1960s for its associated high prevalence of stress susceptibility (Judge et al. 1967, 1968; Briskey 1969; Forrest et al. 1968), and soon afterward for its high prevalence of halothane sensitivity (Jones et al. 1970, 1973; Nelson et al. 1972). In the 1970s, the pattern of spread of the PSS mutation was indicated by national prevalences within the Landrace breed of reactors in the halothane challenge test: approximately 90% in Belgium; 70% in West Germany; 20% in France and the Netherlands; 15% in Sweden, Switzerland, and South Africa; 10% in Britain, Denmark, Finland, and French Canada; and 5% in Norway, Ireland, Australia, and English Canada (Jensen 1979; Webb 1980, 1981; DeRoth et al. 1981; Mitchell and Heffron 1982; Seeler et al. 1984; Kallweit 1985).

Prior to the early 1980s, in marked contrast to the Pietrain, Landrace, and Poland China breeds, positive responders to the halothane challenge test were not reported for Duroc, Large White, and American Yorkshire swine, and Hampshires and Dutch Yorkshire had fewer than 3% responders (Webb 1981).

The rapid spread of the PSS mutation was based on a number of factors other than the conspicuous increase of muscularity and leanness in PSS gene homozygotes. Propagation was, and still is in North America and many other countries, facilitated by pork-packing plants providing financial incentives for carcasses with high lean yields. Consequently, swine breeders emphasized selection for decreased backfat and for increased lean carcass weight. Spread was further propagated by the lack of penalty for production of inferior-quality pork, especially in countries such as Belgium, Germany, Great Britain, and the United States, which were primarily importers of pork, compared with countries that were primarily exporters of pork, such as Denmark and the Netherlands (Kallweit 1985). The speed and pervasiveness of the spread were facilitated by the pyramidal structure of the modern swine industry, which amplifies the genetics of a small proportion of the population into a large proportion of slaughter hogs, and by the rapid national and international exchange of breeding stock. The major impetus for its spread was the intense selection pressure for leanness that began in the mid-1950s and intensified through the early 1970s, resulting in PSS achieving near-epidemic proportions.

There is a noteworthy implication of the rapid spread of the PSS mutation from a single founder animal across numerous breeds in many countries. Crossbreeding must have occurred between supposedly purebred breeds of swine. This is especially evidenced by the high frequency of the PSS gene that developed in Yorkshire, Duroc, and Hampshire breeds (O'Brien 1995), which in the 1970s had been considered to be free of PSS susceptibility (Webb 1981). Furthermore, local swine breeds raised for pork production in areas where modern intensive selection programs have not been used may be free of the PSS mutation, such as in Siberia (Knyazev et al. 1996) or the Guanling pigs in Guizhou, China (ShanHua 1997), or Manchado de Jabugo pig of Portugal (Ramos et al. 2000).

In the 1970s, the relationships of PSS and muscularity and PSE, and the adverse economic impact of mortality and severe PSE pork in homozygotes for the PSS gene, became widely recognized (Topel 1981a; Kallweit 1985). This, and the availability of the halothane challenge test (and blood-typing tests in Europe), led to intense selection against homozygotes for the PSS gene and a rapid and substantial decline in their numbers from the late 1970s and early 1980s (Topel 1981a; Webb 1981; Kallweit 1985; Vögeli et al. 1985), especially in countries with a national swine selection program. From 1978, the percentage of halothane test reactors dropped from 18% to 1% in 1982 in Swiss Landrace; from 18% to 5% in 1984 in French Landrace; from 12% to 5% in 1984 in Finnish Landrace; and from 6% to 2% in 1983 in Norwegian Landrace. In the early 1990s in North America and England, DNA tests of breeding stock indicated that 1–2% of swine, especially Landrace swine, were homozygous for the PSS mutation and therefore likely to be halothane test responders (O'Brien 1995).

Prevalence

Estimates of the prevalence of the PSS mutation in 25,000 swine of various breeds used in breeding programs were made using a DNA-based blood test (O'Brien et al. 1993; O'Brien 1995). Blood was submitted from 200 American swine breeders, of which 50% were from Illinois, Indiana, and Iowa; from 150 Canadian swine breeders, of which 50% were from Ontario; and from 5 British farms. The percentage of swine heterozygous for the PSS mutation varied in different breeds and countries but was highest in England and in the Landrace: in England, 40% of Landrace, 20% of Large White, and 30% of all pigs; in the United States, 40% of Landrace, 35% of Duroc, 25% of Hampshire and of all swine; and in Canada, 30% of Landrace and 15–20% of Yorkshire, Hampshire, Duroc, and all swine. The percentage of swine homozygous for the PSS mutation was 1% in Canada and 2% in the United States and England. In Canada, selection against swine with the PSS mutation over the last 10 years has apparently decreased the incidence of PSS gene heterozygotes by up to 75% (Du 2003).

Mortality is the most conspicuous and dramatic effect of the PSS mutation but is uncommon, typically occurring in substantially fewer than 0.5% of North American and European swine (Tarrant 1993). However, prior to selection against PSS gene homozygotes and improvement of transport conditions (Tarrant 1993), mortality in transported swine was as high as 4–10% (Devloo et al. 1971; Lendfers 1971; Korolija 1979). Mortality from PSS occurs at rates of up to 10–15% of homozygotes for the PSS mutation (Webb and Jordan 1979; Rundgren et al. 1990; McPhee et al. 1994). These deaths may be largely eliminated by not using PSS gene homozygotes as slaughter pigs and by "stress"-free management practices (Topel 1981b). Finnish studies showed that reduction of the prevalence of halothane reactors from 12% to near 0% resulted in a decrease in mortality rates during transport from 0.8% to 0.1% (Kuosmanen and Puonti 1993). In Denmark, where the PSS gene has been largely eradicated, transport death rates are less than 0.02% (Barton-Gade et al. 2003).

The average frequency of PSS gene heterozygotes in North America was approximately twofold higher in tested breeding stock, 20–25% (O'Brien et al. 1993; O'Brien 1995), than in pigs used for slaughter, 11–15% (Pommier et al. 1992; Goodwin 1994a, b; Goodwin and Burroughs 1995; Gibson et al. 1996). This difference probably reflects use of the gene in breeding stock, especially in terminal sire lines, but removal of PSS gene homozygosity from slaughter hogs.

Introduction of the DNA-based test for the PSS mutation has enabled more recent estimates of the frequency of heterozygotes to be made in additional countries, including 28% in Brazil (Bastos et al. 2000), 6% in Japan (Morioka 2002), 9% in Estonia (Sabre et al. 2003), 15% in Korea (EuiKyung and YeonSoo 2002), 28% in Taiwan (Yun et al. 1998), and 11% in Croatia (Lackovic et al. 1997).

Because of possible negative commercial effects, few estimates of the prevalence of PSE pork are published, especially in countries exporting pork (Cassens et al. 1980). Estimates vary depending on the criteria used for defining PSE. In Europe, in the early 1960s, PSE pork was reported in high proportions, in up to 40% of Danish Landrace and 90% of Belgium Pietrain carcasses (Briskey 1964). As previously indicated, the proportion of Landrace swine testing positive in the halothane challenge test was high, and 80% of these swine developed PSE pork (Eikelenboom 1985; Jensen and Barton-Gade 1985). In some countries, such as Switzerland and Finland, where there was intense selection pressure against halothane reactors and where meat quality was used in breeding selection programs, the incidence of PSE pork has decreased. Frequency of PSE pork in Swiss Landrace decreased from 33% in 1978 to 7% in 1983 (Vögeli et al. 1985). In 1998, the incidence of PSE, based on an initial postmortem measurement of semimembranosus pH of less than 6, was reported to be 69% for

Portugal, 23% for the Netherlands, 8% for Italy, and only 2% for Denmark. (Warriss et al. 1998). In contrast, the incidence of PSE pork increased over this time period in Great Britain: in 1964 and 1972–73, 6% of 5000 carcasses were found to have PSE pork as defined by a pH of less than 6 occurring 45 minutes after slaughter; but in 1983, the figure was 13% (Kempster and Cuthertson 1975; Chadwick and Kempster 1983). In two surveys reported in 1981 of 10,000 hogs in Canada, 20% and 22% were found to have PSE pork based on this pH measurement (Thompson 1981). Subjective determinations on swine carcasses of PSE pork scores based on color, firmness, and wetness are apparently little changed in the United States since the early 1960s. A survey of 15,000 swine indicated a prevalence of 18% PSE pork (Briskey 1964). Assessment of more than 10,000 hams at 14 different slaughterhouses in the early 1990s found PSE pork prevalence to average 16% but to vary widely from 6% to 33% (Kauffman et al. 1993; Bäckström and Kauffman 1995). In Ireland in the late 1990s the annual average PSE prevalence was estimated at 26%, although the frequency varied substantially over the year, depending in part on the weather but also on slaughtering rates and variation in resting periods before slaughter (O'Neill et al. 2003).

PATHOGENESIS

The PSS gene causes increased sensitivity and responsiveness of swine and of their isolated skeletal muscle to pharmacologic, neural, anoxic, endocrine, and physical stimulation (Lister et al. 1970; Gronert et al. 1980; Ahern et al. 1985). This muscle hypersensitivity is associated with abnormal intracellular calcium release from the sarcoplasmic reticulum, the organelle primarily regulating intracellular calcium concentration and, therefore, muscle activity. When loading calcium into isolated sarcoplasmic reticulum to study calcium release, release occurred prematurely, especially in the presence of caffeine (Ohnishi et al. 1983; Nelson 1983). Calcium was released in abnormally greater amounts and at faster speeds (Kim et al. 1984). Specifically, the sarcoplasmic reticulum's calcium-release channel, which plays a critical role in the biochemical coupling of muscle stimulation and activity (Ogawa 1994), was activated by lower concentrations of agonists and inhibited by higher concentrations of antagonists than for controls (O'Brien et al. 1985a; O'Brien 1986a). This hypersensitivity of the calcium-release channel causing calcium release at greater speeds and in higher amounts than normal was proposed to result from a submolecular defect that facilitated the opening of the channel or else inhibited its closure (O'Brien 1985; O'Brien 1990). The channel defect arises from a DNA point mutation of cytosine to thymine at the 1843rd nucleotide of the *ryr-1* gene near the centromere of chromosome 6. This causes replacement of arginine by cysteine at the 615th amino acid of

the channel (Fujii et al. 1991). This gene was first referred to as the *Hal* gene in swine, based on linkage studies of halothane sensitivity and blood types (Andresen and Jensen 1977).

Various forms of muscle stimulants activate the hypersensitive calcium-release channel by different mechanisms (O'Brien 1986a; Ogawa 1994). Caffeine and calcium itself are calcium-release channel agonists. Neural and electrical stimulation and depolarizing muscle relaxants depolarize the muscle surface membrane and thereby activate a voltage sensor (itself a vestigial calcium channel) that is coupled to, and regulates, the calcium-release channel. Activation may also occur due to an increased intracellular influx of calcium down its steep concentration gradient into the cell. Nonspecific membrane-perturbing agents, such as volatile anesthetics, increase membrane permeability to calcium (O'Brien 1986a). Stimulation of surface-membrane α-adrenergic or serotonin $5HT_{2A}$ receptors triggers inositol phosphate formation and opening of an associated calcium channel (Scholz et al. 1991, 1993; Gerbershagen et al. 2003). During anoxia, several factors operate to increase calcium influx, including energy depletion, acidosis, free-radical formation, and activation of membrane-degradative enzymes and loss of calcium-sequestration activity by sarcoplasmic reticulum (O'Brien 1986b; O'Brien et al. 1991).

Stress Susceptibility

Stress susceptibility (PSS) is largely restricted to swine homozygous for the PSS gene (see below) and can be attributed to the inappropriate and excessive metabolic and contractile responses of skeletal muscle to stimulation. Hypermetabolism results in accelerated oxygen and muscle glycogen consumption, with release of excessive heat, acids, potassium, carbon dioxide, and muscle proteins into the blood (Berman et al. 1970; Clark et al. 1973; Gronert and Milde 1976; Hall et al. 1980a). Thermogenesis, in conjunction with peripheral vasoconstriction, leads to hyperthermia (Clark et al. 1973; Hall et al. 1976). Rapid rates of aerobic metabolism desaturate venous oxygen, leading to cyanosis (Hall et al. 1976; Gronert 1980). Developing metabolic and respiratory acidosis causes tachypnea and dyspnea. Marked activation of the sympathetic neuroendocrine system causes tachycardia and enhanced cardiac output, but with the developing hypercatecholemia, hyperthermia, hyperkalemia, acidosis, and hemoconcentration, this rapidly progresses to cardiac arrhythmia and eventually arrest (Gronert and Theye 1976; Gronert et al. 1977). The rapid depletion of intramuscular glycogen and adenosine triphosphate (ATP) results in almost immediate onset of rigor mortis (Briskey 1964).

Although sympathetic neuroendocrine responses in PSS-susceptible swine are exaggerated and prolonged, they are clearly consequences and aggravators, rather than initiators, of the exaggerated and prolonged responses of muscle to stimulation (Gronert et al. 1977, 1980). The PSS reaction may be aggravated by sympathetic enhancement of muscle glycogenolysis, facilitation of neuromuscular transmission, vasoconstriction in skin or muscle, leading to decreased heat loss or muscle ischemia (Lister et al. 1970; Gronert et al. 1980) and to direct stimulation of skeletal muscle by alpha-adrenergic receptor activation (Lister et al. 1976; Hall et al. 1977b). Serotonin may also have a secondary role in PSS. Its release in the brain and its serum concentration are increased by stress, may facilitate motor neuron transmission, have a vasoconstrictive effect that impairs oxygenation of ischemic muscle (Komiyama et al. 2004), and directly stimulate skeletal muscle (Löscher et al. 1990, 1994; Gerdes et al. 1992).

Inferior Meat Quality (PSE Pork)

Muscle Characteristics. Formation of PSE pork is due to postmortem glycogenolysis and glycolysis generated by the sudden anoxia and catecholamine, motor nerve, and mechanical stimulation that occur with stunning and exsanguination at slaughter (Lawrie 1960; Briskey 1964; McLoughlin 1971). The combined effects of the resultant increases in acid and heat production cause denaturation of sarcoplasmic and myofibrillar proteins and contraction of the intermyofilament fluid compartment as negative electrostatic repulsion between filaments decreases (Bendall and Swatland 1988). These changes result in loss of water-binding capacity, increased light scattering, altered refractive indices, and sarcomere lengthening, which collectively produce PSE pork (Bendal and Swatland 1988; Swatland 1989, 1993). Furthermore, during the early hypermetabolic state, osmotically active end-products cause a transient influx of water from the extracellular space into the sarcoplasmic fluid compartment (Berman et al. 1970; Frøystein et al. 1984; Janzen et al. 1994).

The PSE pork develops primarily in muscles of the hams and loins, especially the longissimus dorsi, semimembranosus, and gluteus muscles (Ludvigsen 1953; Briskey et al. 1959b; Lawrie 1960; Thoonen and Hoorens 1960). These muscles have a higher proportion of "white" fibers with high glycolytic capacities: 70–85% in the longissimus dorsi, 79–93% in the white semitendinosus, and 81% in the gluteus (Gallant 1980; Rahelic and Puac 1981; Essén-Gustavsson and Lindholm 1984).

Selection for increased muscularity has resulted in domestic swine having skeletal muscle with increased susceptibility to PSE, which is further increased if they have the PSS gene. Compared to wild pigs, their skeletal muscle has more fast-twitch (type II) fibers, and more of these fibers have a high capacity for glycolysis but poor fatigue resistance (Szentkuti et al. 1981; Rahelic and Puac 1981; Essén-Gustavsson and Lindholm 1984). Swine with PSS susceptibility have increased muscle fiber diameter (Dildey et al. 1970; Sair et al. 1972) in association with decreased numbers of capillaries and

oxidative capacity (Essén-Gustavsson et al. 1992; Fiedler et al. 1999), although proportions of fiber types do not differ (Gallant 1980; Heffron et al. 1982; Essén-Gustavsson and Lindholm 1984), or are mildly increased for fast twitch glycolytic fibers (Fiedler et al. 1999), from those of nonsusceptible swine of the same breed. Apparently because of their hypersensitivity to stimulation, muscle fibers from PSS-susceptible swine frequently are supercontracted in histologic preparations (Ludvigsen 1953; Henry et al. 1955; Lawrie 1960), especially the type II fibers (Palmer et al. 1977). Swine with PSS susceptibility also have increased numbers of fibers with internal nuclei and increased numbers of angular fibers and of giant fibers, which may represent accumulation of mild muscle injury (Cassens and Cooper 1969; Palmer et al. 1977; Dutson et al. 1978; Handel and Stickland 1986; Fiedler et al. 1999).

Environmental and Managemental Factors. Because muscle affected by the PSS mutation is hypersensitive to stimulation, postmortem development of PSE pork is more frequent and severe than in normal muscle. However, there are several environmental and swine/carcass management factors that modify the degree of development of PSE pork in swine with the PSS mutation. These factors exert their effect primarily by affecting the degree of muscle stimulation and the amount of muscle metabolic substrate, glycogen. Since the speed and duration of the postmortem glycolytic reaction, and the associated production of acid and heat, are primarily dependent on glycogen content, then preslaughter factors that decrease glycogen concentration will limit the development of PSE pork (Briskey et al. 1959b). If muscle glycogen is substantially reduced prior to slaughter, and the animal given time to normalize any perturbations in acid-base balance, then muscle from PSS swine does not develop PSE. If the glycogen depletion is severe, as with exhaustion or excessive fasting, the opposite to PSE pork may develop, namely, dry, firm, and dark (DFD) pork (Briskey et al. 1959b; Lundström et al. 1989; Bäckström and Kauffman 1995; Gispert et al. 2000). Since swine with the PSS mutation are more sensitive and reactive to muscle stimulation and therefore to initiation of glycogenolysis, they may be more sensitive to development of DFD.

Specific environmental and swine management factors shown to enhance the development of PSE pork are preslaughter transport more than 500 km, high stocking density during transport; increased ambient temperatures of summer and autumn, and stress immediately before slaughter. Factors known to decrease the development of PSE pork are preslaughter transport of 50–300 km; preslaughter fasting for 12–22 hours; preslaughter lairage holding times of 2–3 hours to allow recovery from stresses prior to the abattoir; rubber-textured floor surface allowing stable footing; and preconditioning to stressors such as handling, mixing, and crowding

(Ludvigsen 1954; Scheper 1969, 1976; Lendfers 1969; Barton 1971; Nielsen 1979; Korolija 1979; Grandin 1980b, 1986, 1996; Tarrant 1993; Bäckström and Kauffman 1995; Berg 1998; Guardia et al. 2004). Incidence of PSE was substantially decreased by reduction of stress immediately before slaughter in a French study (Franck et al. 2003). The traditional use of electrical prods and restrainers to drive pigs in single file to the stunning maching was replaced with an automated system of driving small groups of pigs with a sliding door from the piggery to the machine.

Compared with using captive-bolt instruments, carbon dioxide, or low-voltage for stunning for slaughter, muscle stimulation was thought to be reduced and development of PSE pork decreased with the use of short-duration stunning with high voltage (300 V) followed within 30 seconds by bleeding (van der Wal 1971a, b; Ratcliff 1971; Grandin 1980a, 1982; van der Wal and Eikelenboom 1981). Conversely, several more recent studies suggest that high-voltage stunning may produce more PSE pork than when pigs are stunned without restraint and with low voltage or, especially, with carbon dioxide (Bäckström and Kauffman 1995). In a Spanish study, PSE was reduced from 36% to 5% and the incidence of petechiae, ecchymosis, and hematomas was substantially reduced by replacing electrical stunning with carbon dioxide stunning (Velarde et al. 2001). Drip loss was reduced from 7.3% to 5.8% in an Australian study by use of carbon dioxide rather than electrical stunning (Channon et al. 2000).

High rates of postmortem glycolysis stimulated by slaughter and leading to PSE pork are reduced by prior inhibition of neuromuscular transmission with curare (Bendall 1966), nondepolarizing muscle relaxants (Hallund and Bendall 1965), magnesium (Sair et al. 1970; Lahucky et al. 2004), or by prior administration of dantrolene (Yang et al. 1983); whereas rates of postmortem glycolysis are increased by preslaughter administration of epinephrine (Althen et al. 1979). Liquid nitrogen chilling prevents formation of PSE (Borchert and Briskey 1964). Use of rapid chilling within the first half hour postmortem causes decreased rates of pH drop and decreased incidence of PSE, with heterozygotes having normal drip loss (Maribo et al. 1998). However, too rapid a chilling rate is associated with cold shortening of muscle fibers with loss of water binding capacity and development of tough pork (Rosenvold and Anersen 2003).

Hampshire swine have a high prevalence of the *RN* gene, which causes a 70% increase in glycogen content of white muscle (Sair et al. 1963; Monin and Sellier 1985; Le Roy et al. 1990). Consequently, postmortem glycolytic metabolism is prolonged—although at a normal rate—the final pH is abnormally low, and the meat quality is decreased. Carcasses with both the *RN* and *ryr-1* genes are especially susceptible to developing severe PSE pork, because of increased duration and rate of postmortem glycogenolysis (Gibson et al. 1996).

Environmental and swine/carcass management factors may play a more important role than genetic factors in determining the prevalence and severity of PSE pork. Although it has long been known that PSE pork develops in swine without the PSS gene (Mitchell and Heffron 1982), the proportion of PSE pork caused by the PSS gene may be highly variable, depending on the PSS gene frequency, definition of PSE pork used, the severity of the preslaughter stress, and the extent of control over postmortem carcass deterioration. Jensen and Barton-Gade (1985) reported that inclusion of pork of doubtful quality into the category of PSE pork increased the incidence of PSE pork from 5% to 15%, 27% to 38%, and 81% to 90% in swine without, heterozygous for, and homozygous for the PSS gene, respectively. Kauffman et al. (1993) introduced the terms RSE (red, soft, and exudative) and RSN (red, soft, and normal) to classify non-PSE pork of questionable quality and of optimal quality, respectively. Only 15% of pork was considered ideal, with more than 50% being of questionable quality because of exudation despite acceptable color. Barton-Gade found that an increase in preslaughter stress increased the incidence of PSE pork from 0% to 33%, 13% to 33%, and 79% to 100% in swine without, heterozygous for, and homozygous for the PSS gene, respectively (Lundström et al. 1989). The development of the DNA test for PSS allowed a recent study of a slaughterhouse with a high (20–30%) incidence of PSE and revealed that nongenetic causes of PSE pork were twice as important as the PSS gene (Pommier and Houde 1993). Loins deemed by visual appraisal to be PSE pork were objectively assessed for PSE pork using a surface colorimeter. Swine normal, heterozygous, and homozygous for the PSS gene, respectively, had PSE pork frequencies of 54%, 80%, and 91% and produced 68%, 29%, and 4% of the PSE pork at that slaughterhouse. In a Spanish study, meat quality assessed by measuring electrical conductivity in the semimembranosus muscle was unaffected by the heterozygous state (Gispert et al. 2000). However, lack of effect of the heterozygous gene in this study may be related to the slower postmortem rate of decrease in pH in semimembranosus than in longissium muscle for heterozygotes (Fernandez et al. 2002).

Revenue loss related to PSE muscle is caused by increased drip loss during storage, transport, and processing of the carcass and pork. This increased water loss from pork causes shrinkage and weight loss, which decrease its dollar value (Kauffman et al. 1978). Additionally, PSE muscle may be rerouted for processing into less-valuable pork products, such as sausage. Shorter shelf life and, especially, decreased consumer acceptance of PSE pork appearance and taste cause retail loss to the swine and pork industries (Buchter and Zeuthern 1971; Topel 1976; Smith and Lesser 1982; Goodwin 1994a, b; Casteels et al. 1995; Jeremiah et al. 1996). For the swine and pork industries of the United States, estimates of revenue loss due to PSE pork exceed $50 million annually (see below).

Superior Muscularity, Leanness, and Growth Efficiency

The calcium-release channel defect caused by the PSS mutation can plausibly explain the associated muscularity, leanness, and increased growth efficiency, although the physiological mechanisms have not been defined. For the same amount of stimulation as for muscle without the PSS mutation, activity of muscle with the PSS mutation is more frequent, intense, and longer lasting. Because contractile activity is a stimulus for muscle hypertrophy, swine with the PSS mutation develop greater muscularity. This increased demand for muscle growth must also result in increased demand for conversion of feed into lean muscle than into adipose tissue, resulting in greater leanness. And, because the energy content of muscle is lower than that of adipose tissue, less feed is required per unit body weight.

Although a calcium-release channel defect may plausibly explain the phenotypic changes associated with the PSS mutation, it is not implausible that expression of other genes linked to this mutation might modify these phenotypic traits. Several genes with trophic or regulatory effects on skeletal muscle and adipose tissue have been linked to the PSS mutation, including apolipoprotein E, hormone-sensitive lipase, transforming growth factor ß-1, and the extended black (E) locus for the melanocortin 1 receptor for α-melanocyte-stimulating hormone (Vögeli et al. 1993; Mariani et al. 1996). In this regard, it is interesting to note the relationship of the black-spotting phenotype associated with the e-locus and the black coloration of Pietrain and Poland China swine, which have had the highest incidence of PSS, and of their common ancestor, the Berkshire. Recently, the increased muscle mass and decreased fat deposition of the Pietrain compared to Large White pigs has been attributed to similar but separate and noninteractive effects of the PSS mutation and a polymorphism in an imprinted gene linked to the locus for insulin-like growth factor 2 and expressed exclusively from the paternal allele (Nezer et al. 1999). Use of Pietrain lines free of the halothane gene as terminal sires has been reported to decrease incidence of PSE and increase pork quality compared to use of Pietrain sires homozygous for the PSS mutation (Fabrega et al. 2004).

Extramuscular Tissue Effects

Tissues other than skeletal muscle that might be directly affected by the PSS mutation can be deduced from the tissues that express the *ryr-1* gene. Although cardiac and smooth muscle, adipose tissue, and viscera do not express it, the *ryr-1* gene is expressed in the brain, particularly in the thalamus, hippocampus, striatum, and cerebellum, and especially in Purkinje cells (Furuichi et al. 1994; Giannini et al. 1995). Although the physiological relevance of brain *ryr-1* expression is unknown, it may be related in part to the observation of regional abnormalities of neurotransmitter concentrations in brains

from swine with the PSS mutation (Altrogge et al. 1980; Adeola et al. 1993). This interpretation is supported by the association of the mutation of *ryr-1* in swine hippocampus with decreased expression of *ryr-1* and the calcium-binding protein, calsequestrin (Weaver et al. 2000). Alternatively, these alterations in catecholamine and serotonin concentration may be secondary to stress susceptibility. Stress increases the brain release and serum concentration of serotonin, which is a mediator of psychological stress by facilitation of motor neuron excitation, and has a vasoconstrictive effect that impairs oxygenation of ischemic muscle (Komiyama et al. 2004), and directly stimulates muscle (Löscher et al. 1990, 1994; Gerdes et al. 1992).

The increased sensitivity of lymphocytes from individuals with the PSS mutation to halothane-induced increases in intracellular calcium (Klip et al. 1987; O'Brien et al. 1989; O'Brien et al. 1990b) has recently been attributed to the B lymphocyte expressing the *ryr-1* gene (Girard et al. 2001; Sei et al. 2002). There was increased sensitivity to other triggers of *ryr-1*-mediated calcium signaling, including caffeine, and 4-chloro-*m*-cresol. The physiological significance of this lymphocyte hypersensitivity is unknown and has not been associated with any pathophysiology of the immune system or inflammatory response. It is noteworthy, however, that B cells produce inflammatory cytokines, which may elicit a pyrogenic response that could contribute to abnormal temperature regulation in PSS.

In addition to primary involvement of tissues expressing the *ryr-1* gene, there is secondary involvement of other tissues. As described above, the amount and distribution of fat deposition are decreased in swine with the PSS mutation, probably because of their enhanced muscle growth. Also, as described above, PSS is characterized by marked stimulation of the sympathetic neuroendocrine system, causing cardiac arrhythmia and arrest (Gronert et al. 1977). Mild erythrocyte membrane abnormalities (Harrison and Verburg 1973; O'Brien et al. 1985b) and increased sensitivity platelets (Miller et al. 1991; Fink et al. 1992) to halothane-induced increases in cytoplasmic calcium also occur in swine with the PSS mutation. These abnormalities may be secondary to altered muscle metabolism, although a direct effect of the mutation cannot yet be definitively excluded.

Secondary Degenerative Effects

In addition to calcium's role in metabolic and contractile activities, it activates degradative processes, including proteolysis by neutral proteases and free-fatty-acid release from phospholipids by calmodulin-dependent phospholipase A_2 (Cheah et al. 1986; Sensky et al. 1999). Furthermore, as a side-product of increased mitochondrial activity, free radicals are formed and cause lipoperoxidation and further damage (Duthie and Arthur 1993). These processes likely contribute to the postmortem deterioration of pork quality.

INHERITANCE OF THE PSS GENE AND ITS EFFECTS IN THE HETEROZYGOUS STATE

Historically, definition of the pattern of inheritance of the various traits associated with the PSS gene has been controversial. However, with refinement and improved accuracy of methods for detection of the heterozygote, patterns have become more clear. The appearance of the inheritance pattern is dependent upon a number of factors, including nature of the trait being considered, gene dosage needed for the trait to be exhibited, sensitivity and precision with which the trait is measured, presence of exacerbating or obscuring modifying factors, variability in the trait due to other genetic factors, and accuracy with which the genotypes can be separated. Finally, as attention focuses on the heterozygote, it is becoming apparent that there are breed and strain effects modifying the expression of the gene in various live-performance and carcass traits.

Halothane Sensitivity and Stress Susceptibility

Breeding experiments by Christian (1974) and Mabry et al. (1981) using American Yorkshire and Poland China swine first indicated that the pattern of inheritance of reactivity in the standardized halothane challenge test was monogenic and autosomal recessive. This was confirmed in studies of Pietrain (Ollivier et al. 1975; Reik et al. 1983), Pietrain-Hampshire (Smith and Bampton 1977; Webb and Smith 1977), and Dutch (Minkema et al. 1977) and Australian Landrace (McPhee et al. 1979). The average penetrance estimate was high, near 90%, but ranged from 64–130%. Lowered penetrance estimates were caused by false-negative test results (Gallant and Rempel 1987), which in turn were due to various causes, including testing pigs that were less than 8 weeks old (Carden and Webb 1984; Fay and Gallant 1990), in poor body condition, or with poor muscularity (Mabry et al. 1981); using suboptimal halothane exposure (McGrath et al. 1984); and the inherent inaccuracy of the test (Webb and Jordan 1979). Accurate definition of the pattern of inheritance depended on knowledge of the genotype of breeding swine testing negative, which could be determined after mating them with positive responders. Otherwise, offspring from matings of positive with negative responders would frequently yield positive responders and the pattern of inheritance would be confounded (Carden et al. 1983; O'Brien et al. 1985b). Understanding of the pattern of inheritance was further confused by the finding of dominant inheritance when the challenge test was made more vigorous by prolongation of halothane exposure (Williams and Lasley 1977; Britt et al. 1978) or by coadministration of succinylcholine (Webb et al. 1986; Seeler et al. 1984), resulting in identification of heterozygotes.

The pattern of inheritance of susceptibility to PSS has not been well studied but appears recessive. Stress-induced mortality was approximately tenfold higher in halothane test reactors than nonreactors (Eikelenboom et al. 1980a, b). In one study, deaths occurred in none of the PSS gene heterozygotes but occurred in 15% of PSS gene homozygotes (Rundgren et al. 1990). Transport of swine in tropical Australia caused the death of 14% of PSS gene homozygotes, 2.6% of heterozygotes, but only 1.4% of normal swine (McPhee et al. 1994). The adverse effect of the PSS gene on mortality was almost twofold higher in swine selected for rapid lean-growth rates.

Beneficial and Deleterious Carcass Traits

Ollivier (1967, 1980) studied backcrosses of offspring (F1) of Pietrain and Large White matings and was the first to report that increased muscularity in association with the PSS gene was inherited in an autosomal, monogenic, dominant pattern. Heterozygotes had intermediately greater conformation scores for increased muscling, shorter carcass length measurements, and increased ham and loin yields. After the discovery of the halothane test, further studies confirmed these results and showed that positive reactors had shorter carcasses, lower backfat thicknesses, greater ham and loin yields, and increased dressing compared with nonreactors (Eikelenboom and Minkema 1974; Webb and Jordan 1979; Gerwig et al. 1979; Monin et al. 1981) and that heterozygotes typically had intermediate values (Eikelenboom et al. 1980a, b; Kukoyi et al. 1981).

Detection and quantification of the effects of the PSS gene in heterozygotes on carcass characteristics were further facilitated by the development of linked blood markers and the DNA test for the PSS gene. Using these tests, heterozygotes, compared with normal swine, were typically shown to be shorter, leaner, more muscular, and slower but more efficient growers. The effects of the gene varied substantially according to breed and strain but produced up to 4–5% slower daily weight gain, 0.5–0.9% shorter carcasses, 0.5–1% increased carcass weights, 0.5–1.2% increased dressing percentage, 2–6% increased lean yield, 2.5–4% increased daily gain of lean tissue, 2–6% increased ham yield, 3–15% increased loin-eye area, 0–8% decreased backfat, 10–36% decreased marbling, and 2–9% decreased feed consumption per liveweight gain (Jensen and Barton-Gade 1985; Rundgren et al. 1990; Pommier et al. 1992; De Smet et al. 1993; O'Brien et al. 1994; McPhee et al. 1994; Goodwin and Burroughs 1995; Leach et al. 1996; Fabrega et al. 2002). Although these advantageous effects were found in swine heterozygous for the PSS gene in both purebred and various crossbred lines of Hampshire, Berkshire, Duroc, Landrace, Pietrain, Large White, and Yorkshire origin, they were not found in some strains of Yorkshire, Large White, Duroc, and spotted swine. Data from three large studies, each including 1000–3000 swine of various breeds, and in which breeds were not separated, indicated that the only consistent effects of the heterozygous gene in all swine were 0.5–0.6% increased dressing percentage, 8–11% decreased marbling scores, and 2–9% increased loin-eye area (Goodwin 1994a, b; Goodwin and Burroughs 1995; Gibson et al. 1996). A Spanish study of 1300 genotyped swine found that the gene in the heterozygous state increased loin depth by 6% and mean lean content by 1.5%, although other unidentified factors across abattoirs could cause up to 2.5% difference in lean content (Gispert et al. 2000).

Early studies on the inheritance of adverse meat quality due to the PSS gene were inconsistent. MacDougall and Disney (1967) found in crossbreeding studies of Pietrain and British Landrace swine that heterozygotes had intermediate-quality pork, although it was closer to that of normal swine than to that of the PSS homozygous Pietrains. Studies of Dutch Landrace by Eikelenboom et al. (1980a, b) indicated that poor meat quality was a recessive trait; heterozygotes and normal swine carcasses were indistinguishable by subjective scoring. Later studies, in which genotypes could be more accurately distinguished, indicated that heterozygotes for the PSS gene had meat quality characteristics that were intermediate between those of normal and PSS gene homozygotes, but closer to normal. In Danish Landrace, heterozygotes had intermediate meat quality, although it was significantly closer to normal than to that of PSS gene homozygotes (Jensen and Barton-Gade 1985). The frequency of PSE pork in these Danish carcasses was 81% for PSS gene homozygotes, 5% for normal swine, and 27% for heterozygotes. In Spanish commercial swine, incidence of PSE was 25% for heterozygotes and 8% for normal swine (Velarde et al. 2001). Numerous studies found drip loss after 24 hours at 4°C was increased by 5–50% in heterozygous compared with normal loin muscle. Also, intermediate scores for muscle color, firmness, and pH were found in heterozygotes (Jensen and Barton-Gade 1985; Lundström et al. 1989; De Smet et al. 1993; Pommier and Houde 1993; Goodwin 1994a, b; Goodwin and Burroughs 1995; Casteels et al. 1995; Leach et al. 1996; Gibson et al. 1996). Scores for sensory characteristics, such as tenderness and juiciness of cooked pork, and for retail appearance were also found to be intermediate for heterozygotes but closer to normal than to PSS gene homozygotes (Goodwin 1994a, b; Goodwin and Burroughs 1995; Casteels et al. 1995; Jeremiah et al. 1996; Monin et al. 1999; Van Oeckel et al. 2001; Moelich et al. 2003). Untrained consumers, however found no differences in tastiness of pork from heterozygous compared to normal swine (Van Oeckel et al. 2001). Sensory traits of cured-cooked ham, in contrast to fresh meat, was unaffected by heterozygosity for the PSS gene (Fernandez et al. 2002 a, b).

As for beneficial live-performance and carcass traits, the effect of the heterozygous gene on pork quality varied substantially according to breed and strain. All strains were affected at least partially, with Berkshire less affected than other swine, Hampshires more affected than other swine, and Yorkshires more affected than Landrace (O'Brien et al. 1994; Goodwin and Burroughs 1995; Gibson et al. 1996).

Abnormal physiological and biochemical responsiveness of skeletal muscle to stimulation is also inherited in a dominant fashion. Dose-response relationships for heterozygotes are intermediate between those of the homozygotes and those of normal swine for agonist-induced calcium release from isolated calcium-release channels, caffeine-induced contracture of isolated skeletal muscle, and high-energy phosphate depletion and acid production of muscle biopsy specimens (O'Brien 1986a, 1987; Lundström et al. 1989; Fujii et al. 1991; Shen et al. 1992; Geers et al. 1992).

DIAGNOSIS

Visual Appraisal
Visual appraisal by an experienced swine handler may be 40–80% accurate in identification of homozygotes for the PSS gene. The homozygote can frequently be identified by its shorter body, bulging oval hams, thin layer of body fat, and rapid tail tremor when excited.

Necropsy
Postmortem findings after fatal PSS are nonspecific. There may be lesions of acute heart failure, including pulmonary congestion and edema with froth in trachea and bronchi, hepatic congestion, and hydrothorax. In a fresh carcass, rapid onset of rigor mortis and dark blood, due to oxygen desaturation, may be observed. The muscle is pale or gray, watery, and soft-textured with a sour smell (Ludvigsen 1953). Histopathologic examination of muscle frequently reveals hypercontracted fibers, occasional myofiber degeneration, and separation of fibers by edema, especially in longissimus dorsi and semitendinosus muscles (Ludvigsen 1953; Henry et al. 1955; Lawrie 1960). Cardiac muscle may show multifocal myofiber degeneration and fragmentation (O'Brien et al. 1987).

Halothane Challenge Test
In the typical halothane challenge test, 2- to 3-month-old swine are physically restrained and forced to inhale 3–6% halothane in oxygen (2–5 liters/minute) through a face mask for 3–5 minutes or until the development of extensor muscle rigidity (Webb and Jordan 1979; Webb 1981). Those developing rigidity are considered to have a positive response. Rigidity in responders typically starts after 1–3 minutes of exposure (Reik et al. 1983; McGrath et al. 1984; O'Brien et al. 1985b). Halothane exposures of less than 3% for 4 or 5 minutes may cause false-negative responses, whereas exposures of 4% or more only slightly increase frequency of reaction and decrease time of onset but may increase mortality (Webb and Jordan 1979; McGrath et al. 1984). The potency of inhalant anesthetic used is also critical to obtaining an accurate test result, with potency decreasing

in the order halothane, isoflurane, enflurane, desflurane, and methoxyflurane (McGrath et al. 1981b; Wedel et al. 1993).

Sensitivity to halothane is increased by prior exertional (Van den Hende et al. 1976), thermal (Ørding et al. 1985), or pharmacologic stimulation of muscle by caffeine, succinylcholine, and α-adrenergic and serotoninergic agents (Hall et al. 1977b; Chapin et al. 1981; Seeler et al. 1984; Löscher et al. 1990). Halothane sensitivity can be reduced, but not prevented, by poor body condition or muscularity (Mabry et al. 1981), prior tranquillization (Ahern et al. 1977; McGrath et al. 1981a), administration of nondepolarizing muscle relaxants (Gronert and Milde 1981) or magnesium (Flewellen and Nelson 1980), and epidural blockade (Kerr et al. 1975; Gronert et al. 1977; Gronert 1980). However, the reaction can be prevented by administration of dantrolene (Harrison 1975; Gronert and Milde 1976; Hall et al. 1977a) or its analog azumolene (Dershwitz and Sreter 1990).

Responsiveness in the halothane test is also affected by the age of the pig. Pigs homozygous for the PSS gene but less than 8 weeks old had positive tests less frequently, with only 50% of the pigs reacting at age 3 weeks and 75% reacting at 5 weeks (Webb 1981; Carden and Webb 1984). Although the younger pigs did not always develop muscle rigidity, they did develop a nonrigid form of malignant hyperthermia, with increased body temperature and metabolic and respiratory acidosis (Fay and Gallant 1990).

Mortality, occurring within 24 hours of a positive reaction, is an important disadvantage of the halothane test. Rates of mortality among reactors in the halothane test are variable and apparently breed and strain dependent: 0.5% of approximately 360 Dutch Landrace reactors (Eikelenboom et al. 1978) to 9% of 229 Pietrain-Hampshire reactors (Webb and Jordan 1979) and 9% of French and Belgium strains of Pietrain and Landrace (Ollivier et al. 1976). Mortality rates are substantially increased if a more severe challenge is given, such as by prolonging anesthesia or additionally using succinylcholine (Williams and Lasley 1977; Britt et al. 1978; Seeler et al. 1984; Webb et al. 1986). In one Minnesota study of swine of Pietrain or Yorkshire parentage, mortality over an 18-month period averaged 10% of 200 reactors but varied from 4% to 40%, with Pietrain swine dying more often and in hot, humid weather (O'Brien et al. 1985b).

Although the standard halothane challenge test identifies only homozygotes for the PSS gene, used in combination with either progeny testing or blood-typing it has been highly effective at identification of heterozygous swine. However, such time-consuming, labor-intensive tests have been largely replaced with the more accurate and precise DNA-based test, which can be used to identify the PSS genotype in the absence of any pedigree information or ancillary tests.

Serum Enzymes

Early studies of PSS/PSE pork demonstrated that susceptible swine had two- to tenfold greater than normal activities of muscle enzymes in the blood, especially 10–20 hours following stress. These enzymes included the skeletal muscle isozymes of lactate dehydrogenase and creatine kinase (CK), aldolase, aspartate transaminase, malate dehydrogenase, and pyruvate kinase (Hessel-De Heer 1969; Allen et al. 1970b; Woolf et al. 1970; Bickhardt 1971; Duthie and Arthur 1987). Various "CK-tests" for PSS-susceptible swine were subsequently developed, based on measurement of plasma CK activity after a standardized exercise or thermal or pharmacologic stress (Bickhardt et al. 1977; Hwang et al. 1978; Hallberg et al. 1979). Although blood CK activity gained widespread use in screening for PSS susceptibility, its variability and relatively small difference from normal make it inaccurate. Blood CK activity is increased by numerous other factors, including rapid growth phase, increased muscle mass, mild physical injury occurring during routine handling, unaccustomed exertion, and even intramuscular injections (Mitchell and Heffron 1975; Allen et al. 1976). The test was found to be unreliable, especially when the frequency of susceptible swine was low or for identification of heterozygotes (O'Brien et al. 1985b; McDonell et al. 1986).

Clinical Chemistry

Clinical chemistry changes associated with PSS reflect the increased metabolic rate of skeletal muscle (Berman et al. 1970; Gronert and Theye 1976; Hall et al. 1982; Löscher et al. 1994). In a fulminating syndrome, there are marked increases in serum concentration of side-products of metabolism, including phosphate by 3-fold, lactic acid by 25-fold, venous carbon dioxide by 2-fold, potassium by 2- to 3-fold, glucose (from glycogenolysis) by 3-fold, adenosine (vasodilator) by 5-fold, glycerol (from muscle lipolysis) by 2-fold, magnesium by 2-fold, and body temperature by 4–6°C. Blood pH may decrease to 6.6. Because aerobic metabolism is stimulated in addition to anaerobic metabolism, oxygen uptake by muscle is increased 2- to 3-fold and venous blood is two-thirds desaturated of oxygen. Release of potassium and glucose due to glycogenolysis occurs from liver as well as muscle (Hall et al. 1980b). As metabolic end-products accumulate within the muscle cell, its osmotic activity is increased. The resulting influx of water from the extracellular space produces a 30% hemoconcentration (Berman et al. 1970; Frøystein et al. 1984). Due to muscle membrane injury, there may be 20-fold increased leakage of CK into blood. Up to 80-fold increases in epinephrine and norepinephrine develop in association with the endocrine response.

Blood-Typing

Inheritance of PSS susceptibility can be traced through family lines with almost 90% accuracy by haplotype analysis of marker loci linked to the PSS gene, in conjunction with the halothane test (Gahne and Juneja 1985; Vögeli et al. 1985). This method was used extensively in Europe in national breeding selection programs. The locus for the halothane sensitivity gene (Hal or ryr-1) is closely linked to genes for the H blood group system (H; Rasmussen and Christian 1976), suppressing effect on the A-O blood group system (S; Rasmussen et al. 1980), erythrocyte phosphohexose isomerase (Phi; Jorgensen et al. 1976) and 6-phosphogluconate dehydrogenase (6-Pgd; Jorgensen et al. 1976), and serum postalbumin (Po-2; Juneja et al. 1983), which are close to the centromere of chromosome 6 (Davies et al. 1988; Harbitz et al. 1990). However, this accuracy is too low for reliable application of the test to an individual, requires knowledge of the genotypes of the parents, and is substantially more labor intensive and less cost effective than the DNA test. It has poor accuracy when the frequency of halothane responders is low. Furthermore, it requires the halothane challenge test, which may be inaccurate and fatal. Thus, use of blood-typing for diagnosis of PSS susceptibility has been largely replaced by the DNA test.

DNA Testing

Identification of the defective protein responsible for PSS (O'Brien et al. 1985a; O'Brien 1986a, 1987), studies of the molecular biology of this protein in the rabbit by muscle biologists (Takeshima et al. 1989; Marks et al. 1989; Zorzato et al. 1990), and its recognition as a candidate for predisposition to the human form of PSS (McCarthy et al. 1990; MacLennan et al. 1990) precipitated the sequencing of the PSS gene (O'Brien et al. 1990a). Identification of the precise mutation site (Fujii et al. 1991) for PSS defined a now-patented, DNA-based test (MacLennan and O'Brien 1992), which allowed, for the first time, the specific, unequivocal, and direct diagnosis of PSS susceptibility on a wide, cost-effective scale for the eradication or control of PSS (O'Brien et al. 1993).

In this definitive test for PSS susceptibility, DNA is isolated from a small amount of tissue, usually blood collected into a sterile heparinized tube or dropped onto absorbent paper, although hair roots or muscle and adipose tissue have been used. The sequence immediately surrounding the mutation site is copied approximately one million times via the polymerase chain reaction. This amplified DNA is then subjected to restriction fragment length polymorphism (RFLP) analysis, in which it is cut at two sites by a restriction endonuclease enzyme: the mutation site and a site common to both mutated and nonmutated DNA. The number and size of the resulting fragments are determined via agarose gel electrophoresis and a fluorescent stain. The staining pattern unambiguously identifies the PSS genotype (O'Brien et al. 1993).

A patent has been issued in several countries (MacLennan and O'Brien 1992) for the detection of the PSS mutation, and a trademark has been registered for the classification of the PSS genotype of tested animals or their progeny. The trademark is based on the (former) name for the gene locus of the PSS mutation (Hal), on the nucleotide number identifying the site of the single-point mutation (1843), and on additional descriptors that indicate whether the animal is unaffected by the PSS mutation (Hal-1843 nm [nonmutant]), heterozygous for the mutation (Hal-1843 mm [monomutant]), or homozygous for the mutation (Hal-1843 dm [dimutant]).

TREATMENT, PREVENTION, AND CONTROL

In addition to use of the muscle relaxant dantrolene (Harrison 1975) or its analog azumolene (Dershwitz and Sreter 1990), symptomatic treatment of acidosis, hyperthermia, hyperkalemia, hypoxia, and cardiac arrhythmia is necessary (Gronert and Milde 1976). Cooling and intravenous administration of bicarbonate have been effective components of treatment.

Several factors must be considered in developing an optimum strategy for use of the PSS mutation. Whereas it is clear that swine homozygous for the PSS mutation have too high a risk of developing PSS and severe PSE pork to make them economically viable as slaughter pigs, heterozygous swine may offer significant economic advantage under certain conditions. The occurrence of PSE pork in heterozygous swine is not a major deterrent if there is no demerit for pork quality or if swine/carcass management practices are optimized so as to substantially reduce PSE pork in normal and heterozygous swine. Since technology is presently unavailable for rapid online determination of pork quality and for discrimination between genetic and management causes of PSE, producers cannot be penalized for inferior pork quality. In contrast, producers may be paid premiums for decreased backfat, or increased lean yields, which are conferred by the PSS gene. Premiums on lean yield, which may be increased up to several percent in heterozygous swine, significantly increase producer profits because of the narrow profit margins in the swine industry.

Although the producer is not penalized for PSE pork, its occurrence is economically important to the swine industry. Abnormal shrinkage, rerouting to sausage and other less valuable products, and decreased consumer acceptance reduce the value of ham and loin yield by approximately 5%, or $5 per pig ($2 per pound for 50 pounds of ham and loin) (Hall 1972; Kauffman et al. 1978; Brown 1981; Holland 1981; Smith and Lesser 1982). Assuming a PSE pork incidence of 16% (Kauffman et al. 1993) and 90 million pigs slaughtered, PSE pork causes an annual loss of $70 million. Annual losses in each of the U.K. and Australia for the late 1980s were estimated at $20 million (Cassell et al. 1991; Guise 1987). However, less than one-third of heterozygotes usually produce PSE pork (Jensen and Barton-Gade 1985; Lundström et al. 1989), and even when the PSE pork prevalence is high, heterozygotes have produced less than one-third of it, with most of the remainder arising due to effects of management practices on normal swine (Pommier et al. 1992). In comparison, the economic gain from the PSS gene is a 2–6% increase in ham and loin yield, or $2–$6 per pig, depending on breed and strain. Assuming that one-third of heterozygotes develop PSE, the net economic benefit of the PSS gene to the swine and pork industries ranges from approximately $0.3–$4.3 per pig, although benefit to the swine producer, in the present absence of penalties for PSE, is $2–$6 per pig (Pommier et al. 1992; De Smet et al. 1993; O'Brien et al. 1994; McPhee et al. 1994; Goodwin 1994a, b; Goodwin and Burroughs 1995; Gibson et al. 1996).

Accordingly, it may be more advantageous to reduce PSE pork by optimizing management practices than by eradication of the PSS gene and its associated economic benefits. The combination of preslaughter feed restriction to reduce muscle glycogen, reduction of other pre- and perimortem stressors, and rapid chilling of carcasses may dramatically reduce the incidence of PSE pork to an acceptable level in swine with or without the PSS mutation (Borchert and Briskey 1964; Topel 1981b; Grandin 1986, 1996; Tarrant 1993). Short-term dietary supplementation with magnesium oxide may also reduce incidence and severity of PSE (Sair et al. 1970; Ludvigsen 1985; Lahucky et al. 2004), although a study of supplementation with magnesium aspartate (Caine et al. 2000) indicated the effects of magnesium on pork yield and quality were dependent upon diet and genotype. If PSE pork was controlled by such management practices, the prevalence and profit of PSS gene heterozygotes could be increased substantially.

Occurrence of the PSS gene is highly controlled and used to economic advantage in several countries on a wide scale, including Belgium, Germany, Austria, and Norway (Porter 1993; Knap 1996; Burlot and Naveau 2003). An effective strategy for using the PSS gene is to limit it to the sire line to boost performance and carcass quality in the slaughter generation. This strategy requires knowledge of the PSS genotype of replacement breeding stock and payment for testing or royalty costs of the patented testing procedure. However, this should be cost effective given that a breeding boar may produce thousands of slaughter offspring, with each having up to several dollars of added value.

Alternatively to maintaining and controlling the expression of the PSS mutation, it could be eradicated from herds. With the current high prevalence of PSE pork from nongenetic factors, this may be an advantage to the pork-packing and pork-retailing industries and the consumer, although it may be a disadvantage to the swine producer. However, since nearly three-quarters of the top North American breeding stock is free of the PSS mutation, it is clearly not a prerequisite for good muscularity and leanness. Furthermore, as genetic selection for leanness, growth rate, and feed efficiency has continuously improved performance of normal swine, the magnitude of the beneficial effects of the PSS gene may have diminished. This point is made by recent findings for Pietrain swine, in which breed a polymorphism affecting the insulin-like growth factor 2 gene confers increased lean muscle equivalent to that of the PSS gene (Nezer et al. 1999). In use of Pietrain terminal sires, exclusion of the PSS mutation may maintain high yield of lean muscle but decrease PSE in the progeny (Fabrega et al. 2004).

Attempts at eradication of the PSS mutation have been undertaken in some countries, such as Switzerland (Vögeli et al. 1985) and Finland (Kuosmanen and Puonti 1993), with good success and without long-term deleterious effects on swine carcass quantity and pork quality. In the late 1990s, some countries, such as Denmark, and international breeding companies removed the PSS mutation from their selection lines (Rosenvold and Anersen 2003; PIC 2003). In Denmark, the swine population is largely free of the PSS mutation; the percentage of heterozygotes was only 2% (Aaslyng and Barton Gade, 2001). In Canada, the percentage of heterozygotes in Canadian swine has dropped from approximately 20% in the early 1990s (O'Brien 1995) to 5% in 2003 (Du 2003). Eradication has been promoted by the National Pork Producers Council (NPPC: Miller 1996) and is being implemented by the National Swine Registry (NSR 2004) in the United States. However, Germany, Belgium, and Austria use heavily Pietrain boars homozygous for the PSS gene (Burlot and Naveau 2003) and in France, Pietrain and Pietrain crossed (with Large White) boars are still used in some terminal boar production programs (Burlot and Naveau 2003). Elimination of the PSS gene may cause the loss of an easily accessible, predictable, and cost-effective selection criterion for favorable carcass and live-performance characteristics.

REFERENCES

Aaslyng MD, Barton Gade P. 2001. Low stress pre-slaughter handling: Effect of lairage time on the meat quality of pork. Meat Sci 57:87–92.

Adeola O, Ball RO, House JD, O'Brien PJ. 1993. Regional brain neurotransmitter concentration in stress-susceptible pigs. J Anim Sci 71:968–974.

Ahern CP, Milde JH, Gronert GA. 1985. Electrical stimulation triggers porcine malignant hyperthermia. Res Vet Sci 39:257–258.

Ahern CP, Somers CJ, Wilson P, McLoughlin JV. 1977. The prevention of acute malignant hyperthermia in halothane-sensitive Piétrain pigs by low doses of neuroleptic drugs. In Proc 3d Int Conf Production Diseases in Farm Animals, Wageningen, Netherlands, pp. 169–171.

Allen WM, Berrett S, Harding JDJ, Patterson DSP. 1970a. Experimentally induced acute stress syndrome in Pietrain pigs. Vet Rec 87:64–69.

——. 1970b. Plasma levels of muscle enzymes in the Pietrain pig in relation to the acute stress syndrome. Vet Rec 87:410–411.

Allen WM, Collis KA, Berrett S, Belt JC. 1976. Factors which may affect CK estimations in the pig. In Proc 3d Int Conf on Production Diseases Farm Animals, Wageningen, Netherlands, pp. 179–182.

Althen TG, Steele NC, Ono K. 1979. Effects of prednisolone or epinephrine treatment on development of induced pale, soft and exudative pork. J Anim Sci 48:531–535.

Altrogge DM, Topel DG, Cooper MA, Hallberg JW, Draper DD. 1980. Urinary and caudate nuclei catecholamine levels in stress-susceptible and normal swine. J Anim Sci 51:74–77.

Andresen E, Jensen P. 1977. Close linkage established between the HAL locus for halothane sensitivity and the PHI (phosphohexose isomerase) locus in pigs of the Danish Landrace breed. Nord Vet Med 29:502–504.

Bäckström L, Kauffman R. 1995. The porcine stress syndrome: A review of genetics, environmental factors, and animal well-being implications. Agri-Pract 16:24–30.

Barton PA. 1971. Some experience on the effect of pre-slaughter treatment on the meat quality of pigs with low stress-resistance. In Proc 3d Int Conf on Production Diseases Farm Animals, Wageningen, Netherlands, pp. 181–190.

Barton-Gade P, Christensen L, Baltzer M, Fertin C, and Petersen JV. 2003. Investigations into the causes of transport and lairage mortality in Danish slaughter pigs. In Proc 49th ICoMST, Campinas, Brazil, pp 1–3.

Bastos RG, Federizzi J, Deschamps JC, Cardellino R, Dellagostin OA. 2000. Characterization of swine stress gene by DNA testing using plucked hair as a source of DNA. Gen Molec Biol 23:815–817.

Bendall JR. 1966. The effect of pre-treatment of pigs with curare on the post-mortem rate of pH fall and onset of rigor mortis in the musculature. J Sci Food Agric 17:333–338.

Bendall JR, Swatland HJ. 1988. A review of the relationships of pH with physical aspects of pork quality. Meat Sci 24:85–126.

Berg EP. 1998. Critical points affecting fresh pork quality within the packing plant. Pork Facts, Nat Pork Prod Council, pp 1–8. web: http://www.nppc.org.

Berman MC, Harrison GG, Bull AB, Kench, JE. 1970. Changes underlying halothane-induced malignant hyperpyrexia in Landrace pigs. Nature Lond 225:653–655.

Bickhardt K. 1971. Muscle metabolism and enzyme patterns in Landrace strains with different meat quality. In The Condition and Meat Quality of Pigs. JCM Hessel-de Heer, ed. Proc 2d Int Symp, Wageningen, Netherlands, pp. 36–42.

Bickhardt K, Chevalier HJ, Tuch K. 1975. The etiology and pathogenesis of the acute back muscle necrosis of swine. Dtsch Tierärztl Wochenschr 82:475–479.

Bickhardt K, Flock DK, Richter L. 1977. Creatine-kinase test (CK test) as a selection criterion to estimate stress resistance and meat quality in pigs. Vet Sci Commun 1:225–233.

Borchert LL, Briskey EJ. 1964. Prevention of pale, soft, exudative porcine muscle through partial freezing with liquid nitrogen post-mortem. J Food Sci 29:203–209.

Bradley R, Wells GA, Gray, LJ. 1979. Back muscle necrosis of pigs. Vet Rec 104:183–188.

Briskey EJ. 1964. Etiological status and associated studies of pale, soft, exudative porcine musculature. Adv Food Sci 13:89–178.

——. 1969. Pale, soft, exudative muscle. In Recent Points of View on the Condition and Meat Quality of Pigs for Slaughter. W Sybesma, PG van der Wal, P Walstra, eds. Proc Int Symp Zeist, Netherlands. Utrecht: Reproprint, pp. 41–50.

Briskey EJ, Bray RW, Hoekstra WG, Grummer RH, Phillips PH. 1959b. The effect of various levels of exercise in altering the chemical and physical characteristics of certain pork ham muscles. J Anim Sci 18:153–157.

Briskey EJ, Bray RW, Hoekstra WG, Phillips PH, Grummer RH. 1959a. The chemical and physical characteristics of various pork ham muscle classes. J Anim Sci 18:146–152.

Britt BA, Kalow W, Endrenyi L. 1978. Malignant hyperthermia—Pattern of inheritance in swine. In 2d Int Symp on Malignant Hyperthermia. JA Aldrete, BA Britt, eds. New York: Grune and Stratton, pp. 195–211.

Brown FH. 1981. Economic losses. Agenda item 10. In Proc Work Planning Meeting on PSE/DFD, Ottawa. Ottawa: Agric Can, pp. 1–4.

Buchter L, Zeuthern P 1971. The effect of aging on the organoleptic qualities of PSE and normal loins. In The Condition and Meat Quality of Pigs. JCM Hessel-de Heer, ed. Proc 2d Int Symp, Wageningen, Netherlands, pp. 247–254.

Burlot T, Naveau J. 2003. Genetic determination of pig's carcass meat deposition and hypothesis of a major gene. Principles for the organization of selection on this criterion. Anim Sci Papers Reports (Inst Gen Anim Breeding, Jastrzebeic, Poland) 21 (Supp 1) 21:41–47.

Caine WR, Schaefeer AL, Aalhus JL, Dugan MER. 2000. Behavior, growth performance and pork quality of pigs differing in porcine stress syndrome genotype receiving dietary magnesium aspartate hydrochloride. Can J Anim Sci 80:175–182.

Carden AE, Hill WG, Webb AJ. 1983. The inheritance of halothane susceptibility in pigs. Génét Sél Evol 15:65–82.

Carden AE, Webb AJ. 1984. The effect of age on halothane susceptibility in pigs. Anim Prod 38:469–475.

Cassell JF, Dyson S, Reiser PD, Trout JR. 1991. Unlocking the secrets for pork quality. CSIRO, Report on Research 21:79.

Cassens RG, Cooper CC. 1969. The occurrence and histochemical characterization of giant fibers in the muscle of growing and adult animals. Acta Neuropath 12:300–304.

Cassens RG, Marple DN, Eikelenboom G. 1980. Animal physiology and meat quality. Adv Food Sci 24:71–155.

Casteels M, Van Oeckel MJ, Boschaerts L, Spincemaille G, Boucqué ChV. 1995. The relationship between carcass, meat and eating quality of three pig genotypes. Meat Sci 40:253–269.

Chadwick JP, Kempster AJ. 1983. A repeat national survey (ten years on) of muscle pH values in commercial bacon carcasses. Meat Sci 9:101–111.

Channon HA, Payne AM, Warner RD. 2000. Halothane genotype, pre-slaughter handling and stunning method all influence pork quality. Meat Sci 56:291–299.

Chapin JW, Chang CL, Wingard DW. 1981. Coffee (caffeine) and porcine malignant hyperthermia. Anesthesiol 55:A292.

Cheah KS, Cheah AM, Waring JC. 1986. Phospholipase A$_2$ activity, calmodulin, Ca^{2+} and meat quality in young and adult halothane-sensitive and halothane-insensitive British Landrace pigs. Meat Sci 17:37–53.

Christian LL. 1974. Halothane test for PSS—Field application. In Proc Am Assoc Swine Pract, pp. 6–11.

Clark MG, Williams CH, Pfeifer WF, Bloxham DP, Holland PC, Taylor CA, Lardy HA. 1973. Accelerated substrate cycling of fructose-6-phosphate in the muscle of malignant hyperthermia pigs. Nature Lond 245:99–101.

Davies W, Harbitz I, Fries R, Stranzinger G, Hauge JG. 1988. Porcine malignant hyperthermia carrier detection and chromosomal assignment using a linked probe. Anim Genet 19:203–212.

DeRoth L, D'Allaire S, Bélanger M. 1981. Épreuves de susceptibilité au syndrome de stress du porc. Méd Vét Quebec 11:16–30.

Dershwitz M, Sreter FA. 1990. Azumolene reverses episodes of malignant hyperthermia in susceptible swine. Anesth Analg 70:253–255.

De Smet S, Pauwels H, Eeckhout W, Demeyer D, Vervaeke, I. De Bie S, Van De Voorde G, Casteels M. 1993. Relationships between halothane sensitivity, carcass quality and meat quality in Belgian slaughter pigs. In Pork Quality: Genetic and Metabolic Factors. E Puolanne, DI Demeyer, eds. Wallingford: C.A.B. International, pp. 259–272.

Devloo S, Geerts H, Symoens J. 1971. Effect of azaperone on mortality and meat quality after transport of pigs for slaughter. In The

Condition and Meat Quality of Pigs. JCM Hessel-de Heer, ed. Proc 2d Int Symp, Wageningen, Netherlands, pp. 215–224.

Dildey DD, Aberle ED, Forrest JC, Judge MD. 1970. Porcine muscularity and properties associated with pale, soft, exudative muscle. J Anim Sci 31:681–685.

Du W. 2003. Current situation of porcine stress syndrome gene in Ontario. Ont Ministry Agric Food, Sept 2003. website (http://www.gov.on.ca/OMAFRA) report, pp 1–3.

Duthie DD, Arthur JR. 1987. Blood antioxidant status and plasma pyruvate kinase activity of halothane-reacting pigs. Am J Vet Res 48:309–310.

——. 1993. Free radicals and calcium homeostasis: Relevance to malignant hyperthermia? Free Radical Biol Med 14:435–442.

Dutson TR, Merkel RA, Pearson AM, Gann GL. 1978. Structural characteristics of porcine skeletal muscle giant myofibers as observed by light and electron microscopy. J Anim Sci 46:1212–1220.

Eikelenboom G. 1985. Ways to improve meat quality in pigs. In Stress Susceptibility and Meat Quality in Pigs. JB Ludvigsen, ed. Eur Assoc Anim Prod Publ 33, pp. 68–79.

Eikelenboom G, Minkema D. 1974. Prediction of pale, soft, exudative muscle with a non-lethal test for the halothane-induced porcine malignant hyperthermia syndrome. Tijdschr Diergeneesk 99:421–426.

Eikelenboom G, Minkema D, Van Eldik P, Sybesma W. 1978. Production characteristics of Dutch Landrace and Dutch Yorkshire pigs as related to their susceptibility for the halothane-induced malignant hyperthermia syndrome. Livest Prod Sci 5:277–284.

——. 1980a. Results of halothane testing in offspring of Dutch Landrace A.I. boars of different halothane phenotypes. Livest Prod Sci 7:283–289.

——. 1980b. Performance of Dutch Landrace pigs with different genotypes for the halothane-induced malignant hyperthermia syndrome. Livest Prod Sci 7:317–324.

Eikelenboom G, Sybesma W. 1969. Several ways of stunning and their influences on meat quality. In Recent Points of View on the Condition and Meat Quality of Pigs for Slaughter. W Sybesma, PG van der Wal, P Walstra, eds. Proc Int Symp Zeist, Netherlands, Utrecht: Reproprint, pp. 209–212.

Essén-Gustavsson B, Karlström K, Lundström K. 1992. Muscle fiber characteristics and metabolic response at slaughter in pigs of different halothane geneotypes and their relation to meat quality. Meat Sci 31:1–11.

Essén-Gustavsson B, Lindholm A. 1984. Fiber types and metabolic characteristics in muscles of wild boars, normal and halothane sensitive Swedish Landrace pigs. Comp Biochem Physiol 78:67–71.

EuiKyung H, YeonSoo K. 2002. Detection of the ryanodine receptor gene mutation associated with porcine stress syndrome from pig hair roots by PCR-RFLP. Korean J Vet Res 42:65–71.

Fabrega E, Manteca X, Font J, Gispert M, Carrrion D, Velarde A, Ruiz-de-la-Torre; JL, Diestre A. 2002. Effects of halothane gene and pre-slaughter treatment on meat quality and welfare from two pig crosses. Meat Sci 62:463–472.

——. 2004. A comparison of halothane homozygous negative and positive Pietrain sire lines in relation to carcases and meat quality, and welfare traits. Meat Sci 66:777–787.

Fay RS, Gallant EM. 1990. Halothane sensitivity of young pigs in vivo and in vitro. Am J Physiol 259:133–138.

Fernandez X, Gilbert S, and Vendervre JL. 2002a. Effects of halothane genotype and pre-slaughter treatment on pig meat quality. Part 2. Physico-chemical traits of cured-cooked ham and sensory traits of cured-cooked and dry-cured hams. Meat Sci 62:439–446.

Fernandez X, Neyraud E, Astruc T, Sante V. 2002b. Effects of halothane genotype and pre-slaughter treatment on pig meat quality. Part 1. Post mortem metabolism, meat quality indica-

tors and sensory traits of m. *Longissimus lumobrum*. Meat Sci 62:429–437.

Fiedler I, Ender K, Wicke M, Maak S. Lengerken GV, Meyer W. 1999. Structural and functional characteristics of muscle fibers in pigs with different malignant hyperthermia susceptibility (MHS) and different meat quality. Meat Sci 53:9–15.

Fiege M, Wappler F, Weisshorn R, Gergershagen MU, Menge M, Schulte am Esch J. 2003. Induction of malignant hyperthermia in susceptible swine by 3,4-methylenedioxymethamphetamine ("Ecstasy"). Anesthesiol 99:1132–1136.

Fink HS, Hofmann JG, Von Lengerken GH, Till U. 1992. Abnormalities in the regulation of blood platelet free cytosolic calcium in malignant hyperthermia. II. Pig platelets. Cell Calcium 13:157–162.

Flewellen EH, Nelson TE. 1980. In vivo and in vitro responses to magnesium sulphate in porcine malignant hyperthermia. Can Anaesth Soc J 27:363–369.

Forrest JC, Kastenschmidt LL, Will JA, Schmidt GR, Judge MD, Lister D, Nichols R, Briskey EJ. 1968. Homeostasis in animals *(Sus domesticus)* during exposure to warm environment. J Appl Physiol 24:33–39.

Franck M, Svensson M, von Seth G, Josell A, Figwer P, Poirel MT, Monin G. 2003. Effect of stunning conditions on occurrence of PSE defects in hams of rn+/RN⁻ pigs. Meat Sci 64:351–355.

Frøystein R, Grønseth K, Nøstvold SO, Standal N. 1984. Changes in muscle density during malignant hyperthermia syndrome measured by computerized tomography. Z Tierzüchtg Züchtgsbiol 101:198–204.

Fujii J, Otsu K, Zorzato F, de Leon S, Khanna VJ, Weiler JE, O'Brien PJ, MacLennan DH. 1991. Identification of a mutation in the porcine ryanodine receptor associated with malignant hyperthermia. Science 253:448–451.

Furuichi T, Furutama D, Hakamata Y, Nakai J, Takeshima H, Mikoshiba K. 1994. Multiple types of ryanodine receptor Ca^{2+} release channels are differentially expressed in rabbit brain. J Neurosci 14:4794–4805.

Gahne B, Juneja RK. 1985. Prediction of the halothane *(Hal)* genotypes of pigs by deducing *Hal, Phi, Po2, Pgd* haplotypes of parents and offspring: Results from a large-scale practice in Swedish breeds. Anim Blood Groups Biochem Genetics 16:265–283.

Gallant EM. 1980. Histochemical observations on muscle from normal and malignant hyperthermia-susceptible swine. Am J Vet Res 41:1069–1071.

Gallant EM, Rempel WE. 1987. Porcine malignant hyperthermia: False negatives in the halothane test. Am J Vet Res 48:488–491.

Geers R, Decanniere C, Villé H, Van Hecke P, Goedseels V, Bosschaerts L, Deley J, Janssens S, Nierynci W. 1992. Identification of halothane gene carriers by use of in vivo ³¹P nuclear magnetic resonance spectroscopy in pigs. Am J Vet Res 533:1711–1714.

Gerbershagen MU, Wappler F, Fieger M, Kolodzie K, Weishorn R, Szararczynk W, Kudlik C, Schulte am Esch J. 2003. Effects of a $5HT_2$ receptor agonist on anaesthetized pigs susceptible to malignant hyperthermia. Br J Anaesth 91:281–284.

Gerdes C, Richter A, Annies R, Löscher W. 1992. Increase of serotonin in plasma during onset of halothane-induced malignant hyperthermia in pigs. Eur J Pharm 220:91–94.

Gerwig C, Vögeli P, Schwerer D. 1979. Halothane sensitivity in a positive and a negative selection line. Acta Agric Scand 21:441–450.

Giannini G, Conti A, Mammarella S, Scrobogna M, Sorrentino V. 1995. The ryanodine receptor/calcium channel genes are widely and differentially expressed in murine brain and peripheral tissues. J Cell Biol 128:893–904.

Gibson JP, Ball RO, Uttaro BE, O'Brien PJ. 1996. The effects of PSS genotype on growth and carcass characteristics. In Proc Ont Pork Carcass Appraisal Proj Symp. Guelph: Univ Guelph, pp. 35–38.

Girard T, Cavagna D, Padovan E, Spagnoli G, Urwyler A, Zorzato F, Treves S. 2001. B-lymphocytes from malignant hyperthermia-susceptible patients have an increased sensitivity to skeletal muscle ryanodine receptor activation. J Biol Chem 276: 48077–48082.

Gispert M, Faucitano L, Oliver MA, Guarida MD, Coll C, Siggens K, Harvey K, Diestre A. 2000. A survey of pre-slaughter conditions, halothane gene frequency, and carcass and meat quality in five Spanish pig commercial abattoirs. Meat Sci 55:97–100.

Goodwin RN. 1994a. Pork Quality Genetic Evaluation Summary. Nat Pork Prod Council Publ 04103. Des Moines, Iowa.

——. 1994b. Genetic Parameters of Pork Quality Traits. Ph.D. diss. Iowa State Univ., Ames.

Goodwin RN, Burroughs S. (eds.) 1995. Genetic Evaluation: Terminal Line Program Results. Nat Pork Prod Council Publ 04069. Des Moines, Iowa.

Grandin TG. 1980a. Mechanical, electrical and anesthetic stunning methods for livestock. Int J Stud Anim Prob 1:242–263.

——. 1980b. The effect of stress on livestock and meat quality prior to and during slaughter. Int J Stud Anim Prob 1:313–337.

——. 1982. New electric stunning methods. Int J Stud Anim Prob 3:97–99.

——. 1986. Improving pork quality through handling systems. Anim Health Nut, Jul–Aug, pp. 14–26.

——. 1996. PSE problem calls for market changes. PIGS-Misset 12:16–17.

Gronert GA. 1980. Malignant hyperthermia. Anesthesiol 53:395–423.

Gronert GA, Milde JH. 1976. Dantrolene in porcine malignant hyperthermia. Anesthesiol, 44:488–495.

——. 1981. Variations in onset of porcine malignant hyperthermia. Anesth Analg 50:499–503.

Gronert GA, Milde JH, Taylor SR. 1977. Role of sympathetic activity in porcine malignant hyperthermia. Anesthesiol 47:411–415.

——. 1980. Porcine muscle responses to carbachol, α- and ß-adrenoceptor agonists, halothane or hyperthermia. J Physiol 307:319–333.

Gronert GA, Theye RA. 1976. Halothane-induced porcine malignant hyperthermia: Metabolic and hemodynamic changes. Anesthesiol 44:36–43.

Guardia MD, Estany J, Balasch S, Oliver MA, Gispert M, Diestre A. 2004. Risk assessment of PSE condition due to pre-slaughter conditions and RYR1 gene in pigs. Meat Sci 67:471–478.

Guise HJ. 1998. Perceived and Actual Welfare—Pigs. Wheathampstead: UFAW, p. 79–89.

Hall GM. Bendall JR., Lucke JN, Lister D. 1976. Porcine malignant hyperthermia. II. Heat production. Br J Anaesth, 48:305–308.

Hall GM, Lucke JN, Lister D. 1977a. Treatment of porcine malignant hyperpyrexia: The successful use of dantrolene in the Pietrain pig. Anaesth 32:472–474.

——. 1977b. Porcine malignant hyperthermia. V. Fatal hyperthermia in the Pietrain pig, associated with the infusion of alpha-adrenergic agonists. Br J Anaesth 49:855–863.

——. 1980a. Malignant hyperthermia—Pearls out of swine? Br J Anaesth 52:165–171.

Hall GM, Lucke JN, Lovell R, Lister D. 1980b. Porcine malignant hyperthermia. VII. Hepatic metabolism. Br J Anaesth 52:11–17.

Hall GM, Lucke JN, Orchard C, Lovell R, Lister D. 1982. Porcine malignant hyperthermia. VIII. Leg metabolism. Br J Anaesth 54:941–947.

Hall JT. 1972. Economic importance of pork. In Proc Pork Quality Symp. RG Cassens, F Giesler, Q Kolb, eds. Madison: Univ Wisconsin Ext, pp. ix–xii.

Hall LW, Woolf N, Bradley JWP, Jolly DW. 1966. Unusual reaction to suxamethonium chloride. Br Med J 4:1305.

Hallberg JW. Topel DG, Christian LL. 1979. Creatine phosphokinase isoenzymes in stress-susceptible and stress-resistant pigs. J Anim Sci 49:1464–1469.

Hallund O, Bendall JR. 1965. The long-term effect of electrical stimulation on the post-mortem fall of pH in the muscles of Landrace pigs. J Food Sci 39:296.

Handel SE, Stickland NC. 1986. "Giant" muscle fibres in skeletal muscle of normal pigs. J Comp Path 96:447–457.

Harbitz I, Chowdhary B, Thomsen PD, Davies W, Kaufmann U, Kran S, Gustavsson I, Christensen K, Hauge J. 1990. Assignment of the porcine calcium release channel gene, a candidate for the malignant hyperthermia locus, to the 6p11 q21 segment of chromosome 6. Genomics 8:243–248.

Harrison GG. 1975. The prophylaxis of malignant hyperthermia by oral dantrolene sodium in swine. Br J Anaesth 47:62–65.

——. 1994. The discovery of malignant hyperthmia in pigs—Some personal recollections. In Malignant Hyperthermia: A Genetic Membrane Disease. ST Ohnishi, T Ohnishi. Ann Arbor: CRC Press, pp. 29–43.

Harrison GG, Beibuyck FJF, Terblanche J, Dent DM, Hickman R, Saunders SJ. 1968. Hyperpyrexia during anesthesia. Br Med J 3:594–595.

Harrison GG, Verburg C. 1973. Erythrocyte osmotic fragility in hyperthermia susceptible swine. Br J Anaesth 45:131–133.

Heffron JJ, Mitchell G, Dreyer JH. 1982. Muscle fibre type, fibre diameter and ph1 values of *M. longissimus dorsi* of normal, malignant hyperthermia and PSE-susceptible pigs. Br Vet J 138:45–50.

Henry M, Billon J, Haouza G. 1955. Contribution àl'étude de l'acidose des viandes du porc, dites exsudatives. Rev Pathol Gén Comparée No. 669:857.

Hessel-De Heer JCM. 1969. Serum LDH-5 and muscular stress. In Recent Points of View on the Condition and Meat Quality of Pigs for Slaughter. W Sybesma, PG van der Wal, P Walstra. Proc Int Symp Zeist, Netherlands. Utrecht: Reproprint, pp. 179–182.

Holland G. 1981. Processor point of view. Agenda item 4. In Proc Work Planning Meeting on PSE/DFD, Ottawa. Ottawa: Agric Can, pp. 1–3.

Hupka E. 1939. Seuchenhaft auftretenden huhnerfleischahnliche Muskelentartungen unter den Schweinen. Dtsch Tierärztl Wochenschr 47:242–244.

Hwang PT, McGrath CJ, Addis PB, Rempel WE, Thompson EW, Antonik A. 1978. Blood creatine kinase as a predictor of the porcine stress syndrome. J Anim Sci 47:630–633.

Janzen EG, Gareau PJ, Stewart WA, Towner RA. 1994. The use of in vivo magnetic resonance imaging and spectroscopy to study porcine stress syndrome in young, halothane-susceptible pigs: Preliminary results. Can J Anim Sci 74:37–43.

Jensen P. 1979. Incidence of halothane susceptibility in the Danish Landrace breed and its association with meat quality: Preliminary report. Acta Agric Scand 21:427–431.

Jensen P, Barton-Gade PA. 1985. Performance and carcass characteristics of pigs with known genotypes for halothane susceptibility. In Stress Susceptibility and Meat Quality in Pigs. JB Ludvigsen. Eur Assoc Anim Prod Publ. 33, pp. 80–87.

Jeremiah LE, Fortin A, Gibson JP, Ball, RO. 1996. Eating quality of pork. Proc Ont Pork Carcass Appraisal Proj Symp. Guelph: Univ Guelph, pp. 26–30.

Jones EW, Burnap TK, Nelson TE, Anderson IL, Kerr DD. 1970. Preliminary studies of fulminant hyperpyrexia in a family of swine. In Proc Am Soc Anesthesiol pp. 47–48.

Jones EW, Kerr DD, Nelson TE. 1973. Malignant hyperthermia—Observations in Poland China pigs. In Int Symp on Malignant Hyperthermia. RA Gordon, BA Britt, W Kalow. Springfield: Thomas, pp. 198–207.

Jorgensen PF, Hyldgaard-Jensen J, Moustgaard J. 1976. Phosphohexose isomerase (PHI) and porcine halothane sensitivity. Acta Vet Scand 17:370–372.

Judge MD, Briskey EJ, Cassens RG, Forrest JC, Meyer RK. 1968. Adrenal and thyroid function in stress-susceptible pigs *(Sus domesticus)*. Am J Physiol 214:146–151.

Judge MD, Cahill VR, Kunkle LE, Bruner WH. 1959. Pork quality. I. Influences of some factors on pork muscle characteristics. J Anim Sci 18:449–452.

Judge MD, Cassens RG, Briskey EJ. 1967. Muscle properties of physically restrained stressor-susceptible and stressor-resistant porcine animals. J Food Sci 32:565.

Juneja RK, Gahne B, Edfors-Lilja I, Andresen E. 1983. Genetic variation at a pig serum protein locus, Po-2, and its assignment to the Phi, Hal, S, H, Pgd linkage group. Anim Blood Groups Biochem Genet 14:27–36.

Kallweit E. 1985. Selection for stress resistance in pigs in various countries. In Stress Susceptibility and Meat Quality in Pigs. JB Ludvigsen, ed. Eur Assoc Anim Prod Publ # 33, pp.60–67.

Kauffman RG, Cassens RG, Scherer A, Meeker EL. 1993. Variations in pork quality: History, definition, extent, resolution. Swine Health Prod 1:28–34.

Kauffman RG, Wachholz D, Henderson D, Lochner JV. 1978. Shrinkage of PSE, normal and DFD hams during transit and processing. J Anim Sci 46:1236–1240.

Kempster AJ, Cuthertson A. 1975. A national survey of muscle pH value in commercial pig carcasses. J Food Technol 10:73–80.

Kerr DD, Wingard DW, Gatz EE. 1975. Prevention of porcine malignant hyperthermia by epidural blockade. Anesthesiol 42:307–311.

Kim DH, Sreter FA, Ohnishi ST, Ryan JF, Roberts J, Allen PD, Meszaros LG, Antoniu B, Ikemoto N. 1984. Kinetic studies of Ca^{2+} release from sarcoplasmic reticulum of normal and malignant hyperthermia susceptible pig muscles. Biochim Biophys Acta 775:320–327.

Klip A, Ramlal R, Walker D, Britt BA, Elliott ME. 1987. Selective increase in cytoplasmic calcium by anesthetic in lymphocytes from malignant hyperthermia-susceptible pigs. Anesth Analg 66:381–385.

Knap P. 1996. Norway: An organized gene network. Pigs-Misset 12:10–12.

Knyazev SP, Hardge T, Zhuchaev KV. 1996. Molecular genetic screening of Siberian swine populations: Local breeds are free of the genetic load of malignant hyperthermia. Genetika 32:1423–1425.

Komiyama T, Kihara H, Hirose K, Yoshimoto R, Shigematsu H. 2004. AT-1015, a novel serotonin$_{2A}$ receptor antagonist, improves resaturation of exercised ischemic muscle in hypercholesterolemic rabbits. J Vasc Surg 39:661–667.

Korolija S. 1979. Influence of transport, environment and rest on the meat quality of pigs slaughtered for industrial processing. Acta Vet (Beograd) 29:309–326.

Kukoyi EA, Addis PB, McGrath CJ, Rempel WE, Martin FB. 1981. Porcine stress syndrome and postmortem muscle characteristics of two purebreds and three specific terminal crosses. J Anim Sci 52:278–284.

Kuosmanen S, Puonti M. 1993. The eradication of the halothane gene and simultaneous breeding for better carcass quality. In Pork Quality: Genetic and Metabolic Factors. E Puolanne, DI Demeyer. Wallingford: C.A.B. International, pp. 298–299.

Lackovic V, Tadic Z, Vitkovic A, Bosnic A, Balenovic P, Pleli T, Basic A. 1997. Determination of the malignant hyperthermia (MH) gene status in swine in Croatia. Periodicum Biologorum 99:433–435.

Lahucky R, Kuchenmeister U, Bahelka I, Vasicek D, Liptaj T, Ender K. 2004. The effect of dietary magnesium oxide supplementation on postmortem ^{31}P NMR spectroscopy parameters, rate of Ca^{2+} uptake and ATPase activity of *M. longissimus dorsi* and meat quality of heterozygous and normal on malignant hyperthermia pigs. Meat Sci 67:365–370.

Lawrie RE. 1960. Post-mortem glycolysis in normal and exudative longissimus dorsi muscles of the pig in relation to the so-called white muscle disease. J Comp Path 70:273–295.

Leach LM, Ellis M, Sutton DS, McKeith FK, Wilson ER. 1996. The growth performance, carcass characteristics, and meat quality of halothane carrier and negative pigs. J Anim Sci 74:934–943.

Lendfers LHHM. 1969. Transport and meat quality in pigs. In Recent Points of View on the Condition and Meat Quality of Pigs for Slaughter. W Sybesma, PG van der Wal, P Walstra. Proc Int Symp Zeist, Netherlands. Utrecht: Reproprint, pp. 193–199.

——. 1971. Loss of pigs due to death during transport; A one-year survey at an abattoir. In The Condition and Meat Quality of Pigs. JCM Hessel-de Heer, ed. Proc 2d Int Symp, Wageningen, Netherlands, pp. 225–229.

Le Roy P, Naveau J, Elsen JM, Sellier P. 1990. Evidence for a new major gene influencing meat quality in pigs. Genet Res Camb 55:33–40.

Lister D, Hall GM, Lucke JN. 1976. Porcine malignant hyperthermia. III: Adrenergic blockade. Br J Anaesth 48::831–838.

Lister D, Sair RA, Will JA, Schmidt GR, Cassens RG, Hoekstra WG, Briskey EJ. 1970. Metabolism of striated muscle of stress-susceptible pigs breathing oxygen or nitrogen. Am J Physiol 218:102–107.

Löscher W, Gerdes C, Richter A. 1994. Lack of prophylactic or therapeutic efficacy of 5-HT$_{2A}$ receptor antagonists in halothane-induced porcine malignant hyperthermia. Naunyn-Schmiedeberg's Arch Pharmacol 350:365–374.

Löscher W, Witte U, Fredow G, Ganter M, Bickhardt K. 1990. Pharmacodynamic effects of serotonin (5-HT) receptor ligands in pigs: Stimulation of 5-HT$_2$ receptors induces malignant hyperthermia. Naunyn-Schmiedeberg's Arch Pharmacol 341:483–493.

Ludvigsen J. 1953. Muscular degeneration in hogs (preliminary report). 25th Int Vet Cong, Stockholm. 1:602–606.

——. 1954. Undersøgelser over den såkaldte "muskeldegeneration" hos svin I. 272. beretning fra forsøgslaboratoriet, Udgivet af Statens Husdyrbrugsudval, København.

——. 1985. Intermediary metabolism—And calcium metabolism in stress-susceptible pigs EAAP publication No 55, pp. 106–118.

Lundström K, Essén-Gustavsson B, Rundgren M, Edfors-Lilja I, Malmfors G. 1989. Effect of halothane genotype on muscle metabolism at slaughter and its relationship with meat quality: A within-litter comparison. Meat Sci 25:251–263.

Lynch CF. 1914. The lard type of hog: The Poland China. In Diseases of Swine, with Particular Reference to Hog Cholera. Philadelphia: W. B. Saunders, pp. 23–34.

Mabry JW, Christian LL, Kuhters DL. 1981. Inheritance of porcine stress syndrome. J Hered 72:429–430.

MacDougall DB, Disney JG. 1967. Quality characteristics of pork with special reference to Pietrain, Pietrain × Landrace and Landrace pigs at different weights. J Food Technol 2:285–297.

MacLennan DH, Duff C, Zorzato F, Fujii J, Phillips M, Korneluk RG, Frodis W, Britt BA, Worton RG. 1990. Ryanodine receptor gene is a candidate for predisposition to malignant hyperthermia. Nature Lond 343:559–561.

MacLennan DH, O'Brien PJ. 1992. Diagnosis of malignant hyperthermia. South Africa patent 91/10087, 1992; Canada patent 2064091, 1993; USA patent 5358649, 1994.

Mariani P, Moller MJ, Hoyheim B, Marklund L, Davies W, Ellegren H, Andersson L. 1996. The extension coat color locus and the loci for blood group O and tyrosine aminotransferase are on pig chromosome 6. J Hered 87(4):272–276.

Maribo H, Olsen EV, Barton-Gade P, Moller A J, Karlsson A. 1998. Effect of early post-mortem cooling on temperature, pH fall and meat quality in pigs. Meat Sci 50:1115–129.

Marks AR, Tempst P, Hwang KS, Taubman MB, Inue M, Chadwick C, Fleischer S, Nadal-Ginard B. 1989. Molecular cloning and characterization of the ryanodine receptor/junctional channel complex cDNA from skeletal muscle sarcoplasmic reticulum. Proc Nat Acad Sci USA 86:8683–8687.

McCarthy TV, Healy JMS, Heffron JJA, Lehane M, Deufel T, Lehmann-Horn F, Farrall M, Johnson K. 1990. Localization of the malignant hyperthermia susceptible locus to human chromosome 19q12–13.2. Nature Lond 343:562–564.

McDonell WN, Seeler DC, Basrur PK. 1986. Evaluation of a commercial creatine kinase screening test for malignant hyperthermia (porcine stress syndrome). Can J Vet Res 50:494–501.

McGrath CJ, Lee JC, Rempel WE. 1984. Halothane testing for malignant hyperthermia in swine: Dose-response effects. Am J Vet Res 45:1734–1736.

McGrath CJ, Rempel WE, Addis PB, Crimi AJ. 1981a. Acepromazine and droperidol inhibition of halothane-induced malignant hyperthermia (porcine stress syndrome) in swine. Am J Vet Res 42:195–198.

McGrath CJ, Rempel WE, Jessen CR, Addis PB, Crimi AJ. 1981b. Malignant hyperthermia-triggering liability of selected inhalant anesthetics in swine. Am J Vet Res 42:604–607.

McLoughlin JV. 1971. General introduction section 2. Stunning: The death reaction and metabolism post mortem of porcine skeletal muscle. In The Condition and Meat Quality of Pigs. JC M Hessel-de Heer, ed. Proc 2d Int Symp, Wageningen, Netherlands, pp. 123–131.

McPhee CP, Daniels LJ, Dramer HL, Macbeth GM, Noble JW. 1994. The effects of selection for lean growth and the halothane allele on growth performance and mortality of pigs ad libitum fed in a tropical environment. Livest Prod Sci 38:117–123.

McPhee CP. Takken. A. D'Arcy KJ. 1979. Genetic variation in meat quality and the incidence of malignant hyperthermia syndrome in Large White and Landrace boars. Aust J Exp Agric Husb 19:43–47.

Miller D. 1996. Stress gene must go. Nat Hog Farmer, Apr, pp. 8–9.

Miller KE, Brooks RR, Bonk KR, Carpenter JF. 1991. Calcium handling by platelets from normal and malignant hyperthermia-susceptible pigs. Life Sci 48:1471–1476.

Minkema D, Eikelenboom G, van Eldik P. 1977. Inheritance of MHS-susceptibility in pigs. In Proc 3d Int Conf on Production Diseases Farm Animals, Wageningen, Netherlands, pp. 203–207.

MinYung L, IvanChen C, LeCheng C, HuiLiang T, PingCheng Y. 1998. J Chin Soc Vet Sci 24:115–121.

Mitchell G, Heffron JJA. 1975. Factors affecting serum creatine phosphokinase in pigs. J S Afr Vet Assoc 46:145–148.

——. 1982. Porcine stress syndromes. Adv Food Res 28:167–230.

Moelich EI, Hoffman LC, Conradie PJ. 2003. Sensory and functional meat quality characteristics of pork derived from three halothane genotypes. Meat Sci 63:333–338.

Monin G, Larzul C, Le Roy P, Culioli J, Mourot J, RoussetAkrim S, Talmant A, Touraille C, Sellier P. 1999. Effects of the halothane genotype and slaughter weight on texture of pork. J Anim Sci 77:408–415.

Monin G, Sellier P. 1985. Pork of low technological quality with a normal rate of muscle pH fall in the immediate post-mortem period: The case of the Hampshire breed. Meat Sci 13:49–63.

Monin G, Sellier P, Ollivier L, Goutefongea R, Girard JP. 1981. Carcass characteristics and meat quality of halothane negative and halothane positive Pietrain pigs. Meat Sci 5:413–423.

Morioka H. 2002. Prevalence of the ryanodine-receptor mutant gene in breeding and pork pigs on general farms. J Japan Vet Med Assoc 55:149–152.

National Swine Registry. 2004. DNA stress test policy. Rules and Regulations. website: http://www.nationalswine.com/.

Nelson TE. 1983. Abnormality in calcium release from skeletal sarcoplasmic reticulum of pigs susceptible to malignant hyperthermia. J Clin Invest 72:862–873.

Nelson TE, Jones EW, Venable JH., Kerr DD. 1972. Malignant hyperthermia of Poland China swine: Studies of a myogenic etiology. Anesthesiol 36:52–56.

Nezer C, Moreau L, Brouwers B, Coppieters W, Detilleux J, Hanset R, Karim L, Kvaxz A, Leroy P, Georges M. 1999. An imprinted QTL with major effect on muscle mass and fat deposition maps to the IGF2 locus in pigs. Nature Genetics 21:155–156.

Nielsen NJ. 1979. The influence of pre-slaughter treatment on meat quality in pigs. Acta Agric Scand 21:91–102.

O'Brien, PJ. 1985. Membrane Defect in Porcine Malignant Hyperthermai. PhD Thesis, Univ of Minnesota, 134 pp.

——. 1986a. Porcine malignant hyperthermia susceptibility: Hypersensitive Ca-release mechanism of skeletal muscle sarcoplasmic reticulum. Can J Vet Res 50:318–328.

——. 1986b. Porcine malignant hyperthermia susceptibility: Increased calcium-sequestering activity of skeletal muscle sarcoplasmic reticulum. Can J Vet Res 50:329–3376.

——. 1987. Etiopathogenetic defect of malignant hyperthermia: Hypersensitive calcium-release channel of skeletal muscle sarcoplasmic reticulum. Vet Res Commun 11:527–559.

——. 1990. Microassay for malignant hyperthermia susceptibility: Hypersensitive ligand-gating of the Ca channel in muscle sarcoplasmic reticulum causes increased amounts and rates of Ca release. Molec Cell Biochem 93:53–59.

——. 1995. The causative mutation for porcine stress syndrome. Compend Cont Educ Pract Vet 17:257–269, 295.

O'Brien PJ, Ball RO, MacLennan DH. 1994. Effects of heterozygosity for the mutation causing porcine stress syndrome on carcass quality and live performance characteristics. In Proc 13th Int Pig Vet Soc Cong, p. 481.

O'Brien PJ, Fletcher TF, Metz AL, Kurtz HJ, Reed BK, Rempel WE, Clark EG, Louis CF. 1987. Malignant hyperthermia susceptibility: Cardiac histomorphometry of dogs and young and market-weight swine. Can J Vet Res 51:50–55.

O'Brien, PJ, Kalow BI, Ali N, Lassaline LA, Lumsden JH. 1990b. Compensatory increase in calcium extrusion activity of untreated lymphocytes from swine susceptible to malignant hyperthermia. Am J Vet Res. 51:1038–1043.

O'Brien PJ, Kalow BI, Brown BD, Lumsden JH, Jacobs RM. 1989. Porcine malignant hyperthermia susceptibility: Halothane-induced increase in cytoplasmic free calcium in lymphocytes. Am J Vet Res 50:131–135.

O'Brien PJ, Klip A, Britt BA, Kalow BI. 1990a. Malignant hyperthermia susceptibility: Biochemical basis for pathogenesis and diagnosis. Can J Vet Res 54:83–92.

O'Brien PJ, Mickelson JR, Gronert GA, Louis CF. 1985a. Malignant hyperthermia susceptibility: Hypersensitive calcium-induced Ca release mechanism of muscle. Anesthesiol 63:A270.

O'Brien PJ, Rooney MT, Reik TR, Thatte HS, Rempel WE, Addis PB, Louis CF. 1985b. Porcine malignant hyperthermia susceptibility: Erythrocytic osmotic fragility. Am J Vet Res 46:1451–1456.

O'Brien PJ, Shen H, Weiler J, Ianuzzo CD, Wittnich C, Moe GW, Armstrong PW. 1991. Cardiac and muscle fatigue due to relative functional overload induced by excessive stimulation, hypersensitive excitation-contraction coupling, or diminished performance capacity correlates with sarcoplasmic reticulum failure. Can J Physiol Pharmacol 69:262–268.

O'Brien PJ, Zhang X, Shen H, Cory CR. 1993. Porcine stress syndrome: Demonstration of a cost-effective protocol for large-scale, DNA-based diagnosis of the etiologic mutation in 10,000 breeding stock of various breeds. J Am Vet Med Assoc 203:842–851.

Ogawa Y. 1994. Role of ryanodine receptors. Critical Rev Biochem Molec Biol 29:229–274.

Ohnishi ST, Taylor S, Gronert GA. 1983. Calcium-induced Ca^{2+} release from sarcoplasmic reticulum of pigs susceptible to malignant hyperthermia: The effects of halothane and dantrolene. FEBS Lett. 161:103–107.

Ollivier L. 1967. Étude du détermininisme héréditaire de l'hypertrophie musculaire du proc de Pietrain: Premiers résultats. Ann Méd Vét 111:104–109.

——. 1980. Le déterminisme génétique de l'hypertrophie musculaire chez le porc. Ann Génét Sél Anim 12:383–394.

Ollivier L, Sellier P, Monin G. 1975. Déterminisme génétique du syndrome d'hyperthermie maligne chez le porc de Piétrain. Ann Génét Sél Anim 7:159–166.

——. 1976. Frequency of the malignant hyperthermia syndrome (MHS) in some French pig populations: Preliminary results. In Proc 3d Int Conf on Production Diseases in Farm Animals, Wageningen, Netherlands, pp. 208–210.

O'Neill DJ, Lynch PB, Troy DJ, Buckley DJ, Kerry JP. 2003. Influence of the time of year on the incidence of PSE and DFD in Irish pigmeat. Meat Sci 64:105–111.

Ørding H, Hald A, Sjøntoft E. 1985. Malignant hyperthermia triggered by heating in anaesthetized pigs. Acta Anaesth Scand 29:698–701.

Palmer EG, Topel DG, Christian LL. 1977. Microscopic observations of muscle from swine susceptible to malignant hyperthermia. J Anim Sci 45:1032–1036.

PIC. 2003. PICmarq Technology. What is PIC marq and how does PIC use it? PIC Technical Update. Genetics 3 (No 1): 1–7.

Pommier SA, Houde A. 1993. Effect of the genotype for malignant hyperthermia as determined by a restriction endonuclease assay on the quality characteristics of commercial pork loins. J Anim Sci 71:420–425.

Pommier SA, Houde A, Rousseau F, Savoie Y. 1992. The effect of the malignant hyperthermia genotype as determined by a restriction endonuclease assay on carcass characteristics of commercial cross-bred pigs. Can J Anim Sci 72:973–976.

Porter V. 1993. Pigs: A handbook to the breeds of the world. Ithaca: Comstock Publ Assoc, pp. 1–256.

Rahelic S, Puac S. 1981. Fibre types in *Longissimus dorsi* from wild and highly selected pig breeds. Meat Sci 5:439–450.

Ramos AM, Delgado JV, Rangel-Figueiredo T, Barba C, Matos J, Cumbreras M. 2000. Genotypic and allelic frequencies of the RYR1 locus in the Manchado de Jabugo pig breed. In Quality of Meat and Fat in Pigs as Affected by Genetics and Nutrition. Proc joint session of EAAP commission on pig production, animal genetics and animal nutrition. Zurich, Switzerland Wageningen, Netherlands, pp 175–178.

Rasmussen BA, Beece CL, Christian LL. 1980. Halothane sensitivity and linkage of genes for H red blood cell antigens, phosphohexose isomerase (PHI) and 6-phosphodehydrogenase (6-PGD) variants in pigs. Anim Blood Groups Biochem Genet 11:93–107.

Rasmussen BA. Christian LL. 1976. Blood types in pigs as predictors of stress susceptibility. Science 191:947–948.

Ratcliff PW. 1971. Review of papers section 2. Stunning. In The Condition and Meat Quality of Pigs. JCM Hessel-de Heer, ed. Proc 2d Int Symp, Wageningen, Netherlands, pp. 133–137.

Reik TR, Rempel WE, McGrath CJ, Addis PB. 1983. Further evidence on the inheritance of halothane reaction in pigs. J Anim Sci 57:826–831.

Rosenvold K, Anersen HJ. 2003. Factors of significance for pork quality—A review. Meat Sci 64:219–237.

Rundgren M, Lundström K, Edfors-Lilja I. 1990. A within-litter comparison of the three halothane genotypes. 2. Performance, carcass quality, organ development and long-term effects of transportation and amperozide. Livest Prod Sci 26:231–243.

Sabre D, Viinalass H, Varv S. 2003. Molecular diagnostics of porcine stress syndrome and occurrence of porcine stress syndrome in Estonian pig breeding enterprises. Agraarteadus 14:48–53.

Sair RA, Briskey EJ, Hoekstra WG. 1963. Comparison of muscle characteristics and post-mortem glycolysis in three breeds of swine. J Anim Sci 22:1012–1020.

Sair RA, Kastenschmidt LL, Cassens RG, Briskey EJ. 1972. Metabolism and histochemistry of skeletal muscle from stress-susceptible pigs. J Food Sci 37:659–663.

Sair RA, Lister D, Moody WR, Cassens RG, Hoekstra WG, Briskey EJ. 1970. Action of curare and magnesium on striated muscle of stress-susceptible pigs. Am J Physiol 218:108–114.

Scheper J. 1969. Relations between pH value, water-binding capacity and colour of pork after different transport stresses. In Recent Points of View on the Condition and Meat Quality of

Pigs for Slaughter. W Sybesma, PG van der Wal, P Walstra. Proc Int Symp Zeist, Netherlands. Utrecht: Reprographt, pp. 201–208.

——. 1976. Investigations about the frequency of PSE and DFD in pork. In Proc 3d Int Conf on Production Diseases in Farm Animals, Wageningen, Netherlands, pp. 141–143.

Scholz J, Roewer N, Rum U, Schmitz W, Scholz H, Schulte Am Esch J. 1991. Possible involvement of inositol-lipid metabolism in malignant hyperthermia. Br J Anaesth 66:692–696.

Scholz J, Steinfath M, Roewer N, Patten M, Troll U, Schmitz W, Scholz H, Schulte Am Esch J. 1993. Biochemical changes in malignant hyperthermia susceptible swine: Cyclic AMP, inositol phosphates, α_1-, β_1- and β_2-adrenoceptors in skeletal and cardiac muscle. Acta Anaesthesiol Scand 37:575–583.

Seeler DC. McDonell WN, Basrur PK. 1984. Halothane and halothane/succinylcholine induced malignant hyperthermia (porcine stress syndrome) in a population of Ontario boars. Can J Comp Med 147:284–290.

Sei, Y, Brandom BW Bina S, Hosoi E, Gallagher KL, Wyre HW, Pudimat PA, Holman SJ, Venzon DJ, Daly JW, Muldoon S. 2002. Patients with malignant hyperthermia demonstrate an altered calcium control mechanism in B lymphocytes. Anesthesiol 97:1052–1058.

Sensky PL, Parr T, Lockley AK, Bardsley RG, Buttery PJ, Wood JD, Warkup C. 1999. Altered calpain levels in longissimus muscle from normal pigs and heterozygotes with the ryanodine receptor mutation. J Anim Sci 77:2956–2964.

ShanHua W. 1997. Study on stress susceptibility of native Guanling pigs in Guizhou, China. Chinese J Anim Sci 33:29–30.

Shen H. Lahucky R. Kovac L. O'Brien PJ. 1992. Comparison of *HAL* gene status with ^{31}P NMR-determined muscle metabolites and with Ca sequestration activity of anoxia-challenged muscle from pigs homozygous and heterozygous for porcine stress syndrome. Pig News Info 13:105–109.

Smith C, Bampton PR. 1977. Inheritance of reaction to halothane anaesthesia in pigs. Genet Res Camb 29:287–292.

Smith WC, Lesser D. 1982. An economic assessment of pale, soft, exudative musculature in the fresh and cured pig carcass. Anim Prod 34:291–299.

Swatland HJ. 1989. Fluid distribution in pork, measured by x-ray diffraction, interference microscopy and centrifugation compared to paleness measured by fiber optics. J Anim Sci 67:1465–1470.

——. 1993. Paleness, softness and exudation in pork—A review. In Pork Quality: Genetic and Metabolic Factors. E Puolanne, DI Demeyer, eds. Wallingford: C.A.B. International, pp. 273–286.

Sybesma W, Eikelenboom G. 1969. Malignant hyperthermia in pigs. Neth J Vet Sci 2:155–160.

Szentkuti L, Niemeyer L, Schlegel O. 1981. Comparative study on types of muscle fiber in M. longissimus dorsi of domestic and wild pigs using the myosin-ATPase reaction. Dtsch Tierärztl Wochenschr 88:407–411.

Takeshima HS, Nishimura T, Matsumoto T, Ishida H, Kangawa K, Minamino N, Matsuo H, Ueda M, Hanaoka M, Hirose T, Numa S. 1989. Primary structure and expression from complementary DNA of skeletal muscle ryanodine receptor. Nature Lond 339:439–445.

Tarrant PV. 1993. An overview of production, slaughter and processing factors that affect pork quality—General review. In Pork Quality: Genetic and Metabolic Factors. E Puolanne, DI Demeyer, eds. Wallingford: C.A.B. International, pp. 1–21.

Thompson J. 1981. Current research efforts in Canada. Agenda item 5. In Proc Work Planning Meeting on PSE/DFD, Ottawa. Ottawa: Agric Can, pp. 1–6.

Thoonen J, Hoorens J. 1960. Spiernecrose bij varkens. Vlaams Diergeneesk Tijdschr 29:205–209.

Topel DG. 1976. Palatability and visual acceptance of dark normal and pale colored porcine M. *longissimus*. J Anim Sci 41:628–630.

———. 1981a. U.S. overview. Agenda item 4. In Proc Work Planning Meeting on PSE/DFD, Ottawa. Ottawa: Agric Can, pp. 1–4.

———. 1981b. Relationship between stress adaptation traits of swine and management practices with the development of PSE pork and the porcine stress syndrome. Agenda item 7. In Proc Work Planning Meeting on PSE/DFD, Ottawa. Ottawa: Agric Can, pp. 1–12.

Topel DG, Bicknell EJ, Preston KS, Christian LL, Matsushima CY. 1968. Porcine stress syndrome. Mod Vet Practice 40–41:59–60.

Van den Hende C, Lister D, Muylle E, Ooms L, Oyaert W. 1976. Malignant hyperthermia in Belgian Landrace pigs rested or exercised before exposure to halothane. Br J Anaesth 48:821–829.

van der Wal PG. 1971a. Stunning procedures for pigs and their physiological consequences. In The Condition and Meat Quality of Pigs. JCM Hessel-de Heer, ed. Proc 2d Int Symp, Wageningen, Netherlands, pp. 145–151.

———. 1971b. Stunning, sticking and exsanguination as stress factors in pigs. In The Condition and Meat Quality of Pigs. JCM Hessel-de Heer, ed. Proc 2d Int Symp, Wageningen, Netherlands, pp. 153–162.

van der Wal PG, Eikelenboom G. 1981. Stunning of pigs for slaughter: Recent developments in the Netherlands. In Porcine Stress and Meat Quality: Causes and Possible Solutions to the Problems. T Frøystein, E Slinde, N Standal, eds. Ås: Agric Food Res Soc, pp. 298–305.

Van Oeckel MJ, Warnants N, Boucque CV, Delputte, P, Depuydt J. 2001. The preference of the consumer for pork from homozygous or heterozygous halothane negative animals. Meat Sci 58:247–251.

Velarde A, Gispert Ml, Faucitano L, Alonso P, Manteca X, Diestre A. 2001. Effects of stunning procedure and the halothane genotype on meat quality and incidence of haemorrhages in pigs. Meat Sci 58:313–319.

Vögeli P, Bolt R, Fries R, Stranzinger G. 1994. Co-segregation of the malignant hyperthermia and the Arg615-Cys515 mutation in the skeletal muscle calcium-release channel protein in five European Landrace and Pietrain pig breeds. Anim Genet 25:59–66.

Vögeli P, Fries R, Bolt R, Gerwig C, Affentranger P, Künzi N, Bertschinger HU, Stranzinger G. 1993. The significance of blood groups on meat quality. In Pork Quality: Genetic and Metabolic Factors. E Puolanne, DI Demeyer, eds. Wallingford: C.A.B. International, pp. 22–36.

Vögeli P, Schwörer D, Kühne R, Wysshaar M. 1985. Trends in economic traits, halothane sensitivity, blood group and enzyme systems of Swiss Landrace and Large White pigs. Anim Blood Groups Biochem Genet 16:285–296.

Wappler F, Scholz J, Fiege M, Kolodzie K, Kudlik C, Weibhorn R, Schulte am Esch J. 1999. 4-Chloro-m-cresol is a trigger of malignant hyperthermia in susceptible swine. Anesthesiol 90:1733–1740.

Warriss PD, Brown SN, Barton-Gade P, Santos C, Costa LN, Lambooij E, Geers R. 1998. An analysis of data relating to pig carcass quality and indices of stress collected in the European Union. Meat Sci 49:137–144.

Weaver SA, Schaefer AL, Dixon WT. 2000. The effects of mutated skeletal ryanodine receptors on calreticulin and calsequestrin expression in the brain and pituitary gland of boars. Molec Brain Res 75:46–53.

Webb AJ. 1980. The halothane test: A practical method of eliminating porcine stress syndrome. Vet Rec 106:410–412.

———. 1981. The halothane sensitivity test. In Porcine Stress and Meat Quality: Causes and Possible Solutions to the Problems. T Frøystein, E Slinde, N Standal, eds. Ås: Agric Food Res Soc, pp. 105–124.

Webb AJ, Imlah P, Carden, AE. 1986. Succinylcholine and halothane as a field test for the heterozygote at the halothane locus in pigs. Anim Prod 42:275–279.

Webb AJ, Jordan, CHC. 1979. The halothane test in genetic improvement programs: Experiments with Pietrain/Hampshire pigs. Acta Agric Scand 21:418–426.

Webb AJ, Smith C. 1977. Some preliminary observations on the inheritance and application of halothane-induced MHS in pigs. In Proc 3d Int Conf on Production Diseases Farm Animals, Wageningen, Netherlands, pp. 211–213.

Wedel DJ, Gammel SA, Milde JH, Iaizzo PA. 1993. Delayed onset of malignant hyperthermia induced by isoflurane and desflurane compared with halothane in susceptible swine. Anesth 78:1138–1144.

Williams CH, Lasley JF. 1977. The mode of inheritance of the fulminant hyperthermia stress syndrome in swine. In Malignant hyperthermia: Current concepts. EO Henschel, ed. New York: Appleton-Century-Crofts, pp. 141–148.

Wismer-Pedersen J. 1969. The pH-dependent water-binding capacity of pork muscle in relation to processing. In Recent Points of View on the Condition and Meat Quality of Pigs for Slaughter. W Sybesma, PG van der Wal, P Walstra, eds. Proc Int Symp Zeist, Netherlands. Utrecht: Reprorint, pp 53–87.

Woolf N, Hall LW, Thorne C, Down M, Walker R. 1970. Serum creatine phosphokinase levels in pigs reacting abnormally to halogenated anaesthetics. Br Med J 3:386–387.

Yang TS, Hawrysh ZJ, Price MA, Aherne FX. 1983. Effect of dantrolene sodium on pork quality from pigs stunned by captive-bolt. Can J Anim Sci 63:299–302.

Yun S, Gustafsson K, Fabre JW. 1998. Suppression of human antiporcine T-cell immune responses by major histocompatibility complex class II transactivator constructs lacking the amino terminal domain. Transplantation 66(1):103–111.

Zorzato F, Fujii J, Otsu K, Phillips M, Green NM, Lai FA, Meissner G, MacLennan DH. 1990. Molecular cloning of cDNA encoding human and rabbit forms of the Ca^{2+} release channel (ryanodine receptor) of skeletal muscle sarcoplasmic reticulum. J Biol Chem 265:2244–2256.

59 Prolapses

W. J. Smith and Barbara E. Straw

The rectum and vagina are held in place by a complex matrix of fascia, collagen fibers, muscles, and ligaments. This support mechanism may become heavily infiltrated with fat in some animals. In theory, rectal prolapse will occur if the support mechanism is either overcome by pressure or is weakened for some reason. Pressure on the support mechanism may be brought about by straining (proctitis, urethritis, constipation, coughing, and farrowing) or by physical pressure (excessive slope on the floor or increase in abdominal pressure for any reason). Brockman et al (2004) produced rectal prolapse in 10 49–74 kg pigs by insufflating the abdominal cavity with water at pressures of 222–343 mmHg (mean 292 mmHg). In humans, lifting from a flexed position causes intraabdominal pressure to increase to 187 mmHg. Weakness of the support mechanism may be brought about by edema (including that due to mycotoxins), fat infiltration, tumor infiltration, certain drugs, and genetic susceptibility. In most animals, and especially growing pigs, rectal and/or vaginal prolapse is almost an all-or-nothing phenomenon, with the early stages rarely being observed. The prolapse in the growing pig usually protrudes about 10–13 cm. This relatively constant degree of prolapse is probably due to anchorage by the short mesorectum and muscles of the pelvic diaphragm (Hindson 1958; S. H. Done, personal communication, 1990). Although the stockperson is usually presented with a complete rectal prolapse, some pigs have a temporary protrusion of a portion of the rectal mucosa on defecation. This phenomenon is also seen during coughing, and one might conjecture that such pigs might be prime candidates for complete rectal prolapse at a later stage.

The comparative anatomy of the pelvic and perineal regions of several species, including the pig, has been studied by Bassett (1971).

INCIDENCE

Most swine production units experience cases of rectal or vaginal prolapse in swine of various ages. Correction of rectal prolapse is the most commonly performed gastrointestinal surgical procedure in swine (Welker and Modransky 1991). Cases are nearly always sporadic in nature, and most often the cause is not determined. However, outbreaks do occur and may occasionally be prolonged. Kjar (1976) noted that the incidence of rectal prolapse was highest in pigs 6–12 weeks of age and concluded that the cause was unknown but that the incidence, which varied from 1–10%, increased during a change from cold to damp weather.

In a study of one finishing herd over 7 years (total throughput: 56,363 pigs), Garden (1988) noted that the incidence varied from 0.7%–4.7% on an annual basis. In another study in one herd over 6 months, Gardner et al. (1988) noted that 30 (1%) of 2862 pigs of 12–28 weeks of age suffered from rectal prolapse, with a peak incidence between 14 and 16 weeks of age. Becker and Van der Leek (1988) noted an estimated 10–15% prevalence of rectal prolapse over a 12-month period in pigs of 2–4 months of age in a herd of 125 sows (farrow to finish). Perfumo et al (2002) found that rectal prolapse was responsible for 7.7% of deaths that occurred in pigs from weaning to market. In a herd with 8.62% annual emergency-culling mortality, Baumann and Bilkei (2002) found that rectal stricture and rectal prolapse were responsible for 7.5% and 5.9% of the deaths.

Smith has noted (unpublished data) that rectal prolapse was most common in pigs 3–5 months of age; the incidence in three herds of 1000, 600, and 120 sows (all in confinement) was 0.7%, 0.9%, and 0.6%, respectively. The affected pigs ranged from 45 to 180 days of age and from 10–90 kg in weight. Swine were not observed to be ill before prolapse occurred, and the only common factor was mild constipation. Straining was not observed in any of these pigs before prolapse of the rectum occurred, but this clinical sign may have been missed due to the intensity of confinement.

Daniel (1975) noted that rectal prolapse in sows could occur in all sizes of units and that the incidence varied from 0.5%–1%. Two-thirds of the cases occurred around the time of parturition. Although prolapse of the rectum and vagina and/or cervix was not mentioned as a specific reason for culling sows from U.K. pig herds (Anonymous 1964), Jones (1967) reported an 8.9% frequency of culling for rectal prolapse in one herd. In Australia 7.1% of sows culled in a 2500-sow unit were cases of rectal or vaginal prolapse (Penny 1972).

Schulz and Bostedt (1995) noted that vaginal prolapse affected 33 of 523 farrowing sows and was a significant cause of dystocia. Information regarding the incidence of vaginal and uterine prolapse is sparse, apart from outbreaks of vulvovaginitis associated with mycotoxins, when vaginal prolapses can occur in 30% of affected females (McNutt et al. 1928).

CAUSES AND PREDISPOSING FACTORS

Inflammation

Vaginal prolapse is very rare in suckling swine. However, rectal prolapse is sometimes associated with enterocolitis caused by viral, bacterial, parasitic, or mycotic infection (Pfeifer 1984; Straw 1987). In cases where the inflammation is severe and irritation of the rectum occurs, tenesmus results and rectal prolapse may be a sequel. Outbreaks of prolapse have been seen in association with swine fever, although fewer than 0.1% of piglets with diarrhea will suffer from rectal prolapse. Although many outbreaks of colitis, both infectious and noninfectious, have been observed in Scotland, rectal prolapse was not noted as a sequel. In older swine, urethritis and vaginitis from any cause may lead to straining, which may in turn lead to prolapse of the rectum or vagina or both.

Nutritional Factors

P. L. Shanks (personal communication, 1955) observed an outbreak of rectal prolapse in a group of pigs that had been fed waste food material from the floor of a feed mill. He concluded that unusual constituents in the diet led to straining, with resultant prolapse. Morbidity was approximately 30%. More recently, E. N. Wood (personal communication, 1979) described an outbreak of rectal prolapse in early weaned pigs between 2 and 6 weeks of age. Thirty-one of 235 piglets (13.2%) died during the outbreak and all were males. Subsequent investigation revealed the cause of death to be uremia from blockage of the urethra with calculi—a sequel to an unusually high level (2.25%) of calcium in the diet. Partial or complete obstruction of the urethra had caused excessive straining and subsequent prolapse of the rectum. During the outbreak, the piglets fed for short periods only, making frequent visits to the automatic drinker. The food consisted of a mixture of denatured skim milk, dried whey, fish meal, and soya meal.

Sudden changes in the diet (e.g., from meal to whey) may lead to occasional cases of rectal prolapse. Chronic shortage of water will lead to constipation with rectal prolapse as a sequel. Diets that are low in fiber (e.g., those without bran or wheat feed) may also lead to constipation. Constipation produced by this means may also be aggravated by lack of exercise (e.g., sows confined in farrowing crates or dry sow stalls). A higher incidence of rectal prolapse is therefore to be expected in confinement, although the daily feeding of a little straw may help prevent the condition.

In a 250-sow, breeding-to-finishing unit, the author found the number of rectal prolapses in the growing pigs decreased from five to one a week when the barley in the ration was replaced by a variety with a higher fiber content. Reintroduction of the lower-fiber barley and its removal repeatedly worsened or improved the situation, respectively.

In a 300-sow, breeding-to-finishing unit, 15 kg weaners were randomly divided and placed into strawed kennels or second-stage flat decks, both units being contained in the same large general-purpose building. The pigs were fed the same ration and the stocking density in both types of housing was almost identical. Prolapse of the rectum was a chronic problem only in the pigs in the strawed kennels. When the barley straw was replaced with wheat straw from a neighboring farm, the prolapse problem disappeared during the time the wheat straw was used. As soon as the barley straw was reintroduced (three times), the prolapse problem reappeared (Anonymous 1985). It was later postulated that the barley straw might have contained mycotoxins.

Prolapse of the rectum and vagina was a chronic problem in a 400-sow herd in Spain. The sows were housed in level, partly slatted stalls and fed brewers' grains as part of the ration. The grains were kept in an outside pit, which held enough to last about 3 weeks. Prolapses increased toward the end of the 3-week period, by which time the contents were heavily contaminated with fungi. No mycotoxin assays were carried out (E. Marco, personal communication, 1990).

Sudden outbreaks of rectal and vaginal prolapse were noted by the author in pigs over 30 kg every time whey feeding was reintroduced after a few days of absence. The pigs in this 2000-sow herd were normally fed a mixture of meal and whey without access to water. When whey was unavailable (e.g., Christmas holidays), the pigs were fed meal and water, which they did not like and intake dropped markedly. As soon as whey was reintroduced (on a restricted basis), the hungry pigs gorged themselves and the incidence of prolapse rapidly rose to about 1.5% for a short period. Deaths due to torsion also rose.

Muirhead (1989) investigated a chronic problem of rectal prolapse in finishing pigs. The incidence varied from 4–6% at 12–18 weeks of age. Reducing the density of the diet reduced the incidence of prolapse to less than 1%, but this measure also reduced growth rate significantly. In this particular herd most of the prolapses occurred within 1–2 hours of the lights being switched on at 7 a.m.; this observation might be of some significance. Amass et al. (1995) noted that an experimental ration containing a high lysine level was 6.73 times more likely to cause rectal prolapse than a controlled diet. Casper et al. (1991) noted rectal prolapses in sows as a sequel to lupin bean meal toxicosis.

It has to be admitted that many outbreaks of rectal prolapse respond to a change in diet, but the reason for this response is rarely found.

Physical Factors

Injury to the rectum or urethra from service by the boar may also lead to tenesmus and prolapse. In addition, gradual weakening of the pelvic diaphragm may arise as sows age or during pregnancy as the abdominal contents become heaviest. Rupture of one or more of the supporting structures may then occur, with prolapse of either rectum or vagina or both as a sequel.

Outbreaks have been observed when sows are confined in stalls or in tethers with an excessive slope to the floor. When the fall is greater than 1 in 20, increased intraabdominal pressure may overcome the resistance of one or more structures of the pelvic diaphragm, especially as the abdominal contents increase in weight as pregnancy progresses (S. M. Richmond, personal communication, 1979). An outbreak of rectal and vaginal prolapse was also observed in a herd where the dry sows were tethered in stalls with solid floods that were shorter than usual and there was a 13 cm drop from the solid lying area to the dunging passage; the rear end of the sows hung over the dunging passage. Partial or complete rectal or vaginal prolapse was seen in 14%. Sometimes the rectum prolapsed, sometimes the vagina, and in a few cases both. When the sows were recumbent, the first clinical sign was an outward bulging of the vaginal mucous membrane (partial prolapse). In the standing position the prolapse usually disappeared, but as pregnancy progressed and the uterine load increased, the prolapse became more evident when the sow was lying down. Eventually, bacterial contamination occurred, inflammation gradually became more severe, and the partial prolapse became complete. Complete prolapse was prevented by removal of affected animals to a spacious pen with a level, solid floor.

Physical damage to the vaginal tract may also occur during parturition, either by natural means or by human interference. This may damage some of the structures of the pelvic diaphragm or may lead to inflammation, which will cause excessive straining. In either case, vaginal prolapse may result.

Le Bret (1980) noted that sows in five herds from the same origin were most likely to suffer from rectal prolapse at farrowing. These sows were characterized by a particular pelvic conformation shown by measuring different pelvic angles. The larger the angle between the coccygeal vertebrae and the pelvis, the higher the risk of rectal prolapse.

Guise and Penny (1990) noted that rectal prolapses occurred when pigs were transported at high stocking density; no prolapses were noted in the low-stocking-density treatment groups. These authors also reported that haulers had observed prolapses occurring as pigs struggled up steep ramps. V. R. Fowler (personal communication, 1980) noted a high incidence of rectal prolapse in weaner pigs shortly after being tethered in metabolism cages. These cases may have been a sequel to increased abdominal pressure during episodes of struggling.

Drugs

The repeated use of estrogens or any estrogenic substance to stimulate estrus in sows or gilts may lead to excessive swelling of the vulva, with vulvovaginitis and prolapse as sequels. Rectal prolapse has been described in growing pigs fed therapeutic levels of tylosin in the diet. It is not known why this occurs (J. D. Mackinnon, personal communication, 1979), but A. Hogg has suggested (personal communication, 1979) that tylosin may alter the normal bacterial flora of the gut, with overgrowth of fungi such as *Monilia* spp. as a sequel. Moniliasis may cause proctitis and straining, leading to prolapse. Smith has noted (unpublished data) that when Tylasul (tylosin/sulfadimidine) was added to the diet (5 kg/ton) of 10 experimental feeder pigs, 3 suffered from rectal prolapse within 10 days. It was noticeable that the pigs in this group seemed to suffer from a form of anal irritation, manifested as frequent episodes of rapid tail shaking.

Rectal prolapse due to edema has been noted when pigs were medicated with lincomycin. This reaction is frequently observed when swine are first placed on the drug, but clinical signs usually subside within 72 hours (Kunesh 1981).

Genetic Factors

A. Hogg (personal communication, 1979) reported a severe problem characterized by vaginal and uterine prolapse in a large breeding herd in the United States; uterine prolapse occurred both before and after farrowing. Apparently inbreeding had emphasized a recessive genetic factor.

In a commercial swine herd in California, pigs sired by Yorkshire boars were 3.3 times more likely to suffer from rectal prolapse; one Yorkshire boar in particular was 9.4 times more likely to sire affected pigs. In the same herd, sows of low parity (1, 2, and 3) were likely to farrow pigs more susceptible to rectal prolapse, but it was not possible to determine if this was a genetic effect (Gardner et al. 1988). In their studies, Hindson (1958) and Saunders (1974) concluded that hereditary factors were involved. Becker and Van der Leek (1988) concluded that genetic factors were strongly implicated in an outbreak of rectal prolapse in a commercial 125-sow, farrow-to-finish herd.

Environmental Factors

It is generally agreed that rectal prolapse occurs more commonly during winter months; and there is some evidence to support this (Kjar 1976; Wilson 1984; Gardner et al. 1988; Prange et al. 1987). However, in one study over 7 years in a finishing herd (throughput: 56,363 pigs; average incidence: 2.9%), Garden (1988) found no evidence of seasonal effect. It has been suggested that cold weather causes pigs to pile, thus increasing the likelihood of prolapses; no objective data have been produced to support this hypothesis.

Muirhead (1989) reported a problem of rectal prolapse in recently weaned pigs on flat decks. The problem resolved when the climatic environment was improved, particularly temperature and ventilation. Perramón and Muirhead (1998) reported similar findings in another herd in which rectal prolapses were associated only in the winter with a specific building housing 30–60 kg pigs.

Mycotoxicosis

Rectal and/or vaginal prolapse is a common sequel to vulvovaginitis caused by mycotoxicosis (see Chapter 56 for further details).

Other Factors

In a study in one commercial herd, Gardner et al. (1988) noted that male pigs were more likely to suffer from rectal prolapse than females. However, in a study of one herd over a much longer period and with a higher incidence of prolapse, Garden (1988) could find no evidence of a sex effect. In another, very small experimental study, Smith (1980) observed that 6 (32%) of 19 randomly acquired pigs with rectal prolapse were males. On the other hand, Perramón and Muirhead (1998) found 73% of prolapses in females.

Gardner et al. (1988) noted that pigs of low birth weight (less than 1000 g) were more likely to suffer from rectal prolapse later in life. It was hypothesized that low-birth-weight pigs that have fewer muscle fibers at birth have an inherently weaker rectal support mechanism, which may fail when a period of rapid growth occurs. Muirhead (1989) noted that a behavioral aberration, anal nuzzling, in recently weaned pigs led to a rectal prolapse problem (4–6% incidence). Improvement to the climatic environment prevented further cases from arising. An outbreak of anal nuzzling was reported by van Sambraus (1979).

When pigs cough, the rectal mucosa often protrudes temporarily. As with piling, it has been suggested that coughing may precipitate rectal prolapse, but again there are no objective data to support this hypothesis. Indeed, Gardner et al. (1988) could find no relationship between coughing and the prevalence of rectal prolapse. In another study, the prevalence of rectal prolapse was dramatically reduced from 4.7% to 0.7% when weaners (30–35 kg) were placed in a strawed yard for 3 weeks between being held in the second-stage flat decks and the fully slatted finishing accommodation (Garden 1985).

Diarrhea is not a common precursor of rectal prolapse, and in one herd studied by Gardner et al. (1988) an outbreak of transmissible gastroenteritis did not increase the prevalence.

Henry (1983) suggested that lack of anal sphincter control due to infection or trauma of pelvic nerve centers such as might occur after docking (especially short docking) or tail biting could lead to rectal prolapse.

Jennings (1984) noted that a significant number of sows with hypocalcemia suffered from uterine prolapse.

In a survey of sow mortality, Chagnon et al. (1990) noted that uterine prolapse was the cause of death of 6.6% of sows. The average parity was 6.0, and it is possible that some weakness of the support mechanism may have been the main determinant (see Chapter 63).

RECTAL STRICTURES

In the United States, rectal strictures were first reported in Illinois (Gibbons 1967); later outbreaks were observed in Indiana (Lillie et al. 1973) and those authors reported more cases during the coldest months, although in Argentina, the incidence was 10% in the summer months for all-age pigs and in September and December for nursery and grower pigs, respectively (Perfumo et al 2002). Outbreaks have also been noted in the United Kingdom (D. G. Taylor, personal communication 1988). Rectal stricture is considered to be a sequel to rectal prolapse (Saunders 1974; Van der Gaag and Meijer 1974; Häni and Scholl 1976; Von Muller et al. 1980; Prange et al. 1987; Becker and Van der Leek 1988; Jensen 1989). Perfumo et al (2002) reported a mean age for rectal prolapse of 115.8 ± 4.2 days, and that for rectal stricture was 164.2 ± 6.1 days.

In a more detailed study of 25 pigs with rectal prolapses that were allowed to heal naturally without treatment, Smith (1980) noted that 3 developed complete rectal stricture and died; the remainder grew normally, but in every case there was evidence of partial rectal stricture at slaughter (Figure 59.1).

Harkin et al. (1982) considered that a strong genetic component was implicated in the etiology of rectal stricture. Lillie et al. (1973) and Perfumo et al. (2002) reported that routine microbiological procedures failed to demonstrate an infectious agent, and Harkin et al. (1982) failed to detect any salmonellae. However, Wilcock and Olander (1977a) noted that many cases of rectal stricture were preceded by severe enteric disease. *Salmonella typhimurium* was frequently isolated, and ulcerative proctitis, a possible precursor of rectal stricture, was also noted. In later studies Wilcock and Olander (1977b) produced rectal strictures experimentally by injecting chlorpromazine into the cranial hemorrhoidal artery and suggested that rectal prolapses may be a sequel to ischemic proctitis induced by thrombosis associated with salmonellosis.

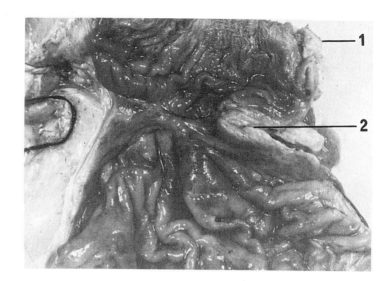

59.1. *Longitudinal section of rectum and anus of a 140 kg pig 9 weeks after resolution of a prolapsed rectum, showing mucocutaneous junction (1) and scar tissue/partial stricture (2).*

TREATMENT AND CONTROL

Apart from treatment and noting any factors peculiar to each case, it is not considered worthwhile to implement any specific control or preventive measures for sporadic cases of rectal prolapse. If an outbreak occurs, however, attempts should be made to identify the causes and predisposing factors. Whatever conclusion is reached, measures taken must be cost effective; for example, if the lack of exercise in farrowing sows is the main factor, the cost of providing that exercise in confinement may be greater than the cost of the disorder. Treatment should also be cost effective. In the United Kingdom it is now common practice to deal with rectal prolapse in feeder pigs by isolation only. No surgical treatment is carried out, and the prolapse is simply left to resolve naturally in 10–14 days. However, this practice is not good welfare, and a simple nonsurgical amputation technique such as described by Douglas (1985) should be considered. Many surgical procedures for treating rectal prolapses have been described (Hindson 1958; Chalmin 1960; Daniel 1975; Ivascu et al. 1976; Kjar 1976; Vonderfecht 1978; Schon 1985; Moore 1989; Kolden 1994; Grosse-Beilage and Grosse-Beilage 1994).

It should be noted that amputation of the uterus often results in high mortality. Prolapse of the uterus is best treated by surgical replacement; a laparotomy technique, which ensures that each horn of the womb can be properly repositioned, has been successful. Surgical techniques for treating the general prolapse have been described by Toth and Huszenicza (1983). Nonsurgical intervention is greatly assisted by general anesthesia and hoisting the hindquarters of the sow with a block and tackle or similar device.

Treatment of rectal stricture is rarely cost effective, but a surgical technique has been described (Boyd et al. 1988).

REFERENCES

Amass SF, Schinckel AP, Clark LK. 1995. Increased prevalence of rectal prolapses in growing/finishing swine fed a diet containing excess lysine. Vet Rec 137:519–520.

Anonymous. 1964. Sow wastage survey, 1962–1963. Pig Industry Development Authority, London.

———. 1985. Scottish Veterinary Investigation Service report. Vet Rec 117:424.

Bassett, E. G. 1971. The comparative anatomy of the pelvic and perineal regions of the cow, goat and sow. NZ Vet J 19:277–290.

Baumann B, Bilkei G. 2002. Emergency-culling and mortality in growing/fattening pigs in a large Humgarian "farrow-to-finish" production unit. Dtsch Tierarztl Wochenschr 109(1) 26–33.

Becker HN, Van der Leek M. 1988. Possible genetic predisposition to rectal prolapse in swine: A case report. Proc Int Pig Vet Soc 10:395.

Boyd JS, Taylor DJ, Reid J. 1988. Surgery in relieving the rectal stricture syndrome. Proc Int Congr Pig Vet Soc 10:403.

Brockman JB, Patterson NW, Richardson WS. 2004. Burst strength of laparoscopic and open hernia repair. Surg Endosc 18(3): 536–539.

Casper HH, Berg IE, Crenshaw JD, Colville JL, Wass WM. 1991. Lupin bean meal toxicosis in swine. J Vet Diag Invest 3:2, 172–173.

Chagnon M, Drolet R, D'Allaire S. 1990. A prospective study of sow mortality in commercial breeding herds. Proc Int Congr Pig Vet Soc 11:383.

Chalmin R. 1960. Rectal Prolapse in Pigs and Its Surgical Treatment. Thèse de Doctorat Vétérinaire. École Nationale Vétérinaire d'Alfort.

Daniel M. 1975. Study of Prolapse of the Rectum in Breeding Sows. Thèse de Doctorat Vétérinaire. École Nationale Vétérinaire d'Alfort.

Douglas RGA. 1985. A simple method for correcting rectal prolapse in pigs. Vet Rec 117:129.

Garden S. 1985. Mortality in feeding pigs. Proc Pig Vet Soc 15:100–107.

———. 1988. Rectal prolapse in pigs. Vet Rec 123:654.

Gardner IA, Hird DW, Franti CE, Glen J. 1988. Patterns and determinants of rectal prolapse in a herd of pigs. Vet Rec 123:222–225.

Gibbons WJ. 1967. Rectal constriction in swine. Mod Vet Pract 48:20.

Grosse-Beilage E, Grosse-Beilage I. 1994. Experiences with the treatment of rectal prolapses in fattening pigs under practical conditions. Deut Tier Wochenschr 101:10 383–387.

Guise HJ, Penny RHC. 1990. Factors influencing the welfare and carcass and meat quality of pigs. 1. The effects of stocking density in transport and the use of electric goads. Anim Prod 49:511–515.

Häni H, Scholl E. 1976. Stricture of the rectum in pigs. Schweiz Arch Tierheilkd 118:325–328.

Harkin JT, Jones RT, Gillick JC. 1982. Rectal strictures in pigs. Aust Vet J 59:56–57.

Henry S. 1983. Vet's view. Pig American, Jan, p. 45.

Hindson JC. 1958. Prolapse of the rectum in the pig. Vet Rec 70:214–216.

Ivascu I, Christea I, Gatina L. 1976. Therapeutical research work on rectal prolapse in swine. Proc Int Congr Pig Vet Soc 4:Z15.

Jennings DS. 1984. Hypocalcaemia in sows. Pig Vet Soc Proc 14:38–40.

Jensen V. 1989. Rectal prolapse in fattened pigs. Dansk Vet 72(10):557–565.

Jones JET. 1967. An investigation of the causes of mortality and morbidity in sows in a commercial herd. Br Vet J 123:327–339.

Kjar HA. 1976. Amputation of prolapsed rectum in young pigs. Proc Int Congr Pig Vet Soc 4:6.

Kolden A. 1994. Rectal prolapse in pigs. Norsk Vet 106:10 731–736.

Kunesh JP. 1981. Therapeutics. In Diseases of Swine, 5th ed. AD Leman, RD Glock, WL Mengeling, RHC Penny, E Scholl, B Straw. Ames: Iowa State Univ Press, p. 724.

Le Bret MV. 1980. Rectal prolapse in sows: Influence of pelvis conformation determined by goniometry. Ann Zootech 29:226–227.

Lillie LE, Olander HJ, Gallina AM. 1973. Rectal stricture in swine. J Am Vet Med Assoc 163:358–361.

McNutt SH, Purwin P, Murray C. 1928. Vulvovaginitis in swine. J Am Vet Med Assoc 73:484.

Moore JC. 1989. A method of replacing rectal prolapse of the sow. Pig Vet J 23:124.

Muirhead MR. 1989. Rectal prolapse. Int Pig Lett 9(1):3.

Penny RHC. 1972. Some current thoughts on lameness in the pig. Vet Annu 13:31–36.

Perfumo CJ, Sanguinetti HR, Giorgio N, Armocida AD, Machuca MA, Massone AR, Risso MA, Aguirre JI, Idiart JR. 2002. Rectal stricture of postmortem examined pigs in a farrow-to-finish units. Considerations about the prevalence, pathology, etiology and pathogenesis. Archivos de Medicina Veterinaria 34(2) 245–252.

Perramón JS and Muirhead MR. 1998. An investigation into a high incidence of rectal prolapses in growing pigs in a commercial herd. Proc Int Congr Pig Vet Soc, p. 208.

Pfeifer CW. 1984. Veterinarians on call. Nat Hog Farmer, Jan 15, p. 64.

Prange H, Uhlemann J, Schmidt A, Gericke R. 1987. Aetiology and pathogenesis of acquired rectal stricture of swine. Monatsh Veterinärmed 42:425–428.

Saunders CN. 1974. Rectal stricture syndrome in pigs: A case history. Vet Rec,94:61.

Schon V. 1985. Rectal prolapse in swine: A simple and rapid surgical technique. Dansk Vet 68:15 772.

Schultz S, Bostedt H. 1995. Bladder flexion and vaginal prolapses as an obstetric problem in sows. Tier-Praxis 23:2 139–147.

Smith WJ. 1980. A study of prolapse of the rectum in swine with naturally occurring resolution. Proc Int Congr Pig Vet Soc 6:356.

Straw B. 1987. Rectal prolapses in swine. Cornell Extension Bull, Fall issue.

Toth MA, Huszenicza G. 1983. Surgery for vaginal prolapse in swine. Magar-Allator-Lapja 38:4 247–248.

Van der Gaag I, Meijer P. 1974. Rectal strictures in pigs. Proc Int Congr Pig Vet Soc 3:v–v3.

van Sambraus HH. 1979. A study of anal massage and subsequent ingestion of faeces in fattening pigs. Deut Tier Wechr 86:58–62.

Vonderfecht HE. 1978. Amputation of rectal prolapse in pigs. Vet Med Small Anim Clin 73:201–206.

Von Muller E, Schoon HA, Schultx LC. 1980. Rectal strictures in pigs. Deut Tier Wochenschr 87:196–199.

Welker B, Modransky P. 1991. Rectal prolapse in food animals. Part 1. Cause and conservative management. Comp Cont Ed Pract Vet 13(12):1869–1873.

Wilcock BP, Olander HJ. 1977a. The pathogenesis of porcine rectal stricture. I. The naturally occurring disease and its association with salmonellosis. Vet Pathol 14:36–42.

——. 1977b. The pathogenesis of porcine rectal stricture. II. Experimental salmonellosis and ischemic proctitis. Vet Pathol 14:43–55.

Wilson MR. 1984. More on rectal stricture. Int Pig Lett 4(5):4.

60 Toxic Minerals, Chemicals, Plants, and Gases

Thomas L. Carson

Although modern confinement facilities, accurately formulated rations, and improved management practices have reduced some risks of poisoning associated with outdoor swine production, cases of poisoning in swine still occur. The occurrence of swine toxicoses associated with the environment, feed, or management practices is frequent enough to warrant their inclusion in differential diagnostic considerations for swine health problems. The following discussion summarizes the impact of potentially toxic agents to which swine may be exposed.

MINERALS

Trace Minerals

Most swine formula feeds are properly fortified with trace elements. However, some trace minerals are deliberately added in excess for various reasons. They include copper (Cu), selenium (Se), and occasionally iron (Fe) and zinc (Zn). The existence of concentrated premixes of these minerals raises the risk of feed mismixes resulting in the accidental feeding of high, potentially toxic levels of these elements.

Copper. Dietary requirements of 5–6 ppm Cu have been established for swine. A dietary level of 250 ppm is generally considered the maximum tolerable level (MTL) of Cu for swine, and ration levels ranging from 300–500 ppm cause reduced growth and anemia. The tolerance to Cu is related positively to dietary levels of Fe and Zn. For example, animals consuming feed containing 750 ppm Cu are essentially normal if also supplemented with 750 ppm Fe and 500 ppm Zn. Icterus, anemia, hemoglobinuria, and nephritis associated with a hemolytic crisis may be observed in swine, although not as commonly as in sheep. Diagnosis can be suggested by clinical signs and a history of feeding excess Cu. Liver and kidney Cu levels greater than 250 and 60 ppm, respectively, on a wet-weight basis are diagnostically supportive.

Iron. The recommended dietary levels of Fe range from 40–150 ppm, the highest requirements being in the youngest pigs. Many factors influence the risk of Fe toxicosis. Elemental Fe and iron oxides are relatively nontoxic, whereas iron salts are more toxic. Dietary phytate, phosphate, cobalt (Co), Zn, Cu, manganese (Mn), and disaccharides competitively depress Fe absorption. Ascorbic acid, sorbitol, fructose, and several amino acids improve Fe absorption, which is facilitated by being chelated with citric, lactic, pyruvic, and succinic acids; Fe chelated by desferrioxamine is poorly absorbed.

Pigs fed 1100 ppm Fe as a salt have shown reduced weight gains. Animals fed 5000 ppm have displayed depressed feed intake and rates of gain as well as rickets characterized by hypophosphatemia and reduced bone ash. The condition has not been prevented by providing 0.92% dietary phosphorus (P). Injections of Fe, usually as the dextran, have caused intoxications characterized by cardiovascular shock and death within hours after administration as well as staining at injection sites and in regional lymph nodes, liver, and kidneys. The incidence of this acute toxicosis appears to be decreasing. High single doses of iron salts will cause gastroenteritis, followed by apparent recovery and then, frequently, collapse and death within 2 days. Diagnosis may be facilitated by consideration of history, clinical signs, and necropsy changes. Feed and serum should be analyzed for Fe. Normal serum Fe levels are approximately 100 mg/dL and will increase during toxicosis. Iron toxicosis should be differentiated from other forms of rickets. There is no practical individual treatment for Fe toxicosis. Desferrioxamine (Desferal) may be used in selected cases. Dietary imbalances should obviously be corrected.

Selenium. The recommended dietary level of Se varies from 0.1 to 0.3 ppm. Selenium, as the selenate or selenite, is approved for addition to swine feeds at up to 0.3 ppm.

Accidental oversupplementation of swine feeds with selenium premixes has been a sporadic problem. When

Se levels of 5–8 ppm have been fed to growing swine, anorexia, alopecia, separation of hooves at the coronary band, and degenerative changes in the liver and kidney have occurred. Liver changes may look remarkably like those seen with vitamin E–Se deficiency. A level of 10 ppm fed to breeding sows has caused retarded conception and pigs dead or weak at birth. Misformulated feeds containing from 10 to 27 ppm Se produced a paralytic disease in growing swine characterized by quadriplegic or posterior paralysis while the pigs remained mentally alert and continued to eat and drink. Focal symmetrical poliomyelomalacia was found in affected swine (Harrison et el. 1983; Casteel et al. 1985).

Several injectable products containing varying concentrations of Se are currently available for treatment or prevention of Se-responsive diseases. Death losses have approached 100% when Se overdose occurred from the mistaken use of a more concentrated product or from miscalculation of the recommended dosage. The minimum lethal dose of injectable Se is about 0.9 mg/kg body weight, with pigs that are Se deficient being the most susceptible to toxicosis (Van Vleet et al. 1974). Weakness and dyspnea progressing to irregular gasps and death occur within 24 hours of the parenteral overdose.

Diagnosis of Se toxicosis in swine can be made by consideration of a history of Se supplementation, clinical signs, necropsy findings, and chemical analysis of tissues and feeds. Liver and kidney Se concentrations greater than 3 ppm (wet weight) are seen with toxicosis.

Zinc. Recommended dietary levels of Zn for swine vary from 15–100 ppm based on age, sex, stage of production, and other ration components. A level of 2000 ppm Zn produced growth depression, arthritis, intramuscular hemorrhage, gastritis, and enteritis. The MTL is probably less than 300 ppm, possibly because zinc salts in large concentration are unpalatable. Zinc interacts competitively for absorption with Fe, Ca, and Cu. Pigs fed 268 ppm Zn developed arthritis, bone and cartilage deformities, and internal hemorrhages. However, feeding 3,000 ppm Zn as zinc oxide for 14 days has shown increased weight gains and reduction of postweaning scours without adverse signs. Diagnostic considerations should include clinical signs, history, and chemical analyses of feed and tissues. Normal kidney and liver levels of Zn are 25–75 ppm (wet weight) and may increase during toxicosis. However, excretion is quite rapid.

Nonessential Minerals

Arsenic. Inorganic arsenicals, which are distinctly different from the phenylarsonic feed additives discussed later, have been used in antiquated ant baits, herbicides, insecticides, and some animal medications. Pigs are relatively resistant to inorganic arsenic (As) poisoning with 100–200 mg/kg body weight of sodium arsenite being a lethal oral dose. This is equivalent to about 2000–4000 ppm in the feed. However, pigs have refused to consume 1000 ppm in the feed. Clinical signs of acute As poisoning colic, vomiting, diarrhea, dehydration, collapse, convulsions, and death within hours to days. Prominent necropsy findings are dehydration and severe hemorrhagic gastritis and enteritis with sloughing of mucosa and edema. Diagnostic considerations should include history, clinical signs, lesions and chemical analyses. Kidney and liver tissues levels of 10 ppm (wet weight) are significant. Prognosis is generally poor and depends on the degree of tissue damage and dehydration.

Fluorine. Fluorosis may be observed in animals consuming water or forages contaminated by nearby industrial plants or eating crops raised on soils high in fluorine (F). A common source is consumption of minerals high in F. Feed-grade phosphates by law must contain no more than one part F to 100 parts P. It is recommended that swine be fed feeds containing no more than 70 ppm F during their lifetime to prevent fluorosis. Sodium fluoride has been used as an ascaricide at levels of 500 ppm; higher levels have caused vomiting. Other signs of acute toxicosis are diarrhea, lameness, tetany, collapse, and death. A tentative diagnosis of chronic fluorosis may be difficult, since the lameness may appear similar to rickets, mycoplasmosis, and erysipelas. Normal bone F levels in swine are 3000–4000 ppm. Higher levels are associated with fluorosis. Normal urine F levels are 5–15 ppm; higher levels are diagnostically significant. Necropsy findings may reveal exostoses on the long bones and tooth mottling. Treatment should be aimed at reducing dietary F and feeding aluminum or calcium (Ca) mineral supplements.

Lead. Swine are quite resistant to elevated lead (Pb) exposure. Consequently, field cases of lead poisoning in swine are extremely rare. Experimentally, pigs fed 35.2 mg lead (as the acetate)/kg body weight for 90 days did not die from lead poisoning despite blood lead concentrations of up to 290 µg/dL (Lassen and Buck 1979). If toxicosis is suspected, a thorough diagnostic workup including kidney and liver analyses should be performed.

Mercury. Mercury (Hg) has been used in paints, batteries, paper, and fungicides, but most uses have been restricted. All mercurial compounds are toxic, but organic forms are the most toxic to all species. Mercury is cumulative, and toxicity depends on form, dose, and duration. Swine have been poisoned after consuming seeds treated with organic mercurial fungicides. Initially, signs of gastroenteritis may be evident, followed by uremia and central nervous system (CNS) disturbance, including ataxia, blindness, aimless wandering, paresis, coma, and death. Mercury toxicosis may be confused with erysipelas, cholera, or poisoning by pigweed or phenylarsonics. Clinical signs, history, necropsy findings, and chemistry should aid in the diagnosis. Kidney and liver normally contain less than 1 ppm Hg but will contain much higher levels following Hg toxicosis. Treatment is usually disappointing.

FEED ADDITIVES

Adverse effects of drug additives are rare except in cases of misuse or misformulation of rations (Lloyd 1978). Details of specific drug effects have been reviewed recently (Adams 1996).

Phenylarsonic Compounds

The phenylarsonic compounds, occasionally referred to as organic arsenicals, have at times been used as growth promotants and to treat swine dysentery and eperythrozoonosis. Arsanilic acid and roxarsone (3-nitro-4-hydroxyphenylarsonic acid) have been approved for use in swine rations, and their sodium salts have been used in drinking water. Arsanilic acid was approved for continuous use in complete swine rations at levels ranging from 50–100 ppm (45–90 g/ton).

Clinical signs of arsanilic acid toxicosis will start within a few days at levels of 1000 ppm, 2 weeks at 400 ppm, and 3–6 weeks at 250 ppm and include ataxia, posterior paresis, blindness, and quadriplegia. Paralyzed animals will continue to live and grow if provided food and water. Swine that receive lower doses for extended periods are prone to develop goose-stepping (a chronic posterior nerve affliction) and total blindness from optic nerve damage. Swine that receive very large doses, for example, 10,000 ppm in the ration, may exhibit a gastroenteritis resembling poisoning by inorganic arsenic compounds.

Roxarsone is approved for continuous use in swine rations at levels of 25–37 ppm and at 200 ppm for 5–6 days. Poisoning may result with feed roxarsone levels of 250 pp or more for from 3–10 days. Clinical signs include uncontrolled urination and defecation as well as muscle tremor and convulsive seizures, all of which are induced by physical stimulation. Ataxia may be observed, although not as severe as the "drunken sailor" incoordination of arsanilic acid toxicosis. In advanced stages, pigs show paraparesis and paraplegia, but will continue to eat and drink.

Clinical signs and a history of administration of arsenicals in feed or water may be the best basis for suspecting phenylarsonic toxicosis. Necropsy findings are generally nonproductive, but histopathologic examination of peripheral nerves, especially the sciatic, may reveal a demyelination.

Chemical analysis of tissues for the specific phenylarsonic compounds may not be helpful, since the compounds are excreted within a few days after withdrawal. However, analysis of kidney, liver, muscle, and feed for As may assist in the diagnosis. Elemental arsenic levels (wet weight) greater than 2 ppm in kidney and liver and 0.5 ppm in muscle are illegal and indicative of excess As intake. Further analyses of feed for the specific phenylarsonic compound will provide more diagnostic evidence.

Deficiencies of B-complex vitamins, especially pantothenic acid and pyridoxine, may cause a similar demyelination of peripheral nerves. Chronic phenylarsonic toxicosis may also resemble rickets. Although water deprivation, organic mercurial poisoning, and viral diseases affect the CNS primarily, they may be confused with phenylarsonic compound toxicosis. Toxicoses are reversible if arsenicals are promptly removed from the feed and water.

Carbadox

Carbadox (Mecadox, Pfizer) is incorporated in feed at 11–27.5 ppm as a growth promotant or at 55 ppm to control swine dysentery or enteritis. A feed level of 100 ppm has caused decreased feed consumption and growth retardation. Higher levels have caused feed refusal and emesis. Mild lesions in the glomerular zone of the adrenal cortex are reported with 50 ppm carbadox in the feed for 10 weeks, while more extensive lesions are seen at feed levels of 100–150 ppm after 5 weeks of consumption (Van der Molen 1988).

When fed a ration containing from 331 to 363 ppm carbadox, recently weaned pigs refused to eat and showed poor weight gains, posterior paresis, the passing of hard, pelleted feces, and death in 7–9 days (Power et al. 1989).

Dimetridazole

Dimetridazole is listed as an antihistomoniasis drug used in turkey rations and for treatment and prevention of swine dysentery in some countries. A level of 1500 ppm has caused no toxicosis, but 17,000 ppm have caused diarrhea in swine. Large overdoses of dimetridazole would cause ataxia, bradycardia, dyspnea, salivation, muscle spasms, prostration, and death. Death or recovery would be rapid.

Monensin

Monensin is marketed as Rumensin for cattle supplements or as Coban, a poultry coccidiostat. Use levels are up to 120 ppm for poultry and 30 ppm in cattle feeds, although some premixes may contain up to 1320 ppm. Swine may be fed monensin by mistake, but the drug is not highly toxic to them. Pigs fed levels ranging from 11 to 120 ppm in the feed for 112 days were not affected as far as feed consumption and weight gains were concerned. Gilts fed 110–880 ppm had a transient anorexia for 14 days; thereafter, only weight gains were depressed. The LD50 of monensin in swine is 16.8 mg/kg. Pigs suffering from monensin toxicosis showed open-mouth breathing, frothing around the mouth, ataxia, lethargy, muscle weakness, and diarrhea. These signs were visible within 1 day of exposure and persisted for about 3 days. Myocardial and skeletal muscle necrosis was present in pigs receiving 40 mg monensin/kg (Van Vleet et al. 1983).

The greatest risk of poisoning from monensin in swine appears to be with the concurrent administration of tiamulin, an antibiotic approved for use in treatment of swine dysentery that potentiates the effect of monensin (Van Vleet et al. 1987). Swine poisoned from this combination show acute massive necrotizing myositis of the skeletal muscles, myoglobinuria, and acute death.

Lasalocid

Lasalocid is a polyether antibiotic marketed as Bovatec for feedlot cattle to improve feed efficiency and weight gains. Swine fed lasalocid at 2.78 mg/kg and 21 mg/kg showed no adverse effects. However, transient muscle weakness occurred at a dose of 35 mg/kg (equivalent to about 1000 ppm of lasalocid in the feed), and death occurred at 58 mg/kg when fed for 1 day.

Sulfonamides

The sulfonamide drugs are antibacterials commonly used in swine medicine. Overdoses will cause crystalluric nephroses. Pigs are not likely to be intoxicated from drinking water containing sulfonamides because of the lack of palatability, but overdosing in the feed, coupled with low water intake, may cause nephrosis and uremia. Nephrotoxic mycotoxicoses such as those caused by citrinin and ochratoxin will predispose sulfonamide toxicoses. Sulfonamide residues in pork are related to persistence of the drugs in feed and excreta and are not a toxicosis.

Urea and Ammonium Salts

Swine may be fed cattle feeds containing nonprotein nitrogen compounds such as urea and ammonium salts. Urea is relatively nontoxic for swine, a level of 2.5% causing only reduced feed intake and growth rate, elevated blood urea nitrogen (BUN), polydypsia, and polyuria. Higher levels of urea should not cause signs of acute toxicosis. Ammonia and ammonium salts are toxic for swine, however, with individual doses of 0.25–0.5 g/kg body weight causing intoxication and doses of 0.54–1.5 g/kg being lethal. Considering that growing swine consume feed equal to 5–10% of their body weights, the expected toxic and lethal levels of ammonium salts are 0.25–1% and 1.5–3%, respectively. Pigs poisoned with ammonia and ammonium salts would be expected to become depressed, have tonoclonic convulsions, and either die or recover within a few hours.

PESTICIDES

Insecticides

Concurrent production of both livestock and crops on the same premises may provide a unique opportunity for exposure of swine to agricultural chemicals. Among the chemicals presenting the greatest potential hazard of poisoning are the organophosphorus (OP), carbamate, and the older chlorinated hydrocarbon insecticides.

Poisoning may occur when insecticides are accidentally incorporated into swine feed. Discarded or unlabeled portions of granular insecticides can be mistaken for mineral mixes or dry feed ingredients and added to swine feeds. When farm equipment used for feed handling is also used for insecticide transportation, contamination of this equipment may result in insecticides being inadvertently mixed into animal feeds. In addition, swine may have accidental access to insecticides when they are stored or spilled on the farm premises. Improperly operating back rubbers and oilers may provide an additional source of these insecticides for livestock.

Miscalculation of insecticide concentrations in spraying, dipping, and pour-on procedures may also result in toxicosis. Re-treating animals with OP or carbamate preparations within a few days' time may result in poisoning.

Organophosphorus and Carbamate Insecticides. The OP and carbamate insecticides are discussed together because of their similar mechanisms of action.

Cholinergic nerves utilize acetylcholine as a neurotransmitter substance. Under normal conditions, acetylcholine released at the synapses of parasympathetic nerves and myoneural junctions is quickly hydrolyzed by cholinesterase enzymes. When the hydrolyzing enzymes are inhibited, the continued presence of acetylcholine maintains a state of nerve stimulation and accounts for the clinical signs observed with poisoning from these insecticides.

Clinical Signs. The clinical syndrome produced by OP and carbamate insecticides is characterized by a rapidly progressing overstimulation of the parasympathetic nervous system and skeletal muscles. Earliest clinical signs of acute poisoning frequently include mild to profuse salivation, defecation, urination, emesis, stiff-legged or "sawhorse" gait, and general uneasiness. As the syndrome progresses, signs observed include profuse salivation; gastrointestinal hypermotility resulting in severe colic, vomiting (especially common in swine), and abdominal cramps; diarrhea; excessive lacrimation; miosis; dyspnea; cyanosis; urinary incontinence; muscle tremors of the face, eyelids, and general body musculature; and acute death. Hyperactivity of the skeletal muscles is generally followed by muscular paralysis, as the muscles are unable to respond to continued stimulation. Swine may exhibit increased CNS stimulation but rarely, if ever, convulsive seizures. More commonly, severe CNS depression occurs.

Death usually results from hypoxia caused by excessive respiratory tract secretions, bronchoconstriction, and erratic, slowed heartbeat. The onset of clinical signs of acute poisoning may appear within a few minutes in severe cases to several hours in milder ones.

Lesions. Lesions associated with acute OP or carbamate toxicosis are usually nonspecific but may include excessive fluids in the respiratory tract as well as pulmonary edema.

Diagnosis. A history of exposure to OP or carbamate insecticides associated with clinical signs of parasympathetic stimulation warrants a tentative diagnosis of poisoning with these compounds.

Chemical analyses of animal tissues for the presence of insecticides are usually unrewarding because of the rapid degradation of OP and carbamate insecticides, resulting in low tissue residue levels. However, finding the insecticide in the stomach contents and the feed or suspect material can be quite valuable in establishing a diagnosis. In addition, the degree of inhibition of cholinesterase enzyme activity in the whole blood and tissue of the suspected animal should be assessed. A reduction of whole-blood cholinesterase activity to less than 25% of normal is indicative of excessive exposure to these insecticides. The cholinesterase activity level in the brain tissue of animals dying from these insecticides will generally be less than 10% of normal brain activity.

Whole-blood and brain samples should be well chilled but not frozen for best laboratory results. Samples of stomach contents as well as the suspect feed or material should be submitted to a laboratory for chemical analysis.

Treatment. Treatment of animals poisoned by OP or carbamate insecticides should be considered on an emergency basis because of the rapid progression of respiratory distress in the clinical syndrome. Initial treatment for poisoned swine should be the intramuscular use of atropine sulfate at approximately 0.5 mg/kg body weight. One-quarter of this dose may be given intravenously for a quick response in especially severe cases. Atropine does not counteract the insecticide-enzyme bond but blocks the effects of accumulated acetylcholine at the nerve endings. Although a dramatic cessation of parasympathetic signs is generally observed within a few minutes after administration of atropine, it will not affect the skeletal muscle tremors. More atropine at approximately one-half the initial dose may be required but should be used only to control recurring parasympathetic signs. Although the use of atropine alone is generally adequate, especially if vomiting has occurred, specific cases may warrant the use of pralidoxime chloride or activated charcoal.

Oral activated charcoal is recommended for treatment of any ingested insecticide to reduce continued absorption of the insecticide from the gut. Although a useful treatment, the need for activated charcoal in swine may be reduced when vomiting helps empty the gut and thereby reduces further absorption of the insecticide.

The use of the oximes (e.g., TMB-4, 2-PAM, pralidoxime chloride) in large animals, although efficacious, may be economically unfeasible. If used, pralidoxime chloride is recommended at a dose of 20 mg/kg body weight. The oximes are of no benefit in treating carbamate toxicoses.

Dermally exposed animals should be washed with soap and water to prevent continued absorption of these compounds.

Morphine, succinylcholine, and phenothiazine tranquilizers should be avoided in treating OP poisoning.

Chlorinated Hydrocarbons. The chlorinated hydrocarbon (CH) insecticides (e.g., toxaphene, chlordane, aldrin, dieldrin, and lindane) produce toxicosis in swine by acting as diffuse but powerful stimulants of the CNS. Even though these are old products that have been restricted from the market for over 30 years, improperly discarded leftover products may become available to animals when older barns or storage areas are cleaned out.

Clinical Signs. Clinical signs often appear 12–24 hours after exposure. Initially, animals may appear apprehensive. A period of hyperexcitability and hyperesthesia characterized by exaggerated responses to stimuli and spontaneous muscle spasms is usually observed. The spontaneous tremors and fasciculation are usually in the facial region and involve lips, muscle, eyelids, and ears, progressing caudally to involve the heavy muscles of the shoulder, back, and hindquarters. These spasms may progress into a tonoclonic convulsive seizure. Abnormal posturing, elevation of the head, and chewing movements may be observed. Varying degrees of respiratory paralysis occur during the seizures, with periods of depression and inactivity between successive seizures.

The rapidity of onset and severity of clinical signs provide a poor index of the prognosis of the episode in individual animals. Occasionally, animals will die during seizures, while others may completely recover following several severe episodes.

Lesions. Specific lesions other than those from the physical trauma of the seizures are not observed.

Diagnosis. Clinical signs of hyperexcitability and tonoclonic convulsive seizures with a known exposure to CH insecticides should yield a tentative diagnosis of toxicosis.

The presence of significant levels of CH insecticide in liver, kidney, and brain tissue is essential for confirming a diagnosis. Samples of these tissues as well as stomach contents and suspect material such as feed or spray should be submitted to a laboratory. Avoid contamination of specimens with hair or gut contents to prevent erroneous analytic results.

Laboratory tests are usually required to differentiate this toxicosis from pseudorabies, water deprivation, or gut edema.

Treatment. Treatment is essentially symptomatic, since there is no specific antidote for the CH insecticides. Animals should be sedated with long-acting barbiturates to control convulsive seizures. Animals with dermal exposure should be washed with warm, soapy water to remove the chemical and prevent continued contact. If the chemical is orally ingested, activated charcoal in a water slurry may be used to prevent further absorption. Oil-based cathartics should be avoided, as they may hasten absorption of the chemicals. Intravenous fluids plus glucose may be needed in protracted cases.

Residues. Because of the persistence of CH insecticides and their concentration in fat deposits of the body, the carcasses of animals dying from CH insecticide toxicosis are a source of contamination for feed ingredients such as tankage, meat and bone meal, and fats. Therefore, proper disposal of contaminated carcasses is very important. Tissue residues of these chemicals in swine surviving an episode of insecticide exposure should be an important consideration in market animals. In some cases the time required for excretion of these residues is too long to make decontamination economically feasible.

Synthetic Pyrethroids. Several synthetic pyrethroids (e.g., permethrin, fenvalerate) are commercially available for fly and external-parasite control. As a class, the synthetic pyrethroids are relatively nontoxic to mammals and are unlikely to produce poisoning in swine.

Formamidines. Amitraz is a formamidine pesticide with insecticidal and acaricidal properties. It is available in the United States as Taktic for control of lice and mange on swine. This compound has low mammalian toxicity and is unlikely to produce toxicosis in swine.

Fungicides

Captan. Captan has been widely used as a seed treatment although some newer fungicides are now being employed. Field corn seed produced commercially in the United States has generally been treated with captan at a level of approximately 1000 ppm. Consumption of captan-treated seed corn represents little hazard of poisoning, as the acute lethal dose of captan for livestock is greater than 250 mg/kg body weight.

Organomercurials. The organomercurials include phenyl mercuric chloride, phenyl mercuric acetate, various aliphatic compounds such as ethyl mercuric chloride, and complex aromatic derivatives like hydroxy mercuric cresol. The toxicoses associated with mercury-based seed treatments are discussed above, in the section on mercury.

Pentachlorophenol. Pentachlorophenol (PCP) has been employed for over 45 years as a wood preservative and fungicide. PCP- or "penta"-treated wood has found application in livestock handling and housing facilities, where wood is in contact with soil, manure, or moisture. Acute poisoning is not a major problem from PCP-treated wood, although toxicosis, including stillborn pigs, may occur when livestock have contact with surfaces that have been freshly treated with PCP preparations (Schipper 1961). A single oral dose of 80 mg/kg was not fatal to a weanling pig. If toxicosis occurs, depression, emesis, muscular weakness, accelerated respiratory rate, and posterior paralysis are clinical signs that may be observed. A problem of greater concern may be the recognition of blood and tissue PCP residues in swine that have been in contact with PCP-treated facilities. Finding from 10 to 1000 ppb PCP in whole blood is apparently unrelated to manifestations of toxicosis.

Chromate–Copper Arsenate. Chromate–copper arsenate (CCA) is widely used as a wood preservative in consumer lumber intended for outdoor use. CCA-treated wood generally presents a negligible hazard to swine, as the metallic salts are bound in the wood fibers. However, the residual inorganic arsenic in the ashes of burned CCA wood can produce poisoning in swine.

Herbicides

Phenoxy Herbicides. 2,4-D; 2,4,5-T; MCPA; and silvex are selective herbicides widely used in crop production and pasture and range management. Because the toxic dose of 2,4-D and 2,4,5-T is greater than 300 mg/kg body weight for several days, the hazard of poisoning by these compounds under normal conditions of use is low. When large doses have been administered experimentally, depression, anorexia, weight loss, muscular weakness, and incoordination have been observed.

Dipyridal Herbicides. Paraquat, a plant desiccant type of herbicide, has found widespread application in no-till farming technology. Accidental, as well as malicious, poisoning of swine with paraquat has resulted in toxicosis. An approximate lethal dose of paraquat for swine is 75 mg/kg.

Acute effects involving necrosis and erosion of the oral and gastric mucosa are attributed to the carrier solvent. The more classic effects, however, occur 7–10 days after ingestion and are characterized by pulmonary congestion and edema. The pulmonary lesions progress to a severe diffuse interstitial pulmonary fibrosis. Initial clinical signs include emesis and diarrhea, and the later stages are characterized by respiratory distress. Once clinical signs suggesting pulmonary involvement develop, therapeutic measures are usually futile.

Rodenticides

The rodenticides are used to control rat and mouse populations in or around farmsteads, feed storage areas, and swine production facilities. Accidental access to these compounds constitutes the usual route of exposure, although malicious poisoning of swine with rodenticides has also occurred.

Anticoagulant Rodenticides. The anticoagulant rodenticides (e.g., warfarin, diphacinone, chlorophacinone, bromadiolone, brodifocoum, pindone) compose the largest group of rodenticides available through retail outlets. Swine are quite susceptible to this class of compound, as evidenced by toxicosis occurring after a single oral dose of warfarin at 3 mg/kg body weight. Repeated oral doses of only 0.05 mg/kg per day for 7 days also produced toxicosis in swine (Osweiler 1978). These rodenticides produce lowered prothrombin levels by interfering with vitamin K utilization. The physiologic result is increased blood-clotting time, which is manifested clinically as mild to severe hemorrhage. The clinical signs—including lameness, stiffness, lethargy, recumbency, anorexia, and dark tarry feces—are related directly to extravasation of blood. Observed lesions include hematoma, articular swelling, epistaxis, intermuscular hemorrhage, anemia, and melena.

A diagnosis of anticoagulant rodenticide toxicosis should include demonstration of a defect in the clotting mechanism as evidenced by increases in clotting time, one-stage prothrombin time, or activated partial thromboplastin time. The chemical detection of the rodenticide in samples of blood, liver, or suspect baits is also helpful.

Injectable vitamin K and oral vitamin K supplements are included in a successful treatment regime. Whole-blood transfusions may be utilized successfully in special cases.

Strychnine. Strychnine, an indole alkaloid, is widely available commercially, often as either a green- or red-dyed pellet or grain or as a white powder. This alkaloid acts by selectively antagonizing certain types of special inhibitory neurons, thereby allowing uncontrolled and relatively diffuse reflex activity to proceed unchecked. The approximate oral lethal dose of strychnine for swine varies from 0.5 to 1 mg/kg body weight. Clinical signs appear within 10 minutes to 2 hours after ingestion and are characterized by violent tetanic seizures that may occur spontaneously or in response to external stimuli such as touch, light, or sound. The intermittent seizures are usually separated by periods of relaxation. Death occurs from anoxia and exhaustion during the seizures, often in less than 1 hour. Diagnosis is best confirmed by detection of the strychnine alkaloid in either the stomach contents or urine. Treatment consists of controlling seizures with long-acting barbiturates and other muscle relaxants.

Cholecalciferol. Rodenticides containing cholecalciferol (vitamin D₃) are commercially available as Rampage, Quintox, or Ortho Rat-B-Gone. Toxic doses of these products produce vitamin D poisoning with hypercalcemia, mineralization of soft tissues, and clinical signs of depression, weakness, nausea, anorexia, polyuria, and polydipsia.

Bromethalin. Bromethalin-based rodenticides, marketed as Assault, Vengeance, or Trounce, produce cerebral edema and signs of rear-leg ataxia and/or paresis and CNS depression. Hyperexcitability, muscle tremors, and seizures may be seen with higher doses of bromethalin in the dog (Dorman et al. 1990).

TOXIC PLANTS

Amaranthus retroflexus (Redroot Pigweed)

A distinct disease syndrome of swine called perirenal edema occurs during the summer and early fall months. Its onset is associated with sudden access to pastures, barn lots, or fencerows containing moderate amounts of *Amaranthus retroflexus* (redroot pigweed).

Clinical signs appear suddenly 5–10 days after access to the pigweed. Initial signs are weakness, trembling, and incoordination. The disease progresses rapidly to knuckling of the pastern joints and finally to almost complete paralysis of the rear legs. Affected pigs usually lie in sternal recumbency, and if disturbed, attempts to walk will be in a crouching gait or with the rear legs dragging. The body temperature is usually normal and the eyes are bright. Coma and death generally occur within 48 hours of the onset of clinical signs, but affected swine may live from 5 to 15 days, with progression from signs of acute nephrosis to those of chronic fibrosing nephritis. In affected herds, new cases may appear for as long as 10 days after removal from the source. Morbidity ranges from less than 5% in some herds to 50% in others, and the mortality is usually about 75–80% in those showing clinical signs.

Gross necropsy findings are dramatic and characterized as edema of the connective tissue around the kidneys. The amount of fluid in the perirenal area varies, at times occupying the greater portion of the abdominal cavity. The edematous fluid may contain considerable blood, although the kidney itself is usually of normal size and pale. Edema of the ventral body wall and perirectal areas as well as ascites and hydrothorax may be observed. Histologic lesions of affected swine are characterized by hydropic degeneration and coagulative necrosis of both proximal and distal convoluted tubules. Glomeruli may be shrunken, with dilation of Bowman's capsules. Proteinaceous casts are numerous in distal and collecting tubules.

As a consequence of severe renal disease, there are elevations in BUN, serum creatinine, and serum potassium. The electrocardiograph of affected swine is characteristic of hyperkalemic heart failure (Osweiler et al. 1969). The changes include bradycardia, a wide and slurred QRS complex, and an increase in magnitude and deviation of the T wave. The probable cause of death is hyperkalemic heart failure.

Immediate removal of affected pigs from the source of the weeds is the only definite therapeutic recommendation that can be made at this time.

Xanthium spp. (Cocklebur)

Cockleburs, including *Xanthium strumarium* and other species, are annual herbs that reproduce only from seed. They may be found throughout the world in cultivated fields, fencerows, and ditches and may heavily infest pastures as a result of being washed in from adjacent cropland.

The greatest potential for cocklebur poisoning arises when the more toxic two-leaf seedling stage or ground seeds are ingested. The unpalatable more mature plant contains less of the toxic principle, carboxyatractyloside. Within 8–24 hours after ingestion, swine develop signs of depression, nausea, weakness, ataxia, and subnormal temperature. Spasms of the cervical muscles, vomiting, and dyspnea may occur. Death occurs within several hours after the onset of symptoms. Lesions typically include ascites with large fibrin strands on the surface of the liver and other viscera and congestion and centrilobular accentuation of the liver. Microscopically acute centrilobular hepatic necrosis is observed (Stuart et al. 1981).

Treatment includes mineral oil per os to delay absorption of the carboxyatractyloside. Intramuscular injection of 5–30 mg physostigmine may produce a dramatic response in some cases (Link 1975).

Solanum nigrum (Black Nightshade)

Even though black nightshade is easily recognized and found in woods, permanent pastures, and fencerows, actual cases of poisoning are rare. The alkaloid solanine is found principally in the leaves and green berries, but the plant is generally not palatable and is usually consumed under conditions of its abundant growth and lack of other suitable forage.

Affected animals display anorexia, constipation, depression, and incoordination. Poisoned swine may vomit. Dilation of the pupils and muscular trembling are neurologic signs observed. Animals may be seen lying on their sides and kicking with all feet, progressing then to coma and death. Necropsy may reveal some degree of gastrointestinal irritation. The toxic alkaloid is rapidly eliminated through the urine (Kingsbury 1964).

Nitrates and Nitrites

As monogastric animals, swine are relatively resistant to the effects of nitrate, especially when compared with cattle. Nitrate or nitrite toxicosis occurs most commonly when these ions accumulate in either plants and/or water sources. Some fertilizers, such as ammonium nitrate or potassium nitrate, may also be a source

of nitrate for animals. Several different plants may accumulate nitrate, depending on varying climatic and soil fertility conditions. Nitrate may accumulate in the lower stalk and perhaps leaves of corn and other plants, but not in the fruit or grain.

The nitrates from both water (see the section on water quality below) and plant sources are additive and should be evaluated together in particular field cases. The nitrate ion (NO3) itself is not particularly toxic and may produce no more than gastrointestinal irritation. However, nitrite (NO_2), the reduced form of nitrate, is quite toxic. The nitrite ion oxidizes ferrous iron in hemoglobin to the ferric state, forming methemoglobin, which cannot accept and transport molecular oxygen. The result is tissue hypoxia from poorly oxygenated blood.

Pigs given single oral doses of greater than 10–20 mg nitrite-nitrogen (as potassium nitrite)/kg body weight developed clinical signs of poisoning but recovered, whereas those given doses greater than 20 mg nitrite-nitrogen/kg body weight died within 90–150 minutes after ingestion (London et al. 1967). Clinical signs became apparent when approximately 20% of the total hemoglobin was present as methemoglobin; death was associated with methemoglobin levels of approximately 80%. Clinical signs observed with acute nitrite toxicosis include increased respiratory rate, salivation, miosis, polyuria, weakness, ataxia, and terminal anoxic convulsive seizures. The blood and tissues are a chocolate brown color from the methemoglobin. Treatment of acute nitrite toxicosis consists of intravenous injection of 10 mg methylene blue/kg body weight in a 4% solution (Link 1975).

WATER QUALITY

Water is one of the most important nutrients for swine. The availability of adequate quantities of good-quality water is essential for successful swine production. Even though it may be easy to incriminate water as the cause of poor performance and vague disease conditions in swine, water evaluation should be part of a thorough diagnostic investigation. A detailed history of the animals as well as the water source, careful clinical evaluation, and submission of representative animal and water specimens should be included in the investigation. Results of water tests should be evaluated in view of existing standards for livestock water quality. Some general guidelines for evaluating water quality parameters for livestock are presented in Table 60.1.

Information about the source of the water should be recorded. Ponds, wells, and regional rural water systems are the most common water sources, and each may influence the quality of the water supplied. The depth of wells may also be helpful, as deeper wells tend to have a higher mineral content, while shallower wells are more likely to have higher nitrate levels and coliform counts.

Table 60.1. Water quality guidelines for livestock

Item	Maximum Recommended Limit (ppm)
Major ions	
Calcium	1000
Nitrate + nitrite	100
Nitrite alone	10
Sulfate	1000
Total dissolved solids	3000
Heavy metals and trace ions	
Aluminum	5.0
Arsenic	0.5[a]
Beryllium	0.1[b]
Boron	5.0
Cadmium	0.02
Chromium	1.0
Cobalt	1.0
Copper (swine)	5.0
Fluoride	2.0[c]
Iron	No guideline
Lead	0.1
Manganese	No guideline
Mercury	0.003
Molybdenum	0.5
Nickel	1.0
Selenium	0.05
Uranium	0.2
Vanadium	0.1
Zinc	50.0

Source: Canadian Task Force on Water Quality 1987.
[a]5.0 if not added to feed.
[b]Tentative guideline.
[c]1.0 if fluoride is present in feed.

Sometimes the age of the well and type of pumping device may suggest certain mechanical problems, including a cracked casing or defective sanitary seal. Estimates of the amount of water consumed may also be helpful when investigating potential water problems.

Microbiologic Standards

Microbiologic examination of water samples determines the general sanitary quality of the sample and indicates the degree of contamination of the water with waste from human and animal sources.

In general, these examinations do not attempt to isolate pathogenic bacteria but detect the presence of indicator organisms. The coliform group of bacteria has traditionally been the indicator used to assess the degree of water pollution and thus the sanitary quality of the particular sample. As an advance in the microbiologic examination of water, the differentiation of fecal coliforms as a subgroup within the general category of coliforms is encouraging. The U.S. Environmental Protection Agency (1973) proposed that acceptable levels for water to be used directly by livestock should not exceed 1000/100 mL. Many believe, however, that as long as animals are allowed to range freely and drink surface waters, these proposed limits will be unenforceable and of doubtful value.

The standard plate count, which enumerates the number of bacteria multiplying at 35°C, is of doubtful significance in evaluating livestock water sources other than helping to judge the efficiency of various water treatment processes.

Salinity

Salinity, or total dissolved solids (TDS), generally expressed in milligrams per liter, is an expression of the amount of soluble salts in a particular water sample and is one of the most important parameters used to evaluate water quality. The ions most commonly involved in saline waters are calcium, magnesium, and sodium in the bicarbonate, chloride, or sulfate form. Hardness is sometimes confused with salinity, but the two are not necessarily correlative. Hardness is expressed as the sum of calcium and magnesium reported in equivalent amounts of calcium carbonate. Although hardness of water may affect the mechanical function of valves and waterers because of the formation of mineral deposits, hardness itself has a minimal impact on animal performance.

Water containing less than 1000 mg soluble salts/L should present no serious hazard to any class of swine. Water containing between 1000 and 5000 mg soluble salts/L may cause mild temporary diarrhea or be refused at first by swine not accustomed to it, although health or performance should not be greatly affected (NRC 1974; Anderson and Strothers 1978; Paterson et al. 1979). Water containing 5000–7000 mg soluble salts/L may present a health risk for pregnant, lactating, or stressed animals. Water containing more than 7000 mg soluble salts/L should be considered unsafe for swine.

In some regions, sulfates are a major portion of the TDS in water. A recent study (Fleck Veenhuizen et al. 1992) demonstrated that except for an increase in fecal moisture content, water containing up to 1800 mg of sodium, magnesium, or a combination of sodium and magnesium sulfate per liter had no effect on nursery pig performance. An epidemiologic study of water on swine farms did not find an association between sulfate concentrations and prevalence of diarrhea, although water sulfate levels increased with the depth of the wells tested (Fleck Veenhuizen 1993). A recent study of water quality on 173 Iowa swine farms found a mean TDS of 343 mg/L (range 100–2,500), but measured no significant effects of elevated TDS on several performance parameters (Ensley 1998).

Nitrates and Nitrites

Nitrates and nitrites are water soluble and thus may be leached from the soil or soil surface into groundwater. Animal wastes, nitrogen fertilizers, decaying organic matter, silage juices, and soils high in nitrogen-fixing bacteria may be sources of contamination through surface-water runoff to adjacent poorly cased, shallow, or low-lying wells or reservoirs.

The upper limit for nitrate in human drinking water is 45 mg nitrate/L (USEPA 1975). This level has the intent of preventing the methemoglobinemia of "blue baby" syndrome in human infants who receive formulas made from high-nitrate waters. Although it has been suggested that neonatal swine are also quite susceptible to elevated nitrates, evidence to support this theory is unavailable. Emerick et al. (1965) concluded, however, that 1-week-old pigs are no more susceptible to nitrite-induced methemoglobinemia than older growing swine. A review of water quality for livestock (NRC 1974) proposed 440 mg nitrate/L as the maximum nitrate that could safely be allowed in livestock water.

Reports of experimental production of a chronic or low-level nitrate-poisoning syndrome in livestock have been extensively reviewed (Turner and Kienholz 1972; Emerick 1974; Ridder and Oehme 1974). The bulk of the evidence indicates that sublethal or chronic effects are extremely rare and difficult to verify. London et al. (1967) fed growing pigs up to 18.3 mg nitrite-nitrogen/kg body weight for 124 days without serious effects developing. No effect on the performance of growing-finishing swine or on reproductive performance of gilts was observed when the drinking water contained 1320 ppm nitrate (Seerley et al. 1965).

MISCELLANEOUS TOXICANTS

Sodium Ion Toxicosis

Sodium ion toxicosis, also called water deprivation or salt poisoning, is a common problem in swine. The occurrence of sodium ion toxicosis is inversely related to water intake and is almost always related to water deprivation caused by inadequate water supply or to changes in husbandry. The likelihood of toxicosis will also increase with increased dietary salt, but the condition may occur when rations contain normal levels of added salt, for example, 0.25–1%. It has also been associated with the feeding of whey and other milk by-products. Sodium ion toxicosis may occur after water deprivation of only a few hours, but in most cases the time exceeds 24 hours.

The initial clinical signs are thirst and constipation, followed by CNS involvement. Intermittent convulsions start within 1 to several days after water deprivation and may be exacerbated by rehydration. The frequency of characteristic tonoclonic convulsions with opisthotonos, often starting from a sitting position, increases. Affected animals may also wander aimlessly and appear to be blind and deaf. Moribund pigs become comatose, often lying on their sides with continuous paddling. Most affected animals die within a few days. Some pigs that appear to be unaffected may succumb later to a subacute polioencephalomalacia. Salt poisoning, from eating excess salt or consuming brine, usually causes vomiting and diarrhea.

Diagnosis is best accomplished by establishing that water deprivation occurred, which may be difficult in some cases. If water deprivation is not evident, other means must be used to aid the diagnosis. Necropsy findings may reveal a gastritis, gastric ulcers, constipation, or enteritis. Chemical analysis of serum and cerebrospinal fluids may confirm a hypernatremia with levels of Na above 160 mEq/L (Osweiler and Hurd 1974). However, after rehydration, normal values of 140–145 mEq/L may exist. Brain sodium levels above 1800 ppm (wet weight) are consistent with a diagnosis of sodium ion toxicosis. Histologic examination of brain tissue, especially cerebrum, will usually reveal the presence of a pathognomonic eosinophilic meningoencephalitis characterized by cuffing of meningeal and cerebral vessels with eosinophils. However, when pigs live several days, the eosinophils may disappear or be replaced by mononuclear cells. Brains of pigs affected subacutely may have a laminar subcortical polioencephalomalacia. Analysis of feed for sodium is usually of limited value. Differential diagnosis should include viral encephalitic diseases such as pseudorabies and hog cholera, chlorinated hydrocarbon insecticide poisoning, and edema disease. In known cases of water deprivation, rehydration should be gradual, but the prognosis is poor.

Coal Tar Pitch

Coal tars are a mixture of condensable, volatile products formed during the destructive distillation of bituminous coal. The phenolic portions of these products have the greatest acute toxicity. Sources of these substances for swine are clay pigeons, lignite tar flooring slabs, tar paper, and tar used in waterproofing and sealing. Because of the rapid clinical course, sudden death is often the first physical sign observed. Weakness, depression, and increased respiratory rate can be observed in animals that may live for several hours or even days. Icterus and a secondary anemia may develop. Necropsy of pigs poisoned by coal tar pitch reveals a greatly enlarged friable liver. The hepatic lobules are very distinct grossly; some are darkened in color, and others are yellowish orange. Microscopically, this lesion is observed as severe centrilobular necrosis with subsequent intralobular hemorrhage. Ascites and large turgid kidneys may also be observed.

There is no specific treatment for this condition. Removal of animals from the source of the coal tar is important to prevent recurrence of poisoning.

Ethylene Glycol

Most permanent antifreeze/coolant mixtures for liquid-cooled engines contain approximately 95% ethylene glycol. A hazard of poisoning exists when animals have accidental access to antifreeze solutions during periods of engine maintenance or when these solutions are used in plumbing systems to prevent freezing. Swine may be poisoned by ingesting 4–5 mL ethylene glycol/kg body weight. Ethylene glycol toxicosis is exhibited in two clinical phases. Initially the glycol may enter the cerebrospinal fluid, producing a narcotic or euphoric state of intoxication. Subsequent clinical signs of acidosis and renal failure are associated with the highly toxic metabolites of the glycol and formation of calcium oxalate crystals in the kidney tubules. Renal tubular blockage with development of uremia is observed 1–3 days after ingestion. Clinical signs generally include emesis, anorexia, dehydration, weakness, ataxia, convulsions, coma, and death. The entire course of illness may be as short as 12 hours following consumption of large quantities of ethylene glycol. Oxalate nephrosis can be demonstrated histopathologically and is characterized by finding pale yellow birefringent oxalate crystals in the tubules. Polarizing filters greatly aid in the detection of oxalate crystals in kidney sections or in impression smears of freshly incised kidney.

Once clinical signs of renal failure are evident, treatment is usually of no avail. If treated within the first 6–12 hours after ingestion, reasonable response has been achieved in ethylene glycol–poisoned dogs by using 5.5 mL/kg body weight of 20% ethyl alcohol intravenously and 98 mL/kg body weight of 5% sodium bicarbonate intravenously.

Gossypol

Cottonseed meal (CSM), a by-product of the cotton fiber and cottonseed oil industries, is an important protein supplement for livestock rations in cotton-producing regions. Its use as a protein supplement for swine, however, is limited by gossypol content, which varies with the strain of the cotton plant, its geographic location, climatic conditions, and the oil extraction procedure used. Gossypol, a polyphenolic binaphthalene, is a yellow pigment in glands of decorticated cottonseed. The toxic "free" gossypol becomes partially inactivated (bound) during the extraction and milling processes, as well as spontaneously in the prepared meal. Toxicity of gossypol depends on the species and age of the animal and on various components of the diet, particularly the protein, lysine, and iron concentrations (Eisele 1986).

Toxicosis only follows prolonged feeding (weeks to months) of CSM with a high content of free gossypol and may be manifested simply as ill-thrift or as an acute respiratory problem followed by death. The main pathologic changes are cardiomyopathy, hepatic congestion and necrosis, skeletal muscle injury, and severe edematous changes throughout the animal. A decrease in hemoglobin total serum, protein concentration, and packed-cell volume is seen in pigs fed a diet containing ≥200 mg of free gossypol/kg (Haschek et al. 1989).

Recommendations for growing and fattening swine include feeding no more than 9% CSM in the diet, with less than 100 mg (0.01%) of free gossypol/kg, in a 15–16% protein diet. Tolerance to gossypol can be induced by adding $FeSO_4$ (≥400 mg/kg) at a 1:1 weight ratio with free gossypol. Increasing the amount of crude protein or supplementing with lysine can also induce tolerance (Pond and Maner 1984).

VENTILATION FAILURE AND TOXIC GASES

Confinement of swine in closed structures increases the risk of potential gas toxicosis and other dynamics dependent upon mechanical ventilation. Fortunately even at relatively low ventilation rates used during cold weather, concentrations of ammonia and hydrogen sulfide, the two most potentially dangerous gases associated with manure decomposition, usually remain below toxic levels. Unfortunately, however, accidents, poor design, and improper operation may result in insufficient ventilation and the concentration of poisonous gases to toxic levels.

The most important gases released by the decomposition of urine and feces either in anaerobic underfloor waste pits or in deep litter or manure packs are ammonia and hydrogen sulfide. Carbon dioxide and methane are also produced but seldom reach significant concentrations. A number of vapors responsible for the odors of manure decomposition are also produced. These include organic acids, amines, amides, alcohols, carbonyls, skatoles, sulfides, and mercaptans. Concentrations of toxic gases are usually expressed as parts of the gas per million parts of air (ppm) by volume.

Ventilation Failure

Even more common than the accumulation of toxic gases are swine deaths associated with failure of a mechanical ventilation system. The failure of ventilation may occur in whole confinement buildings and result in high death losses at any time of the year. Similar dynamics and death losses occur in tightly sealed insulated trucks used to transport young pigs. When ventilation stops because of storms, power outages, or mechanical failure, the dynamics of air, heat, and moisture in the confined space may become critical. The retention of heat and moisture leads to high relative humidity and poor evaporative cooling and consequently hyperthermia as the most critical factor in these confined swine. Death losses may approach 95% under these circumstances. Although there is no method to specifically confirm hyperthermia as a cause of death, a history of ventilation failure, rapid carcass decomposition, a pale "cooked" appearance to the muscles, and blood-tinged foam in the trachea are usually seen.

Ammonia

Ammonia (NH_3) is the toxic air pollutant most frequently found in high concentrations in animal facilities, and production is especially common where excrement can decompose on a solid floor. This gas has a characteristic pungent odor that humans can detect at approximately 10 ppm or even lower. The NH_3 concentration in enclosed animal facilities usually remains below 30 ppm even with low ventilation rates; however, it may frequently reach 50 ppm or higher during long periods of normal facility operation.

Ammonia is highly soluble in water, and as such will react with the moist mucous membranes of the eye and respiratory passages. Consequently, excessive tearing, shallow breathing, and clear or purulent nasal discharge are common symptoms of aerial NH_3 toxicosis.

At concentrations usually found in practical animal environments (<100 ppm), the primary impact of this gas is as a chronic stressor that can affect the course of infectious disease as well as directly influence the growth of healthy young pigs. The rate of gain in young pigs was reduced by 12% during exposure to aerial NH_3 at 50 ppm and by 30% at 100 or 150 ppm (Drummond et al. 1980). Aerial NH_3 at 50 or 75 ppm reduced the ability of healthy young pigs to clear bacteria from their lungs (Drummond et al. 1978). At 50 or 100 ppm, aerial NH_3 exacerbated nasal turbinate lesions in young pigs infected with *Bordetella bronchiseptica* but did not add to the infection-induced reduction in the pigs' growth rate (Drummond et al. 1981a). In another study, aerial NH_3 at 100 ppm reduced the rate of gain by 32% and ascarid infection by 28%; however, effects of the NH_3 and infection, when imposed on the pigs at the same time, were additive, and the rate of gain was reduced by 61% (Drummond et al. 1981b). More extensive reviews of aerial NH_3 and its effect on animal production are provided by Curtis (1983) and the National Research Council (1979a).

Hydrogen Sulfide

Hydrogen sulfide (H_2S) is a potentially lethal gas produced by anaerobic bacterial decomposition of protein and other sulfur-containing organic matter. The source of H_2S which presents the greatest hazard to swine is liquid manure holding pits. Most of the H_2S, which may be continuously produced, is retained within the liquid of the pit. However, agitation of waste slurry to resuspend solids prior to being pumped out causes the rapid release of much of the H_2S that may have been retained within it. Hydrogen sulfide is heavier than air and consequently is found in, and will move to, pits, tanks, and other low areas of a facility. The concentration of H_2S usually found in closed animal facilities (less than 10 ppm) is not toxic, but the release of gas upon agitation may produce concentrations of H_2S up to 1000 ppm or higher within the facility.

Acute H_2S poisoning is directly responsible for more deaths in closed animal facilities than any other gas, with the possible exception of carbon monoxide. Additionally, several human deaths are recorded each year from H_2S accidents associated with animal facilities.

Humans can detect the typical "rotten egg" odor of H_2S at very low concentrations (0.025 ppm) in air. Exposures to these low concentrations have little or no importance to human health, and thus the olfactory response is a useful warning signal of its presence. However, at higher concentrations (greater than 200 ppm), H_2S presents the distinct hazard of a paralyzing effect on the olfactory apparatus, thus effectively neutralizing the warning signal (NRC 1979b).

Hydrogen sulfide is an irritant gas. Its direct action on tissues induces local inflammation of the moist membranes of the eye and respiratory tract. When inhaled, the action of H_2S is more or less uniform throughout the respiratory tract, although the deeper pulmonary structures suffer the greatest damage. Inflammation of the deep lung structures may appear as pulmonary edema. If inhaled at sufficiently high concentrations, H_2S can also be readily absorbed through the lung and can produce fatal systemic intoxication (O'Donoghue 1961).

At concentrations in air exceeding 500 ppm, H_2S must be considered a serious imminent threat to life; between 500 and 1000 ppm, it produces permanent effects on the nervous system. If spontaneous recovery does not occur and artificial respiration is not immediately provided, death results from asphyxia.

Management is the most important part of preventing animal deaths from H_2S. When manure stored in a pit beneath a building is agitated, animals should be moved out of the building if at all possible. When movement of the animals is not possible, other steps should be taken to protect the animals during agitation. In mechanically ventilated buildings, the fans should run at full capacity, even during the winter; in naturally ventilated buildings, manure pits should not be agitated unless there is a brisk breeze blowing. Immediate rescue of affected swine should not be attempted for the rescuer may quickly become a victim of H_2S toxicosis.

Carbon Dioxide

Carbon dioxide (CO_2) is an odorless gas present in the atmosphere at 300 ppm. It is given off by swine as an end product of energy metabolism and by improperly vented, though properly adjusted, fuel-burning heaters. It is also the gas evolved in the greatest quantity by decomposing manure. Despite all this, CO_2 concentration in closed animal facilities rarely approaches levels that endanger animal health (Curtis 1983).

Methane

Methane (CH_2), a product of microbial degradation of carbonaceous materials, is not a poisonous gas. It is biologically rather inert and produces effects on animals only by displacing oxygen in a given atmosphere and thereby producing asphyxiation. Under ordinary pressures, a concentration of 87–90% CH_2 in a given atmosphere is required before irregularities of respiration and eventually respiratory arrest due to anoxia are produced. The chief danger inherent in this material is its explosive hazard as concentrations of 5–15% by volume in air are reached (Osweiler et al. 1985).

Carbon Monoxide

Carbon monoxide (CO), which is produced from the inefficient combustion of carbonaceous fuel and is present in the exhaust fumes of gasoline-burning internal-combustion engines, is also potentially lethal to swine. Poisoning occurs when improperly adjusted and improperly vented space heaters or furnaces are operated in tight, poorly ventilated buildings such as farrowing houses.

Ambient background levels of CO are 0.02 ppm in fresh air, 13 ppm in city streets, and 40 ppm in areas with high vehicular traffic.

Carbon monoxide acts by competing with oxygen for binding sites on a variety of proteins, including hemoglobin, with which most of the compound is associated in the body. The affinity of hemoglobin for CO is some 250 times that for oxygen. When CO becomes bonded to the heme group, forming carboxyhemoglobin, the molecule's oxygen-carrying capacity is reduced. This results in tissue hypoxia.

High concentrations of CO (>250 ppm) in swine farrowing houses can produce an increased number of stillborn piglets. Clinical history generally associated with these stillbirths reveals (1) nonexistent ventilation, (2) inadequate ventilation due to blocked apertures of natural systems or reduction to minimal winter rates for mechanical systems, (3) use of unvented or improperly vented LP gas-burning space heaters, (4) a high percentage of near-term sows delivering dead piglets within a few hours of being put in an artificially heated farrowing facility, (5) sows that appear clinically normal but that produce whole litters born dead, and (6) negative laboratory results for the detection of infectious causes of abortion (Carson 1990).

Exposure to high levels of CO can be confirmed by actually measuring the CO level in the air or by measuring the percentage of carboxyhemoglobin in the blood of the affected animal. In addition to these two parameters, carboxyhemoglobin concentration of greater than 2% in fetal thoracic fluid may be used as an aid in diagnosing CO-induced stillbirth in swine (Dominick and Carson 1983).

Anhydrous Ammonia

On occasion, swine may be exposed to anhydrous ammonia (gas-NH_3) used as an agricultural fertilizer nitrogen source. This gas presents a unique risk of exposure to both animals and people because of its presence on farms and the fact that it is stored, transported, and applied under high pressure. Poisoning with gas-NH_3 is associated with gas release from broken hoses, failure of valves, and errors in operating transport or application equipment. Once released, gas-NH_3 rapidly combines with water and forms caustic ammonium hydroxide. The cornea, mouth, and respiratory tract are high in moisture and especially susceptible to the resulting strong alkali burns. Acute death from laryngospasm and accumulation of fluid in the lungs can occur within a matter of minutes. Blindness from corneal opacity and sloughing epithelium in the respiratory tract may be seen in swine surviving initial exposure. Residual respiratory damage and secondary bacterial invasion may not allow affected animals to regain full productive status.

REFERENCES

Adams HR (ed). 1996. Veterinary Pharmacology and Therapeutics, 7th ed. Ames: Iowa State Univ Press.

Anderson DM, Strothers SC. 1978. Effects of saline water high in sulfates, chlorides, and nitrates on the performance of young weanling pigs. J Anim Sci 47:900–907.

Canadian Task Force on Water Quality. 1987. Task Force on Water Quality Guidelines. Prepared for the Canadian Council of Resource and Environment Ministers.

Carson TL. 1990. Carbon monoxide–induced stillbirth, pp. 186–189. In Laboratory Diagnosis of Livestock Abortion (3d edition). CA Kirkbride, ed. Ames: Iowa State Univ Press.

Casteel SW, Osweiler GD, Cook WO, Daniels G, Kadlee R. 1985. Selenium toxicosis in swine. J Am Vet Med Assoc 186:1084–1085.

Curtis SE. 1983. Environmental Management in Animal Agriculture. Ames: Iowa State Univ Press.

Dominick MA, Carson TL. 1983. Effects of carbon monoxide exposure on pregnant sows and their fetuses. Am J Vet Res 44:35–40.

Dorman DC, Simon J, Harlin KA, Buck WB. 1990. Diagnosis of bromethalin toxicosis in the dog. J Vet Diagn Invest 2:123–128.

Drummond JG, Curtis SE, Simon J. 1978. Effects of atmospheric ammonia on pulmonary bacterial clearance in the young pig. Am J Vet Res 39:211–212.

Drummond JG, Curtis SE, Simon J, Norton HW. 1980. Effects of aerial ammonia on growth and health of young pigs. J Anim Sci 50:1085–1091.

Drummond JG, Curtis SE, Meyer RC, Simon J, Norton HW. 1981a. Effects of atmospheric ammonia on young pigs experimentally infected with Bordetella bronchiseptica. Am J Vet Res 42:963–968.

——. 1981b. Effects of atmospheric ammonia on young pigs experimentally infected with Ascaris suum. Am J Vet Res 42:969–974.

Eisele GR. 1986. A perspective on gossypol ingestion in swine. Vet Hum Toxicol 28:118–122.

Emerick R. 1974. Consequences of high nitrate levels in feed and water supplies. Fed Proc 33:1183.

Emerick R, Embry LB, Seerly RW. 1965. Rate of formation and reduction of nitrite induced methemoglobin in vitro and in vivo as influenced by diet of sheep and age of swine. J Anim Sci 24:221–230.

Ensley SM. 1998. Relationships of swine water quality to cost and efficiency of swine production. Master of Science Thesis, Iowa State University, Ames, Iowa.

Fleck Veenhuizen M. 1993. Association between water sulfate and diarrhea in swine on Ohio farms. J Am Vet Med Assoc 202(8):1255–1260.

Fleck Veenhuizen M, Shurson GC, Kohler EM. 1992. Effect of concentration and source of sulfate on nursery pig performance and health. J Am Vet Med Assoc 201(8):1203–1208.

Harrison LH, Colvin BM, Stuart BR, Sangster LT, Gorgacz EJ, Gosser, HS. 1983. Paralysis in swine due to focal symmetrical poliomalacia: Possible selenium toxicosis. Vet Pathol 20:265–273.

Haschek WM, Beasley VR, Buck WB, Finnell JH. 1989. Cottonseed meal (gossypol) toxicosis in a swine herd. J Am Vet Med Assoc 195:613–615.

Kingsbury JM. 1964. Poisonous Plants of the United States and Canada. Englewood Cliffs, NJ: Prentice-Hall.

Lassen ED, Buck WB. 1979. Experimental lead toxicosis in swine. Am J Vet Res 40:1359–1364.

Link RP. 1975. Toxic plants, rodenticides, herbicides, and yellow fat disease. In Diseases of Swine (4th edition). HW Dunne, AD Leman, eds. Ames: Iowa State Univ Press, p. 861.

Lloyd WE. 1978. Feed additives toxicology. Unpublished data. Iowa State Univ.

London WT, Hendersen W, Cross RF. 1967. An attempt to produce chronic nitrite toxicosis in swine. J Am Vet Med Assoc 150:398–402.

National Research Council (NRC). 1974. Nutrients and Toxic Substances in Water for Livestock and Poultry. National Academy Press, Washington, DC.

——. 1979a. Committee on Medical and Biologic Effects of Environmental Pollutants, Subcommittee on Ammonia. Ammonia. Univ Park Press, Baltimore.

——. 1979b. Committee on Medical and Biologic Effects of Environmental Pollutants, Subcommittee on Hydrogen Sulfide. Hydrogen Sulfide. Univ Park Press, Baltimore.

O'Donoghue JG. 1961. Hydrogen sulfide poisoning in swine. Can J Comp Med Vet Sci 25:217–219.

Osweiler GD. 1978. Hemostatic function in swine as influenced by warfarin and an oral-antibacterial combination. Am J Vet Res 39:633–638.

Osweiler GD, Buck WB, Bicknell EJ. 1969. Experimental production of perirenal edema in swine with Amaranthus retroflexus. Am J Vet Res 30:557–577.

Osweiler GD, Carson TL, Buck WB, Van Gelder GA. 1985. Clinical and Diagnostic Veterinary Toxicology (3rd edition). Dubuque, Iowa: Kendall/Hunt.

Osweiler GD, Hurd JW. 1974. Determination of sodium content in serum and cerebrospinal fluid as an adjunct to diagnosis of water deprivation in swine. J Am Vet Med Assoc 64:165–167.

Paterson DW, Wahlstrom RC, Libal GW, Olson OE. 1979. Effects of sulfate in water on swine reproduction and young pig performance. J Anim Sci 49:664–667.

Pond WG, Maner JH. 1984. Swine Production and Nutrition. Westport, CT: AVI Publishing Co.

Power SB, Donnelly WJC, McLaughlin JG, Walsh MC, Dromey MF. 1989. Accidental carbadox overdosage in an Irish weaner-producing herd. Vet Rec 124:367–370.

Ridder WE, Oehme FW. 1974. Nitrates as an environmental, animal, and human hazard. Clin Toxicol 7:145.

Schipper IA. 1961. Toxicology of wood preservatives to swine. Am J Vet Res 22:401–405.

Seerley RW, Emerick RJ, Embry LB, Olson OE. 1965. Effect of nitrate and nitrite administration continuously in the drinking water for sheep and swine. J Anim Sci 24:1014–1019.

Stuart BP, Cole RJ, Gosser HS. 1981. Cocklebur intoxication in swine: Review and redefinition of the toxic principle. Vet Pathol 18:368–383.

Turner CA, Kienholz EW. 1972. Nitrate toxicity. Feedstuffs 44:28–30.

U.S. Environmental Protection Agency (USEPA). 1973. Proposed criteria for water quality: Quality of water for livestock. Environ Rep 4(16):663.

——. 1975. Primary drinking water proposed interim standards. F.R. 40(51)11990.

Van der Molen EJ. 1988. Pathological effects of carbadox in pigs with special emphasis on the adrenal. J Comp Pathol 98:55–67.

Van Vleet JF, Amstuts HE, Weirich, WE, Rebar AH, Ferrans VJ. 1983. Clinical, clinicopathologic, and pathologic alterations of monensin toxicosis in swine. Am J Vet Res 44:1469–1475.

Van Vleet JF, Meyer KB, Olander HJ. 1974. Acute selenium toxicosis induced in baby pigs by parenteral administration of selenium–vitamin E preparations. J Am Vet Med Assoc 165:543–547.

Van Vleet JF, Runnels LJ, Cook JR, Scheidt AB. 1987. Monensin toxicosis in swine: Potentiation by tiamulin administration and ameliorative effect of treatment with selenium and/or vitamin E. Am J Vet Res 48:1520–1524.

V Veterinary Practice

61 Genetic Influences on Susceptibility to Acquired Diseases

Kin-Chow Chang and Michael J. Stear

The use of genetic information in pig breeding to improve productivity is a successful and an expanding area of research and development, as exemplified by the routine genetic screening, in breeding stock, for the mutant ryanodine receptor allele in malignant hyperthermia (Fujii et al. 1991). The main areas of genetic applications have been on muscle production and reproductive performance (Rothschild et al. 1996; Bidanel and Rothschild 2002). In recent years, there has been increasing focus on the development of genetic markers to be used for enhancement of resistance to porcine diseases in breeding stock. This chapter reviews the current knowledge of porcine genetics and genomics that is relevant to infectious diseases. A consequence of its commercial importance has been the limited amount of publicly available information on specific diseases. Nonetheless, it is anticipated that DNA markers for disease resistance will be in regular use in pig breeding in the not too distant future.

Infectious diseases are realities of pig farming. The demand for improved standards of animal welfare and food safety, as well as farming economics, require that the incidence of disease be minimized. However, modern trends may be increasing the impact of specific diseases. The shift toward more intensive systems of production will reduce soil-transmitted infections such as gastrointestinal nematodes but may exacerbate other conditions like respiratory diseases. With the ban of growth-promoting antibiotics in several countries, there has been some deterioration in animal health, in particular, a rise in the number of gastrointestinal infections in early postweaning piglets, with a concomitant increase in the use of therapeutic antibiotics, which could have the inadvertent and paradoxical effect of promoting antibiotic resistance (Casewell et al. 2003).

Methods to control disease include good management to reduce exposure to pathogens and parasites as well as increasing the ability of animals to resist infection by vaccination and improved nutrition. Genetics also has a role to play in disease control. The identification of resistant or susceptible animals for selective breeding could reduce or prevent outbreaks of disease. A quantitative genetic analysis can indicate how much of the variation among animals in disease incidence is genetic in origin, whereas a study of molecular genetic variation can help identify the mechanisms underlying resistance and susceptibility to disease. Arguably without knowledge of genetic variation, our understanding of the disease process is meager and unsatisfactory. At the very least, genetic studies can target future research more effectively.

DEFINING DISEASE RESISTANCE

In any study of disease, the definition of resistance requires careful consideration. A variety of traits can be used alone or in conjunction, and the most appropriate traits to define disease resistance may vary with the type or nature of disease. Pathogens with different predilection sites of infection (e.g., intestine or lung) will present different clinical signs. However, their systemic effects could be similar, such as pyrexia, inappetance and emaciation (Taylor 1999). With the same pathogen, host responses could vary between individuals, in clinical severity (asymptomatic to peracute), in duration of infection (transient to chronic), and in transmission of infection (no to high infectivity). Hosts could vary in exposure to the disease agent because of differences in behavior. Variation among hosts could also be due to variation in response to infection. The distinction between disease resistance (the ability to prevent infection establishing) and disease resilience (the ability to prevent the infection producing clinical signs or reducing performance) has long been recognized (Albers et al. 1987). However, these terms are commonly used interchangeably. An animal could show disease resistance, in comparison with its exposed cohorts, if it shows no or mild clinical signs, recovers rapidly, or blocks transmission to other pigs. A subclinical infection, compared with a full-blown acute state, with little effect on production could be desirable. Likewise, a clinically affected animal that is able to prevent or reduce horizontal transmission could be regarded as disease resistant and would confer resistance at the herd level. Variation in clinical symptoms could be due to failure of the pathogen or parasite to establish, to rapid clearance by the host innate response, or to effective acquired immune response. Clinical, biochemical, or immunological parameters that can distinguish resistant animals from the rest of the population are phenotypic indicators of disease resistance.

The relationship between disease resistance and production traits is unpredictable and will vary among different environments, diseases, herds, and intensities of infection (Stear et al. 2001). A rational approach to improving disease resistance would be to genetically target improvement of host responses to selected diseases of major economic importance. Any improvement in recovery time and in reduction in mortality, clinical signs, and pathogen shedding in the face of a serious challenge is welcome.

GENETIC CONTRIBUTION TO DISEASE RESISTANCE/SUSCEPTIBILITY

Essentially every disease that has been seriously investigated has shown genetic variation among hosts in disease resistance (Nicholas 1996). Genetic variation could be shown in immune response traits as well as in host responses to direct pathogen exposure. The challenge is to use such information most effectively.

Geneticists divide diseases into different categories depending upon the nature of the genetic variation. Diseases that are entirely caused by the presence or absence of a single abnormal gene are classified as Mendelian diseases. These are subdivided into four categories depending upon the nature of inheritance: autosomal dominant, autosomal recessive, sex-linked dominant, and sex-linked recessive. There are a large number of different Mendelian diseases in pigs, although many are noninfectious (www.morgan.angis.su.oz.au). They are due to mutations in specific genes, either in the coding or regulatory regions. They can be recognized by examining the pedigree of affected animals.

Autosomal dominant diseases are caused by a single copy of a defective gene on one of the autosomes (nonsex chromosomes). They have three characteristic features: They affect approximately equal numbers of males and females. Breeding an affected sire with an affected dam can produce unaffected offspring. If the pedigree of an affected individual is traced back, the disease is present in every generation until the original mutation. Dominant diseases are rare in pigs because breeders do not usually breed from obviously diseased animals. This is an example of deliberate selection. Natural selection will also reduce the frequency of autosomal dominant disorders.

Autosomal recessive diseases occur when both copies of an autosomal gene are defective. They have three characteristic features. They occur in approximately equal numbers of males and females. Crossing an affected sire with an affected dam gives only affected offspring. The disease can also skip generations when tracing the inheritance back to an affected individual, since the offspring is unaffected, although being a carrier, when at least one parent is not a carrier of the defective gene. Autosomal recessive diseases are much more common than autosomal dominant diseases because carriers with only one copy of the disease appear normal.

Sex-linked dominant diseases are caused by a mutation on the X chromosome. The small Y chromosome carries relatively few genes, which include those involved in sex determination. Sex-linked dominant diseases are rare and none are known in pigs. Sex-linked recessive diseases are relatively common and include some hemophilias. They occur at a greater frequency in males than females. All offspring of two affected parents are affected and as with autosomal recessives the disease may skip generations.

If a disease is suspected of being inherited in a Mendelian fashion, the most useful strategy is often to draw up a pedigree and check inheritance against the simple rules outlined above. It can be useful to check whether a similar disease has been shown to be inherited in the same or other species. The simplest way to avoid dominantly inherited diseases is to avoid breeding with affected individuals. The strategy to avoid recessive diseases is to ensure that at least one parent is not a carrier. For many diseases, carriers or noncarriers can be identified among potential parents. Where DNA tests do not exist, crossing a sire with a number of known carriers (females that have given birth to diseased individuals) can indicate whether the sire is a carrier.

Many important diseases are complex: influenced by more than one gene and the environment. A multifactorial model of liability with a threshold describes these diseases. Here statistical methods that utilize the similarity among relatives can indicate what proportion of the variation among individuals in disease prevalence is genetic in origin. This is known as the *heritability* (Nicholas 1996). The heritability is the ratio of the variation due to the average effects of genes divided by the total variation. If the heritability is close to 0 most of the variation is due to nongenetic forces. Conversely, if the heritability is close to 1, most of the variation is genetic in origin.

GENETIC VARIATION IN DISEASE RESISTANCE

Controlling complex diseases by genetic methods is possible and uses the same methods developed by breeders to enhance production traits. A crucial decision is deciding whether to breed for resistance to one disease or for resistance to a range of diseases. For dairy cattle the most economically important disease is mastitis; for sheep the dominant problem is nematode infection. Selective breeding has therefore concentrated on controlling these diseases. For pigs, there is no single overwhelmingly important disease worldwide and research has concentrated on identifying pigs with superior immune responses (Wilkie and Mallard 1999). It may not be possible to breed an animal that is completely immune to all known infectious diseases, but results certainly indicate that animals with enhanced resistance to a variety of important diseases can be identified.

Selection strategies are unlikely to be solely based on clinical symptoms. Selection based on host responses to specific disease challenge is the most direct route to identify resistant animals but is inconvenient and risky in intensive pig production. A sensible approach would be to target responses to diseases of major economic importance. Ideally, phenotypic markers that predict resistance should be detectable in the live animal to facilitate subsequent breeding.

Variation in Immune Responsiveness

Several studies have demonstrated differences in immune traits between individual pigs reared under the same conditions (Edfors-Lilja et al. 1994; Hessing et al. 1995; van Diemen et al. 2002). Immune parameters that were found to vary between individuals included total white blood cell count, neutrophil number and phagocytic capacity, CD2 and CD4 lymphocyte numbers, lymphocyte proliferation rate, antibody level and interleukin-2 (IL-2) production (Edfors-Lilja et al. 1994; Mallard et al. 1998). Differences in immune parameters were also detected between breeds. Several immune traits, like leucocyte number and concanavalin-A induced cell proliferation, were quantitatively different between Large White and Duroc pigs (Nguyen et al. 1998), and C3 complement activity showed breed differences between Duroc and Berlin Miniature pigs (Mekchay et al. 2003). High immune activity is not necessarily a predictor of better protection from disease (Mallard et al. 1998; Visscher et al. 2002).

Variation in Response to Specific Diseases

There are breed differences in neutralization antibody response to vaccination against Aujeszky's disease (Rothschild et al. 1984); Yorkshire and Chester White pigs were found with higher postvaccinated antibody titers than Duroc and Landrace pigs. The humoral response is only part of the immune response, and, as suggested earlier, high postvaccinated titres on their own do not inevitably mean greater resistance to Aujeszky's infection. However, this finding does serve to demonstrate a genetic basis for variation in humoral immune response to vaccination against Aujeszky's disease.

Sarcocystis miescheriana is a coccidial parasite that accumulates as cysts in the skeletal muscle of pigs acting as intermediate hosts. Experimental infection with *S. miescheriana* showed breed differences in host response (Reiner et al. 2002a). Pietrain pigs displayed greater clinical severity and parasite load in skeletal muscles than Meishan pigs.

Finally, a challenge experiment with *Salmonella choleraesuis* was conducted on a reference family bred from full-sister F1 gilts and four selected boars from two commercial lines (van Diemen et al. 2002). Infected pigs showed significant variation in bacterial recovery from liver and spleen, pyrexia response, weight gain, and several immune parameters. The most resistant pigs, as evidenced by low bacterial recovery from liver and spleen and better growth performance, had higher neutrophil numbers and better neutrophil functions (oxidative burst and intracellular killing of *S. choleraesuis*) but lower proliferation rate of lymphocytes and lower antibody response. In this study, it appears that the innate response is more critical than the acquired immune response in deciding on the outcome of *S. choleraesuis* infection.

The above viral, protozoal, and bacterial examples of infection illustrate the range of host response to different types of infection and the genetic contribution to variation in disease response for each type of infection. There is therefore considerable opportunity for genetic improvement of immune capacity since immune traits show wide genetic variation between pigs and moderate heritability (Visscher et al. 2002). However, as exemplified by the *Salmonella* infection experiment (van Diemen et al. 2002), the difficulty lies in the determination of the effective set of innate and/or acquired immune traits to be used as selection markers that are critical in alleviating the severity of a particular disease.

SELECTIVE BREEDING FOR DISEASE RESISTANCE

Unlike muscle and fat traits, which are relatively straightforward to select in breeding programmes (Rothschild 2000; Guldbrandtsen et al. 2002), breeding for disease resistance is more challenging but, in recent years, there has been a noticeable rise in research into porcine disease resistance, conducted in both academia and industry.

Phenotypic Markers

There has been success in selecting pigs for enhanced immunity. Pigs were selected over eight generations for high and low responses in general IgG antibody production and in certain cell-mediated functions (Mallard et al. 1998). Following *Mycoplasma hyorhinis* infection, high responder pigs had reduced pulmonary damage but more severe arthritis, the latter probably due to accumulation of immune complexes. Although protection was incomplete, high responder pigs appeared better equipped than the low responders to deal with *M. hyorhinis*. Additionally, the high response pigs grew more rapidly. As cited earlier, in *S. choleraesuis* infection, the innate immune parameters of neutrophil number and performance seemed able to predict relative resistance (van Diemen et al. 2002).

Genetic Markers

Postweaning Diarrhea: Resistance to Fimbriated F18 *Escherichia coli*. With few exceptions, susceptibility to infectious disease seldom follows a simple pattern of Mendelian inheritance. One such exceptional example of single-gene control of resistance is found in the condition of postweaning diarrhea associated with F18 *E. coli*.

The permissive expression of *E. coli* F18 receptor by the host on its gut lining leads to susceptibility to fimbriated F18 colonization and is controlled by a dominant allele (Meijerink et al. 1997). The gene responsible for F18 bacterial susceptibility has been recently identified as $\alpha(1,2)$-fucosyltransferase (*FUT1*), which exhibits $\alpha(1,2)$fucosylation of glycolipid and glycoprotein acceptors, and is involved in the formation of blood group antigen structures on cell membranes, structures that determine the adherence of F18 bacteria. The causal mutation within *FUT1* has been narrowed to a point mutation at nucleotide position 307 where the residue guanine ($M307^G$), corresponding to a codon for alanine, is replaced by the residue adenine ($M307^A$), coding for threonine (Meijerink et al. 2000). There is a high correlation between the single-nucleotide polymorphism and F18 *E. coli* susceptibility, such that the dominant F18 susceptibility genotypes are homozygous $M307^{GG}$ and heterozygous $M307^{GA}$, where at least one allele has the alanine codon, whereas the recessive F18 resistant genotype is homozygous $M307^{AA}$, where both alleles house the threonine codon (Frydendahl et al. 2003). It should be mentioned that pigs with the resistant $M307^{AA}$ genotype are more, but not completely, resistant to F18 *E. coli* infection as other, as yet undetermined, factors are likely to be involved in the pathogenesis of the disease. Meanwhile, other fimbriated enterotoxigenic *E. coli* will continue to pose a threat for postweaning diarrhea syndrome.

Neonatal Diarrhea: Resistance to Fimbriated F4 *E. coli*. The *E. coli* fimbrial types that are responsible for neonatal diarrhea are F4 (K88), F5 (K99), F6 and F41, of which most is known about type F4. There are three F4 antigenic variants: F4ab, F4ac and F4ad (Python et al. 2002). Like fimbriated F18 in postweaning diarrhea, adherence of F4 *E. coli* to the small intestinal epithelium, leading to host susceptibility, is a dominant trait (S), inherited in a Mendelian manner. Only pigs with the homozygous recessive *ss* genotype are resistant to F4 bacteria challenge (Sellwood 1979). By linkage analysis, a candidate locus, designated *F4bcR*, has been identified that relates to F4ab and F4ac bacteria colonization (Python et al. 2002). The locus is located on chromo-

some 13, and the putative receptor gene involved may be related to a type of transferrin. To date, the gene responsible for the pathogenicity of F4 *E. coli* has not been formally identified, but it is likely to be established in the not too distant future. It would then be interesting to determine the effects of the causal gene at *F4bcR* on the differential binding of the three F4 antigenic variants. Like *FUT1*, its effect is likely to be fimbrial type specific. In the future, there is the real prospect of producing pigs that are resistant to both F18 and F4 fimbriated *E. coli*, which should have a dramatic effect on piglet diarrheas.

Salmonella Resistance: Nramp1. Nramp1 (Natural resistance-associated macrophage protein) is an integral membrane protein that resides in late endocytic vacuoles of macrophages where it removes divalent ions (Fe^{2+} and Mn^{2+}) from the vacuolar compartment (Boyer et al. 2002; Dangl 2003; Kehres and Maguire 2003). An environment deficient in Mn^{2+} and Fe^{2+} is detrimental to bacterial growth, and hence an effective Nramp1 would render greater host resistance to intracellular pathogens, like *Salmonella*. Its function in resisting disease is evident in several animal species. Inbred mice susceptible to infections are associated with a single substitution of aspartic acid for glycine at position 169 of the protein (Vidal et al. 1993). Polymorphisms found in human and poultry Nramp1 are associated with susceptibility to tuberculosis and *Salmonella enteritidis*, respectively (Kramer et al. 2003; Abe et al. 2003). Porcine *Nramp1* has been mapped to chromosome 15 (Sun et al. 1998) and cloned (Zhang et al. 2000). No association study between porcine Nramp1 polymorphism and *Salmonella* resistance has been reported. However, genetic variation in porcine resistance to *Salmonella* infection was recently demonstrated (van Diemen et al. 2002), and a causal relationship between Nramp1 and *Salmonella* resistance may well be found in the near future.

Swine Influenza: Porcine Mx Genes. Swine influenza, caused by influenza A virus, an orthomyxovirus, is a major cause of respiratory disease, and together with porcine reproductive and respiratory syndrome (PRRS) significantly contribute to the problem of postweaning respiratory disease. Additionally, swine influenza has wider significance in the evolution of human and avian influenza viruses. Human and avian influenzas are effectively species specific due to species differences in cell surface sialyoligosaccharides. The pig, however, is potentially susceptible to both human and avian influenzas and could act as an intermediate host to the emergence of new viral strains with the potential to cause devastating epidemics, in the animal or human population (Wentworth et al. 1997). Measures that can reduce the incidence of swine influenza will promote pig welfare as well as carry substantial indirect benefits to human and avian health. One strategic approach to re-

ducing swine influenza in pig herds is to identify and breed from animals that display enhanced resistance to the disease.

The best-documented innate antiviral protein that specifically inhibits influenza virus is encoded by the α/β interferon-inducible *Mx* gene family, whose GTPase protein products are localized either in the nucleus (e.g., murine *Mx1*) or cytoplasm (e.g. human *MxA*). The specific antiinfluenza activity of *Mx1* protein is dependent on its GTPase activity (Melen and Julkunen 1994; Toyoda et al. 1995), but independent of a functioning immune system (Horisberger 1995). Murine *Mx1* protein neutralizes influenza infection by blocking viral mRNA synthesis within the nucleus, probably by interaction with the viral polymerase subunit PB2 (Huang et al. 1992; Stranden et al. 1993). *Mx* proteins also have a broader spectrum of antiviral activity, against vesicular stomatitis virus (VSV), dhori virus, and thogoto virus (Zürcher et al. 1992; Haller et al. 1995; Thimme et al. 1995; Frese et al. 1996). In mice, resistance is inherited as an autosomal dominant trait, conferred by the functional allele $Mx1^+$. The recessive allele $Mx1^-$ is nonfunctional, as a result of a deletion or non-sense mutation. The cDNA and genomic DNA of porcine *Mx1* and *Mx2* have been cloned (Müller et al. 1992; Horisberger 1992). The two porcine genes are arranged in tandem on chromosome 13 (own unpublished data). Early work on the in vitro induction of porcine *Mx* proteins correlated with inhibition of influenza virus and VSV (Horisberger 1992). Three porcine *Mx1* polymorphisms, comprising a silent mutation and a deletion-frame shift mutation, have been identified from several pig breeds (Morozumi et al. 2001; Asano et al. 2002). It will be interesting to see if polymorphisms in *Mx1* or *Mx2* gene are related to differences in influenza susceptibility.

QUANTITATIVE TRAIT LOCI (QTL) AND MARKER-ASSISTED SELECTION

The genetic markers listed above are examples of QTL because they are genetic loci that contribute to variation in the analyzed quantitative (complex) trait of the chosen population. QTL can also be identified by whole genome scans as well as targeted searches on specific areas of the genome. The strength of this approach is that we do not need to make many assumptions about physiological mechanisms. The disadvantage is that preexisting knowledge is not taken into account in the study. Chromosomal regions harboring QTL can be detected by linkage or association analyses, but further work is usually necessary to identify the causative mutation and here a knowledge of physiological mechanisms can be very useful (Segal and Hill 2003). A variety of QTL for disease resistance have been identified including resistance, as assessed by rectal temperature and neurological signs, to the neurological syndrome of Aujeszky's disease (Reiner et al. 2002b). Although all infected pigs

developed fever and nearly all Large White pigs showed neurological signs, none of the Meishans was neurologically affected. QTL for leucocyte counts, neutrophil phagocytosis, lymphocyte proliferation, IL-2 production, virus-induced IFN-α production, and antibody response to F4 *E. coli* vaccination (Edfors-Lilja et al. 2004) were found in 200 F2 wild pig-Swedish Yorkshire crosses.

In summary, in the struggle to minimize the effects of infectious diseases in pig production, there is increasing attention given to the genetic development of disease-resistant animals. The prospects of breeding pigs that are resistant to specific diseases are real and, given current research efforts, many more genetic markers for porcine diseases can be expected in the not too distant future.

REFERENCES

Abe T, Iinuma Y, Ando M, Yokoyama T, Yamamoto T, Nakashima K, Takagi N, Baba H, Hasegawa Y, Shimokata K. 2003. NRAMP1 polymorphisms, susceptibility and clinical features of tuberculosis. J Infect 46:215–220.

Albers GAA, Gray GD, Piper LR, Barker JSF, Lejambre L, Barger IA. 1987. The genetics of resistance and resilience to *Haemonchus contortus* infection in young Merino sheep. Int J Parasitol 17:1355–1363.

Asano A, Ko J, Morozumi T, Hamashima N, Watanabe T. 2002. Polymorphisms and the antiviral property of porcine Mx1 protein. J Vet Med Sci 64:1085–1089.

Bidanel JP, Rothschild M. 2002. Current status of quantitative trait locus mapping in pigs. Pig News Infor 23:39N–54N.

Boyer E, Bergevin I, Malo D, Gros P, Cellier MFM. 2002. Acquisition of Mn(II) in addition to Fe(II) is required for full virulence of *Salmonella enterica* serovar Typhimurium. Infect Immun 70: 6032–6042.

Casewell M, Friis C, Marco E, McMullin P, Philips I. 2003. The European ban on growth-promoting antibiotics and emerging consequences for human and animal health. J Antimicrob Chemother 52:159–161.

Dangl JL. 2003. Molecular call-and-response: How *Salmonella* learns the gospel from its host. Trend Microbiol 11:245–246.

Edfors-Lilja I, Wattrang E, Magnusson U, Fossum C. 1994. Genetic variation in parameters reflecting immune competence of swine. Vet Immunol Immunopathol 40:1–16.

Edfors-Lilja I, Wattrang E, Marklund L, Moller M, Andersson-Eklund L, Andersson L, Fossum C. 2004. Mapping quantitative trait loci for immune capacity in the pig. J Immunol 161: 829–835.

Frese M, Kochs G, Feldmann H, Hertkorn C, Haller O. 1996. Inhibition of bunyaviruses, phleboviruses, and hantaviruses by human MxA protein. J Virol 70:915–923.

Frydendahl K, Jensen TK, Andersen JS, Fredholm M, Evans G. 2003. Association between the porcine *Escherichia coli* F18 receptor genotype and phenotype and susceptibility to colonisation and postweaning diarrhoea caused by *E. coli* 0138:F18. Vet Microbiol 93:39–51.

Fujii J, Otsu K, Zorzato F, de Leon S, Khanna VK, Weiler PE, O'Brien PJ, MacLennan DH. 1991. Identification of a mutation in porcine ryanodine receptor associated with malignant hyperthermia. Science 253:448–451.

Guldbrandtsen B, Lund MS, Nielsen VH, Jensen J. 2002. Detection of QTL for disease resistance, fertility and production in cattle and pig. DIAS Report, Animal Husbandry. 38:105–122.

Haller O, Frese M, Rost D, Nuttall PA, Kochs G. 1995. Tick-borne thogoto virus-infection in mice is inhibited by the orthomyovirus resistance gene-product Mx1. J Virol 69:2596–2601.

Hessing MJC, Coenen GJ, Vaiman M, Renard C. 1995. Individual differences in cell-mediated and humoral immunity in pigs. Vet Immunol Immunopathol 45:97–113.

Horisberger MA. 1992. Virus-specific effects of recombinant porcine interferon-gamma and the induction of Mx proteins in pig cells. J Interferon Res 12:439–444.

——. 1995. Interferons Mx genes and resistance to influenza virus. Am J Respir Crit Care Med 152:567–571.

Huang T, Pavlovic J, Staeheli P, Krystal M. 1992. Overexpression of the influenza virus polymerase can titrate out inhibition by murine Mx1 protein. J Virol 66:4154–4160.

Kehres DG, Maguire ME. 2003. Emerging themes in manganese transport, biochemistry and pathogenesis in bacteria. FEMS Microbiol Rev 27:263–290.

Kramer J, Malek M, Lamont SJ. 2003. Association of twelve candidate gene polymorphisms and response to challenge with *Salmonella enteritidis* in poultry. Anim Genet 34:339–348.

Mallard BA, Wilkie BN, Kennedy BW, Gibson JP, Quinton M. 1998. Immune responsiveness in swine: Eight generations of selection for high and low immune response in Yorkshire pigs. In Proc 6th World Congress on Genetics Applied to Livestock Production 27:257–264.

Meijerink E, Fries R, Vögeli P, Masabanda J, Wigger G, Stricker C, Neuenschwander S, Bertschinger HU, Stranzinger G. 1997. Two a(1,2) fucosyltransferase genes on porcine Chromosome 6q11 are closely linked to the blood group inhibitor (*S*) and *Escherichia coli* F18 receptor (*ECF18R*) loci. Mamm Genome 8:736–741.

Meijerink E, Neuenschwander S, Fries R, Dinter A, Bertschinger HU, Stranzinger G, Vögeli P. 2000. A DNA polymorphism influencing a(1,2)fucosyltransferase activity of the pig FUT1 enzymes determines susceptibility of small intestinal epithelium to *Escherichia coli* F18 adhesion. Immunogenetics 52:129–136.

Mekchay S, Ponsuksili S, Schellander K, Wimmers K. 2003. Association of the porcine C3 gene with haemolytic complement activity in the pig. Genet Select Evol 35:S83–S96.

Melen K, Julkunen I. 1994. Mutational analysis of murine Mx1 protein—GTP-binding core domain is essential for antiinfluenza-A activity. Virology 205:269–279.

Morozumi T, Sumantri C, Nakajima E, Kobayashi E, Asano A, Oishi T, Mitsuhashi T, Watanabe T, Hamasima N. 2001. Three types of polymorphisms in exon 14 in porcine Mx1 gene. Biochem Genet 39:251–260.

Müller M, Winnacker EL, Brem G. 1992. Molecular cloning of porcine Mx cDNAs: New members of a family of interferon-inducible proteins with homology to GTP-binding proteins. J Interferon Res 12:119–129.

Nguyen VP, Wong CW, Hinch GN, Singh D, Colditz IG. 1998. Variation in the immune status of two Australian pig breeds. Aust Vet J 76:613–617.

Nicholas FW. 1996. Introduction to Veterinary Genetics. Oxford University Press, UK.

Python P, Jörg H, Neuenschwander S, Hagger C, Stricker C, Bürgi E, Bertschinger HU, Stranzinger G, Vögeli P. 2002. Fine-mapping of the intestinal receptor locus for enterotoxigenic *Escherichia coli* F4ac on porcine chromosome 13. Anim Genet 33:441–447.

Reiner G, Eckert J, Peischl T, Bochert S, Jäkel T, Mackenstedt U, Joachim A, Daugschies A, Geldermann H. 2002a. Variation in clinical and parasitological traits in Pietrain and Meishan pigs infected with *Sarcocystis miescheriana*. Vet Parasitol 106:99–113.

Reiner G, Melchinger E, Kramarova M, Pfaff E, Buttner M, Saalmuller A, Geldermann H. 2002b. Detection of quantitative trait loci for resistance/susceptibility to pseudorabies virus in swine. J Gen Virol 83:167–172.

Rothschild MF. 2000. Advances in pig molecular genetics, gene mapping and genomics. Itea Production Animal 96A:349–361.

Rothschild MF, Hill HT, Christian LL, Warner CM. 1984. Genetic differences in serum-neutralization titers of pigs after vaccination with pseudorabies modified live-virus vaccine. Am J Vet Res 45:1216–1218.

Rothschild M, Jacobson C, Vaske D, Tuggle C, Wang LZ, Short T, Eckardt G, Sasaki S, Vincent A, Mclaren D, Southwood O, Vandersteen H, Mileham A, Plastow G. 1996. The estrogen-receptor locus is associated with a major gene influencing litter size in pigs. Proc Natl Acad Sci U S A 93:201–205.

Segal S, Hill AVS. 2003. Genetic susceptibility to infectious disease. Trends Microbiol 11:445–448.

Sellwood R. 1979. *Escherichia coli* diarrhoea in pigs with or without the K88 receptor. Vet Rec 105:228–230.

Stear MJ, Bishop SC, Mallard B, Raadsma HW. 2001. The sustainability, feasibility and desirability of breeding livestock for disease resistance. Res Vet Sci 71:1–7.

Stranden AM, Staeheli P, Pavlovic J. 1993. Function of the mouse Mx1 protein is inhibited by overexpression of the PB2 protein of influenza virus. Virology 197:642–651.

Sun HS, Wang L, Rothschild MF, Tuggle CK. 1998. Mapping of the natural resistance-associated macrophage protein 1 (NRAMP1) gene to pig chromosome 15. Anim Genet 29:138–140.

Taylor DJ. 1999. Pig diseases (7th ed). Dr. D.J. Taylor, Glasgow, U.K.

Thimme R, Frese M, Kochs G, Haller O. 1995. Mx1 but not MxA confers resistance against tick-borne dhori virus in mice. Virology 211:296–301.

Toyoda T, Asano Y, Ishihama A. 1995. Role of GTPase activity of murine Mx1 protein in nuclear localization and antiinfluenza virus activity. J Gen Virol 76:1867–1869.

van Diemen PM, Kreukniet MB, Galina L, Bumstead N, Wallis TS. 2002. Characterisation of a resource population of pigs screened for resistance to salmonellosis. Vet Immunol Immunopathol 88:183–196.

Vidal SM, Malo D, Vogan K, Skamene E, Gros P. 1993. Natural resistance to infection with intracellular parasites: Identification of a candiate gene for *Bcg*. Cell 73:437–457.

Visscher AH, Janss LL, Niewold TA, de Greef KH. 2002. Disease incidence and immunological traits for the selection of healthy pigs. A review. Vet Quart 24:29–34.

Wentworth DE, McGregor MW, Macklin MD, Neumann V, Hinshaw VS. 1997. Transmission of swine influenza virus to humans after exposure to experimentally infected pigs. J Infect Dis 175:7–15.

Wilkie BN, Mallard B. 1999. Selection for high immune response: An alternative approach to animal health maintenance? Vet Immunol Immunopathol 72:231–235.

Zhang G, Wu H, Ross CR, Minton JE, Blecha F. 2000. Cloning of porcine *NRAMP1* and its induction by lipopolysaccharide, tumor necrosis factor alpha, and interleukin-1b: Role of CD14 and mitogen-activated protein kinases. Infect Immun 68:1086–1093.

Zürcher T, Pavlovic J, Staeheli P. 1992. Mouse Mx2 protein inhibits vesicular stomatitis virus but not influenza virus. Virology 187:796–800.

62 Preweaning Mortality

Ross S. Cutler, V. Anthony Fahy, Greg M. Cronin, and E. Murray Spicer

Preweaning mortality is a major cause of wastage in pig production. On the best farms with young herds as few as 7% of those born alive die before weaning. Throughout the world on commercial farms preweaning mortality rates generally fall between 10 and 20% (Table 62.1).

In the U.K. the Meat and Livestock Commission (2003) reported a preweaning mortality rate for liveborn piglets of 12.2% in indoor herds and 9.9% in outdoor herds. Some data (MLC 1986) suggested that as litter size born alive has increased, so too has preweaning mortality, but, in 2002 litter sizes in the MLC (2003) study were about 0.5 pigs higher than they were in 1986 and preweaning mortality rates remained steady.

Over half the preweaning deaths occur in the first 4 days of life, and most of these occur in the first 36 hours. The majority of sows successfully rear their litters, but aged sows, sows with large litters, litters with unevenly sized pigs, and sick sows have disproportionately high preweaning mortality (Friendship et al. 1986; Pettigrew et al. 1986; Spicer et al. 1986a, Holyoake et al. 1995).

Although some disease outbreaks have a profound impact on neonatal pig survival, the resolution of day-to-day preweaning mortality problems relates to the attitude, diligence, and skill of the farrowing-house staff in supervising farrowing, providing weak pigs with colostrum, and making sure the piglets are warm. Contributing factors also include the distribution of creep heat, farrowing-crate and farrowing-pen design, the thermal comfort of the sow, disease control, and sow nutrition. Some studies (Dyck and Swiestra 1987) conclude that an inadequate milk supply is the primary factor contributing to piglet deaths and may account for in excess of 85% of the losses.

FACTORS AFFECTING PREWEANING MORTALITY

Birth weight

Birth weight is the single largest predictor of survival in pigs (Stanton and Carroll 1974). It is directly correlated with the energy intake of the sow during pregnancy but there is a considerable variation in response and it is often quite small. Baker et al. (1969) and Libal and Wahlstrom (1977) found that weights of newborn pigs increased as sow gestation energy intake increased but leveled out at about 26.4 MJDE/day. Feeding levels that increase net sow body weight by about 30 kg during gestation will be sufficient to sustain acceptable birth weights.

As litter size increases from ≤ 11 to ≥ 16, birth weight decreases from 1.59 to 1.26 kg, or about 35 g for each piglet born. In these large litters the number of pigs weighing less than 1 kg increases from 7% to 23% of total born. Below 1 kg more than 11% of pigs are stillborn and thereafter more than 17% die in the first 24 hours, compared with 4% and 3%, respectively, in pigs weighing more than 1 kg at birth (Quiniou et al. 2002). Uterine blood flow per fetus and hence fetal nutrition decreases as litter size increases (Pere et al. 1997), so within-litter variation in birth weight is already established by 35 days of pregnancy (van der Lende et al. 1990). In litters of low average birth weight, it is the high variation in birth weight that contributes to reduced survival (Milligan et al. 2002).

Low birth weight pigs have an increased risk of dying from asphyxia during delivery (Herpin et al. 1996). This was directly responsible for the deaths of 5.5% of the liveborn pigs. Nonetheless it does not necessarily follow that pigs of low birth weight will always have higher mortality rates. For example stillbirths and preweaning mortality rates for Jan Xin and Large White breeds are similar, yet the Jan Xin average birth weight is only 50% that of the Large White (0.7 kg vs. 1.4 kg) (Le Dividich citing Bidanel personal communication 1999). Biensen et al. (1998) argued that the growth of Meishan fetuses between day 90 and term depends on a combination of increases in placental size and density of placental blood vessels, whereas Yorkshire fetuses relied exclusively on placental growth to increase the surface area for nutrient exchange between the sow and her litter.

Table 62.1. Preweaning mortality rates from published studies

Country	Author	Data Set	Number Weaned per Litter	Preweaning mortality Rate* (%)
Australia	Cleary et al. 2003	22,000 sows	9.2	13.5
Canada	Friendship et al. 1986	30 farms	8.2	18.6
Canada	PigChamp[1]	69 farms	9.3	12.2
France	Quéméré et al. 1993	53 farms	9.2	14.0
Netherlands	Anon. 1986	36,000 farms (national survey)	8.7	14.2
United Kingdom	MLC 1986	270 farms	9.6	11.5
	MLC 2003		9.7	10.8
	PIC UK 1996	360 indoor herds	9.6	12.2
		122 outdoor herds	9.2	13.3
United States	Cromwell et al. 1989	1080 litters	8.2	16.8
United States	PigChamp[1]	515 farms	9.3	12.2
Venezuela	Gonzalez et al. 1987	461 litters	8.0	12.1

*Rate of pigs born alive.
[1]www.pigchamp.com/overview6.asp and www.pigchamp.com/overview5.asp

Fetal weight gain is most rapid in the last 10 days of pregnancy. More than 50% of fetal energy reserves are deposited in the last month. Moser and Lewis (1981) concluded that supplemental fat in sow diets increased the fat content of milk and colostrum and decreased the preweaning mortality from 18% to 15.4%. Pettigrew (1981) indicated that it was necessary to feed 1 kg/day of fat to the sow in the last 10 days of gestation to demonstrate an effect on the piglets. Improvement in survival is unlikely if the average piglet birth weight is normal (i.e., 1.3–1.4 kg) and preweaning survival is more than 85%.

Although the value of feeding fat in the last 10 days of gestation is equivocal, higher energy intakes for longer periods may be worthwhile. Cromwell et al. (1989) demonstrated that feeding an extra 1.36 kg/day of a maize or sorghum diet (14% protein) from day 90 of gestation resulted in greater sow weight gain to term, more piglets born alive, and, as a consequence, more pigs alive at 21 days. Pigs born to high–feeding-level sows were heavier both at birth and at 21 days of age.

Unlike most newborn mammals pigs do not possess brown adipose tissue so the maturity and hence capacity of skeletal muscle to shiver and preserve body temperature is critical. Indeed explanations for increasing neonatal survival are likely to be found in a higher degree of maturity or fetal development during late gestation (Leenhouwers et al. 2002). Heavier pigs at birth have a lower critical temperature (LCT) and can more readily mobilize their fat or glycogen reserves. Pettigrew et al. (1986) were unable to increase survival solely by feeding corn oil to baby pigs, indicating survival is due more to environmental factors than individual-pig nutrition

Farrowing Crate Design

Where sows are closely confined, neonatal mortality from trauma has generally been reduced compared to sows farrowing in unconfined conditions. The farrowing crate is that portion of the pen that confines the sow. Jones et al. (2003) assessed seven different farrowing systems including nonrestraint systems. They found

that the best and most consistent system was a crate with a fully slatted floor, with a preweaning mortality rate (PWMR) of 11.81%. A nonrestraint system with fully slatted floors and a hinged gate, which when opened allowed the sows to turn around five days postpartum, performed next best (PMWR 15.11%). Nonrestraint systems with straw performed worst (PMWR 20.22%). The research of Weber (1997) indicates that piglet production and survival can be as good in loose pens with straw bedding as in crates, provided genetic selection for careful behavior by sows has occurred and the environmental conditions of the farrowing room are correct.

Spatial Arrangements

Environmental factors influence neonatal mortality. In farrowing pens, two zones can be identified: a safe zone for the piglets, where they can rest free from the sow; and an interaction zone, where the sow and the piglets occupy a common space. The safe zone (creep area) must be attractive and large enough for suckling pigs of all ages, and the piglets must find it comfortable (and prefer it) for resting.

The space requirements of piglets are relative to the thermal environment. In cool conditions piglets huddle and use about 60% of the space they would in warm conditions. Under hot conditions, rectangular creep areas of about 1.3 m² will provide adequate space for about 10 pigs of 3 weeks of age (Baxter 1989).

The interaction zone is the most dangerous area in the farrowing pen. For the piglet, the greatest risk occurs when the sow changes posture (to stand, sit, lie down, or move about), especially during feeding, and when the pen is being cleaned (Svendsen et al. 1986). The danger is compounded because piglets prefer to lie against walls or close to the sow even when the temperatures in the pen are very high.

Danger increases if the sow acts suddenly; gentle, deliberate movements are readily tolerated provided there is enough space within the crate for the sow to change posture. However, movement is often restricted due to the length of the crate, in which case sows adapt their posture or movement but often at the risk of injury to themselves or their piglets (Baxter 1989).

Heating

Curtis (1970) demonstrated that although newborn piglets can mobilize carbohydrate energy reserves in response to cold stress, they utilize it poorly due to physiological immaturity. By 2 days of age the pig can mobilize and use efficiently both glycogen and lipids in response to cold. Thus, the 2-day-old pig has a much better response to cold stress. Protecting the newborn pig is the key priority.

Sows and piglets have different heat requirements. The newborn pig has a LCT of about 30–34°C, whereas the sow's LCT is 15–19°C (Baxter 1989). When the deep body temperature is 39°C at the LCT (34°C), the piglet can generate heat through increased metabolism and conserve heat to a limited degree by piloerection and vasoconstriction. When the environmental temperature falls below 34°C, the single newborn pig is subjected to cold stress and must utilize glycogen and fat reserves to maintain body temperature. Coldness impairs the development of thermostability and induces hypothermia. In farrowing rooms maintained at 17°C, as many as 72% of newborn pigs have rectal temperatures below 37°C. If deep body temperature is reduced by 2°C, piglet vigor is severely reduced. Sucking is less vigorous, and, hence, less colostrum is consumed. As a result, serum IgG levels are lower than in piglets kept warm (Le Dividich and Noblet 1981; Kelley et al. 1982).

Due to their higher surface-area-to-mass ratio, light pigs experience a larger body temperature decrease soon after farrowing than do heavier pigs, further emphasizing the importance of warmth for neonates (Ahlmann et al. 1983). In the creep area, overhead heaters are better than heated pads for lightweight pigs because of the pigs' higher surface area.

Electric or gas heaters are the most common methods of providing warmth for young pigs, but additional comfort factors are required to attract the neonate away from the sow toward the creep area. Large amounts of straw bedding have been the traditional method, but heated floors or heat pads, covered creeps, insulated or heated creep boxes, and carpet have replaced straw on many farms for convenience and safety. Good-quality, deep bedding (sawdust, shredded paper, wood shavings) raises the effective environmental temperature relative to concrete floors by 8°C and is attractive to piglets (Welch and Baxter 1986).

The Importance of Properly Applied Heat. Following birth the piglet has an instinctive desire to remain close to the udder for the first 24–48 hours of life. An extra heat source needs to be provided for this period (Morrison et al. 1983).

With creep areas on both sides of the sow, piglets spent less time lying in the danger zone and mortality was reduced from 19.3% to 6.9% in the first week of life.

Svendsen et al. (1986) reduced mortality in the first week from 7.0% to 1.1% by providing a movable heat source. The addition of a third heat source behind the sow (100 W light bulb) did not further reduce piglet mortality (Ogunbameru et al. 1991). Xin et al. (1996) reported a 19% reduction in piglet mortality for 175 W (5.0%) compared with 250 W radiant heat lamps (6.2%). Piglets subjected to the 250 W heat lamp tended to avoid staying directly under the lamp, an indication of excessive heat. By contrast, piglets under the 175 W heat lamp spread more evenly. In addition, the 175 W heat lamps saved 21% on energy costs and had a 45% lower failure rate than the 250 W lamps. The lower wattage lamps may also benefit the sow, keeping her cooler, due to a narrower radiant beam spread. Where heat sources go unchecked or uncontrolled, very high temperatures have been recorded, as high as 60°C under some heat lamps (Prime et al. 1989).

The effectiveness of electrically heated floor mats (110 W) for piglets after the first day of lactation was compared with 250 W infrared heat lamps by Rousseau et al. (1994). Litters in the heat mat treatment were reported to have a lower level of piglet mortality (6.1% vs. 9.2%), however, 250 W heat lamps were supplied in both treatments: behind the sow during farrowing, then beside the udder for the first day of lactation.

Morrison et al. (1983) also demonstrated the effect of farrowing-house temperature on survival. As farrowing-house temperature was increased from 13.6°C to 20.5°C, liveweight gain to 7 days increased (135 g/day vs. 169 g/day) and 7-day mortality fell (15.1% vs. 10.7%). Ziron and Hoy (2003) tested the effect of a warm flexible piglet nest heating system. Piglets reared in this system weighed 7.72 kg, 0.46 kg heavier at 28 days of age than piglets reared in concrete floored pens with gas heating systems. Pigs reared in the warm nest also had fewer skin lesions than the pigs in the other systems.

Interaction of People and Pigs

Prime et al. (1989) demonstrated how training staff had a positive effect on pigs weaned and how it reduced neonatal mortality. Spicer et al. (1987) described how the successful operation of a crib care system for neonates depended heavily on the diligence of the individual operator. Two operators supervised the care of 600 farrowing sows and their progeny over a 4-week period. Operator A obtained 6.1% mortality (range, 5.5–7.0%) in the first week of life, whereas operator B achieved a piglet mortality of 1.3% (range, 0.95–1.65%) over the same period. Hemsworth et al. (1999) found some moderate correlations between the withdrawal response (as an indicator of fear of humans) of lactating sows at days 16–18 of lactation to an experimenter and stillbirth rate. Sows that were apparently more fearful of humans were more likely to have a higher stillbirth rate. This behavioral variable accounted for about 18% of the variance in stillbirth rate at the farm.

Ravel et al. (1996b) examined personality profiles on independent and integrated farms in Canada. On both types of farm stock people were more reserved, emotionally stable, serious, conscientious, unsentimental, controlled, introverted, and less anxious than the average person in the general population. High levels of self-discipline in the stockperson were associated with high preweaning performance on both integrated and independent farms, whereas poor preweaning performance was associated with exaggerated self-assuredness and boldness (Ravel et al. 1996a).

Tooth Clipping

Sibling fights occur during establishment of the teat order in the first few days and subsequently as piglets defend their teat-order position against littermates (Fraser 1975; Hartsock et al. 1977). Injury may be inflicted to the faces of littermates or the sow's udder and although the occurrence of the latter is generally reported as low to negligible (Robert et al. 1995; Weary and Fraser 1999), serious udder and teat damage occasionally occurs (Wilkinson and Blackshaw 1987). In addition, clipping *per se* can result in injury to gums or infection (Weary and Fraser 1999; Hay et al. 2004).

Piglets are born with eight very sharp, fully erupted "needle teeth" (the deciduous canines and the corner incisors) (Weary and Fraser 1999). To avoid potential problems, on many farms all eight needle teeth are routinely clipped for all piglets during the first 1–2 days after birth (Robertson and Arey 1998).

The tooth consists of a crown (encased in enamel) and a root, with the gum forming a living seal between the crown of the tooth and the root. During tooth clipping, the crown is fractured close to the gum leaving a cross-section of tooth which contains exposed regions of dentine and pulp. Pulp is connective tissue containing numerous nerves. It is therefore sensitive and a potential route of infection to reach the tooth socket and enter the blood stream. In addition, when force is applied to the tooth during the clipping process, there is potential for significant movement in the area where the gum meets the tooth. Poorly performed teeth clipping can result in serrated or splintered teeth and gum damage, which could greatly increase the risk of infection and contribute to morbidity and mortality (Robertson and Arey 1998). The literature is equivocal that tooth clipping is associated with increased incidence of arthritis and mortality (Hay et al. 2004). Nevertheless, care and hygiene are critical factors during the tooth clipping process.

Concern over the potential adverse impacts of tooth clipping on piglet health and welfare has led to questioning of routine tooth clipping and stimulated investigation of alternatives such as selective clipping, partial clipping, and tooth grinding.

Partial clipping was examined by Weary and Fraser (1999). Three clipping treatments were compared: intact, clipped to the gum line, or partial, in which about one-third of the visible tooth was removed. All piglets of a litter received one treatment on one side of the mouth and a different treatment on the other side, with the three treatments balanced over the two sides in different litters. Facial lesions were negligible on the side facing either partially clipped or fully clipped teeth, while lesions on the side facing intact teeth were greater. In the first week after birth, piglets with fully clipped teeth gained the least, those with partially clipped teeth were intermediate and those with intact teeth gained most. There was no effect of treatment however, on later weight gain or the number of piglet deaths.

Fostering

English and Smith (1975) reported that a major factor affecting preweaning mortality was the degree of variation in birth weight. They argued that piglets of average birth weight were not competitive when mixed with larger piglets. Marcatti Neto (1986) found that piglets with a birth weight of 800 g had a preweaning mortality of 62.5% if left on their dam, compared with 15.4% if fostered into groups with equivalent birth weights. Piglets fostered according to weight also grew faster and had half the mortality of piglets fostered without regard to weight.

Straw (1997) cautions against fostering and questions its value, particularly for older piglets. She argues that fostered pigs grow less rapidly than pigs that remain with their dams. Straw's data indicated that although litter weight variation was reduced by fostering, it came at the expense of individual pig performance. Price et al. (1994) reported that 6 hours after being moved to their new dam, fewer than half the pigs fostered after 2 days of age had suckled. Robert and Martineau (1997) reported increased levels of fighting in fostered litters and an increase in lacerations in fostered piglets, in sow aggressiveness, and in nonproductive milk letdowns. Horrell and Bennett (1981) found that piglets fostered at 7 days had reduced weight gains. McCaw and Desrosiers (1997) demonstrated the success of fostering systems if the pigs were fostered only on the first day, only available teat space was filled, pigs were not moved between different rooms, severely sick piglets were euthanized, and no pigs that were doing poorly were moved back to younger age groups. Their program was targeted at porcine reproductive and respiratory syndrome (PRRS) control, but the recommendations apply equally to herds where PRRS is not present. In contrast Kirkwood et al. (1998), in a study of 120 sows, found no advantage in creating litters of uniform bodyweight. They found that mortality rates were always highest in the smallest pigs regardless of uniformity. Nonfostered pigs always had better survival and the light pigs always had higher mortality rates (20%) than heavy pigs (8.7%).

If fostering is to be applied, it must be done on the first day of life. Creating teat space by weaning a good litter early and then filling the teat space with pigs of the same size will alleviate the concerns of those cautious about fostering and those wanting to safeguard small pigs. Fostering piglets after teat order has been established, after a day of age, or from older litters to younger litters is contraindicated.

Hygiene

Good shed hygiene is important in reducing preweaning mortality. It may spell the difference between a microbial challenge that the piglet can cope with and an overwhelming infection. Thorough cleaning and disinfecting of empty sow crates help to reduce environmental microbial burdens and more specifically to reduce pathogens that may be exclusive to newborn piglets. Svendsen et al. (1975) demonstrated that both morbidity and mortality associated with gastrointestinal disease were higher in herds with poor hygiene standards. The prevalence of diarrhea fell from 28 to 5% during the year an organized hygiene program was developed. Ravel et al. (1996a) showed that high preweaning performance was associated with routine washing of farrowing crates between litters. Sanitation programs based on thorough cleaning followed by application of disinfectants effective in the presence of organic matter are preferred.

Field data on litters of unvaccinated gilts indicate that piglets born early in the week take 3–4 days before commencing to scour, whereas piglets born later in the week, when the environmental microbiological load is heavy, may show profuse diarrhea within 24 hours of birth (V. A. Fahy 1997, unpublished data). Studies on coccidiosis in pigs reveal that as hygiene measures lessen in intensity, coccidiosis emerges in herds where it had earlier been controlled, indicating that the severity of the disease reflects the intensity of the challenge dose (Stuart and Lindsay 1985).

SOW FACTORS AFFECTING PREWEANING MORTALITY

Prefarrowing Behavior

Studies investigating the effects of manipulating the environment of the young sow have suggested that, apart from affecting prefarrowing behavior, the environment may also affect the course of parturition, postfarrowing behavior of the sow, and piglet survival (Cronin and Smith 1992; Cronin et al. 1993, 1994, 1998; Thodberg et al. 1999, 2002a, b).

Cronin et al. (1993), McGlone et al. (1996), and Thodberg et al. (2002a) demonstrated that by stimulating nesting behavior in young sows, the sows appeared calmer before parturition, had shorter intrabirth intervals or fewer stillborns. Further, Cronin et al. (1998), who investigated sow behavior and piglet survival in loose farrowing pens, reported that small, narrow farrowing pens appeared to interfere with the sows' prefarrowing nesting behavior, with a consequent increase in sow restlessness during and after farrowing and a reduction in piglet survival.

Litter Size

Litter size increases with parity. Although preweaning mortality increases in numerical terms, more pigs are weaned from the larger litters, including those of older sows, until a plateau is reached between four and six litters. As litter size increases, the number of deaths during parturition increases, birth weight decreases, and the number of small pigs per litter increases (Table 62.2) (Spicer et al. 1986a; Dyck and Swiestra 1987).

Sow Health

Spicer et al. (1986a) indicated that 15% of overlain pigs that died were associated with sow illness. An assessment of sow health using the checklist below is an important part of farrowing-house management.

1. Assess water availability. Sows require up to 40 L/day during hot summer days (R. H. King 1997, personal communication). To consume this amount, they need a drinker flow rate of 1.5–2.0 L/minute.
2. Assess feed intake. The target is an average of 6–7 kg/day (80 MJDE/day) between farrowing and weaning.
3. Observe fecal consistency, urine (color and pus), vulval discharge, vomiting, skin pallor, skin wounds, udder condition, abdominal bloat, and lameness.

Table 62.2. Effects of litter size on stillbirth and birth weight

Litter Size	Number of Litters	Total Born	Preparturient Deaths	Parturient Deaths	Number Weaned	Birth Weight (kg)	Piglets/ Litter <0.8 kg	% Litters with Pigs <0.8 kg	Length of Parturition (minutes)
2, 3	3	2.7 ± 0.3	0	0	1.4 ± 0.3	1.60 ± 0.22	0.0	0.0	53 ± 23
4, 5	15	4.4 ± 0.1	0.07 ± 0.2	0.27 ± 0.6	3.9 ± 0.2	1.56 ± 0.05	0.1	11.1	44 ± 34
6, 7	25	6.7 ± 0.1	0.08 ± 0.3	0.16 ± 0.5	6.1 ± 0.1	1.51 ± 0.04	0.1	8.3	117 ± 18
8, 9	45	8.6 ± 0.1	0.27 ± 0.6	0.31 ± 0.9	7.2 ± 0.2	1.44 ± 0.03	0.2	17.8	79 ± 49
10, 11	69	10.6 ± 0.1	0.41 ± 0.9	0.45 ± 0.6	8.8 ± 0.1	1.35 ± 0.02	0.4	25.0	154 ± 14
12, 13	51	12.4 ± 0.1	0.14 ± 0.4	1.02 ± 1.5	9.7 ± 0.2	1.33 ± 0.02	0.7	45.1	207 ± 40
14, 15	24	14.3 ± 0.1	0.46 ± 0.7	1.08 ± 1.1	11.0 ± 0.3	1.29 ± 0.04	1.1	66.7	158 ± 18
16, 17	6	16.3 ± 0.1	1.50 ± 1.1	0.66 ± 0.8	11.8 ± 0.7	1.26 ± 0.06	1.0	66.7	131 ± 35

Source: Spicer et al. 1986a.

Table 62.3. Number of stillbirths, mummies, and pigs that are small and weak relative to their littermates in 238 litters from one herd

	Average Position in Litter	Average Interpig Interval (minutes)	Average Birth Weight (kg)	Average Time from Birth to First Suck (minutes)
All pigs	5.9 ± 0.1	21 ± 2	1.36 ± 0.01	55 ± 2
Stillbirths	7.9 ± 0.4	70 ± 26	1.17 ± 0.04	
Littermates of stillbirths	6.3 ± 0.2	16 ± 2	1.30 ± 0.01	54 ± 3
Mummies	6.3 ± 0.6	16 ± 4		
Littermates of mummies	6.5 ± 0.2	16 ± 1	1.35 ± 0.01	48 ± 3
Small, weak pigs	5.8 ± 0.7	9 ± 2	0.82 ± 0.07	133 ± 35
Littermates of small, weak pigs	6.3 ± 0.3	34 ± 15	1.29 ± 0.03	63 ± 5

Source: Spicer et al. 1986a.

4. The normal rectal temperature is 39°C ± 0.5°C, but it may exceed 40°C during hot weather.
5. The normal resting respiration rate is 12–30 breaths per minute. Observers should allow for an increase during hot weather.
6. Consider past history, including genetic susceptibility to stress.

Stillbirths

Stillborn pigs represent about one-quarter of all deaths between parturition and weaning. The percentage of pigs born dead varies from 4% to 10%; veterinary intervention is suggested when stillbirths exceed 8%. Approximately 70% of pigs classified stillborn are alive at birth. Although the heart is beating, the piglets are severely anoxic and die within minutes of birth. The anoxia can be related to compression or premature rupture of the umbilical cord during farrowing (Randall 1978). In general, stillborn pigs weigh less than normal pigs and are born after a longer interpig interval (Spicer et al. 1986a) (Table 62.3); however, up to 9% of stillborn pigs may be heavier than average (Evangelista et al. 1996).

Pigs are relatively neurologically mature at birth; hence, a period of anoxia can be serious. As the duration of farrowing increases beyond 4–5 hours, or after 80% of the pigs have been born, the number of stillbirths increases. Most stillbirths occur among the last three pigs born. Svendsen and Andreasson (1980) found that sows kept in stalls during gestation had higher stillbirth rates than sows kept in pens, the difference due to the longer farrowing time in stalls. In fact, the duration of farrowing has a greater impact on stillbirths than parity. Long farrowing times also reduce neonatal survival.

Cutler and Prime (1988) found that about 60% of sows farrowed litters without stillborn pigs; a small percentage of the sows farrowed most of the stillborn pigs. Sows farrowing two or more stillborn pigs per litter delivered 70% of the total number of stillborn pigs, whereas these sows composed only 17.5% of the farrowings. Bilkei-Papp and Papp (1994) found an increase in stillbirths in fat sows in addition to a greater mortality during the first 3 days postpartum.

Parity. As sows age, the duration of parturition increases, and, consequently, the percentage of stillborn pigs farrowed increases. An exception occurs for parity 1 sows, which have a higher percentage of stillbirths than might be expected if the relationship between parity and stillbirths was linear. Parity 1 sows and aged sows (parity 7–10) have the greatest risk of farrowing multiple stillbirths.

Previous History of Stillbirth. It is unusual for a sow to repeatedly farrow stillborn pigs. However, sows that had multiple stillbirths at the previous farrowing have an increased chance of farrowing multiple stillbirths at the next.

Season. The percentage of stillbirths is higher for sows farrowing during summer (7.3%) than winter (6.4%), although the number of affected sows remains the same.

Strategies available to farrowing-house staff to reduce stillbirths include cooling sows in summer, inducing parturition in old sows, and providing close supervision of high-risk sows, including manual assistance after the seventh pig has been delivered and interpig intervals exceed 30 minutes. Attempting to influence stillbirth rates by chemotherapy is generally unrewarding.

Induction of Parturition

Effective supervision of farrowing can reduce stillbirths and preweaning mortality on farms (Holyoake et al. 1995). Several techniques exist for manipulating the timing and duration of parturition. Although parturition can be induced 3 days on either side of the average gestation length for the herd, piglet survival and vigor are highest when farrowing is induced on the due date for the sow. Farrowing sows earlier than day 112 or after day 118 generally results in increased numbers of stillbirths.

Early farrowings can be prevented by daily injections of progesterone (100 mg) from day 112 to 114 or the use of altrenogest (Regumate) at a dose rate of 20 mg from day 110 (Guthrie et al. 1987). Farrowing is most commonly initiated with an intramuscular injection of natural prostaglandin $F_{2\alpha}$ ($PGF_{2\alpha}$) or a synthetic analog

(Dial et al. 1987). Sows farrow 2–44 hours following injection of PGF$_{2\alpha}$, with a mean time of 22–26 hours. This technique has proved valuable where all-in/all-out systems are practiced to ensure that all farrowings occur within a week.

Several authors have used PGF$_{2\alpha}$ injection followed by 20–30 IU oxytocin 18–24 hours later in an attempt to more closely control the time of parturition (Welp et al. 1984; Wilson 1984). This amount of oxytocin can induce uterine spasms in some sows, which increases the number of stillbirths and the number of manual interventions required (Welp et al. 1984). Holtz and Welp (1984) achieved reliable induction of parturition by combining 5 IU oxytocin with 1.5 mg of carazolol, a beta-blocker that effectively blocks adrenaline receptors in the uterus and allows a lower level of oxytocin to initiate parturition. Carazolol shortens farrowing time and can reduce stillbirths, especially in older sows (Bostedt and Rudloff 1983).

Despite attempts to control the time of parturition with PGF$_{2\alpha}$, many sows still farrow overnight, making supervision difficult. To overcome this, Zerobin and Kundig (1980) injected 150 μg of clenbuterol during labor but before the birth of the first piglet and delayed parturition for up to 15 hours. Zerobin (1980) showed that clenbuterol-induced uterine relaxation could be overridden with higher doses of oxytocin (20–40 IU) without uterine spasms. The following schedule using PGF$_{2\alpha}$ to initiate parturition followed by clenbuterol and carazolol/oxytocin has been successful for farrowings needing special supervision: 9:00 a.m., the sows are dosed with 10 mg PGF$_{2\alpha}$; sows not farrowed by 4:00 p.m. are injected with 150 μg clenbuterol to reduce the chance of overnight farrowing; parturition is reinitiated the following morning using 10 IU oxytocin plus 1.5 mg carazolol (Spicer et al. 1986b).

The success of these regimes in improving piglet survival relies heavily on the quality and assistance of the staff during and soon after farrowing. Some caution with oxytocin administration is indicated. Mota-Rojas et al. (2002) found that although oxytocin-treated sows had a significant decrease in farrowing time and expulsion intervals, they also had significantly more stillbirths than the controls.

CAUSES OF PREWEANING MORTALITY ON INTENSIVE PIG FARMS

Several papers have documented the causes of piglet mortality (Nielsen et al. 1974; English and Smith 1975; Glastonbury 1976). These studies have been based mainly on the autopsy of dead piglets. English and Smith (1975), Spicer et al. (1986a), and Dyck and Swiestra (1987) supplemented autopsy findings with case histories or piglet weights so factors predisposing to illness and death could be documented. The causes of preweaning mortality (Table 62.4) are discussed in the light of the authors' experience, from veterinary diagnostic laboratory submissions, and from the documentation of other investigators.

Enteritis

Enteritis is the most common infectious cause of mortality in suckling pigs. Whereas Glastonbury (1977) found that 5% of all deaths were due to enteritis, the Veterinary Investigation Service (Anonymous 1959), Svendsen et al. (1975), and Spicer et al. (1986a) put the figure at 15%. All these data were recorded before the advent of vaccines to control neonatal colibacillosis and effective coccidial chemotherapy. The causative agents of enteritis in suckling pigs are transmissible gastroenteritis virus, porcine adenovirus, porcine epidemic diarrhea virus (coronavirus), rotavirus, calicivirus, Aujeszky's disease virus, enterotoxigenic *Escherichia coli*, *Clostridium perfringens* types A and C, *Salmonella* spp., *Candida* spp., coccidia, and *Strongyloides ransomi*. The

Table 62.4. Causes of preweaning mortality

Cause of Death	Number of Piglets	Deaths (%) of Pigs Born	Age at Death[a] (days)	Birth Weight (kg)
Preparturient deaths	70	2.9		
Parturient deaths	132	5.4		1.15 ± 0.01[b]
Scours	42	1.7	6.5 ± 0.9	1.27 ± 0.04[b]
Overlay	50	2.1	4.2 ± 0.8	1.31 ± 0.50
Small, weak	22	0.9	2.3 ± 0.8	0.82 ± 0.07[b]
Anemia	30	1.2	2.5 ± 0.9	1.24 ± 0.05[b]
Splayleg	11	0.5	2.6 ± 0.4	1.20 ± 0.07[b]
Savaged	27	1.1	0.9 ± 0.3	1.14 ± 0.05[b]
Pneumonia	12	0.5	4.5 ± 0.9	1.30 ± 0.10
Other infections	23	1.0	9.1 ± 1.2	1.39 ± 0.07
Noninfectious	27	1.1	7.7 ± 1.8	1.24 ± 0.07
Nil diagnosis	8	0.3	7.2 ± 2.5	1.33 ± 0.06
Total deaths	454	18.7	4.7 ± 0.4	1.21 ± 0.02[b]

Source: Spicer et al. 1986a.
[a]Mean ± SE.
[b]Significantly (P <0.05) less than the average birth weight of all piglets that survived to weaning (1.39 ± 0.01 kg).

reader is referred to specific chapters on each agent in this text. On a worldwide basis the organisms most commonly causing diarrhea are *E. coli*, *Isospora suis*, and rotavirus. *Clostridium perfringens* and transmissible gastroenteritis, while not cosmopolitan, are nonetheless important causes of enteritis.

Risk Factors. The following factors associated with an increasing risk of enteritis are drawn from Svendsen et al. (1975).

1. *Parity.* Diarrhea was more prevalent in gilt litters, suggesting a lack of specific antibodies.
2. *Litter size.* The incidence of diarrhea increased with litter size, suggesting lack of access to protective milk antibodies. Similarly, there was an increase in enteritis in litters where the sow was ill or dysgalactic.
3. *Season.* There was a higher incidence in winter, probably due to the effect of cold stress, particularly on small piglets.
4. *Hygiene.* A significantly higher level of mortality was associated with low levels of hygiene.
5. *Age.* More than 60% of deaths occurred during the first week of life, with 10.5% occurring in the second week and 1.3% each week thereafter until weaning. The mortality is inversely proportional to age at onset and directly proportional to the duration of diarrhea (Table 62.5). Deaths from enteritis occurring during the first 5 days of life are usually due to colibacillosis. Deaths associated with enteritis from day 5 to weaning are more likely associated with coccidial infection (Driesen et al. 1993) and enterotoxigenic *E. coli* (F4) (Fahy et al. 2003).
6. *Intercurrent disease.* Fifty-three percent of animals that died with enteritis had intercurrent disease or disabilities, such as polyarthritis, respiratory disease, were small or starved pigs, or had been overlain.

Prevention. Immunity to enteric infections is acquired primarily from passive antibodies, which bathe the intestine and prevent attachment and multiplication of pathogens. Piglets must receive adequate antibodies from colostrum and milk. Parenteral vaccination of the dam is effective against neonatal colibacillosis and clostridial infections occurring in the first 5 days of life. Enteric infections occurring after the first week of life are not well controlled by parenteral vaccination as the IgG levels of colostrum have plummeted to about 10% of their original levels by day 7. Oral vaccination of the dam is the most effective way to stimulate lactogenic IgA antibodies, which will protect the pig for the duration of lactation. In this regard oral vaccination of breeders at around 11 weeks of gestation with F4 hemolytic *E. coli* has proven highly effective at preventing diarrhea and death in suckling pigs (Fahy et al. 2003). Supplementary feeding of fostered and small pigs with colostrum will prevent them from scouring and contaminating the en-

Table 62.5. The association between age at onset and duration of diarrhea and preweaning mortality

Piglets	Number of Deaths[a]	Number of % Deaths	Duration of diarrhea (days)
No diarrhea[b]	1648	103	6.3
1	275	24	8.7
2	90	11	12.2[c]
3	93	15	16.1[c]
Age at onset of diarrhea (days)			
1	125	7	5.6
2–4	123	27	22.8[c]
5–7	77	12	15.6
8–11	64	4	6.3
12	64	2	3.1

[a]Includes deaths from all causes.
[b]Excludes piglets that died before 2 days of age.
[c]Significantly (P <0.05) different from no diarrhea.

vironment. In addition to adequate immunity, both warmth and hygiene play pivotal roles in the prophylaxis of neonatal diarrhea. With the advent of vaccination to control fimbriated enterotoxigenic *E. coli*, it is highly unusual to find these strains as a cause of neonatal scour, or indeed to isolate any common enteric pathogens of suckling pigs. The only thing in common with farms that have this problem is inadequate creep heating for newborn pigs. Invariably when this is corrected the problem disappears.

Treatment. Piglets with diarrhea die when they lose approximately 10% of their total body fluid. In addition to specific antimicrobial therapy, piglets should be rehydrated. Although parenteral rehydration can be given by subcutaneous or intraperitoneal injection, oral rehydration via a stomach tube is the preferred method. The volume to be given daily is 10% of total body water, which is 75% of body weight. A 1 kg pig requires 75 ml/day. Piglets will drink water within a few hours from birth, so the provision of electrolytes in troughs is warranted. These troughs should be wall mounted to prevent them becoming contaminated with feces.

Overlay/Trauma

Overlay, the most common noninfectious cause of death for suckling pigs, accounts for the death of up to 20% of all pigs born alive. Most deaths occur within 4 days of birth (see Table 62.4).

Overlays occur more often in larger litters; in sow, rather than gilt, litters (Svendsen et al. 1986); and in free stall crates rather than crates with modifications such as finger-bars, hydraulic rails, and bowed bottom bars (Walker et al. 1996). The risk of overlay is directly proportional to the number of times a sow stands or sits. Edwards et al. (1986) found from video recordings of overlay incidents that even relatively minor movements by the sow, such as sitting up and lying down again, can result in the crushing of healthy, viable piglets. Factors that cause sows to be restless increase the chance of overlay: inadequate water supply, sore teats, too many piglets for the number of active teats, and fear of humans. Highly fearful sows are likely to be restless in the presence of stockpersons.

An increased incidence of postural changes (i.e., from standing to lying and vice versa) and increased time spent standing led, in one set of observations, to a higher incidence of overlays for those sows farrowing during, compared with after or before, the stockpersons' work time (G. M. Cronin 1997, unpublished data). This increased overlay rate may be the direct result of the two feeding sessions that occurred during the stockpersons' work time. Olsson and Svendsen (1989) found that 80% of overlay incidents occurred when the sow was standing or changing posture and that almost 30% of these incidents occurred around feeding times. Since the stockperson may be present during feeding, it is not possible to separate the possible effects of feeding per se from the presence of the stockperson in these studies. Vieuille et al. (2003) found that in outdoor herds, crushing occurred in the evening or at night in the first 12 hours after farrowing.

Spicer et al. (1986a) reported that 44% of deaths due to overlay were secondary to illness in the sow or piglet. Sow illness was associated with overlay in 15% of cases. The illnesses included mastitis, agalactia, purulent vulval discharge, rectal prolapse, and inappetence.

Piglet illness or defect was associated with 26% of overlays. These included enteritis, anemia, splayleg, weakness, and pneumonia. Inadequate creep heating is a common risk factor for overlays. Creep heaters that are too hot or too cold result in piglets lying next to the sow, with consequent risks. It is a common mistake for farrowing house staff to try to make up for inadequate creep heating by raising the temperature of the farrowing house. This may exacerbate the problem by making the sow uncomfortable and hence more restless; it will certainly decrease the lactating sows' feed intake (Muirhead and Alexander 1997.)

Necropsy Findings. Overlain pigs display gross deformity and marked bruising. The pigs are flat sided, with the tongue protruding. Death is caused by suffocation or internal hemorrhage. In the former case there is often extensive bruising and edema of the subcutaneous tissue and muscles, particularly of the head and neck. The lungs are usually edematous and petechial hemorrhages may be present in the upper respiratory tract. In those animals that die of internal hemorrhage, the former lesions may be present in addition to the thoracic or abdominal cavities containing extravasated blood. Skull fractures may be evident.

Prevention. Sows should be monitored closely for the first 48–72 hours after farrowing for signs of illness or restlessness, evidence of mastitis, udder edema, and vulval discharge. Check to determine whether the sow is eating and is passing feces. If there is inappetence, make sure that the water supply is adequate and not overly hot, as can happen when plumbing is exposed to direct sunlight. Conversely, frozen pipes will prevent delivery of water.

Since a disproportionate number of traumatic injuries occur during feeding, particular diligence should be applied at these times. Where splayleg pigs are fostered, the foster mother should be a gilt, for they seem more attentive to the shrieking sounds of an overlain piglet, are more agile, and will stand up to release it.

Walker et al. (1996) identified certain combinations of farrowing-crate design and floor type that were associated with higher incidences of piglet overlay. Producers should therefore consider avoiding the following combinations to prevent overlay: either free stall or finger-bar crate with tri-bar metal floor, and bow-bar crate with either polygrate plastic or rubber-coated expanded metal.

Very Small Pigs

The newborn pig is very susceptible to cold stress and hypoglycemia. Coldness impairs the development of thermostability and induces hypothermia. Glycogen and fat reserves are used as major energy substrates for heat production within the first 24 hours of life (Close 1992). Piglets have no brown fat for thermogenesis (Le Dividich and Noblet 1983). They rely first on an increased metabolic rate and then shivering to maintain warmth (Mellor and Cockburn 1986). In the shivering process muscles initially use glycogen stores. Once these are depleted, they use blood glucose, which in turn is replenished from liver glycogen. However, the liver contains a limited supply of glycogen. In addition, glycogenolysis and glycolysis are poorly developed and cannot keep pace with the demand. To avoid hypoglycemia and hypothermia, the piglet needs an exogenous source of energy. They obtain this from colostrum, which provides lactose and fat. Both play a major role in the supply of energy and in glucose homeostasis in the neonatal pig (Le Dividich et al. 1994). Colostrum supplies 60% of the energy required for heat production.

Piglets feed about 15 times in the first 12 hours of life. They take in 15 ml per feeding (Werhahn et al. 1981) and consume about 7 g of lactose, 16 g of fat, and 19 g of immunoglobulin during this time. Not only does colostrum provide lactose but it also has an enhancing effect on the hormonal and metabolic mechanisms controlling blood glucose levels. A fasting newborn piglet can resist hypoglycemia for 18 hours under favorable conditions (28–32°C). However, this is reduced to 12 hours if the temperature is low (18–26°C) (Mellor and Cockburn 1986). Cold stress of the neonate reduces its acquisition of colostral immunoglobulins and results in increased mortality (Blecha and Kelley 1981). Additionally, a delay in the intake of colostrum after birth will affect the absorption of immunoglobulins: A 4-hour delay in access to colostrum results in 15% of piglets having very low levels of serum immunoglobulin (Coalson and Lecce 1973). Low serum immunoglobulin is associated with higher mortality (Werhahn et al. 1981).

It is against this background that the fate of small pigs weighing less than 800 g is considered. There are two problems: There is a tendency for them to be born weak, and they cannot compete with larger littermates. In the study of Spicer et al. (1986a) pigs less than 800 g had a higher stillbirth rate (25% vs. total stillborn rate of 8.3%), and 62% of those born alive perished, compared with the average of 11.3%. These pigs were assessed as being unable to survive under standard husbandry conditions because they were too weak or small. There was a relationship between birth weight and vitality as determined by the time taken to achieve an adequate first suck (see Table 62.3). The number of small piglets increased markedly in litters with more than 11 piglets; 67% of the litters with more than 13 piglets had some pigs weighing less than 800 g (see Table 62.2). This may reflect a degree of fetal growth retardation due to a small placenta for some of the piglets (Mellor and Cockburn 1986).

The number of mammary glands per pig varies between 8 and 18, with an average of 12. However, 95% of sows have between 10 and 14 glands (Schmidt 1971). The small pig born in a large litter will be the one most likely to miss out. Even if there are enough teats, in older, higher-parity sows with large udders, the top row of teats tends to point upward when the sow is lying down. The small piglet is often unable to reach such teats and will starve to death in the midst of plenty. Because the little pig may be hungry, it is continually at the teat and therefore at a significantly greater risk of being overlain.

Necropsy Findings. Spicer et al. (1986a) found the average age of these small weak pigs at death was 2.3 days; those pigs that survived to that time appeared emaciated and dehydrated. At autopsy there was little, if any, food in the stomach. Glastonbury (1977) found that 17% of 538 dead suckling pigs had empty alimentary tracts. Bille et al. (1974) described a characteristic red-brown color of the striated muscle, which they considered almost pathognomonic for pigs dying of starvation. Often in pigs less than 24 hours of age there are no gross abnormalities, but the size of the pig and absence of food in the stomach prompt a diagnosis of hypoglycemia or hypothermia. Nielsen et al. (1975) reported that 65% of cases of death from septicemia were secondary to low birth weight and starvation and presumably low levels of serum antibody.

Prevention and Treatment. There is much controversy about whether small pigs that are not in excess of func-

tional teats should be fostered. However, where the small pig is in a litter with insufficient functional teats available, it needs to be transferred to a foster sow which has farrowed on the same day and which has an entire litter made up of small pigs. The foster dam also should have a teat line that is accessible to small piglets, hence gilts are favored as foster dams. If a piglet is splaylegged as well as small, a special crate or crib may be required where extra heating is provided. The crib is essentially a temperature-controlled box (30–32°C) where ill or disadvantaged piglets are kept for a limited period of time (usually less than 24 hours) to prevent them from being overlain or dying from hypoglycemia or hypothermia. While they are in the crib, piglets are fed colostrum milked from a sow during farrowing or a commercially available powdered colostrum. Svendsen et al. (1990) found that underweight pigs, both those apparently normal and weak ones, had a greater capacity for absorption of macromolecules, including colostral antibodies, than did apparently normal pigs over 1 kg. The piglets are fed 20 ml of colostrum every 1.5–2 hours using a standard human baby bottle and teat during the period staff are available. Le Dividich et al. (1994) suggested a colostral intake of 12 ml/kg/hour during the first day of life. An electrolyte and a colostrum solution is provided for the piglet to drink overnight. If they do not have a swallowing reflex (or will not drink), they can be fed using a human infant nasogastric tube (French Gauge 8, 40 cm in length). Colostrum can be obtained from the sow by injecting 1–2 ml of oxytocin intramuscularly after one or two pigs have been born; after a few minutes, colostrum can be milked into a wide-necked container and stored at 4°C or frozen until needed.

Piglets selected to be placed in the crib—for example, the small, weak, or splayleg pigs—are those with a high risk of perishing if left in the farrowing pen. Piglets that have survived overlay also respond well to a period in the crib. The rule is, "if in doubt, do not hesitate, place them in the crib." Piglets suffering from hypothermia should be warmed in a bucket of warm water (43°C) for 5–10 minutes, dried, given 20 ml of colostrum via a stomach tube, and placed in the crib.

After receiving nourishment and warmth for 24–48 hours, most piglets can be fostered back to a sow selected for having small nipples and a low teat line to ensure they can readily gain access to milk. Using these approaches small, weak piglet mortality can be reduced to 10–20%, compared with 40–60% under normal husbandry practices.

Neonatal Hemorrhagic Anemia

Spicer et al. (1986a) reported that of 2224 live-born piglets from 238 litters, 4.8% were born anemic (as determined clinically by skin pallor) or became anemic shortly after birth as a result of navel cord bleeding. The preweaning mortality of anemic piglets was 35%, compared with 10% for the remainder of the population.

Anemia was the primary cause of death in 75% of cases and was a major predisposing factor in the death of the remainder. In subsequent studies, using packed-cell volume (PCV) as an indicator, it was found that 6.8% of piglets were anemic (PCV <20%), and 30% of litters had at least one anemic piglet. Statistical analysis indicated that there was a familial effect (Connaughton et al. 1986; Spicer et al. 1986a). Factors contributing to piglet anemia include deficiency of vitamins K or C; toxicity due to mycotoxins, pentachlorophenol, and warfarin; isoimmune thrombocytopenic purpura and isoimmune hemolytic anemia; eperythrozoonosis; and anemia in the sow. Muirhead and Alexander (1997) report that periparturient anoxia will result in excessive retention of blood in the placenta at birth. Martelli et al. (1989) reported that the propensity to bleed is due to a hypofibrinogenemia. Penny (1980) cited data showing that some pale pigs have below-normal levels of platelets. These effects may follow blood loss and the consequent platelet dilution, which accompanies movement of extracellular fluid into the vascular compartment.

Necropsy Findings. Often the umbilical cord is large and fleshy. The skin, muscles, mucous membranes, and internal organs are pale. There is no evidence of internal bleeding, which allows differentiation from pale overlain pigs. PCVs as low as 5% have been recorded.

Treatment. Piglets at risk of bleeding can be identified by their large fleshy umbilical cords; there is also excessive blood on the floor of the farrowing pen. The umbilical cord should be ligated as soon as possible in these pigs. Because they appear to bleed for longer than normal pigs, tail docking and ear notching should be left until 10–14 days of age. Iron is best given orally or in drinking water because excessive bleeding from the injection site follows intramuscular injection. Physical stress of handling should be avoided, for this may greatly increase the tissue demand for oxygen and acute cardiac failure may ensue.

Splayleg

Piglets with splayleg assume a posture in which the hindlimbs or all four legs are laterally extended (Ward 1978). Splayleg is usually evident within 2–4 hours of birth, and the problem has resolved in piglets that survive to 5 days of age. One or several pigs in a litter are usually affected but on occasions the whole litter may be affected. According to van der Heyde et al. (1989), splayleg occurred more often in large than in small litters, with a remarkable breakpoint at eight piglets, and was more than twice as common in male as in female piglets.

Spicer et al. (1986a) demonstrated that splayleg occurred in 5.5% of piglets born alive, and 24% of these died. This is higher than the 0.5% incidence reported by Ward (1978). In the former study afflicted piglets were unable to compete with littermates and died of starva-

tion, hypoglycemia, hypothermia, or overlaying. The death rate was higher (66% vs. 24%) in pigs with both fore- and hindlimbs affected. The average age at death (2.6 days) was similar to that of small weak pigs (2.3 days). There was a greater incidence of splayleg from older sows (0.8/litter) than gilts (0.1/litter).

Splayleg piglets were generally lighter than average (1.20 ± 0.07 kg) and took longer than average to obtain a first suck. Those that survived to weaning had a reduced growth rate to weaning. Offspring from Landrace boars had a 13.7% incidence of splayleg, compared with 4.5% for Large White boars and 3.4% for hybrid boars (P <0.01). Ward (1978) states that in Britain the disease is particularly prevalent within the Landrace and Large White breeds. Identical matings do not always result in splayleg piglets being born (Dobson 1968). The etiology of splayleg is multifactorial, comprising genetic and environmental components (Ward 1978). Slippery floors are an important predisposing environmental factor in the development of splayleg (Kohler et al. 1969). Deficiencies of choline and thiamine may result in splayleg, as does the presence of zearalenone mycotoxin in sow feed, but correction of these problems does not universally eliminate the abnormality.

Treatment and Prevention. The standard treatment for splayleg is to tape (electricians insulating tape) the legs 2–3 cm apart so that they cannot abduct further than in the normal standing position. Where the hindlimbs extend forward beneath the animal after taping, a strip of tape is attached to the middle of the first tape and taken back over the tail to join to a third strip encircling the body in the flank region. A variation of this favored by Gadd (2003) is to tape the hindlimbs in normal position, but to then tape the legs to the body, slightly to one side by placing the tape around the body and the legs just anterior to the pelvis. The animal is left like this for 3–4 hrs and the body tape removed. The theory is that in struggling to get free the muscles regain function much faster than if they are not body-taped. This method will most probably require use of a hospital crib or a creep box in the farrowing pen.

If an animal can move adequately after taping, it can be left with the sow. If, however, they still have difficulty in walking, as is often the case with small piglets that are splayed or piglets splayed in both front and back legs, they need to be transferred to a crib to avoid starvation and crushing. Provision of sows' colostrum is important. Burrin et al. (1995) detected a nonnutrient component of colostrum that has an effect on muscle protein synthesis. By 3–4 days of age the problem has usually resolved. This coincides with the disappearance of histological signs of myofibrillar hypoplasia.

Savaging

Spicer et al. (1986a) found that savaging accounted for 11% of mortalities and was confined predominantly to gilt litters. This is consistent with the finding that a high proportion of gilts attempt to savage at least their first piglet (English et al. 1977). A survey by Harris and Gonyou (2003) of 7 newly constructed pig farms that had exclusively gilt herds recorded that savaging deaths represented 11.2% of preweaning mortality. The proportions of gilts that savaged piglets and piglets that died from savaging varied widely between farms. Some gilts savage the entire litter. Savaging was responsible for increased mortality in piglets born outside the working hours of the piggery staff (13.7% compared with 9.7%) and was the only significant factor in this mortality difference; only 2 of the 27 piglets savaged were born during working hours (Spicer et al. 1986a). The incidence of mortality due to savaging could be reduced outside working hours of the piggery staff, if farrowing rooms were continuously lit (Harris and Gonyou 2003). During savaging the gilt will snap at any piglet that wanders into reach, behavior similar to that of savage sows toward stock people. Cronin and Smith (1992) and Cronin et al. (1994) reported that the level of savaging in gilt litters was higher when animals farrowed in a large pen without straw bedding than when animals farrowed in a standard farrowing crate (with or without straw bedding) or pen with straw bedding.

Necropsy Findings. The lesions of savaging are essentially caused by the crushing effect of the sow's teeth and jaw. In some cases savaged piglets may be difficult to distinguish from overlain pigs. However, the lesions are more focal and the skin is often broken.

Prevention. Little can be done to prevent savaging in the absence of staff. Therefore, if savaging is a problem, induced farrowing will ensure that the majority of gilts farrow when staff is present. Savage gilts may be tranquilized (1–2 mg/kg of azaperone). Piglets can be placed in a small cage in the creep area as they are born. Once farrowing is over, the piglets can be removed from the cage, and the gilt usually makes no further attempt to savage. The birth weight of savaged piglets was significantly lower than the average birth weight of pigs that survived to weaning (see Table 62.4). Gilts that savage their litters were likely to be those mated at lower body weights (Spicer et al. 1985). The lower weights at mating were due to inadequate feed intake between selection and mating of submissive pigs penned in groups of 20. The problem was overcome by periodically drafting off those animals that appeared to be losing weight. It is unusual for dams to savage more than one of their litters; therefore, there is no valid reason to cull them. However, Knap and Merks (1987) and van der Steen et al. (1988) indicate that it is possible to select against aggressiveness in sows. The selection of boars and gilts from mothers with normal behavior will probably be the most efficient procedure.

Pneumonia

Pneumonia is responsible for the death of around 1% of all live-born piglets (Fahmy and Bernard 1971; Bille et al. 1975; Spicer et al. 1986a). The pneumonia is primarily a bronchopneumonia, and gilt litters are more often affected than sow litters. Bille et al. (1975) found a higher incidence in winter, but the pneumonia was unrelated to the indoor climate or level of hygiene. In most cases, only one pig per litter was affected, with an average incidence of 10% per litter. Organisms isolated include *Streptococcus* spp., *Bordetella bronchiseptica, Pasteurella* spp., *Moraxella* spp., *Escherichia coli*, and *Arcanobacterium pyogenes* (Bille et al. 1975), and *Staphylococcus aureus, Pasteurella multocida, Pseudomonas aeruginosa,* and *Citrobacter freundii* (Spicer et al. 1986a).

In a study of pneumonia in 55 baby pigs, Kott (1983) isolated *Haemophilus parasuis, Mycoplasma hyorhinis,* and *Bordetella bronchiseptica*. Pleuropneumonia due to *Actinobacillus pleuropneumoniae* has been reported by Bille et al. (1975) and Cameron and Kelly (1979). Septicemia due to the same organism has been reported in suckling pigs (Thomson and Ruhnke 1965).

Although *Mycoplasma hyopneumoniae* infections are commonly thought to begin in weaned pigs, the organism has been reported from pneumonic suckling pigs; however, microbiological evidence that it is common in such lesions has not been forthcoming (Ross 1986).

Treatment and Prevention. With low mortality levels treatment is probably not a practical procedure due to the difficulty of identifying the affected animals. However, where the problem exceeds a 1% level of mortality, injecting gilts at farrowing with an appropriate antibiotic to lower excretion rate may be warranted. Ensuring piglets adequate access to colostrum is recommended, for the low incidence of the disease and its occurrence in predominantly gilt litters suggest that lack of specific antibodies is a major contributing factor.

Generalized Infections and Septicemia

Field data indicate that as many as 2% of the piglet population die of septicemia (Driesen 1990). Affected piglets were all less than 48 hours of age. Nielsen et al. (1975) surveyed 28,000 live-born pigs and found that 2.1% died from septicemia, 37% of which were primary septicemias, and the remainder were secondary to low-birth-weight starvation or preceding illness; 44% of mortalities occurred before 3 days of age. In a study by Spicer et al. (1986a), septicemias in the first week of life were a secondary manifestation of other causes of mortalities. However, generalized infection was responsible for most deaths in the second and third week of life. Organisms isolated and associated conditions included *Actinobacillus suis*: septicemia, arthritis, peritonitis, and meningitis; *Citrobacter freundii*: septicemia, meningitis, alpha-hemolytic streptococci septicemia: arthritis and meningitis; *E. coli*: septicemia and peritonitis. Glastonbury (1977) and Nielsen et al. (1975) found that *E. coli* and beta-hemolytic streptococci were the most common causes of septicemia in dead suckling pigs.

A major predisposing factor in generalized infection would appear to be the quantity and specificity of maternal antibodies absorbed by piglets. In this regard Nielsen et al. (1975) found (1) a significantly higher incidence in piglets of sows with mastitis and agalactia, (2) an increase in mortality from septicemia with larger litters, (3) a higher incidence in open versus closed herds, and (4) a higher incidence in winter.

Necropsy Findings. Often excess fluid and small amounts of fibrin are found in the serous cavities. Lungs may be edematous and fail to collapse. Jaundice, subserosal petechial hemorrhage, and mild dehydration may be seen.

Treatment and Prevention. The most common isolates are *Streptococcus* spp. and *E. coli*; thus broad-spectrum antibiotics may be of use. Therapeutically the success rate is low (Driesen 1990), but prophylactic treatments are worthwhile. Prevention should be aimed at ensuring adequate intake of colostrum for all piglets and providing adequate heating.

Miscellaneous Causes of Death

This group includes anal atresia, cleft palate, renal hypoplasia, hydrocephalus, and accidental death and accounts for 1.2% of all pigs born alive (Spicer et al. 1986a). A summary of the prevalence of specific congenital defects of pigs is provided by Edwards and Mulley (1999). A summary of their prevalence and etiologies is presented in Table 62.6.

REDUCING PREWEANING MORTALITY

Cutler et al. (1989) reported farm studies where preweaning mortality rates were reduced by paying attention to staff training and attention to detail in the farrowing house. After an intensive period of "hands-on" staff training and demonstration, farrowing-house performance was monitored and preweaning deaths fell by 5–7%. Holyoake et al. (1995) in a study of 250 sows were able to decrease both stillbirths and preweaning deaths by inducing sows to farrow with cloprostenol (250 μg) combined with constant staff supervision from three hours before farrowing to 3 days after. Through supervision, stillbirths were decreased from 0.68 to 0.26 per litter, preweaning deaths per litter decreased from 1.26 to 0.86 and numbers weaned increased from 9.44 to 10.17 per litter. White et al. (1996) reduced preweaning mortality, including stillbirths, by approximately 44% (about a pig per litter) and increased weaning weight in pigs through attending farrowing and implementing a piglet care protocol involving provision of oxygen, drying the pigs, tying the umbilicus, bovine colostrum supplements, and placing the newborn piglets on a teat. In addition to increasing the intensity of staff training and staff awareness, the following measures provide a basis for decreasing neonatal mortality:

1. Provision of written instructions about piglet survival for staff.
2. Thorough hygiene programs for the farrowing house and processing equipment.
3. Creep areas that are draft free and comfortable. Sawdust, wood shavings, shredded paper, or straw are suitable bedding materials.

Table 62.6. Common developmental defects of swine

Defect	Prevalence	Etiology	Diagnosis
Micrencephaly	0.07%	Heat stress midpregnancy	History of heat stress
		Unknown (most cases)	An agent affecting development in early or midpregnancy
Microphthalmia		Vitamin A deficiency	Multiple defects in affected litters; heavy neonatal mortality; history; diet analysis; serum and liver vitamin A analysis
		Hog cholera (HC) infection	HC infection in herd; virus isolation; fluorescent antibody test; serology; congenital tremor AI present in herd
		Heritable	Mode of inheritance uncertain; dominant gene (?)
		Unknown	An agent affecting embryos at 12–16 days of development
Neural tube defects (anencephaly, encephalocele, hydrocephalus, spina bifida)	0.04%	Unknown	An agent affecting embryos at 12–16 days of development
		Vitamin A deficiency (hydrocephalus)	Multiple defects in affected litters; heavy neonatal mortality; history; diet analysis; serum and liver vitamin A analysis
Congenital tremor	0.20%	HC virus (type AI)	HC infection in herd; virus isolation; fluorescent antibody test; serology; affects piglets of all breeds and both sexes; hypomyelinogenesis; cerebellar hypoplasia; neurochemical analysis of myelin lipids of spinal cord; small cross-sectional area of the spinal cord
		Type AII (unidentified virus)	Hypomyelinogenesis of spinal cord; analysis of myelin lipids of spinal cord; small cross-sectional area of the spinal cord
		Type AIII	Monogenic sex-linked gene mutation in Landrace affecting only males and associated with defect in myelin sheath

(continued)

Table 62.6. Common developmental defects of swine (*continued*)

Defect	Prevalence	Etiology	Diagnosis
		Type IV	Autosomal recessive gene in Saddleback affecting both sexes
		Pseudorabies (PR) virus	PR infection in herd; virus isolation; serology
		Neguvon (metrifonate, trichlorfon)	History of dosing sows in midpregnancy; hypoplasia of cerebrum and cerebellum; Purkinje-cell loss; changes in neurotransmitters
Arthrogryposis	0.10%	Tobacco stalks, jimsonweed, poison hemlock, wild black cherry	History of exposure to plants in early to midpregnancy
		Vitamin A deficiency	Multiple defects in affected litters; heavy neonatal mortality; history; diet analysis; serum and liver vitamin A analysis
		HC attenuated vaccine virus	History of vaccination during early pregnancy
		HC infection	HC infection in herd; virus isolation; fluorescent antibody test; serology; congenital tremor AI in herd
		Paramyxovirus infection	Menangle virus infection during pregnancy
		Heritable	Recessive gene (?); autosomal recessive in Yorkshire pigs
		Unknown (most cases)	An agent affecting development in early or midpregnancy
Micromelia	0.10%	Unknown	Possibly caused by limb vascular defects in early pregnancy
Cleft palate/harelip	0.07%	Heritable	Possibly a recessive gene; cleft palate in Poland China pigs probably genetic
		Unknown (most cases)	An agent affecting development in early or midpregnancy
Deformed tail	0.08%	Possibly heritable	Mode of inheritance uncertain; occasionally urogenital defect associated
		Unknown	Often associated with motor defects in hindlimbs; vertebral defects
Myofibrillar hypoplasia	1.05%	Heritable	Most common in Landrace, less in Large White; probably polygenic mode of inheritance; incidence modified by maternal stress, slippery floor, birth weight, maternal nutrition
		Fusarium toxin	Higher mortalities than other forms; feed analysis
Inguinal hernia	0.40%	Heritable	Mode of inheritance uncertain; incidence modified by environment
Umbilical hernia	1.00%	Unknown	Possibly polygenic mode of inheritance
Anal atresia	0.40%	Heritable	Possibly polygenic inheritance or an autosomal recessive or autosomal dominant form of transmission
Hypotrichosis		Heritable in some breeds	Mode of inheritance uncertain
		Iodine deficiency	Stillbirths and high neonatal mortality; enlarged thyroids; skin edematous; feed analysis
Epitheliogenesis imperfecta	0.05%	Heritable	Possibly autosomal recessive gene; hydronephrosis associated
Dermatosis vegetans		Heritable	Autosomal recessive; associated with fatal giant-cell pneumonia
Pityriasis rosea		Probably heritable	Mode of inheritance uncertain; affects young pigs, especially Landrace; benign and self-limiting
Von Willebrand's disease		Heritable	Recessive gene in Poland China pigs; excess bleeding from minor wounds; decrease in factor VIII and platelet retention time
Navel bleeding	0.14–1.2%	Unknown	Cord is edematous, familial linkage
Cardiac defects	0.03%	Unknown	Most cases recognized at 4–8 weeks; mostly males
Cryptorchidism	0.39%	Probably heritable	Polygenic transmission; left testicle most commonly involved
Female genital hypoplasias, duplications	0.68% 0.06%	Probably a heritable component	Mode of inheritance uncertain; genital tract incomplete or duplicated
Male pseudo-hermaphroditism	0.2–0.6%	Heritable	Mode of transmission uncertain; testicles in abdomen together with female tubular tract
True herma-phroditism		Heritable	Mode of inheritance uncertain; testicular and ovarian tissues usually with female tubular tract

4. An additional heat lamp provided toward the rear of the sow during the farrowing period and for 24 hours afterward to reduce the chance of chilling newborn pigs and to provide an extra (lateral) creep area. At birth pigs can be positioned under the heater.

5. Freeing newborn pigs from placenta, drying them, clearing airways of mucus.

6. A heated crib for the care of sick pigs and to house temporarily small pigs (<800 g bodyweight) or pigs from large litters during split suckling sessions.

7. Supervision of pigs to ensure access to colostrum, or supplementation with colostrum substitutes (up to 100 ml/day) or milk replacer by bottle or stomach tube especially for small or weak pigs or for pigs in large litters.

8. An active fostering program based on cross-fostering within 48 hours of birth.

9. Regular inspection of sows and prompt treatments

10. A vaccination program against neonatal colibacillosis.

REFERENCES

Ahlmann K, Svendsen J, Bengtsson AC. 1983. Rectal Temperature of the Newborn Pig. Rep 31. Swedish Univ Agric, Lund, Sweden.

Anonymous. 1959. A survey of the incidence and causes of mortality in the pigs. 1. Sows survey. Vet Rec 71:777–786.

——. 1986. Pig production in the Netherlands. Techni-porc 9:27–28.

Baker DH, Becker DE, Norton HW. 1969. Reproductive performance and pregnancy development in swine as influenced by feed intake during gestation. J Nutr 97:489–498.

Baxter SH. 1989. Neonatal mortality: The influence of the structural environment. In Manipulating Pig Production II.JL Barnett, DP Hennessy, eds. Werribee, Aust.: Australasian Pig Sci Assoc, pp. 102–109.

Biensen NJ, Wilson ME, Ford SP. 1998. The impact of either a Meishan or Yorkshire uterus on Meishan or Yorkshire fetal and placental development to days 70, 90 and 110 of gestation. J Anim Sci 76:2169–2176.

Bilkei-Papp G, Papp GB. 1994. Perinatal losses—General condition of sows. III. Experiences obtained with prednisolone pretreatment. Magyar Allat Lapja 49:680–683.

Bille N, Larsen JL, Svendsen J, Nielsen NC. 1975. Preweaning mortality in pigs. 6. Incidence and cause of pneumonia. Nord Vet Med 27:482–495.

Bille N, Nielsen NC, Larsen JL, Svendsen J. 1974. Preweaning mortality in pigs. 1. The perinatal period. Nord Vet Med 26:294–313.

Blecha F, Kelley KW. 1981. Cold stress reduces the acquisition of colostral immunoglobulin in piglets. J Anim Sci 52:595–600.

Bostedt H, Rudloff PR. 1983. Prophylactic administration of the beta-blocker carazolol to influence the duration of parturition in sows. Theriogenology 20:191–196.

Burrin DG, Davis TA, Ebner S, Schoknecht PA, Fiorotto ML, Reeds PJ, McAvoy S. 1995. Nutrient-independent and nutrient-dependent factors stimulate protein synthesis in colostrum-fed newborn pigs. Pediatric Res 37:593–599.

Cameron RDA, Kelly NR. 1979. An outbreak of porcine pleuropneumonia due to *Haemophilus parahaemolyticus*. Aust Vet J 55:389–390.

Cleary GVC, Philip G, McElhone C. 2003. PigStats 2002. In Australian Pig Industry Handbook, p. 21.

Close WH. 1992. Thermoregulation in piglets: Environmental and metabolic consequences. Neonatal survival growth. Occasional Publ—Brit Soc Anim Prod 15:25–33.

Coalson JA, Lecce JG. 1973. Influence of nursing intervals on changes in serum proteins (immunoglobulins) in neonatal pigs. J Anim Sci 36:381–385.

Connaughton ID, Driesen SJ, Williamson PL, Fahy VA. 1986. The Pale Pig Syndrome. Aust Adv Vet Sci, p. 120.

Cromwell GL, Hall DD, Clawson AJ, Combs GE, Knabe DA, Maxwell CV, Noland PR, Orr DE, Prince TJ. 1989. Effects of additional feed during late gestation on reproductive performance of sows: A cooperative study. J Anim Sci 67:3–14.

Cronin GM Dunsmore B, Leeson E. 1998. The effects of farrowing nest size and width on sow and piglet behaviour and piglet survival. Appl Anim Behav Sci 60:331–345.

Cronin GM, Schirmer BN, McCallum TH, Smith JA, Butler KL. 1993. The effects of providing sawdust to pre-parturient sows in farrowing crates on sow behaviour, the duration of parturition and the occurrence of intra-partum stillborn piglets. Appl Anim Behav Sci 36:301–315.

Cronin GM, Smith JA. 1992. Effects of accommodation type and straw bedding around parturition and during lactation on the behaviour of primiparous sows and survival and growth of piglets to weaning. Appl Anim Behav Sci 33:190–208.

Cronin GM, Smith JA, Hodge FM, Hemsworth PH. 1994. The behaviour of primiparous sows around farrowing in response to restraint and straw bedding. Appl Anim Behav Sci 39:269–280.

Cutler RS, Prime RW. 1988. Reducing stillbirths in pigs. Aust Adv Vet Sci, pp. 111–113.

Cutler RS, Spicer EM, Prime RW. 1989. Neonatal mortality: The influence of management. In Manipulating Pig Production II. JL Barnett, DP Hennessy, eds. Werribee, Aust.: Australasian Pig Sci Assoc, pp. 122–126.

Curtis SE. 1970. Environmental-thermoregulatory interactions and neonatal pig survival. J Anim Sci 31:576–587.

Dial G, Almond, G. W., Hilley, H. D., Repasky, R. R., and Hagen, J. 1987. Oxytocin precipitation of prostaglandin-induced farrowing in swine: Determination of the optimal dose of oxytocin and optimal interval between prostaglandin F2 and oxytocin. Am J Vet Res 48:966–970.

Dobson KJ. 1968. Congenital splayleg of piglets. Aust Vet J 44:26–28.

Driesen SJ. 1990. Intensive care systems for weak piglets: Colostrum substitute and crib system. Report to PRDC. Dep Primary Industries and Energy, Canberra, Australia.

Driesen SJ, Carland PG, Fahy VA. 1993. Studies on preweaning piglet diarrhoea. Aust Vet J 70:259–265.

Dyck GW, Swiestra EE. 1987. Causes of piglet death from birth to weaning. Can J Anim Sci 67:77–89.

Edwards MJ, Mulley RC. 1999. Genetic, congenital and neoplastic diseases. P 696. In Straw BE et al(editors). Diseases of Swine (8th Edition) Iowa State Press, Ames.

Edwards SA, Malkin SJ, Spechter HH. 1986. An analysis of piglet mortality with behavioural observations. Anim Prod 42:470.

English PR, Smith WJ. 1975. Some causes of death in neonatal pigs. Vet Annu 15:95–104.

English PR, Smith WJ, Maclean A. 1977. The Sow—Improving Her Efficiency. Ipswich, U.K.: Farming Press.

Evangelista JNB, Daza A, Gutierrez-Barquin MG. 1996. Mortality of piglets at birth: Factors of variation. Proc Int Pig Vet Soc 14:617.

Fahmy MH, Bernard C. 1971. Causes of mortality in Yorkshire pigs from birth to 20 weeks of age. Can J Anim Sci 51:351–359.

Fahy VA, Driesen S, Moore K, Holyoake T. 2003. Diagnosing the cause of scour in sucker and weaner pigs. In Proc Aust Assoc Pig Vet, Adelaide, pp 149–156.

Fraser D. 1975. The "teat order" of suckling pigs: II. Fighting during suckling and the effects of clipping the eye teeth. J Agric Sci Camb 84:393–399.

Friendship RM, Wilson MR, McMillan I. 1986. Management and housing factors associated with piglet preweaning mortality. Can Vet J 27:307–311.

Gadd J. 2003. Pig Production Problems (1st Ed) Nottingham University Press, United Kingdom, pp. 376–379.

Glastonbury JRW. 1976. A survey of preweaning mortality in the Pig. Aust Vet J 52:272–276.

——. 1977. Preweaning mortality in the pig: Pathological findings in piglets dying between birth and weaning. Aust Vet J 53:310–314.

Gonzalez AC, Necchinacce H, Diaz I. 1987. A comparison of some production traits in gilts and sows. In Informe Anual Inst Prod Anim, Univ Cent Venezuela, pp. 127–128.

Guthrie HD, Meckley PE, Young EP, Hartsock TG. 1987. Effect of altrenogest and lutalyse on parturition control, plasma progesterone, unconjugated estrogen and 13,14-dihydro-15 keto-prostaglandin $F_{2\alpha}$ in sows. J Anim Sci 65:203.

Harris MJ, Gonyou HW. 2003. Savaging behaviour in domestic gilts: A study of seven commercial farms. Can J Anim Sci 83:435–444.

Hartsock TG, Graves HB, Baumgardt BR. 1977. Agonistic behavior and the nursing order in suckling piglets: Relationships with survival, growth and body composition. J Anim Sci 44:320–330.

Hay M Rue J, Sansac C, Brunel G, Prunier A. 2004. Long-term detrimental effects of tooth clipping or grinding in piglets: A histological approach. Anim Welfare 13:27–32.

Hemsworth PH, Pedersen V, Cox M, Cronin GM Coleman GJ. 1999. A note on the relationship between the behavioural response of lactating sows to humans and the survival of piglets. Appl Anim Behav Sci 65:43–52.

Herpin P, Le Dividich J, Hulin JC, Fillaut M, Marco F, de Bertin R. 1996. Effects of the level of asphyxia during delivery on viability at birth and early postnatal vitality of newborn pigs. J Anim Sci 74:2067–2075.

Holtz W, Welp C. 1984. Induction of parturition in sows by prostaglandin-oxytocin programs. Proc Int Pig Vet Soc 8:378.

Holyoake PK, Dial GD, Trigg, T, King VL. 1995. Reducing pig mortality through supervision during the perinatal period. J Anim Sci 73:3543–3551.

Horrell L, Bennett J. 1981. Disruption of teat preferences and retardation of growth following cross fostering of one week old pigs. Anim Prod 33:99–106.

Jones TA, Hunter EJ, Johnson P, Guise J. 2003. Non restraint farrowing system: An industry approach. Pig J 52:124–133.

Kelley KW, Blecha F, Regnier JA. 1982. Cold exposure and absorption of colostral immuno-globulins by neonatal piglets. J Anim Sci 55:365–368.

Kirkwood RN, Zak LJ, Goonewardence LA. 1998. The influence of cross fostering on piglets growth and survival. Proc Int Pig Vet Soc 15:403.

Knap PW, Merks JWM. 1987. A note on the genetics of aggressiveness of primiparous sows towards their piglets. Livest Prod Sci 17:161–167.

Kohler EM, Cross RF, Ferguson LC. 1969. Experimental induction of spraddled-legs in newborn pigs. J Am Vet Med Assoc 155:139–142.

Kott BE. 1983. Chronological studies of respiratory disease in baby pigs. M.S. thesis, Iowa State Univ., Ames.

Le Dividich J. 1999. A review: Neonatal and weaner pig management to reduce variation. In Manipulating Pig Production V11. P Cranwell, ed. Werribee: Australasian Pig Science Association, pp. 135–155.

Le Dividich J, Herpin P, Rosario Ludovino RM. 1994. Utilization of colostral energy by the newborn pig. J Anim Sci 72:2082–2089.

Le Dividich J, Noblet J. 1981. Colostrum intake and thermoregulation in the neonatal pig. Biol Neonate 40:167–174.

——. 1983. Thermoregulation and energy metabolism in the neonatal pig. Ann Rech Vet 14:375–381.

Leenhouwers, J. I., Knol, E. F., and van der Lende, T. 2002. Differences in late prenatal development as an explanation for genetic differences in piglet survival. Livest Prod Sci 78:57–62.

Libal GW, Wahlstrom RC. 1977. Effect of gestation metabolizable energy levels on sow productivity. J Anim Sci 45:286.

Luescher UA, Friendship RM, Lissemore KD, McKeown DB. 1989. Clinical ethology in food animal practice. Appl Anim Behav Sci 22:191–214.

Marcatti Neto A. 1986. Effect of crossfostering on piglet preweaning performance. Arq Brasil Med Vet Zootech 38:413–417.

Martelli P, Manotti C, Rossi L. 1989. Haemorrhagic syndrome (hypofibrinogenaemia) in piglets: Preliminary note. Sel Vet 30:1673–1677.

McCaw MB, Desrosiers R. 1997. Role of extensive cross fostering in PRRS associated disease losses of suckling and nursery pigs. In Proc Am Assoc Swine Pract, Quebec, pp. 451–453.

McGlone JJ, Widowski TM, Stricklen KD, Mitchell D, Curtis SE. 1996. Sow access to tassel prefarrowing: Preliminary evidence of stillbirth rate. J Anim Sci 74(Suppl 1):127.

Meat and Livestock Commission (MLC). 1986. Pig Year Book. U.K.: Milton Keynes.

——. 2003. Pig Year Book. U.K.: Milton Keynes.

Mellor DJ, Cockburn R. 1986. A comparison of energy metabolism in the newborn infant, piglet and lamb. Q J Exp Physiol 71:361–379.

Milligan BN, Fraser D, Kramera D. 2002. Within litter birthweight variation in the domestic pig and its relation to preweaning survival, weight gain and variation in weaning weights. Livest Prod Sci 76:181–191.

Morrison V, English PR, Lodge OA. 1983. The effect of alternative creep heating arrangements at two house temperatures on piglet lying behaviour and mortality in the neonatal period. Anim Prod 36:530–531.

Moser BD, Lewis AJ. 1981. Fat additives to sow diets—A review. Pig News Inform 2:265–269.

Mota-Rojas D, Martinez-Burnes J, Trujillo-Ortega ME, Alonso-Spilsbury ML,, Ramirez-Nechoechea R, and Lopez A. 2002. Effect of oxytocin treatment in sows on umbilical cord morphology, meconium staining and neonatal mortality of piglets. Am J Vet Res 65:1571–1574.

Muirhead MR, Alexander TJL. 1997. Managing Pig Health and The Treatment of Disease (1st ed.) United Kingdom: 5M Enterprises Ltd.,pp. 247, 272.

Nielsen NC, Christensen K, Bille N, Larsen JL. 1974. Preweaning mortality in pigs. 1. Herd investigations. Nord Vet Med 26:137.

Nielsen NC, Riising HJ, Larsen JL, Bille N, and Svendsen J. 1975. Preweaning mortality in pigs. 5. Acute septicaemia. Nord Vet Med 27:129–139.

Ogunbameru BO, Kornegay ET, Wood CM. 1991. Evaluation of methods of providing heat to newborn pigs during and after farrowing. J Anim Sci 69:3939–3944.

Olsson AC, Svendsen J. 1989. Observations at farrowing and mother-offspring interactions in different housing systems. Report 65. Swedish Univ Agric Sci, Lund, Sweden.

Penny RHC. 1980. Navel bleeding and the pale pig syndrome. Vet Annu 20:281–290.

Pere MC, Dourmad JY, Etienne M. 1997. Effect of number of embryos in the uterus on survival and development and on maternal metabolism. J Anim Sci 72:1337–1342.

Pettigrew JE. 1981. Supplemental dietary fat for peripartal sows: A review. J Anim Sci 53:107.

Pettigrew JE, Cornelius SG, Moser RL. 1986. Effects of oral doses of corn oil and other factors on preweaning survival and growth of piglets. J Anim Sci 62:601–612.

PIC UK. 1996. Comparison of indoor and outdoor herds. In Pig Management Yearbook, Incorporating Easicare and Pigtales Data. Oxfordshire, PIC UK, pp. 34–35.

Pomeroy RW. 1960. Infertility and neonatal mortality in the sow: Neonatal mortality and foetal development. J Agric Sci (U.K.) 54:31–56.

Price EO, Hutson GD, Price MI, Borgwardt R. 1994. Fostering in swine as affected by age of offspring. J Anim Sci 72:1697–1701.

Prime RW, Fahy VA, Ray W, Cutler RS, Spicer EM. 1989. On Farm Validation of Research: Lowering Preweaning Mortality in Pigs. Report to PRDC. Dep. Primary Industries and Energy, Canberra, Australia.

Quémeré P, Cousein J, Flament J, Jacob B, Michel G, Poquet P, Richard S, Sibille JC. 1993. Piglet mortality from birth to weaning, a multifactorial approach: A study of 53 farms in North Picardie and results from an experimental centre. Jour Rech Porcine France 25:113–122.

Quiniou N, Dagorn J, Gaudré D. 2002. Variation of piglets' birth weight and consequences on subsequent performance. Livest Prod Sci 78:65–70.

Randall GCB. 1978. Perinatal mortality: Some problems of adaptation at birth. Adv Vet Sci Comp Med 22:53–81.

Ravel A, D'Allaire S, Bigras-Poulin M. 1996a. Influence of management, housing and personality of the stockperson on preweaning performances on independent and integrated swine farms in Quebec. Prev Vet Med 29:37–57.

Ravel A, D'Allaire S, Bigras-Poulin M, Ward R. 1996b. Psycho-demographic profile of stockpeople working on independent and integrated swine breeding farms in Quebec. Can J Vet Res 60:241–248.

Robert S, Martineau GP, eds. 1997. Preliminary observations on the preweaning behaviour of crossfostered piglets. In Proc Am Assoc Swine Pract, Quebec, Canada, pp. 441–442.

Robert S, Thompson BK, Fraser D. 1995. Effect of selective tooth clipping on survival and growth of low-birth-weight piglets. Can J Anim Sci 75:285–289.

Robertson JF, Arey D. 1998. Teeth care for young piglets. A farm guide for the Scottish Pig Industry. Pig Husbandry Guide No. 2, Scottish Agricultural College, Craibstone, Aberdeen.

Ross RF. 1986. Mycoplasmal diseases. In Diseases of Swine, 6th ed. AD Leman, B Straw, RD Glock, WI Mengeling, RHC Penny, E Scholl, eds. Ames: Iowa State Univ Press, pp. 978–1010.

Rousseau P, Chatelier C, Dutertre C, Levêque JC. 1994. Comparaison d'un chauffage par le sol et d'un chauffage par rayonnement pour des porcelets en maternité: Résultats zootechniques et comportementaux, consommation d'énergie. Jour Rech Porcine France 26:47–54.

Schmidt GH. 1971. Biology of Lactation. San Francisco: W. H. Freeman.

Spicer EM, Driesen SJ, Fahy VA. 1986a. Causes of preweaning mortality on a large intensive piggery. Aust Vet J 65:71–75.

Spicer EM, Driesen SJ, Fahy VA, Horton BJ. 1985. Trauma-overlay and savaging of baby pigs. Aust Adv Vet Sci, p. 122.

Spicer EM, Driesen SJ, Fahy, VA, Willamson PL., Connaughton ID. 1987. Preweaning mortality in pigs. Univ Sydney, Post-Grad Comm Vet Sci Proc 95(1):979–985.

Spicer EM, Prime RW, Fahy VA. 1986b. Controlled induction of parturition in swine. Aust Adv Vet Sci, p. 119.

Stanton HC, Carroll JK. 1974. Potential mechanisms responsible for prenatal and perinatal mortality or low viability of swine. J Anim Sci 38:135–146.

Straw BE. 1997. Veterinary practice: Art, science and politics. In Proc Am Assoc Swine Pract, Quebec, pp. 1–31.

Stuart BP, Lindsay DS. 1985. Coccidiosis. In Swine Consultant. Veterinary Learning Systems.

Svendsen J, Andreasson B. 1980. Perinatal mortality in pigs: Influence of housing. Proc Int Pig Vet Soc 6:83.

Svendsen J, Bengtsson AC, Svendsen LS. 1986. Occurrence and causes of traumatic injuries in neonatal pigs. Pig News Inform 7:159–170.

Svendsen J, Bille N, Nielsen NC, Larsen JL, Riising HJ. 1975. Preweaning mortality in pigs. 4. Diseases of the gastrointestinal tract in pigs. Nord Vet Med 27:85–101.

Svendsen LS, Westrom BR, Svendsen J, Olsson AC., Karlsson BW. 1990. Intestinal macromolecular transmission in underprivileged and unaffected newborn pigs: Implication for survival of underprivileged pigs. Res Vet Sci 48:184–189.

Thodberg K, Jensen KH, Herskin MS. 2002a. Nest building and farrowing in sows: Relation to the reaction pattern during stress, farrowing environment and experience. Appl Anim Behav Sci 77:21–42.

Thodberg K, Jensen KH, Herskin MS. 2002b. Nursing behaviour, postpartum activity and reactivity in sows. Effects of farrowing environment, previous experience and temperament. Appl Anim Behav Sci 77:53–76.

Thodberg K, Jensen KH, Herskin MS, Jørgensen E. 1999. Influence of environmental stimuli on nest building and farrowing behaviour in domestic sows. Appl Anim Behav Sci 65:131–144.

Thomson RG, Ruhnke L. 1965. Haemophilus septicaemia in piglets. Can Vet J 4:271–275.

van der Heyde H, De Mets JP, Porreye L, Henderickx H, Calus A, Bekaert H, Buysse F. 1989. Influence of season, litter size, parity, gestation length, birth weight, sex and farrowing pen on frequency of congenital splayleg in piglets. Livest Prod Sci 21:143–155.

van der Lende T, Hazeleger W, de Jager D. 1990. Weight distribution within litters at the early foetal stage and at birth in relation to embryonic mortality in the pig. Livest Prod Sci 26: 53–65.

van der Steen HAM, Schaeffer LR, De Jong H, and De Groot PN. 1988. Aggressive behavior of sows at parturition. J Anim Sci 66:271–279.

Vieuille C, Berger F, le Pape G., Bellanger D. 2003. Sow behaviour involved in the crushing of piglets in outdoor farrowing huts— A brief report. Appl Anim Behav Sci 80:109–115.

Walker PM, Knox RV, Webel SK. 1996. Comparison of selected floor and farrowing crate designs on measures of sow productivity. J Anim Sci 74(Suppl 1):128.

Ward PS. 1978. The splayleg syndrome in newborn pigs: A review. Vet Bull 4:279–295.

Weary DM, Fraser D. 1999. Partial tooth-clipping of suckling pigs: Effects on neonatal competition and facial injuries. Appl Anim Behav Sci 65:21–27.

Weber R. 1997. New farrowing pens without confinement of the sow. *In* R. W. Bottcher and S. J. Hoff (eds). Livestock Environment V. Vol 1. Minneapolis, Minnesota: Amer Soc Agric Engineers, pp. 280–286.

Welch AR, Baxter MR. 1986. Responses of newborn pigs to thermal and tactile properties of their environment. Appl Anim Behav Sci 15:203–215.

Welp C, Jochle W, Holtz W. 1984. Induction of parturition in swine with a prostaglandin analog and oxytocin: A trial involving dose of oxytocin and parity. Theriogenology 22:509–520.

Werhahn E, Klobasa F, Butler JE. 1981. Investigation of some factors which influence the absorption of IgG by the neonatal piglet. Vet Immunol Immunopathol 2:35–51.

White KR, Anderson DM, Bate LA. 1996. Increasing piglet survival through an improved farrowing management protocol. Can J Anim Sci 76:491–495.

Wilkinson FC, Blackshaw JK. 1987. Do day old piglets need to have their teeth clipped? In Manipulating Pig Production; Proc. Inaug. Conf. Australasian Pig Science Assoc., Albury NSW, Nov. 23–25, 1987. JL Barnett et al., eds. Werribee: Australasian Pig Science Association.

Wilson MR. 1984. Synchronisation of farrowing using a combination of oxytocin and prostaglandin administration: An aid to piglet survival rates. Proc Int Pig Vet Soc 8:279.

Xin H, Bundy DS, Zhou, H. 1996. Comparison of 250W versus 175W radiant heat lamps for swine farrowing operation. Iowa Swine Unit, Swine Research Report, Ames, Iowa, pp. 129–132.

Zerobin K. 1980. Possibilities to influence the motility of the uterus during parturition and during puerperium in swine. Proc Int Pig Vet Soc 6:26.

Zerobin K, Kundig P. 1980. The control of myometrial function during parturition with a B2 mimetic compound Planipart (clenbuterol). Theriogenology 14:21–35.

Ziron M., Hoy S. 2003. Effect of a warm and flexible piglet nest heating system—the warm water bed—on piglet behaviour, liveweight management and skin lesions. Appl Anim Behav Sci 80:9–18.

63 Longevity in Breeding Animals

Sylvie D'Allaire and Richard Drolet

Poor sow longevity in commercial breeding herds can lead to economic inefficiency and animal welfare concerns. Thus effective culling strategies should be an essential part of herd health management. Culling policies influence herd economic performance in many different ways. A high sow turnover is generally associated with a shift toward younger females, which are less productive, and with an increase in the number of nonproductive sow days. A high removal rate requires larger replacement gilt pools, which will increase disease risks and the cost of production. Difficulty in supplying replacement animals may also lead to a suboptimum population that will decrease the herd output and disrupt pig flow. On the other hand, an excessively low removal rate, will be associated with a higher proportion of older sows, which are more prone to certain diseases and may have lower production levels.

Evaluation of a culling program should include determination of the average longevity in the herd, reasons for culling and death, nonproductive days associated with removal, lifetime productivity, and risk factors for poor longevity.

MEASURES OF LONGEVITY

Determining the average longevity of animals is the first step in assessing a herd culling program, and several measures have been used to define sow longevity: removal rate, culling rate, replacement rate, percent gilts in the herd, mean parity of females in inventory, and mean parity at removal. Others have proposed the use of more economic indicators, such as pigs weaned per day of life or number of herd days per pig weaned (Culbertson and Mabry 1995; Lucia 1997).

The term "removal rate" covers all types of removal, including culling, natural death, and euthanasia. This rate is defined as the number of animals removed from the herd during a year, divided by the average inventory, and multiplied by 100. Culling and death rates should be analyzed separately; in some instances, the number of euthanasias, which are usually included in the mortality, should also be assessed. Annual removal rates of 35–55% for sows have been reported in different surveys (Dagorn and Aumaitre 1979; Pattison et al. 1980a; Friendship et al. 1986; D'Allaire et al. 1987; Dijkhuisen et al. 1989; Marsh et al. 1992; Paterson et al. 1997a; Boyle et al. 1998).

Because these values represent average rates, higher or lower rates may be found on individual farms, ranging from 20% to 70%. However, high removal rates seem to be more frequent than excessively low rates. A target of 39–40% is recommended: 35–36% for culling and 3–5% for death (Muirhead 1976; Dial et al. 1992). Target values should be adjusted for individual farms, because the removal rate is influenced by many factors, such as herd size, genetic turnover desired, breeds, definition of the average inventory, and population dynamics. Higher rates are to be expected for seed stock herds to ensure genetic improvement and to reduce the genetic lag for commercial producers. Market trends and economic conditions also influence a producer's culling decision and timing (Brandt et al. 1999; Stalder et al. 2004).

A breed difference in longevity has been observed by some authors, with Yorkshire and Large White sows having longer lifetimes than Landrace sows (Dagorn and Aumaitre 1979; Kangasniemi 1996). Others have found no difference between these breeds (Cederberg and Jonsson 1996). In general, purebred sows are less robust than hybrid sows (Kangasniemi 1996; Sehested and Schjerve 1996; Jorgensen 2000); however, this finding might be confounded by the genetic selection occurring in nucleus herds. Nevertheless, several researchers have reported heritability estimates for longevity ranging from 0.05–0.27 (Tholen et al. 1996; Lopez-Serrano et al. 2000; Yazdi et al. 2000; Fortin and Cue 2002). A difference of almost one parity at removal was observed between some genetic lines (Rodriguez-Zas et al. 2003). Collectively these results indicate that selection of a source of breeding stock might impact the producer's ability to improve sow longevity.

Comparisons of sow removal rates between herds or studies are often difficult because the definition of "average female inventory" may be different. The inventory may refer to sows only or to sows and gilts, with gilts being introduced at different times in their production cycle. For a better standardization of terminology, it has been suggested that only mated females be considered in the calculation of the annual removal rate. On some farms, however, culling of gilts introduced into the breeding herd but not yet mated is very high and may require more investigation.

The annual removal rate for the herd is also influenced by specific circumstances, such as a change in the inventory, a change in the culling policies, and the average length of the lactation period. A decrease in the inventory will increase the culling rate for the corresponding year; conversely, an increase in the inventory may decrease the rate if the producer culls less extensively in order to increase the number of females. On some farms, an involuntary cycle is established in culling patterns. For example, a producer realizes that the herd is getting older and reacts by culling more extensively that year. The following year, the rate may be lower because a large proportion of the herd is now very young. This is not counterproductive in itself but it makes production planning more difficult and herd output less constant. Information on such changes in culling policies is needed to evaluate a program. A cycle in culling patterns may also occur in newly established or repopulated herds.

The average length of lactation for the herd may also influence the annual removal rate. Herds with shorter lactation periods tend to have higher removal or death rates even though the mean parity at culling is similar (D'Allaire et al. 1989; Paterson et al. 1997a; Koketsu 2000). A reasonable explanation is that the number of litters per sow per year is higher when the lactation period is shorter. Because a sow has a certain probability of being removed during each farrow-to-farrow interval, more farrowings per year result in a higher annual probability of being removed.

Longevity of sows in the herd can also be evaluated by the replacement rate, which is defined as the total number of animals entering the herd divided by the average inventory and multiplied by 100. The removal rate and replacement rate should be similar in a stable herd if the inventory remains constant. However, in a herd undergoing expansion, the replacement rate may be higher than the removal rate. Conversely, when reduction in herd size occurs, the replacement rate may be lower than the removal rate. Therefore, population dynamics should be considered when analyzing these rates.

The mean parity of sows at removal indicates the average length of time that sows stay in the herd; however, because the mean can be influenced by extreme values, a parity distribution of removed sows is usually more in-

formative. Breeding-life expectancy is low in most swine breeding herds. Several studies reveal that the average parity at removal is between 2 and 5.6, but it can vary from 2 to 8 for a particular herd (Arganosa et al. 1981b; D'Allaire et al. 1987; Stein et al. 1990; Pedersen 1996; Koketsu et al. 1999; Lucia et al. 2000). Sows are removed from breeding herds at a very young age considering that the "natural" longevity would most likely be 12–15 years (Pond and Mersmann 2001).

A high proportion of females are removed in their early parities. Gilts and first-parity females often represent a large proportion of the cullings, with percentages of up to 40%. Considerable losses are involved with such high removals of young females (see section on "Effects of Sow Longevity on Herd Productivity"). Many authors have reported that from 50–69% of the removals occur before the fourth litter (Dagorn and Aumaitre 1979; Arganosa et al. 1981b; D'Allaire et al. 1987; Kangasniemi 1996; Lucia 1997; Paterson et al. 1997a). The probability of being removed is highest for parity 7 and over, followed by parities 0 and 1 (Tiranti et al. 2004). The risk of being removed for some specific reason is also different among parity groups; for example, there is a higher risk of culling for reproductive and locomotor problems in first-parity females and for inadequate performance and old age in advanced-parity sows (Lucia et al. 1996; Paterson et al. 1997a, b; Boyle et al. 1998).

The parity distribution of the herd is also useful to evaluate the longevity, because it indicates when the sows are more likely to be removed. As stated by Dial et al. (1992), it is difficult to recommend a standard parity distribution. The optimum parity distribution for litter size on one farm may be different from that on another farm, considering the breed, the cost of replacement, the type of facilities, and the husbandry skills. The relationship among parities should, however, be optimized to achieve an ideal parity distribution. To obtain an optimum herd maturity, 90% of the gilts that are started in the herd should reach parity 1, and 90% of the parity 1 animals should reach parity 2 (Leman 1992). Other optimal parity distributions of females in commercial breeding herds have been suggested (Table 63.1). To achieve these targets, it is imperative to limit the culling of younger females from the herd.

REASONS FOR REMOVING SOWS

Sows are culled when they are considered unsuitable for further production. A knowledge of the reasons for removal can be beneficial in identifying underlying diseases or management problems. The list of reasons can be as complete as desired, but for the purpose of data analysis, the reasons should be summarized according to a few categories. Although the classification of reasons has varied between studies, there is reasonable agreement and detailed information to allow regrouping and comparison of reasons. Data from different studies reveal

Table 63.1.   Recommendations for optimal parity distribution[a]

Source	Parity								
	0	1	2	3	4	5	6	7	>7
Parsons et al. 1990	30	23	19	14	10	5	2	1	0
Muirhead and Alexander 1997	17	15	14	13	12	11	10	5	3
Morrison et al. 2002	19.1	16.5	16.9	14.1	10.2	8.2	5.1	4.9	4.9

[a]Values within a row indicate the percentage of females that should be in each parity group.

a general pattern of removal in which reproductive failure is the main reason for culling, followed by old age, inadequate performance, locomotor problems, death, and milking problems (Table 63.2). The culling pattern, however, varies slightly over time and according to the country. The predominant causes of removal may also vary among herds and among parities.

Some authors have used the terms "voluntary" (planned) and "involuntary" (unplanned) removal. A strict definition is difficult; ultimately all removals except death are voluntary. In general voluntary removal refers to culling for old age, inadequate performance, poor progeny, and poor milking, for which the producer makes the decision concerning the cause and the time of removal. Involuntary removal refers to other causes, such as locomotor and reproductive problems, for which the producer does not have as much control. Voluntary culling allows minimization of nonproductive days and better planning of the introduction of replacement animals.

Reasons for removal can be analyzed according to two rates: a proportionate rate, which is the percentage of all removals attributable to a specific reason, and a reason-specific removal rate (D'Allaire 1987). The proportionate rate is useful in indicating the relative importance of a given reason in the total culling picture and helps in determining priorities for improving the herd. The reason-specific removal rate is defined as the number of animals removed for a specific reason divided by the average inventory, multiplied by 100, and measures the annual probability of an animal being removed for that specific reason and indicates the extent of a problem. This latter rate is more informative and is not influenced as much by the number of animals removed for other reasons as the proportionate rate is. As an example, two herds, A and B, both have 15% of their removals due to death (proportionate rate). Herds A and B have an annual removal rate of 20% and 60%, respectively. In herd A, the removal rate for death (reason-specific removal rate) is acceptable, at 3% (20% × 15%); in herd B, this rate is three times higher, at 9% (60% × 15%), although the percentage of all removals for this reason is identical. Unfortunately, in most of the literature, only the proportionate rate is used. In Table 63.3, the average and range of reason-specific removal rates and the mean parity at removal are reported for seven reasons.

Reproductive Failure

Reproductive failure is used to define a variety of conditions: no observed puberty in gilts, no observed postweaning estrus, regular and irregular returns to estrus, negative pregnancy diagnosis, failure to farrow, and abortion. Reproductive failure is the predominant reason for culling, representing between 13% and 49% of all removals. The greatest number of nonproductive days since the last weaning is observed for this category (Paterson et al. 1997a). Thus, good reproductive management with an increased awareness of the reproductive state of each sow at all times should be emphasized.

Table 63.2.   Reasons for removing sows and percentage of removals for each reason: Results obtained from 16 studies involving more than one herd

Source	Reproductive Failure	Old Age	Inadequate Performance	Locomotor Problems	Death	Other	No. of Herds or Sows	Country
Lucia et al. 2000	33.6	8.7	20.6	13.2	7.4	16.4	7973 sows	USA
Boyle et al. 1998	29.8	31.3	11.1	11.3	7.4	9.1	25 herds	Ireland
Paterson et al. 1997a	40.3	13.6	4.4	17.6	9.3	15.1	21 herds	Australia
Kangasniemi 1996	28.2	16.8	14.4	13.5	3.2	23.9	1224 herds	Finland
Pedersen 1996	34.5	18.8	4.6	6.1	12.3	23.7	4471 sows	Denmark
Stein et al. 1990	29.6	11.1	9.4	11.0	10.7	28.2	774 sows	USA
Dijkhuizen et al. 1989	34.2	11.0	20.1	10.5	NA	24.2	12 herds	Netherlands
D'Allaire et al. 1987	32.4	16.8	14.0	8.9	11.6	16.3	7242 sows	USA
Friendship et al. 1986	25.8	18.4	14.9	10.2	4.1	26.6	22 herds	Canada
Joo and Kang 1981	32.6	16.7	15.7	9.7	NA	25.3	6 herds	Korea
Stone 1981	12.9	33.4	20.6	14.0	NA	19.1	140 herds	Canada
Jossé et al. 1980	49.1	13.8	4.2	10.6	NA	22.2	593 sows	France
Pattison et al. 1980a	37.5	24.4	13.8	11.8	NA	12.5	60 herds	England
Dagorn and Aumaitre 1979	39.2	27.2	8.4	8.8	6.5	9.9	5118 herds	France
Karlberg 1979	31.3	10.1	8.0	19.7	3.8	27.1	75 herds	Norway
Svendsen et al. 1975	41.4	2.9	16.7	9.7	11.9	17.4	9 herds	Denmark

Note: NA = not available.

Table 63.3. Average and range of reason-specific removal rates and average parity at removal

Removal Reasons	Study A[a]		Study B[b]	
	Reason-Specific Removal Rate (%)	Average Parity at Removal	Reason-Specific Removal Rate (%)	Average Parity at Removal
Reproductive failure	21.3 (5.5–42.0)	2.66	15.1 (0.0–49.5)	2.37
Old age	7.2 (3.0–15.4)	7.32	7.1 (0.0–40.6)	7.11
Inadequate performance	2.3 (0.0–6.2)	4.32	7.7 (0.0–28.0)	5.11
Locomotor problems	9.3 (1.9–14.1)	3.06	4.1 (0.0–18.7)	2.93
Death	5.0 (2.0–8.4)	3.13	5.5 (0.0–14.3)	3.40
Various diseases	3.5 (1.0–5.4)	3.38	0.9 (0.0–30.7)	2.76
Miscellaneous	4.5 (0.0–15.7)	4.14	8.5 (0.0–41.3)	3.13
Total	52.8 (35.3–68.3)	3.71	48.6 (14.5–85.1)	3.77

[a]Study A involved 19 Australian herds with 9096 removed females, including mated gilts. Adapted from Paterson et al. 1996, 1997a.
[b]Study B involved 89 American herds with 7242 females, including selected but unmated gilts. Adapted from D'Allaire et al. 1987.

Young females are more likely than older sows to be culled for reproductive failure (Dagorn and Aumaitre 1979; D'Allaire et al. 1987; Dijkhuizen et al. 1989; Stein et al. 1990; Lucia 1997; Paterson et al. 1997a). The average number of litters produced by these culled sows is between two and four. Inefficient estrous detection, mating at an early age, improper male stimulation, use of young boars that are less mature and can more easily be overused, improper nutrition, infectious or toxic agents, management practices, and environment may be responsible for these high levels of culling for reproductive failure in young females. Older sows that have stayed in the herd also have undergone a selection process and may be less prone to reproductive failure.

Failure to conceive, to maintain pregnancy, or to farrow after a successful mating are the major problems reported. The risk of being removed for failure to farrow was greatest for parity 0 sows (Paterson et al. 1997a). Females that did not conceive are often found only late into their presumed gestation. Sows culled for return to estrus stayed in the herd for an average of 75–79 days, whereas sows removed because they failed to farrow remained for 121–132 days after weaning (Pattison et al. 1980a; Paterson et al. 1997a). It is important to decrease this period of nonproductive days, for it is very costly because of the extra feed and labor required as well as the underutilization of production facilities. To decrease this period, management must differentiate between late loss of pregnancy and late detection of nonpregnant females; these two variables indicate different problems that necessitate different solutions on a farm.

The proportion of females culled because they do not exhibit estrus either at puberty or at weaning is lower than that of sows failing to conceive. However, gilts and first-parity sows are more likely to be removed for anestrus than older sows (Lucia 1997; Paterson et al. 1997a). The acceptable period between introduction or weaning and mating differs among farms and may be partly responsible for the variation in proportion of animals culled. The length of the period allowed is worth investigating; on some farms it might be too short, especially for younger females, which usually have a longer interval from weaning to breeding, thus unnecessarily increasing the number culled. Comparing farmers' decisions to cull with economic model recommendations, Dijkhuizen et al. (1989) found that females culled for absence of estrus were removed too early from the herd, particularly the younger and high-producing sows. The calculated allowable interval from weaning to removal averages 66 days for first-parity sows, whereas the actual interval was 36 days. Abortions do not seem to be a major reason for removal, generally representing less than 3% of all cullings, except in herds experiencing an outbreak of porcine reproductive and respiratory syndrome (PRRS).

When the proportion of culling for reproductive failure is high, a slaughter check may be useful to compare the reasons given by the producer and the physiologic status of the reproductive tracts. Josse et al. (1980) examined 338 reproductive tracts and compared the findings with the reasons for culling reported by producers. The reason for removal could not be substantiated in 36% of the cases. Einarsson et al. (1974) found similar results in a study of genital organs in gilts: of 54 gilts culled for anestrus, 23 had apparently active corpora lutea and 2 were pregnant. Possible explanations for these discrepancies are inefficient estrous detection or pregnancy testing, silent heat, or physiologic changes occurring between the decision of culling and slaughtering.

Old Age

Old age is often the second most likely reason for removal, accounting for 3 to 33% of all removals; the average parity at culling varies between 7 and 9. As the proportion of sows removed for other reasons decreases, the percentage of sows culled because of old age increases. Overlappings between "old age" and "inadequate performance" are likely to occur, for old sows may experience a decrease in productivity. Old age is relative; some producers routinely cull sows as soon as the fifth or sixth parity, and others only after the tenth litter. Some researchers suggest culling older sows when productivity in terms of live-born pigs is comparable with that of gilts. This method, however, takes into account only the number of live-born pigs. According to a model developed by Dijkhuizen et al. (1986), the economic optimal herd life for average-producing sows is generally 10 parities. Rarely is it economically beneficial to cull sows before parity 8, considering the economic losses associated with the cost of replacement, the lower litter size and farrowing rate, and the longer interval from weaning to mating in younger sows. Their model took into account the annual replacement rate, the average parity of farrowing and removed sows, the average slaughter price of culled sows, and the cost of replacement gilts.

Inadequate Performance

This category includes a variety of reasons: small litter size at farrowing or weaning, high preweaning mortality, and low piglet birth or weaning weights. Inadequate performance is usually ranked as the second or third most common reason for culling sows, with a range of 4–21% of removals attributable to this category. Pomeroy (1960) reported that inadequate performance was the main reason for removal, accounting for 33% of all cullings. However, management was different in those years; herds were smaller, usually fewer than 10 sows, and were farrowing outside. The preweaning mortality was also high, up to 48% during certain months of the year.

In a herd with a high level of culling for inadequate performance, a parity analysis is useful. If too many young animals are culled for this reason, action should be taken because it is well known that litter size increases with parity until the third litter. In such a herd, the benefit of culling sows for the purpose of improving productivity might be lost because of a decrease in herd productivity associated with a high proportion of young sows. Culled females will have to be replaced by gilts, which are not very predictable. Dijkhuizen et al. (1986) asserted that parity 1 sows with a litter size of even 50% below average should not be culled on economic grounds. Moreover, the repeatability of litter size is low, which means that predicting the next production from the previous one is very inaccurate.

Locomotor Problems

Locomotor problems refer to a variety of conditions, including osteochondrosis, osteoarthrosis, osteomalacia, arthritis, leg weakness, posterior paralysis, foot rot, foot and leg injuries, and fracture. Dewey et al. (1993) examined 51 sows culled for lameness and found that osteochondrosis, followed by infectious arthritis and foot lesions, was the major underlying cause. The proportion of sows removed for locomotor disorders varies between 9% and 20%; some reports, however, have indicated a percentage as high as 45%. It is imperative when investigating culling for locomotion and leg problems to analyze concurrently the death rate (see section on "Death").

In sporadic cases of very high removal for locomotor disorders, housing and flooring types have often been incriminated (Jones 1967; Smith and Robertson 1971). In general, group housing is associated with more injuries, presumably because several animals of different ages are kept together; whereas individual housing is related to a higher incidence of joint, foot, and leg problems, possibly because of a lower frequency of movement. Housing sows individually during gestation limits the amount of exercise and results in decreased muscle weight. Restricting movement may also cause biomechanical stress (Marchant and Broom 1996).

In swine breeding herds, flooring and housing are closely related, and thus it is often difficult to separate the effects of one from the other. Certain types of housing will rarely be found with certain types of flooring; for example, crates will rarely, if ever, be seen on an earthen floor. There may also be an interaction between the flooring type and the housing type. Levels of culling are also influenced by the housing and flooring types used during the rearing period of the replacement gilts; high density of animals and slatted floors during the finishing period are associated with a greater risk of removal in sows (Dewey et al. 1992).

Flooring can vary in many respects, including design, material, quality, the hygienic conditions associated with it, and other characteristics. The adverse effects of slatted floors have often been associated with foot and leg problems, but most of these reports have pertained to faulty slats that were damaged or were poorly designed with rough edges, too wide apart, or with an improper distribution of nonslippery and nonabrasive materials in the concrete (MAFF 1981; Muirhead 1981; Dewey et al. 1992).

The association between housing and flooring types might be further confounded by the type of feeding system used. For group housing during gestation, longevity was shorter for sows individually fed in an electronic feeding system than for sows fed as a group in individual feeding stalls: 3.0 and 3.9 litters, respectively (Olsson 1996). Competition, queue formation, and aggressive incidents were more frequent around the feeding station in the electronic system and resulted in more injuries.

Proper selection for conformation is essential to improve sow longevity, as buck-kneed forelegs, upright pasterns on hindlegs, and swaying hindquarters have been associated with an increased risk of removal for sows (Grindflek and Sehested 1996; Jorgensen 1996). Some of these conformational traits associated with sow longevity have been shown to be moderately heritable (Rothschild and Christian 1988a; Serenius et al. 2001). Low level of backfat has been associated with leg weakness problems (Rothschild and Christian 1988b), suggesting that the selection against backfat used by seedstock producers might have contributed to the increased locomotor problems recently observed in breeding animals.

The likelihood of a sow being culled for lameness is greater for younger sows, particularly gilts and parity 1 sows (Jovic et al. 1975; Dagorn and Aumaitre 1979; D'Allaire et al. 1987; Dewey et al. 1993; Lucia et al. 1996; Paterson et al. 1997b). Dewey et al. (1992) found that the culling rate due to lameness was higher in start-up than in established herds: 26% and 8%, respectively. Sows culled for locomotor problems produce, on average, only three litters. The reasons that culling for locomotor problems is more frequent in young females are numerous; among the possibilities are marginal nutritional problems, poor selection for conformation and locomotion of gilts, management or environment differing for young females compared with older sows, or a selection process by which sows less prone to problems are kept in the herd. Moreover, clinical signs of osteochondrosis, which is one of the leading causes for removal of lamed sows (Dewey et al. 1993), are mostly observed in animals between 6 and 15 months of age (Grondalen 1974). Some authors have also reported that osteomalacia and osteoporosis are more frequent in first-litter sows (Douglas and Mackinnon 1993). On the other hand, older sows are more likely to have foot problems than younger sows (Dewey et al. 1993).

Sows removed for locomotor problems represent the highest economic losses related to culling (Dijkhuisen et al. 1989). In a study by Paterson et al. (1997b), 25% (range 0–62%) of the sows removed for locomotor problems had to be euthanized for humane reasons; this has an important economic impact due to the loss of the sale value of the animal but also suggests animal welfare problems.

When investigating a problem of high removal rate for locomotor problems, it is important to determine the major causes for lameness and to assess the associated risk factors, for example, housing, flooring, nutrition, genetics, selection process, and management. For more details on risk factors for locomotor disorders, see Chapter 5.

Milking Problems

Milking problems include mastitis, agalactia, low milk production, and poor mothering abilities. This category may overlap with inadequate performance, for milk failure can influence weaning weights and preweaning mortality. The proportion of sows culled for these reasons ranges from less than 1% up to 15%. In some reports, milking problems are included with peripartum problems. In a study from Minnesota (United States), sows culled because of milking problems produced an average of 4.6 litters (D'Allaire et al. 1987). Svendsen et al. (1975) reported that parity 2 sows were more prone to culling for mastitis. Halgaard (1983) observed that the risk of mastitis increased with increasing age up to the third or fourth litter.

Death

Annual death rates of 3–10% are frequently observed; however, they can reach 20% on some farms (Abiven et al. 1998). Recently mortality risks in breeding herds appear to be increasing, especially in the U.S. (Koketsu 2000; Deen and Xue 1999). These high levels of mortality represent significant economic losses and are indicative of compromised welfare. Moreover they are a concern to employees and can affect their morale (Deen and Xue 1999). High levels of death or euthanasia in a herd result in some of the greatest losses per sow (Dijkhuizen et al. 1989, 1990; Paterson et al. 1997a) because of the increased number of nonproductive days, the extra costs (such as veterinary costs before removal and rendering costs), the lack of income associated with unslaughtered sows, or the loss of whole litters, since sow death often occurs around farrowing.

Variation in death rates can be attributed to differences in management, nutrition, environment, and culling policies. Some producers preferably cull their sick sows quickly, hence reducing the death rate. Also, death rate is often negatively correlated with culling rate in order to keep the sow inventory constant within a herd.

In most recording systems, natural death and euthanasia are both included in the mortalities. It is recommended in herds with high mortality that euthanasia rates and reasons be analyzed separately since euthanasia may contribute significantly to the death losses. In a study of 59 herds, the combined death/euthanasia rate was 9%, with 5% for natural deaths and 4% for euthanasia (Paterson et al. 1997a). Similar results were found by Christensen et al. (1995), who reported that among 263 sows submitted to a rendering plant, 36% were euthanized, most of them having locomotor problems. High levels of euthanasia are indicative of a health or welfare problem or a failure to identify and quickly treat sick animals. In that, the work force plays an important role. Employees lacking pig experience and having limited husbandry skills are less likely to recognize sows at risk quickly and institute a prompt and effective treatment before a problem becomes life threatening (Loula 2000). Inappropriate treatments of sows with a product having a long withdrawal period may also preclude the sending of animals to slaughter, hence increasing the euthanasia rate if the health condition of the animals deteriorates. Similarly, a limited availability of transportation as is often observed in large organizations, does not allow timely culling of animals, leading subsequently to euthanasia or death when recovery is not possible.

Christensen et al. (1995) observed that the risk of death for sows was three times higher in herds with more than 100 sows than in herds with fewer than 50 sows. In a study of 130 herds, the death rate was significantly higher in herds with 200 or more sows than in those with fewer than 200 sows: 8% versus 6% (S.

D'Allaire and R. Drolet, 1996 unpublished data). Straw (1984) suggested a target death rate of 3% for herds of 150 sows or less, and 5% for herds of 200 or more sows. Koketsu (2000) observed that as herd size increases by 500 females the mortality risk increases by 0.44%.

Seasonal patterns in sow losses have been observed. In the United Kingdom, Jones (1967, 1968) observed that more than 55% of the dead sows had died during the winter months. These sows were kept inside during winter and outside during summer. A higher incidence of mortality during summer months is reported in studies where herds were kept mainly in total confinement (Chagnon et al. 1991; Drolet et al. 1992; Deen and Xue 1999; Koketsu 2000). A significant percentage of yearly deaths may be associated with thermal stress during periods of warm weather in sows housed indoors (D'Allaire et al. 1996). The annual mortality in Hungarian breeding herds was 5.1% and 12.2% for indoor and outdoor production units, respectively (Karg and Bilkei 2002).

Sows appear to be at risk most during the lactation period (Abiven 1995), and particularly during the peripartum period (Madec 1984; Chagnon et al. 1991; Deen and Xue 1999; Duran 2001). Therefore, particular attention and care should be given to sows during this period of the reproductive cycle to limit sow losses. Older sows are in general at higher risk of dying (Deen and Xue 1999; Koketsu 2000).

The mean parity at death varies between 3.4 and 4.2; the variation among studies and possibly among herds may be a reflection of the relative incidence of certain causes of sow losses, as some of them appear to be age related. Cystitis-pyelonephritis occurs more frequently in older sows (Madec 1984; Paterson et al. 1997a), whereas some locomotor problems seem to be more prevalent in young breeding stock (Spencer 1979; Doige 1982; D'Allaire et al. 1991; Dewey et al. 1993).

Assessing the reasons for death is essential to understand and control the factors influencing sow losses due to mortality. Many conditions responsible for death in sows are often reported by the producers as sudden deaths or rapid deaths associated with some rather nonspecific premonitory clinical signs. When trying to ascertain the causes of death in a particular herd, it is imperative to have a significant number of sows necropsied during the year in order to identify the general pattern of causes of death. Standardized protocols and diagnostic approaches have been proposed to help determine the causes of mortality in herds (Chagnon et al. 1991; Pretzer et al. 2000).

The relative proportions of deaths due to different causes vary between studies, and several factors can be responsible for these differences: the system of recording used, and the size and the number of herds. Environment, management practices, and geographical area also influence the occurrence of certain diseases and may explain some of the variation among herds. The material examined may also not be representative of the entire sow population if investigations are based on submissions to diagnostic laboratories; causes of death that can be readily identified by producers (heat stress, uterine prolapse) are obviously underrepresented. Studies based solely on macroscopic postmortem examinations may introduce bias by excluding some causes of death that need laboratory assistance (microbiology, histopathology, toxicology) to reach a diagnosis.

Although sows die from a variety of causes, some of the causes seem to have a greater incidence. Torsion and other accidents involving abdominal organs, heart failure, and cystitis-pyelonephritis are overall the major causes of natural death in sows, whereas locomotion and leg related problems are the most frequent causes for euthanasia.

Torsions and Accidents Involving Abdominal Organs. Torsions and accidents involving abdominal organs probably are among the most significant causes of death in breeding stock. Gastric, splenic, and hepatic lobe torsions are the most common conditions reported within this category (Figure 63.1). Lethal gastric dilation can also occur without concurrent torsion (Ward and Walton 1980; Sanford et al. 1994). Intestinal accidents such as volvulus are also observed in breeding animals but are less frequent than in growing pigs. In studies on sow mortality published before 1980, torsions of abdominal organs are not reported as significant causes of death. The emergence of these problems, recognized in the early 1980s (Ward and Walton 1980; Morin et al. 1984; Sanford et al. 1984), might have been concurrent

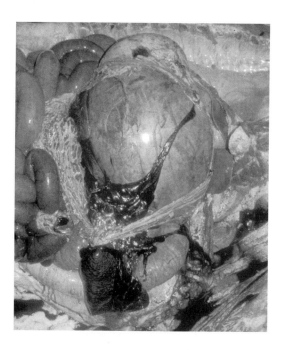

63.1. *Gastric torsion and dilation in a sow; right lateral view. The spleen is displaced, congested, and ruptured. The greater omentum is lacerated.*

with the intensification of swine production and the associated changes in management practices. In one study, the proportion of deaths attributable to torsions of abdominal organs was 20.5% for herds kept indoor compared to 4.1% for outdoor units (Karg and Bilkei 2002). In some herds, these conditions may represent a serious problem.

Torsions of abdominal organs are often found in older sows (Morin et al. 1984; Sanford et al. 1984, 1994; Chagnon et al. 1991; Christensen et al. 1995). Although affected sows are usually pregnant, sows may die at any stage of the reproductive cycle. Rough movements and manipulations, noise, and excitement among sows have been incriminated in the pathogenesis of torsion of abdominal organs (Morin et al. 1984). Feeding management and possibly housing type can influence the incidence of these conditions (Abiven et al. 1998). It has been suggested that any factors that provoke a rapid intake of food and water in excited animals predispose to gastric dilation or torsion; such factors include the number of meals per day, omitting a meal, as often occurs during the weekend, and possibly the fineness of the ground feedstuffs. Gastric contents in these cases are generally abundant and fluid.

Torsions and other accidents involving abdominal organs are usually easily recognized grossly on field postmortem examination without the need for further confirmatory laboratory testing, as is the case for some other conditions, such as septicemia.

Heart Failure. Heart failure has been reported as being among the main causes of death in sows (Senk and Sabec 1970; Svendsen et al. 1975; Smith 1984; Chagnon et al. 1991; D'Allaire et al. 1991; Maderbacher et al. 1993; Abiven 1995; Karg and Bilkei 2002), accounting for up to 31% of the mortalities. However, in several other studies, heart failure per se either is not even reported among the causes of death or is considered of negligible incidence in sows (Jones 1967, 1968; Ward and Walton 1980; Madec 1984; Hsu et al. 1985). The diagnosis of heart failure can be difficult to make, particularly in acute cases and has to rely on all current diagnostic procedures available. Diagnosis should be based on the presence of lesions indicative of heart failure such as cutaneous cyanosis; transudate in the pericardial, thoracic, and abdominal cavities; cardiac chamber changes; pulmonary edema; and passive congestion of lungs and liver, along with the absence of other gross, microscopic, and microbiological findings to carefully exclude other diseases (Figure 63.2).

Some of the predisposing factors for this condition have to be regarded in light of the way pigs often overreact to exogenous factors and, probably more important, of their particularly delicate cardiovascular system. The porcine heart has many anatomic and physiologic peculiarities, namely, low volume and small weight, abnormal systolic-to-diastolic ratio, and exceptional myocar-

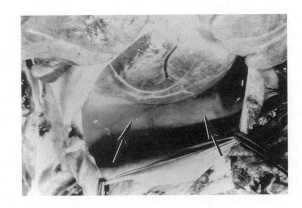

63.2. Hydropericardium (arrows) in a sow dead of cardiac failure.

dial sensitivity to oxygen deficiency. In swine the heart weight to body weight ratio decreases as the size of the animal increases (Stünzi et al. 1959), and in adults, this ratio is considered to be among the smallest of domestic animals (Lee et al. 1975). The swine heart weight to body weight ratio, which is about 0.3% in sows, is much smaller than that of the less sedentary or more athletic species such as the dog, which is about 0.8% (Bienvenu and Drolet 1991). This precarious situation may easily lead to irreversible overload of the circulation and to acute heart failure (Thielscher 1987). The lack of exercise in sows raised in total confinement may also affect cardiovascular fitness. Thus, any factor that requires increased effort from the cardiovascular system in sows may be considered to predispose to heart failure: obesity, parturition, high ambient temperature, and stressful events such as mating, fighting, and transport (Drolet et al. 1992).

Drolet et al. (1992) and Christensen et al. (1995) found that sows that died of heart failure were heavier and fatter than sows dead of other causes. Therefore, in gestation units, sows should be fed properly and not be allowed to put on excessive weight and fat. In a study involving 137 dead sows of which 43 had heart failure, more than 60% of the heart failure deaths occurred during the peripartum period, suggesting that parturition is a demanding event for the cardiovascular system of the sow (Chagnon et al. 1991). Cardiovascular failure associated with high ambient temperatures may be responsible for significant losses in some herds. In a recent study involving 130 breeding herds in which sows were housed indoors, 11% of the yearly deaths occurred during 3 consecutive days of warm weather, which represent only 0.8% of a year (3/365 days) (D'Allaire et al. 1996). Interestingly, only 3 dead sows were submitted for necropsy to the nearby diagnostic laboratory during the week. Causes of death that can be readily identified by producers, such as those occurring on hot days, are underrepresented in submissions to diagnostic laboratories, as was pointed out by Sanford et al. (1994). Sows in total confinement are particularly susceptible to heat stress; they are not allowed to wallow in mud to decrease their body temperature nor are they exposed to winds that would decrease the ambient humidity and increase heat dissipation. Proper ventilation obviously plays a major role within these confinement systems, especially for periparturient females in the farrowing house. When the ambient temperature and humidity are high, the use of portable fans or other cooling system in the farrowing houses may be beneficial for sows. Other precautions may include removing heat sources (e.g., infrared lamp), less handling of animals to limit stress, and modifying the feeding schedule to avoid the heat of the day.

It is important to distinguish heart failure from malignant hyperthermia (porcine stress syndrome), a genetically transmitted disease. In the latter, prevention through selection of resistant animals will decrease the incidence. Many of the predisposing factors associated with heart failure in sows are also considered triggering factors for the development of malignant hyperthermia in pigs. Both conditions also share many clinical and pathological similarities, which make them difficult to differentiate. Lambert et al. (1996) examined, by molecular biology techniques, tissues from 84 sows previously collected by Chagnon et al. (1991) for the presence of the defective gene responsible for malignant hyperthermia. From these selected sows, 42 were identified as having died from heart failure and 42 as having died from various other causes (control group). The majority of the sows dead from heart failure did not possess the halothane gene mutation on any allele, suggesting that these cases were not related to malignant hyperthermia. Furthermore, the proportion of animals carrying at least one mutant allele (monomutant or dimutant) was not significantly different between sows dead of cardiac failure and the control group.

Cystitis-Pyelonephritis. The proportion of all deaths attributable to cystitis-pyelonephritis generally varies between 3% and 15% (Jones 1968; Senk and Sabec 1970; Svendsen et al. 1975; Hsu et al. 1985; Ward and Walton 1980; Chagnon et al. 1991; D'Allaire et al. 1991; Abiven 1995; Christensen et al. 1995). However, in some studies, urinary tract infection represented the major cause of mortality, accounting for up to 40% of all deaths (Jones 1967; Madec 1984; Smith 1984; Karg and Bilkei 2002).

Bacteria most commonly isolated from cases of cystitis-pyelonephritis (Figure 63.3) are *Escherichia coli* and *Actinobaculum suis* (formerly *Actinomyces suis*) (Madec and David 1983; Smith 1984; D'Allaire et al. 1991; Carr and Walton 1993). Other bacteria commonly associated with urinary tract infection include *Proteus* spp., streptococci, enterococci, micrococci, klebsiellae, and *Arcanobacterium pyogenes*.

Determination of urea concentration in ocular fluids can be a useful aid in diagnosing cystitis-pyelonephritis in dead sows, particularly when a complete necropsy is

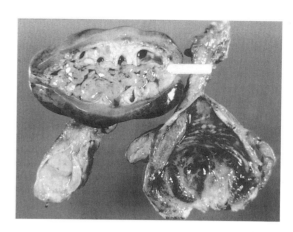

63.3. *Cystitis and pyelonephritis due to* Actinobaculum suis *in a sow. The pelvis and ureter are markedly distended with a mucopurulent exudate.*

not possible or when it is difficult to ascertain that the lesions found in the urinary tract are responsible for death (Drolet et al. 1990). A significantly higher aqueous humor urea concentration was found in sows dead of cystitis-pyelonephritis (45–52 mmol/L) than in those dead of other causes (9–10 mmol/L) (Chagnon et al. 1991; Arauz and Perfumo 2000).

The risk of cystitis-pyelonephritis increases with age (Jones 1967; Madec 1984; Pointon et al. 1990; Chagnon et al. 1991; D'Allaire et al. 1991; Paterson et al. 1997a). The underlying reasons for this age-related susceptibility have not yet been fully investigated. Lack of exercise, limb injuries (Madec and David 1983), and obesity (Smith 1983) appear to be more frequent in old sows and predispose to urinary tract infection. These factors are associated with a decreased frequency of micturition, hence leading to a decreased flushing of bacteria and potentiating microbial growth (Smith 1983; Carr et al. 1991). It has also been reported that restricted water intake is one of the major risk factors for cystitis-pyelonephritis (Madec and David 1983; Carr et al. 1991). Urinary problems are also more common when sows are tethered or kept in stalls, possibly due to the lack of exercise and to hygiene conditions (i.e., confined sows often having to lie in their own feces and urine) (Madec and David 1983; Muirhead 1983; Carr et al. 1991). A flooring type that does not allow easy cleaning and good elimination of urine and feces can also lead to urogenital diseases and serious reproductive problems (Madec and David 1983; Muirhead 1983). For detailed information on cystitis-pyelonephritis, see Chapters 9 and 38.

Locomotor Problems. Locomotor problems are a common cause of euthanasia and may significantly increase the mortality in some herds (Senk and Sabec 1970; Svendsen et al. 1975; Christensen et al. 1995; Karg and Bilkei 2002; Perfumo et al. 2003). When investigating the extent of locomotor problems on a farm, it is important to assess both the death rate and the culling rate associated with these conditions, since culling policies influence both rates, especially for these problems.

Gastric Ulcers. Lethal gastric ulcers are highly prevalent in some herds. Factors responsible for high mortality due to gastric ulceration are not always easy to pinpoint. Gastric ulceration is a multietiologic condition with several recognized risk factors. Most of these factors are related in some ways to housing management–associated stress, to concurrent diseases, or to some feed processing and dietary factors, including feed particle size, feed intake, grain type, and milling process (see Chapter 54).

Infectious Diseases. Proliferative enteropathy and PRRS, among other infectious diseases, may also increase the death rate. But usually, they will appear as outbreaks or will be of short duration. The mortality can reach up to 10% during these episodes (Yates et al. 1979; Halbur and Bush 1997). The incidence of infectious diseases due to pathogens, such as *Haemophilus parasuis*, is higher in start-up herds and in high-health-status herds.

In most studies, endometritis represents less than 9% of all deaths. This condition can be associated with concurrent urinary tract infection or, less frequently, with mastitis (the latter is an uncommon cause of death in sows).

Pneumonia is not a major cause of mortality; it rarely represents more than 5% of all deaths. Pneumonia is often more severe in young growing pigs than in full-grown pigs (Pijoan 1986). This could partly explain why pneumonia is not a frequent cause of death in adult sows and is more likely to affect younger females (Chagnon et al. 1991).

Sow deaths have also been attributed to *Clostridium novyi* in some countries (Walton and Duran 1992; Abiven 1995). The diagnosis of *C. novyi* sudden death (clostridial hepatopathy) is difficult mainly because this organism is a common and early postmortem invader, especially of adult swine in warm weather (Taylor and Bergeland 1992). Different aspects of this disease have been examined by Duran and Walton (1997). They reported that affected sows had generalized edema, subcutaneous infiltration with bubbles, and foul smelling bloody fluid in body cavities. The liver was enlarged and the parenchyma was infiltrated with gas bubbles, giving a spongy appearance. Several deaths in periparturient sows have been attributed to *Clostridium difficile*; sows had been previously treated with enrofloxacin (Mauch and Bilkei 2003). Septicemia and endocarditis have been observed as sporadic causes of death in some earlier studies.

Uterine Prolapse and Complications at Parturition. Uterine prolapses are generally responsible for fewer than 7% of all deaths (Figure 63.4). This condition is

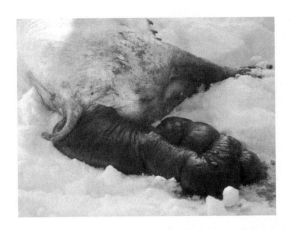

63.4. *Uterine prolapse in a sow.*

mostly observed in old sows, and the reasons for this increased frequency are unclear. Among possibilities are large pelvic inlet, long and flaccid uterus, and excessive relaxation of the pelvic and perineal region, which are probably mostly encountered in full-grown females (Roberts 1986).

Although dystocia or complications at parturition are occasionally reported as causes of death, we must be careful not to ascribe every death occurring in the peripartum period to these causes. As mentioned previously, sows are most at risk of dying during the peripartum period, due to a variety of causes. They may be apathic or suffer from exhaustion or downer sow syndrome which may be interpreted as a difficult farrowing by the producer.

EFFECTS OF SOW LONGEVITY ON HERD PRODUCTIVITY

High removal rates can affect herd productivity by causing a shift in the herd age distribution toward younger females, which usually have fewer pigs born alive per litter, a lower conception rate, and a greater number of nonproductive days. They are also more likely to be culled for reproductive failure and locomotor problems. Considerable losses are involved with high removal rates of young females. Kroes and Van Male (1979) reported that the cost per weaner is highest in the first litter and decreases over the next two litters.

The interval between a production event and the removal of a breeding female affects the number of nonproductive days in a herd, which is one of the best biologic predictors of litters per sow per year (Wilson et al. 1986; Duffy and Stein 1988; Dial et al. 1992). A high removal rate is generally associated with an increase in the number of nonproductive sow days. Target values for intervals between different production events and removal have been proposed by Polson et al. (1990). The interval between a production event and culling is determined by two factors: the interval from the production event to the decision to cull, and the period between when the decision to cull is made and the actual culling. An excessively long interval may be due to the manager's inefficiency in identifying animals that will eventually have to be culled or to the manager's holding animals to be removed too long after the decision to cull is made. The time lost from cullings, deaths, and abortions was found to add the equivalent of 11 days to the farrowing interval and to result in a decrease of 0.16 in the number of litters per sow per year (Pattison et al. 1980b). Kroes and Van Male (1979) observed an increase of 6–8 days in the farrowing interval for each increase of 12% over an annual removal rate of 31%, which was considered to be the base value.

Lifetime productivity has traditionally been defined as the parity at removal or as the number of pigs weaned at removal. More recently, Lucia (1997) reported that the number of herd days per pig weaned by removed sows is a better estimator of lifetime productivity since it takes into account the number of nonproductive days as well as the number of pigs weaned. This parameter was evaluated at 20–21 days and was lower for older sows, 16–18 days, and higher for younger sows, 25–27 days.

High annual removal rates decrease herd productivity by influencing the herd age distribution and the number of nonproductive sow days. Many authors have documented that high removal rates are associated with a decrease in litters per sow per year and pigs weaned per sow per year (Dagorn and Aumaitre 1979; Kroes and Van Male 1979; Pattison et al. 1980a).

Using a sow replacement model, the loss by premature removal represented the equivalent of 16% of pig farm income, at an annual removal rate of 50% (Dijkhuizen et al. 1989). From different models, it appears rarely economical to cull a sow before her eighth or ninth parity. Improving longevity is highly profitable when the average parity at removal is low (Dijkhuizen et al. 1990; Sehested 1996). For example, increases in average parity at removal from 2.8 to 3.8 and from 3.8 to 4.8 improve the income per sow per year by US$25–35 and US$20–25, respectively (Dijkhuizen et al. 1990). Similarly, improving average longevity by one parity was shown to have the same impact as improving meat lean by 0.5% (Sehested 1996). However, improving longevity above an average value of 5 does not seem as beneficial (Sehested 1996). Several software programs have been developed to determine optimal economic

time to cull sows (Dijkhuizen et al. 1986; Stalder et al. 2003).

LONGEVITY IN BOARS

In herds where artificial insemination (AI) is not used extensively, good boar-culling policies are important, for they facilitate the replacement program. Planning problems associated with boar introduction may be considerable, because boars should be kept in quarantine for a certain period and their full workload is attained only at 1 year of age. High boar removal rates seem to be more frequent than excessively low rates. In a study involving 84 commercial herds, the annual removal rate for boars averaged 59% (D'Allaire and Leman 1990). The lifetime breeding expectancy for boars is estimated at 15–20 months but varies considerably between 0.3 and 38.5 months (Le Denmat et al. 1980; Arganosa et al. 1981a; D'Allaire and Leman 1990).

Overweight and old age, reproductive problems, and locomotor problems are the major reasons for culling boars in commercial herds (Table 63.4). The general pattern of removal may vary according to the breed of the boars: culling for reproductive or leg problems was higher in purebred than in crossbred boars, whereas culling for old age and overweight was more frequent in crossbred than in purebred boars (Le Denmat and Runavot 1980). Accordingly, reasons for culling boars from commercial herds would most likely be different from those in AI centers.

Overweight and Old Age

Since overweight and old age are not always easily distinguishable, they are often grouped into one category to avoid the risk of misclassification. Indeed, some producers use these two reasons interchangeably, because older boars are frequently considered too heavy to appropriately serve younger sows without the risk of injuring them. Both overweight and old age are often in relation to the sow herd. The introduction of many replacement gilts into the herd and the necessary introduction of young boars may require culling older or large boars that are not necessarily aged. This aspect of culling is peculiar to commercial herds; overweight and old age are rarely reported as causes of culling in testing stations or artificial insemination centers (Melrose 1966; Navratil and Forejtek 1978). High rates of removal

Table 63.4.   Reasons for removing boars and percentage of removals for each reason: results obtained from 3 studies involving more than one herd

Source	Reproductive Failure	Old Age and Overweight	Locomotor Problems	Death	Other	No. of Boars	Country
Le Denmat et al. 1980	20	31	20	NA	29	246	France
Le Denmat and Runavot 1980	32	23	32	NA	13	98	France
D'Allaire and Leman 1990	18	47	12	7	16	440	USA

Note: NA = not available.

caused by overweight may also reflect a feeding-management problem, in which case feeding management on the farm should be reviewed and corrected to improve boar longevity.

Reproductive Problems

The proportion of boars culled for reproductive problems is considerably lower in commercial herds than in artificial insemination stations (Melrose 1966; Navratil and Forejtek 1978). These differences may be attributed partly to the fact that semen quality is regularly evaluated for boars from artificial insemination centers. Consequently, boars may be removed more quickly and at a higher rate; the culling rate for poor semen quality can be as high as 23% in these stations (Navratil and Forejtek 1978). In two French studies conducted in commercial breeding herds, reproductive problems represented 20% and 32% of all removals and were considered one of the two major causes of culling (Le Denmat and Runavot 1980; Le Denmat et al. 1980). Breed difference may also be responsible for the variations in the proportion of boars culled for reproductive problems; purebred boars are more likely to be culled for this reason than crossbred boars (Le Denmat and Runavot 1980).

In commercial herds, the reason most frequently reported by producers in this culling category is poor libido or behavioral problems that preclude efficient mating. Culling for low reproductive performance is also reported but to a lesser extent. Low reproductive performance is difficult to confirm for boars in commercial herds. A great amount of information is required to make a valid decision; it takes approximately 50 litters to show a one pig per litter difference from the herd average. Therefore, culling for that reason without sufficient data is rarely justified. On the other hand, by the time this information is available, the boar has often completed his productive life in the herd.

Locomotor Problems

Although locomotor problems are rarely the main cause of culling, the percentage of removal can be very high on certain farms (Einarsson and Larsson 1977; D'Allaire and Leman 1990). In herds with high culling for locomotor disorders, the environment of the boars, such as housing and flooring types, should be evaluated carefully. Attention should be given to selection for locomotion and conformation, particularly in artificial insemination centers, as it has been shown in sows that these traits are associated with longevity (Grindflek and Sehested 1996; Jorgensen 1996). Misclassification between locomotor and reproductive problems may also occur, for locomotor problems often result in poor libido or inability to mate.

Death

Death generally accounts for less than 7% of all removals, giving a herd death rate of lower than 4%

(D'Allaire and Leman 1990). In a study by Senk and Sabec (1970), the causes of death in 30 boars were found to be heart failure (50%), locomotor problems (23%), splenic torsions (10%), gastric ulcer (7%), endocarditis (3%), and unknown (7%).

GENERAL GUIDELINES TO ASSESS REMOVAL POLICIES

Determination of the annual removal rate is the first step in evaluating a culling program. Rates that are too high seem to be more common than excessively low rates. Unusual circumstances, such as a change in inventory or culling policy, may temporarily increase the removal rate. Calculating the mean parity at removal is also useful, but a parity distribution of culled females may be more informative. The removal rate for each category of reasons can indicate the extent of a problem. Analysis of reasons by parity may reveal which group of females is more susceptible or whether some cullings are unjustified, either physiologically or economically. An assessment of the interval between a production event and removal is important because it influences the number of litters per sow per year and pigs weaned per sow per year, and these measures of productivity are important factors in economic loss and gain. Clearly, the failure to identify and remove nonproductive sows at an early stage will increase the number of nonproductive sow days. Factors influencing negatively the longevity of breeding animals should be investigated. They have been reviewed by Stalder et al. (2004). To improve breeding-life expectancy of sows and boars in commercial herds, greater attention to the environment, nutrition, and management should be emphasized.

REFERENCES

Abiven N. 1995. Mortalité des truies: Description des causes de mortalité et facteurs de risque d'un haut taux de mortalité. Mémoire ISPA. Ecole Nationale Vétérinaire de Nantes, France.

Abiven N, Seegers H, Beaudeau F, Laval A, Fourichon C. 1998. Risk factors for high sow mortality in French swine herds. Prev Vet Med 33:109–119.

Arauz SM, Perfumo CJ. 2000. Comparative study of urea concentration in aqueous humour taken from sows that died of cystitis, pyelonephritis and other diseases. Rev Med Vet (Buenos Aires) 81:342–344.

Arganosa VG, Acda SP, Bandian MM. 1981a. Lifetime breeding and reproductive performance of boars. Phil Agric 64:41–47.

Arganosa VG, Acda SP, De Guzman AL. 1981b. Lifetime reproductive performance of sows in selected piggeries in the Philippines. Phil Agric 64:1–20.

Bienvenu JG, Drolet R. 1991. A quantitative study of cardiac ventricular mass in dogs. Can J Vet Res 55:305–309.

Boyle L, Leonard FC, Lynch B, Brophy P. 1998. Sow culling patterns and sow welfare. Irish Vet J 51:354–357.

Brandt H, von Brevern N, Glodek P. 1999. Factors affecting survival rate of crossbred sows in weaner production. Livest Prod Sci 57:127–135.

Carr J, Walton JR. 1993. Bacterial flora of the urinary tract of pigs associated with cystitis and pyelonephritis. Vet Rec 132:575–577.

Carr J, Walton JR, Done SH. 1991. Cystitis and pyelonephritis in the sow. Pig Vet, J 27:122–141.

Cederberg ER, Jonsson L. 1996. Sow culling in Sweden. In Proc Nordiska Jordbruksforskares Forening Seminar 265—Longevity of Sows. V Danielsen, ed. Denmark: Research Centre Foulum, pp. 7–8.

Chagnon M, D'Allaire S, Drolet R. 1991. A prospective study of sow mortality in breeding herds. Can J Vet Res 55:180–184.

Christensen G, Vraa-Andersen L, Mousing J. 1995. Causes of mortality among sows in Danish pig herds. Vet Rec 137:395–399.

Culbertson MS, Mabry JW. 1995. Effect of age at first service on first parity and lifetime sow performance. J Anim Sci 73 (Suppl. 1):21.

Dagorn J, Aumaitre A. 1979. Sow culling: Reasons for and effect on productivity. Livest Prod Sci 6:167–177.

D'Allaire S. 1987. Assessment of culling programs in swine breeding herds. Compend Cont Ed Pract Vet 9:F187–F191.

D'Allaire S, Drolet R, Brodeur D. 1996. Sow mortality associated with high ambient temperatures. Can Vet J 37:237–239.

D'Allaire S, Drolet R, Chagnon M. 1991. The causes of sow mortality: A retrospective study. Can Vet J 32:241–243.

D'Allaire S, Leman AD. 1990. Boar culling in swine breeding herds in Minnesota. Can Vet, J 31:581–583.

D'Allaire S, Morris RS, Martin FB, Robinson RA, Leman AD. 1989. Management and environmental factors associated with annual sow culling rate: A path analysis. Prev Vet Med 7:255–265.

D'Allaire S, Stein TE, Leman AD. 1987. Culling patterns in selected Minnesota swine breeding herds. Can J Vet Res 51:506–512.

Deen J, Xue J. 1999. Sow mortality in the U.S.: An industry-wide perspective. Proc AD Leman Swine Conf 26:91–94.

Dewey CE, Friendship RM, Wilson MR. 1992. Lameness in breeding age swine: A case study. Can Vet J 33:747–748.

——. 1993. Clinical and postmortem examination of sows culled for lameness. Can Vet J 34:555–556.

Dial GD, Marsh WE, Polson DD, Vaillancourt JP. 1992. Reproductive failure: Differential diagnosis. In Diseases of Swine, 7th ed. AD Leman, BE Straw, WL Mengeling, S D'Allaire, DJ Taylor, eds. Ames: Iowa State Univ Press, pp. 88–137.

Dijkhuizen AA, Krabbenborg RMM, Huirne RBM. 1989. Sow replacement: A comparison of farmers' actual decisions and model recommendations. Livest Prod Sci 23:207–218.

Dijkhuizen AA, Krabbenborg RMM, Morrow M, Morris RS. 1990. Sow replacement economics: An interactive model for microcomputers. Compend Cont Ed Pract Vet 12:575–579.

Dijkhuizen AA, Morris RS, Morrow M. 1986. Economic optimization of culling strategies in swine breeding herds, using the "PorkCHOP computer program." Prev Vet Med 4:341–353.

Doige CE. 1982. Pathological findings associated with locomotory disturbances in lactating and recently weaned sows. Can J Comp Med 46:1–6.

Douglas RGA, Mackinnon JD. 1993. Leg weakness in weaned first litter sows. Pig Vet J 30:77–80.

Drolet R, D'Allaire S, Chagnon M. 1990. The evaluation of postmortem ocular fluid analysis as a diagnostic aid in sows. J Vet Diagn Invest 2:9–13.

——. 1992. Some observations on cardiac failure in sows. Can Vet J 33:325–329.

Duffy SJ, Stein TE. 1988. Correlations between production, productivity, and population factors in swine breeding herds. Proc Int Pig Vet Soc 10:345.

Duran CO. 2001. Sow mortality. Comp Cont Educ Pract Vet 23:S76–S83.

Duran CO, Walton JR. 1997. *Clostridium novyi* sudden death in sows: Toxaemia or postmortem invader? Pig J 39:37–53.

Einarsson S, Larsson K. 1977. Hallbarhet och utslagsorsaker hos galtar i en bruksbesattning. Sven Vet Tidn 29:595–597.

Einarsson S, Linde C, Settergren I. 1974. Studies of the genital organs of gilts culled for anoestrus. Theriogenology 2:109–113.

Fortin F, Cue RI. 2002. A genetic study of longevity in swine. J Anim Sci 85:89.

Friendship RM, Wilson MR, Almond GW, McMillian RR, Hacker RR, Pieper R, Swaminathan SS. 1986. Sow wastage: Reasons for and effect on productivity. Can J Vet Res 50:205–208.

Grindflek E, Sehested E. 1996. Conformation and longevity in Norwegian pigs. In Proc Nordiska Jordbruksforskares Forening Seminar 265—Longevity of Sows. V Danielsen, ed. Denmark: Research Centre Foulum, pp. 77–84.

Grondalen T. 1974. Osteochondrosis and arthrosis in pigs. II. Incidence in breeding animals. Acta Vet Scand 15:26–42.

Halbur PG, Bush E. 1997. Update on abortion storms and sow mortality. Swine Health Prod 5:73.

Halgaard C. 1983. Epidemiologic factors in puerperal diseases of sow. Nord Vet Med 35:161–174.

Hsu FS, Chung WB, Hu DK, Yang PC, Shen YM. 1985. Incidence and causes of mortality in growing-finishing pigs and sows on the large-scale intensive pig farms. J Chin Soc Vet Sci 11:93–101.

Jones JET. 1967. An investigation of the causes of mortality and morbidity in sows in a commercial herd. Br Vet J 123:327–339.

——. 1968. The cause of death in sows: A one year survey of 106 herds in Essex. Br Vet J 124:45–54.

Joo HS, Kang BJ. 1981. Reproductive performance on intensive swine farms in Korea. J Korean Vet Med Assoc 17:40–43.

Jorgensen B. 1996. The influence of leg weakness in gilts, on their longevity as sows assessed by survival analysis. Proc Int Pig Vet Soc 14:545.

——. 2000. Longevity of breeding sows in relation to leg weakness symptoms at six months of age. Acta Vet Scand 41:105–121.

Josse J, Le Denmat M, Martinat-Botté F, Vanier P, Vaudelet JC. 1980. A propos d'une enquête sur les causes de réforme des truies. Schweiz Arch Tierheilkd 122:341–349.

Jovic M, Varadin M, Nikolic P. 1975. The length of reproduction of breeding sows at intensive piglet production and the chief reasons of their elimination from the breeding herd. Veterinaria (Yugoslavia) 24:17–23.

Kangasniemi R. 1996. Reasons for culling of sows in the Finnish sow recording scheme. In Proc Nordiska Jordbruksforskares Forening Seminar 265—Longevity of Sows. V Danielsen (ed). Denmark: Research Centre Foulum, pp. 17–27.

Karg H, Bilkei G. 2002. Causes of sow mortality in Hungarian indoor and outdoor pig production units. Berl Münch Tierärzlt Wochr 115:366–368.

Karlberg K. 1979. Utrangeringsarsaker hos avlspurker. Norsk Vet Tidsskr 91:423–426.

Koketsu Y. 2000. Retrospective analysis of trends and production factors associated with sow mortality on swine-breeding farms in USA. Prev Vet Med 56:249–256.

Koketsu Y, Takahashi H, Akachi K. 1999. Longevity, lifetime pig production and productivity, and age at first conception in a cohort of gilts observed over six years on commercial farms. J Vet Med Sci 61:1001–1005.

Kroes Y, Van Male JP. 1979. Reproductive lifetime of sows in relation to economy of production. Livest Prod Sci 6:179–183.

Lambert AJ, Houde A, Drolet R, D'Allaire S. 1996. Determination of halothane gene mutation associated with malignant hyperthermia in sows dead of cardiac failure. J Vet Diagn Invest 8:513–515.

Le Denmat M, Runavot JP. 1980. Premiers résultats d'une enquête sur l'âge, la durée d'utilisation et les causes de réforme des verrats en service dans les élevages de production. Journ Rech Porcine France 12:149–156.

Le Denmat M, Runavot JP, Albar J. 1980. Les caractéristiques de la population des verrats en service dans les élevage de production: Résultats d'une enquête sur 293 troupeaux. Techni-Porc 3:41–48.

Lee JC, Taylor JFN, Downing SE. 1975. A comparison of ventricular weights and geometry in newborn, young, and adult mammals. J Appl Physiol 38:147–150.

Leman AD. 1992. Reducing breeding costs and increasing sow longevity. In Pig Production Proc, 186. Sydney Post-Grad Foundation, pp. 181–188.

Lopez-Serrano M, Reinsch R, Looft H, Kalm E. 2000. Genetic correlations of growth, backfat thickness and exterior with stayability in Large White and Landrace sows. Livest Prod Sci 64:121–131.

Loula T. 2000. Increasing sow longevity: The role of people and management. In Proc AD Leman Swine Conf, pp. 139–142.

Lucia T. 1997. Lifetime Productivity of Female Swine. Ph.D. diss. Univ Minnesota, St. Paul.

Lucia T, Dial GD, Marsh WE. 1996. Patterns of female removal. I. Lifetime productivity for reproduction and performance-related culls. Proc Int Pig Vet Soc 14:540.

——. 2000. Lifetime reproductive performance in female pigs having distinct reasons for removal. Livest Prod Sci 63:213–222.

Madec F. 1984. Analyse des causes de mortalité des truies en cours de période d'élevage. Rec Méd Vét 160:329–335.

Madec F, David F. 1983. Les troubles urinaires des troupeaux de truies: Diagnostic, incidence et circonstances d'apparition. Journ Rech Porcine France 15:431–446.

Maderbacher R, Schoder G, Winter P, Baumgartner W. 1993. Causes of pig losses in a pig breeding unit. Dtsch Tierarztl Wochenschr 100:468–473.

Marchant JN, Broom DM. 1996. Factors affecting posture-changing in loose-housed and confined gestating sows. Anim Sci 63:477–485.

Marsh WE, Van Lier P, Dial GD. 1992. A profile of swine production in North America: I. PigCHAMP breeding herd data analysis for 1990. Proc Int Pig Vet Soc 12:584.

Mauch CP, Bilkei G. 2003. Illness in periparturient sows, caused by *Clostridium difficile*. Folia Vet 47:210–211.

Melrose DR. 1966. A review of progress and of possible developments in artificial insemination of pigs. Vet Rec 78:159–168.

Ministry of Agriculture, Food, and Fisheries (MAFF). 1981. Injuries caused by flooring: A survey in pig health scheme herds. Proc Pig Vet Soc 8:119–125.

Morin M, Sauvageau R, Phaneuf JB, Teuscher E, Beauregard M, Lagacé A. 1984. Torsion of abdominal organs in sows: A report of 36 cases. Can Vet J 25:440–442.

Morrison R, Larriestra A, Yan J, Deen J. 2002. Determining optimal parity distribution with a push model of gilt supply. Proc AD Leman Swine Conf 29:173–177.

Muirhead MR. 1976. Veterinary problems of intensive pig husbandry. Vet Rec 99:288–292.

——. 1981. A comparison of different systems of sow housing and management. Proc Pig Vet Soc 8:18–28.

——. 1983. Pig housing and environment. Vet Rec 113:587–593.

Muirhead MR, Alexander TJL. 1997. Managing Pig Health and the Treatment of Disease. Sheffield, UK: 5M Enterprises Ltd.

Navratil S, Forejtek P. 1978. The reasons for culling boars from artificial insemination centers. Veterinarstvi 28:354–355.

Olsson AC. 1996. Longevity and causes of culling of sows: Comparative studies in two housing systems for sows in gestation. In Proc Nordiska Jordbruksforskares Forening Seminar 265—Longevity of Sows. V Danielsen, ed. Denmark: Research Centre Foulum, pp. 59–64.

Parsons TD, Johnstone C, Dial GD. 1990. On the economic significance of parity distribution in swine herds. Proc Int Pig Vet Soc 11:380.

Paterson R, Cargill C, Pointon A. 1996. Investigations into deaths and excessive culling of sows in Australian pig herds. In Proc Nordiska Jordbruksforskares Forening Seminar 265—Longevity of Sows. V Danielsen, ed. Denmark: Research Centre Foulum, pp. 34–45.

——. 1997a. Epidemiology of reproductive failure and urogenital disease. In Proc Pig Production—The A. T. Reid Course for Veterinarians. Post-Grad Foundation Vet Sci, Univ Sydney, pp. C223–244.

Paterson R, Cargill C, Pointon A. 1997b. Lameness in breeding stock. In Proc Pig Production—The A. T. Reid Course for Veterinarians. Post-Grad Foundation Vet Sci, Univ Sydney, pp. C247–300.

Pattison HD, Cook GL, Mackenzie S. 1980a. A study of culling patterns in commercial pig breeding herds. In Proc, Br Soc Anim Prod. Harrogate, pp. 462–463.

——. 1980b. A study of natural service, farrowing rates and associated fertility parameters. In Proc Br Soc Anim Prod, Harrogate, p. 452.

Pedersen PN. 1996. Longevity and culling rates in the Danish sow production and the consequences of a different strategy of culling. In Proc Nordiska Jordbruksforskares Forening Seminar 265—Longevity of Sows. V Danielsen, ed. Denmark: Research Centre Foulum, pp. 28–33.

Perfumo CJ, Sanguinetti HR, Idiart JR, Massone AM, Vigo G, Machuca M, Muredo F, Giacoboni G, Quiroga JA. 2003. Pathological findings associated with sows death in two indoor intensively managed farms. Rev Med Vet (Buenos Aires) 84:84–88.

Pijoan C. 1986. Respiratory system. In Diseases of Swine, 6th ed. AD Leman, B Straw, RD Glock, WL Mengeling, RHC Penny, E Scholl, eds. Ames: Iowa State Univ Press, pp. 152–162.

Pointon AM, Ruen PD, Dial GD. 1990. Vulvar discharge syndrome: How to conduct a clinical investigation. Proc Minn Swine Conf Vet 17:280–281.

Polson DD, Dial GD, Marsh WE, Nimis G. 1990. The influence of nonproductive days on breeding herd productivity and profitability. In Proc Am Assoc Swine Pract, pp. 61–67.

Pomeroy RW. 1960. Infertility and neonatal mortality in the sow I. Lifetime performance and reasons for disposal of sows. J Agric Sci (Cambridge) 54:1–17.

Pond WG, Mersmann HJ. 2001. Biology of the Domestic Pig. Ithaca, New York: Cornell University Press, pp. 148–150.

Pretzer SD, Irwin CK, Geiger JO, Henry SC. 2000. A standardized protocol to investigate sow mortality. J Swine Health Prod 8:35–37.

Roberts SJ. 1986. Veterinary Obstetrics and Genital Diseases (Theriogenology), 3rd ed. Woodstock, Vt.: S. J. Roberts.

Rodriguez-Zas SL, Southey BR, Knox RV, Connor JF, Lowe JF, Roskamp BJ. 2003. Bioeconomic evaluation of sow longevity and profitability. J Anim Sci 81:2915–2922.

Rothschild MF, Christian LL. 1988a. Genetic control of front-leg weakness in Duroc swine. I. Direct response to five generations of divergent selection. Livest Prod Sci 19:459–471.

——. 1988b. Genetic control of front-leg weakness in Duroc swine. II. Correlated responses in growth rate, backfat, and reproduction from five generations of divergent selection. Livest Prod Sci 19:473–485.

Sanford SE, Josephson GKA, Rehmtulla AJ. 1994. Sudden death in sows. Can Vet J 35:388.

Sanford SE, Waters EH, Josephson GKA. 1984. Gastrosplenic torsions in sows. Can Vet, J 25:364.

Sehested E. 1996. Economy of sow longevity. In Proc Nordiska Jordbruksforskares Forening Seminar 265—Longevity of Sows. V Danielsen, ed. Denmark: Research Centre Foulum, pp. 101–108.

Sehested E, Schjerve A. 1996. Aspects of sow longevity based on analyses of Norwegian sow recording data. In Proc Nordiska Jordbruksforskares Forening Seminar 265—Longevity of Sows. V Danielsen, ed. Denmark: Research Centre Foulum, pp. 9–16.

Senk L, Sabec D. 1970. Todesursachen bei Schweinen aus Grobbetrieben. Zentralbl Veterinaermed, B17:164–174.

Serenius T, Sevon-Aimonen AM, Mantysarri EA. 2001. The genetics of leg weakness in Finnish Large White and Landrace populations. Livest Prod Sci 69:101–111.

Smith WJ. 1983. Cystitis in sows. Pig News Info 4:279–281.

——. 1984. Sow mortality—Limited survey. Proc Int Pig Vet Soc 8:368.

Smith WJ, Robertson AM. 1971. Observations on injuries to sows confined in part slatted stalls. Vet Rec 89:531–533.

Spencer GR. 1979. Animal model: Porcine lactational osteoporosis. Am J Pathol 95:277–280.

Stalder KJ, Knauer M, Baas TJ, Rothschild MF, Mabry JW. 2004. Sow longevity. Pig News Info 25:53N–74N.

Stalder KJ, Lacy RC, Cross TL, Conatser GE. 2003. Financial impact of average parity of culled females in a breed-to-wean swine operation using replacement gilt net present value analysis. J Swine Health Prod 11:69–74.

Stein TE, Dijkhuizen A, D'Allaire S, Morris RS. 1990. Sow culling and mortality in commercial swine breeding herds. Prev Vet Med 9:85–94.

Stone MW. 1981. Sow culling survey in Alberta. Can Vet J 22:363.

Straw B. 1984. Causes and control of sow losses. Modern Vet Pract 65:349–353.

Stünzi H, Teuscher E, Glaus A. 1959. Systematische Untersuchungen am Hlerzen von Haustieren. 2. Mitteilung: Untersuchungen am Herzen du Schweines. Zentralbl Veterinaermed 6:640–654.

Svendsen J, Nielsen NC, Bille N, Riising HJ. 1975. Causes of culling and death in sows. Nord Vet Med 27:604–615.

Taylor DJ, Bergeland ME. 1992. Clostridial infections. In Diseases of Swine, 7th ed. AD Leman, BE Straw, WL Mengeling, S D'Allaire, DJ Taylor, eds. Ames: Iowa State Univ Press, pp. 463–464.

Thielscher HH. 1987. The pig's heart—A problem of pathophysiology. Pro Veterinario 3:12.

Tholen E, Bunter KL, Hermesch S, Graser HU. 1996. The genetic foundation of fitness and reproduction traits in Australian pig populations. 1. Genetic parameters for weaning to conception interval, farrowing interval, and stayability. Aust J Agric Res 47:1261–1274.

Tiranti K, Dufresne L, Morrison R, Deen J. 2004. Description of removal patterns in selected herds. Proc Int Pig Vet Soc 18(2):592.

Walton JR, Duran CP. 1992. Sow deaths due to *Clostridium novyi* infection. Proc Int Pig Vet Soc 12:296.

Ward WR, Walton JR. 1980. Gastric distension and torsion and other causes of death in sows. Proc Pig Vet Soc 6:72–74.

Wilson MR, Friendship RM, McMillan I, Hacker RR, Pieper R, Swaminathan S. 1986. A survey of productivity and its component interrelationships in Canadian swine herds. J Anim Sci 62:576–582.

Yates WDG, Clark EG, Osborne AD, Enweani CC, Radostits OM, Theeds A. 1979. Proliferative hemorrhagic enteropathy in swine: an outbreak and review of literature. Can Vet J 20:261–268.

Yazdi MH, Rydhmer L, Ringmar-Cederberg E, Lundeheim N, Johansson K. 2000. Genetic study of longevity in Swedish Landrace sows. Livest Prod Sci 63:255–264.

64 Effects of the Environment on Productivity and Disease

Harold W. Gonyou, Stéphane P. Lemay, and Yuanhui Zhang

Environment is a very broad term referring to all factors that impinge upon the animal. It can be divided into two major aspects, the physical and the biological, which in turn can be further subdivided. Not only is the environment complex, but the means by which animals interact with the environment is beyond the simple stimulus-response paradigm. Moberg (1985) outlined the response of animals to environmental stressors as consisting of three general levels of response. The least costly response is behavioral. But if behavioral responses are not capable of alleviating the stress, a change in biological function occurs. Such changes may involve a redirection of energy or substrates from what we view as productive functions, such as growth or reproduction, to defense strategies. One such change in biological function involves the activation of the pituitary-adrenal axis, resulting in release of corticosteroids. A result of this change in function is an altering of the immune response, making the animal more susceptible to some pathogens (Kelley 1982). Moberg (1985) indicates that if the environment is stressful enough, the animal enters a pathological state (Figure 64.1).

Webster (1988) has divided the means by which the environment contributes to pneumonia into three components. First, the environment includes factors that affect the level of pathogens to which the pig is exposed. Second, the environment affects mechanisms by which the pig resists the invasion of pathogens, such as clearance from the lungs. Finally, the environment affects the immune system and how well it can resist the pathogen load. The resulting complexity means that diseases must be viewed as multifactorial in terms of causative factors (Hartung 1994) and in terms of response and susceptibility.

The model presented in Figure 64.1 moves beyond the responses outlined by Moberg (1985) to include the predisposition of the animal (Gonyou 1993). Each animal will respond differently to environmental stressors because of its unique genetic and experiential makeup. Species have different behavioral and physiological characteristics. Some species, such as pigs, react strongly to repel unfamiliar individuals, while others, such as sheep, do not. Some species, such as cattle, react to high environmental temperatures by sweating, while others, such as pigs, do not. But within a species, within a genetic line, or even among genetically identical individuals, predispositions will differ due to experience. Behavior is greatly affected by learning, and physiology may adapt to the environment by relatively permanent changes in pelage, fat cover, and energy partitioning. Changes in the immune system brought about by "experience" with a pathogen are recognized in our immunization programs. Thus the impact of the environment on the animal is a complex combination of environmental features, the predisposition of the animal, and a variety of possible responses.

The multifactorial nature of the relationship of the environment and productivity and disease is illustrated in a series of papers by McFarlane et al. (1989a, b) and McFarlane and Curtis (1989). Using chicks as a model they demonstrated that five different environmental stressors were capable of reducing productivity and affecting physiological and immune responses. When applied in combination, the stressors affected these responses in an additive manner. An extension of this model to swine using high temperatures, crowding, and unstable social conditions confirmed the additive response to multiple stressors (Hyun et al. 1998). In a review of environmental factors recognized to contribute to various pathological conditions in swine, Whittemore (1993; Table 64.1) indicates that several diseases are affected by more than one environmental factor. In assessing the possibility that the environment is contributing to a clinical condition, the practitioner must expect that multiple factors are involved (Curtis and Backstrom 1992) and will likely suggest several changes to the environment in order to remedy the situation. For example, Done (1991) suggests 20 environmental factors to consider when treating for pneumonia. In any one case it is unlikely that only one such factor applies.

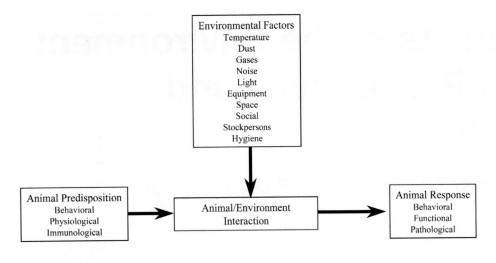

64.1. *The animal/environment inter-action. (Adapted from Moberg 1985, and Gonyou 1993.)*

Although each case of reduced productivity or disease may have multiple environmental factors contributing to it, it is necessary to understand each factor adequately to determine the likelihood that it is involved and how it might be corrected.

THERMAL ENVIRONMENT

The pig is a homeothermic animal with a deep body temperature of 39°C (Baxter 1984). Because the pig's environment is generally lower in temperature than its body, the pig loses heat. Heat is lost through various mechanisms: convection with ambient air; conduction to pen floor, walls, and other pigs; radiation to surrounding surfaces; and evaporation into ambient air. By physiological and behavioral means the pig modifies its heat production to balance heat losses.

The thermoneutral zone is defined as the interval of the thermal environment, usually characterized by temperature, within which an animal's total heat production is approximately constant for a given energy intake (CIGR 1984). Total heat production is at a minimum and independent of ambient temperature in the zone of thermoneutrality (Verstegen et al. 1982; Baxter 1984). According to Bruce and Clark (1979), below the thermoneutral zone heat production is increased, and this

can occur in the growing pig only if energy is diverted from productive purposes.

Lower Critical Temperature

The thermoneutral zone is limited by the lower and upper critical temperatures. Swine buildings are not usually provided with a cooling system, and therefore the reduction of inside temperature during the summer is not possible. A properly designed ventilation system will maintain the indoor air temperature less than 3°C above the ambient temperature. In most commercial buildings, no further control of high indoor temperatures can be achieved and the upper critical temperature is thus of lesser concern in the following discussion. With a temperature colder than the lower critical temperature (LCT), the pig uses a larger proportion of its feed intake energy to increase its total heat production. It is therefore important to define the limits of the thermoneutral zone to minimize wastage of energy intake through higher heat losses.

The LCT is calculated with the thermoneutral total heat production and the minimum latent heat production. It depends upon the heat losses of the pig and consequently the pig body weight, feed intake, air velocity, radiative temperature of surrounding surfaces, type of floor, and the number of pigs. Bruce and Clark (1979)

Table 64.1. Environmental factors associated with diseases in swine

| Disease | Environmental Factor | | | | | | |
	General	Temperature	Crowding	Hygiene	Social	Gases	Dust
Colibacillosis	+	+	+	+			
Swine dysentery	+		+				
Mycoplasma pneumonia	+	+	+		+	+	+
Atrophic rhinitis	+		+	+		+	+
Actinobacillus pleuropneumonia	+		+	+			
Mastitis				+			
Leptospirosis				+			
Streptococcal meningitis		+	+				

Source: Adapted from Whittemore 1993.

developed an extensive model to predict the LCT of pigs. Recently, Brown-Brandl et al. (1998) demonstrated that current design criteria derived from Bond et al. (1959) underestimate heat production at thermoneutral conditions (18–24°C) by approximately 26%, probably due to the increase of lean tissue deposition for the modern high-lean genetic lines. Even if heat production levels increased over time, the pig still dissipates heat through the same mechanisms, and the Bruce and Clark (1979) model continues to be a relevant tool to describe the impact of the thermal environment on the animal's performance and well being.

With an air velocity of 0.15 m × s⁻¹, a feeding level three times the maintenance energy requirement, and a concrete floor, the LCT of a 20 kg pig in a group of 15 pigs is 16°C. The value for a 100 kg pig in the same conditions is 9°C. A reduction of the feeding level to twice the maintenance requirement increases the LCT of 20 and 100 kg pigs to 21°C and 14°C, respectively.

For a 20 kg pig fed three times the maintenance requirement in a group of 15 pigs housed on concrete slatted floors, the LCT increases from 15°C to 18°C when air velocity increases from 0.15 to 0.55 m × s⁻¹ (Baxter 1984). A higher air velocity increases pig heat losses and consequently the LCT as well. The heavier the pig, the better the pig can tolerate lower temperatures (Nicks and Dechamps 1985). CIGR (1992) indicates that with an air velocity of 0.15 m × s⁻¹ and the same feeding level, the LCT decreases from 21°C to 11°C as the pig grows from 20 kg to 60 kg.

The thermal resistance between the pig body temperature and the floor temperature is influenced by the type of floor. Verstegen and Van Der Hel (1974) mentioned that the effective critical temperature of animals weighing 40 kg is 11–13°C on straw bedding, 14–15°C on asphalt, and 19–20°C on concrete slats. A single 34 kg pig fed 3.3 times the maintenance requirement has an LCT of −5°C when it is 70% embedded in straw (Sällvik and Wejfeldt 1993). A group of 16 pigs has an LCT of −20°C in the same conditions. A group of pigs will huddle in the cold (Bruce and Clark 1979), which explains the lower LCT. In fact, postural behaviors can be used to classify the thermal environment of pigs. Shao et al. (1997) captured pictures of postural behaviors of early weaned pigs submitted to four different air temperature regimes varying from 24.4°C to 31.1°C. As their neural network analysis was capable of properly classifying 78% and 96% of testing and training images, their work demonstrated that a picture of animal behavior can be used as an input variable for an environmental controller instead of the conventional approach of using air temperature.

From a production point of view, the LCT is of prime interest. It is the temperature at which the pig will divert some feed energy to produce more heat. However, air temperature alone is insufficient to characterize pig thermal comfort. To choose the right temperature set-

point ensuring the animal's well being and optimal performance, all the parameters previously mentioned should be considered.

Performance

To define the effect of temperature on pig performance, it is necessary to make a distinction between restricted and ad libitum feeding levels. With restricted feeding it appears that the optimum rate of gain is recorded around 20°C, and feed conversion (feed/gain) is minimal from 20–25°C (Verstegen et al. 1978). At similar feed intakes, the rate of gain decreases by 14.3 g × day⁻¹ × °C⁻¹ as the temperature drops from 20°C to 12.5°C (Le Dividich et al. 1985). The growth rate can be maintained constant by an additional supply of food of 38 g × day⁻¹ × °C⁻¹. When pigs are housed at a constant number of degrees below thermoneutrality, the reduction in gain is 14 g × day⁻¹ × °C⁻¹ during the growing period from 25–60 kg (Verstegen et al. 1982). Between 60 kg to 100 kg, the decrease is between 8 and 18 g × day⁻¹ × °C⁻¹ below thermoneutrality. For both growing periods pigs need 25 and 39 g × day⁻¹ of feed to compensate for each degree lower than the thermoneutral zone, respectively.

With pigs fed ad libitum, the maximum growth rate is obtained at an air temperature of 20°C (Nichols et al. 1982; Nienaber et al. 1987a). However, there is no statistical difference in gain observed between 10°C and 20°C or in feed conversion between 15°C and 25°C. As the temperature drops from 10°C to 5°C, the reduction in gain varies from 4 to 21 g × day⁻¹ × °C⁻¹. During summer months, elevated barn temperature reduces animal growth rate by decreasing feed intake (Nienaber et al. 1987a; Lopez et al. 1991; Nienaber et al. 1997). This negative effect on pig performance lengthens the growth period and reduces the productivity level. Experiments showed that when ambient temperature was increased from 20°C to 30°C, the rate of gain was reduced by 17.6–40.0 g × d⁻¹ × °C⁻¹ (Lopez et al. 1991; Nichols et al. 1982; Nienaber et al. 1987a; Massabie et al. 1997). Massabie et al. (1998) measured growth performance of grower-finisher pigs at 17°C and 24°C and at three feed intake levels. For pigs fed ad libitum, the average daily gain of pigs at 17°C (981 g × day⁻¹) was 8% higher than at 24°C (907 g × day⁻¹, reduction of 10.6 g × day⁻¹ × °C⁻¹). However, feed conversion ratio and the percentage of muscle in the carcass were similar at both temperatures.

Diet formulation can have an impact on how pigs will cope with elevated housing temperatures. Bellego et al. (2002) submitted barrows from 27–100 kg body weight and studied the combined effect of reducing the crude protein content of the diet with two housing temperatures (29°C versus 22°C). Overall, increasing the temperature from 22°C to 29°C resulted in a 15% reduction in average daily feed intake and 13% lower average daily gain. The results indicate that a 4-percentage unit reduction of dietary crude protein level does not affect growth and carcass composition as long as the ratio between essential amino acids and net energy is kept optimal. They also concluded that diets with reduced crude protein limit the effect of high ambient temperature on average daily feed intake.

Previous data suggest that, to maximize growth rate and minimize feed conversion rate, grower-finisher pigs should be housed between 15°C and 20°C. It is apparent that the optimum environmental temperature is a temperature zone in which performance and heat production are not significantly different (Nienaber et al. 1987a).

Health Status

Except in extreme cases, a cold air temperature alone cannot precipitate health problems (Nicks and Dechamps 1985). Outbreaks of respiratory diseases can occur only when the microbial agents are present (Tielen 1987). However, fast air temperature fluctuations can trigger a disease outbreak by changing pathogen supply or animal resistance. For example, the results of Narita et al. (1992) indicate that the stress induced by fluctuating temperatures from 4°C to 30°C enhanced the progress and severity of Aujeszky's disease in pigs.

In an experiment by Hessing and Tielen (1994), weaned pigs exposed to draft and low environmental temperature had more pronounced clinical disease signs (i.e., diarrhea, coughing, sneezing, and cyanosis of the ear) than the control group. Le Dividich and Herpin (1994) recommend a stable ambient temperature for piglets penned on a perforated floor. They conclude that data suggest a complex effect of weaning, level of food intake, and nonoptimal climatic conditions on the health status of the weaned pig.

For grower-finisher pigs, there is evidence that the incidence of respiratory problems can be exacerbated by varying air temperature (Christison 1988). Considering the mortality and the incidence of coughing and tail biting, the air temperature for pigs less than 50 kg should be between 17°C and 25°C, with the allowance of an increasing day-night air temperature variability toward the end of this period (Geers et al. 1988). Above 50 kg liveweight, the air temperature should not be higher than 24–26°C, and day-night air temperature fluctuations should be small. In fact, Nienaber et al. (1987b) submitted growing-finishing pigs to constant temperatures of 5°C and 20°C and to similar average temperatures with ±12°C daily cycles in a sine wave pattern. No effect of cyclic temperature was observed for growing pigs, but the results indicated that cycles of ±12°C were stressful to finishing pigs.

Other research has shown limited adverse effects of lower or fluctuating temperature on either piglets or grower-finisher pigs. Nienaber and Hahn (1989) reported that a reduced nocturnal temperature regimen of 6°C resulted in an increased feed intake for nursery pigs.

No performance difference was measured when young piglets were subjected to ambient temperature as low as 15°C (Jacobson et al. 1984). Nursery piglets from 4–8 weeks of age that had been exposed to a fluctuating diurnal air temperature showed no performance difference on daily gain and feed efficiency (Jacobson et al. 1988). Shelton and Brumm (1986) measured slightly improved performance on pigs that were exposed to a nocturnal temperature that had been lowered by 9°C compared to daytime level.

Brumm et al. (1985) conducted an experiment to expose pigs weaned at 23 ±2 days to either a constant regime (30°C for the first week and then decreased by 1.5°C per week for 5 weeks) or a cycling daily temperature regime (the same day temperature as the control, but temperature lowering to 20°C at night during the first week and further reduced by 1°C per subsequent week). Pigs with a reduced nighttime temperature regime grew 6.1% faster as their daily feed intake increased by 7.8%, and feed efficiency was unaffected.

Lemay et al. (2001) conducted two trials over two summers to evaluate the effect of reduced nocturnal temperature on the performance and carcass quality of growing-finishing pigs. Control rooms had a typical temperature setpoint and the temperature setpoint for treatment rooms was 6°C lower. In Saskatchewan, a reduced temperature setpoint resulted in a lower nocturnal room temperature (1.6°C cooler over 8 weeks), but it had no influence on room daytime temperature. The average daily temperature fluctuation in treatment rooms was increased by 2.1°C. During trial 1, pig average daily gain in the treatment room was increased by 5.2%. For trial 2, feed intake was 3.2% higher in treatment rooms, which increased average daily gain by 2.1% on average over 8 weeks. However, no statistical differences were found for pig performance, feed conversion, and backfat thickness (P >0.05). The results suggest that healthy pigs are not negatively affected by a large daily temperature fluctuation (up to 14.8°C) as long as this fluctuation is progressively achieved.

Sow mortality is affected by high environmental temperatures. D'Allaire et al. (1996) examined data from 130 herds and determined sow mortality during a 7-day period with the highest maximum daily temperatures. During one 3-day period, representing less than 0.8% of the year, more than 10% of the annual death loss occurred.

Pigs' health status is not altered by cold air temperature alone. Moreover, some results show that pigs can develop an important mechanism of acclimation to a cold environment (Derno et al. 1995). However, sudden changes in weather have been cited frequently as important factors in the precipitation of disease, and these may be more important than steady extremes of temperature, to which the animal may adapt (Dennis 1986). To maintain a healthy herd, rapid air temperature fluctuations should be avoided.

Setpoint Temperature

The thermal comfort zone of the pig depends on many environmental factors and changes with pig weight. This fact and the results of previous experiments suggest management should be based on temperature intervals rather than a single setpoint value.

Sows and piglets require different temperatures. The farrowing barn should be maintained between 15°C and 21°C (McFarlane and Cunningham 1993). Sows will have a distinct preference for the floor temperature around farrowing. Phillips et al. (2000) concluded that sows showed a pronounced increase in preference for a warm floor (35°C) during 3 days after the start of farrowing. This change in preference may explain why sows tend to avoid metal flooring at the time of farrowing.

Piglets in the first 2 weeks after birth need a 30°C ±2°C temperature to maintain their body temperature and functions (Zhang 1994). Supplemental heat should be provided for piglets. During the first 2 weeks after weaning, Le Dividich and Herpin (1994) recommend an ambient temperature of 26–28°C for piglets penned on a perforated floor. A study by VIDO (1991) suggests that the nursery temperature at weaning should be 27–32°C. Therefore, a temperature of 26–30°C is acceptable for nursery rooms. To choose the best temperature within this range, the pigs' lying behavior should be observed (VIDO 1991). Comfortable pigs lie stretched out on their sides without huddling or piling. Once regular food intake is established, the ambient temperature may be decreased by 2–3°C/week until the finishing-house temperature is reached (Le Dividich and Herpin 1994). Table 64.2 summarizes literature concerning setpoint temperatures for the pig. Because pig thermal comfort depends upon body weight, floor type, air velocity, and the radiant environment as well as temperature, these values should only be used as guidelines and should be refined by observation of the pigs' behavior.

AIRBORNE DUST IN PIG BARNS

Air is a critical factor to living things. People, on average, consume 15 kg of air per day compared to 1 kg of food and 1.5 kg of water. A market size hog breathes about 40 kg of air per day (compared to 2.7 kg of feed and 4 kg of water). People are now beginning to realize how important high quality air is for health and well-being in humans and animals. Of the air quality in pig facilities, airborne dust and toxic gases are two major concerns.

Dust from pig facilities is primarily responsible for health problems in human workers and animals (Zejda et al. 1993, 1994). Toxic gases, especially odorous gases (e.g., ammonia and hydrogen sulfide), are primarily responsible for nuisance smell and for stresses in public relations. These gases can also become major environmental air pollutants in high-density production areas such as the Netherlands and Denmark. Dust tends to be lived with as part of the job and may be ignored until

Table 64.2.   Summary of pig temperature requirements for different stages of production

Stage of Production	Body Mass (kg)	Temperature Range (°C)
Gestation	—	15–24[a,b]
Lactation: sow	—	15–21[b]
Lactation:piglet	—	28–32[a]
Weaning	4–7	25–32[a,c,d]
	7–25	21–27[b]
Growing	25–60	15–24[a,b]
Finishing	60–100	14–21[a,b,e]

[a]Zhang 1994.
[b]McFarlane and Cunningham 1993.
[c]Le Dividich and Herpin 1994.
[d]VIDO 1991.
[e]Midwest Plan Service 1983.

permanent damage is done. Toxic gases cause discomfort (or more dramatic symptoms) that attracts immediate attention and requires quick action to solve the problem.

It is the small dust, or respirable dust, that is responsible for the problems of health and well-being in humans and animals. Dust particles smaller than 10 microns (some say smaller than 5 microns) are called *respirable dust,* because they can be inhaled into respiratory systems of human and animals. Grain dust was once considered to be the largest of all dust particles primarily affecting the airways (nose, throat). However, respirable dust, primarily from fecal materials and other organic compounds, permits more particulate material to reach the lung tissue where it can produce serious health hazards. Very fine particles (smaller than 1 micron) can even penetrate into lung tissues and cause permanent lung damage. Dust particles larger than 10 microns likely bypass a human nose and pose less danger to health (Figure 64.2). To put dust particles into perspective, a naked human eye can only see particles larger than 50 microns in a ray of sunlight. Cigarette smoke contains largely particles ranging from 0.1–1 microns. Dust particles of all sizes suspended in the air are called *total dust.* Thus, air may not be as clean as it appears in a

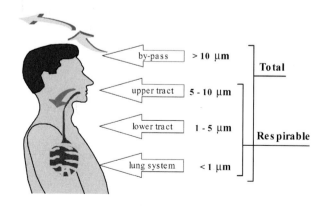

64.2. *Dust particle size and a human respiratory system.*

Table 64.3. Dust sources and microorganisms in swine buildings

Dust Sources	Bacteria and Fungi
Feed particles:	Gram-positive cocci:
Grain dust	*Staphylococcus* spp.
Antibiotics	(coagulase negative)
Growth promotants	*Staphylococcus haemolyticus*
Swine protein:	*Staphylococcus hominis*
Feces	*Staphylococcus simulans*
Urine	*Staphylococcus sciuri*
Dander	*Staphylococcus warneri*
Serum	*Micrococcus* spp.
Other agents:	*Aerococcus* spp.
Bedding materials	*Streptococcus suis*
Endotoxin	(presumptive)
Dust mites	*Enterococcus durans*
Mold	Gram-positive bacilli:
Pollen	*Corynebacterium* spp.
Insect parts	*Corynebacterium xerosis*
Mineral ash	*Bacillus* spp.
Field dust	Gram-negative bacilli:
Building materials	*Acinetobacter calcoaceticus*
Microbial proteases	Nonfermentative gram-
Ammonia adsorbed	negative bacillus
to particles	*Enterobacter agglomerans*
Infectious agents	*Pasteurella* spp.
	Vibrio spp.
	Fungi:
	Alternaria spp.
	Cladosporium spp.
	Penicillium spp.

Source: Adapted from Donham 1986; Martin et al. 1996.

pig barn if it is filled with respirable dust particles because you can not visualize them.

Dusts in pig barns are biologically active and different from ordinary dusts such as field dusts. Swine building dusts are primarily generated from feed grains, fecal materials, animal skin and hair, insects and microorganisms (Donham 1986). They are composed of viable organic compounds, fungi, endotoxins, toxic gases and other hazardous agents (Table 64.3). A dust particle is a very complex mixture with many hazardous agents attached to it. To understand the pathology of health problems caused by dust, it is important to know the dust's microbiological content. Organisms have been isolated and identified as the most important contaminant in swine confinement airspaces (Martin et al. 1996). Some of the organisms such as *Streptococcus suis* and *Alternaria* species are considered particularly hazardous to animals and human beings.

Dust is a carrier of odor. When odor is floated in the air as free molecules, it tends to be diluted quickly into the atmosphere to a less annoying concentration. However, if the odorous molecules are attached to dust particles, they can be carried a long distance and remain present for a long time. For example, a piece of equipment from a pig barn may smell for a couple of months due to the dust adhering to it. Thus, reducing dust con-

centration could have a positive effect on odor reduction. In one study when dust concentration was reduced by 80%, ammonia and hydrogen sulfide were also reduced by 30% and odor was reduced significantly (Zhang et al. 1996).

Threshold values of respirable dust concentration have been recommended to be less than 5 mg/m^3 for workplaces with exposure of 40 hours per week (ACGIH 2003). This threshold limit was established primarily for working environments with inorganic dust, such as the coal-mining industry. A more stringent threshold limit, typically ten times less than that for inorganic dust, has been suggested for pig barn dust concentration because of its biological nature and adverse effects on humans and animals (Donham et al. 1989). High dust concentration is a cause of respiratory problems in pigs, such as bronchitis, coughing, and lung lesions. Dust also has an adverse effect on animal welfare. However, there are few data relating dust concentration to animal performance; one reason is that pigs do not live long enough to develop serious illnesses. Recommendations of threshold limits for dust concentration for animals are not currently available.

The characteristics (e.g., property, behavior and transportation) and pathogenesis of dust in pig barns still remain unclear. However, there is little argument on its adverse effect on the health of people and animals. Therefore, dust in pig barns should be minimized. Improvements to all aspects of swine building design and management practices, such as adding oil to feed have led to a significant reduction in dust (total and respirable) concentration levels in the past decade. The total dust levels in buildings are usually below 3 mg/m^3 compared with the 10 mg/m^3 a decade ago (Barber et al. 1991). However the respirable dust has not been reduced successfully because its origin is primarily the fecal materials and dead microorganisms (Welford et al. 1992). Conventional air cleaning technologies (e.g., fiber and electrostatic filters) for other types of buildings are usually neither efficient nor economical for pig barns due to the high dust concentration. Some new dust control technologies for pig barns have been developed and more research is in process. Dust control strategies involve scrubbing, electrostatic precipitation, ionization, ventilation, filtration and source control technology.

GASES AND HUMIDITY

The primary gases that may affect productivity and the incidence of disease are ammonia, carbon dioxide, hydrogen sulfide (H_2S), methane, and carbon monoxide. Hydrogen sulfide and carbon monoxide may be direct causes of death in pig facilities, whereas the other gases are likely to affect production and health indirectly. For example, ammonia at the levels of 50 and 75 ppm has been shown to reduce the ability of young pigs to clear bacteria from their lungs (Drummond et al. 1978). It is generally recommended, for the comfort of the staff, that ammonia levels be kept at less than 25 ppm. These levels have not been demonstrated to have an effect on the productivity or health status of pigs, but pigs will avoid ammonia levels as low as 10 ppm (Jones et al. 1996).

Under normal barn operation, H_2S concentrations normally stay under 5 ppm. However, manure handling operations within the building, such as pulling plugs to drain pits or power washing rooms, can generate H_2S concentrations many times the levels generally used by occupational health and safety agencies (Chénard et al. 2003). Any manure handling procedure completed in swine facilities should be developed considering the risk associated with H_2S. Readers are referred elsewhere in this volume for more information on these toxic gases (Chapter 60).

Although often ignored as part of the gaseous environment, water vapor is recognized as a contributing environmental factor. Pathogens are best controlled at relative humidity levels between 60% and 80%. Higher or lower levels of humidity result in higher pathogen loads. Respiratory problems are the most commonly observed health problems associated with high levels of humidity. During hot weather high humidity levels may contribute to heat stress because evaporative cooling methods are less effective.

The sources of water vapor include spillage from drinkers, urine, feces, wash water, and water in the feed. Humidity problems are most common during cold weather when ventilation is reduced to conserve heat. Feeding wet feed, particularly on a virtually continuous basis, is a major contributor to humidity problems. The use of water bowls, which waste less water than nipples do, will reduce humidity levels in confinement buildings. The effect of spilled water and of urine will be reduced if the floors are sufficiently sloped for good drainage. Within heated rooms electric heat will result in a drier environment than will gas heaters, which produce water vapor during combustion.

In addition to health concerns, adverse impacts of gases including odor, particulate matter (PM), ammonia (NH_3), hydrogen sulfide (H_2S), carbon dioxide (CO_2), methane (CH_4) and nitrous oxide (N_2O) emitted from animal production facilities have created significant public concerns. These gases are produced by animals or by decomposing manure (Zhang et al. 1992). Current federal and state air quality regulations typically use emission estimates and air dispersion modeling to assess the impact of specific industries or production process on the environment and human health.

Air emissions typically arise from four main sources: the buildings where the animals are confined, outdoor lots where animals are held, manure storage structures, and land application of manure. One of the most effective methods to reduce gas emissions from confinement animal facilities is to reduce the gas concentration in the rooms because most of the gases are emitted via exhaust fans. Many good management practices (power washing, regular cleaning and flushing, sufficient water in the pit) can substantially reduce the odor and gas production and emission in the building, which in turn reduces emission and complaints.

NOISE

Pigs encounter two types of disturbing noises. The first type consists of sudden, startling noises such as sonic booms. The second type of noise is the persistent background noise from fans or other equipment within barns. Sonic booms or other aircraft noises appear to have little effect on the productivity of pigs (Bond 1971), but the noise of burner ignition on low-flying balloons has been claimed to startle animals, sometimes resulting in injury or death (Penny et al. 1995).

Sows and piglets communicate during the nursing/ suckling sequence via grunts and squeals. Loud fan noise (85 decibels) has been shown to interfere with this communication and result in disrupted nursings (Algers and Jensen 1985). Behavioral problems such as tail biting sometimes occur more often near exhaust or recirculation fans. The noise of these fans may contribute to the general discomfort of the pigs, which leads to tail biting. Fan noise may be reduced by regular servicing.

LIGHT

Pigs have been reported to be both diurnal (day-active) (Stolba and Wood-Gush 1989) and nocturnal (Blasetti et al. 1988). The degree of contact with humans may determine which activity pattern is displayed, as shifts from diurnal to nocturnal have been reported during hunting seasons (Hansen and Karstad 1959). Within barns pigs have been reported to perform well in total darkness (Comberg and Doenen 1968, as cited by Curtis and Backstrom 1992). When given the opportunity to control lighting through operant conditioning, pigs will work to obtain as little as 2 min of light a day (Baldwin and Meese 1977). Lighting patterns affect feeding behavior, but not in terms of total intake. Pigs in continuous light evidence a sinusoidal eating pattern, peaking during midday (Gonyou et al. 1992). Pigs on an alternating light/dark cycle display peaks of eating when the lights turn on or off, little eating during darkness, and intermediate levels during midday (Walker 1991; de Haer and Merks 1992). These results suggest that pigs are remarkably adaptable to lighting patterns.

Lighting has been implicated in three areas of production: reproduction, growth, and injuries. Pigs are reported to be short-day breeders (although only moderately so), because the gradually decreasing day length during the summer stimulates the reproductive performance of both boars and sows (Claus and Weiler 1985). Shortening the photoperiod during lactation also improves the return to estrus (Prunier et al. 1994). Longer daylight periods have been demonstrated to increase the growth of suckling pigs (Mabry et al. 1982), primarily through increasing the frequency of nursing (Mabry et al. 1983). One of the few situations in which long photoperiods improve feed intake is during the postweaning period (Bruininx et al. 2002). Although the common recommendation is to use low levels of illumination in grower-finisher barns to reduce activity and aggression, Tuovinen et al. (1992) reported that pigs on farms providing only 48 lx of light had more injuries at the time of marketing than did those on farms providing 77 lx. Christison (1996) reported no differences in postweaning aggression or wound scores under diverse light intensity levels.

EQUIPMENT AND PENNING

A common cause of leg injuries in pigs is slippery floors. Pigs are less likely to slip on concrete floors that are dry and broom- or wood-float–finished than on steel-trowel–finished floors (Applegate et al. 1988). Plastic floors are suitable for creep areas and nurseries but are less desirable for finishing pigs or sows. In addition to slippage, the thermal insulation and comfort value of a floor should also be considered, particularly for young animals. Piglets prefer to lie on plastic-coated metal than on expanded-metal, plastic, or fiberglass slats (Pouteaux et al. 1983). Fully slatted floors are becoming a norm of the industry, even though they are generally recognized to result in more leg problems. A compromise would appear to be flooring with normal slatting around the periphery, where dunging occurs, and a lower percentage of slats in the middle or traffic areas of the pen.

Open penning between pens is also becoming the most common type of pen divider. Such penning is particularly important if convective cooling is heavily relied upon. However, solid walls have advantages in terms of controlling dunging patterns (Hacker et al. 1994) and reducing the movement of manure and pathogens between pens. In general, if convective cooling is desirable, open penning should be used and floors should be fully slatted. In cooler climates in which air movement over the pig is undesirable, solid penning and partially slatted floors work well. Penning materials should be easily cleaned and disinfected. Polyvinylchloride is an easily cleaned material suitable for solid penning.

In general, pens for growing finisher pigs should be 1.5–2.5 times as long as they are wide. This shape facilitates good dunging patterns and easy handling of pigs. Pens should be a minimum of 1.5 times the length of a pig wide (approximately 2 m). This width is necessary to maintain free movement within the pen, particularly if the feeder position requires pigs to stand perpendicular to the pen divisions. If it is compatible with feeder design, in narrow pens feeders should be situated so that pigs stand parallel to pen divisions while eating in order to improve freedom of movement. Pigs perform well on floors with slopes as great as 8%, which facilitates drainage and results in dry sleeping areas (Bruce 1990; Arey and Bruce 1993).

Equipment should be properly sized for the pigs using it. Linear dimensions of the pig, such as length and width, are proportional to body weight $(BW)^{0.333}$. To reduce water wastage (a source of humidity) and injuries, nipple drinkers should be mounted slightly above shoulder level of the pig. The appropriate height for downward-pointing nipples, in centimeters, can be calculated as $18 \times BW^{0.333}$, where weight is in kilograms (Gonyou 1996). The number of pigs that can eat simultaneously from a feeder is dependent on the shoulder width of the pigs rather than the number of dividers in the feed trough. The appropriate width of a feeding space is $67 \times BW^{0.333}$, where width is in centimeters and weight is in kilograms (Baxter 1991). Injuries from feeders are caused by rubbing against parts of the feeder while eating and by feeding-related aggression. Aggression can be reduced by protecting feeding spaces with panels extending back to the shoulder of the pig (Baxter 1991). Injury from feeder contact can be reduced by providing easy access to the feed using a spacious feeding trough and by avoiding sharp edges in construction.

The dimensions of farrowing crates are not as well defined as those for feeders. Even small deviations in the height of the bottom bar or the width of the crate can have significant effects on the behavior of sows and piglets (Rohde Parfet et al. 1989). Studies using existing commercial equipment reported lower piglet mortality for farrowing crates in which the sow was closely confined (Svendsen et al. 1986; Vermeer et al. 1993).

SPACE ALLOWANCE

The allometric relationship for space allowance, a two-dimensional factor, is $k \times BW^{0.667}$, where space allowance is in square meters and body weight is in kilograms (Baxter 1985). Use of an allometric equation for determining space allowance has several advantages over standard tables. An equation allows the producer to determine the space allowance for pigs at the weights they have when they are moved or marketed, rather than extrapolating from a table. This is particularly helpful when market weights are increasing beyond those listed in tables. The k for space used by a lying pig is approximately 0.027 (Baxter 1985). Maximum growth is obtained at k values between 0.034 and 0.039 (Gonyou and Stricklin 1998; Edwards et al. 1988). Growth is depressed approximately 5% when a k value of 0.030 is used. Space allowance should be increased during summer months. The space allowance for a pen should be determined using the average weight of the pigs in the pen when the first pig is removed. For grower facilities this is the average of the pen when they move to the finishing barn. The average weight of the pigs in a pen in the finishing barn is assumed to be approximately 10 kg less than the weight of the largest pig. The weight used for calculating space allowance in finishing facilities should be 10 kg less than market weight.

Overcrowding of pigs results in slower growth and a higher incidence of behavioral problems. Because overcrowding also reduces feed intake, it has been suggested that the performance reduction is due to limited access to the feeding area. If such is the case, increasing the nutrient density of the diet, and thus reducing the time required to consume the feed, should resolve the problem. However, crowding results in similar reductions in intake and growth for pigs that are fed high-density energy (Brumm and Miller 1996), protein (Edmonds et al. 1998), or lysine (Kornegay et al. 1993) diets as well. Chapple (1993) has suggested that stressful conditions may reduce the lean growth potential of pigs, and hence reduce intake. There does not appear to be an effect of crowding on the incidence of stomach ulcers (Eisemann and Argenzio 1999), humoral immune response (Kornegay et al. 1993a), corticosteroid levels, or adrenal weights (Kornegay et al. 1993b). The reduction in growth and feed intake and the increase in behavior problems are indicative of reduced welfare of the animals. However, profitability may be greater under more crowded conditions due to more efficient use of space and capital investment (Edwards et al. 1988; Powell and Brumm 1992). Selection of a space allowance is an ethical decision in which the welfare of the animal must be considered as well as the profitability of the enterprise.

Quality of space refers to how well the space accommodates the behavior of the pig necessary to maintain productivity and comfort. Improving the quality of the space will improve the living conditions of the pigs or at least maintain the quality of life in less space than poor-quality space. Enrichment of the environment is seen as one means of improving the quality of space. Although mechanical toys have not proven to be beneficial (Pedersen 1992), chewable material such as straw or hanging ropes may be useful in reducing behavior problems such as tail biting (Bruce 1990; Feddes and Fraser 1993). Partial partitions in pens for groups of sows allow the formation of subgroups and avoidance of aggressive animals.

SOCIAL

Wild and feral pigs normally live in small groups comprised of closely related individuals (Graves 1984). Even though the animals are related, recognition is based on familiarity rather than genetic similarity (Stookey and Gonyou 1998). When unfamiliar pigs are grouped together, aggression is intense and lasts for several hours. This results in injuries, short-term reduction in growth, and a reduction in immune response. Pigs that are regrouped when young usually recover by the time they

reach market weight. However, when near market weight animals are moved to a new pen and regrouped, they are delayed by 3–5 days in reaching market (Stookey and Gonyou 1994). Regrouping may potentiate susceptibility to other stressors such as crowding (Brumm et al. 2001).

There is some evidence that the composition of a group of pigs can affect their performance. Littermates continue to associate with each other more than with nonlittermates within the same pen throughout the growing-finishing period. However, this association does not confer an advantage on the animals, as small groups of littermates perform just as well as large groups of littermates within the same pen (Gonyou 1997). Pens comprised of very uniform pigs at the time of grouping become more variable as the pigs grow until the within-pen variation is similar to that of highly variable groups (Tindsley and Lean 1984). Within highly variable pens the greatest social stress, as indicated by reduced performance compared to uniform groups, is among the medium-weight pigs (Gonyou et al. 1986). Pens combining pigs of different temperament are more productive than those consisting of pigs with similar personality (Hessing et al. 1994).

Social stress is prevalent in groups of gestating sows that experience the additional stressor of restricted feed intake. Sows added to an established group form a subgroup of their own and are relegated to sleeping in the poorer areas of the pen (Moore et al. 1993). Regrouping during the period of embryonic implantation in bred sows (15–21 days) may result in high return to estrus rates. Social stress in groups of sows can be reduced by providing adequate space (in excess of 2 m²/sow), straw bedding, and partial partitions to allow subgrouping.

STOCKPERSONS

Stockpersons are part of the biological environment of the pig. The importance of the attitude of stockpersons and their interaction with animals on productivity has been reviewed by Hemsworth et al. (1993) and elsewhere in this volume (Chapter 51). Placing greater emphasis on the training of stockpersons and encouraging them to identify and correct problems early are warranted.

HYGIENE

Control of the pathogen load within the pigs' environment is a critical part of management. Management programs such as sourcing of breeding stock, all-in/all-out pig flow, segregated early weaning, and three-site production are discussed elsewhere in this volume (Chapter 68). Within each of these systems of management there is a need for good hygiene to control pathogens. One of the most common sources of pathogens is the feces of other pigs. Solid divisions between pens or smaller rooms are means of restricting movement of material from pig to pig. Frequent cleaning and disinfection of surfaces is the most effective means of reducing pathogen loads in the barn. Morgan-Jones (1987) emphasizes four steps in the cleaning process: removal of gross dirt, particularly organic matter; disinfection; a period of rest before refilling; and fumigation, if possible. Disinfectants include cresols, phenols, quaternary ammonium compounds, iodophors, hypochlorite, and sodium hydroxide (Curtis and Backstrom 1992). Facilities disinfected with cresols should be washed with water once surfaces are dry to prevent skin irritation on pigs. The most effective fumigant for pigs barns is formaldehyde gas, but it must be used carefully due to its toxicity. For most operations the use of all-in/all-out pig flow is the best way to facilitate such cleaning.

REFERENCES

ACGIH. 2003. Threshold Limit Values for Chemical Substances in Work Air. Cincinnati, Ohio: American Conference of Governmental Industrial Hygienists.

Algers B, Jensen P. 1985. Communication during suckling in the domestic pig: Effects of continuous noise. Appl Anim Behav Sci 14:49–61.

Applegate AL, Curtis SE, Groppel JL, McFarlane JM, Widowski TM. 1988. Footing and gait of pigs on different concrete surfaces. J Anim Sci 66:334–341.

Arey DS, Bruce JM. 1993. A note on the behaviour and performance of growing pigs provided with straw in a novel housing system. Anim Prod 56:269–272.

Baldwin BA, Meese GB. 1977. Sensory reinforcement and illumination preference in the domestic pig. Anim Behav 25:497–507.

Barber EM, Rhodes CS, Dosman JA. 1991. A Survey of Air Quality in Saskatchewan Pig Buildings. Can Soc Agric Eng Paper no. 91-216. Ottawa, Ont.: Can Soc Agric Eng.

Baxter M. 1985. Social space requirements of pigs. In Social Space for Domestic Animals. R Zayan, ed. Dordrecht: Martinus Nijhoff, pp. 116–127.

Baxter MR. 1991. The design of the feeding environment for pigs. In Manipulating Pig Production III. ES Batterham, ed. Attwood, Victoria, Australia: Australasian Pig Sci Assoc, pp. 150–177.

Baxter S. 1984. The pig's response to the thermal environment. In Intensive Pig Production: Environmental Management and Design. London: Granada Publishing, pp. 35–54.

Blasetti A, Boitani L, Riviello MC, Visalberghi E. 1988. Activity budgets and use of enclosed space by wild boars (*Sus scrofa*) in captivity. Zoo Biol 7:69–79.

Bond J. 1971. Noise: Its effect on the physiology and behavior of animals. Agric Sci Rev (4th Quarter):1–10.

Bond TE, Kelly CF, Heitman H, Jr. 1959. Hog house air conditioning and ventilation data. Transactions of the ASAE 2:1–4.

Brown-Brandl TM, Nienaber JA, Turner LW. 1998. Acute heat stress effects on heat production and respiration rate in swine. Transactions of the ASAE 41:789–793.

Bruce JM. 1990. Straw-Flow: A high welfare system for pigs. Farm Building Progress 102:9–13.

Bruce JM, Clark JJ. 1979. Models of heat production and critical temperature for growing pigs. Anim Prod 28:353–369.

Bruininx EMAM, Heetkamp MJW, van den Bogaart D, Peet-Schwering CMC, van der Beynen AC, Everts H, den Hartog LA, Schrama JW. 2002. A prolonged photoperiod improves feed intake and energy metabolism of weanling pigs. J Anim Sci 80:1736–1745.

Brumm MC, Ellis M, Johnston LJ, Rozeboom DW, Zimmerman DR. 2001. Interaction of swine nursery and grow-finish space allocations on performance. J Anim Sci 79:1967–1972.

Brumm MC, Miller PS. 1996. Response of pigs to space allocation and diets varying in nutrient density. J Anim Sci 74:2730–2737.

Brumm MC, Shelton DP, Johnson RK. 1985. Reduced nocturnal temperatures for early weaned pigs. J Anim Sci 61:552–558.

Chapple RP. 1993. Effect of stocking arrangement on pig performance. In Manipulating Pig Production IV. ES Batterham, ed. Attwood, Victoria, Australia: Australasian Pig Sci Assoc, pp. 87–97.

Chénard L, Lemay SP, Laguë C. 2003. Hydrogen sulfide assessment in shallow-pit swine housing and outside manure storage. J Agric Safety Health 9:285–302.

Christison GI. 1988. Effects of fluctuating temperatures and of humidity on growing pigs: An outline. In Livestock Environment III, Proc. 3d Int Livest Environ Symp. St. Joseph, Mich.: Am Soc Agric Eng, pp. 101–108.

——. 1996. Dim light does not reduce fighting or wounding of newly mixed pigs at weaning. Can J Anim Sci 76:141–143.

CIGR. 1984. Report of Working Group on Climatization of Animal Houses. Commission Internationale du Génie Rural. Aberdeen: Scottish Farm Building Investigation Unit.

——. 1992. Second Report of Working Group on Climatization of Animal Houses. Commission Internationale du Génie Rural. Ghent, Belgium: Faculty of Agric Sci, State Univ Ghent.

Claus R, Weiler U. 1985. Influence of light and photoperiodicity on pig prolificacy. J Reprod Fert 33 (Suppl):185–197.

Comberg G, Doenen H-D. 1968. Der Einfluss von Fensterlosen, kunstlich beleuchteten Stallen auf die Mast von Schweinen. Schweinezucht Schweinemast 16:209–211.

Curtis SE, Backstrom L. 1992. Housing and environmental influences on production. In Diseases of Swine, 7th ed. AD Leman, BE Straw, WL Mengeling, S D'Allaire, DJ Taylor, eds. Ames: Iowa State Univ Press, pp. 884–900.

D'Allaire S, Drolet R, Brodeur D. 1996. Sow mortality associated with high ambient temperatures. Can Vet J 142:472–485.

De Haer LCM, Merks JWM. 1992. Patterns of food intake in growing pigs. Anim Prod 54:95–104.

Dennis MJ. 1986. The effects of temperature and humidity on some animal diseases—A review. Br Vet J 142:472–485.

Derno M, Jentsch W, Hoffman L. 1995. Effect of long time exposure to different environmental temperatures on heat production of growing pigs. Livest Prod Sci 43:149–152.

Done SH. 1991. Environmental factors affecting the severity of pneumonia in pigs. Vet Rec 128:582–586.

Donham KJ. 1986. Hazardous agents in agricultural dusts and methods of evaluation. Am J Ind Med 10:205–220.

Donham KJ., Haglind P, Peterson Y, Rylander R, Belin L. 1989. Environmental and health studies of workers in Swedish swine confinement buildings. Br J Ind Med 40:31–37.

Drummond JG, Curtis SE, Simon J. 1978. Effects of atmospheric ammonia on pulmonary bacterial clearance in young pigs. Am J Vet Res 39:211–212.

Edmonds MS, Arentson BE, Mente GA. 1998. Effect of protein levels and space allocations on performance of growing-finishing pigs. J Anim Sci 76:814–821.

Edwards SA, Armsby AW, Spechter HH. 1988. Effects of floor area allowance on performance of growing pigs kept on fully slatted floors. Anim Prod 46:453–459.

Eisemann JH, Argenzio RA. 1999. Effects of diet and housing density on growth and stomach morphology in pigs. J Anim Sci 77:2709–2714.

Feddes JJR, Fraser D. 1993. Non-nutritive chewing by pigs: Implications for tail-biting and behavioural management. In Livestock Environment IV. Proc. 4th Int Livest Environ Symp. St. Joseph, Mich.: Am Soc Agric Eng, pp. 521–527.

Geers R, Vranken E, Goedseels V, Berkmans D, Maes F. 1988. Air temperature related behavioural problems and mortality rate of pigs. In Proc 3d Int Livest Environ Symp. St. Joseph, Mich.: Am Soc Agric Eng, pp. 343–348.

Gonyou HW. 1993. Animal welfare: Definitions and assessment. J Agric Envir Ethics 6 (Suppl 2):37–43.

———. 1996. Water use and drinker management: A review. In Annual Research Report. Saskatoon, Sask., Canada: Prairie Swine Centre, pp. 74–80.

———. 1997. Behaviour and productivity of pigs in groups comprised of disproportionate numbers of littermates. Can J Anim Sci 77:205–209.

Gonyou HW, Chapple RP, Frank GR. 1992. Productivity, time budgets and social aspects of eating in pigs penned in groups of five or individually. Appl Anim Behav Sci 34:291–301.

Gonyou HW, Rohde KA, Echeverri AC. 1986. Effects of sorting pigs by weight on behavior and productivity after mixing. J Anim Sci 63 (Suppl 1):163.

Gonyou HW, Stricklin WR. 1998. Effects of floor area allowance and group on the productivity of growing/finishing pigs. J Anim Sci 76:1326–1330.

Graves HB. 1984. Behavior and ecology of wild and feral swine (Sus scrofa). J Anim Sci 58:482–492.

Hacker RR, Ogilvie JR, Morrison WD, Kains F. 1994. Factors affecting excretory behavior of pigs. J Anim Sci 72:1455–1460.

Hansen RP, Karstad L. 1959. Feral swine in the southeastern United States. J Wild Manage 23:64–74.

Hartung J. 1994. Environment and animal health. In Livestock Housing. CM Wathes and DR Charles, eds. Wallingford, U.K.: CAB International, pp. 25–48.

Hemsworth PH, Barnett JL, Coleman GJ. 1993. The human-animal relationship in agriculture and its consequences for the animal. Anim Welfare 2:33–51.

Hessing MJC, Schouten WGP, Wiepkema PR, Tielen MJM. 1994. Implications of individual behavioural characteristics on performance in pigs. Livest Prod Sci 40:187–196.

Hessing MJC, Tielen MJM. 1994. The effect of climatic environment and relocating and mixing on health status and productivity of pigs. Anim Prod 59:131–139.

Hyun Y, Ellis M, Riskowski G, Johnson RW. 1998. Growth performance of pigs subjected to multiple concurrent environmental stressors. J Anim Sci 76:721–727.

Jacobson LD, Boedicker JJ, Janne KA, Noyes E. 1988. Performance and immune response of nursery piglets to fluctuating air temperatures and drafts. In Livestock Environment III: Proceedings of the Third International Livestock Environment Symposium, pp. 109–116. St. Joseph, Mich.: ASAE.

Jacobson LD, Cornelius SG, Jordan KA. 1984. Performance of early weaned piglets as a function of temperature. ASAE Paper No. 84-4019. St. Joseph, Mich.: ASAE.

Jones, J. B., Burgess, L. R., Webster, A. J. F., Wathes CM. 1996. Behavioural responses of pigs to atmospheric ammonia in a chronic choice test. Anim Sci 63:437–445.

Kelley KW. 1982. Immunobiology of domestic animals as affected by hot and cold weather. In Proc 2d Int Livest Environ Symp. St. Joseph, Mich.: Am Soc Agric Eng, pp. 470–482.

Kornegay ET, Lindemann MD, Ravindran V. 1993a. Effects of dietary lysine levels on performance and immune response of weanling pigs housed at two floor space allowances. J Anim Sci 71:552–556.

Kornegay ET, Meldrum JB, Chickering WR. 1993b. Influence of floor space allowance and dietary selenium and zinc on growth performance, clinical pathology measurements and liver enzymes, and adrenal weights of weanling pigs. J Anim Sci 71:3185–3198.

le Bellego L, van Milgen J, Noblet J. 2002. Effect of high temperature and low-protein diets on the performance of growing-finishing pigs. J Anim Sci 80:691–701.

Le Dividich J, Desmoulin B, Dourmad JY. 1985. Influence de la température ambiante sur les performances du porc en croissance-finition en relation avec le niveau alimentaire. Journ Rech Porcine France 17:275–282.

Le Dividich J, Herpin P. 1994. Effects of climatic conditions on the performance, metabolism and health status of weaned piglets: A review. Livest Prod Sci 38:79–90.

Lemay SP, Guo H, Barber EM, Chénard L. 2001. Performance and carcass quality of growing-finishing pigs submitted to reduced nocturnal temperature. Transactions of the ASAE 44(4): 957–965.

Lopez J, Jesse GW, Becker BA, Ellersieck MR. 1991. Effects of temperature on the performance of finishing swine: I. Effects of a hot, diurnal temperature on average daily gain, feed intake, and feed efficiency. J Anim Sci 69:1843–1849.

Mabry JW, Coffey MT, Seerley RW. 1983. A comparison of an 8- versus 16-hour photoperiod during lactation on suckling frequency of the baby pig and maternal performance of the sow. J Anim Sci 57:292–295.

Mabry JW, Cunningham FL, Kraeling RR, Rampacek GB. 1982. Effect of artificially extended photoperiod during lactation on maternal performance of the sow. J Anim Sci 54:918–921.

Martin WT, Zhang Y, Willson PJ, Archer TP, Kinahan C, Barber EM. 1996. Bacterial and fungal flora of dust deposits in a swine building. Br J Occu Environ Med 53:484–487.

Massabie P, Grannier R, Le Dividich J. 1997. Effects of environmental conditions on the performance of growing-finishing pigs. In Livestock Environment: Proceedings of the Fifth International Livestock Environment Symposium, pp. 1010–1016. St. Joseph, Mich.: ASAE.

———. 1998. Incidence de la température ambiante et du niveau de rationnement sur les performances zootechniques du porc en croissance-finition. Journ Rech porcine France 30:325–329.

McFarlane JM, Cunningham F. 1993. Environment: Proper ventilation is key to top performance. Vet Scope 3:6–9.

McFarlane JM, Curtis SE. 1989. Multiple concurrent stressors in chicks. 3. Effects on plasma corticosterone and the heterophil: lymphocyte ratio. Poultry Sci 68:522–527.

McFarlane JM, Curtis SE, Shanks RD, Carmer SG. 1989a. Multiple concurrent stressors in chicks. 1. Effect on weight gain, feed intake, and behavior. Poultry Sci 68:501–509.

McFarlane JM, Curtis SE, Simon J, Izquierdo OA. 1989b. Multiple concurrent stressors in chicks. 2. Effects on hematologic, body composition, and pathologic traits. Poultry Sci 68:510–521.

Midwest Plan Service. 1983. Swine Housing and Equipment Handbook. Ames: Iowa State Univ Press.

Moberg GP. 1985. Biological response to stress: Key to assessment of animal well-being? In Animal Stress. GP Moberg, ed. Bethesda, Md.: Am Physiol Soc, pp. 27–49.

Moore AS, Gonyou HW, Ghent AW. 1993. Integration of newly introduced and resident groups of sows following regrouping. Appl Anim Behav Sci 38:257–267.

Morgan-Jones S. 1987. Practical aspects of disinfection and infection control. In Disinfection in Veterinary and Farm Animal Practice. AH Linton, WB Hugo, AD Russell, eds. Oxford: Blackwell Scientific Publications, pp. 144–167.

Narita M, Nanba K, Haritani M, Kawashima K. 1992. Immunopathology in Aujeszky's disease virus–infected pigs exposed to fluctuating temperatures. J Comp Pathol 107:221–229.

Nichols DA, Ames DR, Hines RH. 1982. Effect of temperature on performance and efficiency of finishing swine. In Proc 2d Int Livest Environ Symp. St. Joseph, Mich.: Am Soc Agric Eng, pp. 376–379.

Nicks B, Dechamps P. 1985. Choix de la température et calcul des besoins de chauffage en porcherie d'engraissement. Ann Méd Vét 129:413–427.

Nienaber JA, Hahn GL. 1989. Cool nighttime temperature and weaning age effects on 3 to 10 week old pigs. Transactions of the ASAE 32(2):691–695.

Nienaber JA, Hahn GL, Eigenberg RA, Korthals RL, Yen JT, Harris KL. 1997. Genetic and heat stress interaction effects on finishing swine. In Livestock Environment V: Proceedings of the Fifth International Livestock Environment Symposium, pp. 1017–1023. St. Joseph, Mich.: ASAE.

Nienaber JA, Hahn GL, Klemcke HG, Becker BA, Blecha F. 1987b. Cyclic temperature effects on growing-finishing swine. In Latest Developments in Livestock Housing. St. Joseph, Mich.: Am Soc Agric Eng, pp. 312–321.

Nienaber JA, Hahn GL, Yen JT. 1987a. Thermal environment effects on growing-finishing swine. Part I, Growth, feed intake and heat production. Transactions of the ASAE 30:1772–1775.

Pedersen BK. 1992. Comprehensive Evaluation of Well-Being in Pigs: Environmental Enrichment and Pen Space Allowance. Ph.D. diss. Univ Illinois.

Penny RHC, Farmer A-MT, Lomas MJ. 1995. "Up and away!" Do hot air balloons scare outdoor pigs? Pig J 34:59–67.

Phillips PA, Fraser D, Pawluczuk B. 2000. Floor temperature preference of sows at farrowing. Appl Anim Behav Sci 67:59–65.

Pouteaux VA, Christison GI, Stricklin WR. 1983. Perforated-floor preference of weanling pigs. Appl Anim Ethol 11:19–23.

Powell TA, Brumm MC. 1992. Economics of space allocation for grower-finisher hogs. J Farm Managers Rural Appraisers 56(1):67–72.

Prunier A, Dourmad JY, Etienne M. 1994. Effect of light regimen under various ambient temperatures on sow and litter performance. J Anim Sci 72:1461–1466.

Rohde Parfet KA, Gonyou HW, Curtis SE, Hurst RJ, Jensen AH, Muehling AJ. 1989. Effects of sow-crate design on sow and piglet behavior. J Anim Sci 67:94–104.

Sällvik K, Wejfeldt B. 1993. Lower critical temperature for fattening pigs on deep straw bedding. In Proc 4th Int Livest Environ Symp. St. Joseph, Mich.: Am Soc Agric Eng, pp. 909–914.

Shao J, Xin H, Harmon JD. 1997. Neural network analysis of postural behavior of young swine to determine the IR thermal comfort state. Transactions of the ASAE 40(3):755–760.

Shelton DP, Brumm, MC. 1986. Energy management in a swine nursery using reduced temperatures, hovers, and reduced nocturnal temperatures. Transactions of the ASAE 29(6):1721–1729.

Stolba A, Wood-Gush DGM. 1989. The behaviour of pigs in a semi-natural environment. Anim Prod 48:419–425.

Stookey JM, Gonyou HW. 1994. The effects of regrouping on behavioral and production parameters in finishing swine. J Anim Sci 72:2804–2811.

———. 1998. Recognition in swine: Recognition through familiarity or genetic relatedness? Appl Anim Behav Sci 55:291–305.

Svendsen J, Bengtsson AC, Svendsen LS. 1986. Occurrence and causes of traumatic injuries in neonatal pigs. Pig News Infor 7:159–170.

Tielen MJM. 1987. Respiratory diseases in pigs: Incidence, economic losses and prevention in the Netherlands. In Energy Metabolism in Farm Animals: Effects of Housing, Stress and Disease. MWA Verstegen, AM Henken, eds. Dordrecht: Martinus Nijhoff, pp. 321–336.

Tindsley WEC, Lean IJ. 1984. Effect of weight range at allocation on production and behaviour in fattening pig groups. Appl Anim Behav Sci 12:79–92.

Tuovinen VK, Grohn YT, Straw BE, Boyd RD. 1992. Feeder unit environmental factors associated with partial carcass condemnations in market swine. Prev Vet Med 12:175–195.

Vermeer HM, Hoofs AIJ, Plagge JG. 1993. Piglet mortality reduction by farrowing crate design. In Proc 4th Int Livest Environ Symp. St. Joseph, Mich.: Am Soc Agric Eng, pp. 820–827.

Verstegen MWA, Brandsma HA, Mateman G. 1982. Feed requirement of growing pigs at low environmental temperatures. J Anim Sci 55:88–94.

Verstegen MWA, Brascamp EW, Van Der Hel W. 1978. Growing and fattening of pigs in relation to temperature of housing and feeding level. Can J Anim Sci 58:1–13.

Verstegen MWA, Van Der Hel W. 1974. The effects of temperature and type of floor on metabolic rate and effective critical temperature in groups of growing pigs. Anim Prod 18:1–11.

VIDO (Veterinary Infectious Disease Organization). 1991. Swine Nursery Design and Management, 2d ed. Saskatoon, Sask., Canada: Univ Saskatchewan.

Walker N. 1991. The effects on performance and behaviour of number of growing pigs per mono-place feeder. Anim Feed Sci Tech 35:3–13.

Webster AJF. 1988. The environmental requirements of tomorrow's livestock. In Proc 3d Int Livest Environ Symp. St. Joseph, Mich.: Am Soc Agric Eng, Suppl 1, pp. S21–S29.

Welford RA, Feddes JJR, Barber EM. 1992. Pig building dustiness as affected by canola oil in the feed. Can Agr Eng 34:365–373.

Whittemore C. 1993. Disease prevention. In The Science and Practice of Pig Production. Harlow, U.K.: Longman Group, pp. 245–279.

Zejda JE, Barber EM, Dosman JA, Olenchock SA, McDuffie HH, Rhodes CS, Hurst TS. 1994. Respiratory health status in swine producers relates to endotoxin exposure in the presence of low dust levels. J Occu Med 36:49–56.

Zejda JE, Hurst TS, Rhodes CS, Barber EM, McDuffie HH, Dosman JA. 1993. Respiratory health of swine producers, focus on young workers. Chest 103:702–709.

Zhang R, Day DL, Christianson LL, Ishibashi K. 1992. A computer model for predicting ammonia release rates from swine manure pits. In ASAE International Winter Meeting. 15. Nashville, Tennessee, 15–18 December.

Zhang, Y. 1994. Swine Building Ventilation: A Guide for Confinement Swine Housing in Cold Climates. Saskatoon, Sask., Canada: Prairie Swine Centre.

Zhang Y, Tanaka A, Barber EM, Feddes JJR. 1996. Effect of frequency and quantity of sprinkling canola oil on dust reduction in swine buildings. Transactions of the ASAE 39:1077–1081.

65 Nursery Pig Management

John R. Pluske, Jean Le Dividich, and David J. Hampson

The young pig is capable of extremely rapid growth after weaning, but unfortunately a number of factors limit the extent to which this inherent genetic potential can be expressed. Whittemore and Green (2001) suggested that growth rates of 100, 200, and 400 g/day in the first, second, and third weeks after weaning, respectively, were commercially acceptable targets under good nutritional, management, disease and environmental conditions. However, it has been recognized for more than 30 years that young, artificially reared pigs (i.e., weaned at 1–2 days of age) given ad libitum access to milk liquid diets can grow in excess of 500 g/day (Hodge 1974; Williams 1976). Excellent growth rates and feed conversion are achievable also in the postweaning period. For example, Pluske et al. (1996) demonstrated that 28-day-old, individually penned weaned pigs fed cow's whole milk every 2 hours for 5 days also grew in excess of 500 g/day and converted milk dry matter to empty body-weight gain at ratios approximating 1.0 (Table 65.1). Williams (2003) commented that if studies such as these were repeated with modern genotypes, young pigs might grow even faster and hence demonstrate a higher potential for lean tissue gain. There is little doubt, therefore, that the commercially reared piglet, both before and after weaning, substantially underperforms relative to what is possible.

Major considerations when discussing overall management and performance of the weanling pig are associations and interactions that occur before and after weaning that can determine future growth. Whittemore and Green (2001) stated that the growth of a pig from birth to maturity is best described by a Gompertz function, which means that the pig has a predetermined growth path and that there are large, fast growing animals and smaller, slower growing animals. The function also means that a larger genotype or a pig with a greater propensity for growth will, at any age, be bigger and grow faster than a smaller genotype, such that pigs heavier at birth and (or) weaning should maintain this advantage as they attain a more mature body size (grow

older) (Williams 2003). The Gompertz function fails, however, to describe the postweaning period where pigs commonly lose weight and then slowly recover. The challenge to people involved in most facets of pig production is to minimize the "growth check" after weaning so that the young pig reestablishes its genetically determined growth path and reaches market weight as quickly as possible.

This chapter commences with a brief description of the variation in piglet weaning age around the world. The chapter then discusses the changes that occur at weaning and is followed by a summary of research concerning the generalized effects of behavior, nutrition and management before weaning on postweaning performance, including the influence of bodyweight at weaning and easing the transition before and after weaning. The chapter concludes with discussion on nutritional and water management and some key nutritional perspectives to promote increased voluntary feed intake and faster gain after weaning.

THE WEANING PROCESS

Weaning generally occurs between 14 and 28 days of age in the major pig producing countries of the world, although key differences exist between and within countries. For example, in the U.S. the majority (60–70%) of pigs are weaned between 16 and 20 days of age, although approximately 15% of the pigs are early-weaned, between 7 and 14 days of age (M. C. Brumm, personal communication) when the passive immunity that the piglet has derived from colostrum and milk is still at a high protective level. In this situation, pigs are moved to off-site facilities or to a nursery physically isolated from older pigs. In contrast, weaning earlier than 21 days of age is banned in the European Union (EU), and legislation might raise this to a minimum of 28 days of age. Moreover, the ban on the use of growth-promoting antibiotics as feed additives in the EU, and legislated reductions in the levels of dietary zinc and copper that can

Table 65.1.   The performance of piglets in the first 5 days after weaning when given either a dry, pelleted starter diet (Starter) offered on an ad libitum basis, or cow's whole milk offered at a calculated maintenance (M) level, a calculated 2.5 times maintenance level (2.5 M), or offered on an ad libitum (Ad Lib) basis.

	Diet Treatment After Weaning				Level of Significance
	Starter	M	2.5 M	Ad Lib	
Bodyweight (BW)					
Weaning	9.0	9.1	9.2	9.2	NS[1]
Slaughter	10.5	9.4	10.5	11.7	NS
Gain, g/day					
BW	288	58	272	514	<0.001
Empty BW[2]	231	49	253	463	<0.001
Dry matter (DM), g/day	286	102	234	400	<0.001
FCR, g DM:g EBWG[3]	1.0	—	1.1	0.9	—

Source: Adapted from Pluske et al. (1996).
[1]NS: not significant at P<0.05.
[2]Empty bodyweight is bodyweight of the pig minus contents of the bladder and the gastrointestinal tract.
[3]EBWG: empty bodyweight gain.

help to control postweaning disorders, have caused an increase in weaning age in countries such as Sweden, where piglets are weaned at closer to 35 days of age. Moreover, in France the issue of saving supernumerary piglets from hyperprolific sows is causing a reexamination of weaning age and practices (Le Dividich et al. 2003).

Regardless of weaning age, the process of weaning is a stressful experience because a number of simultaneous and unique problems not experienced elsewhere in other phases of pig growth occurs. These problems can be classified broadly as nutritional (i.e., change from milk liquid diet to a dry, solid diet differing in texture and composition), environmental (e.g., temperature differences, characteristics of the housing system), social (i.e., separation from the dam, mixing with non littermates) and physical (e.g., transportation, adaptation to new feeding and drinking systems) (Mormède and Hay 2003). Under natural or seminatural conditions, weaning is a progressive process that occurs at 12–17 weeks of age, which is in obvious and stark contrast to commercial pig production. Summaries of the key differences between natural and commercial weaning are described by Brooks and Tsourgiannis (2003).

The collective effect of these actions and events contributes to the postweaning growth check, or lag, which is distinguished by a well-defined period of time in which growth is in deficit (Figure 65.1). The extent of

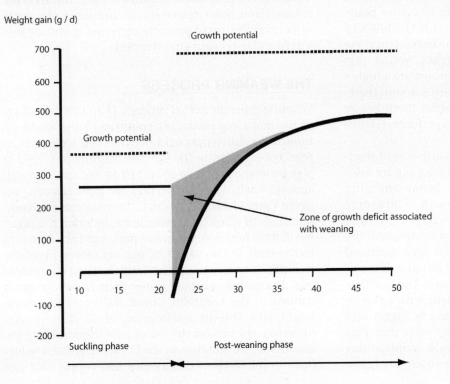

65.1. *The growth potential of piglets and an illustration of the effects of weaning on the growth deficit ("check") that occurs. The least-squares fitted equation of growth rate during the post-weaning phase is as follows:*
$$y = 650\,(\pm 53) - 784\,(\pm 57)\,e^{-0.103\,(\pm 0.02)x},$$
where y = growth rate (g/day), and x = day postweaning (adapted from Le Dividich and Sève 2000).

the growth check appears to be greater the younger the pig is weaned (Dunshea et al. 2002a; Main et al. 2004), partially because of incomplete and hence compromised gastrointestinal development and function (Pluske et al. 2003). Given the nature of the changes imposed it is not surprising that the relative rate of growth of the piglet decreases after weaning. The extent and severity of the growth check depends largely on how resilient the piglet is to the changes and how rapidly it can adjust to its new circumstances and regain homeostasis (Williams 2003).

The extent and duration of the growth check is also highly variable, with some piglets seemingly being unaffected while the condition of others can deteriorate very quickly after weaning. Minimizing the growth check at weaning depends to a large extent on the time taken for a pig to commence eating and the subsequent amount of food eaten, although other factors such as water intake, environmental temperature (see Madec et al. 2003), light schedule (Bruininx et al. 2002a), disease burden and so on must also be considered. Behavioral studies by Bruininx et al. (2001, 2004) and data summarized in Brooks and Tsourgiannis (2003) illustrate that although most pigs in a pen have taken their first meal within 24 hours of weaning, in some pigs it is 50–60 hours before they take their first meal. This causes the variability in performance generally seen in the weaner phase of growth, which can persist through to finishing. Fowler and Gill (1989) calculated that if a pig weaned at 21 days of age was to grow at 280 g/day, a growth analogous to that while sucking the sow, it would need to eat 7.8 MJ of digestible energy (DE) per day. To support this growth rate the piglet would therefore need to eat approximately 500 g of a starter diet containing 15.5 MJ of DE, an intake that is never seen under experimental conditions let alone in commercial practice (Williams 2003).

Commercially, the metabolizable energy (ME) requirement for maintenance is not met until day 3 to 5 after weaning (Le Dividich and Herpin 1994; Bruininx et al. 2002a) (Figure 65.2), and the level of ME intake attained at the end of the first week after weaning accounts for only 60–70% of the preweaning milk ME intake. Usually, 10–14 days are required for pigs to regain their preweaning ME intake. Thereafter, ME intake increases at a rate of 100–120 kJ ME/kg $BW^{0.75}$/day until a plateau is attained at 14–21 days after weaning. Voluntary ME intake attained at the plateau averages 1.5 MJ ME/kg $BW^{0.75}$/day, which is about three times the ME required for maintenance.

Associated with the growth check are changes to the structure and function of the gastrointestinal tract that can predispose to the proliferation of undesirable bacteria (such as enterotoxigenic *Escherichia coli*), leading to general gastrointestinal malaise, diarrhea, morbidity and occasionally mortality. It is not our intention to describe the structural and functional changes occurring in the gastrointestinal tract around weaning because these have been fully and adequately described elsewhere (Hampson 1994; Pluske et al. 1997; Hopwood and Hampson 2003; Miller and Slade 2003; Vente-Spreeuwenberg and Beynen 2003).

The continuous intake of nutrients by the piglet in the immediate postweaning period is generally regarded as being essential to maintain structural and functional integrity of the small intestine (Pluske et al. 1997;

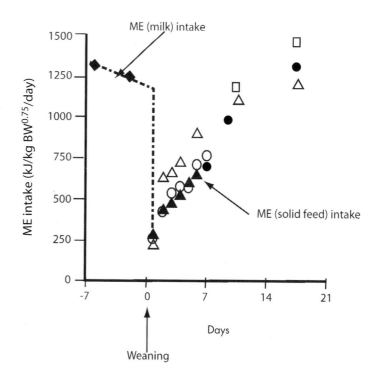

65.2. *The effects of weaning at 21 days of age on the metabolizable energy (ME) intake of pigs fed solid feed. Results were obtained from seven studies. The least-squares fitted equation of ME intake during the postweaning phase is as follows:*

$$y = 1509 \, (\pm 65) - 1479 \, (\pm 80) \, e^{-0.127 \, (\pm 0.02)x}$$

where y = ME intake (kJ ME/kg^{-1} BW$^{0.75}$/day, and x = day postweaning (adapted from Le Dividich and Herpin 1994; Le Dividich and Sève 2000).

Brooks and Tsourgiannis 2003; Vente-Spreeuwenberg and Beynen 2003) and promote large intestinal function (van Beers-Schreuers et al. 1998). Restrictions on the use of antimicrobial agents in some parts of the world however have led to readvocation of restricted feeding to reduce postweaning diarrhea, although some authors (Madec et al. 1998) have reported that higher levels of feed intake after weaning were associated with a reduced risk of diarrhea. Nevertheless, Geary and Brooks (1998) demonstrated the importance of feed intake *per se* in the postweaning period because they calculated that each 50 g per day increase in dry matter intake in the week following weaning increased bodyweight at day 28 postweaning by 0.87 kg. Dry matter intake in the week after weaning accounted for as much variation in bodyweight at 28 days after weaning as any combination of weaning weight, weaning age, gender and diet (Geary and Brooks 1998). Although pigs in this analysis were fed fermented liquid feed that generally promotes a higher level of feed intake than dry feed, the general principles would also apply to pigs eating solid feed.

BEHAVIOR AFTER WEANING

Pigs are rarely kept in their litter groups after they are weaned, but are mixed with pigs from other litters to form the desired group size. Group size for conventional indoor pens that have fully or partially slatted floors has traditionally ranged from 15–30 pigs per pen. Some production systems however, such as outdoor deep-litter hoops, can contain in excess of 250 weanling pigs per pen. Mixing piglets from different litters causes vigorous fighting for the first few hours after weaning and promotes adverse behaviors such as belly-nosing, but eventually a dominance hierarchy and new social order is formed based on dominance-subordination relationships between the pigs in the group. McGlone (1986) commented that social stability is usually observed within 48 hours of weaning, although sporadic fighting events can continue for up to 120 hours after weaning. These behavioral observations have generally been conducted indoors with small group sizes. Housing newly weaned pigs in larger groups in outdoor hoops most likely changes group behavioral dynamics, as has been observed with growing pigs (Morrison et al. 2003a). Unfortunately little or no research appears to have been conducted in this area with weanling pigs.

Associated with these behavioral events are neuroendocrine changes in response to the stress of weaning (Fitko et al. 1992; Mormède and Hay 2003) or to alterations in energy metabolism, although the latter is thought to be of relatively minor physiological importance (Heetkamp et al. 1995). In this respect, regardless of the age at weaning, a transient increase in plasma cortisol or of urinary excretion of cortisol is usually observed (Carroll et al. 1998; Hohenshell 2000; Hay et al. 2001). Changes in the cortisol level are commonly used as an index of stress. Cortisol is also a catabolic hormone, with its secretion being enhanced during periods of feed deprivation (Farmer et al. 1992). Therefore, the increased cortisol secretion could reflect both the weaning stress and the catabolism of energy stores occurring at weaning (see review in Le Dividich and Sève 2000). Urinary excretion of catecholamines are also enhanced after weaning and fasting and implicate low feed intake in altered sympathetic nervous system activity (Young and Landsberg 1977; Hay et al. 2001).

A considerable body of research exists examining ways to ameliorate the stress response at weaning and examine subsequent production effects, mostly with equivocal findings. For example, Pluske and Williams (1996b) attempted to minimize some of the social stress at weaning by comingling (familiarizing) piglets from different litters for the last 14 days of a 28-day lactation period and then grouping these piglets together after weaning. Piglets allowed to familiarize with each other in this manner showed significantly reduced aggressive behaviors after weaning compared to piglets that were mixed directly at weaning. However, this practice showed no lasting stimulatory effects on production indexes such as feed disappearance and daily gain. Other researchers have reported similar findings (Friend et al. 1983; McConnell et al. 1987; Pitts et al. 2000; Weary et al. 2002).

Some of these studies have used alterations in pen design/structure as a means of reducing piglet aggression. For example, McGlone and Curtis (1985) and Waran and Broom (1992) reduced aggressive behaviors and increased growth in the first week after weaning when pigs were provided with "hide or escape areas" in the pen, although long-term positive effects on performance were not evident. It appears that the major advantage of reducing aggression at weaning is on pig welfare.

THE IMPORTANCE OF BODYWEIGHT

Piglet weight at weaning and soon thereafter appears to be a major determinant of the subsequent growth performance, although the manner in which pigs reach a heavier weight also appears crucial. Williams (2003) reviewed numerous studies showing that birth weight is correlated to weaning weight, that weight at 1 week of age is correlated to weaning weight, and that weight at weaning is correlated to subsequent performance after weaning. In addition, Tokach et al. (1992) and Azain (1993) reported that pigs growing well (225–340 g/day) in the first week after weaning reached market weight 10–28 days before pigs exhibiting poor gain in that same week (0–110 g/day). The effects of weight gain (and hence feed intake) in the first week after weaning and weaning weight have been shown to be additive and account for 80% of the variation in body weight on day 20 after weaning and 34% at 118 days of age (Miller et al. 1999; Ilsley et al. 2003). Furthermore, Lawlor et al.

(2002a) commented that the type of diet fed after weaning can affect the significance of the relationship between birth weight and postweaning performance. They recommended feeding a high-density diet after weaning to take advantage of this relationship.

Pigs that are heavier at weaning seem to continue their weaning weight advantage to slaughter weight (Mahan and Lepine 1991; Lawlor et al. 2002a; Dunshea et al. 2003). However, the manner by which a piglet attains that weight, such as higher creep feed intake during the lactation period, appears to have a marked influence on subsequent growth performance. Williams (2003) argued that if food intake is genetically determined to drive growth that is also genetically determined, which it must be, then it is most unlikely that a transient period of higher-than-normal nutrition will change a long-term hypothalamic food "setting." Consequently, any increase in weight caused by an increase in growth would, at best, be maintained and, at worst, disappear with time.

Several data sets support this theory and may help to explain the apparent paradox in the literature surrounding this issue. Wolter et al. (2002a) found that increasing weaning weight by means of supplemental milk replacer during a 21-day lactation had no significant effect on performance to 14 kg after weaning or on performance in the period from weaning to slaughter at 110 kg. On the other hand, piglets that were inherently (genetically) heavier at weaning, partially because they were heavier at birth, ate more and grew faster to slaughter (Table 65.2). Nevertheless, piglets fed milk replacer took 3 days fewer to reach slaughter than piglets not offered milk replacer. Lawlor et al. (2002a) reported a 0.6 kg increase in weaning weight at 28 days, attributable to creep feeding. This weight advantage was lost by day 26 after weaning, whereas pigs inherently heavier at weaning (7.1 vs. 5.8 kg) remained heavier 26 days later (17.5 vs. 15.4 kg) because they ate more feed. These data are consistent with those of Fraser et al. (1994) who estimated that creep feed intake in lactation accounted for only 1–4% of the variation in bodyweight gain after weaning. In another study, Wolter and Ellis (2001) reported that weaning weight had a greater effect on age at slaughter than growth rate in the first 2 weeks after weaning, which was manipulated by offering a liquid milk replacer.

In contrast, Dunshea et al. (1997) found that providing skim milk powder (20% dry matter content) from day 10 of a 20-day lactation not only increased weaning weight (0.7 kg), but had a significant positive effect on bodyweight at 42 and 120 days after weaning compared to piglets that did not receive the milk supplement. These contrasting data sets are difficult to reconcile, but Williams (2003) postulated that consumption of skim milk powder during suckling, with its more favorable protein-to-energy ratio compared to sow's milk for lean tissue gain (Campbell and Dunkin 1982; Williams 1995), might have allowed the piglets to compensate for the inferior quality of sow's milk and hence shifted their preprogrammed growth curve.

Management techniques have also been tried to increase weaning weight. Split weaning is a practice whereby half the litter, or some other proportion, usually the heavier piglets, is weaned. The lighter pigs remain to suck the sow, say for an extra 5–7 days, to obtain more milk. Several workers have shown that the light piglets that remain with the sow grow faster than their counterparts that have to compete with their larger littermates (summarized in Le Dividich 1999). For example, Pluske and Williams (1996a) split-weaned the heavier piglets from litters at 22 days of age and showed that the bodyweight of the remaining lighter piglets could be increased by 60% in the following week because of increased milk intake, relative to counterparts not split-weaned. Lighter piglets in the split-weaned litters weighed 15% more (7.7 vs. 6.7 kg) than their counterparts in the full litters at weaning at 29 days of age. However by 9 weeks of age the difference in weight had disappeared (19.3 vs. 19.3 kg).

MANAGEMENT OF THE PIGLET DURING LACTATION

Associations are believed to occur between the preweaning nutrition and behavior of the piglet and subsequent postweaning performance. The piglet relies predominately on the sow for its nutritional requirements before weaning, at least under modern-day pig husbandry and weaning management systems. Piglets consume colostrum in the first 24–36 hours after parturition and then consume milk at regular intervals during the day and night until weaning (Pluske and Dong 1998). Colostrum intake before closure of the small intestine to immunoglobulins is of critical importance to both the subsequent survival and performance of the young pig, even in the postweaning period (Pluske and Dong 1998; King and Pluske 2003). Giving colostrum to weaker piglets, or to litters where the sow is suffering agalactia,

Table 65.2. The effects of birth weight (Heavy vs. Light), weaning weight and supplementary milk replacer during lactation (Milk vs. No Milk) on voluntary feed intake and growth rate to slaughter.

	Birth Weight		Supplementation in Lactation	
	Heavy	Light	Milk	No Milk
Bodyweight, kg				
Birth	1.83	1.38	1.58	1.58
Weaning (21 days)	6.6	5.7	6.6	5.7
Weaning to 110 kg				
Feed intake, kg/day	1.87	1.78	1.84	1.81
Growth rate, g/day	851	796	827	820

Source: Adapted from Wolter et al. (2002a).

is generally used as a management technique to increase survival rates and weaning weight and possibly reduce the variation in weaning weight (King and Pluske 2003). Alternatively, practices such as split weaning/cross suckling immediately after farrowing offer potential to allow a more equitable transfer of colostral immunoglobulins across the spectrum of weights within a litter (Donovan and Dritz 2000). Many studies show the benefits of colostrum for gut development, as an energy source for thermoregulation of the newborn piglet, a substrate for protein synthesis, and a passive supply of protection against enteric pathogens (Le Dividich and Noblet 1981). Collectively, these functions are important in establishing the pig during lactation and, ultimately, after weaning.

Supplementary Feeding during Lactation

Many studies have investigated the effects of "creep" feeding (i.e., offering a solid diet) during lactation on weaning weight and performance thereafter (reviewed by Pluske et al. 1995; King and Pluske 2003). The major argument for offering suckling piglets supplementary food during lactation is to counteract the growing gap between the piglet's energy requirements and sow milk production as lactation advances. For example, Harrell et al. (1993) calculated that the supply of sow's milk probably begins to limit piglet growth at about 10 days of age and that the sow would need to produce an additional 18 kg of milk per day by day 21 of lactation to support equivalent piglet growth rates. This is clearly not possible. A further argument, although one that is less convincing, is that the consumption of creep feed prepares the gastrointestinal tract for the digestion of complex carbohydrates and plant protein that will be supplied after weaning. However, Chapple et al. (1989) reported that the variation in amylolytic activity in the pancreas of piglets was more a function of the sow (litter of origin) than of the intake of solid feed during lactation and immediately after weaning. Lindemann et al. (1986) and de Passille et al. (1989) found that pepsin and maltase activities in the gastrointestinal tract could not be related to weaning weight or to the duration of creep feeding during lactation. More recently, Bruininx et al. (2002b) reported the lack of any association between creep feed intake before weaning and gut structure at 5 days after weaning.

Finally, creep feeding has been said to familiarize piglets to solid feed so that the transition at weaning will be less stressful, but again, there is no robust evidence to support this sentiment. For instance, Kuller et al. (2004) conducted a study in which sows were either (a) intermittently suckled (IS) for 12 hours/day starting from day 11 to encourage their piglets to become familiar with creep feed before weaning and eat more of it during lactation, or (b) continuously suckled (CS), over a 27-day lactation. They found that although IS piglets consumed more creep feed during and after lactation than

CS piglets, their bodyweights were the same by the seventh day after weaning.

Creep Feed Intake. In spite of the large body of evidence dealing with supplementary feeding, evidence to support the notion that supplying pigs with dry creep food during lactation will improve preweaning and postweaning growth performance is equivocal. Pluske et al. (1995) and Brooks and Tsourgiannis (2003) reviewed a number of studies presented in the literature and found an enormous variation in the intake of creep-fed piglets. Pluske et al. (1995) calculated that the contribution of creep feed to daily energy intake prior to weaning at 21–35 days of age ranged from 1.2–17.4%. Lawlor et al. (2002a) more recently confirmed this level of contribution to overall energy intake of the piglet. The intake of dry creep food during lactation is generally small and variable and unlikely to significantly influence weaning weight, particularly in piglets weaned at 3 weeks of age or younger (King and Pluske 2003). However, Appleby et al. (1991) reported that creep feed intake during a 27-day lactation was enhanced when piglets were provided a feeder with eight spaces compared to two spaces, and that piglets that ate more solid feed before weaning gained more weight in the 14 days after weaning. In spite of this, pigs with the higher intake were also heavier at birth, thereby confounding the effects. In another study, Appleby et al. (1992) found an inverse relationship between birth weight and creep feeding behavior, but by 42 days of age there was no difference in bodyweight between the groups.

Notwithstanding the positive responses of creep feeding observed in some studies, the literature suggests that growth rate after weaning is often poorly related to the intake of creep food before weaning (Barnett et al. 1989; Pajor et al. 1991; Fraser et al. 1994). Creep feed consumption varies tremendously both within litters and between litters. Fraser et al. (1994) estimated that creep feed intake accounted for only 1–4% of the variation in bodyweight gain in piglets in their first 14 days following 28-day weaning, even though there were significant litter effects on the intake of dry feed during lactation. Pluske et al. (1995) and King and Pluske (2003) commented that there is a highly significant effect, 30–60% of the total variance, of litter on weaning weight and subsequent postweaning performance. This indicates that one or more factors before weaning are having a major influence on both weaning weight and subsequent growth rate, with both prenatal and postnatal components likely having an effect. Rooke et al. (1998) reported that the relative importance of these events was 3:1 in favor of the prenatal effects, begging the question of where one begins to investigate the phenomenon of variation in pig weights. These issues currently remain largely unresolved.

One possible reason for the discrepancy seen between published studies is the methodology used to assess intake of creep feed. The consumption of creep feed has generally been measured on either a litter basis or on an individual piglet basis, where litter consumption of the diet is divided by the number of piglets in the litter to achieve a per piglet consumption. The latter method of expression is erroneous because piglets in the same litter will not all consume the same amount of creep feed. In a unique experimental approach, Bruininx and colleagues (2002b) in The Netherlands used fecal Cr_2O_3 as a marker for classifying piglets as "good," "moderate," or "non" eaters of creep feed during lactation. Using this approach, in conjunction with computerized feeding stations that recorded individual feed intake after weaning, Bruininx et al. (2002b) found that pigs classed as "good eaters" preweaning showed less time between weaning and first feed intake compared to the other groups, and consumed more feed in the first 8 days after weaning. By day 34 after weaning the effect of greater creep feed consumption during the lactation period on feed intake was less pronounced, although daily gain was still higher. The methodology used in this study indicated that some individual pigs eat more than others after weaning because of their higher preweaning consumption of dry feed.

In this regard some pork producers, especially those weaning later than 21 days of age, continue to offer high-quality creep diets to suckling pigs irrespective of the general lack of effects seen at the litter level. In some countries, such as Sweden and Denmark, where weaning age is now 28 days of age or greater and the use of growth-promoting antibiotics and antimicrobial agents such as zinc oxide are banned or strictly regulated, the importance of enhancing the intake of solid feed before weaning is not questioned, and is receiving renewed attention.

Liquid Diets to Enhance Feed Intake Before and After Weaning. In contrast to the generally equivocal results reported with the intake of dry creep feed, providing young pigs with liquid feed, either dry diets in a gruel/slurry form or milk liquid diets, would appear to offer more promise as a management tool to increase both weaning weight and postweaning performance. Brooks and Tsourgiannis (2003) argued that in view of the problems the piglet usually encounters in discriminating between hunger and thirst in the immediate postweaning period, then offering a liquid diet has three potential advantages:

1. It provides a diet with a dry matter content more akin to that of sow's milk.
2. It can provide a diet more closely matched to the piglets' needs for nutrients and water.
3. It overcomes some of the issues piglets face in having to learn to satisfy drives for both hunger and thirst.

The feeding of a solid diet in gruel/slurry form allows piglets to associate feed and water together, which in turn could enhance dry matter intake. Toplis et al. (1999) stimulated piglets to consume an average of 374 g/day of gruel (1:2 meal to water ratio) in the last 10 days of a 24-day lactation; yet they weighed 0.2 kg less than piglets allowed to only suck the sow. This practice, however, stimulated performance after weaning, with gruel-fed pigs growing 150% faster (150 vs. 49 g/day) than piglets that ate no creep feed during lactation, and they grew 30% faster (416 vs. 317 g/day) for 5 weeks after weaning. Lawlor et al. (2002b) found no consistent effects of feeding liquid feed or acidified liquid feed to pigs weaned at 28 days of age, while Le Dividich et al. (unpublished data) showed superior performance of 28-day-old weaned pigs fed liquid diets using a programmable, automated liquid feeder. However, long-term advantages of the system on performance were not seen. From a limited number of studies it would appear that benefits derived from feeding weaner diets in liquid (gruel/slurry) form are equivocal.

Many more studies have investigated feeding milk replacer diets to young pigs. For example, Reale (1987) offered cow's whole milk to piglets from 10.00 h each day, adding fresh milk every 2 hours until 23.00 h, from day 7 to day 28 of lactation. Growth was stimulated by 151 g/day (71%) in the fourth week of lactation and by 87 g/day from day 7 to 28. This practice increased weaning weight by 1.8 kg in comparison to controls that were offered a dry creep feed. King et al. (1998) found that piglets offered liquid skim milk powder from day 5 of lactation were 1.6 kg heavier at weaning at 28 days of age than piglets that received no supplemental nutrients. In addition, piglets appeared to still prefer milk from the sow, because the supply of supplemental milk did not reduce the amount of milk that the piglet obtained directly from the sow.

King and Pluske (2003) reviewed a number of studies and reported a weight advantage of 11–35% at weaning in favor of offering a liquid milk replacer during lactation. Heo et al. (1999) reported that 14-day-old weaned piglets fed a liquid milk replacer achieved a growth rate of 470 g/day in the first 7 days after weaning. Kim et al. (2001) showed that feeding 11-day-old weaned piglets a liquid milk replacer through an automated milk machine for the first 14 days after weaning significantly increased weight at 28 days of age by 1.62 kg. This growth advantage was maintained to market weight with no evidence of compensatory gain in the dry-fed control pigs, with the liquid-fed pigs reaching market weight 3.7 days earlier than the dry-fed pigs. These results demonstrate the potential benefit of additional nutrients on weaning weight and a clear benefit of supplemental milk replacer to increase weaning weight. However, Armstrong and Clawson (1980) failed to stimulate growth in piglets offered liquid milk replacer during a 21-day lactation, perhaps suggesting that the sow was providing sufficient milk.

The use of a liquid milk replacer during the weaning

period has also been shown to reduce the severity and extent of the growth check. Dunshea et al. (1997) attempted to alleviate the postweaning growth check by providing extra milk around the time of weaning. Pigs provided with liquid milk replacer, in addition to access to dry starter feed, gained 1.2 kg during the first week after weaning, whereas pigs that received only dry starter feed gained 0.4 kg in the same period. Supply of a liquid milk replacer to piglets both before weaning and in the first week after weaning had an additive effect; pigs that received liquid milk replacer before and after weaning were 10% heavier at 120 days of age than pigs that suckled the sow only and were weaned onto dry starter feed (Dunshea et al. 1997). Much of this improvement was most likely attributable to the extra nutrient intake from supplemental milk replacer prior to and immediately after weaning.

It would appear that offering newly weaned pigs a liquid milk replacer offers the best potential for overcoming the postweaning decline in dry matter intake that occurs and hence increasing growth rate after weaning. Liquid feeding milk-based diets however can be labor intensive and hygiene must be adhered to for the practice to be successful.

Large-Scale Liquid Feeding and Fermented Liquid Feeding for Weanling Pigs. Large-scale, fully automated liquid feeding systems are used commonly throughout the world to feed growing and finishing pigs, especially to take advantage of cheaper co-products and by-products and modulate the bacterial environment in the fermentation vessel and in the pig. Liquid feeding on a similar scale for weaner pigs has met with less success, largely because of problems in maintaining the feed in a palatable and fresh manner, higher labor costs, poor feed hygiene, and feed wastage, particularly in the first week after weaning. Nevertheless, recent technological advances in liquid feeding, a trend for later weaning ages, a greater understanding of fermentation kinetics and the way fermented feed can modulate the gastrointestinal microbiota (e.g., Jensen and Mikkelsen 1998), and some convincing data showing marked improvements in dry matter intake and daily gain (e.g., Russell et al. 1996) offer exciting opportunities for managing the weanling pig in order to improve production and minimize enteric disturbances.

Use of Flavors in Diets

Research has been conducted in an attempt to increase weaning weight and reduce the growth check after weaning by using various sweeteners and aromatic compounds to increase feed consumption (reviewed by Brooks and Tsourgiannis 2003; King and Pluske 2003). Results have generally been variable. Campbell (1976) added a feed flavor into a creep diet and failed to increase creep food consumption or weaning weight, but unexpectedly the pigs that had been weaned from sows given a flavored diet and then given a flavored diet after weaning consumed more feed, particularly in the first 2 weeks after weaning. King (1979) confirmed this interaction on feed intake after weaning and also demonstrated that when the flavor was added to the sow diet, it was detected in milk samples collected from those sows. Madsen (1977) indicated that feed preferences could be transferred from lactating sows to their litter by incorporating a nonmetabolizable substance into both the lactating sow diet and the diet offered to piglets after weaning. Any positive effects of feed flavors observed in young pigs are more likely to be due to this transference of feed preferences via flavors incorporated in sow's milk, or by masking unacceptable tastes to improve the palatability of the creep feed (King and Pluske 2003).

In some regions of the world it is common practice to include flavors/sweeteners in commercial diets for young pigs, both before and after weaning, and various manufacturers actively promote their inclusion in diets. There is very little, if any, peer-reviewed published information relating to the use of flavors/sweeteners and their effects on production before and after weaning, although their continued use in diets suggests they are perceived to be of some benefit.

NUTRITION, NUTRITIONAL MANAGEMENT, AND THE IMPORTANCE OF WATER IN THE POSTWEANING PERIOD

Many review articles, peer-reviewed papers, popular press articles, and book chapters have been written on different aspects of nutrition and nutritional management of the weanling pig. Some of the more recent and comprehensive articles include those by Nelssen et al. (1999), Mavromichalis and Varley (2003) and Tokach et al. (2003). It is not our intention to reiterate this information; however, the principles of a successful nutritional program for the weanling pig will differ around the world according to a variety of factors, such as weaning age, weaning weight as alluded to previously, ingredient availability and cost, physical environment (e.g., indoor pigs kept on fully slatted floors vs. outdoor pigs kept on deep litter), regulations (e.g., restrictions on the use of antimicrobial agents and animal proteins, if any), the system of weaning (e.g., multisite production vs. farrow to finish), method of feeding (e.g., dry diets vs. liquid diets), nutrition during lactation, sow feeding programs, and adoption or not of phase feeding after weaning. For example, Mavromichalis and Varley (2003) commented that in North America the focus after weaning is predominately on reducing production costs, especially for the large integrated operations, by feeding pigs the cheapest diets as soon as possible after weaning (e.g., a phase feeding program; Tokach et al. 2003), whereas the European approach is based more on achieving maximum growth performance and optimum health status after weaning. Consequently a successful transition between lactation and weaning is a multifaceted process that must consider the entire pig production system of any particular enterprise, and not only nutrition.

Campbell (1989) argued that practical nutrition of the young pig at weaning is more of an art than a science and suggested that a dietary regimen that is highly successful and repeatable under research conditions may not apply to commercial practice. This comment presumably reflects the large number of factors that impinge and interact on the piglet at weaning, as outlined previously. Nevertheless, Williams (2003) remarked that high feed intake after weaning, and hence high growth rates, with minimal digestive disturbances can be achieved consistently only with high-density, highly digestible diets. Starter (link) diets are generally required to ease the transition from milk (high-fat, high-lactose) to plant-based diets that are much lower in fat and contain high levels of antinutritional factors, such as nonstarch polysaccharides. Such diets generally need to contain high-quality animal products of milk origin, such as lactose, or products derived from blood. The younger the pig is at weaning the more important this becomes, and this is aptly demonstrated in recent data from Dunshea et al. (2002a). These authors offered piglets a weaner diet containing wheat (550 g/kg), Australian sweet lupins (50 g/kg), soybean meal (50 g/kg), meatmeal (66 g/kg), fishmeal (83 g/kg), skim milk (20 g/kg), blood meal (26 g/kg) and whey powder (100 g/kg), and weaned them at either 14 or 24 days of age. Pigs weaned at the older age gained weight during the first week after weaning; the younger pigs lost weight.

A key factor that has made weaning less problematic in the last 15 years, particularly when weaning at less than 16–18 days of age, is the use of specialized diets containing proteins derived from blood. Products from porcine blood, particularly porcine plasma, are mandatory for diets in parts of the world such as North America because they stimulate voluntary feed intake (Pluske et al. 1995; van Dijk et al. 2001; Tokach et al. 2003). The most favored explanation for this phenomenon is the presence of immunoglobulins, although the exact mechanism(s) of action is/are yet to be elucidated. However, because of the concern about feeding animal proteins to the same species and a ban on the use of plasma/blood proteins in the EU, there is interest in looking at other sources of milk proteins—for example, from cows—to see whether similar effects can be achieved in young pigs.

In New Zealand, Pluske et al. (1999) weaned pigs at 4 weeks of age and found that adding a spray-dried colostrum preparation (containing 150 g/kg IgG) at 50 g/kg diet stimulated food intake by 12% in the first week after weaning. They increased the amount to 10% and stimulated food intake by 25%. This extra food intake boosted growth by 40% and 80%, respectively, so that pigs on the highest level of colostrum grew in excess of

200 g/day in the first week after weaning. King et al. (2001) reported a 25% increase in voluntary food intake in the first 7 days postweaning by adding 60 g/kg of bovine colostrum to a diet after weaning, while Dunshea et al. (2002b) compared porcine and bovine plasma, bovine colostrum and commercially produced skim milk and found relatively little difference between the protein sources in the performance of pigs weaned at 14 days. However, Dunshea et al. (2002b) reported that their studies were conducted in a clean research environment, a factor thought critical in determining whether products such as porcine plasma prove efficacious after weaning (Coffey and Cromwell 1995). Grinstead et al. (2000) indicated that a high protein diet (780 g/kg) with whey protein concentrate provided pig performance comparable to animal plasma in weanling pig diets. More recently, Le Huérou-Luron et al. (2004) found a 22% increase in daily feed intake commensurate with a 33% increase in daily gain in pigs fed a bovine colos-trum preparation in the first week after weaning. It appears, therefore, that high-quality proteins based on colostrum/milk stimulate growth in the immediate postweaning period in a way analogous to porcine plasma, and depending on prevailing price and availability, could be used in regions of the world where blood products are banned or restricted in their use. After the initial phase after weaning, however, plant proteins such as soybean meal, rapeseed meal, peas, beans, and lupins generally form an increasing percentage of diets to minimize the cost per unit gain.

Feeding Management after Weaning

A successful nutritional regimen is one that encourages newly weaned pigs to commence eating as soon as possible after weaning, usually by offering feed on an ad libitum basis, while minimizing feed wastage, simply because diets fed in the immediate postweaning period are expensive. In this chapter, strategies that can be used before and after weaning to promote weight gain have already been discussed, and the intention here is to examine more practical ways to ensure piglets make a good start after weaning. In this regard, Tokach et al. (2003) remarked that the two major keys in management of the feed program are (i) a proper management protocol to encourage feed intake, and (ii) correct adjustment of feeders to reduce wastage.

Mat Feeding after Weaning. Supplying feed on temporary mats and (or) in small trays for several days after weaning has been shown to improve feed intake and growth rate (Mavromichalis and Varley 2003), provided correct management is adhered to. This generally includes adopting a "little but often" feeding policy (100–150 g feed/pig/day in 3–4 feeding episodes) and removing stale and fouled feed regularly. Feed must concurrently be available in self-feeders. Dritz et al. (1996) commented on the importance of trained staff in identifying "starve out" pigs and then managing them properly, for example, by teaching them how to eat. Mavromichalis and Varley (2003) remarked that pellets and blends of pellets with mash (meal) are best because piglets tend to waste more pellets if they are fed alone. Beattie et al. (1999) attempted to increase feed intake after weaning by providing wet feed in a trough in the pen for 5 days after weaning, and although intake was increased, there were no long-term effects on production. Beattie et al. (1999) remarked that the trough containing wet feed incurred additional labor costs.

Management of the Feeder. Proper adjustment of feeders is a labor- and time-consuming process but is key to good feed efficiency and hence lower feed cost per unit gain. Feed wastage is notoriously difficult to measure or estimate, although Mavromichalis and Varley (2003) estimated wastage of 5–7% in properly managed feeders. Mavromichalis and Varley (2003) and Tokach et al. (2003) recommended that the adjustment gate in the feeder must be closed before filling it with feed, because placing pelleted feed into an empty feeder with the adjustment gate open could increase wastage and cause subsequent problems in proper feeder adjustment.

Tokach et al. (2003) recommended managing the flow of feed into the feeder pan to stimulate the development of feeding behavior by allowing only 50% of the pan to be visible in the first few days after weaning. Mavromichalis and Varley (2003) recommended a 66% coverage with feed. Too much feed in the pan can cause the build-up of fines, leading to blockages. Regardless, as pigs become accustomed to feeding, the amount of feed in the pan can be gradually reduced—for example, to 25–33%, which reduces wastage and reinforces feeding behavior. Care also needs to be taken of feeding pellets or mash (meal) because mash diets, particularly if high in milk products, tend to bridge feeders more than pellets. Mavromichalis and Varley (2003) suggested that observing pigs and looking for wastage underneath the pens and around the feeder were the best ways to assess wastage, and that environmental conditions, such as higher humidity, can cause feed to stick to gate openings. The build-up of fines should also be avoided.

The Importance of Water Intake after Weaning

Voluntary or involuntary deprivation of water in the period after weaning can have dire consequences for piglet physiology, health, and performance. Gill (1989), for example, showed that it could take more than a week after weaning for piglets to restore their daily fluid intake to preweaning levels. There are important behavioral components associated with water intake after weaning that presumably influence the extent and volume of water consumed after weaning. Brooks and Tsourgiannis (2003) explained that sucking pigs have been conditioned to consume milk to satisfy their needs for volumetric "fill," and in the early postweaning period may fail to distinguish between the separate drives for hunger and thirst. Having been conditioned to a liquid milk diet, newly weaned piglets may mistakenly believe that water is also a source of nutrients.

Part of the reason for low water intake after weaning is most likely related to piglets' having to locate and use the drinker. There is no convincing evidence that familiarization with water and drinkers before weaning enhances water intake and performance after weaning. Even after weaning, using a drip to try and encourage water consumption has proven largely unsuccessful (Ogunbameru et al. 1991). Rather, factors such as drinker design, placement, height, cleanliness, and number of drinkers per pen have been cited as influencing water intake.

Unfortunately, published data relating these factors to water consumption and then to postweaning performance are both scarce and contradictory. Drinkers placed at an incorrect height and angle or in an appropriate part of the pen will discourage intake of water and could promote its wastage. For example, Gill (1989) showed differences in daily gain and water efficiency use after weaning between drinker types. Torrey and Widowski (2004) demonstrated in 15-day-old weaned piglets that providing water via drinker bowls caused higher apparent feed intake in the first 2 days after weaning and that pigs spent less time engaged in drinking behavior, compared to pigs using a nipple drinker. Overall water use was also lower in piglets drinking from bowls. Pigs allowed access to bowl drinkers also spent less time belly-nosing. Horvath et al. (2000) reported that for the subsequent 8 weeks, piglets weaned at 35 days of age drank more water from a trough placed in each pen versus a nipple drinker. In contrast, Phillips and Phillips (1999) offered water to piglets from a number of dispenser options (nipple, float-controlled bowl with contents replaced daily with fresh water, float-controlled bowl that was not cleaned, or a nipple and float-controlled bowl cleaned daily). They found no differences in performance in the first 4 days after weaning, although they did report lower water intake from nipples on the first day following weaning and more wastage. Anecdotally, the use of bell-shaped turkey drinkers that are placed directly onto the floor of the pen after weaning have purportedly shown good results in terms of both water and feed intake (Brooks and Tsourgiannis 2003).

The rate and velocity of water delivered by the drinker have also been shown to influence feed intake and growth after weaning. Barber et al. (1989) reported a positive correlation between water delivery rate (175–700 ml/min) and voluntary feed intake after weaning, although Celis (1996; cited by Brooks and Tsourgiannis 2003) reported no improvement in performance with an increase in flow rate from 70–700 ml/min in piglets weaned at 28 days of age. Such differences between studies are difficult to explain, but they are most likely related to factors such as drinker design, the number of drinkers and pigs per pen, water quality, drinker cleanliness, and the type of diet(s) fed to pigs. Brooks and Tsourgiannis (2003) remarked, however, that the amount of feed the piglet eats after weaning is determined by the amount of water that it consumes and not the reverse, and so strategies that promote water intake, albeit variable such as the use of sweeteners, can have a positive effect on feed intake after weaning.

FACTORS RELATED TO THE PHYSICAL ENVIRONMENT

Another important consideration regarding management of the weaning pig is the pen structure, which includes flooring materials, feeder and waterer designs, stocking density, and group size. Madec et al. (2003) recently conducted an extensive review of these factors; however, some points require reiteration. Additionally, aspects of the environmental requirements of pigs are covered elsewhere in this book (see Chapter 64).

Feeder Space and Feeder Location

Conventional understanding says that nursery pigs should have sufficient feeder space that allows at least half the pigs in a pen to eat at any one time. In practice this "rule" varies enormously and is not necessarily adhered to. For example, Pluske and Williams (1996c) reported no differences in production indexes in the 28 days after weaning when pigs were offered feed from either a linear trough or a single-space feeder. Laitat et al. (1999) reported similar results comparing a tubetype feeder, allowing piglets to mix feed and water, to a conventional feeder where drinking and water places were separated. Baxter (1989) presented an equation incorporating bodyweight and shoulder width that described the minimum feeding space a pig needs, with a pig weighing 10 kg requiring a minimum feeder space of 13 cm. Commercially, however, this rule is not necessarily followed, particularly in outdoor hoops where feeding behavior patterns can vary dramatically to those for indoor-housed pigs (Morrison et al. 2003b).

In a comprehensive study investigating the interaction between feeder location and group size, Wolter et al. (2000a) used 1,760 17-day-old weaned pigs to examine the effects of three pen designs on pig performance. The designs were (a) large group size (100 pigs/pen) with five two-sided feeders in a single, central location in the pen, (b) large group size (100 pigs/pen) with five two-sided feeders in multiple (five) locations in the pen, and (c) small group size (20 pigs/pen) with a single two-sided feeder in a single central location in the pen. Each feeder provided two 20.3 cm–wide feeding places on each side, and for all treatments, feeder trough space (4 cm/pig) and floor space (0.17 m^2) were the same. A slight yet significant reduction in growth performance (15 g/day) was found due to increased group size, but the approach to providing multiple feeding locations had no effect on production indexes.

Stocking Density

Floor space per pig is usually based on the space required for sternum and fully recumbent resting positions. Using various prediction equations, literature data, and commercial experience on perforated flooring, the current recommendations are 0.25–0.30 m^2 per pig between 5 and 30 kg bodyweight, with pigs on bedded solid floors requiring 20–25% more space (Madec et al. 2003). Extensive housing systems such as hoops on deep litter systems generally provide a more generous space allowance, although there is a dearth of information in this general area relating to the weaning pig.

In a series of studies Wolter et al. (2002b; 2003a, b) investigated the interactive effects of stocking density, feeder trough space, and diet complexity with large numbers of pigs. They reported that although performances to 10–12 weeks after weaning were initially negatively affected by increasing stocking density, reducing feeder space, and feeding a less complex diet, subsequent performances to slaughter at 25 weeks of age were largely unaffected. For example, Wolter et al. (2003b) found that pigs with restricted growth due to low floor space (0.32 m^2 vs. 0.63 m^2) until either 12 or 14 weeks after weaning showed increased growth rate and feed efficiency in the subsequent period to slaughter at 25 weeks postweaning, with only a slight effect on bodyweight and no effect on carcass measures.

Group Size

The optimum group size for maximum performance and efficient feed conversion in the postweaning period is always an area of controversy and interest, particularly in view of the tendency in some countries toward large group sizes (>250 pigs) in outdoor-based, deep-litter housing systems that do not adhere to conventional group size–performance dynamics, as originally proposed by Kornegay and Notter (1984). Moreover, increased group size is sometimes confounded with a decrease in stocking density, so caution needs to be adopted when interpreting data.

In a recent study, Wolter et al. (2000b) used 1,920 weaned piglets weighing 5.3 kg in a 2 x 2 factorially designed study to investigate the effects of group size (20 vs. 100 pigs) and floor-space allowance (calculated requirement vs. calculated requirement minus 50% of free space) on performance after weaning. These authors reported that large groups and reduced floor-space allowance reduced postweaning performance, with pigs in large groups also showing a greater within-pen coefficient of variation in bodyweight at 9 weeks of age. The extent of the difference in bodyweight after 9 weeks of age was less than 5%. In contrast, O'Connell et al. (2001) found no difference in the performance of weaners from 4–10 weeks of age when grouped in pens of 10, 20, 30,

40, or 60 pigs at constant floor space allowances and constant pigs-to-feeder and -drinker ratios. These authors concluded that the group size of pigs could be increased from 10–60 pigs per pen without any adverse effects on performance. From a comprehensive literature review on this subject, Payne et al. (2001) concluded that decreased performance in the weaner phase is not always predictive of decreased or increased performance in the finisher phase or overall performance

In this review, Payne et al. (2001) used statistical regression analysis and surmised that increasing group size from 20–100 pigs per pen appeared to have a small, negative effect on performance of weanling pigs, provided that floor space and the number of feeders and drinkers supplied were adequate. In practice, the economic consequence of increasing group size will depend on relativities between prevailing construction, labor, and feed costs. Housing pigs in large groups decreases construction, maintenance, and cleaning costs, but may increase labor associated with inspection, treatment, and marketing of pigs. Feed efficiency is unlikely to be affected greatly, although slight decreases in growth rate may reduce throughput or sale weight marginally (Payne et al. 2001). These factors must all be considered in any discussion relating group size to postweaning performance.

CONCLUSIONS

The first weeks after weaning are regarded as being crucial in the pork production cycle because they represent a period of adaptation and stress on the young pig. Differences in weaning age, and weaning, housing, and feeding practices worldwide, make it difficult to make *blanket* recommendations for successful feeding management after weaning. However, nutritional and management strategies should be adopted that minimize the stress response and encourage piglets to consume dry matter as soon as possible after the weaning event. A myriad of factors occur that can influence the subsequent performance of pigs and the variability of body-weight gain. Bodyweight at weaning appears to have a major influence on subsequent production indexes; however, the manner in which a pig becomes heavier at weaning—for example, through having a higher birth weight or consuming supplemental nutrients during lactation—appears also to affect postweaning performance. Consequently, responses to various feeding strategies tend to be variable. Supplementation of piglets before and around weaning with liquid milk diets appears to offer the greatest potential to stimulate preweaning growth rate and to eliminate the postweaning check.

REFERENCES

Appleby MC, Pajor EA, Fraser D. 1991. Effects of management options on creep feeding by piglets. Anim Prod 53:361–366.

——. 1992. Individual variation in feeding and growth of piglets—Effects of increased access to creep food. Anim Prod 55:147–152.

Armstrong WD, Clawson AJ. 1980. Nutrition and management of early weaned pigs: Effects of increased nutrient concentrations and/or supplemental liquid feeding. J Anim Sci 50:377–384.

Azain MJ. 1993. Impact of starter on nursery performance. In Swine Report No 86, University of Georgia, pp. 49–54.

Barber J, Brooks PH, Carpenter JL. 1989. The effects of water delivery rate on the voluntary food intake, water use and performance of early-weaned pigs from 3 to 6 weeks of age. Occasional Publication—British Society of Animal Production 13:103–104.

Barnett KL, Kornegay ET, Risley CR, Lindemann MD, Schurig CR. 1989. Characterization of creep feed consumption and its subsequent effects on immune response, scouring index and performance of weanling pigs. J Anim Sci 67:2698–2708.

Baxter SH. 1989. Designing the pig pen. In Manipulating Pig Production II. JL Barnett, DP Hennessy, eds. Melbourne, Australasian Pig Science Association, pp. 191–206.

Beattie VE, Weatherup RN, Kilpatrick DJ. 1999. The effect of providing additional feed in a highly accessible trough on feeding behaviour and growth performance of weaned pigs. Irish J Agric Res 38:209–216.

Brooks PH, Tsourgiannis CA. 2003. Factors affecting the voluntary feed intake of the weaned pig. In The Weaner Pig: Concepts and Consequences. JR Pluske, J Le Dividich, MWA Verstegen, eds. Wageningen: Wageningen Academic Publishers, pp. 81–116.

Bruininx EMAM, Binnendijk GP, van der Peet-Schwering CMC, Schrama JW, den Hartog LA, Everts H, Beynen AC. 2002b. Effect of creep feed consumption on individual feed intake characteristics and performance of group-housed weanling pigs. J Anim Sci 80:1413–1418.

Bruininx EMAM, Heetkamp MJW, van den Bogaart D, van der Peet-Schwering CMC, Beynen AC, Everts H, den Hartog LA, Schrama JW. 2002a. A prolonged photoperiod improves feed intake and energy metabolism of weanling pigs. J Anim Sci 80:1736–1745.

Bruininx EMAM, Peet-Schwering CMC, van der Schrama JW, Vereijken PFG, Vesseur PC, Everts H, Hartog LA, den Beynen AC. 2001. Individually measured feed intake characteristics and growth performance of group-housed weanling pigs: Effects of sex, initial body weight, and body weight distribution within groups. J Anim Sci 79:301–308.

Bruininx EMAM, Schellingerhout AB, Binnendijk GP, van der Peet-Schwering CMC, Schrama JW, den Hartog LA, Everts H, Beynen AC. 2004. Individually assessed creep feed consumption by suckled piglets: Influence on post-weaning food intake characteristics and indicators of gut structure and hind-gut fermentation. Anim Sci 78:67–75.

Campbell RG. 1976. A note on the use of a feed flavour to stimulate feed intake of weaner pigs. Anim Prod 23:417–419.

——. 1989. The nutritional management of weaner pigs. In Manipulating Pig Production II. JL Barnett, DP Hennessy, eds. Melbourne, Australasian Pig Science Association, pp. 170–175.

Campbell RG, Dunkin AC. 1982. The effect of birth weight on the estimated milk intake, growth and body composition of sow-reared piglets. Anim Prod 35:193–197.

Carroll JA, Veum TL, Matteri RL. 1998. Endocrine changes to weaning and changes in post-weaning diet in the young pig. Dom Anim Endocrinol 15:183–194.

Chapple RP, Cuaron JA, Easter RA. 1989. Effect of glucocorticoids and limited nursing on the carbohydrate digestive capacity and growth rate of piglets. J Anim Sci 67:2956–2973.

Coffey RD, Cromwell GL. 1995. The impact of environment and antimicrobial agents on growth response of early-weaned pigs to spray-dried porcine plasma. J Anim Sci 73:2532–2541.

de Passille AMB, Pelletier G, Menard J, Morrisset J. 1989. Relationships of weight gain and behavior to digestive organ weight and enzyme activities in piglets. J Anim Sci 67:2921–2929.

Donovan TS, Dritz SS. 2000. Effect of split nursing on variation in pig growth from birth to weaning. J Am Vet Med Assoc 217:79–81.

Dritz SS, Tokach MD, Goodband RD, Nelssen JL. 1996. Nutritional programs for segregated early-weaned pigs: Part I. Management procedures and nutritional principles. Compend Contin Educ Vet Pract 18:S222–S228.

Dunshea FR, Eason PJ, Kerton DJ, Morrish L, Cox ML, King RH. 1997. Supplemental milk around weaning can increase live weight at 120 days of age. In Manipulating Pig Production VI. PD Cranwell, ed. Australasian Pig Science Association, Melbourne, p. 68.

Dunshea FR, Kerton DJ, Cranwell PD, Campbell RG, Mullan BP, King RH, Pluske JR. 2002a. Interactions between weaning age, weaning weight, sex and enzyme supplementation on growth performance of pigs. Aust J Agric Res 53:939–945.

Dunshea FR, Kerton DJ, Cranwell PD, Campbell RG, Mullan BP, King RH, Power GN, Pluske JR. 2003. Lifetime and post-weaning determinants of performance indices of pigs. Aust J Agric Res 54:363–370.

Dunshea FR, Kerton DJ, Eason PJ, Pluske JR, Moyes T. 2002b. Diets containing high-quality animal proteins increase the growth of early-weaned pigs. Aust J Agric Res 53:779–784.

Farmer C, Petitclerc D, Pelletier G, Gaudreau P, Brazeau P. 1992. Carcass composition and resistance to fasting in neonatal piglets born of sows immunized against somatostatin and/or receiving growth hormone-releasing factor injections during gestation. Biol Neonate 61:110–117.

Fitko R, Rowalski GI, Ziclinski H. 1992. The level of stress hormones in piglets of different hierarchic rank in groups. Med Weteynar 48:666–687.

Fowler VR, Gill BP. 1989. Voluntary food intake of the young pig. In The Voluntary Food Intake of Pigs. JM Forbes, TLJ Lawrence, eds. Occasional Publication No. 13. British Society of Animal Production, Edinburgh, pp. 51–60.

Fraser D, Feddes JJR, Pajor EA. 1994. The relationship between creep feeding behavior of piglets and adaptation to weaning. Effect of diet quality. Can J Anim Sci 74:1–6.

Friend TH, Knabe DA, Tanksley TD. 1983. Behavior and performance of pigs regrouped by three different methods at weaning. J Anim Sci 57:1406–1411.

Geary TM, Brooks PH. 1998. The effect of weaning weight and age on the post-weaning growth performance of piglets fed fermented liquid diets. Pig J 42:10–23.

Gill BP. 1989. Water use by pigs managed under various conditions of housing, feeding and nutrition. PhD thesis, University of Plymouth.

Grinstead GS, Goodband RD, Dritz SS, Tokach MD, Nelssen JL, Woodworth JC, Molitor M. 2000. Effects of a whey protein product and spray-dried animal plasma on growth performance of weanling pigs. J Anim Sci 78:647–657.

Hampson DJ. 1994. Postweaning *Escherichia coli* diarrhoea in pigs. In *Escherichia coli* in Domestic Animals and Humans. CJ Gyles, ed. Wallingford: CAB International, pp. 171–191.

Harrell RJ, Thomas MJ, Boyd RD. 1993. Limitations of sow milk yield on baby pig growth. In Proceedings of the 1993 Cornell Nutrition Conference for Feed Manufacturers. Cornell University, Ithaca, pp. 156–164.

Hay M, Orgeur P, Lévy F, Le Dividich J, Concordet D, Nowak R, Schaal B, Morméde P. 2001. Neuroendocrine consequences of very early weaning in swine. Physiol Behav 72:263–269.

Heetkamp MJW, Schrama JW, de Long L, Swinkels JWGM, Schouten WGP, Bosch MW. 1995. Energy metabolism in young pigs as affected by mixing. J Anim Sci 73:3562–3569.

Heo KN, Odle J, Oliver W, Kim JH, Han IK, Jones E. 1999. Effects of milk replacer and ambient temperature on growth performance of 14-day-old early-weaned pigs. Asian Aust J Anim Sci 12:908–913.

Hodge RMW. 1974. Efficiency of food conversion and body composition of the preruminant lamb and the young pig. Br J Nutr 32:113–126.

Hohenshell LM, Cunnick JE, Ford SP, Kattesh HG, Zimmerman DR, Wilson ME, Matteri RL, Carroll JA, Lay DC. 2000. Few differences found between early- and late-weaned pigs raised in the same environment. J Anim Sci 78:38–49.

Hopwood DE, Hampson DJ. 2003. Interactions between the intestinal microbiota, diet and diarrhoea, and their influences on piglet health in the immediate post-weaning period. In The Weaner Pig: Concepts and Consequences. JR Pluske, J Le Dividich, MWA Verstegen, eds. Wageningen: Wageningen Academic Publishers, pp. 199–218.

Horvath G, Jarabin J, Visnyei L. 2000. Effects of regrouping, feeding and drinking methods on weight gain of weaned piglets. Deut Tierarztl Woch 107:364–367.

Ilsley SE, Broom LJ, Miller HM, Toplis P. 2003. Birth weight and weaning weight as predictors of pig weight at slaughter. In Manipulating Pig Production IX. JE Paterson, ed. Melbourne, Australasian Pig Science Association, p. 31.

Jensen BB, Mikkelsen LL. 1998. Feeding liquid diets to pigs. In Recent Advances in Animal Nutrition. PC Garnsworthy, J Wiseman, eds. Loughborough: Nottingham University Press, pp. 107–126.

Kim JH, Heo KN, Odle J, Han IK, Harrell RJ. 2001. Liquid diets accelerate the growth of easily weaned pigs and the effects are maintained to market weight. J Anim Sci 79:427–434.

King MR, Morel PHC, James EAC, Hendriks WH, Pluske JR, Skilton R, Skilton G. 2001. Inclusion of colostrum powder and bovine plasma in starter diets increases voluntary feed intake. In Manipulating Pig Production VIII. PD Cranwell, ed. Melbourne, Australasian Pig Science Association, p. 213.

King RH. 1979. The effect of adding a feed flavour to diets of young pigs before and after weaning. Aust J Exp Agric Husb 19:695–697.

King RH, Boyce JM, Dunshea FR. 1998. The effect of supplemental nutrients on the growth performance of suckling pigs. Aust J Agric Sci 49:1–5.

King RH, Pluske JR. 2003. Nutritional management of the weaner pig. In JR Pluske, J Le Dividich, MWA Verstegen, eds. The Weaner Pig: Concepts and Consequences. Wageningen: Wageningen Academic Publishers, pp. 37–51.

Kornegay ET, Notter DR. 1984. Effects of floor space and number of pigs per pen on performance. Pig News Info 5:23–33.

Kuller WI, Soede NM, van Beers-Schreuers HMG, Langendijk P, Taverne MAM, Verheijden JHM, Kemp B. 2004. Intermittent suckling: Effects on piglet and sow performance before and after weaning. J Anim Sci 82:405–413.

Laitat M, Vandenheede M, Désiron A, Canart B, Nicks B. 1999. Comparison of feeding behaviour and performance of weaned pigs given food in two types of dry feeders with integrated drinkers. Anim Sci 68:35–42.

Lawlor PG, Lynch PB, Caffrey PJ, O'Doherty, JVO. 2002a. Effect of pre- and post-weaning management on subsequent pig performance to slaughter and carcass quality. Anim Sci 75:245–256.

Lawlor PG, Lynch PB, Gardiner GE, Caffrey PJ, O'Doherty, JVO. 2002b. Effect of liquid feeding weaned pigs on growth performance to harvest. J Anim Sci 80:1725–1735.

Le Dividich J. 1999. The neonatal and weaner pig: Management to reduce variation. In Manipulating Pig Production VII. PD Cranwell, ed. Melbourne, Australasian Pig Science Association, pp. 135–155.

Le Dividich J, Herpin P. 1994. Effects of climatic conditions on the performance, metabolism and health status of the weaned piglets: A review. Livest Prod Sci 38:79–90.

Le Dividich J, Martineau GP, Madec F, Orgeur P. 2003. Saving and rearing underprivileged and supernumerary piglets, and improving their health at weaning. In The Weaner Pig: Concepts and

Consequences. JR Pluske, J Le Dividich, MWA Verstegen, eds. Wageningen: Wageningen Academic Publishers, pp. 361–383.

Le Dividich J, Noblet J. 1981. Colostrum intake and thermoregulation in the neonatal pig in relation to environmental temperature. Biol Neonate 40:167–174.

Le Dividich J, Sève B. 2000. Effects of underfeeding during the weaning period on growth, metabolism, and hormonal adjustments in the piglet. Dom Anim Endocrinol 19:63–74.

Le Huérou-Luron I, Callarec J, Le Roux Th, Le Dividich J. 2004. Supplementation of a weaning diet with bovine colostrum increased feed intake and growth of weaned piglets. J Rech Porcine France 36:33–38.

Lindemann MD, Cornelius SG, El Kandelgy SM, Moser RL, Pettigrew JE. 1986. Effect of age, weaning and diet on digestive enzyme levels in the piglet. J Anim Sci 62:1298–1307.

Madec F, Bridoux N, Bounaix S, Jestin A. 1998. Measurements of digestive disorders in the piglet at weaning and related risk factors. Prev Vet Med 35:53–71.

Madec F, Le Dividich J, Pluske JR, Verstegen MWA. 2003. Environmental requirements and housing of the weaned pig. In The Weaner Pig: Concepts and Consequences. JR Pluske, J Le Dividich, MWA Verstegen, eds. Wageningen: Wageningen Academic Publishers, pp. 337–360.

Madsen FC. 1977. Development of feed preference in young swine. Feedstuffs 49:25.

Mahan DC, Lepine AJ. 1991. Effect of pig weaning weight and associated nursery feeding programs on subsequent performance to 105 kilograms body weight. J Anim Sci 69:1370–1378.

Main RG, Dritz SS, Tokach MD, Goodband RD, Nelssen JL. 2004. Increasing weaning age improves pig performance in a multisite production system. J Anim Sci 82:1499–1507.

Mavromichalis I, Varley MA. 2003. Transition feeding systems post-weaning. In Perspectives in Pig Science. J Wiseman, MA Varley, B Kemp, eds. Loughborough: Nottingham University Press, pp. 405–456.

McConnell JC, Eargle JC, Waldorf, RC. 1987. Effects of weaning weight, co-mingling, group size and room temperature on pig performance. J Anim Sci 65:1202–1206.

McGlone JJ. 1986. Influence of resources on pig aggression and dominance. Behav Proc 12:135–144.

McGlone JJ, Curtis SE. 1985. Behavior and performance of weanling pigs in pens equipped with hide areas. J Anim Sci 60:20–24.

Miller HM, Slade RD. 2003. Digestive physiology of the weaned pig. In The Weaner Pig: Concepts and Consequences. JR Pluske, J Le Dividich, MWA Verstegen, eds. Wageningen: Wageningen Academic Publishers, pp. 117–144.

Miller HM, Toplis P, Slade RD. 1999. Weaning weight and daily live weight gain in the week after weaning predict piglet performance. In Manipulating Pig Production VII. PD Cranwell, ed. Melbourne, Australasian Pig Science Association, p. 130.

Mormède P, Hay M. 2003. Behavioural changes and adaptations associated with weaning. In The Weaner Pig: Concepts and Consequences. JR Pluske, J Le Dividich, MWA Verstegen, eds. Wageningen: Wageningen Academic Publishers, pp. 53–60.

Morrison RS, Hemsworth PH, Cronin GM, Campbell RG. 2003a. The social and feeding behaviour of growing pigs in deep-litter, large group housing system. Appl Anim Behav Sci 82:173–188.

——. 2003b. The effect of restricting pen space and feeder availability on the behaviour and growth performance of entire male growing pigs in a deep-litter, large group housing system. Appl Anim Behav Sci 83:163–176.

Nelssen JL, Dritz SS, Tokach MD, Goodband RD. 1999. Nutritional programs for segregated early weaning. In Diseases of Swine. 8th edition. BE Straw, S D'Allaire, WL Mengeling, DJ Taylor, eds. Oxford: Blackwell Science, pp. 1045–1055.

O'Connell NE, Beattie VE, Weatherup RN. 2001. Influence of group size on the performance and behaviour of 4 to 10 week old pigs. Anim Sci 69:481–489.

Ogunbameru BO, Kornegay ET, Wood CM. 1991. A comparison of drip and non-drip nipple waterers used by weanling pigs. Can J Anim Sci 71:581–583.

Pajor EA, Fraser D, Kramer DL. 1991. Individual variation in the consumption of solid food by suckling pigs and its relationship to post-weaning performance. Appl Anim Behav Sci 32:139–155.

Payne HG, Brumm MC, D'Antuono M, Mullan BP, Pluske JR, Williams IH. 2001. Review of group size effects on performance. Final Report No. 1749. Pig Research and Development Corporation, Canberra.

Phillips PA, Phillips MH. 1999. Technical notes: Effect of dispenser on water intake of pigs at weaning. Trans ASAE 42:1471–1473.

Pitts AD, Weary DM, Pajor EA, Fraser D. 2000. Mixing at young ages reduces fighting in unacquainted domestic pigs. Appl Anim Behav Sci 68:191–197.

Pluske JR, Dong GZ. 1998. Factors influencing the utilisation of colostrum and milk. In The Lactating Sow. MWA Verstegen, PJ Moughan, JW Schrama, eds. Wageningen: Wageningen Press, pp. 45–70.

Pluske JR, Kerton DJ, Cranwell PD, Campbell RG, Mullan BP, King RH, Power GN, Pierzynowski SG, Westrom B, Rippe C, Peulen O, Dunshea FR. 2003. Age, sex and weight at weaning influence the physiological and gastrointestinal development of weanling pigs. Aust J Agric Res 54:515–527.

Pluske JR, Pearson, Morel PCH, King MR, Skilton G, Skilton R. 1999. A bovine colostrum product in a weaner diet increases growth and reduces days to slaughter. In Manipulating Pig Production VII. PD Cranwell. ed. Melbourne, Australasian Pig Science Association, p. 256.

Pluske JR, Williams IH. 1996a. Split weaning increases the growth of light piglets during lactation. Aust J Agric Res 47:513–523.

——. 1996b. Reducing stress in piglets as a means of increasing production after weaning: Administration of amperozide or co-mingling of piglets during lactation? Anim Sci 62:121–130.

——. 1996c. The influence of feeder type and the method of group allocation at weaning on voluntary food intake and growth in piglets. Anim Sci 62:115–120.

Pluske JR, Williams IH, Aherne FX. 1995. Nutrition of the neonatal pig. In The Neonatal Pig—Development and Survival. MA Varley, ed. Wallingford: CAB International, pp. 187–235.

——. 1996. Villous height and crypt depth in piglets in response to increases in the intake of cow's milk after weaning. Anim Sci 62:145–158.

Pluske JR, Williams IH, Hampson DJ. 1997. Factors influencing the structure and function of the small intestine in the weaned pig: a review. Livest Prod Sci 51:215–236.

Reale TA. 1987. Supplemental liquid diets and feed flavours for young pigs. MSc thesis, University of Melbourne.

Rooke JA, Shanks M, Edwards SA. 1998. Maternal and dietary influences on post-weaning piglet growth. In Proceedings of the British Society of Animal Science, Edinburgh, p. 156.

Russell PJ, Geary TM, Brooks PH, Campbell A. 1996. Performance, water use and effluent output of weaner pigs fed ad libitum with either dry pellets or liquid feed and the role of microbial activity in the liquid feed. J Sci Food Agric 72:8–16.

Tokach MD, Dritz SS, Goodband RD, Nelssen JL. 2003. Nutritional requirements of the weaned pig. In The Weaner Pig: Concepts and Consequences. JR Pluske, J Le Dividich, MWA Verstegen, eds. Wageningen: Wageningen Academic Publishers, pp. 259–299.

Tokach MD, Goodband RD, Nelssen JL, Katts LJ. 1992. Influence of weaning weight and growth during the first week post-weaning on subsequent pig performance. In Kansas University Swine Day. Report of Progress No. 667, pp. 15–17.

Toplis P, Blanchard PJ, Miller HM. 1999. Creep feed offered as a gruel prior to weaning enhances performance of weaned piglets. In Manipulating Pig Production VII. PD Cranwell. ed. Melbourne, Australasian Pig Science Association, p. 129.

Torrey S, Widowski TM. 2004. Effect of drinker type and sound stimuli on early-weaned pig performance and behavior. J Anim Sci 82:2105–2114.

van Beers-Schreuers HMG, Nabuurs MJA, Vellenga L, Wensing Th, Breukink HJ. 1998. Role of the large intestine in the pathogenesis of diarrhea in weaned pigs. Am J Vet Res 59:696–703.

van Dijk AJ, Everts H, Nabuurs MJA, Margry RJCF, Beynen AC. 2001. Growth performance of weanling pigs fed spray-dried animal plasma: A review. Livest Prod Sci 68:263–274.

Vente-Spreeuwenberg MAM, Beynen AC. 2003. Diet-mediated modulation of small intestinal integrity in weaned piglets. In The Weaner Pig: Concepts and Consequences. JR Pluske, J Le Dividich, MWA Verstegen, eds. Wageningen: Wageningen Academic Publishers, pp. 145–198.

Waran NK, Broom DM. 1992. The influence of a barrier on the behaviour and growth of early-weaned piglets. Anim Prod 54:485.

Weary DM, Pajor EA, Bonenfant M, Fraser D, Kramer DL. 2002. Alternative housing for sows and litters. Part 4. Effects of sow-controlled housing combined with a communal piglet area on pre- and post-weaning behaviour and performance. Appl Anim Behav Sci 76:279–290.

Whittemore CT, Green DM. 2001. Growth of the young weaned pig. In The Weaner Pig: Nutrition and Management. MA Varley, J Wiseman, eds. Wallingford: CAB International, pp. 1–15.

Williams IH. 1976. Nutrition of the young pig in relation to body composition. PhD thesis, University of Melbourne.

——. 1995. Sow's milk as a major nutrient source before weaning. In Manipulating Pig production V. DP Hennessy, PD Cranwell, eds. Melbourne, Australasian Pig Science Association, pp. 107–113.

——. 2003. Growth of the weaned pig. In The Weaner Pig: Concepts and Consequences. JR Pluske, J Le Dividich, MWA Verste-gen, eds. Wageningen: Wageningen Academic Publishers, pp. 15–35.

Wolter BF, Ellis M. 2001. The effects of weaning weight and rate of growth immediately after weaning on subsequent pig growth performance and carcass characteristics. Can J Anim Sci 81:363–369.

Wolter BF, Ellis M, Curtis SE, Parr EN, Webel DM. 2000a. Feeder location did not affect performance of weanling pigs in large groups. J Anim Sci 78:2784–2789.

——. 2000b. Group size and floor-space allowance can affect weanling-pig performance. J Anim Sci 78:2062–2067.

Wolter BF, Ellis M, Corrigan BP, DeDecker JM. 2002a. The effect of birth weight and feeding of supplemental milk replacer to piglets during lactation on preweaning and postweaning growth performance and carcass characteristics. J Anim Sci 80:301–308.

Wolter BF, Ellis M, Corrigan BP, DeDecker JM, Curtis SE, Parr EN, Webel DM. 2003a. Impact of early postweaning growth rate as affected by diet complexity and space allocation on subsequent growth performance of pigs in a wean-to-finish production system. J Anim Sci 81:353–359.

——. 2003b. Effect of restricted postweaning growth resulting from reduced floor and feeder-trough space on pig growth performance at slaughter weight—A wean-to-finish production system. J Anim Sci 81:836–842.

Wolter BF, Ellis M, DeDecker JM, Curtis SE, Hollis GR, Shanks RD, Parr EN, Webel DM. 2002b. Effects of double stocking and weighing frequency on pig performance in wean-to-finish production systems. J Anim Sci 80:1442–1450.

Young JB, Landsberg L. 1977. Suppression of sympathetic nervous system during fasting. Science 186:1473–1475.

66 Management of Growing-Finishing Pigs

Cornelius F. M. de Lange and Catherine E. Dewey

The main aim in managing growing-finishing pigs is the efficient production of high quality pork meat while considering animal well-being and the potential negative impact of pig production on the environment. With the move toward larger growing-finishing pig units, the impact of relatively minor improvements in production efficiencies will have substantial impact on overall profitability. The main determinant of pork meat production efficiency is lean tissue growth, the accretion rate of dissectible muscle in the pig's body. The pigs' lean tissue growth potential is ultimately under genetic control, and the expression of the pig's lean tissue growth potential is determined by environmental factors such as the presence of disease causing organisms, animal density, the effective environmental temperature, and feeding management. Because feed represents the single biggest cost factor in commercial pork production, close attention should be paid to the development of effective feeding programs and the amount of feed that is consumed by growing-finishing pigs. In this chapter, the importance of accurate production records and monitoring growth and feed intake patterns of growing-finishing pigs is presented briefly. Feeding management and other important aspects of growing-finishing pig management are then addressed.

PRODUCTION RECORDS AND PRODUCTION OBJECTIVES

Both for making meaningful management decisions and to ensure that changes in management result in the anticipated changes in pig performance accurate production data need to be collected. The move towards all-in/all-out production systems has made data collection easier and more accurate. As a minimum the following data is required: cost per feeder pig placed in the barn, number and average body weight of pigs entering the barn and shipped for slaughter, mortality, number of pigs culled or sold as a lightweight pig, total feed usage,

average carcass weight and carcass lean yield, and average carcass value. This will allow for calculation of average daily gain, feed efficiency, feed costs per pig, and a simple estimate of gross margin per pig. The latter can be calculated as carcass value over feed costs and cost of feeder pigs. These production parameters can be adjusted to a common basis such as a constant initial and final body weight and diet nutrient density, which allows for comparison to reasonable production targets (Table 66.1; Tokach and de Lange 2001). Additional useful information relates to seasonal effects on the aforementioned performance parameters, downtime between groups of pigs and variability in final body weight and carcass characteristics. This additional information can serve as a basis for seasonal adjustments to management, to assess space utilization and to relate variation in carcass characteristics to average carcass value and profitability.

An important consideration in managing growing-finishing pig units is the value of average daily gain and barn throughput. When the supply of feeder pigs is unlimited, gross margin per pig may be compromised—for example, by feeding ractopamine to increase preslaughter growth rates or shipping pigs somewhat lighter to optimize gross margin and profit per pig place per year. On the other hand, when the supply of feeder pigs is limited, the production objective in commercial growing-finishing pig units should be to optimize gross margin and profit per pig. In addition, in areas where the potential negative impact of pigs' production on the environment is a concern, reducing nitrogen and phosphorus excretion with manure or controlling the release of odorous compounds from the pig facility should be considered (de Lange 2004). The aforementioned production records allow for benchmarking and some changes to management of growing-finishing pigs. However, to optimize production efficiencies, profits, and nitrogen and phosphorus utilization within individual pig units, more detailed information on lean tissue growth and feed intake patterns is required.

Table 66.1. Feed to gain targets for growing-finishing pigs consuming corn-soybean meal–based diets.[1]

Entry BW, (kg)	Market BW, (kg)	Meal Diets		Pelleted Diets	
		0% fat	5% fat	0% fat	5% fat
18	110	2.92	2.63	2.74	2.47
18	115	2.97	2.67	2.79	2.51
18	120	3.02	2.72	2.84	2.55
23	110	2.97	2.67	2.79	2.51
23	115	3.02	2.72	2.84	2.55
23	120	3.07	2.76	2.89	2.60
28	110	3.02	2.72	2.84	2.55
28	115	3.07	2.76	2.89	2.60
28	120	3.12	2.81	2.93	2.64

[1]Derived from Tokach and de Lange (2001). The values may be adjusted for diets with energy densities that differ from that in a typical corn-soybean meal–based diet (3400 kcal DE/kg), by multiplying the values by 3400 ÷ (actual diet DE content).

BW = body weight.

Table 66.2. Impact of fat-free lean tissue growth potential on growth performance of growing-finishing pigs between 25 and 110 kg body weight.[1]

Lean Tissue Growth Potential	High	Medium	Unimproved
Fat-free lean tissue growth potential, g/day	400	350	300
Maximum body protein deposition rate, g/day	157	137	118
Average daily gain, g	842	794	743
Feed : gain, g/g	2.66	2.82	3.03
Dressing percentage, %[2]	79.1	79.4	79.7
Lean yield, %[2]	60.7	59.0	57.6

[1]Derived from de Lange et al. (2001a). Diets contain 3400 kcal DE/kg and optimum levels of amino acids and other nutrients; feed intake is 90% of voluntary intake according to NRC (1998). A feed wastage of 3% is included.

[2]Canadian carcass grading system.

MONITORING LEAN TISSUE GROWTH AND FEED INTAKE PATTERNS

In growing-finishing pigs, lean tissue growth is closely related to daily gain, feed efficiency, and carcass quality (Schinckel 1994; Table 66.2). Furthermore, lean tissue growth gain is closely related to body protein deposition, the main determinant of dietary amino acid requirements and one of the main determinants of dietary energy requirements (NRC 1998; Schinckel et al. 2002). Across groups of pigs, muscle or lean tissue represents between 28 and 60% of the pigs' body weight (Gu et al. 1992; Quiniou and Noblet 1995). The other main body tissues include visceral organs, fat, integument and bones (de Lange et al. 2001b). The relationships between lean tissue, visceral organs, integument and bones are relatively constant. Therefore, variation in body lean content between groups of pigs is largely influenced by the amount of fat tissue, which can vary between 12 and 30% of the pigs' body weight. Dissectible lean tissue in growing pigs contains about 72% water, 20% protein, and the remainder is made up of lipid, minerals, and some carbohydrates. In contrast, fat tissue contains more than 85% lipid. To minimize feeding costs and optimize carcass value it is thus in the pork producers' interest to optimize carcass lean content in slaughter pigs. Unfortunately, definitions and methods to quantify carcass lean tissue content and lean tissue growth in pigs can vary considerably between countries and individual pig slaughter facilities. For example, the lean tissue content of pigs may be standardized to a fat-free lean tissue content. Alternatively, the trimmed belly that contains fat tissue as well as lean tissue may be considered part of body lean content. Therefore, it is probably more appropriate and objective to characterize groups of pigs in terms of whole body protein deposition rates (Table 66.2). According to NRC (1998) in the

United States fat-free lean tissue can be calculated as body protein deposition × 2.55, but this relationship is likely to vary with pig type and body weight range. The mean average fat-free lean tissue growth rate for groups of growing-finishing pigs may vary between 200 and 450 g/day (NRC 1998; de Lange et al. 2001a).

Estimates of average lean tissue gain for individual groups of growing-finishing pigs may be derived from the average initial and final body weight, the number of days required to grow pigs from initial to final body weight, carcass dressing percentage, and the carcass lean tissue content. Given the relatively low variation in lean tissue content of feeder pigs entering the growing-finishing barn the fat-free lean content of feeder pigs may be estimated from live body weight (NRC 1998).

For the estimation of the pigs' optimum slaughter weight and for the development of the effective multiple phase-feeding programs, the change in lean tissue growth (and feed intake) with increasing body weight needs to be considered as well. In general, there are three segments to a typical lean tissue growth curve. During the early stages of growth, generally up to about 50 kg body weight, the daily lean tissue growth rate increases. Between approximately 50 and 80 kg body weight the daily lean tissue growth rate is relatively constant. Thereafter, the daily lean tissue growth rate starts to gradually decline towards zero when the pigs' mature body weight has been reached. The weight at which pigs are slaughtered generally coincides with the weight at which the daily lean tissue growth rate starts to decline substantially.

Lean tissue growth curves can be established using three different methods: (1) Calculate the average lean tissue growth over the entire growing-finishing periods, as indicated above, and combine this with a standard lean gain curve shape to establish the actual lean gain curves. This is the easiest method and is used in NRC (1998) to estimate nutrient requirements of pigs at the various stages of growth. This is also the least preferred method because it ignores differences in the shape of lean gain curves between different growing-finishing pig units. (2) Establish a growth curve by relating body weight versus time in the barn based on measurements on at least 40 pigs. To do so, make serial B-mode real-time ultrasound measurements at at least four, preferably five, different body weights that are equally spread out over the entire growing-finishing phase on at least 40 pigs. The main sources of error in this approach are the inaccuracies of the real-time ultrasound measurements and the prediction of lean contents of real-time ultrasound measurements at the various body weights. Relationships between real-time ultrasound measurements and body lean content differ between lines of pigs (Hicks et al. 1998). (3) Establish a growth curve, based on at least four equally spread data points that relate body weight to the number of days in the barn and with observations from at least 40 pigs per data point. Combine this information with an actual feed intake curve and diet nutrient content and use mathematical models that represent nutrient utilization for growth to estimate whole body protein deposition (lean tissue growth) as well as whole body lipid deposition (de Lange et al. 2001a). This approach is sensitive to assumptions about maintenance energy requirements and to the accuracy of the feed intake curve.

Care should be taken with the interpretation of lean tissue growth curves. Various factors, including genotype, gender, environmental stresses (health status, crowding) and nutrient intake affect observed lean tissue growth rates. Lean tissue growth has a medium to high heritability and has received considerable attention in pig breeding strategies over the last years (Schinckel and de Lange 1996). In terms of gender, entire male pigs have a higher lean tissue growth potential than gilts, and barrows have the lowest lean tissue growth potential; the differences between genders varies with pig genotype (Schinckel 1994). The presence of subclinical levels of disease can reduce lean growth rates by more than 30% (Williams et al. 1997). Furthermore, lean tissue growth is generally affected by different factors at the various stages of growth. At lower body weights and when daily lean tissue growth are increasing with increasing body weight, lean tissue growth is generally determined by nutrient intake and most often energy intake. To estimate performance potentials of specific groups of growing-finishing pigs, ideally lean tissue growth curves will be established under conditions where nutrient intake is unlikely to limit lean tissue growth. However, because of environmental stressors pigs may not express their full performance potential under commercial conditions (Black et al. 1995). For practical management purposes, the pigs' operation lean tissue growth potential may be considered, which represents the maximum lean tissue growth rates that pigs can achieve under commercial conditions. This implies that for a specific pig genotype the operation lean

tissue growth potential may vary with environmental conditions, and the difference between the actual and operation lean tissue growth potential provides an indication of the ability of particular pig genotypes to deal with environmental stressors. Mathematical models that represent nutrient utilization for growth, such as the NRC (1998) model, may be used to identify whether nutrient intake affects lean tissue growth and to establish whether an increase in nutrient or energy intake would increase lean tissue growth.

Feed intake can have substantial impacts on animal performance, carcass quality, and profits. In growing pigs, up to approximately 50 kg live body weight, energy intake generally limits lean tissue growth. In these pigs the daily energy and feed intake should be maximized. Finishing pigs, especially those with medium or unimproved lean tissue growth potentials and consuming large quantities of feed, consume more energy than what is required for maximum lean tissue growth. In these pigs excessive body fat is deposited and as a result, carcass value is reduced. In finishing pigs with unimproved or average lean growth potentials, carcass value and feed efficiency can be improved by restricting the daily energy intake. It should be pointed out that as lean growth potentials continue to improve, energy intake is likely to determine lean growth rates up to higher body weights. The body weight at which pigs change from a grower pig, where energy intake limits lean growth, to a finisher pig, where energy intake no longer limits lean growth, remains to be determined for the various modern pig genotypes. At least three recent studies suggest that energy intake limits lean growth up to market weight (Schinckel and de Lange 1996).

Feed intakes can vary considerably between groups of pigs and are affected by a whole range of factors associated with the animal (body weight, gender, genotype, health), feed (diet energy density, nutrient imbalances, freshness, presence of toxins, processing), and environment (effective environmental temperature, pig density, feeder design location and management, quality and availability of water, etc.) (NRC 1987). Indeed the accurate prediction and control of voluntary feed intake in specific groups of pigs is one of the main challenges in commercial pork production. Theoretically the pig's feed intake at a particular body weight may be predicted from the pigs' body protein and body lipid deposition rates. This does require, however, accurate estimates of the lipid deposition in the pigs and assumptions about the pigs' maintenance energy requirements (NRC 1987, 1998; Schinckel et al. 2002).

Increasingly on commercial farms feed intake is monitored in representative groups of growing-finishing pigs and the main factors that are known to influence voluntary feed intake are monitored as well: effective environmental temperature, pig health, feeder design and management, pig genotype, water, and feed quality. Reasonable feed intake curves can be established when feed intake is measured accurately in representative monitoring pens over at least a 2-week period and at least three different stages of growth that are equally spread over the growing-finishing period (Schinckel and de Lange 1996). Per body weight range, feed intake and body weight data should be obtained from at least two feeders with at least 40 pigs per body weight range. The highest body weight range should be as close to market weight as possible. Relatively simple and inexpensive devises are now available to measure feed disappearance in individual feeders. As an alternative to measuring feed intake in representative monitoring pens, feed intake may be determined for an entire room or barn if these are managed on an all-in/all-out basis. The latter requires that feed deliveries and inventories, as well as the total number of pigs in inventory, be monitored accurately and frequently. Software packages are now becoming available to aid in collection and interpretation of feed intake data. An additional benefit of continuously monitoring feed intake and in particular water usage is that the onset of disease or changes in the pigs' environment can be identified early, allowing a fast response and reducing the long term impact of these stressors on animal productivity. However, closely monitoring feed and water usage is no substitute for daily inspection of pigs for normal growth, comfort and behavior.

Typical levels of feed intake, feed delivered minus feed wastage, of pigs managed under commercial conditions are about 90% of voluntary feed intake according to NRC (1998; Table 66.3) but may vary between 70 and 100% of NRC (1998). If feed intake levels are below average, check feed quality, feeder type and settings, water availability, environmental temperature, animal health, and pig genotype. Poor feeder designs or improper adjustments of feeders can result in substantial feed intake restrictions or substantial feed wastage (Gonyou and Lou 2000). The effect of gender on feed intake differs between pig genotypes; it may be between 3 and 15% higher in barrows than in gilts, and the gender effect increases with body weight (Schinckel 1994).

FEEDING MANAGEMENT

Establishing Optimum Dietary Nutrient and Energy Intake Levels

Energy, lysine, threonine, other amino acids, and phosphorus contribute generally to more than 80% of the dietary nutrient costs and deserve special consideration when formulating pig diets. However, in some situations specific feed additives that provide health or environmental benefits can increase feed costs substantially. The value of additives should be questioned regularly, considering nonnutritional means to deal with health and environmental issues, solid scientific evidence to support efficacy of feed additives, and costs. The impact of some feed additives, such as synthetic lysine and phytase, on nutrient excretion with manure and feed costs has been amply demonstrated (NRC 1998); for other feed additives the cost effectiveness is not established

Table 66.3. Typical marginal and cumulative average daily gain, daily feed intake and cumulative feed usage for pigs between 25 and 120 kg body weight[1]

Body Weight Range, kg	Average Daily Gain, g		Daily Feed Intake, kg	Feed:Gain	Cumulative Feed Usage, kg
	Marginal	Cumulative			
25–30	679	679	1.337	1.97	9.9
30–35	728	703	1.518	2.09	20.3
35–40	769	724	1.683	2.19	31.2
40–45	804	742	1.835	2.28	42.6
45–50	834	759	1.974	2.37	54.5
50–55	858	774	2.101	2.45	66.7
55–60	878	787	2.218	2.53	79.3
60–65	893	799	2.324	2.60	92.3
65–70	905	809	2.422	2.68	105.7
70–75	912	819	2.511	2.75	119.5
75–80	916	827	2.593	2.83	133.6
80–85	916	834	2.668	2.91	148.2
85–90	913	839	2.737	3.00	163.2
90–95	907	844	2.800	3.09	178.6
95–100	897	847	2.858	3.19	194.6
100–105	884	849	2.910	3.29	211.0
105–110	868	850	2.959	3.41	228.0
110–115	848	850	3.003	3.54	245.8
115–120	826	849	3.044	3.69	264.2

[1]Growth follows the Bridges function (Schinckel and de Lange 1996), and feed intake is equivalent to 90% of voluntary daily feed intake according to NRC (1998) and at a diet-digestible energy content of 3400 kcal/kg. Marginal average daily gain represents growth over the specific 5 kg body weight range. Cumulative average daily gain represents average daily gain from 25 kg body weight. Daily feed intakes and feed usage may be adjusted for changes in diet digestible energy content (Table 66.1).

clearly or does not vary considerably between pig units. Moreover, feed additives, and medication in particular, that are used to treat specific disease problems too often continue to be included in the diet after the problem has disappeared.

The optimum energy content of pig diets will vary with the cost of the various energy yielding feed ingredients such as corn, fat, wheat, barley, and wheat shorts. A good starting point in feed formulation is to determine the dietary available energy content at which the cost per unit of available energy ($ per Mcal or KJ digestible energy) is the lowest, whereby the levels of all other essential nutrients are balanced against available energy. This is the dietary energy density that generally results in the lowest feed costs per kg of body weight gain. However, when throughput and average daily gain have economical value, increasing the energy density in the diet will have additional value. The latter applies in particular to growing pigs up to approximately 60 kg of body weight and to growing-finishing pigs that are under mild heat stress. In these two scenarios either the animals' physical feed intake capacity or the animals' capacity to lose body heat will limit pigs from reaching their desired available energy intake.

The optimum dietary levels of lysine, threonine, other amino acids, and phosphorus should be established based on the pigs' body weight, operational lean tissue growth potential, feed intake level, and dietary energy density (Table 66.4). In addition, the body weight range over which subsequent diets are fed in phase-feeding programs and the marginal cost-benefit response may be considered, which requires the use of dynamic models that represent utilization of dietary nutrients for growth in the pig (Black et al. 1986; de Lange et al. 2001a). The importance of accurate estimates of feed intake and matching dietary feed intake and nutrient levels with pig performance potentials is demonstrated with the simulation results presented in Table 66.5.

These results indicate that the cost of suboptimal feeding programs can be very substantial. The data also suggest that pigs with unimproved lean gain potentials perform well when feed is restricted, and feed intake in pigs with improved lean gain potentials should be maximized.

To closely meet the nutrient requirements of specific groups of pigs the genders may be raised separately and different diets may be fed in sequence with increasing pig body weight. When multiple-phase and split-sex feeding concepts are applied, it is critical that the main factors that determine the optimum dietary available nutrient levels are identified at the various stages of growth and that animal productivity is closely monitored. Establishing feed budgets—i.e., determining the amount of each of the diets that need to be fed—provides an effective means to ensure that diets are switched at the proper time (see Table 66.3). Also, the use of an excessive number of diets in a phase-feeding program makes scheduling feed deliveries more difficult and increases the chance of errors. In general terms, separate feeding of barrows and gilts should be applied when three or more diets are used in a phase-feeding program. Moreover, it is important to realize that the incremental financial benefit of including an additional diet in a phase-feeding program diminishes with the number of diets that are used. For example, if the benefit of changing from feeding a single diet to a two-phase feeding program for growing-finishing pigs is $2.00 per pig, the benefit will be approximately $1.00, $0.50, and $0.25 per pig when the third, fourth, and fifth diet are introduced, respectively. The same principle applies to the impact of phase feeding on nitrogen and phosphorus excretion with manure.

Feed Ingredient Sourcing and Feed Preparation

The following aspects should be considered when sourcing pig feed ingredients: available nutrient content, vari-

Table 66.4. Estimated dietary requirements (%) for true ileal digestible lysine (Lys), true ileal digestible threonine (Thr), and available phosphorus (P) for different pigs with different fat-free lean tissue growth potentials at different levels of feed intake (90% and 80% of voluntary digestible energy intake according to NRC 1998) and at two different body weights.[1]

Fat-free Lean Tissue Growth Potential, g/day	Intake 90% of NRC			Intake 80% of NRC		
	Lys	Thr	P	Lys	Thr	P
	30 kg body weight					
400	0.98	0.60	0.35	0.95	0.59	0.34
350	0.87	0.54	0.30	0.88	0.55	0.31
300	0.77	0.49	0.26	0.81	0.51	0.28
	75 kg body weight					
400	0.72	0.46	0.25	0.74	0.47	0.26
350	0.64	0.42	0.22	0.68	0.44	0.23
300	0.56	0.37	0.18	0.62	0.41	0.21

[1]Adjusted from Tokach and de Lange (2001) and de Lange (2004). Based on diet digestible energy content of 3400 kcal/kg. If diet energy density differs, the target diet nutrient levels may be changed proportionally to diet-digestible energy content.

Table 66.5. Interactive effects of feed intake, pig lean tissue growth potentials, and feeding programs on pig performance and profits.[1]

	Unimproved Pig Type			Improved Pig Type	
Feed allowance, % of NRC	100	80		100	80
Feeding program	Optimal	Optimal	Suboptimal[2]	Optimal	Optimal
Lean tissue gain, g/d	340	290	265	415	330
Daily gain, g	793	643	606	920	714
Average days to market	108	133	141	93	120
Days per rotation	122	147	155	107	134
Feed:Gain	2.97	2.93	3.12	2.54	2.61
Dressing %	80.55	79.75	80.10	79.7	79.23
Carcass lean yield, %	57.48	60.50	59.12	60.68	62.44
Carcass index	104.2	109.4	107.5	109.6	110.95
Feed cost, $/pig	48.07	49.17	50.26	43.65	44.87
Margin, $/pig	−3.48	−0.07	−2.92	5.62	5.22
Margin, $/pig place /year	−10.42	−0.18	−6.87	19.16	14.23

[1]Derived from de Lange et al. (2001a). Based on: performance between 20 and 105.5 kg body weight; 5% feed wastage; 1% mortality; 14 open days per rotation; standard deviations on carcass lean yield and carcass weight of 2% and 4 kg, respectively; weaner pig price $55.00; variable costs per pig $15.00; price per kg carcass at index 100: $1.30; corn ($130/tonne), soybean meal (47.5% CP;$310/tonne) and premix (3% inclusion; $600/tonne) based diets in a 2-phase feeding program; mixed costs are $15/tonne; diets are switched at 65 kg body weight. For all feeding programs, diet soybean meal levels have been adjusted to maximize profit for each pig type and feeding level.

[2]For the suboptimal feeding program, diet soybean meal levels are the same as the optimum diet soybean meal for this pig type at the high feed allowance. Margin ($/pig) is calculated as: carcass value − feed costs − weaner pig price − variable costs per pig. Margin ($/pig place per year) is calculated as: $/pig × 365 ÷ days per rotation. Calculations are conducted using PPGM—Purina Pork Growth Model (1997).

ability, effect on diet palatability, effects on carcass and meat quality, content of antinutritional factors and mycotoxins, storage and handling, availability, and cost.

Tables are available that provide mean contents of available (true or standardized ileal digestible) amino acids, digestible or metabolizable energy, and available phosphorus in a wide range of pig feed ingredients (NRC 1998). For various reasons, such as variation in growing conditions and/or ingredient processing, available nutrient contents of individual batches of feed ingredients can deviate substantially from published means. Routine sampling of ingredients, especially at harvest time, for analyses of dry matter, protein, and fiber contents is recommended. Dry matter content should be considered as part of any nutrient analyses and provides information about potential spoilage during storage. Protein and fiber contents can be used to estimate amino acid and available energy content, respectively. The need for additional analyses will vary with ingredient type and local conditions. Additional analyses may include fat content (high oil corn, full-fat soybeans, and canola seed), ash, calcium and phosphorus (meat meals, mineral sources), and mycotoxins (corn and wheat samples). In order to reduce costs of nutrient analyses, samples of purchased and variable ingredients may be stored in a dark and cool place and analyzed only if problems with animal productivity are observed.

Based on ingredient specific effects on diet palatability (canola meal, peas) and carcass quality (full-fat soybeans and canola seed) the maximum inclusion level in the diet may be restricted. Alternatively, some ingredients or elevated levels of nutrients in the preslaughter diet, such as vitamin E, can enhance pork meat quality (Rosenvold and Andersen 2003).

To establish the actual value of pig feed ingredients, least cost—or best cost—feed formulation systems should be used. These systems provide information on the actual financial value versus the actual cost based on the costs of other available ingredients. Clearly, the price of pig feed ingredients has a substantial impact on feed costs and profit in growing-finishing pig units.

Three key aspects of feed preparation are grinding, mixing, and pelleting. The fineness of grinding of feed ingredients is closely associated with nutrient digestibility and thus feed efficiency. Based on a summary of research at Kansas State University (KSU Swine Nutrition Guide 1997) feed efficiency improves by 1.2% for every 100 micron reduction in average feed particle size. This substantial impact of grinding effectiveness on pig productivity warrants a routine monitoring of mean feed particle size, while the benefits of fine grinding should be weighed against the cost of grinding, flow and dustiness of feed, which is less of a concern when diets are pelleted or when fat is included, as well as increased risks of development of stomach ulcers in growing pigs. A reasonable target mean particle size is between 600 and 800 microns. The adequacy of feed mixing can be assessed based on the variability of nutrient content in 10 or more mixed feed samples. These samples may be analyzed for one or more easily analyzed nutrients, such as sodium or chloride, and the coefficient of variation of nutrient content should be targeted at 10% or less. A coefficient of variation larger than 15% can reduce animal productivity, especially of younger pigs (Patience et al. 1995).

Pelleting of pigs diets can improve feed handling and pig performance and allows the use of a wider range of feed ingredients in the diet. Improved feed efficiency due to pelleting can be attributed to reduced feed wastage, improved nutrient digestibility, and increased available nutrient intake. The benefits of pelleting will vary with feed ingredient composition and pig body weight. In growing-finishing pigs fed corn-soybean meal–based diets feed efficiencies may be improved 5–8%; this value is somewhat higher in diets that contain more fibrous feed ingredients, 7–9% for barley-based diets (Patience et al. 1995; KSU Swine Nutrition Guide 1997). Improvements in average daily gains are slightly smaller than improvements in feed efficiency. These improvements in animal performance should be weighed against the cost of pelleting. A concern with using pelleted diets is pellet quality. Poor pellet quality results in increased amounts of fines in feed, which can reduce feed flow, buildup of fines in the feeder, and increased feed wastage. A recent observation has been that feed pelleting, as well as fine grinding of feed, can influence gut microbiota in pigs in a negative manner (Mikkelsen et al. 2004). In particular the fecal shedding of *Salmonella*, which is a food safety concern, can be reduced by changing from a finely ground pelleted feed to a coarsely ground mash feed. Such a change in feed form will coincide with reductions in pig growth performance.

An important practical consideration is to prepare feed on the farm versus purchasing a complete feed from a commercial feed mill. In this consideration the cost of feed ingredients, feed preparation, ingredient storage, liability, and quality control should be weighed against the cost of purchased feed. Advantages that commercial feed mills can have over on-farm feed preparation facilities include increased access to a wider range of inexpensive feed ingredients, advanced feed processing, better quality control systems, and the use of multiple feed ingredients to reduce the impact of variation in nutrient content of individual ingredients on nutrient content of the complete feed.

GROUP SIZE, SPACE ALLOWANCE, AND MOVEMENT OF PIGS

In North America, growing-finishing pig facilities have traditionally been designed with pens to house groups of 20–30 pigs. In Western Europe group sizes have generally been smaller and close to the size of a large litter of pigs. Recently there has been a renewed interest in accommodating group sizes of more than 100 pigs. Reasons for this move toward larger group sizes include marginally lower construction costs, the potential to increase stocking density, the ability to mix pigs while minimizing aggressive encounters between pigs, and the use of auto-sort technology to separate pigs destined for slaughter (Brumm 2004). The major limitations of handling large groups of pigs are the difficulty of isolat-

ing individual pigs for medical treatment and additional effort or equipment required to select pigs for slaughter. In the Unites States the movement to larger groups of growing-finishing pigs has coincided with the adoption of wean-to-finish technology, where pigs are maintained in the same pen from weaning until slaughter (Wolter et al. 2001, 2002). The latter is driven largely by labor savings, as a result of reduced pig movement and reduced cleaning of facilities, and to a lesser extent by the negative impact of moving and mixing pigs on growth performance. Weaned pigs are typically placed in wean-to-finish pens at double the pig density expected at the end of the finishing phase. When the pigs reach the grower stage, half of the pigs from the pen are moved to a new pen. This allows the producer to make best use of available space without causing pigs to be crowded as finisher pigs.

In contrast to previous beliefs and observations on starter pigs, recent data suggest no reduction in growth performance of finishing pigs managed in larger groups as compared to conventional group sizes of 20–30 pigs per pen, provided that adequate feeder and drinking space is provided (Wolter et al. 2001; Turner et al. 2003; Table 66.6). Increasing group size and total pen space will result in more space per pen not occupied by pigs. This free space is available for eating, drinking, defecation, urination, and sleeping. It also provides more op-

Table 66.6.   Impact of group size on growth performance and carcass characteristics in a wean-to-finish production system.[1]

	Group Size		
	25	50	100
Number of pens	8	8	8
Body weight, kg			
Initial	5.9	5.9	5.9
Intermediate	34.8[a]	33.9[b]	33.9[b]
Final	116.4	116.1	116.2
Variation in body weight (CV), %			
Initial	10.7	11.1	11.1
Final	9.4	9.6	9.8
Daily gain, g			
Initial to intermediate	512[a]	499[b]	498[b]
Intermediate to final	716[ab]	708[b]	733[a]
Overall	655	648	658
Daily feed intake, g			
Initial to intermediate	815	818	821
Intermediate to final	2232	2206	2231
Overall	1759	1755	1759
Gain:Feed			
Initial to intermediate	0.63[a]	0.61[b]	0.61[b]
Intermediate to final	0.32[b]	0.32[b]	0.33[a]
Overall	0.37	0.37	0.37
Mortality, %	3.0	1.5	1.0
Morbidity, %	7.0[a]	3.5[b]	3.9[ab]
Carcass dressing percentage, %	74.9	75.3	75.4
Carcass lean yield, %	53.4	53.7	53.8

[1]Derived from Wolter et al. (2001).

[a,b,c]Values within rows followed by different superscripts differ (P <0.05).

portunity for submissive pigs to avoid dominant pigs and for individual pigs to seek their optimum thermal microenvironment. Pigs show more tolerant behavior in larger groups. In large pens it is apparently possible to introduce new pigs into an existing group without apparent disturbance of the social order (Brumm 2004). Because of the larger amount of total free space, total floor space area per pig may be reduced to 0.65 m² per finishing pig, which is below the typical value of 0.69 m² per pig in the United States for pens with fully slatted floors and the 0.93 m² per pig required to achieve maximum growth rates in finishing pigs between 54 and 113 kg body weight kept on partly slatted floors and with 7 or more pigs per pen (NCR-89 1993). In this extensive study average daily gains and feed efficiencies improved linearly with space allocation from 0.71 kg/day and 0.265 kg/kg at 0.56 m² per pig to 0.80 kg/day and 0.274 kg/kg at 0.93 m² per pig.

The allometric relationship between body weight (BW) and area of a pen per pig can be expressed by $k = A/BW^{0.667}$, where A is the area in m². The constant k represents a critical value relating to productivity. If growing-finishing pigs are raised on fully slatted or partially slatted floors, the critical values for k are 0.0327 and 0.0337, respectively. When k is below this critical value, average daily gain will decrease. The impact of space restriction on productivity is most evident when pigs are close to market weight. To lessen the impact of space restriction, producers may market the fastest growing animals at 5 kg below target weight. This will add 3% to available space, which essentially removes the overcrowding typically observed just prior to marketing the first group of pigs from a barn (Gonyou and Stricklin 1998).

One of the main determinants of space utilization efficiency is within-group variability in pig body weights. In order to meet the target slaughter weights, pigs are usually removed from the growing-finishing unit in three or more uniform body weight groups. In an all-in/all-out production facility, throughput is thus largely determined by the growth rate of the slowest growing or tail-end pigs in the group. In extreme cases and to clean out the pig unit before the planned arrival of the next group of pigs, the tail-end pigs need to be shipped at below-optimal body weight. The latter can have severe implications for carcass value of the tail-end pigs, as well as mean carcass value for the entire group, space utilization efficiency, and profitability. In a survey of seven commercial operations Dewey et al. (2001) reported coefficients of variation of 20–31% for body weights of pigs at different ages, which are substantially higher than values observed under closely controlled studies (Tables 66.6, 66.7). The main determinants of variation in body weight in growing-finishing pigs appear to be presence of diseases in the herd and the use of all-in/all-out versus continuous flow management (de Grau et al. 2001); variation in body weight of feeder pigs that are

Table 66.7. Effect of sorting pig by body weight at placement in the growing-finishing barn on variability in pig body weight after 91 days in the growing-finishing unit.[1]

	Treatment[2]			
	Heavy	Medium	Light	Unsorted
Pig body weight, kg				
Day 0	37.1	34.0	30.2	33.8
Day 91	123.4	117.8	113.2	119.9[3]
Within pen variation in pig body weight (CV), %				
Day 0	3.4	2.3	6.8	9.4
Day 91	6.0	6.5	8.2	7.3
Daily gain, kg	0.94	0.92	0.91	0.94[3]
Daily feed intake, kg	2.67	2.66	2.73	2.70
Feed: Gain	2.85	2.93	3.02	2.88

[1]Derived from O'Quinn et al. (2001).
[2]Treatment represents weight of pigs at sorting on day 0; unsorted represents an equal number of heavy, medium, and light pigs within each pen.
[3]Value for unsorted is different (P <0.05) from the average of the three sorted groups.

placed in the barn and restricted access to good quality feed and water can contribute to this variation as well. Group size and space allocation per pig do not appear to influence within-group variability (Turner et al. 2003).

A common management practice used to be to sort pigs by gender and weight when placing feeder pigs in the growing-finishing unit. Although this practice can be beneficial from a feeding management perspective, it does not result in better overall growth rates and reduced variability in pig body weights at slaughter (O'Quinn et al. 2001; Table 66.7). Apparently, pigs managed in groups have an inherent desire to vary in body weight. The coefficient of variation for within-pen body weight does not change when pigs are placed in pens with a large initial body weight variation, and the coefficient of variation will increase when pigs placed in pens have minimal within-pen initial body weight variation. In units where feeder pigs are placed at a similar age, the practice of sorting pigs for body weight appears to have limited impact on production efficiencies.

EFFECTIVE ENVIRONMENTAL TEMPERATURE AND AIR QUALITY

When pigs are kept dry and in a draft-free environment, the room temperature should be maintained at approximately 18–20°C when feeder pigs first enter the grower barn at approximately 25 kg body weight. Once pigs are adjusted to the new environment and have achieved good levels of feed intake the environmental temperature can be gradually decreased to about 15°C when pigs are approaching market weight (Close 1987; ASAE 1991; Le Dividich et al. 1998). Depending on environmental conditions the actual room air temperature can differ substantially from the effective environmental temperature—i.e., the environmental temperature that the pig actually "feels" (Close 1987). For example, each 0.30 m/s increase in air movement is equivalent to approximately a 1°C reduction in effective environmental temperature for group-housed growing pigs; a cold and wet floor may have a thermal equivalent of 7–10°C. The temperature of walls will influence the radiant heat loss from pigs; in cold climates and in poorly insulated pig facilities a temperature difference between ambient air and walls of 1–2°C is equivalent to a 1°C change in air temperature. In hot environments and when pigs rely largely on heat loss through evaporation of water the negative impact of high relative humidity of the air on pig well-being can be quite substantial.

When the effective environmental temperature is below the pigs' comfort zone, some of the ingested feed will be used to maintain the pigs' body temperature constant, resulting in reduced feed efficiency and growth rates. For example, Close (1987) estimated that pigs at a body weight of 20, 60, and 110 kg body weight will require 14, 32, and 47 g/day, respectively, of extra feed per 1°C below the thermal comfort zone to maintain a constant body temperature. When the effective environmental temperature is too high, feed intake can be reduced substantially. Per 1°C increase in environmental temperature feed intake will be reduced by approximately 2% in pigs around market weight and by approximately 1% in feeder pigs at approximately 25 kg body weight. These reductions in feed intake will be associated with reductions in growth rate of approximately 3 and 1.5%, respectively. Extreme environmental temperatures can also compromise the pigs' immune response and carcass quality. Clearly compromises need to be made in choosing the environmental temperature when pigs at different stages of growth are all kept in a common airspace.

Both mechanical and natural ventilation systems can be used to control the environmental air temperature and air quality (Baxter 1984). Increasingly these ventilation systems are computer-controlled and driven by actual (real-time) versus targeted air temperatures in the pig room and real-time measures of air quality. Mechanical ventilation systems now include several fixed and variable speed fans to control air exhaust from pig barns in incremental steps and air inlets that are all computer-controlled. In cold climates a minimum amount of air in the pig rooms, about 17.6 m³ per hour per pig (1.47 m³/sec or 3 cfm per pig), needs to be replaced with fresh air in order to remove air contaminates, such as ammonia, carbon dioxide, dust and water vapor. In extremely cold environments and when there is limited opportunity to preheat fresh incoming air, additional heat may be provided to maintain air temperature in the pig rooms above minimum levels. On the other hand, in warm climates or during the summer time, the optimum ventilation rate will be determined by the amount of body heat that is produced by pigs and needs to be removed from the pig room. These maxi-

mum ventilation rates will vary with the temperature and humidity of incoming air and may be as high as 150 m³ per hour per pig (12.5 m³/sec or 70 cfm per pig) (Baxter 1984). In well-designed pig facilities, control of air movement can be used to manipulate manuring patterns within pens and thus the comfort and cleanliness of pigs as well as air quality.

CONCLUSIONS AND IMPLICATIONS

With the move toward larger and highly specialized facilities it is becoming increasingly important to refine management within individual growing-finishing pig units, considering profitability, pig well-being, pork meat quality, and the impact on the environment. In order to make effective management changes, accurate production records need to be collected, and special consideration should be given to monitoring the dynamic changes in lean tissue growth, feed intake, and water usage within pig units. In particular, lean tissue growth is related closely to various aspects of pork production efficiency, such as average daily gains, carcass quality, and feed efficiency. As presented in this chapter, suboptimal feeding programs can have substantial impact on pig productivity, carcass quality, profitability, and nutrient excretion with manure. The recent trend toward all-in/all-out, wean-to-finish management of large pig groups represents a means to reduce production costs, while it may enhance growing-finishing pig productivity. A key challenge in any growing-finishing pig production system remains the control and management of variation in within-group pig body weights. The practice of sorting feeder pigs for body weight when moved into the unit has limited impact on within-group pig body weights at the time of slaughter and production efficiencies in units where feeder pigs are placed at a similar age. Improving the health status of pigs appears to be the most effective means to reduce within-group variability of pig body weights, as well as animal productivity. Computer-controlled and automated ventilation systems are used increasingly to ensure that the animals' thermal environment and air quality requirements are met.

The various aspects of growing-finishing pig management, such as feeding program, pig space allocation, and control of the thermal environment are all interconnected. Current developments toward integrated management systems that involve real-time analyses of pig growth and mathematical models that represent nutrient utilization for growth (Green et al. 2004) provide opportunities to truly optimize management in individual pig production units.

REFERENCES

American Society of Agricultural Engineers (ASAE). 1991. Standards. St. Joseph, Michigan, USA: Am Soc Agric Eng (ASAE) p. 435.

Baxter S. 1984. Ventilation. In Intensive Pig Production. Environmental Management and Design. London: Granada Publishing, pp. 79–115.

Black JL, Campbell RG, Williams IH, James KJ, Davies GT. 1986. Simulation of energy and protein utilization in the pig. Res Devel Agric 3:121–145.

Black JL, Davies GT, Bray HR, Chapple RP. 1995. Modelling the effect of genotype, environment and health on nutrient utilization. In Proc IVth Int Workshop on Modelling Nutr Utilization in Farm Animals. A Danfaer, P Lescoat, eds. Tjele, Denmark: National Institute of Animal Science, pp. 85–106.

Brumm M. 2004. Housing decisions for the growing pig. In Building Blocks for the Future. JM Murphy, TM Kane, CFM de Lange, eds. Proc 4th Annual London Swine Conference. Ontario Pork, Guelph, Ontario, Canada, pp. 31–44.

Close WH. 1987. The influence of the thermal environment on the productivity of pigs. In Pig Housing and the Environment. AT Smith, TLJ Lawrence, eds. Occasional publication No. 11. Br Soc Anim Prod, Midlothian, Scotland, pp. 9–24.

de Grau AG, Dewey CF, Friendship RM. 2001. Effect of pig management on weight variation in grower-finisher pigs. Proc Am Assoc Swine Pract, pp. 521–526.

de Lange CFM. 2004. A system approach to represent nitrogen and phosphorus utilization in growing pigs. Proc. 25th Western Nutrition Conference. Department of Animal and Poultry, Science, University of Saskatchewan, Saskatoon, Canada.

de Lange CFM, Birkett SH, Morel PCH. 2001b. Protein, fat and bone tissue growth in swine. In Swine Nutrition. A Lewis, L Southorn, eds. Boca Raton, Florida: CRC Press, pp. 65–84.

de Lange CFM, Marty BJ, Birkett SH, Morel P, Szkotnicki B. 2001a. Application of pig growth models in commercial pork production. Can J Anim Sci 81:1–8.

Dewey C, de Grau A, Friendship B. 2001. Grow/finish variation: Cost and control strategies. Proc Am Assoc Swine Pract, pp. 403–407.

Gonyou HW, Lou Z. 2000. Effects of eating space and availability of water in feeders on productivity and eating behavior of grower-finisher pigs. J Anim Sci 78:865–870.

Gonyou HW, Stricklin WR. 1998. Effects of floor area allowance and group size productivity of growing/finishing pigs. J Anim Sci 76:1326–1330.

Green DM, Parsons DJ, Schofield CP, Whittemore, CT. 2004. Real-time control of pig growth through an integrated management system. Br Soc Anim Sci. (In press.)

Gu Y, Schinckel AP, Martin TG. 1992. Growth, development and carcass composition in five genotypes of swine. J Anim Sci 70:1719–1729.

Hicks C, Schinckel AP, Forrest JC, Akridge JT, Wagner JR, Chen W. 1998. Biases associated with genotype and sex in prediction of fat-free lean mass and carcass value in hogs. J Anim Sci 76:2221–2234.

Kansas State University Swine Nutrition Guide. 1997. Growing-finishing pig recommendations. Kansas State University Agricultural Experimental Station and Cooperative Extension Services. Kansas State University, Manhattan, Kansas.

Le Dividich J, Noblet J, Herpin P, van Milgen J, Quiniou, N. 1998. Thermoregulation. In Progress in Pig Science. J Wiseman, MA Varley, JP Chadwick JP, eds. Thrumpton, Nottingham, U.K.: Nottingham University Press, pp. 229–263.

Mikkelsen LL, Naughton PJ, Hedemann MS, Jenssen BB. 2004. Effects of physical properties of feed on microbial ecology and survival of *Salmonella enterica* serovar Typhimurium in the pig gastrointestinal tract. Appl Env Microbiol 70:3485–3492.

National Research Council (NRC). 1987. Predicting feed intake of food producing animals. Washington, D.C.: National Academic Press.

———. 1998. Nutrient requirements of swine (10th edition). Washington, D.C.: National Academic Press.

NCR-89 (Committee on Confinement Management of Swine). 1993. Space requirements of barrows and gilts penned together from 54 to 113 kg. J Anim Sci 71:1088–1091.

O'Quinn PR, Dritz SS, Goodband RD, Tokach MD, Swanson JC, Nelssen JL, Musser RE. 2001. Sorting growing-finishing pigs by weight fails to improve growth performance or weight variation. J Swine Health Prod 9:11–16.

Patience JF, Thacker PA, de Lange CFM. 1995. Swine Nutrition Guide (2nd ed). Saskatoon, Canada: Prairie Swine Centre Inc.

Quiniou N, Noblet J. 1995. Prediction of tissular body composition from protein and lipid deposition in growing pigs. J Anim Sci 73:1567–1575.

Rosenvold K., Andersen HJ. 2003. Factors of significance for pork quality. Meat Sci 64:219–237.

Schinckel AP. 1994. Nutrient requirements for modern pig genotypes. In Recent Advances in Animal Nutrition. PJ Garnsworthy, DJA Cole, eds. Nottingham, U.K.: Nottingham University Press, pp. 133–169.

Schinckel AP, de Lange CFM. 1996. Characterization of growth parameters needed as inputs for pig growth models. J Anim Sci 74:2021–2036.

Schinckel AP, Smith JW II, Tokach MD, Dritz SS, Einstein M, Nelssen JN, Goodband RD. 2002. Two on-farm data collection methods to determine dynamics of swine compositional growth and estimates of dietary lysine requirements. J Anim Sci 80:1419–1432.

Tokach MD, de Lange CFM. 2001. Lunch bucket approach to on-farm feeding of growing-finishing pigs. In The Pork Industry and Public Issues. JH Smith, CFM de Lange, eds. Proc 1st Annu London Swine Conf. Ontario Pork, Guelph, Canada, pp. 149–165.

Turner SP, Allcroft DJ, Edwards SA. 2003. Housing pigs in large social groups: A review of implications for performance and other economic traits. Livest Prod Sci 82:39–51.

Williams NH, Stahly TS, Zimmerman DR. 1997. Effect of level of chronic immune system activation on the growth and lysine needs of pigs fed from 6 to 112 kg. J Anim Sci 75:2481–2496.

Wolter BF, Ellis FM, Curtis SE, Agspurger NR, Hamilton DN, Parr EN, Webel DM. 2001. Effect of group size on pig performance in a wean-to-finish production system. J Anim Sci 79:1067–1073.

Wolter BF, Ellis FM, DeDecker JM, Curtis SE, Hollis GR, Shanks RD, Parr EN, Webel DM. 2002. Effects of double stocking and weighing frequency on pig performance in wean-to-finish production system. J Anim Sci 80:1442–1450.

67 Animal Welfare

Sandra A. Edwards, Peter R. English, and David Fraser

At the beginning of the 21st century, many of the industrialized countries saw the emergence of new standards for the welfare of farmed animals. For example:

- In 1999, the United Kingdom enacted a ban on keeping pregnant sows individually in tethers or stalls, and the European Union (EU) passed a directive to phase out the standard battery cage for laying hens within 12 years.
- In 2000, a major fast food chain restaurant in the United States (U.S.) announced animal welfare standards that their suppliers would be required to meet, mainly in the slaughter and egg industries.
- In 2001 another fast food chain restaurant in the U.S. adopted a similar program; the EU passed a directive to ban individual stall housing of pregnant sows effective in 2013; and two Washington-based organizations (the Food Marketing Institute and the National Council of Chain Restaurants) began developing a set of food animal welfare standards on behalf of the U.S. grocery and chain restaurant sectors.
- In 2002 the member countries of the World Organization for Animal Health (OIE), which is recognized by the World Trade Organization as the principal standard-setting body in matters of animal health, unanimously voted to begin developing internationally harmonized animal welfare standards.

In these diverse developments covering a period of only a few years, we see a remarkably rapid movement toward explicit animal welfare standards involving a combination of national legislation, international agreements, and corporate standards. These developments raise a number of questions which this chapter will address briefly. First, what is animal welfare, and how did it become such a prominent area of concern? Second, what is the scientific basis of animal welfare research and standards? And third, what are the current animal welfare concerns that need to be considered in swine production?

BACKGROUND

In one sense, the appropriate treatment of animals is one of the long-standing ethical issues of human civilization, which different cultures and religious traditions have addressed in different ways over the centuries (Preece 1999). In the 1800s many industrialized countries created some form of legal protection for animals, particularly to deal with antisocial acts such as deliberate cruelty and gross neglect. In many countries the mid 20th century saw an expansion of legal protection for food animals—for example, through requirements for humane treatment of animals at slaughter plants and humane animal transportation. Throughout the late 20th century, public attention and sympathy toward animals appeared to show a widespread increase, especially in European and English-speaking countries. Many aspects of animal use—including animal-based research, animals in entertainment, and production of animal-based food—were questioned and debated as never before.

During roughly the same period, swine production in the industrialized world underwent profound changes. Average herd size increased steadily, such that fewer and fewer producers operated increasingly large units. Housing and technology also changed in ways that reduced production costs, generally by keeping animals in indoor environments where labor requirements could be reduced and space could be used efficiently. These changes had complex effects on the health and welfare of the animals, but another significant result was a change in public perception of swine production, away from traditional positive images of the small-scale family-run farm with careful attention to individual animals, and toward more negative images of swine production as a depersonalized, industrial activity. With this change came a greater public scepticism over the humaneness of animal production and a greater will to have animal welfare standards imposed on the industry.

WHAT IS ANIMAL WELFARE?

In debate and discussion of animal welfare, three different but overlapping types of concern have been expressed about the quality of life of animals (Duncan and Fraser 1997; Fraser et al. 1997). A traditional set of concerns centers on the basic health and functioning of animals. This includes freedom from disease, parasites, and injury together with normal growth, development, and functioning of the animal's physiological and behavioral systems. A second major concern centers on the affective states of animals—emotions and feelings, especially unpleasant states such as fear, pain, hunger, and distress. Concern arises, for example, over pain caused by castration, over fear caused by rough handling, and over separation distress caused by abrupt weaning or social isolation. A third concern, arising especially over animals kept in very restrictive or barren environments, is that animals be allowed to live reasonably natural lives, in environments that are well suited to the species. For example, philosopher Bernard Rollin (1995) noted that contemporary concern about animal welfare goes beyond issues of pain and suffering and involves respecting the "nature" of animals.

These different views of animal welfare are by no means mutually exclusive. For example, allowing an overheated sow to wallow should be good for her welfare by all three criteria: it will reduce the negative effects of heat stress (a basic health and functioning criterion), it allows her to carry out her natural thermoregulatory behavior (a natural living criterion), and she will presumably feel more comfortable (an affective state criterion). However, the different views can also lead to different conclusions about some issues. For example, those who emphasize basic health and functioning may conclude that housing sows in narrow stalls throughout most of pregnancy is good for their welfare because it prevents fighting-related injuries and promotes uniform weight gain, whereas those who emphasize natural living criteria might conclude that the stalls are incompatible with good welfare because they prevent most forms of natural behavior. Complicating the resolution of such disagreements, the different views of animal welfare tend to be favored by different sectors of the population. Producers and livestock veterinarians tend to interpret animal welfare in terms of basic health and functioning, whereas consumers, together with some small-scale and organic producers, tend to emphasize natural living criteria (te Velde et al. 2002).

Given this diversity, probably no account of animal welfare will be widely acceptable unless it takes all three of the major concerns into consideration to at least some degree. One general description of animal welfare, which nicely combines the different concerns, is the "Five Freedoms" adapted from Webster (1994):

1. Freedom from malnutrition: the diet should be sufficient in both quantity and quality to promote normal health and vigor.

2. Freedom from thermal and physical discomfort: the animal's environment should be neither excessively hot nor cold and should allow normal rest and activity.

3. Freedom from injury and disease: the husbandry system should minimize the risk of injury and disease and facilitate the immediate recognition and treatment of any cases that do occur.

4. Freedom to express most normal patterns of behavior: the physical and social environment should provide the necessary components to enable the animal to carry out behaviors it has a strong motivation to perform.

5. Freedom from pain, fear, and distress.

SCIENTIFIC APPROACHES TO ANIMAL WELFARE

All three perspectives on animal welfare have given rise to productive research to understand, assess, and improve animal husbandry systems. However, each perspective tends to lead to somewhat different approaches and to emphasize different measures to improve animal welfare.

Functioning of Animals: The Physiology of Stress

When animals experience certain welfare challenges, such as physical injury or fear of a dominant penmate, characteristic physiological responses occur that presumably have evolved as adaptive measures to prepare the animal for "fight or flight" (Stephens 1980). Such "stressors" activate both the sympathetic nervous system and the hypothalamo-pituitary-adrenocortical axis. Sympathetic stimulation results in rapid transmission of signals to key organs in the body and secretion of catecholamines (adrenaline and noradrenaline) into the circulation from the adrenal medulla. Concurrent with this immediate response is a more sustained endocrine cascade whereby corticotropin-releasing factor from the hypothalamus causes release of adrenocorticotropic hormone (ACTH) from the anterior pituitary, which, in turn, stimulates the adrenal cortex to secrete corticosteroid hormones (cortisol and other glucocorticoids) into the circulation. Both neural and endocrine responses mobilize body reserves for activity by releasing glucose into the bloodstream, increasing heart rate and directing blood flow to muscles rather than skin and viscera. A negative feedback of plasma corticosteroid on the hypothalamus restores normal conditions when the stressor is removed.

In assessing welfare from a viewpoint of physiological function, measurements of plasma cortisol or ACTH levels are often made to judge the extent of stress experienced by an animal in a given situation. For example, many studies have shown increased plasma cortisol among sows that are kept tethered during pregnancy, although this may have been due to poorly designed tether stalls, which resulted in unresolved aggression between neighboring animals (Barnett et al. 2001). However, there are a number of problems in using these simple measures. Taking a blood sample to assess hormone levels may, in itself, induce a greater adrenal response than any treatment difference under investigation (Moss 1981), and single blood samples are unreliable because corticosteroid release is pulsatile and shows diurnal patterns that can vary with different circumstances (Johnson and Levine 1973). Some of these problems can be overcome by measurement of corticosteroids and their metabolites in saliva, urine, or feces, which can be obtained noninvasively, but these are still subject to temporal fluctuations. Better measures of chronic stress often rely on detection of changes in morphology or function that result from long-term stimulation of physiological pathways or organs. Such measures include the weight of the adrenal glands, the activity of the enzymes controlling catecholamine synthesis (Stanton and Mueller 1976), and the "adrenal function test" whereby a standard amount of ACTH is injected and the resulting blood level of corticosteroid is measured (Ladewig et al. 1986). Interpretation of such results is still difficult because of genetic differences between animals in adrenal response to ACTH (Hennessy et al. 1988) and because some animals in adverse conditions appear to cease adrenal responsiveness after a period.

For short-term challenges it is sometimes simpler to measure the secondary consequences of the stress response rather than the underlying endocrinology. For example, heart rate, which can be monitored noninvasively using skin surface electrodes, increases when animals encounter a fearful situation such as close proximity to a dominant penmate (Marchant et al. 1995), but heart rate also requires careful interpretation because of possible confounding factors such as activity level.

Functioning of Animals: Production, Health, and Animal Welfare

It is often said by veterinarians and producers that good production performance indicates a high level of animal welfare. In support of this argument, the hormonal stress responses just described influence key metabolic and reproductive processes governing production performance. High corticosteroid levels reduce protein synthesis and lean tissue growth (Spencer 1985), resulting in slower growth and poorer conformation. In breeding animals, physiological stress responses also influence the hypothalamo-pituitary-ovarian axis (Arey and Edwards 1998), resulting in delayed onset of estrus, suppressed estrous activity, and development of cystic ovaries. Furthermore, stress in early pregnancy, at the time of implantation, results in increased embryo mortality and reduced litter size. The effects of stress on performance were well illustrated in experiments by Hemsworth and collaborators (1991) on the adverse effects of negative handling of pigs by stockpersons. Unpleasant handling, in comparison with sympathetic handling, resulted in pigs with chronically elevated corticosteroid levels, slower growth rate, a lower pregnancy rate in gilts, and delayed reproductive development in young boars.

A key link between welfare and performance is the maintenance of good pig health. Premature death and poor health are unquestionably indicators of impaired welfare, although the converse may not necessarily be true. Thus, health measures such as the incidence of infectious disease, lameness, or lesions of the skin (Backstrom 1973; de Koning 1985) are useful in assessing welfare in many practical circumstances. Moreover, stressful environmental conditions may increase the susceptibility of pigs to disease, partly because stress influences the immune system (Kelley 1980). In particular, sustained high levels of corticosteroid hormones in the blood can reduce proliferation of lymphocytes and decrease antibody production, thus impairing the ability of the pig to resist infection. Because stressors may reduce immune responsiveness, immune challenge techniques provide another potential measure of animal welfare. For example, sows tethered in a barren environment show a poorer immune response when challenged with a novel antigen, and their piglets also have lower antibody levels (Metz and Osterlee 1981). Thus, stressful conditions would be expected to induce higher corticosteroid levels, which are associated with poorer health, higher mortality levels, poorer growth and food conversion efficiency, and depressed reproductive performance.

In addition to these indirect effects on performance, inadequate environments or husbandry can directly affect both performance and welfare. Examples include lesions and lameness that result from faulty floors or inadequate pen design and aggression and vice resulting from poorly managed groups. Similarly, inadequate environmental temperature and nutrition can affect the welfare and performance of the pig. Close (1987) noted that keeping pigs either below their lower critical temperature or above their upper critical temperature can influence comfort, food intake, growth, food conversion efficiency, health, and viability. Nutritional deficiencies, in addition to predisposing to metabolic diseases and reduced growth and reproductive performance, may also contribute to outbreaks of tail biting (Fraser 1987). Inadequate diets have particularly clear effects on animal welfare in the case of early-weaned pigs, where low-cost diets that are not suited to the immature digestive system can cause severe depression in intake and growth and greatly increase the incidence of scouring and death.

In these various cases, welfare and productivity are correlated, and poor productivity can be a useful indicator of a welfare problem. However, the relationship does not always hold. Low growth rate and food conversion efficiency may, for example, be the result of feeding a low-density diet, which is nevertheless nutritionally adequate and cost-effective in a particular situation. Equally, high productivity does not necessarily indicate a high standard of welfare. For example, the effects of inadequate housing on disease and performance can be masked by the routine use of antibiotics. Similarly, pigs treated with growth hormone or repartitioning agents may deposit lean meat very quickly but at greater risk of metabolic disease, and hyperprolific sow lines carry additional welfare risks for both the lactating sow and her piglets.

Affective States of Animals: Behavioral Measures of Welfare

The behavior of pigs has always been used by stockpersons or veterinarians to identify the onset of problems with health or environment. Simple examples are the apathy of a sick pig or the huddling of a group of pigs that are too cold. Similarly, behavior that results in injury to an animal (such as rooting on inappropriate surfaces) or that inflicts injury on others (such as tail, ear, and flank biting, discussed below) are also generally accepted indicators of impaired welfare.

Behavioral indicators are also used to help understand the "affective states" of animals such as pain, fear, and distress. For example, vocalizations have been used as a metric of separation distress. Piglets that are suddenly separated from the sow call in a pattern so characteristic that experienced pig-keepers immediately recognize the calls as coming from an isolated piglet. The calls begin with quiet grunts made with the mouth closed, progressing to louder grunts made with the mouth open, and then a mixture of loud grunts and squeals. Piglets that are in greater need of being reunited with the sow because they are cold or hungry give more calls, especially more of the high-pitched squeals, and sows respond more vigorously to calls given by such piglets. The calls thus appear to form a communication system which helps reunite sows and isolated piglets, with the number and type of calls reflecting the animals' level of distress at being separated (Weary and Fraser 1995). The calls may be useful for testing ways to reduce separation distress. For example, experiments show that piglets newly separated from the sow vocalize much less if there are several familiar littermates close by. Similar research has used vocalizations to assess pain in piglets when castrated in different ways (Taylor and Weary 2000).

Pig behavior has also been used in experiments designed to assess the needs and preferences of pigs that might contribute to improved welfare (Fraser and Matthews 1997). When given a choice between different circumstances, pigs can express their relative preferences on matters such as diet, floor type, thermal environment, and degree of social contact. However, results of such preference tests must be interpreted with caution, since any preference is relative to the other options available and may be modified by temporary motiva-

tional state and previous experience. A refinement on this approach is the use of instrumental conditioning techniques in which pigs are trained to work for a reward such as food, light, heat, or rooting substrate. The importance of the reward to the pig can then be assessed by measuring the amount of work animals will do to continue receiving that reward. These techniques, when correctly applied, allow the animal to inform us about its relative priorities, and the strength of its motivation to attain them (Ladewig and Matthews 1996). Such knowledge then indicates what we should seek to incorporate in improved husbandry systems.

"Abnormal" behavior has also been interpreted as an indicator of impaired welfare, although the definition of abnormal is not straightforward. Following an international survey of expert opinion, a list of behaviors widely accepted as "abnormal" has been published (Commission of the European Communities 1983). These include vices such as ear, flank, and tail biting, plus stereotypic behaviors as discussed below.

Natural Living: Incorporating Natural Elements into Animal Husbandry

In some cases, the natural behavior of pigs has been used as a guide to improving housing systems for pigs. In a novel approach, Stolba and Wood-Gush (1984) observed pigs that had been turned loose in a hilly, wooded area and identified certain characteristic features of the animals' behavior. In particular, the pigs rooted in the soil, exercised their neck muscles by levering against fallen logs, built nests in secluded areas before giving birth, and used dunging areas well removed from their resting areas. The research also identified certain key stimuli in the environment which were important for these behaviors to be performed. This led to the design of a complex commercial pen which incorporated these key stimuli, with a dunging passage in the front, an area where the pigs could root in soil, a log for levering, separate feeding areas, and secluded areas at the back where sows could be enclosed to farrow. The authors claimed that the animals' welfare was significantly improved by the complex pen. However, because some aspects of basic health and functioning (such as piglet survival) were less good in this system than in more restrictive systems (Edwards 1995), some critics have disagreed with this conclusion.

In contrast to this somewhat radical approach, more conservative approaches have tried to incorporate specific elements of natural behavior into typical commercial production systems in order to solve specific problems. For example, free-living pregnant sows would typically spend much of the day foraging for food. In commercial production they are normally fed a very dense diet which is cheaper to transport and store than a bulky, fiber-rich diet. However, the sow's intake of a dense diet needs to be strictly limited so that the animals do not gain too much weight. The result is that sows may consume their daily ration in a matter of minutes and remain strongly motivated to find food for much of the day (Lawrence and Terlouw 1993). Under these conditions sows often develop stereotypies—repetitive behaviors that are fixed in form and serve no obvious function for the animal—such as the repetitive head-waving and bar-chewing that some sows perform for several hours per day. Some sows also toy with water dispensers to the point of drinking huge quantities of water. Providing sows with straw or other roughage, or providing a fiber-rich diet, can allow the animals to spend a more natural amount of time in finding and consuming food, and the abnormal behavior and water intake can be greatly reduced (Meunier-Salaun et al. 2001).

Although "natural" behavior provides a useful starting point, the relation between natural behavior and animal welfare is complex. Many behavior patterns are responses to the environment in which the animal is kept. The fact that a pig in intensive housing behaves differently from one in the wild is not in itself an indication of impaired welfare but may provide a useful starting point to explore whether the change reflects an animal welfare problem. For example, the stereotyped behavior of pregnant sows in barren environments does appear to indicate a welfare problem because it seems to reflect a state of chronic hunger in the animals (Appleby and Lawrence 1987), and the development of stereotyped behavior has been linked to neural pathology in at least some species (Garner et al. 2003).

In summary, there are many different approaches for assessing and improving the welfare of pigs. Each approach has its own strengths and associated difficulties, and a sensible combination of some or all of the methods outlined is likely to provide a better understanding of animal welfare than the use of any one approach alone.

CURRENT WELFARE ISSUES IN PIG PRODUCTION

With increased public awareness and concern about pig welfare, there is growing pressure to modify or abolish a number of practices that are currently widespread in the pig industry. Unlike most early welfare concerns and legislation, which were designed to penalize deliberate cruelty toward animals, some more recent concerns (and in some countries legislation) have focused on husbandry systems. The debate has highlighted the many difficulties in generalizing about welfare in a given system and the need to balance different welfare considerations, including cases where benefits to some animals occur at the expense of others.

Gestation Housing

The pregnant sow in a gestation stall has little opportunity for exercise and cannot walk or socialize freely with other animals. From a natural living viewpoint, a preferred system is to house pregnant sows in groups in an environment which provides greater freedom to move, explore, and socialize. However, because pregnant sows are offered very limited amounts of concentrate diets, there can be severe competition for feed when group feeding is practiced, with the dominant sows eating too much and the timid (and younger) sows too little. Although group housing can be improved by providing individual feeders to protect the timid sows during feeding, aggression can still occur at other times (Petherick 1989). In particular, competition for space, chronic hunger, and reestablishment of the dominance hierarchy when sows are regrouped can all result in increased aggression (Edwards 1992). Thus greater behavioral freedom for all sows is sometimes achieved at the expense of increased risk of injury and chronic fear in some individuals.

Farrowing Crates

The farrowing sow and her newborn litter provide another case of conflicting interests. The sow is often confined to a crate during and after farrowing to minimize the risk of crushing her piglets, to facilitate beneficial intervention by the stockperson, and to allow specially warmed creep areas to be arranged adjacent to the udder. These areas provide the temperature required by the newborn piglet to minimize the risk of hypothermia and resulting problems of starvation, crushing, and disease (English 1993). However, this system of housing the sow renders her unable to perform the normal farrowing behaviors seen in the wild, especially preparturient locomotion and nest building. When unable to carry out such behavior, sows show indications of stress in the form of increased corticosteroid levels combined with stereotyped behavior such as floor-nosing and bar chewing (Lawrence et al. 1994). Recent data indicate that confinement per se causes bigger problems in the preparturient period than lack of nesting material (Jarvis et al. 2002); hence, the current EU recommendation for provision of nesting material in farrowing crates is at best only a partial solution. However, no system has yet proven capable, under large-scale indoor commercial conditions, of both permitting full behavioral freedom to the sow and safeguarding the survival and welfare of her piglets (Edwards and Fraser 1997).

Early Weaning

Under natural conditions, pigs are weaned in a gradual process that begins at about 3 weeks after farrowing and is not completed until the young are 3–4 months of age (Jensen 1995). Under commercial conditions, economic pressures to maximize sow output have resulted in abrupt early weaning of pigs at 3–4 weeks of age in the EU (where weaning at less than 28 days is restricted to specific situations, and weaning at less than 21 days is generally forbidden) and sometimes at even younger ages elsewhere in the world in segregated early weaning. This practice is designed to improve herd health by restricting transfer of pathogens from older animals to the piglet. When weaned at this young age, the piglet has little experience of solid food intake, and an immature digestive and immune system (Curtis and Bourne 1973; de Passillé et al. 1989). These physiological challenges are accompanied by psychological challenges associated with separation from the mother, first experience of a novel environment and, frequently, social regrouping. The piglets often show both behavioral and physiological indications of reduced welfare. Abnormal oral behaviors such as belly-nosing and ear biting can occur at high levels, particularly with earlier weaning ages, and may continue into later life as tail, ear, and flank biting (Gonyou et al. 1998). There is thus conflict between piglet welfare and the commercial need to maximize sow output.

Space Allowance

The cost of high quality housing creates financial pressure on producers to minimize the amount of space per pig. In many countries there are no minimum legal space allowances, and even in Europe, where space allowance is regulated, the adequacy of the allowance is being increasingly questioned (Ekkel et al. 2003). When pigs are overcrowded, they show higher levels of stress hormones, reduced growth and greater probability of health problems and abnormal behaviors such as tail biting (Meunier-Salaun et al. 1987). However, a degree of overcrowding often yields the best financial returns despite some reduction in individual performance. Here again we see some trade-off between animal welfare and commercial goals.

Bedding and Environmental Enrichment

The provision of adequate, good-quality bedding (usually straw) is frequently cited as contributing to the welfare of pigs of all ages because it helps to provide physical comfort, insulation, and recreation (Day et al. 2002). However, straw can also pose a problem for pig health and welfare by increasing the animals' exposure to microbes, dust, fungal spores, and ammonia in the air. An alternative may lie in providing the benefits of bedding in other ways that do not involve the same drawbacks.

One advantage of straw-based systems is the constant availability of a substrate for the exploratory and manipulative behaviors that comprise a major component of the time budget of pigs under seminatural conditions. In the absence of adequate environmental provision, such behavior can be directed toward penmates and lead to development of injurious behaviors, such as tail biting (van de Weerd et al. 2004). The amount of straw necessary to serve this purpose, and the extent to which alternative bedding materials or toys can replace straw, are still the subject of research. Instrumental conditioning studies indicate that the reward value of full-straw bedding is greater than that of chopped straw or

straw presented in a rack (Ladewig and Matthews 1996). However, a small amount of straw seems effective in providing pigs with recreation (Fraser et al. 1991b; Lyons et al. 1995). Although "toys" (simple enrichment devices such as tires and chains) can provide occupation in the short term, habituation often occurs quite rapidly, and they often provide only 10% of the occupation time provided by full straw bedding, indicating either a lack of the appropriate stimulus properties or inadequate availability to all animals in the group. To attract and maintain interest from pigs, enrichment materials should provide olfactory/gustatory stimulation and respond by changes in form to the chewing behavior of the pigs (Feddes and Fraser 1994; van de Weerd et al. 2003). An ongoing challenge is to develop functional enrichment strategies that meet the needs of pigs but are also practical in large-scale slatted-floor housing.

Invasive Procedures on Piglets: Teeth Clipping, Tail Docking, and Castration

Currently many farms carry out invasive and painful procedures whose long-term benefits are thought to outweigh the transient distress that they cause. Thus, teeth clipping is deemed to be justified because it reduces injury to the faces of littermates during competition for teat position, damage and discomfort to the udder of the sow, and resultant restlessness that might increase the risk of crushing of piglets. Similarly, tail docking is justified on the grounds that it reduces the risk of tail biting in later life, and castration is deemed to be justified because it reduces aggression and harmful sexual behavior in later life while also preventing "boar taint," which renders the meat unpalatable. While such arguments undoubtedly have merit, there is growing public pressure to find alternative methods to achieve the desirable outcomes in less invasive ways. Many farms have found it possible to cease teeth clipping or restrict its use to high-risk litters with temperamental sows, large litter size, or extensive cross-fostering. Castration is more difficult to abolish if pigs are to be slaughtered at heavy weights, but may be superseded in the future by immunological rather than surgical techniques.

Tail biting in growing pigs is a widespread behavioral vice with very significant animal welfare and economic consequences. It is a multifactorial problem, with a variety of identified environmental and nutritional risk factors (Schroder-Petersen and Simonsen 2001). Despite research over many years, the problem has remained intractable in commercial pig production. Where pigs are left with intact tails, serious welfare issues associated with tail biting can be endemic under some environmental conditions (van de Weerd et al. 2004). One reason for the failure to find effective solutions to the vice is that most research into tail biting has involved surveys of only the tail-bitten animals, either on farms or in abattoirs. There is relatively little information on the pigs that actually do the biting and no real understanding of what might initiate the behavior in these individuals, but not others in the same group. Predisposition to tail bite has been shown to have both genetic and metabolic components (Fraser 1987; Fraser et al. 1991a; Breuer et al. 2005), which are exacerbated when pigs are housed in relatively barren environments and subject to other environmental stressors such as overcrowding, extreme temperatures, or drafts. If tail docking is to be rendered unnecessary in the future, a better understanding of the determinants of tail biting is needed to develop effective preventive strategies.

Stockmanship

There is a prevalent and long-held belief that the quality of the stockperson has a more important influence on pig welfare than the choice of production system (Brambell 1965). Increasing scientific evidence suggests that the empathy between stockpersons and the animals in their care is a major factor contributing to animal welfare and performance (English et al. 1992). As highlighted previously, pigs that receive frequent and sympathetic handling are easier to manage and have lower levels of circulating corticosteroid hormones, faster growth rates, and better reproductive performance than those that receive minimal handling or unpleasant handling (Hemsworth et al. 1991). In a comparison of otherwise similar farms, Hemsworth et al. (1981) found that reproductive performance of the unit was higher on those farms where the sows showed little fear of humans. Later work showed that the attitudinal and behavioral profiles of individual stockpersons affected both welfare and performance of their animals (Hemsworth et al. 1989). Legislation in the EU emphasizes the importance of stockmanship, and requires national training programs to be established. However, the quality of stockmanship is still a major limitation on many commercial farms because of the difficulties in attracting and retaining good staff and dealing with the economic pressures to reduce staff time per animal (English et al. 1992).

RESOLVING ANIMAL WELFARE ISSUES

With so many pressures for changes to current practices that are deemed to compromise animal welfare, producers must carefully weigh their future strategy. As detailed previously, a focus on animal welfare should in many cases improve the productivity of farm animals and the quality of their products. In some cases, however, there are likely to be costs associated with conforming to animal welfare standards. For example, requirements to provide straw or to eliminate individual stalls for pregnant sows may create some increase in production costs or at least incur certain expenses during the period of transition. In such cases, producers are understandably concerned about having to compete against lower-priced imports from jurisdictions with less demanding standards.

By the 1990s, debate had arisen about whether countries with high animal welfare standards could block imports from countries lacking equivalent standards. Various mechanisms involving the General Agreement on Tariffs and Trade were proposed, but in each case there are significant difficulties and counter-arguments. The development and acceptance of internationally harmonized standards is an obvious way to avoid conflict among countries over animal welfare standards. As noted above, the World Organization for Animal Health has begun developing international animal welfare standards, initially in the areas of slaughter, killing of animals for disease control, and transport of animals by land and sea. If, and as, standards are adopted, they could help create a level playing field for the industry in different countries. International agreement on contentious production issues, such as minimum weaning age and use of gestation stalls has not yet been attempted outside the European Union.

Resolving animal welfare issues has been made more complicated by the acrimonious and polarized views of modern animal production that are widely presented to the public. On the one hand are thoroughly negative views claiming that confinement systems are inherently bad for animal welfare and for the environment, and that the products of such systems are dangerous for human health. On the other side of the debate are thoroughly positive portrayals of animal agriculture, largely originating from animal producers and their organizations, which claim that modern production is beneficial for animal welfare and the environment, while producing safe and nutritious products (Fraser 2001). With an activity as diverse as swine production, proponents of each of these highly simplified views can cite facts and examples to support their claims.

In this polarized debate, it is sometimes difficult to separate fact from polemic. Some of the modern changes in swine production have had positive effects on animal welfare. The use of indoor housing has eliminated some problems related to predation and cold weather. In some cases confinement has allowed disease prevention through the exclusion of common pathogens. Advances in feeding technology and nutritional knowledge have made it more feasible to meet animals' nutritional needs. Veterinary knowledge and technology allow vaccination, medication, and other disease prevention measures that would not have been possible a half-century ago. However, the changes in production methods have also created a new set of animal welfare problems and dilemmas, as outlined previously. In the midst of the acrimonious debate and the highly charged political environment that has resulted, it will be important for swine producers and veterinarians to retain a constructive focus on animal welfare by building on the positives while solving the problems that current production methods entail.

REFERENCES

Appleby MC, Lawrence A. 1987. Food restriction as a cause of stereotypic behaviour in tethered gilts. Anim Prod 45:103–110.

Arey DS, Edwards SA. 1998. Factors influencing aggression between sows after mixing and the consequences for welfare and production. Livest Prod Sci 56:61–70.

Backstrom L. 1973. Environment and animal health in piglet production. Acta Vet Scand, Suppl 41.

Barnett JL, Hemsworth PH, Cronin GM, Jongman EC, Hutson GD. 2001. A review of the welfare issues for sows and piglets in relation to housing. Aust J Agric Res 52:1–28.

Brambell FWR. 1965. Report of the Technical Committee to Enquire into the Welfare of Animals Kept Under Intensive Livestock Husbandry Systems. Cmnd. 2836. Her Majesty's Stationery Office, London.

Breuer K, Sutcliffe MEM, Mercer JT, Rance KA, O'Connell NE, Sneddon IA, Edwards SA. 2005. Heritability of clinical tail biting and its relation to performance traits. Livest Prod Sci, in press.

Close WH. 1987. The influence of the thermal environment on productivity of pigs. In Pig Housing and the Environment. AT Smith, TLJ Lawrence, eds. British Society of Animal Production, Occasional Publication no. 11, pp. 9–24.

Commission of the European Communities. 1983. Abnormal Behaviours in Farm Animals. Commission of the European Communities, Brussels.

Curtis J, Bourne FJ. 1973. Half lives of immunoglobulins IgG, IgA and IgM in the serum of new-born pigs. Immunology 24:147–155.

Day JEL, Burfoot A, Docking CM, Whittaker X, Spoolder HAM, Edwards SA. 2002. The effects of prior experience of straw and depth of straw bedding on the behaviour of growing pigs. Appl Anim Behav Sci 76:189–202.

de Koning R. 1985. On the well-being of dry sows. Doctoral thesis, Utrecht University, Netherlands.

de Passillé AMB, Pelletier G, Menard J, Morisset J. 1989. Relationships of weight gain and behaviour to digestive organ weight and enzyme activities in piglets. J Anim Sci 67:2921–2929.

Duncan IJH, Fraser D. 1997. Understanding animal welfare. In Animal Welfare. MC Appleby, BO Hughes, eds. Wallingford, UK: CAB International, pp. 19–31.

Edwards SA. 1992. Scientific perspectives on loose housing systems for dry sows. Pig Vet J 28:40–51.

——. 1995. Designing systems to meet behavioural needs: The family pen system for pigs. In Animal Behaviour and the Design of Livestock and Poultry Systems. Northeast Region Agricultural Engineering Service, Ithaca, pp. 115–125.

Edwards SA, Fraser D. 1997. Housing systems for farrowing and lactation. Pig J 39:77–89.

Ekkel ED, Spoolder HAM, Hulsegge I, Hopster H. 2003. Lying characteristics as determinants for space requirements in pigs. Appl Anim Behav Sci 80:19–30.

English PR. 1993. A review of farrowing facilities in relation to the needs of the sow and her piglets and the aspirations of the caring stockperson. Pig Vet J 31:124–142.

English PR, Burgess G, Segundo R, Dunne J. 1992. Stockmanship: Improving the Care of the Pig and Other Livestock. Ipswich, UK: Farming Press.

Feddes JJR, Fraser D. 1994. Non-nutritive chewing by pigs: Implications for tail-biting and behavioural enrichment. Trans Amer Soc Agric Eng 37:947–950.

Fraser D. 1987. Mineral deficient diets and the pig's attraction to blood: Implications for tail biting. Can J Anim Sci 67:909–918.

——. 2001. The "New Perception" of animal agriculture: Legless cows, featherless chickens, and a need for genuine analysis. J Anim Sci 79:634–641.

Fraser D, Bernon D, Ball RO. 1991a. Enhanced attraction to blood by pigs with inadequate protein supplementation. Can J Anim Sci 71:611–619.

Fraser D, Matthews LR. 1997. Preference and motivation testing. In Animal Welfare. MC Appleby, BO Hughes, eds. Wallingford, UK: CAB International, pp. 159–173.

Fraser D, Phillips PA, Thompson BK, Tennessen T. 1991b. Effect of straw on the behaviour of growing pigs. Appl Anim Behav Sci 30:307–318.

Fraser D, Weary DM, Pajor EA, Milligan BN. 1997. A scientific conception of animal welfare that reflects ethical concerns. Anim Welfare 6:187–205.

Garner, JP, Meehan CL, Mench JA. 2003. Stereotypies in caged parrots, schizophrenia and autism: Evidence for a common mechanism. Behav Brain Res 145:125–134.

Gonyou HW, Beltranena E, Whittington DL, Patience JF. 1998. The behaviour of pigs weaned at 12 and 21 days of age from weaning to market. Can J Anim Sci 78:517–523.

Hemsworth PH, Barnett JL, Coleman GJ, Hansen C. 1989. A study of the relationships between the attitudinal and behavioural profiles of stockpersons and the level of fear of humans and reproductive performance of commercial pigs. Appl Anim Behav Sci 23:310–314.

Hemsworth PH, Brand A, Willens PJ. 1981. The behavioural response of sows to the presence of human beings and its relation to productivity. Livest Prod Sci 8:67–74.

Hemsworth PH, Coleman GJ, Barnett JL. 1991. Reproductive performance of pigs and the influence of human-animal interactions. Pig News Info 12:563–566.

Hennessy DP, Stelmasiak T, Johnston E, Jackson PN, Outch KH. 1988. Consistent capacity for adrenocortical response to ACTH administration in pigs. Am J Vet Res 49:1276–1283.

Jarvis S, Calvert SK, Stevenson J, van Leeuwen N, Lawrence AB. 2002. Pituitary-adrenal activation in preparturient pigs (*Sus scrofa*) is associated with behavioural restriction due to lack of space rather than nesting substrate. Anim Welfare 11:371–384.

Jensen P. 1995. The weaning process of free-ranging domestic pigs. Ethology 100:14–25.

Johnson JT, Levine S. 1973. Influence of water deprivation on adrenocortical rhythms. Neuroendocrinology 11:268–273.

Kelley KW. 1980. Stress and immune function: A bibliographic review. Ann Rech Vét 11:445–478.

Ladewig J, Matthews LR. 1996. The role of operant conditioning in animal welfare research. Acta Agric Scand A, S27:64–68.

Ladewig J, Schlichting MC, Beneke B, Von Borell E, Stuhec I, Smidt D. 1986. Physiological aspects of social space in heifers and pigs. In Social Space in Domestic Animals. R Zayan, ed. Dordrecht: Martinus Nijhoff, pp. 151–159.

Lawrence AB, Petherick JC, McClean K, Deans L, Chirnside J, Vaughan A, Clutton E, Terlouw EMC. 1994. The effect of environment on behaviour, plasma cortisol and prolactin in parturient sows. Appl Anim Behav Sci 39:313–330.

Lawrence AB, Terlouw EMC. 1993. A review of behavioural factors involved in the development and continued performance of stereotypic behaviours in pigs. J Anim Sci 71:2815–2825.

Lyons CAP, Bruce JM, Fowler VR, English PR. 1995. A comparison of productivity and welfare of growing pigs in four intensive systems. Livest Prod Sci 43:265–274.

Marchant JN, Mendl MT, Rudd AR, Broom DM. 1995. The effect of agonistic interactions on the heart rate of group-housed sows. Appl Anim Behav Sci 46:49–56.

Metz JHM, Osterlee CC. 1981. Immunologische und ethologische Kritorien für die artgemasse Haltung von Sauen und Ferkeln. Kuratorium Tech Bauwesen Landwirtschaft 264:39–50.

Meunier-Salaun MC, Edwards SA, Robert S. 2001. Effect of dietary fibre on the behaviour and health of the restricted fed sow. Anim Feed Sci Technol 90:53–69.

Meunier-Salaun MC, Vantrimponte MN, Raab A, Dantzer R. 1987. Effect of floor area restriction upon performance, behaviour and physiology of growing-finishing pigs. J Anim Sci 64:1371–1377.

Moss BW. 1981. The development of a blood profile for stress assessment. In The Welfare of Pigs. W Sybesma, ed. The Hague: Martinus Nijhoff, pp. 112–125.

Petherick C. 1989. Feeding regime and the behaviour of group housed non-lactating sows. Appl Anim Behav Sci 22:90.

Preece R. 1999. Animals and Nature: Cultural Myths, Cultural Realities. Vancouver: UBC Press.

Rollin BE. 1995. Farm Animal Welfare: Social, Bioethical, and Research Issues. Ames: Iowa State Univ Press.

Schroder-Petersen DL, Simonsen HB. 2001. Tail biting in pigs. Vet J 162:196–210.

Spencer CSG. 1985. Hormonal systems regulating growth: A review. Livest Prod Sci 12:31–46.

Stanton HC, Mueller RL. 1976. Sympathoadrenal neurochemistry and early weaning of swine. Am J Vet Res 37:779–783.

Stephens DB. 1980. Stress and its measurement in domestic animals: A review of behavioural and physiological studies under field and laboratory situations. Adv Vet Sci Comp Med 24:179–209.

Stolba A, Wood-Gush DGM. 1984. The identification of behavioural key features and their incorporation into a housing design for pigs. Ann Rech Vét 15:287–298.

Taylor AA, Weary DM. 2000. Vocal response of piglets to castration: Identifying procedural sources of pain. Appl Anim Behav Sci 70: 17–26.

te Velde H, Aarts N, van Woerkum C. 2002. Dealing with ambivalence: Farmers' and consumers' perceptions of animal welfare in livestock breeding. J Agric Environ Ethics 15:203–219.

van de Weerd HA, Docking CM, Day JEL, Avery PJ, Edwards SA. 2003. A systematic approach towards developing environmental enrichment for pigs. Appl Anim Behav Sci 84:101–118.

van de Weerd HA, Docking C, Day JEL, Breuer K, Edwards SA. 2004. Longitudinal study of adverse behaviour of undocked pigs in two different housing systems. In The Appliance of Pig Science. JE Thompson, BP Gill, MA Varley, eds. BSAS Publication 31. Nottingham: Nottingham University Press, pp. 165–168.

Weary DM, Fraser D. 1995. Calling by domestic piglets: Reliable signals of need? Anim Behav 50:1046–1055.

Webster J. 1994. Animal Welfare: A Cool Eye Towards Eden. Oxford, UK: Blackwell Science.

68 Swine Disease Transmission and Prevention

Sandra F. Amass and Angela Baysinger

Many factors influence whether an animal will become clinically ill after exposure to a pathogen. Factors affecting host susceptibility include age, immunocompetency, vaccination status, genetic predisposition, concurrent illnesses, stress, environment, management, and nutrition. For example, day-old pigs cleared 50% of a lung bacterial load within 3 hours, whereas 26-day-old pigs cleared 95% of the bacterial load in the same period (Curtis et al. 1976). Moreover, ambient temperatures of 6°C inhibited lung clearance of bacteria in 1-day-old pigs as compared to thermoneutral temperatures, but cold temperatures had little effect on pulmonary clearance in 26-day-old pigs (Curtis et al. 1976). Pertinent characteristics of the organism include pathogenicity, infectiousness, contagiousness, viability inside and outside of the host, and the frequency of host exposure to the pathogen. Additionally, factors that can impact the risk of infection include the source of the pathogen (infected animals, environment, zoonotic) and the route of transmission (direct contact, aerosol, arthropod mediated, ingestion, coit) (Thrusfield 1995).

SOURCES OF INFECTION

Pigs are exposed to organisms either through direct contact with an infected animal or other biological vector, or indirect contact with an animal product, fomite, or contaminated environment. The duration of shedding of pathogens by infected animals and information regarding pathogen survival outside of the host are crucial when preparing protocols to minimize sources of infection. The duration of shedding of a pathogen by an infected animal will vary according to host and pathogen factors; however, scientific reports can be used to approximate this time period. Survival of organisms outside of the host animal is also dependent on a variety of factors. Scientific data regarding organism survival are obtained under experimental laboratory conditions and do not necessarily reflect survival times under natural conditions. However, estimations of pathogen survival

time can be derived from these data. Survival time of select swine pathogens in air, water, manure, and on fomites are listed in Tables 68.1 to 68.4.

Data in Tables 68.1 to 68.4 reflect isolation of viable organisms. Results from other methods such as PCR were not included because the viability or infectiousness of the organism cannot be determined with these techniques. For example, *Mycoplasma hyopneumoniae* was detected in air samples of rooms housing acutely infected pigs using a nested PCR assay; however, survival times and transmission distances could not be determined since the viability of the organisms were not evaluated (Stärk et al. 1998).

Semen

Many swine pathogens have been isolated from semen (Table 68.5). Semen can become contaminated naturally from infected boars or postcollection during processing, storage, or transport (Foley et al. 1971; Thacker 1984). Semen collected using an artificial vagina contained 100–1,000,000 cfu per ml (Koppang and Filseth 1958), whereas semen collected using a gloved hand contained 0–3,800 cfu per ml (Waltz et al. 1968). *Alcaligenes xylosoxydans, Burkholderia cepacia, Enterobacter cloacae, Escherichia coli, Serratia marcescens,* and *Stenotrophomonas maltophilia* of both animal and nonanimal origin were isolated from semen. These bacteria are not porcine pathogens but were spermicidal (Althouse et al. 2000). *Pseudomonas aeruginosa, Proteus,* micrococci, streptococci, enterococci, *Candida, Bordetella, Aerobacter, Corynebacterium,* and *Staphylococcus* have also been isolated from boar semen (Koppang and Filseth 1958; Waltz et al. 1968). Staphylococci, streptococci, *Alcaligenes, Pseudomonas,* and *Corynebacterium* were isolated from semen but not the genital tract of respective boars; therefore, contamination likely occurred during collection (Foley et al. 1971). Semen has inherent cytotoxic and antiviral activity (Richmond 1978). Extension of semen could dilute this natural defense.

Clinically normal boars can shed pathogens in their semen. Classical swine fever virus, foot-and-mouth dis-

Table 68.1. Documented survival times for select swine pathogens in air

Organism	Temperature (°C)	Humidity (%)	Survival Time	Source
Actinobacillus pleuropneumoniae	27–32	60–80	Detected	Torremorell et al. 1997
African swine fever virus	18–23	20–80	At least 1 second	Donaldson and Ferris 1976
	18–23	20–30	At least 5 minutes	
	18–23	>30	<5 minutes	
Bordetella bronchiseptica	NR	NR	Detected	Stehmann et al. 1991
Clostridium perfringens	NR	NR	Detected	Sidorenko 1967
Escherichia coli	15.5–27.2	55–99	At least 1 day	Marshall et al. 1988
	15	<50	14-minute half-life	Wathes et al. 1986
	15	50–87	83-minute half-life	
	30	<50	3-minute half-life	
	30	50–87	14-minute half-life	
Foot-and-mouth disease virus	8.5–18.5	72–100	Up to 5 days in boxes housing infected pigs	Sellers and Parker 1969
Pasteurella multocida	22.6	25–80	At least 45 minutes	Thomson et al. 1992
Porcine respiratory coronavirus	20	47	Up to 6 days after infection in rooms housing infected pigs	Bourgueil et al. 1992
Pseudorabies virus	4	55	43.6-minute half-life	Schoenbaum et al. 1990
	4	85	27.3-minute half-life	
	22	25	18.8-minute half-life	
	22	55	36.1-minute half-life	
	22	85	17.4-minute half-life	
Salmonella spp.	25	88	Detected	Seo et al. 2001
	24	75	At least 2 hours	McDermid and Lever 1996
Streptococcus suis	18–24	20–50	At least 5 minutes	Madsen et al. 2001
Swine Influenza virus	21.1	15	15 hours	Mitchell and Guerin 1972
Swine vesicular disease virus	NR	NR	Up to 3 days in boxes housing infected pigs	Sellers and Herniman 1974

NR: Not reported.

Table 68.2. Documented survival times for select swine pathogens in water

Organism	Temperature (°C)	Survival Time	Source
Bordetella bronchiseptica	37	3 weeks	Porter et al. 1991
Brachyspira hyodysenteriae	NR	Detected	Songer et al. 1978
Clostridium perfringens	NR	Detected	Sidorenko 1967
Escherichia coli	15.5–27.2	3 hours–10 days	Marshall et al. 1988
	NR	Detected	Marshall et al. 1990
Leptospires	3.19–25.4	Detected	Henry and Johnson 1978
Mycoplasma hyopneumoniae	2–7	At least 31 days	Goodwin 1985
Mycobacterium avium	NR	Detected	Ichiyama et al. 1988
Pasteurella multocida	4	14 days	Thomson et al. 1992
	37	24 hours	
	−1.5–13.3	Less than 1 day	Backstrand and Botzler 1986
Porcine reproductive and respiratory syndrome virus	25–27	9–11 days	Pirtle and Beran 1996
Pseudorabies virus	25	2–7 days	Pirtle and Beran 1991
Salmonella spp.	NR	Detected	Letellier et al. 1999
	NR	Detected	Barber et al. 2002
Streptococcus suis	50	60 minutes	Clifton-Hadley and Enright 1984
	60	10 minutes	

NR: Not reported.

ease (FMD) virus, and swine vesicular disease virus were isolated from semen of clinically normal boars (McVicar et al. 1978; de Smit et al. 1999). Pseudorabies virus was also isolated from semen of clinically normal, vaccinated boars (Medveczky and Szabó 1981). A 5 mm loopful of semen from a clinically normal boar naturally infected with brucellosis yielded 800–1000 colonies of *Brucella suis* (Hutchings and Andrews 1946). Shedding of porcine reproductive and respiratory syndrome (PRRS) virus in semen was variable and was not related to the viremic state or the serostatus of the boar (Christopher-Hennings et al. 1995a).

Table 68.3. Documented survival times for select swine pathogens in manure

Organism	Temperature (°C)	Survival Time	Source
African swine fever virus	NR[1]	60–160 days	Strauch 1991
Ascaris suum eggs	NR	Up to 5 years	Strauch 1991
	10–17	<16 weeks	Gaasenbeek and Borgsteede 1998
Brachyspira hyodysenteriae	10	112 days	Boye et al. 2001
	0–10	48 days	Chia and Taylor 1978
	20–22	12 days	
	25	7 days	
Brachyspira pilosicoli	10	210 days	Boye et al. 2001
Classical swine fever virus	5	>6 weeks	Haas et al. 1995
	20	2 weeks	
Erysipelothrix rhusiopathiae	NR	NR: Disease had not been diagnosed for up to 5 years	Wood and Packer 1972
Escherichia coli	6–9	4.8 weeks	Munch et al. 1987
	18–20	0.9 weeks	
Foot-and-mouth disease virus	5	>14 weeks	Haas et al. 1995
	20	2 weeks	
Metastrongylus eggs	12	At least 68 days	Marti et al. 1980
	22	At least 47 days	
Metastrongylus larvae	12	36 days	Marti et al. 1980
	22	At least 47 days	
Oesophagostomum eggs	12	4 days	Marti et al. 1980
	22	7 days	
Oesophagostomum larvae	12	At least 68 days	Marti et al. 1980
	22	11 days	
Pasteurella multocida	4	3 days	Thomson et al. 1992
	37	6 days	
Porcine parvovirus	5 and 20	>40 weeks	Haas et al. 1995
	20	At least 14 weeks	Mengeling and Paul 1986
Porcine reproductive and respiratory syndrome virus	4	2 weeks	Ajariyakhajorn et al. 1997
	25	1 day	
Pseudorabies virus	5	15 weeks	Bøtner 1991
	20	2 weeks	
	25	<1–2 days	Pirtle and Beran 1991
Rotavirus	20–25	4 months	Fu et al. 1989
Salmonella spp.	6–9	1.6–5.9 weeks	Munch et al. 1987
	18–20	0.6–2 weeks	
Streptococcus suis	20	72 hours	Dee and Corey 1993
	0	104 days	Clifton-Hadley and Enright 1984
	9	10 days	
	22–25	8 days	
Strongyloides ransomi eggs	12	7 days	Marti et al. 1980
	22	7 days	
Strongyloides ransomi larvae	12	21 days	Marti et al. 1980
	22	13 days	
Swine influenza virus	5	9 weeks	Haas et al. 1995
	20	2 weeks	
Transmissible gastroenteritis virus	5	>8 weeks	Haas et al. 1995
	20	2 weeks	

[1]NR: Not reported.

Dust

Streptococcus suis (Clifton-Hadley and Enright 1984), rotavirus (Fu et al. 1989), *Mycobacterium avium* (Nel 1981; Ichiyama et al. 1988), *Clostridium perfringens* (Sidorenko 1967), *Salmonella* spp. (Eld et al. 1991; Letellier et al. 1999), and pseudorabies virus (Vannier et al. 1989) have been isolated from dust. The length of time that the organisms survived in dust was only reported for *S. suis*: 30–54 days at 0°C, 1–25 days at 9°C, and less than 24 hours at 22–25°C (Clifton-Hadley and Enright 1984).

Soil

Swine raised outdoors can contact pathogens contaminating soil. Laboratory tests found that *E. coli* and *S. typhimurium* added to liquid manure generally penetrated sand and garden soil columns to a depth of 160 cm. Rarely, organisms penetrated soil to depths greater than 160 cm and this was only under conditions of simulated rainfall, and survival was less than 2 weeks at these depths. Organism survival decreased with increasing soil depth regardless of soil type (Tamasi 1981). Survival

Table 68.4. Documented survival times for select swine pathogens on fomites

Organism	Fomite	Temperature (°C)	Survival Time	Source
Classical swine fever virus	Brick	NR	7 days	Slavin 1938
Cytomegalovirus (Human)	Naturally contaminated fomites	NR	Several hours	Pirtle and Beran 1991
Escherichia coli	Painted wallboard, glass, wood, paper towels, metal, insulation, feed bag	15.5–27.2	≤10 days	Marshall et al. 1988
Foot-and-mouth disease virus	Hay	22	20 weeks	Pirtle and Beran 1991; Cottral 1969
	Barns (brick, adobe, wood)	winter	11 weeks	
	Barns (brick, adobe, wood)	summer	2 weeks	
	Cotton clothing, leather shoes, rubber boots	NR	14 weeks	
Influenza A virus	Steel, plastic	27.8–28.3	48 hours	Bean et al. 1982
	Clothing, paper	27.8–28.3	8–12 hours	Bean et al. 1982
Mycobacterium avium	Bedding	22–45	Detected	Nel 1981
Mycoplasma hyopneumoniae	Paper, cloth	15–26	<96 hours	Goodwin 1985
Porcine parvovirus	Uncleaned room	NR	14 weeks	Mengeling and Paul, 1986
Porcine reproductive and respiratory syndrome virus	Alfalfa, wood shavings, straw, plastic, boot rubber, stainless steel	25–27	<24 hours	Pirtle and Beran 1996
	Plastic, metal, cardboard, styrofoam, concrete, rubber	−2	2–12 hours	Dee et al. 2002
	Plastic, metal, cardboard, styrofoam, concrete, rubber	10 and 20	<1–8 hours	Dee et al. 2003
Pseudorabies virus[1]	Steel, plastic, rubber, straw, concrete, wood, denim, sawdust	25	2–18 days	Schoenbaum et al. 1991; Pirtle and Beran 1991
Salmonella spp.	Boots	NR	Detected	Barber et al. 2002
	Pen flooring	NR	Detected	
Streptococcus suis	Plastic flooring, concrete, painted plywood	20	<20 hours	Dee and Corey 1993
Swine vesicular disease virus	Survived on premises after depopulation and disinfection	NR	11 weeks	Pirtle and Beran 1991
Transmissible gastroenteritis virus	Dried and putrefied ground gastrointestinal tract	19.5–21.1	3 days	Bay et al. 1952
	Ground gastrointestinal tract	−28	At least 3.5 years	

NR: Not reported.

[1]Saline-glucose or saline-moistened fomites.

times for select organisms in soil have been documented (Table 68.6).

Insects

Insects have been reported to carry swine pathogens. *Escherichia coli* was recovered from flies for no more than 8 days after contamination of a barn (Marshall et al. 1988) and from flies exposed to experimentally infected pigs (Marshall et al. 1990). *Mycobacterium avium* (Fischer et al. 2001), *Salmonella* sp. (Letellier et al. 1999), transmissible gastroenteritis (TGE) virus (Gough and Jorgenson 1983), and *Yersinia enterocolitica* (Fukushima et al. 1979) have been isolated from flies in swine herds. African swine fever virus was detected in *Ornithodoros moubata* residing in warthog burrows in Tanzania (Plowright et al. 1969b). The survival times of pseudorabies virus in *Musca domestica* varied with the age of the fly and the ambient temperature but the virus did not appear to replicate in living or dead flies (Zimmerman et al. 1989).

Domestic and Feral Animals

Feral swine can be reservoirs of pathogens (Fritzemeier et al. 2000; Artois et al. 2002). Swine pathogens have

also been isolated from domestic and feral animals other than swine. *Salmonella* sp. and *Brachyspira hyodysenteriae* have been isolated from dogs and cats (Schnurrenberger et al. 1968; Songer et al. 1978; Weber and Schramm 1989; Eld et al. 1991; Barber et al. 2002). *Salmonella* spp. was also isolated from opossums (Schnurrenberger et al. 1968). *Leptospira interrogans* serovar *pomona* was isolated from skunks trapped in and near a swine herd during a leptospirosis outbreak (Kingscote 1986). *Streptococcus suis* has been isolated from dogs, cats, horses, a deer, and a zebra from which there was no contact with swine or contact was not reported (Devriese and Haesebrouck 1992; Devriese et al. 1993; Salasia and Lämmler 1994). Pseudorabies virus was isolated from raccoons and cats found dead on or near farms infected with pseudorabies (Kirkpatrick et al. 1980). *Brucella suis* was isolated from hares in Denmark in the same area as a brucellosis epizootic in swine (Bendtsen et al. 1954). *Toxoplasma gondii* was detected in cat feces collected on swine farms (Dubey et al. 1995). *Trichinella spiralis* has been detected in a farm cat (Hanbury et al. 1986), a red fox, coyotes, raccoons, badger, raccoon dogs, mink, wild boar, wolf, and bear (Hirvelä-Koski et al. 1985; Snyder 1987).

Table 68.5. Documented detection of select swine pathogens in semen from infected boars

Organism	Boar Infection Type	Timing of Detection (Test Used)	Source
Adenovirus	Experimental inoculation	65 DPI (virus isolation)	McAdaragh and Anderson 1975
Brucella suis	Natural infection	Detected (bacteriological isolation)	Lord et al. 1997; Hutchings and Andrews 1946
Classical swine fever virus	Experimental inoculation	7 and 11 DPI (virus isolation)	De Smit et al. 1999; Floegel et al. 2000
	Experimental inoculation	7–63 DPI (RT-PCR); 11, 18, 21, and 53 DPI (virus isolation)	Choi and Chae 2003
Foot-and-mouth disease virus	Exposition to experimentally inoculated pen mates	Up to 9 days post exposure (virus isolation)	McVicar et al. 1978
Porcine circovirus	Natural infection	Detected (multiplex nested PCR)	Kim et al. 2001
	Natural infection	Detected (nested PCR)	Hamel et al. 2000
	Experimental inoculation	Intermittently between 5 and 47 DPI (nested PCR)	Larochelle et al. 2000
Porcine enterovirus	Experimental inoculation	45 DPI (virus isolation)	McAdaragh and Anderson 1975
	Natural infection	Detected (virus isolation)	Phillips et al. 1972
Porcine parvovirus	Natural infection	Detected (virus isolation)	McAdaragh and Anderson 1975
	Natural infection	Detected (multiplex seminested PCR)	Kim et al. 2003
Porcine reproductive and respiratory syndrome virus	Experimental inoculation	2–57 DPI (nested PCR)	Shin et al. 1997
		12–21 DPI (nested RT-PCR)	Christopher-Hennings et al. 1998
		Up to 47 DPI (nested RT-PCR)	Christopher-Hennings et al. 1995b
		Up to 92 DPI (nested RT-PCR)	Christopher-Hennings et al. 1995a
		7 and 8 DPI (swine bioassay-seroconversion)	Swenson et al. 1994a
		43 DPI (swine bioassay-seroconversion)	Christopher-Hennings et al. 1995b
		Up to 43 DPI (swine bioassay-seroconversion and virus isolation)	Swenson et al. 1994b
		7 DPI (virus isolation)	Prieto et al. 1994; Shin et al. 1997
		11 DPI (virus isolation)	Christopher-Hennings et al. 1995b
Pseudorabies virus	Natural infection	Detected (virus isolation)	Medveczky and Szabó 1981
Reovirus	Experimental inoculation	65 DPI (virus isolation)	McAdaragh and Anderson 1975
Swine vesicular disease virus	Exposed to experimentally inoculated pen mates	Up to 4 DPI (virus isolation)	McVicar et al. 1978

DPI: Days postinoculation.
PCR: Polymerase chain reaction; RT-PCR: reverse transcriptase—polymerase chain reaction.

Table 68.6. Documented survival times for select swine pathogens in soil

Organism	Soil Type	Temperature (°C)	Survival Time	Source
Brachyspira hyodysenteriae	Sandy clay soil	10	10 days	Boye et al. 2001
Brachyspira pilosicoli	Sandy clay soil	10	119 days	Boye et al. 2001
Clostridium perfringens	NR	NR	Detected	Hang'ombe et al. 2000
Erysipelothrix rhusiopathiae	Sand, silt, clay	3	35 days	Wood 1973
		12	18 days	
		20	10 days	
		30	2 days	
	Swine pen soils	12	11–16 days	
Escherichia coli	Sand	8	90–131 days	Tamási 1981
	Garden soil	8	37–108 days	
	Sand	20	31–102 days	
	Garden soil	20	8–54 days	
Leptospires	Humus boggy-peaty	NR	Detected	Karaseva et al. 1977
	Lake shore soil	0.5–18.5	Detected	Henry and Johnson 1978
Mycobacterium avium	Soil and ditch mud	NR	Detected	Ichiyama et al. 1988
	NR	NR	Detected	Nel 1981
Pasteurella multocida	Siltic clay loam	−1.5–13.3	<20 days	Backstrand and Botzler 1986
Salmonella spp.	Sand	8	16–131 days	Tamási 1981
	Sand	20	74–131 days	
	Garden soil	8 and 20	76–96 days	
	Agricultural soil	NR	76–96 days	Baloda et al. 2001
Trichuris suis ova	Chalky, flinty	3–22	>2 years	Burden and Hammet 1979

NR: Not reported.

Antibodies to *Toxoplasma gondii* were detected in cats, opossums, raccoons, and skunks that were live-trapped on 19 Iowa swine farms. The authors hypothesized that *Toxoplasma* oocysts from cat feces may be a source of contamination for swine (Smith et al. 1992). *Lawsonia intracellularis* was detected in fecal samples of dogs, calves, hedgehogs, hamster, horse, deer, ostrich, and one giraffe by polymerase chain reaction (Cooper et al. 1997; Herbst et al. 2003). Finally, foot-and-mouth disease virus has been isolated from naturally and experimentally infected deer (Forman and Gibbs 1974).

Rodents

Swine pathogens that have been isolated from rodents or rodent feces include *Bordetella bronchiseptica* (Le Moine et al. 1987; Bemis et al. 2003), *Salmonella* sp. (Davis 1948; Schnurrenberger et al. 1968; Le Moine et al. 1987; Letellier et al. 1999; Barber et al. 2002), *E. coli* (Le Moine et al. 1987; Marshall et al. 1990), rotavirus (Le Moine et al. 1987), *Brachyspira hyodysenteriae* (Joens and Kinyon 1982; Blaha 1983), *Leptospira* spp. (Songer et al. 1983), *Toxoplasma gondii* (Dubey et al. 1995), and *Trichinella spiralis* (Martin et al. 1968; Hirvelä-Koski et al. 1985; Hanbury et al. 1986). Rats and mice have also been shown to seroconvert to TGE virus (Le Moine et al. 1987). Rodents do not appear to be field reservoirs of PRRS virus (Hooper et al. 1994) or pseudorabies virus, even though rats were susceptible to experimental inoculation with pseudorabies virus (Maes et al. 1979).

Birds

Swine pathogens that have been isolated from birds include *Bordetella bronchiseptica* (Farrington and Jorgenson 1976), *Mycobacterium avium* (Bickford et al. 1966), *Streptococcus suis* (Devriese et al. 1994), and *Salmonella* sp. (Schnurrenberger et al. 1968; Eld et al. 1991; Barber et al. 2002; Kirk et al. 2002). Virus isolation from Muscovy ducks, Mallard ducks, guinea fowl, and chickens orally inoculated with PRRSV was attempted on several days from day 0 to 24 postinoculation. The virus was recovered from the feces of guinea fowl on days 5 and 12 postinoculation, from chickens on day 5 postinoculation, and from Mallard ducks on nearly all sample days from day 5 to 24 postinoculation (Zimmerman et al. 1997)

People

Multiple swine pathogens have been detected on people and outerwear including *E. coli*, FMD virus, PRRS virus, *Salmonella* sp., *Mycobacterium avium,* and swine vesicular disease. Two people that entered a barn in which *E. coli* was experimentally aerosolized were sampled. *Escherichia coli* was recovered from their hair for up to 5 hours, clothing for at least 2 hours, and skin for up to 70 minutes after aerosol release (Marshall et al. 1988). Foot-and-mouth disease virus was isolated from the nasal passages of one of eight people at 28 hours, but not at 48

hours, after exposure to infected animals (Sellers et al. 1970). In another study, human nasal carriage of FMD virus was detected in one of four people upon exit of a containment facility after having been exposed to infected animals for the previous 10 hours. Nasal carriage of FMD virus was not detected in any of the four people at time points up to 4 days after exit of the containment facility (Amass et al. 2003b). Porcine reproductive and respiratory syndrome virus has been isolated from contaminated boots and coveralls (Otake et al. 2002b). *Salmonella* sp. have been isolated from boots on a swine farm (Letellier et al. 1999). *Mycobacterium avium* was detected in the sputa of healthy people (Nel 1981). Swine vesicular disease virus was detected in the nasal passages of people that had contacted infected pigs for at least 5 minutes (Sellers and Herniman 1974). The duration of nasal carriage was not reported. Conversely, *Mycoplasma hyopneumoniae* was not detected from the hair of a swine caretaker (Goodwin 1985).

Vehicles

Contaminated vehicles are a potential source of pathogen introduction to farms. Salmonellae were isolated from swab samples of the grain box of 3 of 22 feed delivery trucks (Fedorka-Cray et al. 1997). *Salmonella* and *E. coli* have been isolated from flooring of trailers used to haul pigs. *Salmonella* was isolated from the flooring of 25 of 32 trailers sampled and *E. coli* was isolated from the flooring of all 32 trailers sampled immediately after pigs were unloaded. Trailer contamination with *Salmonella* and *E. coli* was not found to be related to distance traveled hauling pigs or season (Rajkowski et al. 1998). Similarly, *Salmonella* was isolated from the floors of transport trucks before loading pigs. *Salmonella* serovars isolated from transported pigs matched the serovar detected in the truck, but not serovars from the farm of origin. Thus, infection during transport to slaughter is of concern (Gebreyes et al. 2004).

Carcasses

The process of composting swine carcasses in piles was sufficient to kill *Erysipelothrix rhusiopathiae* and pseudorabies virus under experimental conditions. Survival of *Salmonella* varied but most cultures were killed. *Salmonella* cultures placed at the top and bottom of the pile survived (Morrow et al. 1995).

Salmonella sp. have also been isolated from dead swine and manure from dead swine (Letellier et al. 1999).

Animal Feed

Salmonella sp. (Schnurrenberger et al. 1968; Mårtensson et al. 1984; Eld et al. 1991; Fedorka-Cray et al. 1997; Harris et al. 1997; Letellier et al. 1999), *Mycobacterium avium* (Nel 1981) and *Toxoplasma gondii* oocysts (Dubey et al. 1995) have been isolated from samples of feed or feed ingredients. Researchers have not examined whether the number of organisms detected in feed samples were sufficient to or had adversely affected the health of pigs consuming the feed. In contrast, a field survey of six swine farms in Illinois did not detect *Salmonella* in any of 221 feed samples collected. These farms produced most of their own feed and samples were collected from closed feed bags or the top layer of feed in bins (Barber et al. 2002).

Contaminated Foods

Contaminated foods pose a potential risk of introduction of exotic diseases to countries free of those diseases. For example, the 2000 outbreak of classical swine fever (CSF) in the U.K. was thought to have originated from a tourist throwing a CSF-contaminated ham sandwich to a pig (Dudley and Woodford 2002). Some porcine pathogens survive for extended periods in contaminated foods. Swine vesicular disease virus survived for at least 200 days in dry salami, pepperoni sausage, and intestinal casings but not in hams heated to internal temperatures of 68.8°C (McKercher et al. 1974). In one case, swine vesicular disease virus survived in a Serrano ham for 539 days, exceeding the curing time of 365 days (Mebus et al. 1997). Swine vesicular disease virus survived for 90–300 days in Parma hams; however, Parma hams are not considered a risk for introduction of swine vesicular disease because Parma hams are cured for at least 365 days (McKercher et al. 1985). Foot and mouth disease virus survived in salt-cured ham for 89 days, salt-cured bacon for 10 days, and salt-cured sausages for 4 days at 1–7°C (Savi et al. 1962; Cottral 1969). Foot-and-mouth disease virus, African swine fever virus, and CSF fever virus appear to be inactivated by commercial curing processes (Mebus et al. 1993). Classical swine fever virus was detected in Italian salami for up to 75 days of curing (Panina et al. 1992); however, heating ham to 65°C for 30 minutes eliminated all virus (Terpstra and Krol 1976).

ROUTES OF TRANSMISSION

Pathogens are spread by biological, mechanical, and aerosol transmission. Biological transmission can occur from sow to pig or pig to pig or through exposure to infected semen or embryos. Biological transmission of swine pathogens among swine and people is also possible. Mechanical spread of pathogens can occur via contaminated fomites, people, other animals, and pests. The route of transmission traditionally thought to offer the greatest risk of infection is direct contact with an infected animal. However, instances of area spread in which no movement of infected animals was reported have occurred. Alternative methods of area spread such as transmission by aerosol, insects, other animals, vehicles, or people have been hypothesized in these cases.

Sow to Pig

Pathogens can be transmitted from sow to pig in utero (Mengeling et al. 1996), during passage of pig through the vagina or by direct or indirect contact after parturition. Technologies such as cesarean-derived pigs and various modifications of early weaning can assist in minimizing transmission from dam to pig (Young et al. 1955; Meyer at al. 1964; Alexander et al. 1980; Mészáros et al. 1985; Harris et al. 1992). Dam-to-pig transfer of *Actinobacillus pleuropneumoniae*, *Pasteurella multocida*, and in all but one case, *Mycoplasma hyopneumoniae* was prevented by weaning pigs at 14 days of age and rearing pigs with age-matched cohorts. *Streptococcus suis* and *Haemophilus parasuis* were not eliminated from these pigs. Transfer of pseudorabies virus but not PRRS virus was prevented (Clark et al. 1994). Mycoplasmal pneumonia and *A. pleuropneumonia* were eliminated from pigs weaned at 7–10 days of age (Dritz et al. 1996). Many factors will determine the feasibility of using early weaning to prevent sow to pig transmission of pathogens on a commercial farm, including facilities, pig husbandry skills, immune status of herd, pathogen characteristics, and timing of infection. Early weaning can exacerbate some diseases (Pyburn and Schwartz 1995; Fangman and Tubbs 1997; Amass 1998a).

Pig to Pig

Pathogens can be spread when susceptible pigs either contact infected pigs directly or contact the secretions or excretions of infected pigs.

Semen and Embryo Transfer

Some organisms have been reported to be transmissible by semen or embryo transfer. Only three swine pathogens have been proven to be transmissible by semen under experimental conditions: CSF after experimental inoculation of boars (de Smit et al. 1999) and porcine parvovirus (Lucas et al. 1974) and PRRS virus (Prieto et al. 1997b) were transmitted by artificial insemination after experimental inoculation of semen.

Literature regarding interactions between porcine pathogens and embryos is limited; thus, pathogens of interest should be individually tested to determine transmissibility by embryo transfer (Shelton 1987). Porcine reproductive and respiratory syndrome virus was isolated from embryos of experimentally infected gilts at 20 days of gestation but not at 10 days of gestation (Prieto et al. 1997a). However, PRRS virus was not transmitted to embryos, recipient gilts, or resultant piglets when embryos from experimentally infected gilts were transferred to susceptible recipient gilts (Randall et al. 1999). Porcine reproductive and respiratory syndrome virus did not infect the 4- to 16-cell-stage embryos cultured in vitro with PRRSV (Prieto et al. 1996). Porcine parvovirus was not isolated from 4-day-old, 15-day-old, and 32-day-old embryos of experimentally infected gilts (Gradil et al. 1994), but was isolated from the 4- to 8-cell-stage embryos after in vitro incubation with virus (Bane et al. 1990). Pseudorabies virus was not detected in intact or zona pellucida–free 2- to 16-

cell-stage porcine embryos that were exposed to virus in vitro for at least 1 hour (Bolin et al. 1981). However, pseudorabies-neutralizing antibodies were detected at 21 days after embryo transfer in recipients of embryos exposed to pseudorabies virus in vitro or embryos collected from experimentally infected donors (Bolin et al. 1982). African swine fever virus, FMD virus, vesicular stomatitis virus, and CSF virus have been detected on zona pellucida–intact, 4-day-old embryos after exposure to respective viruses in vitro for 2–18 hours followed by washing (Singh et al. 1984; Singh et al. 1986; Singh and Thomas 1987; Dulac et al. 1988).

Aerosol

Evidence points to aerosol transmission in the field under specific conditions of large numbers of pathogens being shed by a large population of animals, low temperatures, high humidity, low wind speeds, smooth topography, and low sunlight (Gloster et al. 1981; Christensen et al 1990; Grant et al. 1994; Stärk 1999). However, the ideal temperatures and relative humidity required for aerosol transmission vary for individual pathogens (Stärk 1999). A Gaussian diffusion model was used to explain an epizootic of pseudorabies virus that affected 10 farms across a 150 km^2 area (Scheidt et al. 1991; Grant et al. 1994). Evidence of aerosol transmission of pseudorabies virus over distances of 15–80 km has been reported (Christensen et al. 1990). Experimental transmission of CSF virus was reported after air was forced by positive pressure from handmade large rectangular metal cans containing pigs inoculated with the virus to cans containing susceptible pigs (Hughes and Gustafson 1960) and under experimental conditions without forced air flow (Laevens et al. 1999). Multiple instances of long distance spread of FMD virus by aerosol have been reported (Sellers and Gloster 1980; Donaldson et al. 1982; Gloster et al. 1982). However, aerosol transmission of FMD virus as a consequence of

burning infected animal carcasses has not been established (Gloster at al. 2001; Champion et al. 2002; Jones et al. 2004). Aerosol transmission of pathogens outside of experimental laboratories cannot be definitively proven due to the variety of confounding factors. Moreover, replicating field conditions for laboratory studies of aerosol transmission is difficult due to the limitation of animal numbers. Porcine reproductive and respiratory syndrome virus did not spread between two buildings located 1 meter apart that housed infected and sentinel pigs, respectively, under controlled field conditions; moreover, PRRS virus was not detected in the air exhausted from the barn containing infected pigs (Otake et al. 2002a). Consequently, pathogens generally travel for short distances by aerosol under experimental conditions (Table 68.7). With the exception of virus, swine pathogens rarely have been reported to travel greater than 3.2 km by air.

People

Biological transmission of swine pathogens by people is possible when zoonotic organisms are considered. Pig-to-person transmission has been documented for zoonotic agents such as *S. suis* and swine influenza virus. *Streptococcus suis* is considered an occupational health hazard for those working in the pork industry in some areas of the world. Over 150 cases of human infection with *S. suis* have been documented (Amass 1998b). However, a pilot study of personnel on five Indiana swine farms did not detect human carriage of *S. suis* (Amass et al. 1998). Similarly, H1N1 swine influenza virus was transmitted to humans after exposure to experimentally infected pigs (Wentworth et al. 1997). Transmission of these pathogens from people back to pigs has little documentation aside from anecdotal evidence. Finally, xenotransplantation of pig organs into human beings offers the potential risk of xenozoonoses (Borie et al. 1998); however, the risk of pig contamina-

Table 68.7. Documented aerosol transmission for select swine pathogens

Organism	Temperature (°C)	Humidity (%)	Distance	Source
Actinobacillus pleuropneumoniae	NR	NR	At least 2.5 m	Jobert et al. 2000
	27–32	60–80	1 m	Torremorell et al. 1997
African swine fever virus	8–25.3	73–100	At least 2.3 m	Wilkinson et al. 1977
Bordetella bronchiseptica	NR	NR	1 m	Brockmeier and Lager 2002
Classical swine fever virus	NR	NR	NR	Laevens et al. 1998
	NR	NR	NR	Hughes and Gustafson 1960
Mycoplasma hyopneumoniae	NR	NR	NR	Czaja et al. 2002
Porcine reproductive and	27–32	60–80	1 m	Torremorell et al. 1997
respiratory syndrome virus	NR	NR	1 m	Brockmeier and Lager 2002
	−5–6.3	84–94	1 m	Kristensen et al. 2004
	4.5–19.3	45–89	1 m	
	−0.7–7.8	84–97	1 m	
Pseudorabies virus	25	NR	NR	Gillespie et al. 2000
Streptococcus suis	NR	NR	40 cm	Berthelot-Hérault et al. 2001

NR: Not reported; if under transmission, transmission was reported but the distance was not specified.

tion by humans with porcine xenotransplants has not been determined.

People can mechanically transmit a pig-infectious dose of certain swine pathogens from infected to susceptible pigs. Contact with contaminated people has been implicated in the spread of CSF virus (Fritzemeier et al. 2000). Transfer of the FMD virus from people to one of four susceptible steers was reported when people exhaled directly into the nasal passages of susceptible steers after showering, but within 30 minutes of contacting FMD virus-infected pigs (Sellers et al. 1971). Similarly, personnel in contact with FMD virus-infected pigs mechanically transmitted an infectious dose to susceptible pigs and sheep (Amass et al. 2003b). Mechanical transmission of *E. coli* (Amass et al. 2003a) and TGE virus of swine (Alvarez et al. 2001) by people from infected to susceptible pigs has been reported under conditions simulating natural field exposure levels. Mechanical transmission by people of PRRS virus from infected to susceptible pigs has been reported when personnel took extraordinary measures to contaminate hands and outerwear with blood, nasal secretions, saliva, and manure, and then allowed pigs direct contact with contaminated outerwear for 24 hours after the exit of personnel from the room (Otake et al. 2002b). Mechanical transmission by people of PRRS virus from infected to susceptible pigs was not demonstrated when contamination of personnel reflected levels found on a typical pork production unit (Amass et al. 2000a). Contact with contaminated boots and clothing did not significantly contribute to the spread of CSF virus (Laevens et al. 1998).

Rodents

Rodents are potential mechanical and biological vectors of disease. Transmission of swine disease by rodents in the field has not been definitively proven; although rodents are considered a risk factor in the spread of swine dysentery and leptospirosis. Pigs exposed to feces from mice that had been experimentally infected with *B. hyodysenteriae* developed clinical swine dysentery after 11–13 days (Joens 1980).

Insects

Insects can act as biological and/or mechanical vectors of swine pathogens (Table 68.8). *Musca domestica* reportedly traveled 1.5 km to adjacent farms (Denholm et al. 1985). Marked mosquitoes (*Anopheles vestitipennis*) were 80.48% faithful in returning to the original animal host for a second blood meal (Ulloa et al. 2002). Most reports of transmission of pathogens by insects are the result of experimental data and may not reflect the actual risk of insects as vectors of these pathogens.

Domestic and Feral Non-Swine Animals

Susceptible non-porcine hosts can act as biological vectors, in which case, the animals would become infected with the pathogen and then shed the pathogen in secretions and excretions to susceptible pigs by direct or indirect contact. Nonsusceptible species can act as mechanical vectors by tracking the pathogen-laden excretions (manure) to areas containing susceptible pigs, which can then become exposed. There is little definitive evidence that non-swine animals are vectors of swine path-

Table 68.8.   Insects experimentally capable of transmitting swine pathogens

Organism	Insect	Source
African swine fever virus	*Ornithodorus* ticks	Plowright et al. 1969a
	Ornithodorus savignyi	Mellor and Wilkinson 1985
	Ornithodorus turicata	Hess et al. 1987
	Ornithodorus marocanus	Endris and Hess 1992
	Stomoxys calcitrans	Mellor et al. 1987
Classical swine fever virus	*Hematopinus suis*	Bernasky 1910
	Tabanus spp.	Tidwell et al. 1972
	Musca domestica	Dorset et al. 1919
	Stomoxys spp.	
	Aedes aegypti	Stewart et al. 1975
Mycoplasma haemosuis	*Stomoxys calcitrans*	Prullage et al. 1993
	Aedes aegypti	
Porcine reproductive and respiratory syndrome virus	[1]*Musca domestica*	Otake et al. 2003
	Aedes vexans	Otake et al. 2002d
Pseudorabies virus	*Musca domestica*	Medveczky et al. 1988
Salmonella sp.	Flies	Barber et al. 2002
	Moth	
	Cockroach	
	Spider	
Streptococcus suis	*Musca domestica*	Enright et al. 1987
Swine pox virus	*Hematopinus suis*	Shope 1940
Vesicular stomatitis virus	*Simulium vittatum* Zetterstedt	Mead et al. 2004

[1]Note: *Musca domestica* are not biting flies. Experimental transmission occurred when flies fed on blood from experimentally scarified areas of skin on the backs of pigs.

ogens. Under experimental conditions, pseudorabies virus was isolated from nasal discharges of pigs 8 days after pigs were fed the viscera of raccoons that were experimentally inoculated with pseudorabies virus (Kirkpatrick et al. 1980). In the field, a watchdog was implicated in the reintroduction of *B. suis* to a swine herd 2 years after the infected herd was depopulated and repopulated with brucellosis-free stock. *Brucella suis* was isolated from the asymptomatic watchdog used to guard the original infected herd, and subsequently the newly populated herd (Körmendy and Nagy 1982). Transmissible gastroenteritis virus was transmitted to pigs that had been fed jejunal material from experimentally infected dogs (Larson et al. 1979). A risk association study in the United States reported that pigs on farms were 6.33 and 6.95 times more likely to be seropositive to *Trichinella* when pigs had access to wildlife and wildlife carcasses (Gamble et al. 1999).

Birds

Introduction of swine pathogens to farms by birds has been hypothesized but not definitively documented. Pigs fed droppings from starlings that were experimentally fed a suspension of transmissible gastroenteritis virus developed clinical signs of transmissible gastroenteritis but virus isolation was not performed (Pilchard 1965). English sparrows mechanically transmitted CSF under experimental conditions (Hughes and Gustafson 1960). An influenza A strain originating in wild ducks was thought to be responsible for an outbreak of influenza in pigs in Belgium. The strains of influenza isolated from the pigs were related to influenza viruses isolated from wild ducks in North America and Germany (Pensaert et al. 1981).

Fomites

Iatrogenic mechanical transmission by use of contaminated needles has been reported for PRRSV (Otake et al. 2002c).

Carcasses

Cannibalism of infected pig carcasses was determined to be the mode of transmission of *Trichinella spiralis* on an Illinois swine farm (Hanbury et al. 1986).

Vehicles

Contact with contaminated vehicles was implicated in the spread of CSF virus (Fritzemeier et al. 2000). Farms with more than two animal transport vehicles per month, greater than 30 rendering trucks per year, and greater than one veterinarian or technician vehicle entering every 2 months had an increased risk of occurrence of two or more respiratory disease outbreaks per year by 5.1, 3.2, and 5.5 times, respectively, than farms with less vehicle entries (Rose and Madec 2002). Under experimental conditions, carriers composed of non-chlorinated well water and snow were injected with $10^{4.4}$ $TCID_{50}$ of PRRSV and attached to the rear wheel wells of a truck to simulate potential transport of PRRSV by a contaminated vehicle in winter. The truck was driven 50 km at temperatures of <0°C to a truck wash. The truck was manually cleaned to ensure that the carriers fell to the cement floor of the truck wash. The carriers were then stepped on. Porcine reproductive and respiratory syndrome virus was recovered by virus isolation from the floor of the truck wash facility in 5 of 10 replicates (Dee et al. 2002). This experiment was repeated in warm weather (10–16°C) using a carrier composed of a ball of soil inoculated with PRRS virus, and the virus was recovered by virus isolation from the floor of the truck wash facility in 6 of 10 replicates (Dee et al. 2003). These experimental conditions might not reflect the level of vehicle contamination that naturally occurs in the field.

ASSESSING RISK OF INFECTION

Assessing the exact risk of infection is difficult because of the numerous factors involved in disease transmission. However, risk can be estimated by using mathematical models. One can estimate the average number of new cases of an infection that would result from the introduction of a single infected animal to the population, given information regarding the pathogen and the specific population of swine. This number is called the basic reproduction number, basic reproduction ratio or basic reproductive rate, and is symbolized by R_0. The basic reproduction number (R_0) is calculated by multiplying the probability of infection after contact with the infectious animal (p), the number of contacts per unit time with the infectious animal (c), and the duration of infectiousness of that animal (D). Thus, $R_0 = pcD$ (Anderson and Nokes 1991). The probability of an epizootic through direct contact is calculated as $P_{epizootic} = 1 - 1/R_0 I_0$, where I_0 is the initial number of infectious animals. The basic reproductive number can also be used to calculate the proportion of susceptible animals that should be vaccinated to prevent an epizootic: $P_{vaccinated} = 1 - (1 \div R_0)$ (Anderson and May 1982; Anderson and Nokes 1991). A major limitation of these equations is that the calculations do not account for indirect contact with the pathogen. However, swine veterinarians can use these formulas as a starting point to estimate risk of infection and subsequent costs. The R_0 of the CSF virus during the 1997–1998 epidemic in The Netherlands was estimated to be 2.9 (Stegeman et al. 1999), whereas the R_0 for CSF under experimental conditions has ranged from 13.7 (Laevens et al. 1999) to 81.3 (Laevens et al. 1998). The R_0 for pseudorabies virus in unvaccinated and vaccinated pigs was 10 and 0.36–0.5, respectively (de Jong and Kimman 1994; Bouma et al. 1995). The R_0 for transmissible gastroenteritis virus was estimated at 2 for the breeding animals and 4 for growing pigs (Hone 1994).

BIOSECURITY: CONTROL OF ENZOOTIC, EPIZOOTIC, AND EXOTIC DISEASES

Location

Increased distance between animal facilities reduced the risk of aerosol infection (Müller et al. 1978). Farms located within 2 km of five or more farms were 2.9 times more likely to experience two or more respiratory disease outbreaks per year than farms located within 2 km of less than five farms (Rose and Madec 2002). Risk factor indices for infection with *M. hyopneumoniae* were developed using characteristics of 55 infected herds and 57 uninfected herds. The most important risk factor for infection was the reciprocal of the square of the distance to the nearest farm. Distances within 3.2 km had the highest risk (Goodwin 1985). Further modeling has suggested that the risk of a noninfected herd becoming infected with *Mycoplasma hyopneumoniae* increased as the distance between that herd and the nearest infected farm decreased (Jorsal and Thomsen 1988; Stärk et al. 1992; Thomsen et al. 1992).

Factors that can be used to prevent aerosol transmission among farms include vaccination of animals to prevent infection and decrease shedding of organisms and selection of a low pig density area. Increasing the distance between the nearest swine farm and manure spreading area is preferable but cannot absolutely prevent airborne infections (Stärk 1999). Within barns, PRRS virus was transmitted among pigs, without direct contact, over short distances in two of five trials. Transmission by aerosol could not be confirmed because experimental design did not prevent the transfer of feed, feces, and urine among pens; however, the authors hypothesized that separation of pens by short distances (46–102 cm) could result in subpopulations of noninfected pigs (Wills et al. 1997). Factors that can be used in general to prevent aerosol transmission within buildings include dust reduction through adding fat to feed, minimizing animal movement, maintaining relative humidity <60%, and optimizing ventilation (Stärk 1999). There was no difference in the concentration of organisms isolated from the air of mechanically ventilated and naturally ventilated swine barns (Predicala et al. 2002).

Introduction of Genetics

Limiting the number of genetic sources can minimize the risk of pathogen introduction to a herd. Danish SPF herds purchasing stock from more than one source per year were 2.7 times more likely to become reinfected with *M. hyopneumoniae* than herds purchasing from a single source (Jorsal and Thomsen 1988). Additionally, introduction of live boars to a herd poses a greater risk of pathogen introduction than bringing in semen (Bouma 2000). However, similar questions should be asked of your semen supplier as of your live animal supplier to determine the health risk posed by the semen source.

Moreover, a boar stud could unintentionally distribute infected semen to large numbers of animals in a wide geographic range; therefore, semen distribution should cease during a disease outbreak in the stud (Bouma 2000). The American Association of Swine Veterinarians has published guidelines for boar studs distributing semen within United States (Althouse et al. 2003). Additionally, procedures to minimize contamination of semen during collection and processing have been published (Althouse et al. 2000). Removal of the preputial diverticulum is a surgical method to decrease contamination of semen (Aamdal et al. 1958).

Veterinarians of the source and the recipient herds should work together to determine the health status and testing procedures to minimize risk of disease introduction. Animals can be tested prior to purchase to determine whether they meet the herd health standards. Animals can then be tested on arrival to establish baseline exposure to disease and any change in health status. Incoming stock can be isolated, monitored for signs of disease, and tested before introduction to the herd. Finally, animals can be retested before exiting isolation facilities. All animals should appear healthy and test negative to diseases of concern, prior to entering the existing herd facilities.

Isolation of incoming animals is one method to lessen the risk of disease introduction to a herd. Isolation provides the opportunity to recognize clinical signs of disease in incoming animals before carrier animals can infect the entire herd. Models have estimated that 6–30 days would elapse before clinical signs of transmissible gastroenteritis virus were detected in a herd after the introduction of a carrier pig (Hone 1994). Isolation also provides an opportunity to test incoming animals for pathogens and acclimatize incoming animals by direct exposure or vaccination before entry to the main herd. The duration of isolation will vary with the pathogen of concern, but it generally lasts at least 30 days.

People

A study of swine herds consisting of greater than 2000 pigs in three California counties reported that swine herds were contacted by people (and vehicles) that had contacted other livestock facilities between 374.9–1239.5 times per month with an average indirect contact rate of 807 times per month (Bates et al. 2001). The ease of transportation in the modern world has resulted in increased frequency of contacts, which could increase the risk of disease transfer.

African swine fever virus was not detected in nasal swabs of people immediately after 30 minutes of exposure to infected pigs (Wilkinson et al. 1977). Moreover, downtimes were not needed to prevent mechanical transmission of *E. coli*, FMD virus (O/UK/35/2001), TGE virus, or PRRS virus by people in experimental trials, provided that the appropriate decontamination methods for each pathogen were implemented (Amass et al.

1998, 2003ab; Alvarez et al. 2001; Otake et al. 2002b). In contrast, nose blowing or washing was not effective in eliminating FMD virus, and cloth or industrial masks were not effective in preventing inhalation of the FMD virus (Sellers et al. 1970). Similarly, use of goggles, gloves, and dust masks were not effective in preventing human infection with swine influenza virus (Wentworth et al. 1997).

Showering and donning clean coveralls, boots, and gloves was sufficient to prevent mechanical transmission of FMD virus (O/UK/35/2001) from infected pigs to susceptible pigs and sheep (Amass et al. 2003b). Hand washing and donning clean outerwear was sufficient to prevent mechanical transmission of FMD virus (O/UK/35/2001) from infected pigs to susceptible pigs, but sheep remained susceptible (Amass et al. 2003b). Pigs are more resistant to FMD virus (O/UK/35/2001) compared to sheep (Donaldson and Alexandersen 2001). Presumably, hand washing and changing outerwear reduced the dose mechanically transmitted by people to that below the infectious dose for swine, but a sheep-infectious dose was still transmitted (Amass et al. 2003b). Similarly, showering and donning clean outerwear was effective in preventing the mechanical transmission of *E. coli* by people from infected to susceptible pigs, while hand washing and donning clean outerwear did not prevent such transmission (Amass et al. 2003a). Hand washing or showering and donning clean outerwear were both effective in preventing a person from mechanically transmitting TGE virus of swine from infected to susceptible pigs (Alvarez et al. 2001). Finally, hand washing or showering and donning clean outerwear were both sufficient to prevent the mechanical transmission of PRRS virus under conditions of extraordinary contamination of people (Otake et al. 2002b).

Scientific studies regarding effective showering procedures are absent, with the exception of those studies cited above wherein showering was used as an intervention for disease transmission. Presumably, showering procedures should ensure that sufficient time is spent to remove all organic material from body surfaces. Similarly, most hand washing studies were performed under experimental or hospital conditions that do not reflect the extent of hand contamination following procedures performed in a swine unit. Both resident and transient bacteria colonize hands. The goal of hand washing is to remove the transient bacteria. The effectiveness of hand washing as a hygiene tool will vary with the contaminant organisms. For example, the percentage reduction in *E. coli* on hands after 10 seconds of hand washing was significantly greater than the percentage reduction of human rotavirus, regardless of the washing media (antimicrobial soap, unmedicated soap, or tap water) used (Ansari et al. 1991). The efficacy of medicated soap in reducing transient bacterial flora after 30 seconds of hand washing varied according to bacterial type, with some medicated soaps more efficacious than others for certain classes of bacteria (Puthucheary et al. 1981).

Current hand washing recommendations for visibly contaminated hands consist of wetting the hands, then using plain or antimicrobial soaps to wash the hands by vigorously rubbing together all hand surfaces for at least 15 seconds. The hands should then be thoroughly rinsed and dried (Centers for Disease Control and Prevention 2002). Fifteen seconds of washing might not be sufficient for grossly contaminated hands; therefore, washing presumably should continue for 15 seconds after the time that hands are visibly free of organic material.

Generally, in cases where hands were not visibly contaminated, use of at least 1–3 ml of an alcohol-based hand antiseptic reduced bacterial counts more than washing with medicated or unmedicated soap and water. Applying less than 0.5 ml of alcohol-based antiseptic to hands was not more effective than washing hands with plain soap and water. The exact volume of alcohol-based solution that is most effective likely varies among products, but generally, hands should still feel wet from the alcohol after rubbing them together for 15 seconds to ensure that a sufficient volume of product was used. Swine care workers should be cautioned that alcohols are not effective on visibly contaminated hands (Centers for Disease Control and Prevention 2002).

Drying hands following washing is an important part of hand hygiene. Drying hands for either 10 seconds with a cloth towel or 20 seconds with an air dryer reduced bacterial transfer from hands to pieces of plastic by 99% when compared to bacterial transfer from wet hands (Patrick et al. 1997). Electric air-drying of hands for 10 seconds was more effective in reducing numbers of both *E. coli* and rotavirus compared to drying hands with a paper or cloth towel for 10 seconds (Ansari et al. 1991).

Wearing gloves can decrease the gross contamination of hands but does not prevent the need for hand washing. Hands can become contaminated through holes in the gloves and/or during glove donning and doffing (Centers for Disease Control and Prevention 2002). Thus, hand washing is recommended following the removal of gloves.

There is little evidence to require restrictions regarding off-farm contact among personnel working at different swine farms to prevent indirect transmission of swine pathogens from farm to farm. Person-to-person transfer of swine pathogens is possible but the frequency of occurrence under field conditions is unknown. Transfer of FMD virus between people was documented after persons in contact with infected animals spoke to unexposed colleagues in a box for 4 minutes (Sellers et al. 1970). Circumstantial evidence of transmission of swine influenza virus among people has been documented but not definitively proven. The 1976 outbreak of swine influenza A at Fort Dix affected at least

230 military personnel and was probably introduced by a new trainee (Top and Russell 1977). However, the initial human source of the virus was never proven and there was no evidence, aside from the viral strain, linking the outbreak to contact with swine (Kendal et al. 1977). Circumstantial evidence exists that a woman attending a county fair in which there was a flulike illness became infected with swine influenza virus from the pigs and subsequently spread the virus to health care workers (Wells et al. 1991). In contrast, an 8-year-old boy that was infected with swine influenza virus and lived on a swine farm did not transmit the virus to his parents or to his five siblings, despite close contact (O'Brien et al. 1977). Notably, definitive evidence of people infected with swine influenza virus transmitting the virus to swine has not been documented, despite some evidence of person-to-person transmission.

Non-Porcine Vectors

Farm management plans should include procedures for the control of wildlife and feral animals that can act as disease vectors.

Insects

Sanitation is the key measure for controlling insects (Williams 1992). From observations of *Musca domestica* in England, it was reported that fly numbers were fairly constant in closed buildings with fly numbers dropping when rooms were cleaned between groups of pigs, but increasing when rooms were restocked (Denholm et al. 1985). Manure, spoiled feed, and wet areas should be removed at least twice a week (Williams 1992). Flies and mosquitoes can be controlled by spraying pigs with insecticides or treating the environments with sprays, fogs, baits, and larvicides (Williams 1992). Persistent use of the same insecticide, especially in houseflies overwintering in indoor buildings was thought to contribute to maintenance of insecticide-resistant fly populations (Denholm et al. 1985). Traps and screens can be used to mechanically rid an area of insects (Williams 1992). Nematodes can be used to control housefly populations. Fewer flies were counted on a farm when baits of the nematode *Steinernema feltiae* were used compared to methomyl baits (Renn 1998).

Cleaning and Disinfection

One route of infection for pigs is through contact with a contaminated environment. Therefore, thorough cleaning and disinfection of all surfaces is crucial to a successful biosecurity program. Swine exposed to a *Salmonella* Typhimurium-contaminated environment for as little as 2 hours became infected (Hurd et al. 2001). Cleaning prior to disinfection is the most important step. All visible organic material (feed, urine, manure, secretions) should be removed from the surface(s) to be disinfected. A general target for the number of aerobic bacteria present following cleaning of surfaces and prior to disinfection is 10^6 cfu/cm^2 (Böhm 1998).

Disinfectants should be applied according to label directions. Extralabel use of most disinfectants is a violation of United States federal law. Disinfectant classes have general properties (Table 68.9) but an individual formulation could have a broader or more limited spectrum of activity (Jeffrey 1995; McDonnell and Russell 1999). Human health risks have been associated with some classes of disinfectants (Table 68.9) (Bruins and Dyer 1995).

The field efficacy of a disinfectant is dependent on a variety of factors, including but not limited to the surfaces to be disinfected, pathogens present, water quality,

Table 68.9.   General properties and human health risks of disinfectants

Disinfectant	Activity against					Human Health Effects
	Bacteria	Virus	Fungi	Spores	Mycobacterium	
Alcohols	bactericidal	virucidal	fungicidal	inhibit sporulation and spore formation	mycobactericidal	
Formaldehyde	bactericidal	virucidal		sporicidal		100 ppm formaldehyde can be life threatening, formaldehyde gas is unstable and can explode, allergenic, potentially carcinogenic
Biguanides	bacteriostatic	virucidal	fungicidal			irritating to skin
Glutaraldehyde	bactericidal	virucidal	fungicidal	sporicidal		allergenic
Halogen releasing compounds	bactericidal	virucidal	fungicidal	sporicidal		irritating to skin and eyes
Phenols	bactericidal	virucidal	fungicidal		mycobactericidal	toxic, irritating to skin
Quaternary ammonium compounds	bactericidal	lipophilic virucidal		sporostatic		
Peroxygen compounds	bactericidal	virucidal	fungicidal	sporicidal		

and organic material. Thus, label claims do not always translate into effectiveness in field situations (Kennedy et al. 1995).

An initial disinfectant choice should be based on disinfectant class properties, label claims, and independent data if available. Disinfectants should be prepared and applied according to label directions. Ideally, the disinfectant should be allowed to dry, or, at minimum, the contact time recommended on the label should elapse. Cleaning and disinfection protocol effectiveness can be determined by sampling the environment for specific pathogens or by using aerobic bacterial counts as a marker for contamination. The target for number of aerobic bacteria present after disinfection is 1 cfu/cm^2 (Tamasi 1995). However, a target of 10^3 cfu/cm^2 has been suggested for disinfection of livestock facilities and transport vehicles (Böhm 1998). Sentinel animals can also be used to monitor for specific pathogens following depopulation of a facility.

Processing Equipment. Dipping processing instruments in disinfectant is a common method of decontaminating instruments between litters of pigs. However, dipping tail clippers in chlorhexidine diacetate solution after a single use did not significantly reduce the mean aerobic bacterial counts on the blade when compared to untreated clippers (Alvarez et al. 2002). Wiping the blade with a clean cloth did significantly reduce the mean aerobic bacterial counts on the clippers (Alvarez et al. 2002). Wiping the blade physically removes organic contamination that dipping does not eliminate. Moreover, dipping instruments in disinfectant does not allow the minimum contact time needed for the disinfectant to work.

Boots. Farms maintain boot baths with the goal of preventing mechanical transmission of pathogens among groups of pigs. Frequently boot baths are grossly contaminated with organic matter as their maintenance is often lacking. They are also inconvenient and people commonly avoid the bath or step through the bath without stopping to clean their boots.

One suggestion for effective utilization of boot baths consisted of cleaning boots in a preliminary bath filled with dilute detergent, followed by immersion of clean boots to a depth of 15 cm, for at least 1 minute, in a second bath filled with detergent (Quinn 1991). Additionally recommendations included that large units prepare new boot baths daily or when visibly contaminated, and small units prepare new boot baths every 3 days (Quinn 1991).

Glutaraldehyde, chlorhexidine, sodium hypochlorite, iodine, phenolic, quaternary ammonium, and peroxygen disinfectants were evaluated utilizing various boot bath protocols. Bacterial counts on boots were not effectively lowered when the boots were contaminated with manure and then dipped in disinfectant (Amass et al. 2001) or soaked in disinfectant for 2 minutes (Amass et al. 2000b, 2001). Bacterial counts were effectively reduced when manure was removed from the boots by either scrubbing off manure in a clean disinfectant boot bath (Amass et al. 2000b, 2001) or scrubbing off manure in water and then dipping boots in a clean disinfectant boot bath (Amass et al. 2001). Contaminated boot baths, even those used only once previously, increased bacterial contamination of the boot (Amass et al. 2000b).

Dipping disposable plastic boots that were experimentally contaminated with PRRS virus into a fresh bath of undiluted 6% sodium hypochlorite for 5 seconds reduced the number of boots that were PCR-positive for PRRS virus as compared to boots that were experimentally contaminated and then dipped in a water bath without disinfectant (Dee et al. 2004). Similar results were reported when this experiment was repeated using fecal contamination in addition to virus contamination of boots (Dee et al. 2004). The disinfectant was not neutralized after sampling in these trials; therefore, the effective contact time likely exceeded 5 seconds. Moreover, virus isolation was not used to determine PRRSV viability.

Laundry. Contaminated clothing is a potential fomite in disease transmission. Poliovirus and vaccinia virus were experimentally transferred from contaminated to sterile fabrics when dry pieces of fabric were randomly tumbled in a jar. Maximum virus transfer occurred between 1 and 30 minutes (Sidwell et al. 1970). Microorganisms were also transferred from contaminated to sterile fabrics during laundering in a washing machine (Wiksell et al. 1973).

The effect of water temperature during laundering varies and is likely dependent on the contaminating pathogens, detergents and laundry chemicals used, and water characteristics such as hardness and pH. Early research recommended that hospital laundry be washed for 13 minutes at 60°C for optimal bacterial reduction (Walter and Schillinger 1975). Later, bacterial counts from hospital towels and sheets laundered at 71°C (160°F) and 22°C (72°F) were reported as not significantly different (Blaser et al. 1984). Washing at 47.8°C (118°F) to 60°C (140°F) with detergent and bleach was just as effective at removing bacteria as washing using similar procedures at 73.9°C (165°F) to 77.2°C (171°F) (Christian et al. 1983). Increased concentrations of bleach could compensate for lower washing temperatures (Christian et al. 1983). In contrast, water temperatures of 54°C to 60°C were more effective at removing poliovirus from contaminated fabrics than laundering at water temperatures of 21°C to 27°C or 38°C to 43°C (Sidwell et al. 1971). Laundering cloth contaminated with enterococci at temperatures of 71°C to 80°C for 3.5–10 minutes was effective even though the enterococci strains used survived for 30 minutes at 85°C under laboratory conditions (Orr et al. 2002). Thus, a correlation cannot always be found between the thermotolerance of an organism and survival during laundering (Orr et al. 2002).

Rinse water discharged from washing machines can contain viable bacteria and viruses. Concentrations of viable bacteria in rinse water were detected at levels from 100–5,000 cfu per ml at wash temperature of 38°C, 12–398 cfu/ml at wash temperature of 49°C, and 3–302 cfu/ml at wash temperature of 60°C. The final rinse had less than or equal to 20 cfu per ml regardless of wash water temperature used (Walter and Schillinger 1975). Viable poliovirus was not recovered from rinse water when laundering at water temperatures of 54°C to 60°C, but it was recovered when water temperatures of 21°C to 27°C or 38°C to 43°C were used (Sidwell et al. 1971).

The target for the number of bacteria adhered to fabric after laundering is 0.2 cfu/cm^2 (Walter and Schillinger 1975). However, quantification of bacteria on fabrics is difficult. Results from impression cultures using RODAC plates (replicate organism detection and counting) do not correlate well with more accurate destructive techniques such as cultures of macerated fabric samples (Nicholes 1970; Wetzler et al. 1971). Thus, the effectiveness of laundry procedures is more accurately determined by culturing fabrics for specific pathogens of concern instead of general quantification of total microorganisms (Wetzler et al. 1971).

Vehicles

Restricting entry of vehicles to farm premises, especially livestock trailers, to those that have been cleaned and disinfected should minimize the chance of pathogen introduction. Farms with parking for pig transport vehicles located within 300 meters of the farm site were 9.28 times more likely to become reinfected with *M. hyopneumoniae* or *A. pleuropneumoniae* than farms with no parking site near the farm (Hege et al. 2002). Cleaning and sanitizing trailers was effective in significantly reducing the numbers of *Salmonella* and *E. coli* on trailer flooring, but it did not eliminate bacterial contamination in all cases (Rajkowski et al. 1998). The principles of vehicle sanitation follow those outlined for facilities and equipment (Poumian 1995). However, cleaning and disinfecting vehicles can be difficult because surfaces are irregular and multiple materials are involved (Böhm 1998). Moreover, low outdoor temperatures prevent adequate decontamination if an indoor washing facility is not available (Böhm 1998). Ideally, vehicles should be decontaminated in an indoor facility at temperatures above 10°C (Böhm 1998). Selection of disinfectants for vehicles should ensure that the disinfectant used is not corrosive.

Water

On-farm water supplies range from freshwater to rural water. They also include sources such as rainwater, including runoff, ground water, rivers, and streams. Re-

ducing the risk of pathogens in water depends on several possible approaches that take into account the source of water, physical treatment (filtration, sedimentation), and chemical treatment (disinfection). Water safety and quality can be determined by bacterial analysis of water samples. Depending on previous history of the water source, a water analysis may need to be done annually at a minimum.

Carcass Disposal

Carcasses of previously ill pigs have the potential to be a source of pathogens. Prompt carcass disposal is recommended for aesthetic as well as biosecurity reasons. Farms storing carcasses inside the perimeter of the farm premises were 3.4 times more likely to experience two or more respiratory disease outbreaks per year than farms that did not maintain carcasses on site (Rose and Madec 2002). Approved carcass disposal options vary according to local regulations. Options for carcass disposal include burial, landfills, composting, rendering, tissue digestion, and incineration (Sander et al. 2002).

Manure

Inactivation of viruses in liquid manure is not practical but could be necessary prior to repopulation after a disease outbreak. Long-term storage of manure for at least 6 months at 4°C without addition of new manure should be effective assuming a virus titer reduction of 1–2 $\log_{10}$ units per month. A directive of the Federal Ministry of Agriculture in Germany recommends the following methods for disinfection of manure: 40% solution of lime hydrate at a concentration of 40–60 liters per cubic meter of liquid manure can be used at temperatures between 0 and −10°C; or a 50% solution of sodium hydroxide at a concentration of 16–30 liters per cubic meter of liquid manure can be used at temperatures between 0 and 10°C. Manure should be stirred prior to, during, and for 6 hours after chemical disinfection. The duration of exposure of manure to chemicals should be at least 4 days and preferably 1 week. Peracetic acid at a concentration of 25–40 liters per cubic meter of liquid manure can be used at temperatures between 0 and 10°C. The exposure time in this case is at least 1 hour and often is not practical due to excessive foaming (Haas et al. 1995).

Feed

Outbreaks of exotic diseases such as classical swine fever have been traced back to swill feeding (Fritzemeier et al. 2000). United States federal law states "No person shall feed or permit the feeding of garbage to swine unless the garbage is treated to kill disease organisms . . ." (9 CFR Ch. 1, Part 166—Swine Health Protection, Section 166.2, 1-1-98 Edition). However, some individual states forbid feeding both treated and untreated garbage. Feed and feed ingredients can be proactively monitored for pathogens and toxins.

Control of Movement

Modifications of pig flow can be used to control disease transmission. Sow-to-pig transmission of certain pathogens can be prevented or minimized by weaning pigs while they still have colostral immunity to their dam's pathogens to a pathogen-free environment with other pigs of similar health status (Clark et al. 1994; Dritz et al. 1996). Strategic medication and vaccination can be used as adjunct procedures for early weaning programs (Alexander et al. 1980; Mészáros et al. 1985; Harris et al. 1992).

Similarly, segregating pigs in groups by age minimizes transfer of pathogens from older to younger pigs. Age-segregated growing pigs can then be moved in cohorts in all-in/all-out fashion by filling and emptying rooms, buildings or sites over a short time frame, and cleaning and disinfecting pig areas between groups of pigs. These procedures are thought to minimize transmission of pathogens from older infected pigs or contaminated environments to susceptible pigs. In contrast, continuous flow systems that continuously commingle pigs of various ages without periodic cleaning of the environment offer increased possibilities of disease transmission from infected to susceptible pigs or through contact with a contaminated environment. The process of age segregation has recently been applied to the breeding herd and designated parity segregation. Parity segregation houses the gilts separately from the existing breeding herd. The gilts are exposed to the sow herd pathogens in the same way as gilts in acclimation. The gilts will farrow at this separate site. They will enter the existing breeding herd after weaning the first litter. This allows a longer "cool down" period for infectious organisms.

Pig Movement

In several countries, a national animal identification plan is used or is being developed to assist tracking pig movement intrastate, interstate, and internationally. In 1924, the Office International des Epizooties (OIE) was formed to encourage and coordinate research for the worldwide monitoring and control of animal diseases. The OIE provides information on the animal disease status of member countries and publishes international animal health standards for import and export of animals and animal products.

People Movement

Limiting visitors to essential personnel is one method of minimizing the risk of pathogen introduction by people. People who have been on farms with disease outbreaks should, at minimum, shower and change clothing before entering a population of susceptible swine. Generally, people movement should flow from healthy pigs to sick or carrier pigs. People flow from young to old pigs is also recommended.

Vaccination and Medication

Strategic vaccination and medication are an essential part of any herd health program. An effective vaccination program should reduce transmission of pathogens within a herd. An experiment to quantify pseudorabies virus transmission among vaccinated and unvaccinated pigs found that the number of secondary cases of pseudorabies per infected pig was 10 in unvaccinated pigs, but only 0.5 in vaccinated pigs (de Jong and Kimman 1994).

Surveillance Testing Programs

Periodic testing can be used to assess herd health status. Tests used will be determined by the pathogens of interest. Sample size will be dependent on expected disease prevalence in the population. Sampling can be simple and random or systematic (Thrusfield 1995). Cross-sectional and longitudinal sampling methods are often used in a complementary fashion. For more detailed information on surveillance programs, see Chapter 69 on disease surveillance in swine populations.

Record Keeping for Surveillance and Regulated Diseases

Morbidity, mortality, reproductive, and growth performance records can be used proactively to identify indicators of pathogen introduction.

Records also become important when regulated diseases are suspected. Information regarding the origin of all animals, animal products (including modified live vaccines, biologicals, and semen), feedstuffs (grain, supplements), equipment, vehicles (for livestock, feed, swine specialists), and people (sales and feed representatives, visitors, veterinarians, technicians, mail delivery personnel, service personnel) that have visited the farm prior to the outbreak is used in "traceback" procedures to identify the source of the pathogen and determine how the pathogen was introduced. Procedures can be implemented to minimize future risk of disease introduction once the source of the pathogen has been identified. Similar information regarding animal and equipment movements off the farm are used in "trace-forward" procedures to determine other premises that possibly received infected animals, animal products, or contaminated equipment.

Maintaining herd records and updated back-up copies of records routinely can assist in both traceforward and traceback procedures when needed. Attempting to acquire information during an outbreak situation is difficult due to the chaotic nature of a disease outbreak. Regular herd records allow the producer to rapidly and accurately produce movement records facilitating the tracking procedures. Moreover, individual animal identification (within sow herds) will enhance the efficiency of tracking procedures. A single individual on each premise should be responsible for maintaining accurate records although every employee should know how to access the records in case of an emergency.

The following are recommendations for records to be kept on a regular basis:

1. Inventory of animals in the herd: number of animals, animal identification, breed, age, species, origin. Animals that die or are culled from the herd should be identified.
2. Animal movement to and from the farm: date, animal identification, origin, destination, reason, driver, vehicle used, previous owners' name and phone number.
3. Visitor: names, phone numbers, reason for visit, time since last contact with livestock, facilities entered. Visitors include all nonemployees: veterinarians, feed salesman, livestock dealers, repairmen, neighbors, etc.
4. Vehicles: driver, dates, origins, destinations. All vehicles other than those recorded in the visitor log should be included, e.g., those used for package delivery, propane trucks, trash pick-up, electric company, etc.
5. Equipment, feed, semen movement: dates, origins, destinations, delivery person, salesman.
6. Manure application/movement: dates, origin, application site, volume, and application method.
7. Vaccination and treatment records: animal identification, date, reason for treatment/vaccination, medication used.
8. Employee records: name, address, phone number, whether the employee has contact with other livestock.
9. Pets and other animals located on the premises.
10. Cull animals sold: number, date, location.

Additional information will be requested in the event of an outbreak of a regulated disease (United States Department of Agriculture 1992). Immediately after a presumptive and/or confirmed diagnosis of a regulated disease, investigators require information regarding all movements of animals (livestock and pets), products (meat), manure, equipment, vehicles, people, and feed to the farm premises for the 21 days preceding the outbreak. Information designated above will be used.

CERTIFICATION PROGRAMS

Certification programs can be used to establish that a herd is free of a specific pathogen. Certification programs can be used on a local level as a transition step for large eradication projects. The Trichinae Certification Program is one example of a program recently initiated to control a pathogen (Pybrun 2003).

ERADICATION PROGRAMS

Eradication programs can be designed on the herd, local, regional, national, or international level. Eradica-

tion can sometimes be achieved through normal replacement of breeding stock. In other cases, programs such as test and removal with or without vaccination, partial depopulation or total depopulation are required.

Emergency vaccination as a tool for eradication of List A diseases has been reviewed (Laddomada 2003). Attempts have been made to eliminate porcine reproductive and respiratory disease virus from swine herds by using test and removal, and nursery depopulation with or without vaccination of the breeding herd (Dee and Joo 1994; Dee et al. 1998, 2001). Transmissible gastroenteritis virus has been eliminated from swine herds by depopulation and test and removal (Gunn 1996). Partial depopulation by removing all animals under 10 months of age from the farm, cleaning and disinfecting facilities, and medicating adult animals was successful in 81% of the attempts to eradicate *M. hyopneumoniae* (Heinonen et al. 1999).

Herd factors will determine the best strategy for eradication. Pseudorabies eradication was used in one decision-making model. Vaccination was preferred in large herds with low seroprevalence in sows and high farm density, partial depopulation was preferred with high seroprevalence in sows, and test and removal was preferred with low seroprevalence in sows. Finally, outdoor operations tended toward depopulation and repopulation (Siegel and Weigel 1999).

Depopulation and repopulation protocols are expensive to implement and require much planning. Briefly, the herd should first be assessed to determine current and desired performance, cost of the enzootic diseases, cost of medications and veterinary care, value of current genetics, labor requirements, antibiotic usage, feed costs, and psychological costs of the disease on personnel. Next, protocols for the timing of depopulation, downtime, cleanup procedures, and methods of repopulation should be investigated to determine whether the plan is feasible (McNaughton 1988). Available data is insufficient to be dogmatic about downtimes needed before repopulation. For example, a review of research on FMD virus survival led to estimates of downtimes of at least 3 months for hot climates (>20°C) and greater than 6 months for cold climates (Bartley et al. 2002).

Depopulation is mandatory for many exotic disease eradication programs. Euthanasia of infected animals and preemptive culling of surrounding susceptible livestock are thought to be the most effective means of controlling a FMD outbreak (Ferguson et al. 2001). In some cases, clinically healthy animals must be euthanized because animal and feed movement restrictions impair their well-being. Animal welfare should be considered when designing and implementing depopulation protocols with a euthanasia component (Whiting 2003). The American Association of Swine Veterinarians and the National Pork Board have published acceptable swine euthanasia options. Additionally, options for euthanasia of large numbers of swine have been published (Lambooy and van Voorst 1986).

REFERENCES

Aamdal J, Hogset I, Filseth O. 1958. Extirpation of the preputial diverticulum of boars used in artificial insemination. J Am Vet Med Assoc 132:522–524.

Ajariyakhajorn C, Goyal SM, Robinson RA, Johnston LJ, Clanton CA. 1997. The survival of *Salmonella anatum*, pseudorabies virus, and porcine reproductive and respiratory syndrome virus in swine slurry. Microbiologica 20:365–369.

Alexander TJL, Thornton K, Boon G, Lysons RJ, Gush AF. 1980. Medicated early weaning to obtain pigs free from pathogens endemic in the herd of origin. Vet Rec 106:114–119.

Althouse GC, Kuster CE, Clark SG, Weisiger RM. 2000. Field investigations of bacterial contaminants and their effects on extended porcine semen. Theriogenology 53:1167–1176.

Althouse GC, Reicks D, Spronk GD, Trayer TP, Burkgren TJ, Waddell JT. 2003. Health, hygiene, and sanitation guidelines for boar studs providing semen to the domestic market. J Swine Health Prod 11:204–206.

Alvarez RM, Amass SF, Anderson CD, Ragland D, Grote LA, Dowell CA, Clark LK, Stevenson GW, Spicer PM. 2001. Evaluation of biosecurity protocols to prevent mechanical transmission of transmissible gastro-enteritis virus of swine by pork production unit personnel. Pig J 48:22–33.

Alvarez RM, Kelly JA, Amass SF, Schneider J, Ragland D. 2002. Evaluating the efficacy of protocols for decontaminating tail-clipping instruments. J Swine Health Prod 10:209–211.

Amass SF. 1998a. The effect of wean age on pathogen removal. Compend Contin Educ Vet Pract 20:S196–S203.

——. 1998b. Review of the literature: *Streptococcus suis* infections of people. J Agromed 5:25–34.

Amass SF, Halbur PG, Byrne BA, Schneider JL, Koons CW, Cornick N, Ragland D. 2003a. Mechanical transmission of enterotoxigenic *Escherichia coli* to weaned pigs by people, and biosecurity procedures to prevent such transmission. J Swine Health Prod 11:61–68.

Amass SF, Kreisle RA, Clark LK, Wu CC. 1998. A pilot study of the prevalence of *Streptococcus suis* in pigs and personnel at five Indiana swine operations. J Agromed 5:17–24.

Amass SF, Pacheco JM, Mason PW, Schneider JL, Alvarez RM, Clark LK, Ragland D. 2003b. Procedures for preventing the transmission of foot-and-mouth disease virus to pigs and sheep by personnel in contact with infected pigs. Vet Rec 153:137–140.

Amass SF, Ragland D, Spicer P. 2001. Evaluation of the efficacy of a peroxygen compound, Virkon® S, as a boot bath disinfectant. J Swine Health Prod 9:121–123.

Amass SF, Stevenson GW, Anderson CA, Grote LA, Dowell BD, Kanitz C, Ragland D. 2000a. Investigation of people as mechanical vectors for porcine reproductive and respiratory syndrome virus. J Swine Health Prod 8:161–166.

Amass SF, Vyverberg BD, Ragland D, Dowell CA, Anderson CD, Stiver JH, Beaudry DJ. 2000b. Evaluating the efficacy of boot baths in biosecurity protocols. J Swine Health Prod 8:169–173.

Anderson RM, May RM. 1982. Directly transmitted infectious diseases: control by vaccination. Science 215:1053–1060.

Anderson RM, Nokes DJ. 1991. Mathematical models of transmission and control. In: Holland WW, Detels R, Knox G (eds). Oxford Textbook of Public Health (2nd ed). Oxford University Press, New York.

Ansari SA, Springthorpe VS, Sattar SA, Tostowaryk W, Wells GA. 1991. Comparison of cloth, paper, and warm air drying in eliminating viruses and bacteria from washed hands. Am J Infect Control 19:243–249.

Artois M, Depner KR, Guberti V, Hars J, Rossi S, Rutili D. 2002. Classical swine fever (hog cholera) in wild boar in Europe. Rev Sci Technique 21:287–303.

Backstrand JM, Botzler RG. 1986. Survival of *Pasteurella multocida* in soil and water in an area where avian cholera is enzootic. J Wildl Dis 22:257–259.

Baloda SB, Christensen L, Trajcevska S. 2001. Persistence of a *Salmonella enterica* serovar Typhimurium DT12 clone in a piggery and in agricultural soil amended with *Salmonella*-contaminated slurry. Appl Environ Microbiol 67:2859–2862.

Bane DP, James JE, Gradil CM, Molitor TW. 1990. In vitro exposure of preimplantation porcine embryos to porcine parvovirus. Theriogenology 33:553–561.

Barber DA, Bahnson P, Isaacson R, Jones CJ, Weigel RM. 2002. Distribution of *Salmonella* in swine production ecosystems. J Food Protection 12:1861–1868.

Bartley LM, Donnelly CA, Anderson RM. 2002. Review of foot-and-mouth disease virus survival in animal excretions and on fomites. Vet Rec 151:667–669.

Bates TW, Thurmond MC, Carpenter TE. 2001. Direct and indirect contact rates among beef, dairy, goat, sheep, and swine herds in three California counties, with reference to control of potential foot-and-mouth disease transmission. Am J Vet Res 62:1121–1129.

Bay WW, Doyle LP, Hutchings LM. 1952. Some properties of the causative agent of transmissible gastroenteritis in swine. Am J Vet Res 13:318–321.

Bean B, Moore BM, Sterner B, Peterson LR, Gerding DN, Balfour HH. 1982. Survival of influenza viruses on environmental surfaces. J Infect Dis 146:47–51.

Bemis DA, Shek WR, Clifford CB. 2003. *Bordetella bronchiseptica* infection of rats and mice. Comp Med 53:11–20.

Bendtsen H, Christiansen M, Thomsen A. 1954. Brucella enzootics in swine herds in Denmark—Presumably with hare as source of infection. Nord Vet Med 6:11–21.

Bernasky. 1910. The louse of the pig as an agent in transmitting infectious diseases of the pig. Vet Rec 23:37–38.

Berthelot-Hérault F, Gottschalk M, Labbé A, Cariolet R, Kobisch M. 2001. Experimental airborne transmission of *Streptococcus suis* capsular type 2 in pigs. Vet Microbiol 82:69–80.

Bickford AA, Ellis GH, Moses HE. 1966. Epizootiology of tuberculosis in starlings. J Am Vet Med Assoc 149:312–318.

Blaha VT. 1983. Zur bedeutung der schadnager für die epizootiologie der schweinedysenterie. Monatsh Veterinaermed 38:606–608.

Blaser MJ, Smith PF, Cody HJ, Wang W-LL, LaForce FM. 1984. Killing of fabric-associated bacteria in hospital laundry by low-temperature washing. J Infect Dis 149:48–57.

Böhm R. 1998. Disinfection and hygiene in the veterinary field and disinfection of animal houses and transport vehicles. Int Biodeterioration Biodegradation 41:217–224.

Bolin SR, Runnels LJ, Sawyer CA, Atcheson KJ, Gustafson DP. 1981. Resistance of porcine preimplantation embryos to pseudorabies virus. Am J Vet Res 42:1711–1712.

Bolin SR, Runnels LJ, Sawyer CA, Gustafson DP. 1982. Experimental transmission of pseudorabies virus in swine by embryo transfer. Am J Vet Res 43:278–280.

Borie DC, Cramer DV, Phan-Thanh L, Vaillant JC, Bequet JL, Makowka L, Hannoun L. 1998. Microbiological hazards related to xenotransplantation of porcine organs into man. Infect Control Hosp Epidemiol 19:355–365.

Bøtner A. 1991. Survival of Aujesky's disease virus in slurry at various temperatures. Vet Microbiol 29:225–235.

Bouma A. 2000. Transmissible virus diseases in porcine reproduction. Reprod Domest Anim 35:243–246.

Bouma A, de Jong MSM, Kimman TG. 1995. Transmission of pseudorabies virus within pig populations is independent of the size of the population. Prev Vet Med 23:163–172.

Bourgueil E, Hutet E, Cariolet R, Vannier P. 1992. Experimental infection of pigs with the porcine respiratory coronavirus (PRCV): measure of viral excretion. Vet Microbiol 31:11–18.

Boye M, Baloda SB, Leser TD, Møller. 2001. Survival of *Brachyspira hyodysenteriae* and *B. pilosicoli* in terrestrial microcosms. Vet Microbiol 81:33–40.

Brockmeier SL, Lager KM. 2002. Experimental airborne transmission of porcine reproductive and respiratory syndrome virus and *Bordetella bronchiseptica*. Vet Microbiol 89:267–275.

Bruins G, Dyer JA. 1995. Environmental considerations of disinfectants used in agriculture. Rev Sci Technique 14:81–94.

Burden DJ, Hammet NC. 1979. The development and survival of *Trichuris suis* ova on pasture plots in the south of England. Res Vet Sci 26:66–70.

Centers for Disease Control and Prevention. 2002. Guideline for hand hygiene in the health-care settings: Recommendations of the Healthcare Infection Control Practices Advisory Committee and the HICPAC/SHEA/APIC/IDSA Hand Hygiene Task Force. Morbidity and Mortality Weekly Report 51:1–34.

Champion HJ, Gloster J, Mason IS, Brown RJ, Donaldson AI, Ryall DB, Garland JM. 2002. Investigation of the possible spread of foot-and-mouth disease virus by the burning of animal carcases on open pyres. Vet Rec 151:593–600.

Chia SP, Taylor DJ. 1978. Factors affecting the survival of *Treponema hyodysenteriae* in dysenteric pig faeces. Vet Rec 103:68–70.

Choi C, Chae C. 2003. Detection of classical swine fever virus in boar semen by reverse transcription-polymerase chain reaction. J Vet Diagn Invest 15:35–41.

Christensen LS, Mousing J, Mortensen S, Soerensen KJ, Stradbygaard SB, Henriksen CA, Anderson JB. 1990. Evidence of long distance airborne transmission of Aujesky's disease (pseudorabies) virus. Vet Rec 127:471–474.

Christian RR, Manchester JT, Mellor MT. 1983. Bacteriological quality of fabrics washed at lower-than-standard temperatures in a hospital laundry facility. Appl Environ Microbiol 45:591–597.

Christopher-Hennings J, Nelson EA, Hines RJ, Nelson JK, Swenson SL, Zimmerman JJ, Chase CCL, Yaeger MJ, Benfield DA. 1995a. Persistence of porcine reproductive and respiratory syndrome virus in serum and semen of adult boars. J Vet Diagn Invest 7:456–464.

Christopher-Hennings J, Nelson EA, Nelson JK, Hines RJ, Swenson SL, Hill HT, Zimmerman JJ, Katz JB, Yaeger MJ, Chase CCL, Benfield DA. 1995b. Detection of porcine reproductive and respiratory syndrome virus in boar semen by PCR. J Clin Microbiol 33:1730–1734.

Christopher-Hennings J, Nelson EA, Nelson JK, Rossow KD, Shivers JL, Yaeger MJ, Chase CCL, Garduno RA, Collins JE, Benfield DA. 1998. Identification of porcine reproductive and respiratory syndrome virus in semen and tissues from vasectomized and nonvasectomized boars. Vet Pathol 35:260–267.

Clark LK, Hill MA, Kniffen TS, Van Alstine W, Stevenson G, Meyer KB, Wu CC, Scheidt AB, Knox K, Albregts S. 1994. An evaluation of the components of medicated early weaning. Swine Health Prod 2:5–11.

Clifton-Hadley FA, Enright MR. 1984. Factors affecting the survival of *Streptococcus suis* type 2. Vet Rec 114:585–587.

Cooper DM, Swanson DL, Gebhart CJ. 1997. Diagnosis of proliferative enteritis in frozen and formalin-fixed, paraffin-embedded tissues from a hamster, horse, deer and ostrich using a *Lawsonia intracellularis*-specific multiplex PCR assay. Vet Microbiol 54:47–62.

Cottral GE. 1969. Persistence of foot-and-mouth disease virus in animals, their products and the environment. Bull Office Int Epizooties 71:549–568.

Curtis SE, Kingdon DA, Simon J, Drummond JG. 1976. Effects of age and cold on pulmonary bacterial clearance in the young pig. Am J Vet Res 37:299–301.

Czaja T, Kanci A, Lloyd LC, Markham PF, Whithear KG, Browning GF. 2002. Induction of enzootic pneumonia in pigs by the administration of an aerosol of in vitro-cultured *Mycoplasma hyopneumoniae*. Vet Rec 150:9–11.

Davis DE. 1948. The survival of wild brown rats on a Maryland farm. Ecology 29:437–448.

Dee SA, Bierk MD, Deen J, Molitor TW. 2001. An evaluation of test and removal for the elimination of porcine reproductive and respiratory syndrome virus from 5 swine farms. Can J Vet Res 65:22–27.

Dee SA, Corey MM. 1993. The survival of *Streptococcus suis* on farm and veterinary equipment. J Swine Health Prod 1:17–20.

Dee SA, Deen J, Pijoan C. 2004. Evaluation of 4 intervention strategies to prevent the mechanical transmission of porcine reproductive and respiratory syndrome virus. Can J Vet Res 68:19–26.

Dee SA, Deen J, Rossow K, Weise C, Eliason R, Otake S, Joo HS, Pijoan C. 2003. Mechanical transmission of porcine reproductive and respiratory syndrome virus throughout a coordinated sequence of events during warm weather. Can J Vet Res 67:12–19.

Dee SA, Deen J, Rossow K, Weise C, Otake S, Joo HS, Pijoan C. 2002. Mechanical transmission of porcine reproductive and respiratory syndrome virus throughout a coordinated sequence of events during cold weather. Can J Vet Res 66:232–239.

Dee SA, Joo HS. 1994. Prevention of the spread of porcine reproductive and respiratory syndrome virus in endemically infected pig herds by nursery depopulation. Vet Rec 135:6–9.

Dee SA, Joo HS, Park BK, Molitor TW, Bruna G. 1998. Attempted elimination of porcine reproductive and respiratory syndrome virus from a seedstock farm by vaccination of the breeding herd and nursery depopulation. Vet Rec 142:569–572.

de Jong MCM, Kimman TG. 1994. Experimental quantification of vaccine-induced reduction in virus transmission. Vaccine 12:761–766.

Denholm I, Sawicki RM, Farnham AW. 1985. Factors affecting resistance to insecticides in house-flies, *Musca domestica* L. (Diptera:Muscidae). IV. The population biology of flies on animal farms in south-eastern England and its implications for the management of resistance. Bull Entomol Res 75:143–158.

de Smit AJ, Bouma A, Terpstra C, van Oirschot JT. 1999. Transmission of classical swine fever virus by artificial insemination. Vet Microbiol 67:239–249.

Devriese LA, Desmidt M, Roels S, Hoorens J, Haesebrouck F. 1993. *Streptococcus suis* infection in fallow deer. Vet Rec 132:283.

Devriese LA, Haesebrouck F. 1992. *Streptococcus suis* infections in horses and cats. Vet Rec 130:380.

Devriese LA, Haesebrouck F, De Herdt P, Dom P, Ducatelle R, Desmidt M, Messier S, Higgins R. 1994. *Streptococcus suis* infections in birds. Avian Pathol 23:721–724.

Donaldson AI, Alexandersen S. 2001. Relative resistance of pigs to infection by natural aerosols of FMD virus. Vet Rec 148:600–602.

Donaldson AI, Ferris NP. 1976. The survival of some air-borne animal viruses in relation to relative humidity. Vet Microbiol 1:413–420.

Donaldson AI, Gloster J, Harvey LDJ. 1982. Use of prediction models to forecast and analyse airborne spread during the foot-and-mouth disease outbreaks in Brittany, Jersey and the isle of Wight in 1981. Vet Rec 110:53–57.

Dorset M, McBryde CN, Mile WB, Rietz IH. 1919. Observations concerning the dissemination of hog cholera by insects. Am J Vet Med 14:55–60.

Dritz SS, Chengappa MM, Nelssen JL, Tokach MD, Goodband RD, Nietfeld JC, Staats JJ. 1996. Growth and microbial flora of nonmedicated, segregated, early weaned pigs from a commercial swine operation. J Am Vet Med Assoc 208:711–715.

Dubey JP, Weigel RM, Siegel AM, Thulliez P, Kitron UD, Mitchell MA, Mannelli A, Mateus-Pinilla NE, Shen SK, Kwok OCH, Todd

KS. 1995. Sources and reservoirs of *Toxoplasma gondii* infection on 47 swine farms in Illinois. J Parasitol 81:723–729.

Dudley JP, Woodford MH. 2002. Bioweapons, bioterrorism and biodiversity:potential impacts of biological weapons attacks on agricultural and biological diversity. Rev Sci Technique 21:125–137.

Dulac GC, Singh EL. 1988. Embryo transfer as a means of controlling the transmission of viral infections. XII. The in vitro exposure of zona pellucida-intact porcine embryos to hog cholera virus. Theriogenology 29:1335–1341.

Eld K, Gunnarsson A, Holmberg T, Hurvell B, Wierup M. 1991. Salmonella isolated from animals and feedstuffs in Sweden during 1983–1987. Acta Vet Scand 32:261–277.

Endris RG, Hess WR. 1992. Experimental transmission of African swine fever virus by the soft tick *Ornithodoros* (*Pavlovskyella*) *marocanus* (Acari: Ixodoidea: Argasidae). J Med Entomol 29:652–655.

Enright MR, Alexander TJL, Clifton-Hadley FA. 1987. Role of houseflies (*Musca domestica*) in the epidemiology of *Streptococcus suis* type 2. Vet Rec 121:132–133.

Fangman TJ, Tubbs RC. 1997. Segregated early weaning. Swine Health Prod 5:195–198.

Farrington DO, Jorgenson RD. 1976. Prevalence of *Bordetella bronchiseptica* in certain wild mammals and birds in central Iowa. J Wildl Dis 12:523–525.

Fedorka-Cray PJ, Hogg A, Gray JT, Lorenzen K, Velasquez J, Von Behren P. 1997. Feed and feed trucks as sources of *Salmonella* contamination in swine. Swine Health Prod 5:189–193.

Ferguson NM, Donnelly CA, Anderson RM. 2001. The foot-and-mouth epidemic in Great Britain: pattern of spread and impact of interventions. Science 292:1155–1160.

Fischer O, Mátlová L, Dvorská L, Švástová P, Bartl J, Melichárek I, Weston RT, Pavlík I. 2001. Diptera as vectors of mycobacterial infections in cattle and pigs. Med Vet Entomol 15:208–211.

Floegel G, Wehrend A, Depner KR, Fritzemeier J, Waberski D, Moennig V. 2000. Detection of classical swine fever virus in semen of infected boars. Vet Microbiol 109–116.

Foley CW, Zehmer RB, Shotts EB, Williams DJ. 1971. Bacterial flora of boar reproductive tract and semen. Am J Vet Res 32:1447–1450.

Forman AJ, Gibbs EPJ. 1974. Studies with foot-and-mouth disease virus in British deer (red, fallow and roe) 1. Clinical disease. J Comp Pathol 84:215–220.

Fritzemeier J, Teuffert J, Greiser-Wilke I, Staubach Ch, Schlüter, Moennig V. 2000. Epidemiology of classical swine fever in Germany in the 1990s. Vet Microbiol 77:29–41.

Fu ZF, Hampson DJ, Blackmore DK. 1989. Detection and survival of group A rotavirus in a piggery. Vet Rec 125:576–578.

Fukushima H, Ito Y, Saito K, Tsubokura M, Otsuki K. 1979. Role of the fly in the transport of *Yersinia enterocolitica*. Appl Environ Microbiol 38:1009–1010.

Gaasenbeek CPH, Borgsteede FHM. 1998. Studies on the survival of *Ascaris suum* eggs under laboratory and simulated field conditions. Vet Parasitol 75:227–234.

Gamble HR, Brady RC, Bulaga LL, Berthoud CL, Smith WG, Detweiler LA, Miller LE, Lautner EA. 1999. Prevalence and risk association for *Trichinella* infection in domestic pigs in the northeastern United States. Vet Parasitol 82:59–69.

Gebreyes WA, Davies PR, Turkson P-K, Morrow WEM, Funk JA, Alter C. 2004. *Salmonella enterica* serovars from pigs on farms and after slaughter and validity of using bacteriologic data to define herd *Salmonella* status. J Food Protection 67:691–697.

Gillespie RR, Hill MA, Kanitz CL, Knox KE, Clark LK, Robinson JP. 2000. Infection of pigs by Aujesky's disease virus via the breath of intranasally inoculated pigs. Res Vet Sci 68:217–222.

Gloster J, Blackall RM, Sellers RF, Donaldson AI. 1981. Forecasting the airborne spread of foot-and-mouth disease. Vet Rec 108:370–374.

Gloster J, Hewson H, Mackay D, Garland T, Donaldson A, Mason I, Brown R. 2001. Spread of foot-and-mouth disease from the burning of animal carcases on open pyres. Vet Rec 148:585–586.

Gloster J, Sellers RF, Donaldson AI. 1982. Long distance transport of foot-and-mouth disease virus over the sea. Vet Rec 110:47–52.

Goodwin RFW. 1985. Apparent reinfection of enzootic-pneumonia-free pig herds: Search for possible causes. Vet Rec 116:690–694.

Gough PM, Jorgenson RD. 1983. Identification of porcine transmissible gastroenteritis virus in house flies (*Musca domestica* Linneaus). Am J Vet Res 44:2078–2082.

Gradil CM, Harding MJ, Lewis K. 1994. Use of polymerase chain reaction to detect porcine parvovirus associated with swine embryos. Am J Vet Res 55:344–347.

Grant RH, Scheidt AB, Rueff LR. 1994. Aerosol transmission of a viable virus affecting swine: explanation of an epizootic of pseudorabies. Int J Biometeorol 38:33–39.

Gunn HM. 1996. Elimination of transmissible gastroenteritis virus from a pig farm by culling and serological surveillance. Vet Rec 138:196–198.

Haas B, Ahl R, Böhm R, Strauch D. 1995. Inactivation of viruses in liquid manure. Rev Sci Technique 14:435–445.

Hamel AL, Lin LL, Sachvie C, Grudeski E, Nayar GPS. 2000. PCR detection and characterization of type-2 porcine circovirus. Can J Vet Res 64:44–52.

Hanbury RD, Doby PB, Miller HO, Murrell KD. 1986. Trichinosis in a herd of swine: Cannibalism as a major mode of transmission. J Am Med Assoc 188:1155–1159.

Hang'ombe BM, Isogai E, Lungu J, Mubita C, Nambota A, Kirisawa R, Kimura K, Isogai H. 2000. Detection and characterization of *Clostridium* species in soil of Zambia. Comp Immunol Microbiol 23:277–284.

Harris DL, Armbrecht PJ, Wiseman BS, Platt KB, Hill HT, Anderson LA. 1992. Producing pseudorabies-free swine breeding stock from an infected herd. Vet Med 87:166–170.

Harris IT, Fedorka-Cray PJ, Gray JT, Thomas LA, Ferris K. 1997. Prevalence of Salmonella organisms in swine feed. J Am Vet Med Assoc 210:382–385.

Hege R, Zimmermann W, Scheidegger R, Stärk KDC. 2002. Incidence of reinfections with *Mycoplasma hyopneumoniae* and *Actinobacillus pleuropneumoniae* in pig farms located in respiratory-disease-free regions of Switzerland- identification and quantification of risk factors. Acta Vet Scand 43:145–156.

Heinonen M, Autio T, Saloniemi H, Tuovinen V. 1999. Eradication of *Mycoplasma hyopneumoniae* from infected swine herds joining the LSO 2000 health class. Acta Vet Scand 40:241–252.

Henry RA, Johnson RC. 1978. Distribution of the genus *Leptospira* in soil and water. Appl Environ Microbiol 35:492–499.

Herbst W, Hertrampf B, Schmitt T, Weiss R, Baljer G. 2003. Diagnosis of *Lawsonia intracellularis* using the polymerase chain reaction (PCR) in pigs with and without diarrhea and other animal species. Dtsch Tierarztl Wochenschr 110:361–364.

Hess WR, Endris RG, Haslett TM, Monahan MJ, McCoy JP. 1987. Potential arthropod vectors of African swine fever virus in North America and the Caribbean basin. Vet Parasitol 26:145–155.

Hirvelä-Koski V, Aho M, Asplund K, Hatakka M, Hirn J. 1985. *Trichinella spiralis* in wild animals, cats, mice, rats and farmed fur animals in Finland. Nord Vet Med 37:234–242.

Hone J. 1994. A mathematical model of detection and dynamics of porcine transmissible gastroenteritis. Epidemiol Infect 113:187–197.

Hooper CC, Van Alstine WG, Stevenson GW, Kanitz CL. 1994. Mice and rats (laboratory and feral) are not a reservoir for PRRSV virus. J Vet Diagn Invest 6:13–15.

Hughes RW, Gustafson DP. 1960. Some factors may influence hog cholera transmission. Am J Vet Res 21:464–471.

Hurd HS, Gailey JK, McKean JD, Rostagno MH. 2001. Rapid infection in market-weight swine following exposure to a *Salmonella* Typhimurium-contaminated environment. Am J Vet Res 62:1194–1197.

Hutchings LM, Andrews FN. 1946. Studies on brucellosis in swine. III. Brucella infection in the boar. Am J Vet Res 25:379–384.

Ichiyama S, Shimokata K, Tsukamura M. 1988. The isolation of *Mycobacterium avium* complex from soil, water, and dusts. Microbiol Immunol 32:733–739.

Jeffrey DJ. 1995. Chemicals used as disinfectants: active ingredients and enhancing additives. Rev Sci Technique 14:57–74.

Jobert JL, Savoye C, Cariolet, Kobisch M, Madec F. 2000. Experimental aerosol transmission of *Actinobacillus pleuropneumoniae* to pigs. Can J Vet Res 64:21–26.

Joens LA. 1980. Experimental transmission of *Treponema hyodysenteriae* from mice to pigs. Am J Vet Res 41:1225–1226.

Joens LA, Kinyon JM. 1982. isolation of *Treponema hyodysenteriae* from wild rodents. J Clin Microbiol 15:994–997.

Jones R, Kelly L, French N, England T, Livesey C, Woolridge M. 2004. Quantitative estimates of the risk of new outbreaks of foot-and-mouth disease as a result of burning pyres. Vet Rec 154:161–165.

Jorsal SE, Thomsen BL. 1988. A cox regression analysis of risk factors related to *Mycoplasma suipneumoniae* reinfection in Danish SPF-herds. Acta Vet Scand (suppl) 84:436–438.

Karaseva EV, Chernukha YG, Sakhartseva TF. 1977. Results of the investigation of soil for contamination with pathogenic leptospires. Folia Parasitol 24:301–304.

Kendal AP, Goldfield M, Noble GR, Dowdle WR. 1977. Identification and preliminary antigenic analysis of swine influenza-like viruses isolated during an influenza outbreak at Fort Dix, New Jersey. J Infect Dis 136:S381–S385.

Kennedy MA, Mellon VS, Caldwell G, Potgieter LND. 1995. Virucidal efficacy of the newer quaternary ammonium compounds. J Am Anim Hosp Assoc 31:254–258.

Kim J, Han DU, Choi C, Chae C. 2001. Differentiation of porcine circovirus (PCV)-1 and PCV-2 in boar semen using a multiplex nested polymerase chain reaction. J Virol Methods 98:25–31.

——. 2003. Simultaneous detection and differentiation between porcine circovirus and porcine parvovirus in boar semen by multiplex seminested polymerase chain reaction. J Vet Med Sci 65:741–744.

Kingscote BF. 1986. Leptospirosis outbreak in a piggery in southern Alberta. Can Vet J 27:188–190.

Kirk JH, Holmberg CA, Jeffrey JS. 2002. Prevalence of *Salmonella* spp in selected birds captured on California dairies. J Am Vet Med Assoc 220:359–366.

Kirkpatrick CM, Kanitz CL, McCrocklin SM. 1980. Possible role of wild mammals in transmission of pseudorabies to swine. J Wildl Dis 16: 601–614.

Koppang N, Filseth O. 1958. The bacterial flora of semen and prepuce in boars. Nord Vet Med 10:603–609.

Körmendy B, Nagy G. 1982. The supposed involvement of dogs carrying *Brucella suis* in the spread of swine brucellosis. Acta Vet Acad Sci Hungaricae 30:1–7.

Kristensen CS, Bøtner A, Takai H, Nielsen JP, Jorsal SE. 2004. Experimental airborne transmission of PRRS virus. Vet Microbiol 99:197–202.

Laddomada A. 2003. Control and eradication of O.I.E. List A diseases the approach of the European Union to the use of vaccines. Developments in Biologicals 114:269–280.

Laevens H, Koenen F, Deluyker H, Berkvens D, de Kruif A. 1998. An experimental infection with classical swine fever virus in weaner pigs. Vet Quart 20:41–45.

Laevens H, Koenen F, Deluyker H, de Kruif A. 1999. Experimental infection of slaughter pigs with classical swine fever virus: transmission of the virus, course of the disease and antibody response. Vet Rec 145:243–248.

Lambooy E, van Voorst N. 1986. Electrocution of pigs infected with notifiable diseases. Vet Quart 8:80–82.

Larochelle R, Bielanski A, Müller P, Magar R. 2000. PCR detection and evidence of shedding of porcine circovirus type 2 in boar semen. J Clin Microbiol 38:4629–4632.

Larson DJ, Morehouse LG, Solorzano RF, Kinden DA. 1979. Transmissible gastroenteritis in neonatal dogs: Experimental intestinal infection with transmissible gastroenteritis virus. Am J Vet Res 40:477–486.

Le Moine V, Vannier P, Jestin A. 1987. Microbiological studies of wild rodents in farms as carriers of pig infectious agents. Prev Vet Med 4:399–408.

Letellier A, Messier S, Paré J, Ménard J, Quessy S. 1999. Distribution of *Salmonella* in swine herds in Québec. Vet Microbiol 67:299–306.

Lord VR, Cherwonogrodzky JW, Marcano MJ, Melendez G. 1997. Serological and bacteriological study of swine brucellosis. J Clin Microbiol 35:295–297.

Lucas MH, Cartright SF, Wrathall AE. 1974. Genital infection of pigs with porcine parvovirus. J Comp Pathol 84:347–350.

Madsen LW, Aalbæk B, Nielsen OL, Jensen HE. 2001. Aerogenous infection of microbiologically defined minipigs with *Streptococcus suis* serotype 2. Acta Pathol, Microbiol Immunol Scand 109:412–418.

Maes RK, Kanitz CL, Gustafson DP. 1979.Pseudorabies virus infections in wild and laboratory rats. Am J Vet Res 40:393–396.

Marshall B, Flynn P, Kamely D, Levy SB. 1988. Survival of *Escherichia coli* with and without ColE1::Tn5 after aerosol dispersion in a laboratory and a farm environment. Appl Environ Microbiol 54:1776–1783.

Marshall B, Petrowski D, Levey SB. 1990. Inter- and intraspecies spread of *Escherichia coli* in a farm environment in the absence of antibiotic usage. Proc National Acad Sci USA 87:6609–6613.

Mårtensson L, Holmberg T, Hurvell B, Rutqvist L, Sandstedt K, Wierup M. 1984. Salmonella isolated from animals and feed stuffs in Sweden during 1978–1982. Nord Vet Med 36:371–393.

Marti OG, Booram CV, Hale OM. 1980. Survival of eggs and larvae of swine nematode parasites in aerobic and anaerobic waste treatment systems. J Environ Quality 9:401–405.

Martin RJ, Schnurrenberger PR, Andersen FL, Hsu C-K. 1968. Prevalence of *Trichinella spiralis* in wild animals on two Illinois swine farms. J Parasitol 54:108–111.

McAdaragh JP, Anderson GA. 1975. Transmission of viruses through boar semen. In Proc 18th Am Assoc Vet Lab Diagn, pp.69–76.

McDermid AS, Lever MS. 1996. Survival of *Salmonella enteritidis* PT4 and *Salm. typhimurium* Swindon in aerosols. Letters Appl Microbiol 23:107–109.

McDonnell G, Russell D. 1999. Antiseptics and Disinfectants: Activity, Action, and Resistance. Clin Microbiol Revi 12: 147–179.

McKercher PD, Blackwell JH, Murphy R, Callis JJ, Panina GF, Civardi A, Bugnetti M, De Simone F, Scatozza F. 1985. Survival of swine vesicular disease virus in "Prosciutto di Parma" (Parma Ham). J Can Inst Food Sci Technol 18:163–167.

McKercher PD, Graves JH, Callis JJ, Carmichael F. 1974. Swine vesicular disease: virus survival in pork products. In Proc Annu Meet US Anim Health Assoc. pp. 213a–213g.

McNaughton CL. 1988. Guidelines for depopulation and repopulation of swine herds. Compend Contin Educ Vet Pract 10:1233–1239.

McVicar JW, Eisner RJ, Johnson LA, Pursel VG. 1978. Foot-and-mouth disease and swine vesicular disease viruses in boar semen. In Proc 81st Annu Meet US Anim Health Assoc. pp. 221–230.

Mead DG, Gray EW, Noblet R, Murphy MD, Howerth EW, Stallknecht DE. 2004. Biological transmission of vesicular stomatitis virus (New Jersey serotype) by *Simulium vittatum* (Diptera: Simuliidae) to domestic swine. J Med Entomol 41:78–82.

Mebus C, Aria M, Pineda JM, Tapiador J, House C, Sánchez-Vizcaíno JM. 1997. Survival of several porcine viruses in different Spanish dry-cured meat products. Food Chem 59:555–559.

Mebus C, House C, Gonzalvo FR, Pineda JM, Tapiador J, Pire JJ, Bergada J, Yedloutschnig RJ, Sahu S, Becerra V, Sánchez-Vizcaíno JM. 1993. Survival of foot-and-mouth disease, African swine fever, and hog cholera viruses in Spanish serrano cured hams and Iberian cured hams, shoulders and loins. Food Microbiol 10:133–143.

Medveczky I, Kovács F, Papp L. 1988. The role of the housefly. *Musca domestica*, in the spread of Aujesky's disease (pseduorabies). Med Vet Entomol 2:81–86.

Medveczky I, Szabó I. 1981. Isolation of Aujesky's disease virus from boar semen. Acta Vet Acad Sci Hungaricae 29:29–35.

Mellor PS, Kitching RP, Wilkinson PJ. 1987. Mechanical transmission of capripox virus and African swine fever virus by *Stomoxys calcitrans*. Res Vet Sci 43:109–112.

Mellor PS, Wilkinson PJ. 1985. Experimental transmission of African swine fever virus by *Ornithodoros savignyi* (Audouin). Res Vet Sci 39:353–356.

Mengeling WL, Paul PS. 1986. Interepizootic survival of porcine parvovirus. J Am Vet Med Assoc 188:1293–1295.

Mengeling WL, Vorwald AC, Lager KM, Brockmeier S. 1996. Comparison among strains of porcine reproductive and respiratory syndrome virus for their ability to cause reproductive failure. Am J Vet Res 57:834–839.

Mészáros J, Stipkovits L, Antal T, Szabó I, Veszely P. 1985. Eradication of some infectious pig diseases by perinatal tiamulin treatment and early weaning. Vet Rec 116:8–12.

Meyer RC, Bohl EH, Kohler EM. 1964. Procurement and maintenance of germ-free swine for microbiological investigations. Appl Microbiol 12:295–300.

Mitchell CA, Guerin LF. 1972. Influenza A of human, swine, equine and avian origin: Comparison of survival in aerosol form. Can J Comp Med 36:9–11.

Morrow WE, O'Quinn P, Barker J, Erickson G, Post K, McCaw M. 1995. Composting as a suitable technique for managing swine mortalities. Swine Health Prod 3:236–243.

Müller W, Wieser P, Kühme H. 1978. Zur frage der ausbreitung von luftkeimen aus tierställen. Zentralbl Veterinarmed B 25:216–224.

Munch B, Larsen HE, Aalbaek B. 1987. Experimental studies on the survival of pathogenic and indicator bacteria in aerated and non-aerated cattle and pig slurry. Biological Wastes 22:49–65.

Nel EE. 1981. Mycobacterium avium-intracellulare complex serovars isolated in South Africa from humans, swine, and the environment. Rev Infect Dis 3:1013–1020.

Nicholes PS. 1970. Bacteria in laundered fabrics. Am J Public Health Nation's Health 60:2175–2180.

O'Brien RJ, Noble GR, Easterday BC, Kendal AP, Shasby DM, Nelson DB, Hattwick MAW, Dowdle WR. 1977. Swine-like virus infection in a Wisconsin farm family. J Infect Dis 136:S390–S396.

Orr KE, Holliday MG, Jones AL, Robson I, Perry JD. 2002. Survival of enterococci during hospital laundry processing. J Hosp Infect 50:133–139.

Otake S, Dee SA, Jacobson L, Torremorell M, Pijoan C. 2002a. Evaluation of aerosol transmission of porcine reproductive and respiratory syndrome virus under controlled field conditions. Vet Rec 150:804–808.

Otake S, Dee SA, Rossow KD, Deen J, Joo HS, Molitor TW, Pijoan C. 2002b. Transmission of porcine reproductive and respiratory syndrome virus by fomites (boots and coveralls). J Swine Health Prod 10:59–65.

Otake S, Dee SA, Rossow KD, Joo HS, Deen J, Molitor TW, Pijoan C. 2002c. Transmission of porcine reproductive and respiratory syndrome virus by needles. Vet Rec 150:114–115.

Otake S, Dee SA, Rossow KD, Moon RD, Pijoan C. 2002d. Mechanical transmission of porcine reproductive and respira-

tory syndrome virus by mosquitoes, *Aedes vexans* (Meigen). Can J Vet Res 66:191–195.

Otake S, Dee SA, Rossow KD, Moon RD, Trincado C, Pijoan C. 2003. Transmission of porcine reproductive and respiratory syndrome virus by houseflies (*Musca domestica*). Vet Rec 152:73–76.

Panina GF, Civardi A, Cordioli P, Massiro I, Scatozza F, Baldini P, Palmia F. 1992. Survival of hog cholera virus (HCV) in sausage meat products (Italian salami). Int J Food Microbiol 17:19–25.

Patrick DR, Findon G, Miller TE. 1997. Residual moisture determines the level of touch-contact-associated bacterial transfer following hand washing. Epidemiol Infect 119:319–325.

Pensaert M, Ottis K, Vandeputte J, Kaplan MM, Bachmann PA. 1981. Evidence for the natural transmission of influenza A virus from wild ducks to swine and its potential importance for man. Bull World Health Org 59:75–78.

Phillips RM, Foley CW, Lukert PD. 1972. Isolation and characterization of viruses from semen and the reproductive tract of male swine. J Am Vet Med Assoc 161:1306–1316.

Pilchard EI. 1965. Experimental transmission of transmissible gastroenteritis virus by starlings. Am J Vet Res 26:1177–1179.

Pirtle EC, Beran GW. 1991. Virus survival in the environment. Rev Sci Technique 10:733–748.

——. 1996. Stability of porcine reproductive and respiratory syndrome virus in the presence of fomites commonly found on farms. J Am Vet Med Assoc 208:390–392.

Plowright W, Parker J, Peirce MA. 1969a. The epizootiology of African swine fever in Africa. Vet Rec 85:668–674.

——. 1969b. African swine fever virus in ticks (*Ornithodoros moubata*, Murray) collected from animal burrows in Tanzania. Nature 221:1071–1073.

Porter JF, Parton R, Wardlaw AC. 1991. Growth and survival of Bordertella bronchiseptica in natural waters and in buffered saline without added nutrients. Appl Environ Microbiol 57:1202–1206.

Poumian AM. 1995. Disinfection of trucks and trailers. Rev Sci Technique 14:171–176.

Predicala BZ, Urban JE, Maghirang RG, Jerez SB, Goodband RD. 2002. Assessment of bioaerosols in swine barns by filtration and impaction. Current Microbiol 44:136–140.

Prieto C, Suárez P, Martín-Rillo S, Simarro I, Solano A, Castro JM. 1996. Effect of porcine reproductive and respiratory syndrome virus (PRRSV) on development of porcine fertilized ova in vitro. Theriogenology 46:687–693.

Prieto C, Suárez P, Sánchez R, Solana A, Simarro I, Rillo SM, Castro JM. 1994. Semen changes in boars after experimental infection with "Porcine Epidemic Abortion and Respiratory Syndrome (PEARS) virus. In Proc 13th Int Pig Vet Soc Congr. p.98.

Prieto C, Suárez P, Simarro I, García C, Fernández A, Castro JM. 1997a. Transplacental infection following exposure of gilts to porcine reproductive and respiratory syndrome virus at the onset of gestation. Vet Microbiol 57:301–311.

Prieto C, Suárez P, Simarro I, García C, Martín-Rillo S, Castro JM. 1997b. Insemination of susceptible and preimmunized gilts with boar semen containing porcine reproductive and respiratory syndrome virus. Theriogenology 47:647–654.

Prullage JB, Williams RE, Gaafar SM. 1993. On the transmissibility of *Eperythrozoon suis* by *Stomoxys calcitrans* and *Aedes aegypti*. Vet Parasitol 50:125–135.

Puthucheary SD, Thong ML, Parasakthi N. 1981. Evaluation of some hand washing and disinfection methods in the removal of transient bacterial flora. Malaysian J Pathol 4:49–55.

Pyburn DG. 2003. The Trichinae Certification Program and the role of swine veterinarians. J Swine Health Prod 11:190–192.

Pyburn DG, Schwartz K. 1995. A review of segregated early weaning. Iowa State Vet 57:56–60.

Quinn PJ. 1991. Disinfection and disease prevention in veterinary medicine. In: Block SS (ed). Disinfection, Sterilization, and Preservation (4th ed). Lea and Febiger, Philadelphia. pp.846–868.

Rajkowski KT, Eblen S, Laubauch C. 1998. Efficacy of washing and sanitizing trailers used for swine transport in reduction of Salmonella and Escherichia coli. J Food Protection 61:31–35.

Randall AE, Pettitt MJ, Plante C, Buckrell BC, Randall GCB, Henderson JM, Larochelle R, Magar R, Pollard JW. 1999. Elimination of porcine reproductive and respiratory syndrome virus through embryo transfer. Theriogenology 51:274–274.

Renn N. 1998. The efficacy of entomopathogenic nematodes for controlling housefly infestations of intensive pig units. Med Vet Entomol 12:46–51.

Richmond JY. 1978. Preadsorption of boar semen with kaolin: Increased efficiency of foot-and-mouth disease virus detection. Am J Vet Res 39:1612–1616.

Rose N, Madec F. 2002. Occurrence of respiratory disease outbreaks in fattening pigs: Relation with the features of a densely and a sparsely populated pig area in France. Vet Res 33:179–190.

Salasia SIO, Lämmler C. 1994. Serotypes and putative virulence markers of *Streptococcus suis* isolates from cats and dogs. Res Vet Sci 57:259–261.

Sander JE, Warbington MC, Myers LM. 2002. Selected methods of animal carcass disposal. J Am Vet Med Assoc 220:1003–1005.

Savi P, Baldelli B, Morozzi A. 1962. Présence et persistence du virus aphteux dans les viandes de porcins et de bovins et dans leurs produits dérivés. Bull Office Int Epizooties 57:853–890.

Scheidt AB, Rueff LR, Grant RH, Teclaw RF, Hill MA, Meyer KB, Clark LK. 1991. Epizootic of pseudorabies among ten swine herds. J Am Vet Med Assoc 199:725–730.

Schnurrenberger PR, Held LJ, Martin RJ, Quist KD, Galton MM. 1968. Prevalence of *Salmonella* spp. in domestic animals and wildlife on selected Illinois farms. J Am Vet Med Assoc 153:442–524.

Schoenbaum MA, Freund JD, Beran GW. 1991. Survival of pseudorabies virus in the presence of selected diluents and fomites. J Am Vet Med Assoc 198:1393–1397.

Schoenbaum MA, Zimmerman JJ, Beran GW, Murphy DP. 1990. Survival of pseudorabies virus in aerosol. Am J Vet Res 51:331–333.

Sellers RF, Donaldson AI, Herniman KAJ. 1970. Inhalation, persistence and dispersal of foot-and-mouth disease virus by man. J Hygiene Camb 68:565–573.

Sellers RF, Gloster J. 1980. The Northumberland epidemic of foot-and-mouth disease 1966. J Hygiene Camb 85:129–140.

Sellers RF, Herniman KAJ. 1974. The airborne excretion by pigs of swine vesicular disease virus. J Hygiene Camb 72:61–65.

Sellers RF, Herniman KAJ, Mann JA. 1971. Transfer of foot-and-mouth disease virus in the nose of man from infected to non-infected animals. Vet Rec 89:447–449.

Sellers RF, Parker J. 1969. Airborne excretion of foot-and-mouth disease virus. J Hygiene Camb 67:671–677.

Seo KH, Mitchell BW, Holt PS, Gast RK. 2001. Bactericidal effects of negative air ions on airborne and surface *Salmonella Enteriditis* from an artificially generated aerosol. J Food Protection 64:113–116.

Shelton JN. 1987. Prospects for the use of embryos in the control of disease and the transport of genotypes. Aust Vet J 64:6–10.

Shin J, Torrison J, Choi CS, Gonzalez SM, Crabo BG, Molitor TW. 1997. Monitoring of porcine reproductive and respiratory syndrome virus infection in boars. Vet Microbiol 55:337–346.

Shope RE. 1940. Swine pox. Archiv Virusforschung Bd 1:457–467.

Sidorenko GI. 1967. Data on the distribution of Clostridium perfringens in the environment of man. J Hygiene Epidemiol Microbiol Immunol 11:171–176.

Sidwell RW, Dixon GJ, Westbrook L, Forziati FH. 1970. Quantitative studies on fabrics as disseminators of viruses. IV. Virus transmission by dry contact of fabrics. Appl Microbiol 19:950–954.

——. 1971. Quantitative studies on fabrics as disseminators of viruses. V. Effect of laundering on poliovirus-contaminated fabrics. Appl Microbiol 21:227–234.

Siegel AM, Weigel RM. 1999. Herd factors affecting the selection and success of intervention strategies in the program for eradication of pseudorabies (Aujeszky's disease) virus from Illinois swine farms. Prev Vet Med 40:243–259.

Singh EL, Dulac GC, Hare WCD. 1984. Embryo transfer as a means of controlling the transmission of viral infections. V. The in vitro exposure of zona pellucida-intact porcine embryos to African swine fever virus. Theriogenology 22:693–700.

Singh EL, McVicar JW, Hare WCD, Mebus CA. 1986. Embryo transfer as a means of controlling the transmission of viral infections. VII. The in vitro exposure of bovine and porcine embryos to foot-and-mouth disease virus. Theriogenology 26: 587–593.

Singh EL, Thomas FC. 1987. Embryo transfer as a means of controlling the transmission of viral infections. XI. The in vitro exposure of bovine and porcine embryos to vesicular stomatitis virus. Theriogenology 28:691–697.

Slavin G. 1938. The resistance of the swine fever virus to physical agencies and chemical disinfectants. J Comp Pathol Therapeutics 51:213–224.

Smith KE, Zimmerman JJ, Patton S, Beran GW, Hill HT. 1992. The epidemiology of toxoplasmosis on Iowa swine farms with an emphasis on the roles of free-living mammals. Vet Parasitol 42:199–211.

Snyder DE. 1987. Prevalence and intensity of *Trichinella spiralis* infection in Illinois wildlife. J Parasitol 73:874–875.

Songer JG, Chilelli CJ, Reed RE, Trautman RJ. 1983. Leptospirosis in rodents from an arid environment. Am J Vet Res 44:1973–1976.

Songer JG, Glock RD, Schwartz KJ, Harris DL. 1978. Isolation of *Treponema hyodysenteriae* from sources other than swine. J Am Vet Med Assoc 172:464–466.

Stärk KDC. 1999. The role of infectious aerosols in disease transmission in pigs. Vet J 158:164–181.

Stärk KDC, Keller H, Eggenberger E. 1992. Risk factors for the reinfection of specific pathogen-free pig breeding herds with enzootic pneumonia. Vet Rec 131:532–535.

Stärk KDC, Nicolet J, Frey J. 1998. Detection of *Mycoplasma hyopneumoniae* by air sampling with a nested PCR assay. Appl Environ Microbiol 64:543–548.

Stegeman A, Elbers ARW, Bouma A, de Smit H, de Jong M. 1999. Transmission of classical swine fever virus within herds during the 1997–1998 epidemic in The Netherlands. Prev Vet Med 42:201–218.

Stehmann R, Mehlhorn G, Neuparth V. 1991. Characterization of strains of *Bordetella bronchiseptica* isolated from animal housing air and of airborne infection pressure proceeding from them. Dtsch Tierarztl Wochenscr 98:448–450.

Stewart WC, Carbrey EA, Jenney EW, Kresse JI, Snyder ML, Wessman SJ. 1975. Transmission of hog cholera virus by mosquitoes. Am J Vet Res 36:611–614.

Strauch D. 1991. Survival of pathogenic micro-organisms and parasites in excreta, manure and sewage sludge. Rev Sci Technique 10:813–846.

Swenson SL, Hill HT, Zimmerman JJ, Evans LE, Landgraf JG, Will RW, Sanderson TP, McGinley MJ, Brevik AK, Ciszewski DK, Frey ML. 1994b. Excretion of porcine reproductive and respiratory syndrome virus in semen after experimentally induced infection in boars. J Am Med Assoc 204:1943–1948.

Swenson SL, Hill HT, Zimmerman JJ, Evans LE, Wills RW, Yoon K-J, Schwartz KJ, Althouse GC, McGinley MJ, Brevik AK. 1994a. Artificial insemination of gilts with porcine reproductive and respiratory syndrome (PRRS) virus-contaminated semen. Swine Health Prod 2:19–23.

Tamasi G. 1981. Factors influencing the survival of pathogenic bacteria in soils. Acta Vet Acad Sci Hungaricae 29:119–126.

——. 1995. Testing disinfectants for efficacy. Rev Sci Technique 14:75–79.

Terpstra C, Krol B. 1976. Effect of heating on the survival of swine fever virus in pasteurized canned ham from experimentally infected animals. Tijdschr Diergeneeskd 101:1237–1241.

Thacker BJ, Larsen RE, Joo HS, Leman AD. 1984. Swine diseases transmissible with artificial insemination. J Am Vet Med Assoc 185:511–516.

Thomsen BL, Jorsal SE, Anderson S, Willeberg P. 1992. The Cox regression model applied to risk factor analysis of infections in the breeding and multiplying herds in the Danish SPF system. Prev Vet Med 12:287–297.

Thomson CMA, Chanter N, Wathes CM. 1992. Survival of toxigenic *Pasteurella multocida* in aerosols and aqueous liquids. Appl Environ Microbiol,58:932–936.

Thrusfield M. 1995. Veterinary Epidemiology (2nd ed). United Kingdom: Blackwell Science Ltd.

Tidwell MA, Dean WD, Tidwell MA, Combs GP, Anderson DW, Cowart WO, Axtell RC. 1972. Transmission of hog cholera virus by horseflies (Tabanidae: Diptera). Am J Vet Res 33:615–622.

Top FH, Russell PK. 1977. Swine influenza A at Fort Dix, New Jersey (January–February 1976). IV. Summary and speculation. J Infect Dis 136:S376–S380.

Torremorell M, Pijoan C, Janni K, Walker R, Joo HS. 1997. Airborne transmission of *Actinobacillus pleuropneumoniae* and porcine reproductive and respiratory syndrome virus in nursery pigs. Am J Vet Res 58:828–831.

Ulloa A, Arredondo-Jiménez JI, Rodriguez MH, Fernández-Salas I. 2002. Mark-recapture studies of host selection by *Anopheles (Anopheles) vestitipennis*. J Am Mosquito Control Assoc 18:32–35.

United States Department of Agriculture, Animal and Plant Health Inspection Service, Veterinary Services. 1992. Foot-and-mouth Disease Emergency Guidelines. Marketing and Regulatory Programs, Maryland.

Vannier P, Madec F, Tillon JP, Monicat F. 1989. Isolation of Aujesky's disease virus from dust in a piggery with infected pigs. In: Wathes CM, Randall JM (eds). Aerosol Sampling in Animal Houses. Commission of the European Communities, Luxembourg. pp.114–116.

Walter WG, Schillinger JE. 1975. Bacterial survival in laundered fabrics. Appl Microbiol 29:368–373.

Waltz FA, Foley CW, Herschler RC, Tiffany LW, Liska BJ. 1968. bacteriological studies of boar semen. J Anim Sci 27:1357–1362.

Wathes CM, Howard K, Webster AJF. 1986. The survival of *Escherichia coli* in an aerosol at air temperatures of 15 and 30°C and a range of humidities. J Hygiene Camb 97:489–496.

Weber A, Schramm R. 1989. The occurrence of *Treponema* in fecal samples from dogs and cats with and without intestinal diseases. Berl Munch Tierarztl Wochenscr 102:73–77.

Wells DL, Hopfensperger DJ, Arden NH, Harmon MW, Davis JP, Tipple MA, Schonberger LB. 1991. Swine influenza virus infections. Transmission from ill pigs to humans at a Wisconsin agricultural fair and subsequent probable person-to-person transmission. J Am Med Assoc 265:478–481.

Wentworth DE, McGregor MW, Macklin MD, Neumann V, Hinshaw VS. 1997. Transmission of swine influenza virus to humans after exposure to experimentally infected pigs. J Infect Dis 175:7–15.

Wetzler TF, Quan TJ, Schatzle K. 1971. Critical analysis of the microflora of toweling. Am J Public Health Nation's Health 61:376–392.

Whiting TL. 2003. Foreign animal disease outbreaks, the animal welfare implications for Canada: Risks apparent from international experience. Can Vet J 44:805–815.

Wiksell JC, Pickett MS, Hartman PA. 1973. Survival of microorganisms in laundered polyester-cotton sheeting. Appl Microbiol 25:431–435.

Wilkinson PJ, Donaldson AI, Greig A, Bruce W. 1977. Transmission studies with African swine fever virus Infections of pigs by airborne virus. J Comp Pathol 87:487–495.

Williams RE. 1992. Control of flies in swine operations. Compend Contin Educ Vet Pract 14:689–692.

Wills RW, Zimmerman JJ, Swenson SL, Yoon K-J, Hill HT, Bundy DS, McGinley MJ. 1997. Transmission of PRRSV by direct, close, or indirect contact. J Swine Health Prod 5:213–218.

Wood RL. 1973. Survival of *Erysipelothrix rhusiopathiae* in soil under various environmental conditions. Cornell Vet 63:390–410.

Wood RL, Packer RA. 1972. Isolation of *Erysipelothrix rhusiopathiae* from soil and manure of swine-raising premises. Am J Vet Res 33:1611–1620.

Young GA, Underdahl NR, Hinz RW. 1955. Procurement of baby pigs by hysterectomy. Am J Vet Res 16:123–131.

Zimmerman JJ, Berry WJ, Beran GW, Murphy DP. 1989. Influence of temperature and age on the recovery of pseudorabies virus from houseflies (*Musca domestica*). Am J Vet Res 50:1471–1474.

Zimmerman JJ, Yoon K-J, Pirtle EC, Wills RW, Sanderson TJ, McGinley MJ. 1997. Studies of porcine reproductive and respiratory syndrome (PRRS) virus infection in avian species. Vet Microbiol 55:329–336.

69 Disease Surveillance in Swine Populations

Peter R. Davies and Katharina D. C. Stärk

Animal disease surveillance is in a phase of rapid evolution and innovation. The impetus for this change arises from several factors including greater recognition of the frequency and impact of emerging diseases, increasing volumes of international trade in animal products, requirements of trading countries and obligations specified under agreements of the World Trade Organization (WTO), ongoing consolidation of animal production worldwide into fewer and larger populations, and the threat of agriterrorism in the wake of September 11. Collectively these factors translate into greater demand among government agencies and other entities for more powerful tools for detecting changing patterns of disease in animal populations. In the contemporary global business environment, efficient disease surveillance provides the foundation for trust in international trade in animals and animal products (Salman et al. 2003). Ongoing advances in communications technology and information management, and technological advances in diagnostics (Risatti et al. 2003), are creating new opportunities for animal disease surveillance.

A recent text edited by Salman (2003) provides a comprehensive overview of the fundamentals of animal disease surveillance and survey systems, principally from the perspective of government agencies responsible for regulated disease control and eradication programs. However, disease surveillance has a growing role in other arenas, particularly at an industry level and in large corporate production systems that make up much of the swine industry of many developed countries (Table 69.1).

Wildlife populations can be important reservoirs for animal diseases (Elbers et al. 2000; Morner et al. 2002), and increased wildlife surveillance has been prompted by increased recognition of the role of wildlife in emerging diseases. At the level of individual commercial herds, disease surveillance has historically involved recording of gross lesions in slaughtered pigs. Readers seeking specific information on slaughter surveillance in swine are referred to the previous edition of *Diseases of Swine* (Pointon et al. 1999). In contrast, due to cost considerations, routine surveillance using laboratory testing has been traditionally less frequent at the herd level. However, demographic changes in the industry (increased herd sizes, consolidation, multiple-site production), improved diagnostic tests, and persistent problems with porcine reproductive and respiratory syndrome (PRRS) in many countries including the U.S., have altered both the need for and feasibility of herd-level surveillance systems (Torrison 1998). In this chapter we attempt to provide an update on current developments in animal health surveillance, and identify opportunities for enhancing surveillance efforts in the context of modern swine production in developed countries.

THE SCOPE OF SURVEILLANCE IN SWINE PRODUCTION

Disease surveillance is a management information tool. In essence, surveillance encompasses activities undertaken to measure disease events in defined populations in order to obtain information of value to decision makers (e.g., producers, veterinarians, industry, government agencies). Surveillance information is applicable to support decisions about health status certification; compliance with customer requirements; compliance with regulatory requirements; and health management decisions, including treatment and preventive measures and altering pig flow. Fundamental objectives of surveillance are to establish the qualitative status of animal populations (groups, sites, pods, companies, regions, or countries) with respect to the presence or absence of a specific disease or agent, or to quantify frequency of disease in affected populations and its distribution in space and time (determining disease trends). Salman et al. (2003) addressed the distinction between monitoring and surveillance that pervades the veterinary literature, and adopted the acronym "MOSS" (designating "monitoring or surveillance system") as an umbrella term to

Table 69.1. Overview of overall objectives and purposes of surveillance activities in different arenas

Arena	Objective	Purpose
National (State)	Demonstrate freedom from disease	Maintain trade access
	Outbreak detection	Facilitate response capability to exotic and novel diseases
	Disease control and eradication	Optimize operational efficiency of regulatory programs
	Monitor notifiable diseases	Gather epidemiologic intelligence to support regulatory decisions
	Monitor zoonotic and foodborne pathogens	Protect public health; maintain trade access
	Monitor emerging diseases	Early detection of novel pathogens
Industry/Corporate	Assure freedom from disease	Breeding stock suppliers; boar studs—protect production pyramids
	Outbreak detection	Protect production pyramids
	Define herd disease status	Inform pig flow decisions
	Monitor endemic production diseases	Epidemiologic intelligence to support health management decisions
	Monitor zoonotic and foodborne pathogens	Public health and trade access; quality assurance and product differentiation
	Indexes of animal welfare	Address consumer concerns; quality assurance
Commercial production	Monitor endemic production diseases	Support health management decisions
	Outbreak detection	Early response to minimize disease impact
Wildlife	Establish disease status	Support regulatory decisions and control programs

discuss the relevant concepts. Similarly, for simplicity we will use the term *surveillance* in a generic sense to include the spectrum of activities that encompass either surveillance or monitoring.

The cornerstone of any epidemiologic endeavor is case definition. Historically the primary focus of animal disease surveillance has been agent-defined infectious diseases, such as diseases listed by the Office International des Épizooties (OIE), or zoonotic or other diseases targeted in national control programs (tuberculosis, brucellosis, hog cholera, pseudorabies). As such, case definition is typically founded on use of agent-specific diagnostic tests (see Chapter 10 on interpretation of laboratory results). Growing concerns about the emergence of apparently novel diseases and of bioterrorism targeting human or animal populations, have led to development of systems for "syndromic" surveillance in both the human and animal arenas (de Groot et al. 2003; Pavlin 2003). Case definition in syndromic surveillance is based on clinical symptoms rather than agent-specific diagnostic testing. For both agent-defined and syndromic surveillance, the precision and accuracy of data are influenced by case definition and other factors and can be enhanced by implementation of standard approaches for quality control (Stärk et al. 2002; Salman et al. 2003).

Although the term *syndromic surveillance* is now very much in mode, both the concept and practice are established pillars of population medicine in food animals. Most of the standard indexes that veterinarians and producers use to assess herd population health and performance are syndromic. Obvious examples are mortality incidence in different age groups of stock, prevalence of stillbirths and mummification in neonatal pigs, and lameness or abortion rates. Typically, fail-

ure to meet predetermined targets triggers further investigation or corrective actions, and these concepts have been widely addressed in the production medicine literature (Deen at al. 2001). For this reason, we will focus our discussion on surveillance opportunities in relation to known and emerging diseases of swine. Because government and regulatory perspectives on surveillance issues have been well covered elsewhere (Salman 2003), our emphasis will be in the arena of modern commercial production, where veterinarians are confronted with rapid change and increasingly complex decisions about disease surveillance in large systems.

COMPONENTS OF A SURVEILLANCE SYSTEM

Surveillance comprises collection, analysis, and interpretation of disease data, coupled with dissemination of the information to decision-makers responsible for implementing appropriate actions (Buehler 1998). At the herd level in traditional farrow-to-finish production, surveillance of pig health has included monitoring of clinical signs, production indexes, and lesions in slaughtered pigs as predominantly syndromic indicators, triggering more specific diagnostic efforts when aberrations were detected. Structural (e.g., multiple-site production in large systems) and operational (e.g., artificial insemination based around boar studs) changes in the industry have ushered in new challenges in surveillance as a tool for managing health risks in swine populations. Veterinarians serving these systems are now confronted with more complex problems of designing sampling and testing programs to obtain the information they require at acceptable cost.

There are many potential sources of surveillance

data, ranging from surveys of producers about animal health to results of diagnostic tests performed in national or international reference laboratories (Doherr and Audige 2001). Inevitably there are trade-offs between the reliability and scope of data, and at a regulatory level diagnostic laboratories have provided the bulk of surveillance data. However, different sources of data provide different (and probably complementary) perspectives on the frequency of health events in herds (McIntyre et al. 2002). Because the utility of disease surveillance is in part determined by timeliness, ideally the processes of data collection and analysis should approach real time, and the value of diagnostic data decays over time (Schlosser and Ebel 2001).

DESIGN ASPECTS OF POPULATION SURVEILLANCE

The principles underlying the use and interpretation of diagnostic testing are reviewed elsewhere in this text (see Chapter 10). It is imperative for veterinarians who confront complex surveillance decisions to have a strong theoretical understanding of the relationships between diagnostic test performance, sampling theory, and disease prevalence that underpin the interpretation of aggregate (herd-level) testing. In evaluating testing strategies for classical swine fever in Denmark, Stärk et al. (2000) list the following factors for consideration in designing testing protocols: diseases to be selected and their epidemiology, unit of analysis (e.g., animal, herd, or region), target population (age group or farm type), test characteristics, and sample size. In recent years, there have been important theoretical advances in diagnostic test interpretation in veterinary medicine, particularly at the aggregate level (Cameron and Baldock 1998; Christensen and Gardner 2000; Greiner and Gardner 2000; Cannon 2001; Johnson et al. 2004). These have led to the development of some practical tools to facilitate quantitative approaches to the design and interpretation of population testing protocols. For example, Survey Toolbox is a suite of software programs designed to support planning and analysis of animal health surveys.[1] One component of this suite is an epidemiological probability calculator (FreeCalc) to support testing to evaluate freedom from disease. FreeCalc has two modules that enable calculation of sample sizes and analysis of test results for freedom from disease. It accounts for imperfections in diagnostic tests and population size and requires inputs for test sensitivity and specificity, population size, minimum expected prevalence of disease (if present). FreeCalc also allows the user to define acceptable error levels. More sophisticated tools are becoming available that extend this approach to incorporate uncertainty in test performance characteristics and expected prevalence (Audige et al. 2001; Johnson et al. 2004). The latter publication explains freely available software (BayesFreeCalc)[2] for

evaluating the probability of freedom from disease allowing for uncertainty in input parameters. A further extension that is required is the incorporation of testing costs as well as the respective costs of misclassification errors (false positive, false negative) that need to be considered when designing surveillance strategies (Greiner 1996; Hilden and Glasziou 1996; Smith and Slenning 2000).

RISK-BASED SURVEILLANCE

The term *risk-based surveillance* is becoming more prevalent in government documents in various countries, and has been applied in relation to residue monitoring, disease surveillance and foodborne hazards. This term conveys the economic axiom that limited surveillance resources need to be applied where risk is greatest and so that the greatest economic return will be realized (Stärk et al., submitted). At any level (farm, company, region, nation), establishing a disease surveillance system is an investment decision for allocating limited financial resources. Logically this requires designing sampling and testing protocols weighted to yield the most valuable mix of disease information. The most topical and controversial example of risk-based approaches to disease is the surveillance options for bovine spongiform encephalopathy (BSE) (Doherr et al. 2001). The strategy of focusing on high-risk population subgroups (older cattle, emergency slaughter, and fallen stock in the case of BSE) to improve the sensitivity of surveillance programs is intuitively obvious. Similarly, swine veterinarians increasingly are sampling nursery pigs for evidence of PRRS virus infection acquired in breeding herds and will usually focus on poor-doing pigs that are assumed more likely to be infected. In the absence of unlimited resources for diagnostic testing, a level of residual risk of disease must be tolerated, and at some point further investment in surveillance becomes unwise because resources would be more effectively allocated to other areas (e.g., improving biosecurity or response capability). The effective implementation of risk-based (or targeted) surveillance strategies is reliant on valid epidemiologic intelligence that accurately reflects the risk profile of the population involved.

In the context of food safety, risk-based approaches are also being developed. The Codex Alimentarius Commission is proposing risk-based systems for meat inspection.[3] In such a system, inspection of carcasses at slaughter may be conducted in alternative ways depending on the health and/or hygiene status of the farm of origin. Surveillance data from farms will be needed at slaughter in order to decide whether a simplified inspection is acceptable or whether intensified inspection with or without laboratory testing is required. This concept has already been included in the new meat hygiene legislation of the European Union.

DEMONSTRATING FREEDOM FROM DISEASE—THE BOAR STUD DILEMMA

Demonstrating freedom of a population from disease is problematic for a number of reasons, recently expounded by Cameron et al. (2003):

- Freedom from disease implies complete absence of disease in the population. This means that a large population may not contain a single infected animal.
- Detection of disease at very low prevalences (e.g., the detection of a single infected animal) is not possible using sampling techniques. To guarantee that a population is free from disease, all animals in the population must be examined.
- The test that is used to detect disease in individual animals must have perfect sensitivity (i.e., always correctly identify diseased animals). Hardly any tests currently available are able to achieve this.
- Because disease may enter a population at any time, it is conceivable that the population has become infected by the time the last animal is tested.

As concluded by those authors, freedom from disease can be guaranteed only if all animals in a population are evaluated simultaneously with a perfectly sensitive test; yet usually herds (and countries) are perpetually exposed to the possibility of disease introduction. The report by Cameron et al. (2003) provides a thorough discussion of issues involved in assuring disease freedom in the context of assessing the status of Denmark with respect to classical swine fever (hog cholera).

Thurmond (2003) provides an insightful discussion of problems derived from temporal delays between the introduction of a disease and its ability to be detected using conventional sampling and testing protocols. This is most relevant to the challenge of surveillance of boar studs to prevent shipment of semen contaminated with PRRS virus. In hog-dense areas in the U.S., introductions of PRRS virus continue to occur despite extensive biosecurity efforts. Given the likely financial consequences of shipping infective semen to multiple breeding farms, considerable investment is warranted to prevent it, both in surveillance and in improving biosecurity of boar studs. From a surveillance perspective, key decisions include the samples to be collected (blood vs. semen), the tests to be applied (e.g., ELISA or PCR), and the frequency and intensity (sample size or census) of sampling. In this scenario, where rapid detection of disease at very low prevalence is desired, serological surveillance is of limited value due to the delay in antibody production following infection. Although PCR testing of semen for PRRS virus is routinely performed in many studs (because sample collection is convenient), the sensitivity of PCR testing of semen for detecting infected animals during the early stages of infection appears to be much lower (approximately tenfold) than PCR testing of serum (Reicks et al. 2004). Ongoing studies point to the future availability of practical approaches for routine blood sampling of boars during semen collection (Darwin Reicks, personal communication).

VETERINARY CLINICAL SURVEILLANCE

While historically focused on diseases under regulatory control, improved surveillance systems can also contribute to improved control of endemic diseases (McIntyre et al. 2002). Concerns about emerging human diseases have led to the development of surveillance systems such as the Rapid Syndrome Validation Project (RSVP) for detecting changing patterns of disease at a broad population level or similar programs involving health care providers (Lombardo et al. 2003). Although veterinarians are the frontline of response to disease problems in food animals, the collective efforts of veterinarians are a virtually untapped resource for epidemiologic intelligence (McIntyre et al. 2003; de Groot et al. 2003).

Consolidation of food animal production (and its veterinary services) together with advances in information technology have increased the potential for harnessing the efforts of veterinary clinicians for purposes of disease surveillance. Pioneering efforts to capture "coal face" food animal disease data from practicing veterinarians have been initiated with dairy cattle veterinarians in New Zealand (McIntyre et al. 2003) and beef veterinarians in Kansas (de Groot et al. 2003). The latter project (RSVP-Animal) is based conceptually on the human RSVP project. Both these veterinary initiatives use palm-held computers for field data capture, integrate data into centralized databases, analyze disease trends, and enable practicing veterinarians to access summary data by location. The Multi-Hazard Threat Database (MHTD) project of the North Carolina Department of Agriculture and Consumer Services represents a significant step forward in integrating veterinary clinical and government regulatory activities. The system, designed to minimize the impact from any disaster or disease on agriculture, integrates information systems of numerous federal, state, and local agencies to offer extensive, real-time information in the event of an emergency, natural disaster, or bioterrorism attack. While primarily designed to support emergency responses, it also provides decision support for veterinarians by enabling web access to real-time maps of endemic disease status (currently PRRS and TGE).

We believe that these initiatives using modern communications technology to capture veterinary activities offer great potential for enhanced surveillance and regional approaches to disease control in the U.S. swine industry. However, there remain numerous issues to address with respect of ownership and confidentiality of data, the sensitivity, specificity of clinical diagnoses, and value (vs. cost) of the information obtained.

SYNDROMIC SURVEILLANCE

Syndromic surveillance is arguably the most novel dimension of contemporary disease surveillance. The key distinction of syndromic surveillance is that, unlike conventional disease reporting, the data collected are not diagnoses of defined diseases, but data on clinical symptoms or other events (e.g., emergency room visits). The Center for Disease Control estimates that syndromic surveillance systems have been implemented by more than 100 public health entities in the U.S., with the goal of achieving earlier detection and public health responses to epidemics (Buehler et al. 2004). The principal motive for syndromic surveillance has been elevated concern about emerging diseases and bioterrorism, and the concept has been enabled through rapid advances in the field of biomedical informatics. The RSVP system exploits Internet connectivity for low-cost capture of data from a network of sentinel physicians who report signs and symptoms, and who are able to view map displays depicting regional disease patterns. Syndromic surveillance systems for public health use statistical tools for cluster detection, such as time series analysis and statistical process control, and may incorporate integrated alarms when threshold levels are exceeded (Reis and Mandl 2003). In common with other diagnostic systems, syndromic systems are evaluated in terms of sensitivity, specificity, and timeliness, and the cost effectiveness of syndromic surveillance as a tool for improving outbreak detection remains to be determined. In order to evaluate the operational performance of syndromic surveillance systems, Duchin (2003) pointed out that it will be necessary to conduct ongoing investigations of clusters identified through syndromic systems. Identifying appropriate epidemiological responses to surveillance signals will depend on effective standardization of methods for the collection, analysis, and interpretation of data (Duchin 2003).

We are aware of two initiatives to apply syndromic surveillance in veterinary medicine. The RSVP-Animal project in Kansas has been developed to enhance detection of emerging diseases in feedlot cattle based on veterinary clinical observations (de Groot et al. 2003). A large companion animal electronic database linking 360 hospitals in 47 U.S. states is being used to detect changes in patterns of clinical signs in dogs and cats (Moore et al. 2004). Syndromic definitions have been defined using CDC descriptions of likely bioterrorism agents, based on the concept that changes in animal health may have sentinel value for the human population.

SURVEILLANCE RELATED TO PUBLIC ISSUES—FOOD SAFETY, ANTIMICROBIAL RESISTANCE, AND ANIMAL WELFARE

Surveillance activities in swine populations already extend beyond the domain of animal health. Over the last 10 years, general advocacy of the concept of preharvest food safety has stimulated efforts to develop suitable surveillance systems for foodborne hazards in animal populations. Although the objective has been to determine the status of animals on farms, for logistic reasons diagnostic testing has been generally confined to samples collected at harvest. The effectiveness of preharvest strategies for reducing foodborne disease risk depends on the efficacy of preharvest interventions for reducing the prevalence of infection in conjunction with post-farm procedures that ensure a low probability of recontamination of animals or food products (Davies et al. 2004). For several decades the Swedish government has maintained *Salmonella* control programs in its swine and poultry industries based on bacteriologic surveillance and regulatory controls (Boqvist et al. 2003). More recently, industrywide serological surveillance of herds for *Salmonella enterica* was implemented in Denmark, and it was subsequently implemented by other European countries (Mousing et al. 1997; Sorensen et al. 2004). Although the use of serological testing has greatly reduced the cost of testing compared with bacteriology, testing costs remain substantial, and considerable research continues to be directed at establishing the validity and reducing the costs of serological testing for *Salmonella* (Alban et al. 2002; Ekeroth et al. 2003; Sorensen et al. 2004). In the U.S., bacteriologic culture of *Salmonella* on swine carcasses is mandated under the Hazard Analysis Critical Control Point/Pathogen Reduction Act of 1995. However, this testing is conducted as part of the evaluation of hygienic measures in slaughter plants rather than for evaluating *Salmonella* in farm animal populations. Serological methods have also been developed for monitoring other foodborne pathogens occurring in swine, including *Trichinella spiralis* (Gamble 1998), *Toxoplasma gondii* (Dubey et al. 1995), and *Yersinia enterocolitica* (Thibodeau et al. 2001). However, routine surveillance for these agents as part of a coordinated control programs is still limited. National surveys conducted by the USDA-National Animal Health Monitoring System in 1990 and 1995 demonstrated a very low and declining prevalence (0.16% and 0.013%, respectively) of antibodies to *T. spiralis* in commercial pigs (Gamble and Bush 1999). Similarly, surveys of domestic and wild pigs in Canada indicate that the parasite is essentially absent from those populations (Gajadhar et al. 1997). Clearly, there is questionable rationale to implementing routine surveillance when infection occurs at low prevalence, and intermittent surveys are to be preferred. In Europe, the Zoonosis Directive (2003/99/EC) is expanding the demands for systematic surveillance of zoonoses and zoonotic agents along the food production chain in member countries.[4] In addition to *Salmonella* spp., the directive now includes—apart from others—also *Campylobacter* spp., verotoxigenic *E. coli,* and antimicrobial resistance surveillance. Results of these surveillance efforts are published as annual reports.

The persistent controversy over the significance of the contribution of antimicrobial use in food animals to the problem of antimicrobial resistance in human pathogens has prompted calls for improved monitoring of patterns of antimicrobial use and of resistance profiles of animal pathogens and commensal organisms (Anderson et al. 2003). Systematic surveillance of antimicrobial use, and of antimicrobial resistance, has yet to be widely implemented in many countries. Again, Danish national surveillance programs set the standard, documenting patterns of antimicrobial use under veterinary prescription (Stege et al. 2003) and trends in antimicrobial resistance in selected animal and human pathogens and commensal organisms (Bager 2000). The Danish swine industry has also implemented a program of surveillance of skin lesions in slaughtered sows assumed to reflect poor welfare conditions on farms, which may provide a basis for classifying farms by welfare status (Cleveland-Nielsen et al. 2004). International recommendations on the surveillance of antimicrobial resistance and antimicrobial usage are available (Anonymous 2003).

FUTURE POSSIBILITIES

Doherr and Audige (2001) state that "the health and safety of the animal and human generations depend on our continuous ability to detect, monitor and control newly emerging or reemerging livestock diseases and zoonoses rapidly." To do so will require scientific approaches that incorporate technological and conceptual advances as well as effective cooperation between stakeholders (government, researchers, industry, clinicians). Over the last 15 years, apparently novel diseases have afflicted the world's swine populations with surprising frequency. However, with few exceptions, our systems for recognizing and responding to these events have not advanced greatly. On a regional scale, disease surveillance efforts in the swine industry are not yet capturing the available technological opportunities. Integration of near real-time clinical disease surveillance with geographical information systems and advanced tools for temporospatial analysis of disease is becoming increasingly feasible, and this has the potential to deliver epidemiologic intelligence that far exceeds existing capability. There is a great opportunity to build upon initiatives such as the MHTD program in North Carolina and the RSVP, a syndromic surveillance system in Kansas, to increase the level of sophistication with which the swine veterinary profession addresses both endemic and emerging diseases.

NOTES

1. http://www.ausvet.com.au/content.php?page=res_software
2. http://www.epi.ucdavis.edu/diagnostictests/
3. www.codexalimentarius.net/download/standards/169/CXP_041e.pdf
4. http://europa.eu.int/eur-lex/pri/en/oj/dat/2003/l_325/l_32520031212en00310040.pdf

REFERENCES

Alban L, Stege H, Dahl J. 2002. The new classification system for slaughter-pig herds in the Danish Salmonella surveillance-and-control program. Prev Vet Med 53:133–146.

Anderson AD, Nelson JM, Rossiter S, Angulo FJ. 2003. Public health consequences of use of antimicrobial agents in food animals in the United States. Microb Drug Resist 9:373–379.

Anonymous. 2003. OIE International Standards on antimicrobial resistance. Paris: Office International des Épizooties (OIE).

Audige L, Doherr MG, Hauser R, Salman MD. 2001. Stochastic modelling as a tool for planning animal-health surveys and interpreting screening-test results. Prev Vet Med 49:1–17.

Bager F. 2000. DANMAP: Monitoring antimicrobial resistance in Denmark. Int J Antimicrob Agents 14:271–274.

Boqvist S, Hansson I, Nord Bjerselius U, Hamilton C, Wahlstrom H, Noll B, Tysen E, Engvall A. 2003. *Salmonella* isolated from animals and feed production in Sweden between 1993 and 1997. Acta Vet Scand 44:181–197.

Buehler JW. 1998. Surveillance. In Modern Epidemiology (2nd edition). KJ Rothman, S Greenland, eds. Philadelphia: Lippincott, pp. 435–457.

Buehler JW, Hopkins RS, Overhage JM, Sosin DM, Tong V. 2004. Framework for Evaluating Public Health Surveillance Systems for Early Detection of Outbreaks: Recommendations from the CDC Working Group. MMWR Recomm Rep, May 7; 53 (RR-5):1–11.

Cameron AR, Baldock FC. 1998. Two-stage sampling in surveys to substantiate freedom from disease. Prev Vet Med 34:19–30.

Cameron AR, Barfod K, , Martin PAJ, Greiner M, Sergeant E. 2003. Documenting disease freedom in swine by combination of surveillance programmes using information from multiple non-survey-based sources. Report to International EpiLab, Danish Institute for Food and Veterinary Research. http://www.dfvf.dk/Files/Filer/EpiLab/P3%20Angus%20Cameron/T1_P3_A.Cameron_final_report.pdf.

Cannon RM. 2001. Sense and sensitivity—Designing surveys based on an imperfect test. Prev Vet Med 49:141–163.

Christensen J, Gardner IA. 2000. Herd-level interpretation of test results for epidemiologic studies of animal diseases. Prev Vet Med 45:83–106.

Cleveland-Nielsen A, Christensen G, Ersboll AK. 2004. Prevalences of welfare-related lesions at post-mortem meat-inspection in Danish sows. Prev Vet Med 64:123–131.

Davies PR, Hurd HS, Funk JA, Fedorka-Cray PJ, Jones FT. 2004. The role of contaminated feed in the epidemiology and control of *Salmonella enterica* in pork production. Foodborne Pathog Dis 1:202–215.

Deen J, Dee SA, Morrison RB, Radostits OM. 2001. Health and production medicine in swine herds. In Herd Health Food Animal Production Medicine (3rd edition). OM Radostits, ed. Philadelphia: W. B. Saunders Company, pp. 635–764.

de Groot BD, Spire, M F., Sargeant JM, Robertson, D.C. 2003. Preliminary assessment of syndromic surveillance for early detection of foreign animal disease incursion or agri-terrorism in beef cattle populations. Proc 10th Symp Int Soc Vet Epidemiol Econom, November 17–21, Vina del Mar, Chile, p. 539.

Doherr MG, Audige L. 2001. Monitoring and surveillance for rare health-related events: A review from the veterinary perspective. Philos Trans R Soc Lond B Biol Sci 356:1097–1106.

Doherr MG, Heim D, Fatzer R, Cohen CH, Vandevelde M, Zurbriggen A. 2001. Targeted screening of high-risk cattle populations for BSE to augment mandatory reporting of clinical suspects. Prev Vet Med 51:3–16.

Dubey JP, Thulliez P, Weigel RM, Andrews CD, Lind P, Powell EC. 1995. Sensitivity and specificity of various serologic tests for detection of *Toxoplasma gondii* infection in naturally infected sows. Am J Vet Res 56: 1030–1036.

Duchin JS. 2003. Epidemiological response to syndromic surveillance signals. J Urban Health 80(2 Suppl 1):i115–116.

Ekeroth L, Alban L, Feld N. 2003. Single versus double testing of meat-juice samples for Salmonella antibodies, in the Danish pig-herd surveillance programme. Prev Vet Med 60:155–165.

Elbers AR, Dekkers LJ, van der Giessen JW. 2000. Sero-surveillance of wild boar in The Netherlands, 1996–1999. Rev Sci Tech 19:848–854.

Gajadhar AA, Bisaillon JR, Appleyard GD. 1997. Status of *Trichinella spiralis* in domestic swine and wild boar in Canada. Can J Vet Res 61:256–259.

Gamble HR. 1998. Sensitivity of artificial digestion and enzyme immunoassay methods of inspection for trichinae in pigs. J Food Prot 61:339–343.

Gamble HR, Bush E. 1999. Seroprevalence of *Trichinella* infection in domestic swine based on the National Animal Health Monitoring System's 1990 and 1995 swine surveys. Vet Parasitol 80:303–310.

Greiner M. 1996. Two-graph receiver operating characteristic (TG-ROC): Update version supports optimisation of cut-off values that minimise overall misclassification costs. J Immunol Methods 191:93–94.

Greiner M, Gardner IA. 2000. Application of diagnostic tests in veterinary epidemiologic studies. Prev Vet Med 45:43–59.

Hilden J, Glasziou P. 1996. Regret graphs, diagnostic uncertainty and Youden's Index. Stat Med 15:969–986.

Johnson WO, Su CL, Gardner IA, Christensen R. 2004. Sample size calculations for surveys to substantiate freedom of populations from infectious agents. Biometrics 60:165–171.

Lombardo J, Burkom H, Elbert E, Magruder S, Lewis SH, Loschen W, Sari J, Sniegoski C, Wojcik R, Pavlin J. 2003. A systems overview of the Electronic Surveillance System for the Early Notification of Community-Based Epidemics (ESSENCE II). J Urban Health 80(2 Suppl 1):i32–42.

McIntyre LH, Davies PR, Alexander G, O'Leary BD, Morris RS, Perkins NR, Jackson R, Poland R. 2003. VetPAD—Veterinary Practitioner Aided Disease Surveillance System. Proc 10th Symp Int Soc Vet Epidemiol Econom, November 17–21, Vina del Mar, Chile, p. 335.

McIntyre LH, Davies PR, Morris RS, Jackson R, Poland R. 2002. The relative value of farmer, veterinary practitioner and diagnostic laboratory records in providing epidemiologically sound endemic disease surveillance. Proc Soc Vet Epidemiol Prev Med, Cambridge, UK, April 2–5 2002. pp. 128–136.

Moore GE, Ward MP, Dhariwal J, Wu CC, Glickman NP, Lewis HP, Glickman LT. 2004. Development of a national companion animal syndromic surveillance system for bioterrorism. In Proc 2nd GISVET conference, Guelph, June 22–24. http://www.gisvet.org/Documents/GisVet04/RegularPapers/Moore.pdf.

Morner T, Obendorf DL, Artois M, Woodford MH. 2002. Surveillance and monitoring of wildlife diseases. Rev Sci Tech 21:67–76.

Mousing J, Jensen PT, Halgaard C, Bager F, Feld N, Nielsen B, Nielsen JP, Bech-Nielsen S. 1997. Nation-wide *Salmonella enterica* surveillance and control in Danish slaughter swine herds. Prev Vet Med 29:247–261

Pavlin JA. 2003. Investigation of disease outbreaks detected by "syndromic" surveillance systems. J Urban Health 80(2 Suppl 1):i107–114.

Pointon AM, Davies PR, Bahnson P. 1999. Disease surveillance at slaughter. In Diseases of Swine (8th edition). BE Straw, S D'Allaire, WL Mengeling, DJ Taylor, eds. Ames: Iowa State Univ Press, pp. 1111–1132.

Reicks D, Munoz-Zanzi C, Christopher-Hennings J, Lager K, Mengeling W, Polson D, Dee SA, Rossow K. 2004. Detection of PRRS virus by PCR in serum and semen of boars during the first six days after infection. Swine Health Prod, (submitted).

Reis BY, Mandl KD. 2003. Time series modeling for syndromic surveillance. BMC Med Inform Decis Mak 23;3:2. http://www.biomedcentral.com/1472–6947/3/2.

Risatti GR, Callahan JD, Nelson WM, Borca MV. 2003. Rapid detection of classical swine fever virus by a portable real-time reverse transcriptase PCR assay. J Clin Microbiol 41:500–505.

Salman MD. 2003. Animal Disease Surveillance and Survey Systems. Ames: Iowa State Univ Press.

Salman, MD, Stärk KD, Zepeda C. 2003. Quality assurance applied to animal disease surveillance systems. Rev Sci Tech 22:689–696.

Schlosser W, Ebel E. 2001. Use of a Markov-chain Monte Carlo model to evaluate the time value of historical testing information in animal populations. Prev Vet Med 48:167–175.

Smith RD, Slenning BD. 2000. Decision analysis: Dealing with uncertainty in diagnostic testing. Prev Vet Med 45:139–162.

Sorensen LL, Alban L, Nielsen B, Dahl J. 2004. The correlation between *Salmonella* serology and isolation of *Salmonella* in Danish pigs at slaughter. Vet Microbiol 101:131–141.

Stärk KDC, Regula G, Hernandez J, Knopf L, Fuchs K, Morris RS, Davies P. Concepts for risk-based surveillance in the field of veterinary medicine and veterinary public health: A novel approach (submitted).

Stärk KDC, Mortensen S, Olsen AM, Barfod K, Bøtner A, Lavritsen DT, Strandbygård B. 2000. Designing serological surveillance programmes to document freedom from disease with special reference to exotic viral diseases of pigs in Denmark. Rev Sci Tech 19:715–724.

Stärk KDC, Salman M, Tempelman Y, Kihm U. 2002. A review of approaches to quality assurance of veterinary systems for health-status certification. Prev Vet Med 56:129–140.

Stege H, Bager F, Jacobsen E, Thougaard A. 2003. VETSTAT—The Danish system for surveillance of the veterinary use of drugs for production animals. Prev Vet Med 57:105–115.

Thibodeau V, Frost EH, Quessy S. 2001. Development of an ELISA procedure to detect swine carriers of pathogenic *Yersinia enterocolitica*. Vet Microbiol 82:249–259.

Thurmond MC. 2003. Conceptual foundations for infectious disease surveillance. J Vet Diagn Invest 15:501–514.

Torrison J. 1998. Application of PCR tests for monitoring large herds. In Proc 25th Allen D Leman Swine Conf, University of Minnesota, pp. 51–53.

70 Anesthesia and Surgical Procedures in Swine

Guy St. Jean and David E. Anderson

ROLE OF THE SURGEON

Veterinarian's roles in the swine industry have changed markedly over the past 20 years. Surgical procedures increasingly conflict with economic goals. The veterinarian must critically evaluate economic benefit versus cost and prognosis of surgery. In most scenarios, services offered by the veterinarian are directed to the need of the enterprise. Surgery on an individual pig is not always cost efficient. However, pigs selected for genetic improvement, show pigs, and pet pigs have individual value, and surgery may be performed with little regard to costs. Some conditions like hernia, prolapse, dystocia, and atresia that can occur in large numbers of animals can be very costly and need to be investigated so that a solution and treatment can be applied. In a commercial swine operation, the veterinarian is often a teacher, showing the manager and experienced personnel how to perform some minor surgical procedures during baby pig processing (castration, ear notching, canine teeth clipping, tail amputation) in a cost-effective fashion. It is the veterinarian's role to make sure that these procedures are done properly.

Among purebred and pet pigs, or pigs used as animal models in biomedical research (because of their anatomic and physiologic similarities to human beings), the individual animal often is of high perceived value, and surgery often is requested. A veterinarian who is able to offer excellent surgical service to swine producers often will have greater credibility as a herd consultant. The purpose of this chapter is to describe clinical swine anesthesia and review baby pig processing, hernia repair, and some common surgical procedures of the digestive, urogenital, and musculoskeletal systems in swine.

ANESTHESIA

Minor surgical procedures (ear notching, teeth clipping, tail amputation, castration) in young swine often are performed without anesthetizing the animal. Performed skillfully, these surgical procedures are tolerated well by young pigs without an anesthetic. Sometimes economics has an influence in the use of an anesthetic. However, public scrutiny of management practices increasingly demands attention to pain and prevention of unnecessary distress. Management of swine anesthesia presents some difficulties. Swine resist mechanical restraint more and are usually more difficult to hold than other species. Strong assistance often is needed. When possible, adult swine should be held off feed for 24 hours before general anesthesia, whereas piglets, which are prone to hypoglycemia, should be held from suckling for only 1–2 hours before anesthetic induction.

Malignant hyperthermia or porcine stress syndrome is a heritable condition in swine that can be triggered in a susceptible pig by any stress and many injectable (acepromazine, ketamine, succinyl choline) and inhalant anesthetics. Susceptible pigs are extremely muscular and usually have reduced subcutaneous fat. Halothane traditionally has been incriminated, but delayed onset of malignant hyperthermia can occur with exposure to isoflurane (Wedel et al. 1993). The clinical signs of malignant hyperthermia can be any of the following: a severe increase in body temperature, muscle rigidity, tachycardia, tachypnea, hypoxemia, cardiac arrhythmias, unstable blood pressure, and myoglobinuria. Death of an affected animal appears to be the result of peripheral circulatory changes that are produced by severe acidosis, vasoconstriction, hyperkalemia, decreased cardiac output, and hypotension. This susceptibility to malignant hyperthermia is due to an autosomal recessive defect in the gene that codes for the ryanodine receptor calcium channel in skeletal muscle (Rosenberg and Fletcher 1994). In response to a trigger, intracellular calcium rises abruptly, which causes muscle contracture and release of heat. Treatment of malignant hyperthermia is largely symptomatic. Early recognition is the key to successful treatment. Whenever malignant hyperthermia is suspected, volatile anesthetics should be discontinued. Aggressive cooling should be instituted using iced packs and alcohol baths. Dantrolene sodium is effective in the treatment of a malignant hyperthermia or as a prophylaxis when given before the anticipated trigger. Suggested doses for swine are 1 to 3 mg/kg IV for treatment and 5 mg/kg orally given prophylactically. (For more information on porcine stress syndrome, please refer to Chapter 58).

Anticholinergics (atropine and glycopyrollate) are recommended before sedation and anesthetic techniques in pigs. Atropine sulfate (0.04 mg/kg IM) or glycopyrollate (0.02 mg/kg IM) will decrease the risk of bradycardia, excessive salivation, bronchoconstriction, and excessive airway secretion. In healthy swine receiving light surgical anesthesia, administration of supportive fluids is not considered necessary, unless the animal was off feed and water for more than 24 hours. However, long general anesthesia is best managed with intravenous fluid support. In swine that are hypovolemic or showing other signs of shock, fluid therapy is essential preferably before or during anesthesia. Fluid therapy is best administered in the ear vein. In the authors' experience, fluid therapy using balanced electrolyte solution before and during anesthesia is essential during cesarean section with dead piglets in utero.

Anesthetic considerations for swine cesarean are important. One needs to remember that sow-fetal drug distribution is quite complete. Therefore, it must be assumed that any drug in the maternal circulation reaches the fetus rapidly in relatively high concentration. Because the fetal blood-brain barrier is extremely permeable, these drugs exert a profound anesthetic effect on the fetus. Also, anesthesia tends to persist after delivery because of the neonate's poorly developed liver enzymes and renal function. Anesthetic agents should be chosen that will minimize fetal depression. General anesthesia will induce greater neonatal depression than regional anesthesia.

Injectable Anesthetics

Injectable agents are most appropriate for field use. With injectable agents, a minimum of equipment is needed, requiring only a small investment. The drugs can be transported easily to the animal, compared to inhalation anesthetics, which are more expensive and can be difficult to transport to a field situation. Pigs have few superficial veins and arteries suitable for catheter placement and intravenous drug administration (Sakaguchi et al. 1996). Also, variation in accessibility of these vessels exists among swine breeds. The auricular (ear) vein is the safest and most accessible vein. It usually is located along the caudal margin of the ear. To inject or place a catheter in the ear vein, the pig can be restrained. The vein is held at the base of the ear by the fingers, forceps, or a rubber band to distend it. Rubbing the ear with alcohol and vigorous massage seem to create better visualization for needle insertion. Inserting a small catheter

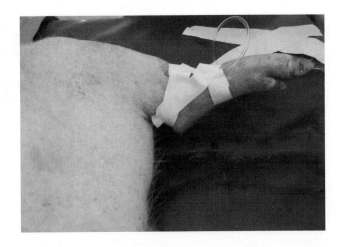

70.1. *Catheterization of medial saphenous vein in a pig.*

(20-gauge) will allow the administration of fluid or injection of additional anesthetic solution intravenously. The medial saphenous vein can be catheterized easily in the anesthetized or well restrained pig (Figure 70.1). Anesthesia can be induced using IM drug protocols or gas anesthetics via face mask followed by catheterization for IV fluids therapy or drug administration. Intramedullary cannulation should be considered when vascular access is vital but an IV catheter has not been established. An 18 gauge cannula can easily be inserted into the greater tubercle of the humerus or via the trochanteric fossa of the femur for intramedullary infusions. Fluid and drug administration is easily done in immature pigs. Older pigs may have sufficient fat and fibrosis of the medullary canal so as to limit administration rate.

Intramuscular injections should be given with a 2 inch needle in the cervical muscles to assure that the drug goes into the muscle and not in the fat. To obtain the maximal effect with the drug the pig should be in a quiet environment if possible. Combinations of anesthetic agents administered in appropriate doses are often superior to any one agent (Table 70.1).

Few drugs currently are approved for use in swine. Practically all anesthetics used are unapproved drugs for swine, and their use is considered extra label (Papich 1996). However, veterinarians often recognize the necessity of relieving pain, anesthetizing a swine for a procedure, or administering a drug as an anesthetic adjunct. Often, no alternative exists to using the drug in an extra label manner. For public protection, steps must be taken to ensure that no harmful residues occur from treated animals by assigning an appropriate withdrawal time before the marketing of meat.

The reader is encouraged to consult the Food Animal Residue Avoidance Data Bank for appropriate withdrawal times in swine (www.farad.org; phone 1-888-873-2723; e-mail farad@ncsu.edu).

Table 70.1. Injectable anesthetic agents for swine

Drug	Dose	Route	Onset (min)	Duration (min)
Pentobarbital	10–30 mg/kg	IV	1–10	15–45
	45 mg/kg	each testicle	10	10
Thiopental	10–20 mg/kg	IV	Immediate	2–10
Acepromazine	0.1–0.5 mg/kg	IM	20–30	30–60
Acepromazine	0.4 mg/kg	IM	5	15–30
and Ketamine	15 mg/kg	IM		
Acepromazine	0.03 mg/kg	IM	2–4	40–50
and Ketamine	2.2 mg/kg			
and Telazol	4.4 mg/kg			
Diazepam	1–2 mg/kg	IM	10	20–40
and Ketamine	10–15 mg/kg	IM		
Midazolam	0.1–0.5 mg/kg	IM	5–10	20–40
and Ketamine	10–15 mg/kg			
Azaperone	2–8 mg/kg	IM	5–15	60–120
Xylazine	0.5–3 mg/kg	IM	5	10
Xylazine	2 mg/kg	IM	7–10	20–40
and Ketamine	20 mg/kg			
Xylazine	2.2 mg/kg/hour	IV	Immediate	As needed
and Ketamine	(see text)			
and Guaifenesin				
Xylazine	4.4 mg/kg	IM	1–2	60
and Ketamine	2.2 mg/kg			
and Telazol	4.4 mg/kg			
Ketamine	20 mg/kg	IM	Immediate	5–30
and Thiopental	6–11 mg/kg	IV		
Medetomidine	80 µg/kg	IM	1–5	60–120
and Butorphanol	200 µg/kg			
and Ketamine	2 mg/kg			
Metedomidine	80 µg/kg	IM	1–5	75–120
and Butorphenol	200 µg/kg			
and Ketamine	10 mg/kg			
Xylazine	2 mg/kg	IM	1–5	60 – 120
and Butorphenol	200 µg/kg			
and Ketamine	10 mg/kg			
Propofol	11 mg/kg/hour	IV	Immediate	Continuous infusion
and Fentanyl	2.5 mg/kg q30 min	IV		

Barbiturates. Barbiturates as a group are poor analgesics. Pentobarbital and thiopental are the most commonly used barbiturates. Pentobarbital is a potent central nervous system depressant and can be administered intravenously, intraperitoneally, and intratesticularly. We do not recommend intraperitoneal injection because of the risk of peritonitis. Because young pigs do not have the hepatic enzymatic capacity of adults, pentobarbital should not be used as a general anesthetic in young piglets.

In adults, an intravenous dose of 10–30 mg per kg will provide 20–30 minutes of relatively safe anesthesia, provided a patent airway is established and maintained until swallowing and other airway protective reflexes have returned. Preanesthetic medication (e.g., diazepam, acepromazine, xylazine) will decrease the amount of pentobarbital required for surgical anesthesia (Table 70.1). Recovery from pentobarbital administration often is prolonged and requires close patient surveillance.

For intratesticular injections, 45 mg per kg of body weight of a 30% solution is injected below the tail of the epididymis in the upper one-third of each testicle. The maximum volume is 20 ml per testicle, the onset of anesthesia is in 10 minutes, and recovery takes 20–40 minutes. Castration must be performed as quickly as possible to prevent continued absorption of the drug and a potentially lethal overdose (Henry 1968). The testes must be disposed of in a safe place. There are reports of fatal poisoning of dogs as a result of eating testes containing the residual drug. Blood on the floor is also dangerous (Henry 1968).

The shorter-acting barbiturate thiopental (10–20 mg/kg) is used sometimes for induction before inhalation anesthesia or for very short procedures. A 2.5–5% solution should be used and one-half of the calculated dose quickly injected. When the pig lies down, incremental amounts are injected until the desired plane of anesthesia is achieved. Apnea often is observed, and means of assisting ventilation should be readily available.

Acepromazine. Acepromazine decreases spontaneous motor activity. Used alone, it usually provides only slight inconsistent sedation in swine. Acepromazine also will predispose to hypotension and hypothermia and should not be used in debilitated pigs. The maximum dose recommended is a total of 10 mg. Acepromazine has been reported to decrease the incidence of malignant hyperthermia (Moon and Smith 1996). It is useful when combined with ketamine or tiletamine-zolazepam (Table 70.1).

Benzodiozepines (Diazepam and Midazolam). Diazepam (1–2 mg/kg IM) can be used in combination with ketamine or xylazine (Table 70.1). Midazolam can be absorbed more rapidly and completely than diazepam because it is water soluble. They both ensure a smooth recovery and have a longer effect then xylazine. The expense associated with these drugs may make them impractical in some swine commercial operations.

Azaperone. Azaperone is a neuroleptic agent and can be given to tranquilize or immobilize swine (Table 70.1). The degree of sedation is dose dependent and should not exceed 1 mg/kg in large boars, because priapism has been reported (Moon and Smith 1996). Azaperone must be given intramuscularly, because intravenous injection often results in excitation. Excessive salivation, hypothermia, sensitivity to noise, and hypotension has been seen in pigs receiving azaperone (Greene 1979). Azaperone is not an analgesic and often is used in combination with other drugs for surgical procedure. Deep tranquilization from azaperone should be obtained before ketamine is given. If azaperone is used alone for surgical procedures, local or regional anesthesia should be administered.

Alpha-2 Receptor Agonists (Xylazine, Medetomidine). Swine are fairly resistant to xylazine compared to other meat-producing animals (Table 70.1). Sedation will result, but animals are aroused easily. Xylazine usually is used in combination with other drugs to produce good muscle relaxation and a smooth recovery. Vomiting has been seen following the use of xylazine in pigs with digestive disturbances.

Medetomidine is a more potent alpha-2 agonist than is xylazine (Sakaguchi et al. 1992). Medetomidine in combination with atropine induces deeper sedation than does xylazine and its effects are enhanced by butorphanol. The anesthetic state is characterized by profound somatic analgesia, but visceral analgesia is poor. Medetomidine, butorphanol, and ketamine induce excellent surgical anesthesia in pigs (Table 70.1). This anesthetic regimen can be reversed by atipamezole (240 μg/kg), a selective and potent alpha-2 antagonist.

Ketamine. Ketamine induces rapid onset of unconsciousness (Thurmon 1986). The anesthetic state is characterized by somatic analgesia, but visceral analgesia is poor. Ketamine has been used as a major component of many regimens to induce chemical restraint or anesthesia in pigs. Ketamine can be given IM, IV, or intratesticularly. Intratesticularly, a combination of ketamine (6 mg/kg) and xylazine (2 mg/kg) has been used successfully for castration (Thurmon 1986). When ketamine is used alone, it exerts some undesirable effects, such as poor muscle relaxation and analgesia-emergence delirium, tachycardia, and hypertension. Ketamine commonly is combined with a muscle relaxant or sedative such as acepromazine, diazepam, xylazine, or droperidol (Table 70.1).

Tiletamine—Zolazepam (Telazol). Telazol provides some muscle relaxation and sedation and also immobilizes swine (Moon and Smith 1996). Telazol requires a smaller volume of injectable compared to ketamine. Telazol frequently is combined with xylazine or acepromazine to provide better muscle relaxation and an easier recovery (Table 70.1).

Propofol. Propofol has recently been used for IV anesthesia in pigs (Martin-Cancho et al. 2004). One dosage regimen reported was 11 mg/kg body weight per hour for abdominal surgery. This was done in combination with fentanyl (2.5 mg/kg IV every 30 min). Compared with pigs anesthetized with isoflurane, propofol-anesthetized pigs required significantly longer to recover consciousness.

Guaifenesin. Guaifenesin is a centrally acting muscle relaxant. Because it produces little analgesia, it should not be used alone. Intravenous infusion of guaifenesin combined with thiobarbiturates and with ketamine and xylazine has been used for induction and maintenance of anesthesia (Thurmon 1986). The authors recommend adding 500 mg of ketamine and 500 mg of xylazine to each 500 ml of 5% guaifenesin in 5% dextrose in water. The mixture is given rapidly in a catheter in the ear vein at a dose of 0.5–1 ml per kg for induction. Anesthesia is maintained by continuous infusion at a rate of 2.2 mg per kg per hour. At the end of the surgery, recovery time may be hastened by administration of yohimbine (0.125 mg/kg) or tolazoline (2.5–5 mg/kg) to reverse the effect xylazine (Thurmon 1986).

Combination Injectable Anesthesia. Combinations of injectable drugs have been used to increase quality, duration, and analgesia of anesthesia when they can be administered safely. A recent study compared three regimes for maintaining anesthesia in pigs induced using azaperone (1 mg/kg, IM) and ketamine (2.5 mg/kg IM). These pigs were divided into three groups: (I) etomidate (200 μg/kg IV) and midazolam (100 μg/kg IV); (II) ketamine (2 mg/kg IV) and midazolam (100 μg/kg IV); (III) pentobarbitone (15 to 20 mg/kg IV) (Clutton et al. 1997). Pentobarbitone provided the least satisfactory anesthesia because of profound respiratory depression, difficulty completing orotracheal intubation, and prolonged time to standing. Another study compared metedomidine-butorphenol-ketamine (MBK: 80 μg/kg–200 μg/kg–10mg/kg, respectively, all IM) with xylazine-butorphenol-ketamine (XBK: 2 mg/kg–200 μg/kg–10 mg/kg, respectively, all IM) (Sakaguchi et al. 1996). MBK was found to provide longer and more satisfactory anesthesia as compared with XBK.

Inhalation Anesthetics

For debilitated swine, for surgical procedures lasting more than 30 minutes, for difficult procedures, or for valuable swine, an inhalation anesthetic provides a more controlled plane of anesthesia. For economic reasons, halothane is the most commonly used inhalation anesthetic in swine. Halothane possesses physical properties and potency consistent with rapid induction, alteration of anesthetic depth, and recovery from anesthesia. Inhalation anesthetics can be administered to small pigs by an open or semiopen method; in larger swine, the semiclosed or closed system is preferred. Swine weighing up to 140 kg can be anesthetized with an anesthetic machine designed for small animals (Tranquilli 1986).

Selection of induction technique and anesthetic protocol depends on the size and special needs of the swine, preference of the veterinarians, and availability of drugs and equipment. Sedation is desirable to reduce the stress of physical restraint before induction of anesthesia (Table 70.1). Swine up to 100 kg can be restrained in a webbed stanchion. Large swine can be restrained in a crate with a head catch or by a snare. Induction of anesthesia can be accomplished with a rapid bolus of injectable agent (barbiturate), by rapid infusions of a combination of drugs (Table 70.1), or by using a face mask delivering a high concentration of anesthetic agent (5% halothane). Tracheal intubation assures a patent airway for delivery of anesthetic and protects the airway from aspiration pneumonia. In the authors' experience, facial, pharyngeal, and laryngeal anatomy of the pig makes endotracheal intubation more challenging than in other meat-producing species. It is often difficult to open the jaws wide enough for good laryngeal exposure, and the pig has a small narrow larynx that deviates ventrally, creating a sharp angle from the pharynx to the tracheal opening. Also laryngeal spasms occur frequently and are induced easily. Occurrence of spasms can be reduced by achieving a sufficient depth of anesthesia prior to intubation or by spraying the larynx with lidocaine.

Following induction, the pig should be placed in sternal recumbency, and the jaws should be held open with small rope. The tongue is pulled forward by an assistant. A laryngoscope and blades of different lengths are needed. For adult swine, the blade length must be at least 25 cm. The blade of the laryngoscope is placed at the base of the tongue and downward pressure is applied

until an unobstructed view of the larynx is provided. Endotracheal tubes should be available in sizes from 3 to 20 mm outside diameter and lengths of 25–50 cm. A malleable metal rod with the first 5 cm bent at a 30° angle is placed inside the endotracheal tube to act as a guide. With the laryngeal opening visualized, the endotracheal tube with the stylet extending slightly beyond the tip is placed into the laryngeal opening. The endotracheal tube is pushed over the tip of the stylet and with a twisting motion is passed through the larynx into the trachea. The tracheal diameter is surprisingly small in the pig. A 50 kg pig often requires only a 7–9 mm tube, and a 10–14 mm tube often is adequate for adult sows (Tranquilli 1986).

Safe maintenance of inhalation anesthesia requires knowledge of the signs associated with anesthetic depth and continual monitoring of the patient and anesthetic equipment. Routinely monitored signs should include pulse quality and rate, respiratory rate, color of mucous membranes, capillary refill time, blood pressure, and electrocardiogram. The body temperature should be evaluated regularly, and appropriate padding should be placed. The pulse can be palpated over the median auricular artery. Direct auscultation of the heart also should be done. The normal heart rate in swine ranges from 60–90 beats per minute and may vary greatly during inhalation anesthesia.

During recovery from inhalation anesthesia, frequent and careful monitoring is necessary, because life-threatening complications can occur (Moon and Smith 1996). Recovery should be in a quiet place, and the pig should be placed in sternal recumbency as soon as possible. The endotracheal tube should be maintained until the pig is spontaneously moving its head or will not tolerate the tube. The pig should not be returned to the herd until it is fully awake.

Local Anesthesia

The use of local anesthesia without additional chemical restraint is limited in swine. Pigs, even in the absence of pain, will resist physical restraint by continuing to struggle. In addition to chemical restraint, infiltration of 2% lidocaine around the surgical site will facilitate surgery involving the skin and superficial underlying tissues. Local infiltration of lidocaine is used commonly for surgical repair of umbilical and inguinal hernias and scirrhous cord removal.

Epidural Regional Anesthesia

Lumbosacral epidural anesthesia is the most commonly used form of regional analgesia in swine (Figure 70.2) (Skarda 1996). Minimal equipment and expense are necessary to perform the procedure during epidural anesthesia. Compared to general anesthesia, the swine is in an awake state so the risk of aspiration pneumonia is minimal. Local infiltration of lidocaine compared to epidural anesthesia has several disadvantages. Infiltra-

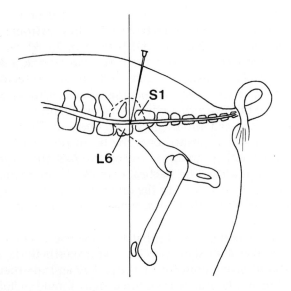

70.2. *The injection site (needle placement) for a lumbosacral anesthesia in swine. L6 is the sixth lumbar vertebra; S1 is the first sacral vertebra.*

tion requires a larger amount of lidocaine and can retard wound healing and muscle relaxation, and analgesia is not as profound. Lumbosacral epidural anesthesia is relatively easy to perform and greatly facilitates cesarean section; repair of rectal, uterine, or vaginal prolapses; repair of hernia; and surgery of the prepuce and penis or rear limbs (Skarda 1996). Lumbosacral epidural anesthesia should be avoided in patients that are in shock or toxemic because of sympathetic blockade and consequent depression of blood pressure (Skarda 1996). Also, general anesthesia may be more appropriate then regional anesthesia when the sow is very aggressive.

Complications that may result from faulty techniques during lumbosacral epidural injection include cardiovascular and respiratory collapse after overdose or subarachnoid injection, meningitis associated with septic technique and tremor, and vomiting and convulsions after injection of the analgesic into the vertebral venous sinus.

The block can best be administered while the animal is standing and restrained with a hog snare, lariat, or head catch. Large hogs can be restrained by placing their heads in the head catch of a cattle chute. The site for injection for epidural anesthesia in the pig is the lumbosacral space. The conus medullaris of the cauda equina of the pig terminates in the region of the first or second sacral vertebra. The filum terminale terminates at the sixth or seventh coxygeal vertebra. Although the meninges extend beyond the lumbosacral articulation, there is only a very slight probability of entering the subarachnoid space. The lumbosacral space is on the midline and identified by drawing a line across the animal's back from tuber coxa to tuber coxa. This line will be just cranial to the point of the stifle joint (Skarda 1996). The

line passes usually through the spinous process of the last lumbar vertebra. The injection site is usually 2.5–5 cm caudal to this transverse line (Figure 70.2).

The site of injection is prepared by clipping or shaving the hair, thoroughly scrubbing the site with a surgical soap, and applying a skin antiseptic. The location is infiltrated with a local anesthetic agent prior to needle insertion. A 6–8 cm 20-gauge needle is used for pigs up to 30 kg. A 10 cm 18-gauge needle is used for pigs between 35 and 90 kg, and a 12–16 cm needle for pigs over 90 kg. The needle is inserted with the level directed cranially and at an angle 10° caudal to perpendicular between the last lumbar and first sacral vertebrae. The needle penetrates the skin, back fat, muscle, and then the fibrous interarticular spinous ligament. The needle passes through a definite area of resistance as it encounters the ligament and a slight pop is felt as the needle passes into the epidural space and drops to the floor of the spinal canal. The lumbosacral space is large in the pig (1.5 × 2.5 cm) and allows for a relatively large margin of error (Skarda 1996). Aspiration should be attempted before injection of the anesthetic to ensure that the subarachnoid space or a blood vessel has not been entered. Little resistance to injection will be encountered if the needle is located properly in the epidural space.

The anesthetic agent most commonly used is 2% lidocaine. The dose is calculated by either weight or length of the pig (Skarda 1996). Generally, a dose of 1 ml/9 kg of body weight is adequate. Analgesia should be present within 10 minutes and last approximately 2 hours. A total dose of 20 ml must not be exceeded regardless of the weight. Four ml per 100 kg and 6 ml per 200 kg of body weight are sufficient for standing castrations (Skarda 1996). Ten ml per 100 kg, 15 ml per 200 kg, and 20 ml per 300 kg have given satisfactory results for cesarean section (Skarda 1996). If the pig is restrained in lateral recumbency, it is important that the head not be placed in extension. In swine with the head extended, the soft palate can occlude the airway, and the patient can suffocate (Benson 1986).

In 28–35 kg pigs, epidural injections of xylazine (2 mg/kg diluted in 5 ml of 0.9% NaCl solution) at the lumbosacral intervertebral space induce immobilization, mild sedation, and regional anesthesia that extends from the anus to the umbilicus within 10 minutes and lasts at least 2 hours (Ko et al. 1992). The injection of a xylazine (1 mg/kg 10% solution) and lidocaine (10 ml, 2% solution) combination into the lumbosacral epidural space has produced excellent anesthesia for cesarean in large sows (Ko et al. 1993). The forequarters in these sows were immobilized by IV injection of 0.003 ml of telazol, mixture containing 50 mg of telazol per ml, 50 mg of ketamine per ml, and 50 mg of xylazine per ml per kg of body weight (Ko et al. 1993). In preparing the telazol, ketamine, and xylazine combination, 2.5 ml of 10% ketamine (250 mg) and 2.5 ml of 10% xylazine (250 mg xylazine) were used as the diluent instead of sterile water. A mean of 3 ml of this combination was given per sow; the sows were quiet and immobilized for an average of 105 minutes (Ko et al. 1993). The sows were able to walk 12 hours after surgery, and the piglets were without signs of sedation or tranquilization. Intravenous tolazoline (2.2 mg/kg) partially reversed the telazol, ketamine, xylazine-induced sedation after surgery but did not antagonize the xylazine-lidocaine epidural effect (Ko et al. 1993).

Epidural analgesia used in combination with general anesthesia allows a light plane of anesthesia with good muscle relaxation distal to the midthoracic region. Medetomidine (0.5 mg/kg diluted in 5 ml of 0.9% NaCl solution) injected epidurally in the lumbosacral space of swine produced sedation and decubitus but minimal analgesia caudal to the umbilicus. The onset of these effects occurred in 10 minutes, and they lasted for less than 30 minutes. Intravenous administration of atipamezole (0.2 mg/kg of body weight) reversed epidurally administered detomidine-induced sedation and immobilization (Ko et al. 1992). Atipamezole had no effect on epidurally administered xylazine-induced sedation and immobilization (Ko et al. 1992).

PAIN MANAGEMENT

Pain management through drug therapy has received relatively little attention in pigs, possibly because of the massive scale of pig operations, because of economics, and because many procedures are done in young pigs at ages where distress can be minimized. One study evaluated postoperative pain and compared transdermal fentanyl patches (25 µg/hour and 50 µg/hour) with buprenorphine (0.1 mg/kg, as needed) (Harvey-Clark et al. 2000). Assessment of analgesia was variable, but 50 µg/hour transdermal patches placed on 26 kg pigs achieved blood concentrations similar to that considered to be in the analgesic range for humans. Another study evaluated the use of isoflurane anesthestic gas for piglet castration at 14 days old (Walker et al. 2004). In that study, piglets castrated under isoflurane gas had significantly fewer reactions to the surgical procedure but stress hormone concentrations after castration were similar among groups. Application of local anesthesia immediately prior to castration of pigs 10–14 days old was associated with less resistance to the procedure (Horn et al. 1999).

GENITOURINARY SURGERY

Castration

Castration of male pigs is routinely performed with the intention to improve performance, feed conversion, and carcass traits (Kiley 1976). Also, management of castrated pigs through finishing may be easier than for intact male pigs. With the onset of puberty, boar meat becomes tainted with an unpleasant odor and taste. However, recommendations for pig age at the time of castration are variable. Stress of castration was evaluated for pigs castrated at 1, 2, 4, 8, 16, and 24 days of age (White et al. 1995). This study indicated that pigs castrated after administration of lidocaine anesthetic subcutaneously and around the spermatic cords had lower heart rate and less vocalization than pigs castrated without local anesthesia. This effect was greatest for pigs castrated after 8 days old. Castration associated behavioral changes were evaluated for pigs castrated at 1, 5, 10, 15, and 20 days old (McGlone et al. 1993). Castration caused reduced suckling, reduced standing, and increased lying time compared with intact male pigs at all ages. Pigs castrated at 14 days old were heavier at weaning and had a higher rate of gain compared with pigs castrated at 1 day old. Administration of aspirin or butorphenol failed to improve castration associated reduction in feeding time and weight gain. Administration of lidocaine anesthesia prior to castration prevented castration-induced nursing behavior suppression (McGlone and Hellman 1988) in 2-week-old pigs. This effect was not observed for pigs castrated at 7 weeks old. Pigs castrated at 2 weeks old had less pronounced behavioral changes than pigs castrated at 7 weeks old. Castrating baby pigs at 2 weeks old minimizes the stress of castration and maximizes performance to weaning.

Castration of 14-day-old pigs is done by suspending the pig by the hind limbs while lying the pig across a smooth rail. The surgical site is wiped clean with alcohol or 2% tincture of iodine. If used, lidocaine anesthetic is injected subcutaneously (0.5 ml per site), overlying each testicle, and over each spermatic cord (0.5 ml per site) in the inguinal canal. A 1 cm long incision is made over each testicle and the testicles pulled from the scrotum. Hemorrhage is minimal at this age. Transfixation ligation of the spermatic cord is recommended for older pigs (see the section on castration of older pigs). Topical antiseptic ointment or spray may be applied at this time. Systemic antibiotics are usually not required, except when castrating older pigs. Castrated baby pigs are placed under a heat lamp in the farrowing crate for convalescence.

Castration of Older Pigs. Pigs are routinely castrated prior to or at 2 weeks old. However, veterinarians may be asked to castrate older pigs that are intended for show or mature boars that are no longer to be used for breeding. Castration of older pigs are best performed with the pig sedated or under general anesthesia (see the section on anesthesia), but manual restraint and local anesthesia may be adequate for pigs weighing 50 kg or less (Becker 1986). The boar is restrained in lateral recumbency and the surgical site aseptically prepared. A 4–6 cm incision is made overlying the testicle at the ventral aspect of the scrotum. The testicle should be removed with the vaginal tunic intact. Inguinal fat and soft tissue are stripped

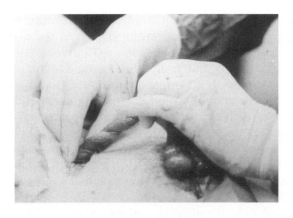

70.3. *Surgical repair of an inguinal hernia showing the tunic and testicle being twisted to force intestines into the peritoneal cavity.*

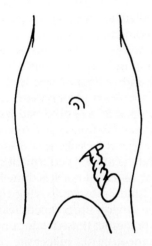

70.4. *Illustration of vaginal tunic twisted to the level of the external inguinal ring for transfixation suture fixation.*

from the spermatic cord and evaluated for the presence of an inguinal hernia. The vaginal tunic and the spermatic cord are twisted until the cord is tightly compressed to the level of the external inguinal ring (Figures 70.3 and 70.4). Two transfixation ligatures (no. 1 chromic gut) are placed securing the vaginal tunic and spermatic cord to the medial aspect of the external inguinal ring. These sutures are intended to close the vaginal tunic and prevent the development of postoperative inguinal hernia. An emasculator may be used, but this method for orchiectomy does not result in closure of the vaginal tunic nor prevent inguinal hernia. Closure of the surgical wound should only be performed if asepsis has been maintained. Subcutaneous tissues may be sutured with no. 0 chromic gut in simple continuous pattern to reduce dead space and minimize postoperative swelling. Skin sutures are placed in a Mayo (Ford) interlocking pattern. We prefer to administer antibiotics for 3 days, beginning the day of surgery, to reduce the incidence of postoperative infection. Also, the barrow should be kept in a clean, dry stall during this period.

Complications of Castration. The most common complications following castration of pigs are hemorrhage, abscess, scirrhus cord, inguinal hernia, and seroma or hematoma formation. Fatal hemorrhagic shock has been reported after castration of 7-week-old pigs by a lay person (Libke 1967). The testicles had been pulled through a 10 cm incision and cut using a knife. Fatal hemorrhage occurred into the pelvic canal and abdomen; thus, the cause of death was not recognized until necropsy. This report emphasizes the need for routine necropsy examination of all deaths for which the cause is not apparent.

Meat inspection of 131 pigs with postcastration abscesses revealed that *Arcanobacterium pyogenes*, ß-hemolytic streptococci, *Streptococcus viridans*, *Staphylococcus aureus*, and *Pasteurella multocida* were the most common bacteria isolated (Százados 1985). Approximately 65% of the abscesses were monomicrobial and 35% were polymicrobial infections. Evidence for bacteremia and septicemia was found in 28% and 11%, respectively. Of the 131 pigs inspected, 11% were judged to be unfit for human consumption. Bilateral hydronephrosis also has been reported as a complication of castration in a Hampshire pig castrated at 8 weeks old (McGavin and Schoneweis 1972). A ventral midline incision was used to remove both testicles and tincture of iodine applied after castration. Infection of the soft tissues occurred and the ensuing infection resulted in progressive occlusion of urethra at the level of the sigmoid flexure. Chronic resistance to urine outflow caused hydronephrosis and the pig died 4 weeks after castration. This case illustrates the importance of adequate ventral drainage after castration.

Unilateral Castration. Indications for removal of only one testicle include testicular trauma, hematoma, seroma, and orchitis or periorchitis (Becker 1986). The damaged testicle may cause enough swelling, heat, and pressure to reduce fertility. The boar is placed under general anesthesia, a 6 cm incision is made over the testicle starting at the most ventral aspect of the scrotum, and the testicle is removed by transfixation ligation and excision. The wound may be left open or closed. Strict asepsis and clean housing are required for closure of the wound to prevent abscess formation. We prefer to leave the wound open for second intention healing. Antiseptic ointment is placed in the defect, antibiotics are administered for 5–7 days, and daily hydrotherapy is used to minimize postoperative swelling. Affected boars may return to productive service 30–60 days after surgery.

Testicular Abnormality (Cryptorchidism, Testicular Atrophy, Ectopic Testicle)

Veterinarians may be presented with barrows demonstrating "boar-like" traits for removal of retained testicular tissues. The testicles of swine descend in the last 30 days of gestation and should be palpable at birth (Van

Straaten et al. 1979). True cryptorchidism (testicle not descended at birth) is a common congenital defect in swine. A homozygous recessive trait involving two gene loci has been postulated based on a breeding trial of cryptorchid Duroc swine (Rothschild et al. 1988). A progeny study of Lacombe and Yorkshire true cryptorchid boars resulted in 10.9% and 31.4% of male progeny being cryptorchid (Fredeen and Newman 1968). Of boars with "late-onset" cryptorchidism (normal at birth but having only one testicle at 42 days old), 3.8% of male progeny were cryptorchid. Cryptorchid testicles are usually intraabdominal and are usually found midway between the ipsilateral kidney and the inguinal ring (Thornton 1972). However, the affected testicle may be located within the inguinal canal and not readily palpable from either the inguinal region or from the peritoneal cavity (Lachmayr 1966). Previous removal of the descended testis makes surgical removal of the retained testis more difficult because the incision is best made over the affected inguinal ring. Often, determination of which testicle has been removed is difficult.

Manual restraint and local anesthesia may be adequate for pigs less than 50 kg, but we prefer to perform cryptorchid surgery with the pig under general anesthesia. A 6 cm incision is made over the appropriate inguinal ring. Laparotomy may be performed by making a 4 cm incision 1–2 cm medial to the inguinal canal (parainguinal incision), or the inguinal ring may be enlarged by starting the incision at the cranial commissure of the external inguinal ring. The fingers of one hand are used to perform an exploration of the abdominal cavity starting at the pelvic brim and searching along the dorsal and lateral abdominal wall until the kidneys are encountered. For show pigs, we prefer to perform laparoscopic exploration and removal of abdominal testes because better cosmesis, fewer incisional complications, and more rapid incisional healing is achieved.

True cryptorchidism should be differentiated from testicular atrophy or degeneration (late-onset cryptorchidism) and ectopic testicular tissue. Pigs affected by testicular atrophy are reported to have palpably normal testicles at birth and weaning but having only one testicle present at 42 days old (Fredeen and Newman 1968). Of 122 cryptorchid studied, 21 had "late onset" cryptorchidism. At slaughter, only one testicle can be found and, occasionally, a small mass of lymphoid tissue or epididymis is identified. Ectopic testicular tissue has been observed in numerous pigs at the time of slaughter (Todd et al. 1968). These tissues occur as smooth, pink or tan nodules on the surface of the liver, spleen, mesentery, and other abdominal viscera. Initially, these masses may be interpreted as metastatic neoplasia, but histology reveals the presence of convoluted seminiferous tubules and interstitial cells. No evidence for neoplasia is seen. Ectopic testicular tissues may be found in castrated or intact male pigs.

Prolapsed Penis

Penile and preputial prolapse have been seen after administration of neuroleptic drugs, but also may occur as a result of trauma to the penis or congenital defect (Figure 70.5). While prolapsed, the penis is at great risk of further injury. The penis and prepuce must be returned to their normal position as soon as possible after prolapse. Treatment of penile prolapse usually required that the boar be placed under general anesthesia. The penis is thoroughly cleaned with cold water and a topical antiseptic ointment applied to the surface of the penis. If a penile wound is present, debridement may be done. Penile wounds typically are not sutured closed unless they have occurred recently (within 2–4 hours) because of the likelihood of formation of an abscess. The penis and prepuce are gently massaged until reduction into the sheath is completed. Use of hydroscopic agents (e.g., anhydrous glycerin) may help reduce the swelling by resolving edema. After the penis and prepuce have been repositioned, a purse-string suture may be used to prevent reoccurrence of the prolapse. The purse string should be removed in 5–7 days. If wounds or abrasions are present, daily preputial lavage or administration of systemic antibiotics and antiinflammatory drugs is indicated. If wounds are not present, sexual rest should be enforced for at least 14 days. If wounds requiring treatment are present, sexual rest should be enforced for 30–60 days (depending on the severity of the wound). Reevaluation of the penile injury is advisable prior to use for mating.

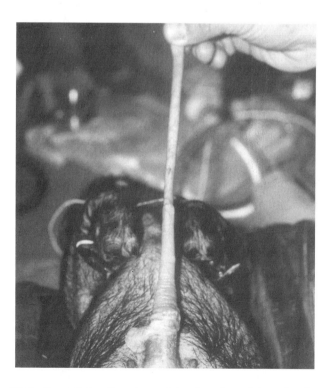

70.5. *Congenital penile and preputial prolapse in a miniature breed pig.*

Preputial Diverticulum

Abnormalities of the preputial diverticulum may cause reproductive unsoundness. Preputial diverticulitis, diverticular ulcers, diverticular stones, urine retention, and penile deviation into the diverticulum may be found (Figure 70.6) (Wieringa and Mouwen 1983; Dutton 1997; Tyler et al. 2000). Preputial diverticulectomy may restore breeding soundness to affected boars. The boar is placed under general anesthesia and prepared for surgery. Any of three procedures for diverticulectomy may be performed:

1. Preputial diverticulectomy via the preputial orifice is done by passing forceps through the preputial orifice, into one lobe of the bilobate diverticulum, gently everting the lobe out through the orifice, and repeating this procedure for the remaining lobe (Figures 70.7 and 70.8). After both lobes of the preputial diverticulum are everted, the diverticulum is excised. Suturing is not required for young boars, but the opening to the diverticulum may be sutured closed in adults.
2. A 6 cm incision is made overlying the lateral aspect of one lobe of the preputial diverticulum. The diverticulum is everted through the preputial orifice, excised, and sutured closed.
3. A 6 cm incision is made as above, but the diverticulum is dissected free from the surrounding soft tissues, excised, and sutured closed (Figure 70.9).

For methods 2 and 3, extreme care must be taken not to perforate the diverticulum prior to removal because contamination will result in incisional infection. Flushing of the preputial diverticulum with antiseptic solutions before surgery is recommended to reduce this possibility. Also, filling the diverticulum with antiseptic solution or gauze pads before surgery makes identification of the diverticulum easier at the time of surgery.

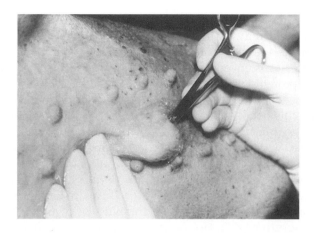

70.7. *Insertion of forceps into one lobe of the preputial diverticulum of an immature boar.*

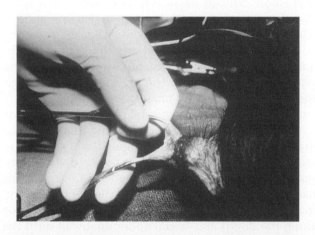

70.8. *Eversion of the preputial diverticulum through the preputial orifice of an immature boar.*

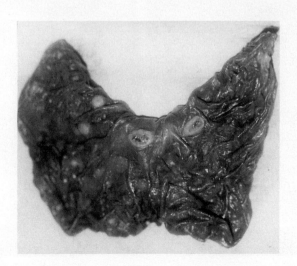

70.6. *Excised preputial diverticulum. Note extensive ulceration of diverticulum.*

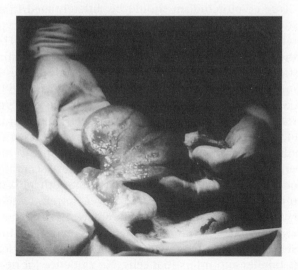

70.9. *Surgical dissection and isolation of the preputial diverticulum in a mature boar.*

Preputial Prolapse

Prolapse of the prepuce may occur with penile prolapse or may result from preputial injury and swelling. If wounds to the prepuce are not present, the prepuce may be repositioned within the sheath, as described for penile prolapse, and a purse-string suture used to maintain the reduction (Schoneweis 1971). Careful evaluation of the preputial swelling should be done to ensure that urination is possible. Preputial edema may be reduced by application of hydroscopic agents (anhydrous glycerin, saturated magnesium sulfate solution). A preputial retaining tube, constructed from rubber or polyurethane tubing, may be placed into the preputial space to prevent prolapse but allow exit of urine. Stay sutures are placed through the tubing and attached to the skin at the preputial orifice. Four sutures are placed 90° from each other suture to maintain the proper position of the tube. Alternatively, a 1.25 cm diameter Penrose drain may be sutured to the tip of the penis (no. 2-0 chromic gut suture) to ensure urine outflow. Often, the prolapsed prepuce has been traumatized and surgical removal of the affected tissues is indicated. Preputial amputation may be performed, but the opening to the urethral diverticulum must be maintained. Alternatively, the preputial diverticulum may be removed at the time of surgery.

The boar is placed under general anesthesia, the prepuce is pulled cranially until normal preputial epithelium is exposed, and stay sutures or crossed pins (7.6 cm, 18-gauge needles) are placed through the exposed prepuce to prevent premature retraction into the sheath. The damaged tissues are amputated and the two layers of the prepuce are sutured closed using an interrupted suture pattern (no. 2-0 chromic gut, PDS, or polyglycolic acid suture). After anastomosis, antiseptic ointment is placed on the prepuce and it is replaced into the sheath. A purse-string suture is placed at the preputial orifice for 7–10 days and sexual rest is enforced for 30–60 days. Systemic antibiotics should be administered perioperatively.

Vasectomy or Epididymectomy

Vasectomy or epididymectomy is done to produce teaser boars used for heat detection in sows for artificial insemination or breeding to valuable boars, or to promote onset of cyclicity in confined gilts (Becker 1986). For vasectomy, the boar is placed in dorsal recumbency under general anesthesia and a 4 cm incision is made over each spermatic cord approximately 6 cm cranial to the ventral aspect of the scrotum. Each spermatic cord is elevated, incised, and the vas deferens isolated. The vas deferens lies next to the spermatic artery, is firm and pale, and an arterial pulse is not present. A 3–4 cm segment of the vas deferens is excised and each end ligated. The incision through the tunic is sutured with no. 2-0 PDS or polyglycolic acid, and the skin is sutured with no. 0 polymerized caprolactam in a Mayo (Ford) interlocking suture pattern. An alternative technique for vasectomizing boars enables the surgery to be done with the boar in lateral recumbency (Althouse and Evans 1997).

Epididymectomy is done by making a 2 cm incision in the scrotum overlying the tail of the epididymis. The tail and 1 cm of the body of the epididymis is isolated. Ligatures are placed between the testicle and the tail of the epididymis and around the exposed portion of the body of the epididymis. The epididymis is excised between these two ligatures. The skin is closed with no. 0 polymerized caprolactam in an interrupted pattern.

Persistent Frenulum

The epithelial attachment of the penis and prepuce atrophies and these tissues separate between 4 and 6 months old in boars. Sexual maturity is achieved by 7–8 months old. Persistence of the frenulum attachment between the penis and prepuce beyond sexual maturity causes failure of breeding soundness and has been observed in boars (Roberts 1986). Surgical removal of the persistent frenulum is performed with the boar under general anesthesia or during a hand mating exercise. Resection of the tissue may be performed with scissors. Ligation is not required in most cases and minimal bleeding is observed after excision. Sexual rest should be enforced for 7–10 days after surgery.

Vaginal Prolapse

Vaginal prolapse occurs as a prepartum event. The cause of vaginal prolapse is unknown, but straining to urinate or defecate may be involved. Sows with lateral deviation of the bladder and difficulty urinating or with inflammation associated with cystitis and urethritis may develop vaginal prolapse because of straining. When the cause can be found, treatment should be aimed at resolving the initial lesion. The vagina is cleaned with cold water, hydroscopic agents (anhydrous glycerin, sugar, etc.) are applied, a towel is wrapped around the prolapsed portion, and constant gentle pressure used to reduce the edema and swelling. The prolapse can usually be reduced in 15–20 minutes. The vagina should be cleansed and topical antibiotic or antiseptic ointments used to reduce the secondary bacterial vaginitis that invariably occurs. Administration of antiinflammatory drugs may reduce straining and shorten convalescence. The bladder should be evaluated to ensure that it is in a normal position (see the section on urinary bladder displacement). Often, partial rectal prolapse accompanies vaginal prolapse. The rectal prolapse should be treated appropriately (see the section on rectal prolapse). A Bühner suture is placed around the vagina to prevent reoccurrence of the prolapse. The sow should be closely monitored and the Bühner suture removed at the first indication of farrowing. If excessive swelling of the soft tissues in the pelvic canal has occurred, a cesarean section is indicated and should be performed early in the process of farrowing.

Bladder Displacement (Lateroflexed)

Displacement of the bladder occurs in multiparous sows in the latter stages of gestation. The bladder is displaced laterally and, occasionally, may become displaced caudally. When this occurs, urination is difficult. The displaced bladder may give the appearance of a vaginal prolapse when the sow is lying down. Affected sows may be seen straining because of the difficulty urinating, and this may lead to true vaginal prolapse. Decompression of the urinary bladder by cystocentesis or catheterization may allow permanent replacement of the bladder. When displacement recurs, an indwelling urinary catheter may be used to allow urination until after parturition. Ascending bacterial cystitis is a complication of the indwelling urinary catheter.

Urethral Obstruction

Urethral obstruction has been observed in miniature pigs most commonly. Clinical signs include signs of abdominal pain, tail flagging, straining to urinate, blood in urine, decreased activity or restlessness, decreased appetite, and teeth grinding. Potential causes of urethral obstruction to be considered include urolithiasis, urethral polyps, and urethral stricture or trauma. Retrograde catheterization of the pelvic urethra and bladder is difficult because of the urethral recess and mucosal flap, which prevent passage of the catheter. Tube cystostomy with positive contrast urethrography was reported to be useful for diagnosis of obstruction of the distal urethra (Palmer et al. 1998). Urethral polyps were reported as a cause of urethral outflow obstruction in Vietnamese potbellied pigs (Helman et al. 1996). Surgical management of urethral outflow obstruction include urethrotomy, cystostomy with normograde flushing, tube cystostomy, perineal urethrostomy, prepubic urethrostomy, and prepubic cystostomy. Prepubic cystostomy was successful in two Vietnamese pigs with urethral injury from castration or urethral stricture (Leon et al. 1997). In these two pigs, the pelvic urethral was exteriorized cranial to the brim of the pelvis and the urethral spatulated and the mucosa sutured to the skin. Both pigs maintained urinary continence. Urethroscopy with laser lithotripsy was used successfully in two potbellied pigs to allieviate urethral obstruction caused by uroliths (Halland et al. 2002).

Tube Cystostomy Procedure. Patients are placed in dorsal recumbency under general anesthesia. An 8–10 cm paramedian approach is made 4 cm lateral to the prepuce and extending from immediately caudal to the preputial orifice to 4 cm cranial to the brim of the pelvis. The bladder is exteriorized and two stay sutures placed near the apex. A cystotomy is performed near the apex, and suction and lavage with saline used to evacuate urine and debris from the bladder. A gallstone scoop may be used to facilitate removal of stones if present. Particular attention is paid to suctioning the region of the trigone and urethral origin to remove debris that may have migrated into the urethra during positioning for surgery. Normograde flushing is attempted to clear the urethra of debris. The cystotomy incision is then closed in two inverting layers using no. 0 or 2-0 absorbable monofilament suture material. A purse-string suture is then preplaced in the ventrolateral aspect of the bladder, near the apex on the same side as the celiotomy incision. A Foley catheter of size appropriate to the animal (range 12–18 F) is placed through a stab incision lateral to the paramedian body wall incision to enter the abdominal cavity. The end of the Foley catheter is then placed through a stab incision in the bladder within the purse-string suture. The purse-string suture is then tied tightly and the catheter balloon inflated with saline. The bladder is pulled close to the body wall using tension on the Foley catheter, which was secured to the skin with a trapping suture pattern. The celiotomy incision is closed routinely using various suture materials, depending on surgeon preference.

Oophorectomy

Removal of the ovaries is rarely indicated in swine. However, oophorectomy may be requested to facilitate research or for pet pigs. For pet pigs, removal of the ovaries is easier, faster, and has less risk of fatal hemorrhage than ovariohysterectomy (OVX). The blood vessels of the broad ligaments of the uterus are extensive and require ligation when OVX is chosen. Both ovaries may be removed from a paralumbar (flank), ventrolateral, paramedian, or ventral midline incision. We prefer to perform ovariectomy via a flank or ventral midline incision. Access to the abdomen is excellent with these incisions, and, in our experience, the risk of postoperative complications (incisional infection, hernia) is less. In either case, we prefer to use general anesthesia while performing the surgery.

For ventral midline approach, the incision may be started immediately caudal to the umbilicus and extended caudally. For a paralumbar approach, the incision is started ventral to the transverse processes of the lumbar vertebrae, midway between the tuber coxae and the last rib. Each ovary is elevated through the incision, two hemostatic forceps are placed on the ovarian pedicle, two ligatures (no. 2-0 polygalactin 910) are placed proximal to the first hemostat, the pedicle is cut between the two hemostats and the ovary removed. Each ovarian artery must be observed for hemorrhage prior to closure. Closure of the ventral midline is done using no. 1 PDS or polyglactin 910 in an interrupted suture pattern. Chromic gut suture should not be used in the linea alba because of the increased risk of postoperative incisional hernia. The skin is closed with no. 2 polymerized caprolactam in a Mayo (Ford) interlocking suture pattern. Paralumbar incisions are closed in three layers (transversus abdominis muscle and peritoneum, internal and external abdominal oblique muscles, and skin).

Ovariectomy, alone, may be performed in pet pigs that have not begun normal estrous cycles. Uterine atrophy is expected to occur after ovariectomy. We recommend OVX in sexually mature pigs because of the potential risk for pyometra in a uterus where the cervix has been open.

Uterus

Hysterectomy. Hysterectomy may be performed as part of cesarean section, and is discussed below. Elective hysterectomy is rarely done in swine. However, hysterectomy may be requested for research purposes or for pet pigs (Figure 70.10). When hysterectomy is performed for pet pigs, the ovaries also are removed. General anesthesia should be used during hysterectomy. The uterus may be removed via a flank, ventrolateral, paramedian, or ventral midline incision. We prefer to perform hysterectomy via either flank or ventral midline incision. The uterus is elevated through the incision, the ovaries are removed as described above, the broad ligament of the uterus is ligated using two to four overlapping simple interrupted sutures for mass ligation of the blood vessels, and transfixation ligatures are placed in the uterine body immediately cranial to the internal os of the cervix. The uterus and ovaries are removed and the incision closed as described above. All sutured pedicles should be checked for adequate hemostasis prior to closure.

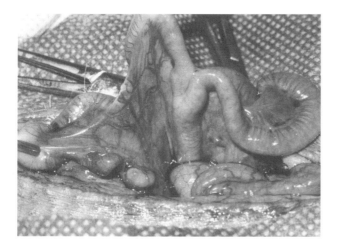

70.10. *Uterus and ovaries exteriorized for ovariohysterectomy in a 4-month-old pet pig.*

Cesarean Section: Indication and Decision Analysis.

Cesarean section is required when transcervical extraction of pigs from the uterus is not possible (complicated dystocia) and to obtain gnotobiotic or specific pathogen free (SPF) pigs. Cesarean section for gnotobiotic pigs is usually performed with the sow under general anesthesia and is discussed below. The most common reported causes of dystocia in swine are uterine inertia, small pelvic size, inadequate dilation of the birth canal, fetal-to-maternal disproportion, fetal malpresentation, and abnormalities of the birth canal (Titze 1977).

Cesarean section for dystocia is usually chosen as a "last-resort" procedure for fetal extraction because of economic pressures. Therefore, the mortality rate among sows and gilts having cesarean section is expected to be higher than for other species. This is not surprising because affected swine suffer extreme physical exhaustion, stress, and shock by the time the decision for cesarean section is made. Interestingly, multiparous sows had a higher frequency of collapse (25.8%) prior to cesarean section compared with primiparous pigs (16.4%) (Dimigen 1972). Owners and veterinarians may become reluctant to perform cesarean section because of expense, previous experiences with fatalities, and the high rate of dead pigs delivered. It is our opinion that unnecessary delays in the decision for surgery is the principle cause of sow and baby pig mortality associated with cesarean section. When the veterinarian is presented with a sow in dystocia, the decision as to whether the owner is willing to incur the costs of cesarean section should be ascertained as early as possible during the initial examination. Other factors influencing the decision for cesarean section includes the cause of dystocia, how long the sow has been in labor, how long the owner has tried to extract the pigs manually, and how swollen or traumatized the sow's pelvic canal has become. Many owners are adept at extracting pigs, and their failure to remove pigs successfully may justify immediate cesarean if the cause of dystocia is not apparent. The most common indications for cesarean section in pigs are undersized pelvic canal, inadequate cervical and soft tissue dilation, prolonged labor (including uterine inertia), fetal-to-maternal disproportion, and trauma to the birth canal (Titze 1977). In our experience, cesarean section performed at the earliest indication has a high success rate for survival of the sow and a higher rate of live pigs obtained (Table 70.2).

Table 70.2. Outcome of cesarean section in sows with respect to duration of labor

Duration of Labor	Number of Sows	% Sows Having >50% Live Pigs	% Sows Having <50% Live Pigs	% Sows Having All Dead Pigs	% Sows Died or Culled
<18 hours	125	66.7	7.9	25.4	13.4
18–48 hours	81	19.7	13.5	66.7	32.1
>48 hours	21	0	4.7	95.3	28.5
Overall	227	43.7	9.7	46.6	21.5

Source: Adapted from Dimigen 1972.

Swine that are physically exhausted, stressed, or in shock must be stabilized prior to cesarean section. Thirteen percent of sows in labor for less than 18 hours died or were salvaged, compared with 60% of sows in labor for more than 18 hours (Dimigen 1972). Among sows necropsied after sudden death, retained fetuses and toxemia were found in approximately 10% (Sanford et al. 1994). Stabilization of the sow often is simple and readily achieved. We routinely place a 16 or 18 gauge, 2-inch intravenous catheter in an ear vein. This catheter is sutured or glued in place and intravenous fluids (0.9% saline or lactated Ringer's solution) administered rapidly (initially 20–40 ml/kg of body weight/hour; then, 4 ml/kg/hour once stabilized) and continued for the duration of the surgery. We prefer to add dextrose (1.25% final solution) and calcium (1 ml/kg) to intravenous fluids after the patient has been stabilized. Further, the shock status of the sow may be improved by administration of dexamethasone (0.5 to 1.0 mg/kg, IV) or flunixin meglumine (1 mg/kg, IV). Because extensive manipulation of the intrauterine environment prior to cesarean section increases the risk for postoperative septic peritonitis, we prefer to administer preoperative antibiotics (procaine penicillin G, ceftiofur HCl, or oxytetracycline).

In severely compromised sows, sedation (see the section on anesthesia section) and local or regional anesthesia may be adequate for surgery. Intravenous fluids should be administered continuously. Epidural anesthesia (lumbosacral level) also may be useful. Overall, we prefer to perform general anesthesia rather than attempt cesarean using physical restraint and epidural anesthesia. In our experience, this causes the least stress on the patient, surgeon, and assistants. The respiratory rate and heart rate should be monitored and supportive therapy adjusted appropriately.

Surgical Approach for Cesarean Section. Multiple surgical approaches have been described for cesarean section. Selection of the surgical approach depends upon the preference of the surgeon, the condition of the patient, and means of restraint and anesthesia used for surgery. The most common approaches are paralumbar fossa, ventrolateral (horizontal low flank), ventral midline, paramedian, or paramammary (Mather 1966; Turner and McIlwraith 1989). With a ventral or paramedian approach, movement by the sow must be prevented because of the risk for contamination of the incision. Also, the mammary veins must be carefully avoided or ligated to prevent excessive loss of blood during the procedure. In our experience, ventral and paramedian incisions have the highest risk for development of postoperative incisional infection (contamination on the floor and trauma from pigs searching for nipples).

The ventrolateral incision is made parallel and ventral to the flank, and lateral to the mammary chain (Mather 1966). The sow is placed in lateral recumbency with the uppermost hind limb tied in adduction and ex-

tension. The incision is started approximately 10 cm cranial to the inguinal region and extended cranially for 15 cm.

For paralumbar fossa incision, the sow is placed in lateral recumbency and the incision is started cranial and ventral to the tuber coxae. The incision is extended ventrally to a point approximately 5 cm dorsal to the cranial skin fold of the flank.

Ventrolateral and paralumbar incisions are relatively easy to perform, have little blood loss during surgery, and are less likely to become infected after surgery. Fewer fat deposits are encountered with ventrolateral incisions, and the meat portion of the flank is left undisturbed. After exteriorizing the closest uterine horn, a 6–8 cm long incision is made parallel with the uterine horn and as close to the bifurcation of the uterine horns as possible. All pigs may not be able to be removed from a single incision in the uterus (Figure 70.11).

Closure of cesarean section incision is based upon the conditions under which the surgery was performed. For a healthy uterus containing live or recently dead pigs, we use no. 1 chromic gut or no. 0 PDS or polyglycolic acid placed in a cushing or Utrecht (modified cushing) pattern for closure of the uterus. Some veterinarians have advocated hysterectomy when performing cesarean section (Schoneweis 1971). This practice allows rapid removal of all pigs soon after entering the abdomen, ensures culling of the sow after the pigs have been weaned, and minimizes surgery time because removal of individual pigs is done by an assistant after removal of the uterus. The uterine arteries are ligated with no. 0 chromic gut, the broad ligaments are divided along the axis of the uterine horns, and the uterine body is ligated using rubber tubing. The rubber tubing may be secured to the uterine body using no. 1 chromic gut suture. Alternatively, sterile 1 cm cotton tape (umbilical tape) suture may be used to perform transfixation

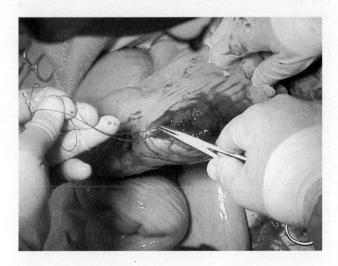

70.11. *Suturing uterus closed after removal of pigs. Sow was positioned in lateral recumbency for a cesarean section via paramammary approach.*

ligation of the uterine body. Then, the gravid uterus is removed. We urge caution with hysterectomy that precise hemostasis must be achieved prior to removal of the uterus. Ligation of abdominal bleeders after removal of the uterus is difficult, and life-threatening hemorrhage may occur if the uterine arteries are inadequately ligated. We close the transversus abdominis muscle and peritoneum, together, and the external abdominal oblique and internal abdominal oblique muscles, together, using no. 2 chromic gut or no. 1 PDS or polyglycolic acid placed in simple continuous pattern. For closure of ventral midline or paramedian incisions, we do not recommend the use of chromic gut because of the higher rate of postoperative hernia formation. We use no. 1 PDS or polyglycolic acid suture placed in simple interrupted or interrupted cruciate pattern. Skin is closed using no. 0 polymerized caprolactam in a Mayo (Ford) interlocking pattern. The sow should remain confined for a minimum of 14 days after surgery.

Gnotobiotic Pigs. The production of gnotobiotic or SPF pigs is an accepted model for scientific research. The selected sow should be placed under general anesthesia and the surgery site aseptically prepared. Several methods have been described for obtaining gnotobiotic pigs including hysterectomy, closed hysterotomy (using a sterile chamber attached to the side of the sow through which surgery is performed), and open hysterotomy with germicidal trap. All methods are expected to have a baby pig mortality rate of less than 15%, except open hysterotomy performed with local anesthesia which may have a 35% baby pig mortality rate (Tavernor et al. 1971; Miniats and Jol 1978). When a hysterectomy technique is selected, baby pig survival is better when the surgery is performed with the sow under general anesthesia rather than euthanized prior to hysterectomy.

Uterine Prolapse. Prolapse of the uterus is occasionally seen in sows during or up to several days after parturition. Excessive straining because of fetal malpositioning, fetal-to-maternal disproportion, or trauma with swelling and inflammation in the birth canal is thought to cause uterine prolapse. Prolapse of the entire uterus has the greatest potential for a life-threatening crisis because of profuse hemorrhage, but partial prolapse also may occur. The sow must be stabilized prior to attempts to replace the uterus into its normal position. If hemorrhage, hypovolemia, or shock (tachycardia, peripheral cyanosis) are present, the sow should be placed into a warm environment, an IV catheter placed into an auricular vein, and intravenous fluids administered. Hypertonic saline may be administered rapidly (5–7 ml/kg body weight, IV over 5–10 minutes) followed by isotonic crystalline fluids (5–10 ml/kg/hour).

For replacement of the prolapse, the sow may be placed on an inclined floor or platform in sternal recumbency with the hindquarters elevated. Epidural anesthe-

sia (administered at the lumbosacral space), sedation, or general anesthesia may be required to eliminate struggling, straining, and agitation of the sow. The uterus is thoroughly cleaned with cold water and assessed for the presence of lacerations and necrosis. Small lacerations may be cleaned, superficially debrided, and sutured closed (no. 0 chromic gut, simple continuous pattern). Hemorrhage may be stopped by ligating affected vessels or by performing en bloc tissue imbrication. Sutures may be placed over stents to increase the region of pressure to control hemorrhage. Then, hydroscopic agents (e.g., anhydrous glycerin, sugar, etc.) may be applied to the uterus to assist in reducing edema. The uterus is wrapped into a towel and gentle pressure applied, starting from the tip of the uterine horn and working toward the body of the uterus. After approximately 15 minutes, the edema should be sufficiently reduced to allow manipulation of the uterine horns. Each horn should be inverted starting with the tip and gradually reduced until the uterine body has been reached.

Often, progress is impeded because of the extensive edema and swelling of the soft tissues of the pelvic canal. When this occurs, left paralumbar fossa laparotomy is indicated (Raleigh 1977). After appropriate preparation of the surgical site and surgeon, a 10 cm long, vertically oriented incision is made in the middle of the left paralumbar fossae. The left arm is passed into the peritoneal cavity and into the everted uterus. One of the uterine horns is grasped and pulled back into the peritoneal cavity. The right arm or an assistant helps by applying gentle pressure on the everted horn from the exterior. After the uterus has been repositioned, all remaining fetuses should be removed. The laparotomy incision should be closed in three layers (transversus abdominis muscle and peritoneum, internal and external abdominal oblique muscles, and skin). Chromic gut (no. 3) or a synthetic absorbable suture (polydioxinone, polyglactin 910, polyglycolic acid) is placed in simple continuous suture patterns in the muscle layers. Polymerized caprolactam (no. 2 braunamide) is placed in a Mayo (Ford) interlocking pattern in the skin. Antimicrobial and antiinflammatory medications are desirable, but strict attention should be paid to drug residues in the meat prior to slaughter. Finally, a Bühner suture should be placed around the vulva to prevent reoccurrence of the prolapse. The Bühner suture (6.4 mm wide sterile cotton tape) should be deeply placed at the junction of the labia and the skin of the perineum to recreate the function of the vestibular sphincter muscle. The Bühner suture may be removed in 7–10 days with minimal risk of prolapse. Oxytocin (20 units) is routinely administered to facilitate contraction and involution of the uterus and cervix. If prolapse reduction using laparotomy is not used as a "last resort" treatment, sows should survive partial prolapse of the uterus (>75% survival), but complete prolapse carries a guarded prognosis (<50% survival).

Amputation of the Uterus. Amputation of the uterus is indicated when excessive bleeding, extensive laceration, trauma, or necrosis of a uterine prolapse is found. The prognosis with uterine prolapse is guarded to poor for survival and affected sows must be provided with supportive care as soon as possible (shelter, IV fluids via ear vein catheter, etc.). Focal lacerations and bleeders can be repaired and the uterus replaced into the abdomen. When severe injury has occurred, amputation of the uterus provides the best option for salvage of the sow. Prior to amputation, the uterus should be closely inspected to ensure that the bladder or small intestine are not entrapped. Hypovolemic or hemorrhagic shock may be present and should be addressed during the course of treatment. If the uterus is swollen, it should be elevated above the pig to encourage drainage of venous congestion. We recommend placing towels around the uterus so that pressure may be applied without further trauma to the wall of the uterus. Hydroscopic agents (e.g., anhydrous glycerin, granular sugar) may be used to help resolve edema of the uterine tissues.

After venous congestion has been reduced, amputation is more easily performed. Transfixation ligatures are placed around the circumference of the uterus. Heavy suture material (0.5 cm sterile cotton tape, no. 3 polymerized caprolactam) is used because the thickness of the uterus requires extreme tension to completely occlude the uterine arteries. Stay sutures or cross pins (using 15 cm long 18 gauge needles) are placed in the vital uterus and the prolapsed portion amputated. Then, any bleeders are ligated with no. 1 chromic gut before the remaining tissues are released and placed back into the pelvic canal. A Bühner suture or purse-string suture should be placed into the labia at the level of the vestibular sphincter to prevent prolapse of the remaining tissues. Affected sows are salvaged as soon as possible or after weaning of the litter.

Mastectomy

Chronic infection of the mammae may result in the formation of abscesses, granulomas, and mammary fistulas (Figure 70.12). The swellings may become large and problematic for the sow. Surgical removal of the mammae is indicated for return of the sow to production soundness. Sows with at least 12 intact mammary glands and that are not in the first week or last 4 weeks of gestation are suitable candidates for surgery (Bollwahn 1992).

The sow is placed under general anesthesia and the affected mammary gland prepared for surgery. An elliptical incision is made approximately 1 cm from the base of the swelling so that enough tissue remains to allow closure of the tissues with minimal tension. A combination of sharp and blunt dissection is used to extirpate the gland, granuloma, and abscesses. The cranial superficial epigastric vein (subcutaneous abdominal vein) should not be compromised, but hemostasis is essential. Hemostasis is ensured by using 2-0 chromic gut ligature

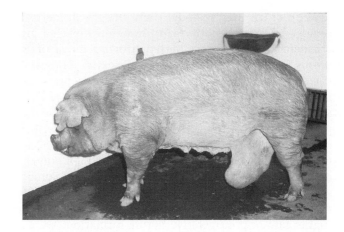

70.12. *Chronic mastitis.*

of transected blood vessels. The wound is closed in three layers: deep subcutaneous, superficial subcutaneous, and skin. Each subcutaneous tissue layer is sutured with a simple continuous suture pattern (no. 0 chromic gut, no. 2-0 PDS or polyglycolic acid). Each suture is anchored to the deeper tissue layer in an attempt to close all dead space, thus minimizing the formation of postoperative seroma, hematoma, and abscess. Administration of perioperative antibiotics is indicated.

ABDOMINAL SURGERY

Umbilical Hernia

Umbilical hernia is a developmental defect of pigs. An umbilical hernia is a discontinuity of the abdominal wall at the umbilicus with protrusion of abdominal content into a hernia sac formed by the skin and surrounding connective tissue (Figure 70.13). In swine herds, the frequency of umbilical hernias ranges from 0.4 to 1.2% and varies with breed and sex (Searcy-Bernal et al. 1994). In addition to heredity, the etiology of umbilical hernia may be navel infection and umbilical abscess. After the umbilical cord is cut at birth, iodine should be applied to decrease the likelihood of infection. Pigs with umbilical hernias may suffer from growth retardation and may die from intestinal strangulation. In one study, pigs sired by American Spotted and Duroc boars were more likely to develop hernia than those sired by Yorkshire, and umbilical hernias often were detected in pigs between 9 and 14 weeks of age (Searcy-Bernal et al. 1994). One possible reason for the recognition of the condition at that age may be the rapid growth of pigs, combined with increased weight of the abdominal contents, leading to a hernia of significant size. Females were at an increased risk of developing umbilical hernia.

As with many other swine surgical conditions, the cost of treatment may preclude surgical correction. In that case, pigs should be consigned to an early slaughter soon (within 1 month) after detection of the hernia, before evisceration or intestinal strangulation or fistula oc-

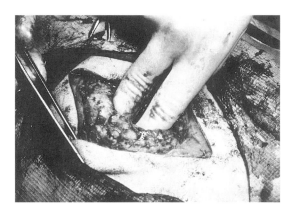

70.13. *Surgical repair of an umbilical hernia in a female. An elliptical incision is made around the hernia sac and the excess skin is discarded.*

curs. A case of intestinal umbilical fistula has been described in a 30 kg castrated male pig (Lewis 1973). The risk of intestinal incarceration and strangulation is more frequent with an umbilical hernia of small dimension, i.e., hernia ring smaller than 8 cm. However, a pig with an umbilical hernia often will be discounted when it goes to slaughter.

Reduced growth rate in untreated pigs with umbilical hernias may encourage surgical correction of the defect. However, whether surgical correction of umbilical hernia will restore the growth potential is unknown. In purebred, show animals and pigs kept as pets, surgical correction often is indicated.

Herniorrhaphy should be performed early in life. Following anesthesia, the pig is restrained in dorsal recumbency in a V-shaped trough. The surgical area then is cleaned and prepared for surgery. If surgical correction is performed on a male, the prepuce, preputial diverticulum, and penis should be reflected posteriorly or to one side. The hernia sac then is isolated, and dissection is performed to the hernia ring. The hernia sac with an abscess, if present, should be removed, and the edges of the ring freshened. If intestinal contents are adhered to the hernia sac, the adhesions are separated and bowel viability is assessed; if judged acceptable, the bowel is replaced in the abdomen. If intestinal viability is compromised, resection and anastomosis of viable intestine should be performed. If no infection is present, the hernia sac also can be inverted into the abdomen. The abdominal defect then is closed using an overlapping or simple continuous pattern. The prepuce, preputial diverticulum, and penis then are repositioned and sutured to the abdominal muscle with absorbable suture material. The skin then is sutured using a simple interrupted pattern of nonabsorbable suture material.

For surgical correction of umbilical hernia in the female, an elliptical incision is made around the hernia sac, and the excess skin is discarded. With a combination of sharp and blunt dissection, the hernia sac then is cut and removed and the abdominal muscle closed, as in the male. The subcutaneous tissue and skin then are closed. Systemic antibiotic should be administered for 5 days, and the skin suture removed in 10 days.

Inguinal or Scrotal Hernia

Inguinal hernia and scrotal hernia are variants of a defect in which intestines or other abdominal organs pass into the inguinal canal. The hernia develops when there is an abnormally large and patent vaginal orifice through which the vaginal process and peritoneal cavity communicate. Scrotal hernia is the more exaggerated form of the defect in that the organs protrude into the scrotum (Vogt and Ellersieck 1990). These hernias are common in swine and have been the most common defect observed in swine (Vogt and Ellersieck 1990). The frequency of scrotal hernia among the porcine population varied between 0 and 15.7% with a realistic number of about 1% (Vogt and Ellersieck 1990). The development of these hernias seems to be genetically influenced. One study indicated that the variation associated with anatomic structures relevant to scrotal hernia is influenced polygenically. In that study, the heritabilities of susceptibility to scrotal hernia development were estimated to be 0.29, 0.34, and 0.34 in Duroc-, Landrace-, and Yorkshire-sired pig groups, respectively (Vogt and Ellersieck 1990). Inguinal and scrotal hernias need to be differentiated from hydrocele, scirrhous cord, and hematoma of the testicle. Taking a good history (e.g., a pig that has been castrated before is more likely to have a scirrhous cord) and direct manipulation often will give the diagnosis. If necessary, ultrasonography and needle aspiration can be used. Inguinal hernias often are encountered at the time of castration. Some of these hernias will reduce spontaneously but recur later. With chronic inguinal hernia, intestinal incarceration and strangulation may be observed.

Surgical repair of an inguinal or scrotal hernia is easier if done before the pig is castrated. With the pig restrained in dorsal recumbency and its rear quarters elevated, the inguinal and scrotal area is thoroughly cleaned and prepared for surgery. An oblique incision is made over the affected external inguinal ring. Once through the skin, the subcutaneous tissue is dissected bluntly. Also by blunt dissection, the tunica vaginalis is isolated. The tunica vaginalis should be kept intact, because this will keep the intestine contained. While external pressure is put on the scrotum, the tunics are gently pulled free from their scrotal attachment. The entire hernia sac is removed through the inguinal incision. The tunic and testicle then are twisted to force the intestines into the peritoneal cavity. The tunics and spermatic cord are transfixated as close to the inguinal ring as possible. The tunic and cord then are cut, and the inguinal ring is closed with interrupted or horizontal mattress suture. The herniorrhaphy then is checked by applying external pressure on the abdomen. The skin then is closed using absorbable sutures. The authors always recommend checking the other side for possible bilateral herniation before performing a castration.

If the surgery was done to repair a large hernia in which marked serum accumulation in the scrotum is expected, an incision in the most ventral aspect of the scrotum should be performed via the inguinal incision before suturing to provide ventral drainage. If intestinal adhesion and incarceration are observed during surgical correction of a scrotal hernia, the vaginal tunic should be opened and the intestine dissected free or an intestinal resection and end-to-end anastomosis performed. If an inguinal hernia occurs after castration, one needs to clean and lavage the herniated bowel, enlarge the inguinal ring and replace the prolapsed intestine (if it is judged to still be viable), and then suture the inguinal ring.

Visceral Torsion or Volvulus

In one series of cases, acute abdominal accidents were characterized clinically by sudden death and were observed more commonly in dry sows (Morin et al. 1984). It was proposed that feeding dry sows in large breeding units once a day or every other day might be an important provoking factor. This feeding method often will make sows ingest large quantity of feed and water rapidly. In swine with gastric torsion, death was preceded sometimes by a short period of anorexia, abdominal distension, shortness of breath, cyanosis, and salivation. At necropsy, clockwise torsions were more common than counterclockwise. The torsions were about the longitudinal axis of the organ and the stomach was distended severely with fluid, gas, and food (Morin et al. 1984). The spleen had rotated with the stomach in some sows; affected spleens were congested severely and some had ruptured, causing hemoperitoneum. Torsion of the liver also was seen occasionally (Morin et al. 1984). In eight sows, intestinal volvulus was observed and it was more common in younger sows. In four sows the entire small intestine was included in the volvulus, the posterior half of the small intestine in one, the small intestine and colon in one, and the cecum and colon in the last one (Morin et al. 1984).

Intestinal Obstruction

In swine with intestinal obstructions from intussusceptions or foreign bodies, clinical signs observed may include depression, vomiting, abdominal distension, and decrease in the amount of feces, sometimes with blood and mucus in it. These two conditions are diagnosed rarely in live animals. If the condition is diagnosed early, a ventral midline celiotomy and an enterotomy are performed for the foreign body obstruction, and an intestinal resection and anastomosis are done for the intussusception. Spiral colon obstruction was diagnosed in an 8-year-old potbellied pig with depression, inappetance, and abdominal distension (Gallardo et al. 2003). Exploratory laparotomy found a stricture at the proximal centripetal loop of the spiral colon and megacolon proximal to the stricture. A side-to-side colonic anastomosis was performed and the pig returned to normal after surgery. A 7-month-old female potbellied pig was diagnosed with idiopathic megacolon based on abdominal palpation, abdominal radiographs, and exploratory surgery (Bassett et al. 1999). A subtotal colectomy was performed and an ileocolonic anastomosis performed. The pig survived and, after a period of diarrhea, stool returned to normal.

Gastric Ulcers

Gastric ulcers are common conditions of the gastrointestinal tract of the pig. Clinical signs are pale mucous membrane (anemia) and dark, tarry feces. In valuable pigs, sometimes gastrotomy can be the best treatment option. With the animal in dorsal recumbency, an incision is made on the ventral midline starting at the xiphoid cartilages. The stomach is isolated from the rest of the abdomen, and the serosal surface is evaluated for changes in color and appearance that would indicate an ulcer. A gastrotomy then is done, and the stomach contents are removed. If an ulcer is found, it can be surgically dissected and the edges electrocoagulated or ligated with some suture material. The wall of the stomach then is closed with a double row of suture material using an inverting pattern. If multiple bleeding ulcers are present, the prognosis is poor even with surgery (see Chapter 54 on gastric ulcers).

Atresia Ani and Rectal Stricture

Atresia ani occurs more frequently in the pig than any other species and is possibly the most important cause of intestinal obstruction. This congenital defect is transmitted genetically. The diagnosis is made by an absence of anal opening, abdominal distension, slower growth rate, and vomiting (Figure 70.14). Because the pigs are able to vomit, the diagnosis of atresia ani may not be made until 3–4 weeks of age. In the female piglet, a fistula may occur between the rectum and vagina, so that the feces may be voided through the vulva. Surgical treatment of atresia ani is necessary for survival. Following anesthesia, a circular piece of skin is excised below the tail over the bulging rectum. Feces usually are discharged immediately. If the rectum is not present at the skin opening, pelvic dissection may be necessary. Depending on the location of the rectum, or if atresia of the rectum is also present, surgical correction may not be possible. In these extreme cases, a celiotomy and colostomy may be necessary but rarely justifiable economically.

Pigs with rectal stricture often show similar clinical signs as pigs with atresia ani, except that they have an anus and are generally older. In one series of cases, pigs with rectal stricture were 16–18 weeks of age (Saunders 1974). After being affected for 2 weeks, these pigs suffered from weight loss compared to their herdmates, no

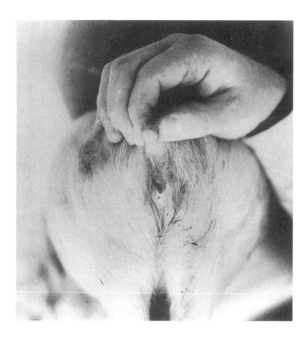

70.14. *Female pig with atresia ani.*

feces were passed, and the abdomen continued to distend. These pigs were slaughtered or killed by other pigs (Saunders 1974). Most cases of rectal stricture are the results of a rectal prolapse that has constricted after repair causing an obstruction. At necropsy, these pigs show a distended cecum and colon. The rectum usually is occluded for 3–5 cm by a band of fibrous tissue. It is speculated that inflammation of the rectal mucosa leads to rectal scar formation with subsequent stenosis and eventually possible complete obstruction (Saunders 1974). Pigs with rectal stricture may respond to celiotomy with colostomy or ileocutaneous anastomosis. Ileocutaneous anastomosis has been successfully performed in pigs as young as 10 days old (Anderson et al. 2000).

Rectal Prolapse and Rectal Amputation

Rectal prolapse is a common occurrence in swine. Prolapse of the rectal mucosa occurs following straining to defecate. The mucosa rapidly becomes edematous and often shows bleeding lesions. Many factors have been associated with the development of rectal prolapse, including genetics, a birth weight of less than 1 kg, being male, diarrhea, coughing, short tails, autumn and winter piling as a consequence of chilling, chronic water shortage, certain antibiotics, zearalenone toxicosis, and a diet containing excess lysine (20% more than required) (Amass et al. 1995). Diagnosis of rectal prolapse is not difficult, but care should be taken that the prolapse does not contain other organs.

The simplest procedure for correction of rectal prolapse is reduction by gentle massage and retention by application of a purse-string suture pattern using umbilical tape. The suture is passed in and out through the skin around the anal opening at a distance of 1 cm from the anus. A one-finger opening should be left when tying the purse string. The suture usually is left in place for 5 days. This should be done only if the rectal mucosa is viable and no laceration is present on close inspection.

If the mucosa is too necrotic to replace, correction of the prolapse can be approached in different ways (Vonderfecht 1978). One technique is a surgical amputation. For this surgery, required instruments are hemostats, blade, scissors, thumb forceps, two 18-gauge needles 8–10 cm long, suture material, and a small-diameter rubber tube. Following anesthesia, the tube is inserted in the rectum until 5 or 8 cm protrude. The tube is fixed in the rectum by inserting the two needles through the rectum at right angles to each other so that they pass through the rectum and tube and emerge from the opposite side. The dissection is started about one centimeter from the mucocutaneous border where the mucosa is still healthy, and the entire circumference of the exposed mucosa of the rectum is cut down to the serosa of the inner wall. Hemorrhaging is usually minor and controlled with gauge until all the layers have been dissected and the dorsal artery of the rectum is cut. Once the dissection is completed around the prolapse, the rectum is held in place because it is attached to the rubber tube with needles. Instead of using tubing and needles, one could use forceps applied at two or three places as the prolapsed rectum is amputated to prevent telescoping into the animal's body (Kjar 1976). To suture the ends of the rectum together, the authors suggest using size 0 absorbable suture material in an inside-out continuous pattern. After the simple continuous pattern has been placed around the rectum, the needles are pulled from the tube, and the tube is removed from the rectum. The rectum then automatically retracts into place.

An alternative method of rectal amputation is to use a prolapse ring, PVC tubing, syringe case, or corrugated tube (Douglas 1985). The ring or tubing is placed in the rectum, and the halfway point on the tube needs to be inserted as far as the anal sphincter. A ligature or rubber band then is applied over the prolapse as near as possible to the anus. The ligature or rubber band must be tight enough to disrupt blood supply to the prolapse. Feces may go through the tube or may block the tube. Usually, the necrotic prolapse falls in 5–7 days with the implant in place, and then fecal production returns to normal.

Three possible complications seen with rectal prolapse are bladder retroversion, eventration of the small intestine, and rectal stricture (Peyton et al. 1980). In a 1-month-old castrated pig, eventration of the small bowel was seen concurrently with a rectal prolapse. The rectal prolapse was 5 cm long, edematous, and purple-black. A small tear was found in the rectum in the pelvic area, and eventration of small intestine was observed. It was speculated that the prolapse was of long duration, allowing necrosis to occur. This provided a friable area, and during straining to defecate, the small intestine perforated this necrotic area (Peyton et al. 1980).

Surgical correction of small intestine eventration in the pig is usually not economically feasible. If treatment is requested, preoperative medical management is often necessary, because these pigs are often in shock. Under general anesthesia, the intestine then is examined and most likely will have to be resected. A ventral midline incision then is made to occlude the lumen of the intestine that remained within the abdominal cavity, and the portion of the intestine that is going to the rectal laceration is resected close to the rectum. The viable end of intestine then is exteriorized through the ventral midline incision, and an end-to-end anastomosis performed (Peyton et al. 1980).

Bladder retroversion with rectal prolapse has been observed in a sow 2 days after normal farrowing (Greenwood 1989). The sow had a grapefruit-sized rectal prolapse with protrusion and tension of the perineal area. The bladder was drained by passage of a polypropylene catheter. One week postpartum, the prolapsed rectum was amputated. The sow reared nine piglets to 6 weeks of age and was sent for slaughter 1 week after weaning the piglets (Greenwood 1989).

MUSCULOSKELETAL SURGERY

Septic Arthritis

Septic arthritis may be caused by bacteremia, direct inoculation of bacteria into the joint, or extension of a local infection into the joint. Bacteremia and polyarthritis are discussed in Chapter 5. Septic arthritis caused by direct inoculation or local extension are treated by wound management, joint lavage, and systemic antibiotic therapy. Infected joints may require daily, or every other day, lavage for 7–10 days or until granulation tissue has covered the wound. Sterile isotonic electrolyte solutions (0.9% saline, lactated Ringer's solution) are lavaged through the joint by inserting an 18- or 14-gauge needle into the joint, injecting the solution under pressure into the joint, and inserting a second needle into the joint with as much separation as possible between the two needles. Approximately 500 ml of the solution are flushed through the joint. After lavage, antibiotics may be instilled directly into the joint to achieve maximal local antibiotic concentration. Success of treatment is assessed by improvement in lameness and wound appearance.

Digit Amputation

Digit amputation is indicated when severe foot abscesses or septic arthritis of the interphalangeal joints have caused unmanageable damage to a single digit. These injuries are most commonly caused by wounds from trauma on concrete flooring or metal side panels. The decision for amputation should not be delayed. If the infection has extended to the fetlock or more proxi-

mally on the limb, digit amputation will not be curative. Also, the soundness of the opposite digit should be assessed to determine if the pig will be able to ambulate on the remaining digit after amputation.

After induction of general anesthesia, the affected digit is cleaned and prepared for surgery. A tourniquet is placed proximal to the surgery site to prevent extensive hemorrhage during surgery. A circumferential incision is made through the skin and soft tissues at a 45° angle to the coronary band, starting at the axial aspect of the digit and continuing proximally to the abaxial surface. The skin is reflected proximal to the site for amputation, and a sterile obstetrical wire is used to amputate the digit. The third phalanx and a portion of the second phalanx is removed by this procedure. The remainder of the second phalanx also should be removed. The remaining tissues are debrided, cleaned thoroughly, and the skin is opposed over the wound. A sufficient opening is left to allow drainage or a Penrose drain is placed into the wound. The foot is placed in a padded bandage for 7–10 days. Then, the foot is cleaned daily with water until the wound is healed. Perioperative antibiotics and antiinflammatory drugs are indicated.

Ankylosis of the Proximal or Distal Interphalangeal Joint

Septic arthritis of the proximal or distal interphalangeal joint is an indication for digit amputation. However, the lateral claw of the hind limb is important to normal ambulation and breeding activity. Salvage of the digit by facilitated ankylosis is an option to preserve normal ambulation. The affected pig is placed under general anesthesia and the digit prepared for surgery. A 1 cm incision is made into the affected joint. The distal interphalangeal joint is approached by placing a 3.75 cm long needle into the joint by inserting the needle immediately proximal to the coronary band and inserting the needle distally. The proximal interphalangeal joint may be located by palpation or insertion of the needle in the midpastern region.

After the arthrotomy has been made, a 4 or 6 mm diameter drill bit is used to destroy the articular surfaces of the joint. Curettes are used to debride the joint and remove all infected subchondral bone. A distinct difference in texture and hardness will be noted between the necrotic (gritty and irregular) and healthy (smooth and hard) bone. Thorough curettage of all infected bone is critical to establishing effective joint ankylosis. The tissues are extensively lavaged with normal saline and antibiotics are administered for 10–14 days. Strict confinement for 6–8 weeks is needed for ankylosis to occur. A cast extending from the ground to the carpus or hock will hasten convalescence.

Fracture Repair

Swine with fracture of long bones are often salvaged because economic considerations preclude treatment.

However, veterinarians may be asked to treat fractures in swine of potential value for genetic improvement. Treatment of fractures can be rewarding and Vaughan (1966) reported clinical experiences with fracture fixation in commercial swine. Fractures were associated with breeding injury (2 pigs), injury on concrete flooring (3 pigs), fighting injury (1 pig), and were of unknown cause in 5 pigs. The most common fractures treated were tibia and fibula (5 pigs), femur (3 pigs), humerus (2 pigs), and tibiotarsal joint luxation with fracture of the fibula (2 pigs). Affected pigs weighed between 64 and 168 kg and were 6 months to 2 years old. Fractures of the tibia and fibula were treated by open reduction and internal fixation using a bone plate and a full limb cast (3 pigs) or by using a full limb cast alone (2 pigs). Fracture of the femur was treated by application of a bone plate (3 pigs). Humerus fractures were treated by confinement (1 pig) or by application of a bone plate (1 pig). Tibiotarsal joint luxation with fracture of the fibula was treated by application of a bone plate and use of a full limb cast (2 pigs). Of these 12 pigs, 10 returned to normal production use and 2 were salvaged; 1 pig with tibiotarsal joint luxation developed *Escherichia coli* osteomyelitis, and 1 pig with humeral fracture repaired by internal fixation suffered permanent radial nerve damage.

Surgical repair of articular fracture of the humeral condyles have been reported for miniature pigs (Figures 70.15 and 70.16) (Payne et al. 1995). The medial humeral condyle was most commonly fractured, but Y-type fractures and supracondylar fractures of the humerus have been found in some miniature pigs. Fractures were repaired using lag screw and Kirschner wire fixation. Five

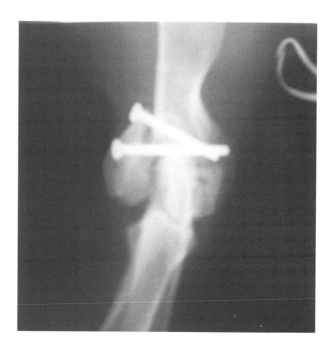

70.16. *Twin cortical bone screw stabilization of medial condylar fracture of the humerus in a pot-bellied pig.*

pigs were reexamined 2 months after surgery and all were walking sound at that time.

Femoral fractures were diagnosed in 20 pigs over a 6-month period (Rousseaux et al. 1981). Nutritional analysis revealed inadequate calcium and phosphorus (both in absolute concentration and calcium to phosphorus ratio) in the feed. Affected pigs were approximately 20 weeks old and weighed between 80 and 90 kg. Pigs walked with a stilted gait and arched back. Necropsy found separation of the proximal femoral epiphysis from the femoral neck. After correction of dietary calcium and phosphorus, clinical evidence of femoral fracture was not observed in any additional pigs. Femoral, pelvic, and vertebral fractures have been found in pigs after accidental electrical shock (Bildfell et al. 1991). Multiple trauma injuries and fractures associated with nutritional deficiency are poor candidates for surgical repair. Fracture of the greater trochanter of the femur also has been identified as causes of lameness in pigs (Blowey 1992, 1994). A simple, oblique fracture of the mid-diaphysis of the femur was successfully repaired in a 10-month-old 150 kg Berkshire boar using a bone plate (Grisel and Huber 1996). The boar returned to normal breeding 190 days after surgery.

CANINE TOOTH (TUSK) REMOVAL AND RESECTION

Removal of the canine teeth of adult boars is challenging because of the long dental root embedded in the mandible. Canine tooth extraction is done with the boar under general anesthesia. The gingiva and perios-

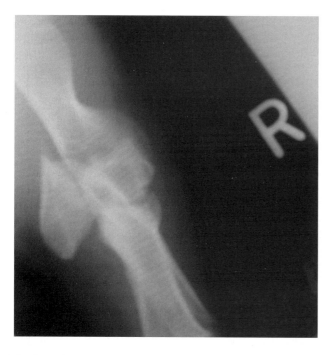

70.15. *Medial condylar fracture of humerus in a Vietnamese pot-bellied pig.*

teum of the mandible are reflected laterally and ventrally using a periosteal elevator. Then the lateral alveolar plate of the tooth alveolus is resected following the course of the tooth root. After the periapical region of the alveolus has been reached, a periodontal elevator is used to disrupt the periodontal membrane around the circumference of the tooth and the tooth is removed. The alveolus is debrided, rinsed, and sutured closed. Alternatively, the alveolus can be left open to heal by second-intention healing.

Resection of the mandibular canine teeth is an easy and rapid method of preventing tusk injuries to personnel and other pigs. The boar is placed under general anesthesia and obstetrical wire is placed around the tooth. The wire is used to saw through the tooth approximately 3 mm above the gingival margin to prevent exposure of the pulp cavity. This procedure is repeated every 6–12 months as needed to restrict growth of the tusks.

REFERENCES

Althouse GC, Evans LE. 1997. A novel surgical technique for vasectomizing boars. J Am Vet Med Assoc 210:675–677.

Amass SF, Schinckel AP, Clark LK. 1995. Increase prevalence of rectal prolapses in growing/finishing swine fed a diet containing excess lysine. Vet Rec 137:519–520.

Anderson DE, Kim JH, Hancock JD, Han IK. 2000. Ileocutaneous anastomosis for collection of ileal digesta in neonatal pigs. Lab Anim Sci 39:26–28.

Bassett JR, Mann EA, Constantinescu GM, McClure RC. 1999. Subtotal colectomy and ileocolonic anastomosis in a Vietnamese pot-bellied pig with idiopathic megacolon. J AM Vet Med Assoc 215:1640–1643.

Becker HN. 1986. Castration, inguinal hernia repair, and vasectomy in boars. In Current Therapy in Theriogenology 2. DA Morrow, ed. Philadelphia: W. B. Saunders Co, pp. 985–987.

Benson GJ. 1986. Anesthetic management of ruminants and swine with selected pathophysiologic alteration. Anesthesia. Vet Clin North Am Food Animal Pract 2:677–692.

Bildfell RJ, Carnat BD, Lister DB. 1991. Posterior paresis and electrocution of swine caused by accidental electric shock. J Vet Diagn Invest 3:364–367.

Blowey RW. 1992. Proliferative osteitis of the femoral greater trochanter and humeral medial epicondyle as a cause of lameness in sows. Vet Rec 131:312–315.

——. 1994. Trochanter fracture and patellar osteochondrosis as causes of lameness in pigs. Vet Rec 134:601–603.

Bollwahn W. 1992. Surgical procedures in boars and sows. In Diseases of Swine (7th ed.). AD Leman, BE Straw, WE Mengeling, S D'Allaire, DJA Taylor, eds. Ames: Iowa State University Press, pp 957–967.

Clutton RE, Blissitt KJ, Bradley AA, Camburn MA. 1997. Comparison of three injectable anesthetic techniques in pigs. Vet Rec 141:140–146.

Dimigen J. 1972. Cesarean section in market pigs. Dtsch Tierarztl Wochenschr 79:235–237.

Douglas, RGA. 1985. A simple method for correcting rectal prolapse in pigs. Vet Rec 117:129.

Dutton DM, Lawhorn B, Hooper RN. 1997. Ablation of the cranial portion of the preputial cavity in a pig. J Am Vet Med Assoc 211:598–599.

Fredeen HT, Newman JA. 1968. Cryptorchid conditions and selection for its incidence in Lacombe and Canadian Yorkshire pigs. Can J Anim Sci 48:275–284.

Gallardo MA, Lawhorn DB, Taylor TS, Walker MA. 2003. Spiral colon bypass in a geriatric Vietnamese potbellied pig. J Am Vet Med Assoc 222:1408–1412.

Greene CJ. 1979. Animal anesthesia. London Lab Anim 187–197.

Greenwood J. 1989. Treatment of bladder retroversion with rectal prolapse in sow. Vet Rec 125:405–406.

Grisel GR, Huber MJ. 1996. Repair of a mid-diaphyseal femoral fracture in a boar. J Am Vet Med Assoc 209:1608–1610.

Halland SK, House JK, George LW. 2002. Urethroscopy and laser lithotripsy for the diagnosis and treatment of obstructive urolithiasis in goats and pot-bellied pigs. J Am Vet Med Assoc 220:1831–1834.

Harvey-Clark CJ, Gilespie K, Riggs KW. 2000. Transdermal fentanyl compared with parenteral buprenorphine in post-surgical pain in swine: A case study. Lab Anim 34:386–398.

Helman RG, Hooper RN, Lawhorn DB, Edwards JF. 1996. Urethral polyps in Vietnamese pot-bellied pigs. J Vet Diagn Invest 8:137–140.

Henry, DP. 1968. Anesthesia of boars by intratesticular injection. Aust Vet J 44:418–419.

Horn T, Marx G, von Borell E. 1999. Behavior of piglets during castration with and without local anesthesia. Dtsch Tierarztl Wochenschr 106:271–274.

Kiley M. 1976. A review of the advantages and disadvantages of castrating farm livestock with particular reference to behavioural effects. Br Vet J 132:323–331.

Kjar HA. 1976. Amputation of prolapsed rectum in young pigs. J Am Vet Med Assoc 168:229–230.

Ko JCH, Thurmon JC, Benson GJ, Gard, J, Tranquilli WJ. 1992. Evaluation of analgesia induced by epidural injection of detomidine or xylazine in swine. J Vet Anaesth 19:56–60.

Ko JCH, Thurmon JC, Benson GJ, Tranquilli WJ, Olson WA. 1993. A new drug combination for use in porcine cesarean sections. Vet Med Food Anim Pract 88:466–472.

Lachmayr VF. 1966. Zum Kryptorchismus des schweines. Wiener Tierarztliche Monatsschrift 53:474–478.

Leon JC, Gill MS, Cornick-Seahorn JL, Hedlund CS, Hosgood G. 1997. Prepubic urethrostomy for permanent urinary diversion in two Vietnamese pot-bellied pigs. J Am Vet Med Assoc 1;210:366–368.

Lewis AM. 1973. An intestinal umbilical fistula in the pig and its surgical treatment. Vet Rec 93:286.

Libke KG. 1967. Gross and histopathologic lesions in a field case of fatal hemorrhagic shock following orchectomy in young pigs. Vet Med Sm Anim Clin 62:551–554.

Martin-Cancho MF, Carrasco-Jimenez MS, Lima JR, Ezquerra LJ, Crisostomo V, Uson-Gargallo J. 2004. Assessment of the relationship of bispectral index values, hemodynamic changes, and recovery times associated with sevoflurane or propofol anesthesia in pigs. Am J Vet Res 65:409–416.

Mather EC. 1966. Lower flank incision for swine cesarean. Vet Med Sm Anim Clin 61:890–891.

McGavin MD, Schoneweis DA. 1972. Porcine bilateral hydronephrosis secondary to castration. Cornell Vet 62:359–363.

McGlone JJ, Hellman JM. 1988. Local and general anesthetic effects on behavior and performance of two- and seven-week-old castrated and uncastrated piglets. J Anim Sci 66:3049–3058.

McGlone JJ, Nicholson RI, Hellman JM. 1993. The development of pain in young pigs associated with castration and attempts to prevent castration-induced behavioral changes. J Anim Sci 71:1441–1446.

Miniats OP, Jol D. 1978. Gnotobiotic pigs—Derivation and rearing. Can J Comp Med 42:428–437.

Moon PF, Smith LJ. 1996. General anesthetic techniques in swine. Anesthesia update. Vet Clin North Am 12(3):663–691.

Morin M, Sauvageau R, Phaneuf JB, Teuscher E, Beauregard M, Lagace A. 1984. Torsion of abdominal organs in sows: A report of 36 cases. Can Vet J 25:440–442.

Palmer JL, Dykes NL, Love K, Fubini SL. 1998. Contrast radiography of the lower urinary tract in the management of obstructive urolithiasis in small ruminants and swine. Vet Radiol Ultrasound 39:175–180.

Papich MG. 1996. Drug residue considerations for anesthetics and adjunctive drugs in food producing animals. Anesthesia update. Vet Clin North Am 12(3):693–706.

Payne JT, Braun WF, Anderson DE. 1995. Articular fractures of the distal portion of the humerus in Vietnamese pot-bellied pigs: Six cases (1988–1992). J Am Vet Med Assoc 206:59–62.

Peyton LC, Colahan PT, Jann HW, Granstedt ME. 1980. Prolapsed rectum and eventration of the small intestine in a pig: Surgical treatment. Agri-practice. Vet Med—Small Anim Clin 75:1297–1330.

Raleigh PJ. 1977. Reduction of uterine prolapse in a sow by laparotomy. Vet Rec 100:89–90.

Roberts SJ. 1986. Infertility in male animals. In Veterinary Obstetrics and Genital Diseases Theriogenology (3rd ed.). SJ Roberts, ed. Ann Arbor: Edwards Brothers, pp. 752–893.

Rosenberg H, Fletcher JE. 1994. An update on the malignant hyperthermia syndrome. Ann Acad Med Singapore 23 (Suppl) 84S–97S.

Rothschild MF, Christian LL, Blanchard W. 1988. Evidence for multigene control of cryptorchidism in swine. J Heredity 79:313–314.

Rousseaux CG, Gill I, Payne-Crosten A. 1981. Femoral fractures in pigs associated with calcium deficiency. Austr Vet J 57:508–510.

Sakaguchi M, Nishimura R, Sasaki N. 1992. Enhancing effect of butorphanol on medetomidine induced sedation in pigs. J Vet Med Sci 54:1183–1185.

Sakaguchi M, Nishimura R, Sasaki N, Ishiguro T, Tamura H, Tekeuchi A. 1996. Anesthesia induced in pigs by use of a combination of metedomidine, butorphenol, and kematine and its reversal by administration of atipamasole. Am J Vet Res 57:529–534.

Sanford SE, Josephson GKA, Rehmtulla AJ. 1994. Sudden death in sows. Can Vet J 35:388.

Saunders CN. 1974. Rectal stricture syndrome in pigs: A case history. Vet Rec 94:61.

Schoneweis DA. 1971. Prolapse of the prepuce and prepucial diverticulum in a boar. J Am Vet Med Assoc 158:1410–1411.

Searcy-Bernal R, Gardner IA, Hird DW. 1994. Effects of and factors associated with umbilical hernias in a swine herd. J Am Vet Med Assoc 204:1660–1663.

Skarda RT. 1996. Local and regional anesthesia in ruminants and swine. Anesthesia update. Vet Clin North Am 12(3):579–626.

Százados I. 1985. Judgment of castration-induced abscesses in pigs at meat inspection. Acta Veterinaria Hungarica 33:177–184.

Tavernor WD, Trexler PC, Vaughan LC. 1971. The production of gnotobiotic piglets and calves by hysterotomy under general anesthesia. Vet Rec 88:10–14.

Thornton H. 1972. Slaughter testicle in the cryptorchid pig. Vet Rec 90:217.

Thurmon JC. 1986. Injectable anesthetic agents and techniques in ruminants and swine. Anesthesia. Vet Clin North Am Food Anim Pract 2(3):567–592.

Titze K. 1977. Obstetrics in pigs with special consideration of cesarean section. Dtsch Tierarztl Wochenschr 84:135–138.

Todd GC, Nelson LW, Migaki G. 1968. Multiple heterotopic testicular tissue in the pig. A report of seven cases. Cornell Vet 48:614–619.

Tranquilli WJ. 1986. Techniques of inhalation anesthesia in ruminants and swine. Anesthesia. Vet Clin North Am Food Anim Pract 2,3:593–619.

Turner AS, McIllwraith CW. 1989. Cesarean section in the sow. In Techniques in Large Animal Surgery (2nd ed.). AS Turner, CW McIllwraith, eds. Philadelphia: Lea & Febiger, pp. 358–359.

Tyler JW, Waver DM, Shore MD, Cowart RP, Branson K, Urdaz J. 2000. Preputial diverticulum stone in a boar. Vet Rec 147:225.

Van Straaten HWM, Colenbrander B, Wensing CJG. 1979. Maldescended testis: Consequences and attempted therapy in pigs. Int J Fertil 24:74–75.

Vaughan LC. 1966. The repair of fractures in pigs. Vet Rec 79:2–8.

Vogt, DW, Ellersieck MR. 1990. Heritability of susceptibility to scrotal herniation in swine. Am J Vet Res 51:1501–1503.

Vonderfecht HE. 1978. Amputation of rectal prolapse in swine. Agri Pract Vet Med/Small Anim Clin 7:201–206.

Walker B, Jaggin N, Doherr M, Schatzmann U. 2004. Inhalation anesthesia for castration of newborn piglets: Experiences with isoflurane and isoflurane/N$_2$O. J Vet Med A 51:150–154.

Wedel DJ, Gammel SA, Milde JH. 1993. Delayed onset of malignant hyperthermia induced by isoflurane and desflurane compared with halothane in susceptible swine. Anesthesiology 78:1138–1144.

White RG, DeShazer JA, Tressler CJ. 1995. Vocalization and physiological response of pigs during castration with or without a local anesthestic. J Anim Sci 73:381–386.

Wieringa W, Mouwen JMVM. 1983. Het ulcus diverticuli praeputialis bij het varken. Tijdschr Diergeneeskd 108:751–760.

71 Drug Therapy and Prophylaxis

Robert M. Friendship and John F. Prescott

This chapter gives an overview of some of the major drugs and biological agents used in swine, with a particular focus on antimicrobial drugs and the basic principles on which effective drug use are based.

USE OF DRUGS: MAJOR CONSIDERATIONS

Managing the effective use of drugs or biological agents for prevention and treatment of disease is an important responsibility of swine veterinarians, which involves detailed knowledge of these agents, including the risks involved in their use and the national and sometimes international regulations governing their use. The major regulatory and industry consideration is the production of safe, uncontaminated meat, followed by considerations of the welfare of the animals, cost, efficacy, and ease of application. However, many other factors need to be considered (Table 71.1) before implementing drug treatment or prophylactic use, with the underlying recognition that all such use involves a calculation that benefits of use exceed the risks involved in using most drugs or biological agents. The underlying goal is to make the minimum use of drugs in swine consistent with the production of healthy animals in a humane, cost-effective, and consumer and environmentally safe manner. Changes in swine production practices have reduced reliance on antimicrobial drugs, but there is still considerable room for further reduction in their untargeted use in many countries.

Routes of Drug Treatment

In general, individual animal treatment through injection is reserved for serious, rapidly developing infections such as acute systemic infections (septicemia, acute pneumonia, or streptococcal meningitis), but mass medication is preferred because of ease, efficacy, and lack of necessity to handle and disturb animals. Intramuscular (IM) injection is preferred for serious infections since it usually results in more complete absorption of drug and higher tissue concentrations than oral

administration. Parenteral therapy of individual animals by IM injection is administered just behind the ear on the lateral side of the neck. This site is chosen in case the drug preparation causes local tissue damage as well as to prevent the possible additional effect of sciatic nerve damage if the ham muscles were used.

Oral medication is easier to apply to groups of pigs and reduces injection-related problems of broken needles, abscesses, and tissue damage. Water medication is a more rapid method of treating a group of sick pigs than feed medication, with the advantages of immediate implementation and that sick pigs will drink when they will not eat. However, the disadvantages are that not all drugs are water soluble, that water may be spilled, and that some drug carriers may block nipple watering systems. Administration of drugs by water is through an in-line proportioner containing a concentrated drug solution or by a water tank containing the appropriately dosed drug. Pigs drink about 8–10% of their body weight daily (Table 71.2), depending on environmental temperature and palatability of the drug. An approximate rule is that pigs should be dosed through water at 5–6 liters (1.32 U.S. gallons) per 60 kg weight (145 lbs).

In-feed medication is the most common route of administration of anthelmintic and antimicrobial drugs. The disadvantage for treatment of acute infections is not only that sick pigs may not eat but also that existing nonmedicated feed needs to be either removed or eaten. For this reason, in-feed medication is often reserved for long term use in the prevention or treatment of chronic infections.

Principles of Treatment

The general principle of treatment is to maximize therapeutic efficacy while minimizing adverse effects such as toxicity, antimicrobial resistance, harmful tissue residues, or adverse environmental impact. This implies a confirmed or reasonable clinical diagnosis with the actual drug chosen according to the required purpose and administered to give optimal effect, consistent usually

Table 71.1. Considerations in drug use in swine

Major Consideration	Further Considerations
Human safety	Direct drug toxicity to user; toxicity to consumer through tissue residues.
Animal welfare	Prevention or reduction of disease; ease of administration for animal.
Host damage and adverse effects	Direct toxicity to pig; tissue damage; adverse drug interactions. Indirect adverse effects: resistance in microorganisms; disruption of microflora.
Regulations	Availability of products; national regulations on use; international regulations for export; extra-label drug use (AMDUCA in U.S.); veterinary-client relationship; withdrawal period.
Efficacy and cost	Assessment of efficacy; cost: benefit of treatment.
Drug dosage and application	Route, ease of administration; physicochemical properties; pharmacokinetic properties; pharmacodynamic properties.
Principles of treatment	Dosage; dosage modification; duration; clinical evidence; drug trial data.
Principles of prophylaxis	Dosage; duration; clinical evidence; drug trial data.
Record keeping	Drug use records.
Stability of drug	Storage conditions.

Table 71.2. Average daily water consumption

Weight or Type of Pig	Liters/Head/Day
7–20 kg body weight	2–4
20–50 body weight	4–6
50–100 body weight	6–8
Pregnant sow	8–12
Lactating sow	16–20

with labeled dosage and always within regulations concerning the use of the drugs. For antimicrobial drugs, discussed below, many of the principles of optimal treatment are well established. Duration of treatment depends on the drug and disease process but should be based on scientific data and/or on clinical experience.

Evaluation of Clinical Trials

The best method for evaluating animal health interventions and to guide clinical decision-making is to conduct on-farm clinical trials (Dohoo et al. 2003). In a clinical trial, exposure to disease occurs naturally and the pigs are housed and managed under normal farm conditions but the treatment is randomly assigned with a second group used as a control population. Clinical trials are difficult to conduct and there is considerable potential for errors in design and misinterpretation of findings. The consequences of these failings may be inappropriate therapeutic recommendations and overall lack of success in treatment programs. Practitioners need to be aware of proper methodology as it relates to design and interpretation in order to evaluate therapeutics either by conducting a trial on a client's farm, or in interpreting claims for a new drug as presented by a pharmaceutical company.

First, a study should have a limited number of objectives, generally one primary and possibly two or three secondary objectives, and these must be clearly stated (Dewey 1999). For example, a trial examining the use of a drug to control pneumonia in a finishing unit might have decreased mortality as its primary objective, and as

secondary objectives the researchers may be interested in improved growth rate and reduced weight variation. The design of the trial would likely be different if the primary objective was reduced weight variation.

Other important elements of a clinical trial include a defined study population, random allocation of subjects, masking or blinding of the observer, thorough follow-up, and appropriate analysis (Dewey 1999). A common error in the design of a trial is to base the statistical analysis on individual pigs but to assign treatments on the basis of pen or even barn. Statistical analysis should be conducted at the smallest level at which the treatment can be applied. Therefore, in a feed trial where all the pigs in a pen are assigned one feed and all the pigs in the next pen are given a second feed, the pen is the unit of concern. The number of animals or pens or barns required to assess whether a drug is beneficial or not can be calculated using formulas that can be found in standard statistics text books. The number of units will depend on the variation you expect and the magnitude of the difference you consider important. For example, if one assumes a coefficient of variation (mean ÷ standard deviation) of 7% for growth rate, one would need approximately 43 pens per treatment to detect a difference in average daily gain of 5%. Whereas it would require only 12 pens per treatment to detect an average daily gain of 10%.

Typically, the confidence interval is chosen to be 95%, implying that the probability that the results were real and not due to chance alone is 95%. The P-value or level of significance is the opposite (i.e., P = 0.05 means there is a 5% chance that the results are due to chance alone). Statistical power is typically set at 80%, implying that there is an 80% probability that we will find a difference when a difference truly exists. Therefore, 20% of the time such a trial will not distinguish a difference between treatment and control when there really is a difference. Statistical power can be increased by increasing sample size.

It is important that bias is minimized wherever possible. Therefore, subjects need to be assigned to a treatment group in a truly random manner, and if this is not possible, an alternatively systematic assignment may be used. The intervention given to the control group needs to be similar to the treatment group. For example, if the treatment group needs to be restrained and injected with a product, the controls need to be handled in a similar manner and given a placebo. Ideally, the animal care givers and whoever records the clinical observations should be kept blind to which animals are in the treatment group and which are in the control group.

Even when animals are assigned in a random manner and trials are carefully designed, confounding factors and other sources of error can be introduced so that a great deal of care is needed in assessing the information gained from a clinical trial, but this is still the best basis to judge efficacy of therapeutic measures, and no amount of in vitro studies can match the value of this type of on-farm assessment.

ANTIMICROBIAL DRUGS

Major Classes of Antimicrobial Drugs
A brief overview of some key aspects of the major classes of antimicrobial drugs, their antimicrobial activities, pharmacokinetic properties, toxic or other adverse effects, and major clinical applications is given in Table 71.3. Further details are available through manufacturer's package inserts or through pharmacology and related textbooks (Prescott et al. 2000).

Antimicrobial Therapy
Rational use of antimicrobial therapy first requires a diagnosis. This may be made clinically and preferably confirmed by laboratory diagnosis, which would include antimicrobial susceptibility testing. Antimicrobial treatment will, however, usually start before laboratory results are available. The selection of a particular drug depends on knowledge of the likely or actual susceptibility of the microorganism, knowledge of factors affecting drug concentration (dosage, pharmacokinetic properties) and activity (pharmacodynamic properties) at the site of infection, knowledge of drug toxicity and factors that enhance it, cost of treatment, and consideration of regulations about drug use, including withdrawal times. The ideal drug is one to which the organism is most susceptible and that achieves effective concentration at the site of infection without damaging the host. Bactericidal drugs are required in serious life-threatening infections, when host defenses are impaired, and in infections of vital tissues such as meninges, endocardium, and bones where host defenses are also not fully functional. In other cases bacteriostatic agents may be equally useful. Where feasible, a narrow spectrum drug may be more appropriate than a broad spectrum antibacterial because the narrow spectrum drug interferes less with the normal microbial flora and is less likely to select for widespread resistance.

To some extent, drug dosage can be tailored to the susceptibility of the organism, the site of infection, and the pharmacokinetic and pharmacodynamic properties of the selected antimicrobial agent. However, in vitro susceptibility data are laboratory-derived and the standardized conditions under which the susceptibility data are generated do not exist at the site of infection. Factors involved in tailoring a dosing regimen include, among other things, the susceptibility of the pathogen in terms of minimum inhibitory concentration (MIC), the concentration of the antimicrobial agent at the site of infection in active form (pharmacokinetic properties of the drug), and the pharmacodynamic properties of the antimicrobial agent. Some antimicrobials (aminoglycosides, fluoroquinolones) are concentration-dependent (optimum action of the drug depends on concentration of the drug above MIC), whereas others (beta-lactams, lincosamides, macrolides, trimethoprim-sulfamethazine) are time-dependent (optimum activity depends on time above MIC). The complex issues involved in optimal antimicrobial therapy are beyond the scope of this chapter although it can be concluded that some dosage recommendations for drugs licensed in the past have not taken modern understanding into account and are suboptimal or inappropriate. Labeled recommendations can therefore be expected to change in the future. In the United States, the Food and Drug Administration's professional flexible labeling approach allows veterinarians to adjust the dose based on the MIC of the pathogen. Although a number of factors determine optimal dosage, the factor that most frequently limits dosage is toxicity. The upper level of the recommended dosage should not be exceeded, because this is often determined by toxicity. Sometimes, however, a drug's antibacterial effects may be limiting and may determine the upper level of dosage. For example, the killing rate of beta-lactam drugs has an optimal concentration, whereas that of the aminoglycosides or fluoroquinolones is proportional to drug concentration. Penicillin G is virtually nontoxic in nonallergenic patients, but its dosage is limited by its antibacterial action. By contrast the dosage of aminoglycoside is limited not by antibacterial effects but by its toxicity.

In terms of duration of treatment, the variables affecting length of treatment have not been defined. Responses of different types of infections to antimicrobial drugs vary, and clinical experience with many infections is important in assessing response to treatment. For acute infections, it will usually be clear within 2 days whether or not therapy is clinically effective. If no response is seen by that time, both the diagnosis and treatment should be reconsidered. Treatment of acute infections should be continued for at least 2 days after clinical and microbiologic resolution of infection. For serious acute infections, treatment should probably last 7–10 days. For chronic infections, treatment will be considerably longer.

Table 71.3. Overview of major classes and identities of antimicrobial drugs used in swine, their antimicrobial activities, pharmacokinetic properties, toxic or other adverse effects, and major clinical applications

Drug Class	Specific Agent or Example of Agents	Antibacterial Activity, Resistance	Pharmacokinetic Properties	Toxic or Adverse Effects	Major Applications
Sulfonamides	Sulfamethazine intermediate acting; others also used	Bacteriostatic; broad-spectrum, gram+, gram− aerobes; anaerobes; acquired resistance very widespread. Active intracellular bacteria, protozoa	Rapidly absorbed from intestine, well distributed in tissues	Violative kidney residues from feed use through recycling, feed contamination if feed not withdrawn 15 days before slaughter	Minor value; largely growth promotional, possible disease prevention
Sulfonamide-diaminopyrimidine combinations	Sulfamethazine-trimethoprim	Bactericidal; gram+, gram− aerobes; anaerobes. *Mycoplasma*, *Leptospira* resistant	Rapidly absorbed from intestine, well distributed in tissues; crosses uninflamed blood-brain barrier	Wide safety margin	Largely IM use for acute infections (pneumonia, streptococcal meningitis). In feed for atrophic rhinitis
Beta-lactam	Penam penicillins, Group 1: Penicillin G	Bactericidal; highly active many gram+, some fastidious gram− aerobe, e.g., *H. parasuis*, *P. multocida*; anaerobes; *Leptospira*. Enteric bacteria and *Mycoplasma* resistant	Poorly absorbed from intestine, relatively poorly distributed in tissues; crosses only inflamed blood-brain barrier. Procaine penicillin is long-acting form for IM use since unconjugated drug rapidly excreted	Safe drug; possible anaphylaxis or procaine-induced excitement	Excellent for IM use in erysipelas, streptococcal infections including meningitis, clostridial infections. Some bacterial pneumonias
Beta-lactam	Penam penicillins, Group 4: ampicillin, amoxycillin	As penicillin G, broader activity against gram− aerobes, but resistance widespread	As penicillin G, but better absorbed orally and distributed through tissues	Safe drug	Similar to penicillin G. Addition of beta-lactamase inhibitors (e.g., clavulanic acid) has resurrected penam penicillins use in other species
Beta-lactam	Group 4, "third generation" cephalosporins; ceftiofur	Bactericidal; gram− aerobes especially, including *E. coli*, *Salmonella*, gram+ aerobes, anaerobes. *Mycoplasma* resistant	Poorly absorbed from intestine, relatively poorly distributed in tissues; crosses only inflamed blood-brain barrier	May predispose to *Clostridium difficile* colitis if used in neonatal pigs. Resistance emerging in *Salmonella* may represent human health hazard	Excellent for IM use in gram− aerobic infections, including colibacillosis, salmonellosis, gram− bacterial pneumonias
Aminoglycoside	Gentamicin, neomycin	Bactericidal; gram− aerobes, including enterics	Poorly absorbed from intestine, relatively poorly distributed in tissues	Nephrotoxic with prolonged parenteral use; persistent kidney residues	Gentamicin IM for neonatal *E. coli* infections; neomycin orally for *E. coli* infection
Aminocyclitol	Apramycin, spectinomycin	Bactericidal; gram− aerobes, including enterics	Poorly absorbed from intestine, relatively poorly distributed in tissues	Nephrotoxic with prolonged parenteral use; persistent kidney residues	Orally for *E. coli* infection
Lincosamide	Lincomycin	Bacteriostatic; gram+ aerobes, anaerobes including *B. hyodysenteriae*; *Mycoplasma*	Well absorbed from intestine and well distributed in tissues	Safe drug in swine	Oral use for control of *Brachyspira*; oral or IM use for control of *Mycoplasma*
Macrolide	Tylosin	Bacteriostatic; gram+ aerobes, anaerobes, some gram− aerobes; *Mycoplasma*	Well absorbed from intestine and well distributed in tissues	Safe drug in swine; IM irritant, may cause edema, pruritis, anal protrusion	Oral use for control of proliferative enteropathy, atrophic rhinitis, possibly leptospirosis

Table 71.3. (*continued*)

Drug Class	Specific Agent or Example of Agents	Antibacterial Activity, Resistance	Pharmacokinetic Properties	Toxic or Adverse Effects	Major Applications
Pleuromutilin	Tiamulin	Bacteriostatic; gram+ aerobes, anaerobes, some gram− aerobes; *Mycoplasma*. More active than tylosin	Well absorbed from intestine and well distributed in tissues	Safe drug in swine	Oral use for control of *Brachyspira, Mycoplasma*, chronic pneumonias, proliferative enteropathy, leptospirosis
Tetracyclines	Oxy-, Chlor-, tetracycline	Bacteriostatic; classically broad-spectrum, gram+, gram− but acquired resistance extremely widespread. *Erysipelothrix, Haemophilus, Leptospira, Pasteurella* are exceptions	Well absorbed from intestine and well distributed in tissues	Safe drugs in swine	Oral use as "feed" drugs for growth promotion and nonspecific disease prophylaxis in countries where allowed. Used in feed, occasionally IM, for treatment of infections caused by bacteria listed as being susceptible

Treatment failure has many causes. The antimicrobial selected may be inappropriate because of misdiagnosis, inactivity at the site of infection, failure to culture infections, inaccurate or inapplicable laboratory results, resistance of pathogens, chronic nature of the infection (which may affect metabolic state of the pathogen), or errors in sampling. These factors are more likely to cause failure than inadequate dosage although this may also be important. It is important that producers comply with dosing instructions. When failure occurs, diagnosis must be reassessed and samples collected for laboratory analysis.

Principles of Prophylaxis
Antimicrobial drugs are administered to swine for the prevention of particular diseases. The generally accepted principles of antimicrobial prophylaxis are:

- Medication should be directed against specific pathogens or diseases.
- Prophylaxis should be used only where efficacy is established. Prophylaxis should be of a duration that is as short as possible consistent with efficacy.
- Dosage should be the same as that used therapeutically.
- Adverse effects itemized earlier should be minimized.

In general, as discussed below, antimicrobial drugs of therapeutic importance in both humans and animals have been markedly overused for both growth promotional and disease prophylactic purposes in swine, in a manner inconsistent with generally accepted principles of prophylaxis. Alternatives to these antimicrobial use practices need to be found, as discussed below.

One reasonable prophylactic practice is that of "pulse medication," whereby a therapeutic level of a specific drug is included in the feed at therapeutic concentrations for a short period for the prevention of endemic diseases, such as proliferative enteropathy or enzootic pneumonia before the predictable onset of these diseases in a particular setting.

Regulations
The use of antimicrobial drugs in animals is regulated by law in many countries, so that veterinarians need to know and abide by the regulations. The regulations involve an approval process of drugs produced by a particular manufacturer only if they meet human and animal safety standards as well as being shown to be efficacious at specified dosages for particular purposes (the labeled dose/purpose). An example of regulated use of antimicrobial drugs, that of the United States, is outlined in Table 71.4. In the United States, failure to comply with the regulations may result in fines or imprisonment.

Antimicrobial Drug Withdrawal
Most antimicrobial drugs must not be used near slaughter, to avoid any significant residues in meat products. The precise period varies with the drug and the dosage. For drugs used at the labeled dosage, this will be specified on the package insert. For extra-label drug use, withdrawal information may be obtained from the manufacturer or in some cases from national or international databases such as, in the United States, the Food Animal Residue Avoidance Databank (toll-free number in the United States, 1-800-USFARAD). Examples of preslaughter medication withdrawal time in the United States are shown in Table 71.5.

Table 71.4. Regulation of antimicrobial drug use for food animals in the United States.

Drug Category or Regulation	Description
Production feed drugs	Growth promotion and feed efficiency including subtherapeutic or therapeutic use for specified purposes in feed. Strict dose, duration, withdrawal period specified. Nonprescription.
Over-the-counter drugs	Drugs for oral or parenteral use available without prescription. Strict dose, duration, withdrawal period specified.
Prescription drugs	Veterinary prescription parenteral use only. Strict dose, duration, withdrawal period specified.
Professional flexible labeling	Approved products have expanded dosage ranges for veterinarian use.
Veterinary Feed Directive	Used in feed only under direction of a veterinarian. Strict recording requirements.
Extra-label use	Regulation under Animal Medicinal Drug Clarification Act (AMDUCA) when actual or intended use of a drug is not in accordance with approved labeling. Only when available labeled products ineffective. Strict recording and other requirements, including prohibited uses.

Table 71.5. Examples of preslaughter withdrawal times from last medication for swine in the United States

Dosage Form	Drug for Labeled Use	Days
Parenteral drug	Ceftiofur	0
	Gentamicin (neonatal pigs only)	40
	Procaine penicillin	7
Oral, water-soluble drugs	Bacitracin	1
	Chlortetracycline	5
	Neomycin	20
	Tylosin	2
Oral, feed forms (maximum time may vary with dose)	Apramycin	28
	Chlortetracycline, procaine penicillin, sulfamethazole	15
	Tiamulin	0–2

The Antimicrobial Resistance Crisis and Its Impact on Antimicrobial Drug Use in Swine

There is both need and considerable scope to reduce the use of antimicrobial drugs in swine. Human medicine is experiencing an antimicrobial resistance crisis because of the surge of resistance in important human pathogens in the last decade. The emergence of this crisis has resulted from many causes, including widespread use and overuse of some drugs for many years, changing social practices including daycare centers and group homes for the elderly, the increasing number of immunosuppressed people, and possibly changes in the drugs being used. As medical science tries to reduce resistance, it again focuses on the widespread use of antimicrobial drugs in farm animals. Agriculture uses about half of all antimicrobials produced, with use in swine being a major component. Why antimicrobials can be administered to animals on a wide scale over long periods to promote growth and prevent endemic disease cannot be understood by physicians desperate to preserve effective antimicrobials. The extent of the contribution of farm animal use to resistance in human pathogens has been the subject of vigorous debate for many years. Although it is easy to document that bacteria, including resistant bacteria, move from farm animals including swine to people, the scale and to some extent the importance of the movement is unclear. The extent and type of resistance in commensal *E. coli* isolated from swine has been shown to be directly proportional to the extent and type of antimicrobial use in pigs (Dunlop et al. 1998). On a broader scale, the use of antimicrobial drugs over many years may not only have selected for resistant bacterial pathogens and an enormous reservoir of resistance genes in commensal bacteria, but it may also have promoted or enhanced the ability of bacteria to move resistance and other genes through enhancement of mobile genetic elements such as transposons, plasmids, and integrons, and thus perhaps to change more rapidly. There is a high frequency of resistance to multiple antimicrobial drugs in porcine enterotoxigenic *E. coli*, with some evidence that the emergence of resistant new serotypes with apparently enhanced virulence may have virulence genes linked to those of resistance (Noamani et al. 2003), so that use of antimicrobial drugs may not only maintain resistant but also virulent bacteria.

In 1999, the European Union banned the use of growth-promoting antimicrobial drugs in food animals. The impetus for the ban on avoparcin, bacitracin, spiramycin, tylosin, and virginiamycin was because of the entry of Sweden into the Union. Sweden had banned these growth promoters in 1986 but, because it needed to harmonize its regulations with those of the EU, it persuaded the EU to change the Union's regulations. This ban was supported by Denmark and Danish pork producers, who had agreed on a voluntary ban shortly before 1999. The impetus for the Danish ban was the convincing evidence that avoparcin use in poultry, swine, and calves was selecting for vancomycin-resistant enterococci (VREs), which were reaching the European population through the food chain (Bager et al. 1997). Vancomycin-resistant enterococci have become major nosocomial pathogens in human hospitals, particularly in the United States. *Enterococcus faecium* are innately highly resistant bacteria for which vancomycin is often the only drug to which they are susceptible; VREs are essentially untreatable infections. The ban on these growth promoters in Denmark led to an over 50% reduction in antimicrobial drug use, a dramatic reduction in enterococci resistant to the growth promoters and a minor increase in the cost of production of swine estimated at about one Euro (World Health Organization 2002).

Numerous reports have recommended that all stakeholders concerned with the use of antimicrobials in both food animals and humans must be involved in an overarching global strategy to contain resistance (e.g., World Health Organization 2000a) and have recommended steps to enhance the prudent use of antimicrobials in animals, including the removal of growth promoters if these drugs are important in human medicine (e.g., World Health Organization 2000b). At the international level, the World Organization for Animal Health (Office International des Epizooties) (2003, 2004) continues to formulate recommendations and options for risk management relating to antimicrobial use in animals. Outside the EU, other countries are in the process of assessing or starting to reassess the use of antimicrobial drugs in food animals based on the importance of the drug in human medicine and the likelihood of exposure of humans to resistant bacteria or resistance genes arising from animals (e.g., Health Canada 2002; Center for Veterinary Medicine, U.S. Food and Drug Administration 2004).

In recent years many countries have started to monitor resistance in both important pathogens (e.g., *Campylobacter jejuni*, *Salmonella*) as well as "indicator" commensal bacteria (e.g., *Enterococcus* species) isolated from animals, foodstuffs, and humans. For example, in the United States the National Antimicrobial Resistance Monitoring System (NARMS) established in 1996 is designed to document emerging resistance problems, as well as to provide data on which public health policy decisions can be made for the use of antimicrobial drugs in food-producing animals. In Canada, the Canadian Integrated Program for Antimicrobial Resistance Surveillance has taken a similar approach to NARMS.

One emerging resistance problem that will likely become of even greater concern in the future is expanded-spectrum cephalosporin resistance in multidrug-resistant *E. coli* and *Salmonella* serovars (Winokur et al. 2001; Zhao et al. 2003), in which the *cmy-2* gene encoding expanded-spectrum cephalosporin resistance may be found on several different plasmids that can readily be transferred through bacterial conjugation (Caratolli et al. 2002).

Prudent Use Guidelines

The widespread concern about antimicrobial resistance and the animal-human resistance link has led most major national veterinary organizations to improve antimicrobial drug use by development of prudent use guidelines. Such guidelines represent first steps in the more judicious use of antimicrobial drugs that may become considerably more complex over time if they address antimicrobial drug choice for particular diseases. An example of such guidelines, that of the American Association of Swine Veterinarians, is shown in Table 71.6.

Drug Selection for Specific Diseases

Table 71.7 contains recommendations for treatment of specific bacterial disease conditions commonly encountered in North America. It is beyond the scope of this

Table 71.6. American Association of Swine Veterinarians Basic Guidelines of Judicious Therapeutic Use of Antimicrobials in Pork Production

(1) Preventive strategies, such as appropriate husbandry and hygiene, routine health monitoring, and immunization, should be emphasized.

(2) Other therapeutic options should be considered prior to or in conjunction with antimicrobial therapy.

(3) Judicious use of antimicrobials, when under the direction of a veterinarian, should meet all requirements of a veterinarian-client-patient relationship.

(4) Prescription, Veterinary Feed Directive, and extra-label use of antimicrobials must meet all the requirements of a valid veterinarian-client-patient relationship.

(5) Extra-label antimicrobial therapy must be prescribed only in accordance with the Animal Medicinal Drug Use Clarification Act amendments to the Food, Drug, and Cosmetic Act and its regulations.

(6) Veterinarians should work with those responsible for the care of animals to use antimicrobials judiciously regardless of the distribution system through which the antimicrobial was obtained.

(7) Regimens for therapeutic antimicrobial use should be optimized using current pharmacological information and principles.

(8) Antimicrobials considered important in treating refractory infections in human or veterinary medicine should be used in animals only after careful review and reasonable justification. Consider using other antimicrobials for initial therapy.

(9) Utilize culture and susceptibility results to aid in the selection of antimicrobials when clinically relevant.

(10) Therapeutic antimicrobial use should be confined to appropriate clinical indications.

(11) Therapeutic exposure to antimicrobials should be minimized by treating only for as long as needed for the desired clinical response.

(12) Limit therapeutic antimicrobial treatment to ill or at risk animals, treating the fewest animals indicated.

(13) Minimize environmental contamination with antimicrobials whenever possible.

(14) Accurate records of treatment and outcome should be used to evaluate therapeutic regimens.

Note: The AASV website elaborates on these basic guidelines listed above (http://www.aasp.org/aasv/jug.html).

Table 71.7. Antimicrobial drug selection for specific bacterial diseases (Warning—These dosages may not conform to government regulations or label instructions.)

Diagnosis	Causative Agent	Comments	Suggested Drug(s)
ENTERIC DISEASES			
Clostridial enteritis	*Clostridium perfringens* type A and C	Treatment of sick piglets affected with type C is not effective. Medicate sows to reduce shedding.	Bacitracin in sow diet (100 gm per ton of feed) Ampicillin (6 mg/kg, oral)
Coccidiosis	*Isospora suis*	Treatment must begin before diarrhea occurs (3- to 6-day-old piglets).	Toltrazuril (20–30 mg/kg, oral) Amprolium 9.6%, (2 ml per piglet/day for days 3–5)
Colibacillosis	*Escherichia coli*	Neonatal piglets must be treated promptly and provision of electrolytes helps minimize effects of dehydration. Post-weaned pigs best treated with antibiotics in water.	*Neonates:* Gentamicin (5 mg per kg, oral) Neomycin (7 mg per kg, oral) Spectinomycin (50 mg twice a day) *Weanlings:* Apramycin (12.5 mg/kg per day, in water)
Colitis	*Brachyspira pilosicoli*	Disease is often mild and responds to change in feed, but if more severe, treat in similar fashion to swine dysentery	
Proliferative enteropathy	*Lawsonia intracellularis*	All-in/all-out management and good hygiene may minimize the need for antibiotics. Feed medication can prevent clinical signs.	Tylosin (100 g per ton of feed) Lincomycin (100 g per ton of feed) Tiamulin (35 g per ton of feed)
Salmonellosis	*Salmonella typhimurium* and other serovars	Antimicrobials may be contraindicated in that they prolong shedding and promote resistance.	
Swine dysentery	*Brachyspira hyodysenteriae*	Resistance against older drugs is common. Treatment for extended period after clinical signs disappear is necessary. Water medicate in acute outbreak.	Tiamulin (200 g/ton of feed to treat) (35 g/ton to prevent) Carbadox (50 g/ton of feed)
MULTISYSTEMIC DISEASES			
Actinobacillus Septicemia	*Actinobacillus suis*	*A. suis* is sensitive to most antibiotics but disease occurs acutely so treatment may not be in time.	Procaine penicillin G 20,000 IU/kg IM
Erysipelas	*Erysipelothrix rhusiopathiae*	Resistance to penicillin does not appear to be a problem.	Procaine penicillin G 20,000 IU/kg IM but also tylosin, tetracyclines, or lincomycin
Glasser's disease	*Haemophilus parasuis*	High dosages, administered parenterally to all members of the affected group. Some resistance to penicillin.	Procaine penicillin G 20,000 IU/kg IM or higher Ceftiofur, 3 mg/kg IM Trimethoprim-sulfadoxine 16 mg/kg IM
Mycoplasma polyserositis	*Mycoplasma hyorhinis*	High dosages, administered parenterally, but results tend to be poor.	Lincomycin 10 mg/kg IM Tylosin 9 mg/kg IM Tiamulin 11 mg/kg IM
Salmonellosis	*Salmonella choleraesuis*	Vigorous treatment early can reduce duration and severity.	Ceftiofur 3 mg/kg IM Trimethoprim-sulfadoxine 16 mg/kg IM
MUSCULOSKELETAL DISEASES			
Foot rot	*Arcanobacterium pyogenes* *Fusobacterium necrophorum*	Improved flooring and sanitation. Topical disinfectants may help. Generally poor response to treatment.	Procaine penicillin G 20,000 IU/kg IM Oxytetracycline 6.6 mg/kg IM
Mycoplasma arthritis	*Mycoplasma hyosynoviae*	Injectable antibiotics and possibly corticosteroids.	Lincomycin 10 mg/kg IM Tiamulin 11 mg/kg IM Tylosin 9 mg/kg IM
Neonatal polyarthritis	*Staphylococcus* spp. *Streptococcus* spp. and others	Treatment is ineffective unless started early.	Procaine pencillin G 20,000 IU/kg IM
Suppurative arthritis	*Arcanobacterium pyogenes*	Treatment is generally ineffective.	Procaine penicillin G 20,000 IU/kg IM Oxytetracycline 6.6 mg/kg IM
NEUROLOGICAL DISEASES			
Edema disease	*Escherichia coli*	Sick pigs eat and drink very little and must be treated parenterally.	Trimethoprim-sulfadoxine 16 mg/kg IM Ceftiofur 3mg/kg IM
Otitis media (Middle ear infection)	*Staphylococci* spp. *Streptococci* spp. *Arcanobacterium pyogenes*	Abscesses can occur and relapses are common.	Trimethoprim-sulfadoxine 16 mg/kg IM Ceftiofur 3 mg/kg
Tetanus	*Clostridium tetani*	Poor prognosis.	

Table 71.7. (*continued*)

Diagnosis	Causative Agent	Comments	Suggested Drug(s)
REPRODUCTIVE DISEASES			
Leptospirosis	*Leptospira* spp.	Antibiotics may not eliminate carrier state.	Streptomycin 25 mg/kg IM Chlor or oxytetracycline at 600–800 g/ton of feed
Mastitis and/or metritis	Generally gram-negative bacteria	Attention needs to be paid to cross-fostering piglets. Treatment varies depending on microorganism and sensitivity.	Ampicillin 6 mg/kg IM
RESPIRATORY DISEASES			
Enzootic pneumonia	*Mycoplasma hyopneumoniae* and secondaries	Preferably sick animals are treated parenterally to achieve high tissue levels.	Oxytetracycline 6.6 mg/kg Trimethoprimsulfadoxine 3 mg/kg IM Ceftiofur 3 mg/kg IM Tulathromycin 2.5 mg/kg IM
Pleuropneumonia	*Actinobacillus pleuropneumoniae*	Parenteral treatment because acutely sick pigs eat and drink very little.	Same as above Tilmicocin (181–363 g/ton of feed)
Progressive Atrophic Rhinitis	*Bordetella bronchiseptica* and toxigenic strains of *Pasteurella multocida*	Responsive to housing/management and vaccination programs.	Oxytetracycline 20 mg/kg IM Sulfamethazine 400–2000 g/ton of feed in nursery ration
SKIN DISEASE			
Exudative epidermitis (Greasy pig disease)	*Staphylococcus hyicus*	May see resistance to penicillin, need to treat fresh wounds topically.	Procaine penicillin G 20,000 IU/kg IM
URINARY TRACT DISEASE			
Cystitis	*Actinobaculum suis* and possibly others	Relapses are common.	Procaine penicillin G 20,000 IU/kg IM Ampicillin 6 mg/kg IM Chlor or oxytetracycline 600–800 gm/ton of feed

text to discuss all product indications and cautions, but the user should always review the information provided by the package insert and the product label. Nor is it within the scope of this text to include all possible treatment options; instead, this table should be considered a general guideline.

ALTERNATIVES TO ANTIMICROBIAL DRUGS

Management and Biosecurity

Modern housing and husbandry methods that tend to segregate age groups, allow for cleaning of the environment between production groups, and minimize the risk of disease introduction through strict biosecurity measures, are the most important methods of reducing the use of antimicrobials and other therapeutic products. Immune system stimulation results in decreased feed efficiency and growth rate whether or not clinical disease occurs. The value of in-feed antibiotics is questionable when high-health status grower-finisher pigs are raised in a clean, biosecure environment (Van Lunen 2003). However, even under ideal management there are circumstances when treatment is required and success of therapy very much depends on the diligence of stockpeople to identify clinical signs of illness early, to treat appropriately, and to provide an environment for the sick pig that promotes healing.

Vaccines

Vaccines are extensively used in swine production, and in fact there are few diseases for which a vaccine is not available. Unfortunately, the fact that a vaccine is licensed and available does not mean it works (Ribble 1990). The usefulness of vaccination varies from disease to disease and even from herd to herd. Despite rapid advances in the fields of immunology and molecular biology there are still diseases for which vaccines have only moderate to poor efficacy (Haesebrouck et al. 2004). Details of the mechanisms of pathogenesis and immune response are covered elsewhere in this text.

There are a number of important considerations that a veterinarian needs to evaluate in order to decide upon a vaccination program for a particular herd. The cost-benefit of vaccination needs to be considered, and this includes estimating the cost of the program, including labor to administer the vaccine; estimating the improvement one would expect from the vaccination program, which requires a knowledge of the vaccines efficacy and an understanding of the disease costs present in the herd; and evaluating the value of alternative control measures. In addition, the veterinarian needs to be aware of possible negative side effects, such as a potential tissue reaction that might lead to trimming losses or a transient loss of appetite that could cause a reduction in growth.

The decision to institute a vaccination program is complex, and unfortunately there is a scarcity of unbiased data regarding the efficacy of vaccines used under practical farm conditions (Moon and Bunn 1993). There are good examples of vaccines that have worked well in controlled experimental infection models but are of no value in the field. Many of the important diseases of swine are a complex of one or more infectious agents and of host, environmental, and management factors.

Swine practitioners are sometimes faced with an unexpected vaccination failure in a situation when using a product that has worked well under similar circumstances in the past. Possible causes of a failure include improper storage and handling of the vaccine, such as failure to refrigerate or protect from light; incorrect administration, such as subcutaneous injection when an intramuscular injection is required; or possibly omitting to vaccinate whole groups of animals. In the case of vaccines administered via the drinking water, there are a number of concerns but possibly the most important is chlorine present in the water, which may kill live attenuated bacteria in vaccines (Kolb 1996).

Timing of a vaccination program is often a problem. In order to maximize compliance and minimize labor, the swine industry prefers to use combination vaccines that require a single injection to be given at a time when animals are ordinarily handled (such as at weaning). Among the problems associated with this approach is the concern that for newly weaned pigs there may still be high levels of passive immunity present to interfere with the stimulation of immunity from vaccination. Therefore, one has to weigh the consequences of vaccinating at a time of greatest convenience versus the extra labor costs and stress to the animals of vaccinating at the most appropriate time to ensure vaccine efficacy.

Passive Immunity

Spray-dried animal plasma has been widely used in diets for newly weaned pigs and is associated with increased growth rates in the order of 27% (van Dijk et al. 2001). The mode of action of spray-dried animal plasma is not fully understood but is assumed to be at least partly due to the presence of immunoglobulins, which may provide a certain level of protection to the newly weaned piglet at a time when the supply of immunoglobulins from sow's milk has ceased. The ability of plasma proteins to neutralize the effect of specific organisms is dependent on the immunizations and disease history of the pigs from which the blood is collected.

Specific antibodies from chicken egg-yolk have been examined as a source of passive immunity for newly weaned pigs as well. Laying hens are vaccinated against specific pig pathogens such as E. coli. Antibodies are secreted into the yolk of the egg (IgY) in large quantities (up to 200 mg/egg) (Marquardt and Li 2001), and dried yolk is incorporated in nursery pig rations. Trials using specific egg-yolk products to prevent postweaning E. coli diarrhea have produced inconsistent results (Chernysheva et al. 2004). Stability of the product during feed processing and passage through the pig's gastrointestinal system are major concerns.

Other Biological Products

Direct-Fed Microbials (Probiotic). Probiotics are defined as live microbials provided in the feed in an attempt to encourage proliferation in the intestine of the specific microorganism fed with the objective of providing health benefits to the host animals (Fuller 1989). The most commonly used probiotics include species of *Lactobacillus*, *Enterococcus*, *Bifidobacterium*, and *Saccharomyces* (Alverez-Olmos and Oberhelman 2001; Holzapfel et al. 2001; Rolfe 2000). Most studies involving probiotics have concentrated on improving intestinal health, particularly during the weaning period when the pig gut microflora undergoes dramatic change.

It is generally accepted that with careful attention to the criteria used to select the particular probiotic strain, there may be a place for probiotics in prevention of enteric disease, but results to date are inconsistent. There are a number of criteria that potential probiotic strains must meet in order to be considered for use as a probiotic, including the ability to demonstrate predictable and measurable health benefits. The screening and selection of a probiotic includes testing in vitro or in vivo of the following criteria:

- It must be nonpathogenic and proven safe.
- It must have stability in an acid environment, in the presence of bile, and resistant to degradation by digestive enzymes.
- It must adhere to gut epithelial tissue and be able to persist in the gastrointestinal tract of the host.

In addition, the microbials used as probiotics must retain viability and stability during commercial production, feed processing, storage, and delivery, and must be cost-effective.

The main mechanisms whereby probiotics exert protective or therapeutic effects are not fully understood, but several ways have been postulated. Probiotics produce antimicrobial substances such as organic acids, fatty free acids, ammonia, hydrogen peroxide, and bacteriocins (Alverez-Olmos and Oberhelman 2001). In addition, probiotics may enhance specific and nonspecific host immunity (Kailasapathy and Chin 2000), and probiotics may prevent colonization of pathogenic microorganisms by competitive inhibition for microbial adhesion sites.

Inconsistent findings have been observed when probiotics have been used in trials to control pig disease or improve growth performance (Conway 1999). It is unlikely they will be capable of replacing antibiotics in the control of disease but they may have a place alongside other techniques for improving the health of the gut microflora and reducing the shedding of pathogens such as *Salmonella*.

There is considerable interest in the use of fermented liquid feed and there appears to be an association between its use and a reduction in *Salmonella* prevalence (van der Wolf et al. 2001). A possible explanation for the beneficial effect of fermented liquid feed is that the reduced pH of the diet and the presence of large numbers of organic acid producing bacteria in the feed have a positive effect on the gut microflora and create an environment unsuitable for *Salmonella* and other coliform bacteria.

Bacteriophages. Bacteriophages or phages are bacterial viruses that invade bacterial cells and in the case of lytic phages, disrupt bacterial metabolism and cause the bacterium to lyse (Sulakvelideze et al. 2001). From a clinical standpoint, phages appear to be innocuous, do not attack normal gut flora, and are extremely common in the environment. In spite of all the positive properties of lytic phages, they are not commonly used prophylactically or therapeutically and their efficacy is still a matter of controversy almost 100 years after their initial discovery.

Nutrients

There are a plentiful supply of physiologically active feed ingredients that can improve pig performance and health by modifying the environment of the digestive tract (Pettigrew 2003). Zinc oxide added to nursery rations at a level of 2500 ppm for 2 weeks will result in increased growth rate and reduced prevalence of diarrhea (Jensen-Waern et al. 1998). In vitro studies have shown that zinc has antimicrobial effects, but in vivo studies show no reduction in *E. coli* numbers and no change in function of circulating neutrophils. There are concerns that high levels of zinc oxide will cause liver toxicity if fed longer than 3–4 weeks.

Likewise, copper sulfate at levels of up to 250 ppm has been added to pig feed to promote growth. However, the combination of zinc and copper does not result in an additive growth response (Hill et al. 2000). In the case of both copper and zinc, there are environmental concerns regarding their use because of the build up of these minerals in manure.

The quest for alternatives to antibiotics in pig feed has caused interest in natural remedies, including herbs, spices, botanicals, and essential oils. These products may improve performance by improving feed palatability and by exerting antibacterial effects, but there needs to be further evidence of their effectiveness (Pettigrew 2003).

Organic acids (fumaric, formic, and lactic) are commonly added to feed or water in order to improve growth and reduce diarrhea during the postweaning period (Tsiloyiannis et al. 2001). Modes of action claimed for the growth-promoting effect of organic acids include decreased gastric pH, reduced coliform population, stimulated pancreatic exocrine secretion, increased pepsin activation, altered gut morphology, and improved intake and digestibility (Partanen 2001).

Response to acidification has been variable and may be attributed to feed and animal factors as well as differences in the properties of the various organic acids. Two problems that are associated with the use of high levels of organic acids are the acids may have a negative effect on palatability and the feed is corrosive to cement and steel in swine housing (Canibe et al. 2001).

An alternative approach to altering the gut microflora is to feed nondigestible material that provide a substrate for beneficial bacteria such as lactic acid-producing bacteria. These products are often referred to as prebiotics. In order for a feed to be classified as a prebiotic it must be neither hydrolyzed nor absorbed in the upper part of the gastrointestinal tract, be a selective substrate for one or a limited number of potentially beneficial commensal bacteria, and induce luminal or systemic effects that are beneficial to the host's health (Roberfroid 2001). Nondigestible oligosaccharides are the most common type of prebiotics, including fructo-oligosaccharides and mannan-oligosaccharides. In general, prebiotics are considered to provide small but positive improvements in growth rate, and are widely used in the swine industry. However, their role in providing health benefits, such as reducing *Salmonella* shedding, needs to be clarified.

Enzymes added to feed to encourage improved feed efficiency and in some cases potential health benefits are used widely. For example, feed can be supplemented with phytase to allow swine to digest plant phosphorus that is in the form of phytate. It has been hypothesized that the use of enzymes may allow the industry to utilize coarse feed particle size as a means of reducing gastric ulcers and the prevalence of *Salmonella* but still maintaining acceptable feed conversion.

There is a possibility that in-feed antimcriobials for growth promotion could be reduced through a combination of feeding manipulations, such as the use of various combinations of liquid feeds or coarse particle size, enzymes, probiotics, prebiotics, and acidifiers.

OTHER THERAPEUTICS

Anesthetics, Tranquilizers

There are few products licensed for use in swine. Most commonly a combination of drugs used in an off-label manner are employed in order to provide satisfactory anesthesia in the field. This has become a controversial area because the swine industry has come under pressure to reduce the potential suffering of pigs during and following routine surgical procedures, such as castration or after a traumatic injury, and yet minimize the use of drugs without proper licensing approval.

Table 71.8. Common swine anthelminitics and dosages

Product	Dosage
Dichlorvos	11.2–21.6 mg/kg body weight in feed with 1/3 of regular ration
Doramectin	300 µg/kg body weight IM
Fenbendazole	9 mg/kg body weight over 3–12 days via feed
Ivermectin	300 µg/kg SQ or 100 µg/kg body weight for 7 days via feed
Piperazine	275–440 mg/kg body weight in feed or water
Pyrantel tartrate	22 mg/kg of body weight as 1 day treatment or 96 g/ton of feed as prophylactic dose

Antiparasitics

In modern confinement operations, there are few parasitic problems (Roepstorff and Jorsal 1989). Under conditions of good hygiene and management, the regular application of anthelminitics may be of little or no benefit (Roepstorff 1997). Ascariasis is generally the main concern, and strategic medication with a wide range of effective products can easily control this parasite.

External parasitism caused by mange mites and lice is no longer a significant problem because of good husbandry practices and effective drugs, particularly the avermectins. Failure to control sarcoptic mange or lice infestation is generally due to a poor understanding of the epidemiology of the organisms and apathy on the part of the herdsman (Cargill et al. 1997). Antiparasitic products and their application are presented in Table 71.8.

Hormones

Oxytocin is widely used as an aid in stimulating parturition and milk letdown. Prostaglandin $F_{2\alpha}$ or a synthetic analog can be used to induce parturition. Puberty can be induced in gilts by treatment with a single injection of 200 IU of human chorionic gonadotropin and 400 IU of equine chorionic gonadotropin. The injection of follicular stimulating hormone at weaning and an injection of luteinizing hormone approximately 72–80 hours later has been shown to induce a predictable ovulation (Barnabe 2002) and can be used in artificial insemination programs where these hormones are licensed for this purpose. Estrus can be synchronized by administering a progestin for 14–18 days. The progestin inhibits follicular maturation until the progestin is withdrawn.

Hormones are also used in certain countries for growth manipulation. Daily injection of porcine somatotropin (PST) strongly influences feed efficiency, growth, and carcass composition. Ractopamine, a phenethanolamine or ß-agonist is used as a feed additive in several countries. Its function is as a repartitioning agent causing improved feed efficiency and a lean carcass at slaughter.

REFERENCES

Alvarez-Olmos MI, Oberhelman RA. 2001. Probiotic agents and infectious diseazees: A modern perspective on a traditional therapy. Clin Inf Dis 32:1567–1576.

Bager F, Aarestrup FM, Madsen M, Wegener HC. 1999. Glycopeptide resistance in *Enterococcus faecium* from broilers and pigs following discontinued use of avoparcin. Microb Drug Resist 5:53–56.

Bager F, Madsen M, Christensen J, Aarestrup FM. 1997. Avoparcin used as a growth promoter is associated with the occurrence of vancomycin-resistant *Enterococcus faecium* in Danish poultry and pig farms. Prev Vet Med 31:95–112.

Barnabe RC, Viana CHC, Candini PH, Gama RD, Carbone A, Stantos ICC, Vianna WL. 2002. Evaluation of a synchronization of ovulation protocol in sows according to the day of oestrous cycle. Rev Brasileira Repro Anim 26:177–179.

Canibe N, Zteien SH, Øverland M, Jensen BB. 2001. Effect of k-diformate in starter diets on acidity, microbiota and the amount of organic acids in the digestive tract of piglets and on gastric alterations. J Anim Sci 79:2123–2133.

Carattoli A, Tosini F, Giles WP, Rupp ME, Hinrichs SH, Angulo FJ, Barrett TJ, Fey PD. 2002. Characterization of plasmids carrying CMY-2 from expanded-spectrum cephalosporin-resistant Salmonella strains isolated in the United States between 1996 and 1998. Antimicrob Agents Chemother 46:1269–1272.

Cargill CF, Pointon AM, Davies PR, Garcia R. 1997. Using slaughter inspections to evaluate sarcoptic mange infestation of finishing swine. Vet Parasitol 70(1–3):191–200.

Center for Veterinary Medicine, US Food and Drug Administration. 2004. Department Guidance for Industry #144— Preapproval Information for Registration of New Veterinary Medicinal Products for Food-Producing Animals with Respect to Antimicrobial Resistance—VICH GL27, Final Guidance, April 27, 2004. See USFDA CVM website.

Chernysheva LV, Friendship RM, Gyles CL, Dewey CE. 2004. The effect of dietary chicken egg-yolk antibodies on the clinical response in weaned pigs challenged with a K88+ *Escherichia coli* isolate. J Swine Health Prod 12:119–122.

Conway PL. 1999. Specifically selected probiotics can improve health and performance of pigs. In Manipulating Pig Production VII. PD Cranwell, ed. Werribee: Australasian Pig Science Association, pp. 220–224.

Dewey CE. 1999. From the editor. Swine Health Prod 7:253.

Dobson KJ, Davies PR. 1992. External parasites. In Diseases of Swine, 7th ed. AD Leman, BE Straw, WL Mengeling, S D'Allaire, DJ Taylor, eds. Ames: Iowa State Univ Press, pp. 668–679.

Dohoo I, Martin W, Stryhn H. 2003. Controlled trials, In Veterinary Epidemiologic Research. Charlottetown: AVC Inc., pp. 185–206.

Dunlop RH, McEwen SA, Meek AH, Clarke RC, Black WD, Friendship RM. 1998. Associations among antimicrobial drug treatments and antimicrobial resistance of fecal Escherichia coli of swine on 34 farrow-to-finish farms in Ontario. Prev Vet Med 34:283–305.

Fuller R. 1989. Probiotics in man and animals. J Appl Bact 66:365–378.

HaesebrouckF, Pasmans F, Chiers K, Maes D, Ducatelle R, Decostere A. 2004. Efficacy of vaccines against bacterial diseases in swine: What can we expect? Vet Microbiol 100:255–268.

Health Canada. 2002. Use of Antimicrobials in Food Animals in Canada: Impact on Resistance and Human Health. Ottawa: Veterinary Drugs Directorate.

Hill GM, Cromwell GL, Crenshaw TD, Dove CR, Ewan RC, Knabe DA, Lewis AJ, Libal GW, Mahan DC, Shurson GC, Southern LL, Veum TL. 2000. Growth promotion effects and plasma changes from feeding high dietary concentrations of zinc and copper to weanling pigs (regional study). J Anim Sci 798:1010–1016.

Holzapfel WH, Haberer P, Geisen R, Bjorkroth J, Schillinger U. 2001. Taxonomy and important features of probiotic microorganisms in food and nutrition. Am J Clin Nutr 73:365–373S.

Jensen-Waern M, Melin L, Lindberg R, Johannisson A, Wallgren PP. 1998. Dietary zinc oxide in weaned pigs—Effects on performance, tissue concentrations, morphology, neutrophil functions, and faecal microflora. Res Vet Sci 64:225–231.

Kailasapathy K, Chin J. 2000. Survival and therapeutic potential organisms with reference to *Lactobacillus acidophilus* and *Bifidobacterium spp*. Immunol Cell Biol 78:80–88.

Kolb JR. 1996. Vaccination and medication via drinking water. Compend Contin Educ Vet Pract S75–S83.

Marquardt RR, Li S. 2001. Control of diarrhea in young pigs using therapeutic antibodies. In Proc AD Leman Swine Conf, St. Paul Minn., pp. 227–239.

Moon H, Bunn TA. 1993. Vaccines against enterotoxigenic *E.coli* infections. Vaccine 11:213–220.

Noamani BN, Fairbrother JM, Gyles CL. 2003. Virulence genes of O149 enterotoxigenic *Escherichia coli* from outbreaks of postweaning diarrhea in pigs. Vet Microbiol 97:87–101.

Partanen K. 2001. Organic acids—Their efficacy and modes of action in pigs. In Gut Environment of Pigs. A Piva, KE Bach Knudsen, JE Lindberg, eds. Nottingham University Press, pp. 201–207.

Pettigrew JE. 2003. Alternative products: Are there any silver bullets? In Proc Amer Assoc Swine Vet, Orlando, pp. 439–441.

Prescott JF, Baggot JD, Walker RD. 2000. Antimicrobial Therapy in Veterinary Medicine, 3rd ed. Ames: Iowa State UnivPress.

Ribble CS. 1990. Assessing vaccine efficacy. Can Vet J 31:679–681.

Roberfroid MB. 2001. Prebiotcs: Preferential substrates for specific germs? Am J Clin Nutr 73:406–409S.

Roepstorff A. 1997. Helminth surveillance as a prerequisite for anthelmintic treatment in intensive sow herds. Vet Parasitol 73:139–151.

Roepstorff A. Jorsal SE. 1989. Prevalence of helminth infections in swine in Denmark. Vet Parasitol 33:231–239.

Rolfe RD. 2000. The role of probiotic cultures in the control of gastrointestinal health. J Nutr 130:396–402S.

Sulakvelidze A, Alavidze Z, Morris, Jr., GJ. 2001. Bacteriophage therapy. Antimicrob Agents Chemotherap 45:649–659.

Tsiloyiannis VK, Kyriakis SC, Vlemmas J, Sarris K. 2001. The effect of organic acids on the control of porcine post-weaning diarrhea. Res Vet Sci 70:287–293.

van der Wolf PJ, Wolbers WB, Elbers ARW, van der Heijden HMJF, Koppen JMCC, Hunneman WA, van Schie FW, Tielen MJM. 2001. Herd level husbandry factors associated with the serological *Salmonella* prevalence in finishing pig herds in the Netherlands. Vet Microb 78:205–219.

van Dijk AJ, Everts H, Nabuurs MJ, Margry RJ, Beynen AC. 2001. Growth performance of weanling pigs fed spray-dried animal plasma: A review. Livest Prod Sci 68:263–274.

van Lunen TA. 2003. Growth performance of pigs fed diets with and without tylosin phosphate supplementation and reared in a biosecure all-in all-out housing system. Can Vet J 44:571–576.

Winokur PL, Vonstein DL, Hoffman LJ, Uhlenhopp EK, Doern GV. 2001. Evidence for transfer of CMY-2 AmpC ß-lactamse plasmids between *Escherichia coli* and *Salmonella* isolates from food animals and humans. Antimicrob Agents Chemother 45:2716–2722.

World Health Organization. 2000a. Global Strategy for Containment of Antimicrobial Resistance. Geneva, Switzerland. See WHO website.

——. 2000b. Global Principles for the Containment of Antimicrobial Resistance in Animals Intended for Food. Geneva, Switzerland. See WHO website.

——. 2002. Impacts of Antimicrobial Growth Promotion Termination in Denmark. Foulum, Denmark. See WHO website.

World Organization for Animal Health (OIE). 2003. Joint First FAO/OIE/WHO Expert Workshop on Nonhuman Antimicrobial Usage and Antimicrobial Resistance: Scientific Assessment. Geneva, Switzerland. See WHO website.

——. 2004. Joint FAO/OIE/WHO 2nd Expert Workshop on Nonhuman Antimicrobial Usage and Antimicrobial Resistance: Management Options. Oslo, Norway. See WHO website.

Zhao S, Qaiyumi S, Friedman S, Singh R, Foley SL, White DG, McDermott PF, Donkar T, Bolin C, Munro S, Baron EJ, Walker RD. Characterization of *Salmonella enterica* serotype Newport isolated from humans and food animals. J Clin Microbiol 41:5366--5371.

Index